The Foundation and Art of Robotic Surgery

Editors in Chief

Pier Cristoforo Giulianotti, MD, FACS
Lloyd Nyhus Professor of Surgery
Chief of the Division of General Minimally Invasive & Robotic Surgery and Vice Department
   Head at the University of Illinois at Chicago
Scientific Director of the SITL (Surgical Innovation and Training Laboratory)
Honorary President and Founder of the Clinical Robotic Surgical Association (CRSA)
Chicago, Illinois

Enrico Benedetti, MD, FACS
Warren H. Cole Chair in Surgery
Professor and Head of the Department of Surgery
Medical Director of the Abdominal Organ Transplant Program
Department of Surgery at UI Health
Chicago, Illinois

Associate Editor

Alberto Mangano, MD
Senior Minimally Invasive and Robotic Surgery Research Fellow and Surgical Instructor
Department of Surgery
University of Illinois at Chicago and Surgical Innovation and Training Laboratory (SITL)
Chicago, Illinois

New York   Chicago   San Francisco   Athens   London   Madrid   Mexico City
Milan   New Delhi   Singapore   Sydney   Toronto

The Foundation and Art of Robotic Surgery

Copyright © 2024 by McGraw Hill LLC. All rights reserved. Printed in Hong Kong. Except as permitted under the United States Copyright Act of 1976, no part of this publication may be reproduced or distributed in any form or by any means, or stored in a data base or retrieval system, without the prior written permission of the publisher.

1 2 3 4 5 6 7 8 9   DSS   29 28 27 26 25 24 23

ISBN 978-1-264-25742-3
MHID 1-264-25742-2

Notice

Medicine is an ever-changing science. As new research and clinical experience broaden our knowledge, changes in treatment and drug therapy are required. The authors and the publisher of this work have checked with sources believed to be reliable in their efforts to provide information that is complete and generally in accord with the standards accepted at the time of publication. However, in view of the possibility of human error or changes in medical sciences, neither the authors nor the publisher nor any other party who has been involved in the preparation or publication of this work warrants that the information contained herein is in every respect accurate or complete, and they disclaim all responsibility for any errors or omissions or for the results obtained from use of the information contained in this work. Readers are encouraged to confirm the information contained herein with other sources. For example and in particular, readers are advised to check the product information sheet included in the package of each drug they plan to administer to be certain that the information contained in this work is accurate and that changes have not been made in the recommended dose or in the contraindications for administration. This recommendation is of particular importance in connection with new or infrequently used drugs.

This book was set in Minion Pro by KnowledgeWorks Global Ltd.
The editors were Sydney Keen Vitale and Christina M. Thomas.
The production supervisor was Richard Ruzycka.
Project management was provided by Radhika Jolly of KnowledgeWorks Global Ltd.
The cover designer was W2 Design.

Library of Congress Cataloging-in-Publication Data
Names: Giulianotti, Pier Cristoforo, editor. | Benedetti, E. (Enrico),
   editor. | Mangano, Alberto editor.
Title: The foundation and art of robotic surgery / editors in chief, Pier
   Cristoforo Giulianotti, Enrico Benedetti ; associate editor, Alberto Mangano.
Description: New York : McGraw Hill, [2024] | Includes bibliographical
   references and index. | Summary: "A comprehensive, illustrated approach
   to operative techniques and instrumentation in robotic general
   surgery"—Provided by publisher.
Identifiers: LCCN 2021049890 | ISBN 9781264257423 (hardcover) | ISBN
   9781264257430 (ebook)
Subjects: MESH: Robotic Surgical Procedures—methods | Robotic Surgical
   Procedures—instrumentation
Classification: LCC R859.7.A78 | NLM WO 505 | DDC
   610.285/63—dc23/eng/20211101
LC record available at https://lccn.loc.gov/2021049890

McGraw Hill books are available at special quantity discounts to use as premiums and sales promotions, or for use in corporate training programs. To contact a representative please visit the Contact Us pages at www.mhprofessional.com.

Contents

Contributors..v
Preface..xi
Introduction..xiii

SECTION I • General Principles 1

CHAPTER 1 • What Robotic Surgery Is 3
Antonio Gangemi, Alberto Mangano, and Pier Cristoforo Giulianotti

CHAPTER 2 • The Basic Principles of Clinical Applications 15
Gabriela Aguiluz, Stephan Gruessner, and Patrice Frederick

CHAPTER 3 • The Assistant's Role in Robotic Surgery 33
Gabriela Aguiluz and Kelly Hoyert

CHAPTER 4 • Robotic Training 45
Alberto Mangano, Valentina Valle, Liaohai Leo Chen, and Antonio Gangemi

CHAPTER 5 • Keys for Success of a Robotic Program 55
Yuman Fong

CHAPTER 6 • Implemented Imaging and Artificial Intelligence 65
Barbara Seeliger, Toby Collins, and Jacques Marescaux

CHAPTER 7 • Fluorescence Imaging: Basics and Clinical Applications 89
Liaohai Chen, Carolina Baz, Natalija Lakic, and Pier Cristoforo Giulianotti

SECTION II • Thyroid Surgery 125

CHAPTER 8 • Gasless Transaxillary Thyroidectomy (Off-Label Indication) 127
Woung Youn Chung and Cho Rok Lee

CHAPTER 9 • Transoral Thyroidectomy (Off-Label Indication) 163
Ji Young You, Dawon Park, and Hoon Yub Kim

SECTION III • Chest Surgery 175

CHAPTER 10 • Nipple-Sparing Mastectomy (Off-Label Indication) 177
Antonio Toesca, Antonia Girardi, and Paolo Veronesi

CHAPTER 11 • Extended Thymectomy for Myasthenia Gravis and Thymoma 197
Hongbin Zhang, Feng Li, and Jens-C. Rückert

CHAPTER 12 • Ivor-Lewis Esophagectomy 209
Andrea Coratti, Francesco Guerra, and Giuseppe Giuliani

CHAPTER 13 • Radical Esophagectomy with Extended Mediastinal Lymphadenectomy 233
Koichi Suda and Ichiro Uyama

CHAPTER 14 • Paraesophageal Hernia Repair 259
Gabriela Aguiluz, Mario Alberto Masrur, and Pier Cristoforo Giulianotti

CHAPTER 15 • Selective Nissen Fundoplication 277
Gabriela Aguiluz, Alberto Mangano, and Pier Cristoforo Giulianotti

CHAPTER 16 • Heller Myotomy with Modified Dor Fundoplication 299
Nicolas Hellmuth Dreifuss, Gabriela Aguiluz, and Pier Cristoforo Giulianotti

CHAPTER 17 • Lung Lobectomies: General Principles and the Total Port, Transfissure Approach (Fissure First) 317
Melani Lighter, Gabriela Aguiluz, Fabio Sbrana, and Pier Cristoforo Giulianotti

CHAPTER 18A • Lung Upper Lobectomies........................... 345
Giulia Veronesi, Pierluigi Novellis, Piergiorgio Muriana, Gabriela Aguiluz, and Francesca Rossetti

CHAPTER 18B • Lung Lower Lobectomies 367
Giulia Veronesi, Pierluigi Novellis, Piergiorgio Muriana, Gabriela Aguiluz, and Francesca Rossetti

SECTION IV • Gastric and Bariatric Surgery 385

CHAPTER 19 • D2 Total Gastrectomy 387
Joong Ho Lee and Woo Jin Hyung

CHAPTER 20 • Sleeve Gastrectomy 407
Chandra Hassan, Alberto Mangano, and Yevhen Pavelko

CHAPTER 21 • Roux-en-Y Gastric Bypass 421
Nicolas Hellmuth Dreifuss, Roberto Bustos, and Mario Alberto Masrur

SECTION V • Intestinal Surgery 435

CHAPTER 22 • Small Bowel Resection 437
Mario Alberto Masrur, Nicolas Hellmuth Dreifuss, Alberto Mangano, and Pier Cristoforo Giulianotti

CHAPTER 23 • Radical Right Colectomy with Complete Mesocolic Excision (CME) 455
Alberto Mangano, Valentina Valle, Colton Johnson, and Pier Cristoforo Giulianotti

CHAPTER 24 • Left Colectomy 479
Alberto Mangano, Valentina Valle, and Pier Cristoforo Giulianotti

Contents

CHAPTER 25 • Total Mesorectal Excision for Rectal Cancer 517
Hye Jin Kim, Alberto Mangano, and Gyu-Seog Choi

CHAPTER 26 • Abdominoperineal Resection 551
Gerald Gantt, Alberto Mangano, Vivek Chaudhry, and Anders F. Mellgren

SECTION VI • Surgery of the Spleen and Pancreas 573

CHAPTER 27 • Splenectomy 575
Valentina Valle, Alberto Mangano, and Pier Cristoforo Giulianotti

CHAPTER 28 • Pancreaticoduodenectomy 599
Pier Cristoforo Giulianotti, Valentina Valle, Roberto Bustos, and Alberto Mangano

CHAPTER 29 • Radical Antegrade Modular Pancreatosplenectomy 635
Rong Liu and Qu Liu

CHAPTER 30 • Spleen-Preserving Distal Pancreatectomy 653
Valentina Valle, Alberto Mangano, Antonio Cubisino, and Pier Cristoforo Giulianotti

CHAPTER 31 • Central Pancreatectomy 673
Antonio Cubisino, Valentina Valle, Nicolas Hellmuth Dreifuss, and Pier Cristoforo Giulianotti

CHAPTER 32 • Enucleation of Pancreatic Tumors 689
Graziano Pernazza and Antonio Cubisino

SECTION VII • Liver Surgery 699

CHAPTER 33 • Right Hepatectomy 701
Eduardo Fernandes, Alberto Mangano, Valentina Valle, and Pier Cristoforo Giulianotti

CHAPTER 34 • Left Hepatectomy 733
Antonio Cubisino, Carolina Baz, Nicolas Hellmuth Dreifuss, and Pier Cristoforo Giulianotti

CHAPTER 35 • Liver Sectionectomies: Left Lateral Sectionectomy 755
Alberto Mangano, Valentina Valle, and Pier Cristoforo Giulianotti

CHAPTER 36 • Segmental and Atypical Liver Resections 769
Francesco Guerra, Carolina Baz, and Alberto Patriti

SECTION VIII • Biliary Surgery 789

CHAPTER 37 • Cholecystectomy 791
Stephan Gruessner, Francesco Bianco, and Pier Cristoforo Giulianotti

CHAPTER 38 • Roux-en-Y Hepaticojejunostomy 809
Eric CH Lai and Chung Ngai Tang

CHAPTER 39 • Bile Duct Injuries Repair 825
Pier Cristoforo Giulianotti, Antonio Cubisino, and Nicolas Hellmuth Dreifuss

CHAPTER 40 • Management of Intrahepatic Biliary Stones 841
Eric CH Lai and Chung Ngai Tang

SECTION IX • Adrenal Surgery 861

CHAPTER 41 • Right Adrenalectomy 863
Francesco Maria Bianco, Yevhen Pavelko, Alberto Mangano, and Pier Cristoforo Giulianotti

CHAPTER 42 • Left Adrenalectomy 879
Francesco Maria Bianco, Yevhen Pavelko, Valentina Valle, and Pier Cristoforo Giulianotti

SECTION X • Hernia Surgery 895

CHAPTER 43 • Inguinal Hernia Repair 897
Francesco Maria Bianco, Yevhen Pavelko, and Pier Cristoforo Giulianotti

CHAPTER 44 • Ventral Hernia Repair (Intraperitoneal onlay mesh with fascial defect approximation) 911
Karl LeBlanc, Patrice Frederick, and Carolina Baz

CHAPTER 45 • Robotic Transversus Abdominis Release (roboTAR) 925
Tiffany Nguyen, Ethan Ballecer, Katherine Hoener, Alice Gamble, and Conrad Ballecer

SECTION XI • Transplant 941

CHAPTER 46 • Donor Nephrectomy 943
Mario Spaggiari, Ivo Georgiev Tzvetanov, and Enrico Benedetti

CHAPTER 47 • Kidney Transplant 963
Pierpaolo Di Cocco, Ivo Georgiev Tzvetanov, Luciano Ambrosini, and Enrico Benedetti

CHAPTER 48 • Pancreas Transplant 983
Pierpaolo Di Cocco, Ivo Georgiev Tzvetanov, Mario Spaggiari, Luciano Ambrosini, and Enrico Benedetti

CHAPTER 49 • Living Donor Hepatectomy 997
Ahmed Zidan and Dieter Broering

SECTION XII • Additional Procedures 1015

CHAPTER 50 • Renal Aneurysm 1017
Valentina Valle, Stephan Gruessner, Alberto Mangano, and Pier Cristoforo Giulianotti

CHAPTER 51 • Single Port Robotic Surgery: Basic Concepts (Procedures still not FDA approved/off-label indication) 1037
Nicolas Hellmuth Dreifuss, Antonio Cubisino, and Francesco Maria Bianco

Index *1067*

Contributors

Gabriela Aguiluz, MD
Minimally Invasive and Robotic Surgery Research Fellow
Surgical Instructor
Department of Surgery
University of Illinois at Chicago
Chicago, Illinois

Luciano Ambrosini, MD
Minimally Invasive and Robotic Surgery Research Fellow
Surgical Instructor
Department of Surgery
University of Illinois at Chicago
Chicago, Illinois

Conrad Ballecer, MD, MS
Clinical Assistant Professor
Creighton University School of Medicine Phoenix Division
Phoenix, Arizona

Ethan Ballecer
Pre-medicine
Arizona State University
Tempe, Arizona

Carolina Baz, MD, FACS
Minimally Invasive and Robotic Surgery Research Fellow
Surgical Instructor
Department of Surgery
University of Illinois at Chicago
Chicago, Illinois

Francesco Maria Bianco, MD, FACS
Associate Professor of Surgery
Department of Surgery
University of Illinois at Chicago
Chicago, Illinois

Dieter Clemens Broering, MD, PhD, FEBS, FACS
Professor
Al Faisal University
Consultant
Transplant & Hepatobiliary Pancreatic Surgery and Executive Director
Organ Transplant Centre of Excellence
King Faisal Specialist Hospital & Research Centre
Riyadh, Saudi Arabia

Roberto Bustos, MD
Minimally Invasive and Robotic Surgery Research Fellow
Surgical Instructor
Department of Surgery
University of Illinois at Chicago
Chicago, Illinois

Vivek Chaudhry, MD, MS, FACS, FASCRS
Clinical Associate Professor
Department of Surgery
University of Illinois at Chicago
Chicago, Illinois

Liaohai Leo Chen, PhD
Professor
Director of Surgical Innovation Training Laboratory (SITL)
Department of Surgery
University of Illinois at Chicago
Chicago, Illinois

Gyu-Seog Choi, MD, PhD
Professor
Colorectal Cancer Center
Kyungpook National University Chilgok Hospital
Kyungpook National University School of Medicine
Daegu, South Korea

Woung Youn Chung, MD, PhD
Professor of Surgery
Department of Surgery
Yonsei University College of Medicine
Seoul, South Korea

Toby Collins, PhD, MSc, MA, Cantab
Director of Research
IRCAD France & Africa Surgical Data Science
The Research Institute against Digestive Cancer (IRCAD) France
Strasbourg, France
The Research Institute against Digestive Cancer (IRCAD) Africa
Kigali, Rwanda

Andrea Coratti, MD
Head of Surgery
Department of General and Emergency Surgery
Misericordia Hospital
Grosseto, Italy

Antonio Cubisino, MD
Minimally Invasive and Robotic Surgery Research Fellow
Surgical Instructor
Department of Surgery
University of Illinois at Chicago
Chicago, Illinois

Pierpaolo Di Cocco, MD, PhD
Assistant Professor in General Surgery
Division of Transplantation
Department of Surgery
University of Illinois at Chicago
Chicago, Illinois

Nicolas Hellmuth Dreifuss, MD
Fellow Minimally Invasive and Robotic Surgery
Department of Surgery
University of Illinois Chicago
Chicago, Illinois

Eduardo Fernandes, MD, PhD, FRCS
Assistant Professor of Surgery
Department of Surgery
University of Illinois Chicago
Chicago, Illinois

Yuman Fong, MD, ScD, FACS
Sangiacomo Chair and Chairman
Department of Surgery
City of Hope Medical Center
Duarte, California

Patrice Frederick, MD, FACS
Assistant Professor of Surgery
Department of Medical Education
University of Central Florida, College of Medicine
Orlando, Florida

Alice Gamble, DO
Resident
Department of surgery
Creighton University
Phoenix, Arizona

Antonio Gangemi, MD, FACS, FASMBS
Associate Professor of Surgery
Department of Medical and Surgical Sciences (DIMEC)
Alma Mater Studiorum – University of Bologna
Bologna, Italy

Gerald Gantt, MD, FACS
Assistant Professor of Surgery
Department of Surgery
University of Illinois at Chicago
Chicago, Illinois

Antonia Girardi, MD, MSc
Breast Surgeon
Division of Breast Surgery
European Institute of Oncology IRCCS
Milan, Italy

Giuseppe Giuliani, MD
Attending Surgeon
Department of General and Emergency Surgery
Misericordia Hospital
Grosseto, Italy

Stephan Gruessner, MD, MPH
General Surgery Resident
Department of Surgery
University of Illinois at Chicago
Chicago, Illinois

Francesco Guerra, MD
Attending Surgeon
Department of General and Emergency Surgery
AUSL Toscana Sud Est - Misericordia Hospital
Grosseto, Italy

Chandra Hassan, MD, FACS, FRCS (Eng.)
Associate Professor of Surgery
Director of Bariatric Surgery Program
Director of Bariatric Surgery and MIS Fellowship
Division of General, Minimally Invasive and Robotic Surgery
University of Illinois Hospital and Health Science Systems
Chicago, Illinois

Katherine Hoener, DO
Resident
Department of Surgery
Creighton University
Phoenix, Arizona

Kelly Hoyert, PA-C
Physician Assistant
Department of Surgery
Division of General, Minimally Invasive & Robotic Surgery
UI Health
University of Illinois at Chicago
Chicago, Illinois

Woo Jin Hyung, MD, PhD
Professor
Department of Surgery
Yonsei University College of Medicine
Seoul, South Korea

Colton Johnson, MD Candidate – Class of 2024
University of Illinois College of Medicine
Rockford, Illinois

Hye Jin Kim, MD
Associate professor
Colorectal Cancer Center
Kyungpook National University Chilgok Hospital
Kyungpook National University School of Medicine
Daegu, Korea

Hoon Yub Kim, MD, PhD, FACS
Professor of Surgery
Department of Surgery
Korea University College of Medicine
Seoul, South Korea

Eric CH Lai, MD
Attending Physician
Department of Surgery
Pamela Youde Nethersole Eastern Hospital
Wan, Hong Kong, China

Natalija Lakic, MB, BCh, BAO Candidate – Class of 2025
Vice President – RCSI Surgical Society
Director of Education – RCSI Student Medical Journal (SMJ)
Royal College of Surgeons in Ireland
Dublin, Ireland

Karl A. LeBlanc, MD, MBA, FACS, FASMBS
Clinical Professor
Department of Surgery
Louisiana State University Health Science Center and
  Sr. Medical Director
Our Lady of the Lake Regional Center
Baton Rouge, Louisiana

Joong Ho Lee, MD
Clinical Assistant Professor
Department of Surgery
Yonsei University College of Medicine
Seoul, South Korea

Cho Rok Lee, MD
Assistant Professor
Department of Surgery
Yongin Severance Hospital
Yonsei University College of Medicine
Seoul, South Korea

Feng Li, MD
Attending Physician
Department of Thoracic Surgery
The First Affiliated Hospital of Zhengzhou University
Zhengzhou, China

Melani Lighter, MD, MSc
Assistant Professor of Surgery
Department of Surgery
University of Illinois at Chicago
Chicago, Illinois

Qu Liu, MD, PhD
Associate Chief Surgeon
Associate Professor
Faculty of Hepatopancreatobiliary Surgery
The First Medical Center of Chinese People's Liberation Army
  (PLA) General Hospital
Organ Transplantation Department
The Three Medical Center of Chinese People's Liberation
  Army (PLA) General Hospital
Beijing, China

Rong Liu, MD, PhD
Director, Chief Surgeon, Professor
Faculty of Hepatopancreatobiliary Surgery
The First Medical Center of Chinese People's Liberation Army
  (PLA) General Hospital
Beijing, China

Jacques Marescaux, MD, FACS, Hon FRCS, Hon FASA, Hon APSA, Hon FJSES, Hon FJSS
President & Founder of IRCAD (Research Institute Against
  Digestive Cancer)
Dr Honoris Causa of: The University of Buenos Aires
  (Argentina); The University of Bucarest (Romania)
The University of Lasi (Romania)
The University of Manitoba (Canada)
Winnipeg, Canada

Mario Alberto Masrur, MD, FACS, FASMBS
Associate Professor of Surgery
Department of Surgery
University of Illinois at Chicago
Chicago, Illinois

Anders Mellgren, MD, PhD, FACS, FASCRS
Turi Josefsen Chair in Surgery
Professor and Chief
Division of Colon & Rectal Surgery
University of Illinois at Chicago
Chicago, Illinois

Piergiorgio Muriana, MD
Attending Physician
Department of Thoracic Surgery
IRCCS San Raffaele Scientific Institute
Milan, Italy

Tiffany Nguyen, MD
General Surgery Resident Creighton University – Phoenix
Department of Surgery
St. Joseph Medical Center
Phoenix, Arizona

Pierluigi Novellis, MD
Attending Physician
Department of Thoracic Surgery
IRCCS San Raffaele Scientific Institute
Milan, Italy

Dawon Park, MD, PhD
Assistant Professor
Department of Surgery
Korea University Medical Center
Seoul, South Korea

Alberto Patriti, MD, PhD
Chief
Department of Surgery
Ospedale San Salvatore
Pesaro, Italy

Yevhen Pavelko, MD
Bariatric Surgery Clinical Fellow
Department of Surgery
University of Illinois at Chicago
Chicago, Illinois

Graziano Pernazza, MD
Chief
Robotic General Surgery Unit
Department of Surgery
San Giovanni Addolorata Hospital
Rome, Italy

Francesca Rossetti, MD
Attending Physician
Department of Thoracic Surgery
IRCCS San Raffaele Scientific Institute
Milan, Italy

Jens-C. Rückert, MD, PhD
Professor of Surgery
Head of Thoracic Surgery
Clinic of Surgery, University Medicine Berlin (Charité)
Berlin, Germany

Fabio Sbrana, MD, FACS
Director of Center for Digestive Health
Director of Center for Robotic Surgery
Director of General Minimally-Invasive Robotic Surgery
Advocate Lutheran General Hospital
Park Ridge, Illinois

Professor of Surgery
Chicago Medical School
Rosalind Franklin University
North Chicago, Illinois

Barbara Seeliger, MD, PhD, FACS
Associate Specialist Surgeon and Senior Researcher
Institute of Image-Guided Surgery
IHU-Strasbourg
Department of Digestive and Endocrine Surgery
Strasbourg University Hospitals
ICube UMR 7357 CNRS
University of Strasbourg / IRCAD
Research Institute Against Digestive Cancer
Strasbourg, France

Mario Spaggiari, MD, FACS
Associate Professor of Surgery
Division of Transplantation
University of Illinois at Chicago

Surgical Director Liver Transplant Program
ASTS Fellowship Program Director
Chicago, Illinois

Koichi Suda, MD, PhD, FACS
Professor & Head
Divisions of GI & HPB Surgery
Department of Surgery
Fujita Health University

Collaborative Laboratory for Research and Development in Advanced Surgical Intelligence
Fujita Health University
Toyoake, Aichi, Japan

Chung Ngai Tang, MBBS (HK), FCSHK, FRCS (Ed), FRCSEd (Gen) & FHKAM (Surgery)
Past President of Clinical Robotic Surgery Association (CRSA)
Founding President of Hong Kong Society of Robotic Surgery (HKSRS)
Senior Consultant (D4) Department of Surgery, Pamela Youde Nethersole Eastern Hospital
Wan, Hong Kong, China

Antonio Toesca, MD
Head
Department of Breast Surgery
Candiolo Cancer Institute FPO-IRCCS
Turin, Italy

Ivo Georgiev Tzvetanov, MD, FACS
Professor of Surgery
Chief Division of Transplantation
Department of Surgery
University of Illinois at Chicago
Chicago, Illinois

Ichiro Uyama, MD, PhD, FACS
Professor
Department of Advanced Robotic and Endoscopic Surgery
Fujita Health University
Collaborative Laboratory for Research and Development in Advanced Surgical Technology
Fujita Health University
Toyoake, Aichi, Japan

Valentina Valle, MD
Minimally Invasive and Robotic Surgery Research Fellow
Surgical Instructor
Department of Surgery
University of Illinois at Chicago
Chicago, Illinois

Giulia Veronesi, MD
Associate Professor
Department of Thoracic Surgery
IRCCS San Raffaele Scientific Institute
School of Medicine and Surgery
Vita-Salute San Raffaele University
Milan, Italy

Paolo Veronesi, MD
Full Professor of Surgery
Department of Oncology and Oncohaematology
University of Milan
Director of Breast Cancer Program and Breast Surgery Division
IRCCS European Institute of Oncology
Milano, Italy

Ji Young You, MD, PhD
Clinical Associate Professor
Division of Breast and Endocrine Surgery
Department of Surgery
Korea University Medical Center
Seoul, South Korea

Hongbin Zhang, MD
Doctoral Candidate of Charité Universität Berlin, Thoracic Surgery
Attending of Thoracic Surgery
Peking University International Hospital, Peking University
Beijing, China

Ahmed Zidan, MD, MSc, PhD
Associate Consultant
Transplant & Hepatobiliary Pancreatic Surgery
Organ Transplant Centre of Excellence
King Faisal Specialist Hospital & Research Centre
Riyadh, Saudi Arabia

Preface

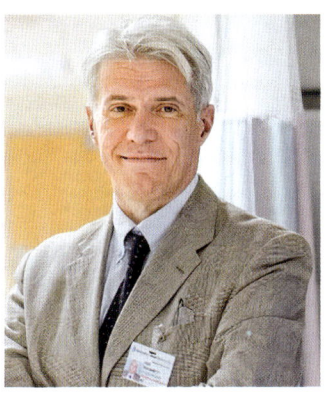

Writing a textbook of medicine in the 21st century may seem like a daunting and obsolete challenge. We live in an age where information travels quickly and becomes outdated even faster.

The rapid evolution of technology makes writing a textbook on robotic surgery even more paradoxical. Since the initial procedures were performed with the Da Vinci at the onset of the 21st century, at least 4 generations of robotic surgical systems have been deployed. The global, logarithmic growth in surgical applications and indications requires a constant reassessment and expansion of the basic knowledge. In addition, new devices continue to emerge in the clinical setting, each with its own peculiar features influencing how procedures are performed.

As robotic surgery has grown so rapidly, there is a lack of scholarly materials and standardized approaches. Today, initial training in robotic surgery mostly consists in familiarizing the surgeon with the system's mechanical controls. I realized, with time and experience, that such an approach will lead many young surgeons to confuse their skills in controlling the robotic system mechanically with the actual know-how associated with performing surgery. The basics are often unclear due to the absence of a standardized, codified approach where steps can be analyzed, measured, and repeated consistently.

The purpose of this textbook is to facilitate students' learning of surgery while applying robotic technology. Each chapter presents a "paradigmatic" procedure, explained step by step, providing notes, suggestions, and insight into common mistakes and approximate timing.

The material includes intraoperative images and video clips to add a visual, sensory dimension to the learning experience, thus facilitating comprehension of the surgical technique.

Great emphasis is placed on the explanation of anatomy and its variants with numerous original drawings included to help with understanding anatomical details.

Past centuries saw the study of anatomy at the center of the surgeon's education. Even more emphasis should be placed on anatomy today, since robotic surgery can also be defined as "image-guided surgery." I often tell my students that good surgery begins with a love for anatomy's beauty. Through that lens, surgery becomes a fascinating journey inside the human body infused with a sacred respect for anatomy's structure and functions.

In the future, robotic surgery may allow us to perform the perfect, dream operation: functional, selective, bloodless, painless, and scarless. The path to achieve such an ideal procedure is still long, but dreaming and anticipating the future is the only way to make it a reality.

The title of this book, *The Foundation and Art of Robotic Surgery*, reflects this dual component, from the basic, scientific concepts toward the perfection of the details, which is typical of art.

A perfect operation becomes like a masterpiece, where the artist is going beyond the basic technical skills, adding personal talent, conceptual insights, harmony, search of beauty, and ethical inspiration. Robotic surgery and artificial intelligence will give us "superhuman powers" and will pave the way to surgical perfection.

I do hope that along this way we'll not lose the ethical commitment, the compassion, the dedication, and the "holy" respect for human life. Even masterpieces may become meaningless without ethical values.

I would like to dedicate this textbook to the surgeons who inspired me at the beginning of my career, Prof Mario Selli and Giovan Battista Sarteschi. And to my family, my wife and beloved companion, Paola, who helped and constantly supported me, and my kids, Lorenzo and Chiara, who grew up waiting for their dad.

—**Pier Cristoforo Giulianotti, MD, FACS**

Introduction

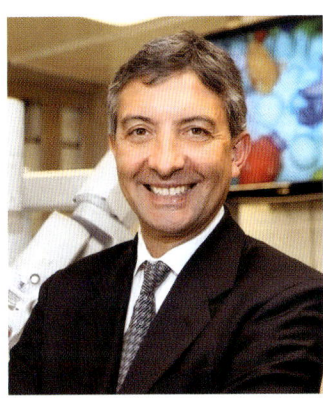

Establishing efficacious techniques for minimally invasive surgery has been one of the greatest progress in modern surgical care. While laparoscopy has opened the way for this impressive trend, robotic surgery has extended the ability to perform minimally invasive surgery in virtually all the procedures, including those of significant technical complexity.

As a surgeon trained in the late 1980s to early 1990s, I witnessed the rapid diffusion of laparoscopic techniques at a time in which attending surgeons were learning and surgical residents were "holding the camera." Since my career has been focused on open case for abdominal organ transplantation, I reached the new millennium with minimal expertise in laparoscopic techniques. All changed when robotic surgery became available in early 2000: I finally had a minimally invasive option in which my open surgery skills could easily transition, with minimal change in surgical strategy. Working closely with one of the most-recognized masters in robotic surgery, Dr. Pier Cristoforo Giulianotti, my coauthor, I have been able to experience firsthand the incredible reach and potential of robotic surgery even in the field of organ transplantation.

Our over 20-years journey in the field of robotic surgery constitutes the basis for this ambitious textbook. Our aim is to provide a modern tool for robotic surgical techniques both for the beginner and the experienced surgeon who is performing a complex robotic procedure for the first time. I believe that the reader will greatly enjoy the accuracy and depth of the anatomical details as well as the precise "step-by-step" technique suggested by the top world experts in the specific procedure.

The spectacular iconography is an integral part of our attempt to provide an authoritative guide to perform robotic surgical procedure in the best and safest way possible. In line with a highly technological field such as robotic surgery, we have integrated the standard drawing and pictures with easily accessible videos, several in 3D format.

The future of surgery is certainly linked to continuously improved technology capable to expand the individual ability of the surgeon with the aim to treat the patients with minimal negative consequence on their function and physical appearance. Robotic surgery is here to stay and, with further technical improvement and cost containment through competition among companies, will soon become accessible to the majority of surgeons operating in highly developed countries. I sincerely hope that all our colleagues, one day, will have the possibility to consider the robotic approach in their armamentarium, regardless the country of origin.

I would like to dedicate this book to my wife, Carla, and my daughter, Eleonora, but also to my loyal friend and the Soul and Leader of Robotic Surgery at the University of Illinois, Pier Cristoforo Giulianotti.

—**Enrico Benedetti, MD, FACS**

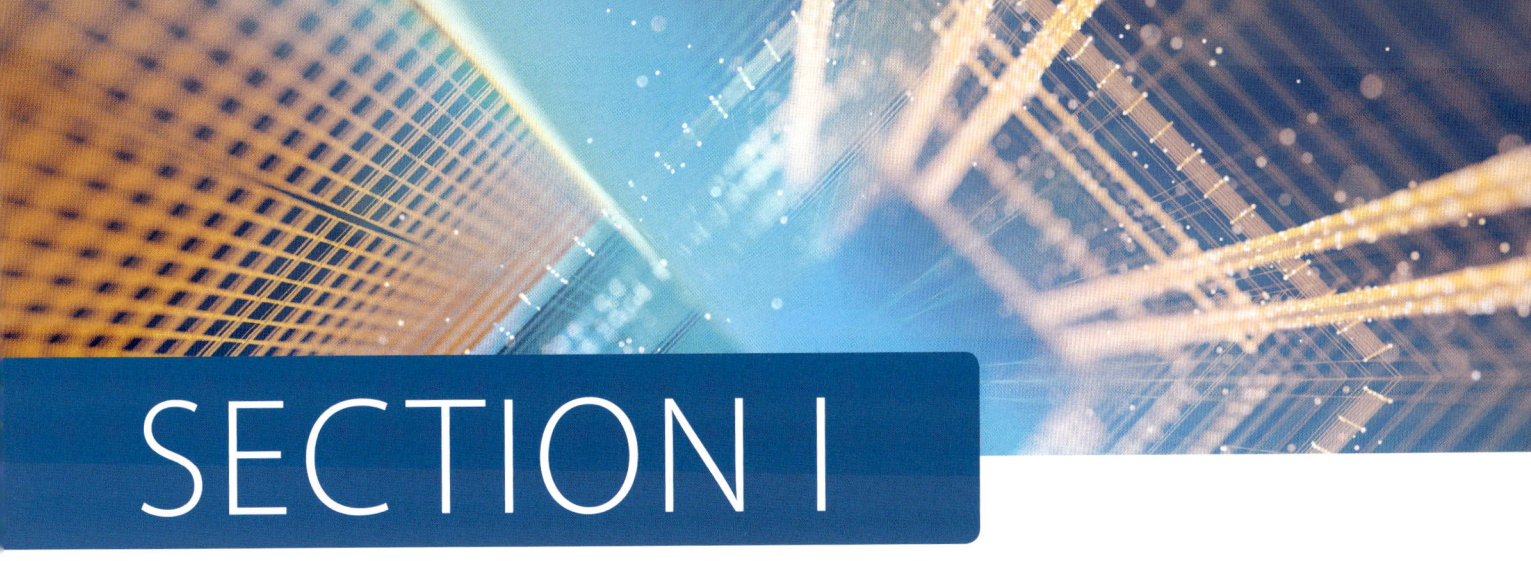

SECTION I

General Principles

Chapter 1 • What Robotic Surgery Is...3
Antonio Gangemi • Alberto Mangano • Pier Cristoforo Giulianotti

Chapter 2 • The Basic Principles of Clinical Applications... 15
Gabriela Aguiluz • Stephan Gruessner • Patrice Frederick

Chapter 3 • The Assistant's Role in Robotic Surgery... 33
Gabriela Aguiluz • Kelly Hoyert

Chapter 4 • Robotic Training... 45
Alberto Mangano • Valentina Valle • Liaohai Leo Chen • Antonio Gangemi

Chapter 5 • Keys for Success of a Robotic Program.. 55
Yuman Fong

Chapter 6 • Implemented Imaging and Artificial Intelligence 65
Barbara Seeliger • Toby Collins • Jacques Marescaux

Chapter 7 • Fluorescence Imaging: Basics and Clinical Applications... 89
Liaohai Chen • Carolina Baz • Natalija Lakic • Pier Cristoforo Giulianotti

"I don't know how long it will take, but certainly robotics will be used by the future surgeon routinely for some operations or some parts of the operations."
—A. Carpentier (1933)

What Robotic Surgery Is

Antonio Gangemi • Alberto Mangano • Pier Cristoforo Giulianotti

HISTORY OF ROBOTIC SURGERY

What is robotic surgery? It is these authors' belief that in order to address this important question, we should make the reader acquainted with the conditions that preceded the conception of this technological advance or, in simpler words, with its *history*.

In less than half a century, the introduction in the surgical field of not 1 but 2 breakthrough technologies occurred: robotic being the most recent and laparoscopy being its predecessor.

Pioneers of laparoscopy surgery, such as Dr. Mouret in France, advocated the adoption of the less invasive laparoscopic approach for treating very common surgical conditions such as gallbladder disease. Their theses were based on considerations of minimized trauma to the surgical tissues, better cosmetic outcomes, less pain, lower rates of wound infections, quicker recovery, and an overall shorter hospital stay.

The advantages of the newer approach became obvious to many in a short time.

Barely 6 years after Dr. Mouret presented the outcomes of his first laparoscopic cholecystectomy, 80% of cholecystectomies were already being performed with the laparoscopic approach, and various surgical disciplines had adopted the newer "technology."

In the following decade, laparoscopy quickly became the gold standard for a wide range of surgical procedures ranging from cholecystectomy to appendectomy, inguinal hernia repair, gastric fundoplication, adrenalectomy, bariatric surgery, colectomy, splenectomy, and nephrectomy.

However, the laparoscopic "revolution" did not come without drawbacks.

The long laparoscopic instruments with wrist-less tips and associated fulcrum effect (i.e., the instrument's end-point moves in the opposite direction to the surgeon's hands; see **Figure 1-1**) and the bidimensional vision of the laparoscopic monitors forced the surgeon to master nonintuitive motor skills and movements and to strain their vision for transferring 3D information (acquired by their brain) into a 2D format (the laparoscopic screen).

The long, steep learning curve and the fatigue resulting from these limitations discouraged many surgeons from adopting the laparoscopic approach or using this approach to perform their most complex procedures. Even the most successful and best-established laparoscopic surgeons could not escape from the physical toll that their body took to compensate for the engineering limitations of this technology.

It is based on these critical considerations that another group of pioneers, a generation later, attempted to combine telerobotic technology and human–machine interfaces with minimally invasive surgery.

Drs. Moll, Freund, and Robert took the lead in the United States by creating *Intuitive Surgical.* (Sunnyvale, California, U.S.) While waiting for the FDA approval in the United States, they began marketing their breakthrough system in Europe in 1999. The platform was named after another Italian pioneer and polymath, who left an indelible mark in the history of humankind thanks to his many extraordinary inventions—Leonardo da Vinci (see **Figures 1-2 A–G**).

Photo from Miguel Medina, Stringer / Getty Images.
Quote reproduced with permission from The Annette and Irwin Eskind Biomedical Library Special Collections. Vanderbilt University Medical Center.

4 The Foundation and Art of Robotic Surgery

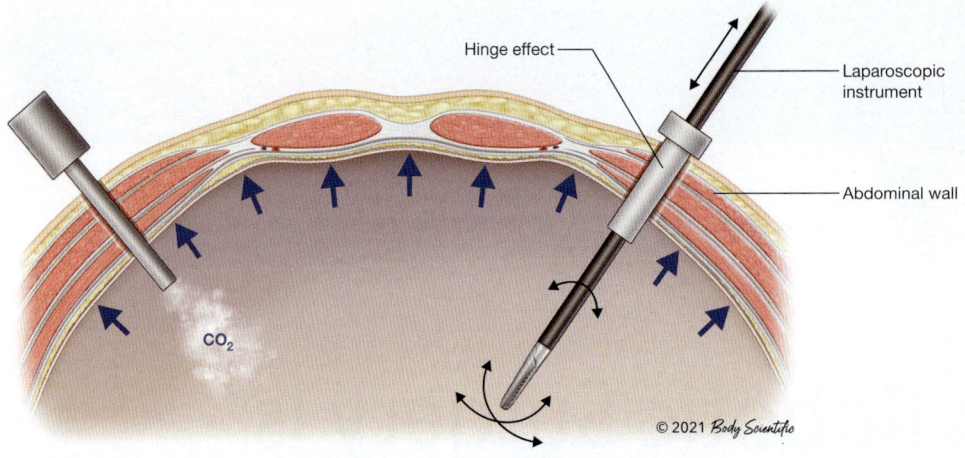

FIGURE 1-1 • The fulcrum effect.

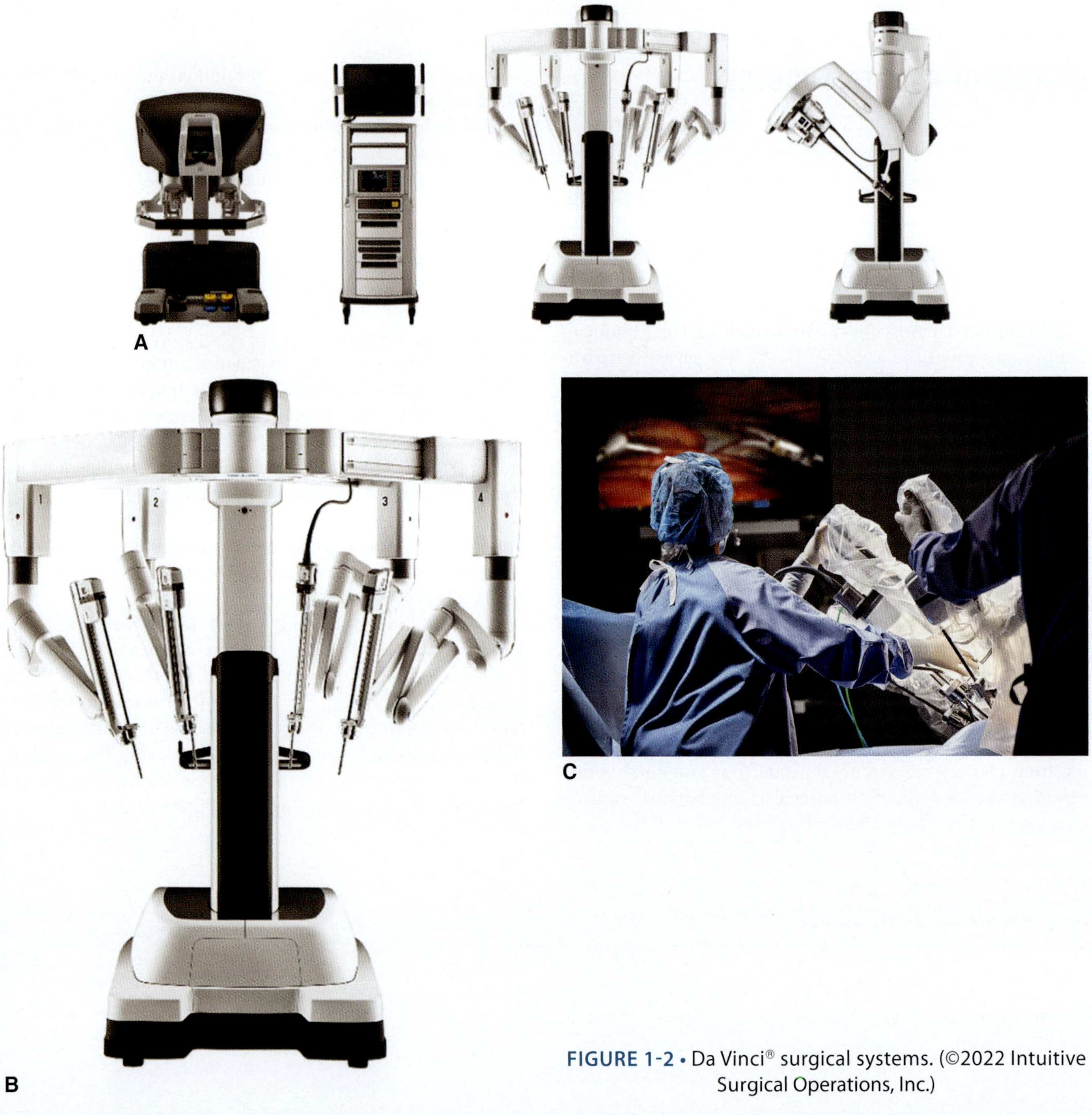

FIGURE 1-2 • Da Vinci® surgical systems. (©2022 Intuitive Surgical Operations, Inc.)

What Robotic Surgery Is   5

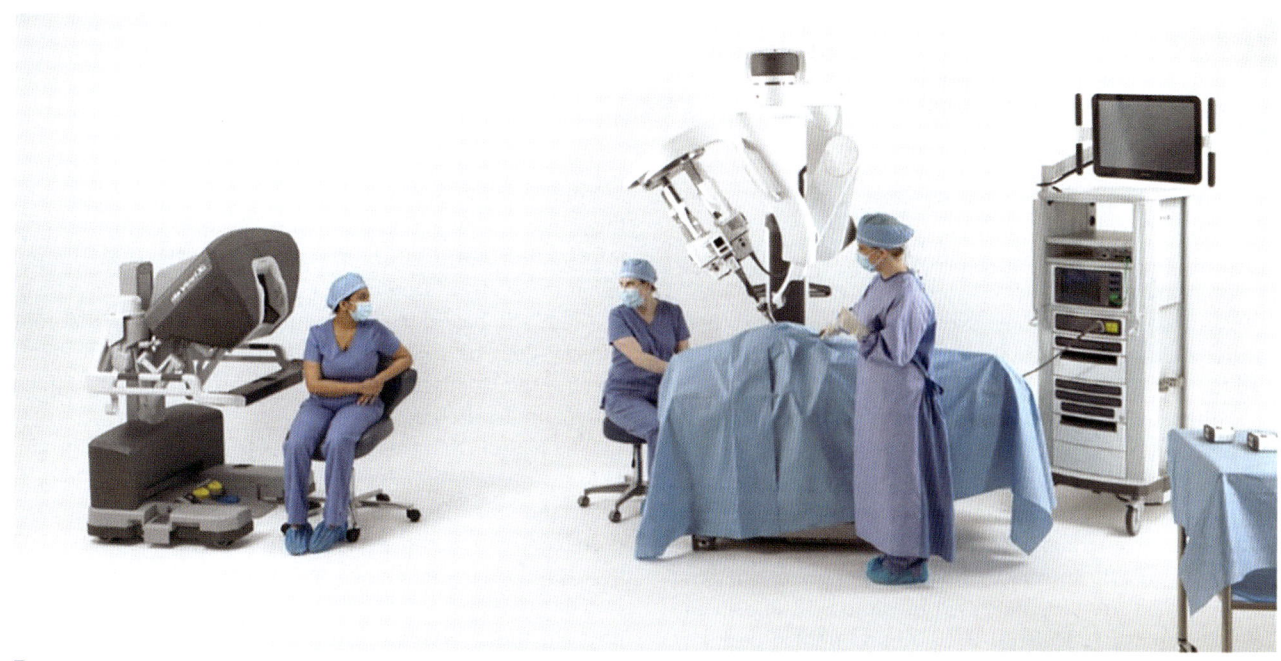

D

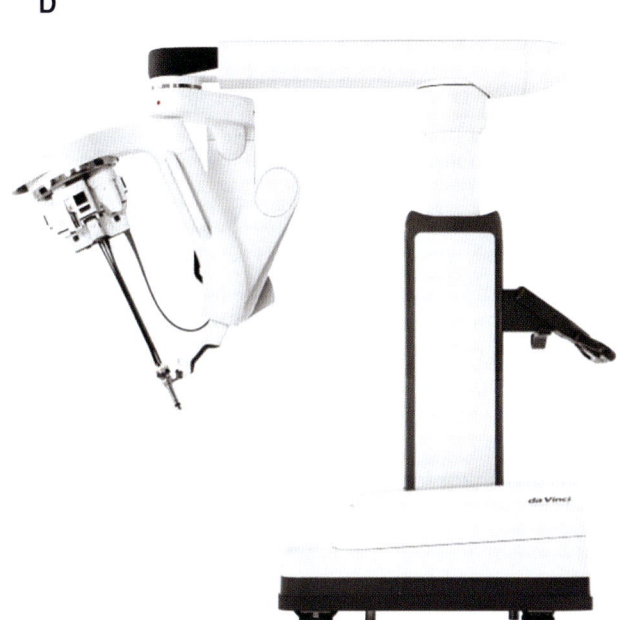

E

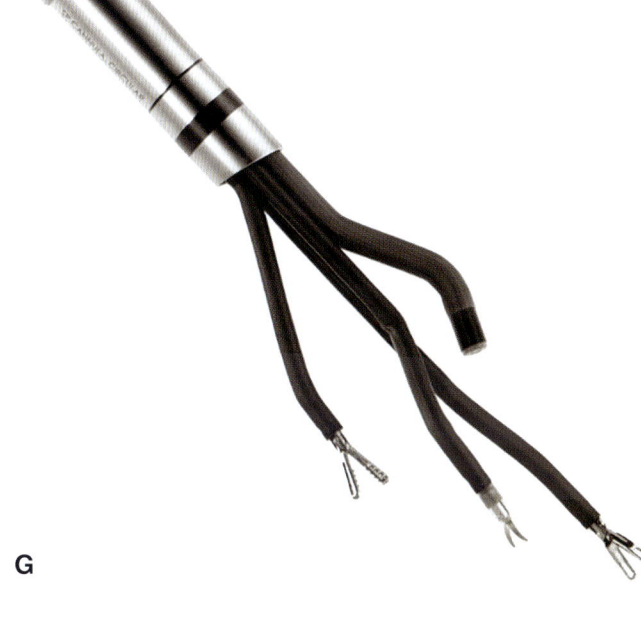

G

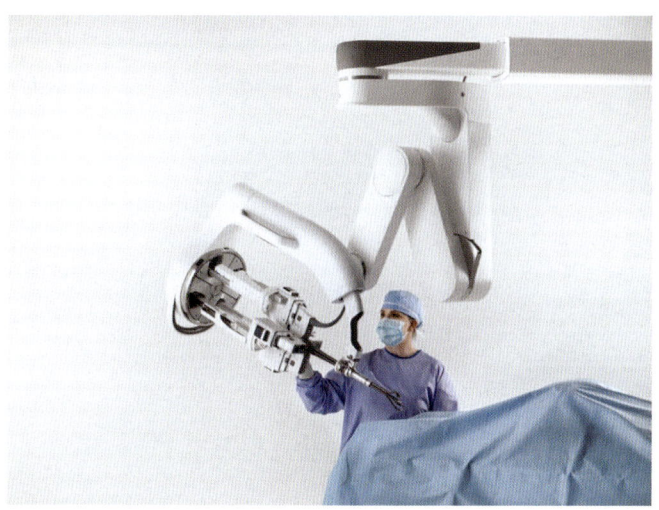

F

FIGURE 1-2 • (*Continued*)

Video 1-1. Da Vinci® Xi™ (©2022 Intuitive Surgical Operations, Inc.)

Video 1-2. Da Vinci® SP™ (©2022 Intuitive Surgical Operations, Inc.)

A year later, the FDA approved the da Vinci® system for surgical use in the United States.

At present day, the fourth generation of the da Vinci® Surgical System is being operated.

It became obvious to almost everyone that robotic surgery had overcome most technical limitations that 2 decades earlier delayed the widespread adoption of laparoscopy.

Since the original patents introduced by Intuitive Surgical (Sunnyvale, California, U.S.) have expired, the rapidly expanding release of newer robotic surgery platforms that we have been witnessing is perhaps the best corroboration of the account. Additionally, there is an ongoing steep increase of the scientific interest in the field of robotic surgery. In fact, the number of scientific articles published per year increased by almost 18-fold in the period 2005–2020 (see **Figure 1-3**, based on PubMed data, key words "robotic surgery").

Telemanipulation and Digital Interaction

For the first time in history, a surgical dogma is being infringed. The surgeon can operate on another human being without any physical contact with the operating instruments and the patient: a new concept of surgical *telemanipulation* is being introduced, and a newer discipline of *tele-* or *remote surgery* is being created.

Who or what made this scientific marvel possible? The same machine that changed and/or affected the life of every human being living in the 20th century: the computer, or *interface* as many experts of computer science would perhaps prefer to call it.

The computer or interface is the link between the surgeon, who manipulates the master grips at their working unit (the *console*), and the remote patient's unit (the *master-slave*) with its robotic arms that manipulate the instruments performing the surgery. These 3 components, by constantly exchanging information, form altogether *the system*, hence a computer-enhanced system (see **Figure 1-4**).

Many still have a hard time fully understanding that robotic surgery goes beyond a mere advance of surgical technology because they focus primarily on the hardware—the platform—and its multiple components.

The truth is that this novel surgical approach has produced a *conceptual revolution* in the surgical field that is yet to be fully witnessed and that has changed forever the way that surgery is conceptualized and perceived. A third player is stepping in between the surgeon and the patient.

The surgeons used to think that to operate on patients, a physical touch was necessary either directly with the hands or through the interposition of surgical instruments. Open surgery, endoscopic or laparoscopic instruments are mere tools that serve only one purpose: to cut, dissect, grasp, hold, retract, or suture when the surgeon's hands hold and use them to manipulate human tissues. Therefore, surgical instruments per se are incapable of providing any "intelligent" aid to the surgeon because they have a passive, inanimate nature.

Even the haptic feedback is no prerogative of the surgical instruments. The surgeon must apply some sort of pressure/force on the surgical *tool* to perceive tactile feedback.

In robotic surgery, these subservient and physically close relationships between surgical instruments and surgeon and between surgeon and patient, respectively, are all subverted as the interface places itself in between these 3 actors generating a bidirectional flow of information from one to the other and vice versa (see **Figure 1-5**).

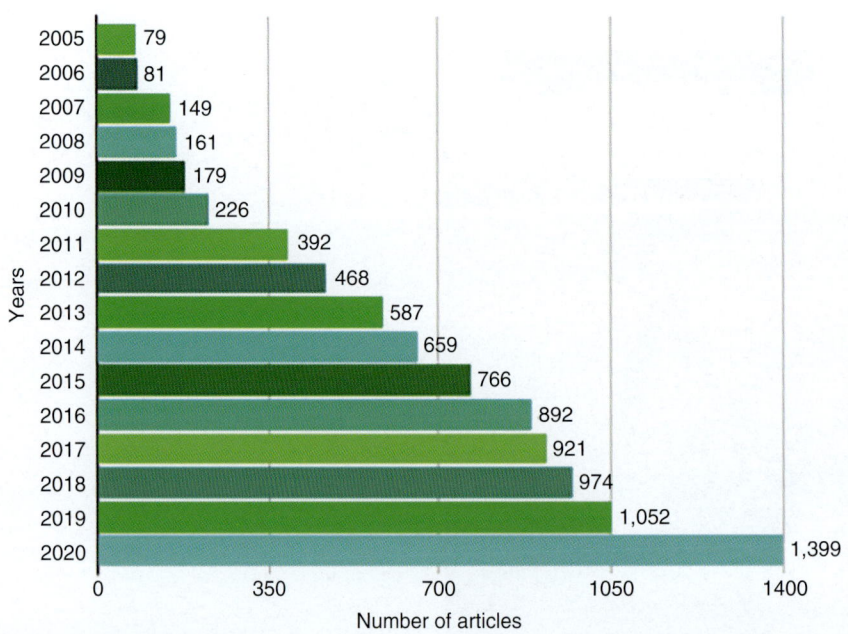

FIGURE 1-3 • The number of scientific articles published per year increased by almost 18-fold in the period 2005–2020.

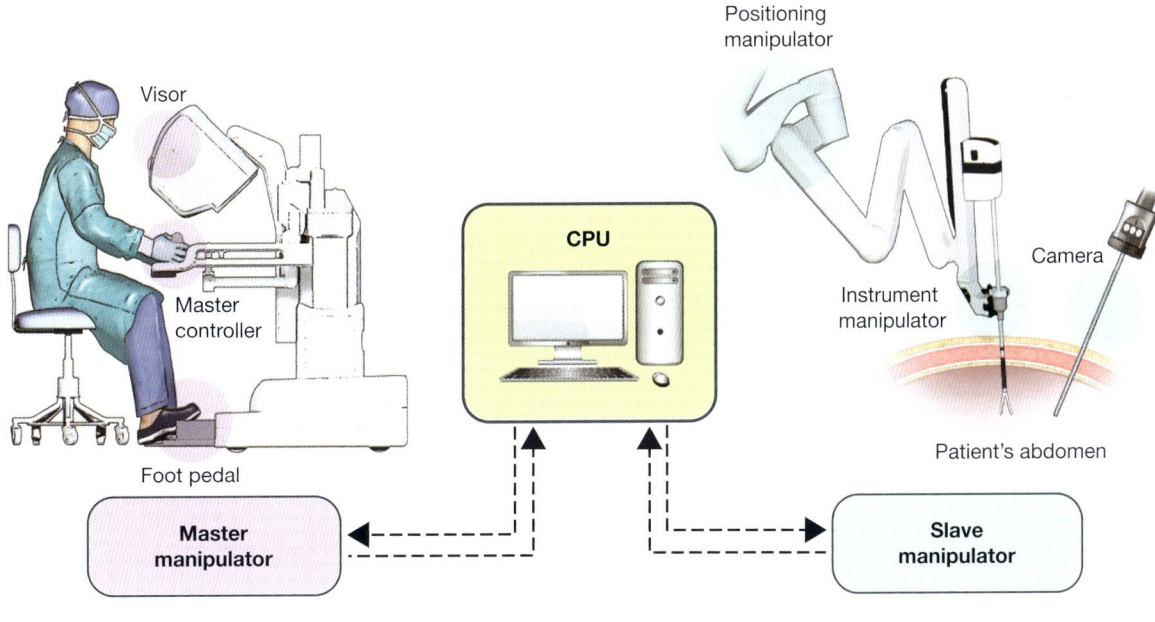

FIGURE 1-4 • The computer-enhanced system.

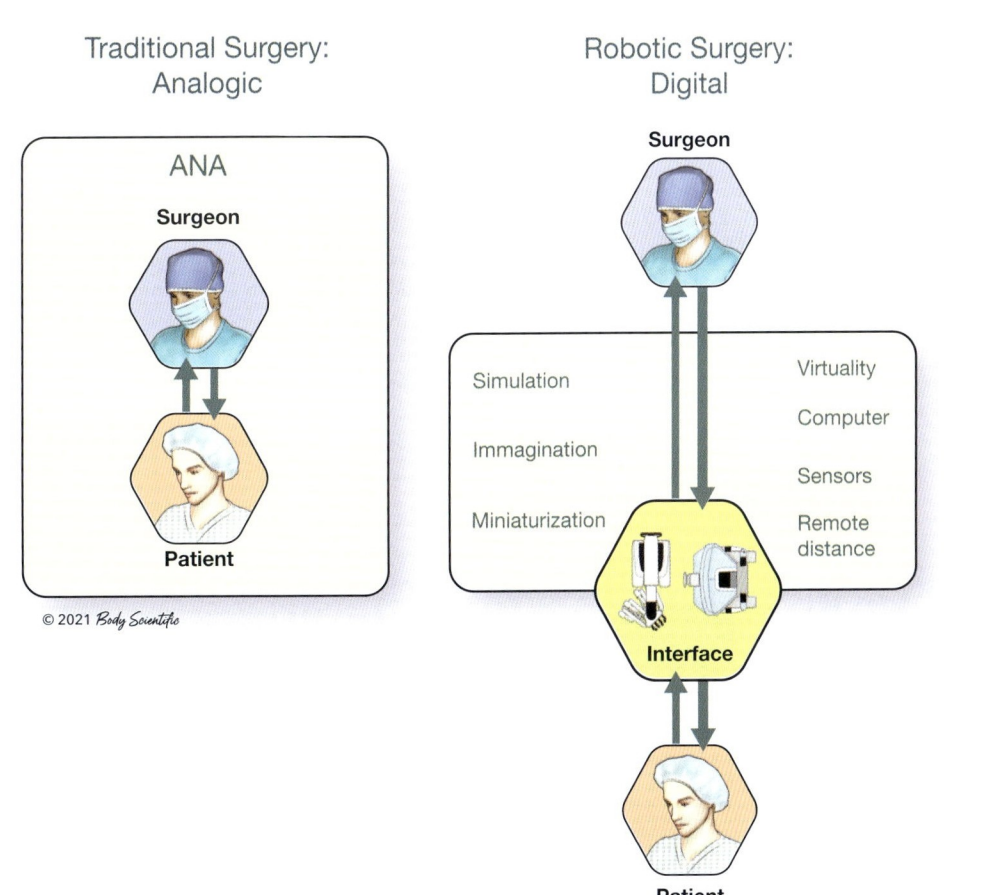

FIGURE 1-5 • Patient–surgeon interface.

Vision could be an example. Undoubtedly, it is the surgical tool—the robotic camera—that captures the images, but it is the robotic tower—the interface—that receives and processes these images, before they can be projected over the binocular screen, and be apprehended by the eyes of the surgeon at the robotic console.

Similarly, the hands of the surgeons have no physical contact with the patient's tissues or with the tools that are touching these same tissues, and any time the hands of the surgeon move the master grip at the robotic console, it is the "brain" of the tower—the interface—that receives the information generated at the console, analyzes it, and then translates it in physical motion of the robotic arms and instruments.

The robotic console and the robotic tower do not even need to be in the same physical space any more, where the master–slave and the patient are located.

As matter of fact, advances in telecommunication technology and high-speed data connection enabled the implementation of remote (transcontinental) robotic surgery. In 2001, Dr. J. Marescaux successfully removed the gallbladder of a patient lying down on the operative table in a hospital in Strasbourg (France) while the surgeon was operating at the robotic console in New York (USA).

The failure of this significant breakthrough to gain widespread popularity is conducible to regulatory and medical–legal considerations, rather than technical constraints. At the beginning, one of the limitations was the delay in transmission. Currently, with high-speed internet and high-speed wireless communication, even for long distances, the delay is <200 ms (which is compatible with the conduction of telesurgery).

Once protocols are built and cooperative agreements on a global scale are reached, patients will potentially never need to travel beyond their local hospital to access specialized care by expert robotic surgeons.

The Platform and the Hardware

Henceforward, the authors are challenged with the difficult task of describing "the robotic platform" knowing that additional and perhaps more complex or versatile platforms or, simply speaking, *different* platforms will be introduced in the years following the publication of this book.

What do current platforms have in common and what characteristics will they almost certainly share even many years from now? It is their multimodular structure that includes the patient cart, the console station, and the interface–tower ("digital interaction").

The surgeon operates at the console. It is through this module that the movements of the surgeon's hands and feet are now and will continue to be translated (in the future) by the interface–tower into movements of the instruments manipulating the patient's tissue. It is these authors' opinion and prediction that the "hardware" is likely to change and evolve over time.

A giant of the medical industry, Medtronic (Minneapolis, MN, USA), has recently released a newer and alternative robotic platform, Hugo™ Robotic-assisted surgery (RAS) system, with a submodular conformation including individual, separate, smaller carts for the camera and each robotic arm (see **Figure 1-6**).

Vision Enhancements of the Robotic Systems

This topic will be discussed in greater detail in Chapter 6, Implemented Imaging and Artificial Intelligence, of this book. Herein, a broad view about general concepts of vision-related and mechanics-related enhancements of the robotic platform is provided.

The Tridimensional Vision

The 3D vision of the surgical field introduced by robotic technology is collectively seen as the new standard, and it is indivisible from future advancement of robotic platforms.

There are currently 2 strategies in place for achieving robotic 3D vision. The first one relies on the use of 2 optics inside the robotic camera converging into one binocular system mounted right below the area of the console where the surgeon places their forehead. The surgeon can adjust the height of the console, armrest, and the location of the pedals, so that they can comfortably sit in the chair with their head and eyes in line with their straight-up torso. The pros of this system are a more "natural" feel, more comfortable position, and better ergonomics; the surgeon is more focused on the intraoperative image with no external distractions; and the 3D quality of the image is perfect due to a combination of the HD technology and magnified images with absolute mechanical stability

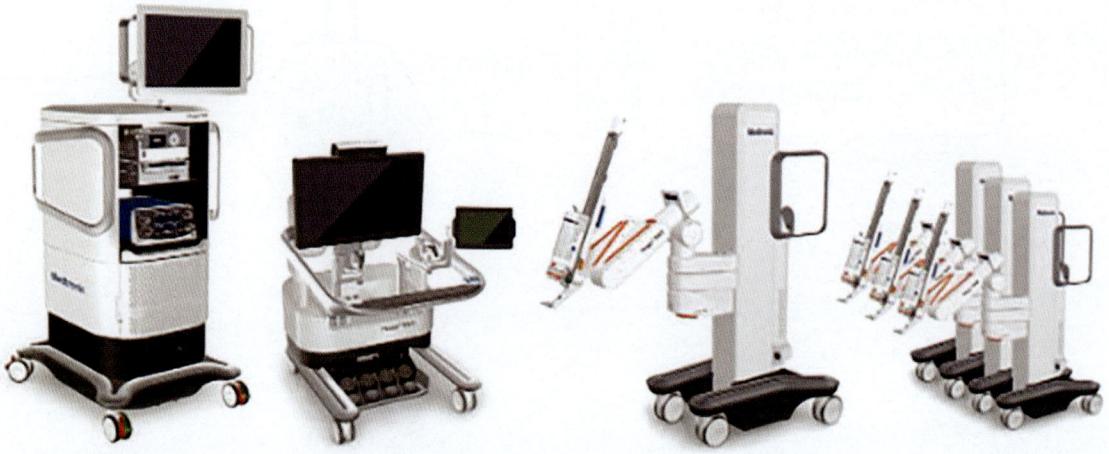

FIGURE 1-6 • Medtronic's new Hugo™ Robotic-assisted surgery (RAS) system. (©2022 Medtronic. All rights reserved. Used with the permission of Medtronic.)

(a considerable advantage over laparoscopy). However, the cons of this technology are limited peripheral vision because the surgeon is looking through binoculars, and there may be some fatigue at the neck level, in particular during long procedures.

A more recent alternative strategy has been adopted. In this system, biocular 3D vision can be presented to the surgeon on a 2D monitor. In order for the user to differentiate the 2 images presented simultaneously, a mediary (typically 3D glasses) is used. These glasses can separate the images in multiple ways:

1. Anaglyph glasses: The old-fashioned red and blue glasses that pioneered the technology.
2. Polarized glasses: Using polarized lenses that restrict light passing through in the opposite polarized direction allows each lens to present a different image. However, this technology typically requires a specific monitor that separates the pixels using an orthogonal polarizing filter.
3. Shutter 3D Glasses: These are currently the most advanced type of 3D glasses on the market to date. These glasses function by alternately dimming each lens rapidly. Using a high refresh rate monitor (e.g., 120 Hz display), the 120 images shown per second display 60 unique images per eye.

These options all allow the surgeon to maintain peripheral vision of the surroundings in the operating room. However, eyestrain and sensations of motion sickness are well-known shortcomings of these kinds of visual aids.

Fluorescence Enhancement

Near infrared indocyanine green (ICG) fluorescence will be described in detail in Chapter 6, Implemented Imaging and Artificial Intelligence, and Chapter 7, Fluorescence Imaging: Basics and Clinical Applications.

The fluorescence-capable robotic camera can now aid the surgeon not only in the recognition of the surgical anatomy, but also with the intraoperative identification of biliary structures or with real-time assessment of the blood supply to the tissues being surgically manipulated.

The near-infrared ICG dye is injected into the patient prior to the start of the operation, or during the procedure, and it reaches the target tissue that is being manipulated by the surgeon. At this point, the laser source inside the robotic camera will excite the ICG to fluoresce, and the tissue that has previously absorbed the dye will turn into a bright, intense green. The surgeon is in full control, and can switch back and forth from the white light imaging mode (powered by the LED light source placed inside the camera) to the fluorescent (green) light mode by the touch of a button at the robotic console (see **Figure 1-7** and Chapters 6 and 7 for more details).

Augmented Reality and Virtual Reality Enhancement

Implemented images and augmented reality will be more extensively described in detail in Chapter 6. Herein, a general preliminary introduction about the basic principles and potential future applications will be provided.

The old adage that surgical planning is the first step of a successful surgical procedure still holds true. However, the 2 were once physically and chronologically separated. The enhancement of the vision enabled by this feature of the robotic system—augmented reality—is destined to infringe this dogma. But before digging deeper into the possible applications and benefits of this technology, some words of elucidation are required. What is *augmented* reality and how does this differentiate from *virtual* reality? The former adds to (augmented comes from the Latin *augēre* "to increase") reality, while the latter recreates it.

Thanks to the augmented reality feature, the interface can, for instance, store and then project in real time the preoperative imaging over the surgical field at the robotic console (see **Figure 1-8**). With this technique of intraoperative augmented reality, 3D virtual models of tumors can be obtained from preoperative magnetic resonance imaging (MRI) or computed tomography (CT) scans, and then be superimposed on the surgical field while the robotic surgeon is performing the resection. Liver and adrenal tumors relying on the superimposed images have been already successfully resected by some

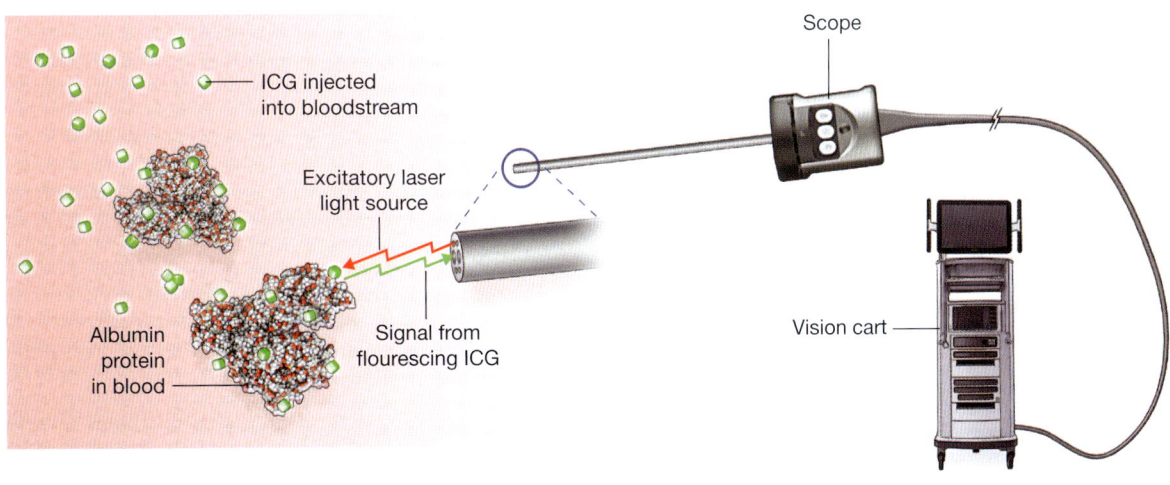

FIGURE 1-7 • Fluorescence imaging vision system.

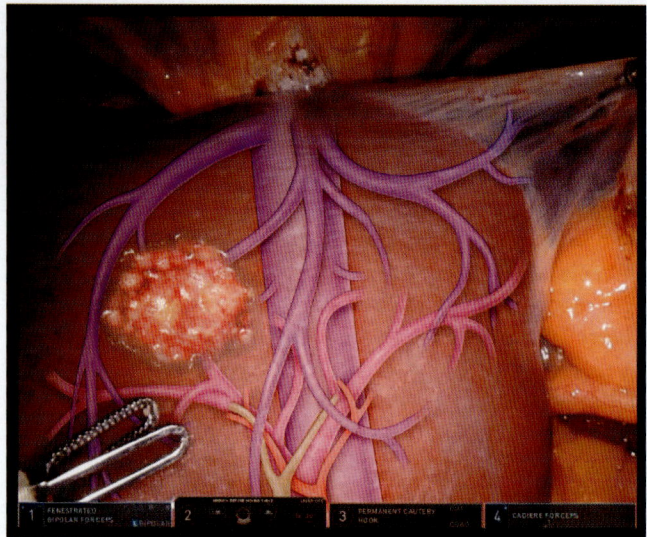

FIGURE 1-8 • This is an example of how an augmented reality system may potentially work in the future. The location of the tumor and its anatomical relationships with the surrounding anatomy will be superimposed in real time during the surgical operation on the actual intraoperative images (here, for paradigmatic purposes, the vessels and the tumor are represented by a drawing, not by an augmented reality system based on actual imaging data. Whereas, the intraoperative image is from an actual surgical case).

pioneer centers across the globe, and this technology will soon be widely available.

Virtual reality goes one step further because it recreates reality. Soon, patient-specific 3D models will be created and implemented into a robotic surgery simulator. This will enable the surgeon, before even setting a foot inside the operative theater, to simulate and field test their intended surgical approach in a virtual reality and risk-free environment.

Integrated Information Enhancements

The interface can hold a much larger amount of information and data than even the most gifted human brain could. In the future, if surgeons will encounter a very unusual and technically challenging situation (that they might not have seen or treated before), they may be getting real time access to an entire video library on technical tips and tricks to deal with that specific technical challenge by the simple clicking of a button, and without moving their eyes off the binocular of the robotic console.

Sooner than later, all the various robotic platforms will have integrated information systems as described.

Mechanical Enhancements

Perhaps the best way to summarize the "mechanistic" benefits of the robotic systems is to say that they do provide a human hand with all its associated advantages, but without its limitations.

The EndoWrist®

It is these authors' opinion that another functional element of the hardware destined to remain unchanged potentially forever is the robotic *wrist*, which is modeled after its human equivalent (the EndoWrist®, if we go by the original and branded name of the leading industry at the time of writing; see **Figures 1-9 A, B**).

The 7 degrees of freedom of the robotic *wrist* enable the surgeon—one will still have to work through their own learning curve—to potentially perform any complex surgical tasks at ease, without suffering the mechanical stress on their own joints that is inevitably associated with the 4 degrees of freedom of laparoscopic instruments, while getting additional degrees of freedom that the human wrist would be otherwise not capable of.

 Video 1-3. Da Vinci EndoWrist® (©2022 Intuitive Surgical Operations, Inc.)

However, the progression of miniaturization is likely going to result in the availability of smaller and more flexible robotic wrists, perhaps even in the elimination of the multiwire system that is currently supporting the mechanics of their "joints."

Stability—Lack of Tremor and Down Scaling

Understandably, a tremor is a peculiar feature and intrinsic limitation of even the finest surgeon's hand. This intrinsic limitation can impinge on the accuracy of the surgical manipulation. This is an especially important consideration in the setting of microsurgery where the highest degree of accuracy is expected.

A common denominator of all robotic-aided technology is the stability and *lack of tremor*.

The physical separation created by the robotic platform between the tremor-encumbered initiator (the surgeon's hand maneuvering the master grips at the console) and the tremor-free effector (the robotic instrument being held by the robotic arms) of the manipulation allows filtering of the motion. Similarly, the amplitude of surgical motion has represented a major obstacle to the further expansion of microsurgery. Even the smallest millimetric movement of the human hand can be disproportionately larger than the *micron*-size of some human tissues that are the target of surgical manipulation (e.g., the retinal membrane or the microvasculature of a solid organ). This discrepancy between the hand-generated motion and the motion at the output greatly curbs the accuracy of some microsurgery procedures and averts the technical feasibility of others.

The interface of the robotic platform can modulate the amplitude of the hand motion to various degrees (for the leading industry platform this would be a ratio of 1 to 7) causing the motion at the output to be a fraction of the hand motion. The surgeon can then carry out larger motions with greater accuracy. These 2 features of the robotic platform (lack of tremor

What Robotic Surgery Is   11

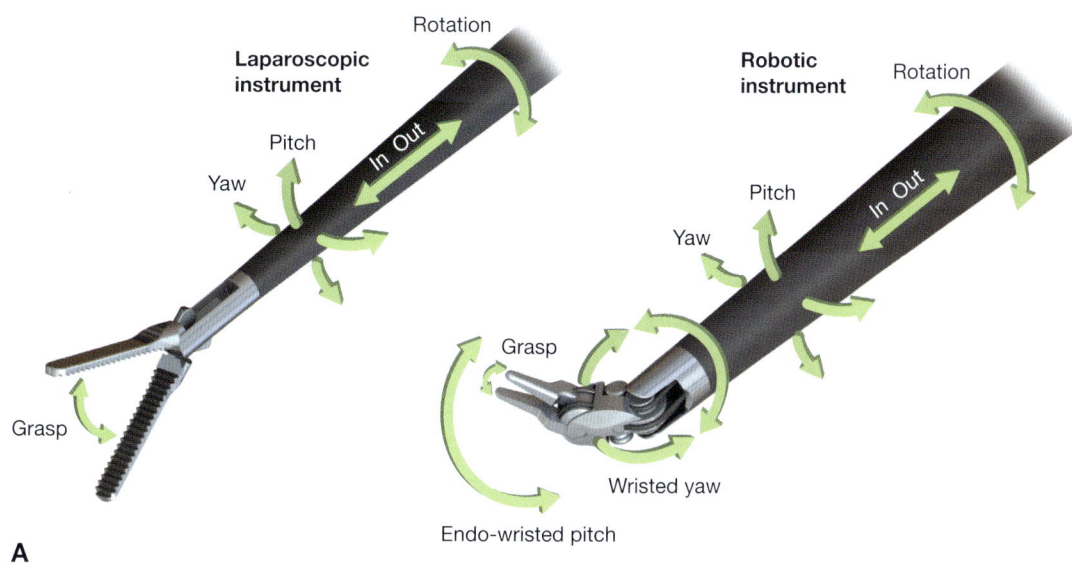

A

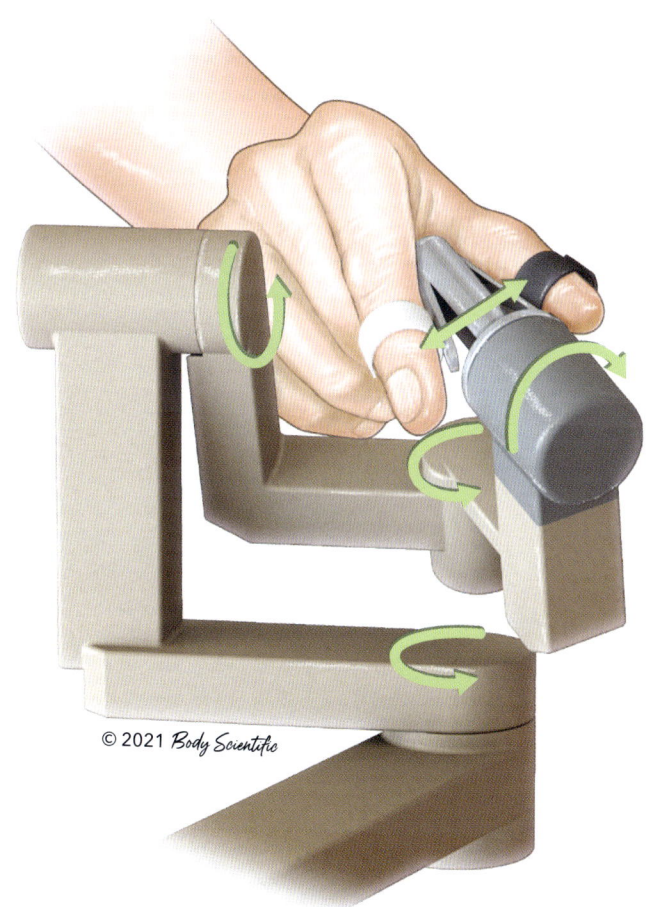

B

FIGURE 1-9 • **A.** Laparoscopic versus robotic instruments. **B.** Robotic wrist.

and downscaling) have opened the way to new surgical procedures that until not long ago would have been considered unthinkable in the traditional minimally invasive surgical setting; for example, the robot-assisted kidney transplant and the procurement of partial graft from living donors. Robotic-assisted retinal surgery is another area of possible expansion in the future. The border of what is feasible microsurgically will be pushed farther and farther away over the next few decades and will allow surgery at even a cellular level (*nano surgery*).

The Role of AI: General Principles, Current Limitations, and Future Perspectives

For more details about augmented reality/implemented images and artificial intelligence (AI), please see Chapter 6, Implemented Imaging and Artificial Intelligence. Herein, the fundamental basic principles and potential future applications will be provided.

If it is true that computers will continue to evolve, progress, and advance, then potentially endless opportunities and applications of the *computer-enhanced* robotic technology can be foreseeable. It is therefore an arduous task for these authors to anticipate all possible scenarios of further technological expansion. However, the recent and successful application of AI has inspired a fast-growing alliance between tech giants, academic institutions, and surgical companies. This will soon empower and further speed up the evolution and potential clinical applications of AI.

AI can be defined as a multidisciplinary field composed of several subdomains (e.g., machine learning, neural networks, computer vision, natural language processing, Bayesian methods), with the common purpose of creating algorithms to make machines capable of executing cognitive tasks (e.g., words/image recognition, problem solving, or even making decisions). In other words, AI uses various technologies to create intelligent machines able to accomplish specific goals.

Over the last 15 years, in the scientific literature, there has been a steep increasing trend regarding the applications of AI in surgical context. In particular, between 2018 (132 articles) and 2020 (812 articles), there has been an over 6-fold increase in the amount of scientific literature production (see **Figure 1-10**).

The potential surgical applications of AI will be evident during the preoperative, intraoperative, and postoperative periods.

During the ***preoperative*** **period,** some future applications of AI will potentially be:

1. Tracking/storage of data (e.g., diet, physical activity, weight) on the patient's smartphone/smart watch may be integrated into the electronic medical record and managed by AI algorithms.
2. Improvement of preoperative imaging results.
3. AI-personalized prediction of the preoperative overall risk.

In terms of **future *intraoperative* applications of AI**, the robotic platform will be one of the most effective tools to utilize and further develop the technology. If integrated into the robotic platform, AI will be combined with several synergistic technological features; for example, near-infrared ICG fluorescence or 3D stereotactic vision-system implemented with tailored image-guided surgery. Some of the possible intraoperative applications of AI include:

1. Global OR coordination: anesthesia (ventilation, IV fluids), surgical bed control, OR environment and lighting, integration of diagnostic tools, automatic docking, help in port positioning, and OR communication.

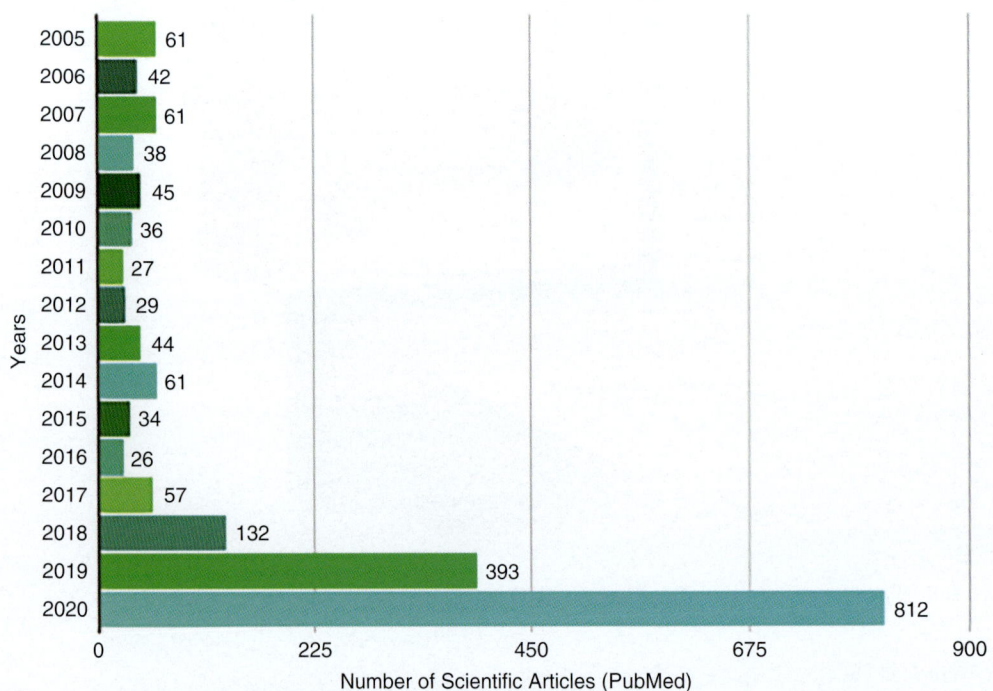

FIGURE 1-10 • The number of articles available on PubMed from 2005 to 2020; keywords "artificial intelligence" and "surgery."

2. Intraoperative correct recognition of the anatomy and differential diagnosis.
3. Evaluation of tissue perfusion (e.g., a score estimating the chances of anastomotic leakage).
4. Intraoperative diagnosis of complications.
5. Predictions of postoperative complications.
6. Assistance in surgical decision-making.
7. Providing patient clinical information intraoperatively.
8. Identification of specific steps of the surgical procedure, and possible alarms/warnings when an iatrogenic injury is about to happen or when a standardized step is missing.
9. Counting surgical instruments or assessing suturing performance.
10. Checking on the patient's vital parameters.
11. Integrated surgical instruments (e.g., energy-based devices with real-time data on their thermal lateral spread around neural structures).
12. Digital pathology.
13. Virtual fixtures enhancement. The surgeon predraws a safe region delimited by lines along specific structures in the surgical field and then programs the *interface* (computer) to apply resistive force to the robotic instruments anytime they will try to get into the forbidden area. This technology will probably have useful applications in training. In the foreseeable future, AI may take over this role, and draw the lines in place of the attentive and guiding eye of a human expert.
14. Automated surgery.

Finally, during the **postoperative period**, AI will have multiple applications, including:

1. Constant and tailored monitoring, via the patient's smart devices (smartphone, smart watches), may be useful during the follow-up period: weight loss tracking or physical activity trends after bariatric procedures.
2. Prognostic markers.
3. Cost reduction and unburdening clinicians from administrative tasks.
4. Prevention of malpractice

AI: Current Limitations and Future Perspective

In spite of the vast potential of AI, there is an intrinsic limitation related to data accuracy (e.g., systematic bias, wrong labeling/classification). This may hamper pattern detection and the reliability of AI-based predictions. In other words, AI learns by assessing preexisting evidences; hence, data quality is crucial for finding meaningful results.

Clinicians have a key role in evaluating AI estimations and framing the outputs in the proper context. To direct the progress of AI and achieve the most useful clinical applications, teamwork among different professionals will be essential (e.g., medical professionals such as surgeons, oncologists, radiologists, and pathologists, and also computer scientists and engineers).

AI will increasingly be used in a varied range of clinical fields. The clinician will have an essential function in evolving, guiding, and evaluating AI progression in order to achieve the most relevant clinical needs. On the one hand, the robotic platform is one of the most appropriate tools for fostering the evolution of, assessing, and improving AI. On the other hand, AI will play a major and pivotal role in the development of the next generation of surgical robots and in redefining the role of the surgeon inside the operating room.

AI and robotics are part of our present world. Despite this, we are still far from involving AI in the entire OR work. The robot is a powerful tool, but it is surrounded by old-fashioned technology, and currently, most processes are still performed manually. It is possible to imagine a "smart" AI-integrated OR with partial automatization of some surgical tasks in the near future.

The robotic surgeon of the future will likely have a supervisory role as the physical execution of those critical portions of the surgical procedure that require extreme precision and the finest motor skills will be carried out by the surgical robot. How far this concept of autonomy is going to get is a matter of further future dissertation and speculation.

Suggested Readings

1. Giulianotti PC, Coratti A, Angelini M, et al. Robotics in general surgery: personal experience in a large community hospital. *Arch Surg.* 2003;138(7):777-784. doi: 10.1001/archsurg.138.7.777
2. Ghezzi TL, Corleta OC. 30 years of robotic surgery. *World J Surg.* 2016;40(10):2550-2557. doi: 10.1007/s00268-016-3543-9
3. Johnson KB, Wei WQ, Weeraratne D et al. Precision medicine, AI, and the future of personalized health care. *Clin Transl Sci.* 2021;14(1):86-93.
4. Hashimoto DA, Rosman G, Rus D, et al. Artificial intelligence in surgery: promises and perils. *Ann Surg.* 2018;268(1):70-76.
5. Topol, E. *Deep Medicine: How Artificial Intelligence Can Make Healthcare Human Again.* Basic Books; 2019.
6. Yao RQ, Jin X, Wang GW, et al. A machine learning-based prediction of hospital mortality in patients with postoperative sep-
7. Skrede OJ, De Raedt S, Kleppe A, et al. Deep learning for prediction of colorectal cancer outcome: a discovery and validation study. *Lancet.* 2020;395(10221):350-360.
8. Mangano A, Valle V, Dreifuss NH, et al. Role of artificial intelligence (AI) in surgery: introduction, general principles, and potential applications. *Surg Technol Int.* 2020;38:17-21.
9. Handelman A KY, Livny E, Barkan R, Nahum Y, Tepper R. Evaluation of suturing performance in general surgery and ocular microsurgery by combining computer vision-based software and distributed fiber optic strain sensors: a proof-of-concept. *Int J Comput Assist Radiol Surg.* 2020;1359-1367. doi: 10.1007/s11548-020-02187-y
10. Hashimoto DA, Rosman G, Witkowski ER, et al. Computer vision analysis of intraoperative video: automated recognition of operative steps in laparoscopic sleeve gastrectomy. *Ann Surg.* 2019;270(3):414-421.

11. Giulianotti PC, Mangano A, Bustos RE, et al. Educational step-by-step surgical video about operative technique in robotic pancreaticoduodenectomy (RPD) at University of Illinois at Chicago (UIC): 17 steps standardized technique-Lessons learned since the first worldwide RPD performed in the year 2001. *Surg Endoscop.* 2020; 34(6):2758-2762.
12. Rimmer L, Howard C, Picca L, Bashir M. The automaton as a surgeon: the future of artificial intelligence in emergency and general surgery. *Eur J Trauma Emerg Surg.* 2021;47(3):757-762.
13. Carpentier A, Loulmet D, Aupècle B, et al. Computer assisted open heart surgery. First case operated on with success. *C R Acad Sci III.* 1998;321(5):437-442.
14. Diana M, Soler L, Agnus V, et al. Prospective evaluation of precision multimodal gallbladder surgery navigation: virtual reality, near-infrared fluorescence, and x-ray-based intraoperative cholangiography. *Ann Surg.* 2017;266(5):890-897.
15. Gangemi A, Danilkowicz R, Elli FE, Bianco F, Masrur M, Giulianotti PC. Could ICG-aided robotic cholecystectomy reduce the rate of open conversion reported with laparoscopic approach? A head-to-head comparison of the largest single institution studies *J Robot Surg.* 2017;11(1):77-82.
16. Marescaux J, Smith M K, Fölscher D, et al. Telerobotic laparoscopic cholecystectomy: initial clinical experience with 25 patients. *Ann Surg.* 2001;234(1):1-7. doi: 10.1097/00000658-200107000-00001

"Get the fundamentals down and the level of everything you do will rise."
—Michael Jordan (1963)

The Basic Principles of Clinical Applications

Gabriela Aguiluz • Stephan Gruessner • Patrice Frederick

THE IMPORTANCE OF A FOUNDATION IN GENERAL SURGICAL PRINCIPLES

While robotic surgery is a significant innovation over open and laparoscopic surgery, the core principles are built on the foundation set forth by traditional surgery. Before becoming proficient in robotics, these principles should be understood:

- First and foremost, every surgery should have an organized, logical, and patient-focused approach. This can be done by segmenting the procedure into easy-to-remember steps and optimizing the surgical approach.
- The surgeon should have a detailed understanding of the anatomy. This includes the relative location of pertinent anatomy, and the variations, texture, and strength of the respective tissues. Identifying the distinct embryological planes and pedicels must guide the dissection.
- Traction and countertraction should be used effectively to dissect tissue along natural planes.
- Each instruments indications, capabilities, and drawbacks should be perfectly comprehended. The instruments should become an extension of the surgeon's hand and be used intuitively.
- Proper exposure is vital to any surgery. This is achieved by multiple, coordinated actions like retracting with the nondominant hand, utilizing gravity, and guiding the assistant's work.
- Basic hemostatic techniques should be mastered and applied based on the severity and source of bleeding.

Incorporating Laparoscopic Knowledge and Skills

Many of the surgeons being trained today are advancing to robotic surgery without the experience gained by years of laparoscopic surgery. While this is possible due to the intuitive nature of the robotic platform, they may ultimately lose out on fundamental knowledge and skills necessary for mastery. The usual environment for robotic surgery is the laparoscopic one. This means that a laparoscopic background facilitates overcoming the learning curve.

Common problems such as fogging of the camera, loss of pneumoperitoneum, hinge effects, inadvertent bowel injuries, CO_2 emphysema, and adhesions can also happen in robotic surgery. A mature laparoscopic experience helps in adopting tricks in creative troubleshooting. Also, maintaining laparoscopic skills (such as dissection and suturing) may be necessary for hybrid situations. An initial laparoscopic adhesiolysis to create the proper working space is an example of a hybrid situation. Also, in case of conversion for a mechanical breakdown of the system, the surgeon should be able to finish the operation in a minimally invasive way.

The following sections introduce and expand on some of these core concepts and translate them to robotic surgery.

Proper Patient Positioning

The surgical suite utilized for the robotic platform must accommodate the movement of the patient cart. Once the room is set up, the next step is to ensure proper patient positioning. An optimal position of the surgical table from the beginning is important to avoid inefficiencies. Anytime a position change is required, the robotic cart needs to be undocked and redocked unless a synchronized table is used. The patient's position must also maximize the benefits of gravity, which aid in the natural retraction of tissue and allow the surgeon and the assistant to access targeted anatomy during critical steps of the procedure. For example, in robotic cholecystectomy, the patient is placed in a reverse Trendelenburg and a slight left lateral decubitus position (**Figure 2-1A**). However, in the pelvic step of robotic

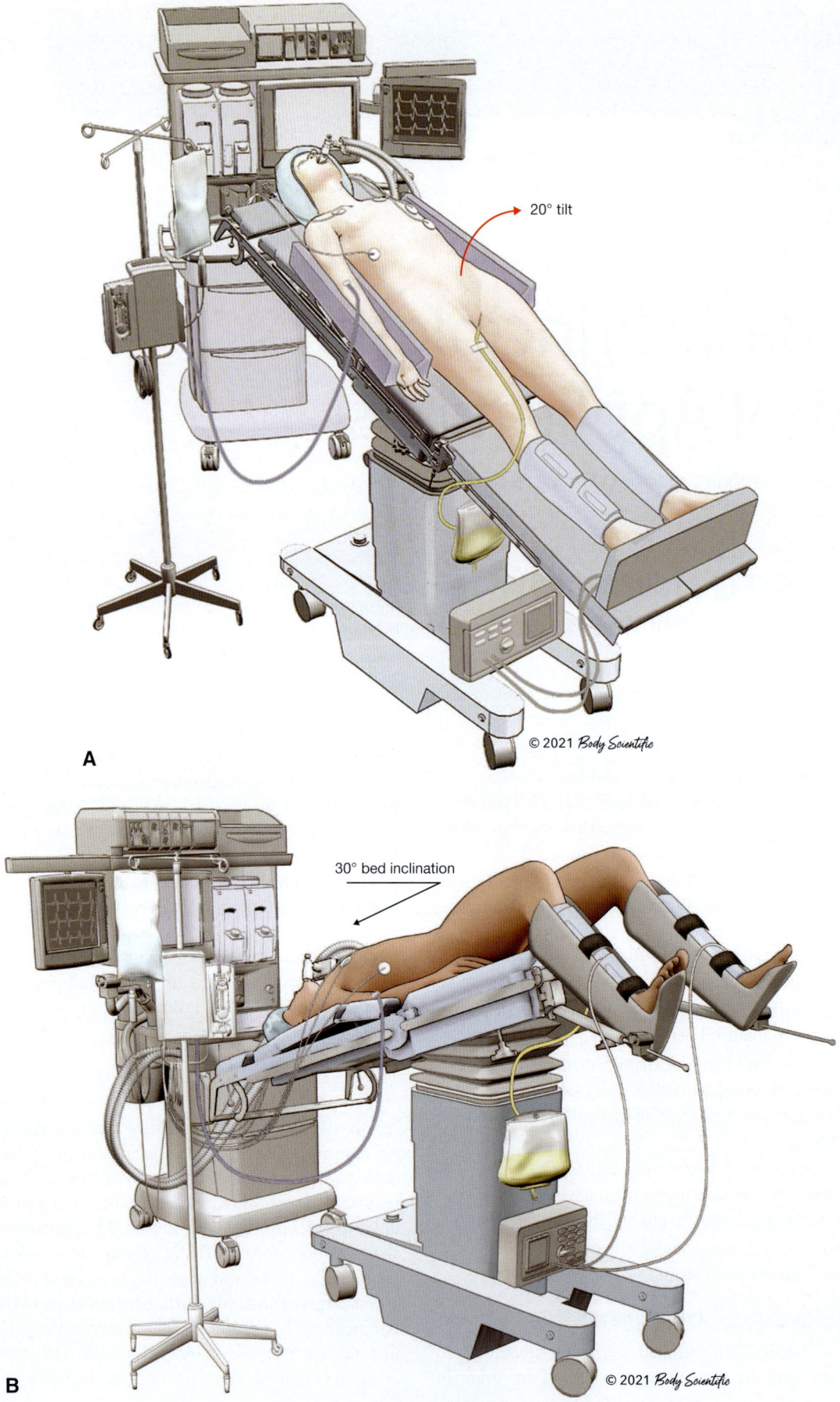

FIGURE 2-1 • A. Patient positioning for upper quadrant abdominal surgery. **B.** Patient positioning for lower quadrant abdominal surgery.

sigmoidectomy, the patient is positioned in a steep Trendelenburg and lithotomy position (**Figure 2-1B**).

Integrated OR tables that synchronize motion with the robotic cart are available. The synchronization has the benefit of adjusting the patient's position when the robot is docked. However, for significant changes such as reverse-to-steep Trendelenburg for rectal surgery, the cart should still be redocked for safety reasons.

The final port position is required before docking the robot. Once the patient has been positioned, the robotic arms are adjusted to limit conflict between the arms, the patient cart, and the OR table. Also, the arms need to be adjusted to avoid potential conflicts during instrument manipulation and insertion or injury to the patient can occur. Communication with the OR staff is essential to ensure that all potential objects are adjusted away from the patient cart as the patient cart is moved for docking to avoid large collisions.

Establishing the Pneumoperitoneum

The initial entry into the abdomen must be performed safely. Over half of complications in minimally invasive surgery occur during initial port entry. Multiple options exist, including open and closed techniques. Open techniques involve Hasson and direct optical entry. Closed techniques include Veress needle insertion and gasless trocar insertion. Many factors contribute to the choice of initial entry: previous surgery, abdominal distention, body habitus of the patient, hepatosplenomegaly, the presence of abdominal hernias, and the surgeon's preference and experience.

The Veress technique is possibly the most flexible and versatile way to induce pneumoperitoneum in different body habitus, including obesity. Veress needle entry is preferred in the left upper quadrant (LUQ). A modified Palmer's point insertion is performed within 1 cm of the subcostal region and lateral to the midclavicular line (**Figure 2-2A**). When placing the needle close to the subcostal area, the fascia is fixed, and the abdominal wall layers are thinner, even in obese patients, allowing greater success of entry. When the needle is inserted lateral to the midclavicular line, there is less risk of puncturing the colon, stomach, liver, or spleen. The stomach should be decompressed preoperatively by the anesthesiologist with a naso- or orogastric tube. Hepatosplenomegaly could be a contraindication to this approach. Most adhesions typically present medially, so the lateral insertion will be safer if the patient has had previous abdominal surgery. While rare, there is a

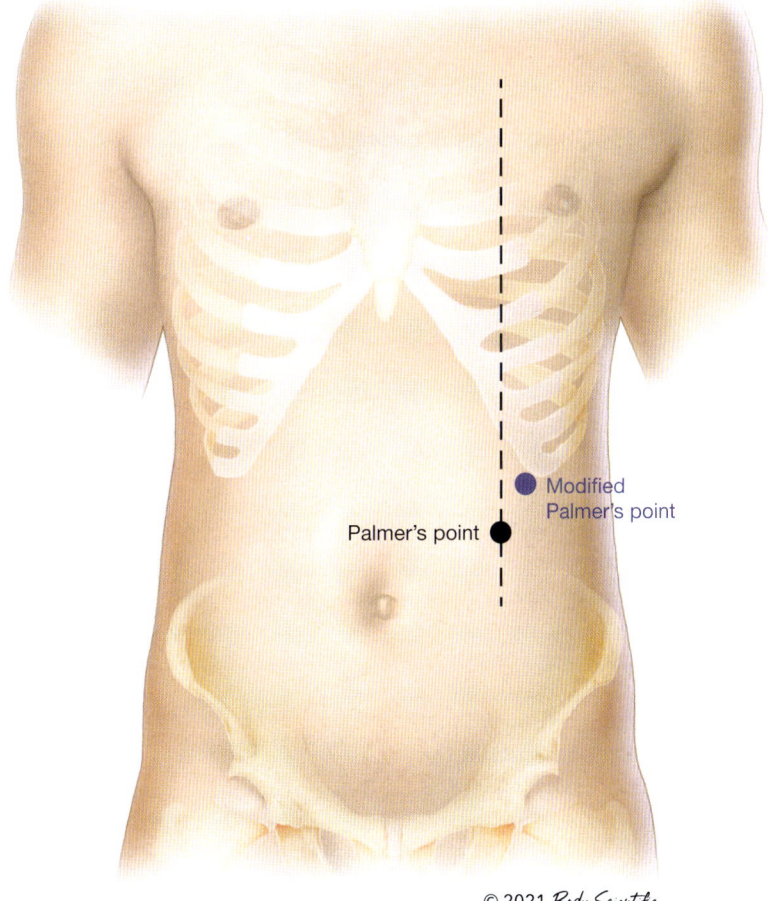

FIGURE 2-2 • **A.** Modified Palmer's point.

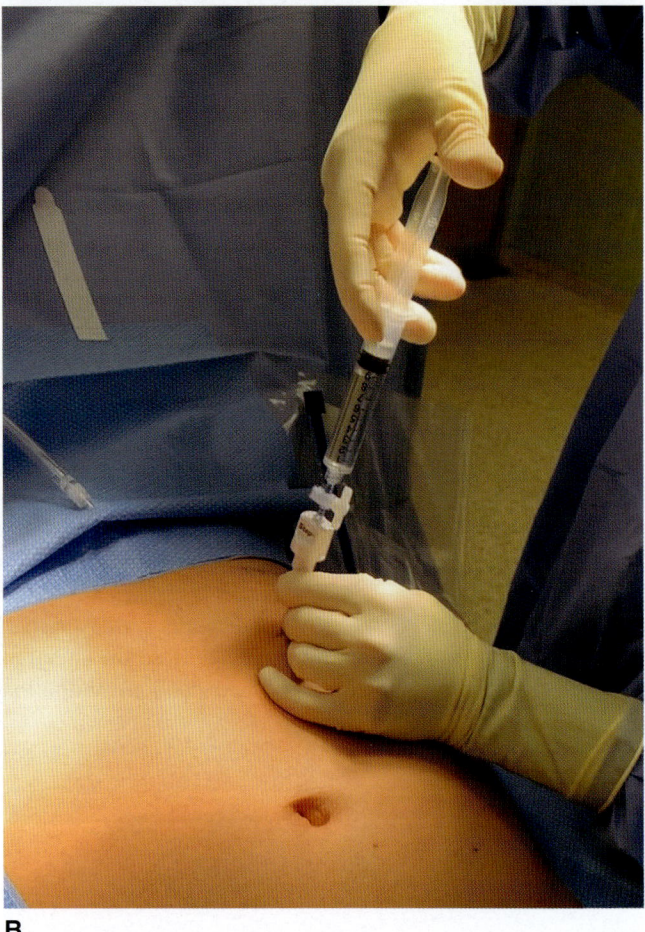

FIGURE 2-2 • (Continued) B. Saline drop test.

concern of injuring the great vessels, which a lateral insertion should prevent.

After insertion of the needle, a saline drop test is done (**Figure 2-2B**). A syringe with saline is attached to the Veress needle and aspirated, looking for any organic material such as blood. Then, a small amount of saline is injected into the needle to determine if it freely drops into the abdomen. At this point, the initial intraperitoneal pressure is checked upon the insufflation of CO_2. If the initial intra-abdominal pressures are >8 mm Hg, the Veress needle may be malpositioned. After confirming the adequate placement of the Veress needle, insufflation is allowed to reach maximum pressure, routinely 12–15 mm Hg. Then, the first port is inserted by direct optical entry. This technique allows the abdominal wall layers to be visualized through a transparent trocar with the endoscope.

After 3 failed Veress attempts in the LUQ, the needle is moved to the umbilicus. The umbilicus can be strongly lifted with a towel clamp, and the Veress needle is inserted in the infraumbilical area with another saline drop test. If this proves to be unsuccessful, the use of an optical trocar in the lateral LUQ with the gasless technique is suggested. Direct optical entry without prior insufflation with CO_2 should be done preferably in the lateral LUQ, but other locations are feasible depending on patient variables such as previous operations, presence of scars, hepatosplenomegaly, and port placement planning. However, the insertion should be extremely careful, considering the anatomy underneath in the potential trajectory of the port.

The final method, the Hasson technique, involves direct visualization and dissection of the preperitoneal tissues, followed by the incision of the peritoneum and a blunt trocar insertion. This technique is typically done by making a 10-mm incision above the umbilicus, where the abdominal wall is thinner but can be used in any quadrant if the patient has a normal body mass index (BMI). The subcutaneous tissue is then dissected under direct visualization, and the fascia is divided. The peritoneum is grasped with a pair of hemostats, elevated, and carefully opened with a scalpel. Stay sutures are placed in the fascia. A blunt trocar is inserted into the peritoneum under direct visualization, and the balloon is inflated to decrease the air leak.

The Concept of Triangulation and the Priorities of Port Placement

When planning the initial port placement, the primary goals are to optimize triangulation for enhanced visualization and dexterity. The purpose of triangulation is to reconstruct the natural way that humans are interacting with the environment. Just like how our eyes are directed toward an object while 2 hands are manipulating it on both sides, the robotic camera is directed toward the target anatomy between 2 instruments. This creates a triangle, with the peak signifying the target anatomy,

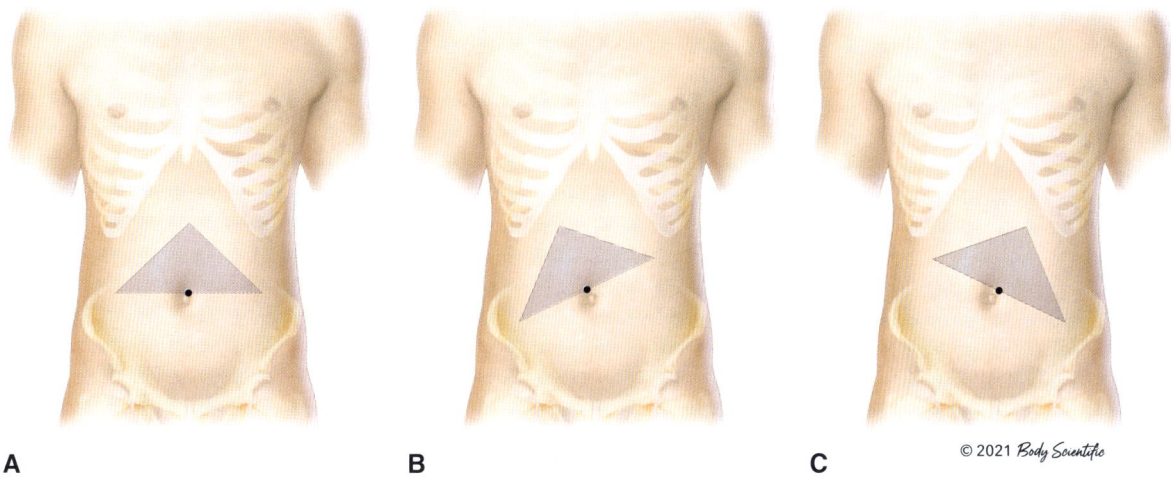

FIGURE 2-3 • Triangulation.

and 2 corners as the instrument trocars (**Figures 2-3 A–C**). This creates an ergonomic setting, where the actions reproduced by the system match the intuitive way that the surgeon interacts with its environment.

With many surgeries requiring multiquadrant dissection, it can be challenging to shift the focus of the rigid system from a narrow target to a wide area without sacrificing visualization and dexterity. For this reason, proper planning is paramount to overcoming this limitation. By carefully planning the position for each trocar and assistant port, a surgeon can repurpose each trocar when redocking the robotic arms and camera.

The trocars must be inserted considering their hierarchical importance, maximizing triangulation.

1. The most critical trocar that will be placed is the camera trocar. Robotic surgery is first and foremost a visually based surgery. One of the most powerful features of the robot is the unparalleled visualization resulting from high-definition picture, 3-dimensionality (3D), stability of the camera, and magnification. These empower the surgeon's skills by offering a greater ability to recognize the nuances of the anatomical details. While dexterity and cosmesis are important, adequate visualization of the target anatomy should be paramount. As the surgeon at the console loses the sensation of pressure and tension on tissue, proper visualization is needed to avoid crushing or tearing the tissue. By inspecting with the camera first, the surgeon will visualize the surgical field and plan accordingly for the subsequent trocars to optimize dexterity and reduce collisions. In the following chapters, the camera port site will be denoted as "Scope" (S).

    The angle of visualization depends on the position scope trocar, the distance from the target, and the height of the abdominal wall. The perfect choice of this port site is fundamental. Optimally, the camera should observe the tissue from a 45° angle. A lower viewing angle is like looking at a mountain range. Just like how the complexity of the topography will hide detail, a surgeon will be unable to fully see his target anatomy by the contours of the tissue. Alternatively, if the viewing angle of the surgeon is vertical (90°), it can be comparable to looking down from a parachute, unaware of depth perception. It will be difficult for the surgeon to differentiate the height of tissues in relation to one another, and the contours of the 3D anatomy will be lost. There are also several differences between using a 30° forward-oblique endoscope versus a 0° forward-viewing one. The 30° endoscope can bypass obstacles to identify anatomy (e.g., duodenum for visualization of the hilum of the liver) and can circumvent the instruments themselves, blocking the target anatomy. The 30° can also provide a wider view of the surgical field and visualize relatively inaccessible regions simply by changing the setting from 30° up-down to 30° down-up (e.g., dome of the liver, adhesions of bowel against the wall). Alternatively, the 0° forward-viewing camera can function in a long tunnel. Examples include operating in the mediastinum, axillary access to the thyroid, or narrow pelvis. A surgeon should be knowledgeable of both scopes and know when each serves the needs of the surgical field.

2. The second priority is unrestricted working arms to take advantage of the powerful EndoWrist® of the robotic instruments. Internal and external conflicts should be avoided evaluating the extension of the surgical field in advance. The position of the working ports largely determines the range of motion of the instruments within the surgical field. The robotic port incisions should have a 6–10-cm distance between them (approximately the length of a fist). However, some close surgical targets may require increased spacing between trocars, and distant targets may need decreased spacing. The importance of the 2 working arms depends on the dominant hand of the surgeon. Therefore, the depiction of trocar placements for each procedure will show the surgeon's right hand as "R1," and left hand as "R2" (considering that the majority of surgeons are right-handed).

3. The third arm, which provides dynamic retraction during the case, should have the proper port site after the

2 working arms. It should be placed in such a way as to minimize the risk of collision and maintain dexterity of the working arms. To do this, the surgeon should recognize the actions that the third arm will need to perform. Many surgeons, at the beginning of their learning curve, underestimate the third arm as an asset and will either not use it or forget it during the procedure. In the following chapters, the third arm port will be depicted as "R3."

4. Lastly, when needed, the assistant's trocars are placed. While maneuverability and comfort of the assistant are important, the most fundamental principle is that the assistant enhances but does not impede the vision or dexterity of the surgeon. The importance of this port may take precedence over the third arm, depending on the complexity of the case or the need for more rapid assistance. An example is in a small bowel resection, where a flexible assistant can be more important than static retraction. Generally, the assistant should receive 2 ports to assist the surgeon best. Just like a surgeon wouldn't operate with a hand behind his back, the assistant should have control of 2 instruments. If the scope is between both assistant trocars, the triangulation will help create a comfortable environment for the assistant to act. Exceptions to having 2 assistant trocars should only include maintaining cosmesis, operating in a restricted space, and avoiding collisions.

Due to the population's increasing BMI worldwide, some chapters will include illustrations showing the recommended port placement for normal wide/obese abdomens (**Figures 2-4 A, B**). As a patient's BMI will likely fall within or outside the range shown in the models, it is important not to memorize the recommended locations, but to understand how shifting the trocars adapts to the body habitus of the patient to allow better visualization and dexterity. An example of this is when using the umbilicus as a trocar landmark. In patients with a low–healthy BMI, it can be a helpful marker, but in patients with a high BMI, the umbilicus can be suprapubic or shift the perceived midline drastically when the table is tilted.

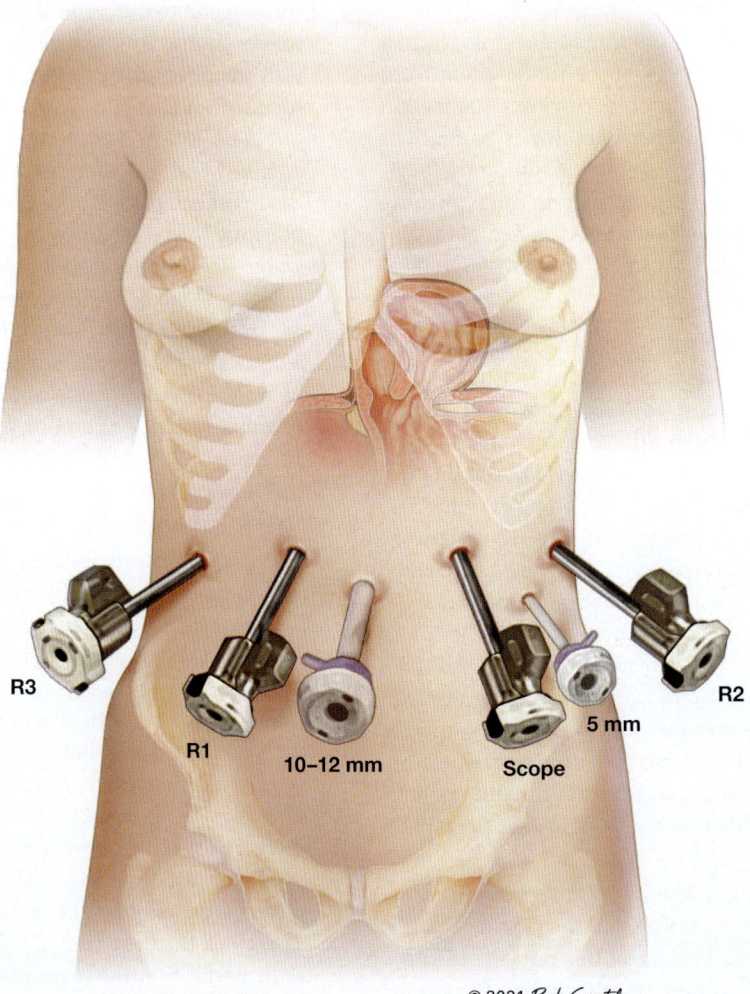

FIGURE 2-4 • Port placement for Heller myotomy: **A.** Normal abdomen.

The Basic Principles of Clinical Applications   21

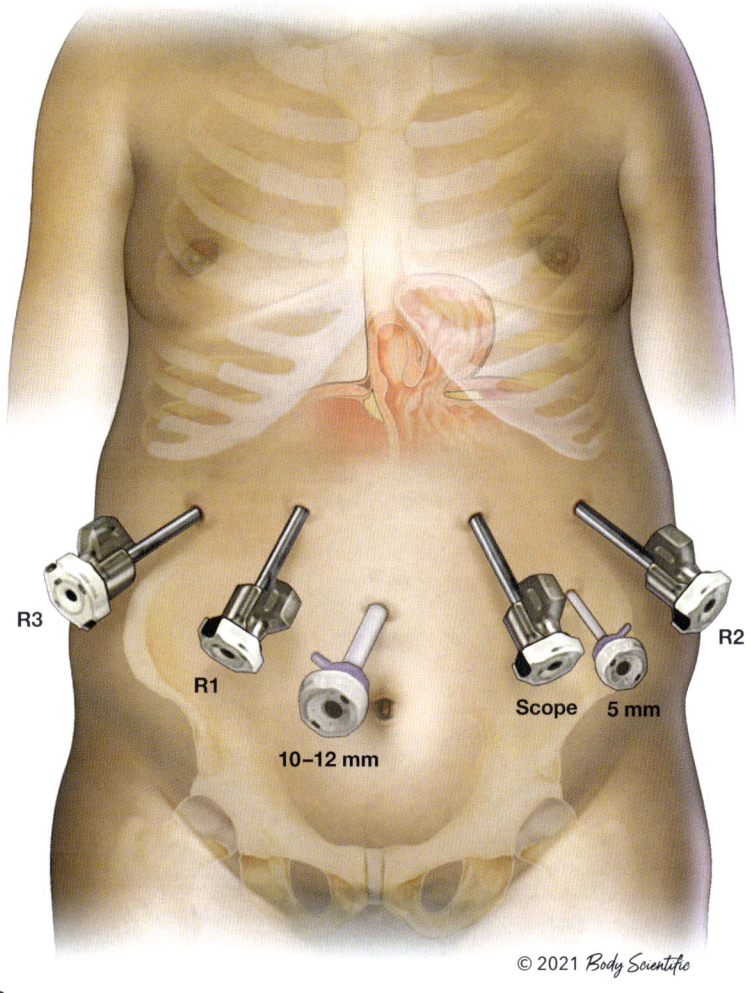

Wide abdomen

FIGURE 2-4 • (*Continued*) **B.** Wide abdomen.

> **EDITORIAL COMMENT**
>
> Before completing the final robotic ports setting, there are multiple reasons that make a preliminary laparoscopic exploration necessary.
> - To confirm the diagnosis
> - To detect reasons for changing the operative strategy (cancer spread)
> - To find concomitant pathologies that might interfere with the operation (e.g., peritoneal adhesions that require adhesiolysis for a proper port placement)
> - To optimize the port line depending on the anatomy of the surgical field (distance/width)

Obtaining the Optimal Exposure

There are 4 levels of retraction that provide exposure in robotic surgery.

1. The first level is the static forces, which include gravity and pneumoperitoneum. The surgeon can utilize these forces to their advantage by positioning the patient at the beginning of the case and adjusting the pneumoperitoneum pressure. Understanding the relationship between the direction of gravity and the surrounding structures in any procedure is fundamental to optimizing exposure. An example of the use of gravity is in a rectal dissection. Without tilting the table (Trendelenburg), the bowel will frequently fall into the pelvis and obstruct the operation.

2. The second level of retraction is that of the R3. The R3 can act as a static or active force as needed but primarily works against gravity to provide fundamental exposure. For example, when performing a cholecystectomy, the R3 can retract segment 4b of the liver cranially with minor adjustments needed throughout the case (**Figure 2-5A**). The R3 also has an active role in single port surgery. With the narrow working space of all instruments, the R3 will typically remain in the visual field and require more frequent readjustments to provide effective retraction.

3. The third level is the assistant's laparoscopic retraction (**Figure 2-5B**). It can be the most versatile of the levels, because the assistant can use forceps and suction devices

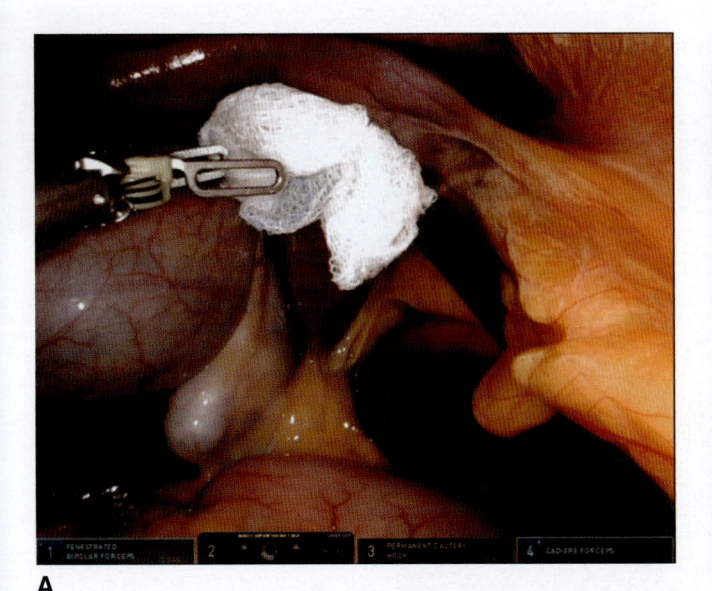

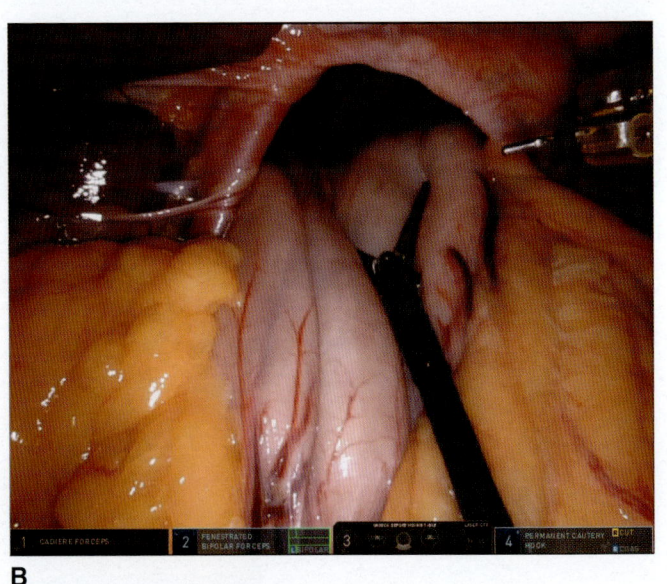

FIGURE 2-5 • **A.** Exposure for dissection of triangle of Calot: lifting of the segment 4 and left lobe of liver with the R3. **B.** Retraction of herniated stomach by the bedside assistant.

to clear the target anatomy of blood and fluid. This level is below that of the static forces and the R3 because both of those forces allow the assistant to retract effectively. Because prolonged retraction may be necessary for even hours at a time, the first 2 levels can provide most of the exposure, and free the assistant to focus on more fine/precise actions. While the first 2 levels are under the control of the console surgeon, the third level relies on the experience and skills of the assistant.

4. The final level is provided by the nondominant hand of the surgeon. The nondominant hand can utilize forceps to apply precise and delicate retraction of tissue obscuring target anatomy. An example is when the surgeon uses the forceps to gently grasp the adventitia of a vessel to prepare for an anastomosis.

Principles for Specimen Extraction (Service Incision)

The extraction incision should be planned in advance and reflect the overall strategy of the operation. When planning the incision, multiple factors should be considered:
- Cosmesis
- Previous surgical scars
- Usage of the incision for specimen retrieval exclusively or for multitasking access (e.g., introduction of instruments, clamps, staplers, hand-assistance, extracorporeal suture anastomosis)
- Size of specimen, and possibility of morcellation
- Obesity (the most favorable incision is in the midline, epigastric area, above the umbilicus, where the pannus is thinner and the incision is limited to the opening of the fascia without incising the muscle)
- Redundant suprapubic pannus may contraindicate a Pfannenstiel incision

Pfannenstiel Incision

The Pfannenstiel incision is one of the preferred extraction sites, not only for cosmetic reasons but also for the low rate of long-term incisional hernias. If done correctly, there is no destruction of muscle fibers, and there is a strong overlapping of layers opened with different directions. It starts with a transverse incision, 2 inches above the pubis, dividing the subcutaneous tissue transversally and exposing the anterior rectus abdominis fascia. The incision length depends on the abdomen configuration, thickness of the subcutaneous tissue, and the size of the specimen. In the same way, a long transversal cut is made in the fascia. The 2 rectus muscles are revealed underneath and are gently retracted, exposing the aponeurosis which is then separated from the pyramidalis and rectus muscles. The peritoneum is picked up and incised longitudinally. The opening can be enlarged to allow the position of a wound retractor, the specimen is extracted contained in a Endobag (see **Figure 2-6**).

Virtual Tactile Feedback

One of the benefits of open surgery lost in robotics and partially in laparoscopy is haptic feedback. Haptic feedback can be explained in two categories: force feedback (kinesthetic) and tactile feedback (cutaneous) (**Figures 2-7 A, B**). Force feedback is the signal conveyed to the surgeon of the degree of force required to close and open graspers or the movement of an instrument against resistance. On the other hand, tactile feedback is more delicate and precise, providing the details of the distribution of pressure over a surface (e.g., palpating the borders of a mass within normal tissue). Significant advancements in force feedback have been made in modern systems; however, there is no tactile feedback for robotic instruments. It is a technological and cost limitation, due to the complexity of integrating sensors on the instrument tips.

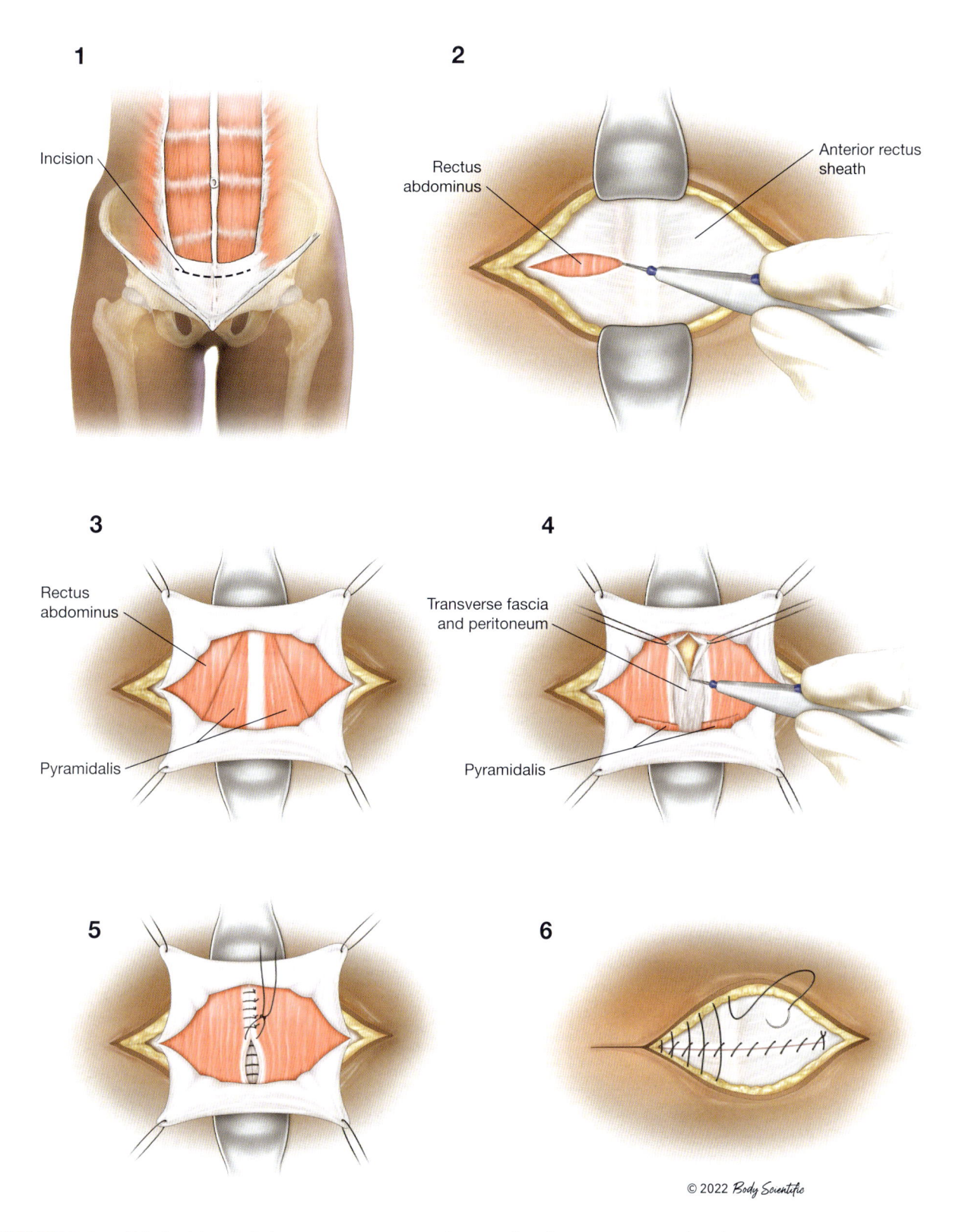

The Basic Principles of Clinical Applications   23

FIGURE 2-6• 1. Skin incision **2.** Subcutaneous tissue is dissected and anterior rectus sheath is incised. **3.** Fascia is separated from the rectus muscle. **4.** The transverse fascia and peritoneum are incised longitudinally. **5.** Upon finalization, after peritoneum closure, the rectus muscle are approximated with sutures. **6.** The anterior rectus sheath is approximated with a continuous suture followed by the approximation of the subcuticular tissue and the skin.

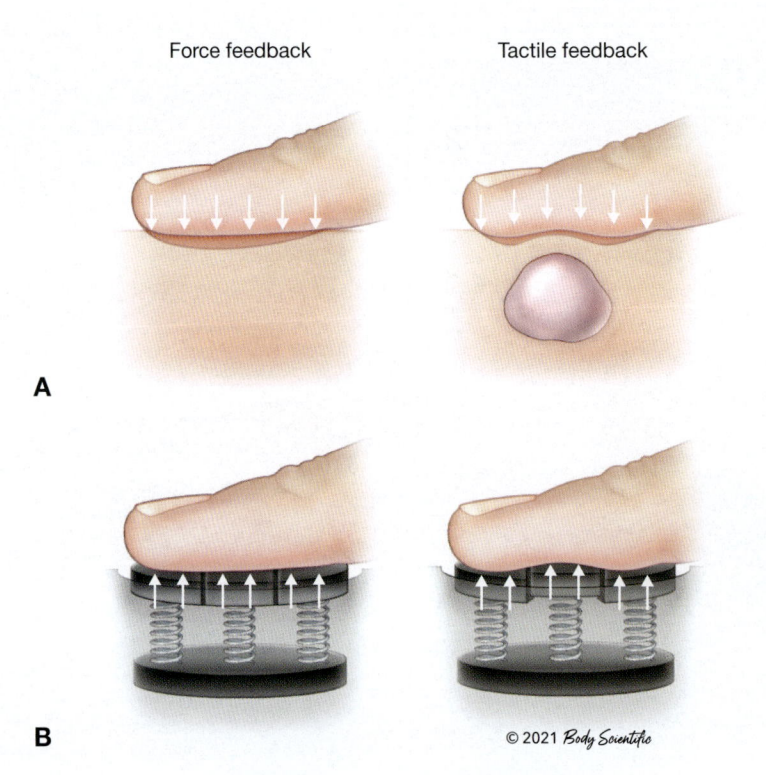

FIGURE 2-7 • Haptic feedback.

One of the ways that surgeons have overcome limited haptic feedback is using visual feedback. In open surgery, the force exerted on tissue is visually matched with the perceived distortion of that tissue. In this way, an understanding of the physical characteristics and texture of the anatomy is developed. This skill can carry over to laparoscopy and robotic surgery, where the visual distortion of tissue can provide more information than the perceived force applied. This is useful in preventing excessive force on tissue and appreciating the relation of tissues with their surroundings.

By brushing against tissue with an instrument or slowly increasing the tension, obscured anatomy distorts the overlying tissue being acted upon. This distortion can be recognized innately by its characteristics (e.g., lymph nodes create an oval distortion, blood vessels from a cord-like distortion). With further training, the surgeon creates an anatomic blueprint in their mind. By actively moving and manipulating the tissue, the surgeon can refine this skill and observe how different structures interact with each other just like they would if they were being palpated in open surgery. When an advanced surgeon operates on extremely delicate and fragile tissue, mastery of visual feedback can become more useful than haptic feedback in preventing injury. A good example of this is when a surgeon is performing a pancreaticoduodenectomy. The small details from manipulating the duct reveal how the surrounding parenchyma is affected. Control of the force applied in this situation is critical to avoid injury to the pancreas. Even though it is desirable to have tactile feedback as an added feature, it is not a priority now. New generations of sensors will be more important, providing more information (e.g., digital instant pathology).

Understanding the Surgical Instruments

Like with open and laparoscopic surgery, every surgeon should know the capabilities and functions of the instruments at their disposal (**Figures 2-8 A–D**). However, robotic instruments are not only tools, but also the surgeon's fingers. While the surgeon's visual feedback of the distortion of tissue can assess an excessive quantity of applied force, many instruments have been engineered to fit their necessary actions. The double fenestrated grasper and bowel grasper are designed to prevent bowel trauma, and therefore have the lowest maximal grip strength distributed over a large area. The Cadière and Maryland forceps have a greater grip strength and are primarily used to grasp tissue. They are more versatile and can be combined with bipolar/monopolar energy to aid dissection and hemostasis. The difference between the two is that the Maryland forceps have a pointed tip, which can penetrate and bluntly dissect tissue. The ProGrasp™ forceps look identical to the Cadière but are designed for greater grip strength than their counterpart. The needle driver has the greatest grip strength of the forceps, but it is not recommended for grasping delicate tissue. The small focus of force is designed to control a suture needle through resistance and can easily crush tissue. SutureCut™ needle drivers should be cautioned in beginner's hands, because inadvertent cutting of the suture before tying can waste a considerable amount of time, especially when creating an anastomosis.

The robotic platform also has multiple instruments for dividing tissue and maintaining hemostasis. Each tool has its advantages and limitations, and intimate knowledge of each one will contribute to the procedure's safety. The monopolar hook is among the most versatile tools. It can divide tissue and provide effective hemostasis allowing for a 360° operating

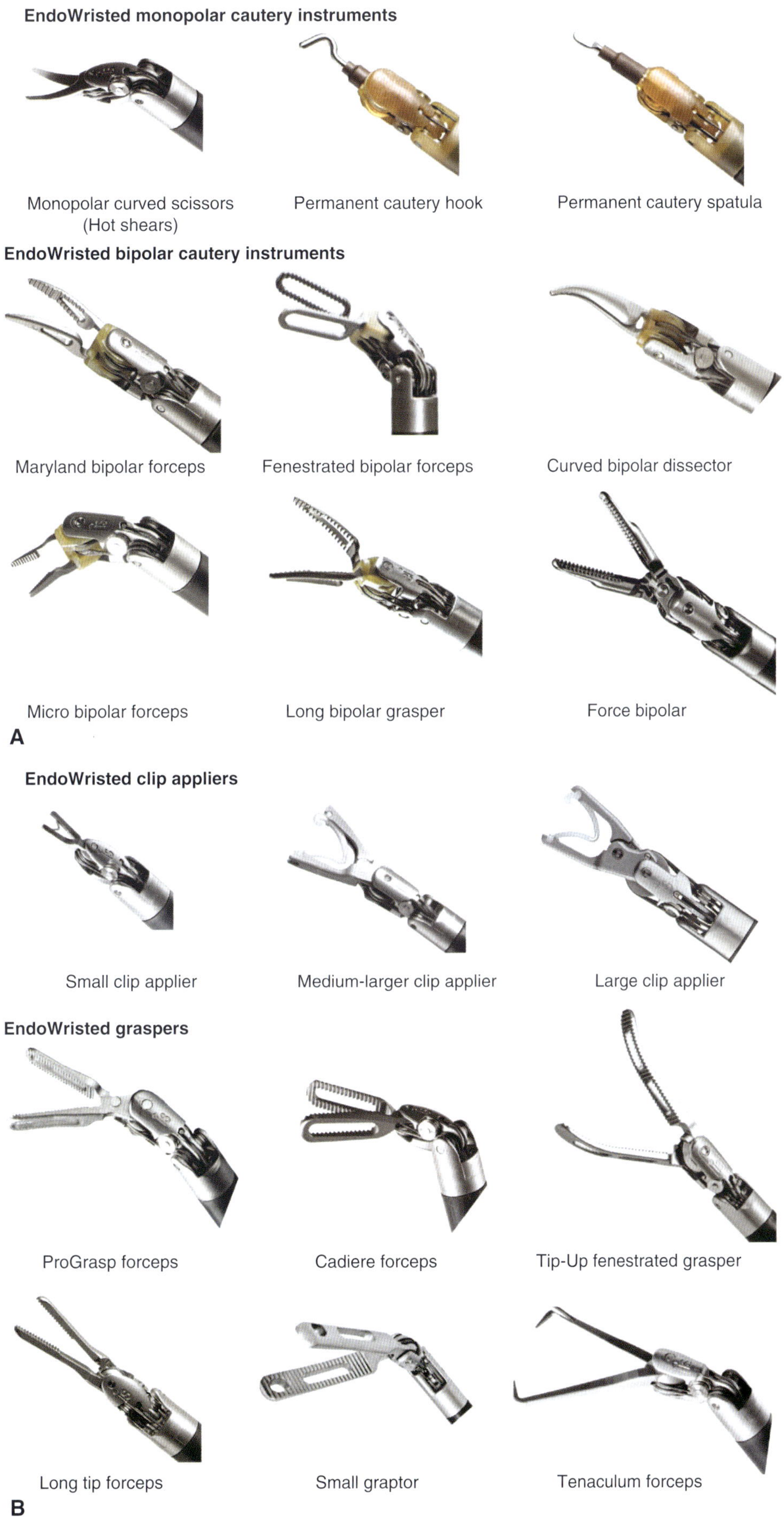

The Basic Principles of Clinical Applications

EndoWristed monopolar cautery instruments

Monopolar curved scissors (Hot shears) | Permanent cautery hook | Permanent cautery spatula

EndoWristed bipolar cautery instruments

Maryland bipolar forceps | Fenestrated bipolar forceps | Curved bipolar dissector

Micro bipolar forceps | Long bipolar grasper | Force bipolar

A

EndoWristed clip appliers

Small clip applier | Medium-larger clip applier | Large clip applier

EndoWristed graspers

ProGrasp forceps | Cadiere forceps | Tip-Up fenestrated grasper

Long tip forceps | Small graptor | Tenaculum forceps

B

FIGURE 2-8 • Robotic instruments.

26 The Foundation and Art of Robotic Surgery

EndoWristed needle drivers (ND)

Large ND   Large SutureCut ND   Mega ND   Mega SutureCut ND

EndoWristed scissors

Round tip scissors   Potts scissors

Harmonic ACE curved shears   **Vessel sealer**

C

Specialty instruments

Resano forceps   Small atrial retractor   Dual blade retractor

Black diamond micro forceps   Cardiac probe grasper

Synchroseal   **Suction irrigator**

D

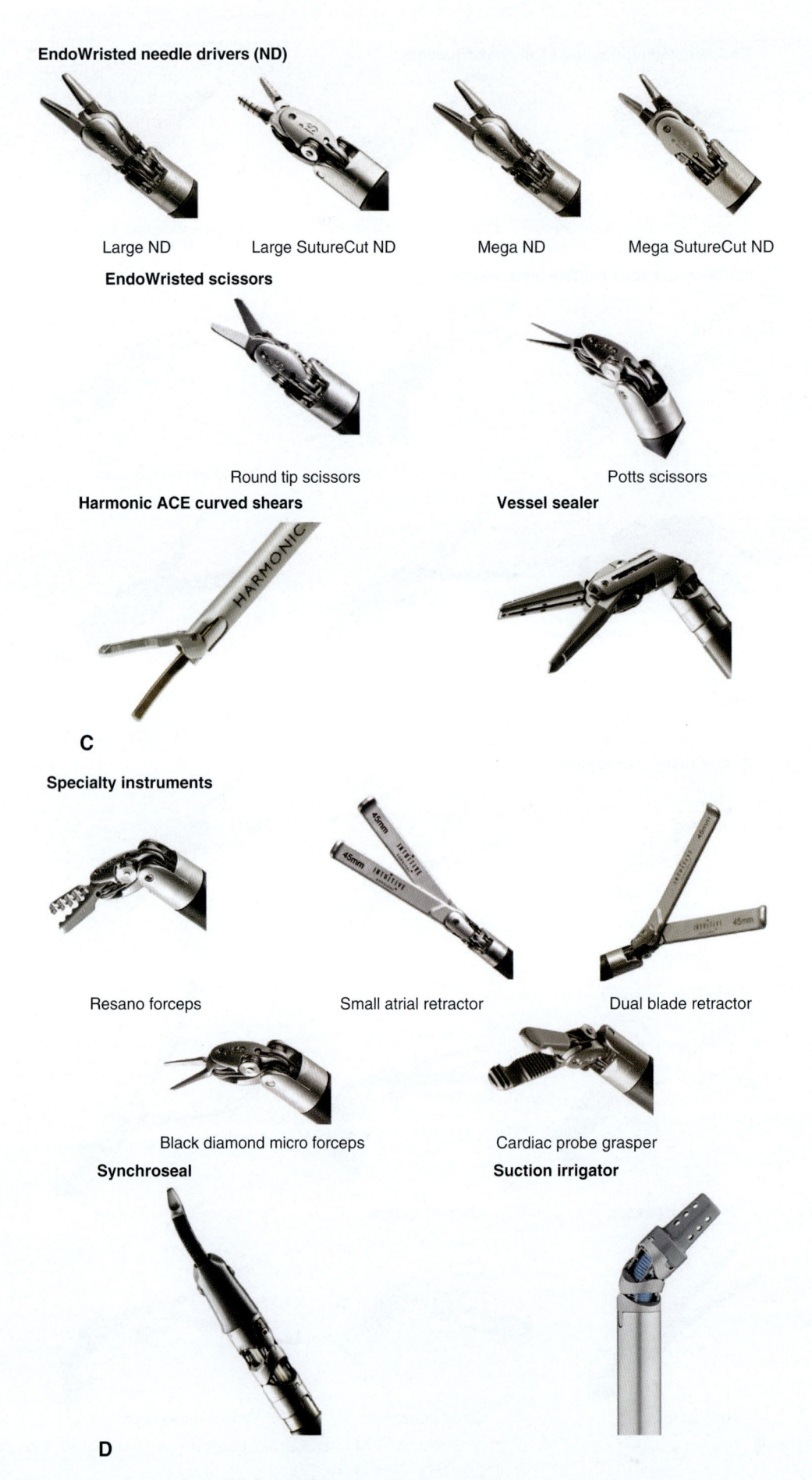

FIGURE 2-8 • (*Continued*)

angle. A pull and push technique can be utilized to take full advantage of its unique shape. While using the tip of the hook, tissue can be pulled away from critical structures and safely divided using pinpoint electrocautery without risk of surrounding thermal injury. The back of the hook can apply energy to the tissue under tension by a noncontact spark gap (fulguration), rapidly dissecting within a tissue plane. While it is less controlled with a higher thermal spread, it allows for efficient dissection in permitting stages of the surgery. Even when using both methods, the tissue being acted upon requires a high water content for the electrocautery to function effectively. For this reason, fibrotic and ligamentous tissue will resist the actions of the hook. While the scissors are less versatile in dissection, they can be beneficial in these situations. The monopolar hook is ideal when dissecting within a tissue plane; however, when the surgeon is required to divide tissue planes to reach the target anatomy, the Harmonic scalpel/vessel sealer and scissors may provide better efficiency.

When dividing parenchymal tissue, advancements in technology have many options over classic hand-tying techniques. In many instances, a robotic stapler can be utilized, or a laparoscopic stapler can be inserted through an assistant port to safely divide tissue, secure potential sources of bleeding, and create an anastomosis. However, in hepatic parenchymal transection, 3 common options exist with pros and cons: the Harmonic scalpel, the vessel sealer, and the Cavitron Ultrasonic Surgical Aspirator (CUSA®). The Harmonic scalpel is a versatile instrument in which ultrasonic energy is converted to mechanical energy by a rapidly vibrating blade creating a high-grade frictional force. The tissue is spontaneously divided between the jaws of the instrument, while being sealed. It provides reliable hemostasis to vessels up to 5 mm in diameter. Unfortunately, the instrument is non-endowristed, and the entrance port restricts the angle of action. The vessel sealer is another option; it is an endowristed instrument utilizing bipolar energy in conjunction with the pressure of the instrument's jaws, sealing larger tissue areas and vessels up to 7 mm in diameter. Unfortunately, its insertion inside of the parenchyma is traumatic, and it is a reason of bleeding before the action of the jaws is activated. The CUSA® is a laparoscopic instrument that utilizes ultrasonic frequencies to separate parenchymal tissue while simultaneously irrigating and aspirating the fragmented tissue. It has a unique feature; it spares and exposes vascular and ductal structures during dissection. This allows the surgeon to identify and ligate vessels and ducts through various techniques (e.g., suture, clips, etc.). Unfortunately, there is no equivalent robotic instrument that matches the function of the CUSA®. Therefore, this technique requires a 2-surgeon approach. A skillful surgeon at the bedside will determine the resection line and advance the CUSA®, in coordination with the surgeon at the console, responsible for clipping, ligating, and dividing skeletonized vessels and biliary ducts. Consequently, this will assign the lead role as the primary surgeon during the transection step to the bedside surgeon, relegating the console surgeon. Clear communication between the surgeons is crucial.

The Diverging Models of Robotic Surgery

The robotic platform allows the organization of different work models in the OR. The first original idea was to develop a solo surgery unit where the surgeon (using multiple robotic arms) and a robotic scrub nurse could perform operations without the presence of other team members. This model is already feasible for simple operations, and innovations in the field hope to push this model further. Research is currently being done to create automated scrub technicians to facilitate instrument switching. Ideally, the model has the benefit of significantly reducing surgical costs by minimizing necessary staff but may also aid surgeons in routinely performing remote surgeries (telesurgery), potentially alleviating some of the problems associated with the shortage of surgeons.

Moving in the opposite direction of solo surgery, the complex surgery model requires the presence of 2 surgeons: a console and a bedside surgeon. The need for a second surgeon at the patient's bedside depends on multiple variables: the complexity of the procedure, the experience of the console surgeon, and the skills of the assistant. An example of this is in robotic hepatic resections with the CUSA®. The surgeon guides the dissection, quickly sutures, and cuts as needed, while the assistant uses the CUSA® to divide the hepatic tissue laparoscopically.

Nowadays, most operations of medium complexity fall in a third category where a qualified assistant is sufficient at the patient's bedside (see Chapter 3, The Assistant's Role in Robotic Surgery, for more details).

The Robotic Platform and Change in OR Organization

Despite being functional with minimal assistance, the robotic OR has many moving parts, all of which need to work seamlessly. The surgeon is at the console, performing the surgery while guiding the team through the case. The assistant provides the exposure necessary for the surgeon to perform the surgery as effectively as possible. The surgical technician is at the bedside with the assistant and is responsible for preparing the sterile surgical environment and providing the instruments as needed. The circulating nurse works outside the sterile setting and maintains documentation regarding the patient, staff, instruments, specimens, and key events throughout the surgery (see Chapter 3, The Assistant's Role in Robotic Surgery).

The anesthesiologist and certified registered nurse anesthetists are co-leaders in the OR with the surgeon. They need to be familiar with the physiologic differences between open and robotic surgery. The need for constant communication between anesthesia and the surgical team cannot be overemphasized. Communication is essential when repositioning and administrating specific medications. For example, when using biofluorescence, the correct dosage and timing of indocyanine green needs to be communicated efficiently between the anesthesia team and the surgeon. Additionally, patient relaxation should remain static throughout the case to avoid port malposition and extreme fluctuations of pneumoperitoneum while not overmedicating and/or delaying extubation. Respiratory mechanics that fluctuate due to patient positioning have been well documented, and the anesthesiologist is required to adjust for changes in pulmonary function.

Each surgical staff member is vital to ensure a safe environment for the patient and the completion of a successful operation.

The Role of Robotic Training

The learning curve of robotic surgery has been cited as a common drawback to the widespread adoption of the technology. The learning curve can be divided into conceptual surgical knowledge and mechanical skills. As stated earlier, much of the learning curve can be overcome with a solid foundation in open and laparoscopic surgery tenets. This experience will greatly impact the conceptual surgical knowledge and lessen the training needed to become a robotic surgeon. However, those who lack an extensive background in open and laparoscopic surgery will have a more significant learning curve to overcome.

Alternatively, mechanical skills can be quickly learned. The ability to telemanipulate objects is not new, because videogames have been training a new generation in this skill for decades. However, overcoming the conceptual and mechanical learning curve is necessary to become an effective surgeon. While many will find this challenging to overcome, many options are available to advance skills toward proficiency (for more details, see Chapter 4, Robotic Training).

A stepwise approach to mastery allows the surgeon and OR team to overcome learning challenges together. This will allow improved efficiency in docking, instrument switching, and troubleshooting.

Efficiency and Outcomes Optimization

There are many strategies to optimize the financial strain for hospitals considering purchasing a robotic system or upgrading to a new model. The upfront cost of a system may seem insurmountable to many; however, alternative pricing strategies, such as leasing, have been introduced to help with affordability.

The robotic system's return on investment (ROI) is primarily increased by the number of billable cases and reduced length of hospital/ICU stay. With the volume of cases being an important driver, increasing the utilization rate of the system will make a significant impact on reimbursement. As surgeons overcome learning curves, total operative and turnover time will decrease, thereby increasing the potential number of procedures on any given day.

As the daily number of cases increases, a slight change in material utilization can significantly affect the revenue spent. When utilizing the system daily, it is essential to remember that each instrument has a limited life span before it is no longer usable. The number of available uses is recorded in each instrument and can be checked during the procedure. Proper planning, removal of redundant tools, and standardization of case equipment can minimize instrument utilization, hence minimizing the direct material cost. For this reason, each chapter will include the essential required instruments that can be considered for decreasing the direct material cost of any given procedure.

Some of the additional drivers that will improve the ROI include:

- Efficiency of the OR (turnover/equipment)
- Defining appropriate use of the system
- Extending the daily scheduled use of the system (e.g., increasing the volume of cases)
- Multispecialty program
- Avoidance of hybrid techniques
- Short track postoperative recovery program
- Marketing/differentiation from competitors

Knowing the Machine and General Troubleshooting

When a challenge occurs during robotic surgery, it is important to consider that the robotic team is split into the bedside team and the surgeon at the console. This requires communication with all team members and an effort to define the problem clearly. For example, the surgeon may remark that an instrument is not moving correctly or feels limited. The assistant at the bedside may notice the arms collisions, and adjustments can be made to free the instruments' mobility. Lack of instrument motion can be due to inadvertent switching to the R3. Other examples include instrument fault, which can be noted by a flashing light on the arm and patient cart screen. Additional tips on how to handle collisions can be read in Chapter 3, The Assistant's Role in Robotic Surgery.

Some problems that arise frequently can be mitigated by proper planning. A good example of this is fogging of the camera. This is due to the discrepancy in temperature between the camera and abdomen combined with the humidity of the pneumoperitoneum. This can be avoided by warming the scope prior to insertion, moving the insufflation away from the camera port (to reduce cold CO_2 blowing at the camera), or using warmed insufflation.

However, when a difficult challenge occurs, delegating is not enough. Just like a commander must know his ship, a surgeon must know the robotic system. There can be times when a small error can become a nightmare if not rectified efficiently. Being humble and taking every minor troubleshooting event as an opportunity to grow and better understand the system are advised.

CLINICAL CHALLENGES

Bleeding

A well-trained robotic surgeon should always keep in mind a strategy for the prevention and management of bleeding. This strategy must bear 4 important components: prevention, anticipation, control, and repair (PACR).

Prevention

The surgeon needs to have a perfect understanding of the anatomy, surgical planes, and vascular pedicles to prevent bleeding. The dissection should be done meticulously with the utmost precision.

Bleeding can blur the surgical planes, increasing the chances of additional bleeding. When the avascular plane is lost, chances to enter another wrong plane are increased. Bleeding can flood the surgical field and decrease illumination, mainly in narrow areas such as the chest, where a small amount of blood can darken the field.

Bleeding prevention is critical in any kind of surgery. But in robotic surgery it is even more important, because dealing with complex situations is more challenging. The open surgeon can use their hands or different size vascular clamps to control a bleeding spot, while simultaneously suturing, an option that doesn't exist in robotics. Emergency conversion to open may require time and perfect coordination with the bedside team. In some areas, such as the chest, a few minutes delay in converting to thoracotomy might endanger the patient's safety.

Anticipation

As the dissection proceeds around a risky vessel, which might be injured or torn, the area for potential risk should be anticipated. For example, when dissecting along the portal vein, the surgeon should understand if there are adhesions, encasement, or infiltration of the vessel.

If the surgeon is aware of dissection at high risk of bleeding, precautions must be taken in advance. Technical anticipation should suggest actions with the goal of minimizing the bleeding. The proximal and distal preparation on loops of the vessel at risk, and the preliminary introduction of small clamps in the surgical field, will decrease the reaction time.

Additionally, a crucial component of anticipation is proper team communication. The team should be informed of the potential risk of bleeding so that each member can react appropriately. The anesthesiologist should be aware of the patients' baseline hemodynamic status and the potential measures needed to be taken (e.g., checking proper IV lines are in place, lowering the central venous pressure before the surgeon approaches the vena cava, having units ready in the room for transfusion, and evaluating the administration of additional vasoactive medications). The team should have prepared gauzes, suction and energy devices, sutures, stapler loads, and a back table for emergency conversion. The need for an additional assistant's port or upsizing a 5-mm port to a 10–12-mm port should be evaluated.

Control

Control involves actions to manage the situation and minimize the hemorrhage once it happens. The use of sponges to compress the bleeding area, mainly if it is venous, could be part of a first reaction. The sponge can be managed by an assistant with laparoscopic forceps or the surgeon at the console with their nondominant hand. A simple gesture such as using the back of a forceps to apply light pressure on a bleeding spot could momentarily decrease the blood loss and allow maintenance of the continuous visualization and allow the team to prepare the required instruments and materials for the repair.

Grasping the bleeding vessel directly with the robotic instruments (forceps, needle driver) to control the hemorrhage should be avoided. There is only partial force feedback, and mainly the arteries can be severely damaged by the grasping action of the robotic instrument. It is important not to react under the pressure of panic. The magnification and the narrow field usually overestimate the entity of the bleeding. It is essential to remain calm and direct the team with precise and logical instructions.

Robotic surgery is based on proper visualization; if the camera lens is blurred, control cannot be achieved. The scope must be appropriately positioned to avoid blood sprinkles, causing a waste of time to clean up the lenses and more bleeding.

The team should be trained for fast removal, cleaning, and reintroduction of the camera. Clear directions to the bedside assistant should be given to aid with control, to use a precise and effective suction while maintaining retraction and exposure. The scrub nurse or second assistant might be necessary to help in changing instruments and introducing sutures and materials, while the first assistant is busy with exposure and suctioning.

Repair

Surgeons must take advantage of the precise suturing that the robot platform allows. Suturing is the most critical skill and should be mastered by all surgeons; surgeons should be able to handle different types of tissues, needles, and sutures without breaking them, understand the type of suture needed, and possess the most impeccable technique. The surgeon should be trained to effectively suture in different bleeding conditions (e.g., narrow deep fields, wet/flooded surface, fragile tissue, instrument crowded spaces, pulsatile sprinkles, breathing dynamics, distant edges, arm collisions, etc.).

Additionally, the surgeon must have complete knowledge and understanding of the entire armamentariums available for use and when each tool is effective and necessary. For example, a bleed might be temporarily controlled with a clip for quick control, followed by a precise suturing. A vessel sealer might be able to control a stump. Staplers might be used inside the liver to control deeper segments.

▶ Video 2-1. Bleeding Control

Adhesions

Loose adhesions with long, hanging meso are easy to dissect laparoscopically. Conversely, in complex cases with mesh adhesion and bowel loops plastered to the anterior abdominal wall, it is challenging to reach them with laparoscopic instruments limited by their hinges.

In such cases, the adhesiolysis is difficult, because the dissection line is very thin, and straight, rigid instruments coming with an angle can cause injury. Such cases are even tricky in an open approach. The endowristed instruments of the robot allow working parallel to the abdominal wall. The microdissection capabilities, steadiness, magnified vision, and 30° down/up scope allow for an enhanced dissection under perfect visualization. These conditions prevent serosal injuries, and if they happen, one can microsurgically repair them immediately without taking the risk of missing the injury point when the repair is done later on during the procedure.

Operations that require complex adhesiolysis should be considered as a 2-step approach. The first step is the adhesiolysis, and the second one is the intended operation. When complex adhesions are present in the anterior abdominal wall, an initial single port for the camera using an optical trocar (OptiView™, VisiPort®) can be introduced using a gasless technique avoiding bowel injury. Carefully, the scope's tip can be used to steadily do blunt dissection and create enough space to place a second trocar, close and parallel to the first one. A pair of scissors or a grasper can then be introduced to continue enlarging the space for a third port dedicated to a bipolar forceps for hemostasis and retraction. Two or three 8-mm trocars can be placed in a small space of a few inches, similar to the trocar placement for thyroid access. Once the scissors and the bipolar forceps are inside, one has the tools to free the entire anterior abdominal wall.

Once this step is finished, the second step dedicated to the intended final operation starts. The ideal port setting for the target anatomy is placed. One might use some of the initial ports used during the adhesiolysis, only if the position coincides with the proper one. The ideal port setting for the target operation should not be compromised, and suboptimal ports should be abandoned or used by the assistant.

Conversely, simple adhesiolysis that does not compromise the ideal port setting becomes a part of the intended operation. In these situations, the adhesions are not involving the ideal line of port setting, and the adhesiolysis can be done with the same ports used for the target operation. This is often the case with enteral adhesions not involving the anterior abdominal wall.

Video 2-2. Adhesiolysis

Conversion

Sometimes, one needs to convert to a laparoscopic or open procedure. There are 2 types of conversion: elective and emergent. Elective conversions can be subdivided into laparoscopic, open, or hybrid. Laparoscopic conversions may be utilized by surgeons more familiar with laparoscopic techniques to overcome some of the challenges of a difficult robotic procedure. An example of this in the mobilization of the left colonic flexure in an anterior rectal resection. An open conversion may be needed due to the size of the lesion or vascular encasement requiring reconstruction (e.g., portal vein encasement in pancreatic cancer) or to safely complete the procedure. A hybrid procedure may involve a mini-laparotomy for hand assistance.

In emergencies, such as bleeding or swift hemodynamic changes in the patient, conversion to open procedures may be necessary for the patient's safety (**Figure 2-9**). The threshold

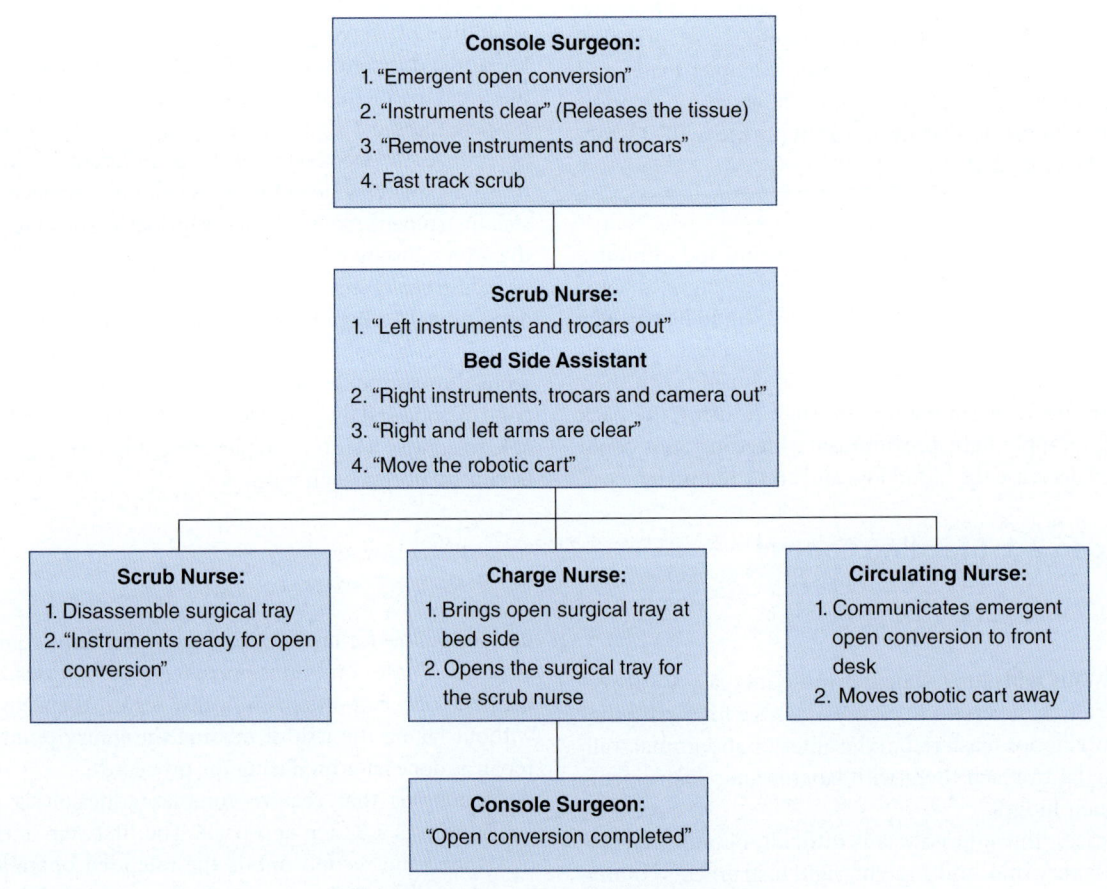

Console Surgeon:
1. "Emergent open conversion"
2. "Instruments clear" (Releases the tissue)
3. "Remove instruments and trocars"
4. Fast track scrub

Scrub Nurse:
1. "Left instruments and trocars out"

Bed Side Assistant
2. "Right instruments, trocars and camera out"
3. "Right and left arms are clear"
4. "Move the robotic cart"

Scrub Nurse:
1. Disassemble surgical tray
2. "Instruments ready for open conversion"

Charge Nurse:
1. Brings open surgical tray at bed side
2. Opens the surgical tray for the scrub nurse

Circulating Nurse:
1. Communicates emergent open conversion to front desk
2. Moves robotic cart away

Console Surgeon:
"Open conversion completed"

FIGURE 2-9 • Open conversion algorithm.

of conversion should be taken in the context of the surgeon's skills. A more experienced surgeon can overcome an obstacle without converting, whereas a more junior surgeon may convert early. The act of converting in an emergency should not be seen as a failure. Ultimately, the patient's safety is the highest priority, and delaying conversion when not fully understanding one's own limitations can put that at risk.

When the decision to convert is made, the entire team must work cohesively to maximize efficiency. Depending on the conversion, all team members must know their roles in safely undocking the robot and preparing the surgical field.

Knowing the Roles in an Emergency Code

As the surgical teams embark upon robotic training with the different components of the robotic platform, simulated scenarios to train the team in case of a code blue or emergent open conversions should be included. In these scenarios, each team member should recognize their role and avoid overlapping to maximize efficiency. An example of an algorithm trained at the University of Illinois at Chicago is shown below (see **Figure 2-10**). With tasks assigned for each member of the team and the necessary verbal communication between team members optimized, safe outcomes can be achieved for the patient.

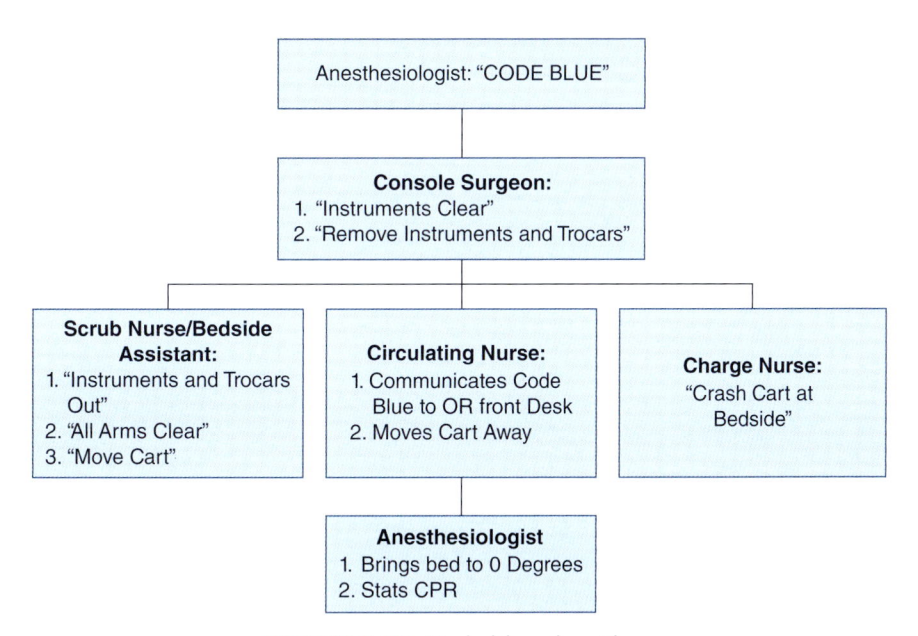

FIGURE 2-10 • Code blue algorithm.

Suggested Readings

1. Da Vinci Instruments. Intuitive. 2022. Accessed February 18, 2022. https://www.intuitive.com/en-us/products-and-services/da-vinci/instruments
2. Giulianotti PC, Coratti A, Angelini M, et al. Robotics in general surgery: personal experience in a large community hospital. *Arch Surg*. 2003;138(7):777-784. doi: 10.1001/archsurg.138.7.777
3. Gheza F, Esposito S, Gruessner S, Mangano A, Fernandes E, Giulianotti PC. Reasons for open conversion in robotic liver surgery: a systematic review with pooled analysis of more than 1000 patients. *Int J Med Robot*. 2019;15(2):e1976. doi: 10.1002/rcs.1976
4. Mangano A, Gheza F, Giulianotti PC. Virtual reality simulator systems in robotic surgical training. *Surg Technol Int*. 2018;32:19-23.

3

"Coming together is a beginning, staying together is progress, and working together is a success."

—Henry Ford (1863–1947)

The Assistant's Role in Robotic Surgery

Gabriela Aguiluz • Kelly Hoyert

INTRODUCTION

Robotic surgery requires the primary surgeon to step outside the sterile field and relinquish control to the team at the patient's bedside. As a result, having a well-trained assistant becomes critical.

The robotic system may allow different and divergent modalities of organization in the OR.

The robotic platform can act as a solo system for simple procedures. This allows the surgeon to operate alone, in an almost autonomous fashion, using 3 robotic instruments and switch between them independently.

We can easily imagine future scenarios of solo surgery in remote locations or even in outer space.

For complex surgeries, a 2-surgeon model becomes necessary. Intricate laparoscopic maneuvers and skills are required for difficult operations, therefore, a second surgeon usually fulfils this role. However, a majority of procedures will fall somewhere between a solo and a 2-surgeon model. In this setting, a specialized robotic surgical assistant can play a critical role.

A successful bedside assistant should have a strong surgical background with sophisticated laparoscopic skills, technological competence with a deep understanding of the robotic software and troubleshooting, and leadership abilities to coordinate and communicate effectively with the bedside team.

The assistant's qualifications can vary, and the definition of who can fill that role is evolving. The American College of Surgeons (ACS) defines a surgical assistant as "a trained individual who can participate in and actively assist the surgeon in completing the operation safely and expeditiously by helping to provide exposure, maintain hemostasis, and other technical functions" (see suggested reading #1). Robotic surgery is becoming more popular, and the demand for a highly trained surgical first assistant is increasing. While a qualified surgeon, fellow, or resident can certainly cover this role, it is suitable to have other nonphysician specialties, with additional surgical training instead, to allow physicians to work independently and perform more cases. These include, but are not limited to, physician assistants (PAs), certified surgical first assistants (CSFAs), certified surgical assistants (CSAs), surgical assistant certified (SA-Cs), and registered nurse first assistants (RNFA). Each position provides unique qualifications, and it is up to the individual institutions to determine which type of surgical assistant is best suited for their practice. By having a designated surgical assistant replacing a cosurgeon, there is a positive impact on general costs and productivity.

Prepping the OR

The role of the assistant begins even before the patient enters the OR. A PA or an advanced practice nurse (APN) in this role will have access to the medical history of the patient that may impact the surgical plan. Body habitus, surgical history, and hemodynamic status are examples of circumstances resulting in a deviation from the standard surgical procedure or preference card. Knowledge of the scheduled operation is usually enough to prep accordingly.

Once the assistant enters the OR, they should verify the room layout. This includes noting the position of the robotic cart, the surgical technicians' back table, and the surgical monitors. This will ensure that the room setup coincides with the surgeon's preference and the unique circumstance of the procedure or patient. If changes need to be made, these should be promptly communicated with the OR staff to avoid delays. The assistant should also verify the robotic cart's placement in

---

Photo source: Hartsook, photographer. Henry Ford, head-and-shoulders portrait, facing slightly left, 1919 (?). Prints and Photographs Division, Library of Congress. Reproduction Number LC-USZ62-111278.

Quote reproduced with permission from Price A, Price D. Introducing Leadership: A Practical Guide. London: Icon Books, Ltd; 2013.

34 The Foundation and Art of Robotic Surgery

the room, because different procedures may benefit from a different docking orientation. Suggested OR setup and patient's positioning are illustrated in each of the following chapters. For example, during left colon resections, it may be especially helpful to have the robotic cart approaching from the patient's left side (**Figures 3-1 A–D**). This will allow more space for the surgical technician and the assistant to operate without interference from the robotic system.

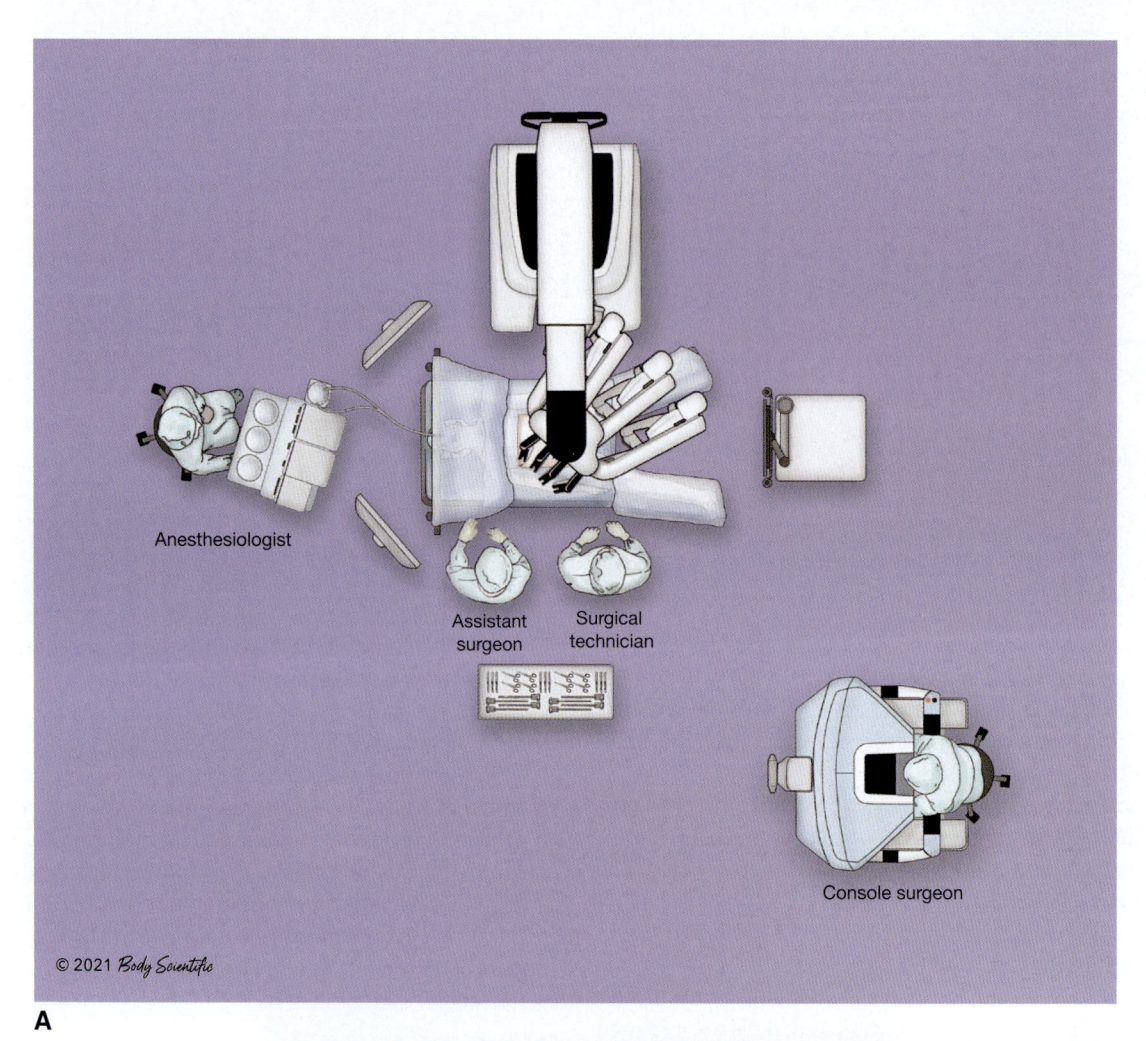

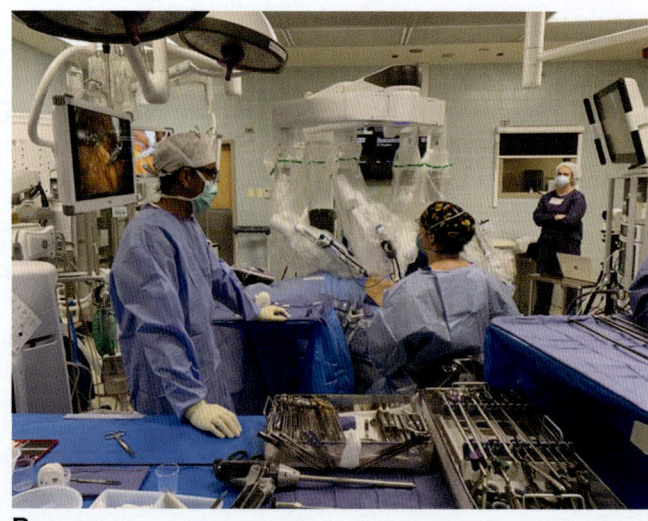

FIGURE 3-1 • OR setup for the left colon resection. The robotic cart should approach from the patient's left side because this allows for more room for the assistant as well as unrestricted access to the surgical technician. **A, B.** Correct setup, cart docked from patient's left side, assistant and technician on the right side.

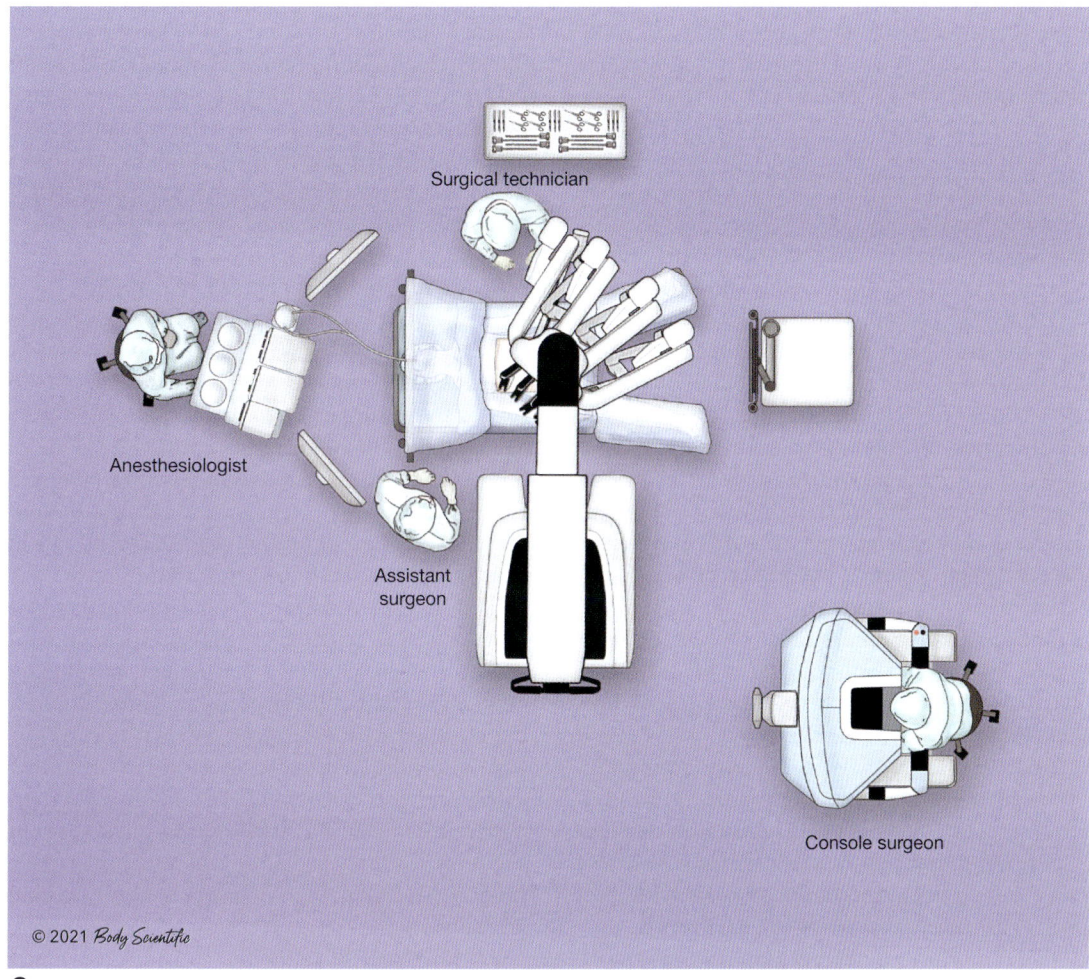

C

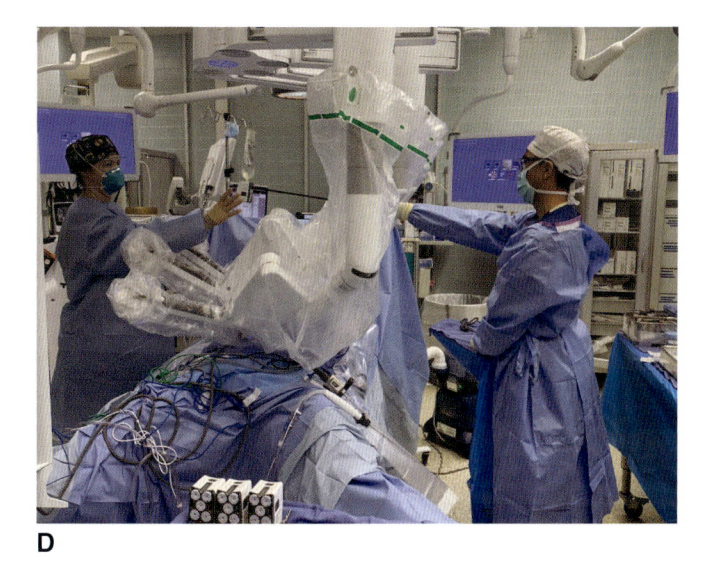

D

FIGURE 3-1 • (*Continued*) **C, D.** Wrong setup, cart docked from patient's right side, assistant and technician at opposite side of the patient. Increased risk of contamination.

Checking that the room is equipped with the proper operating table is also an important task. Verifying that the table can accommodate the patient's body habitus, or sometimes extreme positioning may be required for the procedure. Taking the time for appropriate preparation can significantly facilitate the flow of the operation, improve patient safety, and reduce unnecessary frustrations among the team.

Prepping the Patient

Once a patient is intubated on the operating table, the assistant should actively participate and oversee this process. Careful positioning is one of the first measures that should be utilized to prevent iatrogenic injury. This should be a collaborative effort between the circulating nurse, surgical assistant, and anesthesiologist. Depending on the procedure being performed, different positioning will be required to allow gravitational retraction, access for docking of the robotic system, full range of motion for the robotic arms, and space for the assistant to stand. Since the priority must always be patient safety and injury prevention, the assistant must also be mindful of the interaction between the robotic arms' movements and the patient's body. For example, having the patient's arms safely tucked helps minimize obstacles around the patient and allows for the robotic arm's maximum range of motion. However, attention must be given when tucking the patient's arms to protect the ulnar nerve and IVs using gauze, foam, gel padding, or other appliances available. Avoiding excessive pressure on bony prominences is crucial in preventing injury during longer surgeries. Throughout the positioning process, it is essential to maintain clear communication with the anesthesiologist. Before sterile prep and draping, both parties must ensure that the IVs continue to flow freely and have access to the lines if needed. This will help prevent disruption during the case.

Integrated table motion (a feature inclusive to some tables) allows for repositioning of the patient while the robotic system is docked to the patient, at least for minor changes. Unless the hospital has such an operative table with integrated table motion, once the robot is docked, the table cannot be repositioned unless the robotic system is disconnected. Therefore, in some cases, it may be warranted to test the extreme positioning with either Trendelenburg or reverse Trendelenburg. This will determine if the patient can hemodynamically tolerate the positioning and is well fixed and properly aligned. Once the patient is positioned, the assistant can sometimes laparoscopically verify that the optimum position has been achieved. For example, during table adjustments for pelvic operations, where a steep Trendelenburg is required, the assistant can check with the laparoscopic camera that most of the small bowel has been cleared from the pelvis by gravity, and target anatomy can be visualized. Necessary adjustments can be made before the robotic cart is redocked (**Figures 3-2 A–D**).

Naturally, the robotic platform has been designed to allow the primary surgeon to operate comfortably at the console. However, the same consideration can be taken to ensure that the assistant can operate comfortably at the patient's bedside. For upper abdominal procedures, it can help to have the patient in a spread leg, or so-called French position, through stirrups or leg spreaders. This allows room for the assistant to stand, or sit closer to the patient, minimizing strain and fatigue throughout the procedure (**Figure 3-3**). This positioning also orients the surgical assistant toward the target anatomy, allowing for a more active role during the surgery. An assistant that is oriented off to the side will often have a more passive role. Active assistance may include complex stapling, suctioning, and the dynamic maintenance of exposure. In contrast, passive assistance might be just for exchanging needles and sponges.

By lowering the table, the assistant can remain seated for much of the procedure. This can be especially advantageous

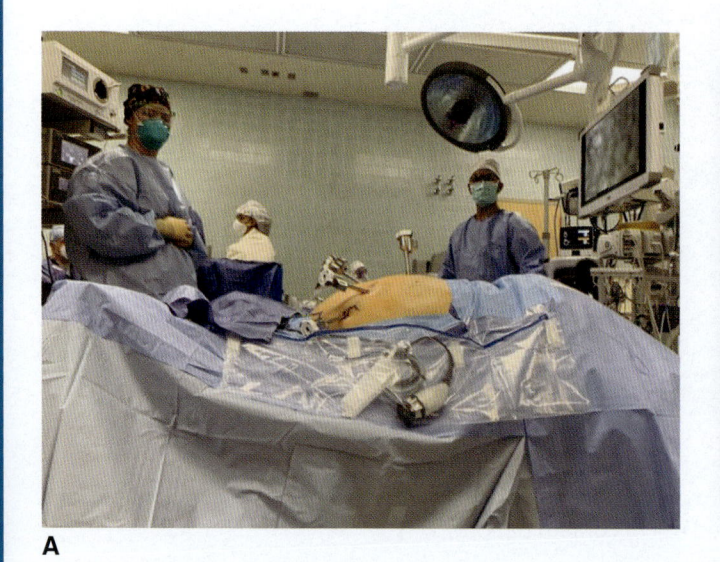

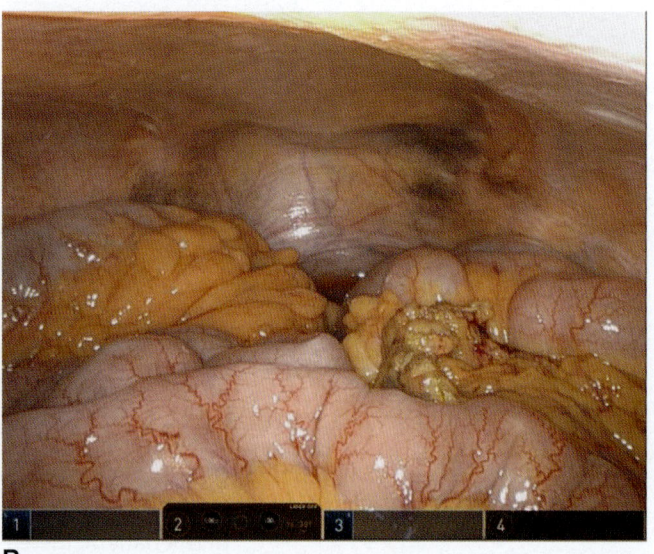

FIGURE 3-2 • **A.** Patient in supine position. **B.** Small bowel fills the pelvis, obstructing the operative field.

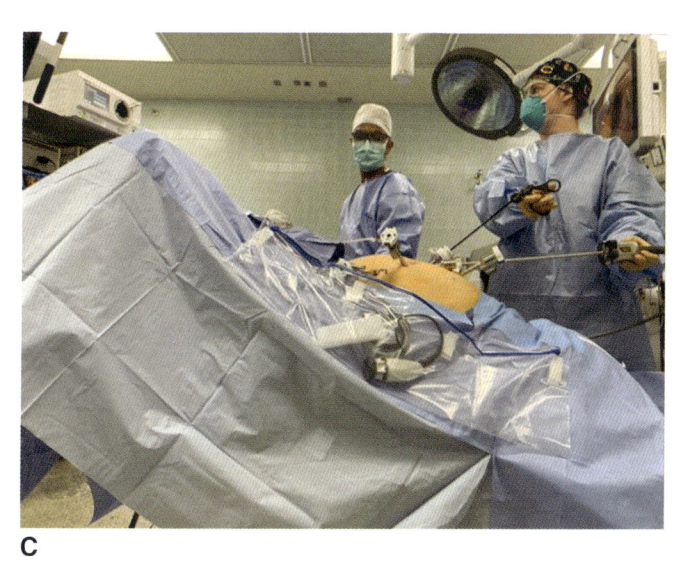

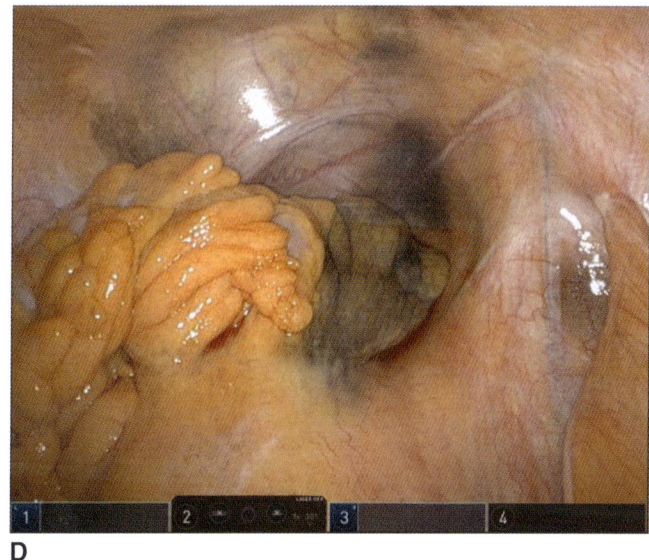

FIGURE 3-2 • (*Continued*) **C.** Patient in steep reverse Trendelenburg. **D.** Small bowel displaced away from the pelvis, optimizing the surgical field.

for longer operations, decreasing the assistant's strain as a result of prolonged standing (**Figures 3-4 A, B**). Ensuring that the table height is appropriately set allows the assistant to maximize the range of arm motion while minimizing the amount of back and shoulder strain. This concept is analogous to changing the bed's height (raising) during open operations to prevent back injuries.

An increased number and strategic positioning of surgical monitors can make orchestrating at the bedside easier. Multiple monitors must be available. If the assistant is required to look away from the screens to the Mayo stand or the back table, visualization can be maintained as to what is occurring laparoscopically. These monitors should be strategically positioned immediately after docking for maximum efficacy. Multiple appropriately placed monitors can also decrease neck or shoulder strain.

Other devices are being investigated, such as optical see-through head-mounted displays, to facilitate the team's visualization capabilities. These wearable electronic glasses can offer the assistant real-time, high-quality 3D vision comparable to what is seen by the surgeon in the robotic console while keeping the background environment perception. The assistant can sit or stand while maintaining a neutral neck and spine position, minimizing the strain usually encountered with mounted surgical monitors. More clinical experience is needed to validate the impact of head-mounted devices (**Figures 3-5 A–C**).

Instrumentation

The assistant must review the instrumentation available for the procedure and anticipate any unique circumstances that might be encountered. As a cost-saving measure, the assistant can instruct the operative team on instrumentation needed open on the sterile field and available on standby. Standby instrumentation should be easily accessible to avoid wasted time and resources during the procedure. For example, these can be placed in a designated cabinet within the OR for robotic supplies or on a side table easily accessible to the circulating nurse. Standby instrumentation must also include instruments for emergent conversion to an open procedure. For instance, vascular clamps in the case of bleeding should be promptly

FIGURE 3-3 • Assistant positioned in between patient's legs.

38   The Foundation and Art of Robotic Surgery

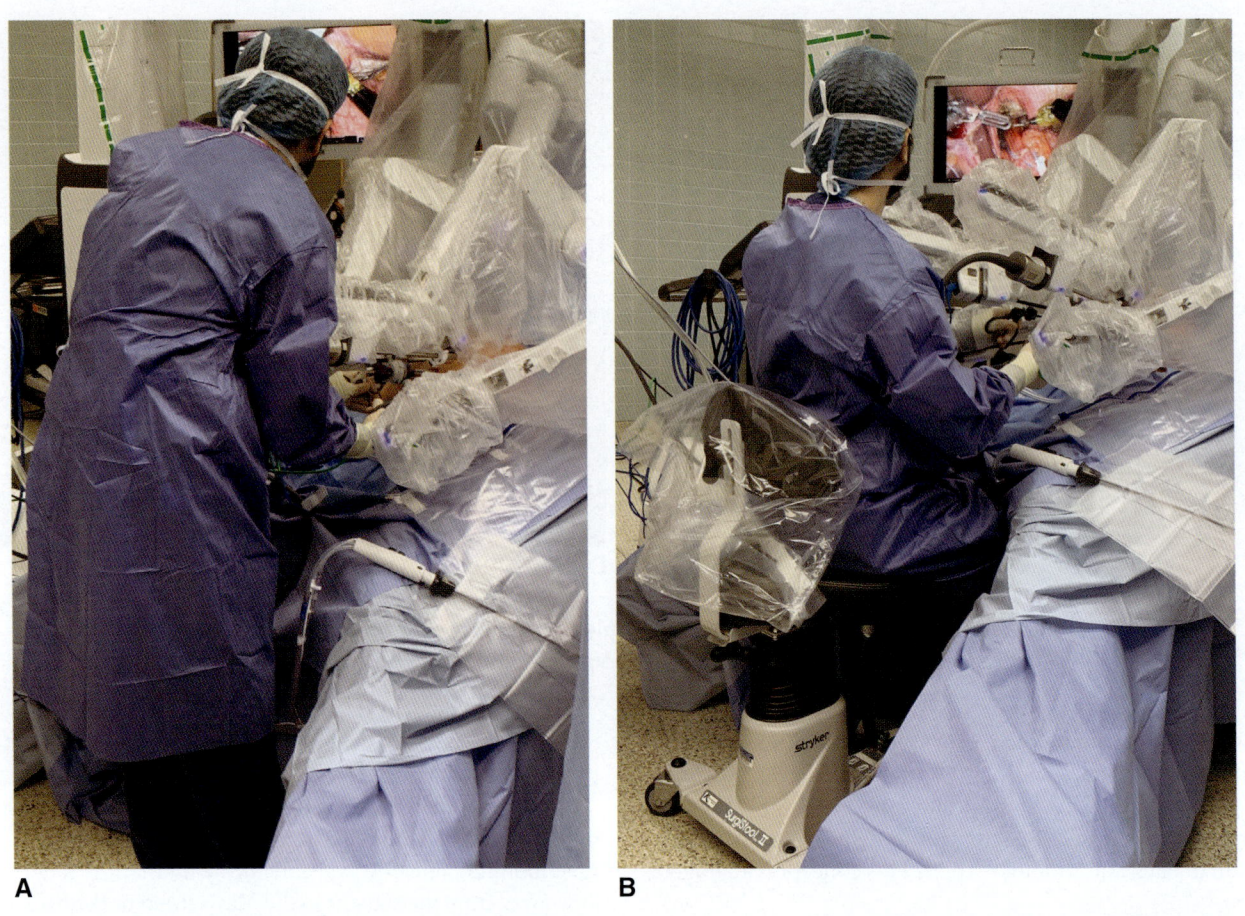

FIGURE 3-4 • Assistant's ergonomic positioning. They are orientated toward target anatomy. When positioned between the patient's legs, all 4 robotic arms are easily accessed. **A.** The surgical bed has a low height, and assisting while standing is not ergonomic. **B.** A seated position is advised to reduce fatigue.

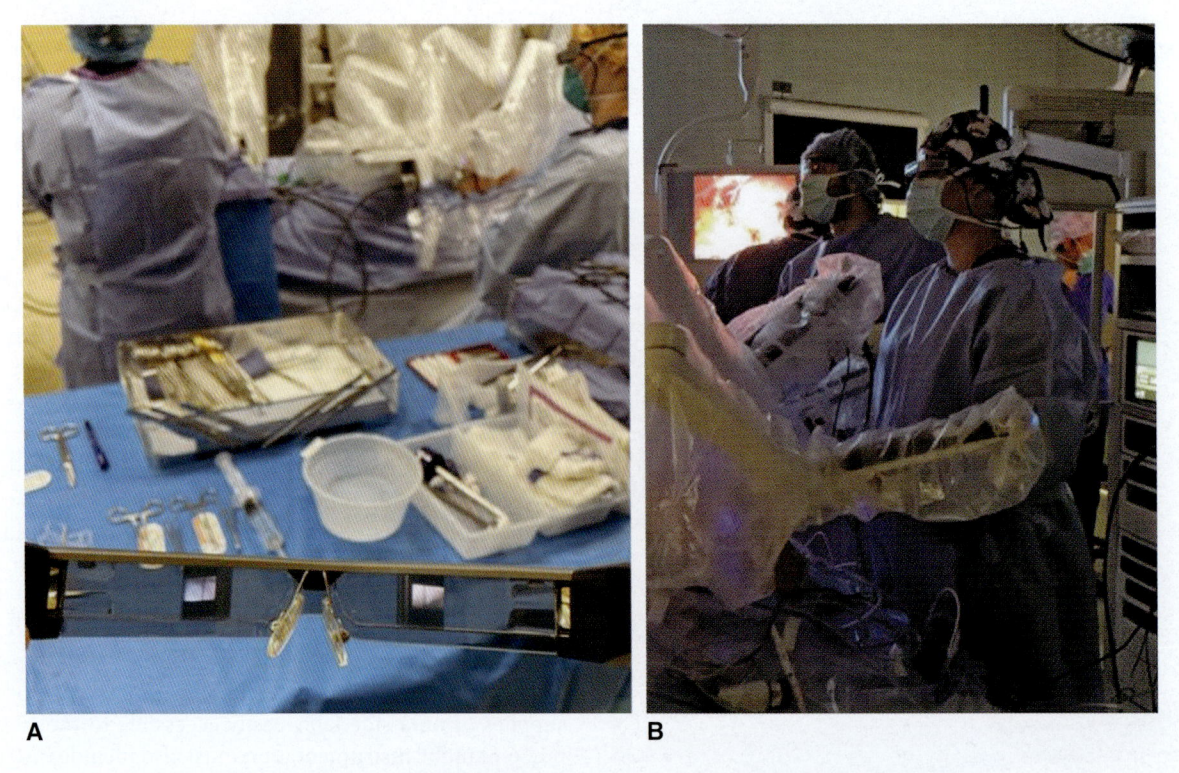

FIGURE 3-5 • Head-mounted display. Second generation of glasses with 3D vision. **A.** Intraoperative image shown at the center of the glasses. **B.** Bedside assistant using the glasses during surgery.

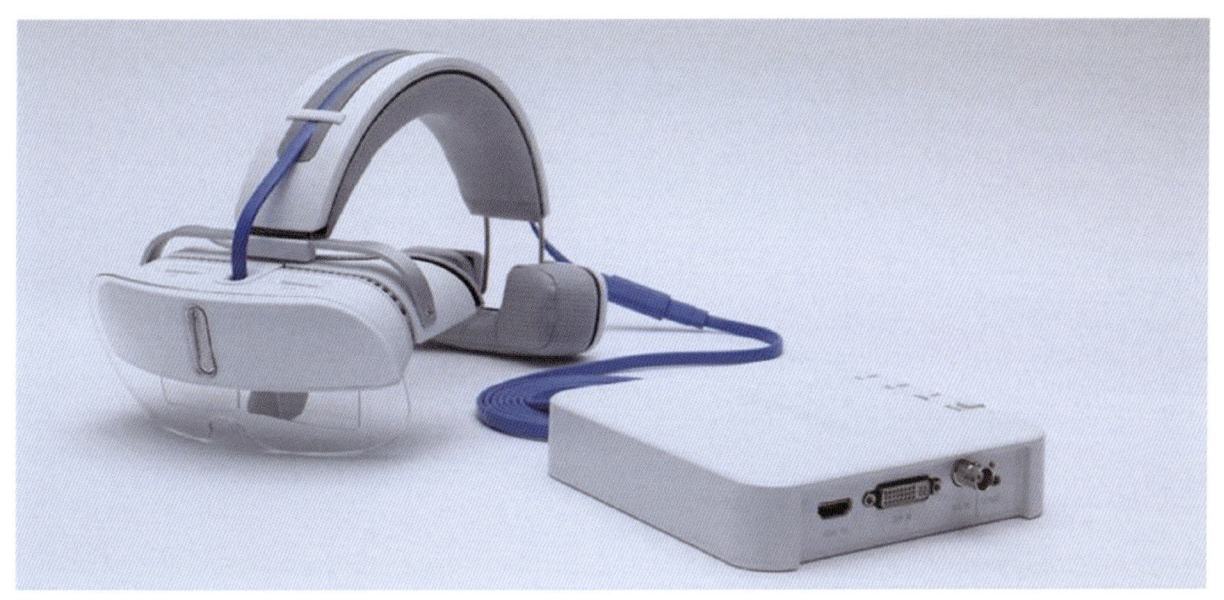

FIGURE 3-5 • (*Continued*) **C.** Third-generation headset for 3D vision. ScopEYE® (Reproduced with permission from Medithinq Co, Seongnam-si, Gyeonggi-d, South Korea.)

available. Minimizing these small-time delays may decrease the overall operating time and may result in potential cost savings. Extra robotic supplies should also be made readily available in case of malfunction or contamination. These include but are not limited to robotic instruments, drapes, and trocars. Basic sutures (preferred by the surgeon) should already be open on the field. Having these sutures ready, whether during the operation or the closing, will be a significant time-saver. If vascular sutures are already opened and can be quickly accessed, the overall blood loss of a procedure can also be decreased.

▶▶ **TIPS**

A second Mayo stand for robotic instruments can be placed where the assistant can easily access it. If bleeding is encountered, this can be especially helpful. The stand allows the assistant to access and exchange the instruments independently, and the surgical technician can prepare the sutures and loads. This allows the entire exchange to occur more quickly and efficiently (**Figure 3-6**).

This will naturally differ based on the surgeon's preference, but as the assistant and the surgeon continue to work together, the surgeons' needs can be anticipated.

For most robotic cases, there are standard laparoscopic instrumentation that should be available. A blunt grasper can safely manipulate bowel and other tissue or insert and remove surgical sponges and specimens. A needle driver is preferred instead of a grasper, for the insertion and removal of sutures and needles. This allows one to grasp the suture more securely and avoid misplacing needles during the case.

If a needle is lost, it should be communicated with the surgeon and immediately retrieved. Depending on the complexity of the case, a suction-irrigation device should also be included to help maintain visualization of the entire surgical field. Procedure-specific instrumentation will be outlined in the following chapters.

The Robotic System and Troubleshooting

Having an experienced robotic team can optimize robotic performance. However, depending on the institution or time of day, that team may not always be available. Instead, it is helpful to have an assistant who is proficient with all aspects of the robotic platform and who can provide the surgical team with detailed instructions as needed. This is not only

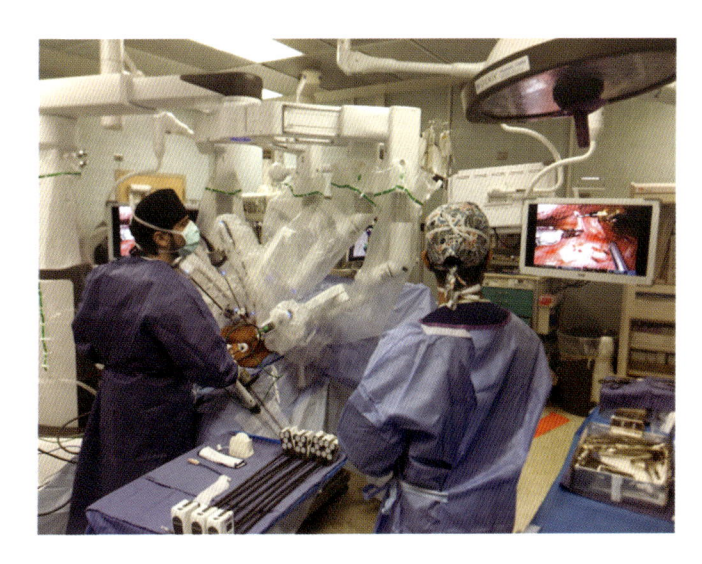

FIGURE 3-6 • Second Mayo stand.

for docking but also for undocking protocol in the case of an emergency. Docking of the robotic system requires clear and constant communication with the circulating nurse. The first assistant will specifically indicate where to maneuver the robot to avoid collisions with external structures in the OR, the bed, and the patient.

> ▶▶ **TIPS**
>
> It is often helpful to give directions in relation to the patient (for example: toward the patient's head or feet), versus saying "right" or "left," to avoid confusion.

▶ Video 3-1. Perform Targeting

The primary surgeon is responsible for planning the placement of the trocars. This will be determined based on the surgical procedure, target anatomy, and patient's body habitus. During this process, there are special considerations that can be evaluated. For instance, 2 assistant ports for more complex procedures allowing for active assistance, with at least one of these ports being 12 mm. This allows for easier exchanging of needles and sponges, and removing small specimens, such as lymph nodes. If the assistant uses a laparoscopic stapler, the 12-mm trocar's positioning should allow for the optimum angle to be achieved. If stapling is not a factor, this trocar can be located on the side of the assistant's dominant hand, which is more actively utilized. However, this cannot always be accommodated, and it is still essential that the assistant be laparoscopically skilled with both hands. Procedure-specific port placement will be illustrated in each chapter.

Once the patient cart is in position and the targeting sequence has been completed, the assistant can adjust each of the robotic arms at the patient's bedside. Doing this will provide an unrestricted range of motion. This can be achieved by starting with the uppermost joints, or flex, of the arm and progressing downward to the joints that provide the finer movements and patient clearance. The robotic joints' range of motion is

The circulating nurse should carefully guide the laser lines of the robotic patient cart (Da Vinci Xi System) to the robotic cannula that will function as the endoscopic port. While the robotic system provides a rough blueprint for positioning the system based on the regional anatomy of the surgery, the assistant needs to recognize when this may need to be adjusted to maximize the space and range of motion of the robotic arms. This includes vertical clearance of the robotic system in relation to the patient. The assistant must first perform an initial targeting sequence by aligning the endoscope with the target anatomy. Then the assistant must press and hold the target button on the endoscope, while supporting the cannula with the other hand.

clearly indicated on the patient cart. The assistant should aim to adjust the arm to maximize each one's range of motion. In a patient with smaller body habitus, sacrifices to the range of motion may sometimes be required because the optimum space between port sites cannot be achieved. In this instance, priority should be given to the camera and primary operating arms. In this case, the third arm is often providing stationary retraction and may not require as much range of motion as the primary operating arms (**Video 3-2**). Naturally, repositioning the robotic arms may become necessary during a procedure if external or internal collisions occur. The first assistant must communicate any external collision, but most should be anticipated and prevented. External collisions that occur on the front end of the robotic arm, resulting in arm-to-arm interference, can be corrected by making minor adjustments to the flex joints and uppermost joints. External collisions can also occur near the patient clearance joint, resulting in back-end interference of the robotic arm. If this occurs, those joints can be adjusted using the patient clearance buttons located on each arm's back. More information and online courses regarding the robotic system and docking process specific trainings to the Da Vinci system can be accessed by logging in to https://learning.intuitive.com (see suggested reading #2).

▶ Video 3-2. Optimal Docking

Given the system's lack of tactile feedback, the range of motion limitations should be communicated by the surgeon, which are most likely the result of internal collisions. Prompt communication can help prevent damage to the robotic instrumentation. The safest and most efficient way to correct collisions is first to disengage the robotic instrument. This will prevent any unintentional internal injury while manipulating the robotic arm. Next, the arm can be repositioned safely at any of the available joints, allowing for the desired range of motion. The robotic instrument can then be reengaged and safely advanced back into the surgical field. Dynamically readjusting the robotic arms throughout a procedure can help maintain maximum range of motion and avoid placement of extra trocars. The assistant can easily adjust the patient clearance joint without disengaging any instrumentation. Even minor adjustments can significantly improve the surgeon's range of motion.

Multiquadrant procedures may also require repositioning of the robotic arms. If the patient's position and cannula used for the endoscope do not change, the patient cart can be entirely at the bedside. With all the robot arms undocked, the assistant can use the rotation button located on the back of arms 1 and 4. These buttons allow the patient cart to be rotated 180°. The robotic arm can then be reattached to the cannula for the endoscope and the targeting sequence can be repeated. If the patient's position or the cannula used for the endoscope changes, the circulating nurse can readjust the patient cart as needed. To safely reposition the patient, the patient cart may need to be withdrawn and then readvanced after repositioning is complete.

Once the robotic arms are docked and in position, it is time for the installation and insertion of the robotic instruments. The assistant should be familiar with basic troubleshooting measures. As the instruments are installed into the robotic cart, the assistant must recognize and address the different reasons for instrumentation failure. First, any error messages that the vision cart may be displaying should be checked. If an error with the instrument's installation occurs, the assistant can first try to remove and then reengage the instrument. If it continues to fail, the instrument should be removed again ensuring that the robotic drape was applied correctly. If an error message continues, the instrument may be expired or damaged and it should be replaced. If the energy source of an instrument is not functioning, the assistant should communicate with the circulating nurse to ensure that all the energy and vision cables are connected properly to the vision cart. If the electrocautery continues to not function, a replacement cable or instrument may be necessary. This equipment should be readily available on standby as part of presurgical preparation.

> ▶▶ **TIPS**
>
> The robotic instruments' remaining uses or lives must always be checked at the beginning of the procedure. Overtime, instruments can become damaged or dull. Therefore, when minimal uses are remaining, backup instruments should be readily available.

The initial introduction of the instruments should always be done under direct visualization. The assistant can perform some basic maneuvers during the initial setup that can improve exposure for the surgeon. Lifting of the robotic cannula away from the patient, also referred to as "burping," results in a tenting of the tissue that can provide improved visualization with increased operating space. This tenting maneuver can be adjusted to obtain an optimum ~45° vision angle to the target anatomy, allowing the surgeon to utilize the robotic 3D vision to its full capacity. This can be especially helpful in patients with a narrow abdomen, giving the surgeon a wider field of vision (**Figures 3-7 A–D**).

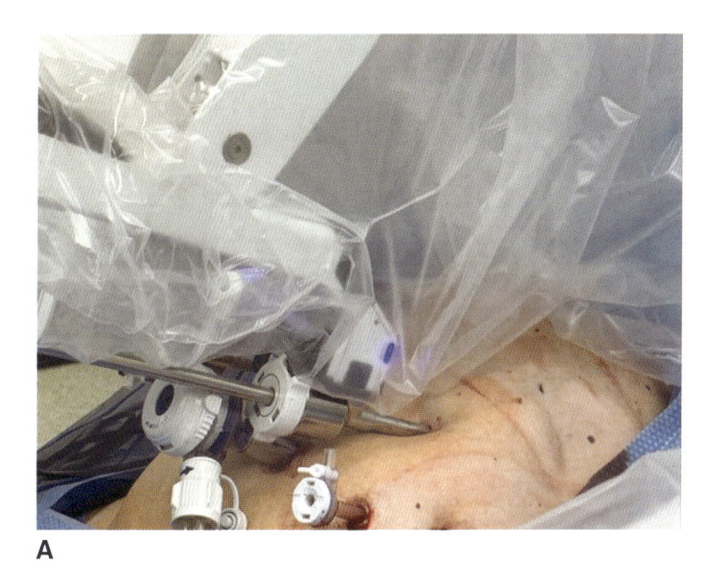

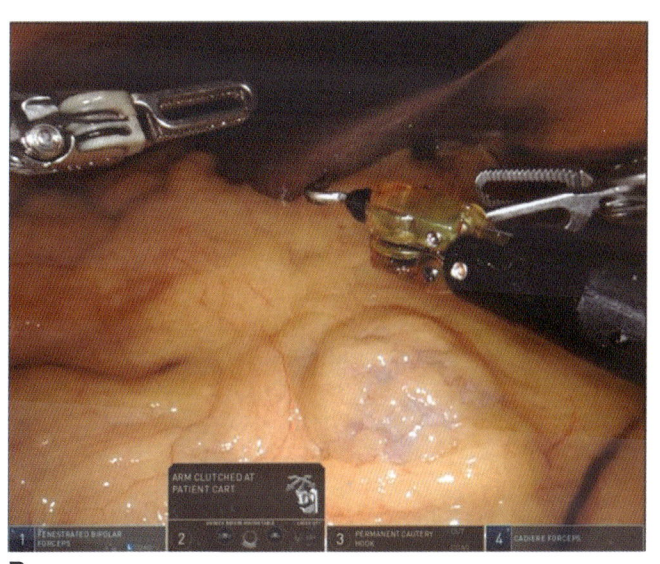

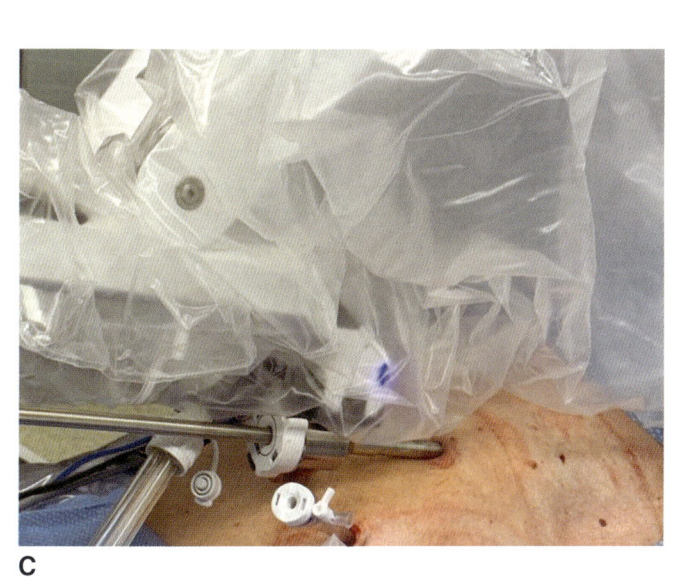

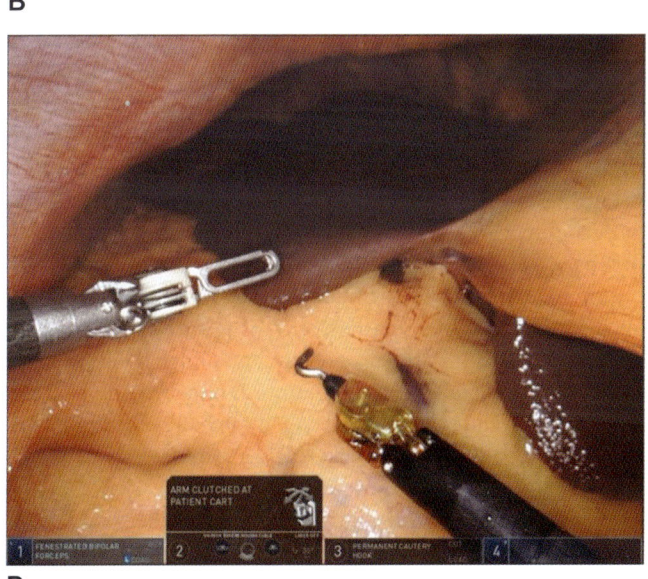

FIGURE 3-7 • Camera port adjustment. Lifting the robotic camera to optimize surgical field. **A.** Camera neutral position. **B.** Narrow surgical field. **C, D.** Camera lifted/tented, providing wider field of vision.

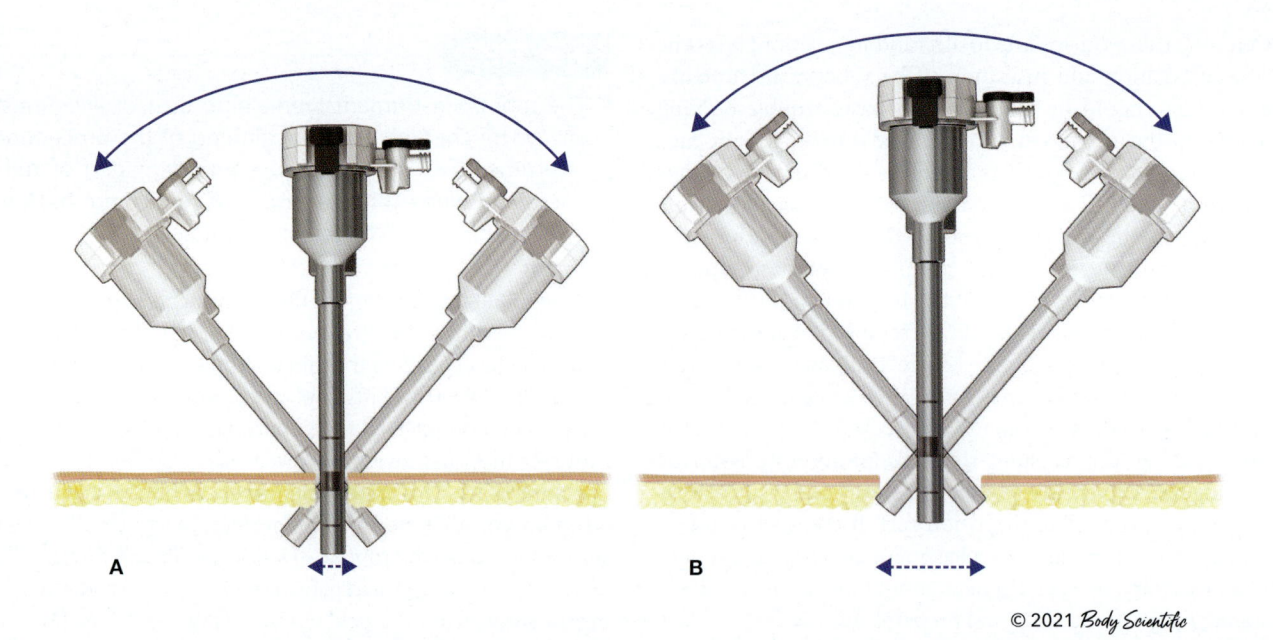

FIGURE 3-8 • Mechanical effect of the remote center placement. Placement outside of the abdominal wall produces lateral movement of the cannula, causing enlargement of the incision, air leak, pain, and additional complications (hematoma, incisional hernia). **A.** Correct placement. **B.** Wrong placement.

The assistant needs to be vigilant, not only of the ongoing surgery, but of the entire surgical field. At the patient's bedside, the assistant must make sure that robotic cannulas are correctly placed, not only at the start of the procedure, but throughout the surgery and as conditions change. First, the correct positioning of the cannula's remote center should be verified, as indicated by the robotic cannula's markings. The remote center of the cannula is marked by a thick black line (**Figures 3-8 A, B**). By maintaining this line within the patient's fascia plane, the remote center allows the robotic arm to move freely without causing trauma to the tissue, resulting in less postoperative pain and better cosmesis. However, throughout the surgery, this will require adjustments to allow for a greater range of motion for the surgeon. Sometimes the cannula may need to be advanced to allow the surgeon to reach distant anatomy, and the assistant must know how to achieve this. Safely removing the robotic instrument before advancement is the safest approach. The assistant would then advance the cannula to the desired depth and then reengage the instrument and advance it into the surgical field. It is possible to advance the cannula with the instrument still engaged, but the assistant must first pull back the instrument while maintaining visualization without disengaging. The instrument's tip should then be aimed up and away from vital structures, such as toward the abdominal or chest wall. This will help prevent any injury while advancing the instrument. Then, the entire robotic arm and cannula should be advanced as one unit. Again, this must be done with great caution and under direct visualization.

By maintaining an awareness of the surgical field at the patient's bedside, the assistant can ensure that the robotic cannulas do not withdraw into the subcutaneous tissue, because subcutaneous emphysema can occur. The assistant can correct the cannula's position by first communicating the issue with the surgeon and then removing the robotic instrument. Once the instrumentation is removed, the cannula and robotic arm can be repositioned safely.

> ▶▶ **TIPS**
>
> It is often easier and faster to reposition the cannula without the robotic arm attached. Using the obturator can be helpful to find the previous track. Blind maneuvers can be risky and should be performed under direct visualization when possible.

Prompt recognition of withdrawn cannulas and correction is important, because continuous insufflation into the subcutaneous space can impose upon the surgical field, thus making visualization more difficult. In severe subcutaneous emphysema, respiratory distress can occur, which can be a reason for open conversion. The assistant can communicate with the anesthesiologist so that they can anticipate respiratory changes and prompt intervention can be taken. Decreasing the intraabdominal pressure level maintained by the insufflation machine may also be considered.

> ▶▶ **TIPS**
>
> Having the robotic arms lifted takes advantage of the ability of the robot to maintain the electronic hinge. The working space can be preserved even when decreasing the intraabdominal pressure. This results in a gasless-like technique. The cannula is shifted upward by burping the robotic arm at the port clutch button, consequently lifting the entire arm and "tenting" the abdomen.

Video 3-3. Arm-to-Arm Troubleshooting

Laparoscopic Assisting

A first assistant must be knowledgeable of the surgical procedure and its regional anatomy and possess a strong laparoscopic skill set. An active *versus* a passive assistant is responsible for implementing and maintaining exposure of the surgical field. Recognition of the surgical planes and critical structures is imperative, as knowing which tissues are appropriate to grasp and with what pressure, as well as being mindful to avoid damage to surrounding vasculature. Knowledge of the surgical procedure allows assuming a more active role in the surgery. A more passive role would be just passing sutures, retrieving tissue samples, and exchanging the robotic instrumentation. An active assistant can anticipate the next steps of the procedure and provide the appropriate exposure. Often, the surgeon will first provide stable retraction through the use of the third robotic arm; for example, lifting and stabilizing the liver for upper abdominal procedures. The assistant can then provide a secondary, more generalized retraction. This allows the surgeon to utilize both operative arms for fine delicate retraction and dissection. The less the surgeon has to stop and instruct the assistant on where to grasp and retract, the faster and smoother the procedure can proceed. This fluid and intricate maneuvering between the assistant and the surgeon can decrease overall operating time and potential cost to the patient.

With the surgeon in control of the robotic scope, it is sometimes necessary for the assistant to perform blind laparoscopic maneuvers. Therefore, it is crucial to be an expert in regional anatomy. Knowing not only where structures are within view, but also outside the field of vision will help prevent inadvertent injury to the tissue. This is constantly changing throughout the procedure with manipulation of structures. Therefore, caution should always be taken with the introduction and replacement of robotic and laparoscopic instruments into the surgical field. The assistant must immediately recognize when there is resistance with the introduction of the robotic instrument and not force any movements.

> ▶▶ **TIPS**
>
> When there is resistance, the advancement of an instrument should never be forced. The trocar might have become withdrawn into the subcutaneous tissue or anatomy could be blocking the introduction. When there is doubt, it should be communicated to the surgeon so that the cannula can be visualized.

If there is concern that potential damage has been caused to tissue outside of the surgeon's view, it must be immediately communicated to the primary surgeon. The surgeon can then assess the tissue and determine if corrective action needs to be taken.

Applying appropriate tension and retraction to the tissue exposes the correct surgical plane, facilitating the surgeon's dissection and preventing tissue damage. Without the tactile feedback, the surgeon relies heavily on its superior 3D vision. Therefore, the assistant should assume responsibility for recognizing the tactile tension of the tissue and adjusting as necessary. If the tissue is very friable or there is concern about grasping tissue, a surgical sponge can be used to provide a protective buffer between the laparoscopic grasper and the tissue.

Diligent suctioning and irrigation should be used to maintain visualization of the surgical field. The suction device should act as a dynamic instrument, because it can be used for suctioning and retraction. In instances of bleeding, this maneuvering allows for the assistant to quickly alternate between suctioning and retraction without exchanging laparoscopic instruments.

> ▶▶ **TIPS**
>
> The suction device can serve a dual purpose, for suctioning and retraction. Retraction with the suction device can be achieved by gently pressing down or lifting the tissue with the instrument.

Reduced visibility can occur when there is an abundance of light-absorbing red (blood) in the surgical field, and this should be removed whenever possible. White is more reflective, so by placing a clean surgical sponge into the field, the vision can often be improved. Of course, the sponge must be exchanged as needed to maintain proper vision. When saturated, they should be promptly removed, not only for visualization purposes but also to be accounted for. The suction device can also be used to reduce contamination of the surgical field. Minimally invasive procedures typically help decrease infection rates postoperatively. Therefore, the assistant should take great care to minimize contamination within the field, such as bowel or gastric content through suctioning.

Depending on surgeon preference, the first assistant can also perform laparoscopic stapling. The need for stapling during a procedure should be determined starting from the placement of the trocars. As discussed earlier, the 12-mm laparoscopic trocar usually provides the assistant with the most appropriate angle. An 8-mm or 15-mm trocar may be utilized depending on the type of stapler and size of the reload. With the surgeon able to provide precise and controlled exposure, the assistant can place the stapler with ease. After stapling is completed, the surgeon can continue operating or suture as needed without delay.

Video 3-4. Laparoscopic Assistance Techniques

Communication

As described previously, clear and concise communication is of the utmost importance, at every step during robotic surgery. The primary surgeon is without direct control at the patient's bedside and is outside the sterile field. As a result, the first assistant must maintain communication with the surgeon, circulating nurse, surgical technician, and anesthesiologist. This includes communication with the surgical technician to have specific sutures, vessel loops, and umbilical tape cut to specific lengths, ready and available. With experience, other nonverbal cues between the surgeon and the assistant can develop. For example, a surgeon may lift tissue indicating the need for retraction. ORs can often be high-stimuli environments. These nonverbal forms of communication can become increasingly important, especially in the robotic setting. Without the entire operating team within the sterile field, visual and auditory cues can be difficult to interpret and the potential for a breakdown of communication can occur. The first assistant can alleviate this burden by acting as a liaison between the surgeon and the remaining operative team, promoting a collaborative and more harmonious working environment.

Training for Robotic Assistants

Technological advancements in the surgical field have resulted in more ORs using robotic systems to execute delicate surgeries. As the robotic surgical platform continues to evolve, and more complex procedures are being readily performed, it will become necessary for standardized robotic first assistant courses to be developed. These courses should focus on generalized laparoscopic and robotic techniques as companies introduce other competitive platforms into the market (see suggested reading #3). Currently, the first assistants often receive only basic training during their education; otherwise, it is primarily on-the-job training, and the training received during their education can vary greatly. The assistant's experience depends upon the location of clinical sites, caseload, and the preceptor. Hospitals in rural locations may have a narrow focus and small caseload when compared to a larger university setting. As a result, the assistant may not have as much exposure to a large number and variety of surgeries. It may be in surgical practices' interest to invest time in training their robotic first assistant on the job to evolve the dynamic working relationship between the surgeon and assistant. Concerning technical training in specific robotic platforms, some robotic companies offer self-directed online informational courses. However, these courses are not required by all hospitals. A competent and efficient assistant can improve the overall surgical performance and decrease operating time. This results in reduced costs and improvement of postoperative outcomes. With time, hospitals and surgical practices worldwide will discover that a skilled and well-educated robotic first assistant can be an indispensable member of the surgical team.

Suggested Readings

1. American College of Surgeons statements on principles. *Bulletin of the American College of Surgeons.* 2016; 19-34. Accessed January 15, 2021. https://www.facs.org/~/media/files/publications/bulletin/2016/2016%20september.ashx
2. Intuitive. https://learning.intuitive.com
3. Guideline statement for the surgical assistant in robotic surgery. Association of Surgical Assistants. 2021. Accessed January 15, 2021. https://www.surgicalassistant.org/about/guidelines/files/Guidelines_Surgical_Robotics.pdf
4. Giulianotti PC, Coratti A, Angelini M, et al. Robotics in general surgery: personal experience in a large community hospital. *Arch Surg.* 2003;138(7):777-784. doi: 10.1001/archsurg.138.7.777

"It's not practice that makes perfect. It's perfect practice that makes perfect."
—Vince Lombardi (1913–1970)

Robotic Training

Alberto Mangano • Valentina Valle • Liaohai Leo Chen • Antonio Gangemi

INTRODUCTION

As of this day, a standardized, comprehensive, diversified, and well-validated path for robotic training is still to be established.

Recent literature, investigating policies from 42 American hospitals geographically spread across the country, indicates that most centers relied solely on a defined number of proctored cases as a surrogate for proficiency and requirement for initial credentialing. Moreover, only 31% of the training courses offered at these institutions had a cadaveric or animate laboratory component, while a dismal 21% specified a minimum passing score (see suggested reading #1).

These negative data are supported by expert opinions, as confirmed by a recent consensus conference gathering 28 national robotic surgery experts. After review of available institutional policies and discussion, the group unanimously agreed that there is a need for standardized robotic surgery credentialing criteria across institutions that promote surgeon proficiency.

One area of wide-ranging consensus is represented by the multistep approach to robotic training. It is simply unconceivable, based on the modern standards of surgical care, that one could start operating on patients without transitioning through some form of supervised training in a controlled environment.

The ideal *controlled environment* should be a dedicated *training laboratory*, where trainees can acquire proficiency with the robotic platform, without exposing the patient to the inherent risks of being operated by an untrained robotic practitioner. It is not difficult to envision a large consensus of expert opinions on this argument.

However, things start to get more convoluted when a definition of *controlled* is being endeavored. The first attribute of such definition is the *training model,* and the second is the *curriculum* implemented on that specific model. Both topics will be addressed in the following sections of this chapter that will be concluded by a forward-looking outline of the robotic privileging and credentialing process.

TRAINING MODELS

Should training start on inanimate models? Live tissues? Animal models? In the virtual reality environment of robotic simulators? All of the above? And, if it is assumed that they are all critical for a steadfast and reliable learning curve, which one should be the starting point?

Inanimate Training Models

The boost of virtual reality (VR) simulators witnessed over the last decade has halted interest for the development of inanimate models. The inanimate training model developed for the Fundamentals of Robotic Surgery (FRS) stands to this day as a solid exception to this negative trend.

This multispecialty, proficiency-based curriculum of basic technical skills was developed by over 80 national/international robotic surgery experts, behavioral psychologists, medical educators, statisticians, and psychometricians.

The experts recruited to develop this curriculum represented all the major surgical specialties performing robotic-assisted surgical procedures in the United States.

A specific physical and inanimate model (DOME) was developed to train and assess the psychomotor robotic skills of the FRS (**Figure 4-1**).

Later, a VR version of the physical model was introduced and has been recently validated for its use in some robotic simulators (**Figure 4-2**).

Remarkably, the training model was conceived as "agnostic" of a specific robotic system, and could therefore be used with different robotic platforms in the future.

A prior multicenter effort known as the Fundamental Inanimate Robotic Skills Tasks (FIRST) validated a multilayered inanimate model—(1) Penrose tube, (2) clover pattern cut, (3) semispherical plastic dome and pegs, (4) circular needle target—created by using robotic prostatectomy as the model procedure, and to assess many basic psychomotor

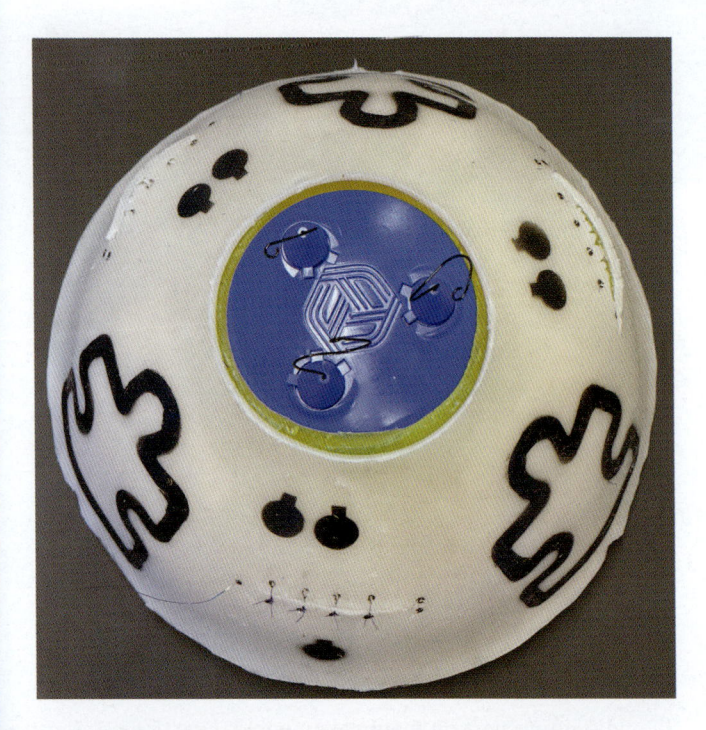

FIGURE 4-1 • 3D-printed FRS physical DOME.

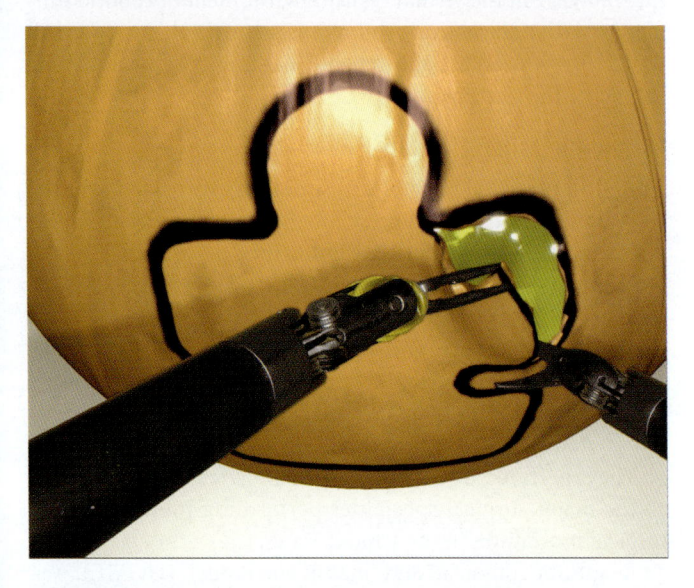

FIGURE 4-2 • Simbionix RobotiX Mentor. (Reproduced with permission from Surgical Science, Göteborg Sweden.)

skills that the expert panel deemed to be essential for robotic surgery (**Figures 4-3 A–D**).

However, the model has failed to gain wide acceptance, mainly due to its specialty-specific derivation and shortage of transferability to a VR platform.

Aside from these 2 aforementioned endeavors, the only other area of development, that has interested inanimate models, is represented by the box trainers which simulate the insufflated abdomen to allow the apprenticeship of ports placement and robotic docking (**Figures 4-4** and **4-5**).

Virtual Reality–Based Training Models

The future is already here: no other adage could be more appropriate to describe the importance and ascendancy of VR-based training in robotic surgery.

The realism (the simulation expert would call it the *face validity*), expressed by the software and the hardware of robotic simulators, has been exponentially improving.

The list of available VR robotic simulators has been solidly growing over the last decade or so. At first, various standalone simulators were introduced, and then they had been validated, on solid scientific ground, for their face and content validity (**Figures 4-6** and **4-7**).

The surge of interest for robotic simulation, coupled with the fast-moving pace of product innovation and an ever-increasing need for brand expansion, have created an extremely competitive market that has forced some of the more traditional "stand-alone" simulators out of business and encouraged others to seek merging with complementary companies (Mimic & Surgical Science) (**Figure 4-8**).

More recently, robotic simulators that can be integrated with the robotic surgeon's console have been introduced by the larger players of the robotic industry who have the necessary resources, and operational capability, to create this kind of product. For instance, the da Vinci Skills Simulator [also known as the *backpack* for the possibility to be connected to the back of the da Vinci Si (see **Video 4-1**) or da Vinci Xi console (see **Video 4-2** for an example of a robotic cholecystectomy simulation)] allows trainees to practice, and refine, their robotic skills in a VR environment while sitting at the actual da Vinci surgical console (**Figure 4-9**).

Video 4-1. Si Exercises

Video 4-2. Simulation of a Robotic Cholecystectomy

Both basic and more advanced, as well as procedure-specific, psychomotor robotic skills can be trained, and assessed, on robotic simulators. There is already a good-sized body of scientific literature proving that basic and procedural robotic surgical skills can be successfully transferred from the simulator to the OR.

Furthermore, hybrid platforms are also being created where the trainees can use the VR robotic instruments to interact with the superimposed anatomy of video-recorded surgical procedures from the OR. The introduction of this technology has greatly improved the ability of available robotic simulators to train and assess trainees' familiarity and decision-making skills for various surgical procedures such as nephrectomy, hysterectomy, inguinal hernia repair, prostatectomy (**Figure 4-10**), cystectomy, and lymph nodal dissection (**Figure 4-11**).

Additionally, some robotic simulators allow team training thanks to a separate (laparoscopic) hardware unit that allows the

Robotic Training 47

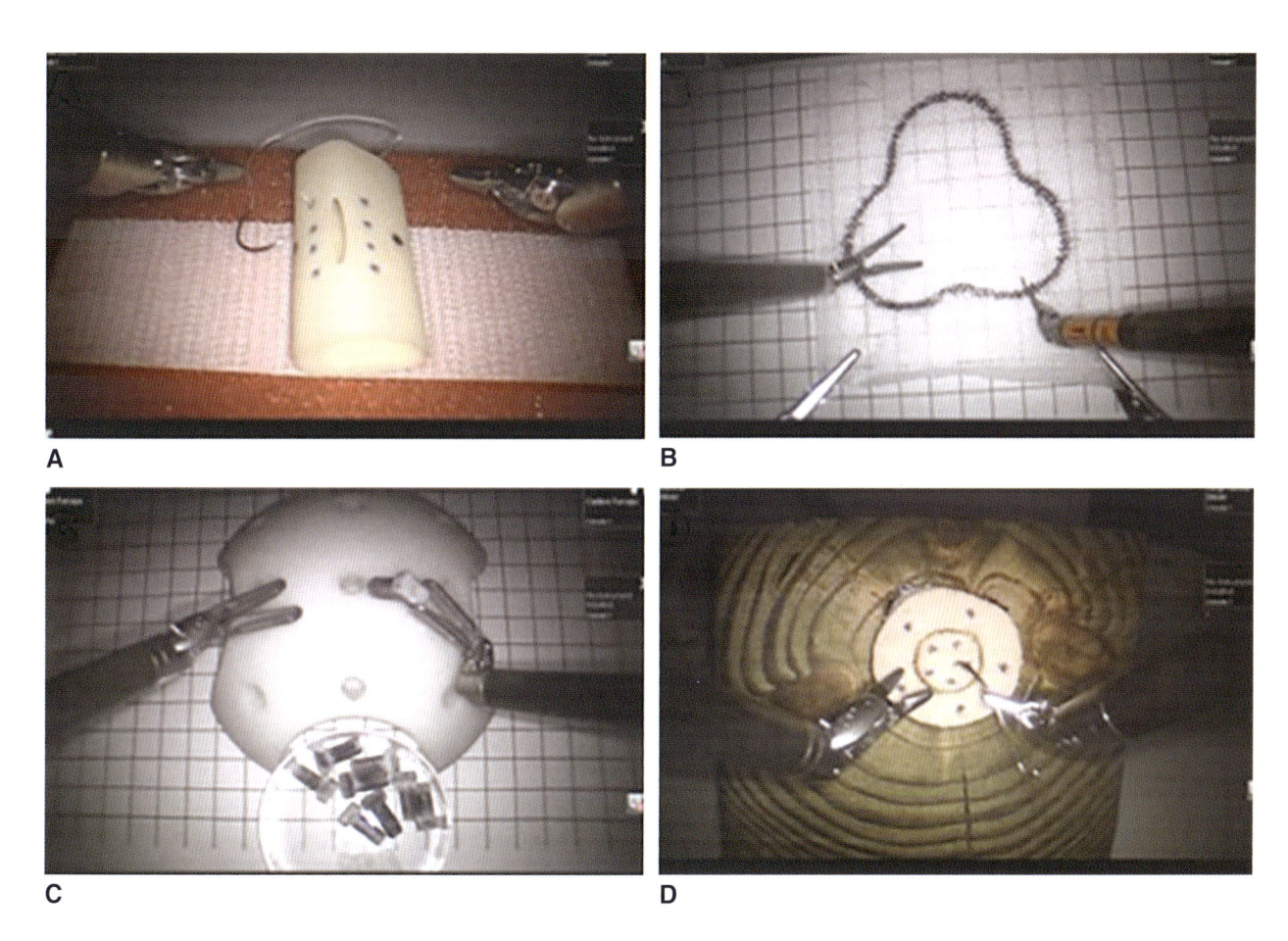

FIGURE 4-3 • FIRST. **A.** Horizontal mattress. **B.** Clover pattern cut. **C.** 3D and peg. **D.** Circular needle target. (Reproduced with permission from Goh AC, Aghazadeh MA, Mercado MA, et al. Multi-institutional validation of fundamental inanimate robotic skills tasks. *J Urol*. 2015;194(6):1751-1756.)

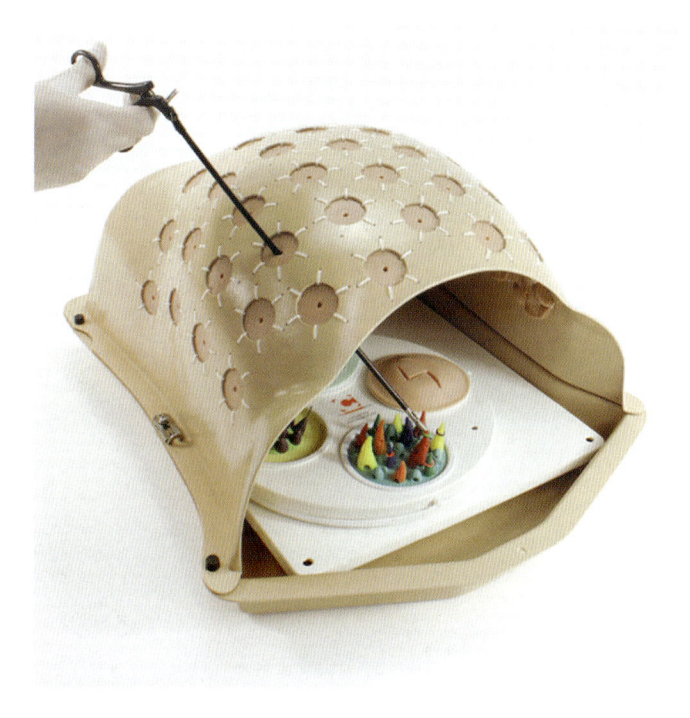

FIGURE 4-4 • Insufflated abdomen with ports. (Reproduced with permission from The Chamberlain Group, LLC. Great Barrington, MA.)

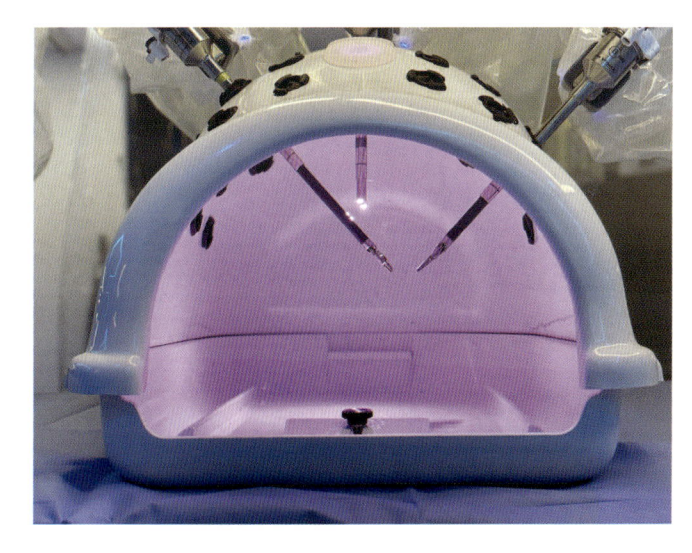

FIGURE 4-5 • Abdomen-like box developed by Intuitive Surgical (Sunnyvale, CA) but not commercially marketed.

48 The Foundation and Art of Robotic Surgery

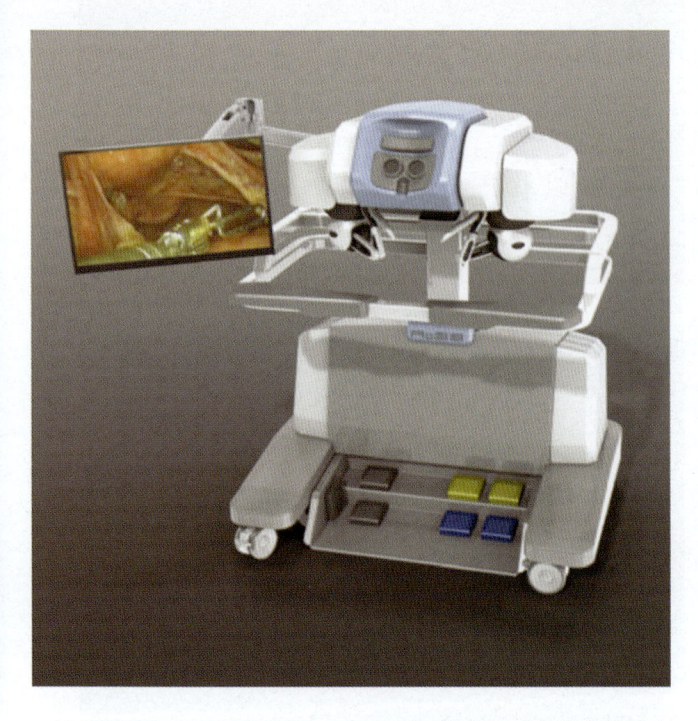

FIGURE 4-6 • RoSS II. (Reproduced with permission from Simulated Surgical Systems, LLC. San Jose, CA.)

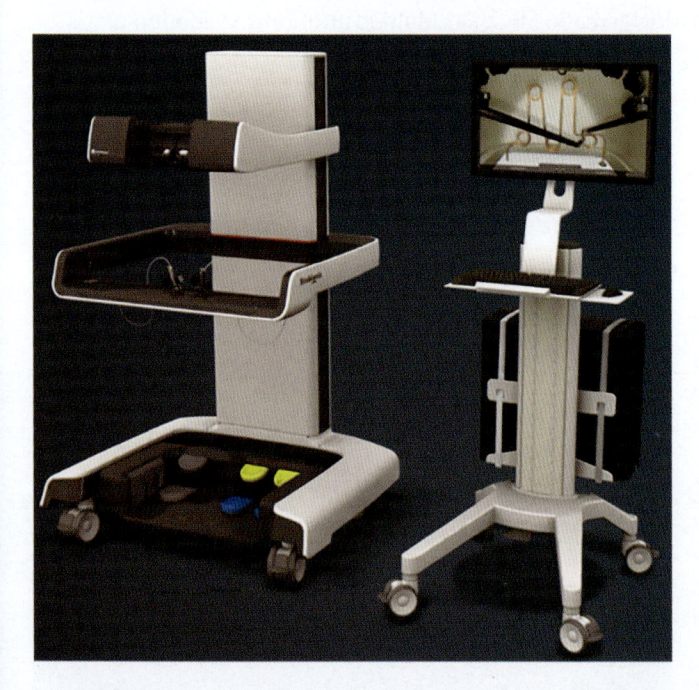

FIGURE 4-7 • Simbionix RobotiX Mentor (3D Systems). (Reproduced with permission from Surgical Science, Göteborg Sweden.)

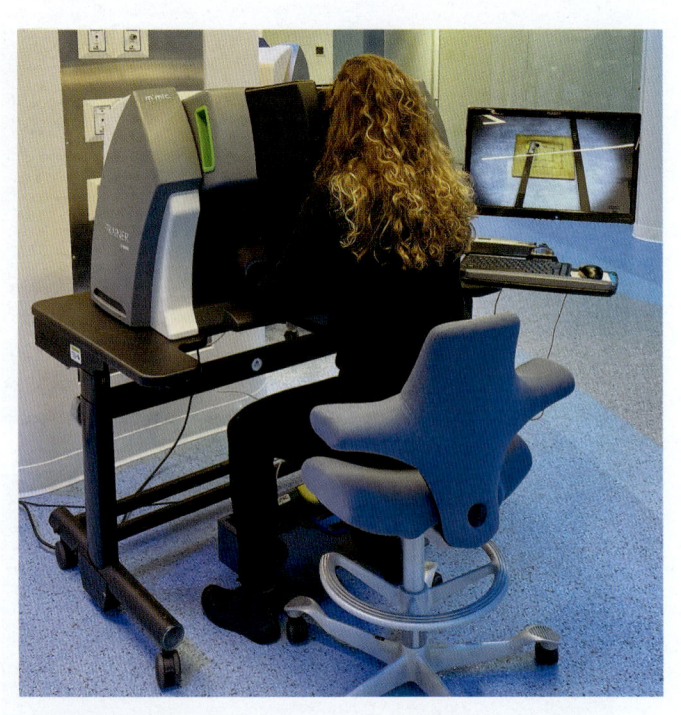

FIGURE 4-8 • Mimic dV-Trainer (Surgical Science, Göteborg, Sweden.)

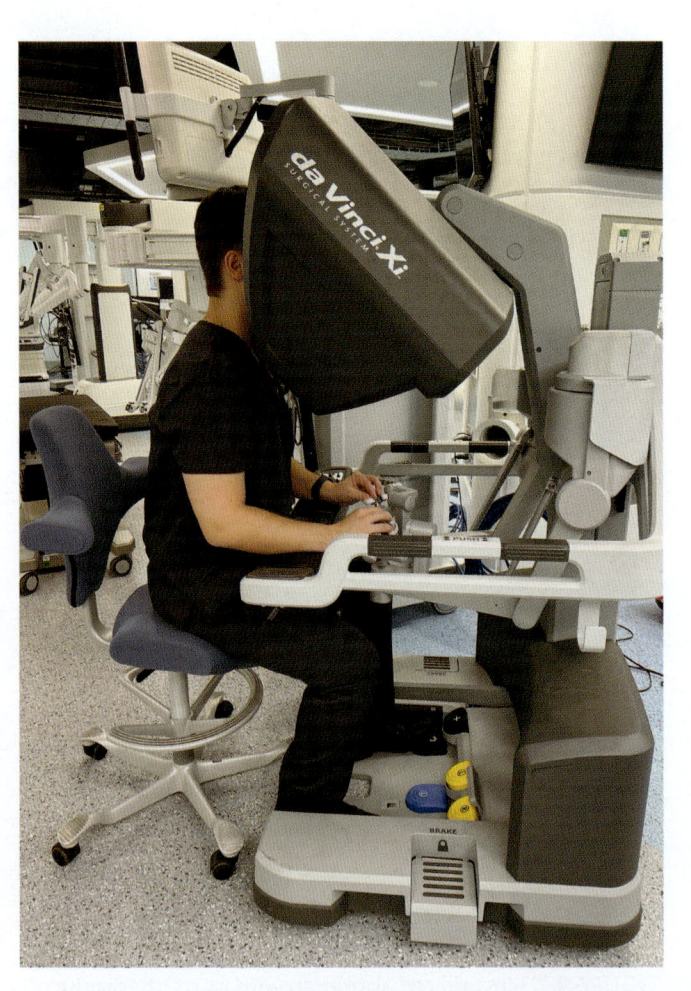

FIGURE 4-9 • The da Vinci Xi (Intuitive Surgical, Sunnyvale, CA.)

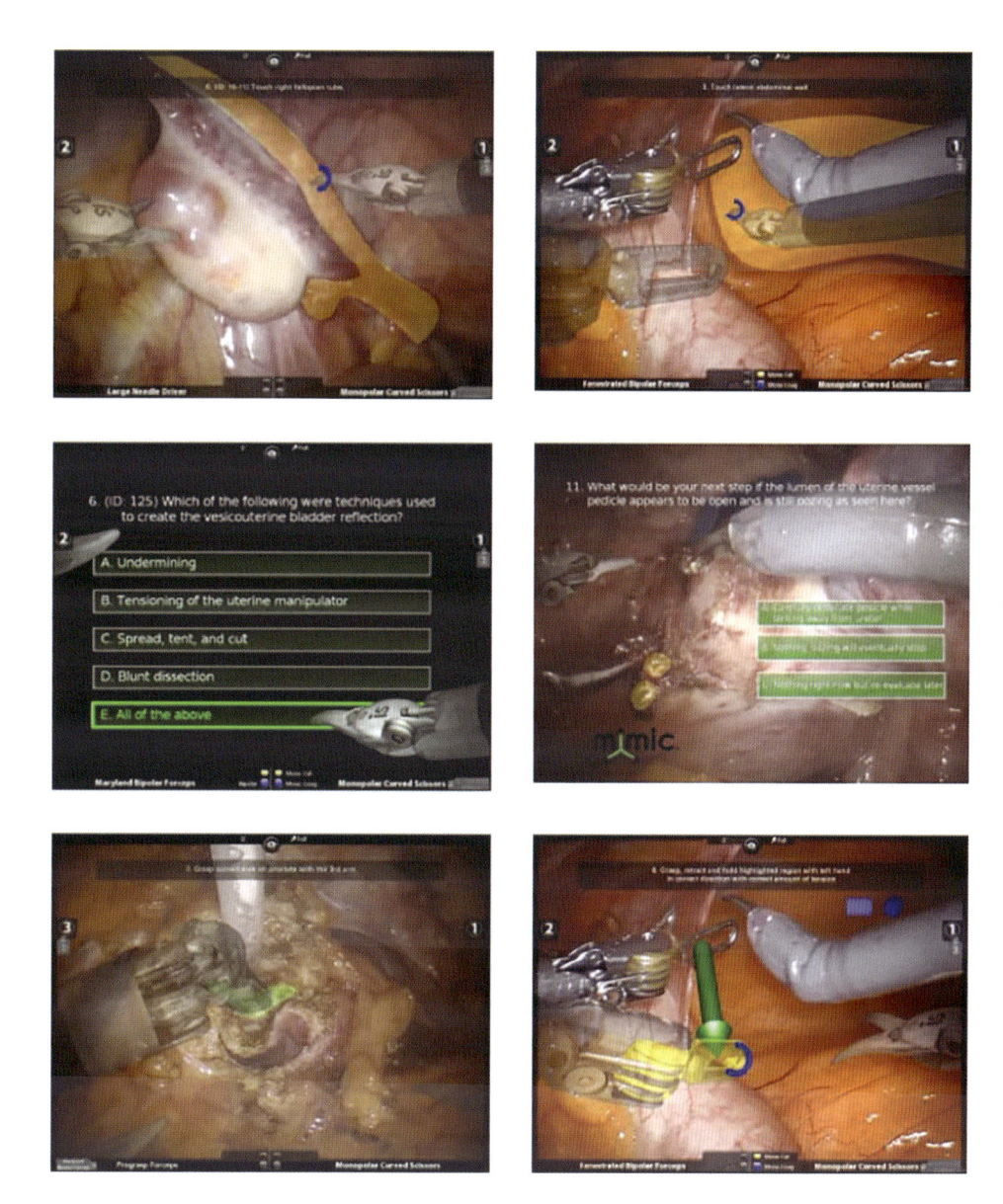

FIGURE 4-10 • Procedure-specific learning in 3D augmented reality (MaestroAR Mimic dV-Trainer simulator). (Reproduced with permission from Surgical Science, Göteborg Sweden.)

laparoscopic assistant to interact in the same VR environment of the trainee sitting at the console (**Figures 4-12** and **4-13**).

Also, all the major companies of the robotic simulation industry are offering cloud-based portals, where both trainees and trainers can track down training performance and progress in real time.

An interesting product is the SimNow™ simulator by Intuitive which is designed for the da Vinci surgical systems (da Vinci Si, X, Xi, and SP systems).

SimNow™ allows the learning process to be supported over time with a library including procedure-based training exercises, as well as VR. The system is very realistic and provides a simulated surgical field.

Additionally, SimNow™ allows the assessment of the users' performance and customizable curricula.

SimNow™ has automatic on-line software upgrades, real-time data transfer and the possibility to connect to smart devices or computers.

The definition of proficiency benchmarks, and the validation of metrics, are certainly the area where there is the greatest room for advancement and further investigation.

Preliminary evidences indicate a positive correlation between human evaluators and simulator metric scoring on basic simulator tasks, and between simulator scores and dry laboratory performances among trainees.

However, it is yet to be completely established how accurately the proficiency on the robotic simulators reflects on important clinical outcomes, such as: operative time, intra- and perioperative morbidity, estimated blood loss, length of hospital-stay, and many others. Nevertheless, VR simulators are being increasingly integrated into training curricula.

It is to be expected that the role of robotic simulators will continue to expand beyond the initial privileging and credentialing process. As technology advances, transitioning into an era of *continued surgical education*, robotic simulators will likely play a pivotal role for *maintenance of robotic certification*

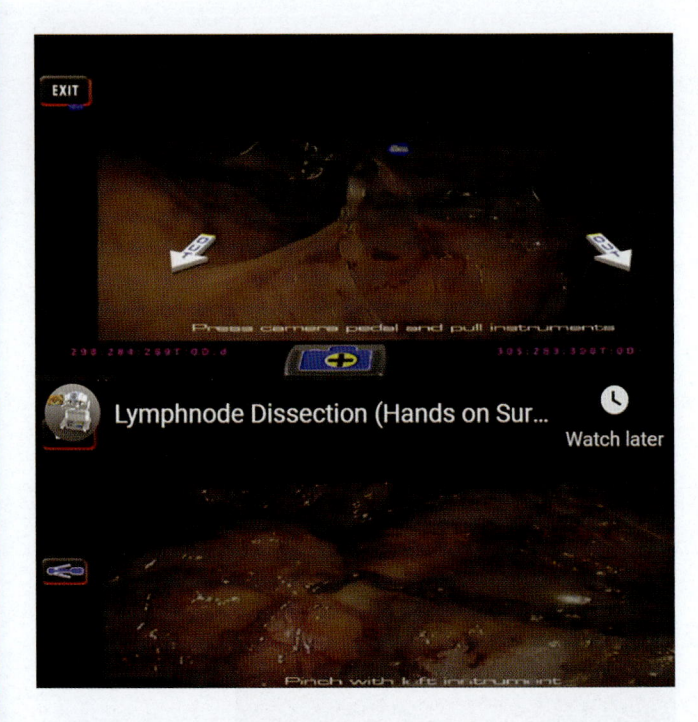

FIGURE 4-11 • Haptics-assisted procedure-specific learning (HOST RoSS simulator). (Reproduced with permission from Simulated Surgical Systems, LLC. San Jose, CA.)

or for its reacquisition, likely paralleling the trend witnessed by the civilian and military aviation fields.

Animal Models

Currently, this training model has a greater realism than even the most advanced VR simulator. For instance, the hemorrhage encountered in a heart-beating specimen, and the way this reflects on its hemodynamics and on the management of general anesthesia, is something that cannot be fully reproduced in the current VR simulators. Real live tissues appear different and react

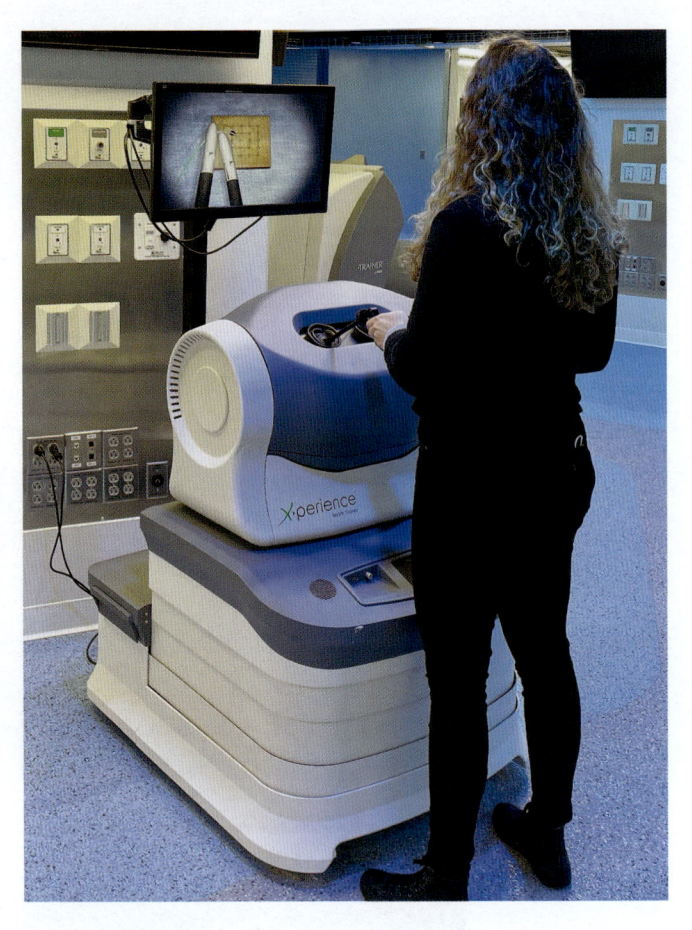

FIGURE 4-12 • Mimic X-perience team trainer (Surgical Science, Göteborg, Sweden.)

more realistically to the touching, the grasping, the cutting, the suturing and the pulling compared to the tissues created by the software engineer in the VR environment existing at present time.

Also, the trainee's psychomotor skills are challenged by the awareness of performing surgery on a living being. This

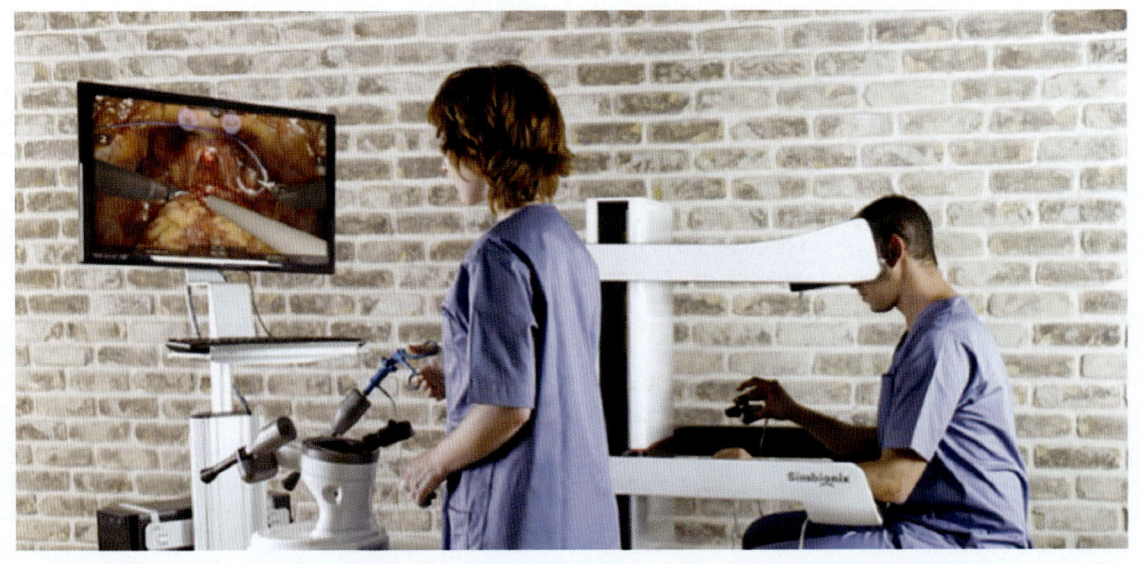

LAP Mentor Express

RobotiX Mentor

FIGURE 4-13 • Simbionix RobotiX Mentor team trainer. (Reproduced with permission from Surgical Science, Göteborg Sweden.)

psychological pressure is something that the future surgeons will have to face once they move to the OR, and it is not present when performing the same tasks in a robotic simulator environment.

Furthermore, this model allows trainees to practice more realistically the robotic port setting and docking, which can play an important role in preventing the possible need to convert to the open approach if, for instance, the robotic surgeon encounters internal (between the robotic instruments inside the surgical cavity being operated on) or external (between the robotic arms reaching to the trocars) collisions. Even the direction of trocars placement, through the abdominal or thoracic wall, is important in preventing excessive torquing on the joints of the robotic arms and, most importantly, on the skin and muscle layers of a patient. The latter technical pitfall can significantly increase the peri- and postoperative pain experienced by the patient over the robotic trocar sites and/or increase the risk of wound complications (such as hematoma or skin damage or incisional hernias). Current VR simulators lack these attributes.

The porcine model is among the most frequently used in robotic surgery training.

Nevertheless, live animals are quite expensive, and their treatment and handling mandate compliance with stringent regulatory requirements, as well as on-site availability of proper facilities and trained veterinarian staff. Therefore, only a small number of academic institutions can or are willing to offer this kind of training model. An interesting development, which can partly offer a solution to the resources limitation problems encountered with animal facilities, is the "hybridization" of animal parts with mechanical supporting systems: KindHearth™ has realistic CAD model of body and organs which are made utilizing silicone and urethane casting. Additionally, this product is designed to be modular, with multiple possible surgeries set-ups, and it is able to hold porcine tissue recreating some of the features of the traditional animal models. KindHearth™ can be standardized and it may be more easily available even in centers without an animal facility already in place.

In recent years, the growing pressure from animal rights advocates has persuaded many medical schools to abandon animal models and shift towards other solutions (see previous and next sections).

Cadaver Model

In the future, cadavers will probably completely replace live animals for the purpose of robotic training. This model demonstrates unparalleled anatomical realism, as they overcome the artificial tissue handling and imprecise anatomy of current robotic simulators and animal models.

Furthermore, the lack of blood flow to the organs traditionally associated with the cadaver is not anymore an insuperable hurdle, because strategies for integrating perfusion to mimic blood flow are being developed. Perfusion techniques restoring blood flow and pressure in the fresh human cadaveric model are available and applicable to procedure-based specialties. In these techniques, the cannulation of the femoral vessels and the infusion of a technique-specific perfusate by a vortex centrifugal pump and pulmonary ventilation are successfully established, resulting in a mean arterial pressure of 80 mm Hg and venous pressure of 15 mm Hg (**Figures 4-14 A–C**).

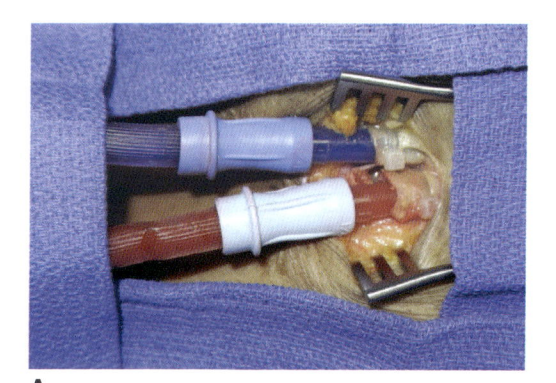

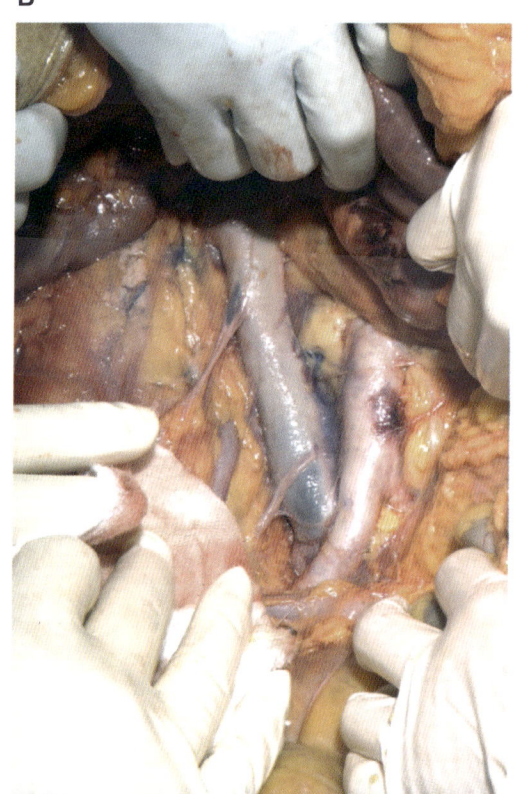

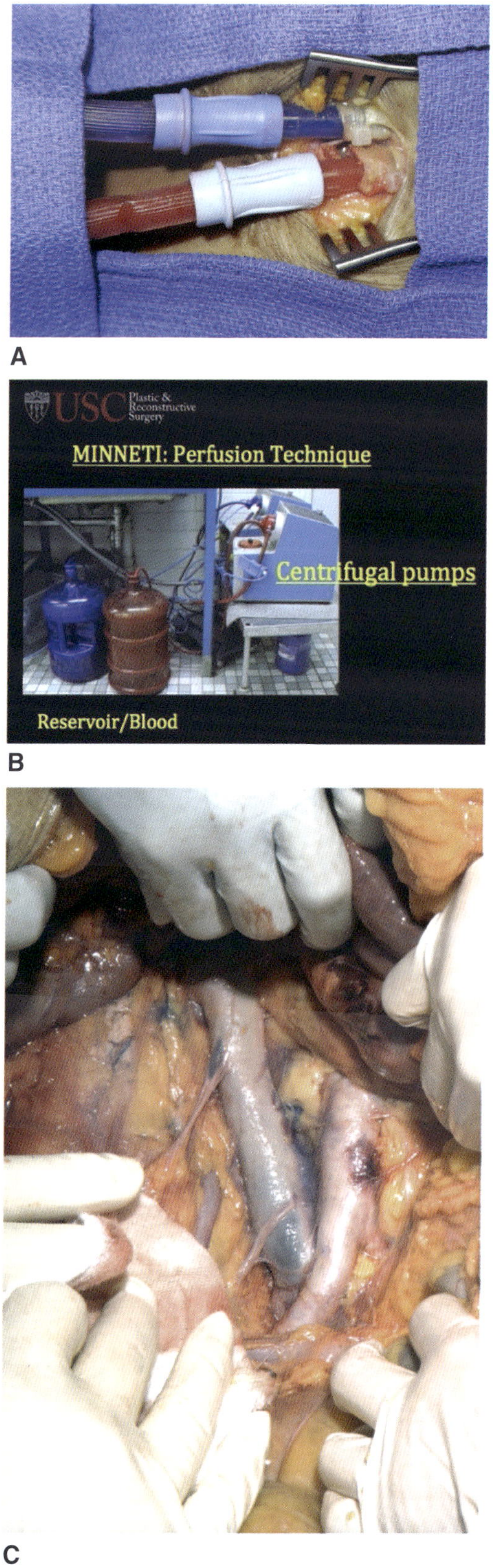

FIGURE 4-14 • **A.** Cannulation of the femoral artery/vein. **B.** Arterial and venous circuits connecting the arterial and venous femoral cannulas with the centrifugal pumps. **C.** Pressurized abdominal aorta and inferior vena cava. (Reproduced with permission from Carey JN, Minneti M, Leland HA, et al. Perfused fresh cadavers: method for application to surgical simulation. *Am J Surg.* 2015;210(1):179-187.)

A significant improvement of trainee confidence with the adoption of these perfused models has been reported.

Based on these technical advancements and a relatively easy sourcing of cadavers from body donation programs (that are being established by the medical school of major academic institutions across the globe), it is possible that the perfused fresh cadaver will soon become the gold standard of robotic simulation in the *wet lab* setting.

> **EDITORIAL COMMENT**
>
> The perfused fresh cadaver model has advantages but also some limitations. The most important drawbacks are the cost, and the fact that fresh cadavers are not always easily available everywhere, and the model has to be prepared on site, and it requires considerable resources.

CURRICULA

Currently, a comprehensive, multilevel, standardized, and proficiency-based curriculum spanning through the VR simulator, the robotic dry, the wet lab, and the OR is still to be established. However, multiple, isolated, and often limited efforts have been successfully implemented by individual training programs, national consensus networks, or robotic system companies.

Part of the reason is the lack of compulsory and detailed guidelines by the surgical governing bodies about if and when to start robotic surgery training during the residency. However, some preliminary reports suggest that early robotic training is well perceived and received by the newer generations of surgical residents as early as in their first or second year of residency.

So far, the FRS curriculum (introduced in the inanimate training models section) has represented the widest reaching and most validated effort, although it does lack any data about predictive validity because the performance of the participants in the OR was not assessed during its validation trial. Furthermore, some other important components of the robotic training need to still be addressed, such as bedside assisting, team training, or specialty-specific or procedural training.

In general, the FRS and the other curricula that have been proposed so far share all or some of the following components: (1) cognitive (didactics), (2) psychomotor (skills at the console), and (3) intraoperative (using a wide array of simulation modalities such as VR, dry, and wet laboratory).

As novel robotic systems enter the market, the development of standardized and validated curricula will be increasingly important. It has been suggested that robotic surgery curricula will have to be held to the same levels of regulations, and international standards, adopted for the training model of airline pilots to attain a global standardization of training, accreditation, and certification. In fact, the 2 fields share many similarities: technical and procedural instructions, as well as a multistep and gradual approach to training and nontechnical training focused on crisis management, decision making, leadership, and communication.

Some surgical societies such the Clinical Robotic Surgery Association (CRSA) and the Society of American Gastrointestinal and Endoscopic Surgeons (SAGES) are actively and currently engaging targeted efforts for developing a unified approach, and standards, for basic robotic training.

THE ROLE OF ARTIFICIAL INTELLIGENCE

Information about the role of artificial intelligence (AI), in its main surgical applications, can be found in Chapter 1, What Robotic Surgery Is, and Chapter 6, Implemented Imaging and Artificial Intelligence. This section is specifically focused on the use of AI in robotic training. In this field, AI is still in its infancy. Thus, much of the contents presented in this chapter will have to rely on expert knowledge to predict the further development and future role of AI in robotic training.

The review of surgical performance by peers and/or experts is time- and resource-consuming because the individuals involved with the assessment will have to be physically present and observe the trainee in real time, or will have to assess trainees' performance retrospectively by reviewing video-recordings (*crowdsourcing*). Additionally, inconsistencies related to inter-rater reliability, or agreement among the individuals performing the assessment, are inevitable due to the variability among human raters.

Machine learning algorithms (MLAs) are being developed to process large volumes of automated performance metrics (APMs) captured directly from the robotic console. For instance, a trained MLA developed at University of Southern California has already successfully predicted clinical outcomes of robot-assisted radical prostatectomy by using APMs only.

The collaboration between computer scientists and surgical educators has been so far the main limiting factor for a speedier implementation of this technology in the robotic field. Prior isolated efforts, executed by engineers, lacked clinical relevance and applicability. On the other side, surgical educators usually lack the required computer science background to implement efforts of this kind that will translate in an educational/training benefit, or a clinical application.

Assuming a strengthening of this collaboration, and a parallel/sustained growth of robotic surgery and machine learning models, it is reasonable to believe that within the next 10 years, the level of training and/or the robotic surgery expertise of a specific individual will be routinely and accurately measured through the acquisition of processed automated data by an *intelligent* machine learning model.

> **EDITORIAL COMMENT**
>
> AI software (SuPR, *Intuitive*™) is able to review segments of the procedure. Such a technology may impact the assessment of surgical performance quality. As a consequence, by the institutional review process, it may be decided, for example, that a surgeon may need more training in specific areas/skills (e.g., suturing).

Credentialing–Privileging

As discussed in the prior section of this chapter, over the last 10 years, there has been a surge of initiatives at a local or regional level, as academic and nonacademic institutions are trying to establish their own curricula.

In most cases, these efforts have not been backed up by solid data validation and lacked centralization and coordination, because the governing bodies of the respective surgical disciplines have provided, at the best, only general guidance.

The gap left behind by the academia has been partially filled in by the robotic surgery industry that started offering training courses at their own facilities and within their premises. Healthcare institutions would then grant the surgical practitioner robotic surgery privileges based on the acquisition of this certificate released by the industry and under the condition that an initial (and usually small) number of cases would be performed under the guidance of a proctor identified by the same establishment.

This trend created a peculiar anomaly as many practicing robotic surgeons started their practice without any formal training during their residencies and fellowships. Then board certification and sufficient experience measured by surgeons' volume would justify procedural privileges.

A nonnegligible number of adverse events reported to the publicly available MAUDE database (maintained by the US Food and Drug Administration), and various legal rulings of lawsuit against the robotic surgery industry and/or the hospitals who adopted and oversighted this novel technology, raised serious concerns about the adequacy of robotic credentialing policies in ensuring patients' safety.

Ever since, many hospitals have appointed dedicated robotic surgery committees to oversee and assist with the institution's robotic credentialing/privileging process and policies.

More recently, an expert consensus panel was gathered, and a detailed set of criteria for robotic credentialing was released. Among the 76 items that achieved consensus, experts agreed that "privileges should be granted based on video review of surgical performance and attainment of clearly defined objective proficiency benchmarks." One hundred percent consensus was achieved on 4 specific criteria for initial credentialing: (1) basic cognitive training in robotic surgery, (2) basic robotic technical skills training, (3) robotic device–specific technical training, and (4) objective procedure-specific performance benchmarks met the proficiency demonstrated outside the OR.

However, the recommendations of the expert panels, and of the surgical governing bodies, are not mandatory or legally binding (unlike airline pilots who are subject to continuous learning with recertification through benchmarked high-stake tests). Likewise, the whole aviation training model, including its curricula, simulation devices, and even training centers and instructors, is held to high, internationally recognized, and legally binding standards.

If the robotic surgery community and the healthcare system will adopt the aviation training methods, the challenges that we are currently facing will become an opportunity to make the robotic training more effective, more efficient and likely safer at a global level.

> **EDITORIAL COMMENT**
>
> There are 2 main components of the surgical competence credentialing and privileging:
>
> 1. **Mechanical skills.** Like suturing, mechanical skills can be easily measured by a reviewer and in the future by AI. Also, these skills may be developed/improved by attendance to courses, by getting basic certificates (like the manufacturing companies already do), or reviewing the VR models and scores. This aspect is similar to what it is currently done in the aviation field.
> 2. **Procedure-specific competence (i.e., the ability to perform a surgical procedure).** The evaluation of these surgical knowledge components is more sophisticated and it is difficult to assess. This entails the knowledge of the surgical anatomy and the physiology, the correct understanding of the surgical planes, and of the correct tools. This is a very sophisticated process. At the moment, there is no effective simulation, or tool, to replace the human assessment by the proctors, by the supervisors and by the surgical department head. The lack of surgical knowledge is a source of potential problems and iatrogenic complications. It is not advisable to give privileges just by reviewing surgical videos: from a mere video analysis, for example, it is difficult to assess how a specific surgical complication is managed. These decisions entail ethical and legal responsibilities. The "mechanical" proficiency at the console does not necessarily equate to clinical performance.

Suggested Readings

1. Huffman EM, Rosen SA, Levy JS, Martino MA, Stefanidis D. Are current credentialing requirements for robotic surgery adequate to ensure surgeon proficiency? *Surg Endosc.* 2021;35(5):2104-2109. doi: 10.1007/s00464-020-07608-2
2. Stefanidis D, Huffman EM, Collins JW, Martino MA, Satava RM, Levy JS. Expert consensus recommendations for robotic surgery credentialing. *Ann Surg.* 2020, Nov 17. doi: 10.1097/SLA.0000000000004531
3. Satava RM, Stefanidis D, Levy JS, et al. Proving the effectiveness of the Fundamentals of Robotic Surgery (FRS) skills curriculum: a single-blinded, multispecialty, multi-institutional randomized control trial. *Ann Surg.* 2020;272(2):384-392. doi: 10.1097/SLA.0000000000003220
4. Martin JR, Stefanidis D, Dorin RP, Goh AC, Satava RM, Levy JS. Demonstrating the effectiveness of the Fundamentals of Robotic Surgery (FRS) curriculum on the RobotiX Mentor Virtual Reality Simulation Platform. *J Robot Surg.* 2021;15(2):187-193. doi: 10.1007/s11701-020-01085-4
5. Goh AC, Aghazadeh MA, Mercado MA, et al. Multi-institutional validation of fundamental inanimate robotic skills tasks. *J Urol.* 2015;194(6):1751-1756. doi: 10.1016/j.juro.2015.04.125
6. Alshuaibi M, Perrenot C, Hubert J, Perez M. Concurrent, face, content, and construct validity of the RobotiX Mentor simulator for robotic basic skills. *Int J Med Robotics Comput Assist Surg.* 2020;16:e2100.
7. Abboudi H, Khan MS, Aboumarzouk O, et al. Current status of validation for robotic surgery simulators: a systematic review. *BJU Int.* 2013;111(2):194-205.
8. Perrenot C, Perez M, Tran N, et al. The virtual reality simulator dV-Trainer® is a valid assessment tool for robotic surgical skills. *Surg Endosc.* 2012;26:2587-2593.
9. Seixas-Mikelus SA, Stegemann AP, Kesavadas T, et al. Content validation of a novel robotic surgical simulator. *BJU Int.* 2010;107:1130-1135.
10. Almarzouq A, Hu J, Noureldin YA, et al. Are basic robotic surgical skills transferable from the simulator to the operating room? A randomized, prospective, educational study. *Can Urol Assoc J* 2020;14(12):416-422. doi: 10.5489/cuaj.6460
11. Raison N, Harrison P, Abe T, Aydin A, Ahmed K, Dasgupta P. Procedural virtual reality simulation training for robotic surgery: a randomised controlled trial. *Surg Endosc.* 2020. doi: 10.1007/s00464-020-08197-w.
12. Dubin AK, Smith R, Julian D et al. A comparison of robotic simulation performance on basic virtual reality skills: simulator subjective versus objective assessment tools. *J Minimally Invasive Gynecol.* 2017;24(7):1184-1189.
13. Newcomb LK, Bradleyn MS, Truong T, et al. Correlation of virtual reality simulation and dry lab robotic technical skills. *J Minimally Invasive Gynecol.* 2018;25(4):689-696.
14. Carey JN, Minneti M, Leland HA, et al. Perfused fresh cadavers: method for application to surgical simulation. *Am J Surg.* 2015;210(1):179-187.
15. Vetter MH, Green I, Martino M, Fowler J, Salani R. Incorporating resident/fellow training into a robotic surgery program. *J Surg Oncol.* 2015;112(7):684-689. doi: 10.1002/jso.24006
16. Breslera L, Perez M, Hubert J, Henryd JP, Perrenot C. Residency training in robotic surgery: the role of simulation. *J Visceral Surg.* 2020;157(3):S123-S129.
17. Intuitive Surgical, Inc DaVinci Surgery Community. Accessed June 5, 2021. https://www.davincisurgerycommunity.com
18. Alzahrani T, Haddad R, Alkhayal A, et al. Validation of the da Vinci Surgical Skill Simulator across three surgical disciplines: a pilot study. *Can Urol Assoc J.* 2013;7(7–8):e520-e529.
19. Gangemi A, Dunham T, Gheza F et al. Robotic training in general surgery residency: how early can we begin? *J Surg Surgical Res.* 2016;2(1):021-024. doi: 10.17352/2455-2968.000025
20. Collins JW, Wisz P. Training in robotic surgery, replicating the airline industry. How far have we come? *World J Urol.* 2020;38(7):1645-1651. doi: 10.1007/s00345-019-02976-4
21. Hung AJ, Chen J, Gill IS. Automated performance metrics and machine learning algorithms to measure surgeon performance and anticipate clinical outcomes in robotic surgery. *Review JAMA Surg.* 2018;153(8):770-771. doi: 10.1001/jamasurg.2018.1512
22. Alemzadeh H, Raman J, Leveson N, Kalbarczyk Z, Iyer RK. Adverse events in robotic surgery: A retrospective study of 14 years of FDA data. *PLoS ONE.* 2016;11(4):e0151470.
23. Pradarelli JC, Campbell DA, Dimick JB. Hospital credentialing and privileging of surgeons. A potential safety blind spot. *JAMA.* 2015;313(13):1313-1314. doi: 10.1001/jama.2015.1943
24. Mangano A, Gheza F, Giulianotti PC. Virtual reality simulator systems in robotic surgical training. *Surg Technol Int.* 2018;32:19-23.
25. Giulianotti PC, Coratti A, Angelini M, et al. Robotics in general surgery: personal experience in a large community hospital. *Arch Surg.* 2003;138(7):777-784. doi: 10.1001/archsurg.138.7.777

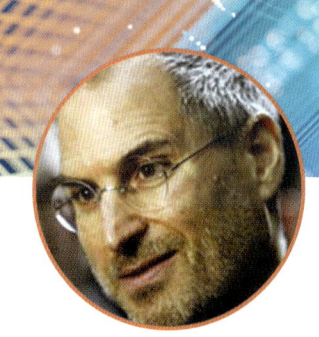

"The only way to do great work is to love what you do."
—Steve Jobs (1955–2011)

Keys for Success of a Robotic Program

Yuman Fong

INTRODUCTION

Robotic surgery has come a long way since the launch of the Zeus® robotic system (Computer Motion, Inc., Santa Barbara, CA) and the Intuitive Surgical Robot (Intuitive Surgical, Inc., Sunnyvale, CA) in the early 2000s. Millions of operations have been performed using the various generations of robots from Intuitive Surgical, Inc. Many other surgical robots have entered the field including orthopedic joint replacement robots (MAKO SmartRobotics™, Stryker Corp), endoluminal robots (Ion™, Intuitive surgical Inc.; Monarch™, Auris Health Inc.), natural orifice robots (Hominis®, Memic Innovative Surgery Ltd.), and soft tissue robots (Hugo™, Medtronic Inc.; Versius®, CMR Surgical Ltd.; Senhance®, Asensus Surgical Inc.; Enos™ single access surgery system, Titan Medical Inc.; Vicarious Surgical System™, Vicarious Surgical Inc.; Flex® Robotic System, Medrobotics Corp.) (**Figures 5-1** to **5-3**).

In the thorax and abdomen, the procedures that are influenced by robotics include not only simple single-field operations such as prostatectomies, but also multifield operations, complex multiorgan resections, and reoperative surgical procedures. No longer is robotic surgery perceived as experimental, but it is now considered at the forefront of minimally invasive surgery in most specialties. The robot is no longer just the instrument of pioneers but is now an instrument for day-to-day surgical care. The goal of this chapter is to present some principles underlying success of any clinical program but particularly tailored for robotic programs (**Table 5-1**).

Financials

With most hospitals in the United States running at fairly thin financial margins, making sure that the robotics program is a revenue-generating program is extraordinarily important. No ongoing money-losing program can be tolerated. Losses may be accepted during the ramp-up phase of a program. However, as each program matures, it must produce profits for the institution.

Case Volume

The most important factor in the financials is adequate utilization of the robotic platform. The goal should be to perform at least 40 operations per month per robot. A multimillion-dollar machine that sits idle represents huge losses for an institution. The best way to ensure utilization is to have a group of surgeons committed to robotic surgery from many different disciplines. Coordinating use from surgeons in many fields including urology, gynecology, general surgery, colorectal surgery, thoracic surgery, otolaryngology, pediatrics, endocrine, and transplant surgery ensures high-volume utilization of the robot (**Table 5-2**).

It is best to have robotic surgeons committed to this field who are willing and able to schedule multiple cases on a single day. These surgeons should have an assigned block time, along with dedicated robotic nurses and bedside assistants. These established robotic teams are the keys to full and efficient utilization of an expensive resource. In some countries, like China, the surgical robot is used more than 20 hours in a day in order to maximize the number of cases performed.

A surgeon early in their robotic experience may use the robot only intermittently. Adequate resources should be applied to helping those committed to robotic surgery to ramp up to high-volume robotic utilization. Those who don't increase the number of cases should be encouraged to remain open or laparoscopic surgeons. This would ensure ease of scheduling and a full program.

Photo reproduced with permission from O'Reilly T. Steve Jobs (1955-2011). Nature. 2011;479(7371):42.

Quote reproduced with permission from Marmotti A, Peretti GM, Mangiavini L, et al. Tips and tricks for writing a scientific manuscript. J Biol Regul Homeost Agents. 2020;34(4 Suppl. 3): 441-449.

56 The Foundation and Art of Robotic Surgery

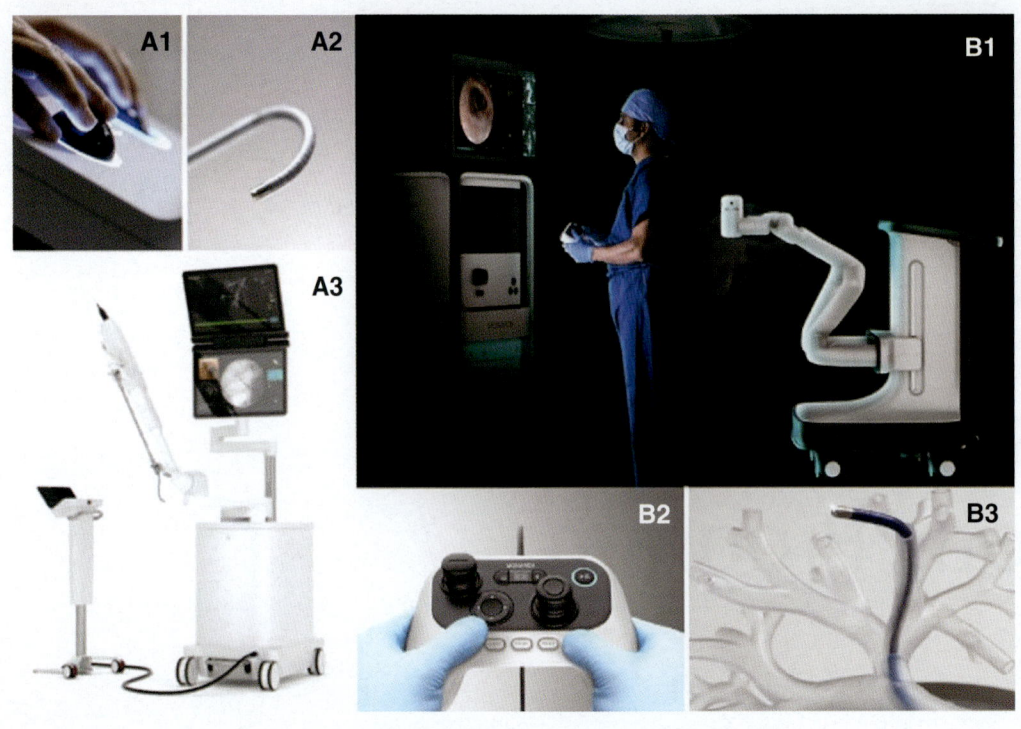

FIGURE 5-1 • Other surgical robots. **A1–3.** Ion platform. (©2022 Intuitive Surgical Operations, Inc.) **B1–3.** Monarch platform. (©Auris Health, Inc. 2022. Reproduced with permission.)

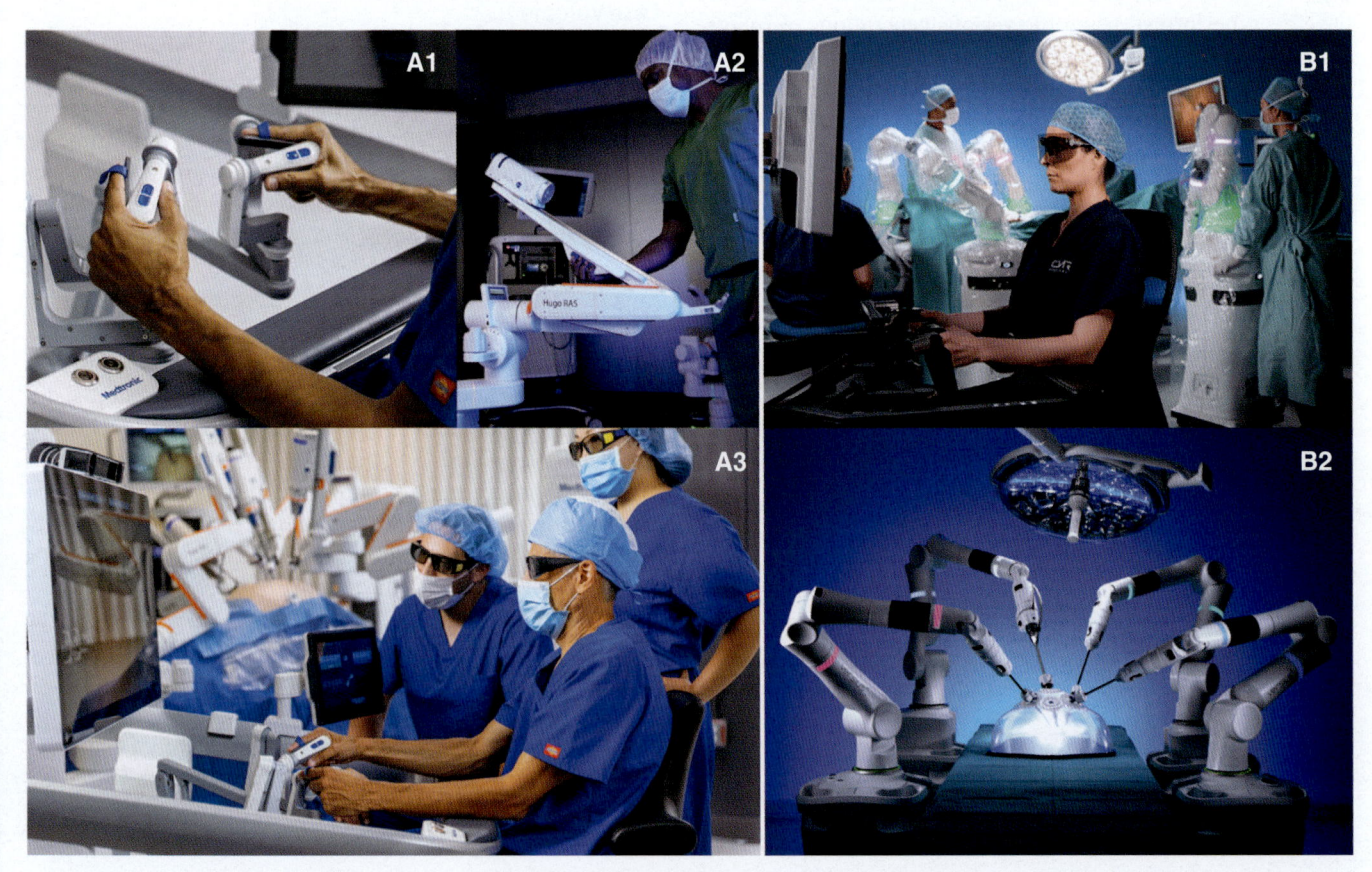

FIGURE 5-2 • Other surgical robots. **A1–3.** Hugo. (©2022 Medtronic. All rights reserved. Used with the permission of Medtronic). **B1–2.** Versius. (Reproduced with permission from CMR Surgical. Cambridge UK.)

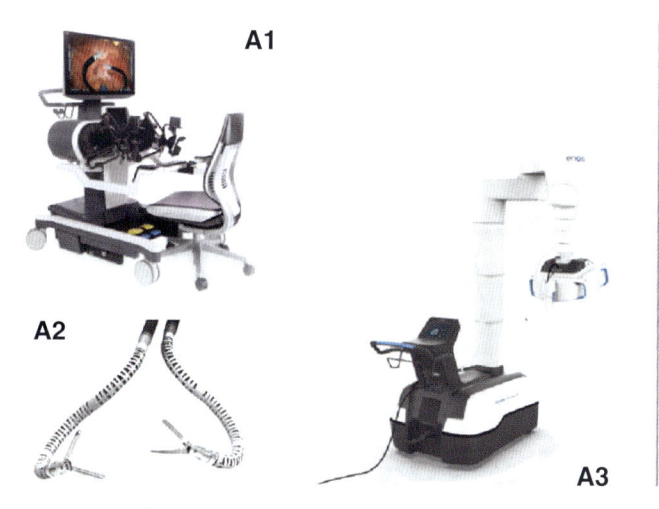

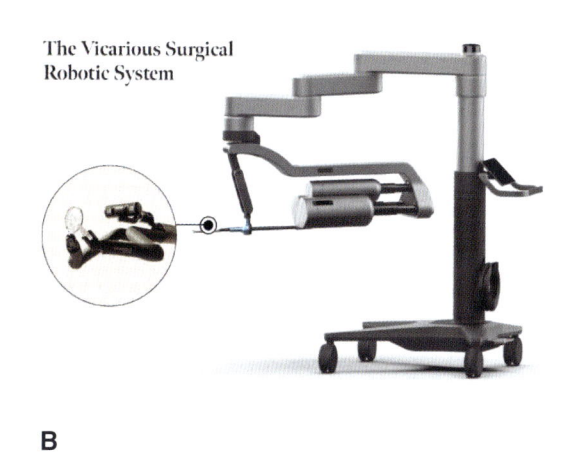

FIGURE 5-3 • Other surgical robots. **A1–3.** Enos single access surgery system. (Reproduced with permission from Titan Medical. Chapel Hill, NC.) **B.** Vicarious Surgical System. (Reproduced with permission from Vicarious Surgical. Waltham, MA.)

Cost Tracking

Tracking utilization of disposables is routine in most institutions for all surgeries. In robotic surgery, such cost accounting is particularly important. Most instruments that are activated by the robot have a limited number of uses (lives). Optimization of instrument use is a combination of minimizing numbers of instruments and eliminating those ones used marginally for a brief period of time. Adopting excessive numbers of instruments is highly inefficient, difficult for the bedside assistant, and expensive. By having the various surgeons in each discipline, optimized instrumentation and standardized use will not only improve supply chain performance but also control cost. Limiting hybrid approaches, laparoscopic, and robotic in the same operation is a way of containing costs and decreasing the numbers of utilized instruments. Clear examples of hybrid operations are the adhesiolysis at the beginning of the procedure or the mobilization of the left colonic flexure in rectal surgery.

Making the surgeons aware of the cost of various robotic instruments is also important. Staple loads, sealers, and suction devices represent particularly high-cost items because they are

TABLE 5-1 • Keys for Success

- **Financials**
  - Volume
  - Cost
  - Revenue
- **Value**
  - Patient
    - Better outcome
    - More patients eligible for MIS treatment
  - Hospital
    - Revenue generating (profit)
    - Increased number of patients
    - Better payor contracting
  - Surgeon
    - Less work-related musculoskeletal disorders
    - Less stress
    - Longer professional life span
  - Payors
    - Shorter hospital stays
    - Less cost
- **Safety**
  - Less complications
  - Less readmissions
- **Robotic team**
  - Increased efficiency
- **Academics**

TABLE 5-2 • Financials of Robotic Surgery

- **Volume**
  - Number of cases per month: goal >40 procedures/robot/month
  - Need surgeons committed to robotic surgery
  - Need many disciplines sharing robots
    - Urology, gynecology, general surgery, colorectal, thoracic, ENT, transplant, pediatrics, endocrine
- **Cost tracking**
  - Robotic instruments
  - Disposables
  - OR time
  - Ancillary (smoke evacuation, retrieval bags, etc.)
- **Value proposition for robotic surgery**
  - Cases that can easily be done laparoscopically
    - Value in teaching
    - Resident and fellow console time
    - Graduated responsibility
      - Gallbladder, ovary, uterus, intestine, lung, pancreas, liver
  - Cases that are more comfortable robotically
    - Value is for surgeon
  - Cases that transform surgery if done robotically
    - Adoption, feasibility
- **Patient outcome: Safety, cases that need a lot of sewing**

single-use disposable instruments. There are also other disposables that are not attached to the robot that should be considered. Smoke evacuators, specimen retrieval bags, and suction irrigation devices must all be accounted for. The total cost of each operation should be tracked including robotic instruments, disposable instruments, personal costs, and OR costs. These should be balanced against the reimbursement for each procedure.

Reimbursement should be examined, including professional and facilities fees. A savvy organization would also figure out by payer which disposable instruments may be reimbursable. Rules for reimbursement for disposables also differ depending on whether the procedure is an inpatient operation, extended-stay procedure, or an outpatient one. Procedures that can be delivered in either the inpatient or outpatient setting should be assessed as to financial reimbursement for each. While patient outcomes should always be the most important determinant of delivery of care, if outpatient or inpatient workflow results in the same patient outcome, financials may drive which is operationalized at an institution.

For most hospitals, the hourly cost of an OR is the most expensive commodity in these calculations. There must be auditing of operative times for various practitioners for specific operations. If multiple surgeons do the same type of operations, comparing their OR times allows identification of inefficiencies. Sometimes, it is a matter of just adding a better bedside assistant or making sure that the right instrumentation arrives in the OR for that operation that will decrease OR times. In other instances, a surgeon may need mentoring or assistance to optimize their workflow.

Slow speed of a surgeon during the ramp-up period is expected and should be tolerated. However, the occasional robotic surgeon who takes a very long time is a huge financial drain and subjects their patients to excessive anesthesia and likely poor outcome. Ultimately, the robot should be for patient benefit and not for surgeon benefit. A rule of thumb is that a surgeon should be reimbursed approximately 10 relative value units (RVUs) per OR hour. If the RVUs resulting from the sum of the codes of the performed procedure divided by number of hours spent do not approximate 10, then analysis should be performed to try to help increase efficiency of the particular surgeon.

Ideally, all procedures performed robotically should be profitable or cost neutral. No program can tolerate too many money-losing procedures. Decreasing operative time and lowering cost of all procedures, as experience increases, are important. Lowering cost to make the procedure increasingly profitable is essential for long-term sustainability of a program.

Value

Every successful program should assess for value and be able to articulate the value proposition of robotics to patients, colleagues, payers, and administrators.

Value for Patients

Robotic programs must provide value for patients. The most important benefit of any minimally invasive surgery is to spare the patient a large incision. In most open laparotomy incisions, the disability that is associated with the incisions results in necessary hospitalization for days and necessary recovery for weeks. Laparoscopic and thoracoscopic procedures offer the possibility of decreasing this disability. Operations that could be easily performed by straight instruments such as cholecystectomy and gynecologic procedures for benign disease converted open operations with extended stay into outpatient procedures with quick recovery. While more intricate laparoscopic and thoracoscopic procedures including liver resections, esophageal resections, and rectal surgeries are now routinely performed by expert surgeons, the majority of these operations nationwide are still being performed as open surgeries. Robotic surgery offers easier adoption for a minimally invasive surgical approach for intricate procedures. Thus, it offers a potential for a much larger subset of patients to benefit from minimally invasive surgery (**Figure 5-4**).

Many procedures that were only attainable by highly talented laparoscopic masters can now be performed by many surgeons.

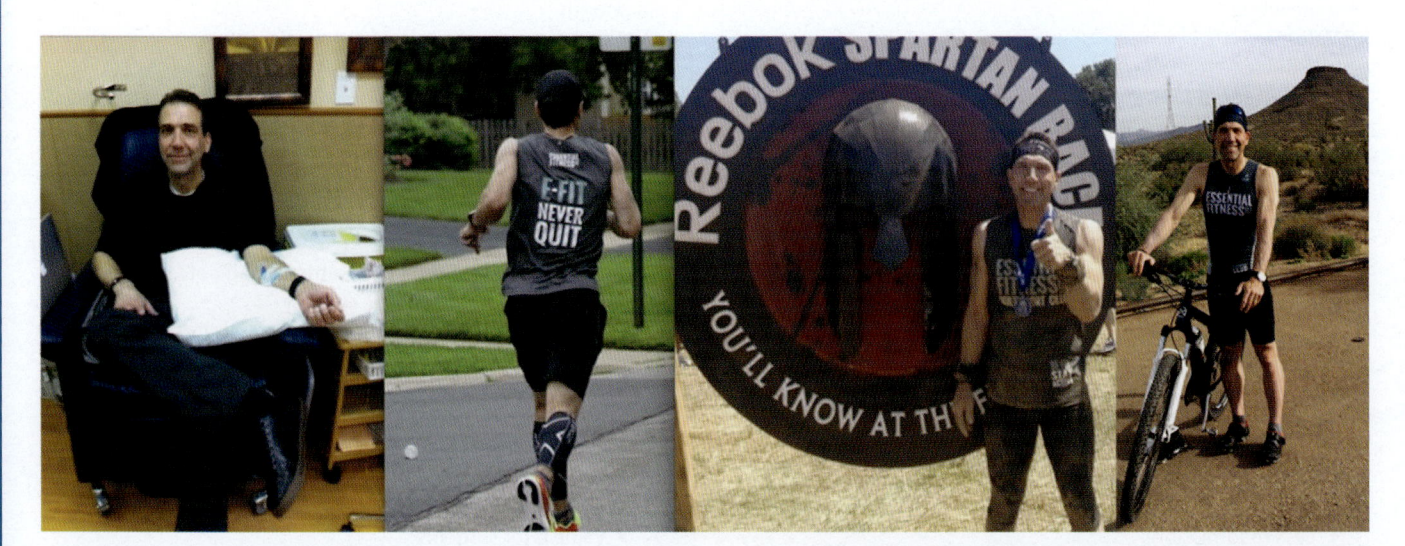

FIGURE 5-4 • Value for patients: Patient that underwent robotic pancreaticoduodenectomy at the University of Illinois at Chicago (UIC) for malignancy who later participated in a spartan race.

Sewing in laparoscopy is an expert skill, while sewing in robotics is a competency. Thus, injury to a major vascular structure in laparoscopy likely means conversion while the same injury encountered robotically usually is repaired robotically.

Ultimately, the best procedures performed robotically are those that have their outcome in the open surgery determined mainly by the large incision but are hard to reach by straight laparoscopy instruments. Resections of superior and posterior sections of the liver fall into this category. This is why there are a number of papers documenting clinical benefit in patient outcome for such resections. In one of these series, use of robotics has converted resections of posterior hepatic tumors with extended stay into outpatient surgery. These procedures are often reimbursed in a bundle payment for 4–5 days of hospital stay. This shift in patient outcome and in length of hospital stay to a median of 1–2 days would benefit both patients and hospitals.

Usually, if a medical procedure, drug, or device can be proven to benefit patients, the financials will follow. There are now ample data that minimally invasive colorectal, gastric, liver, biliary, lung, and esophageal surgery is beneficial for patients. What has been harder to get are data from randomized trials proving that robotics is superior to laparoscopy. This is not surprising since robotic surgery is just computer-aided laparoscopic surgery. The decrease in morbidity and in recovery should be the same. Advocates of laparoscopy point out that laparoscopic surgery when completed laparoscopically is not inferior to robotics and is less expensive. There are growing data showing an increased adoption of robotic surgery compared to laparoscopy for open surgeons. Since most major gastrointestinal surgery is currently performed by open techniques, robotics will clearly contribute to patient benefit by encouraging a greater adoption of a minimally invasive surgical approach. In addition, there are data that conversion to open surgery is less likely with robotic surgery. Conversion negates many of the benefits of a minimally invasive surgical approach. There will also be fewer converted cases even in the early experience of a young surgeon. Thus, if a robotic procedure is profitable and it attracts more patients to the hospital, the robotic program will not only be justified but will be robust.

Value for Surgeons

There are also ample data that robotic surgery is ergonomically easier for the surgeon than laparoscopy. A large amount of data has emerged documenting ergonomic advantages of robotic surgery compared to laparoscopy. Arthritic hand injuries are common when performing laparoscopy. There are more musculoskeletal injuries in laparoscopy and open surgery. An injured surgeon is unlikely to be able to perform surgery optimally and may not be able to perform surgery at all. Thus, the beneficial effects of robotic surgery in alleviating work-related injuries must be accepted as an important value for robotic surgery. It is easy to imagine that professional life can be prolonged, and this aspect in an era anticipating a shortage of surgeons has an important financial and social value (**Figures 5-5 A, B**).

Value for Trainees

Even for cases that could be easily performed by straight laparoscopic instruments, robotic surgery has value. These are perfect training cases for residents, fellows, and novice robotic surgeons to gain the skills necessary to perform high-intricacy robotic surgical cases. Trainees performing cholecystectomies, oophorectomies, and hysterectomies gain important technical skills that allowed them to graduate into intestinal, pulmonary, pancreatic, and liver operations. In addition, there are emerging data that robotic cholecystectomy may have a lower conversion rate and a lower length of hospital stay than laparoscopy.

Safety

Safety of all robotic procedures is essential. Robotic surgery is considered minimally invasive surgery. A patient coming for minimally invasive surgery expects good outcome, rapid recovery, and no readmission. Serious major complications or deaths can shut down an entire program or stop referral of patients. Therefore, the reputation of any robotic program is only as good as its weakest surgeon. Rigorous peer review with

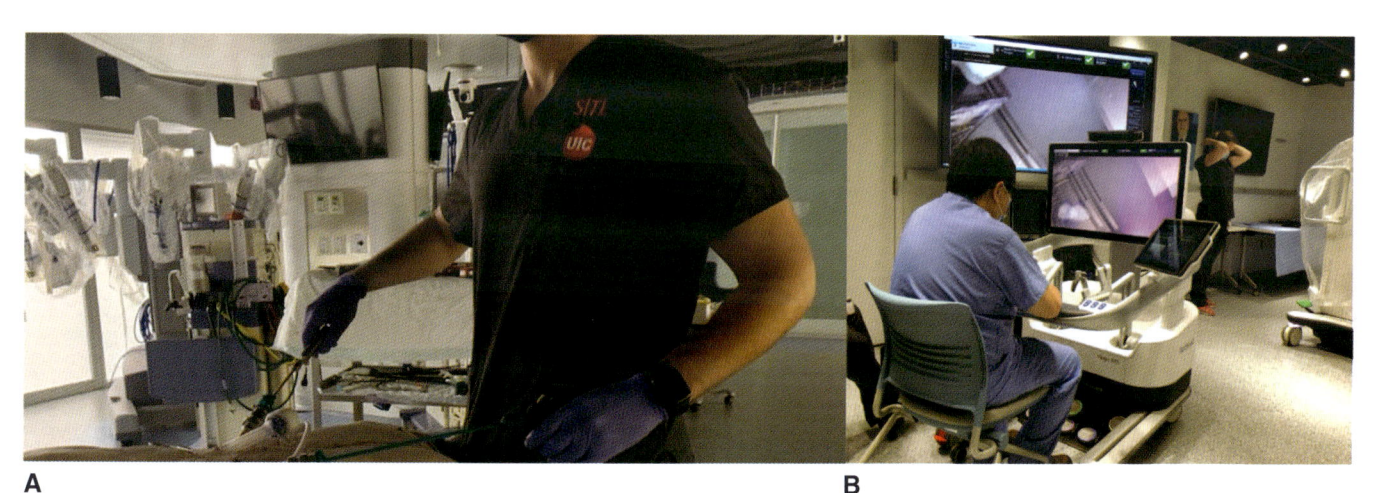

FIGURE 5-5 • Value for surgeons. Surgeon position during: **A.** Laparoscopic and **B.** Robotic procedures.

constructive coaching of poor performers is therefore important for success and reputation of the program.

Education, Credentialing, and Auditing
For each individual surgeon, achieving optimal outcome for robotic surgery requires good patient and case selection, good technical skills, experience, and a good support team to assist the patient in recovery. For each hospital engaged in robotic surgery, achieving good outcome requires hiring and assembling an effective robotic surgical team, sufficiently rigorous credentialing, supervision of young and inexperienced faculty, and regular auditing of results.

Preparing for Emergencies
No major surgical program can be without complications including major complications such as intraoperative hemorrhage. The key is to make sure that there is a system in place for rescue of major intraoperative misadventures. In the OR, it is highly recommended that each robotic team, on each surgical day, engage in a robotic emergency timeout. Contingencies should be made for having blood for transfusion. This timeout should also verify that essential vascular instruments and self-retaining retractors are immediately available, and review responsibilities of each team member in an urgent conversion to open surgery. These steps are essential for rescue in case of a major hemorrhage during robotic surgery (**Figures 5-6 A, B**).

Remote Monitoring for Complications after Discharge
The outcomes of robotic surgery have sufficiently improved such that many patients are discharged from the hospital very shortly after the procedure. For prostatectomies and even for major surgery such as liver resections, it is not uncommon for patients to have these surgeries as outpatients or as extended-stay operations. Recognizing when someone is getting sick at home and instituting rescue for complications are essential for good outcomes. One approach for finding the patients who are getting sick has been to call them at home shortly after their discharge and at other times in the first week after the patient is home. This approach is labor intensive.

A most exciting area of study is the use of telemedicine and novel sensors for tracking patient progress and setbacks at home after discharge. In pilot studies, investigators have used step-trackers and patient-reported symptoms transmitted over a smartphone app to detect early complications and rescue patients before major complications set in. There are now a number of prospective trials of such technology coupled to delivery of minimally invasive and robotic surgery to define the 21st-century workflow for care of the surgical patient (**Figure 5-7**).

Rolling Out New Robotic Systems
The last few years have seen new robotic systems enter the market, including the Senhance® (Asensus Surgical Inc., Durham, NC), Ion™ (Intuitive Surgical Inc., Sunnyvale CA), Monarch™ (Johnson and Johnson Ltd., New Brunswick, NJ), Hominis® (Memic Innovative Surgery Ltd., Ft. Lauderdale, FL), CorPath® GRX (Corindus Vascular Robotics Inc., Waltham, MA), and the Velys™ (DePuy Synthes Inc., Raynham, MA). The near future will also see the Hugo™ (Medtronic Inc., Dublin, Ireland) and the Ottava™ (Johnson & Johnson Ltd.) arriving in the US market. Hospitals and health systems are going to be considering acquisition of new robotic technology. Also facing the leadership of hospitals will be decisions on how to train and credential surgeons for use of new robotic systems.

Leaders in surgery are also gathering to achieve consensus as to training pathways for robotic systems. For general, hepato pancreatobiliary, thoracic, and other robotic procedures, consensus statements and guidelines are being published. For liver and pancreatic surgery, a consensus panel study using a Delphi process recently concluded that the training for new robots should be different for open surgeons with little robotic experience versus the training for robotic surgeons experienced on current systems. Experienced robotic surgeons committed to robotics need much less education to be facile on new systems (**Figure 5-8**). There is no need to teach the science and application of robotic surgery. Training is mainly to understand the new robot's buttons and controls and the

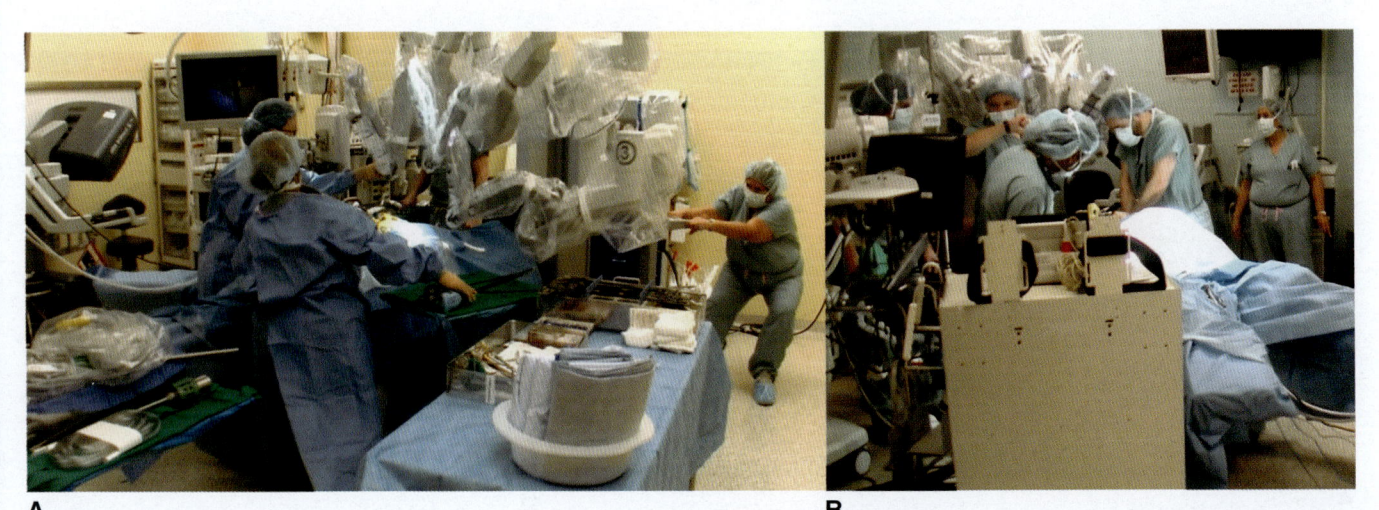

FIGURE 5-6 • Code training in robotic surgery at the University of Illinois at Chicago (UIC). (Reproduced with permission from Dr. Antonio Gangemi.)

POSTOPERATIVE PATIENTS RECOVERING AT HOME

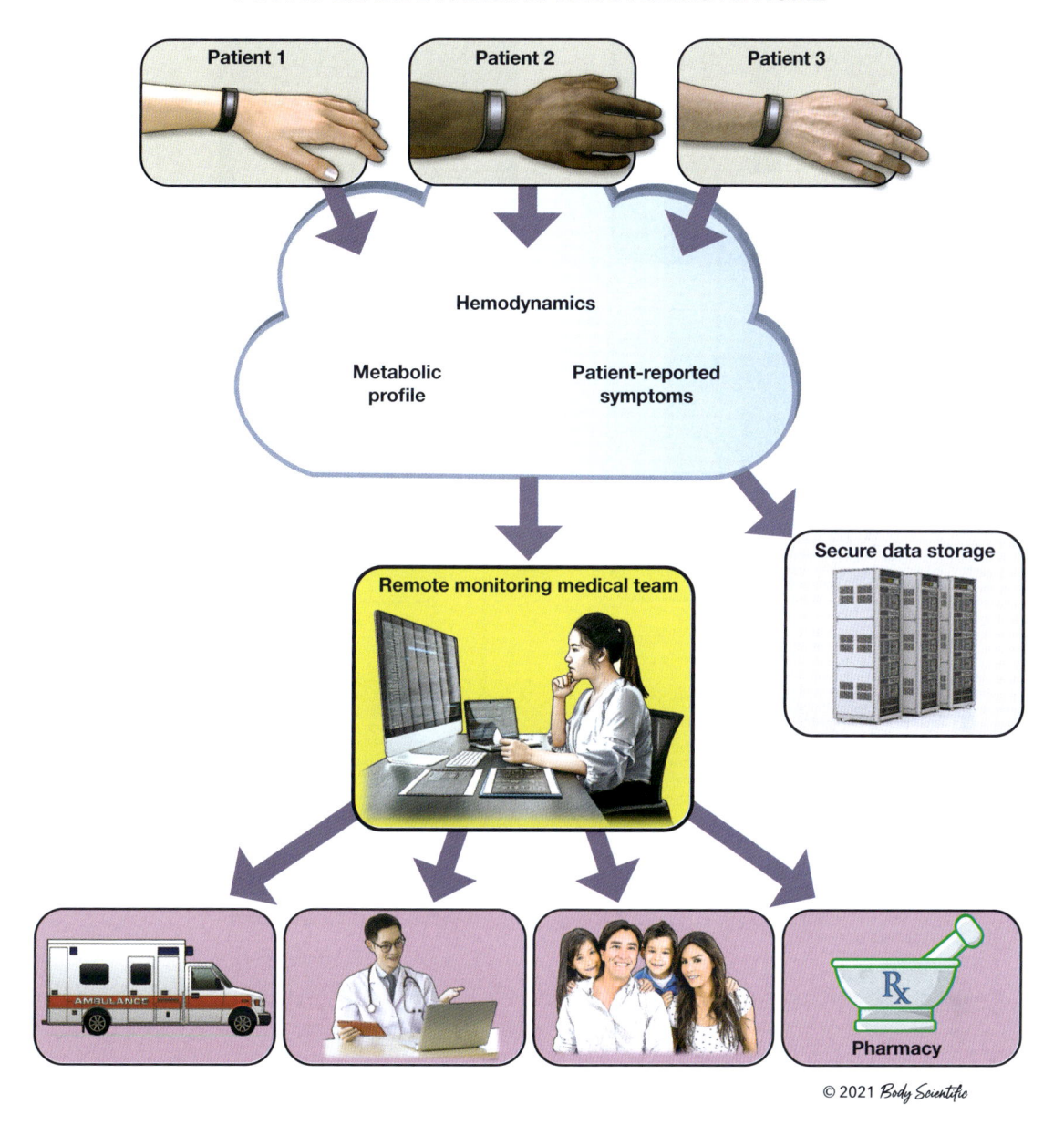

FIGURE 5-7 • Monitored prehabilitation and recovery program. A model of home postoperative monitoring being tested is illustrated. Patients with wearable sensors and using smartphone apps will send intermittent data (symptoms, hemodynamics, and metabolic profile) to a remote monitoring team. The monitoring team assisted by artificial intelligence (AI)-driven algorithms can triage course of action: (1) no action, (2) call family, (3) call primary care team to intervene, and (4) call ambulance.

new robot's capabilities and to develop a new workflow. The need is to teach the new system and not all of robotic surgery. Engaging experienced robotic surgeons is the ideal strategy for rolling out new robotic systems because this group will likely use the new robot and help establish efficient workflow.

Engaging open operative surgeons with little robotic experience in the first wave of early adoption of the newer robots results in higher risk to the patient, to the hospital, and to the robotic platform. The inexperienced surgeon requires teaching of not only the new robot, but also robotic principles in general. They are usually noncommitted and only occasionally perform robotic surgery. Therefore, they are much more likely to interrupt a fluid schedule in robotic ORs than to contribute with many cases, which is essential for success of a new program. They are also the surgeons most likely to be at risk for poor outcomes and to unduly hurt the reputation of the new robotic platform.

Robotic Team

Robotic OR Coordinator

The robotic team is much more than the surgeon and the bedside assistant. It must include an OR coordinator that helps with inventory for instruments and disposables, tracks instrument usage, tracks instrument wastage, verifies credentialing, and helps in scheduling (**Table 5-3**). Such a coordinator is very helpful to enhance efficient sharing of resources among

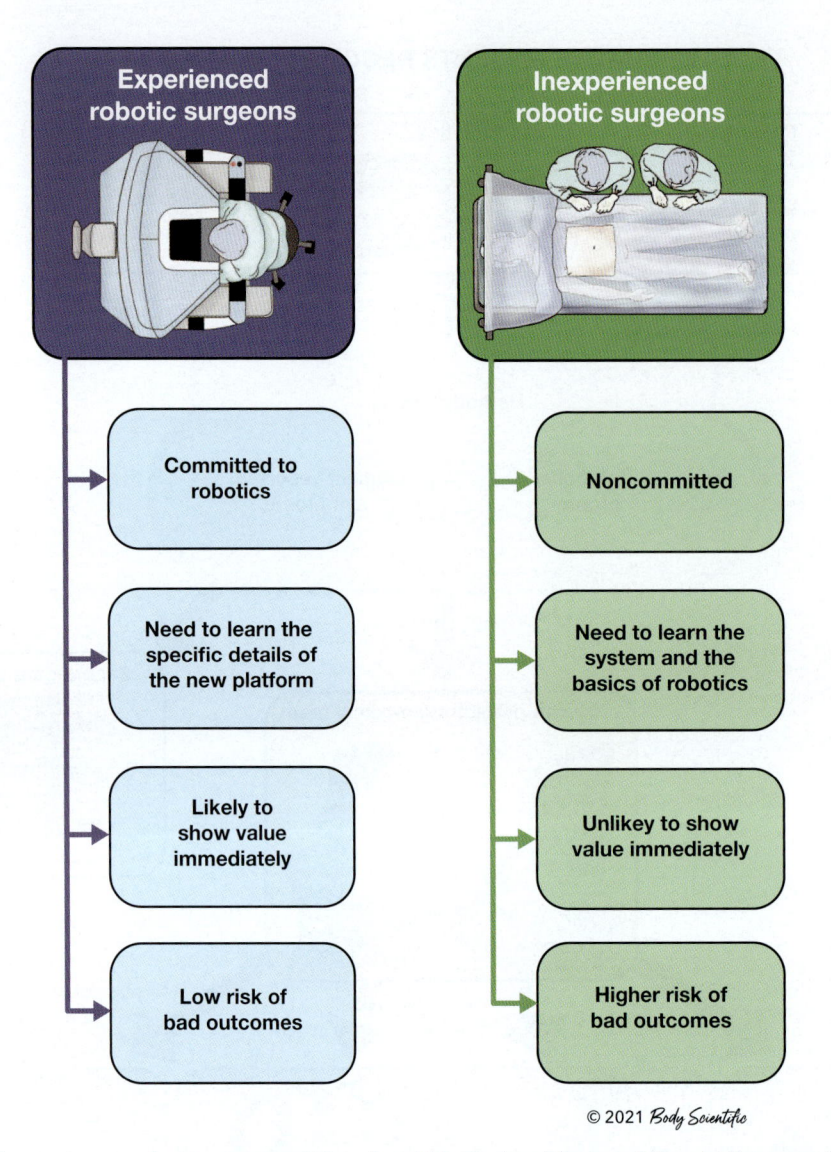

FIGURE 5-8 • Rolling out new robotic systems. Who should be trained first and the challenges of involving immediately traditional open-operative surgeons.

different divisions and departments using the same robot. Such a professional is also important for educating the entire team as to the availability of new instrumentation as well as obsolescence of existing instruments.

Nursing/Technician Team

The team must also include nurses experienced in robotic surgery and robot setup. Organizing for a robotic procedure involves room setup, patient table preparation including pads and harnesses, and arranging the instrument tray. It also involves preparing and testing ancillary instrumentation like ultrasounds, energy, and smoke evacuation equipment. These nurses and technicians should be experienced in preparing sutures for robotic sewing including modification of lengths of sutures for various uses. Slings and sutures for suspension of adjacent organs to facilitate exposure of the surgical field is another setup need for many complex robotic operations.

Bedside Assistant

A well trained bedside assistant can save time by improving exposure through retraction and can keep the surgical field clear using suction. The bedside assistant is essential for insertion and retrieval of needles when sewing is required. Stapling and use of ultrasonic dissectors are also important tasks that could be accomplished by the first assistant to speed up an operation. Finally, a skilled bedside assistant during an urgent conversion for hemorrhage may be lifesaving (see also Chapter 3, The Assistant's Role in Robotic Surgery).

Communication Among Team Members

Good communications among team members can ensure success of the robotic program. Prior to surgery, communication of the desired room setup and instrumentation can save time on the day of surgery. Having the appropriate setup and the correct instruments and supplies shortens an operative time to significantly decrease cost.

TABLE 5-3 • OR Team and Communications

- **Team members**
  - OR coordinator
  - Nurses/technicians
  - Bedside assistant
  - Surgeon/fellows/residents
- **Team communications**
  - Controlling cost by team communications
    - Save OR time
    - Correct OR setup
    - Correct instrumentation and supplies
    - Saves on disposables
    - Saves on blood bank costs
    - Tracking costs
      - Spend
        - Disposables
        - Instruments used
      - Waste
        - Disposables opened and not used
        - Instruments opened and not used
  - Communications essential for safety
    - Preparation for possible hemorrhage
      - Make available
        - Vascular access
        - Instruments including vascular
        - Retractors including self-retaining
        - Sutures and staplers
    - Rehearsal
    - Emergency time out to define roles and check availability of above

Having a strong, cohesive team is particularly important during times of crisis in the OR. In times of urgent conversions, knowing that you can rely on having equipment already nearby for operative salvage of hemorrhage or other emergencies, and knowing that there is a team member responsible for blood availability in the OR are essential.

In order to hire and retain a good robotic surgical team, the robotic OR must be a good workplace. Everything to optimize work conditions should be done, including predictable and reasonable work hours, atmosphere of mutual respect, and an atmosphere of teamwork and trust.

Academics

A successful program should have a good national and international reputation. Contributing academically to the field is one way to increase the prominence of a robotic program. Publications on favorable patient outcomes, favorable financial outcomes, or innovations in technology can be leveraged for publicity and enhance program reputation (**Figure 5-9**). Scientific studies on devices, workflows, and perioperative care can set new standards for the field. Leading such trials or participating in such national/international studies could also greatly enhance the reputation of the program and its surgeons.

Training, proctoring, and credentialing new robotic surgeons is essential for the growth of the field. Surgeons that participate in these processes not only improve the reputation of their program, but also develop a link to the next generation of robotic surgeons. Thus, running training courses or participating in national/international societal training courses, while not an obligation, should be a desire for any leader in robotic surgery.

In summary, the field of robotic surgery is now a highly successful academic and clinical field. For ongoing growth and improvement, there must be a commitment by the hospitals and the robotic team for quality, safety, sound finances, and education. Success should be defined by proven patient benefits, sound fiscal outcome, academic excellence of the program, and morale of the surgical team.

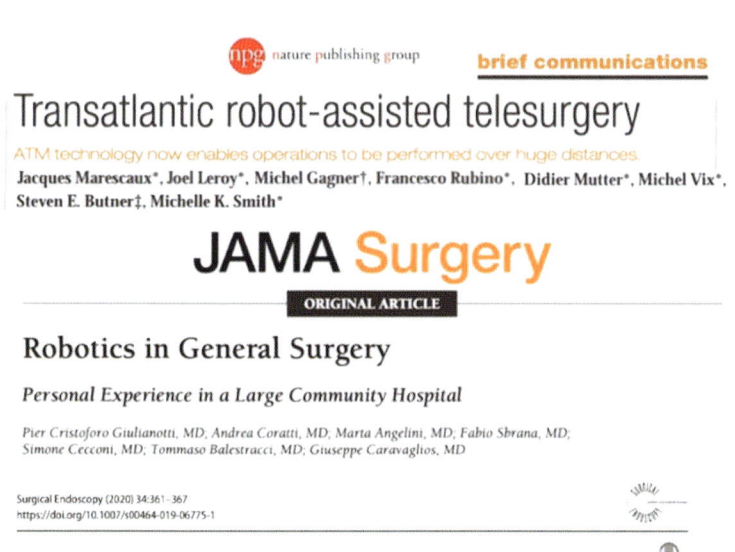

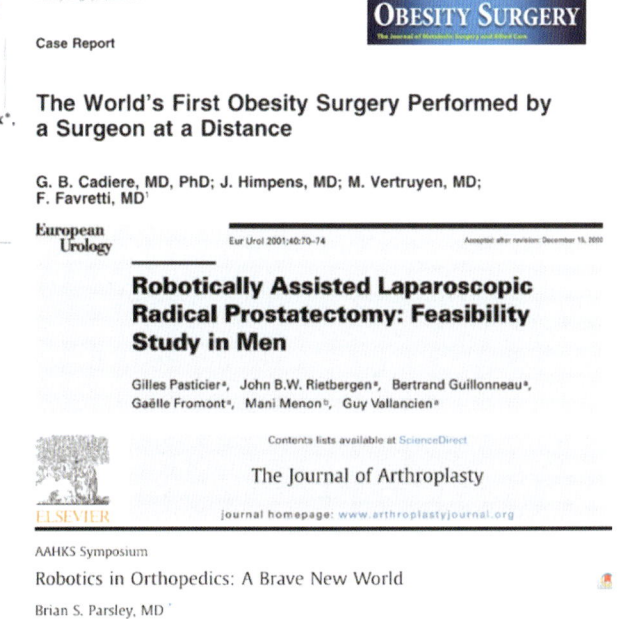

FIGURE 5-9 • Academic contributions.

Suggested Readings

1. Fong YWY, Hyung WJ, Lau C, Strong VE. *The SAGES Atlas of Robotic Surgery*. Springer; 2018.
2. Peters JH, Ellison EC, Innes JT, et al. Safety and efficacy of laparoscopic cholecystectomy. A prospective analysis of 100 initial patients. *Ann Surg*. 1991;213:3-12.
3. Wright JD, Ananth CV, Lewin SN, et al. Robotically assisted vs laparoscopic hysterectomy among women with benign gynecologic disease. *JAMA*. 2013;309:689-698.
4. Buell JF, Cherqui D, Geller DA, et al. The international position on laparoscopic liver surgery: the Louisville Statement, 2008. *Ann Surg*. 2009;250:825-830.
5. Haisley KR, Abdelmoaty WF, Dunst CM. Laparoscopic transhiatal esophagectomy for invasive esophageal adenocarcinoma. *J Gastrointest Surg*. 2021;25:9-15.
6. Wang X, Cao G, Mao W, Lao W, He C. Robot-assisted versus laparoscopic surgery for rectal cancer: a systematic review and meta-analysis. *J Cancer Res Ther*. 2020;16:979-989.
7. Tsung A, Geller DA, Sukato DC, et al. Robotic versus laparoscopic hepatectomy: a matched comparison. *Ann Surg* 2014;259:549-555.
8. Nota CL, Woo Y, Raoof M, et al. Robotic versus open minor liver resections of the posterosuperior segments: a multinational, propensity score-matched study. *Ann Surg Oncol*. 2019;26:583-590.
9. Nota CL, Rinkes IH, Molenaar IQ, van Santvoort HC, Fong Y, Hagendoorn J. Robot-assisted laparoscopic liver resection: a systematic review and pooled analysis of minor and major hepatectomies. *HPB (Oxford)*. 2016;18:113-120.
10. Melstrom LG, Warner SG, Woo Y, et al. Selecting incision-dominant cases for robotic liver resection: towards outpatient hepatectomy with rapid recovery. *Hepatobiliary Surg Nutr*. 2018;7(2):77-84.
11. Stewart CL, Ituarte PHG, Melstrom KA, et al. Robotic surgery trends in general surgical oncology from the National Inpatient Sample. *Surg Endosc*. 2019;33(8):2591-2601.
12. Konstantinidis IT, Ituarte P, Woo Y, et al. Trends and outcomes of robotic surgery for gastrointestinal (GI) cancers in the USA: maintaining perioperative and oncologic safety. *Surg Endosc*. 2020;34(11):4932-4942.
13. Stewart C, Raoof M, Fong Y, Dellinger T, Warner S. Who is hurting? A prospective study of surgeon ergonomics. *Surg Endosc*. 2022;36(1):292-299.
14. Zarate Rodriguez JG, Zihni AM, Ohu I, et al. Ergonomic analysis of laparoscopic and robotic surgical task performance at various experience levels. *Surg Endosc*. 2019;33:1938-1943.
15. Gofrit ON, Mikahail AA, Zorn KC, Zagaja GP, Steinberg GD, Shalhav AL. Surgeons' perceptions and injuries during and after urologic laparoscopic surgery. *Urology* 2008;71:404-407.
16. Catanzarite T, Tan-Kim J, Menefee SA. Ergonomics in gynecologic surgery. *Curr Opin Obstet Gynecol*. 2018;30:432-440.
17. Tao ZE VS, Pham T, Augustine MM, Guzzetta A, Huerta S. Outcomes of robotic and laparoscopic cholecystectomy for benign gallbladder disease in Veteran patients. *J. Robotic Surg*. 2021;15(6):849-857.
18. Dobbs RW, Nguyen TT, Shahait M, et al. Outpatient robot-assisted radical prostatectomy: are patients ready for same-day discharge? *J Endourol*. 2020;34:450-455.
19. Melstrom LG, Warner SG, Woo Y, et al. Selecting incision-dominant cases for robotic liver resection: towards outpatient hepatectomy with rapid recovery. *Hepatobiliary Surg Nutr*. 2018;7:77-84.
20. Ojeda PI, Kara A. Post discharge issues identified by a call-back program: identifying improvement opportunities. *Hosp Pract (1995)*. 2017;45:201-208.
21. Sun V, Dumitra S, Ruel N, et al. Wireless monitoring program of patient-centered outcomes and recovery before and after major abdominal cancer surgery. *JAMA Surg*. 2017;152:852-859.
22. Melstrom LG, Rodin AS, Rossi LA, et al. Patient generated health data and electronic health record integration in oncologic surgery: a call for artificial intelligence and machine learning. *J Surg Oncol*. 2021;123(1):52-60.
23. Collins JW, Levy J, Stefanidis D, et al. Utilising the Delphi process to develop a proficiency-based progression train-the-trainer course for robotic surgery training. *Eur Urol*. 2019;75:775-785.
24. Fong Y, Buell JF, Collins J, et al. Applying the Delphi process for development of a hepatopancreaticobiliary robotic surgery training curriculum. *Surg Endosc*. 2020;34:4233-4244.
25. Veronesi G, Dorn P, Dunning J, et al. Outcomes from the Delphi process of the Thoracic Robotic Curriculum Development Committee. *Eur J Cardiothorac Surg*. 2018;53:1173-1179.
26. Giulianotti PC, Coratti A, Angelini M, et al. Robotics in general surgery: personal experience in a large community hospital. *Arch Surg*. 2003;138(7):777-784.

"We are leaving behind the golden age of surgery in which procedures were performed directly by hand. We are stepping into a new era where computers, micromachines, human interface technologies and virtual reality will converge to enhance both the manual and cognitive abilities of physicians through computerized equivalents."

—Jacques Marescaux (1948)

Implemented Imaging and Artificial Intelligence

Barbara Seeliger • Toby Collins* • Jacques Marescaux*

INTRODUCTION

The introduction of minimally invasive approaches transformed surgery beyond the level of surgical techniques. In the days of open surgery, the expert surgeon was the only person who constantly saw or felt the relevant anatomy. Consequently, dissection in the ideal and embryological planes was virtually reserved to their inner circle. Neither spectators in an auditorium nor even tableside assistants had a view of the procedure as a whole. Nowadays, endoscopic approaches allow everyone to observe what is done at any given surgical step. Video-assisted procedures rely on endoscopic imaging systems, which share the primary surgeon's view with the entire operating room (OR) and allow transmission of live surgical procedures into auditoriums across the world. This has been a crucial first step toward teaching expert techniques to surgical trainees and providing continuous surgical education.

Operative video recording and analysis pave the way for the next step, namely to define the standard of care and provide quality control, as well as a video library of educational procedures. The definition of universal standard of care criteria via surgical video analysis allows the dissemination of educational material and the implementation of video-based evaluation for surgical accreditation. Robotic operative techniques and approaches can be unified worldwide. For this purpose, international recommendations based on expert consensus conferences will further integrate the emerging artificial intelligence–based analysis of global data sets.

There is considerable potential in eliminating substandard operative techniques that result in diverse outcomes and quality of life for the same disease, depending on the locally available expertise. Dissection in the proper plane is a key factor to optimize outcomes in oncological surgery. Inadequate dissection and resection (e.g., in complex operations such as rectal cancer surgery with total mesorectal excision) increase recurrence rates and deteriorate functional results. For complex surgical procedures, preoperative simulation becomes a valuable adjunct. It integrates critical surgical steps, as well as individual anatomical variants. Three-dimensional (3D) reconstruction of patient imaging studies provides a digital clone where normal and aberrant anatomy can be visualized. Additionally, entire procedures can be rehearsed on these virtual patient models with adequate software capacities. Rehearsals can be repeated as required for an optimal preparation and this approach should be mandatory for any complex procedure to avoid inadequate resections and prevent complications.

Robotic surgical platforms already integrate a variety of tools for intraoperative assistance that exceed manual control. Advanced vessel-sealing devices sense tissue electrical impedance and adjust their energy delivery to achieve the desired effect on the tissue. Similarly, automated stapling devices monitor tissue compression and automatically adjust during firing to deliver consistent staple lines in variable tissue thickness. When using the first generations of da Vinci systems (Intuitive Surgical, Sunnyvale, California, USA), the patient-side cart had to be undocked and redocked for adjustments of the OR table. With an integrated table motion update, the most recent da Vinci Xi Surgical System connects with a designated operating table (TruSystem™ 7000dV, Trumpf Medical [Saalfeld, Germany]). The wireless connection allows adaptation of

---

Photo reproduced with permission from Dr. Jacques Marecaux.

Quote reproduced with permission from Marescaux J. What is surgery? 2006(Suppl):88(10).

Barbara Seeliger and Toby Collins contributed equally.

robotic arms during table movement, hence allowing for the repositioning of the patient throughout the procedure without a need for undocking and redocking.

> **EDITORIAL COMMENT**
>
> The integrated table motion update works at its best for minor adjustments. For major changes of positioning (e.g., from reverse Trendelenburg to steep Trendelenburg), it is still necessary, for safety reasons, to undock and redock. However, with expert teams, this process only takes a few minutes.

As a navigation tool, the computer interface of robotic platforms allows to visualize virtual patient models within the surgeon console display.

Guidance based on image analysis is the principal axis for further progress in surgery. Robotic surgical systems enable capabilities reaching far beyond sensors, actuators, and telemanipulation. In addition to the mechanical advantages of steering a platform with advanced instrumentation, integrated imaging modalities provide an enhanced visualization and valuable guidance for various complex procedures.

There is great potential in computer-aided intraoperative data acquisition, information processing, and integration of decision support systems. Virtual reality (VR), augmented reality (AR), and artificial intelligence (AI)-based technologies are increasingly integrated into our daily lives and their incorporation into minimally invasive surgery is equally underway. The digitized interface between the surgeon and the patient gives access to smart systems and tools. Large amounts of data are created and collected, and data analytics allow us to process this abundance of information and to convey relevant information back to the surgeon. All of these factors, including AI algorithms for automatized assessments, are mandatory steps in the ultimate quest for the automation of robotic surgery. Next-generation robotic surgical systems will be sophisticated machine vision/AI digital surgery platforms. In the present chapter, an overview regarding the numerous applications of integrated imaging and AI in robotic surgery will be provided (**Figure 6-1**).

Implemented Imaging

Minimally invasive surgery is based on the insertion of an optical device into a body cavity, such as laparoscopy for intra-abdominal procedures, thoracoscopy for intrathoracic procedures, and endoscopy for intraluminal procedures.

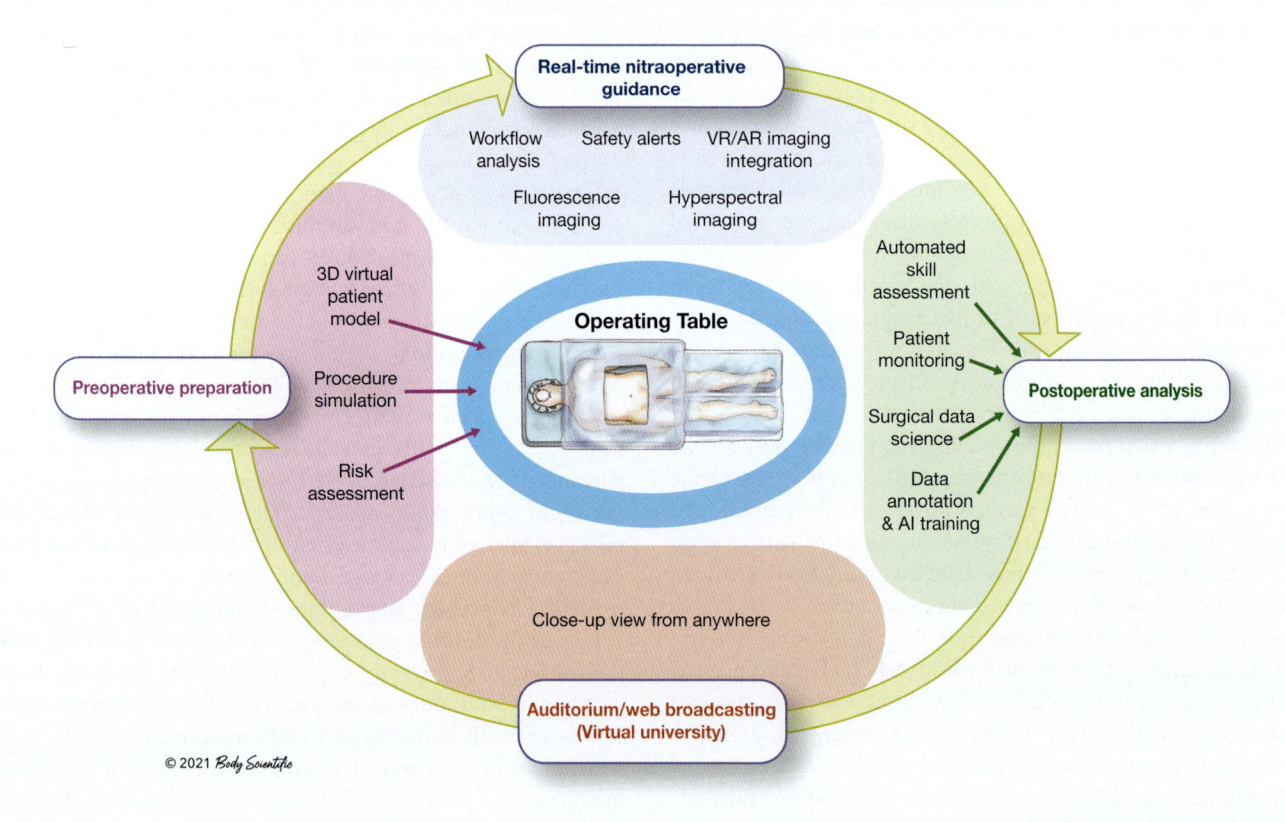

FIGURE 6-1 • Virtuous cycle highlighting the impact of implemented imaging and AI on surgery, enhancing the historical auditorium setup.

Because the interior of a human body is visually inaccessible without dedicated devices, the eyesight of surgeons is only as good as the imaging system that they use. The implementation of advanced imaging systems can boost the vision of surgeons beyond human abilities. Robot-assisted procedures rely on a computer interface for endoscopic telemanipulation and surgical instrumentation. As long as robotic platforms lack the sense of touch and partly of force feedback, the surgeon is compelled to visually assess tissue deformation during its manipulation in order to estimate its consistency and resistance. When a view beyond the organ surface is required to anticipate the next surgical step and the course of a procedure, preoperative tomographic imaging studies represent a valuable support. For additional intraoperative assistance, in select hospitals, there is a hybrid OR, which is defined as a facility that is equipped as an OR with integrated intraoperative guidance systems (including imaging modalities such as computed tomography [CT], magnetic resonance imaging [MRI], ultrasound, and fluoroscopy).

In analogy to the success of flight assistance systems in the field of aviation, computer assistance in surgery aims to overcome "human factor" limitations. In many complex fields, such as medical interventions, a decline in task performance is observed during high workloads, including time pressure and distractions. Advanced technology has the potential to reduce intraprocedural mental workload. Robotic platforms are human–machine interfaces that will allow to integrate the forthcoming assistance systems. Integrated imaging solutions are the next step toward a new generation of surgical robots. Currently, the most widely used platform is the da Vinci Surgical System (Intuitive Surgical). The integrated imaging modalities are 3D image reconstruction (Iris®) and fluorescence imaging (Firefly®). The CE-marked and FDA-cleared VISIBLE PATIENT™ solution for enhanced surgical planning provides highly detailed virtual 3D models of patient CT or MRI scans. This spin-off company originated from the Institute for Research against Digestive Cancer (IRCAD) based in Strasbourg, France, and recently entered into a strategic agreement with Ethicon Inc., within the Johnson & Johnson (New Brunswick, New Jersey, U.S.) Medical Device Companies. The upcoming surgical robotic platform Ottava (Johnson & Johnson) targets a comprehensive digital surgery system for thoracoabdominal procedures, as well as interventional and endoluminal procedures. Its interdisciplinary usability will additionally integrate simulation, machine learning, data analytics, and connectivity to advanced robotic instrumentation.

3D Image Reconstruction and Virtual Reality

Data from preoperative CT or MRI contain relevant anatomical details that are key for each patient's individual procedure. Anatomical variants are quite frequent throughout surgical domains. However, they can be missed in conventional views. Traditionally, surgeons consulted tomographic imaging studies before starting an operation by scrolling through the slices, or perhaps for adjustment during a procedure. However, it is cumbersome to walk to a computer in sterile clothing and ask for assistance to visualize the images. Consequently, integrated solutions with direct surgeon control are most welcome.

> **CONCEPTUAL HIGHLIGHTS**
>
> The field of robotic surgery is continuously evolving. Preoperative and intraoperative imaging as well as comprehensive image analysis are the next crucial steps for further transformation in minimally invasive precision surgery.

Dedicated software allows generation of 3D reconstructions of these imaging studies. Direct volume rendering (DVR) is integrated into radiological workstations and provides a simultaneous visualization of all slices resulting in a 3D view. This surface rendering (SR) technique can be achieved with several software solutions and modeling workstations or via distant services for 3D modeling. DVR allows viewing organ borders without preprocessing. However, it does not allow for the computation of organ volumes or simulation of resections. To do so, a special preprocessing has to be performed. It is called segmentation and consists in the delineation of anatomical and pathological structures within the images. The labor-intensive manual delineation of anatomical structures is now replaced by computer algorithms using machine learning, and in particular deep neural networks, by training them on a large data set of validated segmentations. These deep learning approaches significantly reduce segmentation time. From approximately 4 hours of semiautomatic annotation time, the AI-based approach developed by the Visible Patient (Strasbourg, France) company in 2020 allowed to reduce abdominal organ segmentation time down to 9 minutes (**Figure 6-2**). As a result, the productivity of specially trained experts is augmented, because they need to perform fewer and fewer manual corrections to validate the accuracy of a model. 3D reconstructions of various organs are shown in **Figure 6-3**.

In robotic consoles, individual 3D models from the simulation environment can be displayed intraoperatively. Using the connection of a mobile device, the surgeon can navigate in the virtual model throughout the procedure as demonstrated with the software developed by the IRCAD research team. The computer interface of robotic systems allows for a side-by-side view of the VR model and a live video feed within the surgeon console and for the OR team via an auxiliary screen (**Figure 6-4**). Intuitive Surgical recently integrated Iris®, a proprietary visualization service generating individual patient 3D models from deidentified CT scans by providing segmentation and labeling of anatomical structures. Independently from the 3D model provider, the reconstructed images can be shown in a dual view within the console using da Vinci's TilePro™ and they can be manipulated on connected devices such as tablets.

In patient-specific virtual models, it is easier to recognize normal, variant, and pathological findings. Navigational tools allow the user to rotate the 3D model, zoom in and out, and selectively show chosen structures with transparency settings. In such VR models, the interactive visualization is advantageous over traditional viewing techniques. Consequently, the interest in 3D reconstructions has grown over previous decades to support diagnosis and treatment planning. Virtual surgical

68 The Foundation and Art of Robotic Surgery

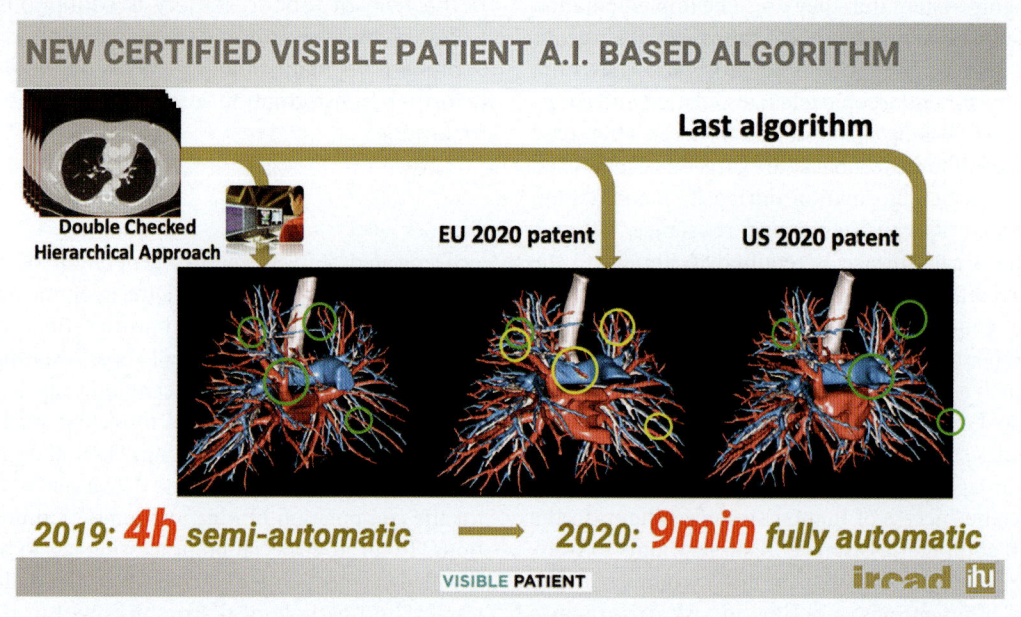

FIGURE 6-2 • AI-based segmentation significantly reduces 3D reconstruction time.

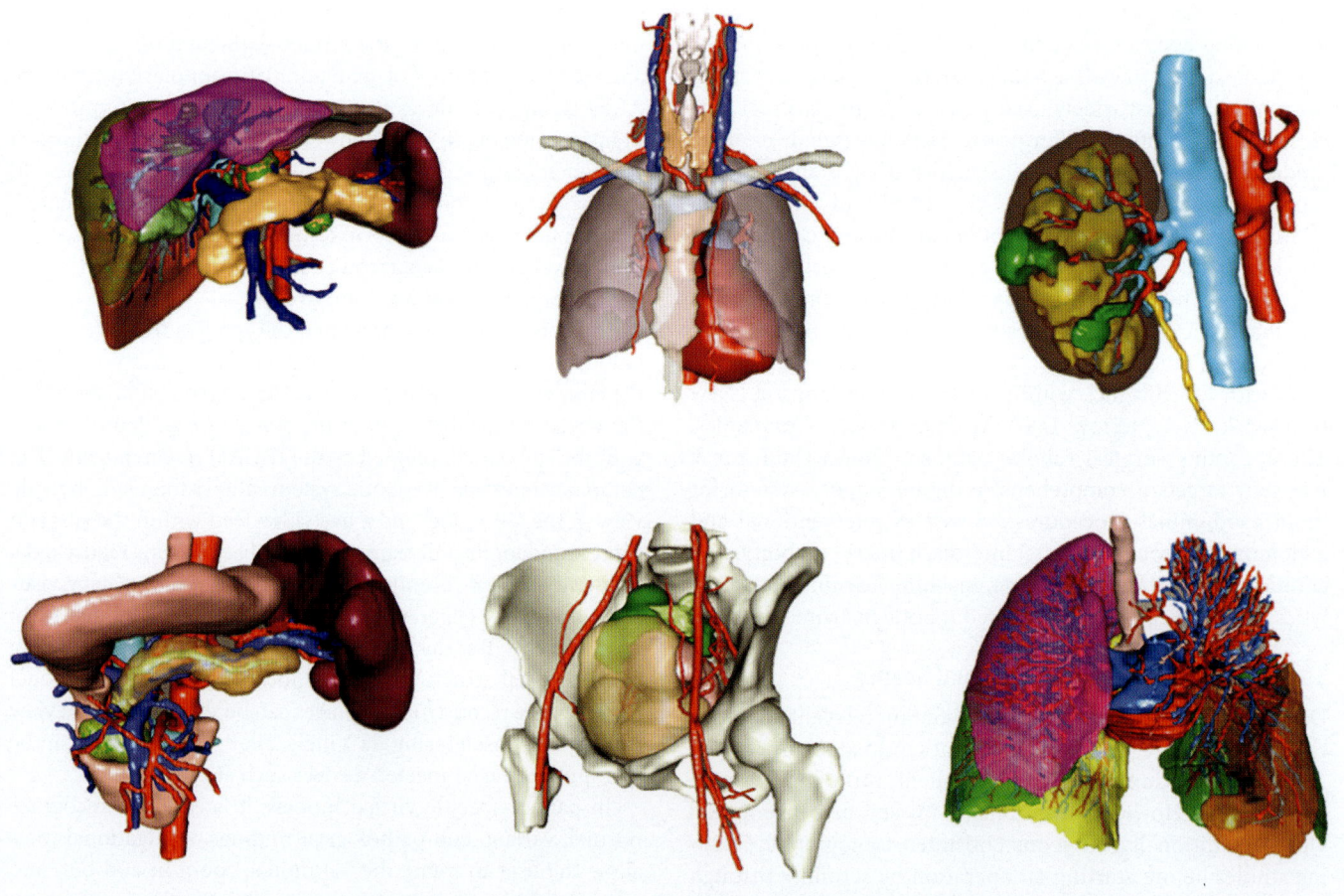

FIGURE 6-3 • Virtual patient models make it possible to clearly understand normal anatomy, individual variants, and pathological conditions throughout the various organ systems. Image courtesy of Visible Patient®.

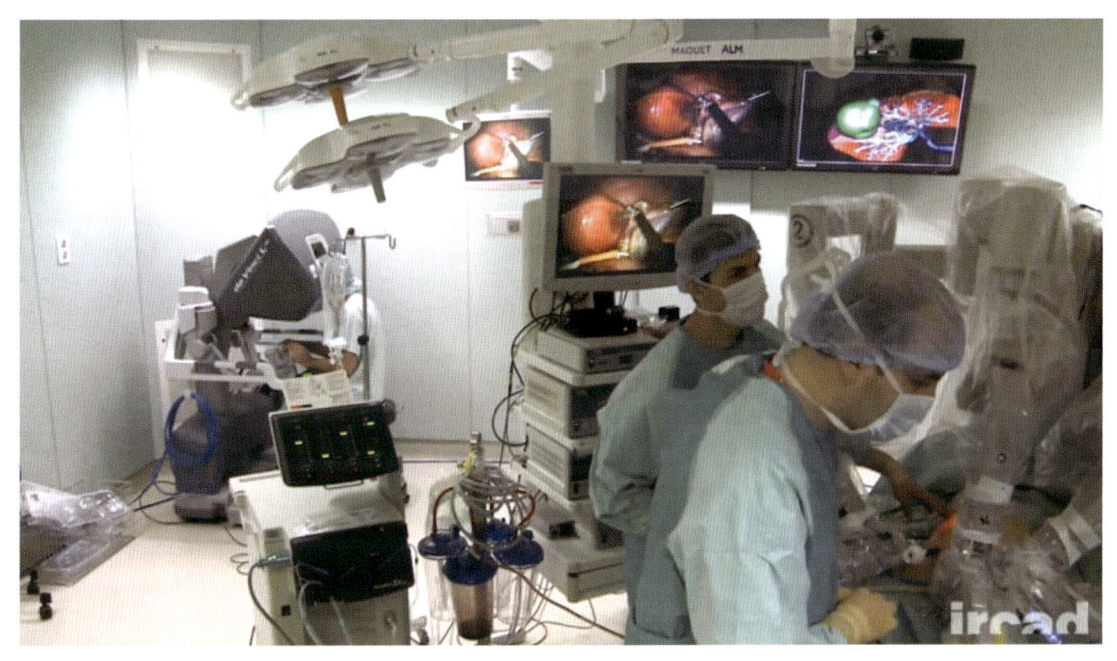

FIGURE 6-4 • AR-guided robotic liver segmentectomy. (Reproduced with permission from Pessaux P, Diana M, Soler L, et al. Towards cybernetic surgery: robotic and augmented reality-assisted liver segmentectomy. *Langenbecks Arch Surg.* 2015;400[3]:381-385.)

explorations in 3D models include the simulation of an individual procedure with an organ volume reconstruction technique that allows resections and the calculation of remnant volumes. Virtual surgical tools such as selective vascular clamping allow identification of liver tumors in relation to the respective segments. Occasionally, in standard tomographic images, a liver tumor appears to be located in one segment, whereas segmental vessel occlusion in the virtual model reveals that the affected segment is indeed a different one. Consequently, resections can be simulated and optimized for an organ-sparing approach with safe margins. Surgical planning based on a virtual model provided valuable assistance and led to a change in operative strategy in approximately 10% of liver resections (**Figures 6-5** and **6-6 A, B**).

> ### 🔍 CONCEPTUAL HIGHLIGHTS
>
> **3D images** provide a virtual clone of the patient. The virtual model can be manipulated in order to best visualize the relevant anatomy, including anatomical variants and pathological findings. **VR** provides a simulation environment for surgical procedures and can be displayed intraoperatively for guidance. When the virtual model is overlaid onto the real-time intraoperative images, an **AR** view is obtained.

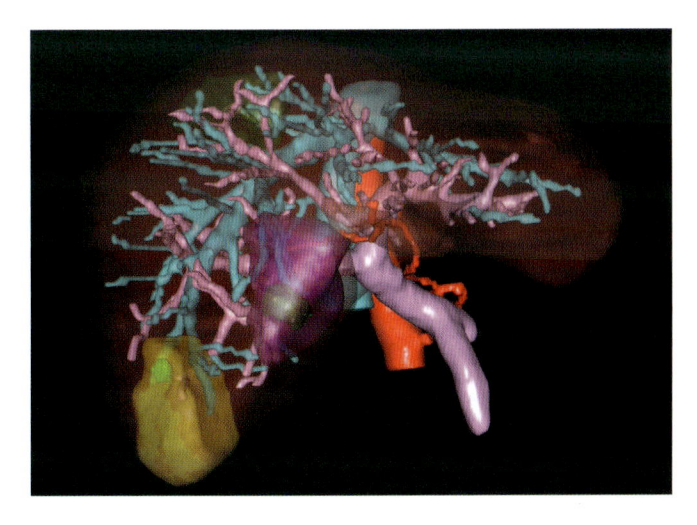

FIGURE 6-5 • Virtual surgical explorations in 3D models.

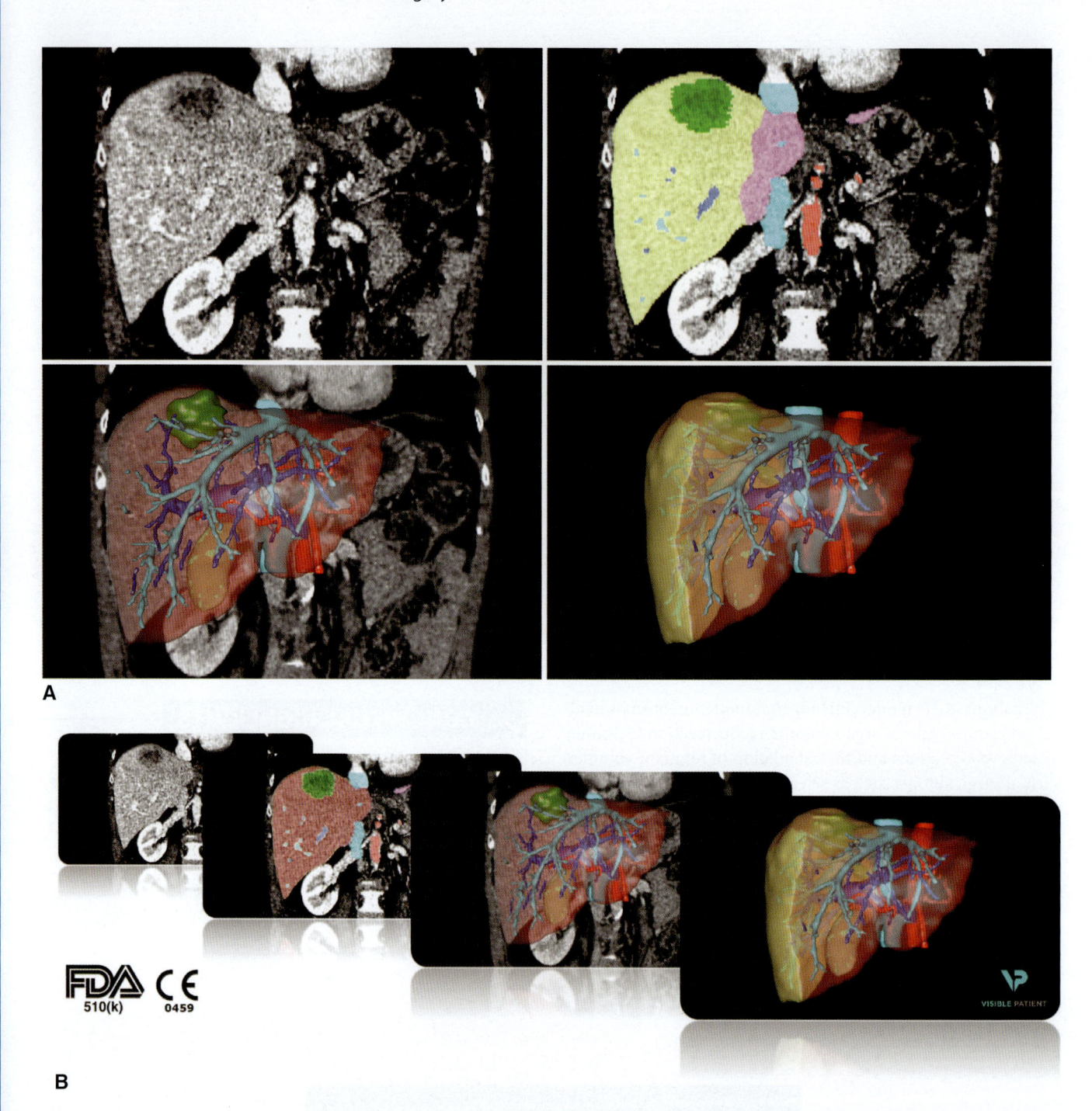

FIGURE 6-6 • Virtual surgical explorations in 3D models.

Fluorescence Imaging

Fluorescence image-guided surgery (FIGS) is an optical surgical navigation modality based on the use of light sources in the near-infrared (NIR) spectrum (wavelength between 700 and 900 nm). Fluorescence imaging can guide human eyes beyond their natural limit. The NIR window allows for a light penetration into the tissue of several millimeters, which enables to see behind the tissue surface. FIGS requires an intravenously or locally administered NIR fluorescent agent (called a fluorophore), and an imaging system capable of both exciting the fluorophore and detecting the signal it emits to display it on the screen intraoperatively, in real time. Indocyanine green (ICG) is the most frequently used fluorophore in surgery. It is a sterile tricarbocyanine dye that absorbs light between 790 and 805 nm and reemits light at a wavelength of 835 nm. Fluorescence can be visualized after a few milliseconds, which is an advantage over other emerging imaging techniques, such as Raman spectroscopy or optical coherence tomography, which require more time to visualize the same field of view.

Most systems merge fluorescence signals with normal RGB color signals, allowing for a direct anatomical orientation. These camera systems are equipped with specific filters for the optimal detection of NIR fluorescence and white light through the laparoscope. The augmented view displays an overlay of the NIR light onto the white light image. When using the da Vinci Firefly® system, the switch from standard light to NIR mode is controlled by the surgeon in the console menu. The image augmentation system offers adjustable viewing modalities that can be selected based on the surgeon's preferences. FIGS is increasingly used in a variety of surgical conditions to achieve improved visualization of vessels, organ perfusion, bile ducts, or the lymphatic basin of tumors. Operative videos regarding the use of robotic ICG-based imaging are accessible in multiple chapters of this book (see Chapter 23, Radical Right Colectomy with Complete Mesocolic Excision (CME), and Chapter 33, Right Hepatectomy, among others). The integration of fluorescence imaging into several other manufacturers' robotic systems is underway.

Imaging modalities can be complementary, as demonstrated by the combined use of intraoperative AR-guided navigation based on preoperative VR magnetic resonance cholangiopancreatography (MRCP) biliary tree models, near-infrared cholangiography (NIR-C), and x-ray intraoperative cholangiography (IOC) during robotic cholecystectomy (**Figures 6-7 A–L**). The assessment of the 3D-reconstructed MRCP-based biliary tree model ruled out choledocholithiasis in all patients and detected anatomical variants, of which some had been missed in the radiology reports. The 3 modalities resulted in the identification of the cystic duct junction with the common bile duct prior to the dissection of Calot's triangle (VR: 100%, NIR-C: 98.15%, IOC: 96.15%) and might subsequently prevent bile duct injuries.

A feasibility study in robot-assisted rectal cancer surgery coupled intraoperative stereotactic real-time navigation with fluorescence imaging. The da Vinci TilePro™ feature allowed the user to simultaneously display the various image sources. Navigation within a deformable soft tissue environment still represents a considerable challenge. However, there is significant potential in the use of an enhanced operative environment integrating imaging-based advances and robotic surgical platforms.

The benefit of fluorescence imaging still remains a subject of controversy within the scientific community. On the one hand,

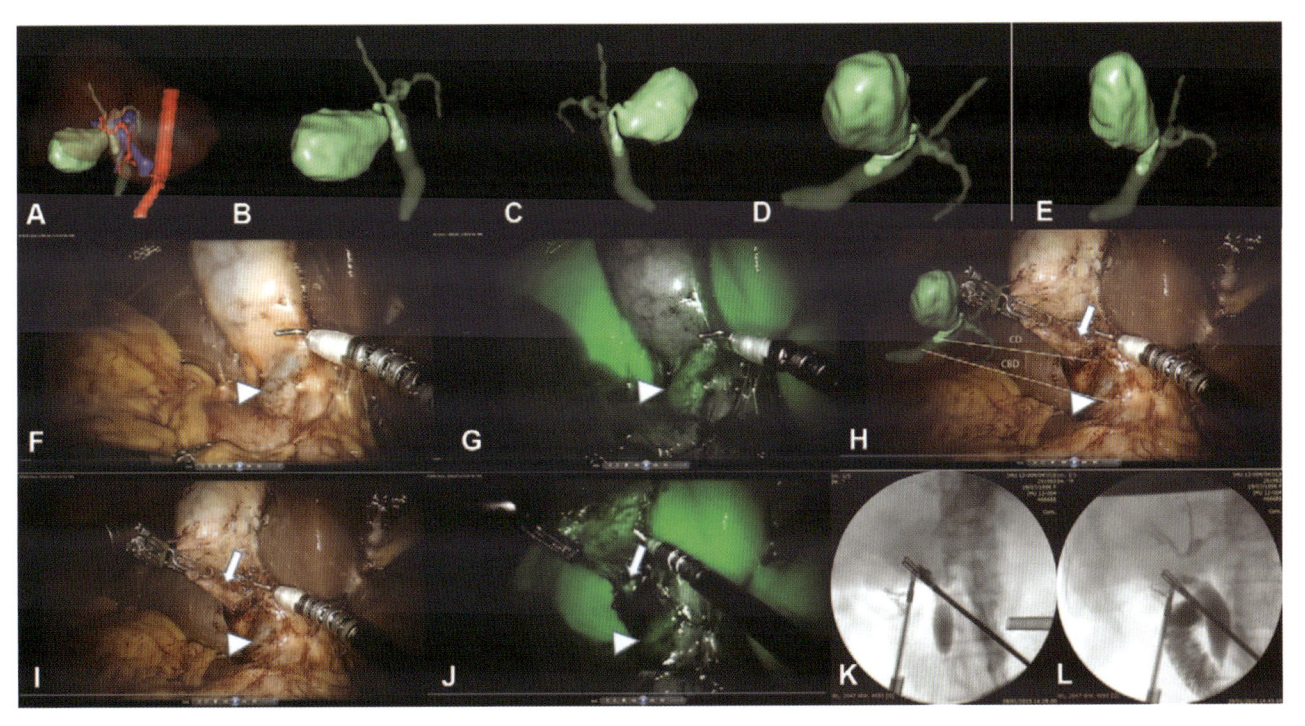

FIGURE 6-7 • Precision multimodal gallbladder surgery navigation: Virtual reality (VR), near-infrared fluorescence, and x-ray-based intraoperative cholangiography. **A.** 3D VR model showing biliary anatomy, the portal vein, and hepatic arteries. **B–E.** 3D VR model of the main biliary tree from different angles, showing that the cystic duct (CD) enters the common bile duct (CBD) from behind with a narrow angle. **F.** White light imaging showing an inflamed gallbladder, tightly adherent to a large tubular structure, which is interpreted as the CBD (*arrowhead*). **G.** Same image in near-infrared mode. **H, I.** The 3D model is displayed onto the operative field and rotated in 3D to help the surgeon identify the CD–CBD junction. The peritoneal sheet is opened and the CD (*arrow*) is detached from the inflamed tissue and exposed. **J.** Same image in near-infrared mode. **K, L.** Intraoperative cholangiography (IOC) confirms the biliary anatomy and shows the CD–CBD junction. (Reproduced with permission from Diana M, Soler L, Agnus V, et al. Prospective evaluation of precision multimodal gallbladder surgery navigation: virtual reality, near-infrared fluorescence, and X-ray-based intraoperative cholangiography. *Ann Surg*. 2017;266[5]:890-897.)

CONCEPTUAL HIGHLIGHTS

Fluorescence imaging provides a view beyond the visible surface. Injection of a fluorescent dye can be used to assess organ perfusion, to delineate segments within organs, and to highlight critical anatomical structures relevant to various procedures. Its integration into robotic systems, such as the da Vinci Firefly®, facilitates its application. Ongoing developments in objective signal analysis via computer assistance and AI algorithms will provide additional insight and intraoperative guidance.

expert users promote its use for real-time guidance in a broad variety of procedures. On the other hand, there is a lack of an objective standard for the interpretation and evaluation of fluorescent signals. Fluorescent signal intensity decreases with the camera-to-target distance (a closer camera position showing a higher signal intensity) and the fluorescent area changes over time (fluorophores even diffuse into ischemic areas after a while).

In order to minimize interobserver variability and optimize the use and applications of fluorescence imaging, approaches to quantitatively measure fluorescence intensity over time were proposed by IRCAD, as well as other groups. Quantitative fluorescence imaging allows for objective measurements with the speed of fluorophore arrival as a surrogate marker of tissue perfusion, and analysis of additional contrast uptake for reinjections of fluorescent dyes. Quantitative assessment of fluorescence signal dynamics in real time with a subsequent overlay onto laparoscopic images opens a new field of perfusion evaluation. The IRCAD/IHU group achieved a simultaneous laparoscopic and transanal endoluminal view of segmental colonic ischemia in an experimental model. The chosen thresholds were displayed on the intraoperative view and marked on the serosal surface with a surgical marker. In the procedure series with creation of an ischemic distal colonic segment, the same perfusion threshold delineated a significantly larger mean ischemic zone on the mucosal side than on the serosal one. Bowel ischemia extent can be underestimated from the serosal side alone (**Figure 6-8**).

Clinical studies further determine objective perfusion thresholds to ensure a safe resection and anastomotic healing. In a quantitative colon perfusion pattern analysis based on ICG angiography during laparoscopic colorectal surgery, slow perfusion was an independent factor for anastomotic complications. The ratio of *time from first fluorescence increase to half maximum intensity* ($T_{1/2MAX}$) divided by the *time from first*

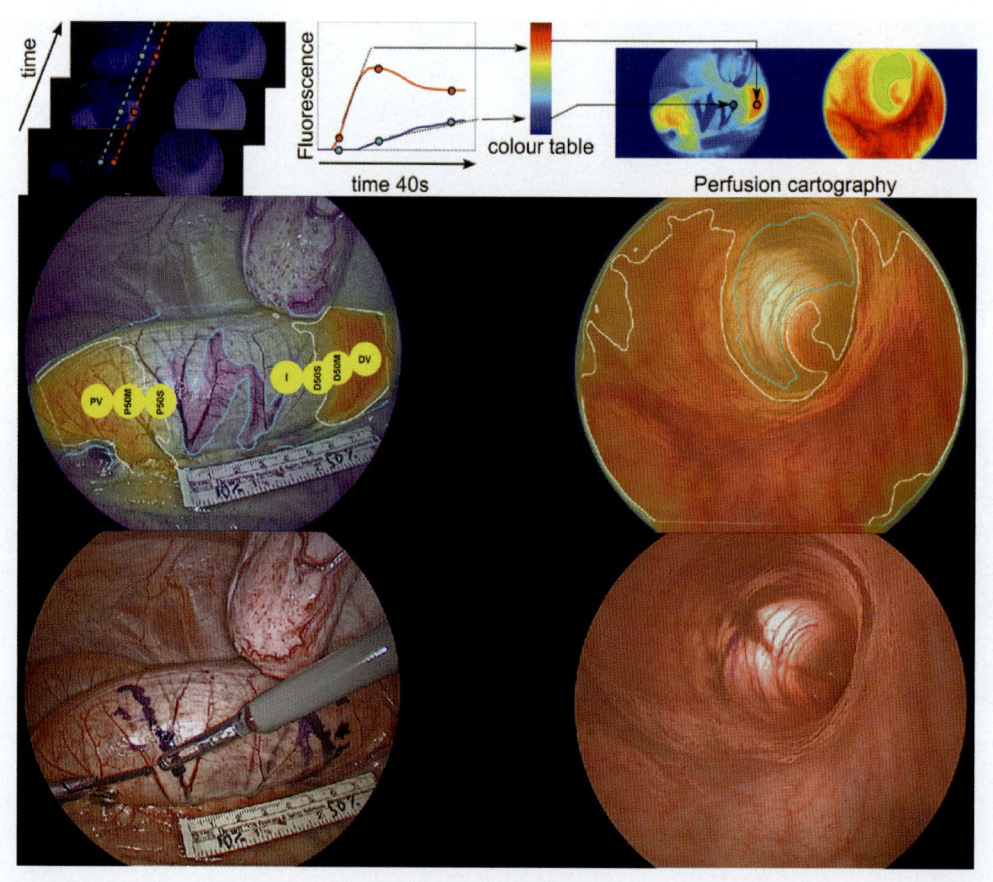

FIGURE 6-8 • Simultaneous laparoscopic and transanal quantitative fluorescence imaging. The speed of fluorescence signal arrival is translated to a color-coded perfusion cartography. Arbitrary thresholds can be chosen and displayed on the real-time intraoperative view to assess the ischemia extent from the serosal and mucosal side at the same time. (Reproduced with permission from Seeliger B, Agnus V, Mascagni P, et al. Simultaneous computer-assisted assessment of mucosal and serosal perfusion in a model of segmental colonic ischemia. *Surg Endosc*. 2020;34[11]:4818-4827.)

fluorescence increase to maximum intensity (T_{MAX}) was identified as the most reliable predictor of perfusion and anastomotic complications.

An AI-based ICG perfusion analysis was performed using a self-organizing map network using unsupervised learning, and results were compared with the previous quantitative parameters (such as the time ratio above). Using multiple graphs of ICG fluorescence intensity over time within each laparoscopic video, the training data set was acquired via the preprocessing of ICG videos from a patient cohort with 200 regions of interest per image, totaling 10,000 ICG curves. Videos of a separate cohort were used for testing. The AI-based real-time microcirculation analysis outperformed the conventional parameter-based quantitative method, showing a more accurate and consistent performance. In favorable colonic perfusion as documented via a steep increase in the ICG curve, the AI-based risk classification was consistent with previously defined conventional quantitative parameters. However, when a stepped rise was observed, the conventional parameter accuracy decreased whereas the AI-based classification consistently maintained accuracy. As a result, AI analysis was considered to be the most accurate to predict the risk of anastomotic complications. When compared to the existing computer-assisted quantitative fluorescence assessment, an AI-based analysis has the advantage of processing a large number of ICG curves in a short amount of time. With this approach, preprocessing, ICG curve pattern classification, and display of the result with a color map on the colon in enhanced reality took less than a minute, which is easy to integrate into any OR workflow.

In another recent study, intraoperative tissue classification based on indocyanine green fluorescence imaging was achieved based on AI algorithms. The AI model was developed and trained on white light and NIR fluorescence multispectral intraoperative videos of normal mucosa, as well as benign and malignant colorectal lesions within 30 cm from the anal verge. The dynamic perfusion assessment after fluorophore injection demonstrated distinct NIR fluorescence intensity changes over time for the different regions of interest. The resulting AI real-time tissue tracking and categorizing model based on NIR fluorescence data to discriminate normal, benign, and malignant lesions was tested intraoperatively within the reported series. This prototype allowed for data acquisition, AI analysis, and tissue classification of operator-selected regions of interest within 10 minutes. This approach has ample potential by exploiting the altered vascular architecture in neoplastic lesions with characteristic fluorophore uptake and distribution patterns, in order to help with the identification and delineation of tumors as opposed to benign and normal tissue throughout various organ systems.

> **CONCEPTUAL HIGHLIGHTS**
>
> Fluorescence image-guided surgery can be combined with 3D VR/AR models for additional intraoperative guidance. Quantitative fluorescence imaging and AI-based analysis of fluorescence signal dynamics provide intraoperative support for perfusion assessment and tissue classification and will further encourage adoption of fluorescence image-guided surgery.

> **EDITORIAL COMMENT**
>
> The possibility of recognizing different patterns of ICG microperfusion and delineating the tissue vascular architecture with AI may open the way to perform digital pathology intraoperatively.

AUGMENTED REALITY AND IMAGE-BASED AI IN SURGERY

Overview

AI technologies have an enormous potential to improve surgery and its outcomes in all stages of care (see also Chapter 1, What Robotic Surgery Is, for the preliminary basic principles about AI). The benefits of surgical AI in the preoperative stage include early automated cancer detection from medical images or blood tests, personalized surgery risk assessment, and 3D surgery planning. Intraoperatively, it provides decision-making support including augmented reality, real-time complication risk assessment, and automation of intraoperative tasks with robotics. Perioperatively, surgical AI supports patient monitoring in intensive care and emergency wards, monitoring using wearable or implantable sensors for an early detection of postoperative complications in the ward or at home for early discharge, as well as a more efficient patient movement and hospital coordination. AI is also likely to have a major impact on surgical education and training, including the automated and objective assessment of skills and learning curve, and personalized educational resources.

Medical images play a pivotal role in preoperative planning and intraoperative guidance in minimally invasive and robot-assisted surgery. Consequently, medical image data is at the core of most advances in AI and surgery. In the past, research progressed at a fast rate for several years, mainly driven by the astounding accomplishments of deep learning approaches to automatic image analysis and interpretation. This has been accelerated by the renaissance of convolutional neural networks (CNNs), which have proven to be very successful when trained in large, annotated data sets via powerful computers that have become widely available over the last decade. Additionally, it is more accessible than ever before to train deep neural networks using high-quality and open-source software libraries including TensorFlow by Google (Mountain View, CA, USA) and PyTorch by Meta (Menlo Park, CA, USA – formerly know as Facebook). Nevertheless, the integration of AI tools into routine surgical practice has been very slow, as a result of important regulatory and ethical barriers combined with inherent challenges in applying AI technologies to surgical data.

This section discusses the recent advances and work from IRCAD/IHU, starting with AR-guided surgery, which is an important surgical navigation tool to visualize hidden structures. Nowadays, AR techniques increasingly use deep learning methods to solve image registration and tracking. Some of the other main applications of image-based AI in surgery will then be addressed, including 3D endoscopic reconstruction and measurement, surgical workflow analysis, safety alert systems, and education/competency assessment. Major clinical translation barriers of using AI-based tools in surgical practice will be highlighted, as well as the recent work to overcome them from both academia and the industry. Armed with this knowledge, it is possible to have a clear understanding of the state of surgical AI progress today and to separate the hype from reality. This section concludes with a broader perspective on the longer-term integration of AI into routine surgical practice.

AR is a technological concept that combines computer-generated virtual models with real images or videos to enhance visual perception. Surgical AR is the application of AR technologies to enhance the surgeon's visual perception using patient-specific virtual models aligned (or registered) intraoperatively in real time (**Figure 6-9**). The virtual content is generated from a different imaging modality than the surgical camera, such as CT or ultrasound. It can be structural (e.g., 3D models of liver vasculature) or functional (e.g., perfusion models acquired from fluorescence imaging). The system shown in **Figure 6-9** provides real-time visualization of liver vasculature developed at IRCAD with the University of Zaragoza. The system works in 2 phases. In phase 1, a 3D reconstruction of the liver and abdominal cavity is created using a dense SLAM method. A preoperative virtual liver model is then aligned (registered) to the 3D reconstruction using surface-based registration. In phase 2, the liver is automatically tracked in the laparoscopic video using ORB-SLAM, allowing the virtual model to be visualized in real time.

The challenge in AR techniques is the precise overlay (registration) within the enhanced view. In contrast to rigid bone structures where an accurate overlay is relatively easy, the constant deformation of soft tissue requires a continuous adaptation of registration throughout respiratory movements, intraperitoneal insufflation, or during direct organ deformation via surgical manipulation. The retroperitoneum is relatively stable when compared to other intra-abdominal organs. Consequently, the IRCAD team was able to first use AR assistance in a laparoscopic adrenalectomy. Both the external camera view of the patient and the laparoscopic view were merged with the virtual model. The external AR view demonstrated the anatomical landmarks for an access to the adrenal gland. Using an additional video screen, the AR view complemented the standard laparoscopic view throughout the procedure. A remote operator performed the overlay with a video mixer, guided by an interactive dialogue with the surgeon. As the transparency of the virtual image can be adjusted, it supported the identification of dissection planes by highlighting landmark structures with the relevant vasculature, the adrenal gland, and the Conn's adenoma. Subsequently, IRCAD's VR and AR approach was applied to various minimally invasive procedures and clinical settings, including endocrine, colorectal, hepatobiliary, and pancreatic surgery.

Many different surgical AR systems are currently investigated because they incorporate machine learning components to solve some of the core technical challenges concerning 3D modeling and registration.

Augmented Reality Workflow

Surgical AR systems are implemented differently depending on specific applications and hardware and software technologies. However, all surgical AR systems share the same 8-step computation workflow (**Figure 6-10**). Understanding this workflow allows us to comprehend the general principle behind any surgical AR system.

> **🔍 CONCEPTUAL HIGHLIGHTS**
>
> All surgical AI systems include 8 main workflow stages illustrated in **Figure 6-10**. These stages give the main principles behind any AR system.

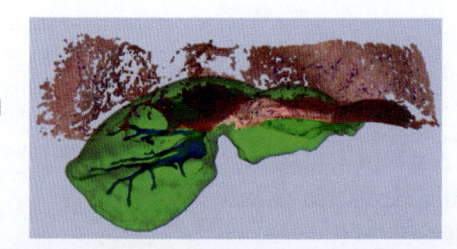

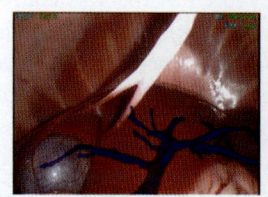

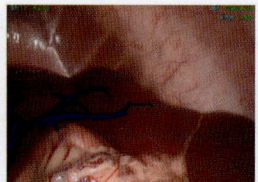

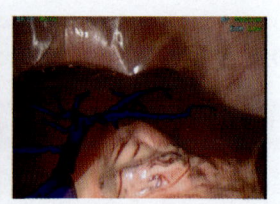

FIGURE 6-9 • Surgical AR system for real-time visualization of liver vasculature.

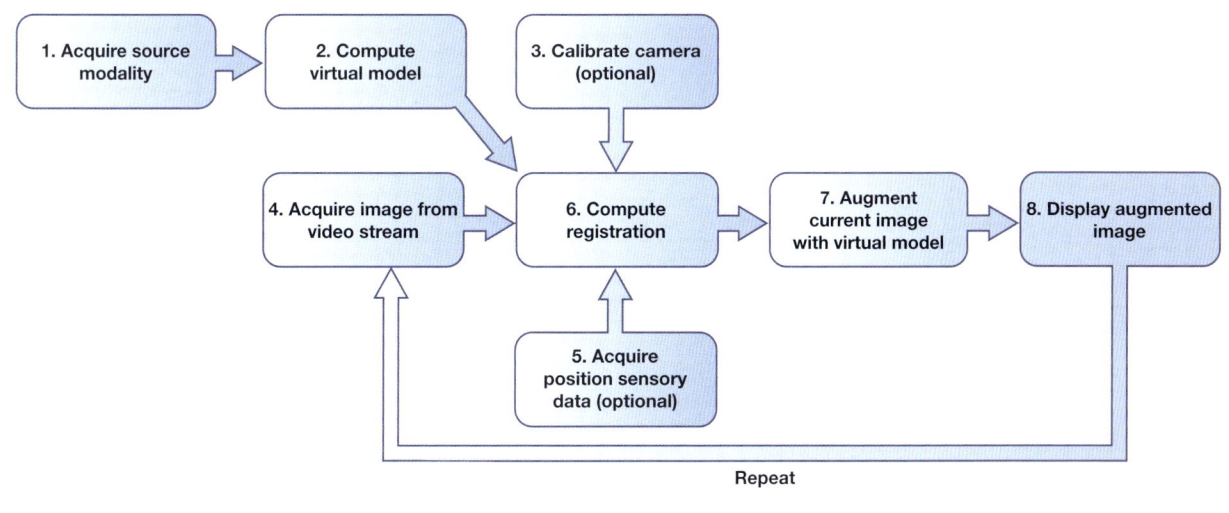

FIGURE 6-10 • The main components of any surgical AR system.

Step 1. Acquire source modality
The source modality is data from which the virtual model is extracted. The most common source modalities include preoperative CT and MRI, or intraoperative ultrasound and fluorescence.

Step 2. Compute virtual model
The virtual model consists in digital information that will be visually overlaid with the camera's video stream. The virtual model can be structural (e.g., a vascular surface model from CT), or functional (e.g., perfusion measured by means of fluorescence). Computing structural virtual models has advanced significantly over recent years due to automatic and semiautomatic methods that use deep neural networks (see subsection "3D Image Reconstruction and Virtual Reality").

Step 3. Calibrate camera (optional)
Camera calibration provides information about the physical parameters of the camera, such as its zoom, which the surgeon may change during the procedure. These parameters are required to correctly align the virtual models with the camera images. When the camera device has a fixed lens, which is typical of robotic laparoscopes, and any zooming can be achieved digitally, camera calibration is not necessary during the procedure and it can be performed just once in the factory. In other settings, it must be performed using a short calibration process during the surgery setup.

Step 4. Acquire image from video stream
The laparoscopic image that is to be augmented is acquired from the camera device.

Step 5. Acquire position sensory data (optional)
Position sensors such as robot joint angle measurements, gyroscopes, and electromagnetic tracking equipment can be used to provide extra information about the camera or instrument 3D positions. This information significantly helps with the registration of rigid structures. However, this sensor data does not have much value to register strongly deforming structures.

Step 6. Compute registration
A registration is the geometrical alignment between the virtual model and the camera image for a correct visual fusion and AR visualization. Computing registration is usually not trivial, particularly when the virtual model must undergo soft tissue deformation. Registration misalignment can lead to visualization errors. Consequently, the software to perform registrations is a critical component.

Step 7. Augment current image with virtual model
The registered virtual model is combined with the current video stream using image fusion software. Typically, a transparent visualization effect is used, where the virtual model is blended to give the impression of seeing through the tissue to observe hidden structures (**Figure 6-9**). This kind of visual fusion is made using a renderer, which is the same computer graphics software used in computer games.

Step 8. Display augmented image
The augmented image is then displayed onto a hardware device. Various display systems can be used depending on the application. In most robotic surgery cases, the display system is the console display. In AR applications using an external camera, the display system can be a handheld tablet, AR glasses, or a standard 2D monitor.

Repeat
Steps 4 to 8 are then repeated using the next image from the video stream until the AR system is no longer required by the surgeon.

The most demanding technical challenge in a surgical AR system is Step 6 (registration), followed by Step 2 (computing the virtual model). In recent years, AI, and in particular deep learning, have contributed to substantial advances in both challenges. Step 2 using structural models has already been discussed in the subsection "3D Image Reconstruction and Virtual Reality." In this section, the technical challenges associated with registration in laparoscopic AR surgery are discussed, as well as solutions that the IRCAD/IHU team and other groups have proposed.

A **B**

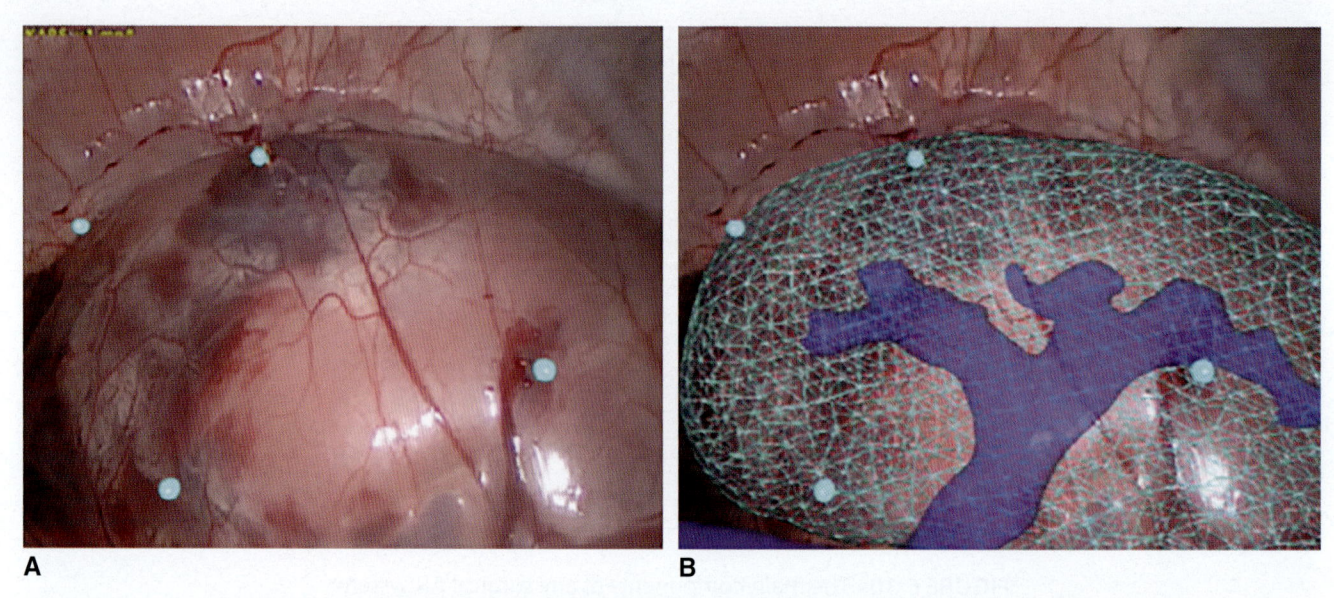

FIGURE 6-11 • Marker-based approach for organ registration to enable AR-guided surgery. (Reproduced with permission from Kong SH, Haouchine N, Soares R, et al. Robust augmented reality registration method for localization of solid organs' tumors using CT-derived virtual biomechanical model and fluorescent fiducials. *Surg Endosc.* 2017;31[7]:2863-2871.)

Registration

Registration algorithms can be broadly categorized into **marker-based** and **image-based** methods. Marker-based methods are mainly used for registration in open surgery via fiducials positioned on an organ surface. In laparoscopic surgery, fluorescent markers have been used because they allow effective marker identification even in low light (**Figures 6-11 A, B**). Marker-based approaches simplify registration because markers are highly distinct and easy to recognize by a computer. However, they are also quite impractical to deploy. The small number of markers used in practice restricts this approach to rigid registration, because it is impossible to recover strong 3D deformation from only a few makers.

> ⚠ **CHALLENGES AND POTENTIAL PITFALLS**
>
> Registration is the main technical challenge to achieve surgical AR. For soft-body organs that can deform significantly, registration of a preoperative model using only laparoscopic camera images is very hard. There are still no algorithms that have been verified in clinical trials or certified for medical use yet.

In contrast, image-based approaches solve registration issues using the rich visual organ shape information contained in the camera view, thereby allowing for deformable registration (**Figure 6-12**). Image-based methods prevent the need for manually placing and removing fiducials. However, they are technically much more challenging than marker-based methods, requiring a computer vision system capable of comprehending organ position and shape from the camera view. Consequently, there are no medically approved products yet available that perform image-based registration in laparoscopic AR, and research is ongoing.

Much research in image-based registration has been conducted in abdominal surgery, and particularly for liver, uterine, and renal procedures. In collaboration with the University of Zaragoza, the IRCAD group has created a novel image-based registration system using simultaneous localization and mapping (SLAM) techniques. The approach is divided into 2 main phases (**Figure 6-9**). In phase 1, a reconstruction algorithm is used to reconstruct the abdominal cavity and the anterior liver surface in 3D, using a video clip lasting less than a minute, captured with a monocular or stereo laparoscope. A preoperative virtual liver model (from CT or MRI) is then aligned (registered) to the 3D reconstruction using surface-based registration and a modified iterative closest point (ICP) algorithm. In phase 2, the liver is automatically tracked in the laparoscopic view using ORB-SLAM that detects small natural features on the liver surface, allowing the virtual model to be visually augmented in real time.

The registration method of phase 1 was improved at IRCAD/IHU in collaboration with the EnCoV group to handle soft tissue deformation (**Figure 6-12**). This operates by iteratively deforming the virtual model so that its surface aligns with the 3D reconstruction while also respecting an elastic tissue model implemented as a mass-spring system. The benefit of this approach is to handle the strong organ deformation induced by an intraoperative posture change and intraperitoneal insufflation when compared to the preoperative virtual model. This method has also been used to automatically register the 3D reconstruction with an external abdominal view from a depth camera viewing the patient from above (**Figure 6-13**). This technique can guide port placement and percutaneous interventions. Another approach to AR-guided liver surgery using DVR (**Figure 6-14**) is based on IRCAD/IHU's hybrid OR with an interventional CT and optical or electromagnetic tracking equipment for dedicated 3D tracking of the laparoscope. Here, the virtual model is the unmodified intraoperative CT image that is visualized directly using DVR. This approach is effective to visualize vasculature and tumors using a novel

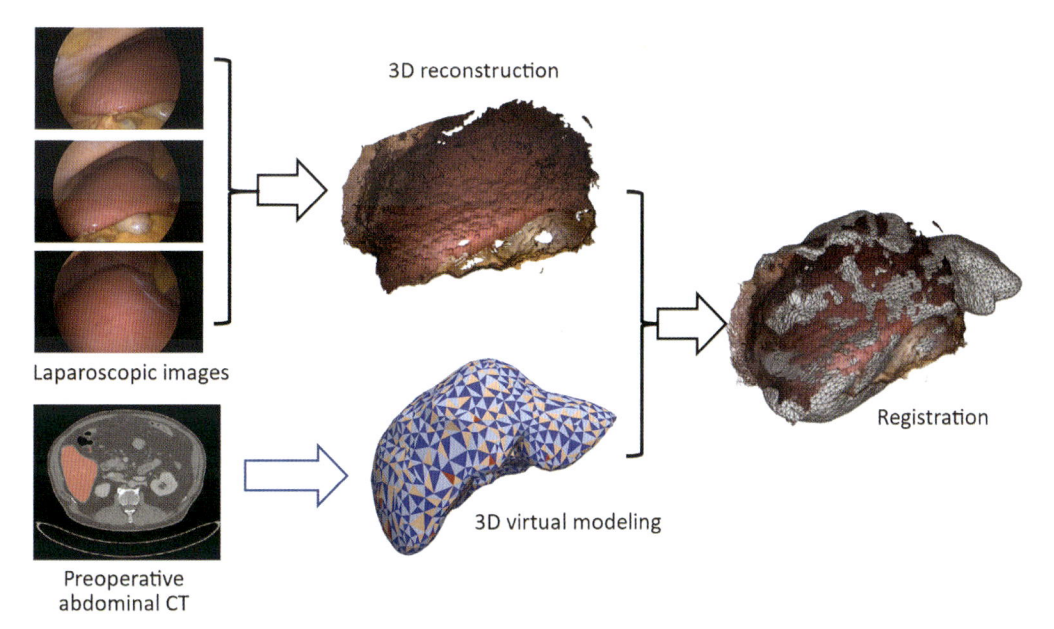

Implemented Imaging and Artificial Intelligence 77

FIGURE 6-12 • Image-based registration system to align the liver from a preoperative CT to the laparoscopic view.

"cone visualization," where a virtual cone is cut out of the liver parenchyma. Using appropriate DVR transfer functions, this approach does not require a 3D virtual model of the patient.

Registration Challenges

There are great expectations for the use of AR technologies to improve surgical practice. However, it is key to understand the technical challenges involved in registration, because they often impose fundamental limits on what can be achieved or expected in real clinical use.

The first factor that determines the feasibility of registration is the amount of soft tissue deformation of the structure. This can be put into 3 categories: (I) rigid registration, where the structure does not deform significantly, (II) deformable registration where the structure deforms but remains intact, and (III) deformable registration with an incised nonintact structure (e.g., the liver during tumor resection).

Rigid registration is the simplest one because it only requires the estimation of the 3D position and orientation of the structure relative to the camera, which may be achieved with as few as 3 natural or artificial landmarks on the organ surface. In contrast, deformable registration involves the deformation of the virtual model, and as a result, its shape matches with the organ shape during surgery. To handle dissection, the virtual model has to undergo some significant adaptation, which is highly complex. Despite research efforts in this area, there is no registration software that can reliably handle category III today.

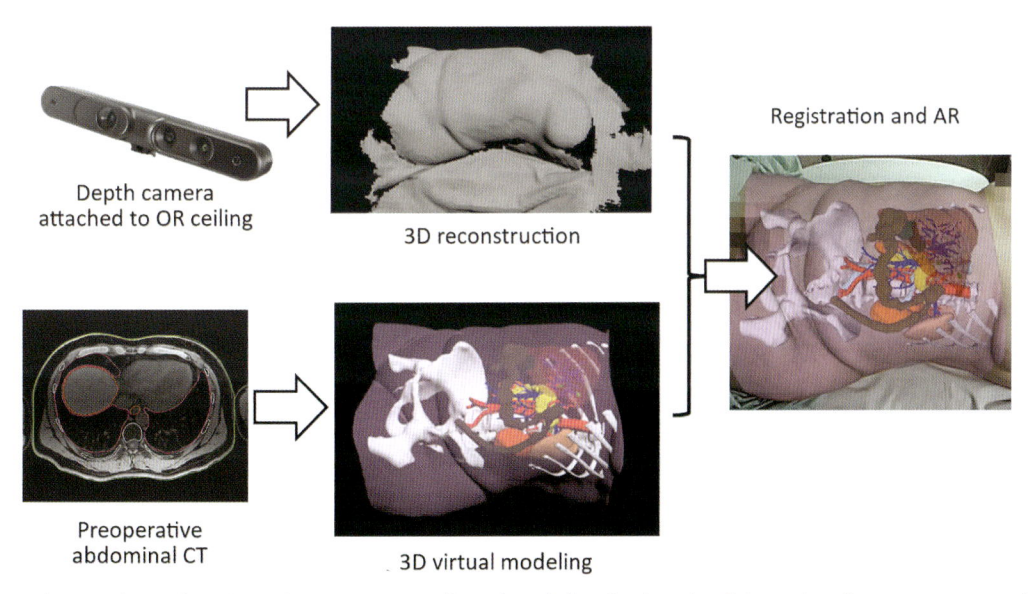

FIGURE 6-13 • Image-based registration system to align the abdominal and pelvic region from a preoperative CT to an external view. (Reproduced with permission from Frangi AF, Schnabel JA, Davatzikos C, et al. *Medical Image Computing and Computer Assisted Intervention—MICCAI 2018.* Cham, Switzerland: Springer; 2018.)

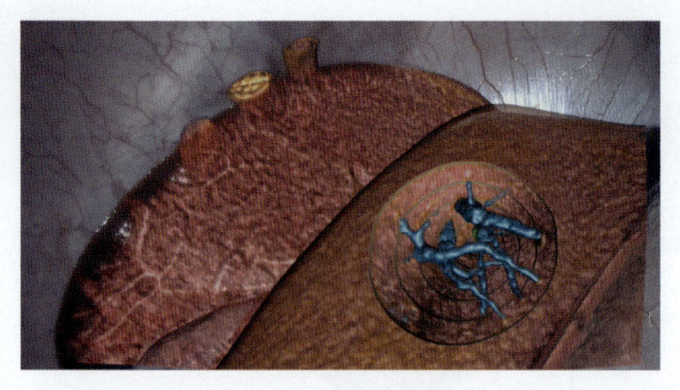

FIGURE 6-14 • Real-time AR-guided liver surgery using DVR developed in the IRCAD/IHU LASAR2 project. A novel "cone visualization" has been developed to virtually inspect the inside of the liver parenchyma to reveal an important vasculature. Virtual contours are added to the cone to assist depth perception, similarly to elevation contours on a geographic map.

also automatically detect and match natural landmarks in images and segment laparoscopic images to detect liver and kidney, to distinguish which regions of the image should be aligned with the virtual model (**Figure 6-15**). The left column of **Figure 6-15** shows sample images from a laparoscopic partial nephrectomy. The middle column shows corresponding predicted segmentations color-coded according to structure type, from the IRCAD's competition submission using a CNN-based approach based on DeepLab. The right column shows segmentations that have been annotated manually by a trained expert. These approaches are still in the research phase, but they are expected to be crucial to allow for the clinical translation of AR systems in the coming years.

OTHER INTRAOPERATIVE AI APPLICATIONS

3D Endoscopic Modeling and Measurement

Endoscopic cameras are either monocular (single lens) or stereo (dual lens). Stereo endoscopes are used in most robotically assisted procedures and have the advantage of providing 3D perception. However, neither of them produces 3D data, such as a 3D measurement of a lesion's diameter directly from endoscopic images. 3D conversion of the endoscopic images to a 3D surface that can be measured is first required (**Figure 6-16**), and this may also be useful for other applications such as AR registration. In **Figure 6-16**, 3 laparoscopic images in a laparoscopic transabdominal preperitoneal (TAPP) repair are shown (left). On the right, a 3D reconstruction of a partially dissected Triangle of Doom is shown with automatic 3D measurements to assess if the dissection is sufficient for mesh placement.

Methods based on deep learning produce exceptional results that surpass previous approaches by far. For stereo cameras, 3D reconstruction requires an algorithm that computes *parallax*, which is the relative displacement of each pixel from left to right images. The depth at the pixel is directly proportional to the amount of parallax (triangulation). The best performing reconstruction methods use CNNs where 2 stereo images are inputted into the CNN, which outputs the depth of each pixel (the depth-map). 3D measurements between 2 pixels can then be made interactively using the information from the depth-map. One of the main challenges is that the depths associated with stereo images (i.e., the labels) are unknown, which prevents the use of supervised learning. Instead, it is possible to train the CNN without labeled data using unsupervised learning. In this process, the CNN learns to predict depth-maps using a different learning function, such as pixel similarity.

3D reconstruction from monocular endoscopes is considerably harder to achieve as compared to stereo endoscopes. IRCAD has developed state-of-the-art algorithms using SLAM, discussed earlier. This has several applications, including its use for registration and 3D measurement (**Figure 6-16**).

Surgery Workflow Analysis

Surgery workflow analysis is about automatically monitoring and assessing the progress of a procedure using AI models. Workflow analysis using surgical videos has been an area of research for over a decade, and mature algorithms have now entered commercial products such as Medtronic's Digital

Rigid registration can be applied to orthopedic surgery, or for soft organs prior to surgical manipulation. This provides a visual appreciation of the subsurface anatomy with surgical AR before starting any significant manipulation. For deformable registration, the main challenge is that the organ deformation must be inferred from only the region of its surface visible to the camera. For the liver, this region can be as small as 15% of the total surface (**Figure 6-9**, phase 1), which provides limited information to assess the position of nonsuperficial structures. Mechanical modeling is used to account for this data limitation, where the most probable position of the structure is estimated based on mechanical tissue properties. The uncertainty of this approximation increases with the depth of the structure. It remains uneasy to achieve an accurate registration of the liver when it is strongly manipulated, and more research is required to both make more accurate registrations and to convey the degree of uncertainty in the prediction to the surgeon.

The second main factor that determines the difficulty of registration is whether the 3D model is constructed from a preoperative medical image (a *preoperative model*) or constructed from an intraoperative image (an *intraoperative model*). The main advantage of a preoperative model is that it does not require a hybrid OR, which is not available in most hospitals, and which is usually not compatible with a bulky robotic equipment. Its main disadvantage is that registration must compensate for changes between the preoperative and intraoperative status (mainly pneumoperitoneum and postural changes). In contrast, an intraoperative model simplifies registration because it represents the current status. However, after the intraoperative model has been created, soft tissue deformation is challenging to handle, which may require repeated intraoperative acquisitions to make sure that the model retains the current status.

AI-based solutions solve certain aspects of image-based registration. Deep learning has been used to efficiently compute physical deformations of a virtual model in real time, replacing previous methods requiring computationally slow physics-based simulators. Deep learning–based methods can

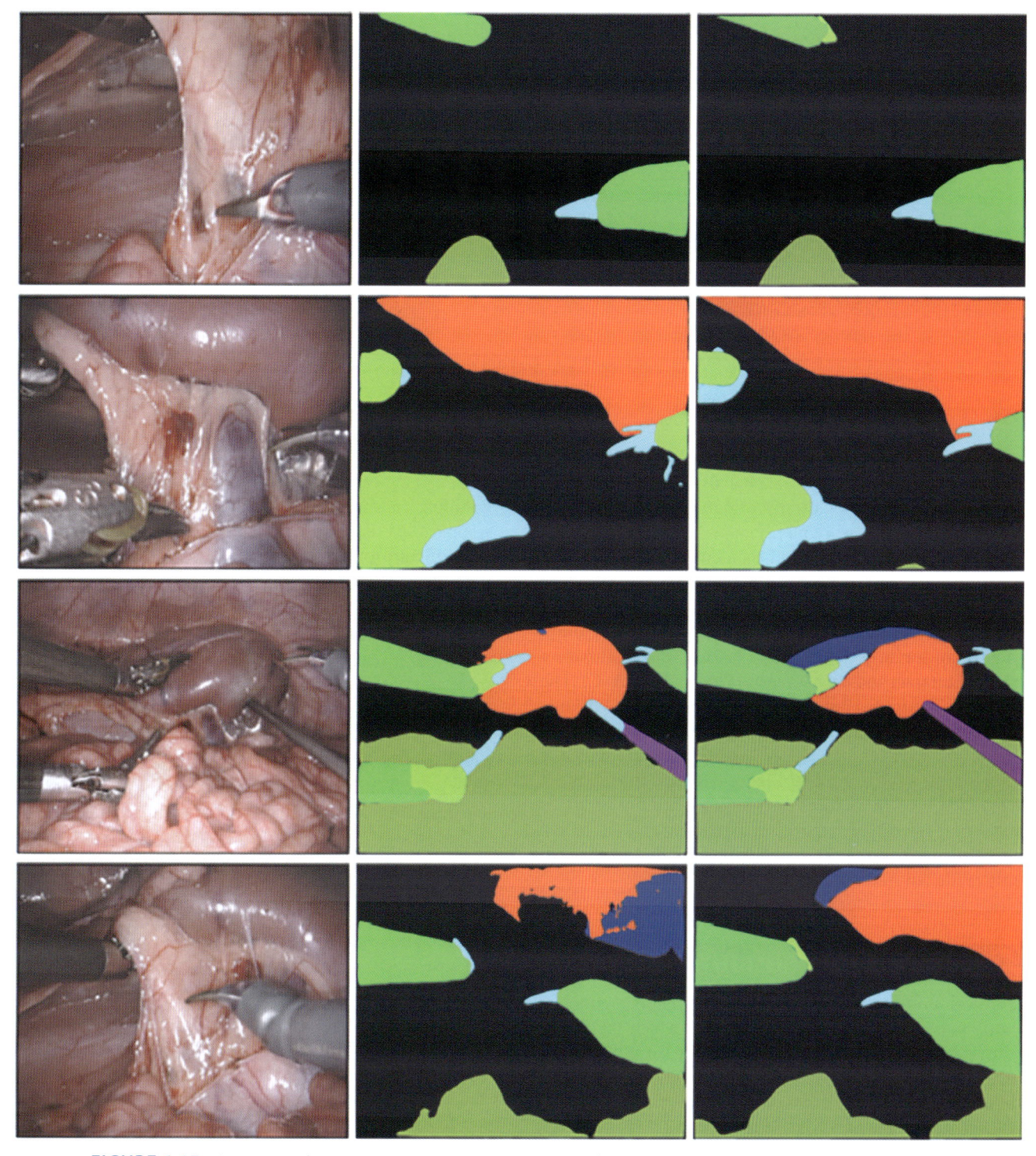

FIGURE 6-15 • Automatic laparoscopic image segmentation from the Robotic EndoVis 2017 Instrument Segmentation Challenge.

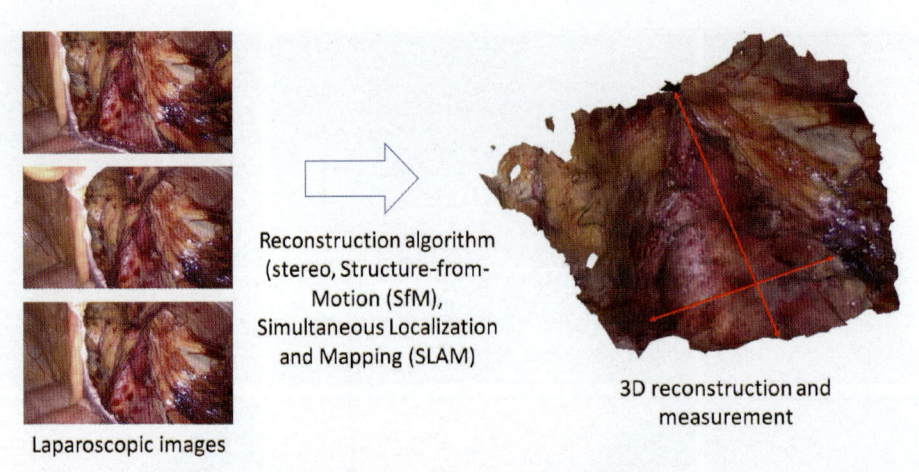

FIGURE 6-16 • AI and 3D measurement.

Surgery, Johnson & Johnson's C-SATS, and Intuitive Surgical's Orpheus. One of the central objectives of surgery workflow analysis is to automatically recognize the major steps (or phases) during a procedure. Pioneering work in laparoscopic cholecystectomy allowed to identify its main steps. This has been driven to a large extent by the public release of the Cholec80 data set constituting videos with the durations of each step labeled by a surgeon. Today, step recognition systems have been developed for a broad range of surgeries including cataract and hernia repair (**Figures 6-17 A–C**). The 3 images in **Figure 6-17** are taken at different timepoints during a bilateral TAPP hernia repair. **Figure 6-17A** is before the laparoscope has been introduced "no step," **Figure 6-17B** is during hernia dissection, and **Figure 6-17C** is during mesh deployment. On the right of each image is a set of bars that give the time spent in each step up to the current time (seconds). The white circle shown on one of the bars indicates the currently predicted step.

> **CONCEPTUAL HIGHLIGHTS**
>
> Surgical step recognition (also called "phase recognition") means to automatically identify which surgical step is performed during a procedure. The surgical video is the main source of data for the recognition software, but it can also include other data such as video from the OR ceiling camera and vital signs.

From a technical perspective, automatic surgical step recognition is considered one of the simplest tasks in surgical AI, and it is the basis for a more advanced AI comprehension of surgery. Step recognition is solvable using modern AI with methods based on deep learning provided that adequate high-quality annotated training data is available. It has several major uses that help patients either directly or indirectly. Its main uses are as follows:

Detection of difficulties and risk of complications: A critical step that takes an unusually long amount of time could well indicate that the surgeon is experiencing difficulties as well as an increased risk of complications. Consequently, step durations can be fed into a second AI model to predict the complication risk, or to automatically alert the senior surgeon of a difficulty for a resident.

Procedure standardization: For well-standardized procedures such as laparoscopic cholecystectomy or TAPP hernia repair, an alert can signal if the executed steps deviate from standardized workflow. However, such a standardization is mandatory for step recognition to have clinical value.

Performance analytics and learning curve assessment: Time taken to achieve surgical steps is an important indicator of technical competency. A descriptive statistical analysis software can use this information to measure the learning curves of surgeons and to compare performance with peers.

Improving OR efficiency: The ability to automatically determine when a procedure is nearing completion can increase OR efficiency and reduce hospital costs, by automatically notifying the ward to prepare for the next patient and cleaning staff.

Education and Skills Assessment

Surgical skills are based on training and experience, and they influence procedure outcomes. However, surgeons' skills are difficult to assess, particularly due to the amount of time needed for expert assessment during a procedure or for reviewing video footage. With an interobserver variability in skills assessment and a limited resource of experts available for single or plural evaluations, attempts emerged to automatize an objective surgical skills assessment using machine learning.

Simulators are used increasingly outside of the OR for training, assessment, and certification, such as the Fundamentals of Laparoscopic Surgery (FLS), the Fundamentals of Robotic Surgery (FRS), and the Fundamentals of Endoscopic Surgery (FES). FES uses a flexible endoscopy virtual simulator, and an exam pass is mandatory for general surgery board certification. Basic scoring metrics (time and errors) are used; yet the definition of errors can be subjective. For

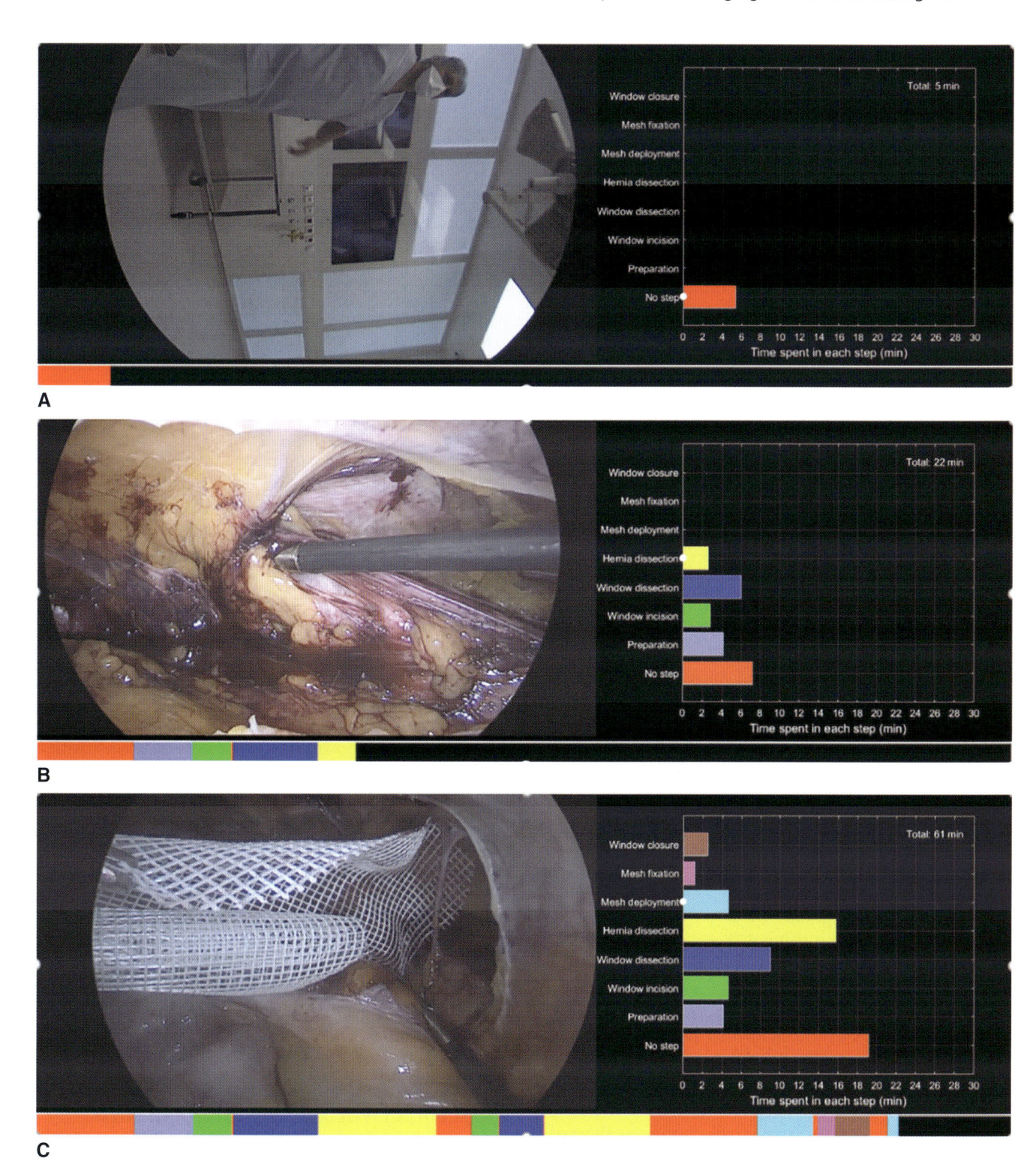

Implemented Imaging and Artificial Intelligence   81

FIGURE 6-17 • Automatic surgical step recognition system for hernia repair with AI.

FLS, there is considerable cost associated with proctors, as well as a time-consuming and labor-intensive need for task apparatus to be sent away for visual inspection. To overcome the limitations of manual scoring, automatic objective scoring using machine learning has been developed. Proposed solutions use the procedure video, the 3D movements of instruments (kinematic data) including velocity, rotation, and position information, or a combination of video and kinematic data. Kinematic data is substantially simpler to use as compared to video data, which requires advanced computer vision techniques to extract relevant information, such as the detection and tracking of instruments or sutures. These techniques usually require intensive data preparation to construct training data sets involving instrument detection delineated by hand (annotation). Crowdsourcing is an effective strategy to reduce the annotation cost using a workforce of laymen annotators organized online.

The Johns Hopkins University and Intuitive Surgical, Inc. Gesture and Skill Assessment Working Set (JIGSAWS) is a widely used data set to prototype autonomous scoring systems. Surgical videos and kinematic data were recorded of surgeons with 3 skill levels (expert, intermediate, and novice) using a da Vinci robot and a benchtop model to perform fundamental tasks (suturing, knot-tying, and needle passing). Scoring approaches using various machine learning tools including CNNs, recurrent neural networks (RNNs), and Markov chains have been attempted with excellent results in classifying 3 skill classes with an overall accuracy of 98.7%.

Automatic skills assessment from real surgical videos has also been studied. Jin et al. expanded the Cholec80 data set to include instrument annotations (the m2cai16-tool-locations) to train deep learning models to track tool motion. Instrument usage and movement patterns were found to correlate well with the Global Operative Assessment of Laparoscopic Skills (GOALS) rating system that assesses depth perception, bimanual dexterity, efficiency, and tissue handling. However, testing was limited to a few videos and a descriptive analysis. Recently, Lavanchy et al. proposed a method to automatically rate skills into 5 categories using automatic instrument tracking and logistic regression (see suggested reading #21). In a private cholecystectomy video data set, the system distinguished good versus poor surgical skills with an accuracy of 87 ± 0.2%. Further research is necessary to achieve both a finer-grained assessment of skills and to convey more relevant information to the user beyond a single skill rating. This could be implemented using explainable AI methods such as Grad-CAM to identify sections of the video that most contributed to the skills rating.

In the future, improved automatic objective skills assessment will have a profound impact on surgical education, quantitative learning curve assessment, as well as on the evaluation of residency programs. Other important uses of AI tools in surgical education that are likely to be introduced in the coming years include automatic retrieval of relevant previous surgical videos to prepare for surgery, and automatic video curation for online learning platforms such as WebSurg. For example, a user will automatically be presented with a custom set of educational videos, each one augmented with personalized educational information including AR visualizations and anatomical labeling with automatic recognition. Telemetry measurements and data transfer promote the evaluation of surgeon performance and proficiency. Video storage provides a logbook of cases that can be assessed for technical improvements. Procedure analysis on a high level allows benchmarking against best practice worldwide and promotes the reproducibility of best techniques. Digital intraoperative guidance has the potential to reduce the cognitive burden of surgeons, prevent mistakes or complications, and promote operator independence.

Safety Alerts

Human error is a major, yet preventable cause of complications and poor surgery outcomes. The 2019 Baylor College of Medicine study found that more than half of adverse events within 6 months of surgery were caused by human performance deficiency. In response, AI systems capable of detecting or anticipating human errors in surgery are intensively investigated.

Several studies focus on the automatic visual verification of established safety guidelines using deep learning. For example, bile duct injury after laparoscopic cholecystectomy can lead to life-altering complications, and rates of injury have increased to approximately 3 per 1000 procedures. The Critical View of Safety (CVS) was introduced to prevent injury, by ensuring a correct identification of the cystic duct and cystic artery. Automatic verification of the CVS has been recently attempted with CNNs as a safety alert system. Other studies aim to automatically identify safe and unsafe ("No Go") zones, which, combined with instrument tracking, can produce a safety alert system for unsafe dissection. Madani et al. developed a system for laparoscopic cholecystectomy that identifies safe ("Go") zones (areas within the hepatocystic triangle with a low risk of bile duct injury) and unsafe ("No Go") zones (see suggested reading #15). This was implemented using semantic segmentation CNNs, producing a mean Intersection over Union (IOU) score of 0.54 for "Go" zones and 0.71 for "No Go" zones. These results are encouraging. However, they are not sufficiently accurate for clinical practice. The main difficulty stems from inherent challenges to precisely identify anatomical structures in surgical videos and annotation subjectivity.

It may seem that errors in such safety systems are less critical as compared to errors in a surgical decision-making system. However, they carry important risks associated with an *automation bias*, the term used to describe an over-reliance on a decision-making support system. In the case of CVS for example, if a system fails to warn a surgeon of an incomplete critical view, we may think that no extra harm is done by the system (the surgeon would have made a mistake without using the system anyway). However, this is false when the surgeon becomes overreliant on the system's recommendation. Consequently, education is of paramount importance to ensure that surgeons understand the capabilities and limitations of the system to avoid an overreliance on imperfect technology. It is expected that surgery competency assessment programs will need to adapt to include the assessment of appropriate reliance on AI tools.

THE CHALLENGES OF SURGICAL AI AND PATHS TO ADOPTION

Despite much interest surrounding surgical AI, there are several key challenges that must be overcome for a broader adoption. In addition to legal, ethical, and regulatory considerations associated with creating any medical device including one that uses AI technology, there are 4 other main barriers to adopting surgical AI tools in clinical practice:

1. Surgical data acquisition and management
2. Data labeling and data quality
3. Explainable and trustworthy AI
4. Reproducibility

Surgical Data Acquisition

Surgical data is key to training and evaluating surgical AI systems. The data required by a surgical AI system depends on the exact application, which can range from preoperative CT or MR images, patient questionnaires, Electronic Health Record (EHR) data, intraoperative endoscopic videos, OR ceiling cameras, to postoperative wearable device data. Today, only a small proportion of this data is routinely stored, organized, and prepared in a way that it is suitable to train an AI system. However, to fully realize the potential of surgical AI, access and structuring of this heterogeneous data from multiple devices at different stages of the treatment path is essential. In addition, the stored data must be appropriately organized and accessible to AI systems to train them and to evaluate their performance in controlled conditions. There are major legal and regulatory issues with doing this correctly that protect the privacy and rights of patients and medical staff.

> **CONCEPTUAL HIGHLIGHTS**
>
> To fully realize the potential of surgical AI, access and structuring of heterogeneous patient data from multiple devices at different stages of the treatment pathway are essential. Because this is challenging from technical, regulatory, and ethical perspectives, shorter-term progress will be made using limited data (e.g., just the endoscopic video, which may be sufficient for simpler objectives such as step recognition).

There are now some significant advances toward introducing data capture and management systems into the OR from the industry, such as GE's Edison platform, the Surgical Black Box, and Karl Storz's OR1, as well as upcoming robotic platforms integrating data acquisition, storage, and management. This is driven by the high value seen by these companies in providing a key data service, and in the intrinsic value of the data. A broader use of these systems in the coming years will drive surgical AI innovation and adoption. Nevertheless, there are associated risks with using such systems, even those that fully adhere to all regulatory, legal, and ethical requirements. The main risk is a "walled garden" approach to data collection, where a closed ecosystem is built by a corporation that has a powerful influence on the control of data, using, for example, proprietary standards that are only compatible with the corporation's hardware. This element may stifle innovation, by making it more difficult to access data by independent academic institutes to develop and test surgical AI systems. There are several major projects initiated with collaborations between academia and the industry to develop open standards and OR data management systems to avoid a walled garden approach.

The Connected Optimized Network and Data in Operating Rooms (CONDOR) project, led by BPI France partnered with IRCAD, IHU Strasbourg, the University of Strasbourg, and the University of Rennes and Harmonic, is one such initiative. This project extends the DICOM standard to real-time video (DICOM-RTV), data capture from heterogeneous OR devices, to create publicly accessible annotated data sets, and AI systems to predict adverse events and complications from surgical videos. Another important open initiative is OR 4.0 from the University of Heidelberg in partnership with Karl Storz (Tuttlingen, Germany).

> **EDITORIAL COMMENT**
>
> UIC is working, in partnership with Argonne National Laboratory, on perioperative mass data acquisition (both surgical videos and surgeon kinematic data) and machine learning with the aim of achieving an AI-powered surgical context awareness system for automatic procedure step recognition. This line of research, in the long term, may be used for making evaluation and providing feedback for personalized training, and pave the way toward a smart surgical warning/correcting system, and eventually semi or fully automatic robotic surgery.

There are also important research efforts to train surgical AI systems using data from different centers where the patient data never leaves each hospital's secure network. This approach is known as federated learning, which is in contrast to the traditional approach of centralizing all data in one place. Federated learning can also be combined with differential privacy (DP), which is a technique that makes it practically impossible to know whether a patient's data contributed to training an AI model, even if one has complete access to the model's parameters (e.g., the neural network's weights). Federated learning and DP have only recently been applied to train surgical AI systems, for example at King's College London, in collaboration with NVIDIA (Santa Clara, CA, USA) and the NHS using the Clara AI platform.

Data Labeling and Data Quality

Most surgical AI models are trained using data and supervised learning, which involves careful data preparation and a data labeling process (also known as annotation). The annotation is used to teach an AI model to make predictions from previous examples (training data). In surgical step recognition, the data is the surgical video and the labels are the surgical steps associated with each image in the video. Other labels may include 30-day mortality, or readmission, required to predict complications. The time and cost associated with acquiring labeled data and ensuring that it is correct is often one of the strongest barriers to the adoption of AI. The difficulty of acquiring labeled data depends on the task at hand and the skill required to label the data. In addition, labels can have errors or be subjective, particularly for tasks that are difficult to annotate by expert surgeons, such as labeling the quality of a procedure from a surgical video or rating a surgeon's performance for AI-based competency assessment. The most basic of surgical AI applications should be considered in order to detect smoke in the images during robot-assisted laparoscopic surgery. A basic clinical application is to automatically engage the aspiration to prevent loss of visibility and maintain safety, which could save time and reduce cognitive load. Training this model can be performed with a set of laparoscopic images with one label per image (the presence or absence of smoke). Gathering this data may seem straightforward because it is simple for most humans to detect smoke in a laparoscopic image, and it has been shown that CNNs can do well at this basic task. However, problems are encountered quickly. Indeed, it is not the presence or absence of smoke that should trigger the aspiration, but merely the moment prior to reducing visibility. Consequently, instead, it is necessary to label each image in terms of visibility rather than the presence or absence of smoke. However, this is more challenging because "sufficient visibility" is not quantified and has confounding factors (e.g., endoscope illumination, dirt on the endoscope, image focus, etc.). As a result, even the most mundane surgical AI task may be difficult to annotate. This problem grows substantially for more challenging tasks, such as assessing the adequacy of a colonic anastomosis.

> **CONCEPTUAL HIGHLIGHTS**
>
> "Annotated data" and "labeled data" are synonymous. They mean data coupled with one or more variables that we want the machine to predict.

> **CHALLENGES AND POTENTIAL PITFALLS**
>
> The time and cost associated with acquiring high-quality labeled data are often the strongest barriers to the adoption of surgical AI tools.

The challenges associated with acquiring annotated data can be reduced substantially using better annotation tools that can evaluate consistency, and to reduce the need for large annotated data sets. In the latter case, transfer learning has emerged as a very important solution. This involves first training a deep neural network on a larger data set that is not directly associated with the target application. The network's features (specifically the weights that connect the network's neurons) are then copied onto a second neural network that is slightly adapted to solve the target application using a smaller training data set. It may be surprising to learn that, in surgical AI using video data, the original deep neural network is usually trained on the ImageNet data set, which consists of over 1 million nonmedical images of buildings, plants, and cats. A neural network trained on this kind of data can learn to extract general purpose image features that are also good at discriminating structures in other domains, including medical videos. Transfer learning can reduce the amount of required annotated data with several orders of magnitude, and it is possible to train some applications with a few hundred images. It is used in most if not all AI health care systems that involve deep learning today.

> **CONCEPTUAL HIGHLIGHTS**
>
> Transfer learning is one of the essential tools to create surgical AI systems with limited data sets. It involves the reuse of components of deep learning models trained on larger related data sets.

Another major step forward is the development of easy-to-use annotation software tools, which can significantly reduce the amount of time required to annotate surgical images and improve annotation quality. IRCAD/IHU have developed a web-based annotation platform called Indexity (**Figure 6-18**), which allows surgical video annotation with quality control checks. In addition, it supports collaborative AI annotation, where an expert can validate automatically generated annotations produced by means of a machine learning model, hence substantially reducing the time and cost of annotation.

Explainable and Trustworthy AI

The high risks associated with the use of AI systems to influence treatment processes require strict regulatory processes and clinical validation to make sure that the technology is safe and reliable. This can be especially hard with AI technologies that are highly complex computation systems, the reliability of which can be difficult to predict. Indeed, today, the most successful form of AI to process medical image data is deep learning, which is a powerful, yet particularly "opaque" form of AI using a computational network arranged in a hierarchical structure to resemble the arrangement of biological neurons. Its exceptional performance can rival or exceed expert level human performance across many tasks. However, deep learning models are extremely hard to understand and, nowadays, they do not provide sufficient mechanisms to explain or justify their decisions, nor do they communicate adequately when they may fail to make an accurate prediction. It is also difficult to clearly explain what biases may have been learned from data. For example, a system trained from data in one hospital to assess the adequacy of a surgical dissection may not work well on data from another hospital because of differences in customs or surgical approaches. As a result, it is dangerous to use such a system without understanding the biases learned in the data. In summary, the problem of *explainability* is a strong barrier preventing trust and adoption of surgical AI in routine clinical use.

To overcome this barrier, there is great interest in developing explainable AI (XAI) systems for surgical decision-making support. XAI is the subfield of AI to allow the results of a machine learning model to be understood and interpreted by humans, and it follows 3 principles: transparency, interpretability, and explainability. XAI contrasts "black box" AI models (i.e., nonexplainable models), shown in **Figure 6-19**, where the machine outputs a prediction only. The designers of a "black box" model normally cannot easily explain why a model produces a decision, nor answer the following important questions:

- Why should the model's outputs be trusted?
- Why did the model make a certain decision?
- What drives model predictions?

There is ongoing progress among XAI research to create models that can answer these questions. XAI can be implemented in several ways and a common approach is illustrated in **Figure 6-19** to predict the likelihood of adverse events such as complications or readmissions using demographic clinical parameters. However, if the system only produces a prediction,

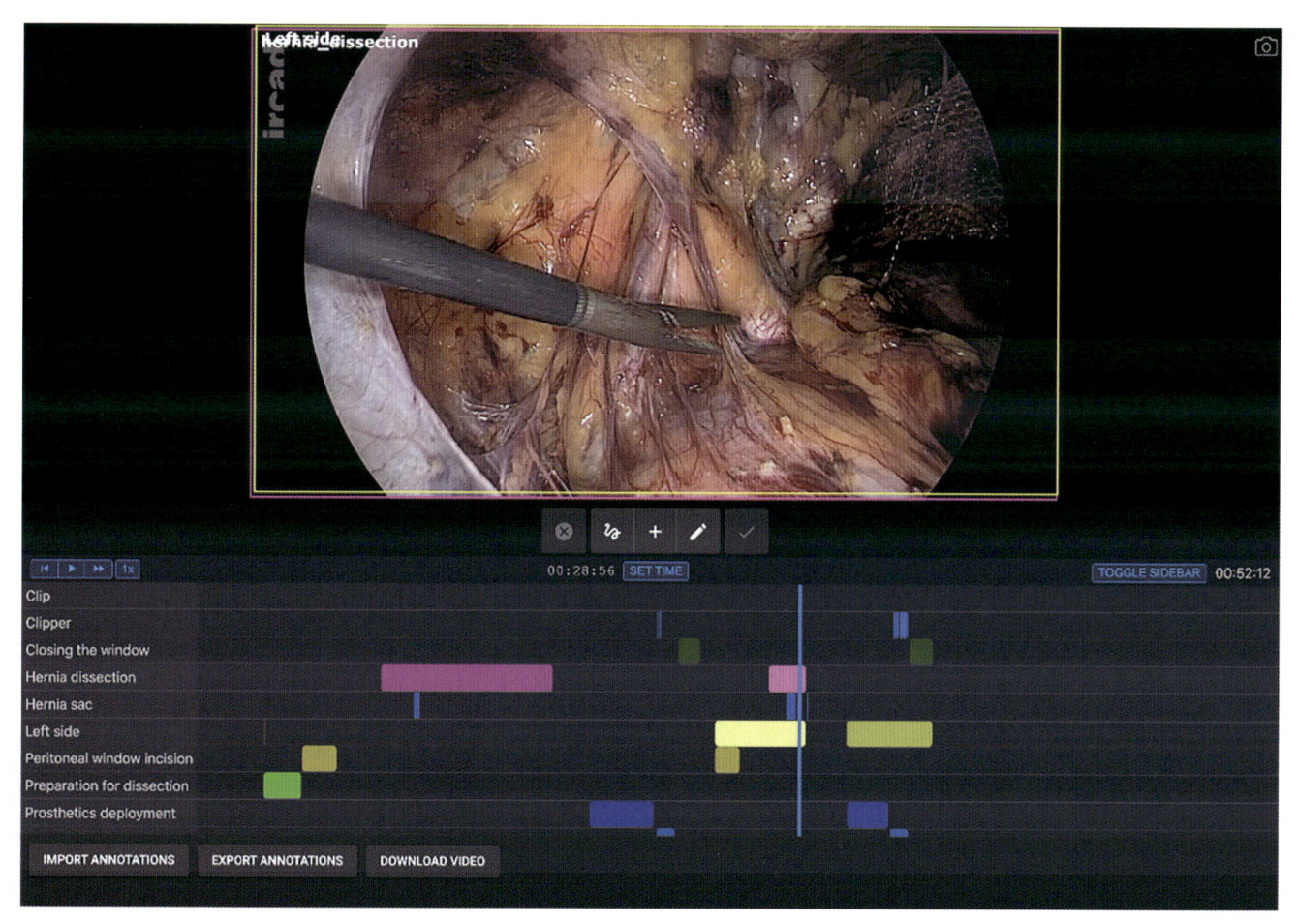

Implemented Imaging and Artificial Intelligence 85

FIGURE 6-18 • The Indexity web-based annotation platform.

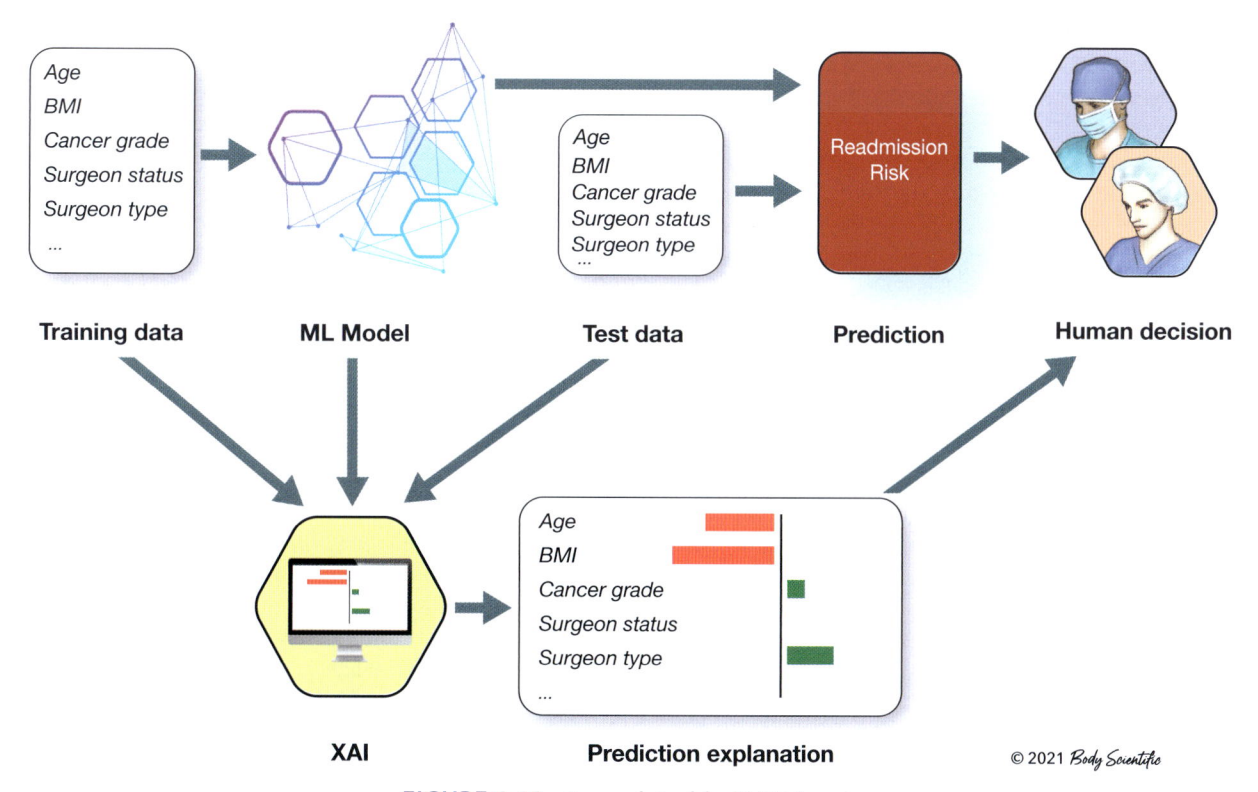

FIGURE 6-19 • An explainable AI (XAI) system.

its value is limited to both the surgeon and patient, because the AI model does not supply an explanation for its prediction. In contrast, in XAI, each feature is associated with a degree-of-influence on the prediction. A red bar indicates that a feature contributed to a low-risk prediction (a longer bar indicating a higher contribution). A green bar indicates that a feature contributed to a high-risk prediction. This information can help to convey the justification for an AI model's decision.

Some XAI systems such as Local Interpretable Model-Agnostic Explanations (LIME) and Shapely Additive Explanations (SHAP) explain the prediction by revealing what specific characteristics of the test data lead to the decision. The main idea behind LIME is that, given a complex AI model, its behavior for a specific prediction can be adequately approximated by a simpler and interpretable model such as a logistic regression model, giving the relative importance of the features (i.e., their influence on the prediction). However, XAI tools such as LIME and SHAP do not supply a complete explanation, such as data biases and confounders, and more research work is required to automatically detect them.

Reproducibility

The prediction of a surgical AI system is determined by 3 main factors: *data* (for training the system and for making the prediction), *software* (in particular the machine learning model architecture design, the learning algorithm, and its associated parameters), and computer *hardware* (for running the software to train and test the model, which is usually not run on the same computer). Many key choices must be made when designing an AI system particularly related to data (e.g., how to divide data into training and testing sets, and how to annotate data), and software (e.g., setting the number of neural network layers, the learning rate, and the choice of loss function). These choices do not represent an exact science and reproducibility is becoming a major issue in surgical AI research and AI research in general. According to the American Statistical Association (ASA), "A study is reproducible if you can take the original data and the computer code used to analyze the data and reproduce all of the numerical findings from the study." Measures to assure that surgical AI research is reproducible is essential for scientific progress and for trusting AI systems in the clinic. A worthwhile way is to apply data science best practices, which include code and data versioning to allow a complete history of changes and updates to be recorded during project development and product improvements. Additionally, many journals such as the ones in the Nature portfolio are now promoting reproducible research by requiring data to be publicly available and code to be available to reviewers during peer review. This combats the problem that it is usually impossible to replicate an AI study from its description in an academic paper because it is unfeasible to document all data and software decisions in a manuscript. However, code and data availability are not fully guaranteed to ensure that a study is reproducible. It is because most methods using deep learning involve randomized variables (e.g., the initialization of network weights is usually randomly selected, and training batches are drawn randomly). If one is not careful, running exactly the same software twice with no software changes may not produce identical results.

This can be controlled for the most part by ensuring that all random variables are similar for every software execution (by setting the random seeds). However, this is still not totally sufficient for reproducibility. Differences in hardware and versions of software libraries used to train the system may also yield slightly different results. It is subsequently difficult to ensure exact reproducibility unless all software and hardware configurations are documented and tightly controlled. To handle such challenges, journals and conference societies such as Medical Image Computing and Computer-Assisted Intervention (MIC-CAI) demand a reproducibility checklist with each submission, which includes a description of the measures adopted to obtain good, if not perfect, reproducibility.

SURGICAL AI BROADER PERSPECTIVES

Today, the impact and benefits of surgical AI research has been only scratched at its surface. This is mainly due to the above challenges that create tough clinical translation barriers. In the short run, surgical AI tools will, and have already, emerged to help with relatively basic and low-risk tasks that include automatic surgical step recognition, smart camera control in robotic laparoscopic surgery, tools to detect human errors such as a failure to achieve the CVS in laparoscopic cholecystectomy, and learning curve assessment.

These short-term goals are pursued by research groups, not because of lack of ambition, but for pragmatic and feasibility reasons. They are the kind of tools that stand the quickest route to clinical use because of the lower patient risk associated with system failures. Nevertheless, there are risks associated with any autonomous decision aid because of *automation bias*. Surgery automation with robotics and AI carries greater risks than a correctly used clinical decision-making support system, especially because of the difficulty that state-of-the-art deep learning algorithms have to adapt to dynamic and unpredictable environments. Laparoscopic intervention represents one of the hardest possible environments for the autonomous planning, execution, assessment, and adaptation of surgical actions, requiring a high dexterity and precise motor control. Other forms of surgery such as percutaneous surgery, where the effect of the needle on the patient is spatially localized to a small zone and easier to predict, stand a much greater chance of full automation in the coming decade, because it is simply more technically feasible.

The ongoing translation of basic surgical decision-making support AI tools should demonstrate measurable value to the patient. Their use should also pave the way for more streamlined data collection that will serve other more ambitious AI goals. Virtually all of the AI tools built today use only a small portion of the patient's data (e.g., only the laparoscopic video, ignoring other major parameters that contribute to surgical decisions and outcomes). Thanks to the increasing connectivity of devices and health care IT systems, the data will and should be drawn from a wide range of sources including images, lab reports, genetics, patient history, wearable technologies, and psychological parameters to incorporate patient sentiment and emotion. This will allow a personalized treatment strategy with associated risks clearly communicated with explainable AI backed up by reproducible research. Despite all attempts for standardized treatment recommendations including sophisticated algorithms and analysis of all available data, the final therapeutic decision remains a deeply personal one. Data analysis will allow for a technically optimized operation and treatment plan. However, with the patient understanding the disease and treatment options, value-based health care integrates informed consent tailoring any therapeutic approach to each patient's individual priorities. Even with the most advanced technological achievements, patient care including surgery relies on empathy and shared decision-making.

Suggested Readings

1. Atallah S (ed.). *Digital Surgery*. Springer; 2021. doi: 10.1007/978-3-030-49100-0
2. Mascagni P, Longo F, Barberio M, et al. New intraoperative imaging technologies: Innovating the surgeon's eye toward surgical precision. *J Surg Oncol*. 2018;118(2):265-282. doi: 10.1002/jso.25148
3. Pessaux P, Diana M, Soler L, Piardi T, Mutter D, Marescaux J. Towards cybernetic surgery: robotic and augmented reality-assisted liver segmentectomy. *Langenbecks Arch Surg*. 2015; 400(3):381-385. doi: 10.1007/s00423-014-1256-9
4. Diana M, Soler L, Agnus V, et al. Prospective evaluation of precision multimodal gallbladder surgery navigation: virtual reality, near-infrared fluorescence, and x-ray-based intraoperative cholangiography. *Ann Surg*. 2017;266(5):890-897. doi: 10.1097/SLA.0000000000002400
5. Seeliger B, Agnus V, Mascagni P, et al. Simultaneous computer-assisted assessment of mucosal and serosal perfusion in a model of segmental colonic ischemia. *Surg Endosc*. 2020;34(11): 4818-4827. doi: 10.1007/s00464-019-07258-z
6. Kong SH, Haouchine N, Soares R, et al. Robust augmented reality registration method for localization of solid organs' tumors using CT-derived virtual biomechanical model and fluorescent fiducials. *Surg Endosc*. 2017;31(7):2863-2871. doi: 10.1007/s00464-016-5297-8
7. Atallah S, Parra-Davila E, Melani AGF, Romagnolo LG, Larach SW, Marescaux J. Robotic-assisted stereotactic real-time navigation: initial clinical experience and feasibility for rectal cancer surgery. *Tech Coloproctol*. 2019;23(1):53-63. doi: 10.1007/s10151-018-1914-y
8. Gimenez M, Gallix B, Costamagna G, et al. Definitions of computer-assisted surgery and intervention, image-guided surgery and intervention, hybrid operating room, and guidance systems: Strasbourg International Consensus Study. *Ann Surg Open*. 2020;1(2):e021. doi: 10.1097/AS9.0000000000000021
9. Son GM, Kwon MS, Kim Y, Kim J, Kim SH, Lee JW. Quantitative analysis of colon perfusion pattern using indocyanine green (ICG) angiography in laparoscopic colorectal surgery. *Surg Endosc*. 2019;33(5):1640-1649. doi: 10.1007/s00464-018-6439-y
10. Park SH, Park HM, Baek KR, Ahn HM, Lee IY, Son GM. Artificial intelligence based real-time microcirculation analysis system for laparoscopic colorectal surgery. *World J Gastroenterol*. 2020;26(44):6945-6962. doi: 10.3748/wjg.v26.i44.6945
11. Cahill RA, O'Shea DF, Khan MF, et al. Artificial intelligence indocyanine green (ICG) perfusion for colorectal cancer intra-operative tissue classification. *Br J Surg*. 2021;108(1):5-9. doi: 10.1093/bjs/znaa004
12. Hashimoto DA, Rosman G, Meireles OR. *Artificial Intelligence in Surgery: Understanding the Role of AI in Surgical Practice*. McGraw-Hill Education; 2021.
13. Bernhard S, Nicolau S, Soler L, Doignon C. The status of augmented reality in laparoscopic surgery as of 2016. *Med Image Anal*. 2017;37:66-90. doi: 10.1016/j.media.2017.01.007
14. Mascagni P, Vardazaryan A, Alapatt D, et al. Artificial intelligence for surgical safety: automatic assessment of the critical view of safety in laparoscopic cholecystectomy using deep learning. *Ann Surg*. 2020 Nov 16. doi: 10.1097/SLA.0000000000004351
15. Madani A, Namazi B, Altieri MS, et al. Artificial intelligence for intraoperative guidance: using semantic segmentation to identify surgical anatomy during laparoscopic cholecystectomy. *Ann Surg*. 2020 Nov 13. doi: 10.1097/SLA.0000000000004594
16. Modrzejewski R, Collins T, Bartoli A, Hostettler A, Marescaux J. Soft-*Body Registration of Pre-operative 3D Models to Intra-operative RGBD Partial Body Scans*. Springer International Publishing; 2018:39-46. doi: 10.1007/978-3-030-00937-3_5
17. Allan M, Shvets A, Kurmann T, et al. 2017 robotic instrument segmentation challenge. *arXiv preprint*. 2019; arXiv:190206426.
18. Twinanda AP, Shehata S, Mutter D, Marescaux J, De Mathelin M, Padoy N. Endonet: a deep architecture for recognition tasks on laparoscopic videos. *IEEE Trans Med Imaging*. 2016;36(1):86-97. doi: 10.1109/TMI.2016.2593957
19. Gao Y, Vedula SS, Reiley CE, et al. Jhu-isi gesture and skill assessment working set (JIGSAWS): a surgical activity dataset for human motion modeling. 2014. https://cirl.lcsr.jhu.edu/wp-content/uploads/2015/11/JIGSAWS.pdf
20. Yanik E, Intes X, Kruger U, et al. Deep neural networks for the assessment of surgical skills: a systematic review. *The Journal of Defense Modeling and Simulation*. 2022;19(2):159–171. doi: 10.1177/15485129211034586
21. Lavanchy JL, Zindel J, Kirtac K, et al. Automation of surgical skill assessment using a three-stage machine learning algorithm. *Sci Rep*. 2021;11(1):5197. doi: 10.1038/s41598-021-84295-6
22. Maier-Hein L, Vedula SS, Speidel S, et al. Surgical data science for next-generation interventions. *Nat Biomed Eng*. 2017;1:691-696. doi: 10.1038/s41551-017-0132-7
23. Giulianotti PC, Coratti A, Angelini M, et al. Robotics in general surgery: personal experience in a large community hospital. *Arch Surg*. 2003;138(7):777-784. doi: 10.1001/archsurg.138.7.777

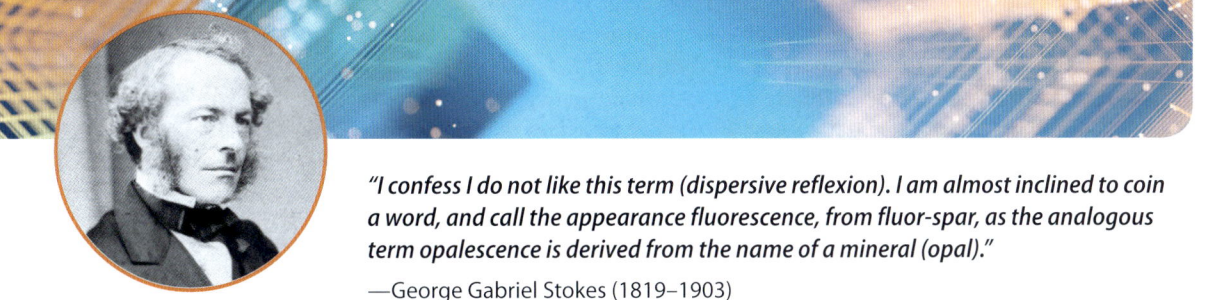

"I confess I do not like this term (dispersive reflexion). I am almost inclined to coin a word, and call the appearance fluorescence, from fluor-spar, as the analogous term opalescence is derived from the name of a mineral (opal)."

—George Gabriel Stokes (1819–1903)

Fluorescence Imaging: Basics and Clinical Applications

Liaohai Chen • Carolina Baz • Natalija Lakic • Pier Cristoforo Giulianotti

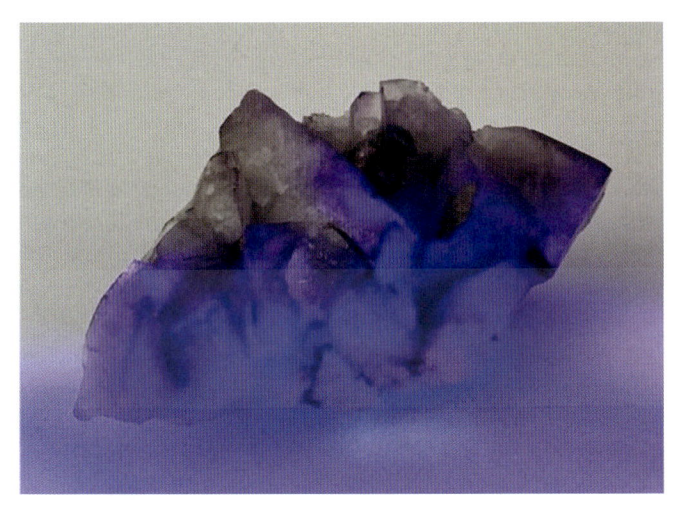

Fluorite—Seen under long-wave UV light.

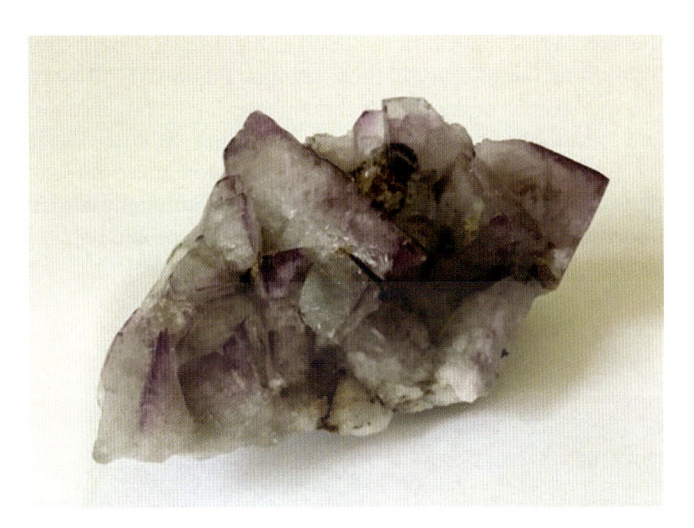

Fluorite—Viewed with visible light only.

BASICS OF FLUORESCENCE IMAGING

One unique feature of robotic surgery is the physical separation of the surgeon and the patient by a robotic platform. As surgeons cannot see the surgical field directly, they rely on an endoscopic camera to view the anatomy of the surgical plane and to perform the surgery. Common endoscopic cameras use white-light imaging, which is formed based on the light absorption and scattering contrasts. Tissues with large differences in absorption and scattering profiles can be clearly viewed by white-light imaging. However, some other tissues such as early-stage lesions have similar scattering and absorption properties as those in the surrounding area, making them hard to be differentiated, and requiring additional optical contrasts to view them decisively. Fluorescence imaging has the capability of providing such additional contrasts.

Fluorescence is an optical process that involves electrons being excited into a higher energy state (excited state) after certain molecules (fluorophores) absorb the light. These excited electrons lose some of the acquired light energy through

Photo from Hulton Archive / Stringer. Getty Images.
Quote reproduced with permission from Stokes GG. On the change of refrangibility of light. Philos Trans R Soc Lond B Biol Sci. 1852;142(1852):463-562.

vibrational relaxation and then settle to a lower-level state. As electrons start dropping from the lowest energy state to their ground state, they release the rest of the energy gained in the excitation process through a form of light known as fluorescence. Compared to the excitation light, fluorescence has lower energy and therefore it is normally observed at wavelengths that are longer than the excitation one (i.e., red-shifted). Such a light turn-on process at the fluorescence detection wavelength has a higher signal-to-noise ratio due to the dark background. As a result, fluorescence imaging has better sensitivity than regular white-light imaging—up to 3 orders of magnitude more, theoretically.

Based on this mechanism, the fluorescence intensity of a tissue sample is proportional to the excitation light intensity, the fluorescence quantum yield of the fluorophore inside the tissue (the percentage of photons emitted over the photons received), the ability of the fluorophore to absorb light (extinction coefficient), and the fluorophore concentration. To image a target surrounded by normal tissues via fluorescence, the fluorescence intensity contrast between the target and surrounding tissues needs to be sufficiently large. Normal tissues, which are mainly made from water, blood, proteins, lipids, and nucleic acids, have lower fluorescence quantum yields, but larger extinction coefficients in the ultraviolet-visible (UV-Vis) region (<650 nm) and the short-wavelength infrared (SWIR) band (>1500 nm), thus have strong fluorescence in those regions (**Figure 7-1**). To view the endogenous or exogenous fluorophores in the target tissue, and to minimize the interference of normal tissue fluorescence (i.e., so-called background fluorescence or autofluorescence), an optical window in the 650–1500-nm region is commonly used in target tissue fluorescence imaging unless the fluorophore has a very large fluorescence quantum yield. In addition, as the depth of light penetration is proportional to the light wavelength, fluorophores that absorb and emit light in the 650–1500-nm optical window are preferred since their fluorescence can penetrate deeper in tissues than those in the UV-Vis region, thus having the potential to image a target underneath the tissue surface.

Currently, 3 fluorescence dye molecules are approved by the FDA (Food and Drug Administration) for *in vivo* medical applications: fluorescein, methylene blue, and indocyanine green (ICG). Among them, ICG is the most commonly used dye due to its near-infrared (NIR) absorption and emission wavelengths, which render less tissue background fluorescence and deeper tissue penetration.

Structure-wise, ICG belongs to the cyanine dye family with electron donor and acceptor motifs linked by polymethine scaffolds. Like many other cyanine dyes, its photoinduced intramolecular charge transfer nature makes ICG fluorescence sensitive to the polarity of the medium it resides in. Most cyanine dyes have a strong tendency to aggregate in water, and their aggregates display distinct changes in their absorption and emission spectra compared to their monomeric form. The same principle applies to ICG; the presence of a shoulder peak at 780 nm in the ICG absorption spectrum in water is due to the formation of H-aggregates (face-to-face stacking of ICG molecules), which yield weak or no fluorescence due to the existence of a forbidden exciton transition state. As a result, ICG has a fluorescence quantum yield of 0.12 in dimethyl sulfoxide as monomers, but only 0.04 in water due to the presence of many H-aggregates. On the other hand, the sharp and strong absorption peak at 900 nm with a higher extinction coefficient indicates the formation

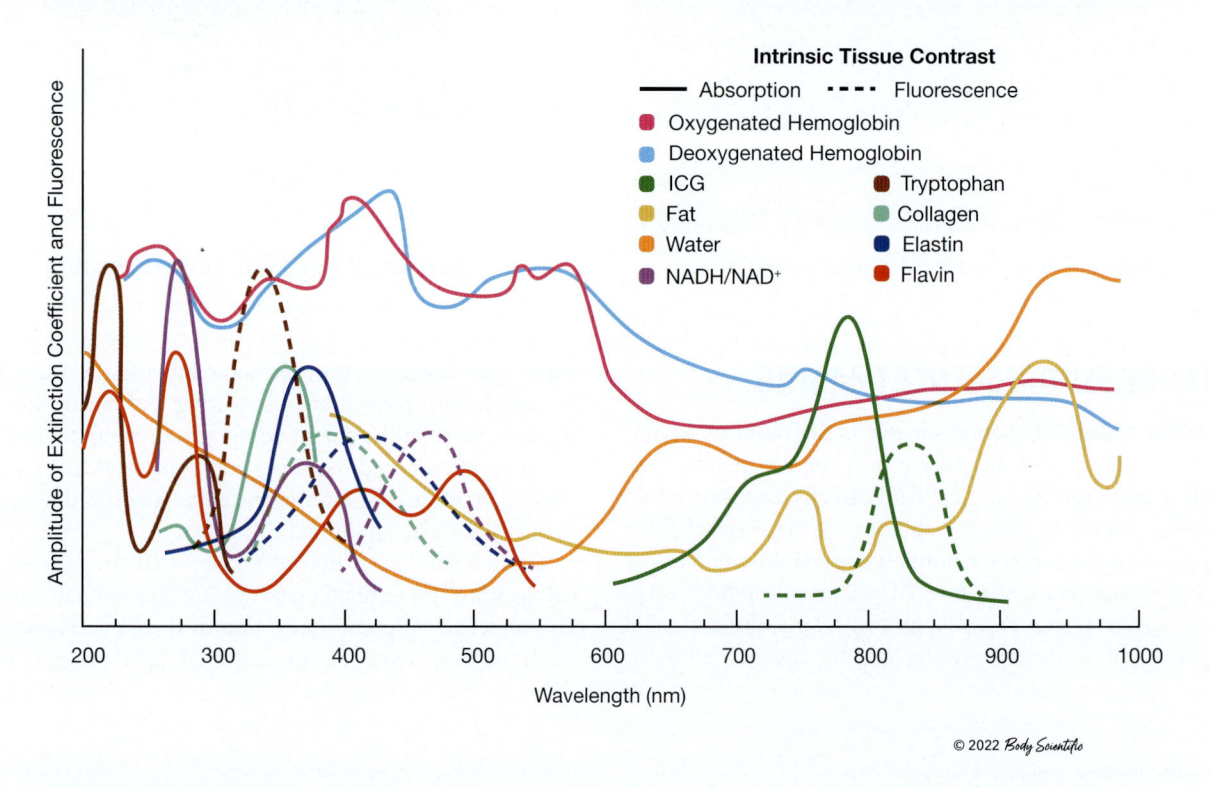

FIGURE 7-1 • Absorption and emission spectra of the tissue components and indocyanine green (ICG) dye.

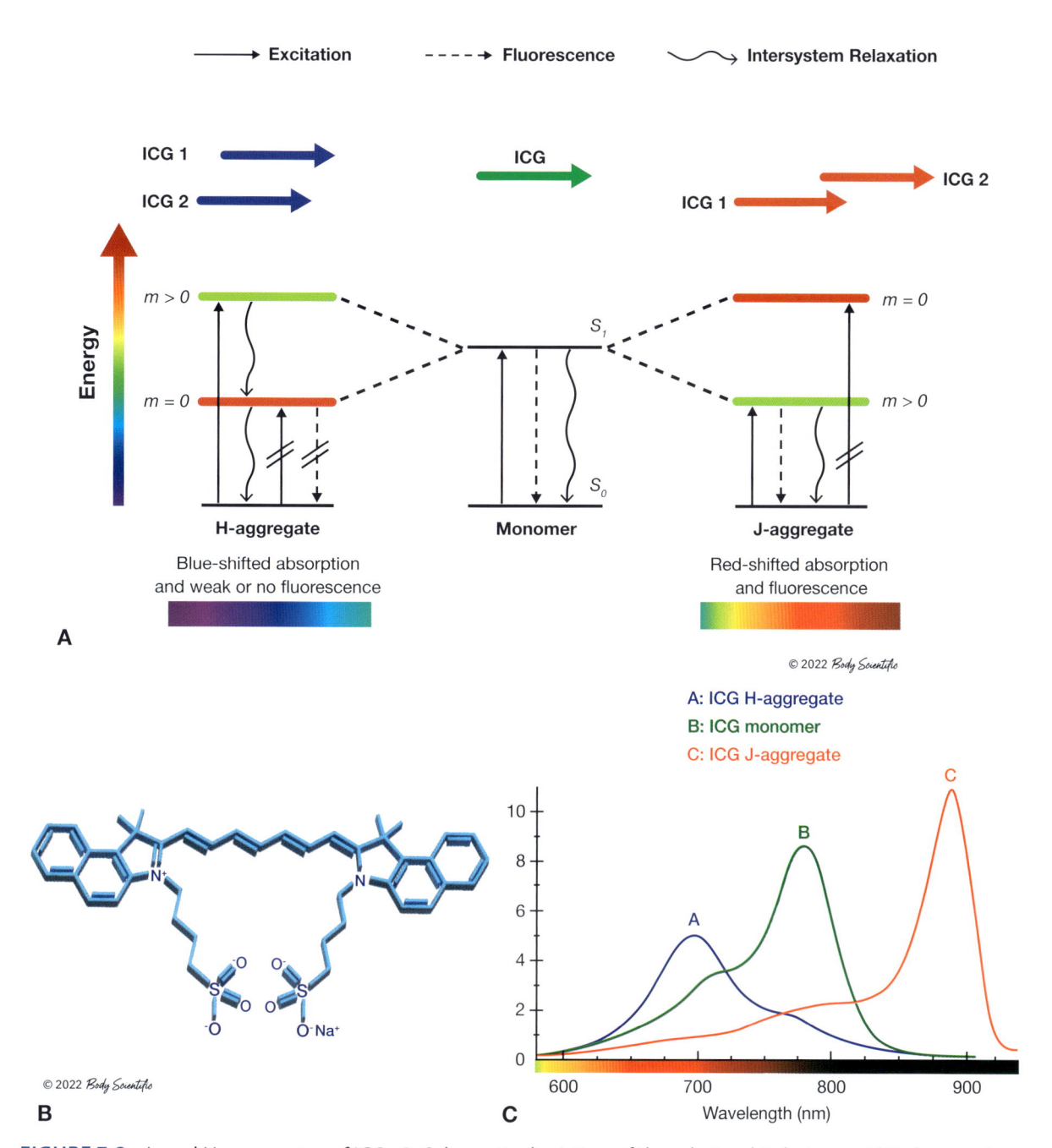

FIGURE 7-2 • J- and H-aggregates of ICG. **A.** Schematic depiction of the relationship between ICG chromophore orientation and the energy changes in allowable excitation and fluorescence on the formation of H- and J-aggregates from ICG monomers based on the molecular exciton theory. **B.** Chemical structure of ICG. **C.** Absorption spectra of ICG and its H- and J-aggregates.

of J-aggregates (head-to-tail stacking of ICG molecules), which can be formed after cooling a warmed ICG solution (**Figures 7-2 A–C**). Since J-aggregates of cyanine dyes theoretically can emit red-shifted fluorescence, ICG has been explored for fluorescence imaging at a wavelength above 1000 nm with better tissue penetration and less background autofluorescence (see "Perspectives" section).

Another unique property of ICG that enables its clinical application, despite its complicated photophysical properties, is its ability to specifically interact with human serum albumin (HSA) protein with binding affinity constants at the micromolar range. The binding pocket of ICG in HSA is in the hydrophobic area of the protein and only allows 1 ICG binding to 1 HAS (**Figure 7-3**). Thus, when ICG is administered intravenously, the high concentration of HSA in the blood keeps most of the ICG molecules in their monomeric form. This interaction of ICG with HSA is sustained throughout the circulation process until ICG is eventually cleared out through the bile ducts. This renders strong ICG fluorescence with minimal aggregation *in vivo*. However, when ICG is applied topically, its aggregation behaviors and the corresponding self-quenching fluorescence properties (due to the formation of H-aggregates) need to be considered. ICG also has 3 other favorable pharmacokinetic and pharmacodynamic properties: (1) a short plasma

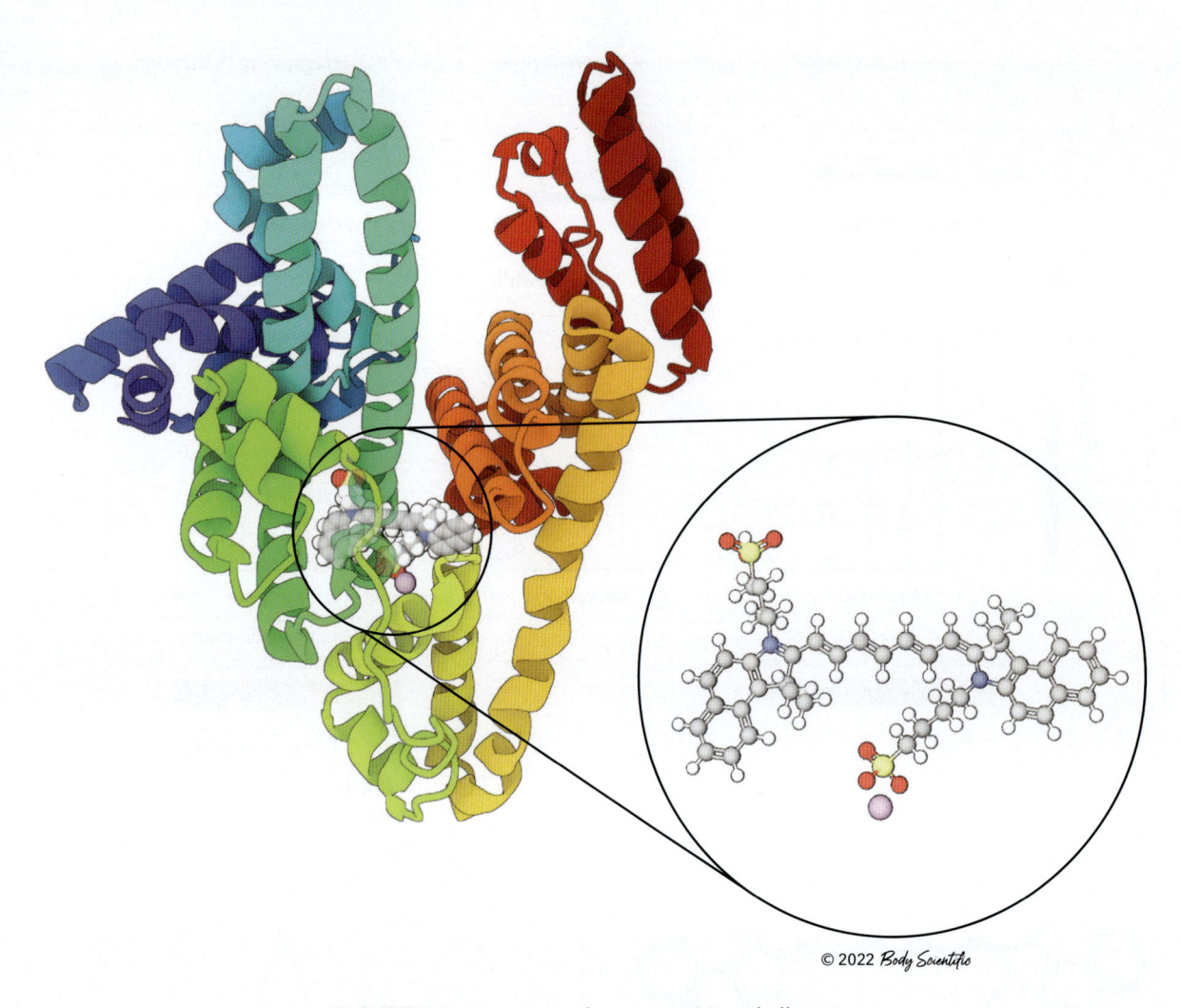

FIGURE 7-3 • Interaction between ICG and albumin.

life (3–5 minutes); (2) an extremely low toxicity and high safety index (1:300,000 adverse reaction rate; 2 mg/kg maximal recommended dose); and (3) a dominated biliary excretion pathway (10–15 minutes). All these features make ICG the most used fluorophore for anatomy visualization, perfusion assessment, and tumor imaging.

There are approximately 4 strategies to image a target tissue using fluorescence:

1. **Exploiting the intrinsic fluorescence properties of the target tissue.** Targets containing distinguished fluorophore profiles can be imaged as their fluorescence outstands the autofluorescence of surrounding tissues. For example, some specific tissues and some pathological ones have higher concentrations of riboflavin, lipofuscin, flavin adenine dinucleotide (FAD), or porphyrin fluorophores. This quantitative fluorophore increase can exhibit enough fluorescence contrast against the autofluorescence of normal tissues. While the advantage of this strategy is the avoidance of any dye molecules to be administered to the patients, the major limitation is the weaker fluorescence contrast of the target. In addition, the fluorescence wavelengths is in the UV Vis region, thus having much less depth penetration. One exception is the autofluorescence of the parathyroid glands, which has a fluorescence above 800 nm, therefore has been used for parathyroid imaging during robotic thyroidectomy.

2. **Following a fluorescent tracer.** This strategy involves the introduction of a fluorescence dye, a fluorescent tracer, into the patient. As the tracer disperses throughout the body, its fluorescent path can be imaged. Depending on the pharmacokinetic and pharmacodynamic properties of the tracer, as well as the properties of the tissue target, it can specifically accumulate in the target, thus highlighting the location and morphology of the target. For example, ICG has been routinely used for revealing blood vessel networks and bile ducts as it travels through the circulation and during its later excretion. It is also widely used to assess tissue perfusion by quantifying the fluorescence intensities as ICG disperses through the micro-vascular structures.

3. **Monitoring a fluorescence probe.** A fluorescent probe can be specifically designed and synthesized against a target so that it can be recruited and light up the target via fluorescence. This strategy takes advantage of ligand-receptor or antibody-antigen interactions by anchoring a dye molecule to a ligand or an antibody. Due to the unique expression or overexpression of a receptor or antigen in the target tissue,

the fluorescence probe can accumulate in the target due to the ligand-receptor or antibody-antigen interactions, thus providing a fluorescence contrast in the target against the surrounding normal tissues. For example, Cy5 fluorophore has been conjugated onto nerve-specific peptide NP41 (NTQTLAKAPEHT) that binds to laminins along the epineurium. The resulting Cy5-peptide probe can highlight peripheral nerves intraoperatively in live animal experiments.

4. **Using a fluorophore inducer**. In this strategy, a fluorescence inducer acting as an endogenous or exogenous fluorophore precursor is administered to the patient; it is based on a mechanism in which the fluorophore synthetic pathway is enhanced in the target tissue. Upon reaching the target, the inducer will either lead to the overproduction of the fluorophore or interact with other fluorophore precursors to form the fluorophore. The flourescence of the overformed fluorophores can therefore light up the target. For example, it is well established that the porphyrin synthesis pathway is enhanced in many types of solid tumors. By giving the patient 5-aminolevulinic acid (ALA), the first compound in the porphyrin synthesis pathway, before surgery, ALA will lead to the selective accumulation of the fluorophore of protoporphyrin IX (PpIX) in tumor cells. PpIX fluoresces strongly at 635 nm when excited by 405-nm light. Such a red–pink fluorescence contrast in tumors provides surgeons with real-time feedback of the surgical field and can be used to facilitate tumor resection.

One of the most common and pursued fluorescence applications is tumor imaging and margining. The key challenge in this application is the development of high-performance, tumor-specific imaging reagents. Tumor specificity can be achieved through the use of tracer (passive) or probe (active) tactics. In the passive approach, an imaging tracer such as ICG without a targeting motif is used. Since normal and tumoral tissues differ both in hemodynamic and metabolic properties, these differences in vascularization and excretion pathways allow, in many cases, a distinct accumulation of ICG in tumors. This will lead to a fluorescence contrast between the tumor and normal tissues, thus enabling the fluorescence visualization of the lesion. In the active approach, 2 types of imaging probes are used: the first type of target-specific probe consists of a tumor affinity reagent (such as an antibody, peptide, or small-molecule ligand against a cancer biomarker) conjugated with a NIR fluorescence dye. Following the administration to the patient, the imaging probe circulates through the body and builds up in the tumor due to the specific interactions between the probe and the tumor. Such a molecular imaging approach has shown better sensitivity and specificity. For example, an imaging probe of ICG-labeled trastuzumab has been used in the lab to image breast, stomach, gastroesophageal, ovarian, bladder, endometrial, pancreatic, and non–small cell lung cancers. Several target-specific probes have been under active clinical trials and the results have so far indicated that the imaging probe can guide a better dissection by delineating the tumor mass.

The second type of target-specific probe carries a unique "on-off" feature so that it is nonfluorescent during circulation or in normal tissues, but fluoresces in the tumoral tissue. Common designs for such an activable imaging probe include a NIR dye-linker-quencher triad architecture. The fluorescence is quenched due to the presence of a quencher in the triad probe. The linker is specifically structured as the substrate for a proteinase that is overpresented in tumors. The proteinase cleaves the linker, leading to dissociation of the quencher from the probe and resumption of the dye's fluorescence in tumors. For example, ICG has been conjugated to the quencher molecules through a short peptide that can function as the substrate for multiple cysteine cathepsins. In colorectal tumors, cathepsins are overexpressed by tumor-associated macrophages. Thus, the peptide linker can be effectively cleaved by the overexpressed cathepsins in the tumor. As a result, ICG-labeled cathepsin-activated imaging probes can highlight gastrointestinal lesions by fluorescence imaging. The advantage of this approach is that the probe fluorescence only turns on in colorectal tumors and does not produce fluorescent signals in normal mucosa, leading to improved tumor-to-background ratios. It also allows for imaging without a lengthy washout period of the probe in normal tissues, thus enabling intraoperative applications.

Another actively pursued research area in fluorescence is nerve imaging. Iatrogenic nerve injury is one of the causes of morbidity in patients undergoing surgery. Current methods for identifying nerves in real time involve neurophysiologic nerve stimulation, which only monitors nerve integrity without providing visual guidance; therefore, they are not feasible for imaging-guided surgery. There are 2 approaches for nerve visualization: using a dye molecule that has a different retention time in nerves and surrounding tissue; or deploying a nerve-specific imaging probe, in which an affinity reagent such as a peptide or antibody specific to nerves is labeled with fluorophores. For the first approach, ICG has been explored for visualizing the prostatic neurovascular bundle, the inferior hypogastric plexus, and other peripheral nerves using a negative contrast approach (see "Clinical Applications of Fluorescence Imaging in Robotic Surgery" section). At the same time, other fluorophores such as styryl pyridinium, tricarbocyanine, or oxazine have been found to bind to nerves specifically, showing noticeable sensitivity and nerve specificity in the lab. Current efforts have been focused on tuning the structure of these dyes to emit at the NIR region, while still maintaining their ability to cross the blood–nerve barrier and bind to nerves specifically. In the second approach, anti-ganglioside antibodies or nerve-specific peptides, including sodium channel selective peptide and nerve growth factor, have been labeled with NIR dyes to function as imaging probes for intraoperative nerve imaging (Nervelight™). In both cases, imaging reagents can be administered systemically and enriched in the peripheral nerves for intraoperative imaging of nerves.

APPARATUS FOR FLUORESCENCE IMAGE ACQUISITION

An overall apparatus for fluorescence imaging consists of (1) an excitation light source(s), (2) optics to direct the excitation light to the target, (3) optics to collect and direct the fluorescence light of the target to the detector, (4) a fluorescence detector/camera system, and (5) computer hardware and software for processing and displaying the image. Factors related to each component can affect the overall sensitivity of the image acquisition and thus need to be finely tuned individually and systematically. These include (1) the intensity of the light source, (2) the selection of an excitation wavelength, (3) optical efficiencies and parameters (including the field of view size, field depth, lens f-number, and lens-target distance), (4) the performance of the optical components such as long or short wavelength pass filters that are used to prevent the excitation and background light leak to the detector, and (5) the quantum efficiency of the detector in the fluorescence wavelength window. As the dominant surgical robot manufacturer currently in the market, Intuitive uses a Firefly™ fluorescence camera in their da Vinci surgical robots to record and display the fluorescence of ICG. Specifically, it uses an 805-nm laser light as the excitation source and an emission filter with an 815-nm wavelength cut-off to remove the excitation light and collect the fluorescence. The camera has a working distance of approximately 2–20 cm with an upper field of view (FOV) size of about 15×12 cm^2 for better sensitivities. Regarding the detector, the Firefly™ fluorescence camera for Si has a detector on its proximal end of the camera instrument as a separate unit, while the Xi Firefly™ system uses a Complementary Metal Oxide Semiconductor (CMOS) sensor located at the tip of the camera instrument. This arrangement can lead to a fully wristed flexible camera such as the one used in the latest da Vinci SP system (**Figure 7-4**). For image processing, the early version of Si Firefly™ has 2 modes of fluorescence display—unprocessed and processed fluorescence imaging—while Xi Firefly™ only possesses the processed fluorescence imaging mode. As a result, the Si camera can be used to obtain fluorescence images from other dyes as long as these dyes can be excited, whereas Xi can only be used for ICG or a dye with similar absorption and fluorescence profiles as ICG. In the newer Xi systems, a sensitive firefly mode is added to enable visual detection of lower concentrations of fluorescent imaging agents. This is accomplished by turning off the illumination used to create the gray scale (black and white) background view observed in regular mode. Since both visible and NIR fluorescent images share a single optical channel, by turning off the illumination, the gain applied to the fluorescent image can be increased, resulting in a more vibrant fluorescent image. On the other hand, Medtronic EleVision™ IR Platform (likely to be used in their Hugo robot), utilizes 2 separated optical channels for the NIR fluorescence and visible light images. This allows one to tune and optimize the gains and focus of both NIR fluorescence and visible light images at the same time, thus helping to display focused and sharp white light and fluorescence imaging at the same time.

Given that the fluorescence emission for ICG peaks at 820 nm, which is invisible to the human eye, the ICG camera systems process the raw signals and display the fluorescence images in green color, to which human eyes are most sensitive. The fluorescence image can be viewed on its own or superimposed onto the white-light image, thus highlighting organ perfusion and areas of relevant anatomy in real time.

CLINICAL APPLICATIONS OF FLUORESCENCE IMAGING IN ROBOTIC SURGERY

Taxonomic classification of fluorescence imaging applications in robotic surgery can be based on the following: (1) organ-specific surgical procedures and (2) purposes of the applications that include revealing the anatomy of the tissue (such as vessels, bile ducts, lymph nodes, or lesions), and evaluating the tissue's physiological properties (such as perfusion). To serve better as an application manual for surgeons in the different surgical fields, and to match the rest of the book chapters, this section takes the first taxonomic classification and arranges the applications based on organ-specific surgical procedures.

ICG is provided as a kit containing a vial of 25 mg of sterile, lyophilized green powder with no more than 5% sodium iodide (to promote its solubility in water) and one 10-mL aqueous solvent ampule. Under sterile conditions, one 25-mg vial of ICG will be reconstituted using one 10-mL sterile water ampule. After reconstitution by shaking the ICG vial gently, a 25-mg vial of ICG contains 2.5 mg of dye per mL of solution, so a 1.0-mL injection contains a 2.5-mg dose of ICG. The reconstituted ICG solution should be used within 6 hours to avoid aggregation and degradation. Since it contains sodium iodide, caution should be taken in patients who have a history of allergy to iodides.

Once a dose of ICG is injected intravenously, it immediately binds to plasma proteins and joins into the systemic circulation. The ICG concentrations, at the target tissue, will vary in 4 phases: arterial, venous, washout, and balanced phases. During the arterial and venous phases, the ICG concentration peaks rapidly due to the first cardiac passing and then decreases as mixing proceeds with the total blood volume, followed by relatively flat concentration changes as perfusion in the tissue progresses. Subsequently, in the washout phase, ICG concentrations will further decrease as the dye is metabolized and removed from the circulatory system by the liver and secreted through the bile ducts. Finally, during the balanced phase, some remaining ICG will enter the lymphatic circulation, and some will stay in the tissues, depending on the nature of the tissues with different ICG retention times. Since the fluorescence intensity is proportional to the ICG concentration, the observed fluorescence intensities at the target tissue will follow the ICG concentration curves. This will allow one to visualize and identify vital vessel structures in the arterial and venous

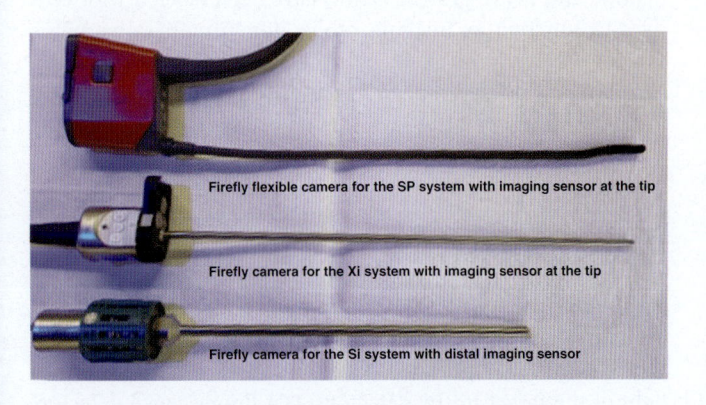

FIGURE 7-4 • Intuitive Firefly™ cameras.

phases, to show the bile duct and liver anatomy in the washout phase, to conduct tumor margining and lymphatic mapping during the balanced phase, and to assess tissue perfusion by evaluating the rate of the fluorescence intensity changes in the arterial and venous phases.

Fluorescence imaging can be used in the following applications: (1) fluorescence-aided anatomy visualization, which mainly includes imaging biliary ducts, hepatic segments, blood vessels, lymphatic networks and lymph nodes, nerves, and parathyroids; (2) lesion visualization and margining; and (3) tissue perfusion assessment. While the first 2 areas of applications can be qualitative with the expectation of "yes or no" answers, the latter requires a quantitative analysis to be objective. Depending on the applications, ICG can be administered before operations (mostly for tumor imaging and margining) or intraoperatively (predominantly for anatomy visualization and perfusion assessment). It can be injected either intravenously (systemic administration) or topically (local administration, mainly for lymphatic mapping). Most of the time, positive contrast (brighter fluorescence contrast to the surrounding normal tissues) will be expected for anatomy visualization, but negative contrast (very weak fluorescence or darker contrast to the surrounding normal tissues) could be encountered in tumor imaging, liver section visualization, and nerve revelation. Since fluorescence intensity is proportional to the amount of fluorescent dye diffused in the tissue, which is further determined by tissue vascularization, fluorescence intensity can function as a quantitative biomarker to gauge tissue perfusion objectively. Depending on the organs, some procedures include all types of applications (anatomy visualization, lesion margining, and perfusion assessment), while others only cover selected applications.

Fluorescence Imaging Application in Cholecystectomy

Cholecystectomy, one of the most performed surgeries, is commonly considered a safe procedure. However, the cystic duct can be misidentified as the common hepatic duct or the common bile duct, which may lead to a bile duct injury. It is a serious complication with an incidence of 0.3–0.7% and the main cause is the misinterpretation of biliary anatomy (71–97%) (see suggested readings #9, 10). The anatomical variations of the biliary tree are a possible cause of iatrogenic lesions, but obesity, previous surgery on the biliary tract, and underlying liver disease may also play an important role. Although conventional x-ray contrast-enhanced cholangiography can accurately depict the biliary anatomy, it requires a surgical dissection for the injection of the contrast agent, which by itself could create some injuries if the initial perception of the anatomy was wrong. In addition, it involves more organizational resources, is time consuming, and exposes patients and health care professionals to radiation.

ICG fluorescence imaging provides an alternative intraoperative cholangiography that is less invasive, does not require radiation, and is not time and resource consuming. After being administered into the circulation, ICG accumulates in the liver and is subsequently secreted into the bile. This allows for the visualization of the bile duct, offering a simple navigation tool for obtaining a biliary roadmap. Unlike x-ray–enhanced cholangiography, which involves using a C-arm, fluorescence cholangiography can be performed on-demand during the surgery, making the procedure easier. It has a short learning curve, as its use only requires switching between standard and NIR vision. Not surprisingly, "ICG-enabled" fluorescence cholangiography has become one of the most common and reliable applications in robotic surgery.

In practice, a dose of 2.5–5 mg ICG is used for intraoperative fluorescence cholangiography. It is injected intravenously at least 45 minutes before the procedure, excreted into the bile within a few minutes of the injection and reaches its maximum concentration within 2 hours. Once the exposure of the triangle of Calot is achieved, the extrahepatic biliary ducts can be viewed under the fluorescence mode as shown in **Figures 7-5 A, B**.

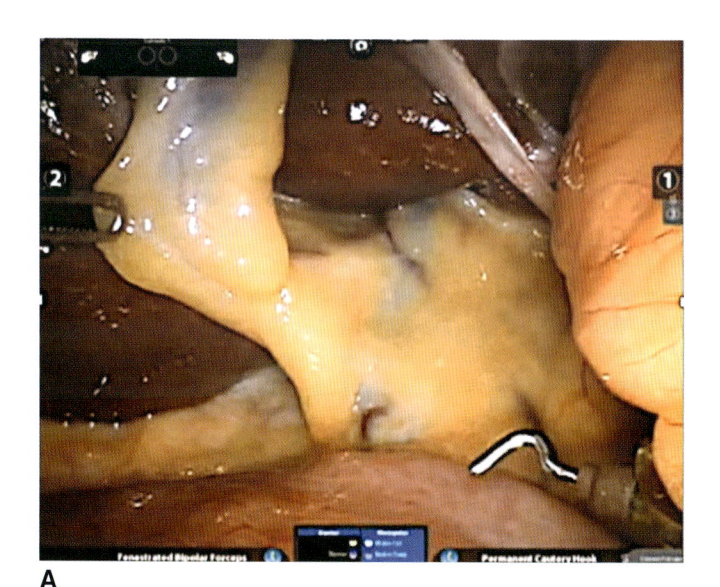

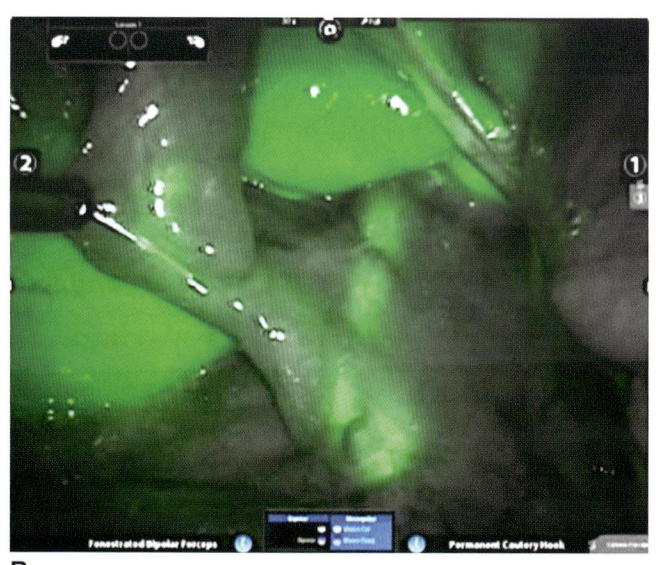

FIGURE 7-5 • Biliary structures.

▶ Video 7-1. Cholecystectomy. Biliary Structures

Since ICG fluorescence cholangiography enables real-time guidance for the cystic duct clipping and boundary delineation between the gallbladder and liver bed, it has become a standard practice in many institutes for cholecystectomies either laparoscopically or robotically. For example, among hundreds of robotic cholecystectomy cases conducted, with the aid of fluorescence cholangiography, at the University of Illinois at Chicago, there were no biliary injuries. In addition, the percentage of identified biliary anomalies was up to 2% (see suggested reading #11) (**Figures 7-6 A–D**; **Videos 7-2** and **7-3**).

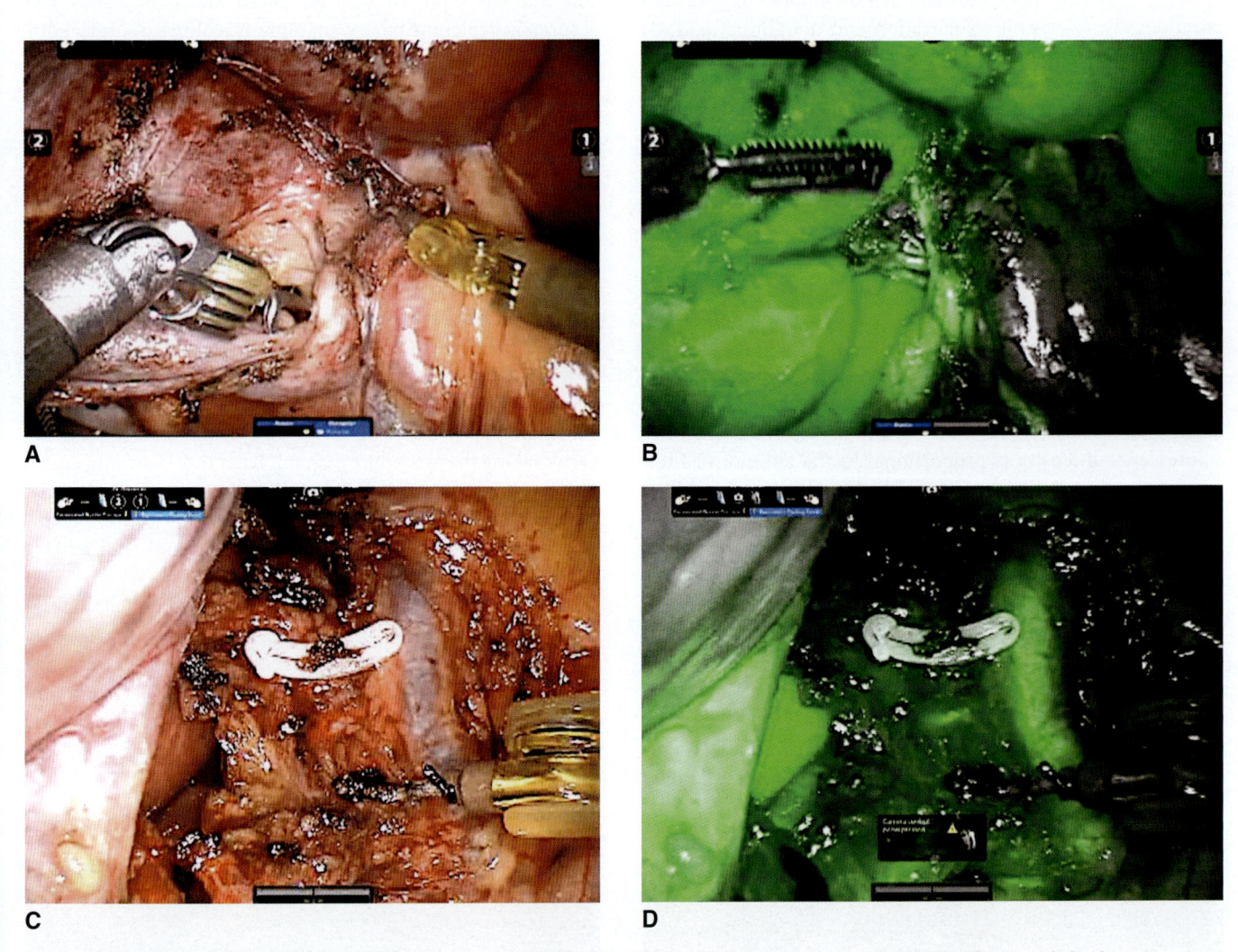

FIGURE 7-6 • Anomalies during cholecystectomies. **A–B.** Aberrant duct to segment 5. **C–D.** Aberrant bile duct to the caudate lobe.

▶ Video 7-2. Aberrant Duct to Segment 5

▶ Video 7-3. Aberrant Bile Duct to the Caudate Lobe

Moreover, fluorescence cholangiography may facilitate the identification of biliary leaks (Luschka ducts/iatrogenic injuries) and biliary structures in challenging situations such as reoperations where adhesions and distorted anatomy hinder the dissection (**Figures 7-7 A, B** and **7-8 A, B**; **Videos** 7-4 and 7-5).

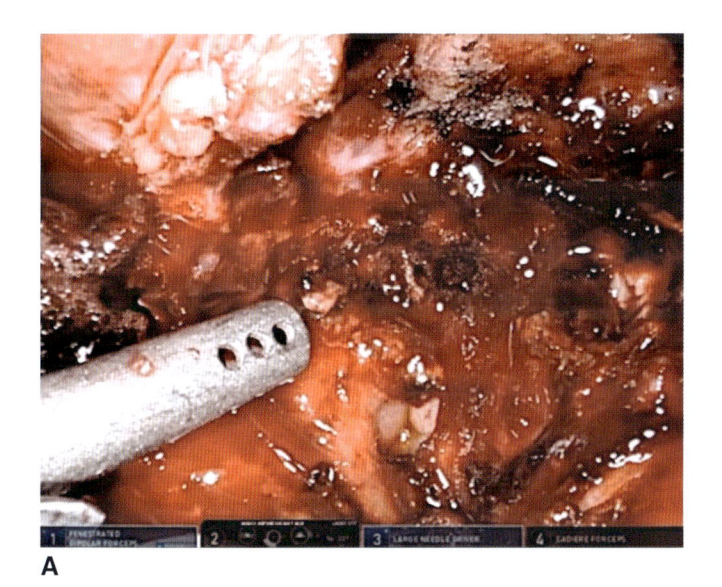

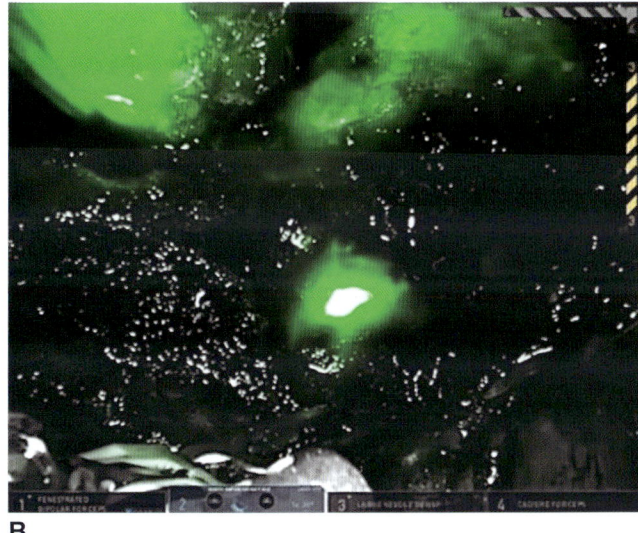

FIGURE 7-7 • Bile leak identification in acute cholecystitis.

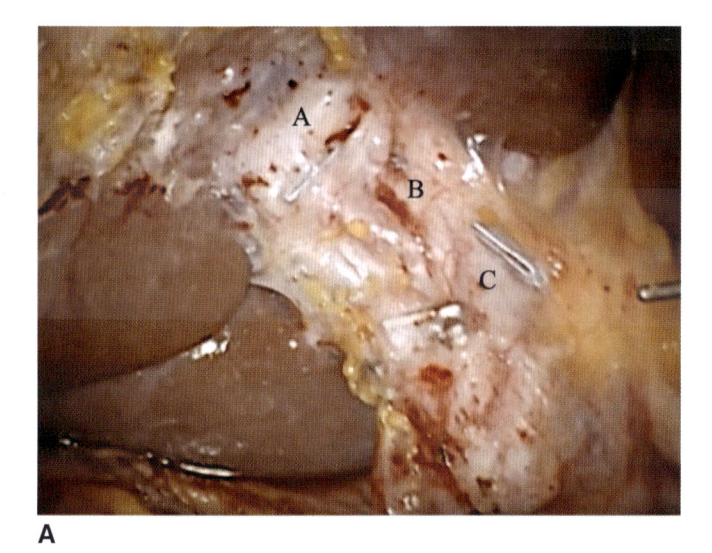

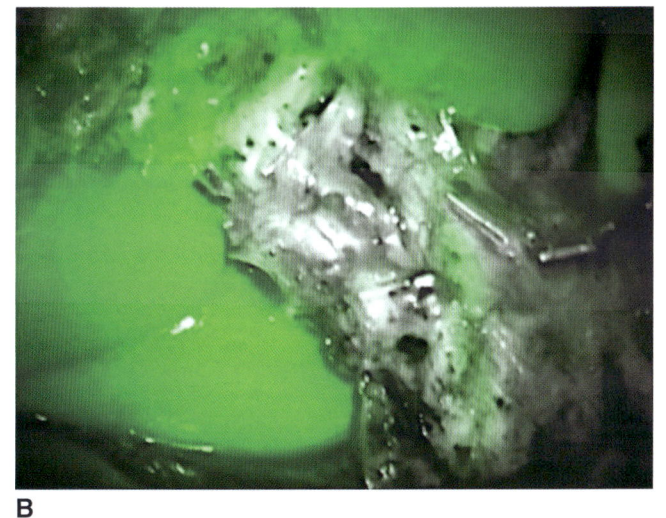

FIGURE 7-8 • Dissection of the hilum in iatrogenic injury after cholecystectomy. **A.** Position of the strictured stump of the right hepatic duct. **B.** Left hepatic duct. **C.** Common bile duct. (Reproduced with permission from Daskalaki D, Aguilera F, Patton K, et al. Fluorescence in robotic surgery. *J Surg Oncol.* 2015;112(3):250-256.)

▶ **Video 7-4. Bile Leak Identification and Repair after Cholecystectomy for Acute Cholecystitis**

▶ **Video 7-5. Hepatic Hilum Dissection in Iatrogenic Injury after Cholecystectomy**

98   The Foundation and Art of Robotic Surgery

Due to the retention of ICG in the liver, its high background fluorescence could interfere with the fluorescence imaging of the bile duct. Strategies to mitigate such interference, for better bile duct identification, include the administration of ICG as far in advance as possible before surgery to minimize liver retention, a prudent predissection of the hepatoduodenal ligament to remove the fat tissue covering the bile duct, and adjustment of the angle of the scope to avoid the interference from the fluorescence in the caudate lobe.

Another limiting factor of fluorescence cholangiography, compared to x-ray enhanced cholangiography, is the inability to detect endoluminal defects like common bile duct stones. Also, the common bile duct is not always identified due to the limited penetration depth of approximately 1 cm of light in the NIR fluorescence. To rule out choledocholithiasis, x-ray–enhanced cholangiography is still necessary. Obesity, inflammation, and scar tissue are all factors that can decrease the visualization capabilities of ICG cholangiography.

> ▶▶ **TIPS**
>
> The retention of ICG in the liver can cause a significant background fluorescence signal that hinders the differentiation between bile ducts and liver tissue. To overcome this drawback, prolonged interval (at least 1 hour) between ICG injection and intraoperative fluorescence cholangiography provides better contrast.

> ⚠ **PITFALLS**
>
> The visualization of the biliary anatomy depends on the uptake of ICG by the liver and its excretion into the bile; therefore, it will be affected by impaired liver function or bile secretion. The delayed secretion can be compensated by anticipating the IV injection of the contrast (at least 2–3 hours in advance).

Fluorescence Imaging Application in Liver Surgery

Hilum and Segment Imaging

The unique feature of liver catabolism of ICG provides a convenient tool for real-time visualization of the hepatic segments, vascular structures, and bile ducts, enabling more accurate anatomical hepatic resections (**Figures 7-9 A–D**; **Video 7-6**). Both positive and negative contrast techniques have been used to identify hepatic segments. The positive contrast technique is achieved by the transhepatic injection of ICG under the intraoperative robotic ultrasound (IUS) guidance. In brief, an infusion set connected to a syringe containing the ICG solution is introduced through a trocar and aimed at the portal vein branch of the target hepatic segment area. Under IUS guidance, the surgeon at the console inserts the needle carefully into the portal vein at the hepatic hilum. The bedside assistant will then inject 1–2 mg ICG. Special attention must be paid to avoid the dye entering other hepatic lobes. The portal vein branches and the specific segment can be visualized immediately under the fluorescence mode.

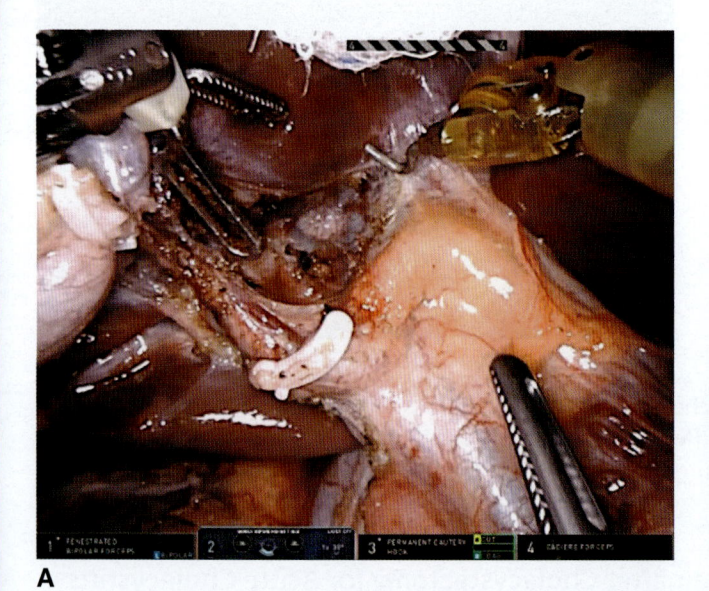

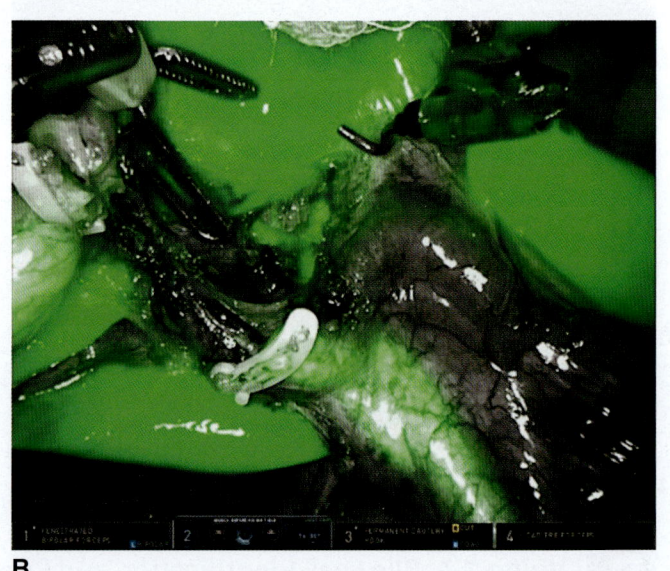

FIGURE 7-9 • The hepatic dissection during robotic right hepatectomy.

C **D**

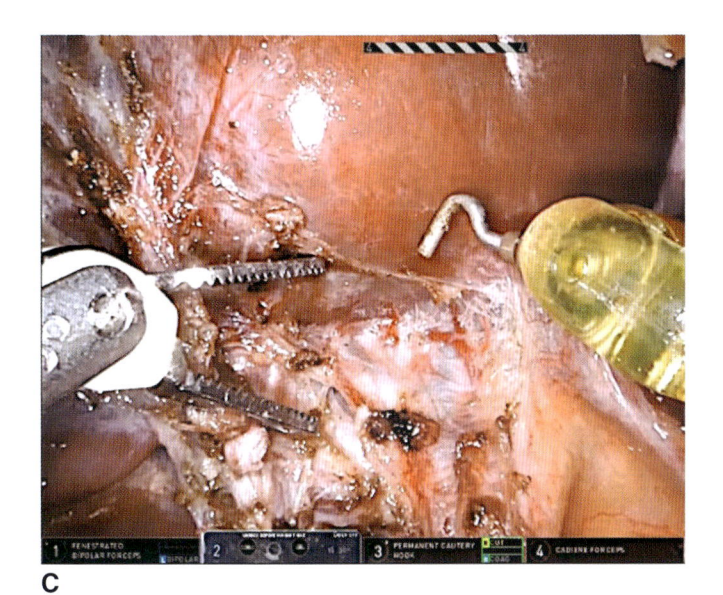

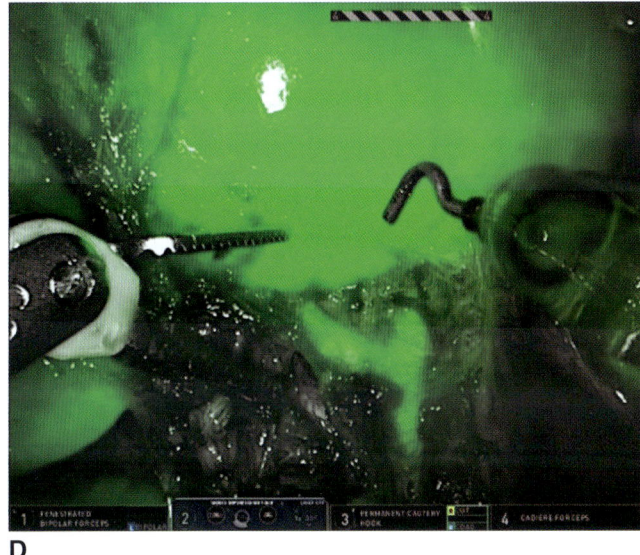

FIGURE 7-9 • (*Continued*)

▶ **Video 7-6.** Hepatic Hilum Dissection

On the other hand, the negative contrast technique has also been explored by occluding the portal vein mainly by intraoperative selective clamping. The hepatic parenchyma to be resected can be identified due to the lack of fluorescence after intravenous injection of 5 mg ICG. The segment can be distinguished as a dark contrast zone while the surrounding tissue fluoresces strongly (negative contrast).

> ▶▶ **TIPS**
>
> It is necessary to avoid any preoperative injection of ICG if the objective is to obtain a negative contrast segmental visualization.
>
> The fluorescent dye in the segment being resected gradually disappears and the selectiveness of both positive and negative techniques decreases over time due to progressive recirculation of ICG.
>
> Repeated injections of ICG in the pedicle might be useful even though the definition of the images tends to diminish.

The resection can then be performed based on the demarcation between fluorescing and nonfluorescing areas, which will be the boundaries of the hepatic segments.

Tumor Imaging

Although tremendous research efforts have been made to develop tumor-specific fluorescence contrast agents, and some of them are currently under clinical trials, none have been approved by the FDA for robotic surgery so far. Currently, in the operating room, ICG fluorescence imaging plays an exclusive role in intraoperative tumor imaging, based on the different uptake and retention times of ICG between the tumor and surrounding normal tissues. The lack of target-specific molecular imaging motifs limits the ICG fluorescence imaging mainly for large lesion visualization to help define the tumor margins.

For liver surgery, fluorescence imaging might aid in the identification of tumors and adequate resection margins, thus allowing better oncological results while avoiding the unnecessary resection of unaffected liver parenchyma. It has been reported that lesions as deep as 10 mm from the liver surface can be visualized and their proximity to vascular or biliary structures can also be assessed.

Two ICG administration approaches are used to visualize a liver tumor: (1) intraoperatively and (2) preoperatively. In the first approach, a dose of 2.5–5 mg ICG is given intravenously to the patient right before the tumor resection. After 2–5 minutes, the tumor may be visualized as a dark mass surrounded by normal fluorescent tissue, as shown in **Figures 7-10 A–D** and **Videos** 7-7 and **7-8**.

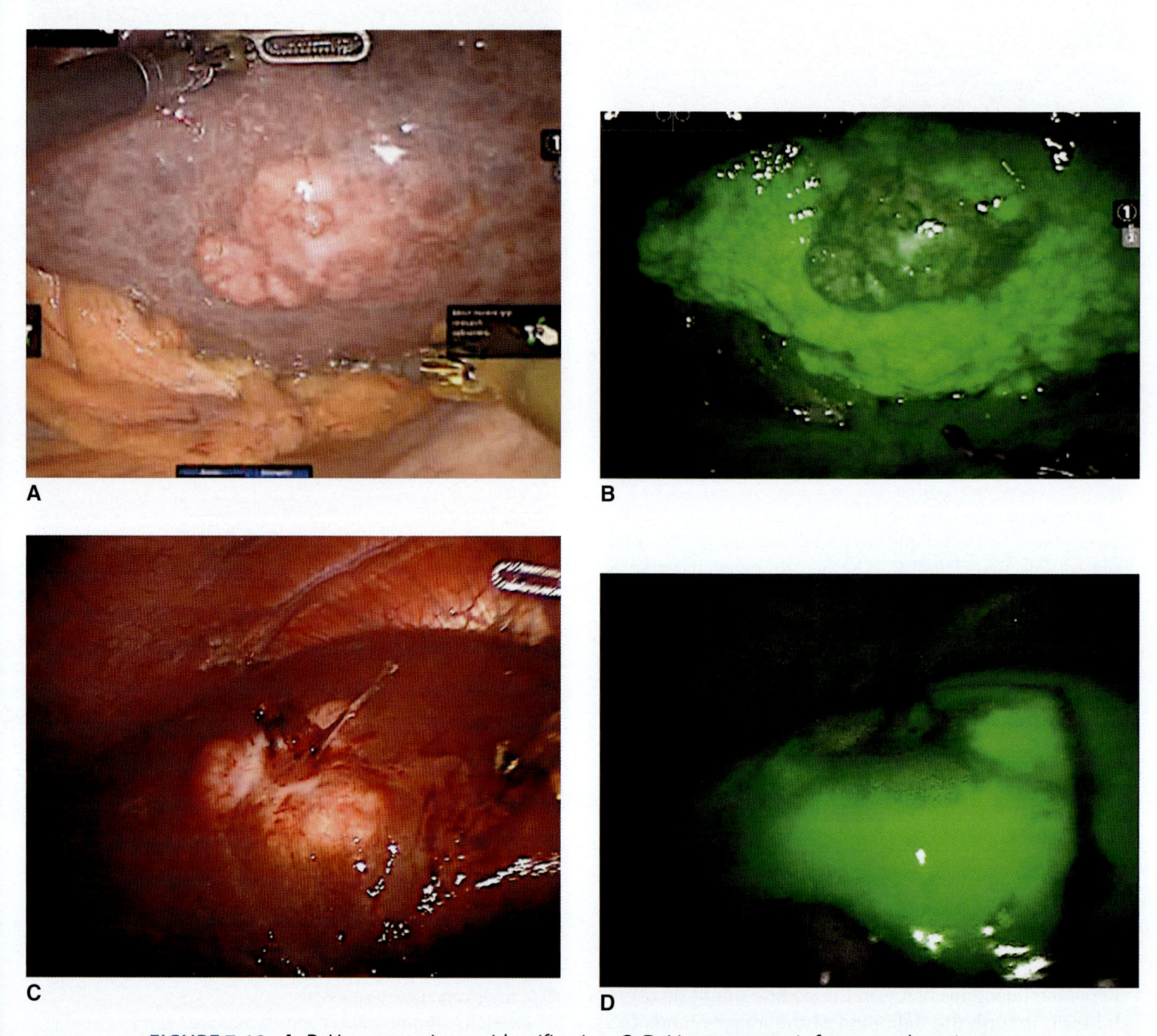

FIGURE 7-10 • **A–B.** Hepatocarcinoma identification. **C–D.** Liver metastasis from rectal carcinoma.

▶ **Video 7-7.** Hepatocarcinoma Identification

▶ **Video 7-8.** Liver Metastasis from Rectal Carcinoma

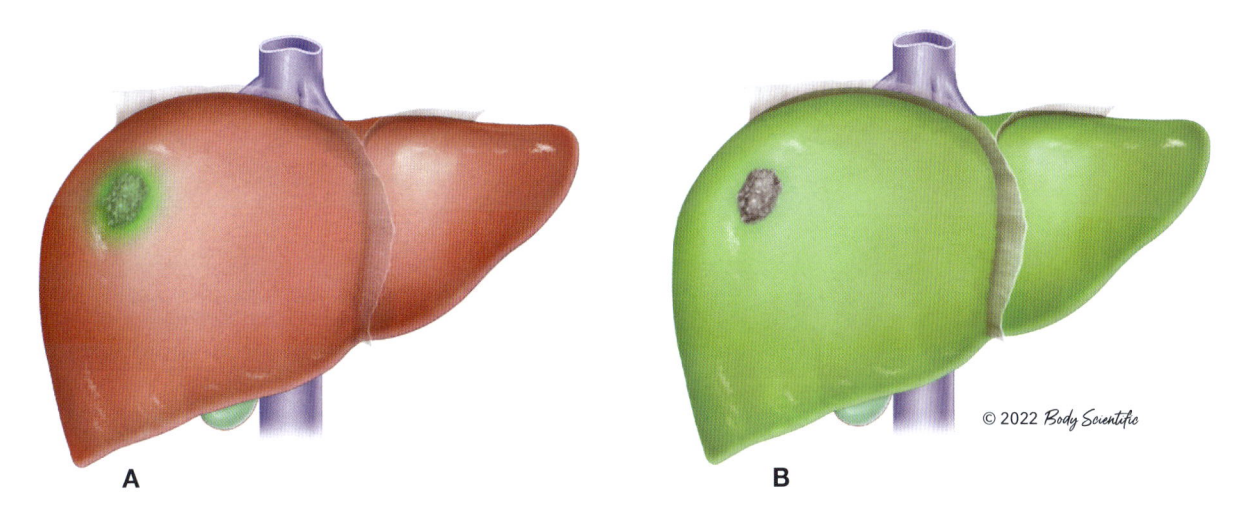

FIGURE 7-11 • **A.** Illustration of ICG fluorescence imaging of a tumor mass in positive contrast. Since ICG is administered preoperatively, ICG molecules in the normal tissue are already cleared, while ICG molecules in the tumor mass are retained due to the longer retention time of ICG in the tumoral tissue. ICG fluorescence in the lesion stands out from the normal tissue background under the intraoperative fluorescence mode. **B.** Illustration of ICG fluorescence imaging of a tumor mass in negative contrast. When administered intraoperatively, ICG molecules are distributed in the normal tissue before being cleared from the bloodstream by the liver but rationed much less in the tumor mass due to its abnormal vasculature. This leads to a dark contrast in ICG fluorescence against normal tissues under the intraoperative fluorescence mode.

For the preoperative administration approach, a single dose of 5–10 mg ICG is given within 2–5 days before the surgery. During the operation, the tumor can be identified as a bright mass surrounded by nonfluorescent tissue as shown in **Figures 7-11 A, B**.

The mechanism of fluorescence contrasts of tumors in the liver with different timings of ICG administration has not been fully understood. It has been hypothesized that the retention of ICG in tumor cells is linked to the expression levels of organic anion transporting polypeptides (OATPs) and the organic anion transporters (OATs). A well-differentiated hepatocarcinoma (HCC) cell has higher levels of OATPS and OATs, which leads to the retention of more ICG, thus showing a brighter fluorescence contrast. But this hypothesis couldn't explain well the dark contrast of tumors when ICG is administered intraoperatively. Another hypothesis for the mechanism of different fluorescence contrasts is based on the role of the tumor stroma–extracellular matrix and specialized connective tissue cells surrounding the tumors. All tumors have stroma for nutritional support, which plays a key role in tumor formation and metastasis. It has been established that a tumoral mass has a hypoxic physiological nature with poor blood circulation (normal tissues have an oxygenation level of around 40 mm Hg, but tumors have regions of tissue with oxygenation levels below 10 mm Hg). The poor vesiculation properties of the tumors cause less ICG accumulation compared to normal tissues, yielding the negative fluorescence contrast before ICG is cleared by the body. On the other hand, the tumor stroma controls the tumor cell-host interactions with enhanced vascular permeability to circulating macromolecules. This leads to the leakage of plasma proteins (such as albumin) to the tumor stroma area, where ICG can bind tightly, thus showing bright fluorescence in tumor stroma (**Figures 7-12 A–C**).

If ICG is injected intraoperatively, and if the tumor is located shallow enough, the lesion will most likely show a dark contrast because the fluorescence of the stroma and the surrounding normal tissue will be the same, i.e., the contrast pattern is bright (normal tissues)-bright (stroma) and dark (tumor). In case of ICG is injected preoperatively, the fluorescence contrast between the stroma and the normal tissue will become different as ICG in normal tissue will be depleted due to the blood circulation and its metabolism in the liver. However, the presence of plasma proteins and cross-linked extravascular fibrin in the stroma area will retain ICG. The contrast pattern becomes dark (normal tissues)-bright (stroma) and dark (tumor). Since fluorescence imaging is a visualization tool, the stroma on the top of the tumor will make the entire lesion show bright contrast under 2D fluorescence imaging. Several histological studies of dissected tumor slides using a fluorescence microscope confirmed that ICG fluorescence signals were indeed from the cells in tumor margin areas, and there was no fluorescence in the central tumor mass. This rim type of fluorescing pattern explains well the different contrast of tumoral lesions when ICG is injected intraoperatively (darker contrast) versus preoperatively (brighter contrast). Further research studies need to be conducted to prove the proposed mechanism.

> ⚠ **PITFALLS**
>
> The limited penetration of up to 10 mm of tissue prevents the visualization of deeper lesions.
>
> ICG removal from noncancerous tissue can be insufficient in patients with impaired liver function, creating false-positive nodules. Benign lesions can also emit fluorescence, making it difficult to determine the tumor-free margins.

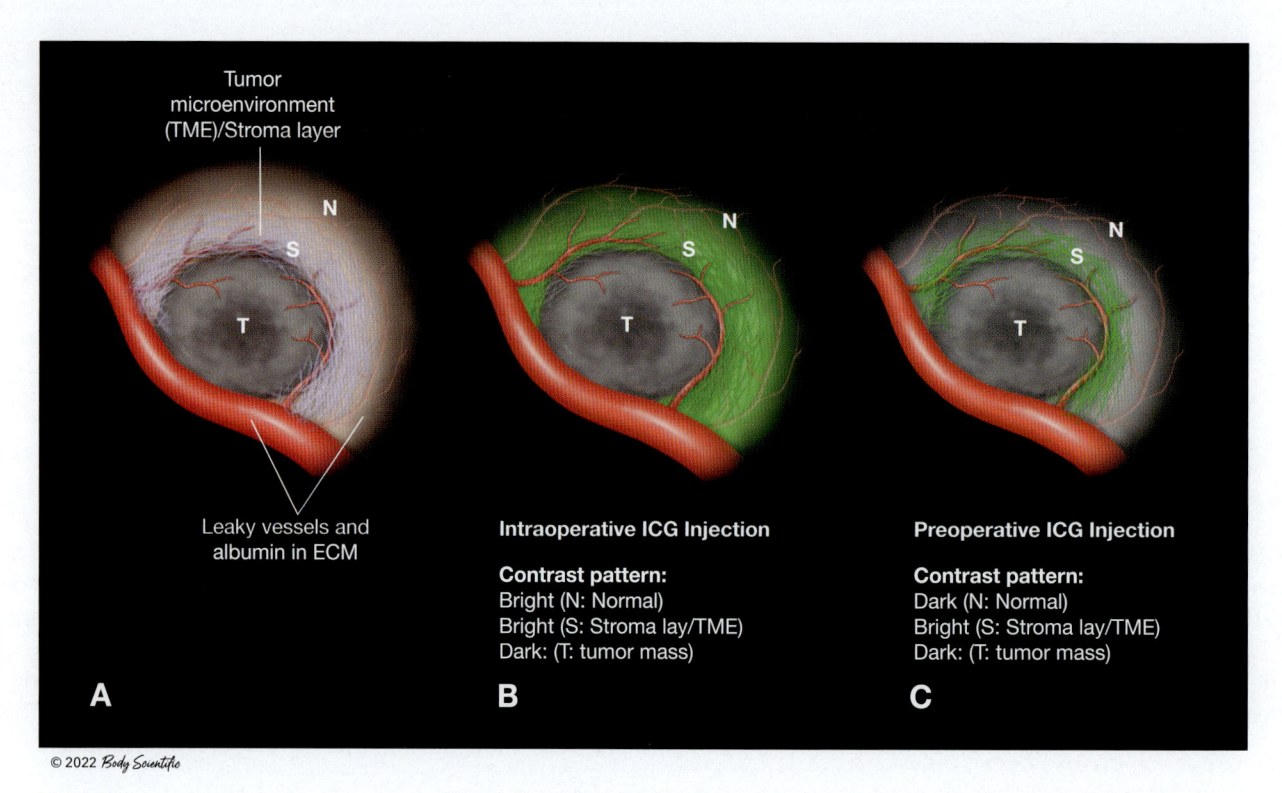

FIGURE 7-12 • Potential mechanism of ICG interaction with a tumor mass. **A.** Depiction of a tumoral structure and surrounding stroma. **B.** Fluorescence pattern among the tumor, stroma, and the normal tissue shortly after the intravenous administration of ICG. **C.** Fluorescence pattern among the tumor, stroma, and the normal tissue when ICG is administered 1 day before the surgery.

Fluorescence Imaging Applications in Bowel Surgery

Perfusion Assessment

Another major application of fluorescence imaging is the assessment of blood perfusion in tissues. As perfusion is a critical element related to the function of an injured, resected, or transplanted tissue, it is essential to have the capability of assessing tissue blood flow quantitatively, so that it can help to change the strategy or technique accordingly. Currently, the quality of tissue perfusion is judged using a conventional colorimetric method by visually examining changes in serosal color, grade of peristalsis, pulsation, and bleeding from tissue margins under white light imaging, all of which are highly subjective and vary with each surgeon's experience. Quantitative fluorescence imaging analysis can tackle this problem and gauge tissue perfusion objectively. Fluorescence intensity is proportional to the amount of fluorescent dye present in the tissue, and the ICG molecules are brought into the tissue by the blood. Consequently, the fluorescence intensity of ICG can function as a quantitative biomarker of tissue perfusion.

One of the most common perfusion assessments is to judge the blood flow status in the stumps before the anastomosis during colorectal or small bowel procedures. Anastomotic leakage is a severe complication, and hypoperfusion is an important risk factor. Fluorescence imaging with ICG has been used to assess intestinal perfusion by intravenous administration of 2.5–5 mg ICG to the patient, followed by watching the brightness of the fluorescence or the rise of its intensity in the stumps that will be used for the anastomosis. As shown in the intraoperative pictures and videos, as the intensity of fluorescence is associated with the grade of perfusion, the lack of brightness implies poor vascularization, thus it is necessary to modify the transection line until well-perfused margins are observed (**Figures 7-13 A–J**; **Videos 7-9 to 7-13**).

> ⚠ **PITFALLS**
>
> Perfusion, when estimated purely based on fluorescence intensity, in a static fashion and without considering the diffusion of ICG in the tissue over time, can result in an overestimation. A well-perfused area observed from further away with the scope may seem less intensively fluorescent than a poorly perfused one observed from more closely.
>
> After repeated injections, ICG persists in the lymphatic system, thus showing constant fluorescence. This persistence of the tracer can be confused with adequate perfusion.

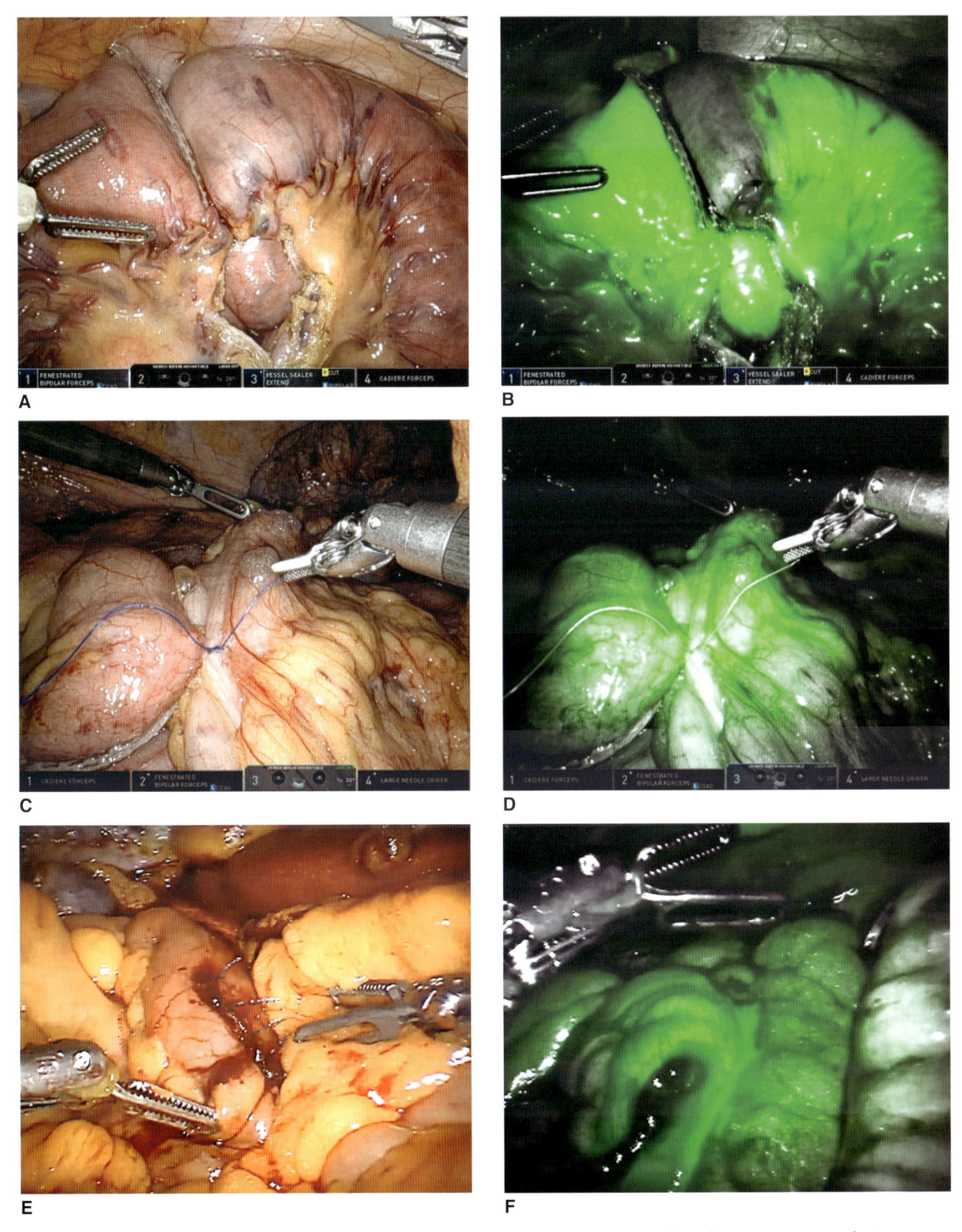

FIGURE 7-13 • **A–B.** Small bowel viability during a central pancreatectomy. **C–D.** Ileocolonic anastomosis during a left colectomy. **E–F.** Right colon stump during a right colectomy.

104 The Foundation and Art of Robotic Surgery

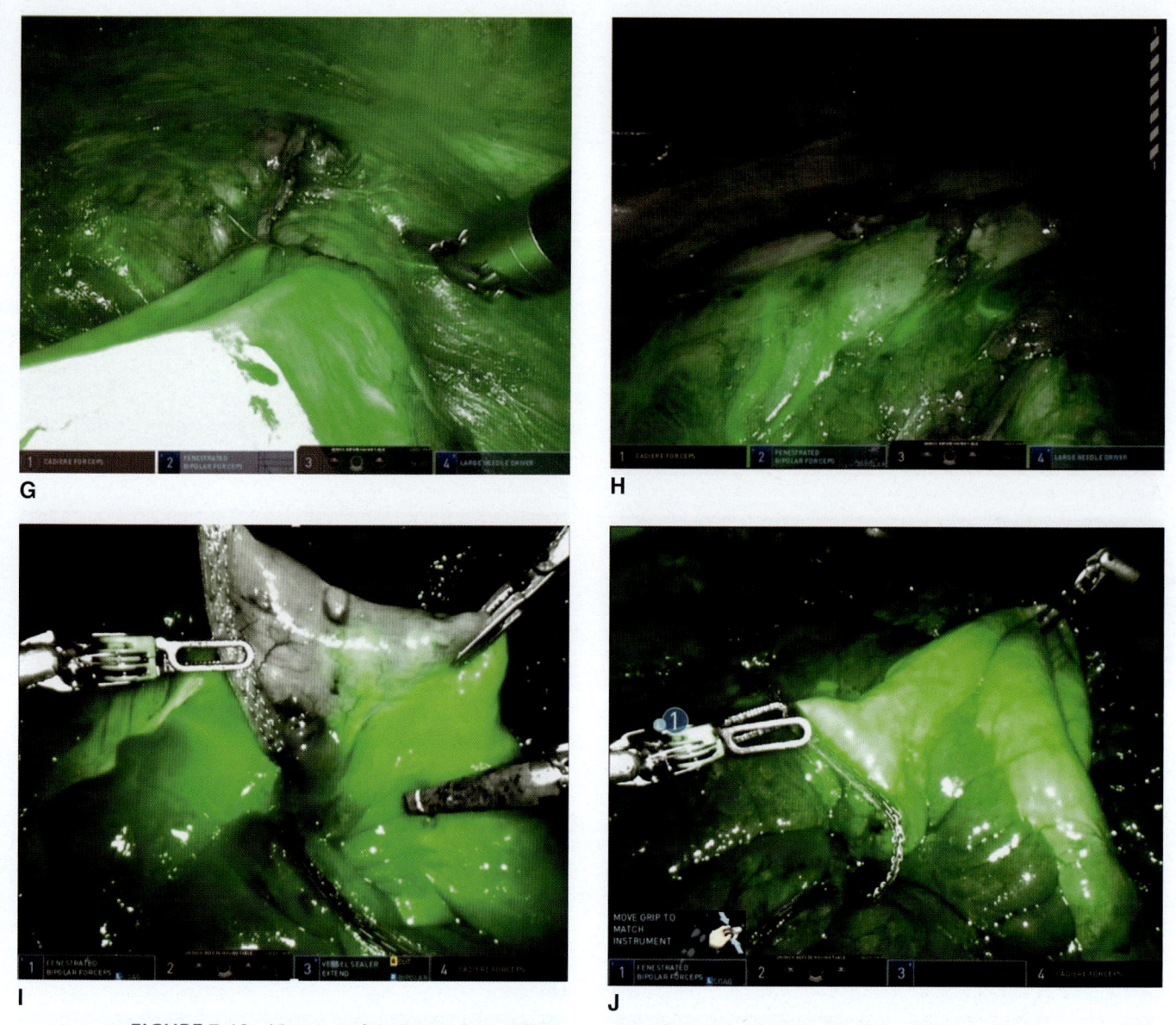

FIGURE 7-13 • *(Continued)* **G.** Rectosigmoid anastomosis after rectum resection for rectal carcinoma. **H.** Mesocolon blood flow. **I–J.** Small bowel stump. Absence of fluorescence in proximal stump. A new resection is made following the ICG line of demarcation.

▶ **Video 7-9.** Small Bowel Viability during a Central Pancreatectomy

▶ **Video 7-10.** Ileocolonic Anastomosis during a Left Colectomy

▶ **Video 7-11.** Right Colon Stump during a Right Colectomy

▶ **Video 7-12.** Colorectal Anastomosis and Mesocolon Blood Flow

▶ **Video 7-13.** Small Bowel Stump

The advantage of using ICG fluorescence is that it enables an objective perfusion assessment. It is more sensitive than color demarcation, which is not always reliable, as subtle color changes in tissue might take hours to happen. It is easier than the use of Doppler, which requires specific training not only to manipulate the transducer appropriately, but also to interpret the visualized images, and it helps to modify the surgical procedure according to real-time visualization of the blood flow. As this technique is a practical way to assess perfusion, it might aid in decreasing the leak rate.

Unfortunately, the current fluorescence-based perfusion assessment is still qualitative. Similar to the colorimetric estimation under the white-light images, it is based on the surgeon's visual evaluation of how bright the fluorescence becomes in the tissues after the dye is administered. Such an empirical assessment can be subjective or misleading, especially for new surgeons, which may lead to making an anastomosis in a less perfused area than assumed. To overcome this, efforts of quantifying fluorescence intensity to yield perfusion objectively have been actively pursued. One of the approaches is to read out the pixel intensity of fluorescence images and depict their changes by plotting the relative intensity as a function of time. Laparoscopic ICG fluorescence cameras such as Stryker's Spy™ Elite™ camera or Medtronic Envision IR™ camera already implemented such a function, and hopefully, the new generation of Intuitive Firefly™ camera and Medtronic Envision IR™ camera will come with this fluorescence intensity read-out function as well. However, although fluorescence intensity is proportional to the concentration of fluorescent dye, it is also dependent on other parameters including light path length and the measurement constant that accounts for the distance between the light source and the target, detection angles, etc. These parameters are not uniform across the surgical field. Therefore, fluorescence intensities among the pixels in the surgical field (pixel intensities) may not truly reflect ICG concentration at each pixel. One way to address such a disparity is to calculate the rate of fluorescence intensity change (i.e., the slopes of the intensity-over-time curves) at each pixel and reconstruct the fluorescence image as a color-coded image based on this change. Such an image can lead to a more accurate determination of the differences in tissue perfusion across the surgical field (see Chapter 6, Implemented Imaging and Artificial Intelligence in Robotics). A threshold based on fluorescence intensity changing rate that determines the status of the tissue perfusion can be defined after validation, which will enable a more objective assessment.

Identifying the Sentinel Lymph Node and Mapping Lymph Nodes

The identification of the sentinel lymph node and lymph node mapping are other major applications of fluorescence imaging. This approach provides a feasible, safe, time-efficient, and reliable method with better detection rates, enabling an adequate lymphadenectomy, which could improve oncological outcomes. Furthermore, it may facilitate the recollection of small fluorescent lymph nodes, that otherwise wouldn't be identified with usual methods, increasing the number of lymph nodes resected. While some ICG can enter the lymphatic circulation when injected intravenously, to achieve a reliable lymph nodal mapping and sentinel lymph node identification, ICG should be administered locally near the tumor. Once injected, ICG is drained through the lymphatic network reaching the first lymph node in 10–15 minutes and the regional lymph nodes in 1–2 hours, staying in the lymphatic network for about 24–48 hours. These time frames could guide the lymph node mapping and the sentinel lymph node identification, respectively. Lymph nodes will appear as bright ICG fluorescence emitting green spots under the fluorescence mode due to the uptake and retention of ICG. An endoscopic procedure before the day of the surgery provides a convenient way for local administration of ICG, although it can be also administered during the actual procedure. For intraoperative administration during a colorectal operation, a dose of 1–2 mg ICG is injected submucosally or subserosally in the periphery of the tumor. This is accomplished by inserting an infusion set connected to a syringe containing the ICG solution through a trocar. The console surgeon inserts the needle carefully into the subserosa around the tumor. The bedside assistant then injects the ICG slowly and the needle is retrieved while retracting the syringe plunge to prevent ICG from leaking into the peritoneum. The fluorescent sentinel lymph node and the lymphatic station can be viewed under the fluorescence mode in 10–15 minutes and 1–2 hours, respectively. In case that ICG is administered preoperatively through colonoscopy, usually 24–48 hours in advance, a dose of 2–5 mg ICG is used and the lymph node networks are visible under the fluorescence mode throughout the surgery (**Figures 7-14 A–F**; **Video 7-14**).

After 10–15 minutes of ICG

After 1–2 hours of ICG

A

B

C

D

E

F

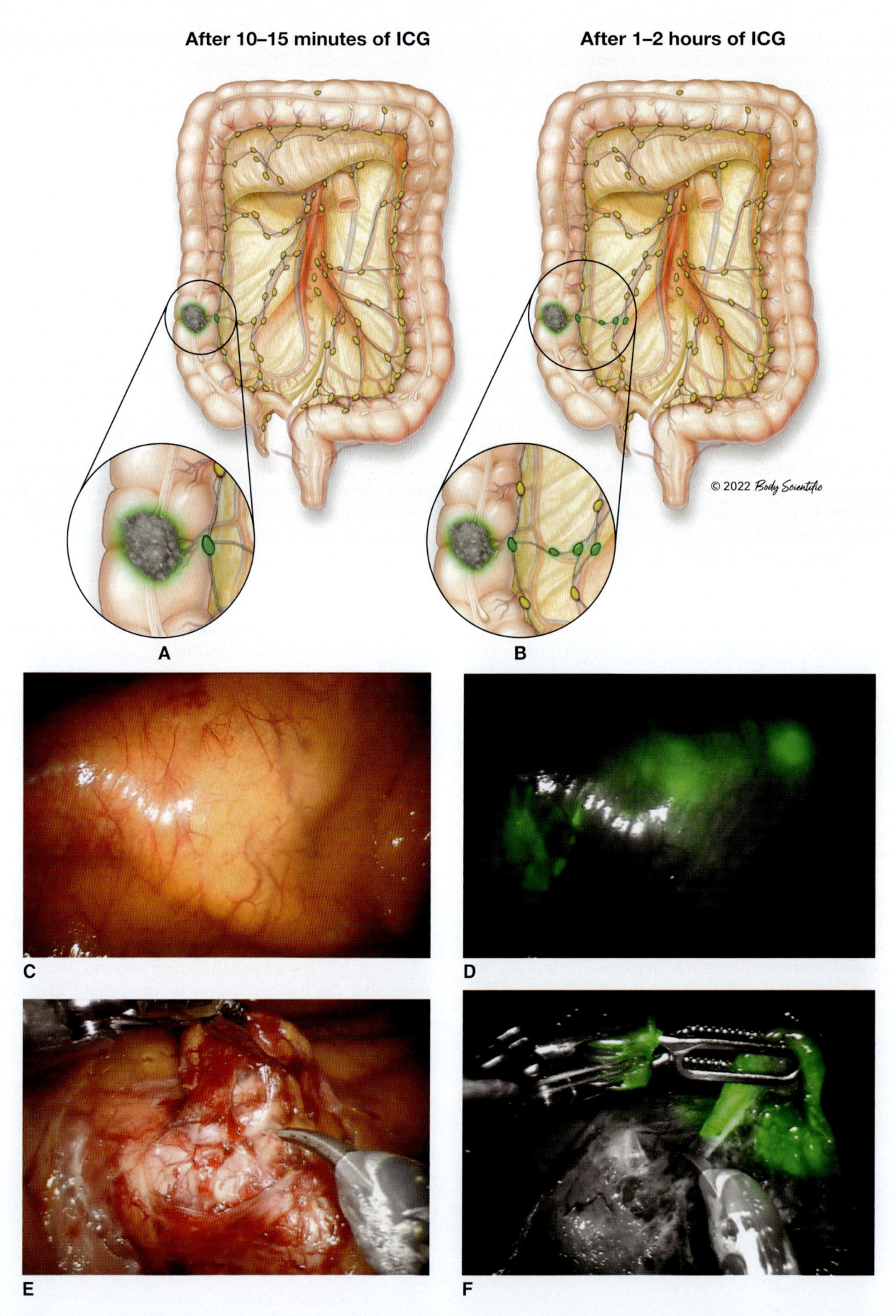

FIGURE 7-14 • A. Sentinel lymph node visualization after 10–15 minutes of ICG injection. **B.** Lymphatic station visualization after 1–2 hours of ICG injection. **C–F.** Mesenteric lymphography during a left colectomy.

▶ **Video 7-14.** Mesenteric Lymphography during a Left Colectomy

> **EDITORIAL COMMENT**
>
> The endoscopic injection of ICG has some inconveniences—the patient needs to be admitted 1 day earlier; the distension of the bowel after CO_2 insufflation during the endoscopy can be persistent in some patients. This persistance may interfere with the robotic operation. In addition, mainly for rectal cancer, the needle could go through the rectal wall and ICG might spread not specifically in the mesorectum, thus impeding the nodal mapping technique.

Nerve Imaging During Colorectal Surgery

Iatrogenic nerve injuries during colorectal surgery are a significant cause of morbidity and may lead to an altered urogenital and pelvic floor function, resulting in a reduced quality of life. Although a nerve-specific fluorescence probe for intraoperative nerve-sparing guidance has not been clinically approved, ICG has been explored for nerve visualization in colorectal surgeries, especially during nerve-sparing lymph node dissection or total mesorectal excision (TME). Since the superior hypogastric plexus around the inferior mesenteric artery (IMA) is accompanied by lymphatic channels strings, ICG fluorescence imaging of lymph nodal mapping can be repurposed for the hypogastric plexus visualization in a negative contrast approach. In this scenario, the nerve is surrounded by lymph node–rich tissues, which can retain the ICG, thus showing brighter fluorescence signals, while the nerve itself has very weak fluorescence due to the lack of ICG retention.

Practically, 2–5 mg ICG is administered locally in the tumor area under the guidance of colonoscopy 24 hours before the surgery. During the procedure, while dissecting along the mesentery and exposing the avascular plane, different tissues and structures can be differentiated under the fluorescence imaging mode. Specifically, the pelvic plexus can be identified in gray contrast, surrounded by the mesorectum in green (mainly from fluorescent lymph nodes) and the IMA in black. Such a negative contrast imaging of the nerves can enhance the success of nerve-preserving TME techniques (**Figures 7-15 A, B; Video 7-15**).

A B

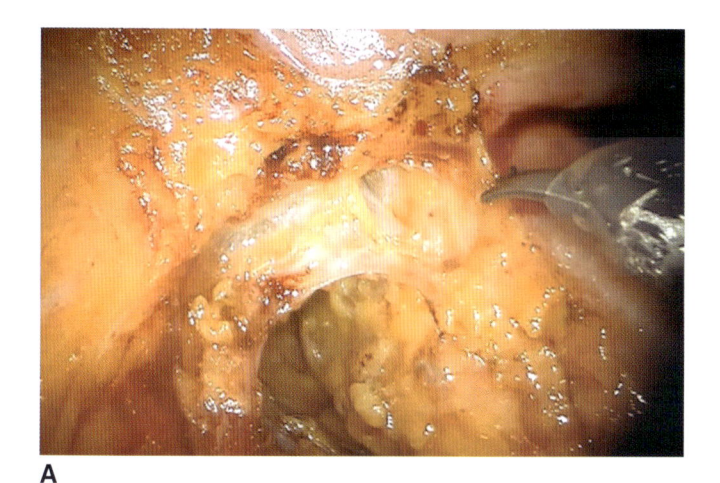

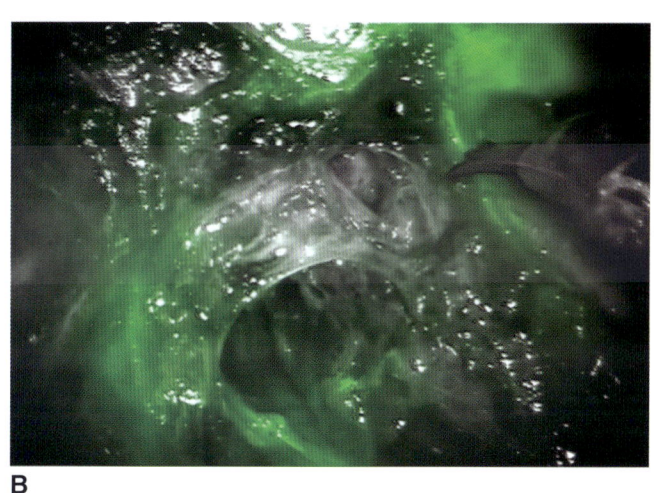

FIGURE 7-15 • The plexus identification during the TME.

▶ **Video 7-15.** The Pelvic Plexus Identification in TME

Fluorescence Imaging Applications for Gastric Surgery

Perfusion Assessment

Anastomotic leakage is an infrequent but severe postoperative complication in gastric surgery. Several contributing factors are: poor blood perfusion, infection of the suture line, treatment with nonsteroidal anti-inflammatory drugs and steroids, and technical pitfalls, despite advancements in staple formation and the general improvement in surgical technology. Among these factors, it has been suggested that inadequate blood supply to the stumps is the most relevant one. Either the gastric or jejunal stumps, in case of gastroenteric anastomosis, can have problems of micro blood supply, and the construction of the anastomosis can make the situation even worse creating small side patches of ischemia. The use of ICG fluorescence imaging to evaluate the perfusion in real time offers a convenient way to obtain a more reliable assessment and thus may decrease the potential development of leaks associated with ischemia. The blood supply network of the stomach and the bowel can be visualized immediately under the fluorescence mode after intravenous injection of 2–5 mg ICG.

Mapping Lymph Nodes and Identifying the Sentinel Lymph Node

As lymph node involvement in gastric cancer is associated with poor prognosis, lymphadenectomy is considered a fundamental step for staging during radical gastrectomy. The lymph nodal mapping can decrease the adverse effects of extended lymphadenectomy while achieving the same statistical capability for reaching a proper staging with a smaller number of dissected lymph nodes. Conventionally, lymph node mapping is performed using blue dye and/or radioisotope (Tc^{99m}). However, blue dye injection bears potential risks of necrosis and allergic reactions, while isotope tracer exposes patients and healthcare professionals to radiation. By utilizing an upper endoscope for a local administration of ICG near the tumor area, ICG fluorescence imaging can enable the intraoperative visualization of the lymph nodes, thus helping to achieve a complete lymphadenectomy, avoiding blue-dye complications, and radiation exposure. Briefly, 2–3 mg ICG is injected into 4 quadrants of the submucosa layer of the primary lesion using an endoscopic puncture needle 1 day before the surgery. During the procedure, after dividing the gastrocolic ligament, the lymph nodes with the directions of the lymphatic flow can be visualized from the stomach under the fluorescence mode (**Figures 7-16 A–F; Video 7-16**).

> ⚠ **PITFALLS**
>
> Massive infiltration of the submucosa (*linitis plastica*) might occlude the lymphatic vessels and prevent ICG diffusion along the lymphatic network.

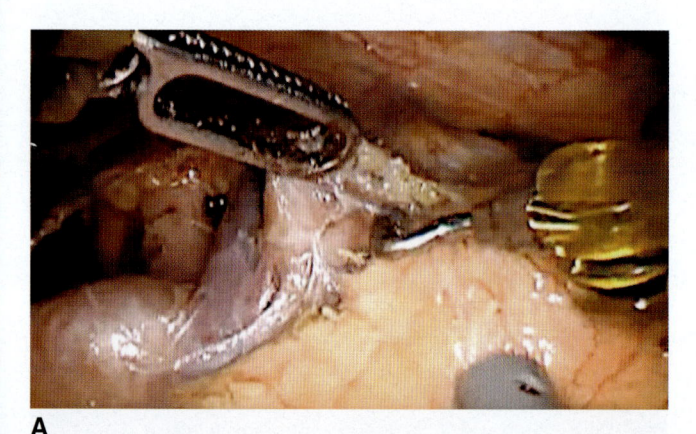

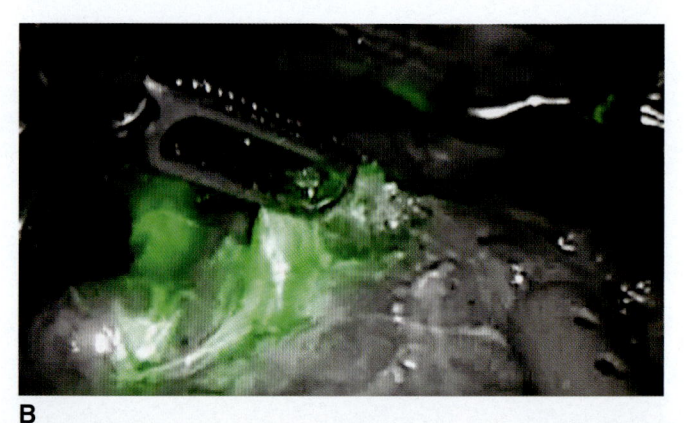

FIGURE 7-16 • Gastrectomy with ICG-guided lymphadenectomy.

C   D

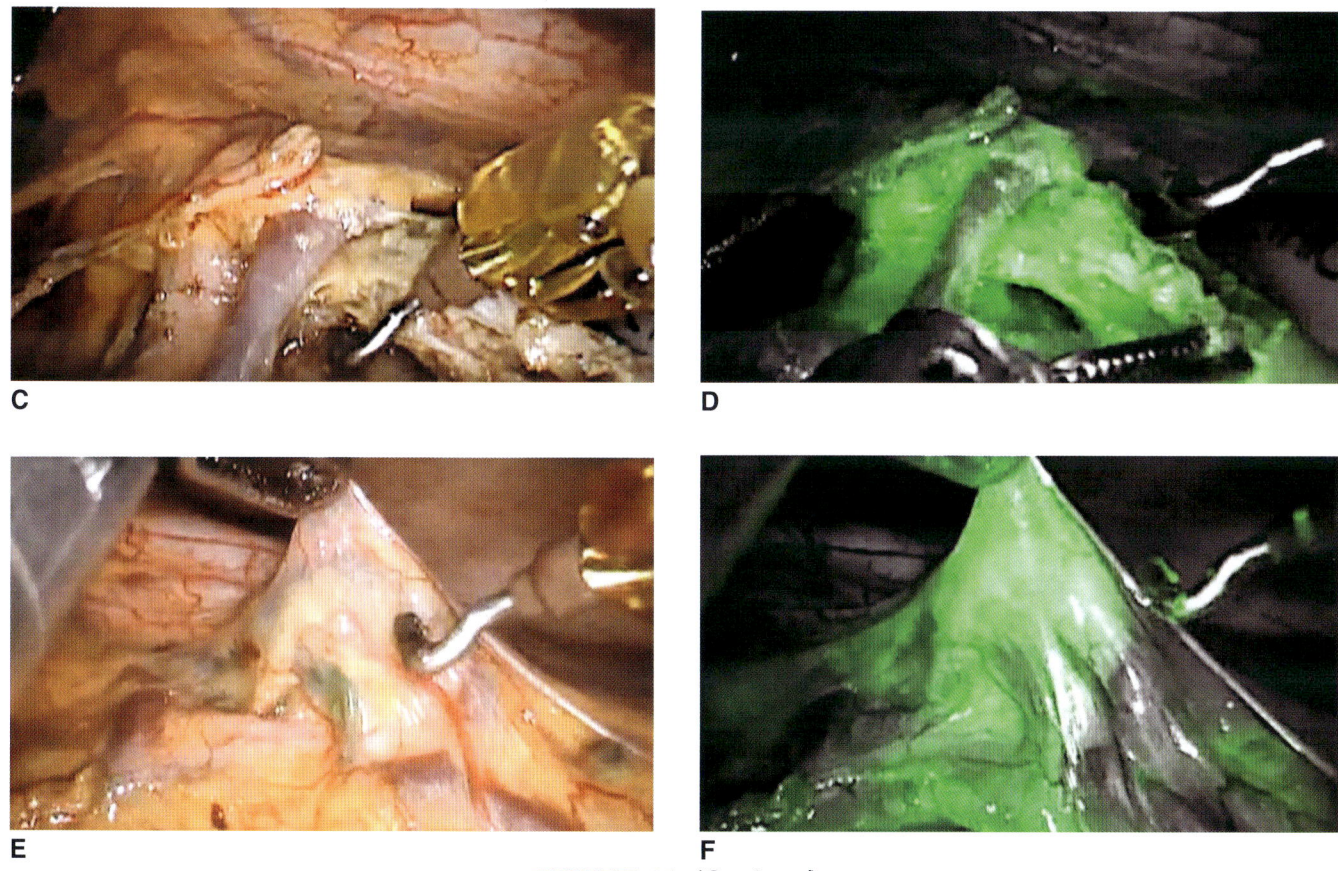

E   F

FIGURE 7-16 • (Continued)

▶ **Video 7-16. Gastrectomy with ICG-Guided Lymphadenectomy**

A lymph node map with the proximal border from the fatty tissue attached to the stomach wall, the distal one from the front of the bright fluorescent node most caudal from the stomach, as well as the number and direction of the lymphatic basins, can all be obtained. Such an improved visualization of the lymph nodes allows tailored dissections, which may improve the procedure's outcomes.

Fluorescence Imaging Applications for Esophageal Surgery

Perfusion Assessment

With a 10–20% leakage rate of esophagogastric anastomosis and graft necrosis, which leads to higher mortality, reoperations, and increased hospital stay, a reliable perfusion assessment of the gastric conduit is critical to ensure an adequate blood supply as ischemia is one of the specific factors that may contribute to the failure of the esophageal anastomosis (see suggested reading #31). ICG fluorescence imaging has been used to evaluate blood perfusion of the gastric conduit in real time, thereby enabling a precise delineation of the ideal site for the anastomosis with the esophagus. To assess perfusion, 2–5 mg ICG is injected intravenously during the surgical procedure and the fluorescence signal is detected immediately after the injection. As shown in **Figures 7-17 A–D**, the blood supply network of the stomach can be visualized under the fluorescence mode within a minute after the ICG administration (**Videos 7-17** and **7-18**).

110 The Foundation and Art of Robotic Surgery

A

B

C

D

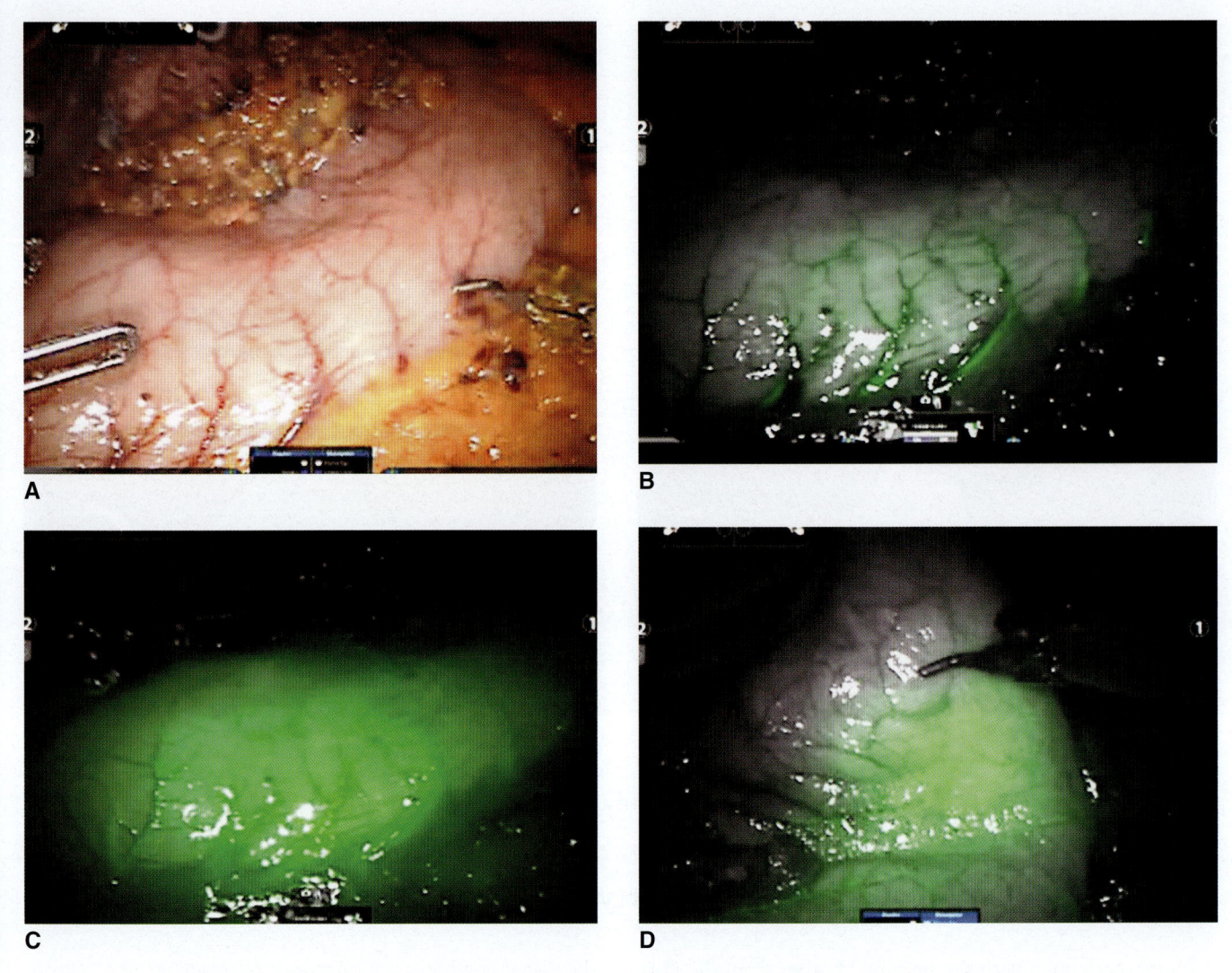

FIGURE 7-17 • The stomach blood supply visualization during robotic-assisted esophagectomy.

▶ **Video 7-17. The Stomach Blood Supply Visualization during Robotic-Assisted Esophagectomy**

▶ **Video 7-18. The Stomach Perfusion Visualization during Robotic-Assisted Esophagectomy**

Although ICG fluorescence imaging allows a feasible assessment of perfusion, again, the lack of objectivity and of a threshold for adequate perfusion are major limitations. Quantification of the fluorescence intensity and the rate of its change will overcome this limitation when correlated to anastomotic leakage and graft necrosis.

> **▶▶ TIPS**
>
> ICG fluorescence imaging might correctly identify anomalies in the blood supply of the proximal stomach, helping in a good preparation of the conduit. Furthermore, the assessment of the blood supply to the tip of the gastric conduit is fundamental, being the less perfused area and where the anastomosis is usually placed.
>
> Absence of fluorescence after a certain time can suggest arterial insufficiency of the right gastric/gastroepiploic arteries.
>
> Fluorescence delay might indicate a slow inflow or venous congestion, leading to ischemia.

> **EDITORIAL NOTE**
>
> In case of venous congestion, ICG fluorescence after a slower appearance finally displays an enhanced gastric conduit coloration as arterial flow is intact.

Imaging Sentinel Lymph Node, Lymph Nodes, and the Thoracic Duct

It is quite common that esophageal cancers exhibit multidirectional lymphatic flows from the primary tumor site, as well as random patterns of lymph node metastasis. This can require an extended lymphadenectomy and radical esophagectomy, which is prone to significant complications. As described in gastric cancer section, the sentinel lymph node mapping may become a reliable option, to tailor the procedure according to the particular lymph node enhancement. ICG fluorescence imaging has been successfully used to identify the sentinel lymph node and lymphatic stations; it can be achieved by injecting 2–3 mg ICG along the submucosal layer at 4 points around the tumor during the endoscopy for its localization on the day before surgery.

One of the possible complications after an esophagectomy is the thoracic duct injury with an estimated incidence between 0.6 and 9% (see suggested reading #31). Intraoperative identification of the thoracic duct can be challenging, especially for learning surgeons. The conventional methods of identifying the thoracic duct, including a diet rich in fat components the day before the procedure or the administration of milk/cream by nasogastric tube, are not reliable. The difficulty to detect its location and the chyle leakage make intraoperative ICG lymphography an interesting technique, especially in reoperations and in patients after radiation therapy where the anatomy is altered and anatomical landmarks may be absent.

In practice, 2–3 mg ICG is injected subcutaneously in both inguinal regions approximately 30 minutes before the surgery. During the procedure, real-time fluorescence lymphography can be achieved, usually allowing one to locate and eventually spare or ligate the thoracic duct. Moreover, the thoracic duct may have branches that cannot be identified without fluorescence, and if they are not ligated, they may be the source of the leakage. ICG enables the detection of these branches, thus potentially improving surgical outcomes (**Figures 7-18 A, B**).

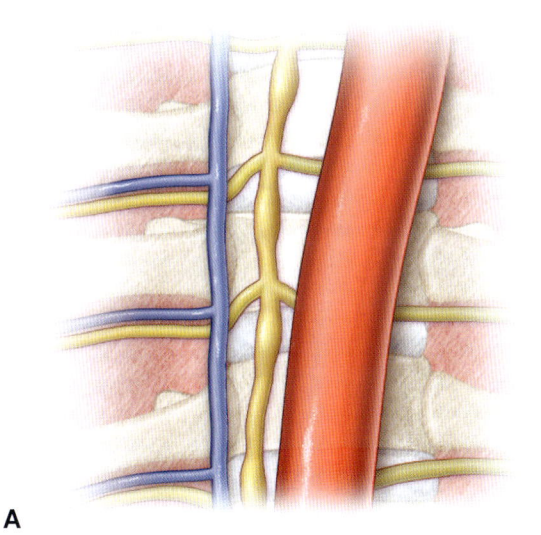

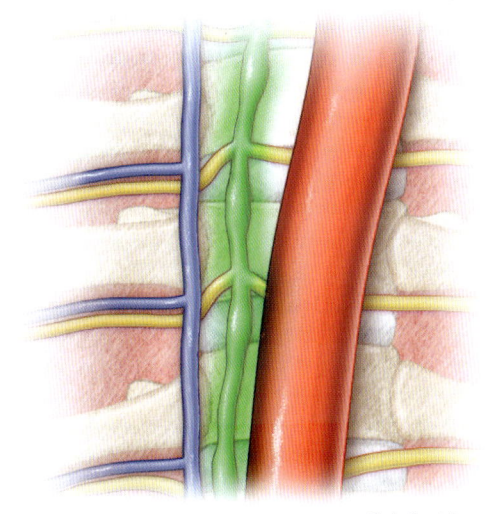

FIGURE 7-18 • Thoracic duct identification with ICG.

Fluorescence Imaging Applications for Kidney Surgery

Renal Artery Identification

ICG fluorescence can be used during partial nephrectomy to identify the renal artery, evaluate parenchymal perfusion, and facilitate super-selective arterial clamping. This not only allows preservation of the renal parenchyma uninvolved by the tumor but also ensures adequate margins for resection and reduces ischemia and perfusion/reperfusion injury. The tumor and the immediate surrounding parenchyma remain dark while the rest becomes fluorescent.

After the injection of 5 mg ICG, the fluorescent flow can be observed through the main renal artery, and subsequently the renal vein in approximately 1–2 minutes (**Figures 7-19 A, B**).

In addition, the enhanced visualization of the renal artery anatomy can also aid in aneurysm repair. The IV administration of 5 mg ICG allows immediate visualization of both the renal artery and the aneurysm site, making easier the identification of the vessels and the position of the aneurysm. At the end of the reconstruction, the ICG injection can be repeated, verifying the normal restoration of the blood flow (**Figures 7-20 A–D; Video 7-19**).

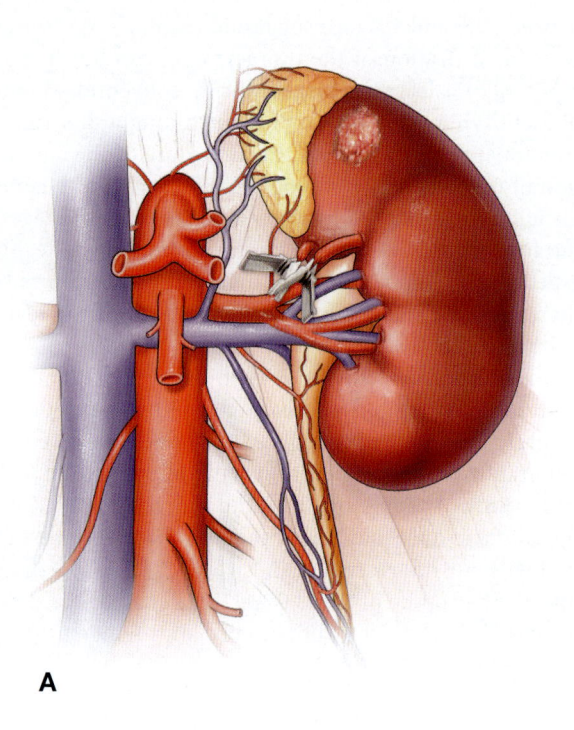

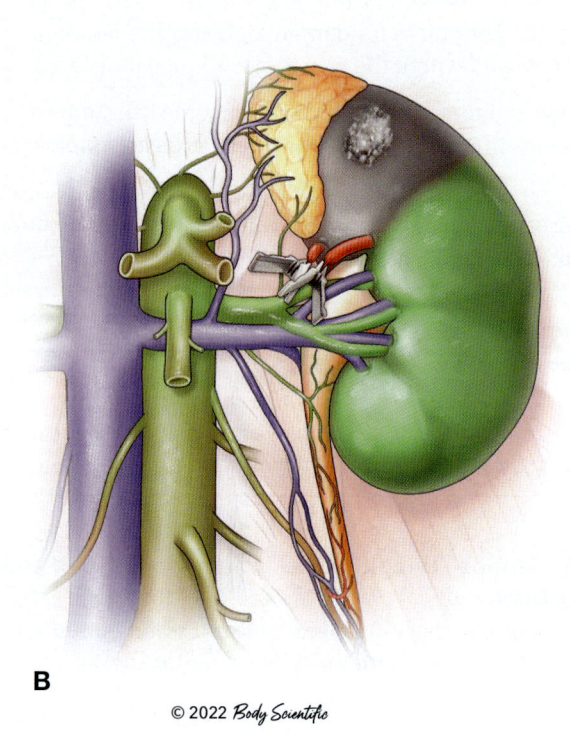

FIGURE 7-19 • Parenchymal perfusion evaluation with ICG after selective arterial clamping. **A.** After selective arterial clamping without ICG. **B.** After selective arterial clamping with ICG.

Fluorescence Imaging: Basics and Clinical Applications   113

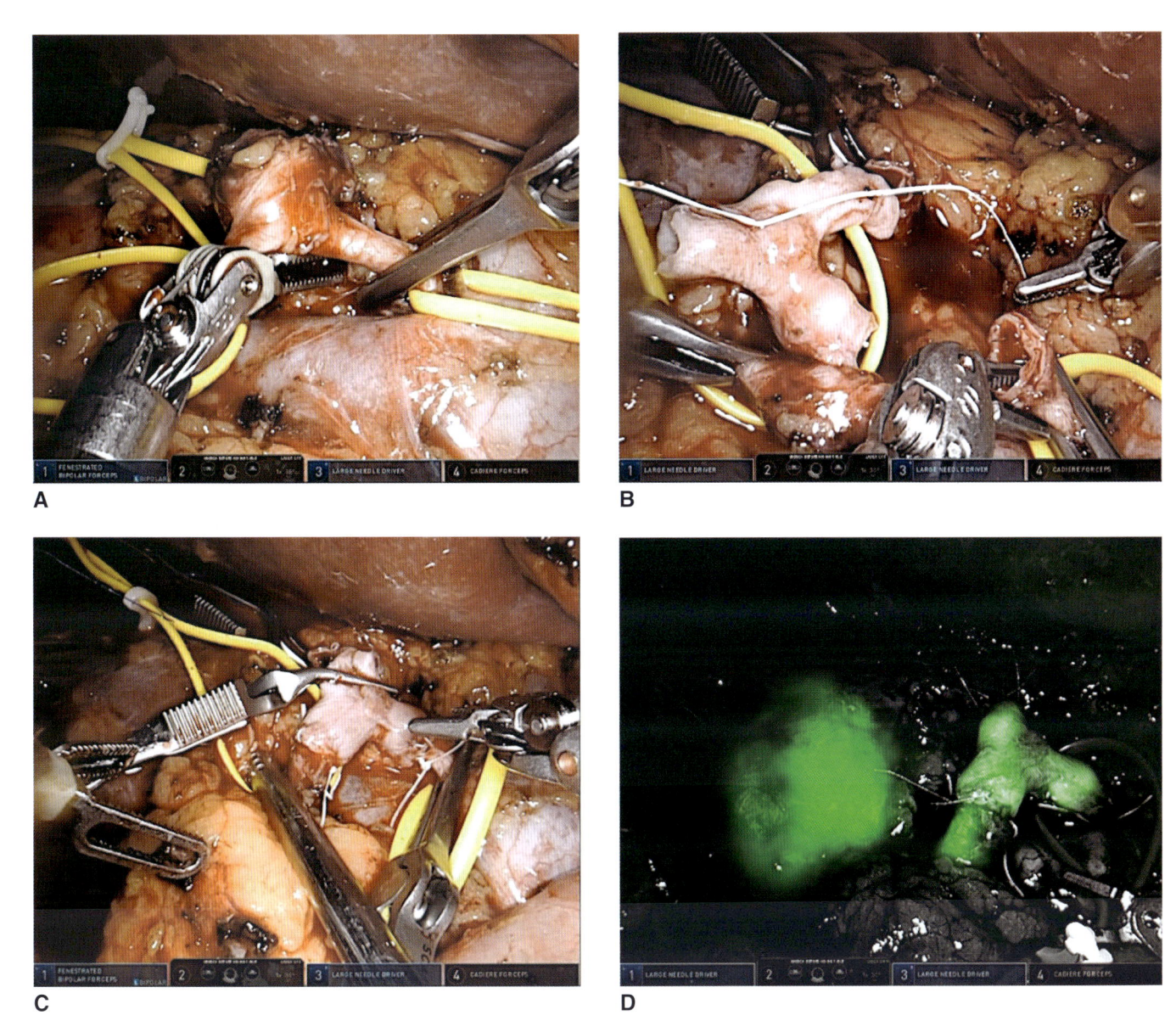

FIGURE 7-20 • Right renal artery aneurysm repair.

▶ Video 7-19. Right Renal Artery Aneurysm Repair

Perfusion Confirmation for Transplanted Kidney
During the kidney transplant procedure, a fundamental step is to confirm an adequate blood flow from the patient's artery to the allograft renal artery, circulating throughout the entire grafted kidney, and exiting through the allograft renal vein to the patient's vein. Even though Doppler ultrasound can give information on the blood flow status, the technique may be hindered by artifacts—it is operator dependent and does not provide information about the entire organ. ICG fluorescence, on the other hand, is not operator dependent, and it allows a real-time and comprehensive evaluation of vascularization with good spatial and temporal resolution. It helps to assess the integrity of the vascular anastomosis and the overall blood supply of the transplanted kidney. After completion of the allograft venous and arterial anastomosis, the recipient IV administration of 5 mg ICG followed by unclamping the bulldog forceps, allows visual evaluation of the perfusion (**Figures 7-21 A–D; Videos 7-20** and **7-21**).

> ▶▶ **TIPS**
>
> Identifying perfusion defects in real time allows a quick understanding also of the causes with eventual corrective actions before irreversible damage can occur.

114 The Foundation and Art of Robotic Surgery

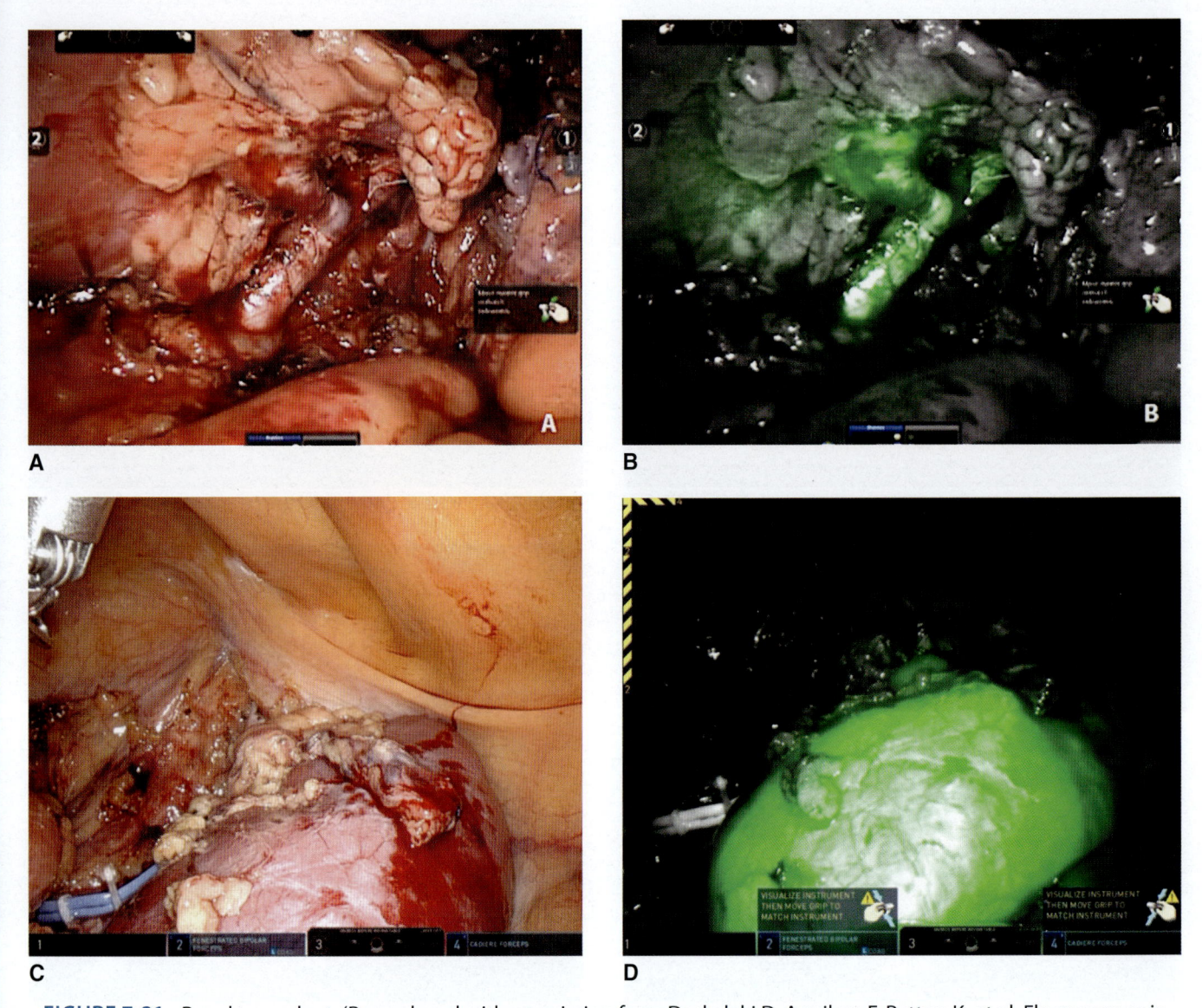

FIGURE 7-21 • Renal transplant. (Reproduced with permission from Daskalaki D, Aguilera F, Patton K, et al. Fluorescence in robotic surgery. *J Surg Oncol*. 2015;112(3):250-256.)

Video 7-20. Renal Transplant: Vascular Flow

Video 7-21. Renal Transplant

Fluorescence Imaging Applications for Pancreatic Surgery

Pancreatic Tumor Imaging and Margining

ICG allows enhancement of hypervascular pancreatic lesions such as neuroendocrine tumors. The common approach is to administer ICG preoperatively and use the positive contrast strategy to visualize the lesion. In practice, 5–10 mg ICG is intravenously injected into the patient 1 day before the procedure. During the surgery, the standing-out ICG fluorescence in the lesion facilitates the exact localization of pancreatic neuroendocrine tumors, allowing one to spare unaffected parenchyma and to achieve a resection with clean margins (**Figures 7-22 A–E**; **Videos 7-22 and 7-23**).

▶▶ **TIPS**

ICG fluorescence technique is also useful to identify small, superficial neuroendocrine tumors that are highly hypervascular and helps in performing selective enucleations.

ICG fluorescence intensity is poor for the identification of cystic neoplasms given their vascularization is lower than that of the surrounding pancreatic parenchyma.

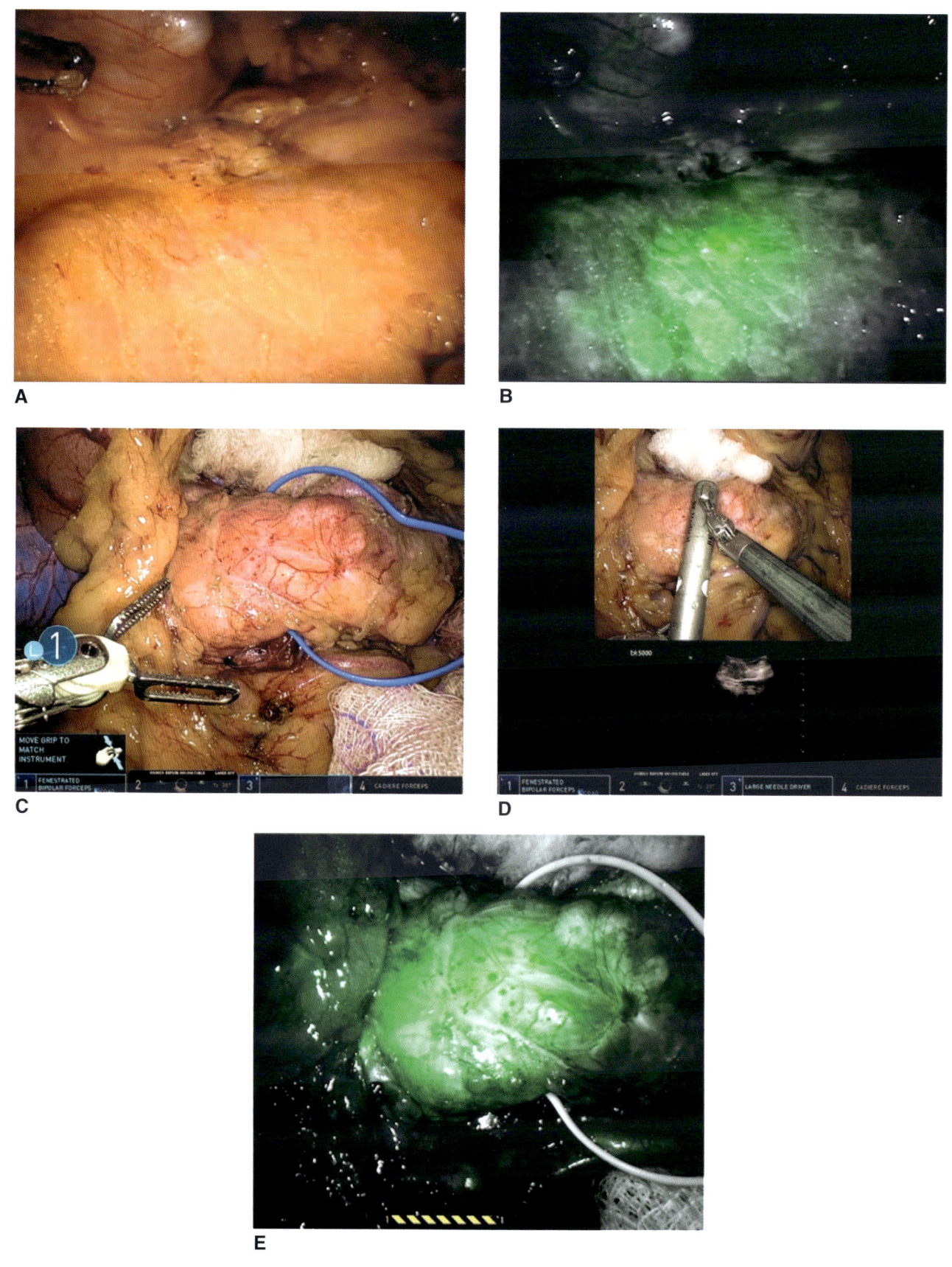

Fluorescence Imaging: Basics and Clinical Applications 115

FIGURE 7-22 • Pancreatic neuroendocrine tumor.

Video 7-22. Pancreatic NET

Video 7-23. Pancreatic NET

Spleen Vessel Imaging and Perfusion Assessment

During a distal pancreatectomy, when indicated, it is important to preserve the spleen not only to reduce postsurgical morbidity, but also to avoid altering the patient's immune system. One of the possible intraoperative complications of the spleen-preserving pancreatectomy is thrombosis of the splenic vein, which might lead to other complications such as gastric varices or the risk of splenic rupture when the short gastric vessels are taken down. ICG fluorescence can be used to assess splenic vessel anatomy and perfusion. The intraoperative IV administration of 5–10 mg ICG shows the splenic artery and vein along with the perfusion of the spleen as shown in **Figures 7-23 A–C** and **Videos 7-24** and **7-25**.

A

B

C

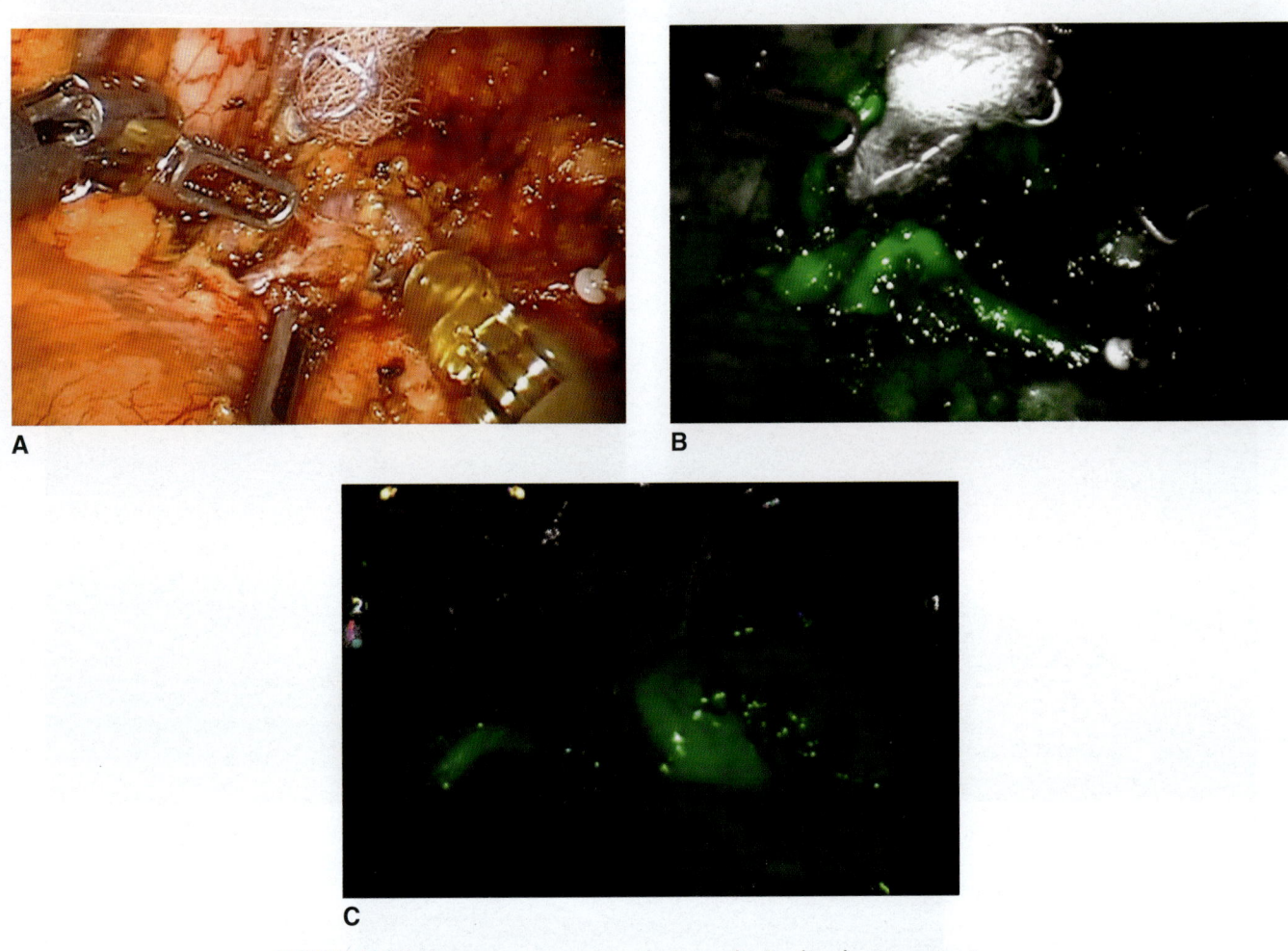

FIGURE 7-23 • Spleen preservation during robotic distal pancreatectomy.

▶ Video 7-24. Spleen Preservation in Distal Pancreatectomy

▶ Video 7-25. Spleen Preservation in Distal Pancreatectomy

Both ICG fluorescence intensity and the rate of its changes can be used to evaluate spleen perfusion. Such intraoperative fluorescence results can help to decide between preserving the spleen given adequate blood flow or removing it if weak or lack of fluorescence is observed.

The clear view of the splenic vessel anatomy with ICG fluorescence technique also facilitates splenic artery aneurysm repair as described for the renal ones. As shown in **Figures 7-24 A–D**, both the splenic artery and the aneurysm site can be observed under the fluorescence mode during the surgery (**Video 7-26**).

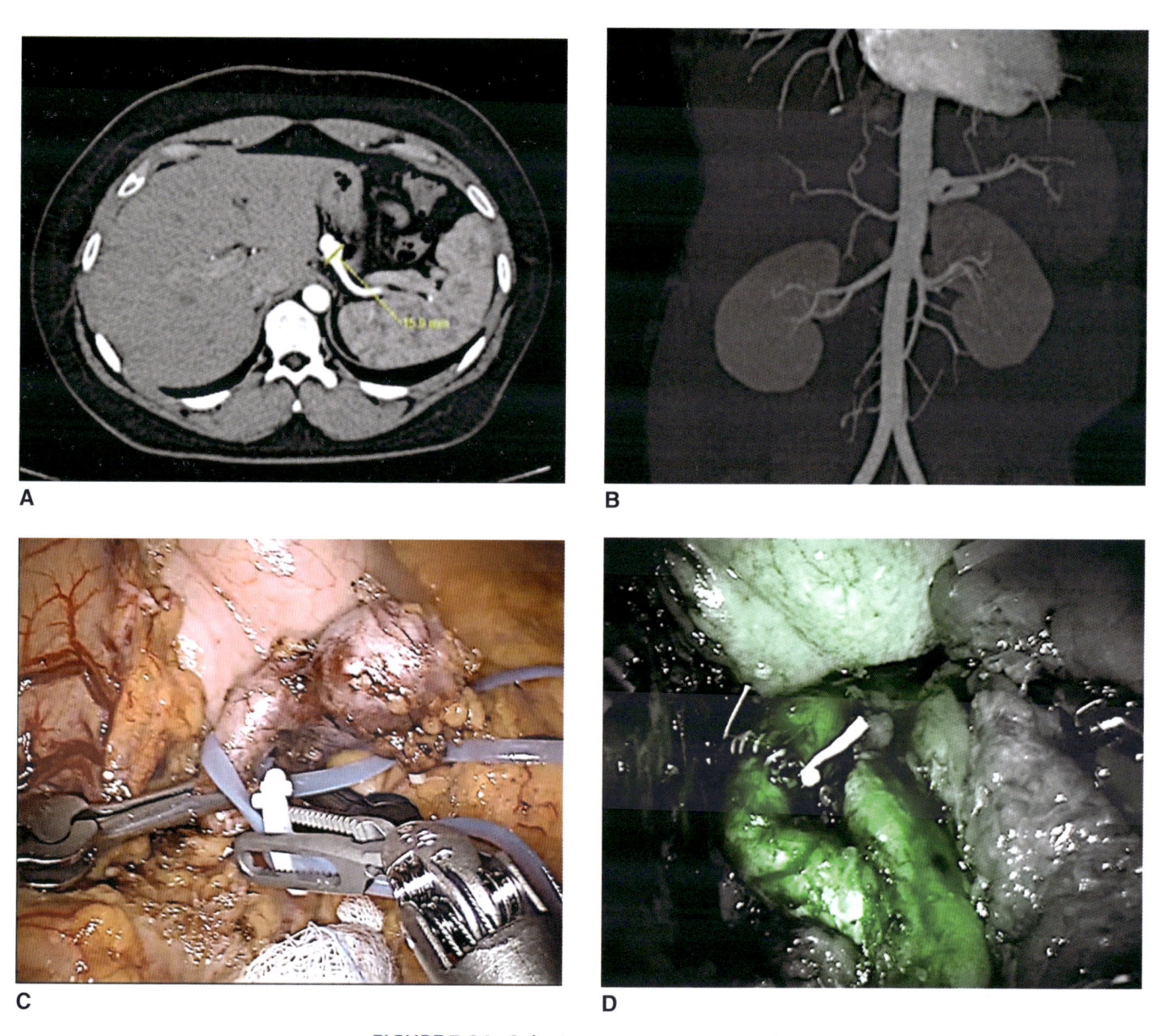

FIGURE 7-24 • Splenic artery aneurysm repair.

Video 7-26. Splenic Artery Aneurysm Repair

Fluorescence Imaging Application for Adrenal Surgery

The primary utility of ICG fluorescence in adrenal surgery is to guide a more precise operation by delineating the margins of resection. By taking advantage of the highly vascular nature of the adrenocortical tissue compared to the less vascular retroperitoneal one, more ICG will be accumulated in the adrenal gland, and the strong positive fluorescence contrast will help to obtain a precise dissection with identification of the boundaries of the adrenal gland. In addition, when partial adrenalectomy is indicated, it can guide parenchymal sparing surgery by showing the plane between the normal adrenal tissue and the tumor, as in some pheochromocytoma resections (**Figures 7-25 A, B**; **Video 7-27**).

A B

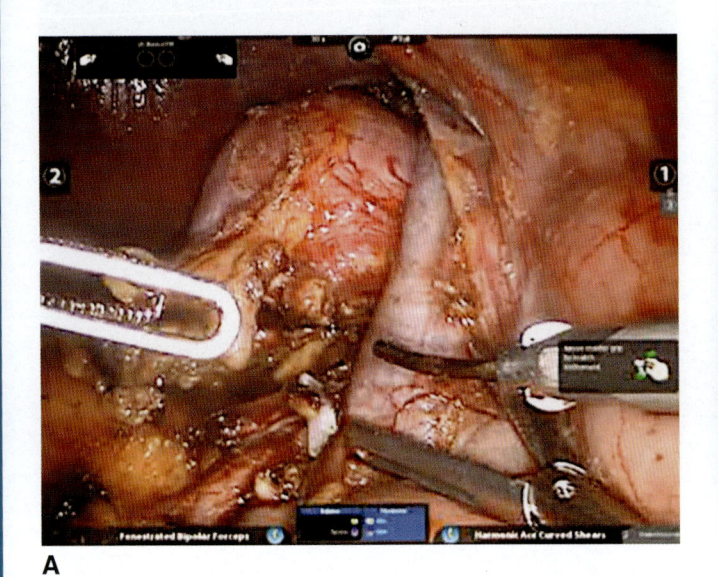

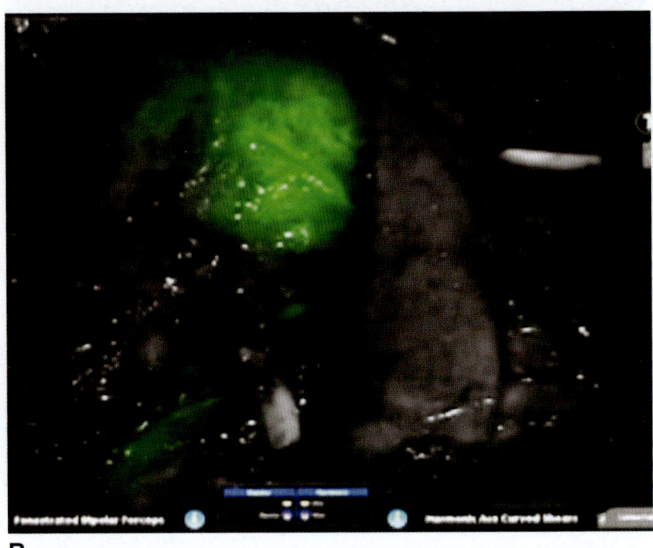

FIGURE 7-25 • Pheochromocytoma identification.

Video 7-27. Pheochromocytoma Identification

Fluorescence Imaging Applications for Parathyroid Surgery

Accurate identification and preservation of healthy parathyroid glands are key to prevent hypoparathyroidism and hypocalcemia in thyroid surgery. While large, abnormal glands can be visualized under white light imaging, small glands, especially those in unusual locations, are very difficult to see, even for experienced surgeons. Two different fluorescence imaging techniques have been used to tackle this challenge: (1) using ICG as a contrast agent to visualize the parathyroid glands and (2) taking advantage of the unique autofluorescence property of the parathyroid glands.

During a thyroidectomy, the poor perfusion of the thyroid lesion, and the good vascularization of the parathyroid glands, will yield less ICG in the diseased thyroid and more ICG in the parathyroid. This will make the fluorescence of the parathyroids stand out from the background thyroid ICG fluorescence. As a result, the parathyroids can be visualized as green dots under the fluorescence imaging mode. In practice, 5–10 mg ICG is administered intravenously after the retraction of the strap muscles and the exposure of the thyroid gland. The enhancement of the parathyroids can be observed after 2 minutes and the imaging can last up to 20 minutes. ICG should be injected slowly and progressively to allow the parathyroid glands to be differentiated from the thyroid gland; if the injection is too fast, both parenchymas will light up simultaneously and strongly. The strap muscle dissection should be performed carefully to prevent bleeding from the surrounding structures, such as the thyroid capsule and central lymph nodes. Otherwise, the visualization of the parathyroid glands could be hampered due to the masking effect of the blood.

On the other hand, for a mechanism that is still under investigation, parathyroid glands exhibit spontaneous and immediate emission at 820–830-nm wavelength (2–11-fold signal enhancement over that of the surrounding tissue) when excited with light at 785–800-nm wavelength. The autofluorescence can be detected using the NIR camera, thus allowing the visualization of parathyroid glands under the fluorescence imaging mode. NIR cameras for open surgery such as Fluobeam® (Fluoptic) or PTeye™ Parathyroid Detection System (Medtronic) have been successfully used for imaging the autofluorescence of the parathyroid glands, but camera systems specifically optimized for ICG fluorescence imaging in laparoscopic and robotic surgeries are less effective in observing the parathyroid's autofluorescence due to the use of a different excitation light source at 805-nm wavelength. It is expected that the next generation of fluorescence cameras for robotic surgery could include this function (**Figures 7-26 A, B**).

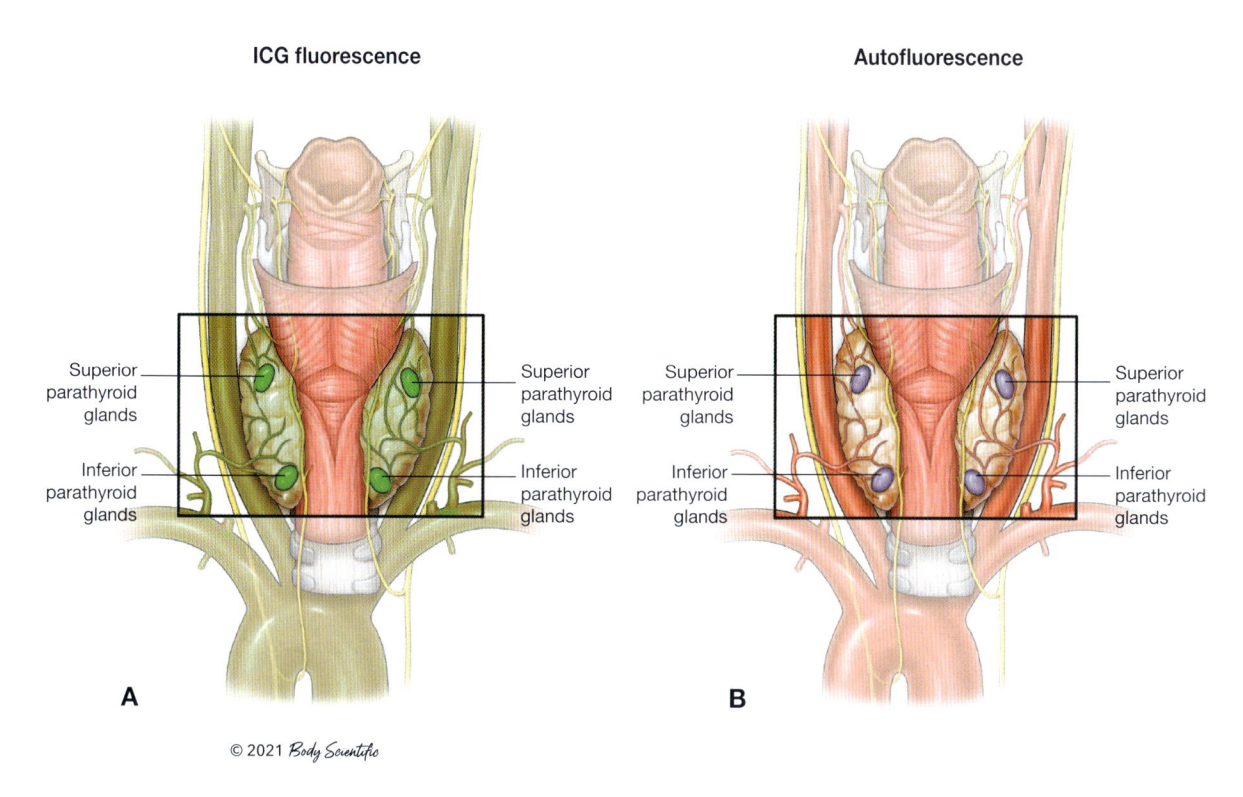

FIGURE 7-26 • Visualization of the parathyroid glands. **A.** ICG fluorescence. **B.** Autofluorescence.

Fluorescence Imaging Applications for Thoracic Surgery

With the advances in surgical robotic platforms, thoracic surgery has been progressively spread worldwide, particularly for thymectomy and lobar resections. The fluorescence imaging technique has been applied to these procedures to maximize safety and improve surgical outcomes.

Vasculature and Nerve Imaging in Thymus Surgery

Robotic thymectomy for the treatment of thymic tumors and the management of myasthenia gravis has been progressively adopted due to encouraging oncological outcomes and the trends of myasthenia gravis improvement and remission rates. During thymectomy, a high level of accuracy is needed with complete resection of the gland and avoidance of intraoperative morbidity. The identification of the phrenic nerves, mainly the contralateral to the access site, may be difficult and time-consuming. ICG can aid to localize the periardiophrenic vessels surrounding the phrenic nerve, thus facilitating the identification of the nerve itself. To identify the contralateral phrenic nerve bundle, 5–10 mg ICG is injected intravenously, and the pericardiophrenic vessels and nerve bundle can be visualized within 1 minute. In case ICG needs to be injected repeatedly, it should be done at least 5 minutes after the previous injection to allow enough time for the dye to be cleared.

Thoracic Tumor Imaging

Fluorescence imaging is useful for detecting lung nodules during lobectomies or sublobar resections. The latter ones have become a feasible alternative to lobectomy in high-risk patients and with early-stage lung cancer as it enables a complete resection of the tumor and has comparable survival outcomes. The robotic approach has the advantage of expedited recovery, the avoidance of chest wall trauma from a thoracotomy, and the negative impact on respiratory mechanics. However, unlike open surgeries, where the detection of pulmonary nodules can be carried out with finger palpation, most of the lesions cannot be detected using this method in the current surgical robot platforms where virtual tactile feedback is not yet available. Therefore, the precise localization of the lesion, and an adequate surgical margin for a wedge resection are more challenging to obtain. Fluorescence imaging can help to localize the nodules and to expose the intersegmental plane.

For nodule identification, 5–10 mg ICG is intravenously injected into the patient 1 day before the surgery and the positive contrast strategy is used to visualize the lesion. In addition, nodules can also be marked with ICG via a bronchoscopic needle during the bronchoscopic examination, and these fluorescently marked nodules can be identified during the surgery. The recent computer-aided bronchoscopic platforms such as

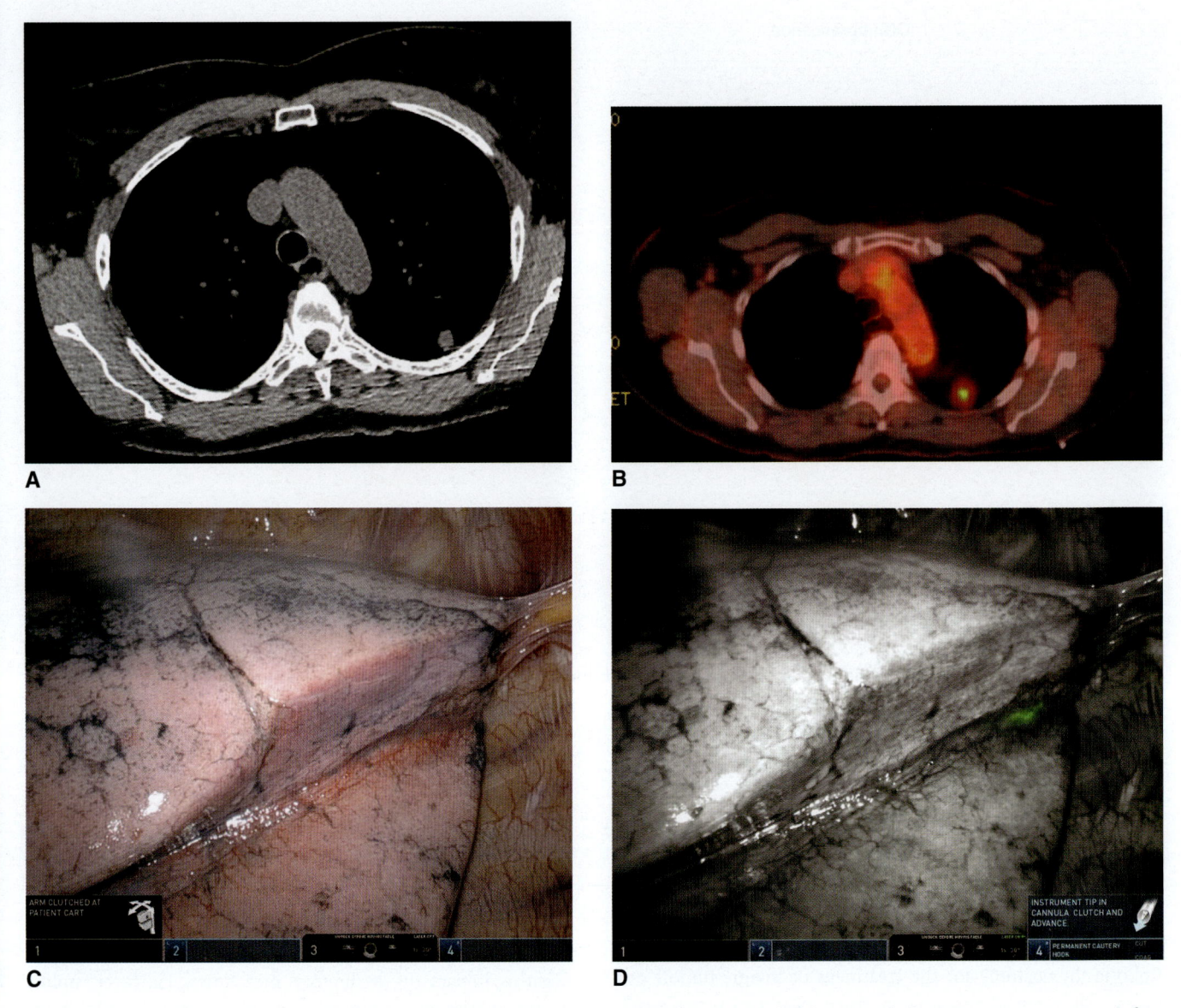

FIGURE 7-27 • Lung nodule visualization. **A–B.** Preoperative images of an upper-left lung nodule. **C.** During an upper-left lobectomy without ICG. **D.** During an upper-left lobectomy with ICG.

ION™ (Intuitive) and MONARCH™ (J&J) may allow preoperative selective ICG nodule injection in sequential combination with the following robotic operations, thus facilitating the intraoperative localization of the tumor (**Figures 7-27 A–D**).

Revealing the Intersegmental Plane

Segmental resection consists of transecting the corresponding vein, artery, and bronchus, and dividing the lung parenchyma. During the parenchymal division, the intersegmental plane has to be identified to achieve an appropriate tumor margin. Although the intersegmental plane can be identified by inflating/deflating the tissue, it is practically difficult and prone to errors due to air diffusion ICG fluorescence imaging can help to reveal the intersegmental plane. After IV injection of ICG, it binds to HSA and is confined to the vascular compartment. This allows to delineate the intersegmental plane after the ligation of the segmental artery. More recently, transbronchial ICG injection has been introduced, thus enabling ICG fluorescence imaging to determine the surgical margins for pulmonary sublobar resections in patients with early-stage lung cancer. Briefly, after positioning a bronchoscope to the target bronchus, a balloon catheter is inserted, and the balloon is inflated at the orifice of the bronchus. 2.5 mg ICG (10-fold diluted with autologous blood) is diffused to the target subsegmental bronchus, followed by the introduction of 300–400 mL of air to the bronchus to spread the ICG to the peripheral regions. A double-lumen endobronchial tube is inserted and maintained by 5–10 cm H_2O of positive end-expiratory pressure ventilation. During the procedure, the target segmental bronchus and the corresponding segmental bronchial tree can be visualized under the fluorescence mode. This will help to define the segmental borders to facilitate the resection. The previously mentioned bronchoscopic robotic platforms (ION™ and MONARCH™) may help in the further development of these sophisticated techniques of lung planes and nodule mapping.

PERSPECTIVES

Fluorescence imaging, integrated with white-light imaging, has been proven to enable real-time assessment of vessel structures, blood flow, tissue perfusion, bile duct exposure, and visualization of lesions and lymph nodes during robotic surgery. Although fluorescence imaging based on tissue intrinsic fluorescence properties without administering any imaging reagents to the patient is desirable, it currently has very limited applications and most intraoperative fluorescence imaging procedures are still conducted by using a tracer and a probe as the contrast agent. Remarkable progress has been made to develop new fluorescence imaging contrast agents in the laboratory, with high fluorescence quantum yields, good target specificity, and better target-to-background ratios. However, considered as a drug under the FDA regulation, any new fluorescence contrast agents will face a lengthy and expensive approval process before reaching the clinical use. Thus, it is expected that ICG will be the dominating fluorescence tracer for a long time, despite its low fluorescence quantum yield. On the other hand, its rich photophysical properties could enable the exploration of new applications of ICG from different disciplinary angles. A promising recent development is to move fluorescence imaging to the short-wave infrared (SIR) (900–1500 nm) region. Such a movement holds great potential for higher contrast, sensitivity, and penetration depths compared to conventional NIR fluorescence imaging. This effort has been facilitated by advances in detectors, specifically the emergence of indium gallium arsenide-based SIR cameras (versus silicon-based NIR cameras). ICG J-aggregate, which has an absorption peak at 900 nm, should exhibit red-shifted fluorescence in the SIR region theoretically. Recent studies have demonstrated that both ICG and its derivative, IRDye® 800CW, can be used for SIR fluorescence imaging at clinically relevant doses to visualize blood and lymph vessels as well as lesions in the lab, with better contrast compared to NIR fluorescence imaging.

With the breakthroughs in the imaging software and hardware, as well as the ever-progressing computational powers, computer-aided imaging analysis and transformation can overcome some limitations of fluorescence imaging and further improve the image clarity of the target tissue. Specifically, through computer-aided deep and sequential analysis of an ongoing surgical video, a content-aware subtraction feature can be created, so that unwanted objectives can be removed from the target fluorescence images in real time. For example, a computer equipped with state-of-the-art hardware and developed software can temporally aware the objectives in the surgical field. This will enable one to automatically remove the fluorescence of the liver parenchyma and analyze frames over time to fill the fluorescence on any overlay pixels between the liver and bile duct, thus yielding a clarified image of the bile duct without the background fluorescence from the liver. At the same time, artificial intelligence (AI) will play a critical role in both fluorescence imaging probe development (AI-assisted design and synthesis) and imaging process and analysis. Chapter 6, Implemented Imaging and Artificial Intelligence, delineated the current progress, especially in the area of quantitative fluorescence imaging for objective perfusion assessment, which can be validated and applied to clinics in a short time. Another area of interest is machine-learning-based tumor margining from spectroscopic fluorescence imaging or fluorescence lifetime (the time the fluorophore's electrons spend in the excited state before emitting photons and returning to their ground state) imaging. It takes advantage of the fact that the fluorescence spectrum and fluorescence lifetime of many endogenous and exogenous fluorophores are very sensitive to minute chemical/physical changes in their environment. As a result, they can be used to detect subtle biochemical and biophysical changes in tumor tissues. With the use of a pixel addressable imaging detector/method for spectroscopic fluorescence imaging or fluorescence lifetime imaging, the distinct spectrum and/or lifetime signatures of the fluorophores on tumor and surrounding tissues can be obtained across longitudinal and transverse directions in both spatial and temporal dimensions. These massive signature data associated with alterations in tumor structure and biochemical profiles can be fed to machine learning algorithms under a supervised or unsupervised mode. Such an entirely data-driven approach can lead to the differentiation of the tumor from surrounding tissues at the molecular levels, thus capable of margining tumors more precisely. It is expected that the combination of new fluorophores, high-throughput optics, advanced imaging detectors, and imaging processes supported by AI will further increase the use of fluorescence imaging as an intraoperative guidance tool to enhance the safety and accuracy of robotic surgery.

Molecular imaging modalities such as PET-CT, MRI, and ultrasound imaging can all yield 3D tomography images, yet intraoperative fluorescence imaging currently remains at the 2D level. By taking advantage of better tissue penetration of NIR light, a 3D construction of fluorescence imaging in centimeter scales should be possible. Given the current layout of the surgical robot platforms, conventional fluorescence tomography methods with a geometry of a rotating detector or a detector ring may not be feasible. However, with recent developments in ultrafast imaging cameras and optics, time-of-flight imaging or fluorescence image correlation technologies could potentially reveal the depth information of a fluorescence probe/tracer, thus outputting a 3D fluorescence image. For example, with the advent of ultrafast cameras with high quantum efficiency, fluorescence stacks with time resolutions in the microsecond or even nanosecond ranges can be obtained. By computing spatiotemporal correlations and machine learning, fluorophore distribution and their dynamics in different depths can be reconstructed. This could render a 3D map of small lesions or other important anatomies that fluorophore resides beneath the tissue surface when using a NIR or SWIR fluorescence tracer or probe.

In conclusion, fluorescence imaging allows earlier recognition of anatomical variants, reducing the risk of inadvertent damage, and enabling successful anastomosis and precise lesion resections with negative margins. By revealing the anatomy of vital structures during surgery, fluorescence imaging can also help decreasing the learning curve in robotic surgery, especially for advanced and complicated procedures.

ACKNOWLEDGMENTS

The authors would like to thank Pauline Ostoja-Starzewski and Krishna Shah for their help with the figures in the chapter.

The authors are also grateful to Dr. Giuseppe Spinoglio for providing **Figures 7-14 C–F** and **7-15 A, B**, and the videos regarding mesenteric lymphography and nerve identification in TME.

Suggested Readings

1. Mishra A, Behera RK, Behera PK, et al. Cyanines during the 1990s: a review. *Chem Rev.* 2000;100(6):1973-2012. doi: 10.1021/cr990402t
2. Carr JA, Franke D, Caram JR, et al. Shortwave infrared fluorescence imaging with the clinically approved near-infrared dye indocyanine green. *PNAS*, 2008;115(17):4465-4470.
3. Sano K, Mitsunaga M, Nakajima T, et al. In vivo breast cancer characterization imaging using two monoclonal antibodies activatably labeled with near infrared fluorophores. *Breast Cancer Res.* 2012;14:R61.
4. Yim JJ, Tholen M, Klaassen A, Sorger J, Bogyo M. Optimization of a protease activated probe for optical surgical navigation. *Molecul Pharmaceut* 2018;15(3):750-758.
5. Liu X, Lovell P, Cruz, DR, et al. Novel intra-operative peripheral nerve agent for fluorescence guided imaging. *Proceedings of the SPIE.* 2020;11225(8).
6. Van Manen L, Handgraaf HJM, Diana M, et al. A practical guide for the use of indocyanine green and methylene blue in fluorescence-guided abdominal surgery. *J Surg Oncol.* 2018;118:283-300.
7. Meershoek P, KleinJan GH, Van Willigen DM, et al. Multi-wavelength fluorescence imaging with a da Vinci Firefly—a technical look behind the scenes. *J Robotic Surg* 2020;s11701-020-01170-8
8. Daskalaki D, Aguilera F, Patton K, Giulianotti P. Fluorescence in robotic surgery. *J Surg Oncol.* 2015;112(3):250-256. doi: 10.1002/jso.23910
9. Ishizawa T, Bandai Y, Ijichi M, et al. Fluorescent cholangiography illuminating the biliary tree during laparoscopic cholecystectomy. *Br J Surg.* 2010;97(9):1369-1377. doi: 10.1002/bjs.7125
10. Pesce A, Palmucci S, La Greca G, Puleo S. Iatrogenic bile duct injury: impact and management challenges. *Clin Exp Gastroenterol.* 2019;12:121-128. doi: 10.2147/CEG.S169492
11. Gangemi A, Danilkowicz F, Elli FE, et al. Could ICG-aided robotic cholecystectomy reduce the rate of open conversion reported with laparoscopic approach? A head to head comparison of the largest single institution studies. *Robot Surg.* 2017;11(1):77-82. doi: 10.1007/s11701-016-0624-6
12. Daskalaki D, Fernandes E, Wang X, et al. Indocyanine green (ICG) fluorescent cholangiography during robotic cholecystectomy: results of 184 consecutive cases in a single institution. *Surg Innov.* 2014;21(6):615-621. doi: 10.1177/1553350614524839
13. Ambe P, Plambeck J, Fernandez-Jesberg V, Zarras K. The role of indocyanine green fluoroscopy for intraoperative bile duct visualization during laparoscopic cholecystectomy: an observational cohort study in 70 patients. *Patient Saf Surg.* 2019;13:2. doi: 10.1186/s13037-019-0182-8
14. Agnus V, Pesce A, Boni L, et al. Fluorescence-based cholangiography: preliminary results from the IHU-IRCAD-EAES EURO-FIGS registry. *Surg Endosc.* 2020;34(9):3888-3896. doi: 10.1007/s00464-019-07157-3
15. Onda N, Kimura M, Yoshida T, Shibutani M. Preferential tumor cellular uptake and retention of indocyanine green for in vivo tumor imaging. *Int J Cancer* 2016;139:673-682.
16. Tashiro Y, Aoki T, Hirai T, et al. Pathological validity of using near-infrared fluorescence imaging for securing surgical margins during liver resection. *Anticancer Res.* 2020;40:3873-3882.
17. Nakaseko Y, Ishizawa T, Saiura A. Fluorescence-guided surgery for liver tumors. *J Surg Oncol.* 2018;118(2):324-331. doi: 10.1002/jso.25128
18. Kobayashi K, Kawaguchi Y, Kobayashi Y, et al. Identification of liver lesions using fluorescence imaging: comparison of methods for administering indocyanine green. *HPB (Oxford).* 2021;23(2):262-269. doi: 10.1016/j.hpb.2020.06.006
19. Lim C, Vibert E, Azoulay D, et al. Indocyanine green fluorescence imaging in the surgical management of liver cancers: current facts and future implications. *J Visc Surg.* 2014;151(2):117-124. doi: 10.1016/j.jviscsurg.2013.11.003
20. Kobayashi Y, Kawaguchi Y, Kobayashi K, et al. Portal vein territory identification using indocyanine green fluorescence imaging: technical details and short-term outcomes. *J Surg Oncol.* 2017;116(7):921-931. doi: 10.1002/jso.24752
21. Boni L, David G, Dionigi G, Rausei S, et al. Indocyanine green-enhanced fluorescence to assess bowel perfusion during laparoscopic colorectal resection. *Surg Endosc.* 2016;30(7):2736-42. doi: 10.1007/s00464-015-4540-z
22. Wada T, Kawada K, Takahashi R, et al. ICG fluorescence imaging for quantitative evaluation of colonic perfusion in laparoscopic colorectal surgery. *Surg Endosc.* 2017;31(10):4184-4193. doi: 10.1007/s00464-017-5475-3
23. D' Urso A, Agnus V, Barberio M, et al. Computer-assisted quantification and visualization of bowel perfusion using fluorescence-based enhanced reality in left-sided colonic resections. *Surg Endosc.* 2021;35(8):4321-4331. doi: 10.1007/s00464-020-07922-9
24. Mangano A, Fernandes E, Gheza F, et al. Near-infrared indocyanine green-enhanced fluorescence and evaluation of the bowel microperfusion during robotic colorectal surgery: a retrospective original paper. *Surg Technol Int.* 2019;34:93-100.
25. Mangano A, Gheza F, Chen LL, Minerva EM, Giulianotti PC. Indocyanine green (ICG)-enhanced fluorescence for intraoperative assessment of bowel microperfusion during laparoscopic and robotic colorectal surgery: the quest for evidence-based results. *Surg Technol Int.* 2018;32:101-104.
26. Mangano A, Masrur MA, Bustos R, Chen LL, Fernandes E, Giulianotti PC. Near-infrared indocyanine green-enhanced fluorescence and minimally invasive colorectal surgery: review of the literature. *Surg Technol Int.* 2018;33:77-83.
27. Liberale G, Bohlok A, Bormans A, et al. Indocyanine green fluorescence imaging for sentinel lymph node detection in colorectal cancer: a systematic review. *Eur J Surg Oncol.* 2018;44(9):1301-1306. doi: 10.1016/j.ejso.2018.05.034
28. Huh YJ, Lee HJ, Kim TH, Choi Y. Efficacy of assessing intraoperative bowel perfusion with near-infrared camera in laparoscopic gastric cancer surgery. *J Laparoendosc Adv Surg Tech A.* 2019;29(4):476-483. doi: 10.1089/lap.2018.0263
29. Baiocchi G, Molfino S, Molteni B, Quarti L. Fluorescence-guided lymphadenectomy in gastric cancer: a prospective

western series. *Updates Surg.* 2020;72(3):761-772. doi: 10.1007/s13304-020-00836-0
30. Okubo K, Uenosono Y, Arigami T, et al. Quantitative assessment of fluorescence intensity of ICG in sentinel nodes in early gastric cancer. *Gastric Cancer.* 2018;21(5):776-781. doi: 10.1007/s10120-018-0816-z
31. Thammineedi S, Patnaik S, Saksena A, et al. The utility of indocyanine green angiography in the assessment of perfusion of gastric conduit and proximal esophageal stump against visual assessment in patients undergoing esophagectomy: a prospective study. *Indian J Surg Oncol.* 2020;11(4):684-691. doi: 10.1007/s13193-020-01085-8
32. Slooter M, de Bruin D, Eshuis W, et al. Quantitative fluorescence-guided perfusion assessment of the gastric conduit to predict anastomotic complications after esophagectomy. *Dis Esophagus.* 2021;34(5). doi: 10.1093/dote/doaa100
33. Yang F, Zhou J, Li H, et al. Near-infrared fluorescence-guided thoracoscopic surgical intervention for postoperative chylothorax. *Interact Cardiovasc Thorac Surg.* 2018;26(2):171-175. doi: 10.1093/icvts/ivx304
34. Bibas B, Costa-de-Carvalho R, Pola-dos-Reis F, et al. Video-assisted thoracoscopic thoracic duct ligation with near-infrared fluorescence imaging with indocyanine green. *J Bras Pneumol.* 2019;45(4). doi: 10.1590/1806-3713/e20180401
35. Mishra P, Saluja S, Ramaswamy D, et al. Thoracic duct injury following esophagectomy in carcinoma of the esophagus: ligation by the abdominal approach. *World J Surg.* 2013;37(1):141-146. doi: 10.1007/s00268-012-1811-x
36. Vecchiato M, Martino A, Sponza M, et al. Thoracic duct identification with indocyanine green fluorescence during minimally invasive esophagectomy with patient in prone position. *Dis Esophagus.* 2020;33(12). doi: 10.1093/dote/doaa030
37. Gadus L, Kocarek J, Chmelik F, et al. Robotic partial nephrectomy with indocyanine green fluorescence navigation. *Contrast Media Mol Imaging.* 2020;2020:1287530. doi: 10.1155/2020/1287530
38. Diana P, Buffi N, Lughezzani G, et al. The role of intraoperative indocyanine green in robot-assisted partial nephrectomy: results from a large, multi-institutional series. *Eur Urol.* 2020;78(5):743-749. doi: 10.1016/j.eururo.2020.05.040
39. Rother U, Gerken A, Karampinis I, et al. Dosing of indocyanine green for intraoperative laser fluorescence angiography in kidney transplantation. *Microcirculation.* 2017;24(8). doi: 10.1111/micc.12392
40. Shirata C, Kawaguchi Y, Kobayashi K, et al. Usefulness of indocyanine green-fluorescence imaging for real-time visualization of pancreas neuroendocrine tumor and cystic neoplasm. *J Surg Oncol.* 2018;118(6):1012-1020. doi: 10.1002/jso.25231
41. Kawasaki Yi, Maemura K, Kurahara H, et al. Usefulness of fluorescence vascular imaging for evaluating splenic perfusion. *ANZ J Surg.* 2018;88(10):1017-1021. doi: 10.1111/ans.14364
42. Paras C, Keller M, White L, et al. Near-infrared autofluorescence for the detection of parathyroid glands. *J Biomed Opt.* 2011;16(6):067012. doi: 10.1117/1.3583571
43. Zhang C, Lin H, Fu R, et al. Application of indocyanine green fluorescence for precision sublobar resection. *Thorac Cancer.* 2019;10(4):624-630. doi: 10.1111/1759-7714.12972
44. Ferrari-Light D, Geraci TC, Sasankan P, Cerfolio RJ. The utility of near-infrared fluorescence and indocyanine green during robotic pulmonary resection. *Front Surg.* 2019;6:47. doi: 10.3389/fsurg.2019.00047
45. Sekine Y, Itoh T, Toyoda T, et al. Precise anatomical sublobar resection using a 3D medical image analyzer and fluorescence-guided surgery with transbronchial instillation of indocyanine green. *Semin Thorac Cardiovasc Surg.* 2019;31(3):595-602. doi: 10.1053/j.semtcvs.2019.01.004

SECTION II

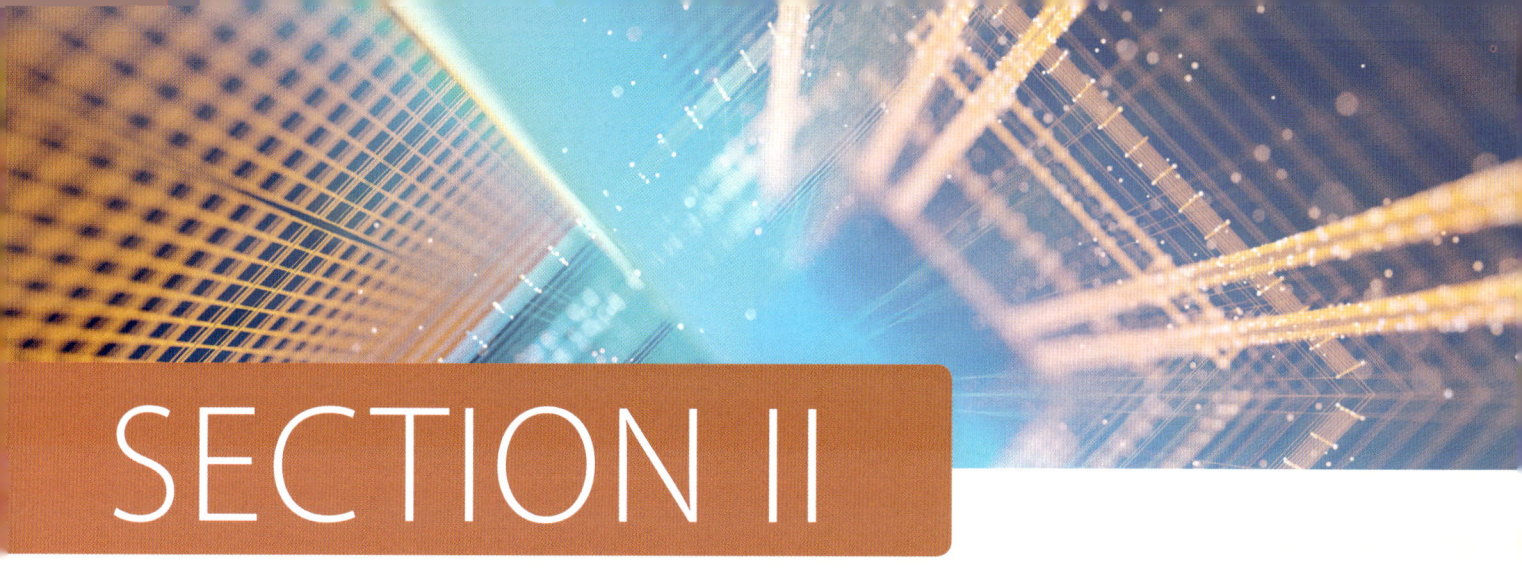

Thyroid Surgery

Chapter 8. Gasless Transaxillary Thyroidectomy (Off-Label Indication) 127
Woung Youn Chung • Cho Rok Lee

Chapter 9. Transoral Thyroidectomy (Off-Label Indication) 163
Ji Young You • Dawon Park • Hoon Yub Kim

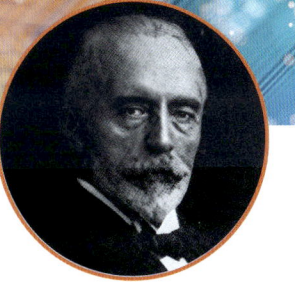

"Surgical treatment underwent a vast expansion. ... It has become possible within less than half a century to expose all the organs of the body. ... But it was just this ability to make all the organs accessible to direct observation ... that broadened our knowledge of the physiology of the body extraordinarily."

—Emil Theodor Kocher (1841–1917)

Gasless Transaxillary Thyroidectomy
(Off-Label Indication)

Woung Youn Chung • Cho Rok Lee

INTRODUCTION

Robotic thyroidectomy has provided some functional advantages over open thyroidectomy and has shown safe and effective surgical results. Many years have passed since the launch of the gasless transaxillary approach, and multiple advances have been made regarding this topic.

The improvement of cosmetic outcomes after thyroidectomy has been increasingly at the center of the scientific investigation. Robotic thyroidectomy, besides being as safe, feasible, and effective as conventional cervical and endoscopic thyroidectomy, also shows superior cosmetic results by avoiding scars in visible areas.

Indications and Relative Contraindications to the Robotic Approach

The initial indications of robotic thyroidectomy were restricted to: (1) well-differentiated thyroid cancer without thyroid capsular invasion, (2) a lesion <4 cm in size, and (3) follicular neoplasms <5 cm in size. Conversely, the contraindications were considered: (1) a history of previous head and neck surgery

EDITORIAL COMMENT

On the market, there are other similar retractors which have interesting features: for example, the UIC retractor (Automated), which has a strong lifting power, and it is particularly fit for larger BMI patients.

INSTRUMENT REQUIREMENTS

The suggested main robotic instruments/tools can be listed as follows:
- 30° endoscope
- Maryland dissector
- ProGrasp forceps
- Harmonic curved shears

Supplemental materials:

Patient position:
- Neck pillow (**Figure 8-1A**)
- Arm board (**Figure 8-1B**)

Creation of the skin flap:
- Fiberoptic retractor (2) (replaceable to headlight) (**Figure 8-1C**)
- Army-Navy retractors (**Figure 8-1D**)
- Monopolar cautery pen with short, medium, and long tips (**Figure 8-1D**)
- Vascular DeBakey or Russian forceps (**Figure 8-1D**)

Maintenance of the working space:
- Chung's external retractor system/similar autostatic retractor (**Figure 8-1E**)
- Elevator and lifter set

Robotic procedures:
- Endoscopic rolled gauzes
- Endoscopic suction irrigator
- Endobags
- Medium-large clips (for modified radical neck dissection)
- Closed-suction drain (3 and 5 mm)

128 The Foundation and Art of Robotic Surgery

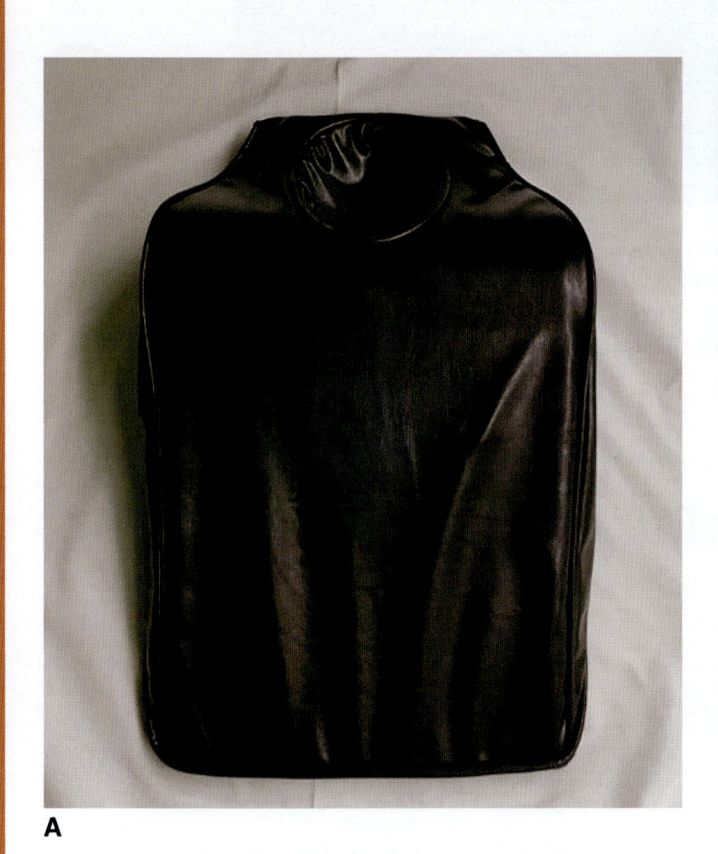

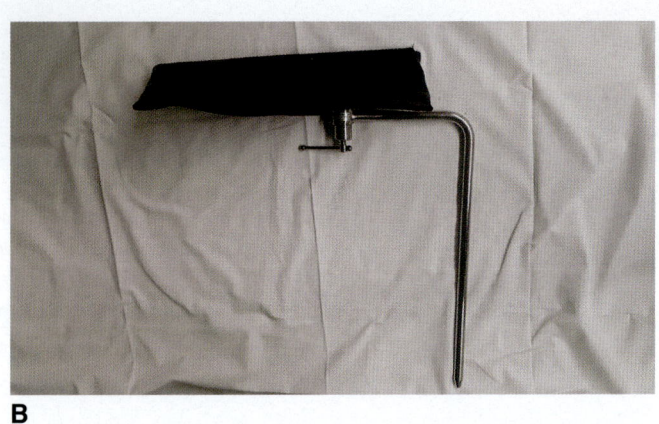

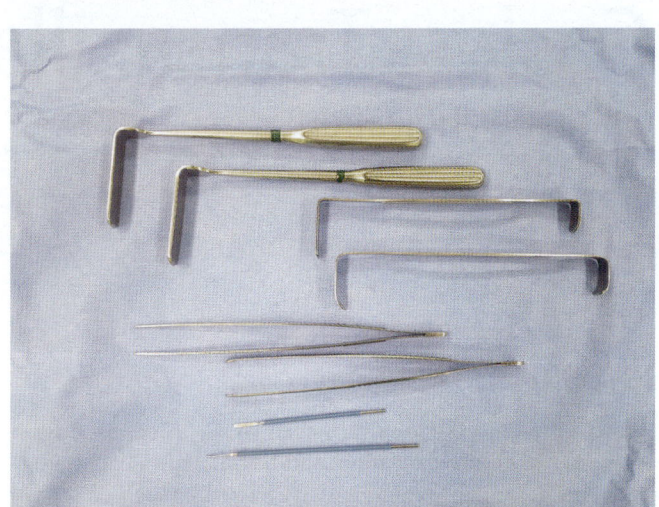

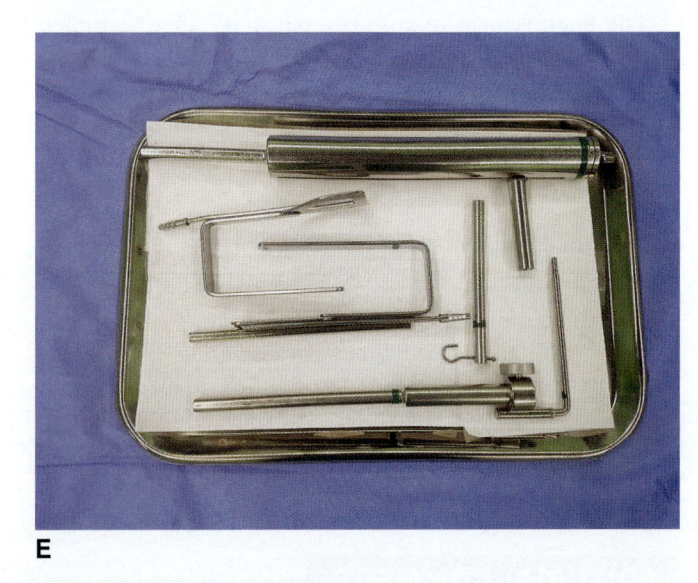

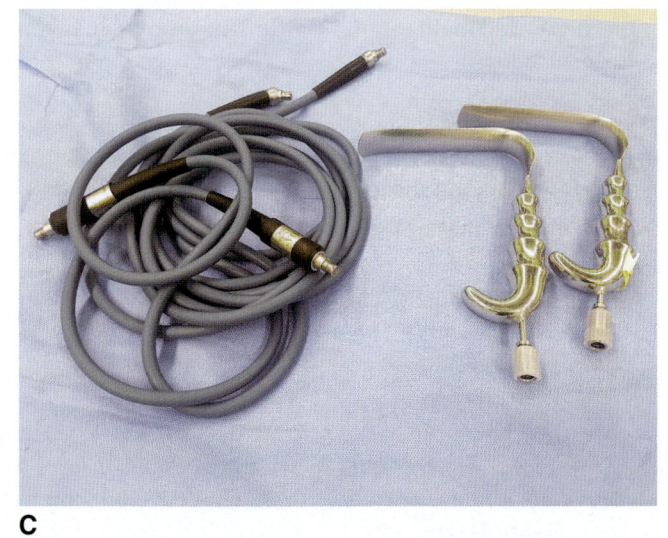

FIGURE 8-1 • Instruments for gasless transaxillary robotic thyroidectomy. **A.** Neck pillow. **B.** Arm board. **C.** Fiberoptic retractor. **D.** Army-Navy retractors, monopolar cautery pen with different tips, vascular DeBakey and Russian forceps. **E.** Chung's external retractor system/similar autostatic retractor.

or irradiation (and radioactive iodine treatment), (2) uncontrolled thyrotoxicosis, (3) lesions located in the dorsal thyroid area, especially in the region adjacent to the tracheoesophageal groove (because of possible injury to the trachea, esophagus, or recurrent laryngeal nerve [RLN]), (4) unrelated pathologic conditions of the neck or shoulder, and (5) an extremely high body mass index (BMI).

As the experience in robotics gradually increased, surgery of more advanced lesions (e.g., strap muscle invasion, multiple central compartment lymph node metastases) has become possible. Furthermore, even if superficial cancer invasion is present in the RLN, trachea, and neck vessels, it can be removed by a "shaving technique" with robotic scissors. In addition, Graves' disease of large multinodular goiter can be managed robotically.

THYROIDECTOMY

Patient Positioning, OR Setup, and Port Setting

Under general anesthesia, the patient is placed in supine position on a small neck pillow with the neck slightly extended.

The arm homo-lateral to the lesion is raised to minimize the distance between the axilla and anterior neck (**Figure 8-2A**). This setup rotates the clavicle, lowering its medial aspect and providing excellent access to the thyroid gland.

Occasionally, in cases where there is difficulty in raising the shoulder straight or in obese individuals, the shoulder should be lifted to expose the axilla homo-lateral to the lesion. After that, the elbow should be bent at a 90° angle, and the arm padded and fixed to an arm board overlying the forehead (**Figures 8-2 B, C**). This modified position avoids transient traction injuries of the brachial plexus (neuropraxia). The patient's arm should not be hyperextended.

>> **TIPS**

The basic principle of the patient positioning is to reduce the distance between the axilla and the anterior neck as much as possible.

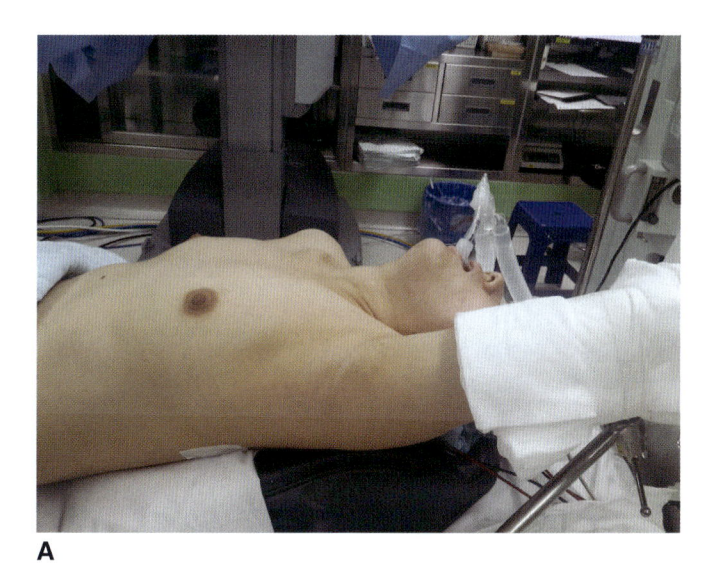

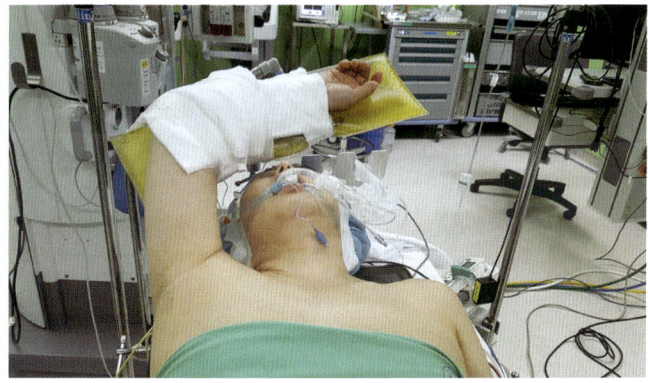

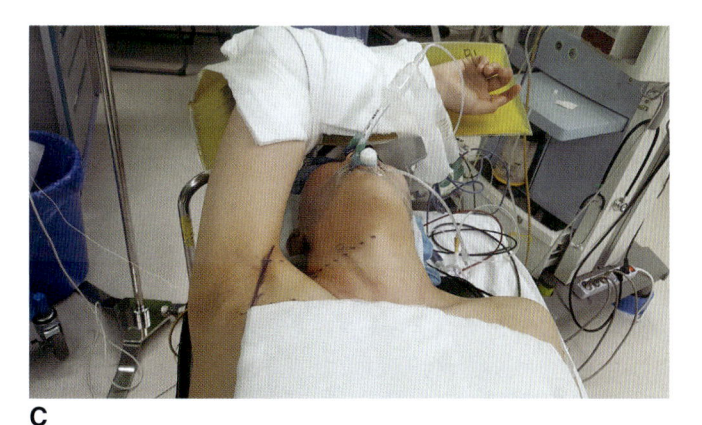

FIGURE 8-2 • Patient positioning. **A.** Standard position. **B, C.** Modified arm position.

Creation of the Working Space

Drawing the Incision Lines (Figure 8-3)

The following lines have to be drawn to define the dissection in the surgical field:

- An oblique line from the thyroid cartilage to the clavicle (passing the thyroid upper pole) and a parallel line from the clavicle to the axillary fold.
- A parallel line from the sternal notch to the axillary fold.
- A vertical incision line on the axilla, located about 5–6 cm along the lateral border of the pectoralis major muscle.

> ►► **TIPS**
>
> After drawing the incision lines and positioning the arm, it must be reassessed that the drawing is still in the correct direction in order to approach the tunnel.
>
> The patient positioning must facilitate as much as possible the creation of the tunnel between the axilla and the anterior neck.

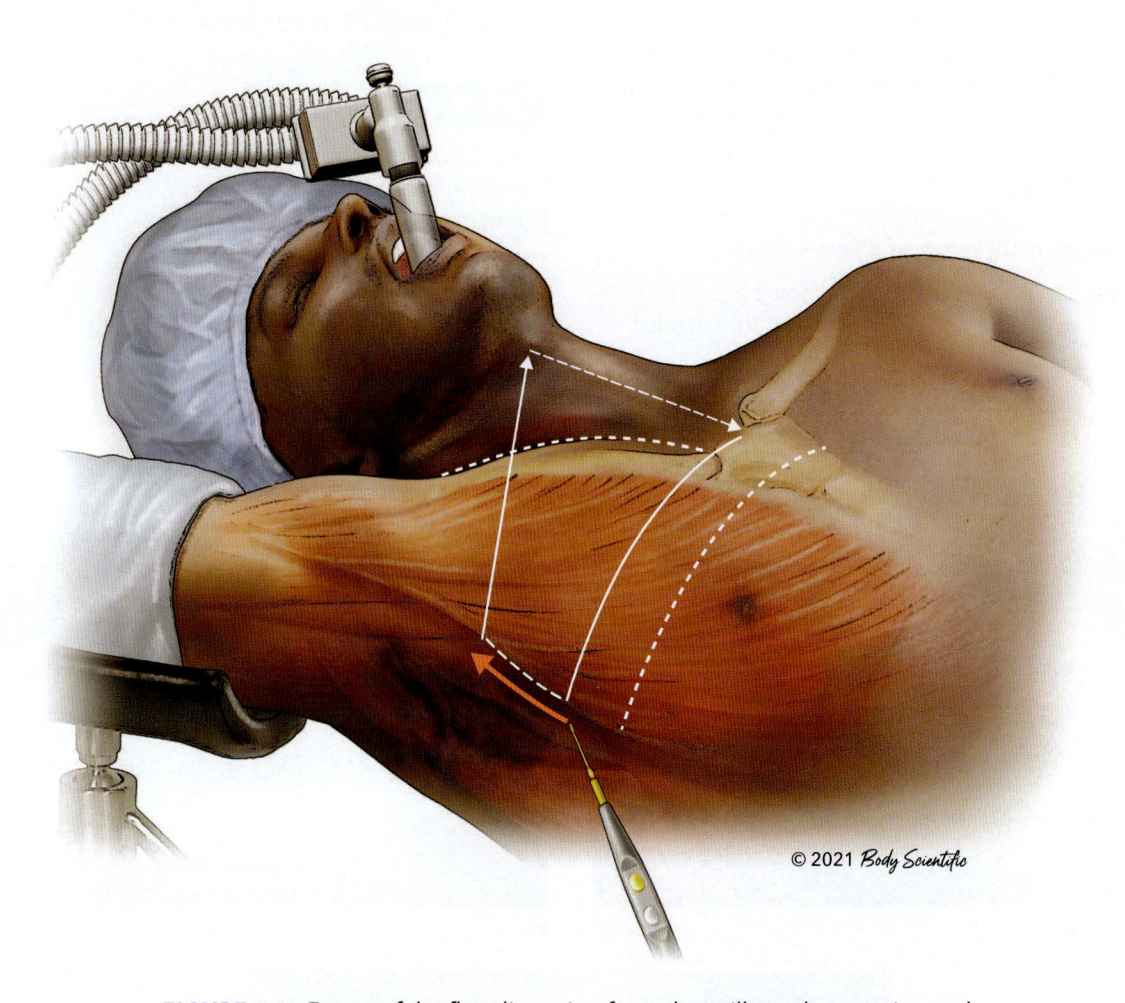

FIGURE 8-3 • Extent of the flap dissection from the axilla to the anterior neck.

Creation of the Working Space

The working space is prepared, under direct vision, by electrocauterization over the anterior surface of the pectoralis major muscle from the axilla to the clavicle and the sternal notch (**Figures 8-4 A, B**).

A subplatysmal skin flap is performed beyond the clavicle to the point of the bifurcation of the sternocleidomastoid (SCM) muscle (**Figure 8-4C**). The subplatysmal skin flap dissection should be continued until the posterior neck area is exposed (**Figure 8-4D**).

> ⚠ **PITFALLS**
>
> During the posterior neck area exposure, sometimes a burn in the skin flap can occur. The surgeon should proceed being well-aware of the depth of the flap.

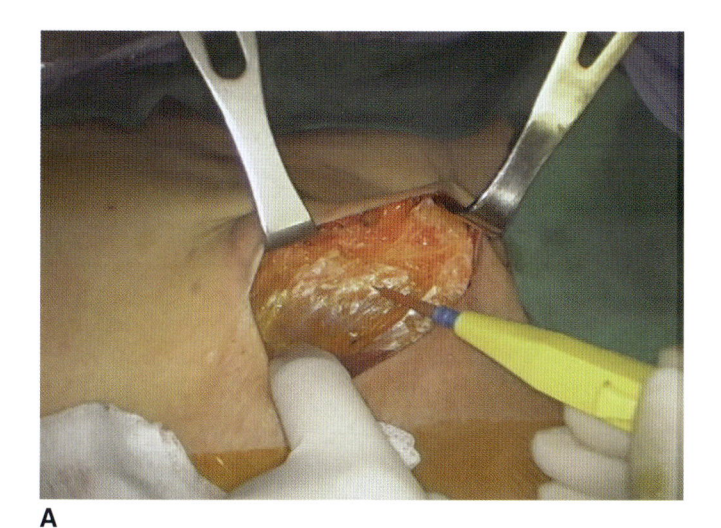

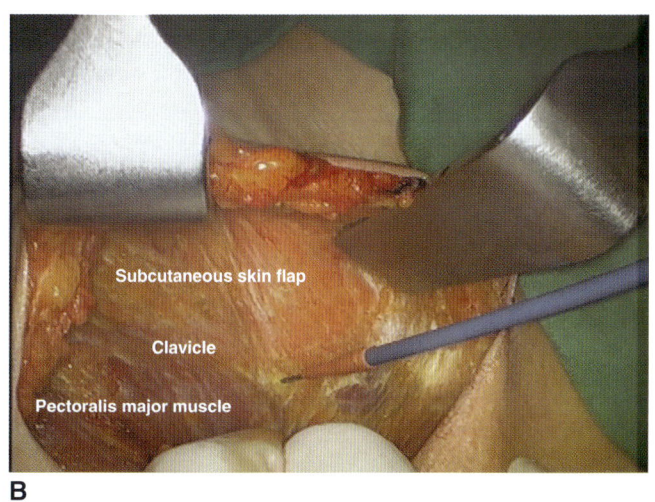

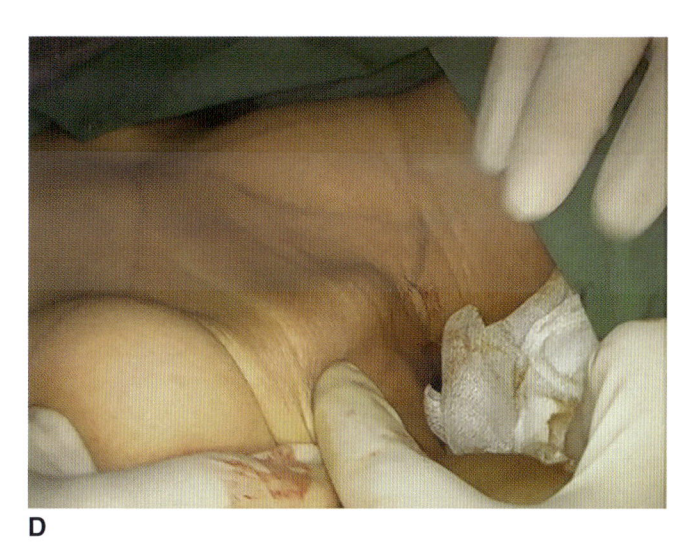

FIGURE 8-4 A–D • Creation of the working space. **A.** Subcutaneous skin flap elevation. **B.** Subcutaneous skin flap elevation over the pectoralis major muscle's anterior surface to the clavicle and the sternal notch. **C.** Subplatysmal skin flap elevation. **D.** Checking of the posterior neck area exposure status.

132 The Foundation and Art of Robotic Surgery

The dissection is approached through the avascular space of the 2 heads of the SCM muscle and beneath the strap muscles (**Figure 8-4E**). From this point, a fiberoptic retractor is better than using shorter retractors to show the inside of the flap in progress.

The omohyoid muscle is retracted superficially and posterolaterally after the dissection (**Figure 8-4F**).

The carotid sheath and the internal jugular vein (IJV) are separated from the strap muscles, taking care not to injure the IJV and the common carotid artery (CCA) (**Figure 8-4G**).

The strap muscles should be carefully detached from the lateral aspect of the thyroid gland in order to expose its full lateral aspect; then, they are separated from the anterior surface of the thyroid gland and are lifted until the contralateral lobe of the thyroid gland is exposed (**Figure 8-4H**).

The blades of the external retractor system are inserted through the skin incision in the axilla and maneuvered to lift the skin flap, sternal head of the SCM, and the strap muscles together, to maintain the working field for the robotic procedure.

In the da Vinci SP system, a narrow external blade is used to raise the working space (**Figures 8-4 I, J**).

Incision lines drawing and creation of working space total average time frame: 20–30 min

> ▶▶ **TIPS**
>
> Sufficient exposure of the posterior neck area, and enough dissection between the 2 heads of the SCM muscle, are important to develop an appropriate working space.

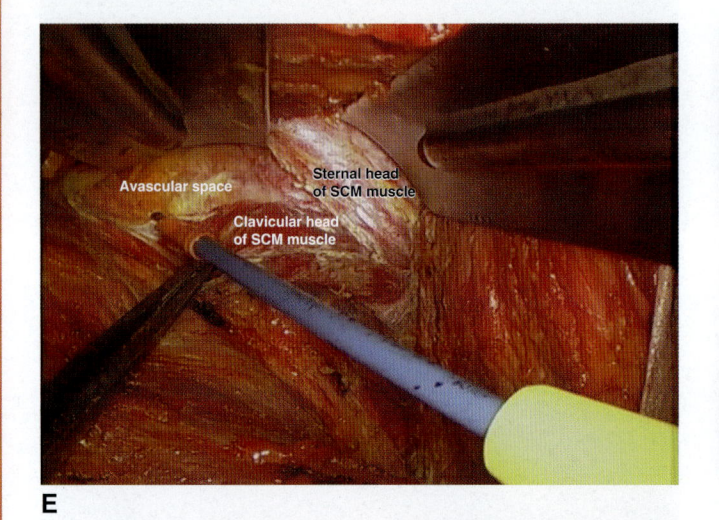

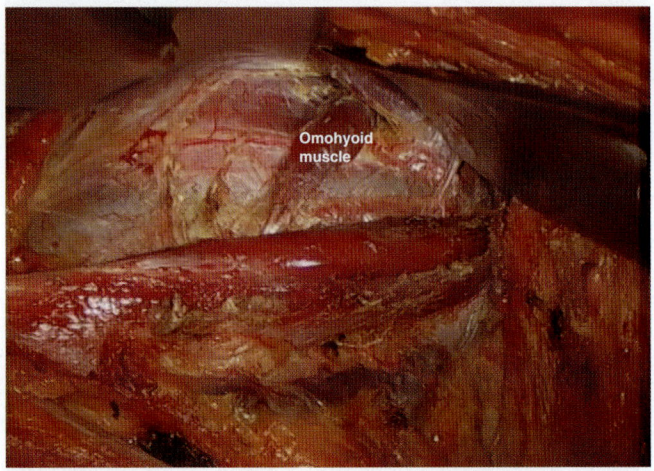

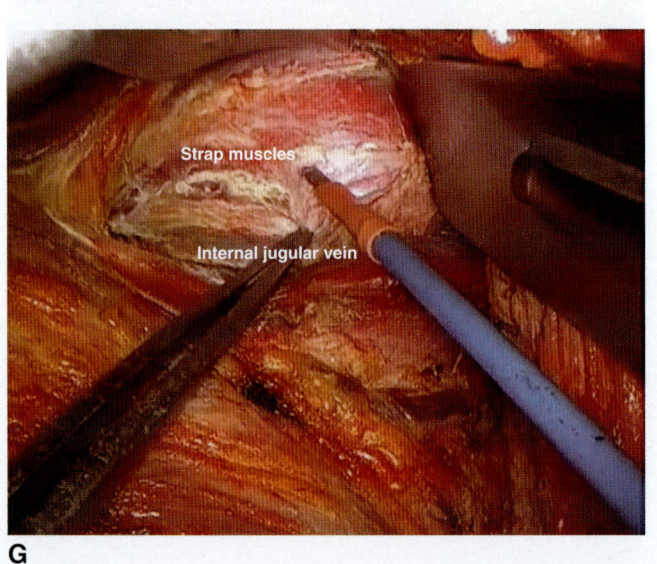

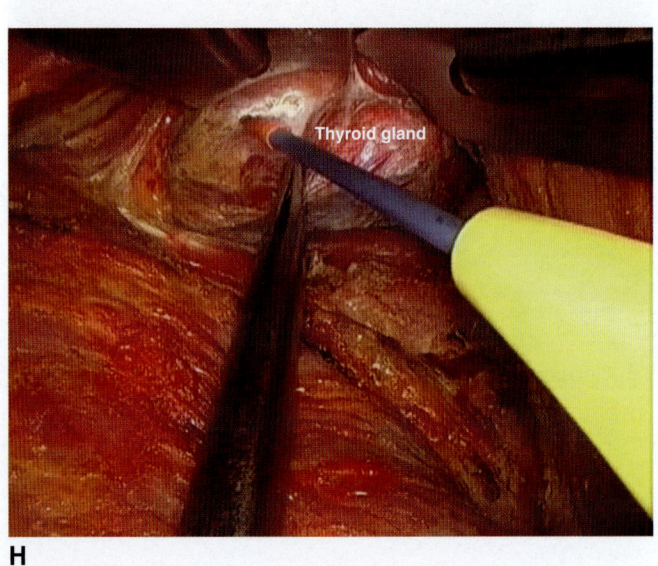

FIGURE 8-4 E–H • Creation of the working space. **E.** The dissection approaching through the avascular space of the two heads of the SCM. **F.** Omohyoid muscle mobilization. **G.** Separation of the carotid sheath and the IJV from the strap muscles. **H.** Thyroid gland exposure.

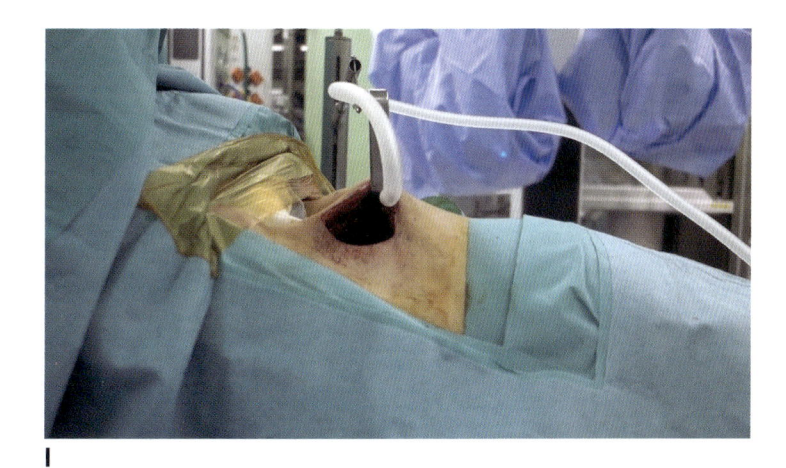

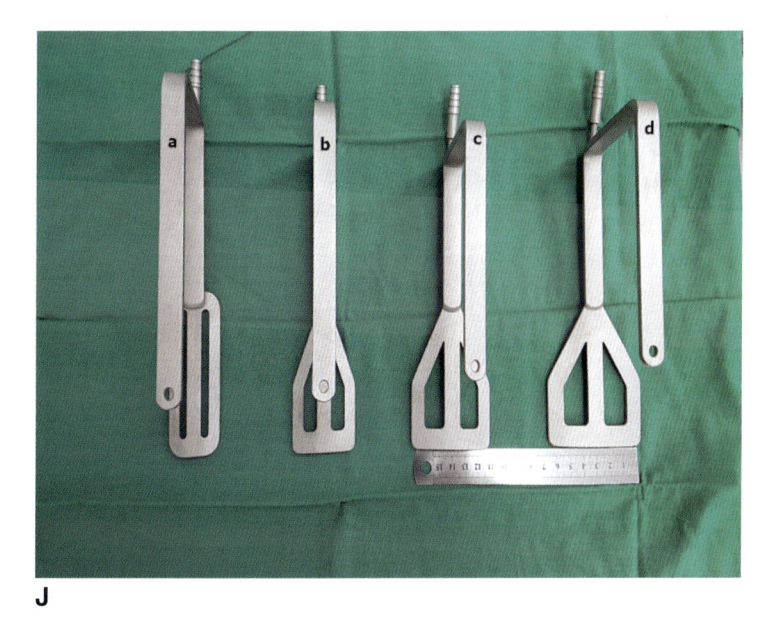

FIGURE 8-4 I, J • Creation of the working space: external retractor and blades. **I.** External retractor blade insertion. **J.** External blades for robotic thyroid surgery: **a, b** for the SP system, **c** for the thyroidectomy, and **d** for modified radical neck dissection (mRND).

134 The Foundation and Art of Robotic Surgery

> ▶▶ **TIPS**
>
> Checkpoint/landmarks of adequate exposure of the thyroid gland:
> - Superior thyroid artery visualization
> - Central compartment node area control
> - Contralateral lobe with about 30% exposure
>
> Checkpoints of sufficient working space:
> - Axillary incision entrance height: the distance from the external blade's lower pole to the incision line should be >4 cm (**Figure 8-5A**).
> - A distance >1 cm between the blade and the anterior aspect of the thyroid has to be maintained (**Figure 8-5B**).
> - The contralateral side strap muscles should be lifted after the external blade is inserted (**Figure 8-5C**).

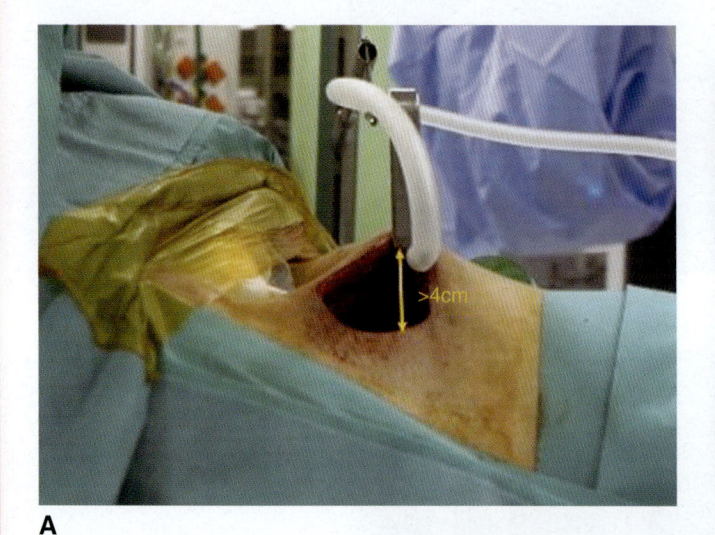

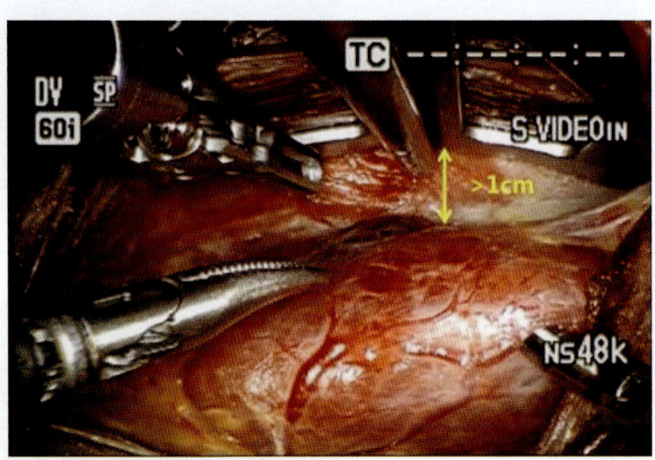

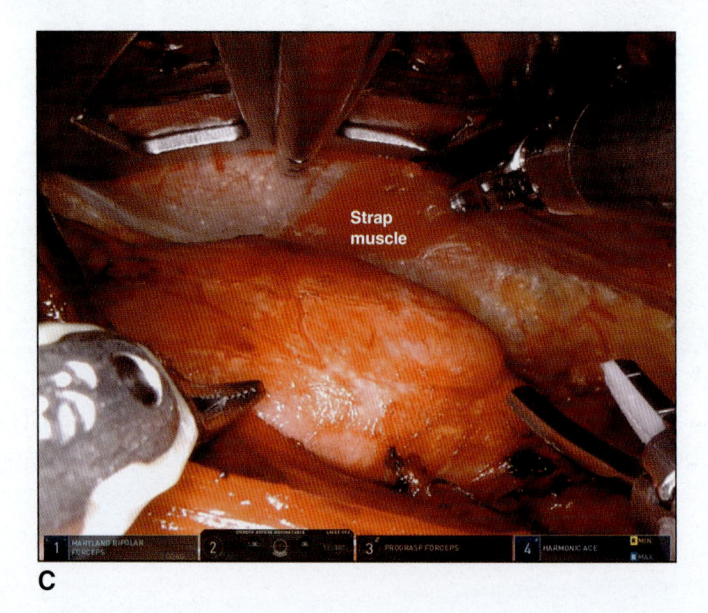

FIGURE 8-5 • Verification of adequate working space. **A.** Axillary incision entrance height >4 cm. **B.** Retractor blade >1 cm away from the anterior surface of the thyroid gland. **C.** The contralateral side strap muscles are lifted.

Gasless Transaxillary Thyroidectomy 135

Patient Positioning, OR Setup, and Port Setting with Different Robotic Systems (S, Si, Xi and Sp)

Da Vinci S, Si System

The patient cart is placed contralateral to the location of the incision, aligning the center column of the cart with the line of the retractor. The operative table is positioned slightly oblique to the direction of the robotic column to allow direct alignment between the axis of the robotic camera arm and the operative instruments (**Figure 8-6A**).

A 12-mm trocar for the camera and the 30° robotic scope should be positioned in the middle of the incision, such that the camera arm is in line with the camera cannula and the center column of the patient cart. The camera is inserted in an upward direction (30° up); the external third joint should be placed in the lowest part (floor) of the incision entrance, and the camera tip should be directed upward (**Figure 8-6B**).

An 8-mm trocar for the ProGrasp forceps is then positioned beneath the anterior part of the skin incision, parallel to the suction tube of the retractor blade. The ProGrasp forceps must be located as close as possible to the ceiling of the working space (the retractor blade).

The 5-mm cannula for the Harmonic curved shears is placed lateral to the camera, and the 5-mm cannula of a Maryland dissector is then positioned on the opposite edge of the incision. Therefore, all three instruments and the camera are inserted through the axillary incision (**Figure 8-6C**).

> ▶▶ **TIPS**
>
> The angle and the position of the robot arm's joint should be optimized to avoid collisions among robotic instruments and to provide unobstructed access to the thyroid bed.

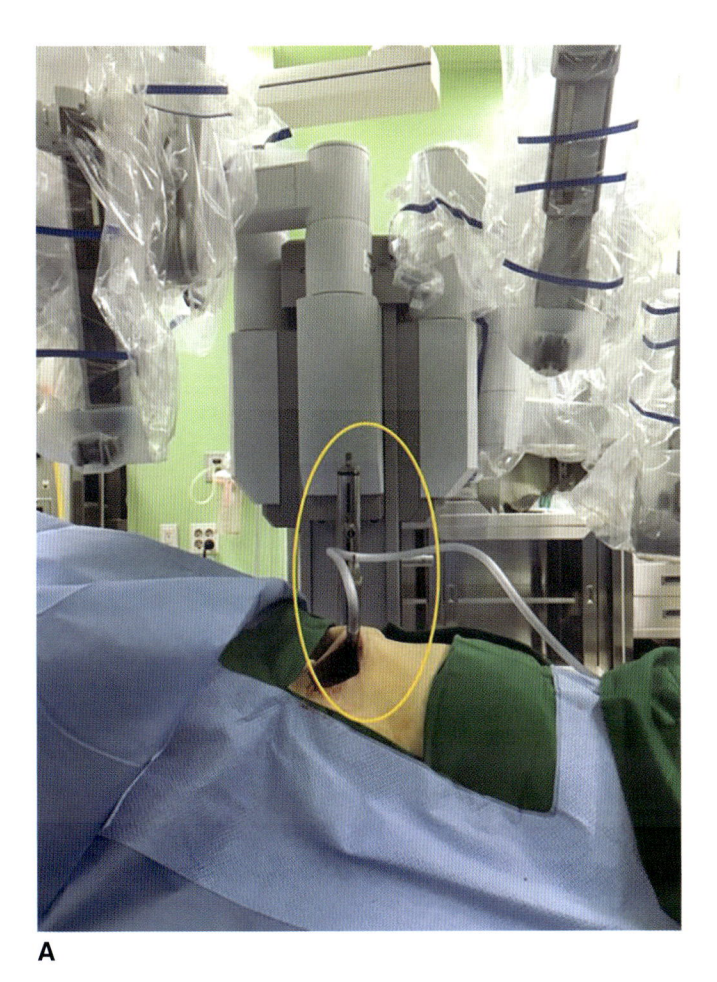

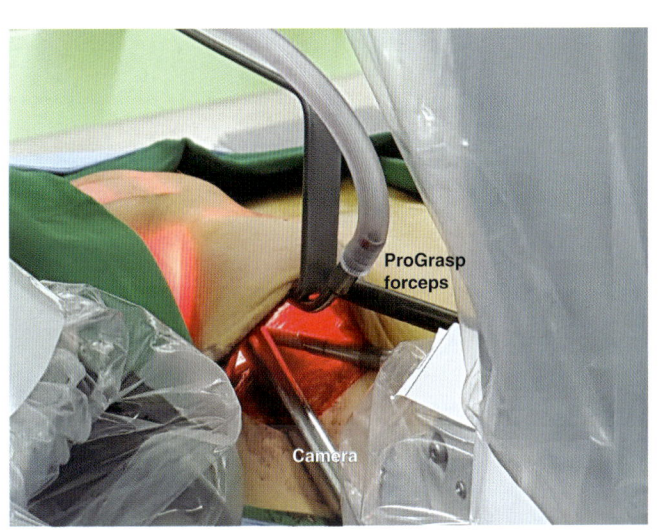

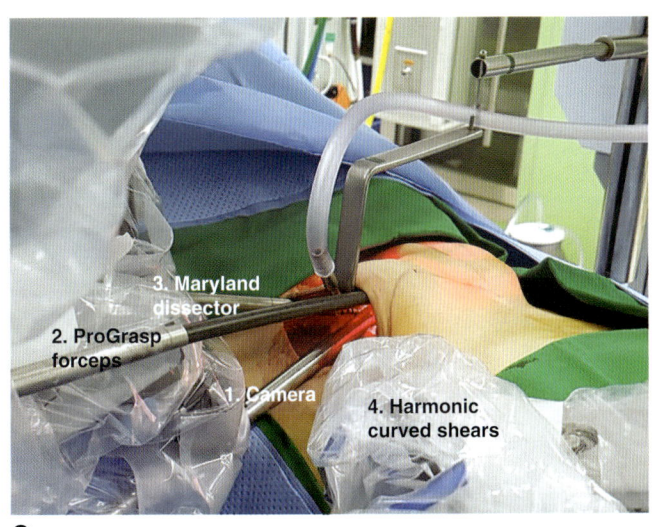

FIGURE 8-6 • S and Si systems robotic cart positioning and docking **A.** Axis of alignment between the robotic cart and the external retractor. **B.** Placement of endoscope and ProGrasp forceps. **C.** Placement of all robotic trocars.

Video 8-1. Creation of a Working Space for Thyroidectomy

Da Vinci Xi System

The patient cart position is on the contralateral side of the incision. There is no need to move the patient table to create an alignment, but rotating the boom, the correct setting of the arms can be achieved with any direction of the cart. The boom is centered until the laser point is visible on the external retractor (**Figure 8-7A**).

The locations of the 4 robotic arms are almost the same as those of the S or Si system. Adjustment of the robotic arms, or instrument insertion distance, is needed to avoid collision (**Figure 8-7B**).

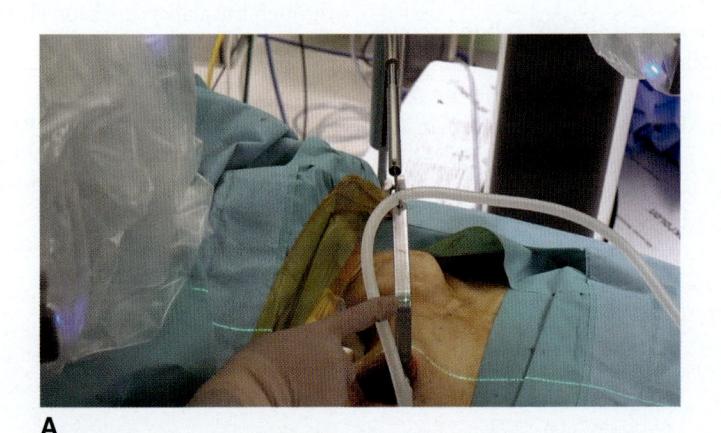

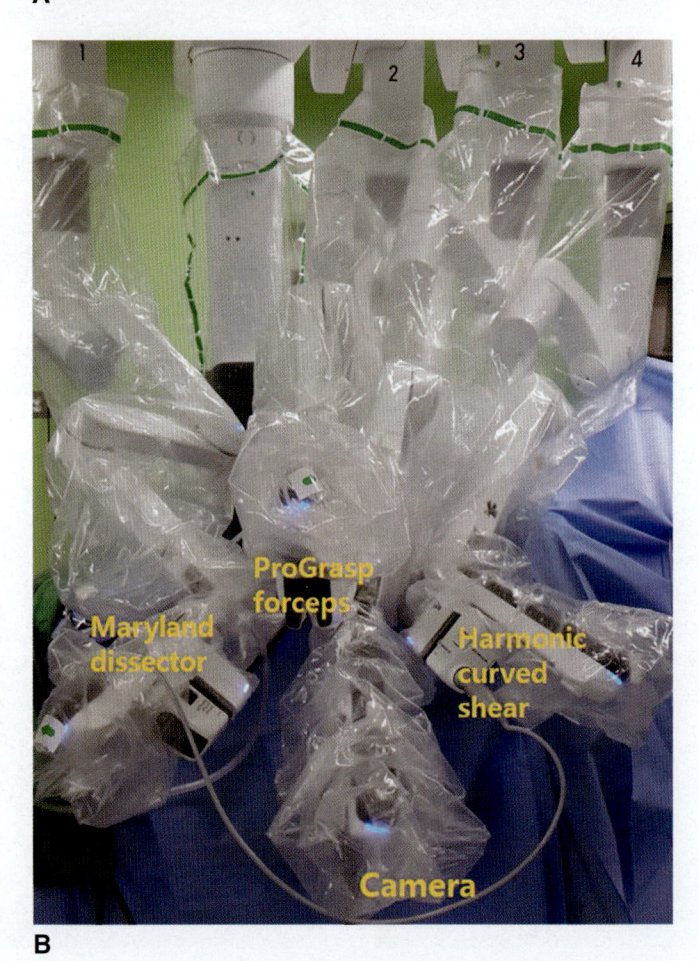

FIGURE 8-7 A, B • Xi system robotic cart positioning and docking. **A.** Axis alignment using the crosshair laser on the external retractor. **B.** Placement of the 4 robotic instruments.

Da Vinci SP System

In the SP system, before docking the SP cannula, the arm homo-lateral to the lesion is stretched laterally and abducted.

The cannula of the single robotic arm is introduced through the axilla incision (**Figure 8-7C**).

In the cannula, the camera is placed at the bottom (bottom-up), and a Maryland dissector with bipolar and spatula (or scissors) with monopolar electrocautery are placed on both lateral-side arms. In addition, a grasper is placed on top with the guidance of an entry guide tool. The entire robotic arm is introduced in an upward direction just below the horizontal plane of the patient.

Average time frame: 3–5 min

▶▶ **TIPS**

Before docking the SP cannula, the patient's arm homo-lateral to the lesion is stretched laterally and abducted to expose more effectively the upper thyroid pole (**Figure 8-7D**).

C

D

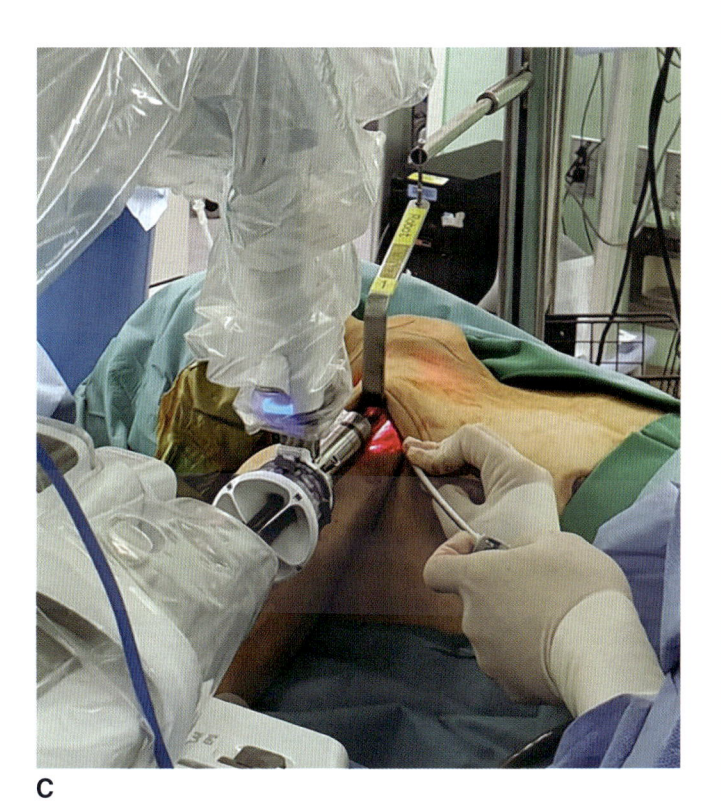

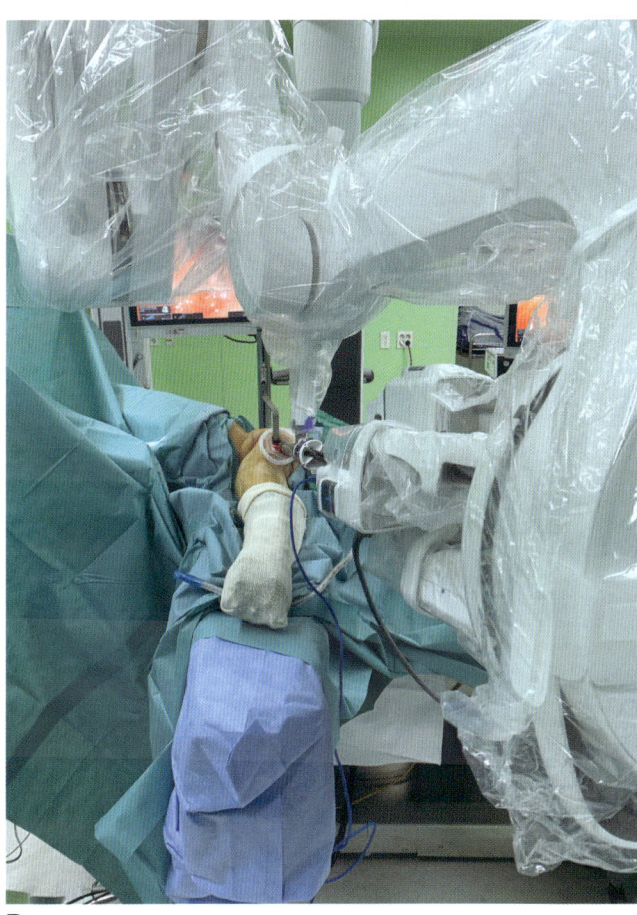

FIGURE 8-7 C, D • SP system positioning and docking. **C.** The cannula is inserted through the axillary incision. **D.** The arm is positioned to better expose the upper pole of the thyroid.

THYROIDECTOMY FOR CANCER

After the docking is completed, the thyroidectomy is performed in the same manner as conventional open thyroidectomy. The thyroid gland is retracted using ProGrasp forceps in the fourth robotic arm, and the dissection is carried out using Harmonic curved shears and a Maryland dissector. This procedure allows the surgeon to use 3 robotic arms during thyroidectomy.

> **ANATOMICAL HIGHLIGHTS**
>
> A detailed knowledge of the anatomy and the numerous anatomical variations is essential to achieve successful outcomes and to minimize potential complications. A particular focus should be put on the following aspects:
>
> - Vascular anatomy (**Figures 8-8 A, B** and **8-9**).
> - Neural anatomy: RLN (**Figures 8-10 A, B**) variations such as the nonrecurrent laryngeal nerve (**Figures 8-11 A–D**). [For more information, see suggested reading #19.]
> - The anatomical relationships between the RLN and the inferior thyroid artery (**Figures 8-12 A–C**).
> - The external branch of the superior laryngeal nerve (EBSLN) (**Figure 8-13**). There are multiple classifications pertaining to the EBSLN variations. The most internationally recognized is the one described by Cernea et al. [see suggested reading #20], which relates to the risk of neural iatrogenic injury during thyroid surgery. It classifies the EBSLN in relation to the superior thyroid vessels and the superior edge of the superior thyroid pole. [For more information, see suggested readings #21–23.]
> - Parathyroid glands standard anatomy (**Figure 8-14**) and their anatomical variations (**Figures 8-15 A–G** and **8-16**). [For more information, see suggested reading #24.]

Gasless Transaxillary Thyroidectomy 139

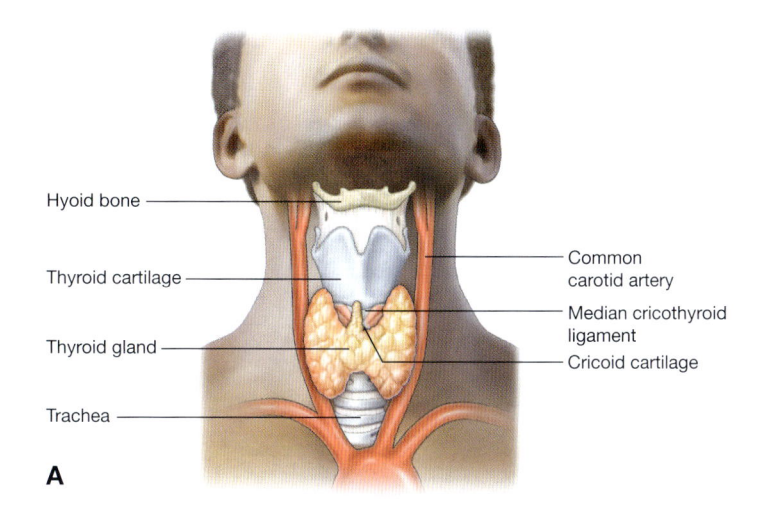

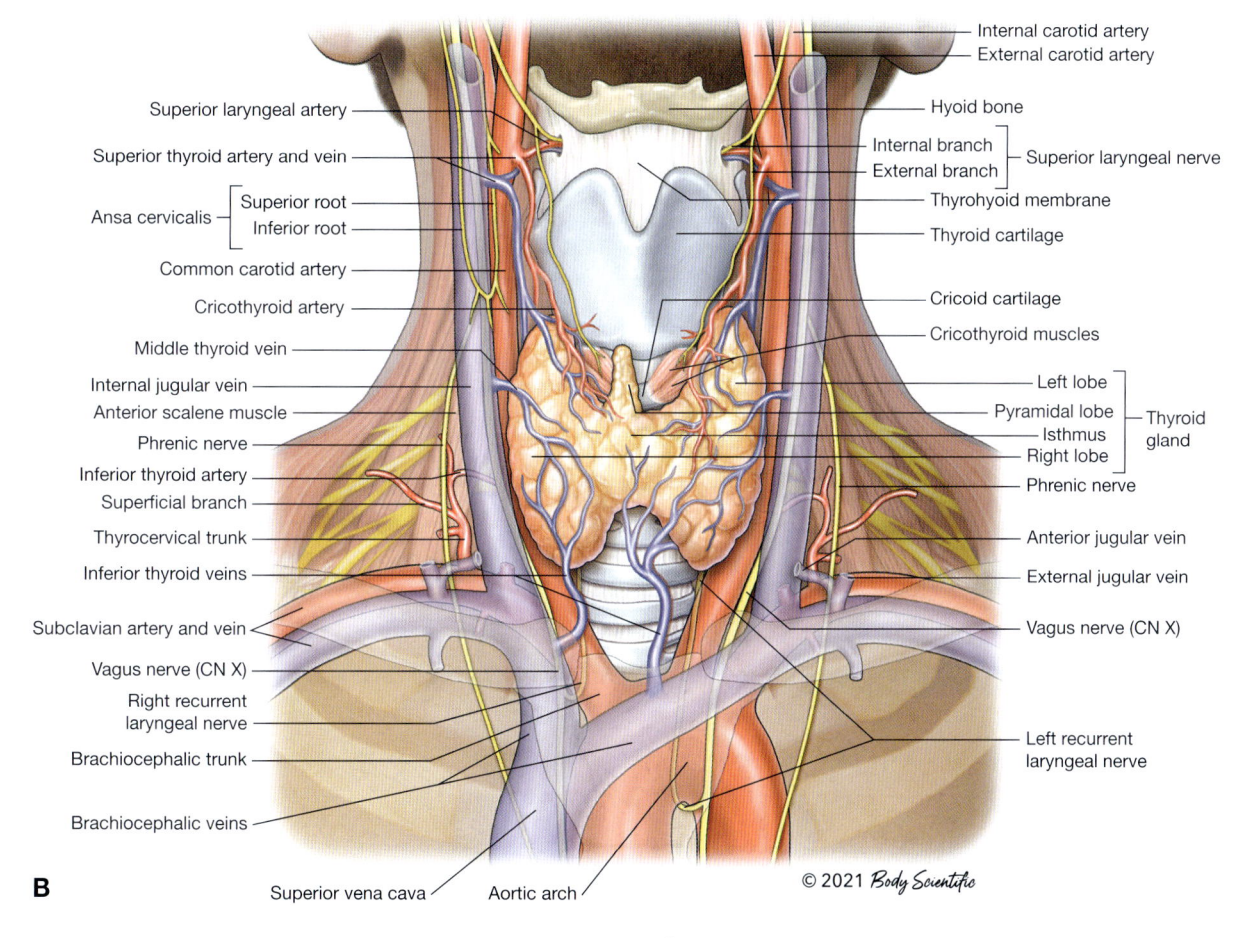

FIGURE 8-8 • Vascular anatomy.

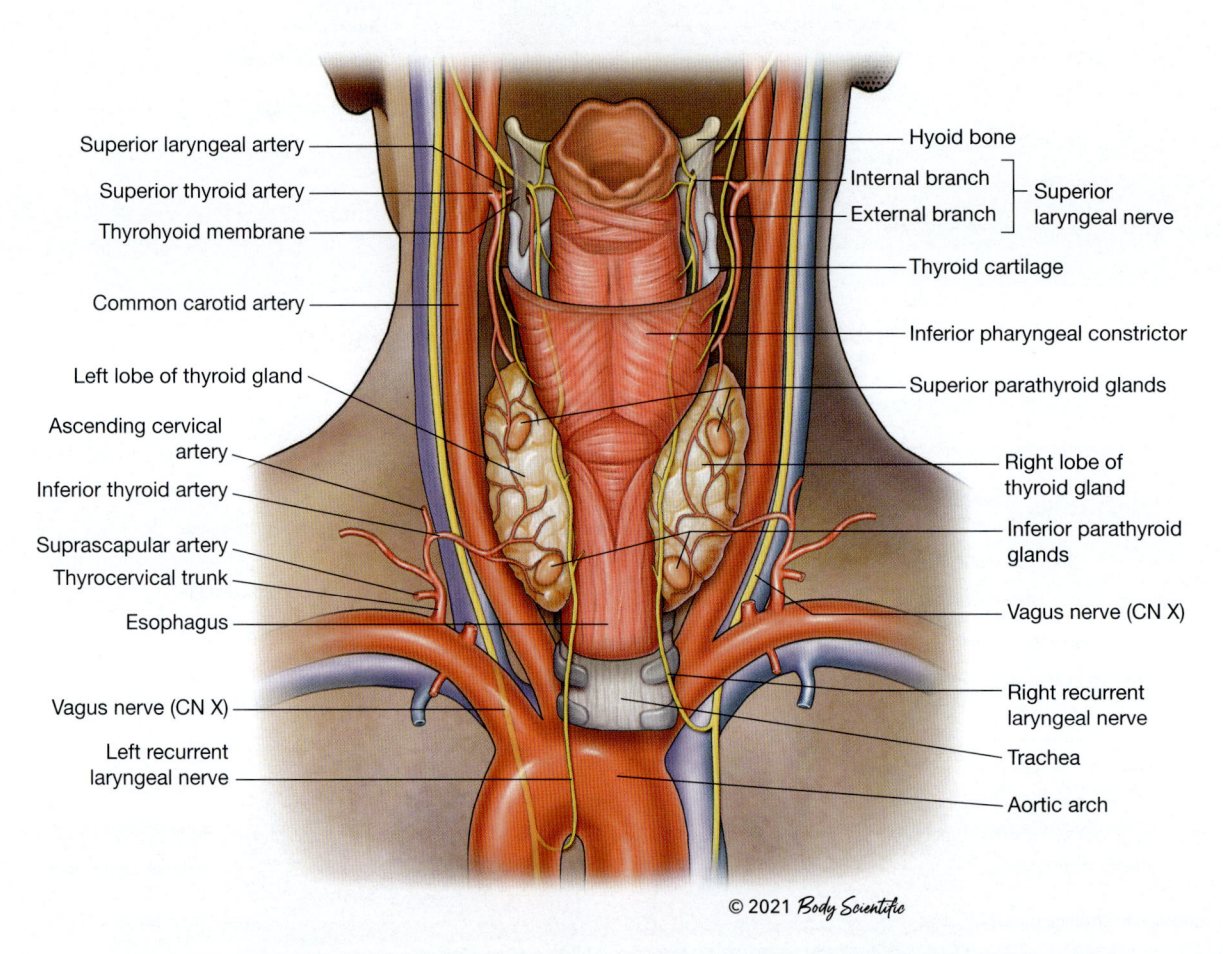

FIGURE 8-9 • Posterior view of the thyroid, the parathyroid with vascular and neural anatomy.

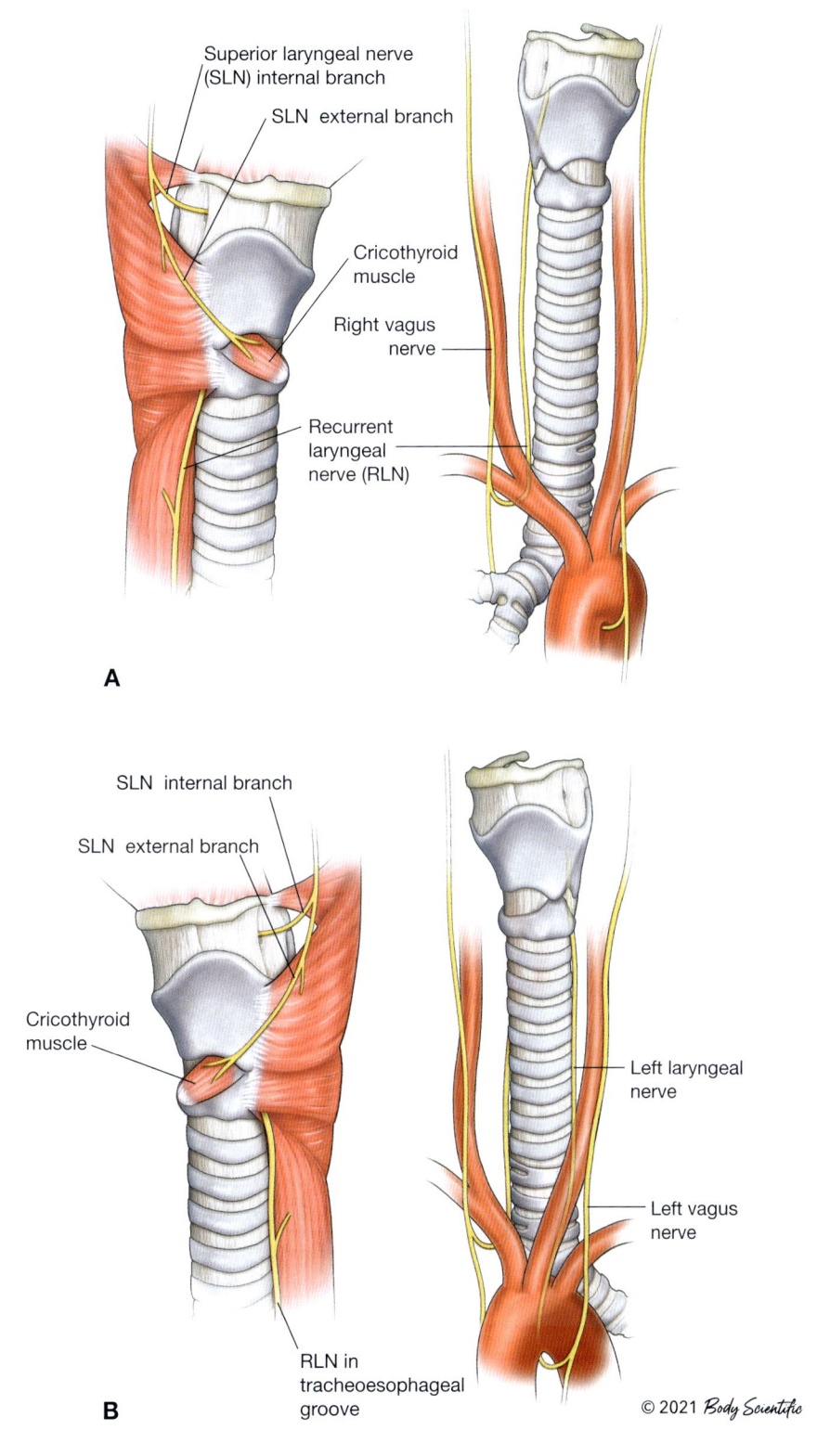

FIGURE 8-10 • Standard course of the recurrent laryngeal nerve across the right (**A**) and left (**B**) paratracheal area. [For more information about the parathyroid glands and variations, see suggested readings #19, 24.]

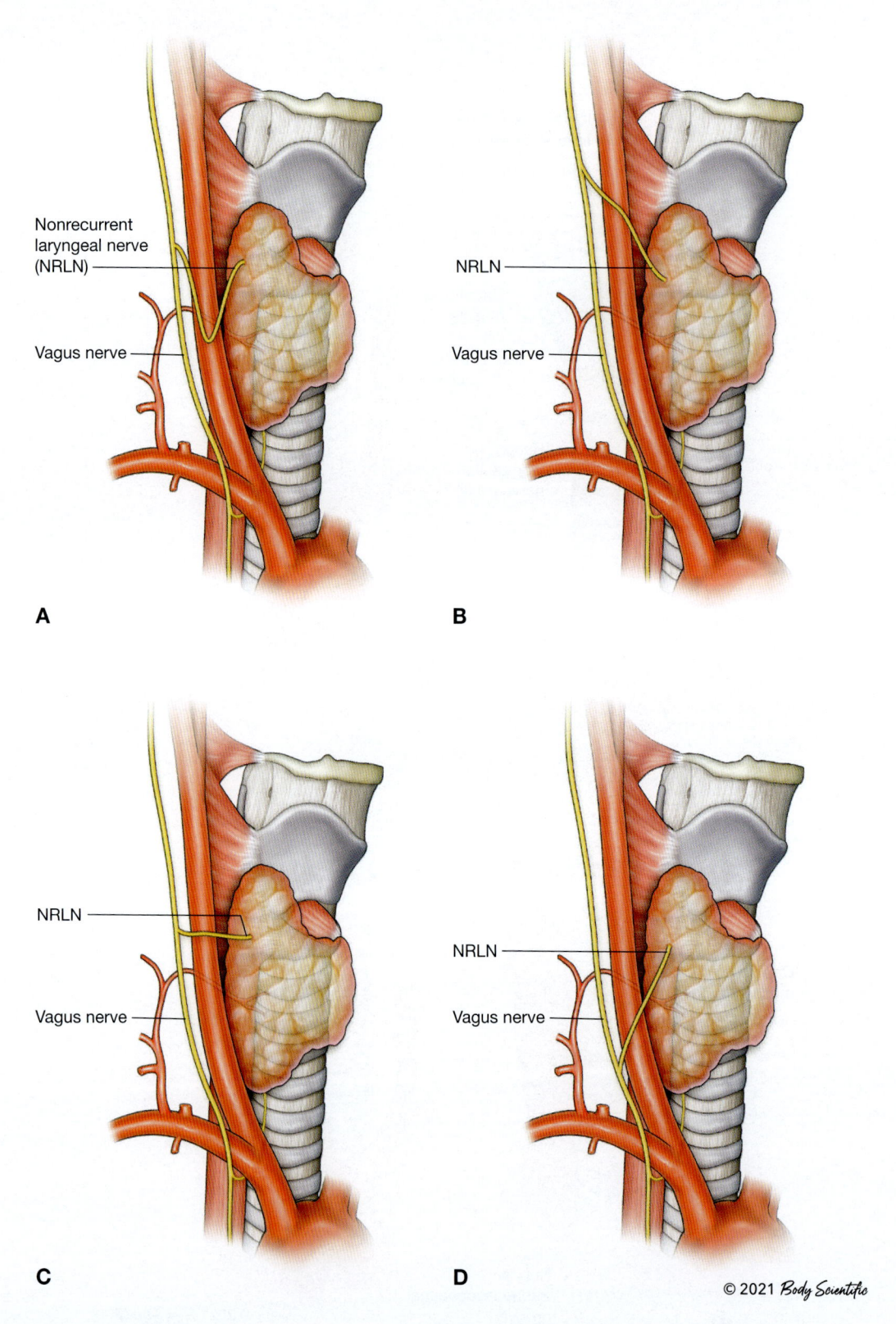

FIGURE 8-11 • Four different scenarios of nonrecurrent laryngeal nerve (NRLN). **A.** U-shaped, first coursing down and then cranially toward the cricothyroid joint. **B.** The NRLN courses directly downward, branching from the vagus nerve. **C.** The NRLN courses horizontally, toward the cricothyroid joint. **D.** The NRLN courses in a caudal-to-cranial fashion, toward the cricothyroid joint. [For more information, see suggested reading #26.]

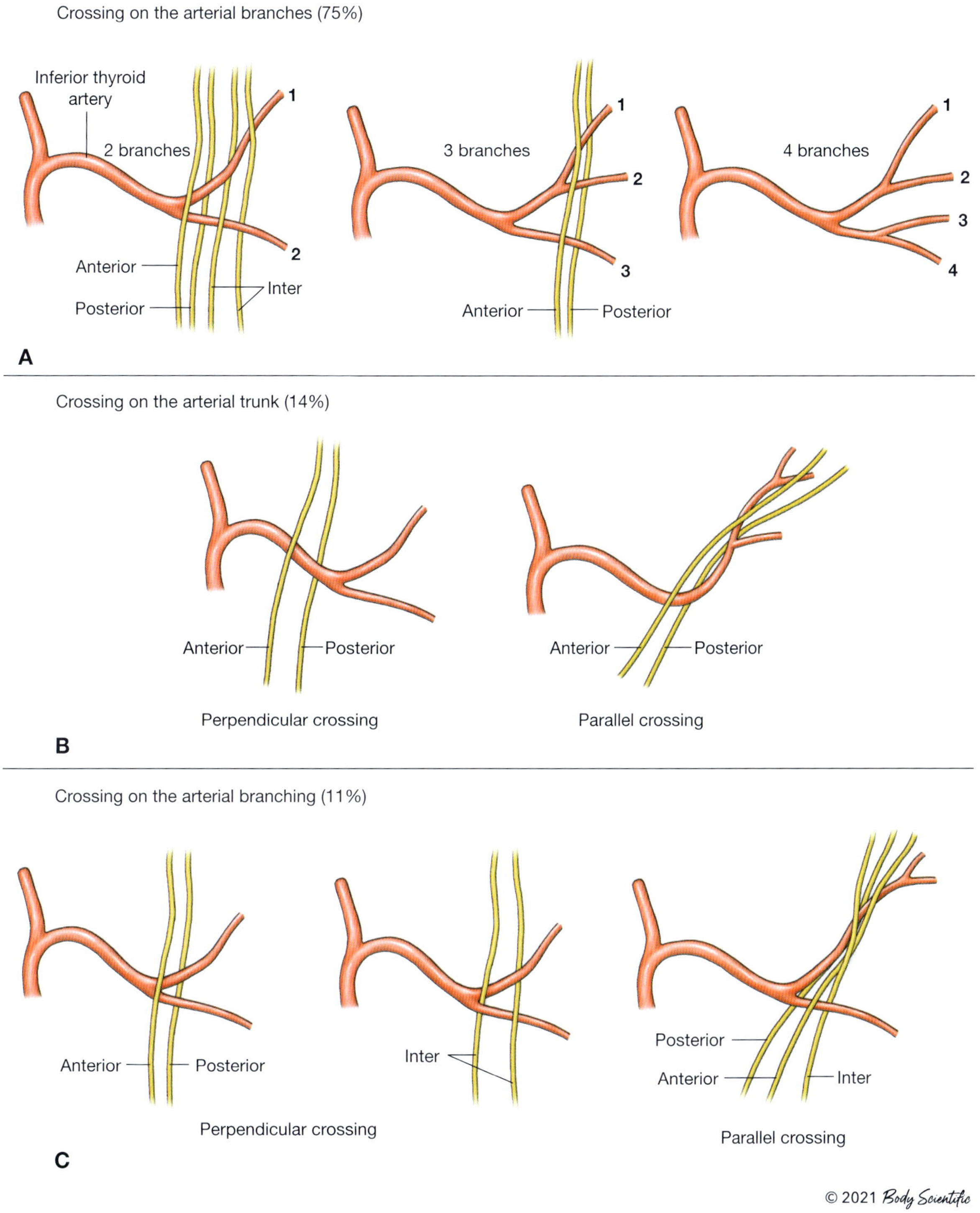

Gasless Transaxillary Thyroidectomy 143

FIGURE 8-12 • The inferior thyroid artery and the recurrent laryngeal nerve: the most frequent anatomical relationships are reported. **A.** Crossing on the arterial branches (75%), 2, 3, or 4 branches. **B.** Crossing on the arterial trunk (14%). Perpendicular crossing or parallel crossing. **C.** Crossing on the arterial branches (11%). Perpendicular crossing or parallel crossing. [For more information, see suggested reading #28.]

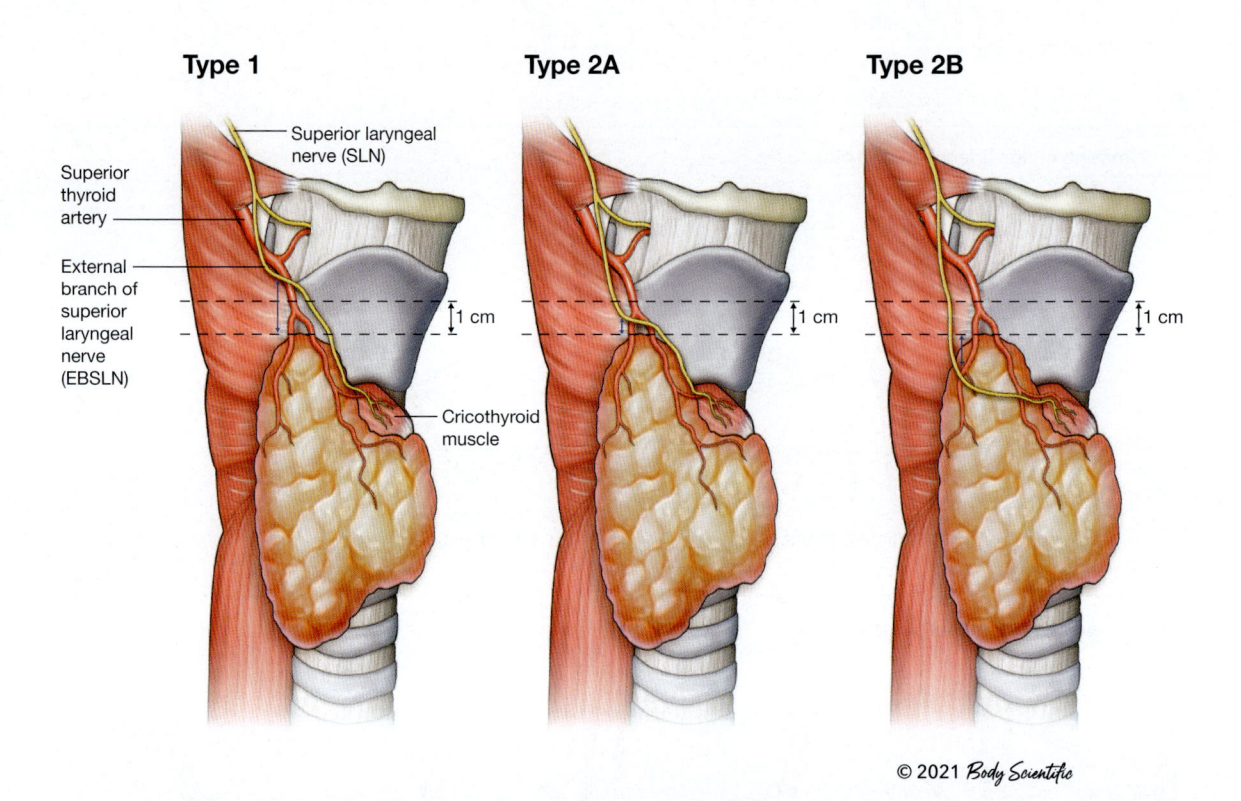

FIGURE 8-13 • EBSLN Cernea classification: Type 1, Type 2A, and Type 2B. Types 2A and 2B, because they present a more caudal course, are more at risk of iatrogenic injury while dissecting or ligating the superior thyroid vessels. [For more information, see suggested readings #20–23.]

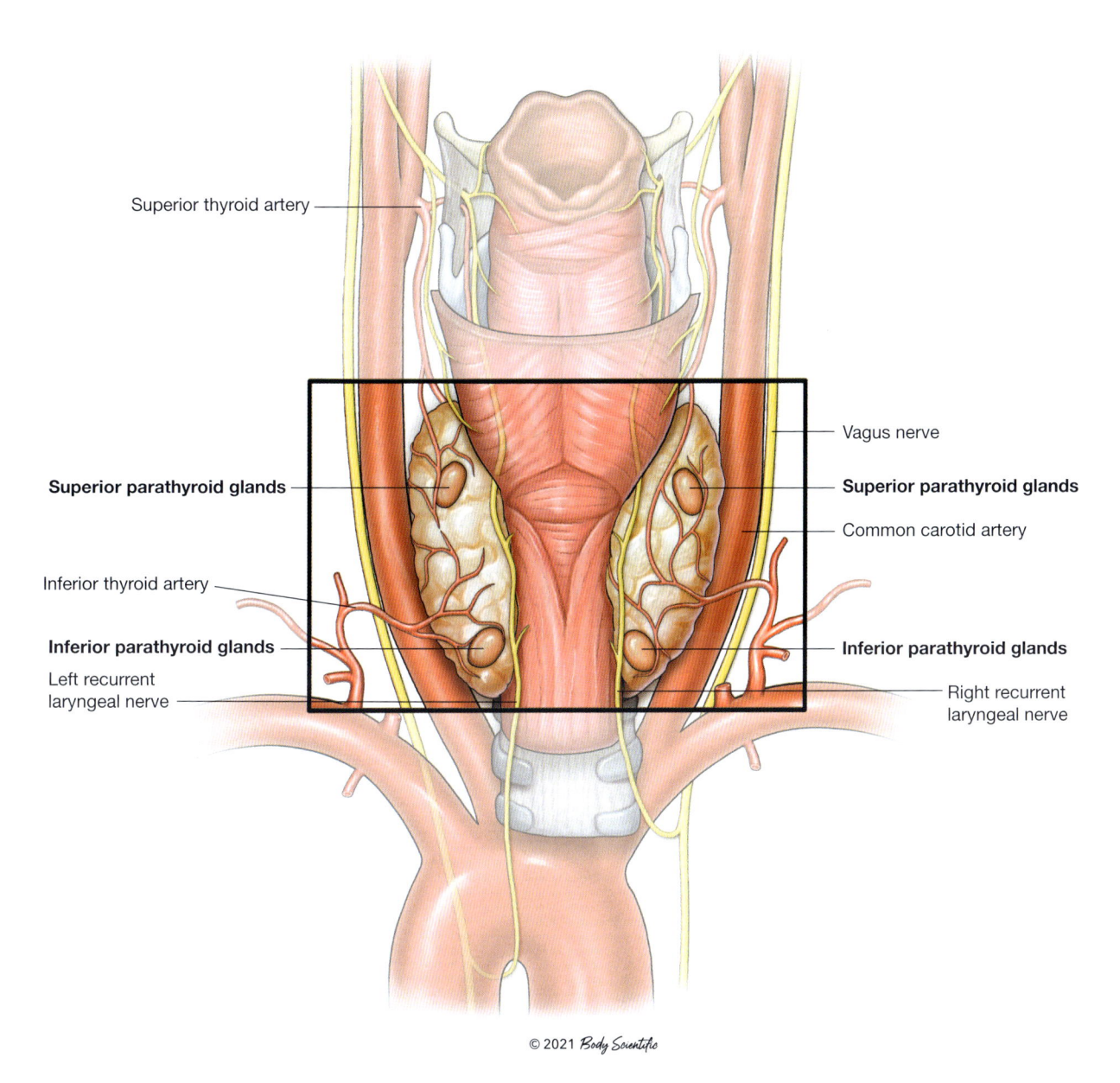

FIGURE 8-14 • The parathyroid glands: standard anatomy.

Distribution of inferior parathyroid glands

Ectopic (2%) | Juxtathyroidal (15%) | Intrathymic (2%, 39%) | Lower thyroid (42%)

Thymic tongue (39%)
Mediastinal (2%)

A   B   C   D

Distribution of superior parathyroid glands

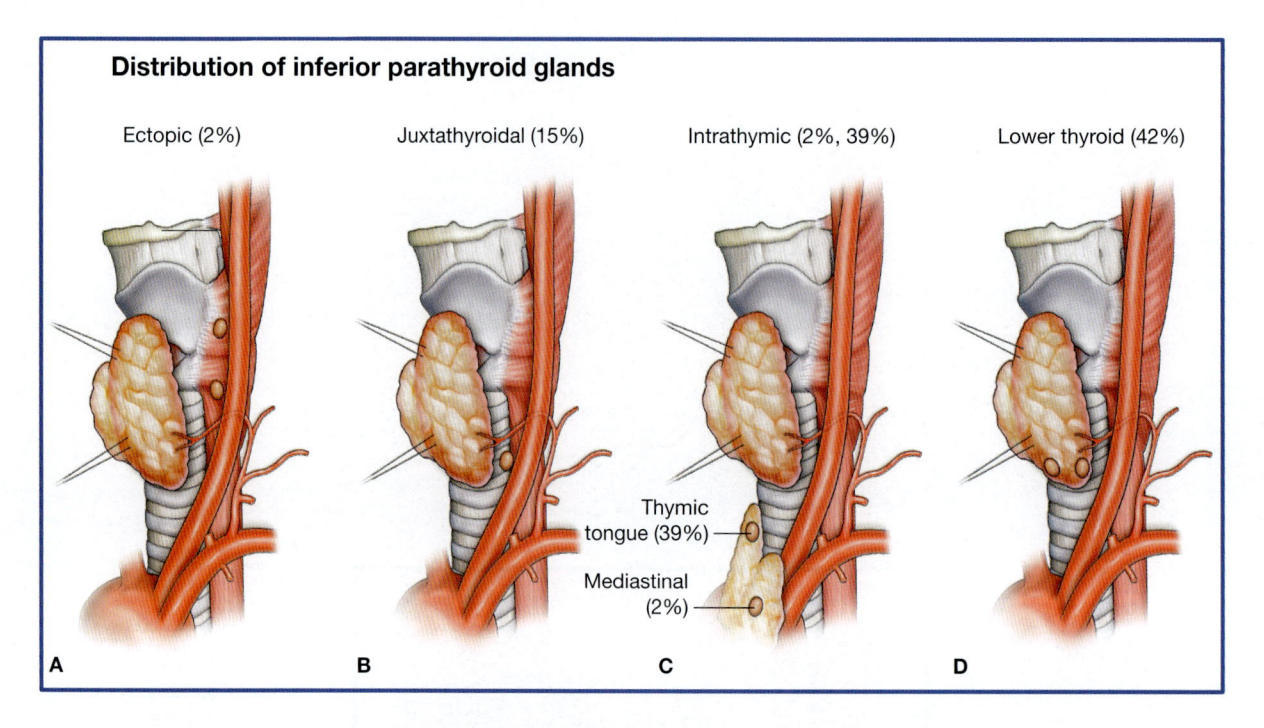

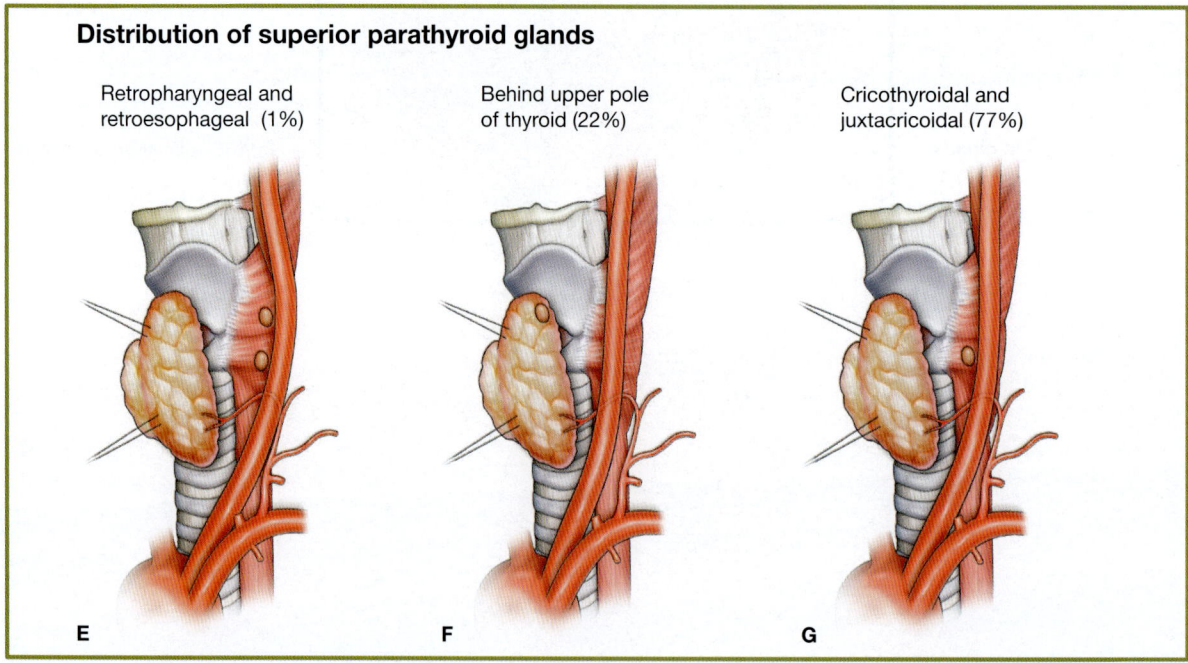

Retropharyngeal and retroesophageal (1%) | Behind upper pole of thyroid (22%) | Cricothyroidal and juxtacricoidal (77%)

E   F   G

© 2021 Body Scientific

FIGURE 8-15 • Anatomical variations in the location of the inferior (**A–D**) and superior (**E–G**) parathyroids. [For more information, see suggested readings #24, 27.]

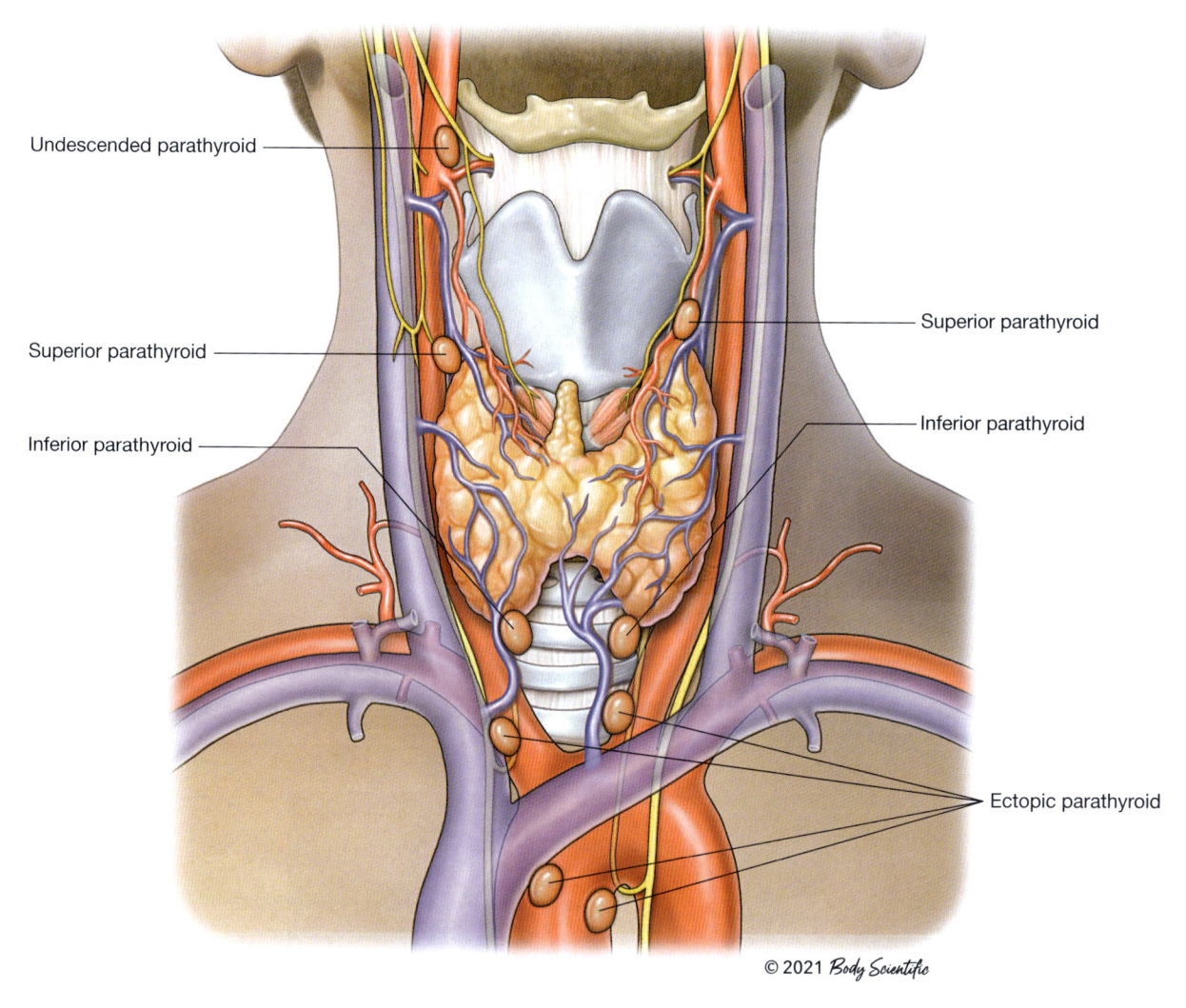

FIGURE 8-16 • The parathyroid glands and possible ectopic locations.

Step 1. Upper pole dissection

The ProGrasp forceps exerts traction on the thyroid upper pole in a medio-inferior direction.

The superior thyroid artery and vein are individually divided (**Figure 8-17A**).

The upper pole of the thyroid gland is pulled steadily with the ProGrasp forceps for countertraction. Gentle dissection of the superior thyroid vascular pedicle is initiated along the long axis of these vessels (**Figure 8-17B**).

The thyroid gland is peeled from the cricothyroid muscle, allowing the identification and preservation of the superior parathyroid gland (**Figure 8-17C**).

The upper pole dissection is continued until the superior part of the Zuckerkandl tubercle is exposed, and great care is taken around the RLN insertion site.

Step 1 average time frame: 10–15 min

⚠ PITFALLS

Lesion of the superior laryngeal nerve is possible if the upper pole dissection is performed above the merging of the superior thyroid artery and vein.

▶▶ TIPS

The first assistant provides additional contralateral traction during dissection, places sponges into the working space, makes suction, removes the specimen, and irrigates the field.

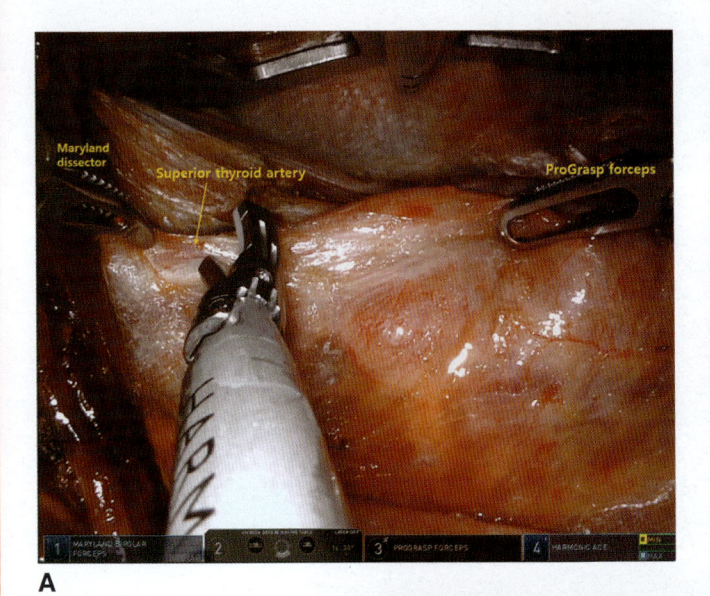

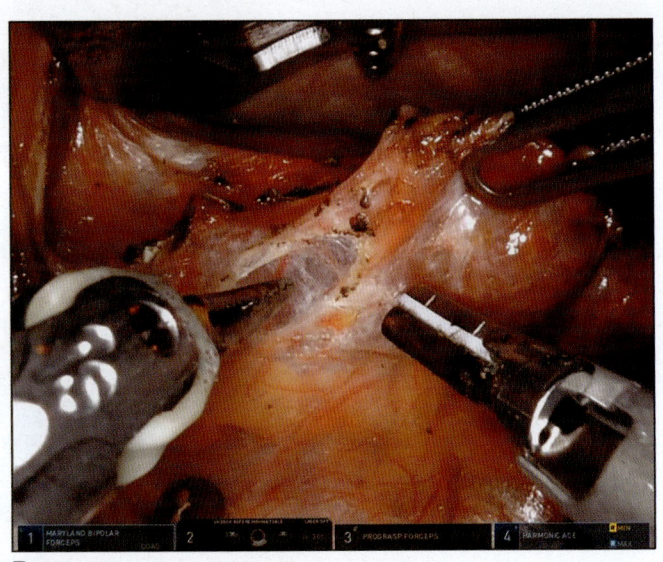

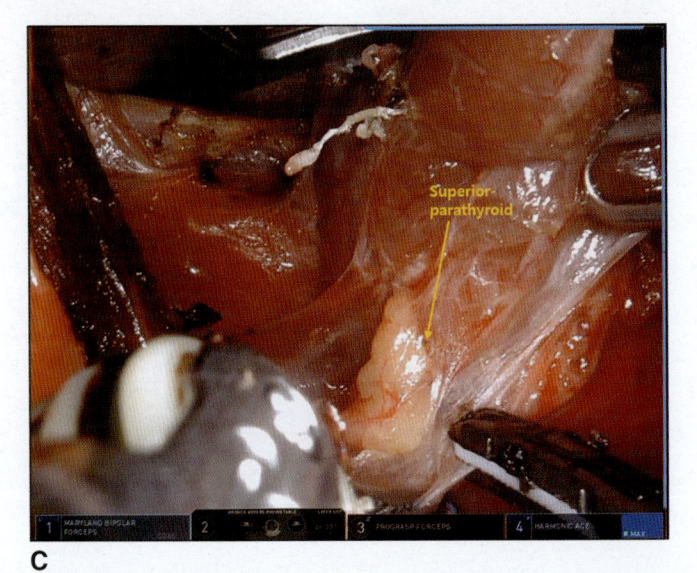

FIGURE 8-17 • Step 1. Upper pole dissection. **A.** Ligation of the superior thyroid vessels. **B, C.** Countertraction of the upper pole of the thyroid gland.

Step 2. Central compartment node dissection (CCND)

The lower pole of the thyroid gland is pulled in a superior and medial direction using the ProGrasp forceps, and the lateral side of the CCND is performed from the CCA to the inferior thyroid artery superiorly, and to the substernal notch inferiorly (**Figure 8-18A**). Gentle fascial dissection along the medial aspect of the carotid in the cephalocaudal direction (along the long axis of the nerve) allows for the inspection of the paratracheal lymphatics, and initial visualization of the RLN and inferior parathyroid gland (**Figures 8-18 B–F**).

Step 2 average time frame: 15–20 min

▶▶ **TIPS**

While performing the right-side CCND, due to the collision of the ProGrasp forceps and Harmonic curved shears, the surgeon can experience a problematic movement restrictions. To avoid the collision, the first assistant should move the camera and the ProGrasp forceps cephalad.

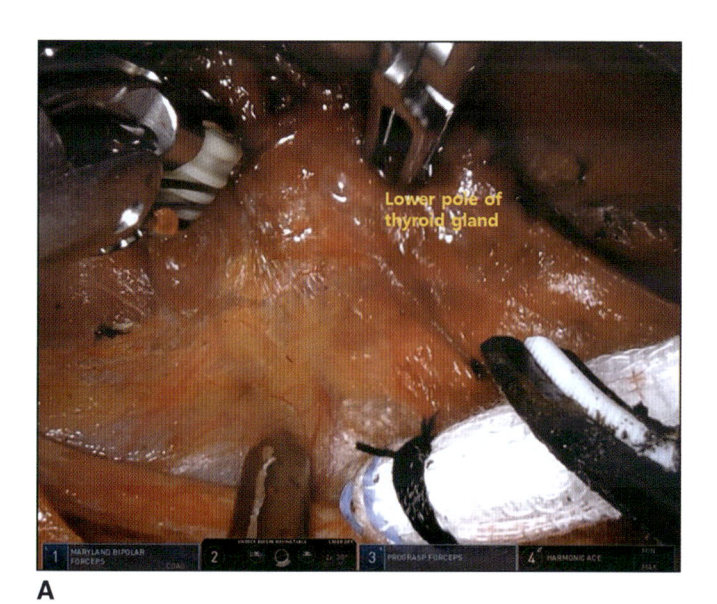

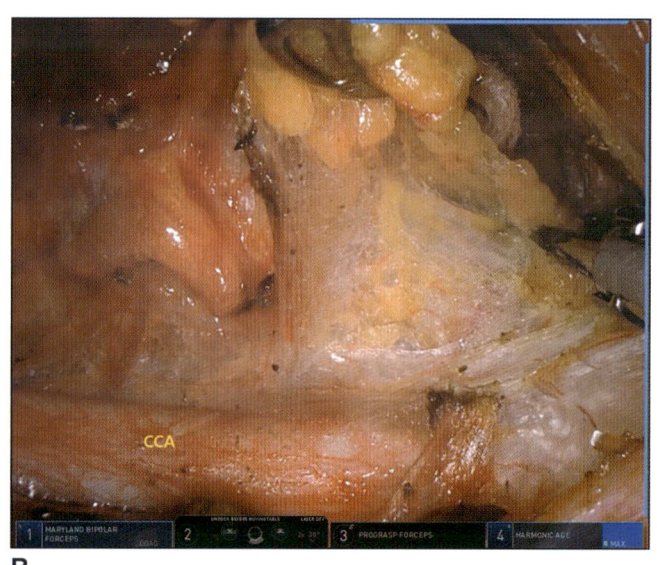

FIGURE 8-18 • Step 2. Central compartment node dissection. **A.** Pulling of the lower pole to expose the central compartment lymph nodes. **B.** Fascial dissection along the medial aspect of the carotid sheath.

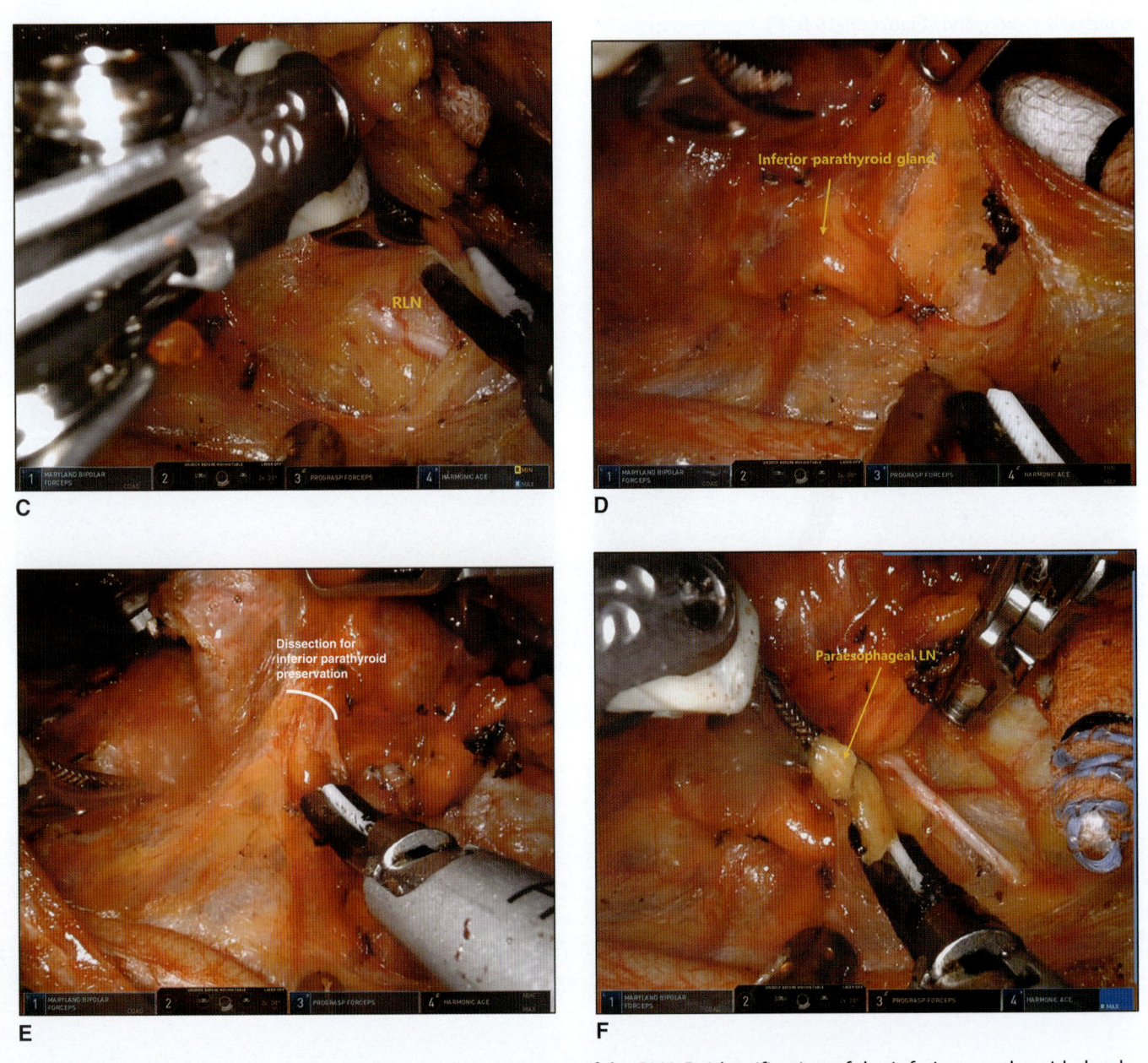

FIGURE 8-18 • *(Continued)* **C.** Identification and preservation of the RLN. **D.** Identification of the inferior parathyroid gland. **E.** Direction of the dissection to preserve the inferior parathyroid gland. **F.** Parathyroid lymph node dissection.

Gasless Transaxillary Thyroidectomy 151

Step 3. Completion of the ipsilateral lobectomy

Once the RLN and the inferior parathyroid have been identified, the entire inferior and lateral mobilization of the thyroid gland is completed along the thyroid capsule. In the Berry ligament region, great caution is required to prevent direct or indirect thermal injury to the RLN using the Harmonic curved shears (**Figures 8-19 A, B**).

Along the side of the isthmus, contralateral to the lobe that is being dissected, the isthmus is transected and 1 lobe of the thyroid gland is delivered.

Step 3 average time frame: 10–15 min

> ⚠ **PITFALLS**
>
> Using Harmonic curved shears can rarely cause a tracheal perforation during the dissection of the Berry ligament and the isthmus. Great caution is required while using an energy-based device.

> ▶▶ **TIPS**
>
> Frequent repositioning of the ProGrasp forceps would allow optimal exposure of the thyroid gland.
>
> The use of roll gauze is helpful to prevent the thermal injury of the RLN.

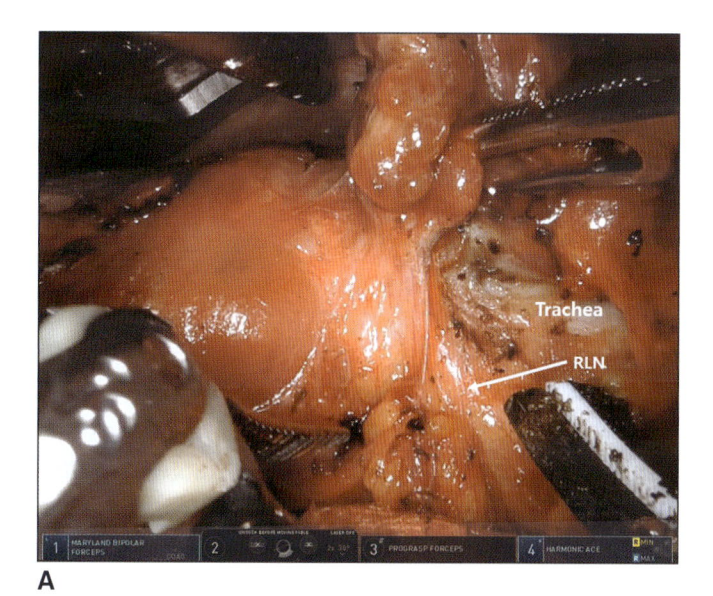

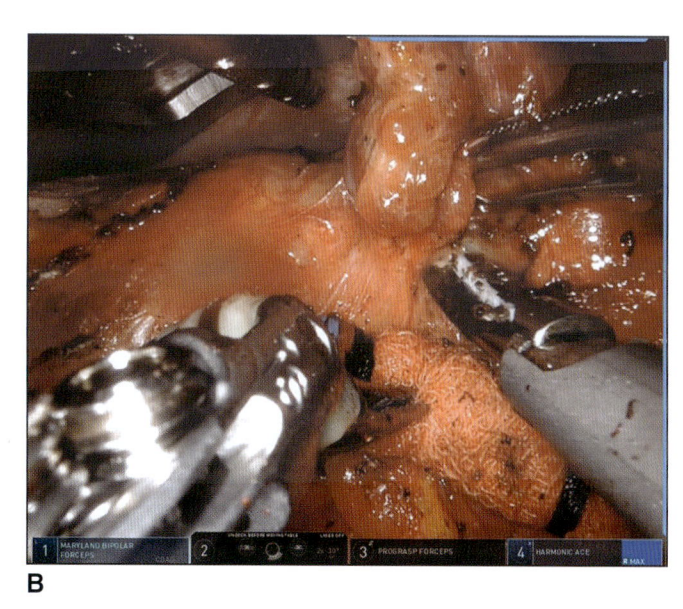

FIGURE 8-19 • Step 3. Completion of the ipsilateral lobectomy. **A.** Thyroid detachment and mobilization from the trachea with the preservation of the RLN. **B.** Indirect or direct thermal injury to the RLN must be prevented.

Step 4. Completion of the contralateral lobectomy

For a total thyroidectomy, the contralateral lobe is similarly excised via a capsular or subcapsular approach. The contralateral strap muscles dissection from the thyroid gland anterior capsule should be performed first.

The upper pole of the thyroid gland is pulled steadily with the ProGrasp forceps for countertraction. Gentle dissection of the superior thyroid vascular pedicle is initiated along the long axis of these vessels (**Figure 8-20A**).

The thyroid gland is peeled from the cricothyroid muscle, with identification and preservation of the superior parathyroid gland (**Figure 8-20B**).

The subcapsular dissection is performed along the thyroid gland, while preserving the inferior parathyroid gland, and ligating the inferior thyroid vessels. The inferior parathyroid gland is lateralized with its vascular pedicle, and the RLN is dissected more distally toward its laryngeal insertion (**Figure 8-20C**).

The Berry ligament is divided close to the thyroid capsule, using Harmonic curved shears, while retracting laterally and taking care of preserving the RLN.

Step 4 average time frame: 15–20 min

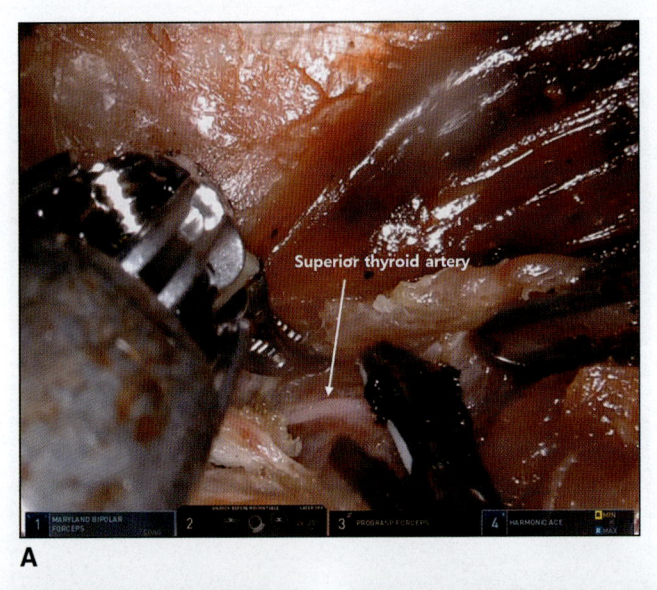

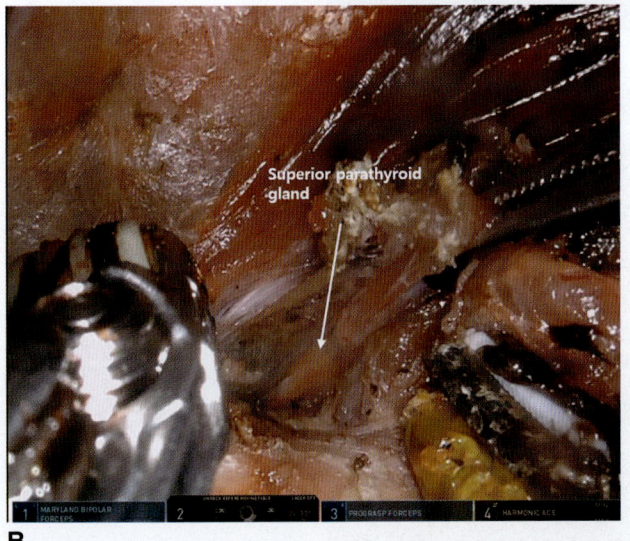

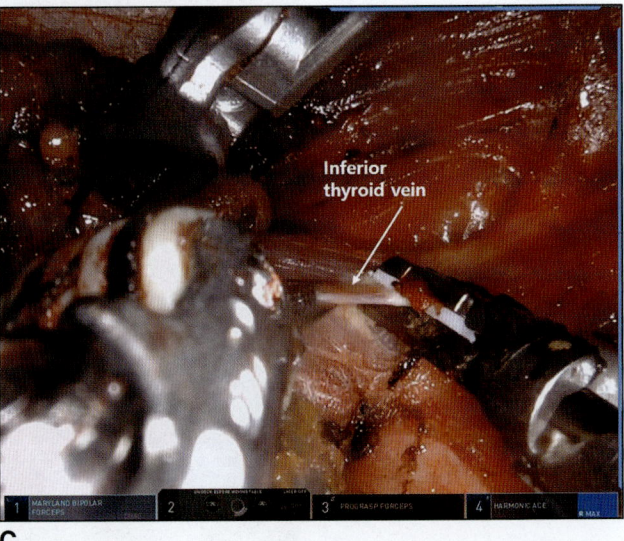

FIGURE 8-20 • Step 4. Completion of the contralateral lobectomy. **A.** Ligation of the superior thyroid vessels. **B.** Identification and preservation of the superior parathyroid gland. **C.** Subcapsular dissection performed along with the thyroid gland, preserving the inferior parathyroid gland and ligation of inferior thyroid vessels.

> ⚠ **PITFALLS**
>
> The transection of the vessels running to the lower pole should be done cautiously, during or after the exposure of the RLN, which is located deeper than it may appear in the ipsilateral side view.

> ▶▶ **TIPS**
>
> In a patient with a prominent trachea and a deeply located contralateral thyroid gland, the surgical table can be tilted by 10–15°; this provides optimal exposure of the contralateral tracheoesophageal groove.

> **EDITORIAL COMMENT**
>
> The identification of the counterlateral RLN is not always easy and feasible. It depends on the anatomy of the trachea and on the position of the nerve. The dissection of the counterlateral thyroid lobe should always be subcapsular to minimize the risk of nerve and parathyroid injury. The strong action of lifting the lobe, and the creation of a good working space, allowing this vertical/medial lifting, is paramount.

▶ Video 8-2. Step 4. Bilateral Total Thyroidectomy with Central Compartment Node Dissection

Step 5. Specimen extraction and wound closure

After the extraction of the specimen through the axillary skin incision, irrigation can be performed to clean the operative field. The robotic cart is undocked.

A 3-mm closed-suction drain is inserted through a separate skin incision below the axillary access.

Wounds are closed cosmetically, and the axillary incision scar is completely covered when the arm is in its natural position.

Step 5 average time frame: 5–10 min

> ▶▶ **TIPS**
>
> **Thyroidectomy with SP System:**
>
> The thyroidectomy with the SP system has the same steps of the already described procedure with the Xi. All the dissections and the vessel ligations are performed by a monopolar electrocautery and Erbe (Erbe USA Inc, Marietta, GA) with SWIFT COAG mode and power level 1 to 4 in the vision cart. There is no Harmonic instrument with the SP.
>
> *Average time frame: 50–80 min*

MODIFIED RADICAL NECK DISSECTION

Indications for and Relative Contraindications to the Robotic Approach

To perform this complex procedure the surgeon needs to have an extensive experience with the transaxillary robotic thyroidectomy. The indications for modified radical neck dissection (mRND) can be listed as follows: (1) well-differentiated thyroid carcinomas with LN metastases; (2) the primary tumor size <4 cm; and (3) minimal tumor invasion into the anterior thyroid capsule and strap muscles.

The contraindications are as follows: (1) tumor invasion to an adjacent organ such as the RLN, esophagus, major vessels, or trachea; (2) conglomerated lymph nodes involved by cancer; or (3) any evidence of perinodal infiltration of lymph nodes to the adjacent structures (IJV, CCA, vagus nerve, or RLN).

Accurate knowledge of the anatomical classification of the zones of the neck and lymph nodes is essential (**Figures 8-21 A, B**).

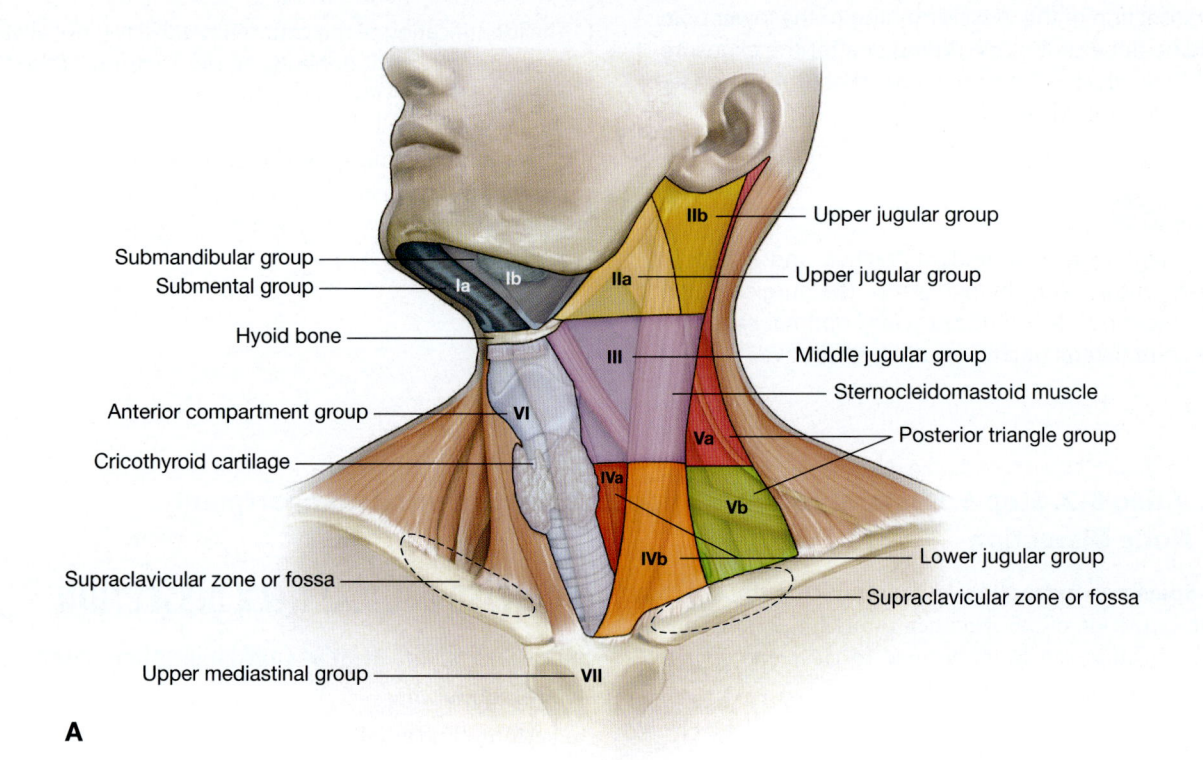

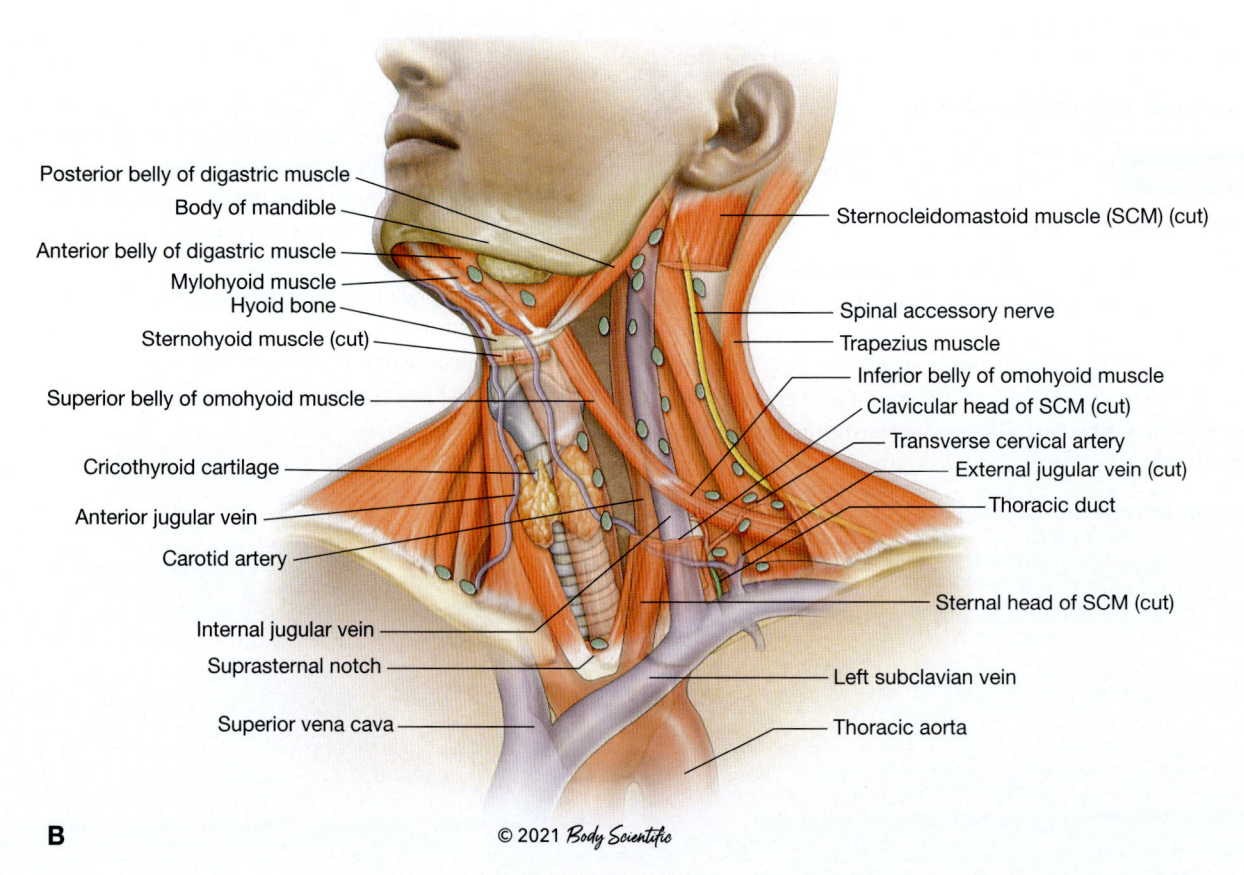

FIGURE 8-21 • The zones of the neck and lymph nodes.

Gasless Transaxillary Thyroidectomy 155

Patient Positioning, OR Setup, and Port Setting

Under general anesthesia, the patient is placed in a supine position on a neck pillow with the neck slightly extended.

The arm homo-lateral to the lesion is stretched laterally and abducted by about 80° from the body. The head is tilted and rotated to expose the axilla and the lateral neck (**Figure 8-22**).

The surgical pad is placed under the shoulder homolateral to the lesion, such that the level of the thyroid gland and shoulder can be adjusted.

Creation of Working Space

Incision Line Drawing (Figure 8-23)

The inferior border of the mandible and the submandibular gland must be marked.

The following lines should be drawn:
- from the thyroid cartilage to the sternal notch.
- along the border of the trapezius muscle from the ear to the clavicle and extended to the axilla (lateral border of the pectoralis major muscle).
- from the sternal notch to the axilla (lateral border of the pectoralis major muscle). A 7–8 cm skin incision is made in the axilla along the anterior axillary fold, and the lateral border of the pectoralis major muscle.

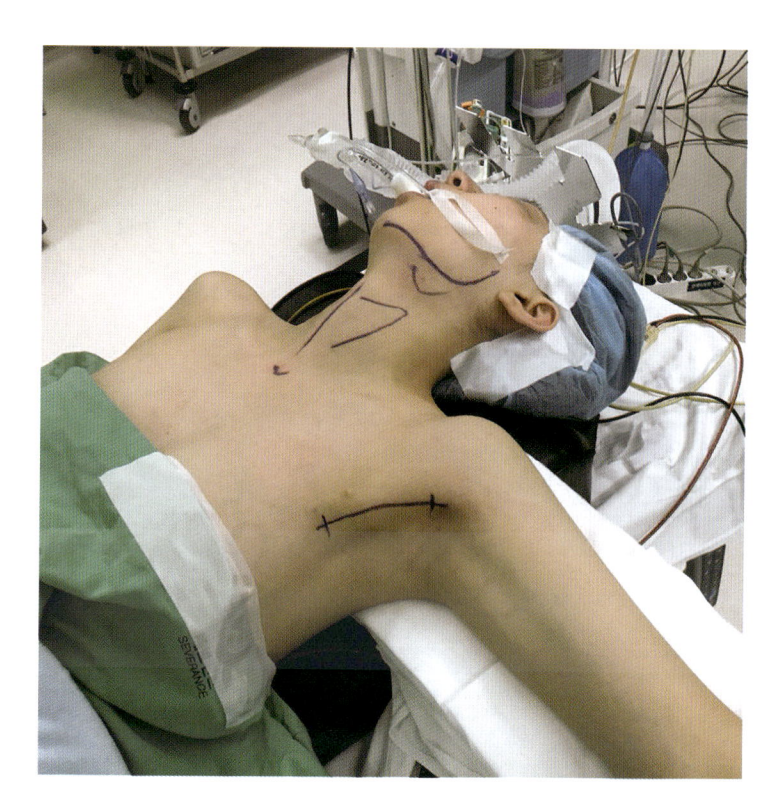

FIGURE 8-22 • Patient positioning for robotic mRND.

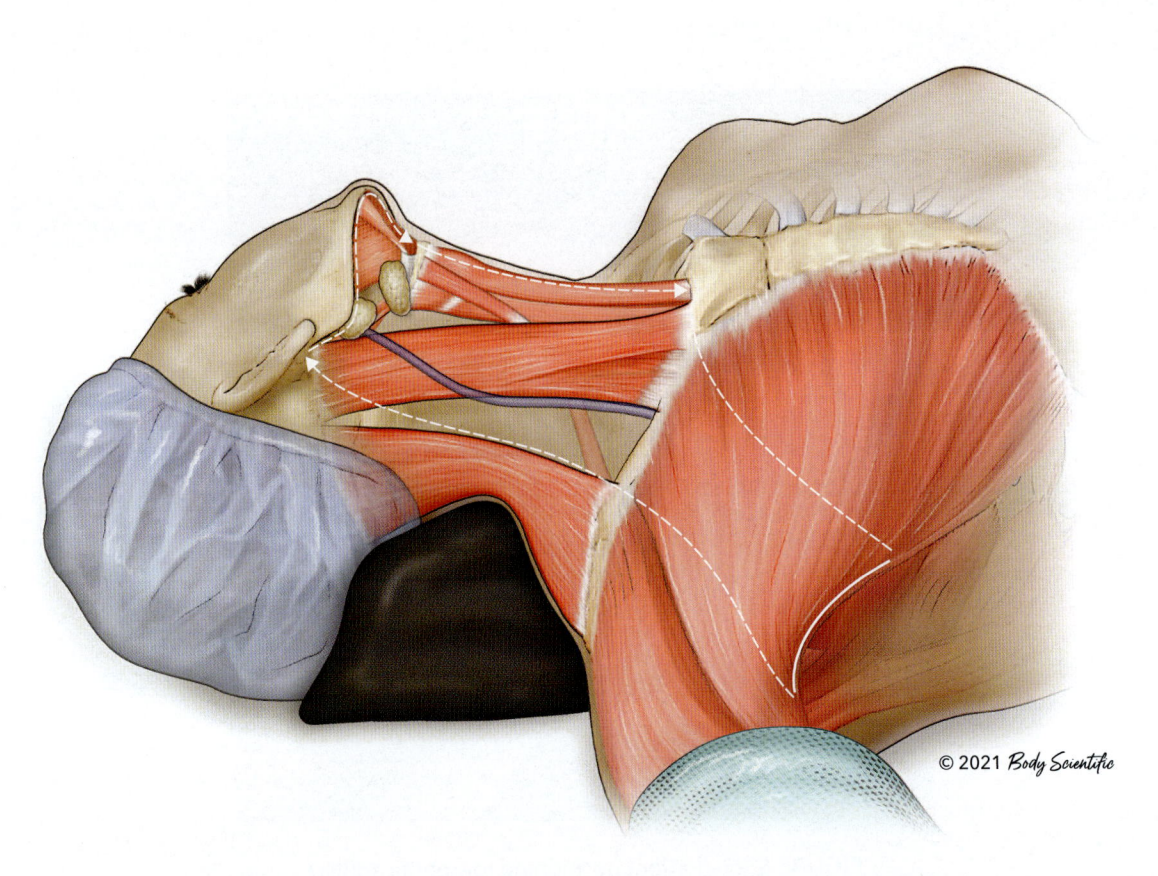

FIGURE 8-23 • Extent of flap dissection from the axilla to the anterior neck.

Creation of the Working Space

The working space is created under direct vision by electrocauterization over the anterior surface of the pectoralis major muscle and the clavicle from the axilla to the midline of the anterior neck.

After exposing the clavicle, the subplatysmal flap dissection proceeds to the midline of the anterior neck medially, to the upper point where the external jugular vein and the great auricular nerve cross the lateral border of the SCM superiorly, and to the trapezius muscle posteriorly (**Figure 8-24A**). The external jugular vein is ligated at the crossing point of the SCM muscle.

Laterally, the trapezius muscle is identified and dissected upward along its anterior border. During flap dissection, in the posterior neck area, the spinal accessory nerve is identified and exposed along its course (**Figure 8-24B**).

After finishing the subplatysmal flap dissection, soft-tissue detachment from the lateral border of the SCM is continued (**Figure 8-24C**). The dissection proceeds upward along the posterior surface of the SCM, through the avascular space between the carotid sheath and the strap muscles, until the thyroid gland is exposed.

To expose the level II area, the dissection proceeds until the submandibular gland and the posterior belly of the digastric muscle are exposed superiorly.

After finishing the flap dissection, the patient's head is returned to the neutral position. A (mRND) blade of the external retractor system is inserted through the axillary skin incision, located between the anterior surface of the thyroid and the strap muscles. The retractor is then used to raise and tent the skin flap at the anterior chest wall, SCM, and strap muscles to create a working space (**Figure 8-24D**).

Incision lines drawing and creation of working space total average time frame: 50–70 min

> ▶▶ **TIPS**
>
> The spinal accessory nerve is identified along the anterior border of the trapezius muscle, roughly 2–4 cm superior to the clavicle, and dissected free from the surrounding tissue to the posterior border of the SCM. A perfect understanding of the anatomy makes the dissection safer and faster.

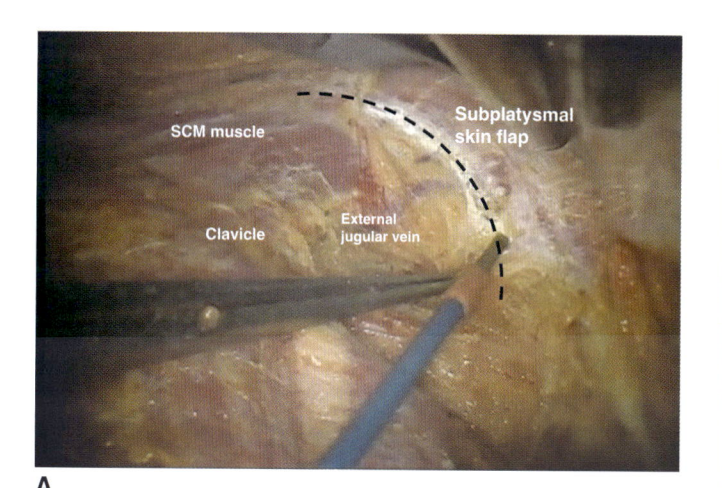

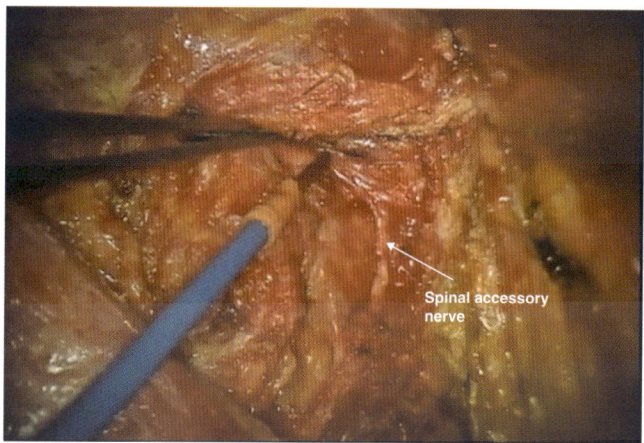

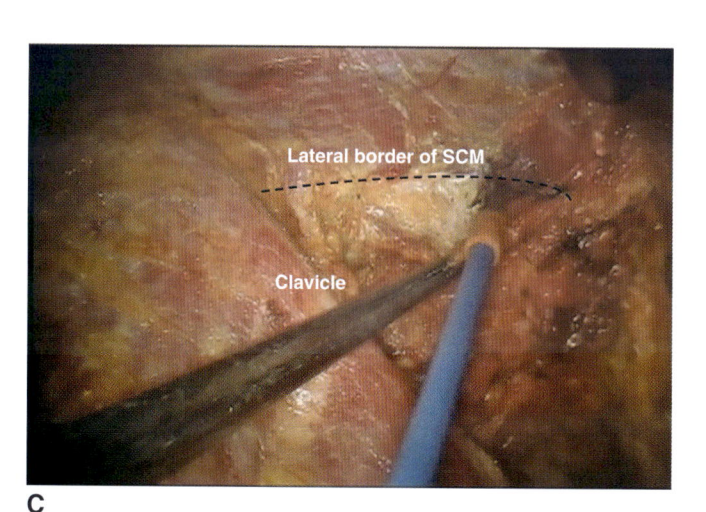

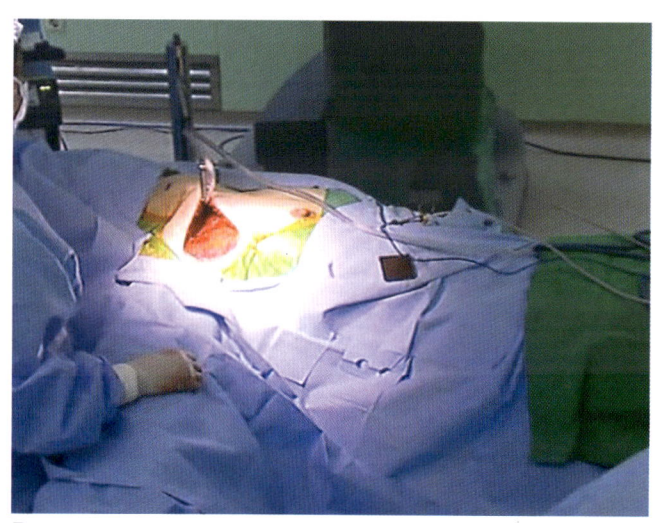

FIGURE 8-24 • Step 2. Creation of the working space. **A.** Margin of the subplatysmal skin flap. **B.** Spinal accessory nerve identification and exposure. **C.** Soft-tissue detachment from the lateral border of the SCM; the dissection proceeds along the posterior surface of the SCM. **D.** External retractor blade insertion.

Robot Positioning and Docking (2-Stage)

The following description is for the da Vinci Si, S, and Xi systems. The thyroidectomy with the central compartment lymphadenectomy is completed in the stage 1 (already described).

Lateral Neck Lymph Nodes Dissection of Level III, IV, and V

The patient cart and the operative table are located in the same direction as for the thyroidectomy, and the position of the 4 robotic arms is also similar (**Figure 8-25A**).

Lateral Neck Lymph Nodes Dissection of Level II

The external retractor is reinserted through the axillary incision and directed toward the submandibular gland. The operative table should be repositioned more obliquely with respect to the direction of the robotic column; this allows for the same alignment between the axis of the robotic camera arm and direction of the retractor blade insertion (**Figures 8-25 B, C**). The position of the 4 robotic arms remains the same as that in the first stage.

Average time frame (re-docking/repositioning): 10–15 min

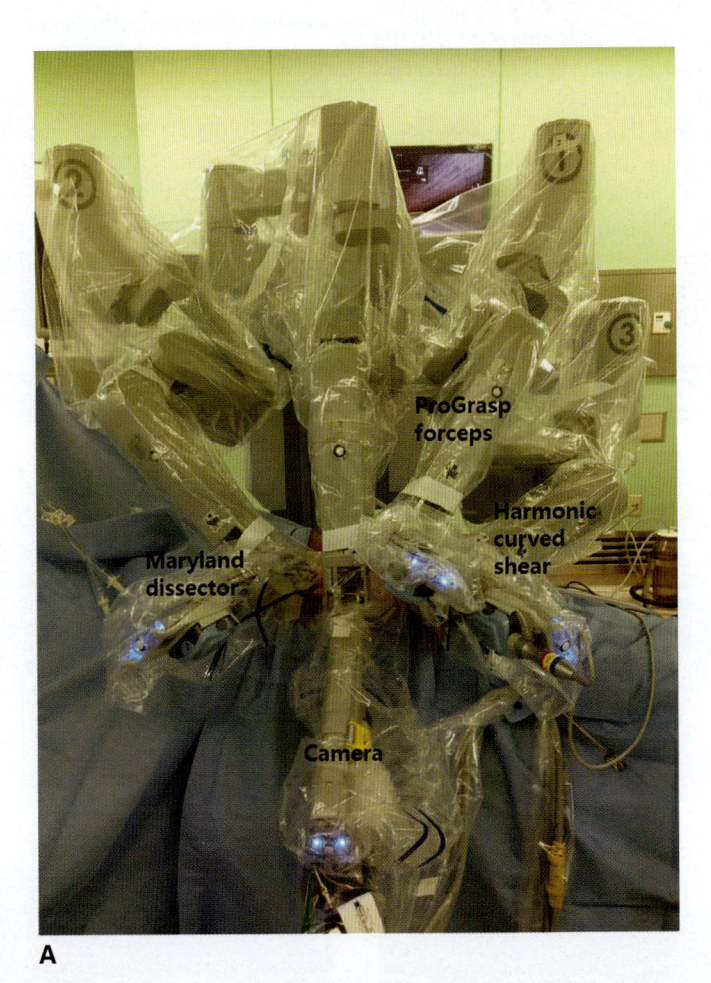

FIGURE 8-25 • Robot positioning and retractor placement. **A.** Initial placement of robotic arms.

B **C**

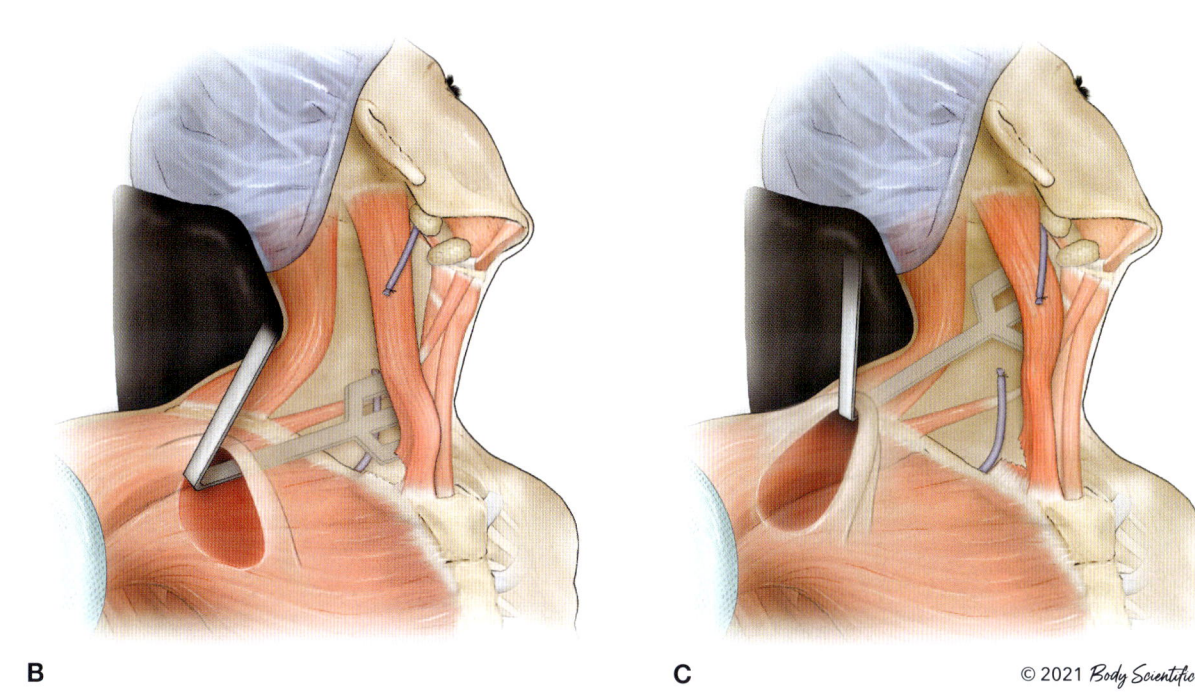

FIGURE 8-25 • (Continued) **B.** External retractor insertion: initial position for thyroidectomy and neck dissection for the levels III, IV, and Vb. **C.** External retractor repositioned for level II dissection.

Video 8-3. Creation of the Working Space for Modified Radical Neck Dissection

Modified Radical Neck Dissection (mRND)

Step 1. Level III and IV dissection

The lateral neck dissection is started from the level III and IV area around the IJV. This vessel is pulled medially using the ProGrasp forceps, and soft tissues and lymph nodes are pulled laterally using a Maryland dissector. The lymph nodes are then detached carefully from the anterior surface of the IJV to the posterior aspect of it until the CCA and vagus nerve are identified (**Figures 8-26 A, B**).

Dissection of the IJV is continued upward from level IV to the upper level III area. Packets of lymph nodes are then drawn superiorly using the ProGrasp forceps, and the lymph nodes are meticulously detached from the junction of the IJV and subclavian vein. If there is difficulty in reaching this point with nonarticulated Harmonic curved shears, increasing the height of the external third joint of the robotic arm, equipped with the Harmonic curved shears, is likely to resolve this problem and allow the target point to be reached.

In general, the transverse cervical artery courses laterally across the anterior scalene muscle and anterior to the phrenic nerve. Using this anatomic landmark, the phrenic nerve and the transverse cervical artery can be preserved (**Figures 8-26 C, D**).

The inferior belly of the omohyoid muscle is cut where it meets the trapezius muscle. The distal external jugular vein is then clipped and divided at its connection with the subclavian vein.

> ▶▶ **TIPS**
> The transverse cervical artery can be used as an anatomical landmark; all tissues are resected anterior to the phrenic nerve and transverse cervical artery.

> ⚠ **PITFALLS**
> The thoracic duct of level IV (especially left mRND) should be approached cautiously. Injury of the thoracic duct can be managed with clipping and sometimes with suturing.

Step 2. Level Vb dissection

The level Vb dissection, in the posterior neck area, is carried out along the spinal accessory nerve in the superomedial direction. This is followed by the level IV dissection, while also preserving the brachial nerve plexus, the phrenic nerve, and the thoracic duct (**Figure 8-26E**).

The dissection proceeds by making turns at levels Vb, IV, and III, and then by continuing upward to the level IIa area. The individual nerves of the cervical plexus are sensory, and

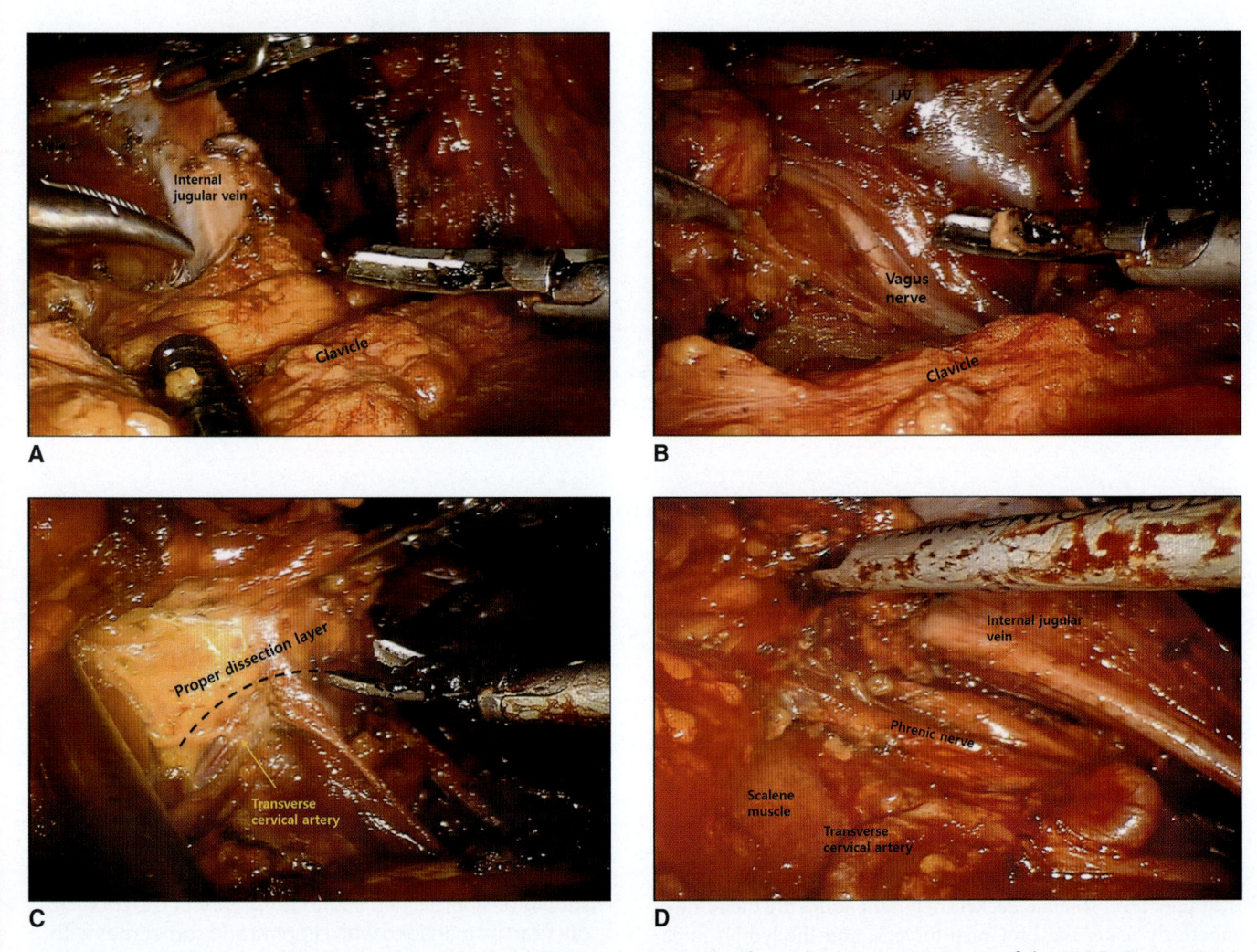

FIGURE 8-26 A–D • Level III and IV dissection. **A.** Lymph node dissection from the posterior aspect of the IJV. **B.** Preventing injury of the common carotid artery and vagus nerve. **C.** Dissection of the deep cervical fascia avoiding injury to the transverse cervical vessels. **D.** Dissection layer of the deep cervical fascia avoiding injury to the phrenic nerve.

when encountered during dissection, some may be sacrificed to ensure a complete node dissection, while preserving the phrenic nerve and the ansa cervicalis.

Step 3. Level II dissection
After finishing the levels III, IV, and Vb node dissection, re-docking is needed to better expose the level II area.

By pulling the specimen tissue inferolaterally, the soft tissues and lymph nodes are detached from the lateral border of the sternohyoid muscle, the submandibular gland, the anterior surface of the carotid artery, and the IJV (**Figure 8-26F**).

After superiorly exposing the posterior belly of the digastric muscle, the level II node dissection is completed.

> ⚠ **PITFALLS**
>
> The external retractor's direction should be toward the submandibular gland. In the wrong direction, the robotic arms cannot properly reach the level II area. (Right side: Maryland dissector, Left side: Harmonic curved shears)

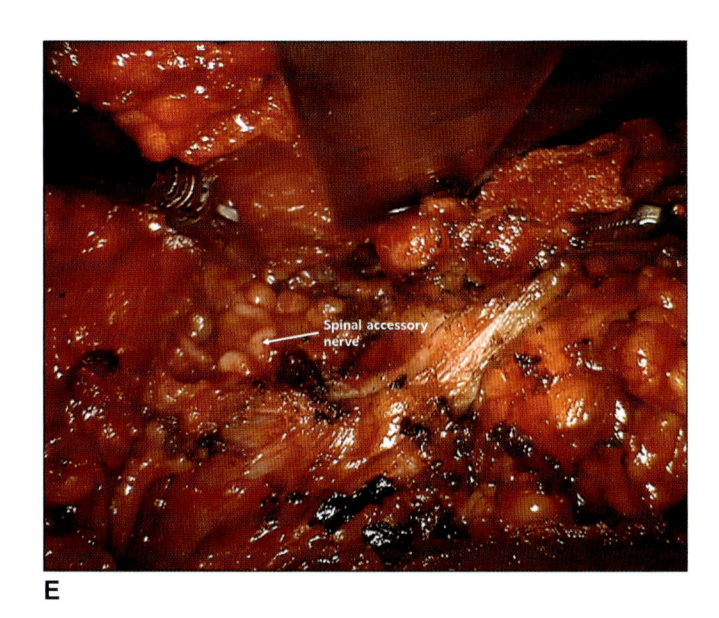

FIGURE 8-26 E • Level Vb dissection preserving the spinal accessory nerve.

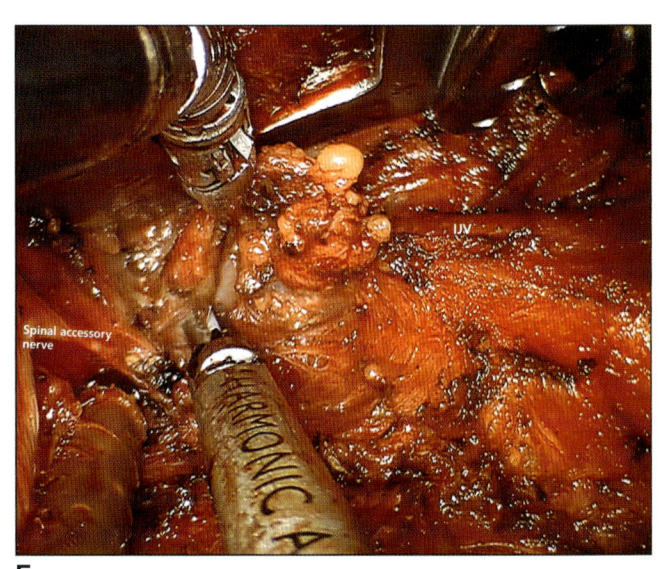

FIGURE 8-26 F • Level II dissection proceeding to the posterior belly of the digastric muscle and the submandibular gland.

▶ **Video 8-4. Step 3. Modified Radical Neck Dissection**

Step 4. Specimen extraction and wound closure
After extraction of the specimen through the axillary skin incision, irrigation can be performed to clean the operative field. The robot is undocked.

A 5-mm closed-suction drain is inserted through a separate skin incision below the axillary one.

A surgical pad is placed under the shoulder of the lesion, such that the level of the thyroid gland and shoulder can be adjusted. The wound is closed.

Average time (total thyroidectomy with mRND): 150–180 min

> ▶▶ **TIPS**
>
> The repositioning of the operative table should be more oblique, with respect to the direction of the robotic column, to allow the same alignment between the axis of the robotic camera arm and the direction of the retractor blade insertion.

Suggested Readings

1. Kang SW, Jeong JJ, Nam KH, et al. Robot-assisted endoscopic thyroidectomy for thyroid malignancies using a gasless transaxillary approach. *J Am Coll Surg.* 2009;209:e1-7.
2. Lee S, Ryu HR, Park JH, et al. Excellence in robotic thyroid surgery: a comparative study of robot-assisted versus conventional endoscopic thyroidectomy in papillary thyroid microcarcinoma patients. *Ann Surg.* 2011;253:1060-1066.
3. Kang SW, Lee SH, Ryu HR, et al. Initial experience with robot-assisted modified radical neck dissection for the management of thyroid carcinoma with lateral neck node metastasis. *Surgery.* 2010;148:1214-1221.
4. Kim MJ, Lee J, Lee SG, et al. Transaxillary robotic modified radical neck dissection: a 5-year assessment of operative and oncologic outcomes. *Surg Endosc.* 2017;31:1599-1606.
5. Bae DS, Koo do H, Choi JY, et al. Current status of robotic thyroid surgery in South Korea: a web-based survey. *World J Surg.* 2014;38:2632-2639.
6. Kim MJ, Nam KH, Lee SG, et al. Yonsei experience of 5000 gasless transaxillary robotic thyroidectomies. *World J Surg.* 2018;42:393-401.
7. Ban EJ, Yoo JY, Kim WW, et al. Surgical complications after robotic thyroidectomy for thyroid carcinoma: a single center experience with 3,000 patients. *Surg Endosc.* 2014;28:2555-2563.
8. Lee S, Lee CR, Lee SC, et al. Surgical completeness of robotic thyroidectomy: a prospective comparison with conventional open thyroidectomy in papillary thyroid carcinoma patients. *Surg Endosc.* 2014;28:1068-1075.
9. Son H, Park S, Lee CR, et al. Factors contributing to surgical outcomes of transaxillary robotic thyroidectomy for papillary thyroid carcinoma. *Surg Endosc.* 2014;28:3134-3142.
10. Lee J, Kang SW, Jung JJ, et al. Multicenter study of robotic thyroidectomy: short-term postoperative outcomes and surgeon ergonomic considerations. *Ann Surg Oncol.* 2011;18:2538-2547.
11. Tae K, Song CM, Ji YB, et al. Comparison of surgical completeness between robotic total thyroidectomy versus open thyroidectomy. *Laryngoscope.* 2014;124:1042-1047.
12. Lee J, Nah KY, Kim RM, et al. Differences in postoperative outcomes, function, and cosmesis: open versus robotic thyroidectomy. *Surg Endosc.* 2010;24:3186-3194.
13. Park JH, Lee J, Hakim NA, et al. Robotic thyroidectomy learning curve for beginning surgeons with little or no experience of endoscopic surgery. *Head Neck.* 2015;37:1705-1711.
14. Lee J, Yun JH, Choi UJ, et al. Robotic versus endoscopic thyroidectomy for thyroid cancers: a multi-institutional analysis of early postoperative outcomes and surgical learning curves. *J Oncol.* 2012;2012:734541.
15. Kim K, Kang SW, Kim JK, et al. Robotic transaxillary hemithyroidectomy using the da Vinci SP robotic system: initial experience with 10 consecutive cases. *Surg Innov.* 2020;27:256-264.
16. Jackson RN, Yao L, Tufano RP, Kandil EH. Safety of robotic thyroidectomy approaches: meta-analysis and systematic review. *Head Neck.* 2014;36(1):137-143. doi: 10.1002/hed.23223
17. Kang SW, Jeong JJ, Yun JS, et al. Robot-assisted endoscopic surgery for thyroid cancer: experience with the first 100 patients. *Surg Endosc.* 2009;23:2399-2406.
18. Park JH, Lee CR, Park S, et al. Initial experience with robotic gasless transaxillary thyroidectomy for the management of graves disease: comparison of conventional open versus robotic thyroidectomy. *Surg Laparosc Endosc Percutan Tech.* 2013;23:e173-177.
19. Randolph G, ed. *The Recurrent and Superior Laryngeal Nerves.* Springer; 2016:125-128. doi: 10.1007/978-3-319-27727-1
20. Cernea C, Ferraz AR, Nishio S, Dutra Jr A, Hojaij FC, dos Santos LR. Surgical anatomy of the external branch of the superior laryngeal nerve. *Head Neck.* 1992;14:380-383.
21. Barczyski M, Freeman JL, Cernea CR. External branch of superior laryngeal nerve (EBSLN) anatomic classification. In: Randolph G, ed. *The Recurrent and Superior Laryngeal Nerves.* Springer; 2016:187-195. doi: 10.1007/978-3-319-27727-1_16
22. Cernea CR, Ferraz AR, Furlani J, et al. Identification of the external branch of the superior laryngeal nerve during thyroidectomy. *Am J Surg.* 1992;164:634-639.
23. Kierner AC, Aigner M, Burian M. The external branch of the superior laryngeal nerve: its topographical anatomy as related to surgery of the neck. *Arch Otolaryngol Head Neck Surg.* 1998;124:301-303.
24. Taterra D, Wong LM, Vikse J, et al. The prevalence and anatomy of parathyroid glands: a meta-analysis with implications for parathyroid surgery. *Langenbecks Arch Surg.* 2019;404(1):63-70. doi: 10.1007/s00423-019-01751-8
25. Fundakowski CE, Hales NW, Agrawal N. Surgical management of the recurrent laryngeal nerve in thyroidectomy: American Head and Neck Society consensus statement. *Head Neck.* 2018;40(4):663-675. doi: 10.1002/hed.24928
26. Le VQ, Ngo QD, Ngo XQ. Nonrecurrent laryngeal nerve in thyroid surgery: frequency, anatomical variations according to a new classification and surgery consideration. *Head Neck.* 2019;41(9):2969-2975. doi: 10.1002/hed.25771
27. Standring S, ed. *Gray's Anatomy: The Anatomical Basis of Clinical Practice.* 42nd ed. Churchill Livingstone-Elsevier; 2020.
28. Tran Ba Huy P. Tiroidectomie. *Encyclopedie Medico-Chirurgicale I 46-460.* Editions Scientifiques et Médicales Elsevier; 2001.
29. Giulianotti PC, Coratti A, Angelini M, et al. Robotics in general surgery: personal experience in a large community hospital. *Arch Surg.* 2003;138(7):777-784. doi: 10.1001/archsurg.138.7.777

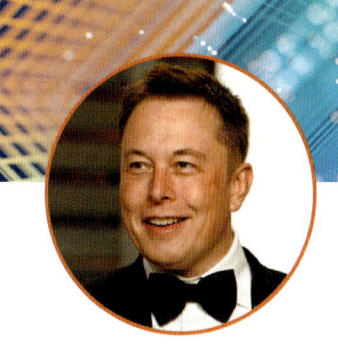

"Innovation often doesn't come through one breakthrough idea, but through a relentless focus on continuous improvement."

— Elon Musk (1971)

Transoral Thyroidectomy
(Off-Label Indication)

Ji Young You • Dawon Park • Hoon Yub Kim

INTRODUCTION

The transoral thyroidectomy technique has a unique advantage of accessing the thyroid gland from a natural orifice, which leads to a good cosmetic appearance. Furthermore, the transoral approach is less invasive in terms of working space than other types of remote access thyroidectomy. The proximity to the thyroid gland from the oral mucosa allows this technique to have a minimized flap dissection that fulfills the idea of true minimally invasive surgery. Transoral thyroidectomy also provides a top-down operative view, and therefore, bilateral lobe access and central neck dissection can be performed easily up to level VII. It has been reported that the central compartment inspection and dissection with complete lymphadenectomy are feasible and safe in the transoral approach.

Indications and Contraindications to the Robotic Approach

The patients must meet the following inclusion criteria: (1) an ultrasonographically (US)-estimated thyroid gland diameter ≤10 cm, (2) a US-estimated thyroid volume ≤45 mL, (3) a US-estimated main nodule size ≤5 cm, (4) presence of a benign tumor such as a thyroid cyst or a uni- or multinodular goiter, (5) follicular neoplasm, or (6) papillary microcarcinoma of the thyroid without evidence of metastasis.

Patients should be excluded if they: (1) are unfit for surgery; (2) cannot tolerate general anesthesia; (3) underwent previous radiation therapy in the head, neck, and/or upper mediastinum; (4) had a previous neck surgery; (5) have a recurrent goiter; (6) have a thyroid volume >45 mL; (7) have a dominant nodule size >5 cm; (8) show evidence of lymph nodal or distant metastases; (9) have a locally advanced cancer with tracheal/esophageal invasion; (10) have recurrent laryngeal nerve (RLN) palsy;

INSTRUMENT REQUIREMENTS

The suggested main robotic instruments/tools can be listed as follows:
- 30° endoscope
- Maryland bipolar forceps/dissector
- ProGrasp™ forceps
- Harmonic ACE+ curved shears
- Needle driver
- Monopolar hook cautery
- PreCise™ bipolar forceps

Supplemental materials:

Patient position:
- Neck pillow
- Arm board

Creation of a skin flap:
Tunneler
- Monopolar Cautery Pen with short, medium, and long tips
- Harmonic scalpel

Robotic procedures:
- Clip applier
- Endoscopic rolled gauzes
- Endoscopic suction irrigator
- Endoscopic Plastic Bag
- Medium–large clips

Thyroid surgery:
- NIM™ System
- Jackson-Pratt drain
- Fibrin glue
- Antiadhesive agent
- V-Loc™ absorbable suture 3-0

Photo from Alberto E. Rodriguez / Getty images.
Quote from Wall Street Journal's CEO conference 12/8/2020.

164 The Foundation and Art of Robotic Surgery

(11) have a biochemical sign of hyperthyroidism; or (12) have an oral abscess. Patients with poorly differentiated or undifferentiated cancer, posterior extrathyroidal extension and/or N1b differentiated thyroid cancer, a huge goiter, and Graves' disease are therefore not candidates for the transoral approach.

Patient Positioning, OR Setup, and Port Setting

Patient Positioning and Draping

▶ **Video 9-1. Preparation**

The patient is positioned supine and intubated with an electromyogram tube (Medtronic, Minneapolis, MN) for intraoperative nerve monitoring. After general anesthesia is induced, the patient's neck is placed in a slightly extended position. Draping is performed to expose the patient's upper chest, bilateral axillae, and lower lip. Subsequently, the oral cavity is irrigated with a solution of chlorhexidine and povidone-iodine (**Figure 9-1**).

▶ **Video 9-2. Skin Marking**

Incision and Flap Creation

After injection of 10 mL of a diluted epinephrine-saline solution (1:200,000) into the lower lip down the tip of the chin, 3 incisions are made in the gingival-buccal sulcus: one inverted U-shaped 1-cm midline incision approximately 2 cm above the *frenulum labii inferioris*, and two 0.5-cm bilateral incisions near the angle of the mouth (**Figure 9-2A**). The midline incision is made first. After the identification of the mandibular periosteum through the midline incision, a submental subplatysmal pocket is formed by blunt dissection with mosquito and Kelly forceps. Next, 30–50 mL of epinephrine-saline solution is injected into the subplatysmal space to create a tunnel from the edge of the mandible to the lower neck. Subsequently, blunt dissection with an 8-mm vascular surgical tunneler is gently performed down to the sternum to separate the platysma from the strap muscles (**Figure 9-2B**).

Once an adequate flap is created, the 8-mm trocar is inserted and carbon dioxide (CO_2) insufflation is maintained through

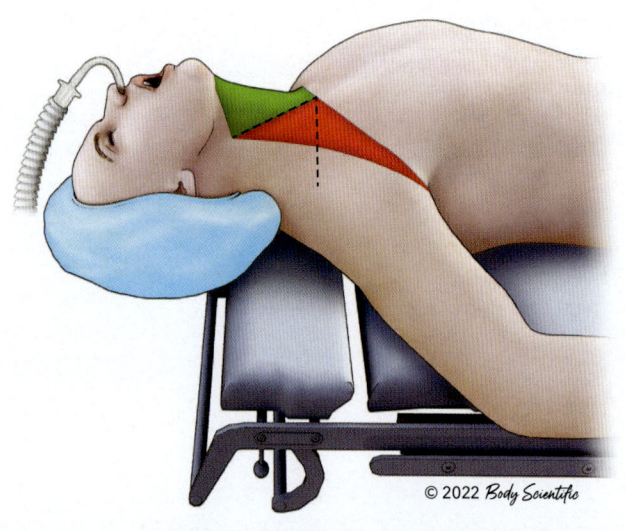

FIGURE 9-1 • Patient positioning.

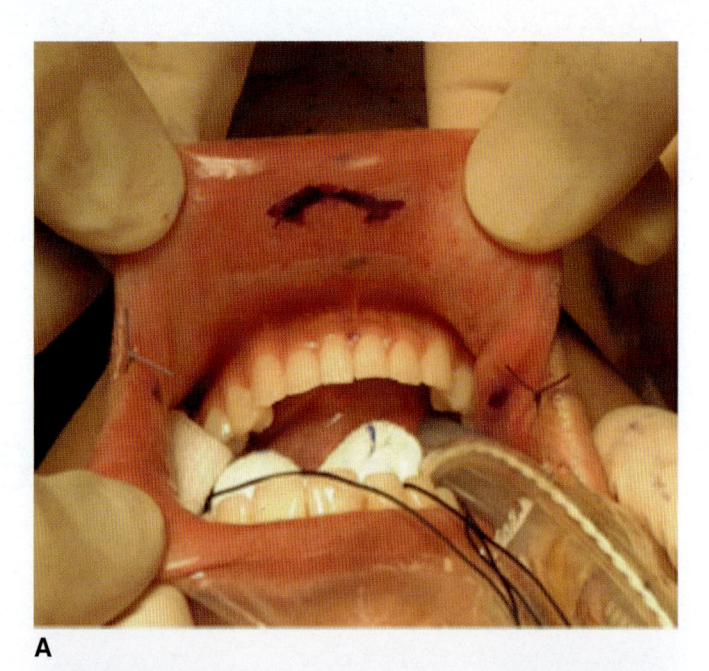

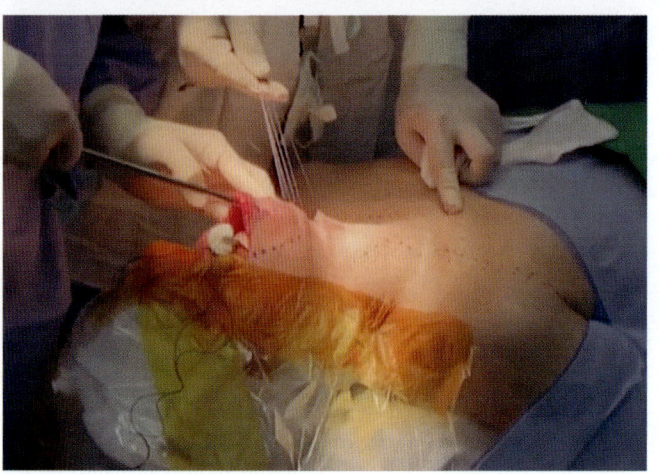

FIGURE 9-2 • Outer operative views before the insertion of the trocars. **A.** Intraoral incision sites. **B.** Blunt dissection with vascular surgical tunneler.

> **EDITORIAL COMMENT**
>
> A certain amount of CO_2 is continuously leaking throughout the surgery. However, the operative space is maintained with several flap traction sutures and the leakage is essential to evacuate the smoke and particles during the operation.

the midline port at the maximal pressure of 5–7 mm Hg. Similar blunt dissection is performed through both lateral incisions to insert the 8-mm trocars in each side (**Figure 9-3A**).

The platysma is then elevated superiorly to the level of the mandible, inferiorly to the sternum, and laterally to the sternocleidomastoid muscles using a suction electrocautery and ultrasonic energy device (Harmonic Ace™+, Ethicon Endo-Surgery, Cincinnati, OH) through the lateral ports (**Figure 9-3B**).

An additional 8-mm trocar is inserted through an incision made along the right anterior axillary fold for countertraction with the R3 and the subsequent insertion of the closed-suction drain.

Several synthetic absorbable sutures are used to retract the subplatysmal flap superiorly in order to create a larger working space.

Average time frame: 30–50 min

▶ **Video 9-3. Trocar Insertion**

A B

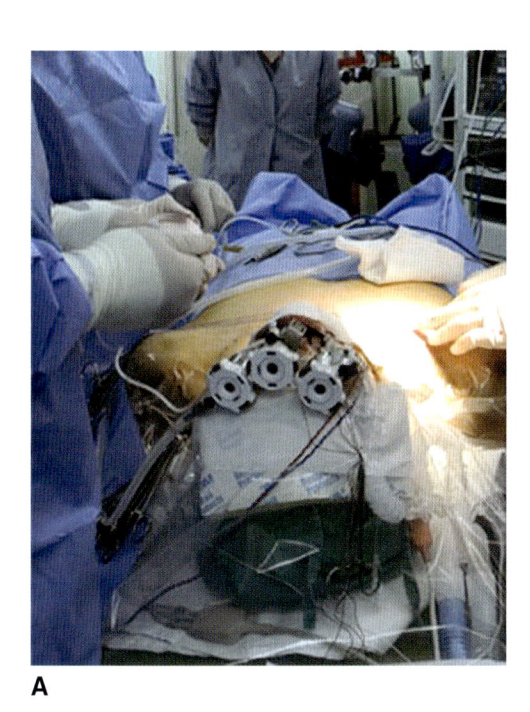

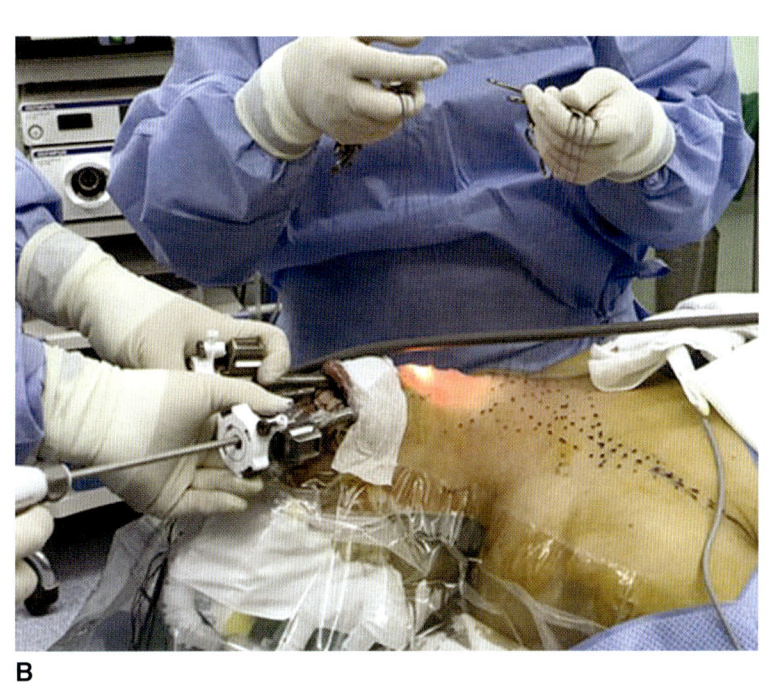

FIGURE 9-3 • Outer operative views after insertion of the trocars. **A.** Intraoral trocar positions. **B.** Subplatysmal dissection using a suction electrocautery and ultrasonic shears.

▶ **Video 9-4. Flap Formation**

⚠ PITFALLS

If the incision is too close to the bone, the mental nerve injury may occur.

Although flap perforation is a rare complication, flap burn is relatively common. Great caution is required when using energy devices for dissection.

▶▶ TIPS

After the modification of the incision for ports placement, by increasing the distance from the periosteum, the mental nerve injuries are less likely to occur (**Figure 9-4**).

🔍 ANATOMICAL HIGHLIGHTS

In the transoral thyroidectomy, the trocars are inserted in front of the jaw through the vestibular incision, and the mental nerve can be encountered during this process (**Figure 9-5A**).

⚠ PITFALLS

Mental nerve injury can cause sensory deficits in the lower lip and lower chin. The mechanism of occurrence is due to oral vestibular mucosa and muscular tearing (**Figures 9-5 B, C**).

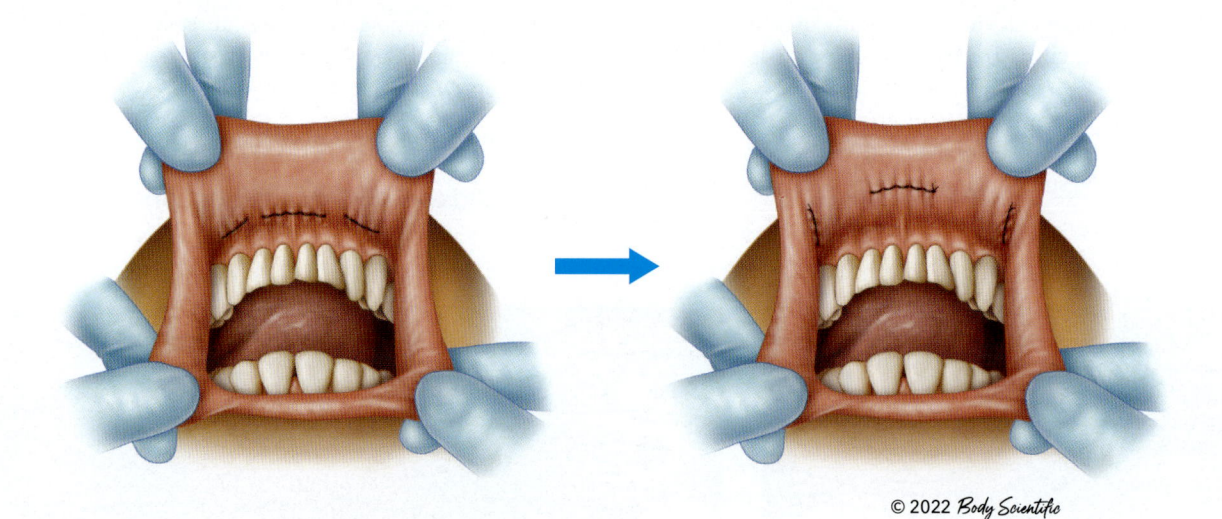

FIGURE 9-4 • Modification of the incision for ports placement.

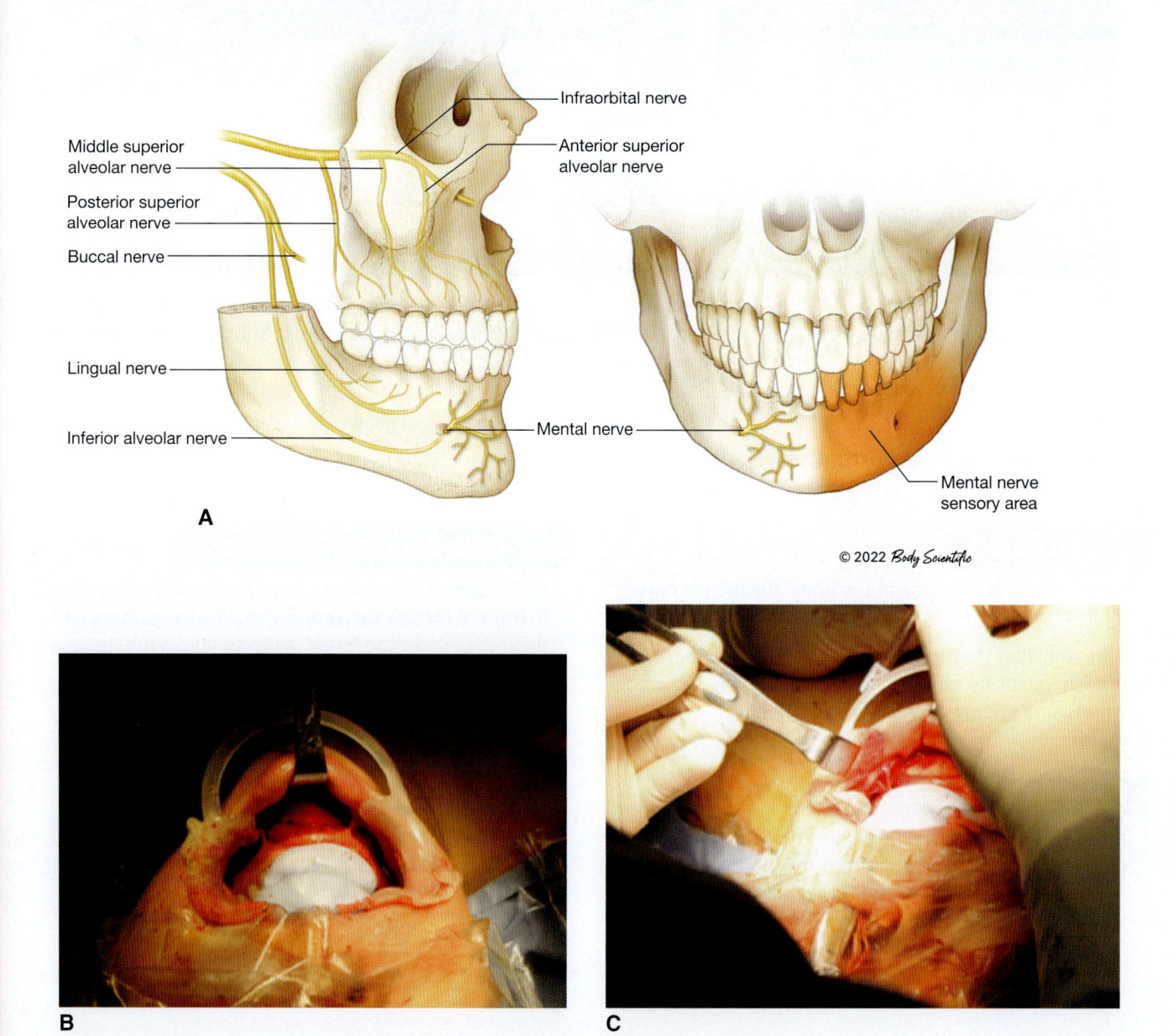

FIGURE 9-5 • **A.** Anatomy of the mental nerve. **B.** Midline incision. **C.** Vestibular approach for tunneling.

Xi Docking

Once the working space is completely formed, the patient is placed in the Trendelenburg position. Then, the da Vinci Surgical System (Xi) is docked left laterally to the patient using a laser pointer in the overhead boom targeted to 1-cm right lateral to the cricoid cartilage (**Figures 9-6 A, B**).

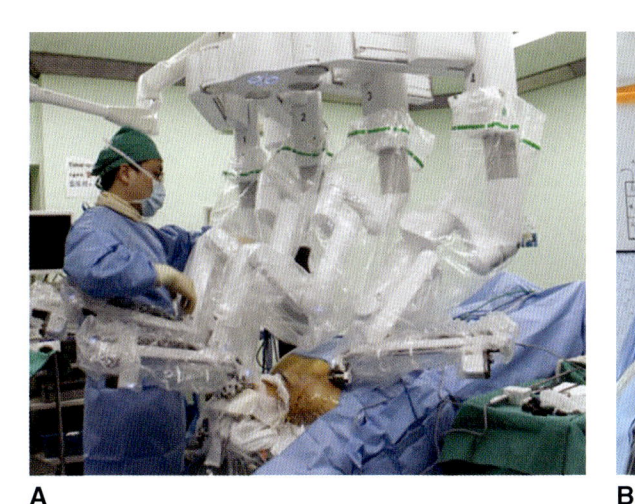

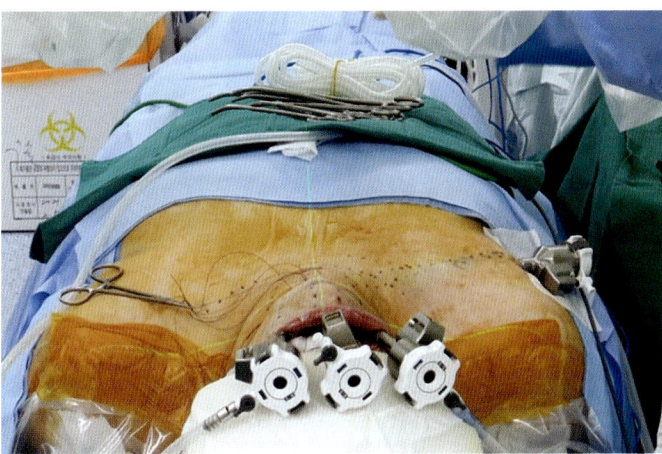

FIGURE 9-6 • Docking of Xi Robotic System.

Video 9-5. Docking

Subsequently, the robotic arms are connected to the ports, starting with the central endoscope cannula (30°, down facing). A Maryland bipolar forceps and the Harmonic scalpel are inserted through the left and right operative ports, respectively. For countertraction, an 8-mm ProGrasp™ bipolar forceps is connected with the R3 to the right axillary port.

Average time frame: 5–10 min

> **EDITORIAL COMMENT**
>
> The Maryland forceps are introduced through the axillary port for the right lobectomy and through the intraoral ports for the left lobectomy.

> ▶▶ **TIPS**
>
> **Pros and cons of additional axillary arm for TORT**: Transoral robotic thyroidectomy (TORT) can be done either using just 2 robotic arms for the instruments and 1 for the endoscopic camera or using 3 robotic arms for the instruments (R3 through the axilla) and 1 for the camera.
>
> The R3 through the additional axillary port is mainly responsible for countertraction of the strap muscles and the thyroid tissue. The additional axillary port tract is also an excellent passage for the specimen removal with lower risk of disruption or fragmentation. The implementation achieved with the R3 through the axilla allows the TORT to be performed safely in a wider range of patients.
>
> One of the issues with the axillary access is that it leaves a cutaneous scar. The retraction of the strap muscles through the subcutaneous stitches applied after establishing the working space may make up for the lack of countertraction if there is no access in the axilla.

Si Docking

The patient is placed with parted legs flexed on stirrups (lithotomy position) to allow the docking of the robotic cart in between the legs (**Figures 9-7 A, B**).

Differently from the Xi system, which can be docked from any direction, the Si cart should be aligned with the longitudinal axis of the surgical field and usually it can be placed in between the patient's legs (**Figure 9-7A**) or left laterally to the patient where there is less interference with the overall surgical work (**Figures 9-8 A–C**).

Average time frame: 10–15 min

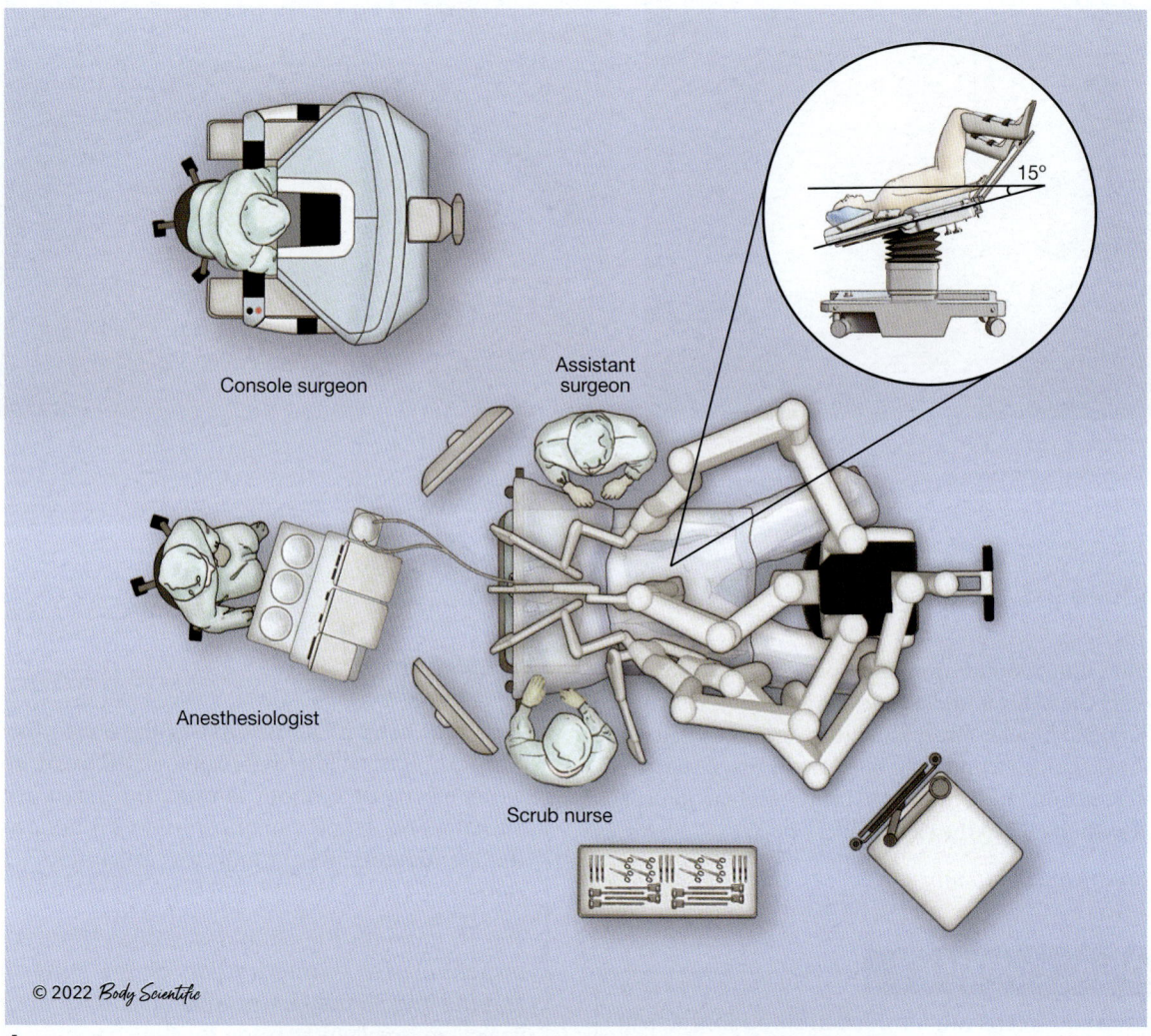

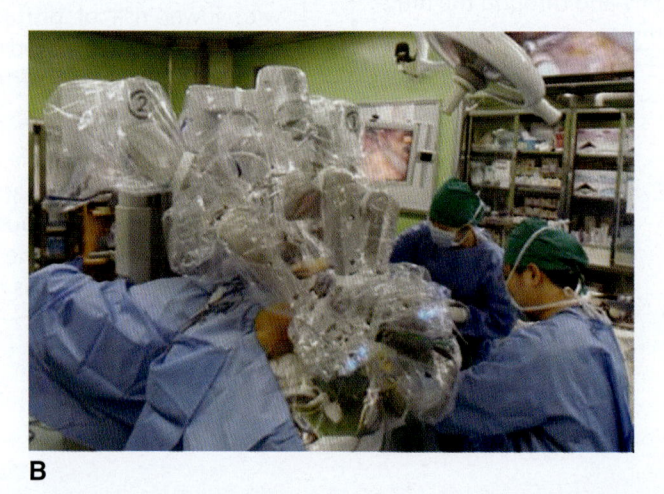

FIGURE 9-7 • Patient position and docking of da Vinci Si system. **A.** OR setting of the Si system. **B.** Patient placed in the lithotomy position with the Si system. (Reproduced with permission from Kim HK, Kim HY, Chai YJ, et al. Transoral robotic thyroidectomy: comparison of surgical outcomes between the da Vinci Xi and Si. *Surg Laparosc Endosc Percutan Tech*. 2018;28[6]:404-409.)

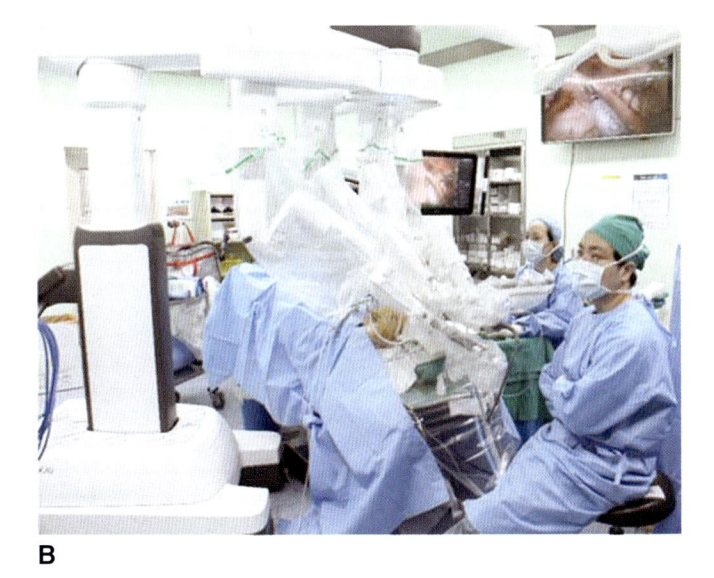

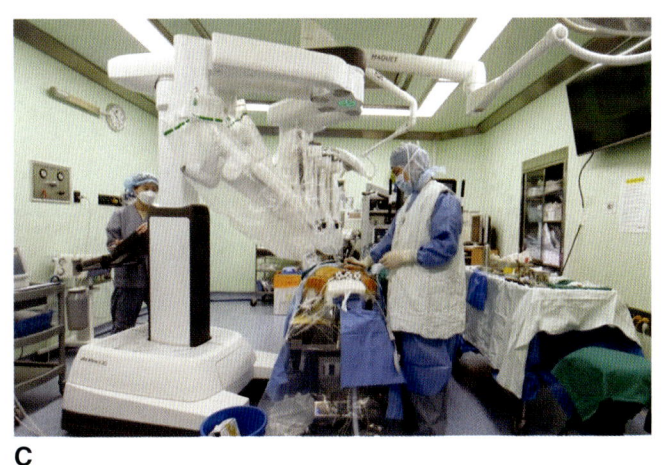

FIGURE 9-8 • Patient position and docking of da Vinci Xi system. **A.** OR setting of the Xi system. **B, C**. Patient placed in the supine position with the Xi system. (Reproduced with permission from Kim HK, Kim HY, Chai YJ, et al. Transoral robotic thyroidectomy: comparison of surgical outcomes between the da Vinci Xi and Si. *Surg Laparosc Endosc Percutan Tech*. 2018;28[6]:404-409).

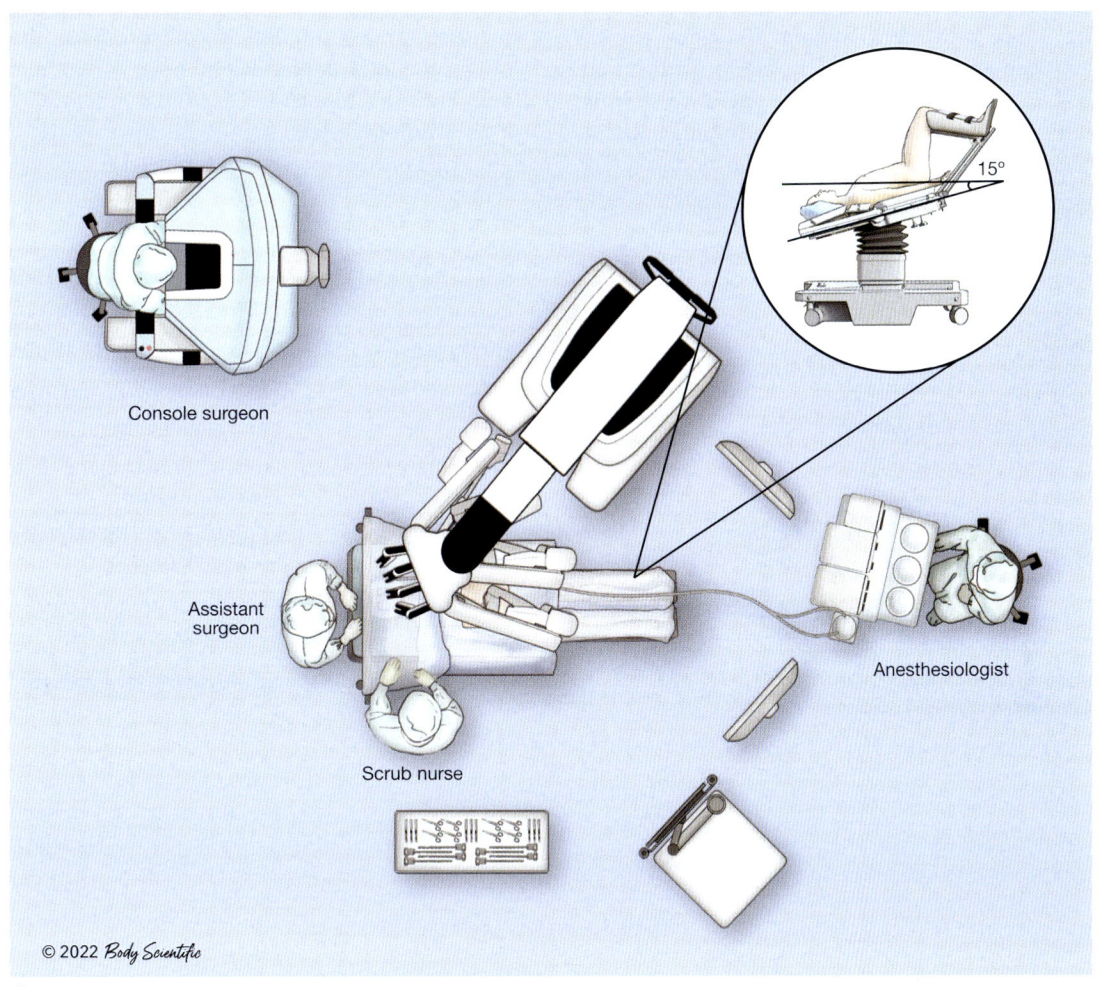

Operative Instruments for Xi and Si Systems

With the Si system, a 12-mm midline camera port, 5-mm lateral working ports, and an 8-mm axillary port are used, whereas all 4 ports are 8 mm with the Xi system. A 12-mm camera in the Si system and an 8-mm camera in the Xi platform are used through the intraoral middle port for operative viewing. Harmonic ACE+ curved shears (Ethicon Endo-Surgery, Cincinnati, OH), a needle driver, and a monopolar hook cautery, through the intraoral right lateral port, are used for dissection and coagulation. For thyroid manipulation, a 5-mm Maryland dissector is used for the Si system, and an 8-mm Maryland dissector or 8-mm ProGrasp™ forceps for the Xi platform through the intraoral left lateral port. For countertraction, an 8-mm PreCise™ bipolar forceps and 8-mm ProGrasp™ forceps (or an 8-mm Maryland bipolar forceps) are used through the right axilla port, respectively (**Table 9-1**).

TABLE 9-1 • Differences in Surgical Instruments According to the Robotic Systems

Incision	Main Function	da Vinci Si	da Vinci Xi
Intraoral midline	Camera	12-mm endoscope, 30 degrees	8-mm endoscope, 30 degrees
Intraoral right lateral	Dissection	5-mm Harmonic ACE+ curved shears	8-mm Harmonic ACE+ curved shears
	Coagulation	5-mm needle driver	8-mm needle driver
		5-mm monopolar hook cautery (also as nerve stimulator)	8-mm monopolar hook cautery (also as nerve stimulator)
Intraoral left lateral	Thyroid manipulation	5-mm Maryland dissector	8-mm Maryland bipolar forceps/8 mm ProGrasp™ forceps
Right axilla	Countertraction	8-mm PreCise™ bipolar forceps	8-mm ProGrasp™ forceps/8 mm Maryland bipolar forceps

Reproduced with permission from Kim HK, Kim HY, Chai YJ, et al. Transoral robotic thyroidectomy: comparison of surgical outcomes between the da Vinci Xi and Si. Surg Laparosc Endosc Percutan Tech. 2018;28(6):404-409.

Surgical Technique

Step 1. Midline incision and division of the isthmus

First, the midline raphe is dissected to separate the strap muscles using the monopolar hook cautery. The pyramidal lobe and Delphian nodes are dissected off the thyroid cartilage, and the isthmectomy is subsequently performed (**Figure 9-9**).

Step 1 average time frame: 10–15 min

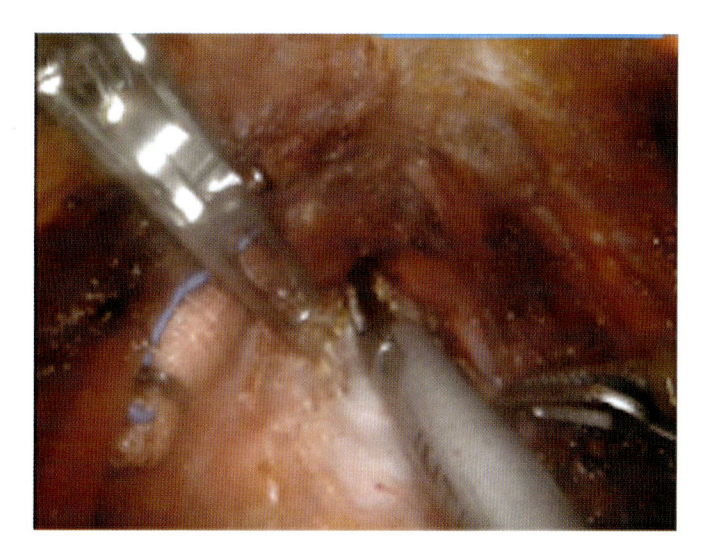

FIGURE 9-9 • Division of isthmus.

Step 2. Superior pole dissection

The posterior surface of the isthmus is detached from the trachea, and the strap muscles are dissected off from the thyroid gland exposing the right lobe. Once it is partially freed from the trachea in its medial attachments, the superior pole is addressed. The sternothyroid muscle is retracted laterally by the Maryland bipolar forceps through the axillary port and the superior pole is lifted up using ProGrasp™ forceps. Careful dissection of the superior lobe is performed and the vessels are ligated one at a time using the Harmonic ACE+ curved shears (**Figure 9-10**). The endoscopic metal clips may be applied to the engorged superior thyroid vessels.

Step 2 average time frame: 15–20 min

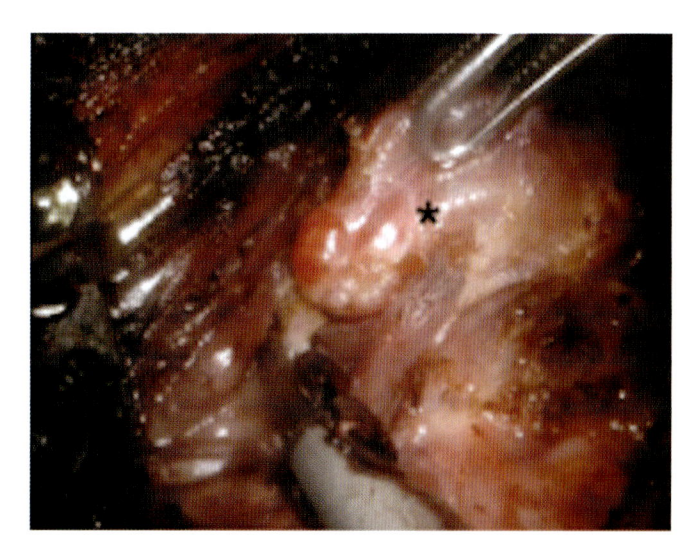

FIGURE 9-10 • Ligation of the superior thyroidal vessels of the left thyroid gland.

Video 9-6. Superior Pole Dissection

> **TIPS**
>
> In the conventional endoscopic thyroid surgery, the superior pole dissection may be particularly difficult mainly in male patients due to the acute angle of the thyroid cartilage. The robot-assisted transoral technique achieves a wider and better exposure of the upper pole of the thyroid even in particularly high locations.

> **ANATOMICAL HIGHLIGHTS**
>
> **External Branch of Superior Laryngeal Nerve (EBSLN):** The EBSLN involved in high pitch sound is one of the most important structures to pay attention to during the dissection of the upper pole of the thyroid (**Figure 9-11**). EBSLN seems at relatively lower risk of injury in TORT compared with open thyroidectomy. This is because the nerves can be seen better under the magnified 3D vision of the robot and lifting up of the superior pole is easier in the transoral approach.

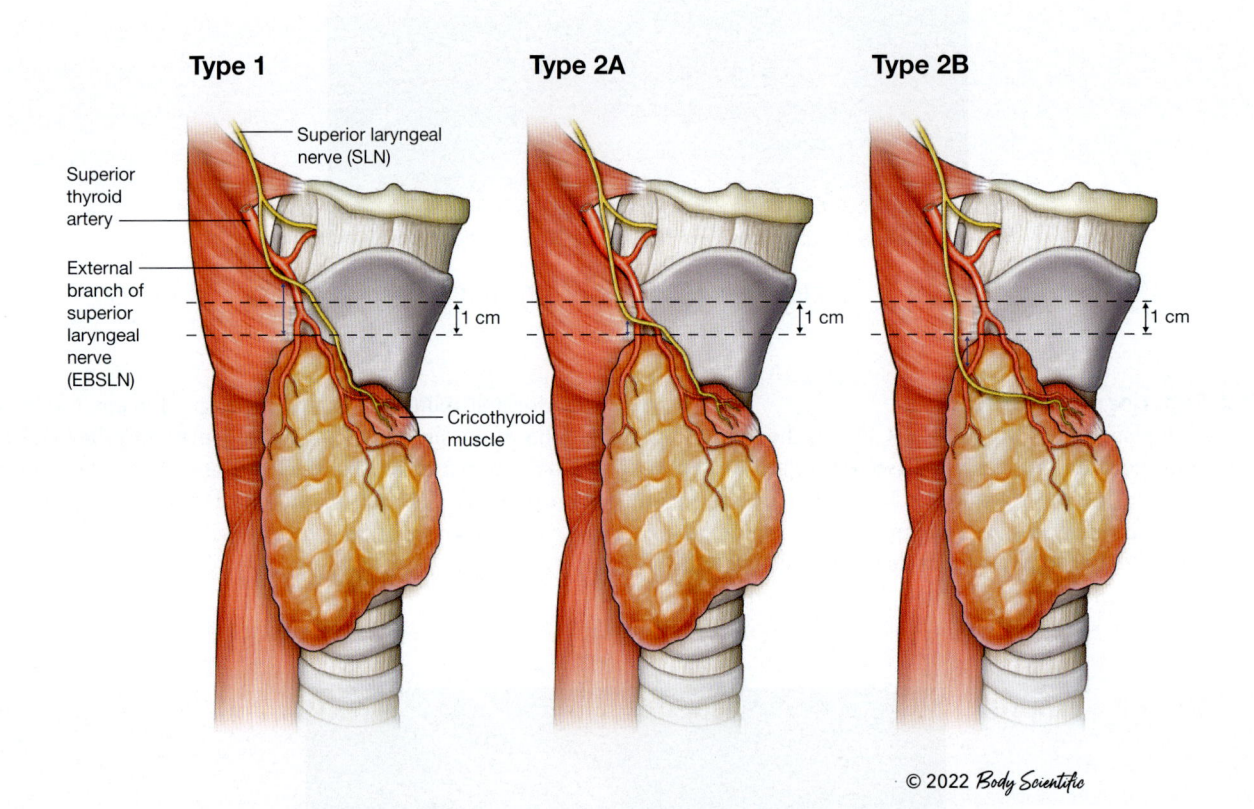

FIGURE 9-11 • EBSLN Cernea Classification: Type 1, Type 2A, and Type 2B.

Step 3. Preservation of the recurrent laryngeal nerve and the parathyroid glands

The superior parathyroid gland is identified first and then dissected downward carefully (**Figure 9-12**). The thyroid gland is retracted medially and sometimes inferiorly, and the ligament of Berry is dissected using a needle driver to identify the RLN at its entry point to the cricothyroid articulation (**Figure 9-13**). The monopolar hook cautery is connected to the NIM™ 3.0 Response System (Medtronic, Minneapolis, MN) to be used as the nerve stimulator for intraoperative nerve monitoring to confirm the location and integrity of the RLN. The dissection is then performed inferiorly to identify and preserve the inferior parathyroid gland. (For standard anatomy of the parathyroid glands, see Chapter 8, Gasless Transaxillary Thyroidectomy [Off-Label Indication].)

Step 3 average time frame: 10–15 min

> **EDITORIAL COMMENT**
>
> The parathyroid glands recognition could be facilitated by the utilization of ICG fluorescence (for more details, see Chapter 7, Fluorescence Imaging: Basics and Clinical Applications).

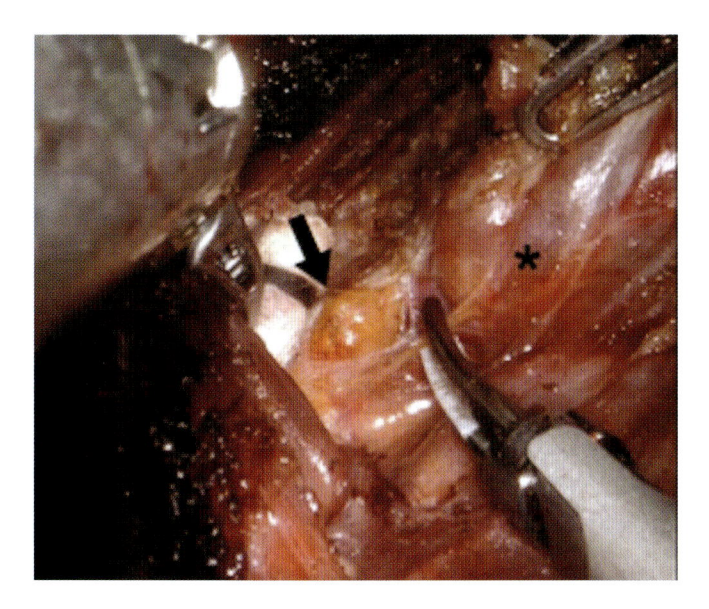

FIGURE 9-12 • Identification and preservation of the left superior parathyroid gland (black arrow). Asterisk represents the thyroid gland.

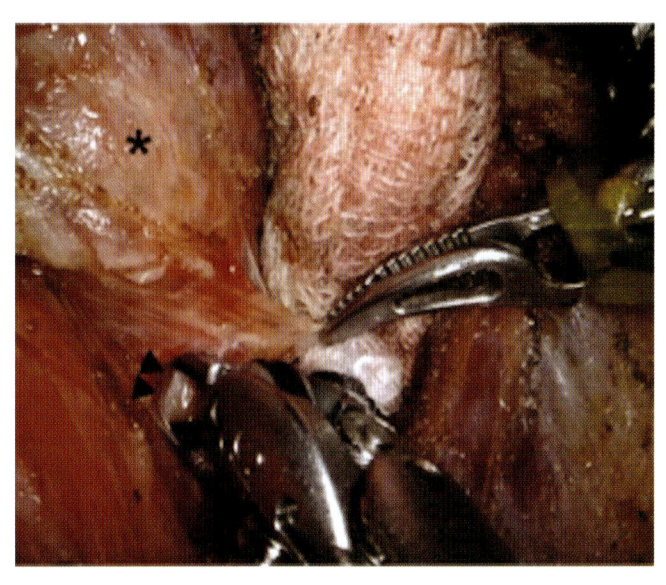

FIGURE 9-13 • Identification of the right recurrent laryngeal nerve (arrowhead). Asterisk represents the thyroid gland.

Video 9-7. Preservation of the RLN and the Parathyroid Glands

ANATOMICAL HIGHLIGHTS

Recurrent Laryngeal Nerve (RLN): Preservation of the recurrent laryngeal nerve during thyroidectomy is a fundamental issue. (For standard course of the RLN, see Chapter 8.)

PITFALLS

Damage of the RLN: There are several possible causes of RLN injury, including stretching, "thermal lateral spread", clamping, ligature, transection, and a constrictive band of connective tissue. As with the EBSLN, the use of intraoperative neuromonitoring (IONM) might help in decreasing the risk of damage to the RLN.

▶▶ TIPS

For RLN preservation in TORT:

- The upper parathyroid gland has to be identified first laterally, then the RLN with dissection of Berry's ligament medially should be recognized.
- The nerve encountered first can be the sensory branch of RLN. It is advisable to test it with IONM to define the motor function of the nerve. If the electromyogram signal cannot be obtained from it, the motor branch of RLN should be searched more medially.
- The medial attachment of RLN should be dissected off and the nerve gently retracted away from the thyroid capsule using a cotton swab.

Step 4. Completion of the right lobectomy, central neck dissection, and specimen removal

The right lobectomy is completed in a cephalad-to-caudal direction while tracing the RLN. A prophylactic ipsilateral central compartment node dissection is performed while preserving the lower parathyroid gland, and the lympho-adipose tissue is retrieved *en bloc* with the resected thyroid lobe. The specimen is removed in an endoscopic plastic bag through the axillary incision. The integrity of the RLN is tested again.

Step 4 average time frame: 15–20 min

▶ **Video 9-8.** Completion of the Lobectomy, CND, and Specimen Removal

▶ **Video 9-9.** Oral Mucosa Incision Closure

Step 5. Left lobectomy
The left lobectomy of the thyroid gland is performed in a similar way without any additional incision following the same steps of the right lobe.

Step 5 average time frame: 40–50 min

Step 6. Closure of the midline incision
After meticulous hemostasis, the wound is irrigated and the fibrin glue is applied. Subsequently, a Jackson-Pratt drain is inserted through the axillary port and the middle raphe of the strap muscles is re-approximated with a V-Loc™ 3-0 absorbable suture. An antiadhesive agent is applied to the subplatysmal space. The robotic cart is undocked and the intraoral vestibule incisions are closed in a single layer with absorbable sutures. A compression dressing is applied across the neck and chin after the patient is extubated.

Step 6 average time frame: 5–10 min

ACKNOWLEDGEMENT
The editors thank Dr. Carolina Baz for reviewing the manuscript, adding anatomical drawings, and providing the editorial notes.

Suggested Readings

1. Chang EHE, et al. Overview of robotic thyroidectomy. *Gland Surg.* 2017;6(3):218-228.
2. Tae K, et al. Robotic and endoscpic thyroid surgery: evolution and advances. *Clin Exp Otorhinolaryngol.* 2019;12(1):1-11.
3. Kim HK, et al. Transoral robotic thyroidectomy for papillary thyroid carcinoma: perioperative outcomes of 100 consecutive patients. *World J Surg.* 2019;43(4):1038-1046.
4. Dionigi G, et al. Transoral thyroidectomy: why is it needed? *Gland Surg.* 2017;6(3):272-276.
5. Dionigi G, et al. Transoral endoscopic thyroidectomy via a vestibular approach: why and how? *Endocrine* 2018;59(2):275-279.
6. Russell JO. Transoral thyroid and parathyroid surgery vestibular approach: a framework for assessment and safe exploration. *Thyroid* 2018;28(7):825-829.
7. Anuwong A. Transoral endoscopic thyroidectomy vestibular approach (TOETVA): indications, techniques and results. *Surg Endosc.* 2018;32(1):456-465.
8. Lee HY, et al. The safety of transoral periosteal thyroidectomy: results of swine models. *J Laparoendosc Adv Surg Tech A.* 2014;24(5):312-317.
9. Lee HY, et al. Robotic transoral periosteal thyroidectomy (TOPOT): experiences of two cadavers. *J Laparoendosc Adv Surg Tech A.* 2015;25(2):139-142.
10. Lee HY, et al. Transoral periosteal thyroidectomy: cadaver to human. *Surg Endosc.* 2015;29(4):898-904.
11. Chae YJ, et al. Comparative analysis of 2 robotic thyroidectomy procedures: transoral versus bilateral axillo-breast approach. *Head Neck.* 2018;40(5):886-892.
12. Kim HY, et al. Trnasoral robotic thyroidectomy: lessons learned from an initial consecutive series of 24 patients. *Surg Endosc.* 2018;32(2):688-694.
13. Anuwong A, et al. Safety and outcomes of the transoral ensocopic thyroidectomy vestibular approach. *JAMA Surg.* 2018;153(1):21-27.
14. Lee HY, et al. The efficacy of intraoperative neuromonitoring during robotic thyroidectomy: a prospectice, randomized case-control evaluation. *J Laparoendosc Adv Surg Tech A.* 2015;25(11):908-914.
15. Witzel K, et al. Transoral access for endoscopic thyroi resection. *Surg Endosc.* 2008. 22(8):1871-1875.
16. Benhidejeb T, et al. Natural orifice surgery on thyroid gland: totally transoral video-assisted thyroidectomy (TOVAT): report of first experimental results of a new surgical method. *Surg Endosc.* 2009;23(5):1119-1120.
17. Benhidejeb T, et al. Natural orifice surgery on thyroid gland: totally transoral video-assisted thyroidectomy (TOVAT): report of first experimental results of a new surgical method. *Surg Endosc.* 2009;23(5):1119-1120.
18. Richmon JD, et al. Transoral robotic-assisted thyroidectomy: a preclinical feasibility study in 2 cadavers. *Head Neck.* 2011;33(3):330-333.
19. Richmon JD, et al. Transoral robotic thyroidectomy (TORT): procedures and outcomes. *Gland Surg.* 2017;6(3):285-289.
20. Anuwong A. Transoral endoscopic thyroidectomy vestibular approach: a series of the first 60 human cases. *World J Surg.* 2016;40(3):491-497.
21. You JY, et al. Transoral robotic thyroidectomy versus conventional open thyroidectomy: comparative analysis of surgical outcomes in thyroid malignancies. *J Laparoendosc Adv Surge Tech A.* 2019;29(6):796-800.
22. Richmon JD, et al. Transoral robotic-assisted thyroidectomy with central neck dissection: preclinical cadaver feasibility study and proposed surgical technique. *J Robot Surg.* 2011;5(4):279-282.
23. Kim HY, et al. The pros and cons of additional axillary arm for transoral robotic thyroidectomy. *World J Otorhinolaryngol Head Neck Surg.* 2020;6(3):161-164.
24. Kim HK, et al. Transoral robotic thyroidectomy: comparison of surgical outcomes between the da Vinci Xi and Si. *Surg Laparosc Endosc Percutan Tech.* 2018; 28(6):404-409.
25. Giulianotti PC, Coratti A, Angelini M, et al. Robotics in general surgery: personal experience in a large community hospital. *Arch Surg.* 2003;138(7):777-784. doi: 10.1001/archsurg.138.7.777

SECTION III

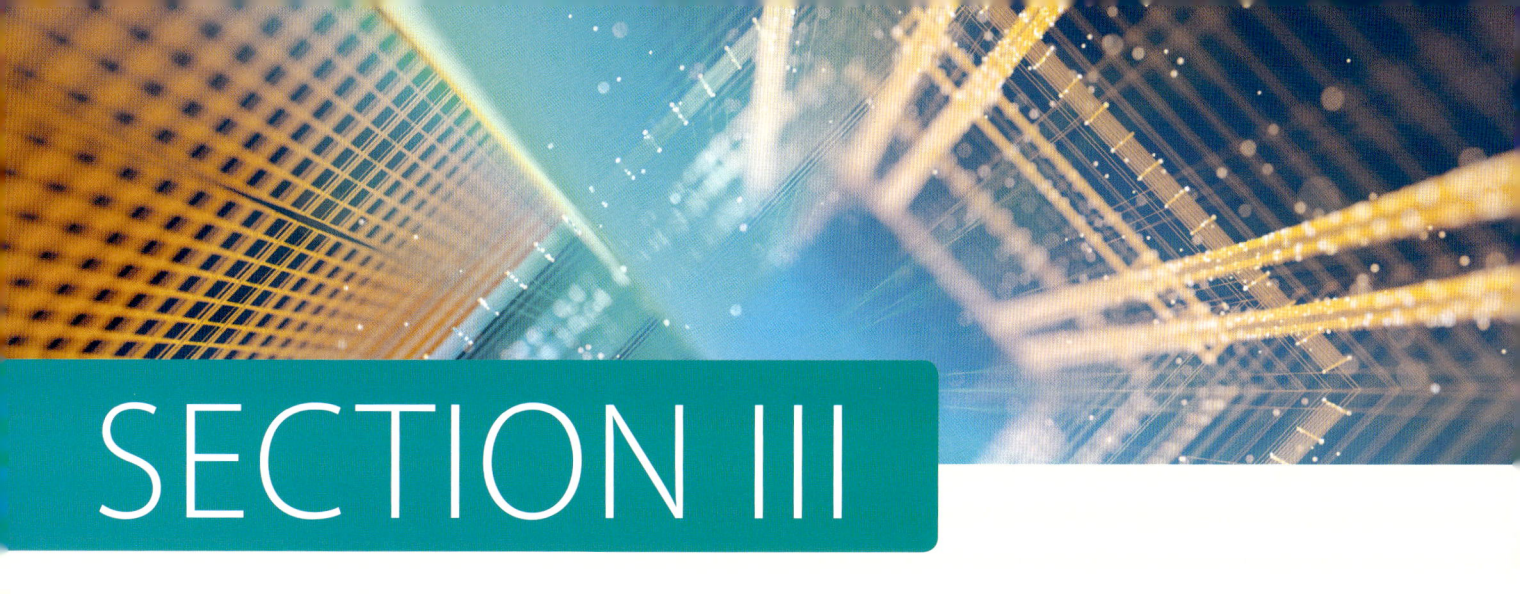

Chest Surgery

Chapter 10 • Nipple-Sparing Mastectomy (Off-Label Indication) 177
Antonio Toesca • Antonia Girardi • Paolo Veronesi

Chapter 11 • Extended Thymectomy for Myasthenia Gravis and Thymoma 197
Hongbin Zhang • Feng Li • Jens-C. Rückert

Chapter 12 • Ivor-Lewis Esophagectomy 209
Andrea Coratti • Francesco Guerra • Giuseppe Giuliani

Chapter 13 • Radical Esophagectomy with Extended Mediastinal Lymphadenectomy 233
Koichi Suda • Ichiro Uyama

Chapter 14 • Paraesophageal Hernia Repair 259
Gabriela Aguiluz • Mario Alberto Masrur • Pier Cristoforo Giulianotti

Chapter 15 • Selective Nissen Fundoplication 277
Gabriela Aguiluz • Alberto Mangano • Pier Cristoforo Giulianotti

Chapter 16 • Heller Myotomy with Modified Dor Fundoplication 299
Nicolas Hellmuth Dreifuss • Gabriela Aguiluz • Pier Cristoforo Giulianotti

Chapter 17 • Lung Lobectomies: General Principles and the Total Port,
Transfissure Approach (Fissure First) 317
Melani Lighter • Gabriela Aguiluz • Fabio Sbrana • Pier Cristoforo Giulianotti

Chapter 18A • Lung Upper Lobectomies 345
Giulia Veronesi • Pierluigi Novellis • Piergiorgio Muriana • Gabriela Aguiluz • Francesca Rossetti

Chapter 18B • Lung Lower Lobectomies 367
Giulia Veronesi • Pierluigi Novellis • Piergiorgio Muriana • Gabriela Aguiluz • Francesca Rossetti

"From a 'maximum tolerable' to a 'minimum effective' treatment."
—Umberto Veronesi (1925–2016)

Nipple-Sparing Mastectomy
(Off-Label Indication)

Antonio Toesca • Antonia Girardi • Paolo Veronesi

INTRODUCTION

The nipple-sparing mastectomy (NSM) is increasingly performed for the treatment and prevention of breast cancer and has acceptable oncologic outcomes in appropriately selected patients. The strong interest in maximizing the natural appearance of the breast has led to the development of the nipple-sparing mastectomy. Owing to superior cosmetic results and oncologic safety, the use of the nipple-sparing mastectomy has increased in recent years, replacing the total mastectomy, which entails the removal of the nipple-areola complex.

Since there are no data from randomized controlled trials comparing nipple-sparing mastectomy with total mastectomy, there were concerns that a procedure sparing the nipple-areola complex could lack oncologic safety. The potential risk of local recurrence in residual glandular tissue may result in an occult involvement of the nipple-areola complex. However, recent evidence has shown that the overall the disease-free survival and the local recurrence do not differ significantly between these 2 procedures. The evolutionary concept is to preserve the healthy tissues and to reduce scars while maintaining oncologic validity.

To achieve desirable aesthetic outcomes in patients with breast cancer, many surgeons have introduced various methods of oncoplastic surgery with breast reconstruction after partial or total mastectomy, but a large visible scar often remains after the operation. Because the breast is an organ that symbolizes femininity, a large visible scar can be worrisome for female cancer survivors. The conventional open surgical approach for nipple-sparing mastectomies is limited by higher rates of nipple necrosis with the periareolar access incision and by compromised exposure of the superior breast pole with access from the inframammary fold.

Robotic nipple-sparing mastectomy was developed in 2014 to allow for enhanced visualization and more precise dissection of tissue planes difficult to reach with the open technique. Moreover, considering distributional patterns, directions, and arrangements of the arteries participating in the blood supply of the nipple-areola complex, the access for the robotic approach was intentionally planned to lessen the vascular compromise

INSTRUMENT REQUIREMENTS

The suggested main robotic instruments/tools can be listed as follows:
- 0° or 30° scope
- Monopolar Cautery: Monopolar curved scissors or permanent cautery spatula/vessel sealer
- Grasper: ProGrasp forceps or Cadiere forceps
- Bipolar Cautery: Fenestrated bipolar forceps or Maryland bipolar forceps

The suggested main laparoscopic instruments/tools can be listed as follows:
- Needle drivers
- Grasper
- Suction-irrigation

Supplemental materials:
- Monoport device: Access Transformer OCTO™
- Gauzes, sponges
- Drain
- Blunt tunneler/Metzenbaum scissors
- Endobag™
- Sutures: Vicryl™ 2-0; Monocryl™ 3-0 and 4-0

Photo from Mondadori Portfolio / Contributor, Getty Images.
Quote reproduced with permission from Veronesi U, Stafyla V, Luini A, et al. Breast cancer: from "maximum tolerable" to "minimum effective" treatment. Front Oncol. 2012;2:125.

> **🔍 ANATOMICAL HIGHLIGHTS**
>
> The lateral and medial vascular pedicles regularly provide dominant arteries reaching the lateral hemi-circumference of the nipple-areola complex through superficial branches deriving from the lateral thoracic artery and the internal mammary artery (**Figure 10-1**).

to the nipple skin, while using a cosmetically more favorable location of the breast.

The feasibility and safety of the robotic technique have been outlined in several prospective studies that consistently report a low complication rate, and no local failure at short-term follow-up. Robotic mastectomy has been reported to be safe and feasible and has acceptable short-term oncologic outcomes. Although this technique seems secure in terms of technical and surgical outcomes, robotic mastectomy still remains experimental. In fact, there is a need to evaluate long-term oncologic and patient-reported outcomes in future prospective comparative and randomized studies.

During the 15th St Gallen International Breast Cancer Conference, the robotic mastectomy was recognized as an option in selected patients. However, the use of robotic breast surgery is not currently approved by the US Food and Drug Administration (FDA), which issued a statement in February 2019 warning that safety and effectiveness of robotic devices for mastectomy had not been established.

The world scientific community has felt the need to publish several opinion manuscripts reiterating that robotic-assisted mastectomy should be considered only in the context of a well-designed, randomized trial evaluating patient selection, patient safety, surgical complications, and oncologic outcomes with a concomitant cost analysis. Any paradigm shift in the standard of care deserves an ethical evaluation of non-inferiority. Following these opinion papers, a systematic review was conducted: this includes 8 articles, reporting on 249 robot-assisted nipple-sparing mastectomies in 187 women. This analysis showed that robot-assisted nipple-sparing mastectomy is feasible with acceptable short-term outcomes, but it still remains in the assessment phase, considering that locoregional recurrences were not observed, and longer follow-up is necessary to clarify long-term oncologic results.

An international multicenter pooled analysis using prospective and retrospective studies is ongoing and the aim is to evaluate surgical and oncologic outcomes after robotic nipple-sparing mastectomy and immediate reconstruction. In this protocol, raw data for robotic versus conventional

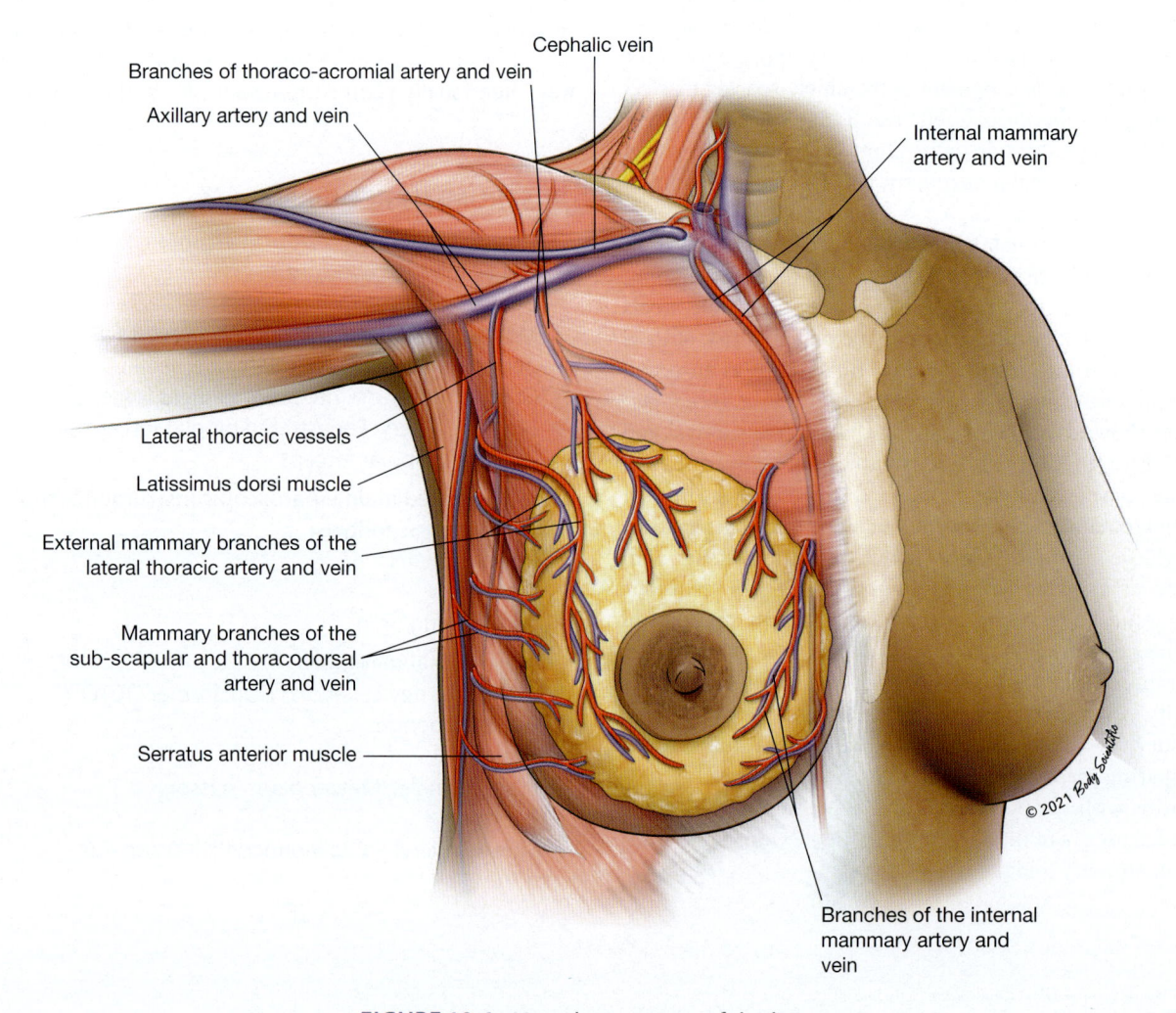

FIGURE 10-1 • Vascular anatomy of the breast.

nipple-sparing mastectomy from Severance Hospital and Samsung Medical Center in Seoul, the European Institute of Oncology in Milan, Changhua Christian Hospital in Taiwan, and Gustave Roussy in Paris were collected to assess clinicopathologic variables including operation times, hospital stay, medical history, smoking history, family history, body mass index (BMI), menopausal status, specimen weight, TNM stage, grade, histologic type, estrogen receptor, progesterone receptor, HER2, Ki-67, and perivascular involvement. The objective was to evaluate postoperative complications within 30 days, locoregional recurrence-free survival, and local and systemic recurrences. The estimated sample size for this study originating from the 4 institutions is about 300 cases for robotic nipple-sparing mastectomy and matched cases for conventional nipple-sparing mastectomy. Results of this study are under analysis.

At the end of 2019, the first early oncologic follow-up data on consecutive patients undergoing robotic mastectomy from June 2014 to January 2019 were published. In 56 cancer patients, there was no local relapse after 19 months of median follow-up.

In June 2020, a consensus statement was published to self-regulate robotic mastectomy clinical trials and clinical practice. The results of the Consensus Statement on Robotic Mastectomy-Expert Panel from the International Endoscopic and Robotic Breast Surgery Symposium (IERBS) 2019 were that robotic mastectomy is a promising, safe/feasible technique and could well be the future of minimally invasive breast surgery. This first consensus statement on robotic mastectomy from an international panel of experts is an extremely important milestone, and provides recommendations for breast surgeons keen to embark on this technique (inside of a clinical trial evaluating also oncologic outcome).

In this scenario, as the use of robotic nipple-sparing mastectomy continues to rise, improved understanding of the surgical, oncologic, and quality of life outcomes is imperative for appropriate patient selection and counseling, as well as for regulatory authorities to better understand indications, limits, advantages, and risks.

At the beginning of 2017, a phase 3, open-label, single-center, randomized controlled trial, comparing conventional open nipple-sparing mastectomy with robotic nipple-sparing mastectomy started at the European Institute of Oncology in Milan. The aim of the study was to determine how surgical technique affected rates and types of complications, health-related quality of life, and patient satisfaction outcomes at 1 year. A secondary objective was to evaluate the long-term oncologic outcomes. Version 2 of BREAST-Q, a validated patient-reported outcome measure consisting of a health-related quality of life and a satisfaction domain, was completed preoperatively and also at 1 month, 6 months, and 1 year postoperatively. The preoperative and postoperative scales were linked psychometrically to measure change over time and between the 2 groups.

The Hopwood body image scale (BIS), a 10-item monofactorial questionnaire designed to capture and compare distress and symptoms related to body image in cancer patients, was administered 12 months postoperatively. Patient satisfaction with the nipple-areola complex and subjective nipple sensitivity were evaluated, at 12 months postoperatively, using a specific questionnaire. Preliminary results were presented in the general session at the 20th Annual Meeting of the American Society of Breast Surgeons in Dallas in 2019. On average, robotic procedures were 1 hour and 18 minutes longer than open surgery. No differences in terms of absolute number and severity of complications between robotic and open technique were observed. Women undergoing robotic surgery developed multiple complications less frequently, and were less likely to suffer postmastectomy axillary web syndrome. The robotic procedure decreased the body image disturbance related to mastectomy (Hopwood BIS). Women undergoing robotics had values of satisfaction with the breast, physical well-being, psychological well-being, and sexual well-being unchanged compared with the preoperative period, whereas those who underwent open surgery experienced a worsening of their condition (Breast-Q).

Indications and Relative Contraindications to the Robotic Approach

Robotic breast surgery is not currently approved by the FDA, so subjects should be enrolled in a registered clinical trial. With this premise, women with invasive breast cancer, with ductal carcinoma in situ (DCIS), with genetic predisposition to breast cancer (i.e., pathogenic BRCA1 or BRCA2 mutation), aged 18 years or older, or who are candidates for nipple-sparing mastectomy followed by immediate breast reconstruction are potentially eligible to participate in hypothetical clinical trials. Multifocal and multicentric cancers can be allowed; however, tumors have to be located at a distance from the nipple-areola complex greater than 1 cm as assessed by clinical examination and breast imaging (similarly to open classical nipple-sparing mastectomy). Patients with inflammatory breast cancer; evidence of tumor involvement in skin or the nipple-areolar complex; Paget's disease; mesenchymal, inflammatory, or recurrent breast cancer; or history of previous thoracic radiation therapy should not be eligible. Additionally, patients should not be included if they are pregnant, have a high American Society of Anesthesiologists (ANA) score (>2), have uncontrolled diabetes

> **EDITORIAL COMMENT**
>
> The vessel sealer should be considered, when dealing with bigger arteries, while posteriorly detaching the mammary gland from the pectoral fascia. The use of this instrument can decrease the risk of bleeding, hematomas, and seromas.

> **▶▶ TIPS**
>
> The best instrument for dissection is monopolar curved scissors. This instrument is very versatile: it can work as a sharp instrument (without energy) to avoid burns of the breast skin (mastectomy flap), or it can be used as a cautery for small superficial veins and arterioles inside the subcutaneous suspensory breast ligaments.

mellitus, are prior or current heavy smokers (>20 cigarettes/day), or have large breast volume (greater than cup D breast).

Patient Positioning and Operating Room Setup

Before surgery, while the patient is awake and standing, landmarks are marked according to the general and plastic surgeon's preference and to the specific patient's procedure plan. Usually, the borders of the breast, the projection of the anterior edge of the naturally hanging ipsilateral arm on the lateral thorax, the anterior axillary line, and the midaxillary line are marked, in order to serve as reference points during mastectomy and reconstruction. The patient is placed in supine position, under general anesthesia, and intubated with an endotracheal tube. For the right mastectomy, the edge of the right chest is positioned at the edge of the table allowing the patient's arm to drop alongside the operating table rail (same for the left side). This will provide maximum exposure of the chest/axilla and allows better movements of the robotic arms (**Figure 10-2**).

A gel pad or towel roll may be placed under the right (or left) shoulder to elevate the breast. The patient's arm is off the table, and it is secured in a towel sling.

> ▶▶ **TIPS**
>
> For bilateral mastectomy, the positioning of the patient's arms in towel slings is completed for both sides before the start of the procedure. This can speed up the transition between sides, saving time, and better preserving the sterility of the operating field.

> ⚠ **PITFALLS**
>
> Attention should be paid not to stretch the brachial plexus while changing the position of the patient on the table edges.

Alternatively, the patient can be placed in a flat supine position, with the ipsilateral arm above the head, with internal rotation and 90° abduction. The forearm should be supported with a table arm board approximately 15 cm above the patient's face. The adaptor should be mounted to the bed, opposite to the operative side, such as in open thoracic surgery. This setting requires a change in position during bilateral mastectomy, when passing from one side to the other.

For bilateral nipple-sparing mastectomy, the operating room is configured so that the patient cart will approach the patient table with an oblique angle coming over the patient's shoulder, centered approximately at the patient's thorax, to allow for the operating platform of the patient cart to be rotated to reach either breast, while not interfering with the anesthesia workstation or access by the patient-side assistant (**Figures 10-3 A, B**).

The assistant surgeon is on the patient's side, opposite to the patient cart. A scrub nurse is at the patient's feet, opposite to the patient cart. At least 1 video monitor showing the endoscopic view is located in front of the assistant.

For unilateral nipple-sparing mastectomy, the operating room can be alternatively configured so that the patient cart will approach the patient table perpendicularly, centered approximately at the patient's thorax.

> **EDITORIAL COMMENT**
>
> A precise angle of cart docking is necessary only for the da Vinci Si and X systems because of the mechanical structure of the arms, which are mounted on a column. The da Vinci Xi system, with its capacity for boom rotation, allows the robotic cart to be set in any position, based on the available space and on the needs of the team.

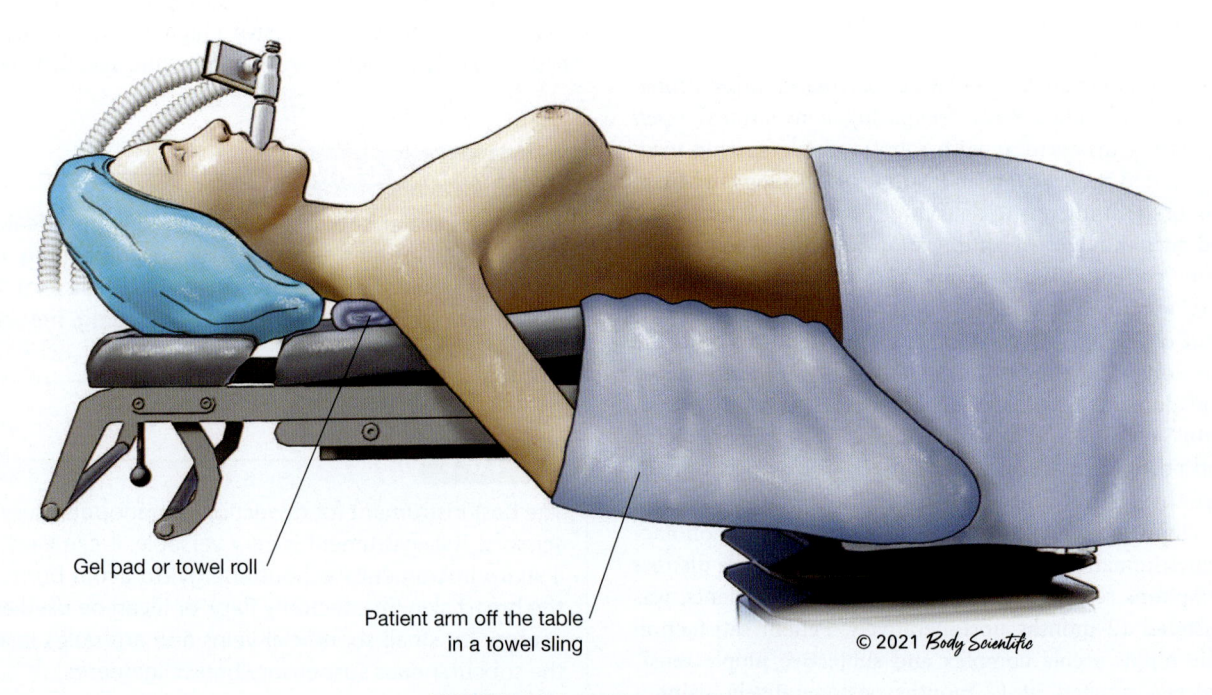

FIGURE 10-2 • Patient positioning.

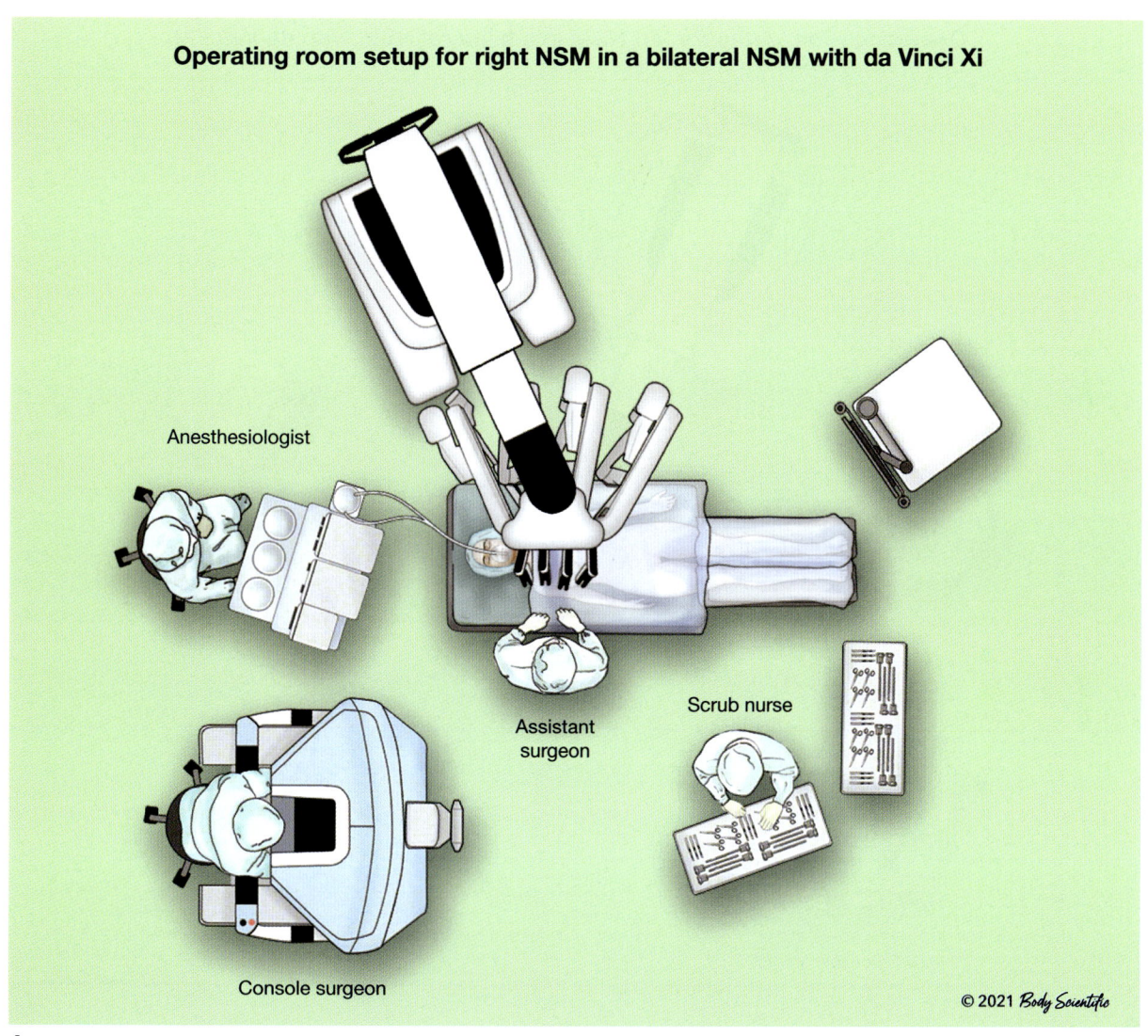

FIGURE 10-3 • **A.** Operating room setup for right side bilateral nipple-sparing mastectomy (NSM).

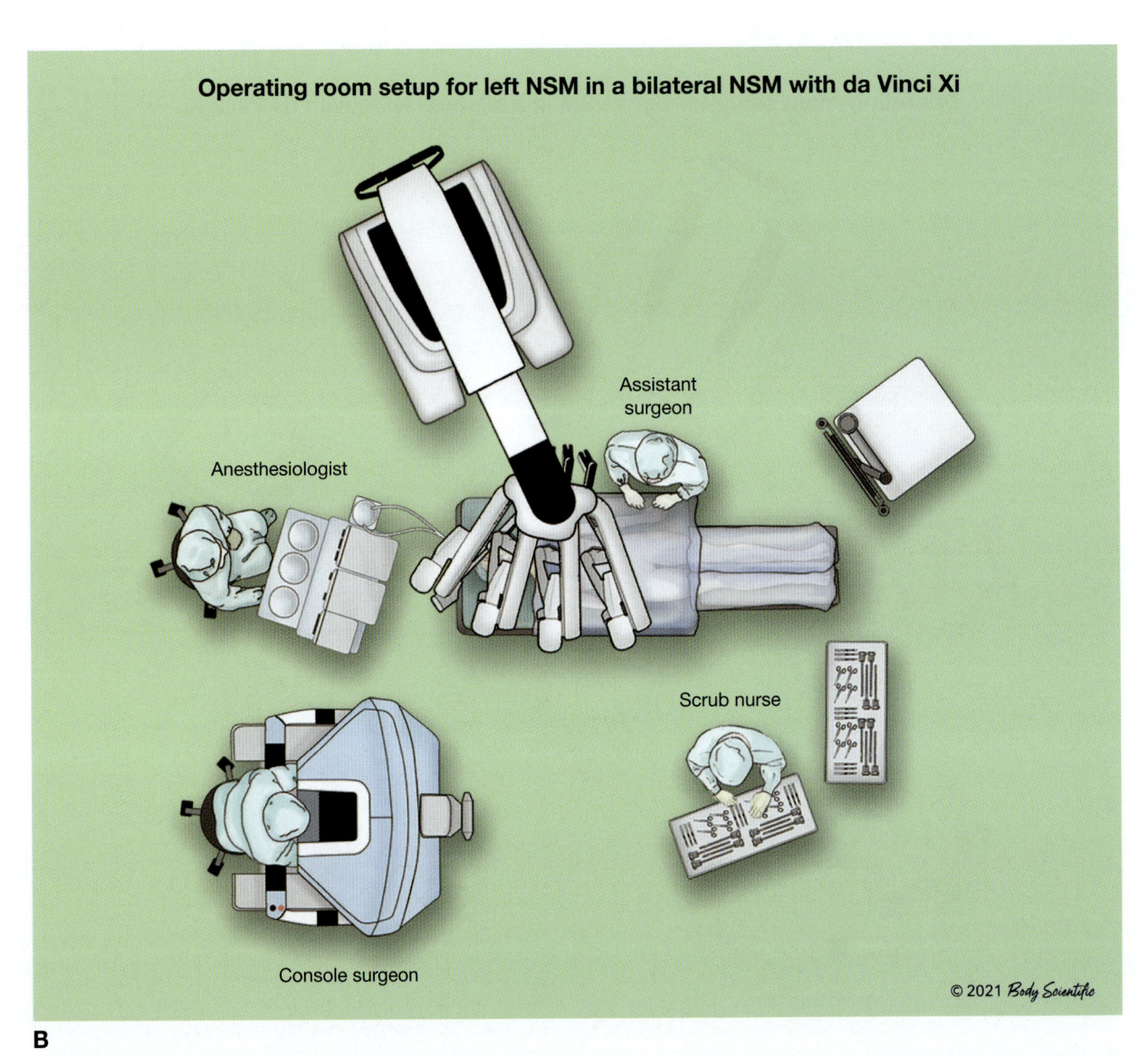

FIGURE 10-3 • (*Continued*) **B.** Operating room setup for right side bilateral nipple-sparing mastectomy (NSM).

Surgical Technique

▶ Video 10-1. Robotic Nipple-Sparing Mastectomy – Entire Procedure

Step 1. Open axillary access

The surgical area is sterilely prepared and draped. According to the surgeon's preference, the borders of the breast may be marked trans- or subcutaneously with medical blue dye, or similar, as some surgeons also do in open procedures, in order to facilitate identification of the borders when viewed endoscopically.

An approximately 3-cm incision line along the anterior axillary line, at the nipple-areola complex level, should be marked (the incision level is dependent on the patient's habitus and might be toward the midaxillary line in some patients) (**Figure 10-4**).

The incision can be occasionally extended up to 5 cm in cases of larger breast (cup D). The incision length is dependent on breast volume, or cup size, and dictates which specific OCTO™ Port Access size to use. A 3-cm port is the standard device. A 5-cm port is also available with the same characteristics. In any case, a dotted line must be drawn to mark circularly around the center of the port incision with a radius of approximately 5 cm. This dotted line marking indicates the extent of subcutaneous dissection needed to place the wound protector for the surgical access port.

During the first phase of the procedure, through the 3-cm incision, the subcutaneous flap is dissected with classic electrocautery scalpel, under direct vision in a 5-cm area, to obtain a subcutaneous working space for the introduction of the single port in order to overcome the blind spots, and to start the robotic phase of the mastectomy (**Figure 10-5**).

Sentinel node biopsy/axillary dissection can be performed according to the clinical indication. In case of axillary surgery, the procedure can be performed using an open technique and utilizing the same 3–5 cm incision (**Figure 10-6**).

Step 1 average time frame: 15–20 min

> ▶▶ **TIPS**
>
> At least 1 assistant may be needed to help with retraction of the skin flap during the subcutaneous dissection.

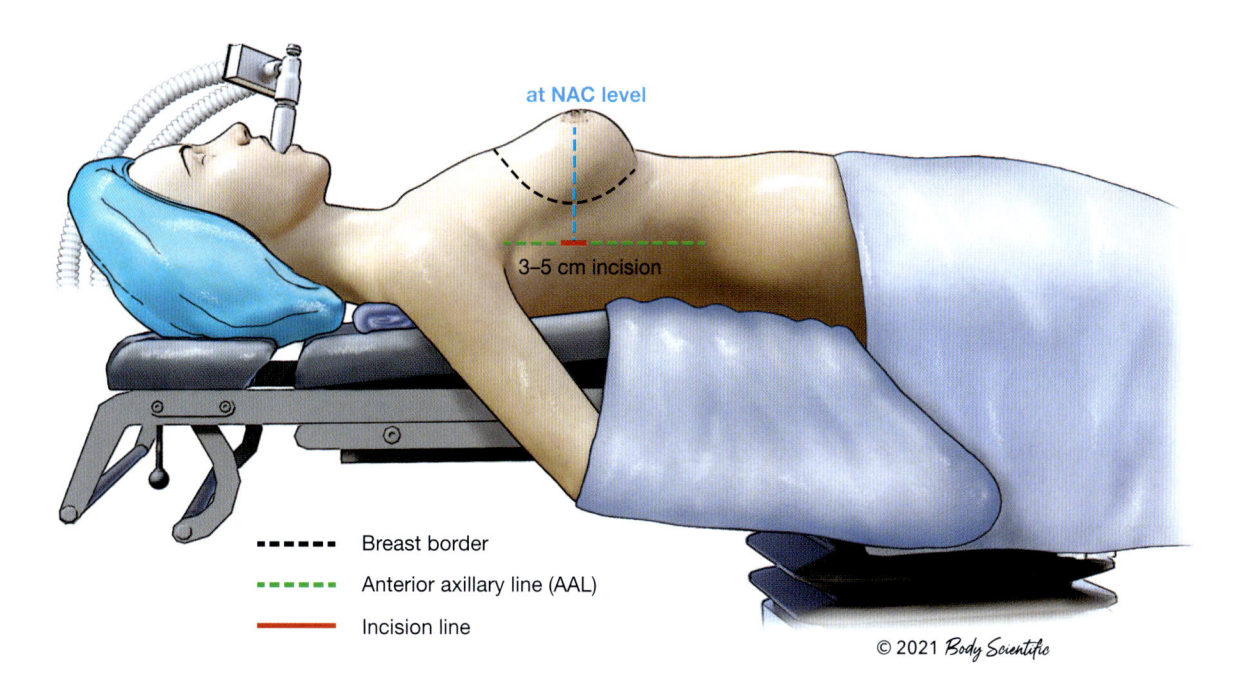

FIGURE 10-4 • Incision placement.

184 The Foundation and Art of Robotic Surgery

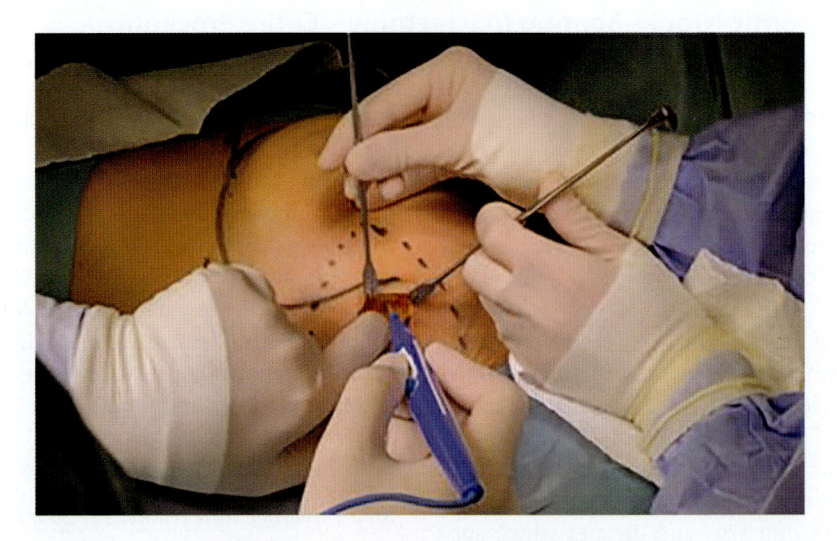

FIGURE 10-5 • Subcutaneous flap dissection.

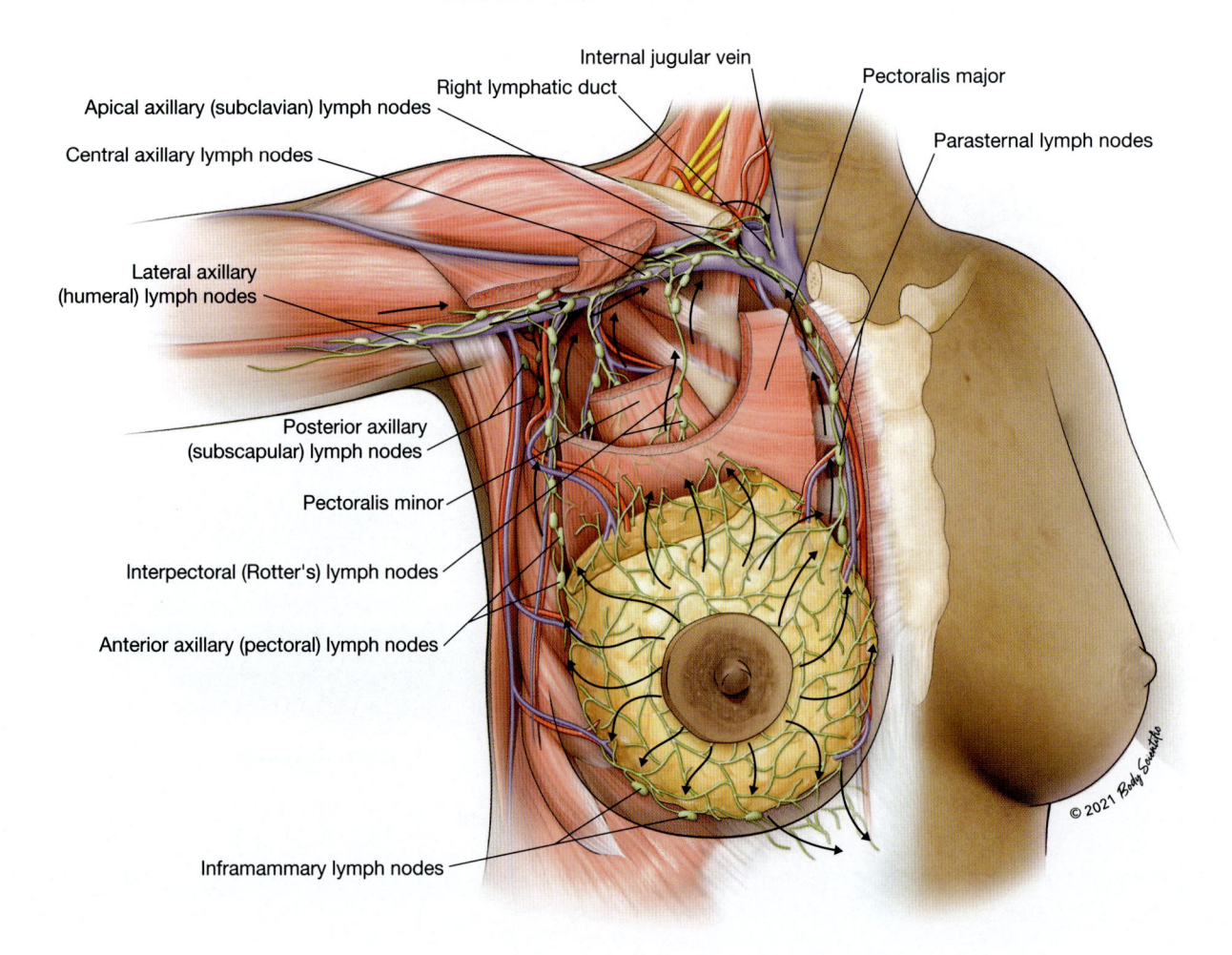

FIGURE 10-6 • Lymphatic drainage of the mammary gland.

Step 2. Tumescent injection and tunneling technique

After performing the skin flap dissection circularly around the incision using standard electrocautery and after preparation of the subcutaneous 10-cm diameter, tumescent injection per surgeon's preference may be performed subcutaneously to initiate a bloodless anterior mammary gland tunnel dissection plane (**Figure 10**-7).

After the tumescent injection, the anterior dissection of the mammary gland, with blunt technique using long Metzenbaum scissors or blunt tunnelers, is performed to create a subcutaneous tunnel network (tunneling technique) (**Figure 10**-8). This step allows the gas to diffuse into the subcutaneous plane and to create a virtual cavity that can be used for the endoscopic phase.

Step 2 average time frame: 5–10 min

> ▶▶ **TIPS**
>
> A finger should be used to confirm that the area of skin flap dissection matches the dotted circular marking, which will allow the insertion of the wound protector of the surgical access port.

> ⚠ **PITFALLS**
>
> When creating subcutaneous tunnels, blunt instruments should be used, like Metzenbaum scissors, with closed jaws or smooth tunnelers. This blunt technique prevents the instruments from entering the deeper mammary gland and creating a false dissection plane. An incorrect technique may cause bleeding or may leave fragments of mammary tissue attached to the skin, thus compromising the oncologic radicality.

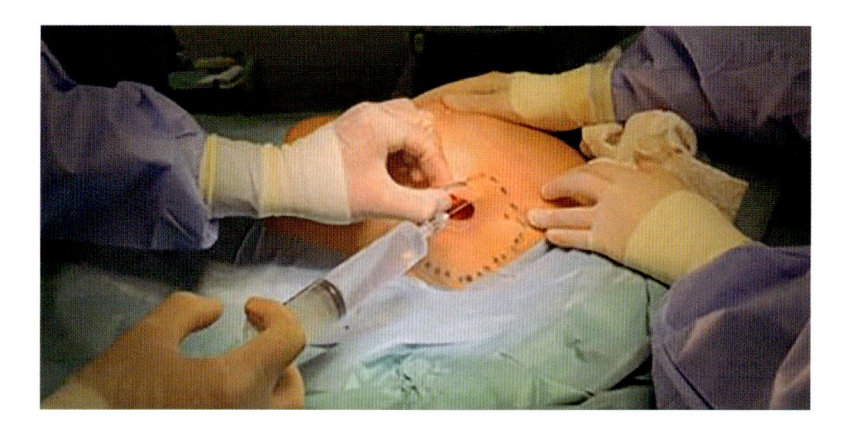

FIGURE 10-7 • Tumescent injection.

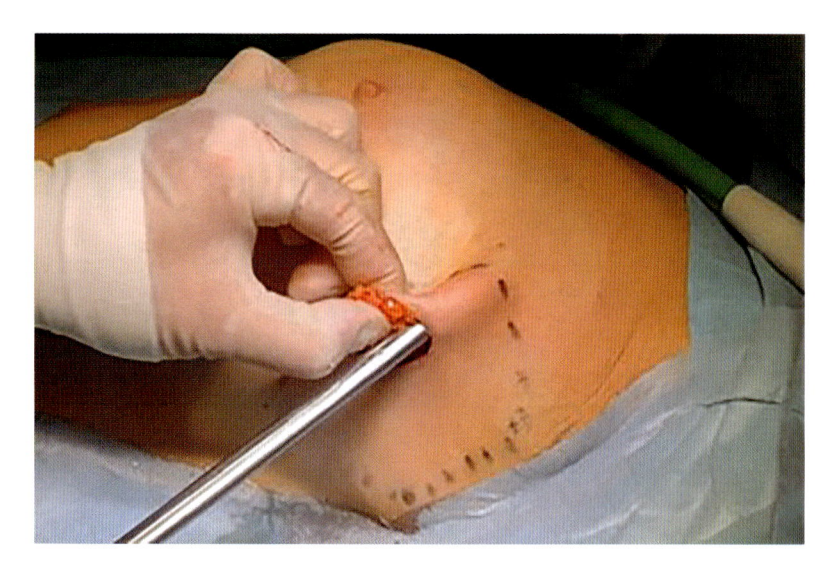

FIGURE 10-8 • Tunneling technique.

Step 3. Monoport placement

Since no specific robotic port for mastectomy has been developed yet, it can use a sterile, single-patient access system device, designed for laparoscopic surgery (Access Transformer OCTO™; Seoul, Korea), consisting of 4 plastic 5–12 mm accesses for the camera and instruments, gas valve, and silicon gas pipe (**Figure 10-9**).

First, the wound protector of the surgical access port must be inserted through the incision and, according to the manufacturer's instructions, then the surgical access port to obtain 4 insertion tubes of the surgical access port is assembled.

CO_2 must be insufflated with a pressure of 8 mm Hg to create the surgical workspace in the breast.

> ⚠ **PITFALLS**
>
> Higher CO_2 pressure could create subcutaneous emphysema. This resolves spontaneously some hours later but can be unpleasant.

A three 8-mm da Vinci Xi cannula should be inserted through the access tubes of the surgical port. If necessary, this should be rotated for the appropriate orientation. A grounded cannula should be used for the endoscope and for each arm on which the use of monopolar energy is planned.

Step 2 average time frame: 3–5 min

> ▶▶ **TIPS**
>
> In contrast to the classical robotic technique, in nipple-sparing robotic mastectomy, an important distinction is that the tip of the trocar is not located inside the surgical cavity but remains outside. The fulcrum point remains external to the skin. The tips of the 3 trocars are inserted inside the monoport device, which maintains the pneumocavity.

> **EDITORIAL COMMENT**
>
> In reality, this concept is already well known in other kinds of robotic surgery such as transaxillary thyroidectomies and transanal or transoral procedures. It became very common with the single port (SP) platform in order to increase the operative space of the working arms (floating dock).

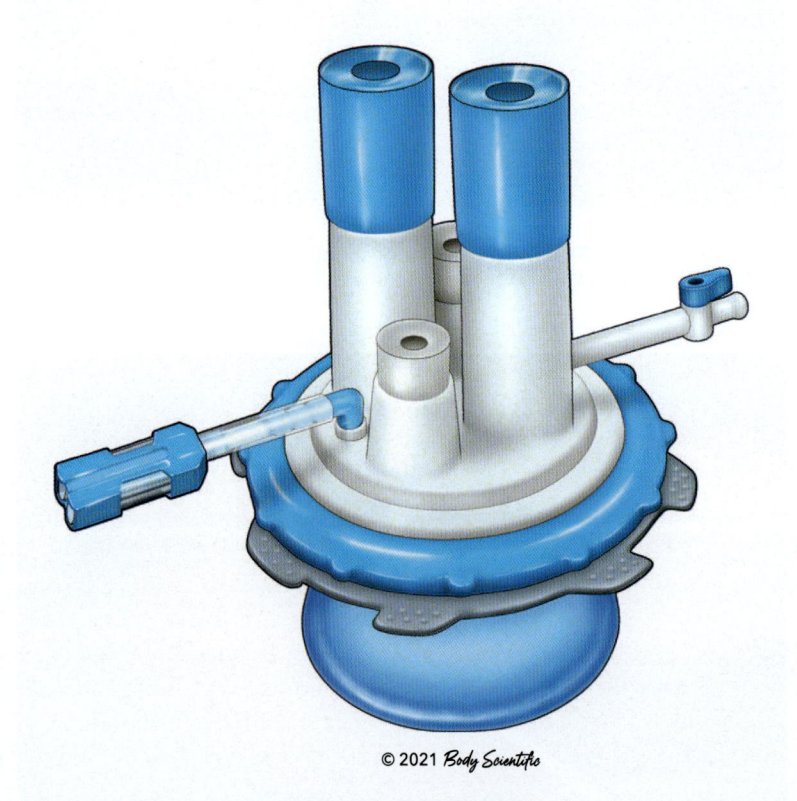

FIGURE 10-9 • Port device.

Step 4. Docking

The robotic cart (X/Si) should approach the patient table coming from the opposite side of the breast involved, centered on the transverse mammillary line, and perpendicular to the patient side (**Figures 10-10 A–C**).

The arm holding the scope should be set first in the middle of the theoretical surgical field, and with the arm stretched to minimize collisions with the operative arms. The central column of the robotic cart and the arm holding the scope should be aligned with the transverse mammillary line.

The R1 and R2 are set parallel to the arm holding the scope with the joints arranged in a way to maximize the ranges of motion of the instruments.

Once the arms are set, the scope should be inserted in the disposable cannula and plugged. The position of the scope should be at the apex of a virtual triangle with the corner sides for the operative cannulas/instruments.

Step 4 average time frame: 7–10 min

Si Model **Xi Model**

A

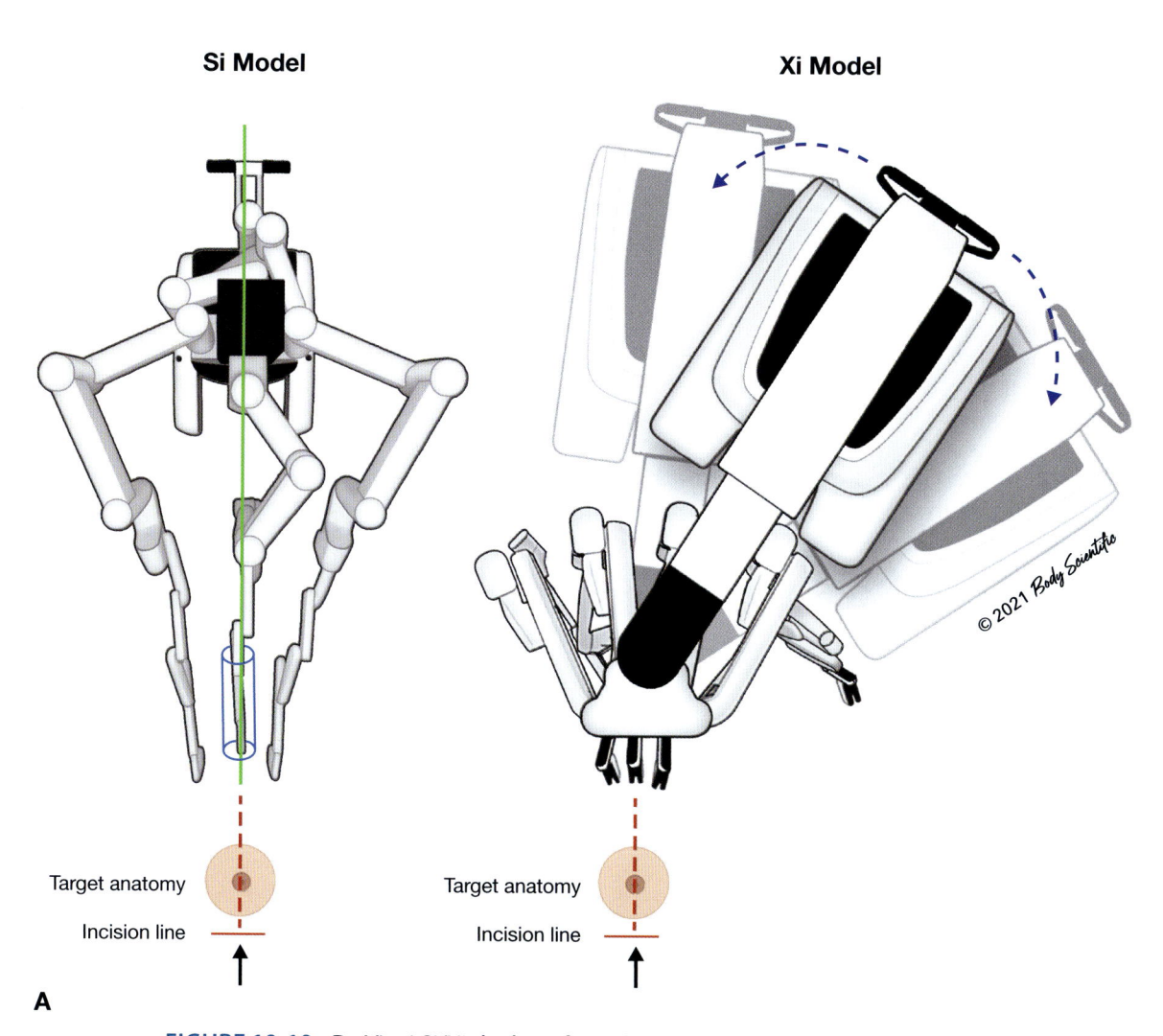

FIGURE 10-10 • Da Vinci Si/Xi docking for right mastectomy from patient left side.

B

C

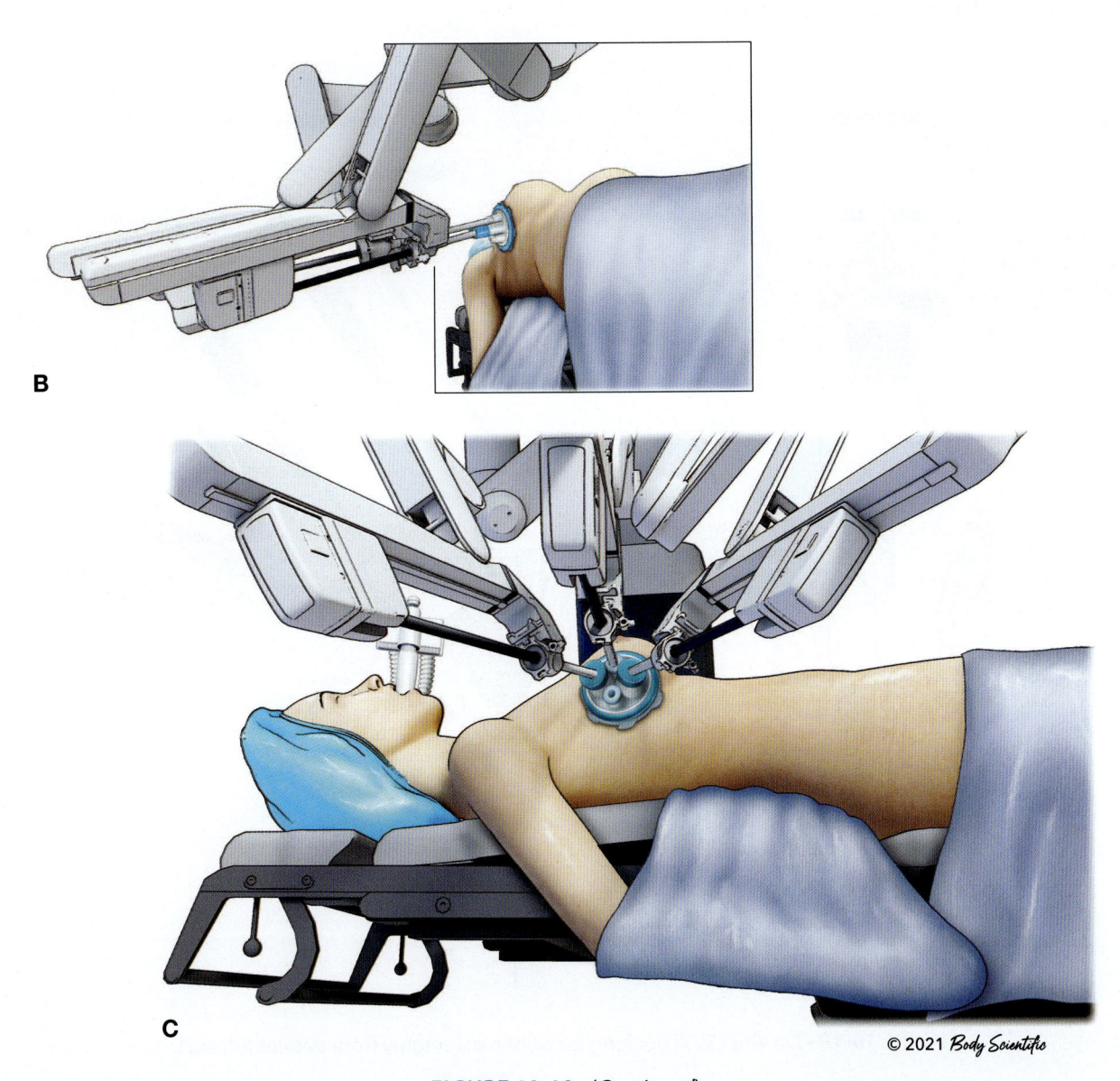

FIGURE 10-10 • (Continued)

Step 5. Robotic dissection

The endoscopic view can be observed through a 0° or 30° rigid camera installed between the 2 operative arms to enable a central view.

> **▶▶ TIPS**
>
> Considering that the surgical cavity volume is limited, a 0° view may be sufficient to see all the cavity walls. The choice of a 30° scope is optional, according to the surgeon's preference or availability. The 30° camera, with the 30° up setting, may allow better control of the anterior plane.

The dissection is performed with monopolar curved scissors, or with a 5-mm monopolar cautery with cautery spatula tip, used on the R1. Traction and countertraction, along with maintaining excellent exposure and stretching out the tissue, are performed with a ProGrasp fitted on the R2.

The assistant surgeon and nurse are at the operating table to orient the surgeon along the different quadrants of the breast. Their important role is to minimize conflicts between robotic arms, to avoid the risk of patient decubitus lesions with the mechanical parts of the robot, and to check, through transillumination of the skin flap (**Figure 10-11**), the position of the instrument tip during the dissection. This feedback coming from the bedside team helps the console surgeon to maintain the orientation.

The robotic nipple-sparing procedure requires a superficial dissection of the gland, moving from the axillary toward the nipple-areola complex (**Figure 10-12**); it then continues below the nipple-areola complex up to the breast fold along the lateral, inferior, and internal margins (**Figures 10-13 A–C**).

First, the axillary tail, that was mobilized from the musculature during preparation, should be identified and used as reference point.

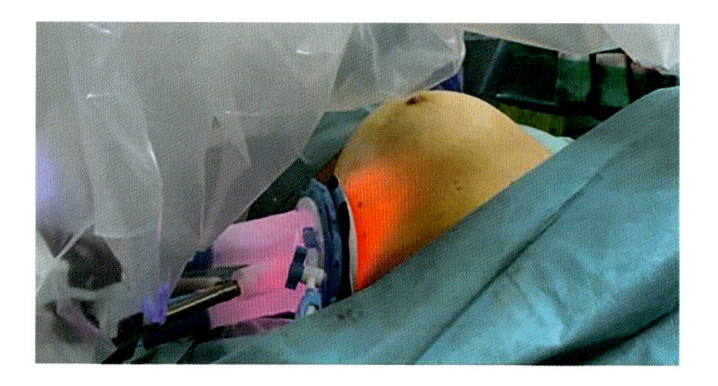

FIGURE 10-11 • Transillumination of the skin flap.

The breast tissue has to be retracted with ProGrasp forceps to provide countertraction, and monopolar curved scissors should be used to dissect the septa between the skin flap and mammary gland (**Figure 10-14**). The septa were created by blunt dissection with Metzenbaum scissors/tunnelers during the initial preparation.

> **🔍 ANATOMICAL HIGHLIGHTS**
>
> The septa created by blunt dissection with Metzenbaum scissors during preparation (tunnels) correspond to suspensory ligaments of the breast, also called crests of Duret (**Figures 10-15 A, B**).

The appropriate skin flap thickness is kept by the surgeon following the same anterior plane created during the preparation. A perfect evaluation of the 3-dimensional endoscopic images is fundamental to maintain the perfect plane during the dissection.

> **▶▶ TIPS**
>
> Skin flap thickness is important. A flap too thick may leave residual breast tissue, and potentially disease, within the skin, whereas a flap too thin increases the risk of necrosis. The superficial fascia is the main anatomical plane that should be followed during skin flap dissection, but its thickness may vary between breasts and between different parts of the same breast (from <1 mm to 29 mm). A single specific universal thickness for mastectomy skin flaps cannot be recommended currently as in open technique.

In all cancer cases, the retroareolar ducts can be excised and the sample examined intraoperatively by frozen section.

The operation proceeds with the deep layer dissection. The plane starts from the posterior part of the gland along the major pectoral fascia. The breast tissue is pulled up to create a sufficient working space along the major pectoral fascia (**Figure 10-16**).

The dissection of the last attachment from the inferior breast fold is completed, thus fully mobilizing the gland for extraction. The gland can be oriented with landmarks prior to extraction. The specimen is then removed entirely en bloc through the 3-cm axillary skin incision.

Step 5 average time frame: 100–120 min

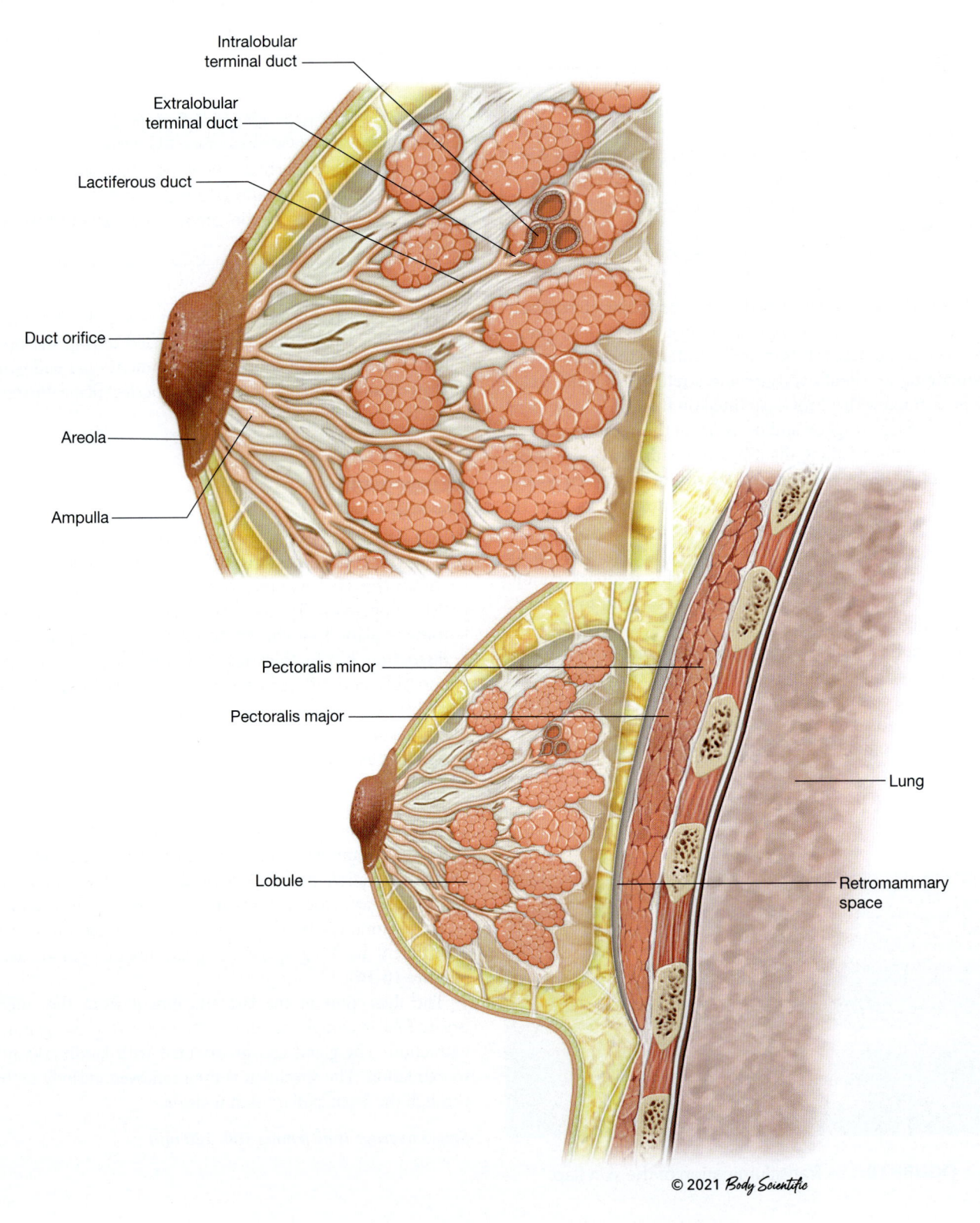

FIGURE 10-12 • Anatomy of the nipple and mammary gland.

Nipple-Sparing Mastectomy   191

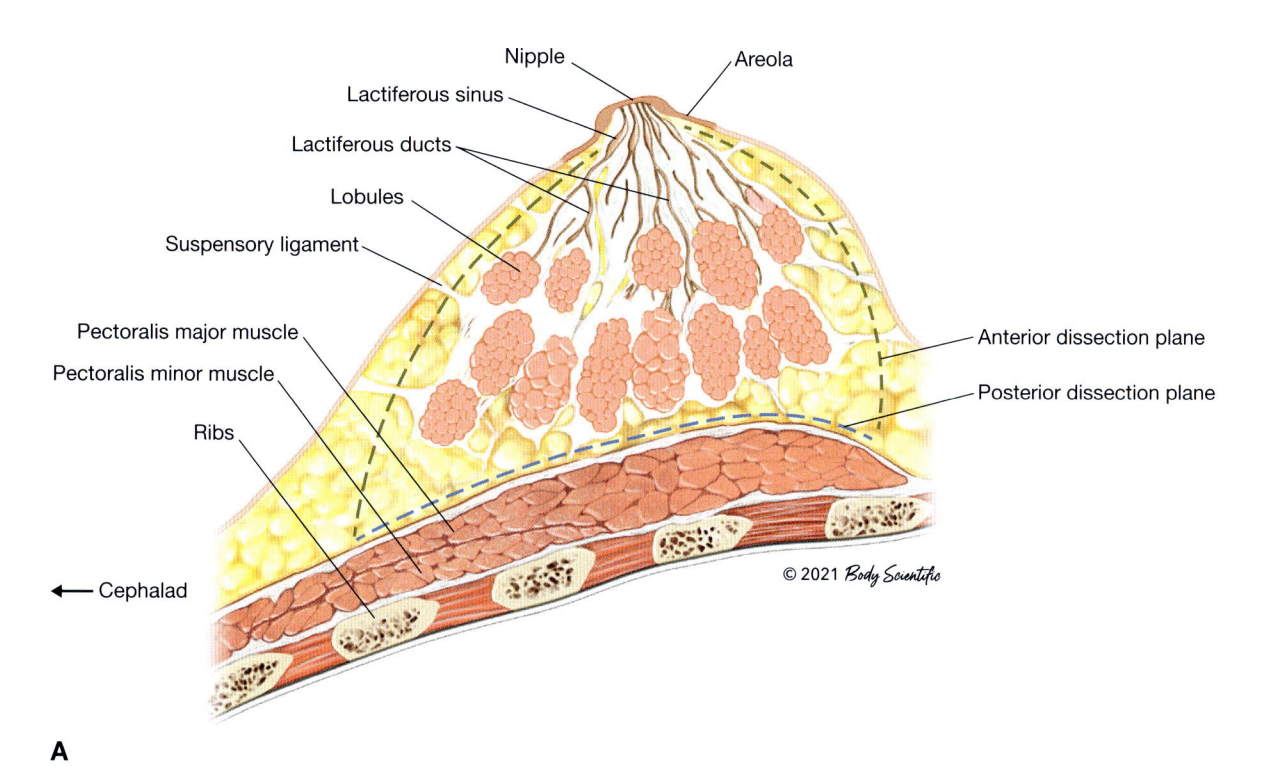

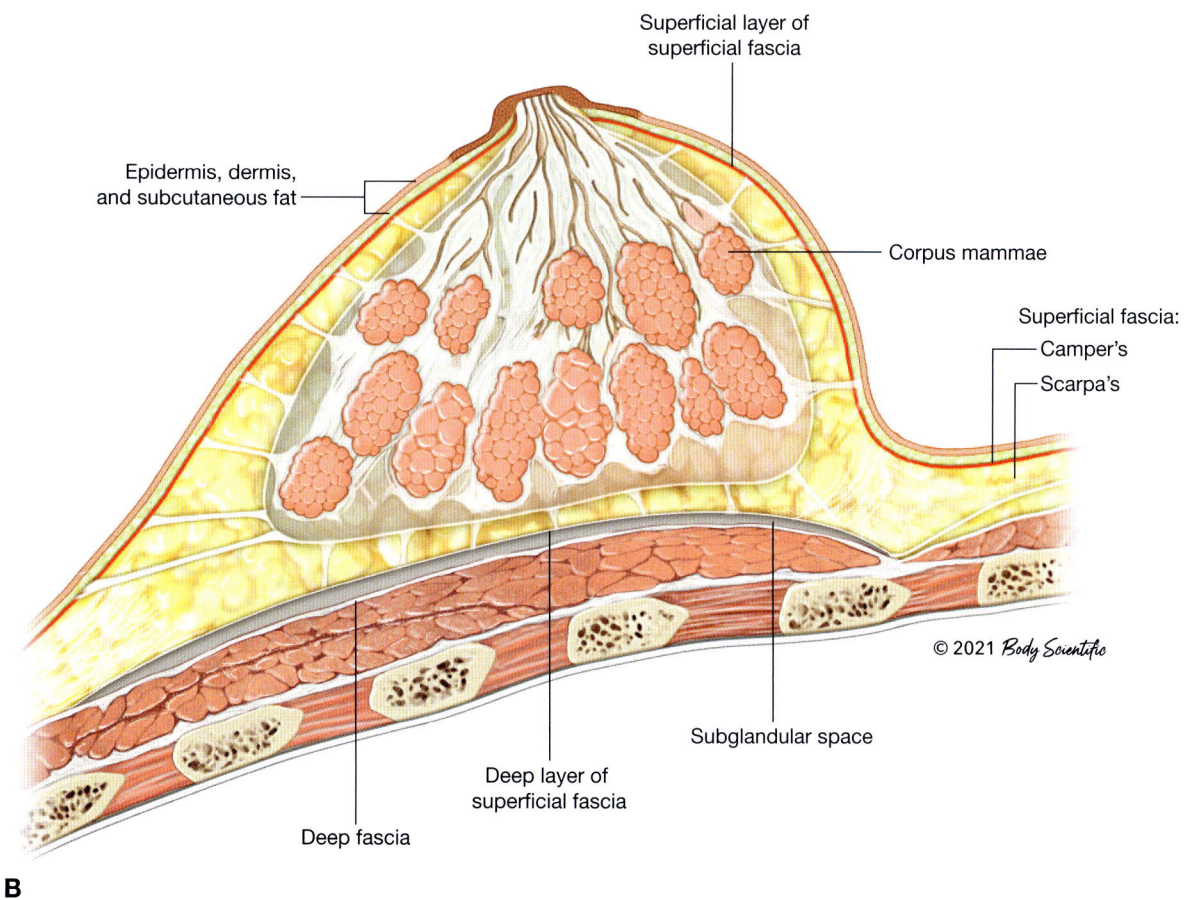

FIGURE 10-13 • Dissection planes and superficial fascia system.

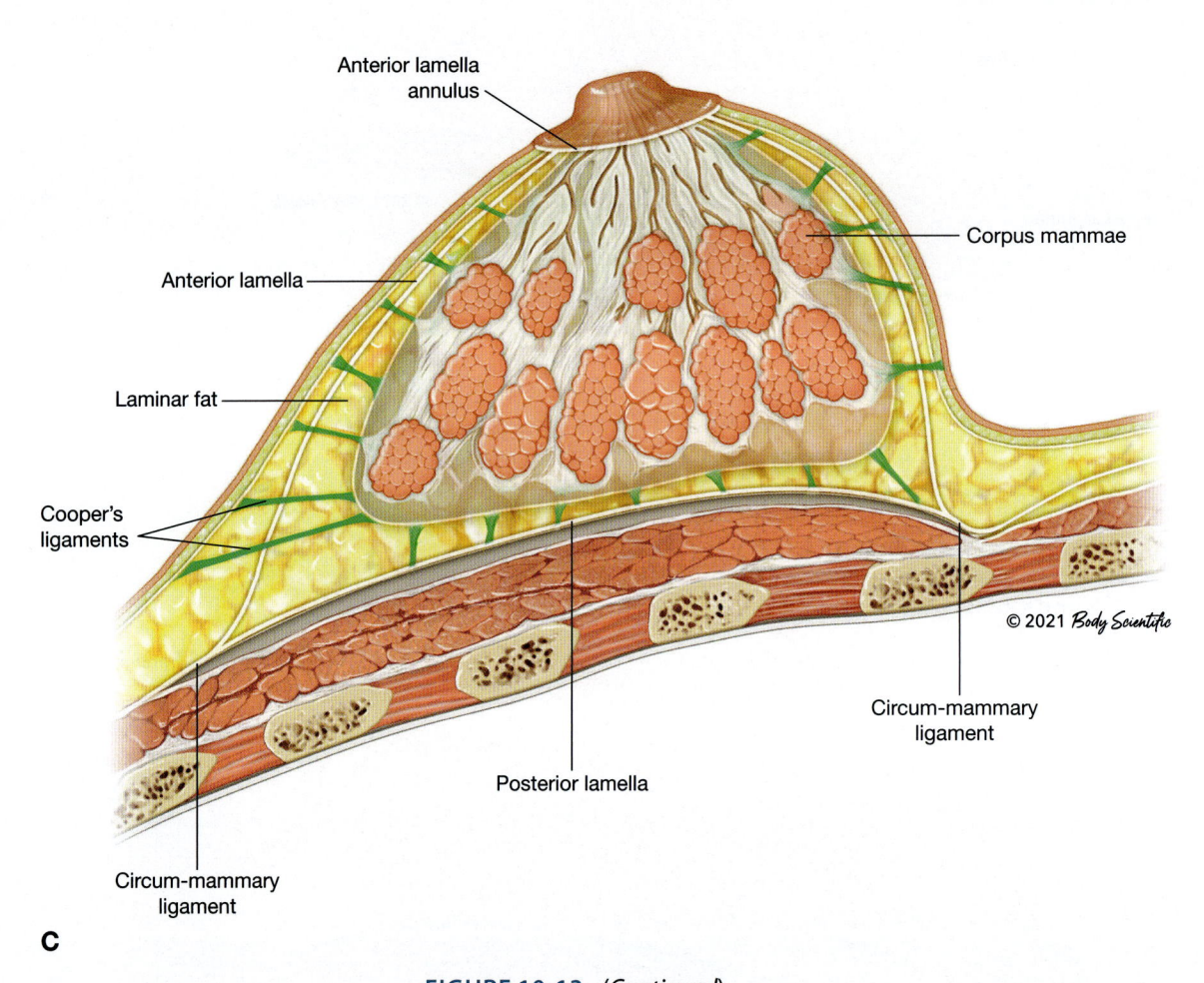

FIGURE 10-13 • *(Continued)*

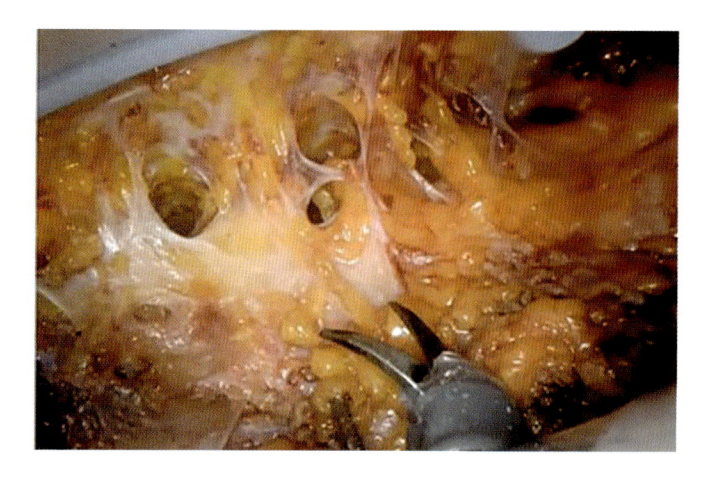

FIGURE 10-14 • Tunnels/dissection planes.

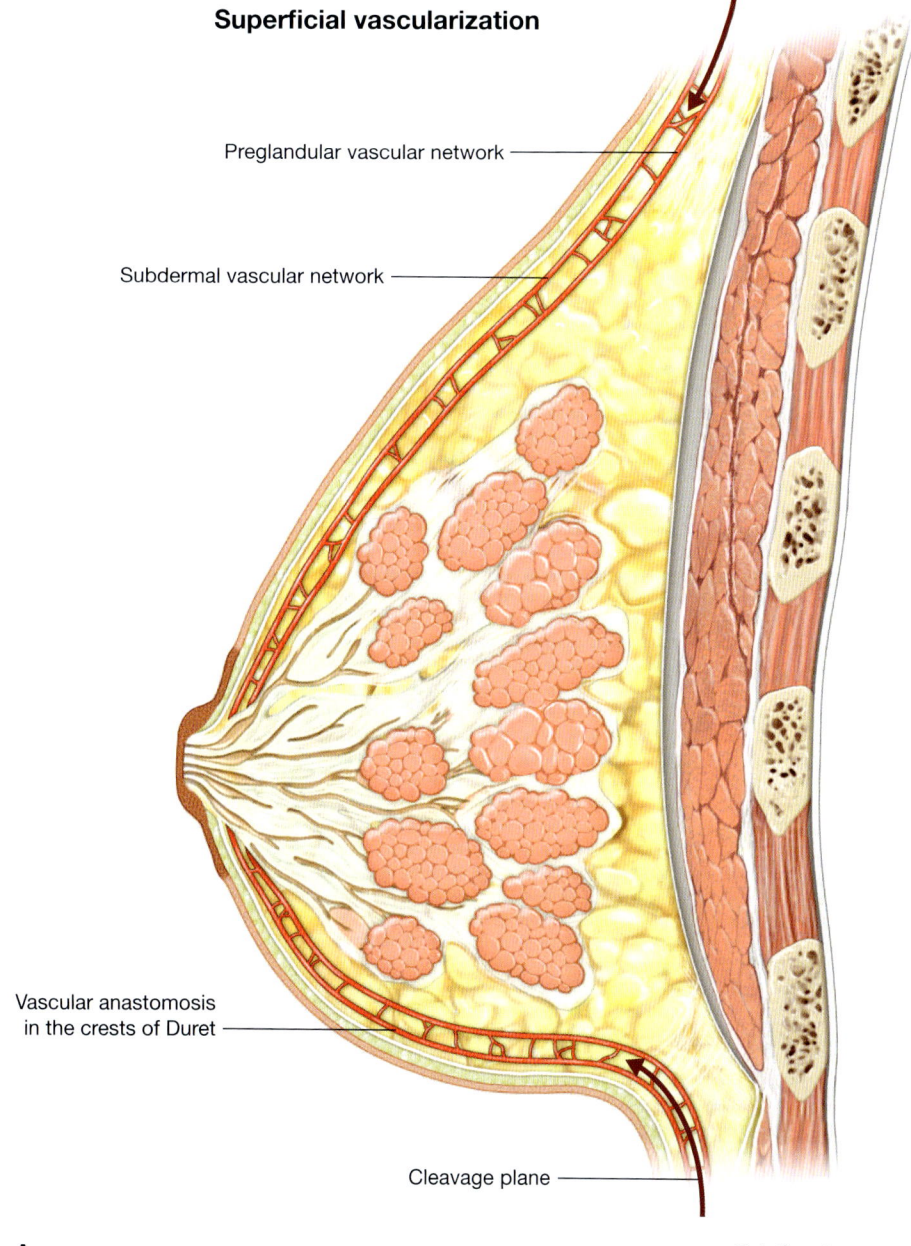

Superficial vascularization

- Preglandular vascular network
- Subdermal vascular network
- Vascular anastomosis in the crests of Duret
- Cleavage plane

© 2021 Body Scientific

A

FIGURE 10-15 • **A.** Superficial vascularization of the mammary gland.

Deep vascularization and vascular bridges

Superficial vascular network

Intraglandular network

B

Posterior vascular network

© 2021 Body Scientific

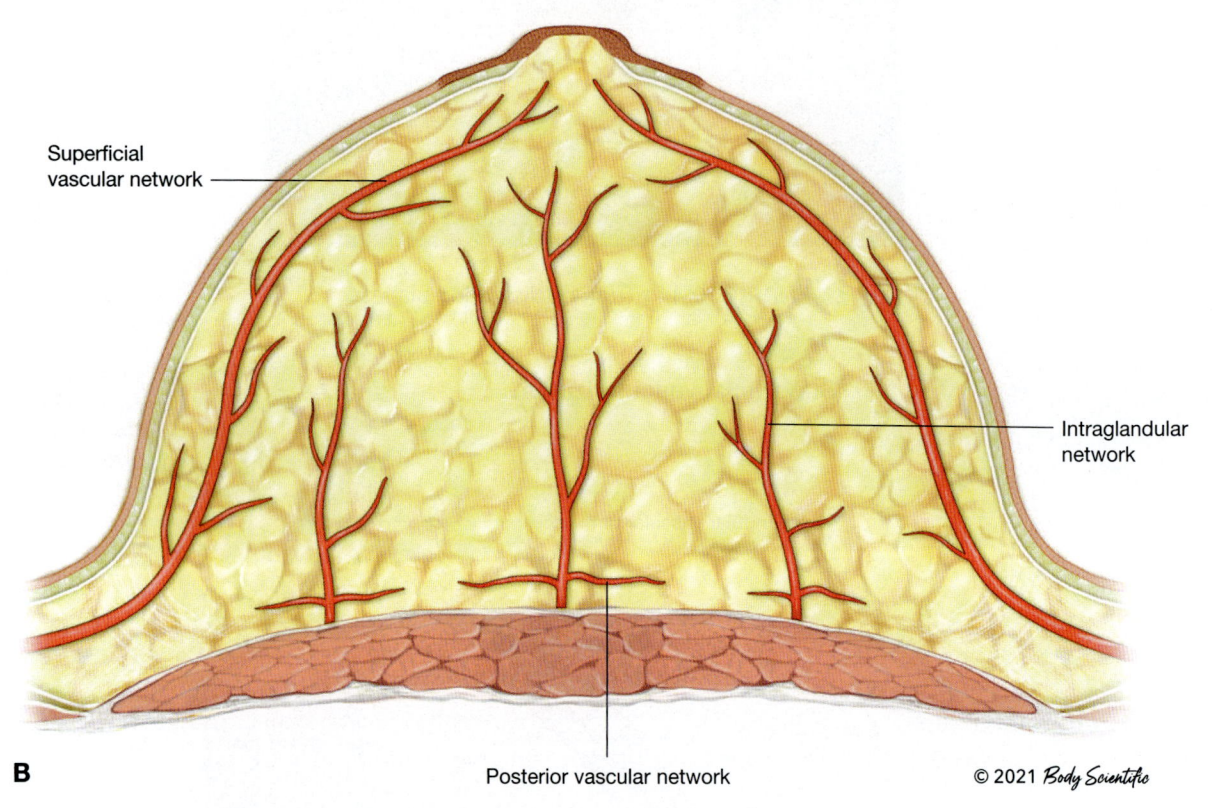

FIGURE 10-15 • (*Continued*) B. Deep vascularization of the mammary gland.

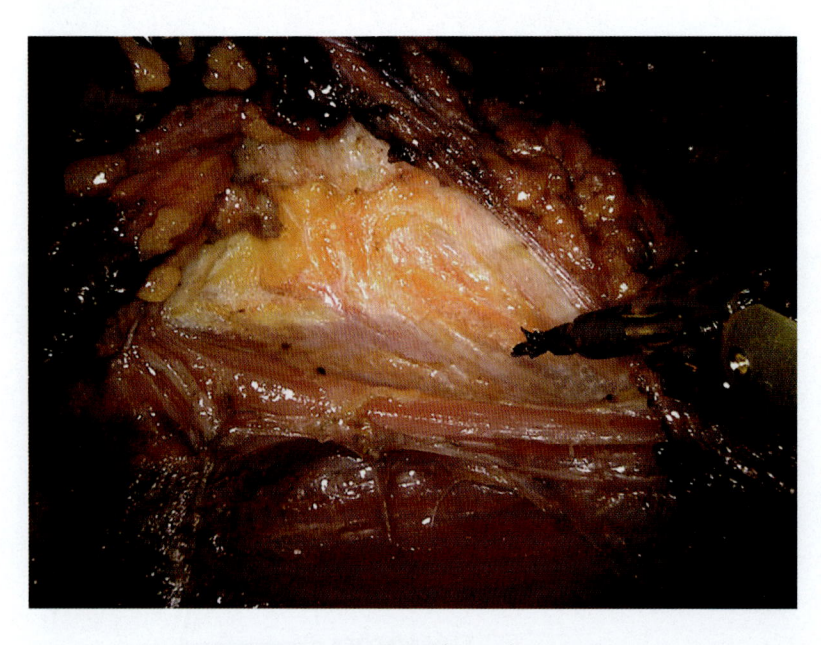

FIGURE 10-16 • Deep layer dissection.

Nipple-Sparing Mastectomy

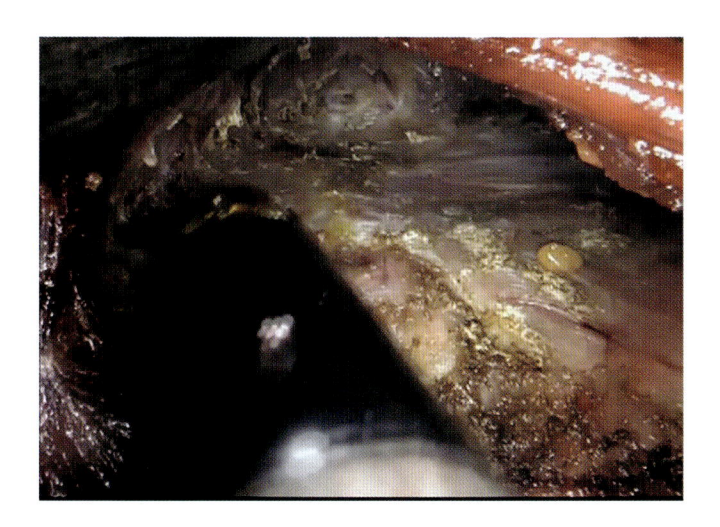

FIGURE 10-17 • Retropectoral reconstruction.

Step 6. Robotic reconstruction

In case of prepectoral implant reconstruction (more frequent), the implant is positioned manually, through the lateral incision without the help of the robotic system. For retropectoral reconstruction, the lateral border of the pectoralis major muscle can be elevated. In this phase, the gas pressure is not high enough to elevate the pectoralis major muscle. For this reason, the monoport can be removed, and a long and narrow standard retractor can be used to lift the muscle, while maintaining the same axillary access, and the same robotic instruments. The submuscular pocket can be dissected inferiorly and medially (**Figure 10-17**).

Inferiorly, the dissection continues reaching the inframammary fold and sternum, taking care to completely release the pectoralis major muscle from the chest wall, allowing for adequate muscular distension. At the same time, the pectoralis major muscle attachment to the skin flap is spared in order to guarantee an adequate implant cover.

The implant can be placed in a retropectoral or prepectoral space manually, through the initial working incision, according to the plastic surgeon's preference. Drains are manually placed, and the subcutaneous and cutaneous suture is performed by the standard technique. The entire operation is carried out involving a 3-cm hidden axillary incision in case of cup A–C size or a 5-cm incision for cup D size.

Step 6 average time frame: 70–90 min

Postoperative Outcome Evaluation

All postsurgical adverse events should be recorded for at least 3 months after the operation. Complications should be classified according to validated methods, in order to be compared in different trials, by using a multiple-level severity grading. Perioperative technical outcome measures should include total surgery time, blood loss, conversion rate to open mastectomy, and length of hospital stay. Patient satisfaction outcomes and cosmetic results should be also registered for clinical trials with measures and photos (**Figure 10-18**).

Early results of ipsilateral breast tumor recurrence and disease-free and overall survival rate should be recorded, analyzed, and shared with the scientific community.

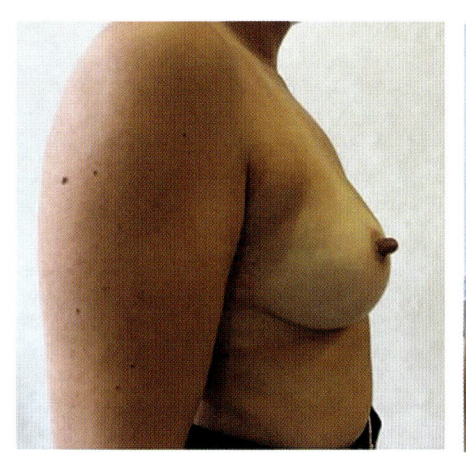

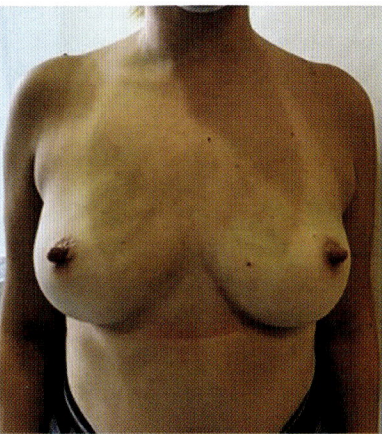

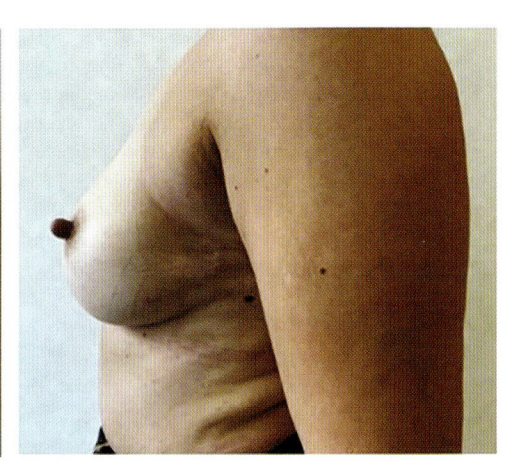

FIGURE 10-18 • Six months postoperative outcome.

Suggested Readings

1. Headon HL, Kasem A, Mokbel K. The oncological safety of nipple-sparing mastectomy: a systematic review of the literature with a pooled analysis of 12,358 procedures. *Arch Plast Surg.* 2016;43(4):328-338.
2. Galimberti V, Morigi C, Bagnardi V, et al. Oncological outcomes of nipple-sparing mastectomy: a single-center experience of 1989 patients. *Ann Surg Oncol.* 2018;25(13):3849-3857.
3. Yang JD, Lee J, Lee JS, Kim EK, Park CS, Park HY. Aesthetic scarless mastectomy and breast reconstruction. *J Breast Cancer.* 2021;24(1):22-33. doi: 10.4048/jbc.2021.24.e11
4. Toesca A, Manconi A, Peradze N, et al. 1931 Preliminary report of robotic nipple-sparing mastectomy and immediate breast reconstruction with implant. *Eur J Cancer.* 2015;51(3):S309.
5. Toesca A, Peradze N, Galimberti V, et al. Robotic nipple-sparing mastectomy and immediate breast reconstruction with implant: first report of surgical technique. *Ann Surg.* 2017;266(2):e28-e30. Epub 2015.
6. Park HS, Lee J, Lee H, Lee K, Song SY, Toesca A. Development of robotic mastectomy using a single-port surgical robot system. *J Breast Cancer.* 2019;23(1):107-112.
7. O'Dey DM, Prescher A, Pallua N. Vascular reliability of nipple-areola complex-bearing pedicles: an anatomical microdissection study. *Plast Reconstr Surg.* 2007;119(4):1167-1177.
8. Houvenaeghel G, Bannier M, Rua S, et al. Robotic breast and reconstructive surgery: 100 procedures in 2 years for 80 patients. *Surg Oncol.* 2019;31:38-45. doi: 10.1016/j.suronc.2019.09.005. Epub 2019 Sep 10.
9. Toesca A, Invento A, Massari G, et al. Update on the feasibility and progress on robotic breast surgery. *Ann Surg Oncol.* 2019;26(10):3046-3051.
10. Sarfati B, Struk S, Leymarie N, et al. Robotic prophylactic nipple-sparing mastectomy with immediate prosthetic breast reconstruction: a prospective study. *Ann Surg Oncol.* 2018;25(9):2579-2586.
11. Lai HW, Chen ST, Mok CW, et al. Robotic versus conventional nipple sparing mastectomy and immediate gel implant breast reconstruction in the management of breast cancer—a case control comparison study with analysis of clinical outcome, medical cost, and patient-reported cosmetic results. *J Plast Reconstr Aesthet Surg.* 2020;73(8):1514-1525.
12. Park HS, Lee J, Lee DW, et al. Robot-assisted nipple-sparing mastectomy with immediate breast reconstruction: an initial experience. *Sci Rep.* 2019;9(1):15669.
13. Toesca A, Peradze N, Manconi A, et al. Robotic nipple-sparing mastectomy for the treatment of breast cancer: feasibility and safety study. *Breast.* 2017;31:51-56.
14. Lai HW, Chen ST, Lin SL, et al. Robotic nipple-sparing mastectomy and immediate breast reconstruction with gel implant: technique, preliminary results and patient-reported cosmetic outcome. *Ann Surg Oncol.* 2019;26(1):42-52.
15. Morigi C. Highlights from the 15th St Gallen International Breast Cancer Conference 15-18 March, 2017, Vienna: tailored treatments for patients with early breast cancer. *Ecancermedicalscience.* 2017;11:732.
16. Margenthaler JA. Robotic mastectomy-program malfunction? *JAMA Surg.* 2020;155(6):461-462.
17. Kopkash K, Sisco M, Poli E, Seth A, Pesce C. The modern approach to the nipple-sparing mastectomy. *J Surg Oncol.* 2020;122(1):29-35.
18. Selber JC. Robotic nipple-sparing mastectomy: the next step in the evolution of minimally invasive breast surgery. *Ann Surg Oncol.* 2019;26(1):10-11.
19. Struk S, Qassemyar Q, Leymarie N, et al. The ongoing emergence of robotics in plastic and reconstructive surgery. *Ann Chir Plast Esthet.* 2018;63(2):105-112.
20. Toesca A, Peradze N, Manconi A, Nevola Teixeira LF. Reply to the letter to the editor "Robotic-assisted Nipple Sparing Mastectomy: A feasibility study on cadaveric models" by Sarfati B. et al. *J Plast Reconstr Aesthet Surg.* 2017;70(4):558-560.
21. Angarita FA, Castelo M, Englesakis M, McCready DR, Cil TD. Robot-assisted nipple-sparing mastectomy: systematic review. *Br J Surg.* 2020;107(12):1580-1594. doi: 10.1002/bjs.11837
22. NIH US National Library of Medicine. Surgical and oncologic outcomes after robotic nipple sparing mastectomy and immediate reconstruction (SORI). https://clinicaltrials.gov/ct2/show/NCT04108117
23. Lai HW, Toesca A, Sarfati B, et al. Consensus statement on robotic mastectomy—expert panel from International Endoscopic and Robotic Breast Surgery Symposium (IERBS) 2019. *Ann Surg.* 2020;271(6):1005-1012.
24. National Institutes of Health, US National Library of Medicine. Robotic nipple-sparing mastectomy vs conventional open technique. https://clinicaltrials.gov/ct2/show/NCT03440398
25. Pusic AL, Klassen A, Scott A, Klok J, Cordeiro PG, Cano SJ. Development of a new patient reported outcome measure for breast surgery: the BREAST-Q©. *Plast Reconstr Surg.* 2009;124(2):345-353.
26. Hopwood P, Fletcher I, Lee A, Al Ghazal S. A body image scale for use with cancer patients. *Eur J Cancer.* 2001;37(2):189-197.
27. Van Verschuer VM, Mureau MA, Gopie JP, et al. Patient satisfaction and nipple-areola sensitivity after bilateral prophylactic mastectomy and immediate implant breast reconstruction in a high breast cancer risk population: nipple-sparing mastectomy versus skin-sparing mastectomy. *Ann Plast Surg.* 2016;77(2):145-152.
28. Sarfati B, Toesca A, Roulot A, Invento A. Transumbilical single-port robotically assisted nipple-sparing mastectomy: a cadaveric study. *Plast Reconstr Surg Glob Open.* 2020;8(5): e2778. doi: 10.1097/GOX.0000000000002778. PMID: 33133886; PMCID: PMC7572180.
29. Morrow M. Robotic mastectomy: the next major advance in breast cancer surgery? *Br J Surg.* 2021 Mar 16:znab010. doi: 10.1093/bjs/znab010. Epub ahead of print.
30. Giulianotti PC, Coratti A, Angelini M, et al. Robotics in general surgery: personal experience in a large community hospital. *Arch Surg.* 2003;138(7):777-784. doi: 10.1001/archsurg.138.7.777

"… science is knowledge reduced to principles; art is knowledge reduced to practice."

—Sir Samuel Wilks (1824–1911)

Extended Thymectomy for Myasthenia Gravis and Thymoma

Hongbin Zhang • Feng Li • Jens-C. Rückert

INTRODUCTION

It has been more than 100 years since the first thymectomy for myasthenia gravis (MG) was performed by Sauerbruch in 1911. The debate on the efficiency of thymectomy for MG had never stopped until the randomized controlled MGTX study published in 2016, see suggested reading #1. Over 3 years of follow-up, compared to the medication group, the thymectomy plus medication group recorded a lower requirement of prednisone or immunosuppression. Furthermore, the subsequent 5-year follow-up data obtained a consistent result. Irrespective of the different techniques, an extended thymectomy including the thymus gland and surrounding adipose tissue, is necessary for MG patients and it is recommended for thymoma patients as well. With initially questionable resectability, a multimodal treatment including neoadjuvant chemotherapy may shrink the tumor and provide a better chance of complete resection.

As many as 14 different approaches for thymectomy have been described; their advocators all declared acceptable neurologic or oncologic outcomes. However, transsternal thymectomy remained the standard and it is the only one certified by a randomized controlled trial. However, most experienced centers have adopted minimally invasive approaches to thymectomy since growing evidence has shown the safety and feasibility of robotic-assisted thymectomy (RAT). Moreover, compared with extended transsternal thymectomy, neurologic outcomes for MG and medium-term oncologic outcomes for thymoma have also shown encouraging results. RAT has a special indication because of the narrow cavity of the mediastinum and the need of entering the neck, as well as the anatomic region of the cardiophrenic angle. Compared to conventional thoracoscopic surgery, RAT has shown to possibly have a higher complete stable remission rate for MG patients. This procedure may have an increased acceptance due to the superior dexterity

INSTRUMENT REQUIREMENTS

The suggested main robotic instruments/tools can be listed as follows:
- 30° scope
- Harmonic shears or vessel sealer
- Bipolar forceps or Maryland bipolar forceps
- Cautery hook/monopolar scissors
- Medium/large clip applier
- Cadière forceps/tip-up grasper (4 arm variation)
- Needle drivers (pericardial patch or vascular dissection/reconstruction)
- Cardiac scissors (for phrenic nerve neurolysis)

The suggested main laparoscopic instruments/tools can be listed as follows:
- Needle drivers
- Scissors
- Graspers
- Suction-irrigation

Supplemental materials:
- Gauzes, sponges
- Vessel loops
- Endobag™
- Medium–large clips
- Sutures: Prolene™ 3-0, 4-0 (optional)

Photo reproduced with permission from Banerjee AK. Sir Samuel Wilks: a founding father of clinical science. J R Soc Med. 1991;84(1):44-45.
Quote reproduced with permission from Wilks S. Introductory to part of a course on the theory and practice of medicine. Lancet. 1866;87(2221):307-309.

198 The Foundation and Art of Robotic Surgery

combined with milder incisional pain, high aesthetic value, reduced hospital stay, lower complication rate, and better postoperative pulmonary function.

Patient Positioning, OR Setup, and Port Setting

The left-sided unilateral approach for most cases of RAT is favored except for a right-sided thymoma that would indicate the right-sided approach (**Figure 11-1**). Although thymectomy can be safely performed from either sides, in consideration of the anatomy of the thymus and its variations, the left-sided approach is regarded as a more rational option. First, the left lobe of the thymus is almost always larger and frequently extends laterally beyond the left phrenic nerve, sometimes even in a wrapping manner. This is rarely, if ever, seen at the right side around the phrenic nerve. Moreover, the aortopulmonary window can be dissected easier from the left side, which ensures a safer radical resection of the adipose tissue where ectopic thymus frequently resides in. It is reported that even merely 2 grams of thymic residue can cause an incapacitating myasthenic weakness. More advantages of dissection beneath, around, and above the innominate vein, as well as the neck dissection, are associated with a left-sided approach.

For obese patients, or the ones with small thoracic cavities, the right-sided approach can be an option. In such situations, the increased space in the right hemithorax and direct view of the superior vena cava allows proximal control.

Double lumen intubation is routinely applied for anesthesia. When preparing for a left-sided approach, the patient is positioned at the left edge of the operating table on a beanbag (**Figure 11-2**). The left arm is placed at a lower position to allow for all movements of the robotic arms. The position of the trocars should be adapted to the individual anatomy; they are mostly placed between the 3rd and 5th intercostal spaces along the submammary fold, also permitting a cosmetic incision (**Figure 11-3**). The operative field should be prepared and draped from the left posterior axillary line to the right middle axillary line to ensure enough exposure for additional contralateral or subxiphoid trocar insertion, as well as any other modification including conversion to median sternotomy. The working trocars should always be placed under direct vision with the 30° optic. In case of a high

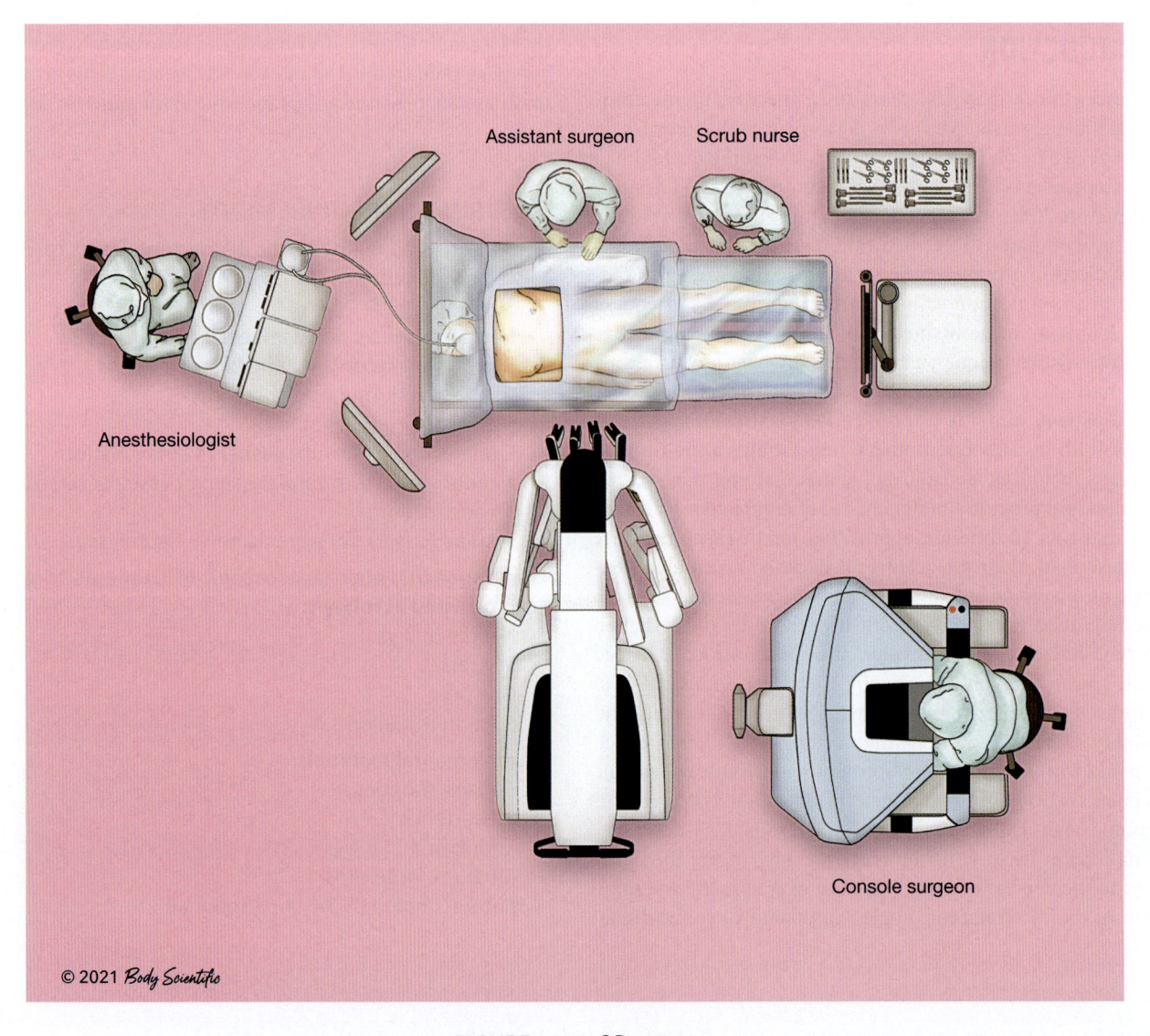

FIGURE 11-1 • OR setup.

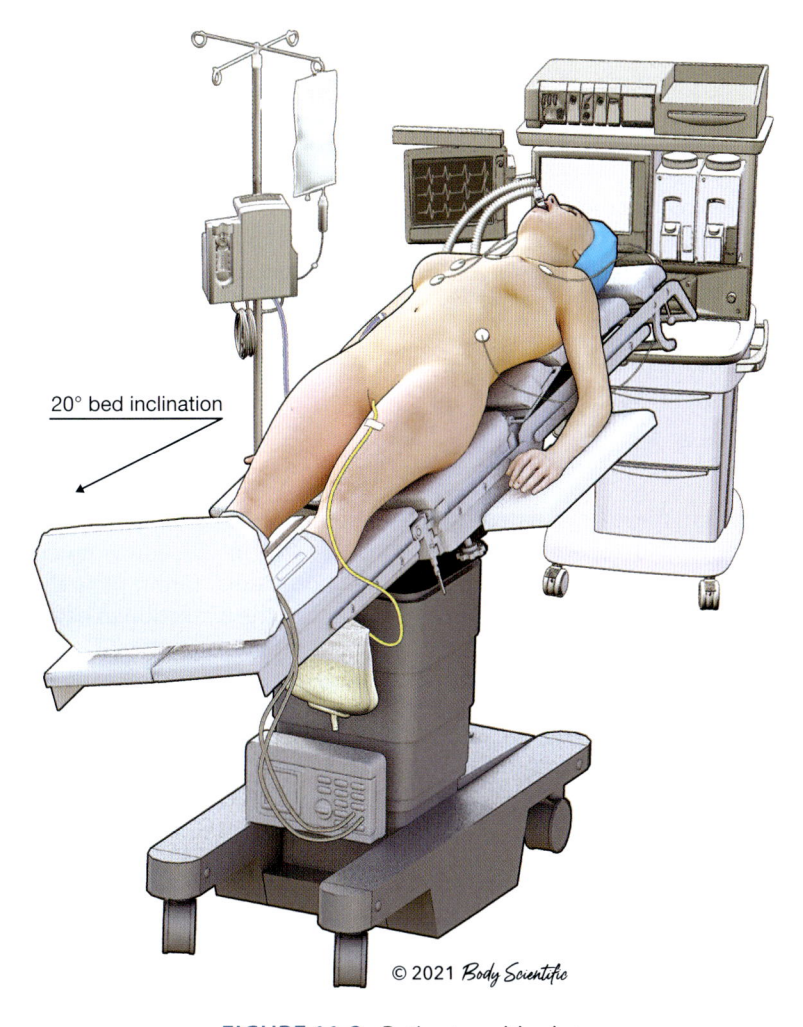

FIGURE 11-2 • Patient positioning.

body mass index (BMI) patient or reoperation, where the pleural cavity might be extremely narrow or severely adhesive, a direct dissection with scissors is useful to install the first trocar. Then an early use of CO_2 insufflation can help to avoid unexpected injury to the lung or the pericardium. In case of a large thymoma, an additional 5-mm trocar could be inserted to facilitate the dissection, or an additional subxiphoid incision could be done to extract the specimen.

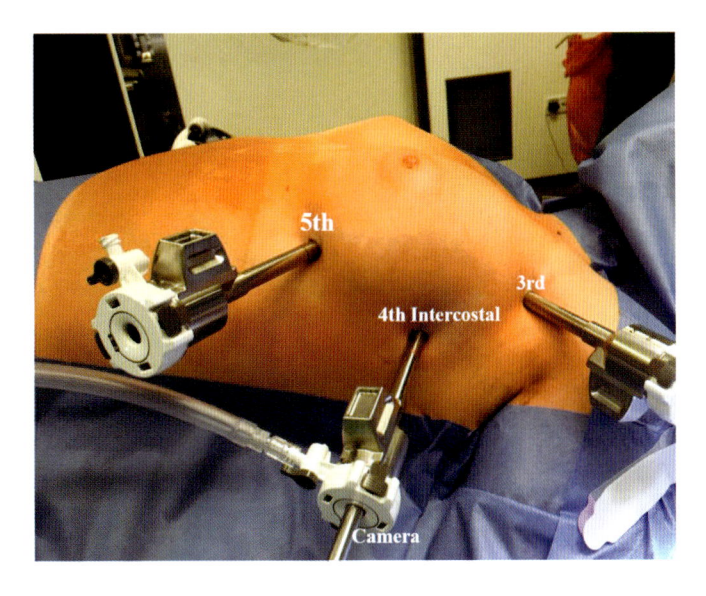

FIGURE 11-3 • Three trocars approach.

Surgical Technique

▶ **Video 11-1.** Extended Thymectomy for Myasthenia Gravis and Thymoma – Full Procedure

Prior to dissection, an essential element for a successful progression is an in-depth knowledge of the anatomy from all angles. Some anatomical reminders are depicted in **Figures 11-4 to 11-7**.

Step 1. Early dissection

Dissection usually starts at the caudal part of the pericardium medial to the phrenic nerve (**Figure 11-8**). In most cases, the phrenic nerve can be easily identified. In elderly and/or obese patients, this area is frequently covered by fatty tissue; therefore, immediate CO_2 insufflation can be applied to get a better view.

Step 1 average time frame: 10–15 min

> ▶▶ **TIPS**
>
> The insufflation of CO_2 is helpful to maintain a better exposure and to enlarge the operative field, especially for cases associated with additional narrowing of the mediastinal space. Such situations include cases with high BMI, extensive adhesions, or large thymomas. Normally, CO_2 insufflation is started after the incision of the jugular pleural fold, but for the conditions mentioned above, an earlier use is preferred.
>
> Keeping the contralateral (right) pleural cavity intact during the CO_2 insufflation is crucial. Intentional opening of the contralateral (right) pleural space is only necessary at the end of the dissection to harvest the right cardiophrenic fat pad. Besides, after the CO_2 insufflation, the original position of the pleura could change, and the proper dissection plane should be identified with caution.

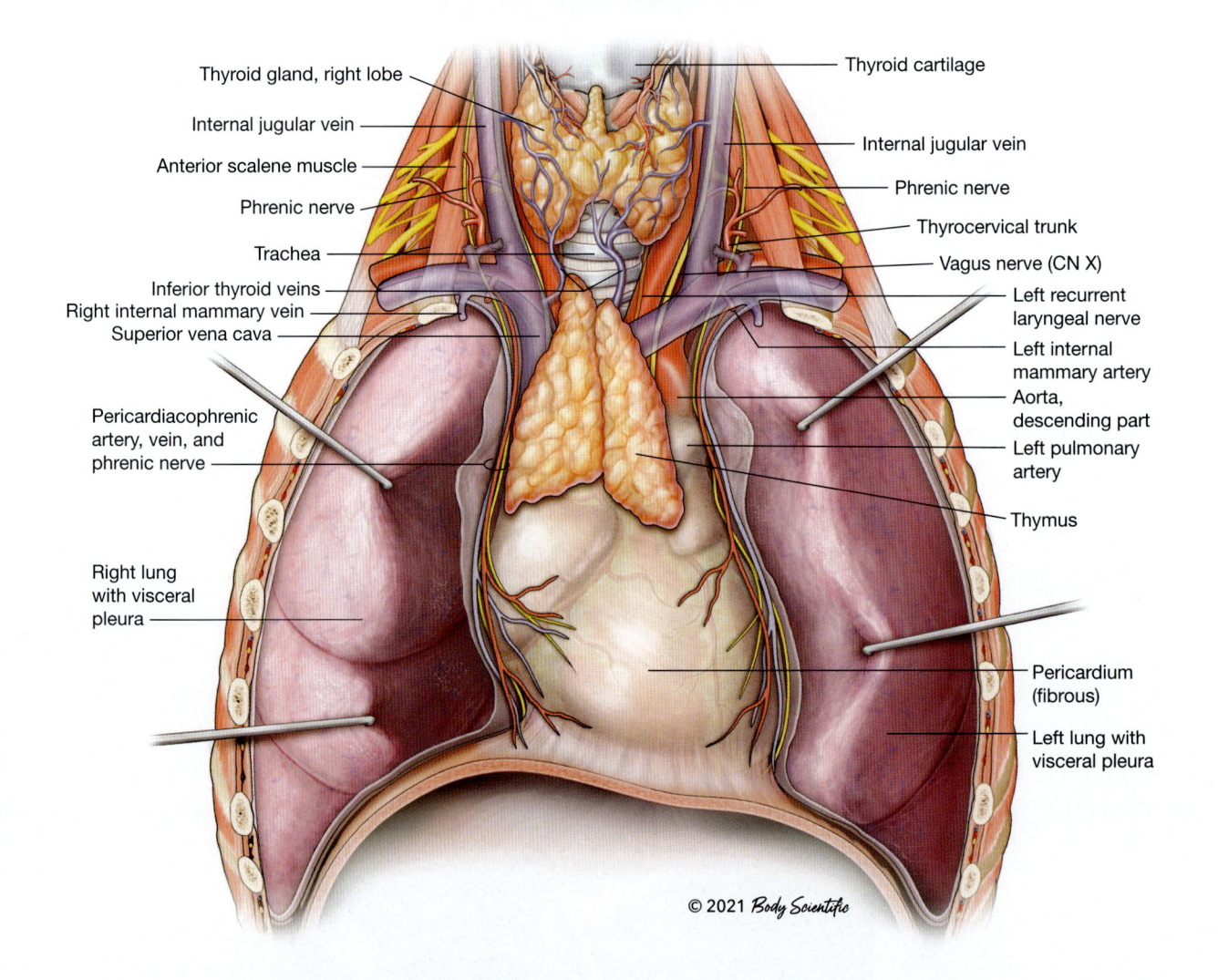

FIGURE 11-4 • Anterior thymus anatomy.

▶▶ TIPS

With higher BMI or highly hypertrophic thymus, and due to anatomic variations, the left phrenic nerve might be hidden in the adipose tissue or be surrounded by the thymus. In such cases, isolation of the phrenic nerve bundle is necessary, and meticulous dissection is mandatory to avoid injury of the phrenic nerve and the vagus nerve in the aortopulmonary window.

⚠ PITFALLS

Attention should be paid to the hemodynamic monitoring. The CO_2 insufflation at 8–10 mm Hg is safe for most patients, but attention should be paid to patients in a hypovolemic state and/or with poor left ventricular function. Meanwhile, right-sided pneumothorax was reported to be associated with more impact on the vena cava and right atrium, which leads to the reduction of venous return and a low cardiac index.

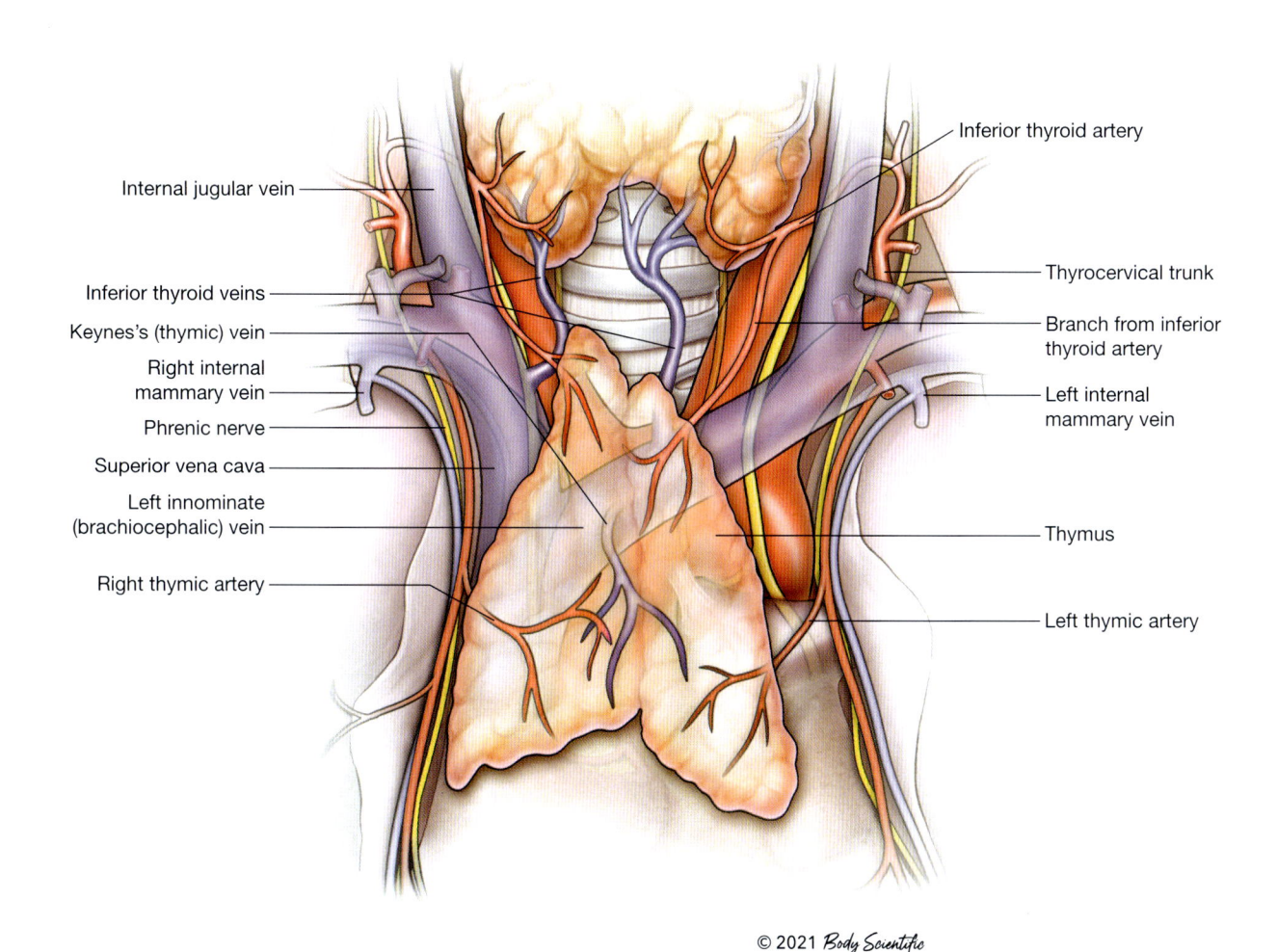

FIGURE 11-5 • Anterior thymus vasculature.

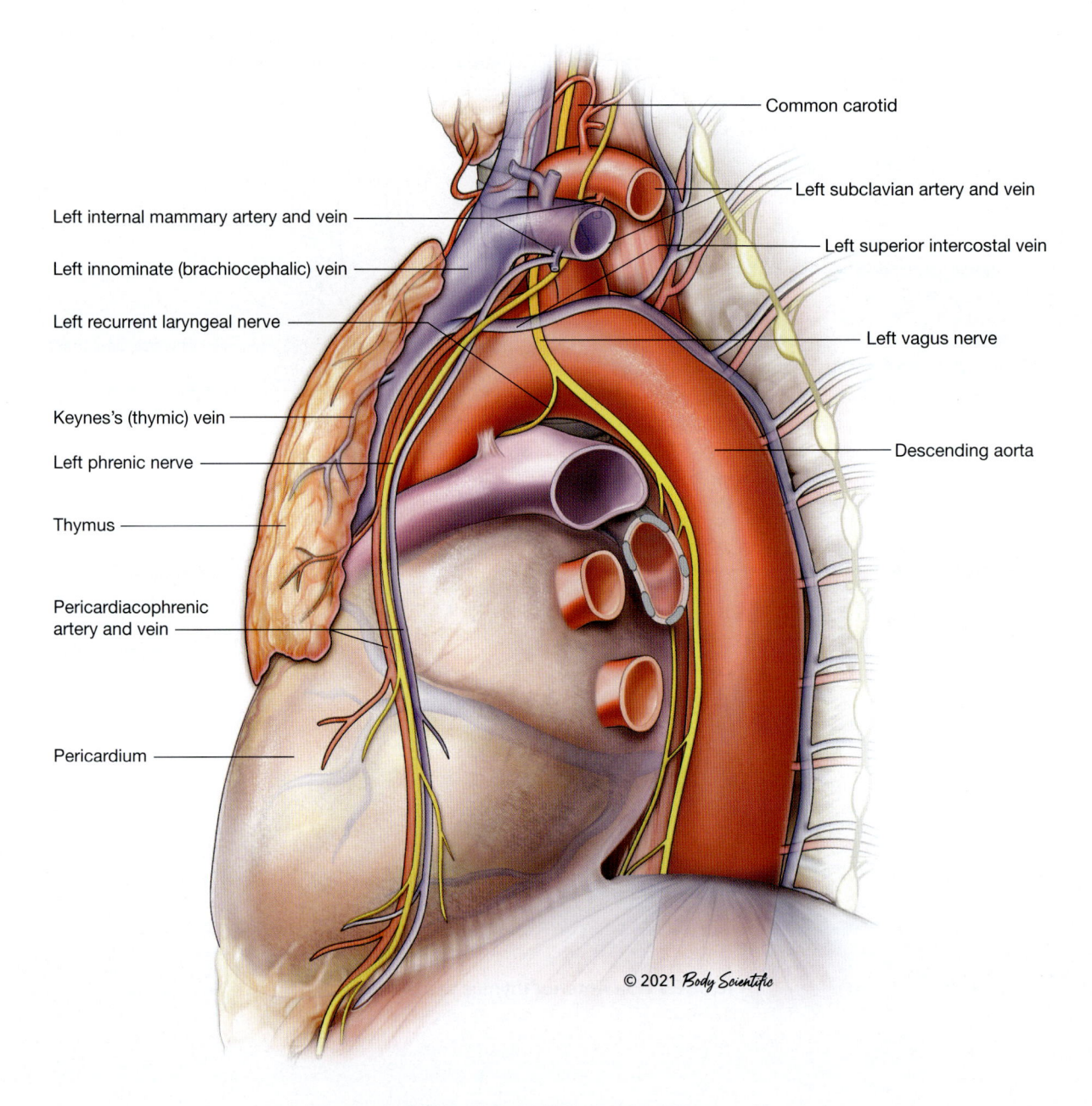

FIGURE 11-6 • Left thymus anatomy.

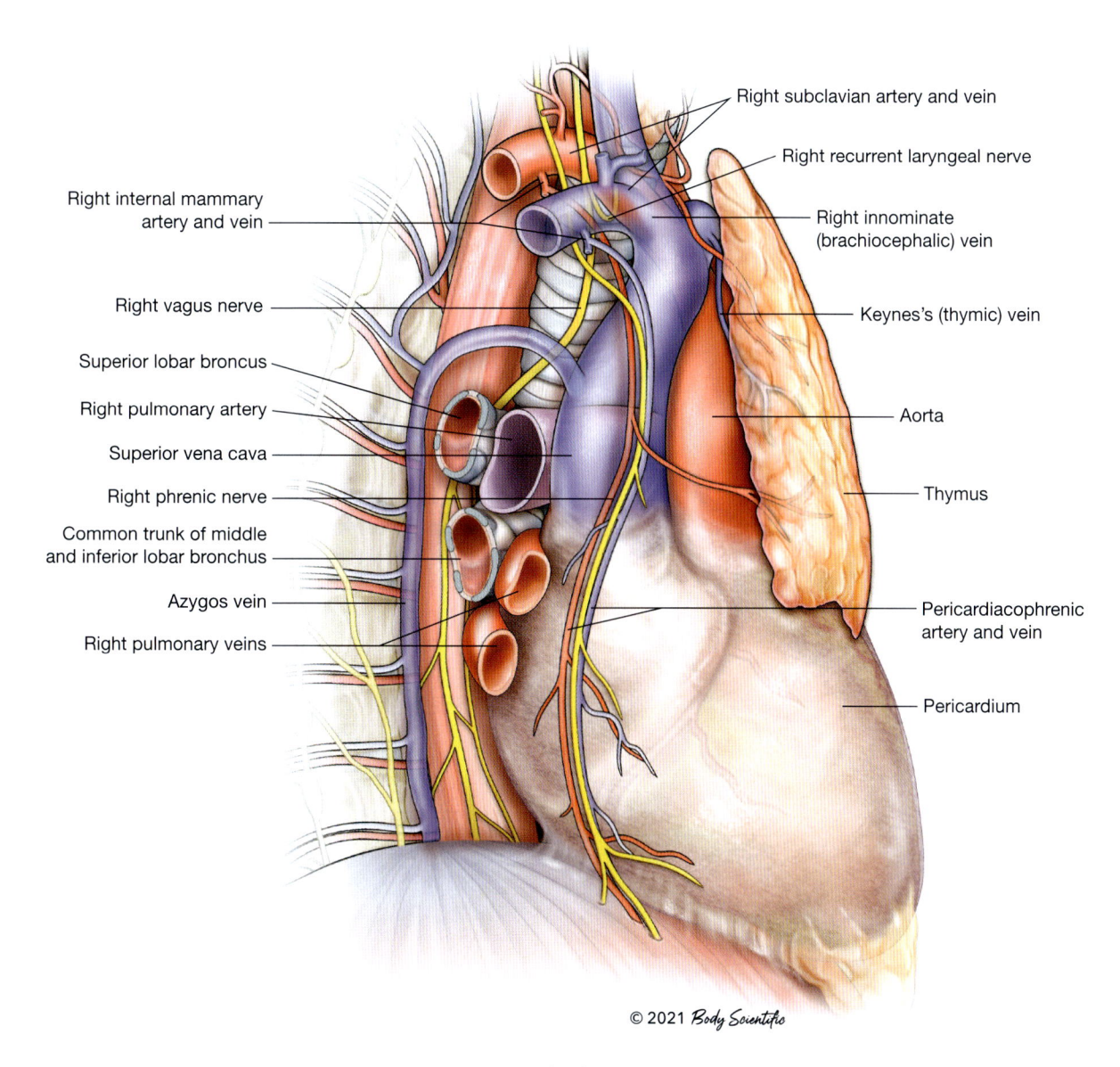

Extended Thymectomy for Myasthenia Gravis and Thymoma 203

FIGURE 11-7 • Right thymus anatomy.

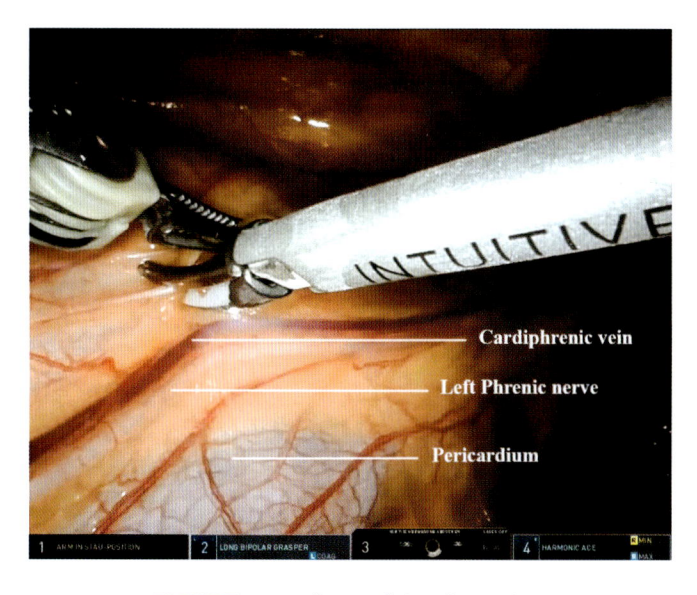

FIGURE 11-8 • Start of the dissection.

Step 2. Innominate vein identification as an anatomic landmark

The dissection along the left phrenic nerve continues cranially until the innominate vein is exposed after the incision of the pleural fold. The innominate vein serves as an important landmark (**Figure 11-9**). A precise dissection of the innominate vein is crucial for many of the essential steps of robotic thymectomy.

Step 2 average time frame: 5–10 min

> ⚠️ **PITFALLS**
>
> In robotic thymectomy, the innominate vein is the most common site of bleeding irrespective of the left-sided or right-sided approach.

> 🔍 **ANATOMICAL HIGHLIGHTS**
>
> The anterior wall of the innominate vein runs medial to the left phrenic nerve. Depending on the amount of fat in the anterior mediastinum, the innominate vein may run directly underneath or at a distance of more than 5 mm from the mediastinal pleura.

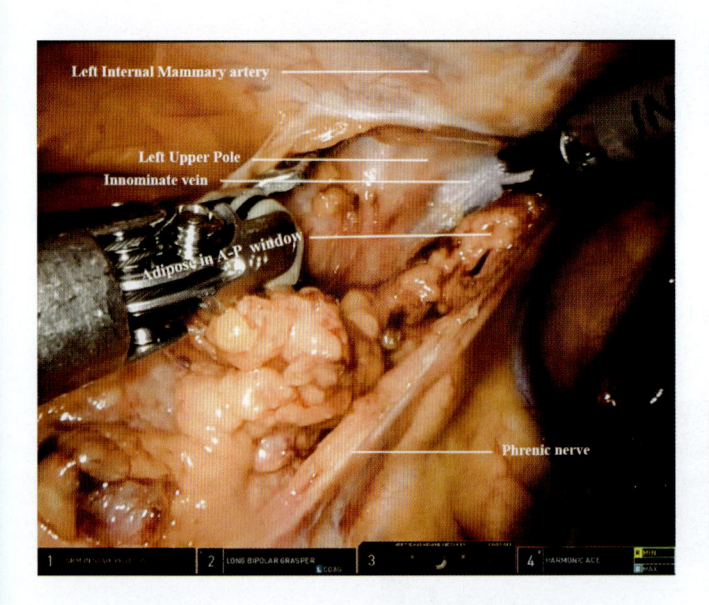

FIGURE 11-9 • Innominate vein as a landmark.

Step 3. Dissection of the aortopulmonary window

The aortopulmonary window (**Figure 11-10**) is a common site of ectopic thymus, either macroscopically or microscopically. The adipose tissue should be retracted gently with a long bipolar grasper in the left hand, and the whole piece of the fat tissue should be removed.

Step 3 average time frame: 10–15 min

> ⚠️ **PITFALLS**
>
> When isolating the phrenic nerve bundle, injury to the adjacent vagus nerve on the left can occur.

> 🔍 **ANATOMICAL HIGHLIGHTS**
>
> There are many different sites where ectopic thymic tissue may be present. The anterior mediastinal perithymic fat is the most common, followed by the pericardiophrenic angles, the aortopulmonary window, the pretracheal fat, the lateral to phrenic nerves, the aortocaval groove, and behind the innominate vein (**Figure 11-11**).

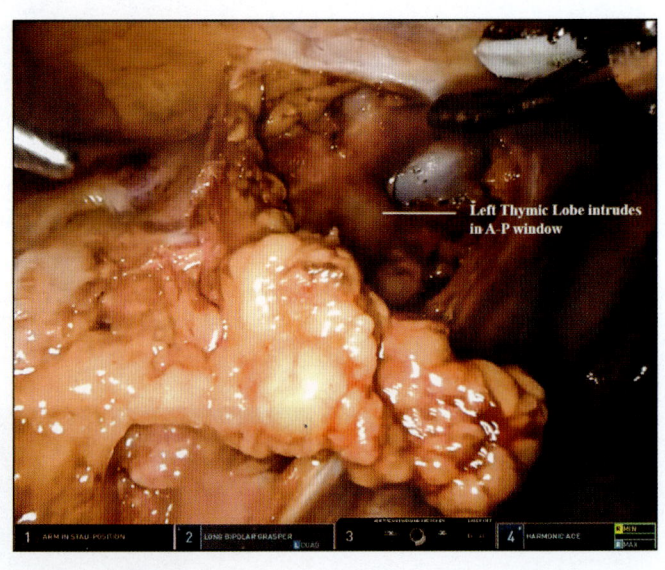

FIGURE 11-10 • Aortopulmonary window.

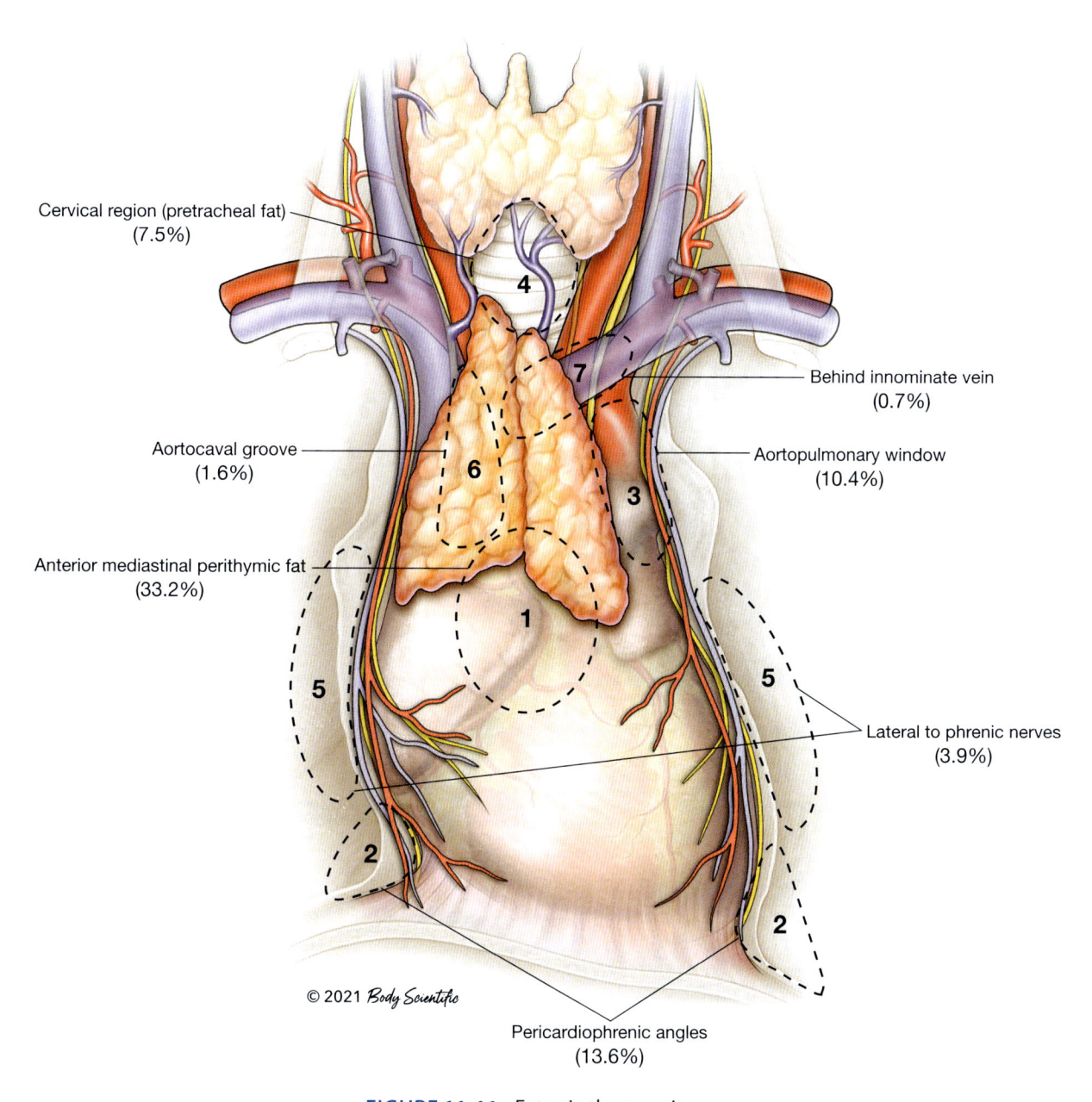

Extended Thymectomy for Myasthenia Gravis and Thymoma | 205

FIGURE 11-11 • Ectopic thymus sites.

Step 4. Dissection of the cervical pleural fold and exposure of the upper pole

This step is started from the exposed innominate vein and the dissection is extended to the mediastinal retrosternal line. The upper pole (**Figure 11-12**) can be identified on the innominate vein in most cases. It extends in a great variety into the neck.

Step 4 average time frame: 5–10 min

> **🔍 ANATOMICAL HIGHLIGHTS**
>
> The cervical part of the thymus may be partially or completely located between the innominate vein and aortic arch.

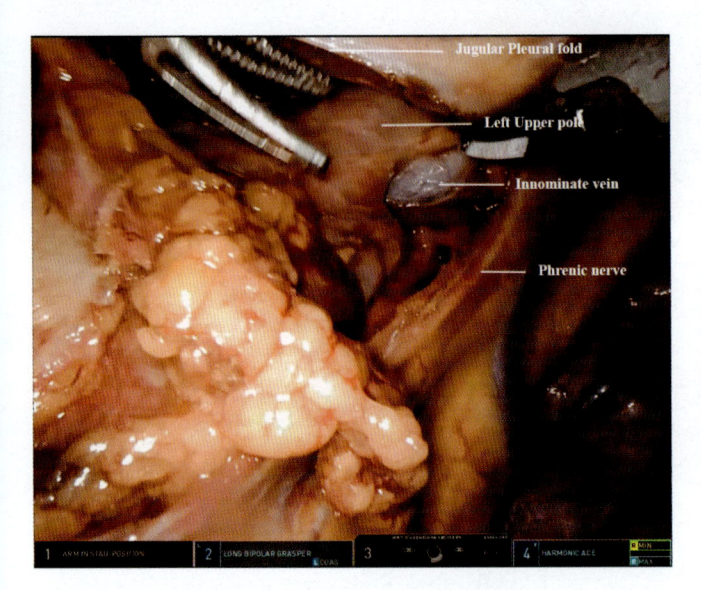

FIGURE 11-12 • The upper pole.

Step 5. Dissection of the main thymic lobes

The dissection proceeds to the right mediastinal pleura and caudally until the subxiphoid fold.

The dissection is carried out to the right side until the right lung is visible and then extends caudally until the subxiphoid pleural fold is reached. The tissue anterior to the pericardium is also dissected with Harmonic shears cranially and contralaterally until the innominate vein plane and right pleura, respectively.

Step 5 average time frame: 7–10 min

> **▶▶ TIPS**
>
> Attention should be paid to keep the right parietal pleura intact, which maintains the positive CO_2 pressure. In case the pleura is opened, the pressure of the CO_2 insufflation should be reduced to have less interference with the ventilation of the right lung.

Step 6. Managing the left upper pole

The capsule of the left upper pole is carefully dissected using two grasping instruments for retraction in an alternating fashion (the long bipolar grasper in the left hand, the Harmonic shears in the right one). The surrounding adhesions are dissected bluntly, and the supplying vessels are divided with the ultrasonic shear. After proper dissection, the thyrothymic ligament (**Figure 11-13**) can be visualized and severed with the ultrasonic shears.

Step 6 average time frame: 10–15 min

> **▶▶ TIPS**
>
> Retraction should be gentle, the surrounding adipose tissue should be dissected off, and the upper pole should be severed with an energy-based device rather than blunt retraction.

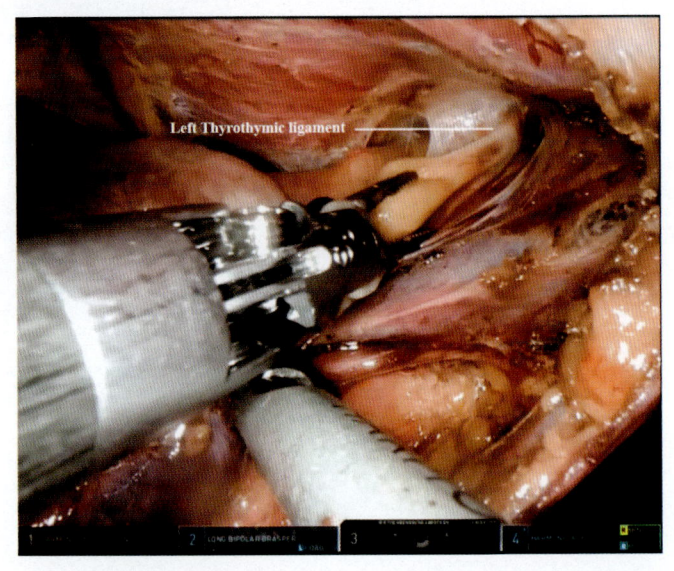

FIGURE 11-13 • Left thyrothymic ligament.

Extended Thymectomy for Myasthenia Gravis and Thymoma   207

Step 7. Dissection of the right upper pole and surrounding adipose tissue

With a left bipolar grasper retracting the left upper pole caudally, the cervical adipose tissue between the upper poles is dissected, where ectopic thymus might be located. Care should be taken, during the dissection not to injure the vena thyroidea ima. After the whole median retrosternal tissue is mobilized, the right thymic lobe and the surrounding fat tissue can be visualized. With the same dissecting methods as that handling the left upper pole, the right thyrothymic ligament should be visualized and divided with the ultrasonic shears.

Step 7 average time frame: 10–15 min

Step 8. Dissection of the thymic veins

Usually, 2 to 4 thymic veins are found to drain into the left innominate vein (**Figure 11-14**). But occasionally, a single central vessel (Keynes vein) collects all venous blood from the thymic gland and drains into the innominate vein. After being prepared, all the thymic veins should be divided in between clips.

Step 8 average time frame: 5–10 min

> **EDITORIAL COMMENT**
>
> Even though thymic veins can be controlled and sealed with the vessel sealer, clips have a more stable action. A bleeding from the innominate vein may be challenging and requires the addition of more ports for assisting instruments like suction device and the introduction of sutures.

> **▶▶ TIPS**
>
> The innominate vein should be dissected with clear exposure that can help to identify the thymic veins. At least 1 vessel should always be expected to be found directly at the venous confluence.

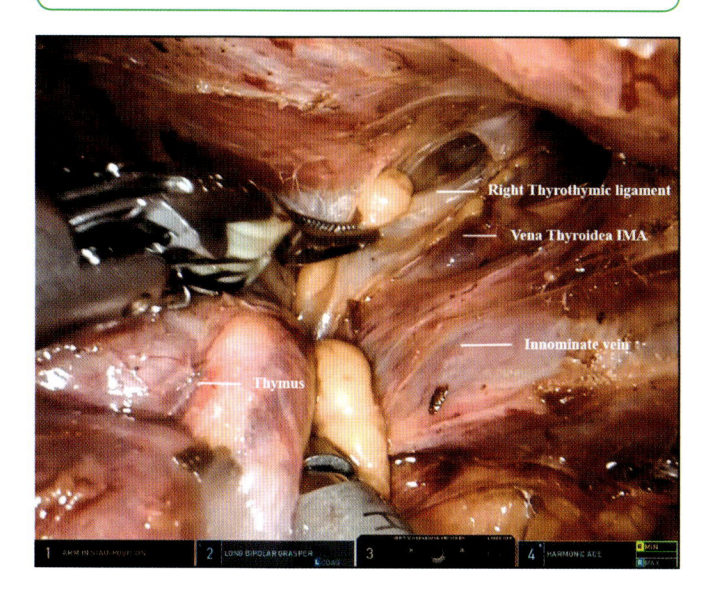

FIGURE 11-14 • Right thyrothymic ligament and adjacent structure.

Step 9. Mobilization of the tissue in the aortocaval groove

The dissection is continued along the innominate vein. If no thymic vein branches arise, the surgeon should expect a major thymic vein draining directly at the venous confluence. This anatomical conformation may increase the risk of bleeding if it is not properly anticipated and recognized (**Figure 11-15**).

Step 9 average time frame: 10–15 min

> **🔍 ANATOMICAL HIGHLIGHTS**
>
> After retracting down the right upper pole, the right internal mammary vein is visible. Adjacent to its entrance into the venous confluence, the right phrenic nerve is always at the lateral side of the superior vena cava.

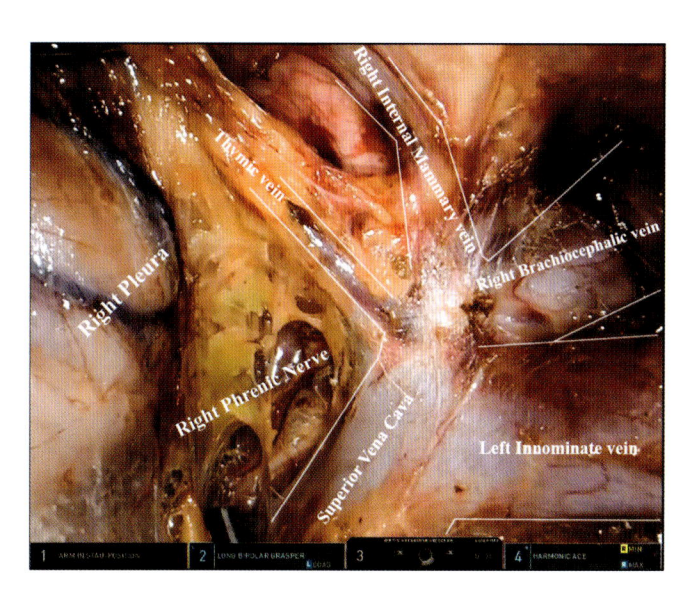

FIGURE 11-15 • Right phrenic nerve in the aorta cava groove.

Step 10. Resection of the cardiophrenic fatty tissue on the right side

En bloc dissection of the mediastinal adipose tissue is the next step, from the left cardiophrenic angle to the subxiphoid area and proceeding to the right cardiophrenic area. At this point, the dissection continues to the adjacent pleura, the right pleura is opened here, and then the retrosternal fat tissue cranially is dissected until the innominate vein plane. Then, as the last maneuver, the dissection turns caudally along the right phrenic nerve to resect the right pleura adjacent to the thymus gland.

Step 10 average time frame: 10–15 min

Step 11. Completion of the dissection and hemostasis
A final exploration of the operative field is routinely conducted for hemostasis and to ensure that no thymic residue or additional thymic is lobe present.

Step 11 average time frame: 5–10 min

Step 12. Specimen extraction
The whole specimen is taken out through the camera trocar incision after changing the instruments and weighed immediately after the removal. After that, it is placed on a surgical tray and positioned as *in situ* to be photographed before being sent to the pathologist.

Step 12 average time frame: 10–15 min

> ▶▶ **TIPS**
>
> In case of a big thymoma, an additional subxiphoid incision is suggested to retrieve the specimen within a large retrieval bag.

Suggested Readings

1. Wolfe GI, et al. Randomized trial of thymectomy in myasthenia gravis. *N Engl J Med.* 2016;375(6):511-522.
2. Masaoka A. Staging system of thymoma. *J Thorac Oncol.* 2010;5(10 Suppl 4):S304-S312.
3. Jaretzki A 3rd, Wolff M. "Maximal" thymectomy for myasthenia gravis. Surgical anatomy and operative technique. *J Thorac Cardiovasc Surg.* 1988;96(5):711-716.
4. Ruckert JC, Swierzy M, Ismail M. Comparison of robotic and nonrobotic thoracoscopic thymectomy: a cohort study. *J Thorac Cardiovasc Surg.* 2011;141(3):673-677.
5. Li F, et al. Unraveling the role of ectopic thymic tissue in patients undergoing thymectomy for myasthenia gravis. *J Thorac Dis.* 2019;11:4039-4048. doi: 10.21037/jtd.2019.08.109
6. Schumacher EJMC. Thymektomie bei einem fall von morbus basedowi mit myasthenie grenzgeb. 1912;25:746-765.
7. Detterbeck FC, Zeeshan A. Thymoma: current diagnosis and treatment. *Chin Med J (Engl).* 2013;126(11):2186-2191.
8. Mi W, Silvestri NJ, Wolfe GI. A neurologist's perspective on thymectomy for myasthenia gravis: current perspective and future trials. *Thorac Surg Clin.* 2019;29(2):143-150.
9. El-Dawlatly AA, et al. Right vs left side thoracoscopic sympathectomy: effects of CO2 insufflation on haemodynamics. *Ann Chir Gynaecol.* 2001;90(3):206-208.
10. Sonett JR, Jaretzki A 3rd. Thymectomy for nonthymomatous myasthenia gravis: a critical analysis. *Ann N Y Acad Sci.* 2008;1132:315-328.
11. Ye B, et al. Surgical treatment of early-stage thymomas: robot-assisted thoracoscopic surgery versus transsternal thymectomy. *Surg Endosc.* 2014;28(1):122-126.
12. O'Sullivan KE, et al. A systematic review of robotic versus open and video assisted thoracoscopic surgery (VATS) approaches for thymectomy. *Ann Cardiothorac Surg.* 2019;8(2):174-193.
13. Cakar F, et al. A comparison of outcomes after robotic open extended thymectomy for myasthenia gravis. *Eur J Cardiothorac Surg.* 2007;31(3):501-504; discussion 504-505.
14. Kang CH, et al. Robotic thymectomy in anterior mediastinal mass: propensity score matching study with transsternal thymectomy. *Ann Thorac Surg.* 2016;102(3):895-901.
15. Renaud S, et al. Robotic-assisted thymectomy with Da Vinci II versus sternotomy in the surgical treatment of non-thymomatous myasthenia gravis: early results. *Rev Neurol (Paris).* 2013;169(1):30-36.
16. Buentzel J, et al. Thymectomy via open surgery or robotic video assisted thoracic surgery: can a recommendation already be made? *Medicine (Baltimore).* 2017;96(24):e7161.
17. Marulli G, et al. Surgical and neurologic outcomes after robotic thymectomy in 100 consecutive patients with myasthenia gravis. *J Thorac Cardiovasc Surg.* 2013;145(3):730-735; discussion 735-736.
18. Ashton RC Jr, et al. Totally endoscopic robotic thymectomy for myasthenia gravis. *Ann Thorac Surg.* 2003;75(2):569-571.
19. Ooi A, Sibayan M. Uniportal video assisted thoracoscopic surgery thymectomy (right approach). *J Vis Surg.* 2016;2:13.
20. Giulianotti PC, Coratti A, Angelini M, et al. Robotics in general surgery: personal experience in a large community hospital. *Arch Surg.* 2003;138(7):777-784. doi: 10.1001/archsurg.138.7.777

12

"For no field in surgery presented more dangers and difficulties; in none was the challenge taken up with more persistent endeavour in the face of repeated failures."

—Ivor Lewis (1895–1982)

Ivor-Lewis Esophagectomy

Andrea Coratti • Francesco Guerra • Giuseppe Giuliani

INTRODUCTION

The last decade has seen an exponential diffusion of minimally invasive esophagectomy, mainly due to the growing experience of surgical teams and the availability of new technologies. In this context, robotic esophagectomy has also been rapidly expanding, and several referral centers dedicated to esophageal surgery are currently reporting excellent outcomes.

In this chapter, the operative technique of robotic Ivor Lewis esophagectomy is described.

Indications and Relative Contraindications to the Robotic Approach

After many years from its initial introduction, the robotic Ivor-Lewis has become the preferred approach in many centers for patients with resectable malignancies of the distal esophagus (Siewert tumors type I and II). As for the conventional thoracolaparoscopic technique, there are no absolute contraindications to the procedure, except for the inability to tolerate pneumoperitoneum. However, a history of gastric resection or previous open chest surgery is generally considered a relative contraindication to the minimally invasive approach.

INSTRUMENT REQUIREMENTS

The suggested main robotic instruments/tools can be listed as follows:
- 30°/0° scope
- Tip-up fenestrated grasper/Cadière forceps
- Maryland bipolar forceps
- Monopolar curved scissors/permanent cautery monopolar hook
- Needle drivers (round tip or macro)
- Vessel sealer
- SureForm™ Robotic Stapler: green cartridge (gastric conduit creation), white cartridge (division of azygos vein), and blue cartridge (esophagogastric anastomosis).
- Bipolar forceps
- Clip applier

The suggested main laparoscopic instruments/tools can be listed as follows:
- Graspers
- Scissors
- Needle drivers
- Suction-irrigation
- Alternative: Laparoscopic 60-mm stapler: green cartridge (gastric conduit creation)

Supplemental materials:
- Gauzes, sponges
- Hem-o-lok™ clips
- Sutures: PDS™ 3-0, Prolene™ 3-0/4-0, and V-Loc™ 3-0, and Ti-Cron™ 2-0
- Penrose drain

Photo reproduced with permission from Morris-Stiff G, Hughes LE. Ivor Lewis (1895-1982)-Welsh pioneer of the right-sided approach to the oesophagus. Dig Surg. 2003;20(6):546-552.
Quote reproduced with permission from Lewis I. The surgical treatment of carcinoma of the oesophagus; with special reference to a new operation for growths of the middle third. Br J Surg. 1946;34:18-31.

Abdominal Phase

Patient Positioning, OR Setup, and Port Setting

The patient is placed supine, with the legs apart. A 30° reverse Trendelenburg position is given, and the robot is positioned on the right side of the patient (**Figure 12-1**).

The assistant surgeon stands between the patient's legs. The pneumoperitoneum is obtained using the Veress needle in the left hypochondrium. Three 8-mm robotic cannulas and a 12-mm robotic port (R2, right pararectal line, for the robotic stapler) are placed along a straight line in the upper quadrants. Two laparoscopic assistant ports are placed, one 12 mm and one 5 mm, on both sides of the scope at a lower level as illustrated in **Figure 12-2**.

The robot is docked, and targeting is done pointing at the esophageal hiatus (**Figure 12-3**).

The tip-up fenestrated grasper/Cadière forceps is installed in the R3, the Maryland bipolar forceps/robotic stapler in the R2, and the R1 is used to maneuver the monopolar scissors, the large needle driver, or the vessel sealer as needed during the dissection. The scope is placed between the R1 and the R2 at the intersection of the mamillary line.

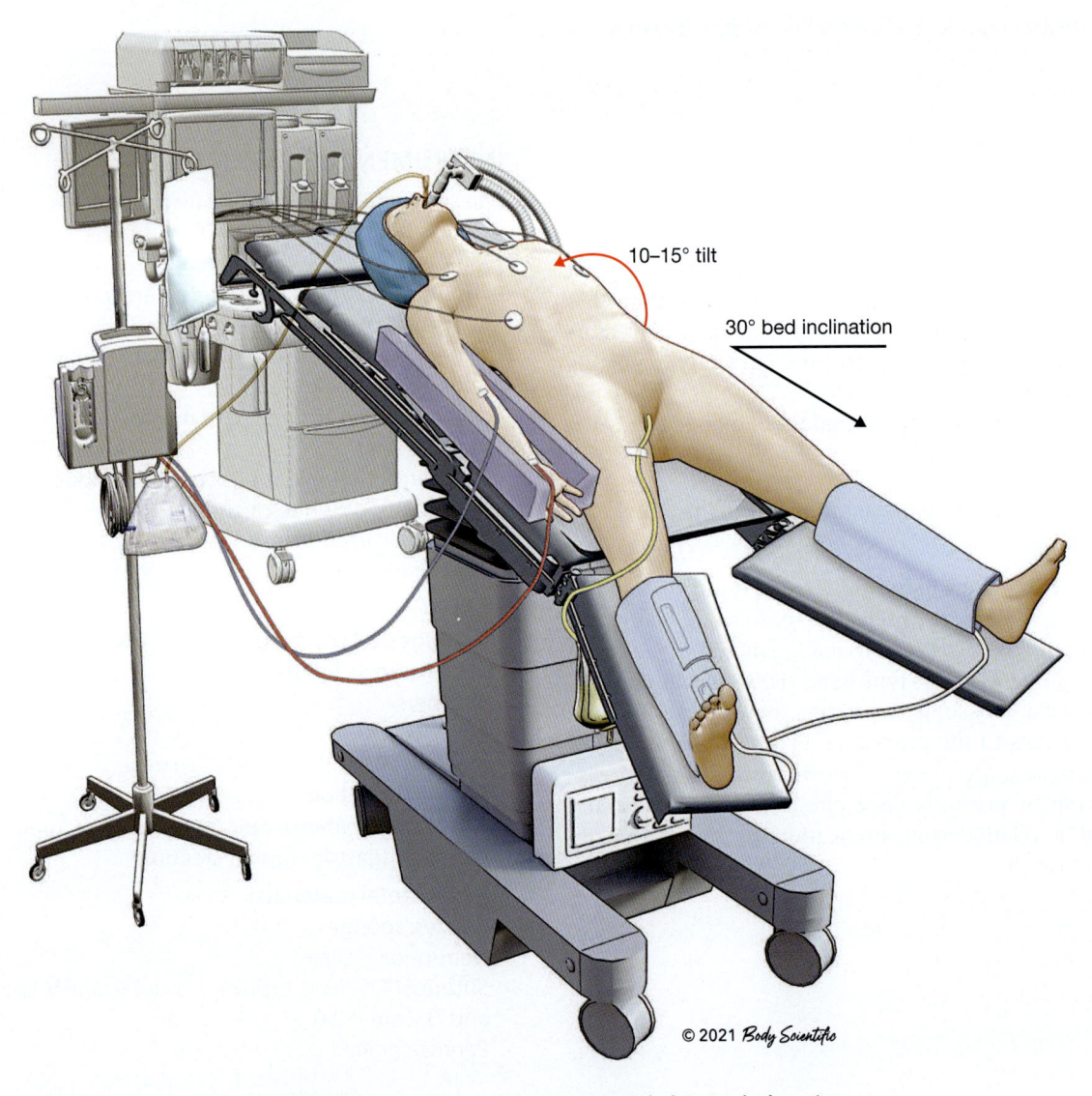

FIGURE 12-1 • Patient positioning (abdominal phase).

Ivor-Lewis Esophagectomy   211

▶▶ **TIPS**

The robotic ports are generally placed along a horizontal line passing through the center of the abdomen, which often corresponds to the level of the umbilicus. Depending on the conformation of the abdomen, ports may be placed more cranially (for more details see Chapter 2, The Basic Principles of Clinical applications). A careful evaluation of the internal abdominal anatomy is performed for an accurate robotic port placement. Especially for the optic trocar position, it is important to consider the height of the esophageal hiatus.

Although a 30° camera is mostly used during the operation, the 0° scope is performing better during the transhiatal mediastinal dissection, improving the visualization. The operative field becomes a kind of long tunnel at this point and the 0 scope has a better positioning in this narrow space.

EDITORIAL NOTE

An extra assistant port could be placed on the right side, between the scope and the R2. This will allow the bedside assistant to work with 2 hands and to use the laparoscopic stapler (during the gastric conduit creation) with a more favorable angle.

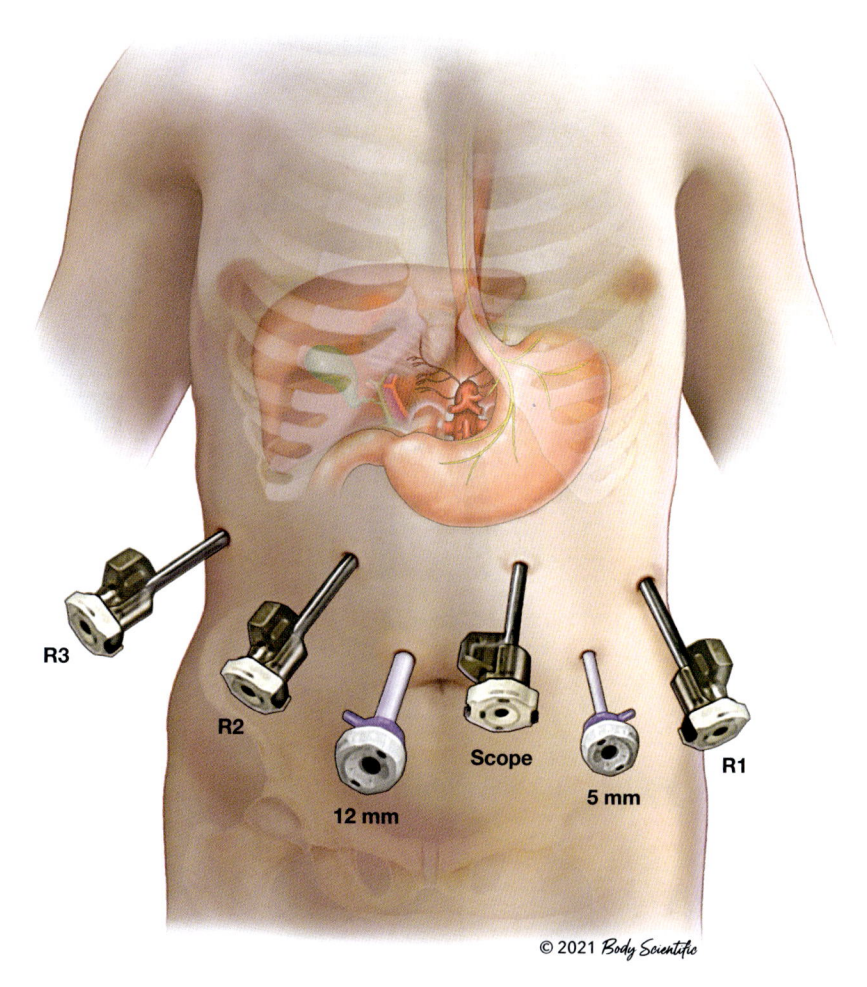

FIGURE 12-2 • Port setting (abdominal phase).

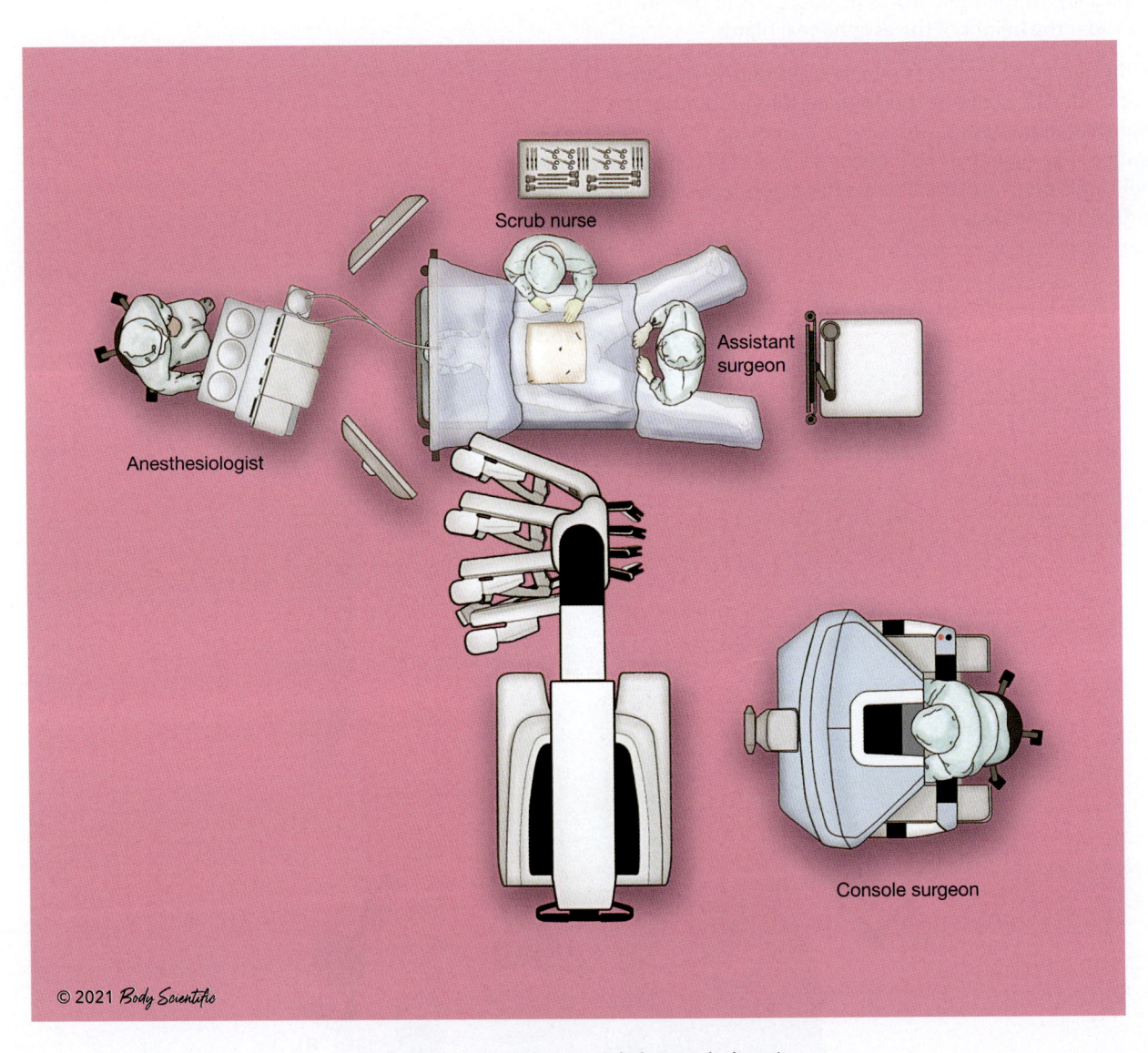

FIGURE 12-3 • OR setup (abdominal phase).

Surgical Technique

Step 1. General exploration

On entering the peritoneal cavity, a careful inspection is carried out to rule out any evidence of disseminated disease. It is mandatory to perform a meticulous examination and confirm resectability before performing any irreversible step. In case of lower esophagus tumors, special attention should be paid to rule out carcinomatosis in the area of the hiatus and of the celiac trunk.

Step 1 average time frame: 3–5 min

Step 2. Preliminary dissection of the hiatus

▶ **Video 12-1. Esophageal Hiatus Dissection**

Before starting formal dissection of the stomach, it is always convenient to anticipate the hiatus dissection to confirm resectability (mainly for advanced or bulky tumors). To expose the hiatus, the liver's left lobe is lifted and retracted to the right by using the tip-up grasper or the Cadière forceps with a sponge (R3). The assistant surgeon retracts the stomach downward to facilitate the dissection.

The gastrohepatic ligament is divided, and the dissection is carried out toward the right diaphragmatic crus. The paracardial lymph nodes (station 16) are left attached to the esophagogastric junction. The hiatus is entered, and the anterior phrenoesophageal membrane (Laimer-Bertelli membrane) is divided. The dissection proceeds anteriorly, and the peritoneal reflection between the diaphragm and the abdominal esophagus is opened. Afterward, the left diaphragmatic crus is dissected. The paracardial lymph nodes on this side are also left attached to the specimen.

The esophagogastric junction is released circumferentially from its peridiaphragmatic attachments, and it is encircled with a tape to facilitate its traction. At this point, the tip-up forceps (R3) is used to expose the inferior mediastinum lifting and retracting the right pillar. A preliminary dissection is conducted in front of the aorta just enough to understand the extension of the cancer. This step ends here to avoid the risk of opening the pleura, which can worsen the patient's ventilation and lead to bulging of the diaphragm dome into the abdomen. The complete lymphadenectomy of the lower mediastinum will be part of a later step of the procedure. The goal of this phase is to confirm the tumor's resectability and to identify landmarks that will facilitate the following steps. In particular, this will help with the takedown of the short gastric vessels closest to the esophagogastric junction.

Step 2 average time frame: 15–20 min

> ▶▶ **TIPS**
>
> Lesions of the lower esophagus extending beyond the esophageal wall require an en bloc resection of periesophageal tissue for oncologic safety. If the lesion involves the diaphragmatic pillars, a partial resection of them may be necessary.
>
> If the hiatus needs to be enlarged to facilitate the passage of the gastric conduit, it is better to divide the left crus instead of the right because it is more distant from the thoracic duct.

> ⚠ **PITFALLS**
>
> - Postoperative hiatal hernia due to an excessive opening of the hiatus.
> - There is risk of thoracic duct injury at the level of esophageal hiatus during a too lateral/posterior dissection on the right side.

Step 3. Opening of the gastrocolic ligament

Video 12-2. Opening of the Gastrocolic Ligament, Right Colonic Flexure Mobilization, and Kocher Maneuver

By using the tip-up grasper in the R3, the stomach is lifted by gentle traction on the anterior aspect of the greater curvature. Paying attention to preserve the right gastroepiploic artery, the gastrocolic ligament is divided with the vessel sealer, and the lesser sac is entered. The stomach is now retracted ventrally and superiorly, and the dissection continues to the right toward the duodenum.

Step 3 average time frame: 10–15 min

> **ANATOMICAL HIGHLIGHTS**
>
> - Gastric arterial supply (**Figure 12-4**).
> - Anatomical variations of the gastroepiploic arcade (**Figures 12-5 A–D**). (Multiple anatomical variations can occur, and these can be classified in different ways; for more information, see suggested reading #2.)

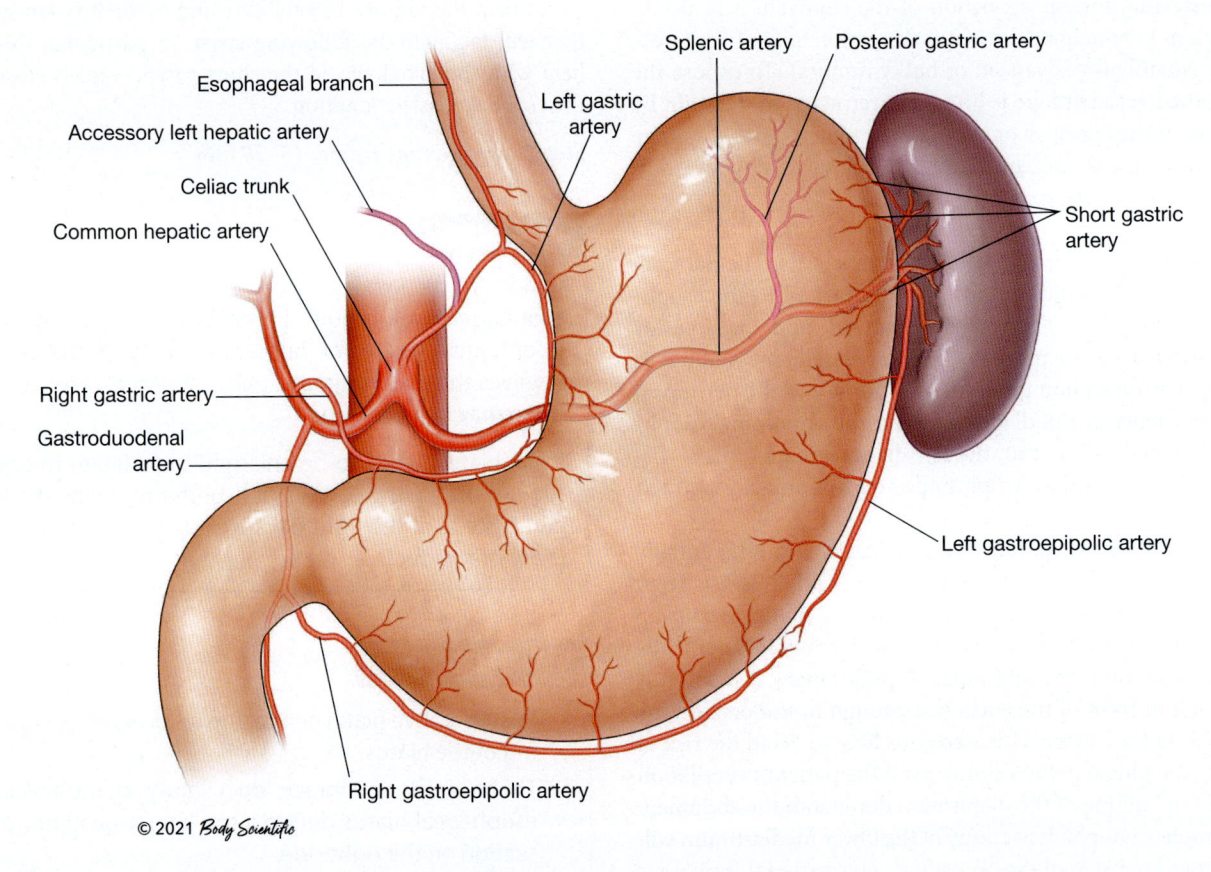

FIGURE 12-4 • Gastric arterial supply.

Ivor-Lewis Esophagectomy 215

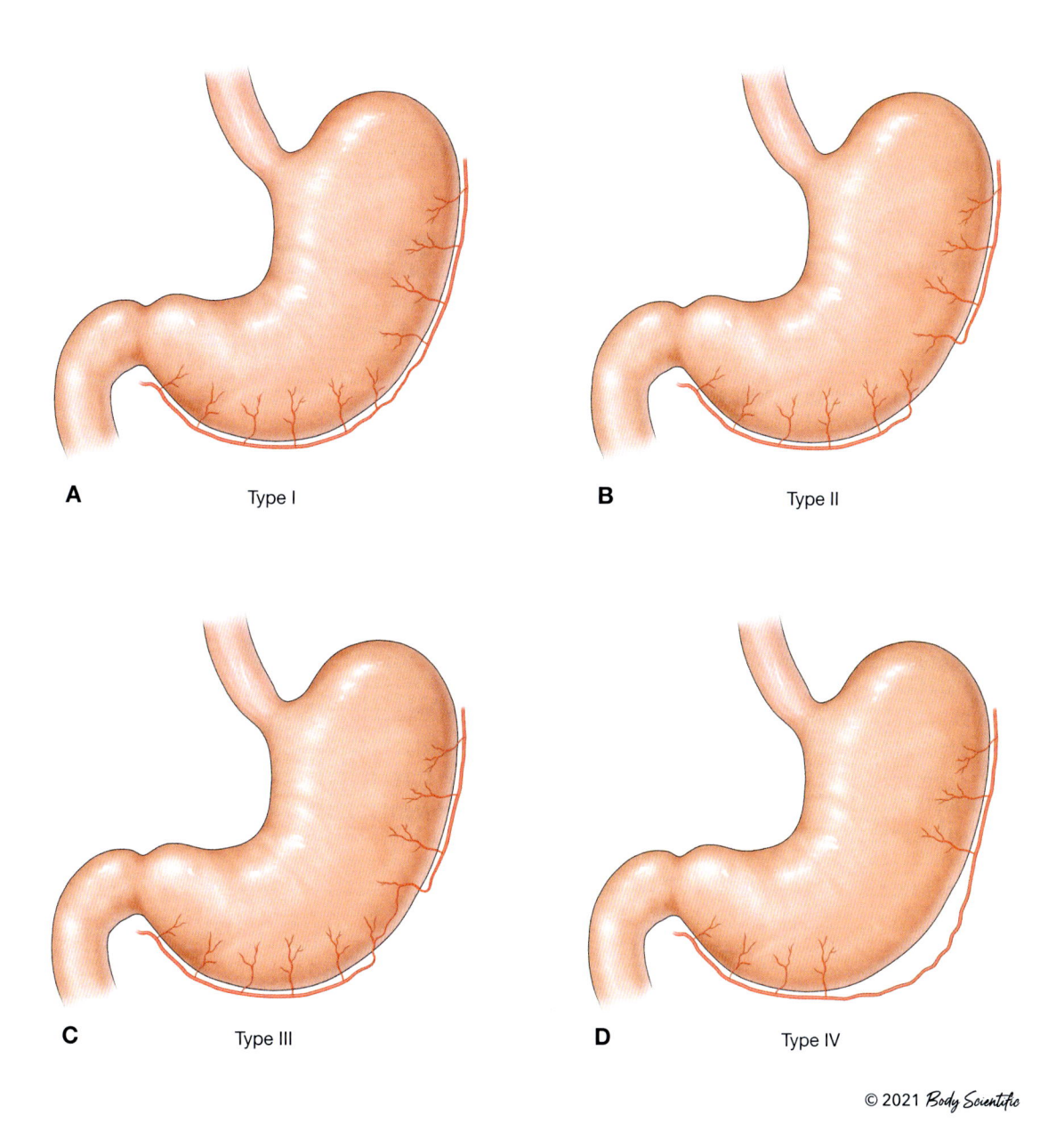

A Type I

B Type II

C Type III

D Type IV

© 2021 Body Scientific

FIGURE 12-5 • Anatomical variations of the gastroepiploic arcade.

Step 4. Right colonic flexure mobilization and Kocher maneuver

The right colic flexure is detached. With an atraumatic grasper, the assistant surgeon helps by retracting the colon downward and medially. The right colic flexure is partially mobilized to expose the second portion of the duodenum.

At this point, a partial Kocher maneuver is performed to lift the pylorus to the level of the esophageal hiatus. The second portion of the duodenum is retracted medially, and the peritoneal reflection immediately lateral to the duodenum is incised starting from the Winslow foramen. The avascular plane between the inferior vena cava and posterior surface of the duodenum/head of the pancreas is carefully dissected. The mobilization is completed after resecting the peritoneal attachments on the corner between the second and third portion of the duodenum.

Step 4 average time frame: 10–15 min

> **▶▶ TIPS**
>
> The Kocher maneuver must be adequate enough to mobilize the pylorus up to the hiatus. This will increase the length of the gastric conduit and, if needed, will allow resection of its upper portion (most prone to vascular insufficiency).

Step 5. Short gastric vessel dissection

The dissection of the gastrocolic ligament is continued to the left. Special care must be taken to avoid injuring the right gastroepiploic artery and the gastroepiploic arcade, which represents the main blood supply of the gastric conduit. To do so, the dissection is performed a few centimeters away from the greater curvature. After meeting the first short gastric vessel, the arcade is usually absent, and the dissection can become closer to the stomach's greater curvature. In this way, the short gastric arteries are divided with a longer stump on the splenic side to decrease the chances of delayed bleeding. This concept and the anatomical variations of the left gastroepiploic artery are illustrated in **Figures 12-6 A–D**.

The short gastric vessels are dissected to the level of the left diaphragmatic pillar (previously exposed in Step 2) using the vessel sealer mounted in the R1.

In most cases, the short gastric vessel's dissection can be performed in 1 step. In some instances, where the pericardial gastric vessels are very short, the dissection can be completed after the division of the left gastric artery and the celiac lymphadenectomy. This maneuver allows stretching of the posterior fundus and better control of the spleno-pancreato-gastric corner.

Step 5 average time frame: 20–30 min

> **🔍 ANATOMICAL HIGHLIGHTS**
>
> Anatomical variations of the left gastroepiploic artery (**Figures 12-6 A–D**). (For more information, see suggested reading #2.)

> **▶▶ TIPS**
>
> During this phase, an omental flap may be prepared by preserving 1 or 2 omental branches of the upper gastroepiploic arcade. This will be used as a buttress to cover the intrathoracic esophagogastric anastomosis.

> **⚠ PITFALLS**
>
> - Bleeding or thermal injury to the gastric wall during the short gastric vessel dissection.
> - Delayed bleeding from an unstable hemostasis on very short gastric vessel stumps (transfixing stitches of Prolene™ 3/0 may be indicated).

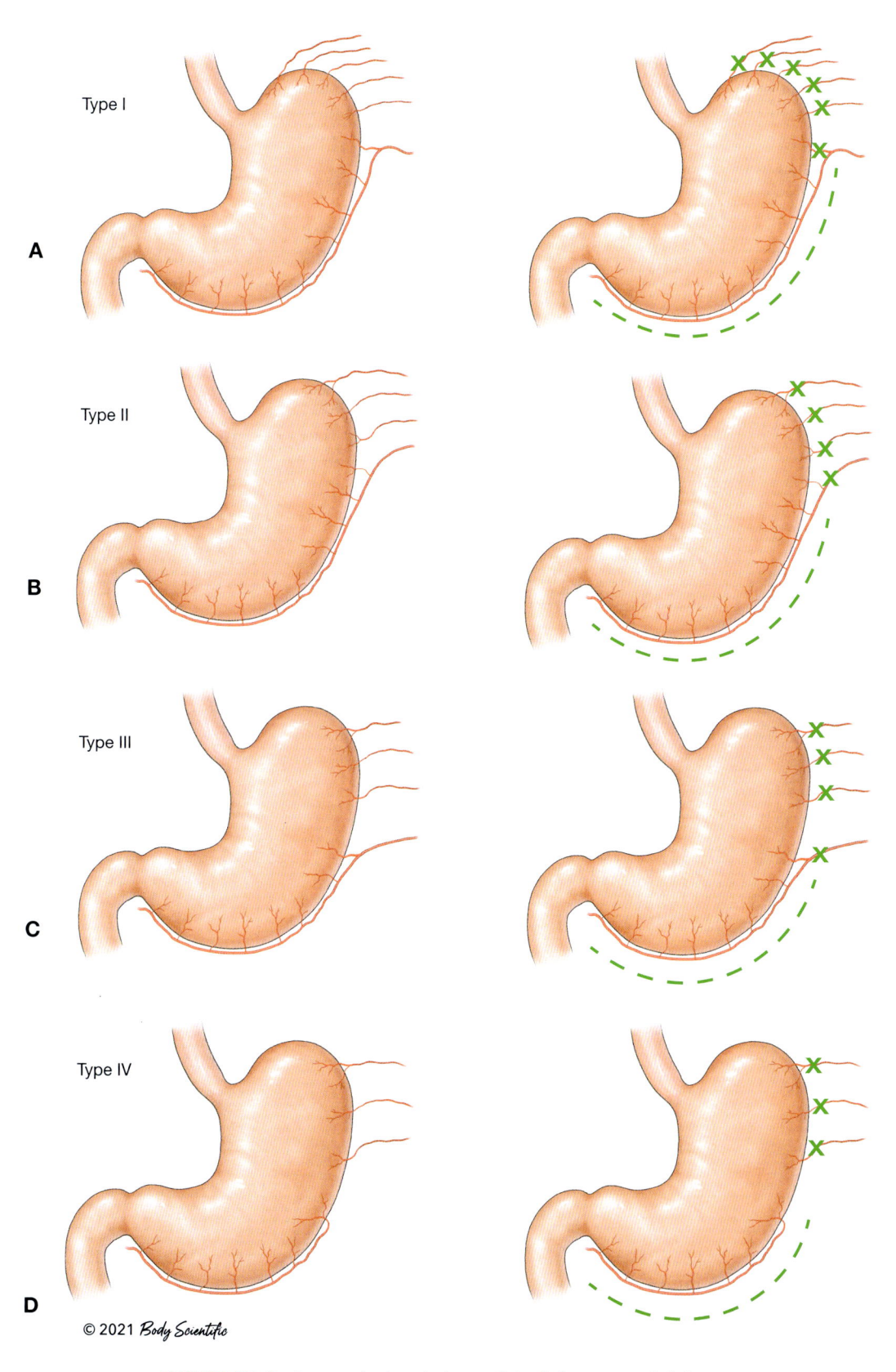

FIGURE 12-6 • Anatomical variations of the left gastroepiploic artery.

Step 6. Celiac lymphadenectomy

▶ **Video 12-3. Celiac Lymphadenectomy**

By using the tip-up grasper in the R3, the posterior wall of the stomach is lifted. This maneuver will put under tension the peritoneum covering the left gastric artery and vein. This peritoneal fold will join the pancreas in a T-shape configuration.

The lymphadenectomy is started coming down from the hepatic hilum following the proper hepatic artery. The right gastric artery is identified and resected. The common hepatic, left gastric, and splenic arteries are visualized. The common hepatic artery is prepared, and the lymph nodes along its superior border (station 18) are dissected toward its origin on the celiac trunk. In a similar way, the proximal part of the splenic artery is skeletonized to harvest its lymph nodes (station 19). Afterward, the left gastric vein is identified, dissected toward its base, and divided between sutures. The left gastric artery is typically found just cephalad to the coronary vein. The lymph nodes around the artery are dissected and swept upward into the specimen (station 17). The left gastric artery is divided with the vascular stapler (R2) at its origin in the celiac trunk.

Finally, the fatty and nodal tissue around the celiac trunk (station 20) and between the left gastric artery stump and diaphragmatic crus is removed to complete the lymphadenectomy.

Step 6 average time frame: 15–20 min

> 🔍 **ANATOMICAL HIGHLIGHTS**
>
> Lymph nodal stations map for esophageal cancer (**Figures 12-7 A–C**).

> ▶▶ **TIPS**
>
> To dissect the left gastric pedicle, a vertical lifting of the stomach with the tip-up grasper (R3) may be a useful maneuver. It allows a better identification and an easier dissection at the base of the artery and vein.

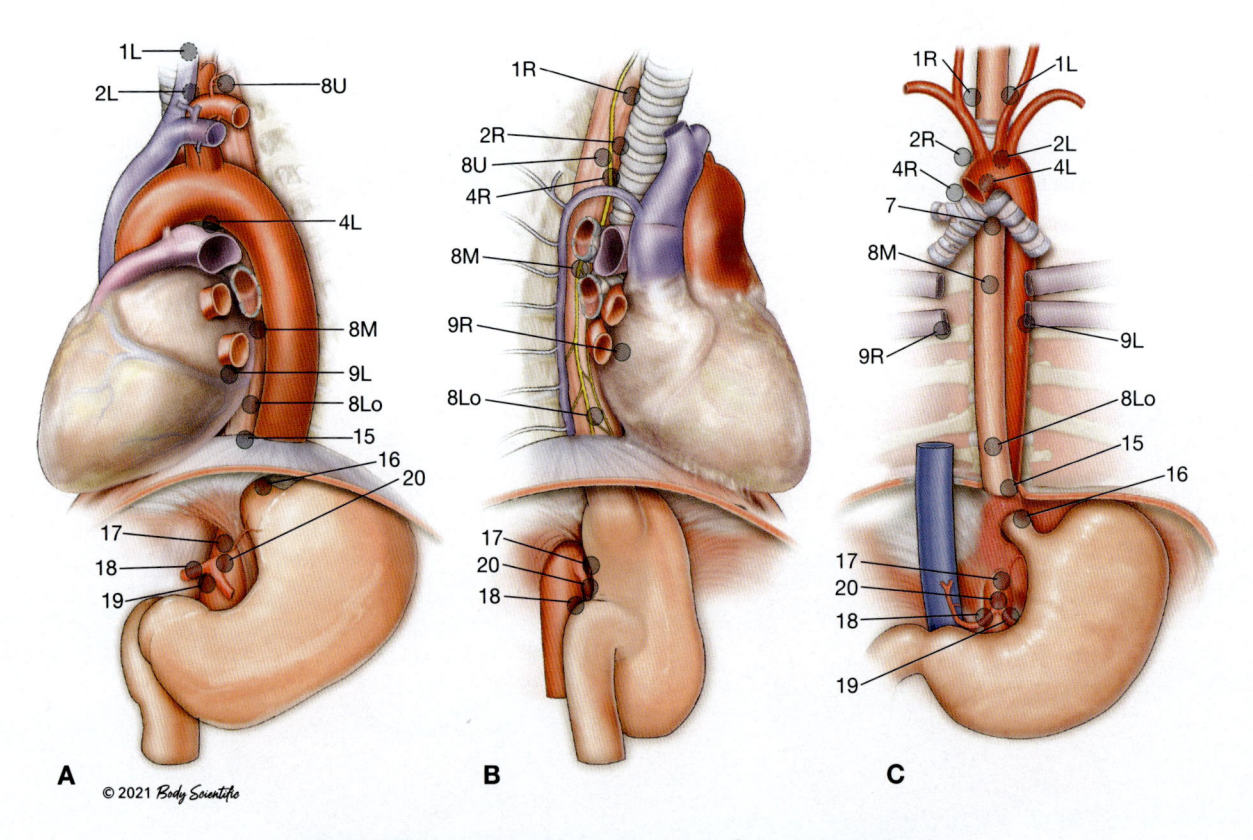

FIGURE 12-7 • Lymph nodal stations map for esophageal cancer.

Step 7. Division of the lesser curvature

▶ **Video 12-4.** Division of the Lesser Curvature, Gastric Conduit Creation, Mediastinal Dissection, and Pyloric Release (Feeding Jejunostomy)

The *incisura angularis* along the lesser curvature is skeletonized. Afterward, the robotic stapler is introduced through the R2. Alternatively, the laparoscopic stapler can be used through the 12-mm assistant port on the right side. The first gastric section is performed horizontally, staying approximately 5–6 cm proximal to the pylorus. The perigastric lymph nodes along the upper portion of the lesser curvature are left attached and removed with the specimen. This maneuver will separate the oncologic segment from the gastric conduit.

Step 7 average time frame: 5–10 min

Step 8. Gastric conduit creation and transhiatal mediastinum dissection completion

A 4–5-cm wide gastric conduit is created by means of sequential sections toward the gastric fundus. Care must be taken to keep the staple line as straight as possible by stretching the stomach from the fundus tip (**Figures 12-8 A–D**).

Before the last stapling, the transhiatal mediastinum dissection is completed. The Penrose drain helps with the distal esophagus retraction to allow a circumferential dissection into the mediastinum. The transhiatal dissection is completed when the aorta and pericardium are exposed.

Indocyanine green (ICG) fluorescence is used to check adequate perfusion of the conduit (**Figure 12-8B**). Intersection points of the staple line along the gastric conduit are reinforced with Prolene™ sutures 3/0. After the gastric conduit is completely transected, it is anchored with mattress sutures to the specimen to facilitate the pull-up into the chest and to maintain its correct orientation (**Figure 12-8D**). An alternative way is to leave a short bridge of gastric tissue connecting the specimen to the conduit that will be divided later in the chest.

Step 8 average time frame: 30–50 min

> **ANATOMICAL HIGHLIGHTS**
>
> Gastric conduit creation (**Figures 12-8 A–D**).

> **▶▶ TIPS**
>
> The creation of the gastric conduit starts 5–6 cm proximal to the pylorus, at the lesser curvature, and continues cranially to the 3° or 4° parietal branch of the right gastric artery (depending on the anatomy). The right gastric vascularization of the antrum-pyloric region is preserved.
>
> During this step, the distance between the cardia and the upper portion of conduit must be considered, especially for Siewert type II tumors, to ensure an adequate distal margin.
>
> If a laparoscopic stapling technique is utilized for the creation of the gastric conduit, an assistant port in the right quadrant is usually necessary. This allows a better orientation of the stapler for the first horizontal staple line.

> **⚠ PITFALLS**
>
> - A too wide gastric conduit (>5 cm) may entail a higher risk of delayed gastric emptying.
> - A too narrow gastric conduit (<4 cm) may increase the technical challenge of constructing the esophageal-gastric anastomosis and be the reason for postoperative digestive complains.
> - The oversewing of the staple line, with running sutures or figure 8 interrupted stitches, should be avoided because they may shorten the length of the conduit. If it is necessary to add sutures for hemostasis, single Prolene™ 3/0 stitches are the best option.

220 The Foundation and Art of Robotic Surgery

A

Surgical specimen
Left gastric artery (cut)
Gastric tube
5 cm

© 2021 Body Scientific

B

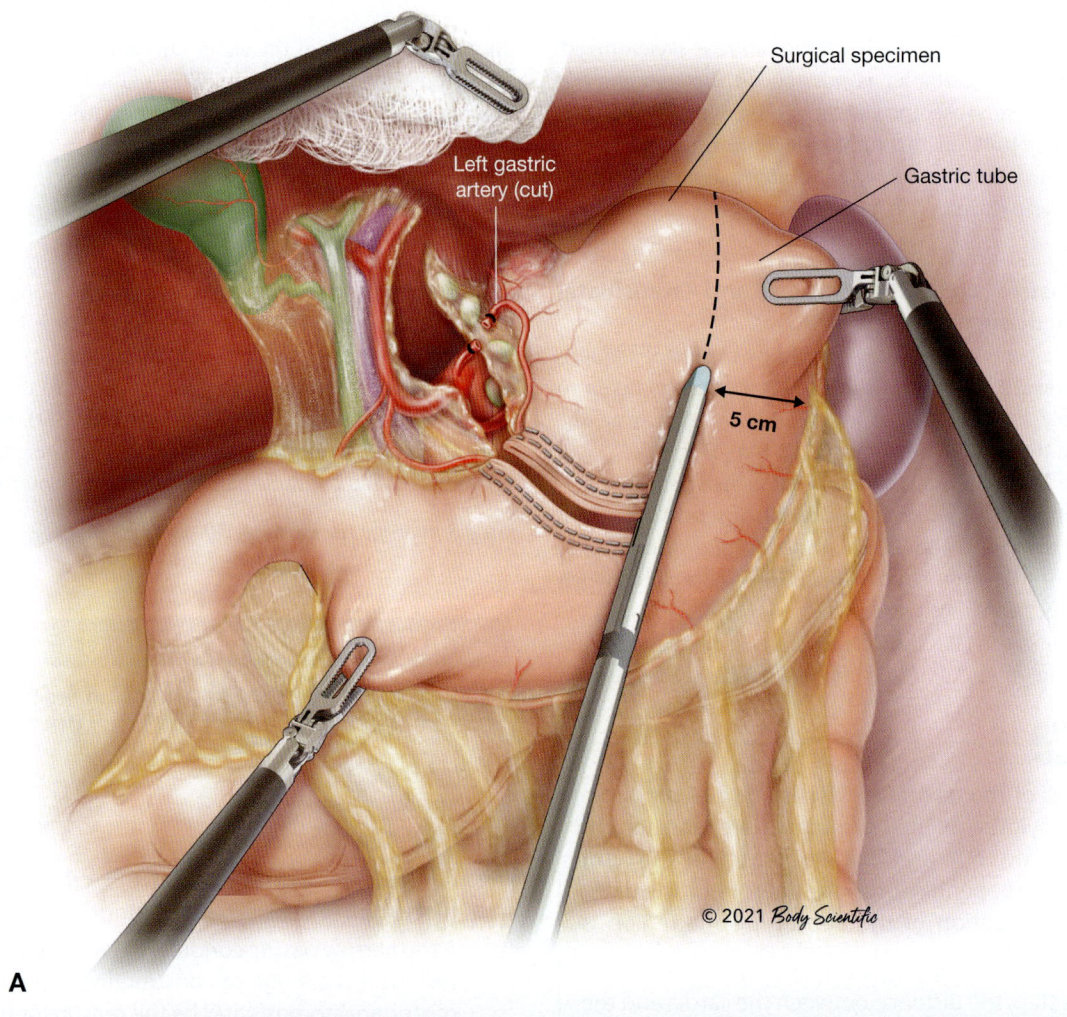

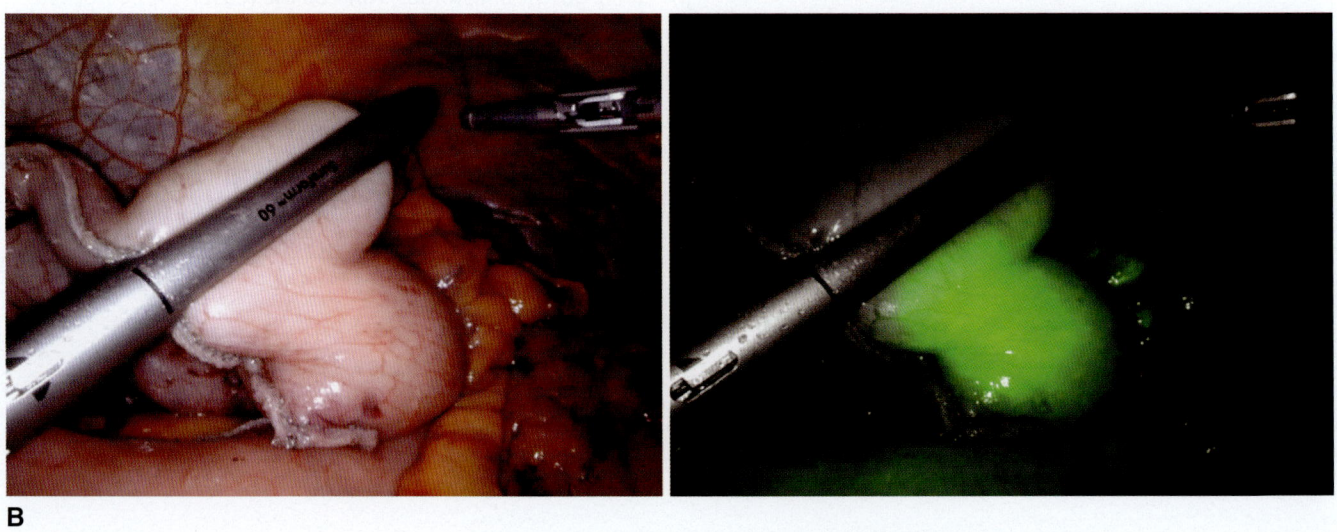

FIGURE 12-8 • Gastric conduit creation.

Ivor-Lewis Esophagectomy 221

C

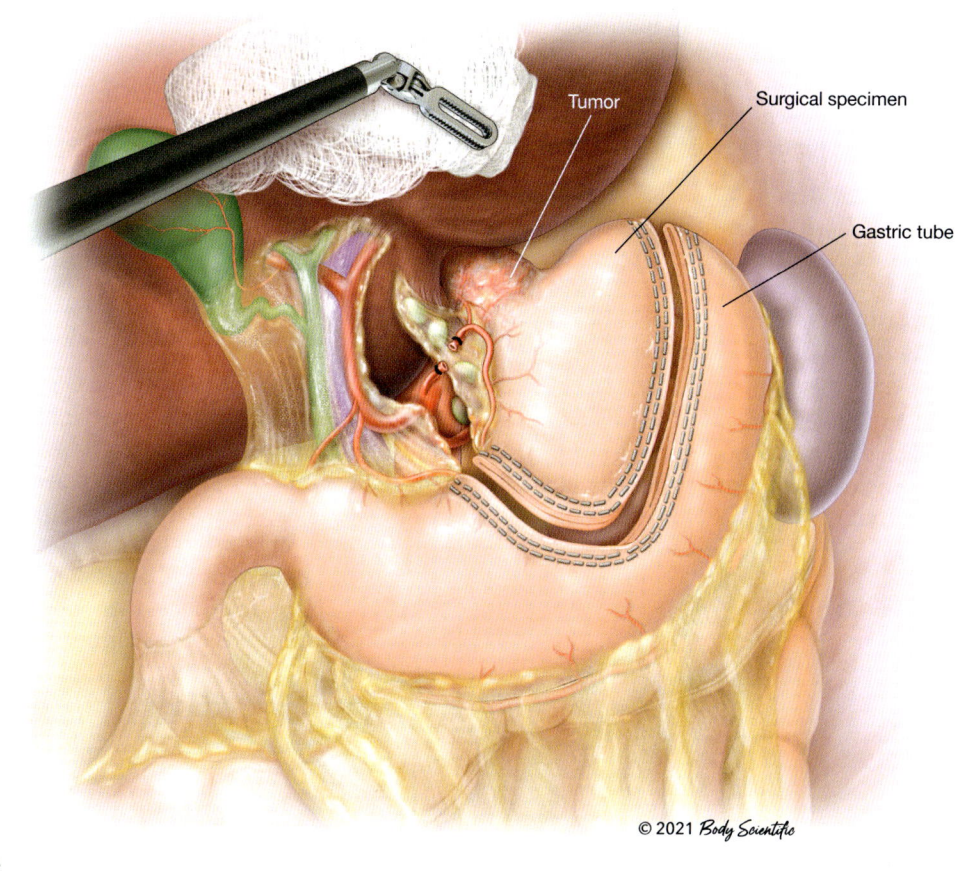

D

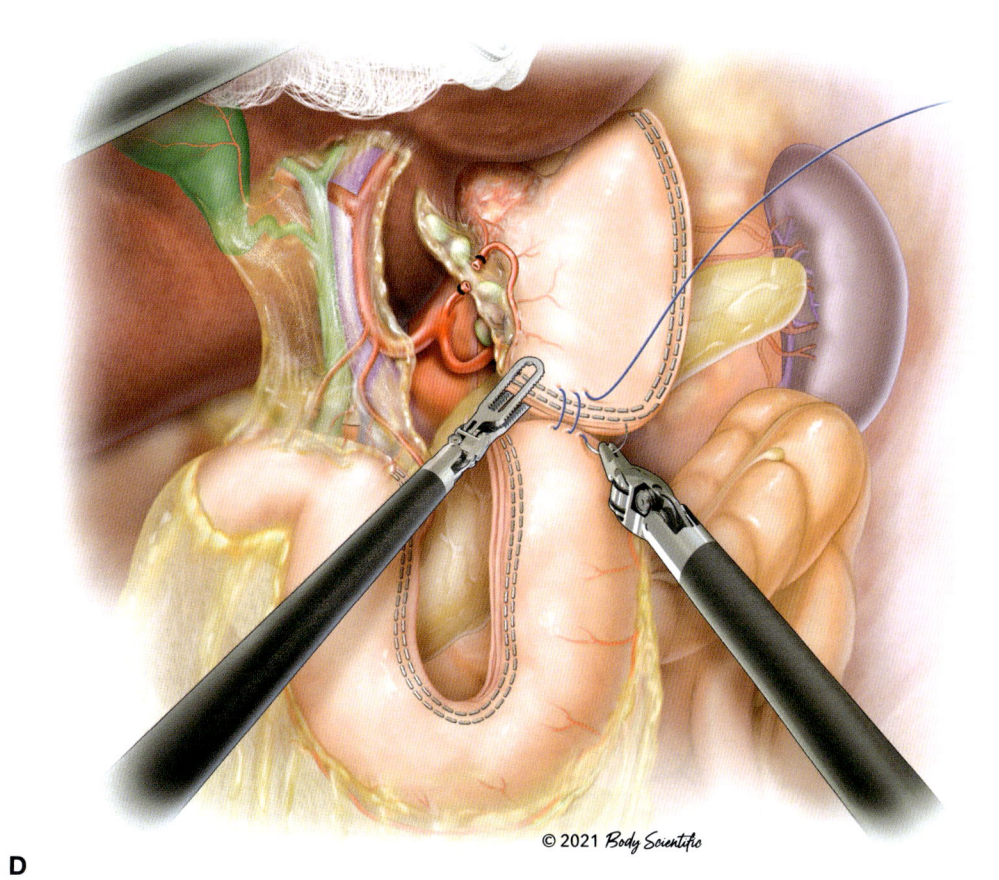

FIGURE 12-8 • *(Continued)*

Step 9. Pyloric release and feeding jejunostomy

Botulinum toxin type A injection may be used for the pyloric release. Finally, a feeding jejunostomy is created (when necessary), and brought out through the robotic port in the left lateral upper quadrant. The abdomen is thus deflated and the port sites are closed in a conventional fashion.

Step 9 average time frame: 20–30 min

> ▶▶ **TIPS**
>
> - Chemical pyloroplasty is performed by injecting botulinum toxin type A (100 UI in 5-mL sterile solution, divided in 4 boluses) in the 4 cardinal locations.
> - During the feeding jejunostomy creation, a trocar-in-trocar technique is used introducing the R1 in the assistant trocar to increase the distance between the cannula and the target.

> **EDITORIAL NOTE**
>
> The utility of pyloric drainage procedures (botulinum toxin injection, pyloroplasty, or pyloromyotomy) in the setting of esophageal resections is controversial. Advocates for routine pyloric drainage argue that it prevents early gastric outlet obstruction (associated with pyloric denervation) and reduces the risk of pulmonary aspiration, and anastomotic leaks. On the contrary, other authors suggest that gastric outlet obstruction is a rare event and pyloric drainage might result in additional complications such as those related to biliopancreatic reflux.
>
> **Feeding jejunostomy:** Adequate postoperative enteral nutrition has been shown to improve the outcomes of patients undergoing esophagectomy. A feeding jejunostomy is selectively placed in patients who underwent preoperative radiotherapy, who are malnourished, or who are at high risk of postoperative complications. It is important to notice that jejunostomies are not free of morbidity risks like dislodgement, leakage and obstruction.

Ivor-Lewis Esophagectomy 223

Thoracic Phase

Patient Positioning, OR Setup, and Port Setting

The patient is now placed in a left-sided (45°) semiprone position for the thoracoscopic step of the procedure. During this phase, a low-pressure pneumothorax of 6–8 mm Hg is maintained. The port setting for the thoracic phase of the procedure is shown in **Figure 12-9A**.

> **EDITORIAL NOTE**
>
> An alternative port setting, following a more transverse line along the base of the chest, is shown in **Figure 12-9B**. This configuration has the advantage of less instrument collision, mainly in the upper chest above the azygos vein where the dissection, lymphadenectomy, and potential suturing for the handsewn anastomosis might be necessary.

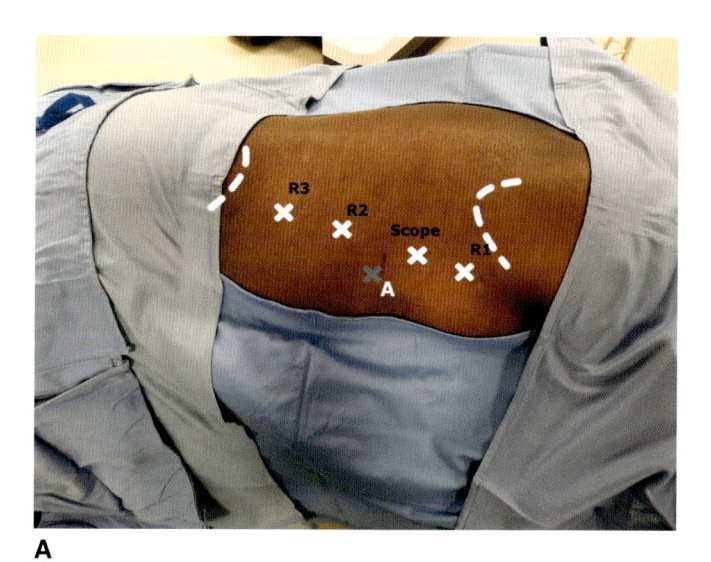

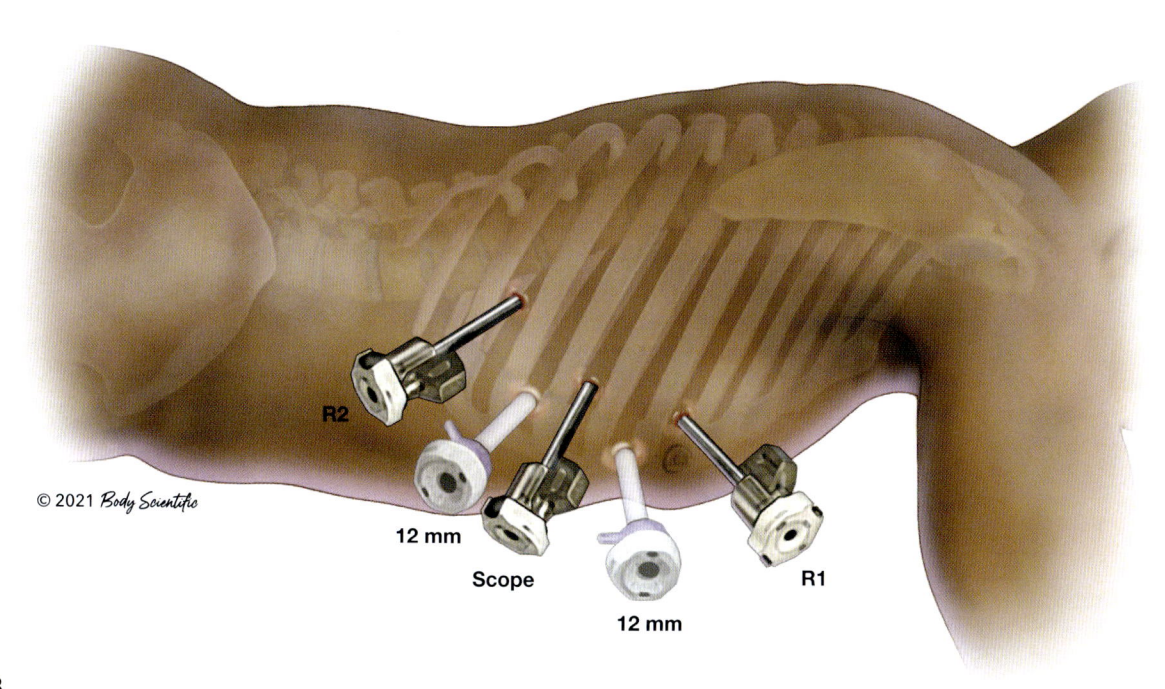

FIGURE 12-9 • Port setting (thoracic phase).

224 The Foundation and Art of Robotic Surgery

Targeting is performed pointing at the level of the azygos vein, a few centimeters below its arch. The tip-up fenestrated grasper, Maryland bipolar forceps/robotic stapler, and monopolar scissors are mounted on the R3, R2, and R1, respectively. On the R1, the large needle driver, or the vessel sealer, can replace the monopolar scissors as needed. The OR setup for the thoracic phase is shown in **Figure 12-10**.

> ▶▶ **TIPS**
>
> The robotic port placement follows an oblique line, extending from the 11th intercostal space at the level of the scapular line to the 4th intercostal space, just ventral to the scapula. A minimal 6-cm spacing should be maintained between the ports.
>
> The semiprone position has some advantages over the full prone or lateral one:
> 1. It provides faster patient positioning and a larger area for port placement.
> 2. It allows for a rapid conversion into an open procedure, if needed.
> 3. Single lung ventilation may be avoided.

> ⚠ **PITFALLS**
>
> Suboptimal trocar positioning or inadequate robotic cart targeting will significantly hinder the procedure by limiting instrument maneuverability and proper visualization.

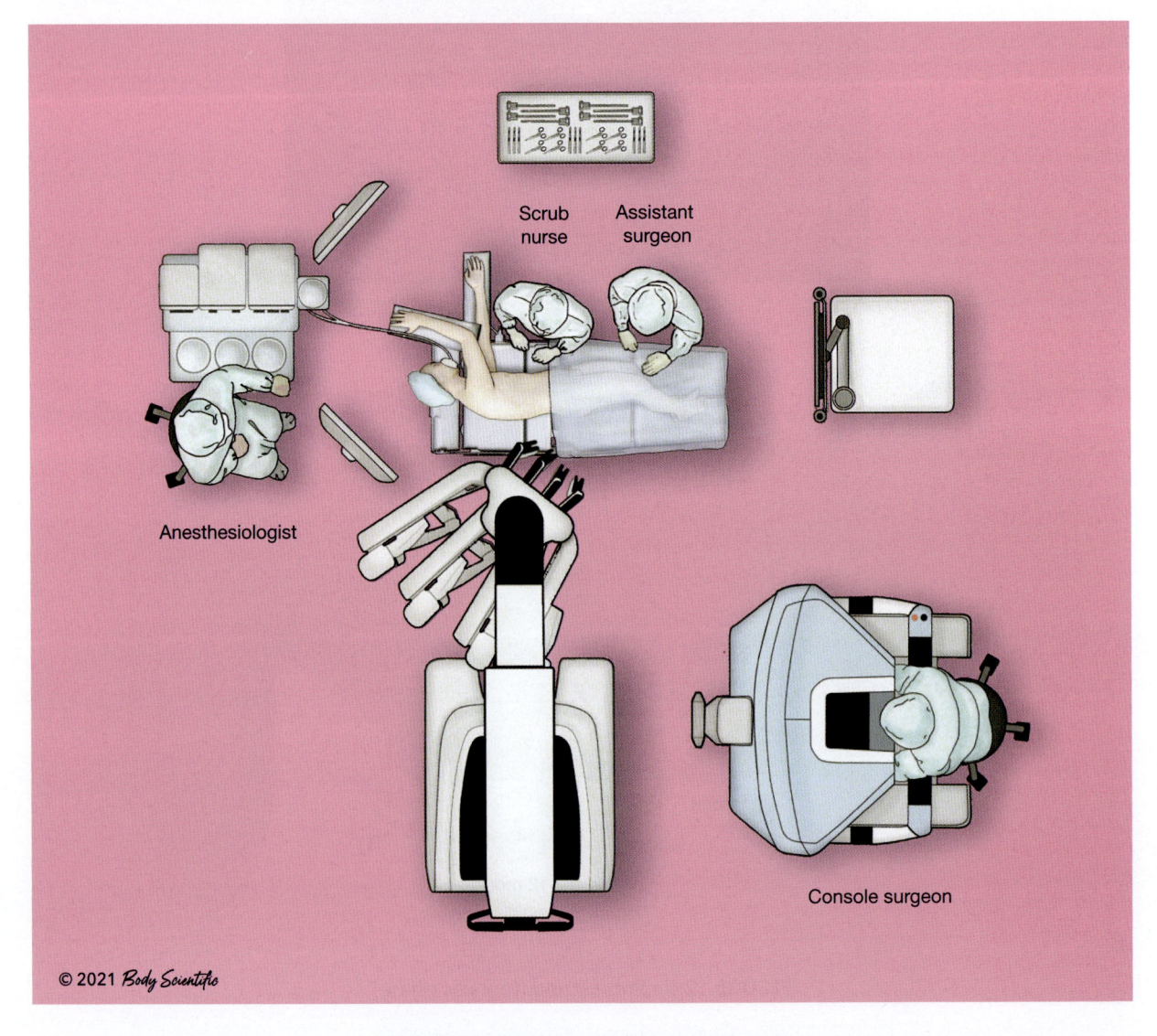

FIGURE 12-10 • OR setup (thoracic phase).

Step 10. Mobilization of the inferior pulmonary ligament and retraction of the lung

▶ **Video 12-5.** Mobilization of the Inferior Pulmonary Ligament, Opening of the Mediastinal Pleura, and Azygos Vein Division

The thoracic phase of the procedure starts with the division of the inferior pulmonary ligament with monopolar energy. At this point, the pulmonary ligament lymph nodes are resected (station 9).

Step 10 average time frame: 15–20 min

Step 11. Opening of the mediastinal pleura and azygos vein division

The mediastinal pleura between the thoracic esophagus and pericardium is retracted ventrally and divided in a caudal-to-cranial fashion. The dissection continues along the plane between the esophagus and the pericardium up to the carina; the right vagus nerve is sectioned under the homolateral bronchus. The arch of the azygos vein is next prepared and divided with the robotic stapler using a vascular cartridge. Afterward, the procedure continues with the division of the right bronchial artery (constantly located behind the arch of the azygos).

Step 11 average time frame: 15–20 min

▶▶ **TIPS**

The use of the robotic stapler may facilitate the control of the azygos and decrease the risk of injury of the vein connected with unexperienced handling of thoracoscopic instruments. The angle and the space to go around the azygos vein are very limited, and the rigidity of the intercostal space may further limit the maneuverability of straight instruments.

Step 12. Esophageal dissection, subcarinal mediastinal lymphadenectomy, and en bloc mesoesophagus removal

▶ **Video 12-6.** Esophageal Dissection, Subcarinal Mediastinal Lymphadenectomy, and En Bloc Mesoesophagus Removal

The pleura along the azygos vein is subsequently opened in a cranial-to-caudal direction. The descending aorta is then exposed. The esophagus is now encircled with a tape below the level of the carina, away from the area of the cancer, to facilitate downward retraction and exposure (**Figure 12-11**).

The procedure continues with the section of the mesoesophagus up to the diaphragm; the left mediastinal pleura and the aorta represent the deep limit of dissection during this step (if necessary for oncologic radicality, left pleura may be resected en bloc). Any esophageal branches from the aorta and lymphatics encountered during retroesophageal mobilization should be clipped or selectively ligated. The esophagus is thus mobilized en bloc with the paraoesophageal lymph nodes (station 8). This step ends with the resection of the subcarinal lymph nodes (station 7).

The thoracic duct if recognized, may be ligated and divided in the supradiaphragmatic area, as it emerges through the aortic hiatus, where less anatomic variations and branching are present.

Step 12 average time frame: 30–40 min

▶▶ **TIPS**

- The tape that encircles the esophagus facilitates the dissection and the resection of the mesoesophagus.
- Mediastinal dissection must start between the esophagus and the pericardium, which is the simplest and safest plane.
- It is advisable to separately perform the carinal lymphadenectomy because the en bloc esophagectomy is more complex, and may increase the risk of left bronchus injury.

⚠ PITFALLS

- Risk of thermal injury to the membranous wall of the airways: during subcarinal nodal dissection, judicious use of energy is crucial.
- Use of the Hem-o-lok™ clips on the arch of the azygos should be avoided: cases of transmural migration in the gastric conduit and trachea have been reported.
- Risk of aortic bleeding: prevention with selective control of little vessels using the Maryland bipolar forceps/robotic vessel sealer/selective Prolene™ 3/0-4/0 suturing.

EDITORIAL NOTE

Prophylactic thoracic duct ligation (TDL) during esophagectomy has been proposed to reduce the rates of postoperative chylothorax, an uncommon complication with a reported incidence of 0.6–9% (see suggested reading #7). However, several studies have shown inconsistent results regarding its effectiveness. Only ligation in the presence of intraoperative injury is universally accepted as a way of treating the chylothorax.

It also needs to be considered that TDL may have side effects that may negatively impact the normal immune function (T lymphocytes), fluid balance, nutritional status, and also the oncologic outcomes.

Injection of ICG in the groin is a technique that may help in visualizing the thoracic duct and avoid its injury during the mediastinal dissection.

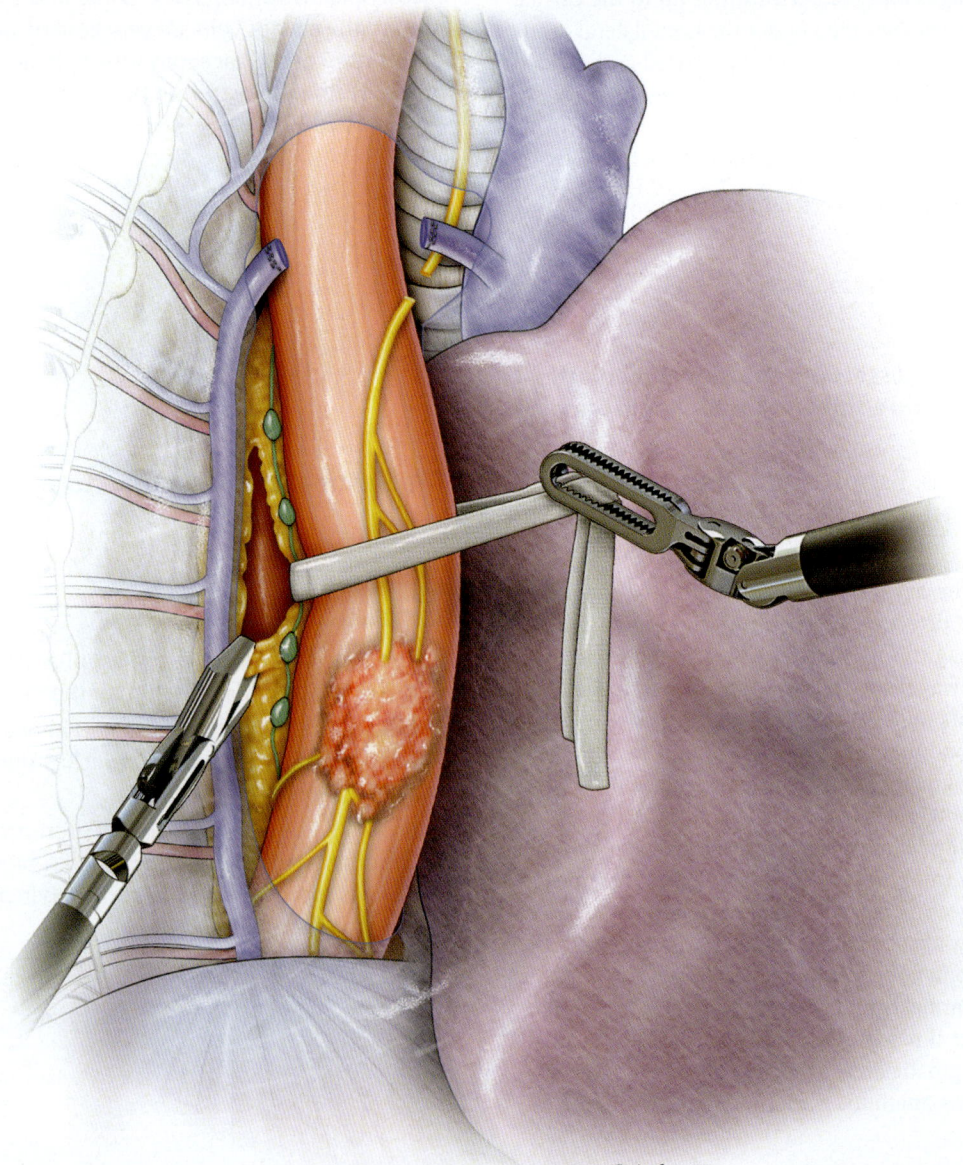

FIGURE 12-11 • Mediastinal dissection.

Step 13. Supracarinal lymphadenectomy

▶ **Video 12-7. Supracarinal Lymphadenectomy, Esophageal Transection, and Esophagogastric Anastomosis**

The procedure continues with the mobilization of the supracarinal esophagus up to 2–3 cm above the arch of the azygos vein. The lower paratracheal lymph nodes (station 4R) are removed en bloc. The proximal esophagus, above the azygos vein, is fully mobilized. Dissection must proceed very cautiously to avoid traction or direct damage to the left recurrent laryngeal nerve that passes under the aortic arch. According to the margins required, further cranial mobilization may be necessary: if concerns about the extent of the tumor exist, an intraoperative endoscopy may be considered before proceeding further.

In selected cases, lymphadenectomy is extended in the upper mediastinum (right and left paratracheal nodes, stations 2R/2L).

Step 13 average time frame: 20–30 min

▶▶ **TIPS**

The upper thoracic esophagus must be well mobilized, almost up to the superior mediastinum, not only to complete the lymphadenectomy but also to facilitate the anastomosis. This mobilization must be completed before the esophageal transection, to avoid subsequent maneuvers to free up the stump that are more difficult and may require multiple grasping of the proximal esophagus with risk of damages.

Step 14. Esophageal transection and esophagogastric anastomosis

Once completely free, the specimen with the anchored conduit is delivered into the thorax (**Figure 12-12**).

Attention must be paid to ensure that the longitudinal staple line is appropriately oriented to avoid twisting of the conduit. The esophagus is dissected circumferentially and transected using monopolar scissors between the carina and the arch of the azygos vein (**Figure 12-13**).

If necessary, a frozen section line of the margins can be sent. The distal margin of the esophagus is then sutured. The specimen is separated from the gastric conduit by dividing the sutures placed during the abdominal phase or dividing the connecting bridge. At this point, the perfusion of both, the gastric conduit and the esophageal stump, is again assessed with ICG fluorescence (**Figure 12-14**).

A side-to-side stapled anastomosis is usually performed. The gastric conduit is located between the upper esophagus (widely mobilized) and the trachea. The apex of the gastric conduit is anchored to the posterior esophageal muscular layer with 2 interrupted, untied nonabsorbable stitches (Ti-Cron™ 2-0). Afterward, the lumen of the esophageal stump is fixed to the gastric conduit with an absorbable suture (PDS™ 3-0). A 2-cm transverse gastrotomy (on the posterior wall of the gastric conduit, anteriorly of the operative field) is performed, at least 2 cm away from the lateral staple line (**Figure 12-15A**). The robotic stapler (R2) is inserted through the transected esophagus and the gastrotomy. At this point, the stapler is fired, creating a 3-cm side-to-side esophagogastric anastomosis (**Figure 12-15B**). The nasogastric tube is advanced through the anastomosis into the gastric conduit and the remaining enterotomy is closed transversally with 2 semicontinuous running barbed sutures (V-Loc™ 3-0) or PDS 3/0 (**Figure 12-15C**). The anastomosis is completed with a few interrupted PDS™ 3-0 stitches. It is not a real second layer: these are only stitches placed to reduce the tension of the continuous suture.

After the esophagogastric anastomosis is completed, a methylene blue test is performed, and a portion of the greater omentum, transposed with the conduit, is used to cover the anastomosis (**Figure 12-17**).

Step 14 average time frame: 20–30 min

EDITORIAL COMMENT

The esophagogastric anastomosis creation is one of the most critical steps of the Ivor-Lewis operation. The most commonly used anastomotic techniques include the following:

- **Side-to-side linear stapled anastomosis** is wider and less prone to strictures.
- **Transthoracic circular stapled end-to-end anastomosis (EEA)** is less time consuming but needs a skilled bedside assistant to position and deploy the stapler. In patients with narrow intercostal spaces, it might be challenging to insert the shaft.
- **Transoral anvil (OrVil™) EEA** may avoid the need of a purse-string if the proximal stump was stapled.
- **Handsewn EEA** requires expertise because it is more technically challenging. It is especially useful for high intrathoracic anastomosis and shorter conduits (**Figures 12-16 A–D**).

EDITORIAL COMMENT

Barbed sutures have the advantage of maintaining the approximation of the anastomotic edges but the disadvantage of not allowing a perfect visualization of the corners since the suture cannot be momentarily loosen to appreciate the details of the anatomy.

228 The Foundation and Art of Robotic Surgery

> ▶▶ **TIPS**
> - The suture used to anchor the upper part of the gastric conduit and the esophageal lumen facilitates the alignment of the stumps for the stapled anastomosis.
> - The robotic technique, allowing a direct control by the console surgeon, makes the placement of the stapler easier compared with the conventional thoracoscopic technique.

> ⚠ **PITFALLS**
> - Difficult alignment of the esophageal stump and gastric conduit due to a limited mobilization of the upper thoracic esophagus.
> - A gastrotomy too close to the gastric conduit's staple line might increase the risk of microischemia on this side of the anastomosis.

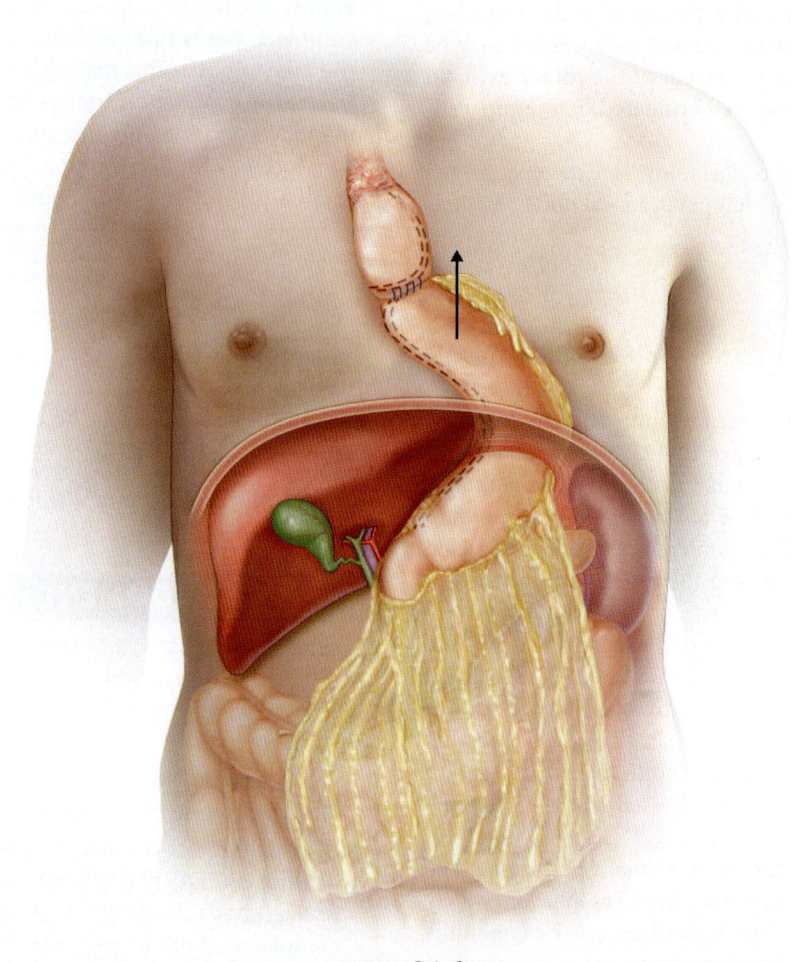

FIGURE 12-12 • Gastric pull-up.

Ivor-Lewis Esophagectomy 229

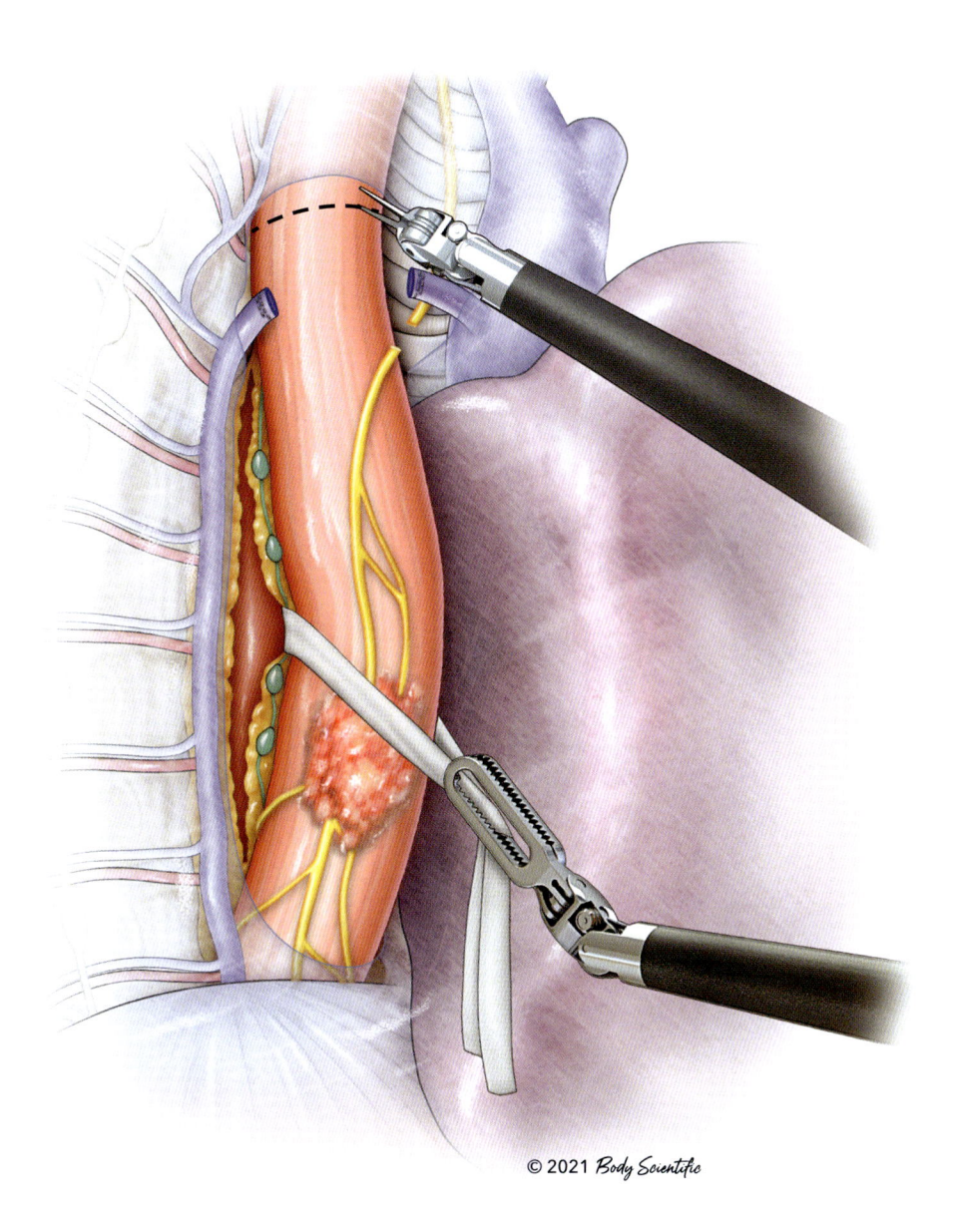

FIGURE 12-13 • Esophageal transection.

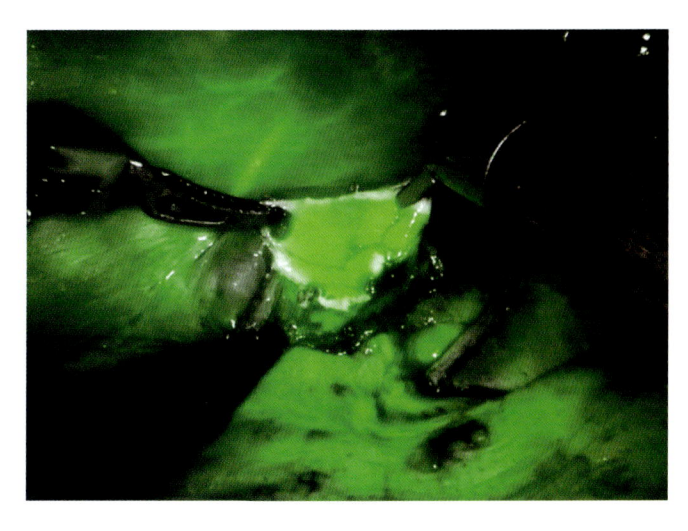

FIGURE 12-14 • ICG perfusion assessment.

230 The Foundation and Art of Robotic Surgery

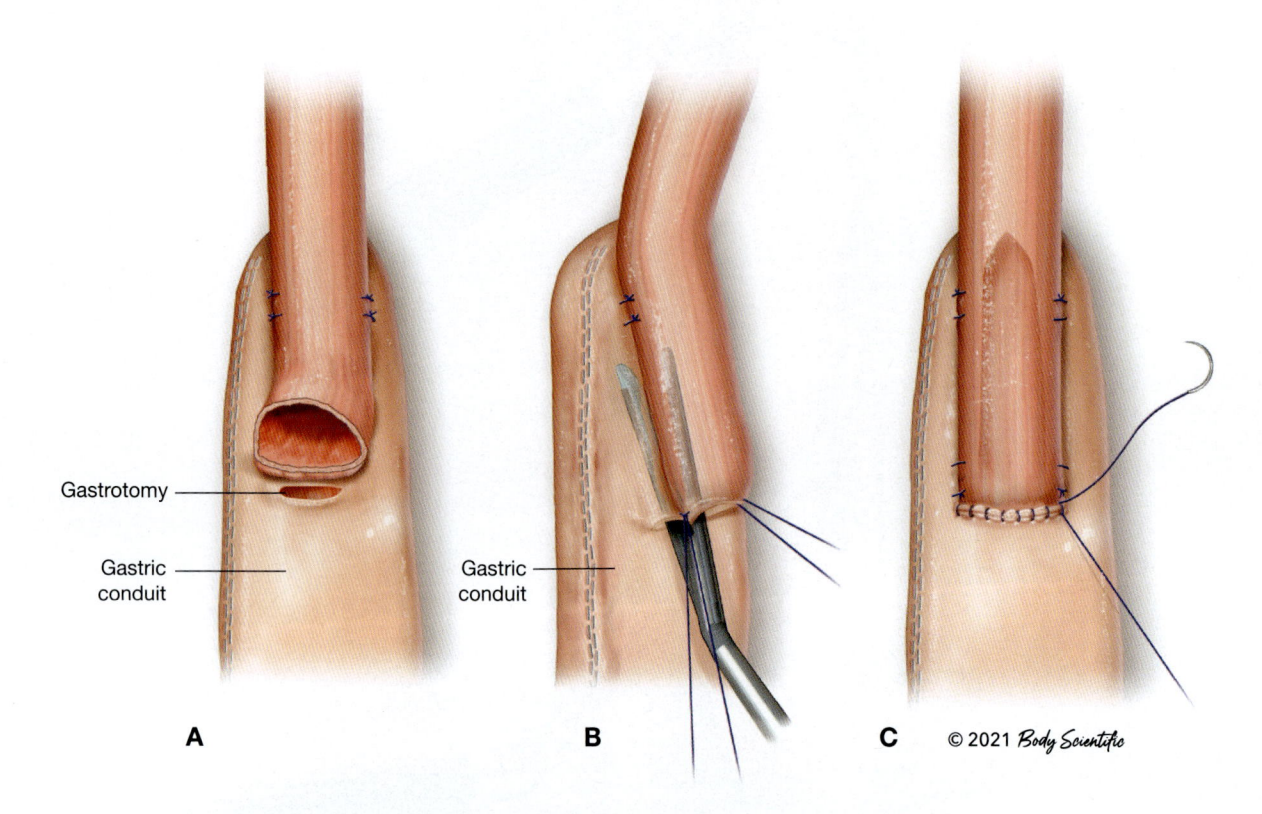

FIGURE 12-15 • Side-to-side esophagogastric anastomosis.

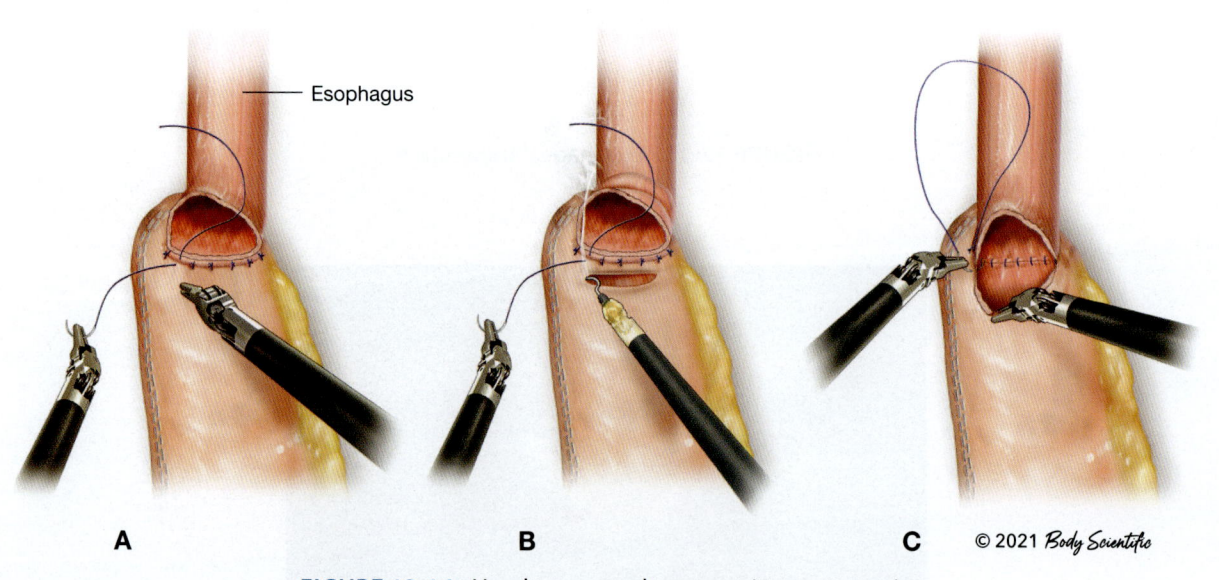

FIGURE 12-16 • Handsewn esophagogastric anastomosis.

D

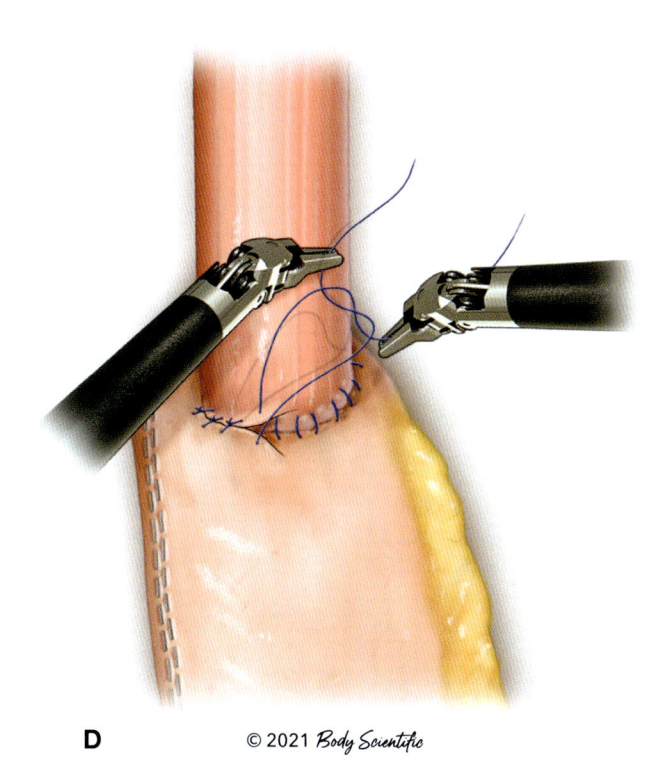

FIGURE 12-16 • (Continued)

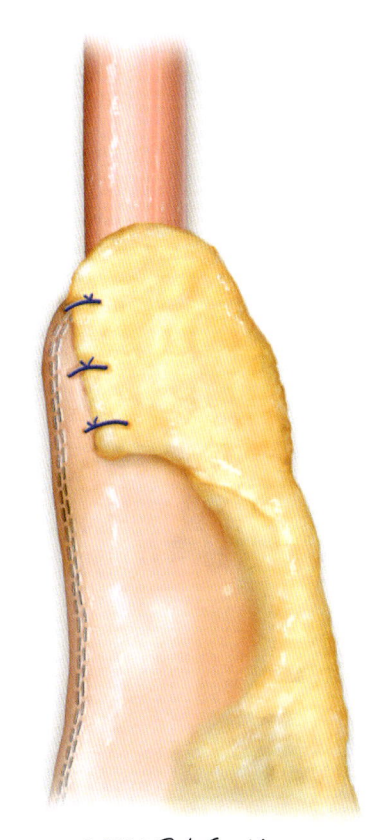

FIGURE 12-17 • Omental patch.

Step 15. Specimen extraction

A 5-cm thoracotomy is created, at the level of the assistant trocar, and protected using an Alexis® wound retractor (Applied Medical, Rancho Santa Margarita, CA). The specimen is delivered out of the chest, and the thoracotomy is temporarily covered closing the Alexis®.

The chest is generously irrigated and the hemostasis is checked. Two chest tubes are usually placed into the right chest (a 28 Fr at the apex for the lung expansion and a curved 32 Fr for the base to collect serous-hemato-lymphatic secretions), and the lung is reinflated. The thoracic ports and the thoracotomy are closed in a conventional fashion.

Step 15 average time frame: 15–20 min

Suggested Readings

1. Koskas F, Gayet B. Anatomical study of retrosternal gastric esophagoplasties. *Anat Clin.* 1985;7(4):237-256. doi: 10.1007/BF01784641
2. Prudius V, Prochazka V, Pavlovsky Z, et al. Vascular anatomy of the stomach related to resection procedures strategy. *Surg Radiol Anat.* 2017;39(4):433-440. doi: 10.1007/s00276-016-1746-2
3. Rice TW, Ishwaran H, Ferguson MK, et al. Cancer of the esophagus and esophagogastric junction: an eighth edition staging primer. *J Thorac Oncol.* 2017;12(1):36-42. doi: 10.1016/j.jtho.2016.10.016
4. Arya S, Markar SR, Karthikesalingam A, et al. The impact of pyloric drainage on clinical outcome following esophagectomy: a systematic review. *Dis Esophagus.* 2015;28(4):326-335. doi: 10.1111/dote.12191
5. Lei Y, Feng Y, Zeng B, et al. Effect of prophylactic thoracic duct ligation in reducing the incidence of postoperative chylothorax during esophagectomy: a systematic review and meta-analysis. *Thorac Cardiovasc Surg.* 2018;66(5):370-375. doi: 10.1055/s-0037-1602259
6. Hou X, Fu JH, Wang X, et al. Prophylactic thoracic duct ligation has unfavorable impact on overall survival in patients with resectable oesophageal cancer. *Eur J Surg Oncol.* 2014;40(12):1756-1762. doi: 10.1016/j.ejso.2014.05.002
7. Thammineedi S, Patnaik S, Saksena A, Ramalingam P, et al. The utility of indocyanine green angiography in the assessment of perfusion of gastric conduit and proximal esophageal stump against visual assessment in patients undergoing esophagectomy: a prospective study. *Indian J Surg Oncol.* 2020;11(4):684-691. doi: 10.1007/s13193-020-01085-8
8. Pointer DT Jr, Saeed S, Naffouje SA, et al. Outcomes of 350 robotic-assisted esophagectomies at a high-volume cancer center: a contemporary propensity-score matched analysis. *Ann Surg.* 2020; Nov 16. doi: 10.1097/SLA.0000000000004317
9. Kingma BF, Grimminger PP, van der Sluis PC, et al; UGIRA Study Group. Worldwide techniques and outcomes in robot-assisted minimally invasive esophagectomy (RAMIE): results from the Multicenter International Registry. *Ann Surg.* 2020; Nov 9. doi: 10.1097/SLA.0000000000004550
10. Giulianotti PC, Coratti A, Angelini M, et al. Robotics in general surgery: personal experience in a large community hospital. *Arch Surg.* 2003;138(7):777-784. doi: 10.1001/archsurg.138.7.777
11. Okusanya OT, Sarkaria IS, Hess NR, et al. Robotic assisted minimally invasive esophagectomy (RAMIE): the University of Pittsburgh Medical Center initial experience. *Ann Cardiothorac Surg.* 2017;6(2):179-185. doi: 10.21037/acs.2017.03.12
12. Guerra F, Vegni A, Gia E, et al. Early experience with totally robotic esophagectomy for malignancy. Surgical and oncological outcomes. *Int J Med Robot.* 2018;14(3):e1902. doi: 10.1002/rcs.1902
13. Morse CR. Minimally invasive Ivor Lewis esophagectomy: how I teach it. *Ann Thorac Surg.* 2018;106(5):1283-1287. doi: 10.1016/j.athoracsur.2018.09.001
14. Ali AM, Bachman KC, Worrell SG, et al. Robotic minimally invasive esophagectomy provides superior surgical resection. *Surg Endosc.* 2020; Nov 10. doi: 10.1007/s00464-020-08120-3
15. Kordzadeh A, Charalabopoulos A, Lorenzi B. Transmural migration of azygous vein Hem-o-lok clip causing food bolus 3 months following uneventful minimally invasive oesophagectomy. *Acta Chir Belg.* 2018;118(4):270-271. doi: 10.1080/00015458.2018.148718

"The operation for carcinoma of the esophagus, I feel certain, will gain friends very quickly, now that the way has been shown for its successful management."
—Franz John A. Torek (1861–1938)

Radical Esophagectomy with Extended Mediastinal Lymphadenectomy

Koichi Suda • Ichiro Uyama

INTRODUCTION

Thoracic esophageal carcinoma (EC) is frequently associated with extensive lymph node metastasis in the cervical, mediastinal, and upper abdominal regions. It is a common practice that a right thoracotomy with esophagectomy and lymphadenectomy of the cervical, mediastinal, and upper abdominal regions is carried out in patients with clinical T1b-SM2- 3, or more advanced disease. Complete lymph node dissection (LND) along the recurrent laryngeal nerves (RLNs), which are among the most commonly involved lymph nodes especially in squamous cell carcinoma, has been considered beneficial for postoperative prognosis; however, it is technically demanding and even microscopic injury of the RLNs deteriorates laryngopharyngeal function postoperatively.

The outermost layer of the autonomic nerves is the thin, loose, connective-tissue layer between the autonomic nerve sheaths of the major anatomical structures and the adipose tissue bearing lymphatic tissue. The target tissue bearing the mediastinal lymph nodes sits at the outermost part of the autonomic nerves, including the vagus nerves (VNs) and RLNs surrounding the heart, bronchi, trachea, aorta, subclavian arteries, and common carotid arteries, suggesting that mediastinal LND could be safely and appropriately conducted along their outermost layers.

The technical aspects of semiprone radical esophagectomy (RE) using the outermost layer-oriented approach are presented in this chapter.

INSTRUMENT REQUIREMENTS

The suggested main robotic instruments can be listed as follows:
- 30° scope
- Maryland bipolar forceps
- Fenestrated bipolar forceps
- Cadière forceps
- Vessel sealer
- EndoWrist suction irrigator
- Permanent cautery monopolar hook
- Small clip applier
- Medium-large clip applier
- Large suture-cut needle driver
- Large needle drivers (qty 2)

The suggested main thoracoscopic/laparoscopic instruments can be listed as follows:
- Tri-Staple reloads loading units (Medtronic)
- Needle driver
- Graspers
- Scissors

Supplemental materials:
- Clips
- Vessel loops
- Sutures: 3-0 coated Vicryl™ SH-1, 3-0 V-Loc™ PBT
- ForceTriad energy platform (Medtronic)
- NIM™ intraoperative neuromonitoring system (Medtronic)

Photo courtesy of the History of Medicine Division at the U.S. National Library of Medicine.
Quote reproduced with permission from Torek F. The first successful resection of the thoracic portion of the esophagus for carcinoma: preliminary report. JAMA. 1913;60(20):1533.

Indications and Relative Contraindications to the Robotic Approach

RE has currently been applied to most of the operable patients with resectable esophageal cancer (EC), including locally advanced EC after neoadjuvant chemo- or chemoradiotherapy. Some conditions, including clinical T4 tumor, severe intrathoracic adhesions, and 1-lung ventilation failure, are considered to be excluded from the indications for RE.

Cervical Dissection and Nerve Monitoring

The patient is initially placed in the supine position under general anesthesia. Left cervical oblique incision is created between the trachea and the left external jugular vein 1–2 cm cranial to the clavicle. The sternal head of the sternocleidomastoid muscle is encircled and taped (**Figure 13-1A**). Once the omohyoid muscle is circumferentially mobilized, the carotid sheath appears (**Figure 13-1B**). The left part of the anterior cervical

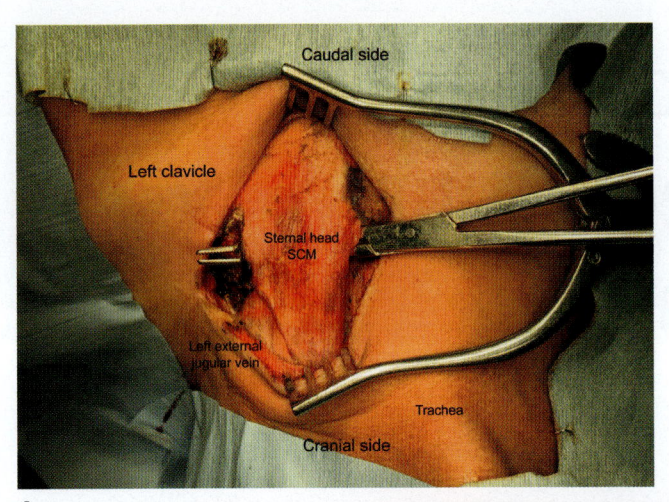

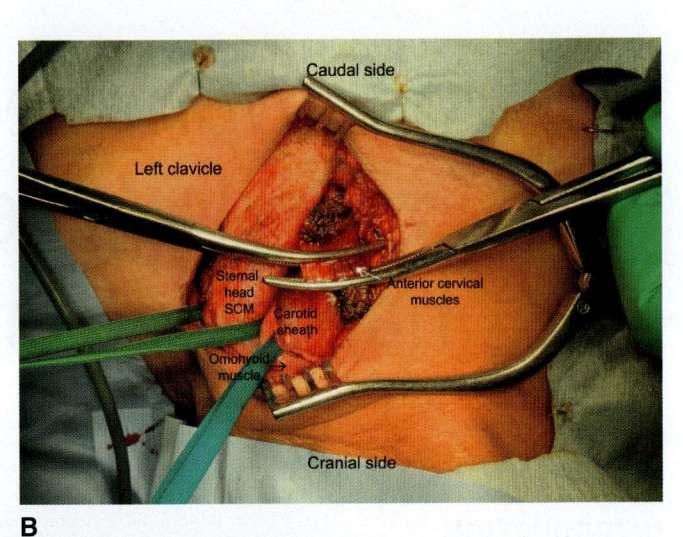

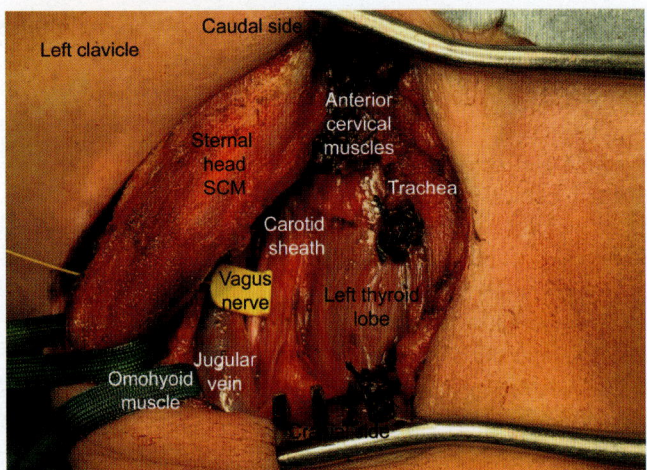

FIGURE 13-1 • Neck dissection and electrode placement on the left vagus nerve.

D

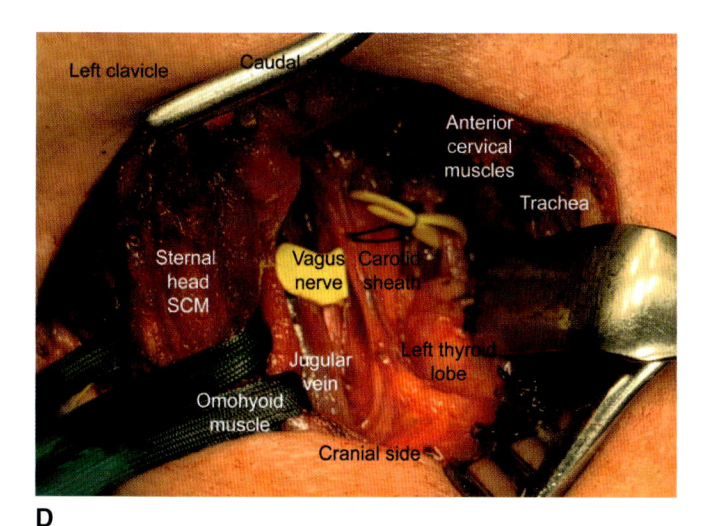

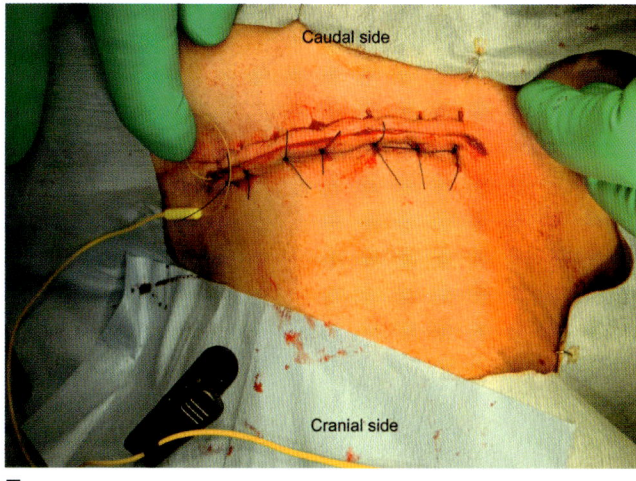

E

FIGURE 13-1 • (Continued)

muscles (prethyroideal) is divided into 2 layers; each layer is dissected, and the lower pole of the left thyroid lobe shows up. The carotid sheath is opened, the jugular vein is gently mobilized laterally, and the main trunk of the left vagus nerve is exposed. The electrode of the continuous NIM™ intraoperative neuromonitoring system (NIM™, Medtronic) is attached to the left vagus nerve (**Figure 13-1C**). The lateral aspect of the lymphatic chain including the left cervical paraesophageal lymph nodes (station 101L) as well as the dorsal aspect of the cervical esophagus is mobilized on the dissectable layer along the carotid sheath, which is connected to the prevertebral fascia. Then, under the guidance of the intermittent NIM™, the medial aspect of the lymphatic chain including the station 101L is mobilized from the trachea and the cervical esophagus at the lower pole of the left thyroid lobe, and the cranial margin of the station 101L is taped using yellow Vessel Loops (**Figures 13-1 D, E**). The wound is temporarily closed, and the patient is repositioned.

Thoracic Phase: Patient Positioning, OR Setup, and Port Setting

The assistant surgeons and a scrub nurse stand according to **Figures 13-2 A, B**. The patient is turned over to a semiprone position with the face placed toward the right, to facilitate suction of the saliva by bronchial scope and to avoid increasing ophthalmic pressure (**Figure 13-2C**). A muscle relaxant is not administered to maintain the activity of the vocal cords, which is monitored with NIM™ during the thoracic phase of RE. The right lung is collapsed using CO_2 insufflation (8–10 mmHg) but not with bronchial blockers.

A

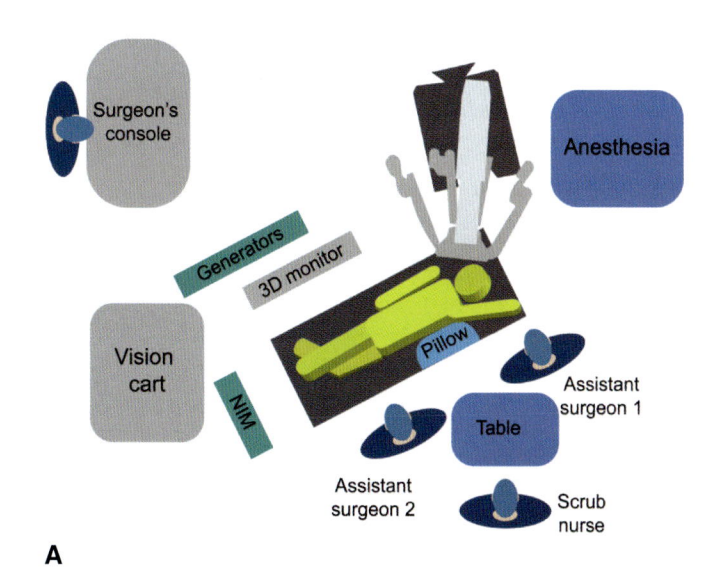

FIGURE 13-2 • OR setup. **A.** OR setup showing the placement of the additional generator and NIM™ intraoperative neuromonitoring system.

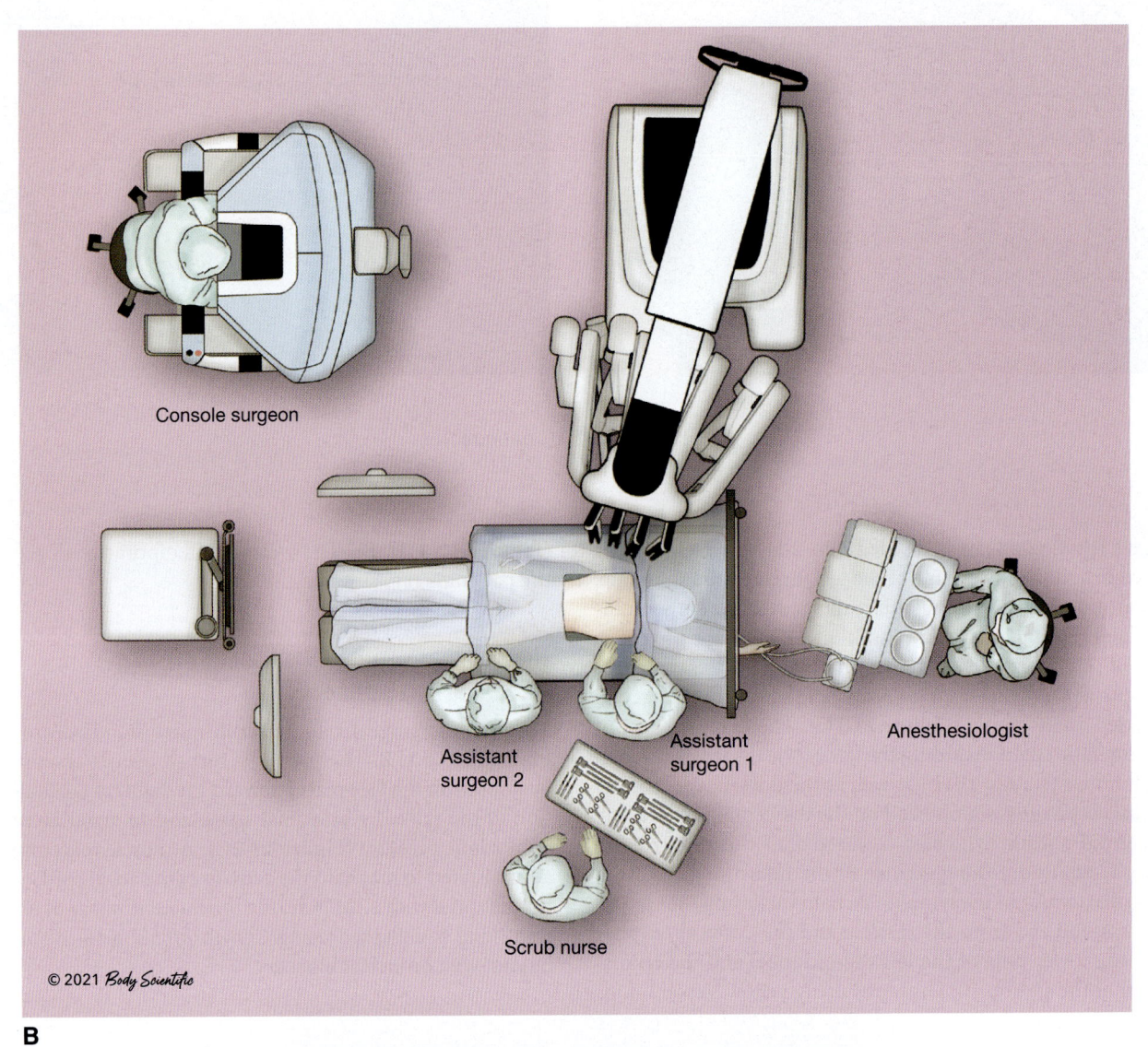

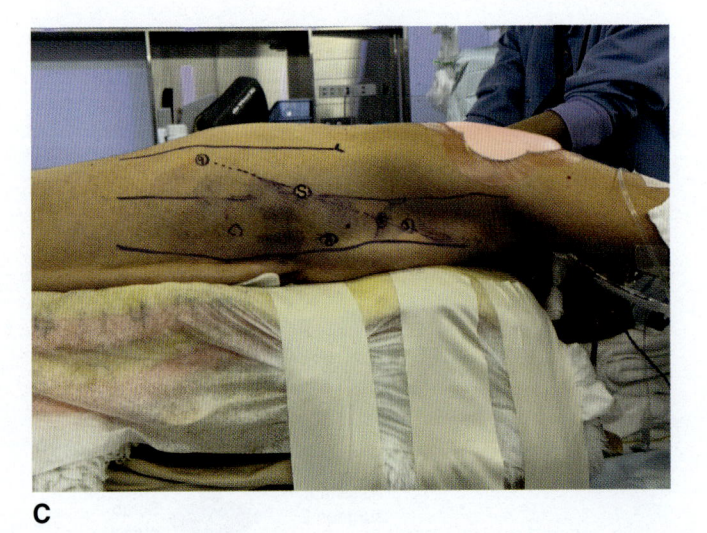

FIGURE 13-2 • (*Continued*) **B.** OR setup. **C.** Patient in semiprone positioning.

The right arm is raised cranially to expose the right axillar fossa. A disposable inflatable pillow (Zimmer Biomet™) is inflated under the right chest to create sufficient semiprone position, making the right subscapular angle and the nipple visible from the patient's right side (**Figure 13-3A**). The trocar placement is planned, and the center of the parallelogram formed by the subscapular angle line (SAL) and the anterior axillary line (AAL) between the 2nd and the 12th ribs is marked as "S" (scope) (**Figure 13-3A**). Four 8-mm da Vinci trocars (R1, R2, R3, and Scope) are placed on the straight line through the "S" and the 3rd intercostal space (ICS) behind the AAL (**Figure 13-3B**). An 8-mm da Vinci trocar ("S") for the thoracoscope is inserted into the 7th ICS on the posterior axillary line (PAL), carefully confirming the absence of pleural adhesion. Then, the 3 remaining 8-mm da Vinci trocars are placed under thoracoscopic guidance at the 9th ICS behind the PAL (R2), the 5th ICS below the PAL (R1), and the 3rd ICS behind the AAL (R3), respectively. The distance between each trocar must be longer than 7 cm. In addition, 1 or 2 12-mm trocars for an assistant surgeon are placed at the 5th ICS (A1, on the AAL) and 8th ICS (A2, below the PAL). Finally, the patient cart is docked targeting the caudal edge of the azygos arch. The ports are interchangeable, and the scope and the operative arm positions can be modified during the procedure.

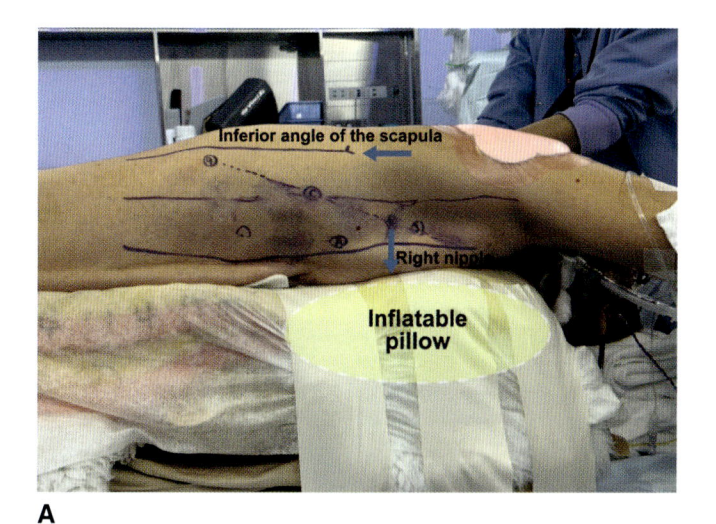

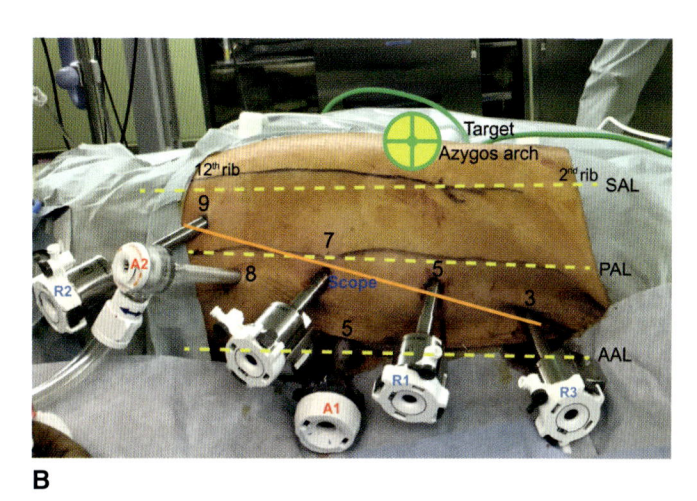

FIGURE 13-3 • **A.** Patient semiprone positioning. **B.** Trocar placement. AAL, anterior axillary line; PAL, posterior axillary line; SAL, subscapular angle line.

Surgical Technique

> **▶▶ TIPS**
>
> The "double bipolar" method is preferred, which is characterized by simultaneous use of right-hand Maryland bipolar forceps and left-hand fenestrated bipolar forceps (connected to VIO dV®, bipolar soft coagulation, level 6). In particular, the Maryland bipolar forceps is connected to the ForceTriad™ energy platform (Macrobipolar mode, 60W). When this bipolar forceps is used with a thick bite, the grasped tissue is coagulated; in contrast, when this forceps is used with a thin bite, a spark cuts the grasped tissue.

Step 1. Mobilization of the middle and lower mesoesophagus

The right lower pulmonary ligament is dissected, and the mediastinal pleura overlying the ventral aspect of the lower and middle thoracic esophagus is opened up to the caudal edge of the right bronchus. The ventral aspect of the lower and middle thoracic esophagus with mesoesophagus is widely mobilized on the outermost layer (**Figure 13-4**) on the dorsal aspect of the pericardium, exposing the left mediastinal pleura (**Figure 13-5A**).

Then, the mediastinal pleura is dissected along the caudal edge of the azygos arch and the ventral aspect of the azygos vein. The dorsal aspect of the middle and lower thoracic esophagus with the mesoesophagus is mobilized on the dissectable layer preserving the thoracic duct in a craniocaudal direction, until the descending aorta and the aortic arch are exposed (**Figure 13-5B**).

Step 1 average time frame: 50–60 min

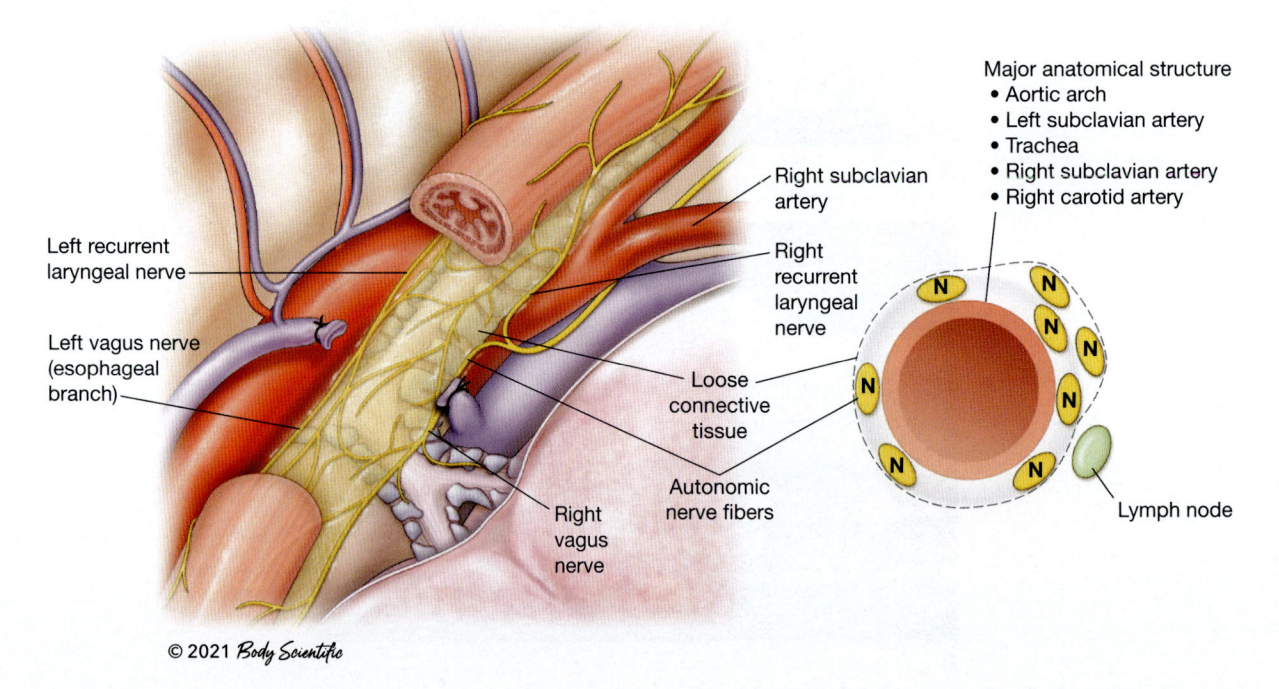

FIGURE 13-4 • The outermost layer in the posterior mediastinum. The targeted lymphatic tissue should be removed on the dissectable layer (as shown by the *dashed line*), where all the autonomic fibers are preserved along the major anatomical structures.

> **⚠ PITFALLS**
>
> Injury of the pulmonary veins.

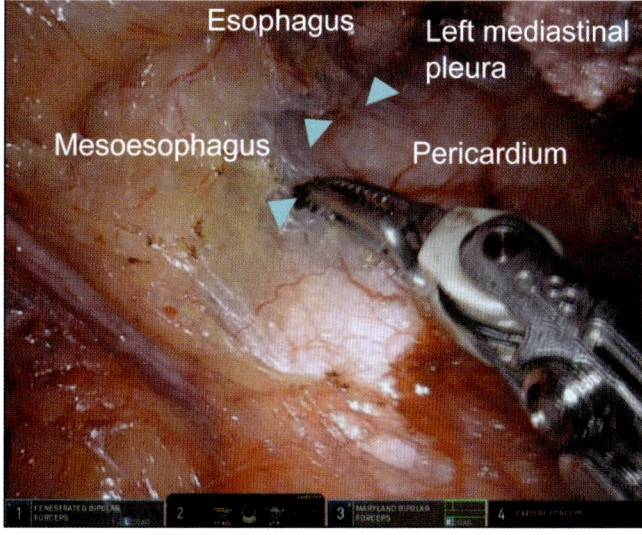

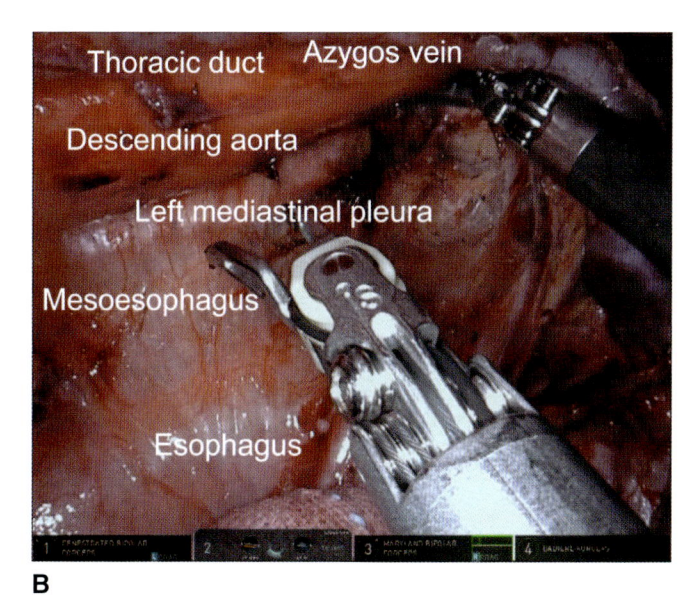

Radical Esophagectomy with Extended Mediastinal Lymphadenectomy

FIGURE 13-5 • Step 1. Mobilization of the middle and lower esophagus. *Blue arrowheads* indicate the outermost layer.

> ▶▶ **TIPS**
>
> The dissectable layer preserving the thoracic duct should be explored between the middle and lower esophagus to avoid thoracic duct injury. At the more cranial site, the thoracic duct runs closer to the azygos vein.

240 The Foundation and Art of Robotic Surgery

🔍 ANATOMICAL HIGHLIGHTS

The thoracic duct runs between the azygos vein and the descending aorta (**Figure 13-6**). Thoracic duct anatomical variants are shown in **Figures 13-7 A–F**.

Table 13-1 outlines the Japanese classification of esophageal cancer (**Figure 13-8**).

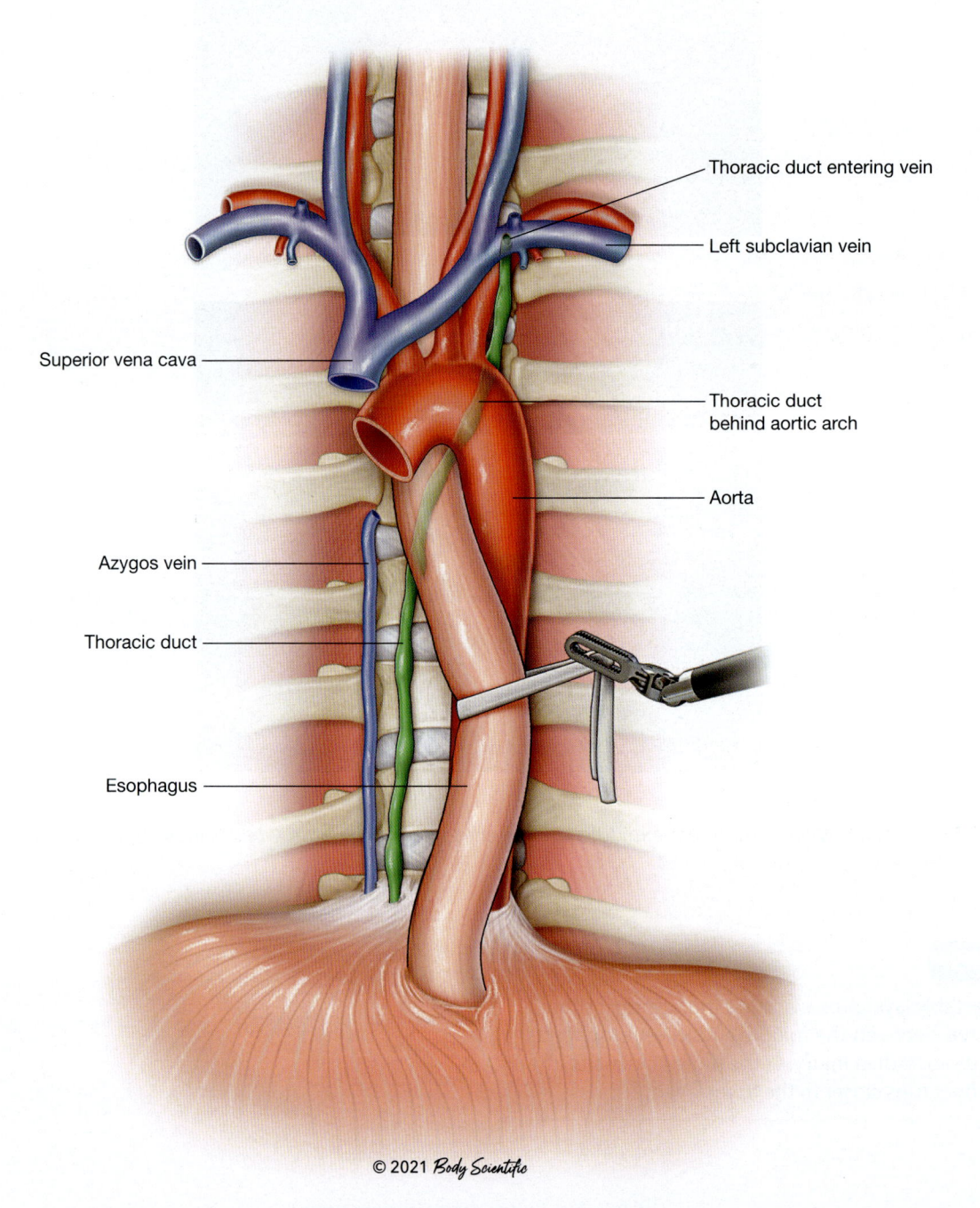

FIGURE 13-6 • Thoracic duct anatomy.

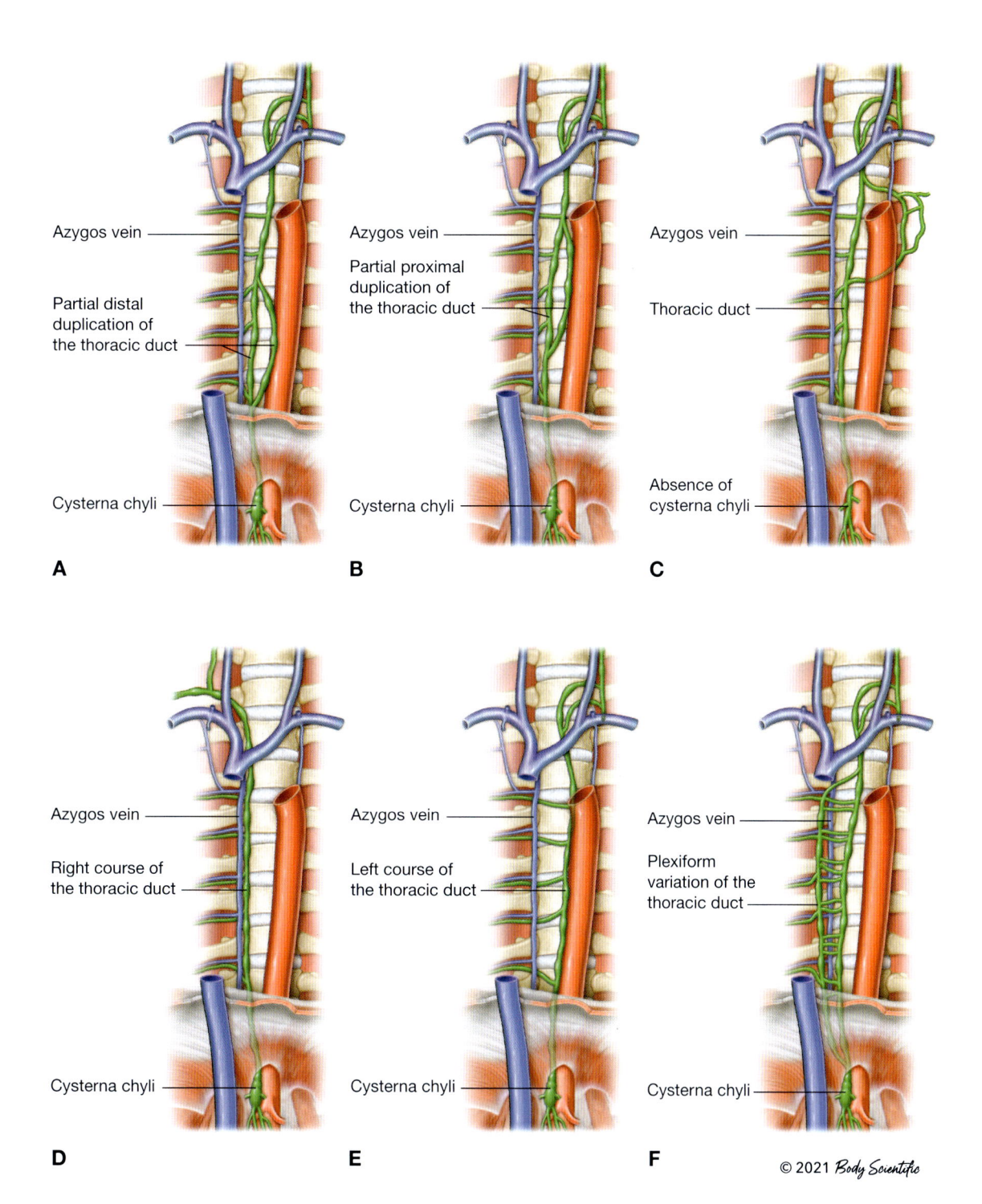

Radical Esophagectomy with Extended Mediastinal Lymphadenectomy   241

FIGURE 13-7 • Thoracic duct anatomical variants.

TABLE 13-1 • Numbers and Naming of Regional Lymph Nodes
Cervical lymph nodes
No. 100 Superficial lymph nodes of the neck
No. 100spf Superficial cervical lymph nodes
No. 100sm Submandibular lymph nodes
No. 100tr Cervical pretracheal lymph nodes
No. 100ac Accessory nerve lymph nodes
No. 101 Cervical paraesophageal lymph nodes
No. 102 Deep cervical lymph nodes
No. 102up Upper deep cervical lymph nodes
No. 102mid Middle deep cervical lymph nodes
No. 103 Peripharyngeal lymph nodes
No. 104 Supraclavicular lymph nodes
Thoracic lymph nodes
No. 105 Upper thoracic paraesophageal lymph nodes
No. 106 Thoracic paratracheal lymph nodes
No. 106rec Recurrent nerve lymph nodes
No. 106recL Left recurrent nerve lymph nodes
No. 106recR Right recurrent nerve lymph nodes
No. 106pre Pretracheal lymph nodes
No. 106tb Tracheobronchial lymph nodes
No. 106tbL Left tracheobronchial lymph nodes
No. 106tbR Right tracheobronchial lymph nodes
No. 107 Subcarinal lymph nodes
No. 108 Middle thoracic paraesophageal lymph nodes
No. 109 Main bronchus lymph nodes
No. 109L Left main bronchus lymph nodes
No. 109R Right main bronchus lymph nodes
No. 110 Lower thoracic paraesophageal lymph nodes
No. 111 Supradiaphragmatic lymph nodes
No. 112 Posterior mediastinal lymph nodes
No. 112aoA Anterior thoracic para-aortic lymph nodes
No. 112aoP Posterior thoracic para-aortic lymph nodes
No. 112pul Pulmonary ligament lymph nodes
No. 113 Ligamentum arteriosum lymph nodes (Botallo lymph nodes)
No. 114 Anterior mediastinal lymph nodes

(Continued)

TABLE 13-1 • Numbers and Naming of Regional Lymph Nodes (Continued)
Abdominal lymph nodes
No. 1 Right paracardial lymph nodes
No. 2 Left paracardial lymph nodes
No. 3a Lesser curvature lymph nodes along the branches of the left gastric artery
No. 3b Lesser curvature lymph nodes along the 2nd branches and distal part of the right gastric artery
No. 4 Lymph nodes along the greater curvature
No. 4sa Lymph nodes along the short gastric vessels
No. 4sb Lymph nodes along the left gastroepiploic artery
No. 4d Lymph nodes along the right gastroepiploic artery
No. 5 Suprapyloric lymph nodes
No. 6 Infrapyloric lymph nodes
No. 7 Lymph nodes along the left gastric artery
No. 8a Lymph nodes along the common hepatic artery (anterosuperior group)
No. 8p Lymph nodes along the common hepatic artery (posterior group)
No. 9 Lymph nodes along the celiac artery
No. 10 Lymph nodes at the splenic hilum
No. 11 Lymph nodes along the splenic artery
No. 11p Lymph nodes along the proximal splenic artery
No. 11d Lymph nodes along the distal splenic artery
No. 12 Lymph nodes in the hepatoduodenal ligament
No. 13 Lymph nodes on the posterior surface of the pancreatic head
No. 14 Lymph nodes along the superior mesenteric vessels
No. 14A Lymph nodes along the superior mesenteric artery
No. 14V Lymph nodes along the superior mesenteric vein
No. 15 Lymph nodes along the middle colic artery
No. 16 Lymph nodes around the abdominal aorta
No. 16a1 Lymph nodes in the aortic hiatus
No. 16a2 Lymph nodes around the abdominal aorta (from the upper margin of the celiac trunk to the lower margin of the left renal vein)
No. 16b1 Lymph nodes around the abdominal aorta (from the lower margin of the left renal vein to the upper margin of the inferior mesenteric artery)
No. 16b2 Lymph nodes around the abdominal aorta (from the upper margin of the inferior mesenteric artery to the aortic bifurcation)
No. 17 Lymph nodes on the anterior surface of the pancreatic head
No. 18 Lymph nodes along the inferior margin of the pancreas
No. 19 Infradiaphragmatic lymph nodes
No. 20 Lymph nodes in the esophageal hiatus of the diaphragm

The left side (L) and the right side (R) should be distinguished for 101, 102, 104, 106rec, 106tb, 109, and 112pul. Reproduced with permission from Japan Esophageal Society. Japanese Classification of Esophageal Cancer, 11th Edition: part I. Esophagus. 2017;14(1):1-36.

244　The Foundation and Art of Robotic Surgery

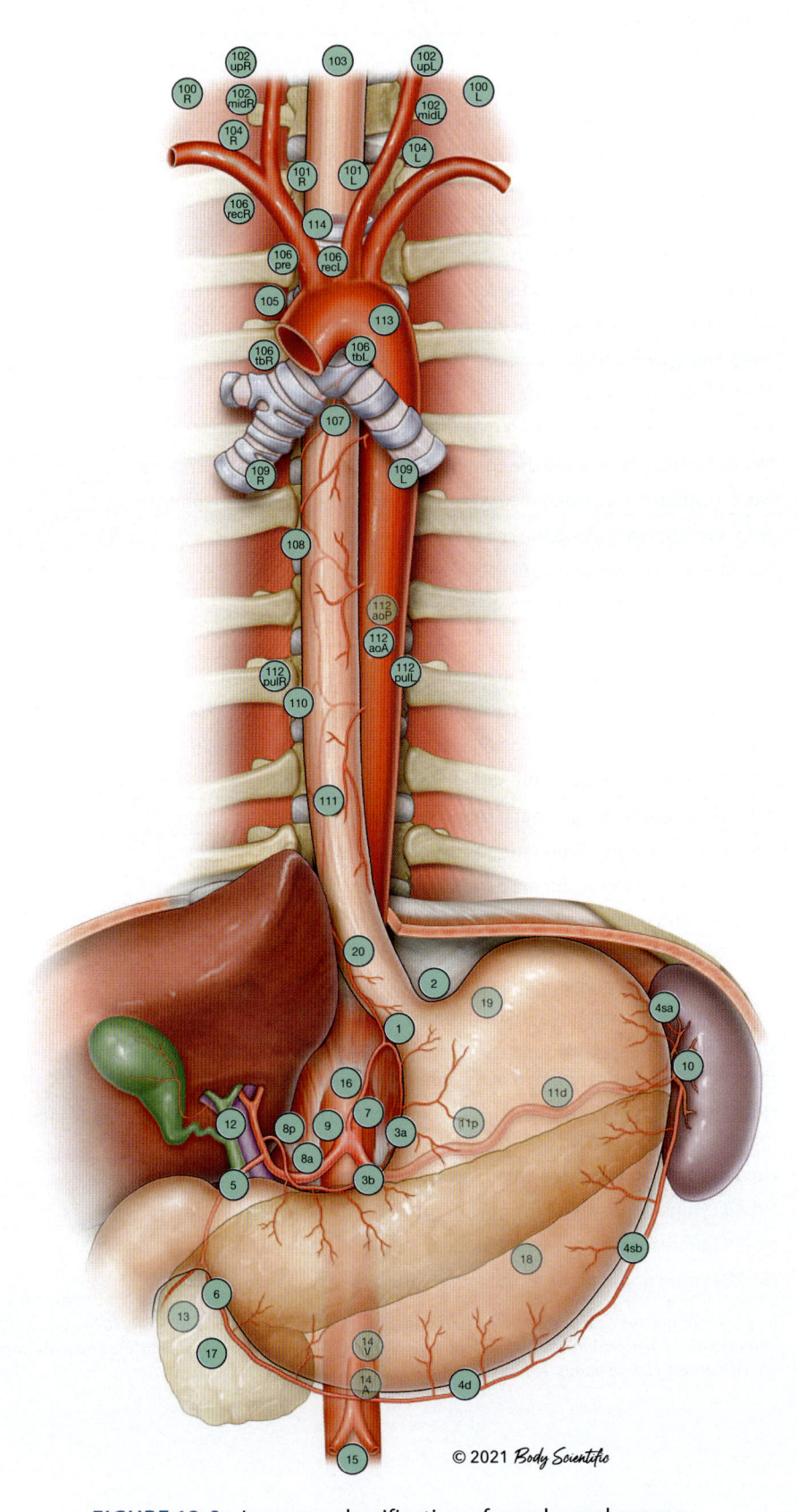

FIGURE 13-8 • Japanese classification of esophageal cancer.

During this procedure, proper esophageal arteries are transected at their origin. Finally, supradiaphragmatic lymph nodes (station 111) are dissected along the diaphragmatic crus, which is circumferentially exposed. At this step, middle and lower mediastinal periesophageal tissue (mesoesophagus) is fully mobilized, with as much adipose tissue bearing the posterior thoracic para-aortic lymph nodes (station 112aoP) attached to the specimen.

> ### 🔍 ANATOMICAL HIGHLIGHTS
> Mesoesophagus: thick vascular fascia between the aorta and the left aspect of the esophagus.

Step 2. Middle mediastinal lymph node dissection
The ventral aspect of the main bronchus and subcarinal nodes (station 107+109) are mobilized on the outermost layer of the pericardium, while the cranial edges of the pulmonary veins are exposed. As the dissection of the station 109L nodes on this layer continues, the membranous portion of the left main bronchus becomes evident (**Figure 13-9A**).

The upper thoracic paraesophageal lymph nodes (station 105) are dissected on the outermost layer of the right main bronchus along the pulmonary branches of the right vagus nerve, exposing the main trunk of the right vagus nerve behind the azygos arch. Then, the station 109R nodes are dissected on the outermost layer of the right main bronchus along the pulmonary branches of the right vagus nerve (**Figure 13-9B**). The esophageal branches of the right vagus nerve are transected at their origin, and the ventral aspect of the upper thoracic esophagus is mobilized on the outermost layer of the tracheal carina. In the middle of this process, the distal side of the right bronchial artery is divided and transected. Finally, the ventral border of the subcarinal lymph nodes (station 107) is determined, and station 107+109 dissection is completed.

Step 2 average time frame: 25–30 min

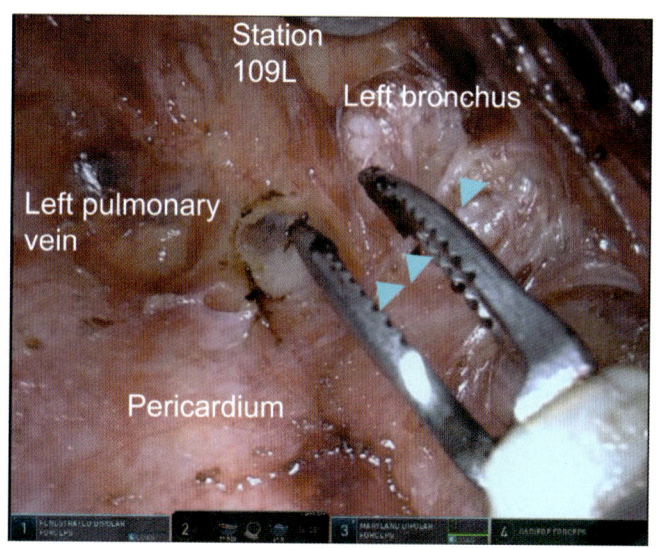

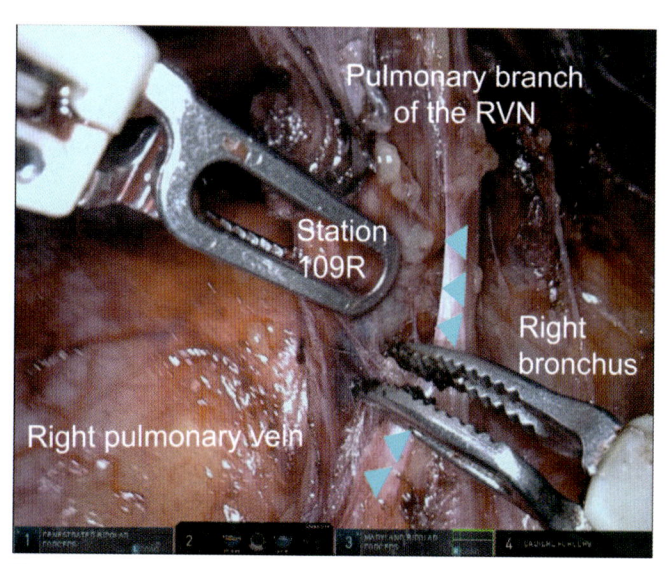

FIGURE 13-9 • Step 2. Middle mediastinal lymph node dissection. *Blue arrowheads* indicate the outermost layer. RVN, right vagus nerve.

Video 13-1. Step 2. Middle Mediastinal Lymph Node Dissection

> **TIPS**
> By dissecting the station 107+109 on the outermost layer, preserving the autonomic nerve fibers attached to the trachea and the bronchi, 2 goals are achieved: (1) sufficient lymph node dissection is achieved with a small amount of blood loss, and (2) intraoperative trachea and bronchial injury is avoided.

ANATOMICAL HIGHLIGHTS
Bronchial arteries and their variations (**Figures 13-10 A–C**).

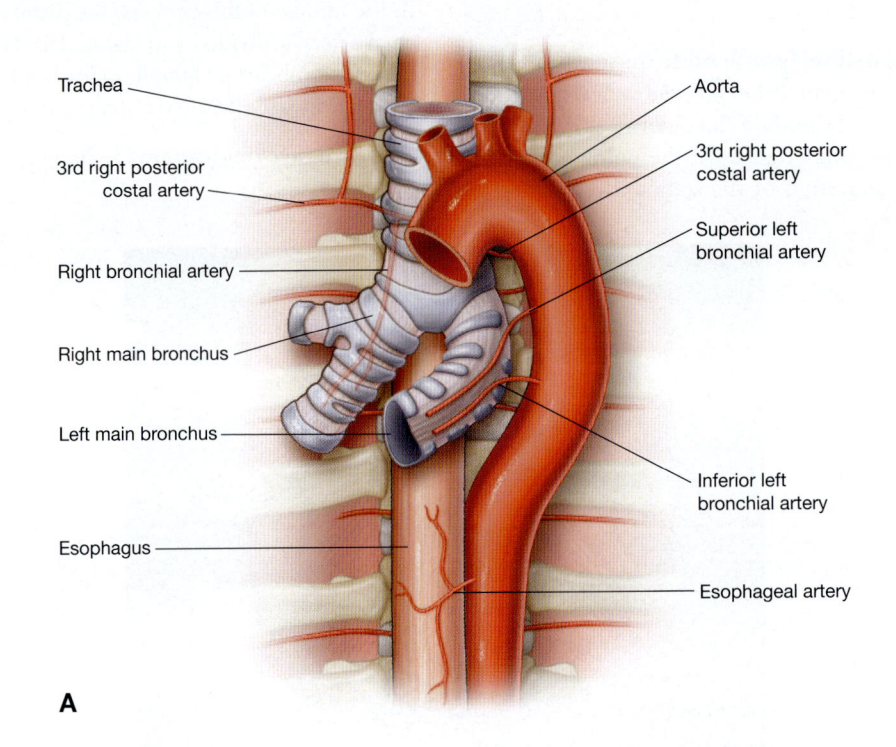

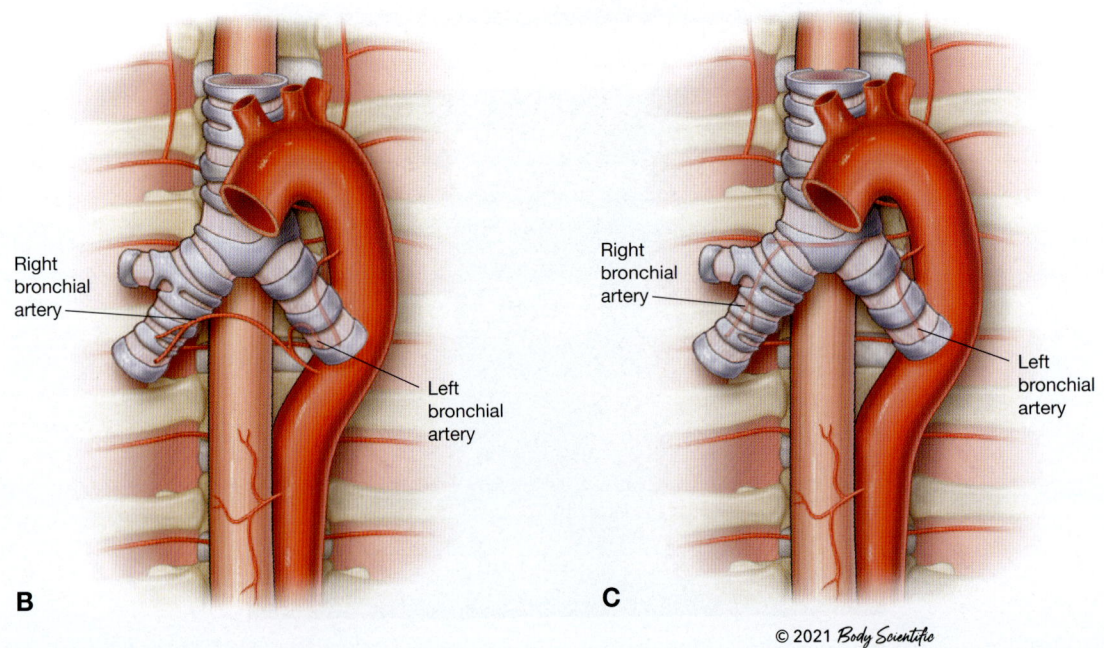

FIGURE 13-10 • Bronchial arteries and their variations. **A.** Common anatomy: 2 bronchial arteries for the left bronchus and 1 for the right bronchus. **B.** A single stem for right and left bronchial arteries. **C.** A single bronchial artery for each bronchus.

Step 3. Exposure of the 3 dissectable layers along the dorsal aspect of the upper esophagus

Before transecting the azygos arch and moving on to upper mediastinal dissection, the following 3 independent dissectable layers should be exposed: the layer along the aortic adventitia on which the thoracic para-aortic lymph nodes (station 112ao) are dissected, the one along the adipose tissue surrounding the thoracic duct, and the interpleural ligament (Morosow's ligament). In particular, the layer on the interpleural ligament can consistently be found behind the azygos arch above the upper esophagus (**Figures 13-11 A, B**).

Step 3 average time frame: 5 min

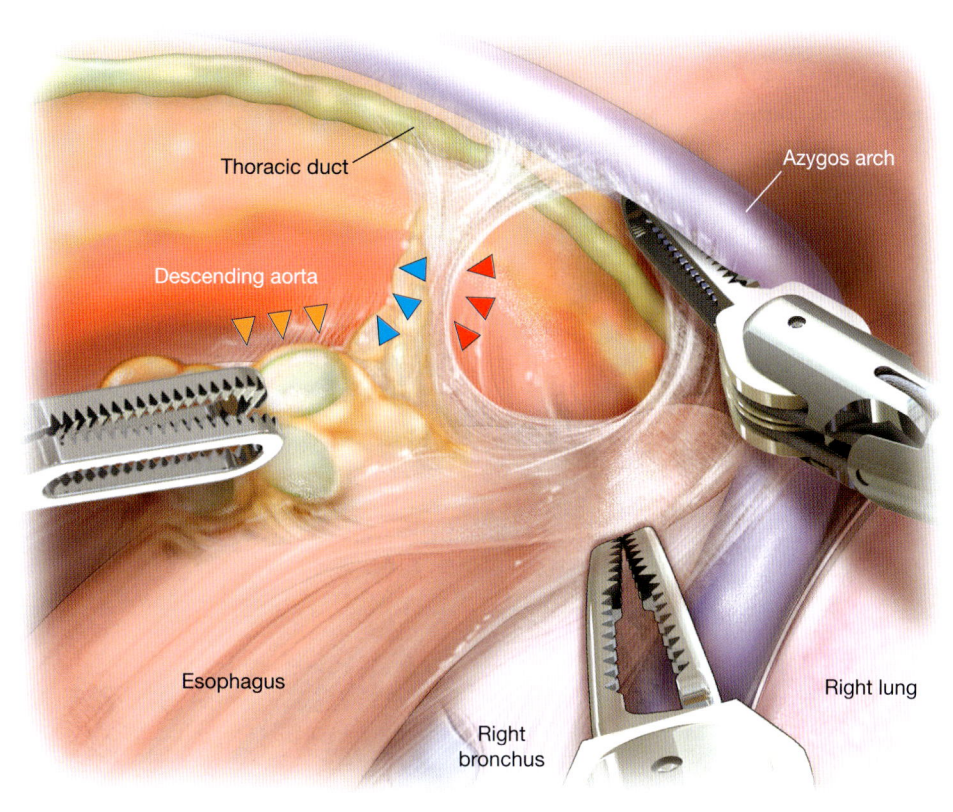

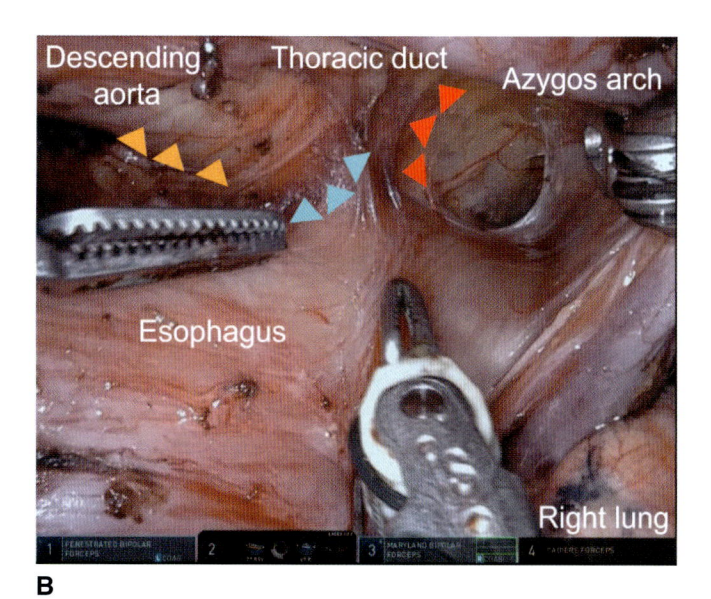

FIGURE 13-11 • Step 3. Exposure of the 3 dissectable layers. *Orange arrowheads,* the dissectable layer along the aortic adventitia on which the thoracic para-aortic lymph nodes (station 112ao) are dissected; *blue arrowheads,* that along the adipose tissue surrounding the thoracic duct; *red arrowheads,* that on the interpleural ligament (Morosow's ligament).

> **TIPS**
> By recognizing these 3 dissectable layers, preservation or combined resection of the thoracic duct could be easily conducted, and postoperative chylothorax may be avoided.

> **TIPS**
> By keeping the outermost layer of the trachea along the right vagus nerve trunk and its branches, the trachea could be well preserved and the right RLN may be easily found.

Step 4. Mobilization of the upper esophagus on the outermost layer of the right vagus nerve

The arch of the azygos vein is transected with a linear stapler and the distal edge is pulled to the back with a stitch. The ventral aspect of the upper esophagus is mobilized on the outermost layer of the trachea along the right vagus nerve trunk and its branches covering the membranous portion of the trachea in the caudocranial direction toward the neck, and the mediastinal pleura is opened along the right vagus nerve trunk. Then, the right RLN appears laying on the right subclavian artery (**Figures 13-12 A, B**).

Step 4 average time frame: 25–30 min

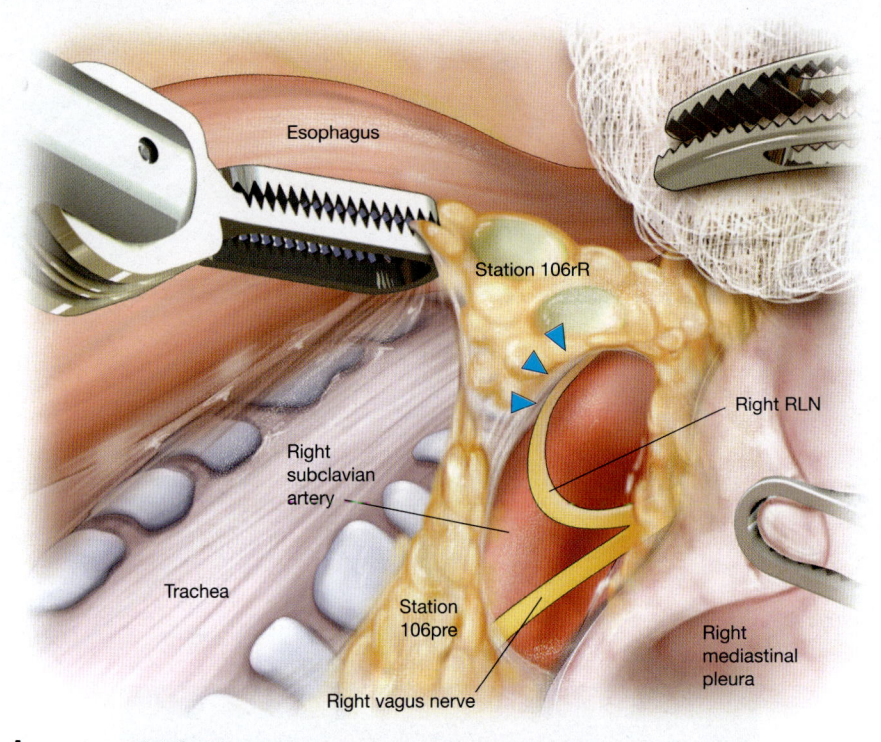

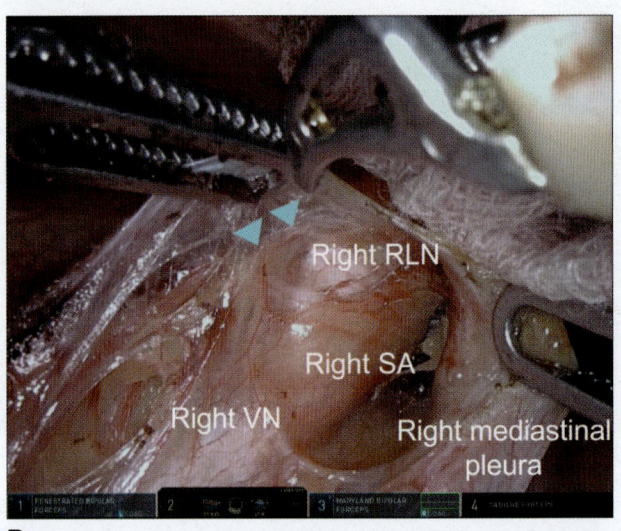

FIGURE 13-12 • Step 4. Mobilization of the upper esophagus. *Blue arrowheads,* the outermost layer along the right RLN. RLN, recurrent laryngeal nerve; SA, subclavian artery; VN, vagus nerve.

Radical Esophagectomy with Extended Mediastinal Lymphadenectomy

▶ **Video 13-2.** Step 4. Mobilization of the Upper Esophagus on the Outermost Layer of the Right Vagus Nerve

Step 5. Mobilization of the dorsal aspect of the upper esophagus on the dissectable layer along the interpleural ligament

The dorsal aspect of the upper esophagus is mobilized on the interpleural fascia in a caudocranial direction beyond the thoracic inlet, with the mediastinal pleura being opened. Dissection on the interpleural fascia is extended toward the right aspect of the cervical esophagus behind the right upper mediastinal mesoesophagus. Then, the interpleural fascia is mobilized from the dissectable layer on the adipose tissue surrounding the thoracic duct, and the fascia is dissected along the left aspect of the upper esophagus, resulting in sufficient mobilization of the left upper mediastinal periesophageal tissue (mesoesophagus). At this stage, the yellow Vessel Loop, which shows the cranial margin of the lymphatic chain of station 101L at the lower pole of the left thyroid lobe, is visible. The origin of the right bronchial artery is divided during this step in between clips using Maryland bipolar forceps (**Figures 13-13 A, B**).

Step 5 average time frame: 10–15 min

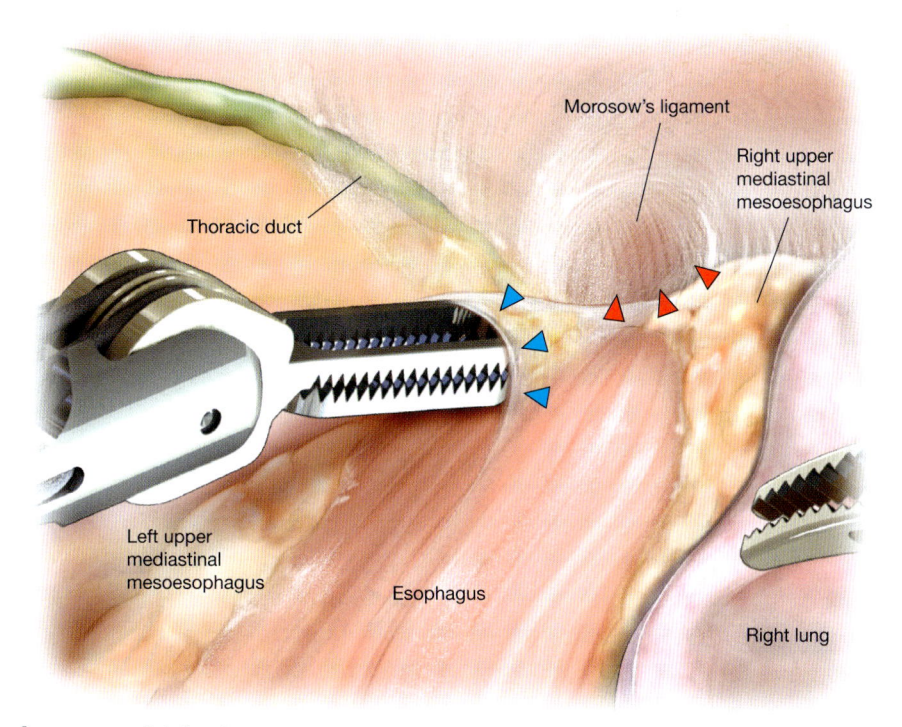

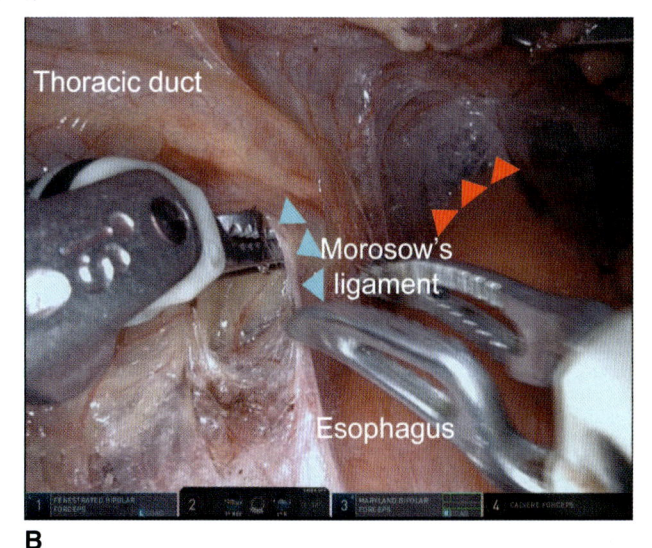

FIGURE 13-13 • Step 5. Mobilization of the dorsal aspect of the upper esophagus. *Blue arrowheads,* the dissectable layer along the adipose tissue surrounding the thoracic duct; *red arrowheads,* that on the interpleural ligament (Morosow's ligament).

Video 13-3. Step 5. Mobilization of the Dorsal Aspect of the Upper Esophagus on the Dissectable Layer Along the Interpleural Ligament

Step 6. Dissection of the right recurrent nerve and cervical paraesophageal lymph nodes

The right upper mediastinal periesophageal tissue (mesoesophagus) is mobilized on the outermost layer of the trachea, and the medial border of the lymph nodes around the right RLN (station 106recR+101R) is determined. The lateral border of the station 106recR+101R is defined on the outermost layer of the right subclavian artery and the right carotid artery. The bottom of the station 106recR+101R is prepared on the dissectable layer along the right RLN, with its esophageal branches being divided in between clips or bipolar coagulated with the Maryland forceps (**Figures 13-14 A, B**).

Step 6 average time frame: 25–30 min

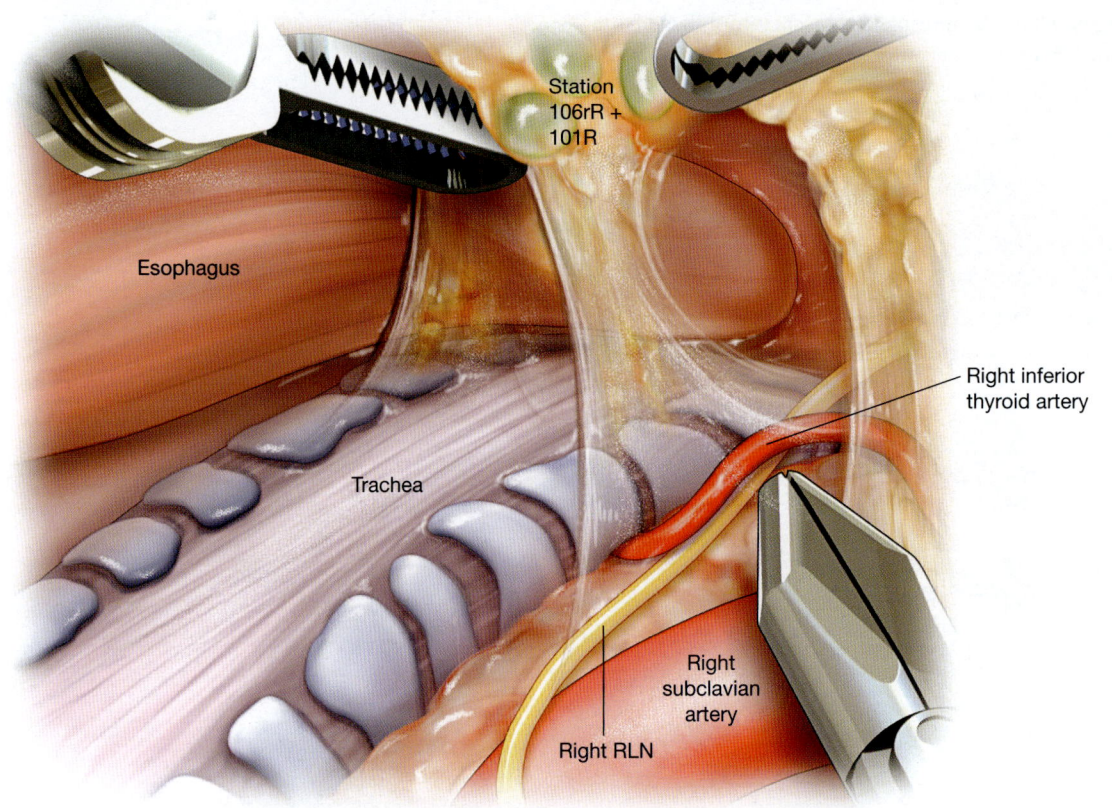

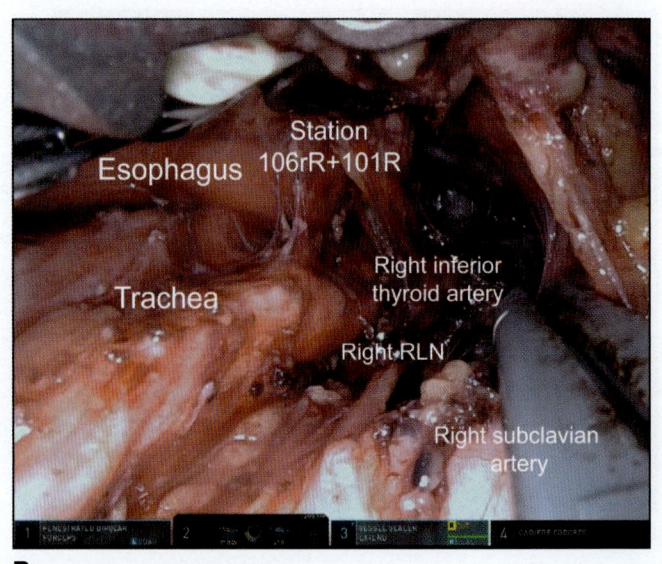

FIGURE 13-14 • Step 6. Dissection of the right recurrent nerve and cervical paraesophageal lymph nodes.

Radical Esophagectomy with Extended Mediastinal Lymphadenectomy | **251**

> ▶▶ **TIPS**
> To avoid postoperative right RLN palsy, the right RLN should not be freed from the right subclavian artery.

> 🔍 **ANATOMICAL HIGHLIGHTS**
> Recurrent laryngeal nerve anatomy (**Figures 13-15 A, B**). Nonrecurrent laryngeal nerve anatomical variations (**Figures 13-16 A–D**).

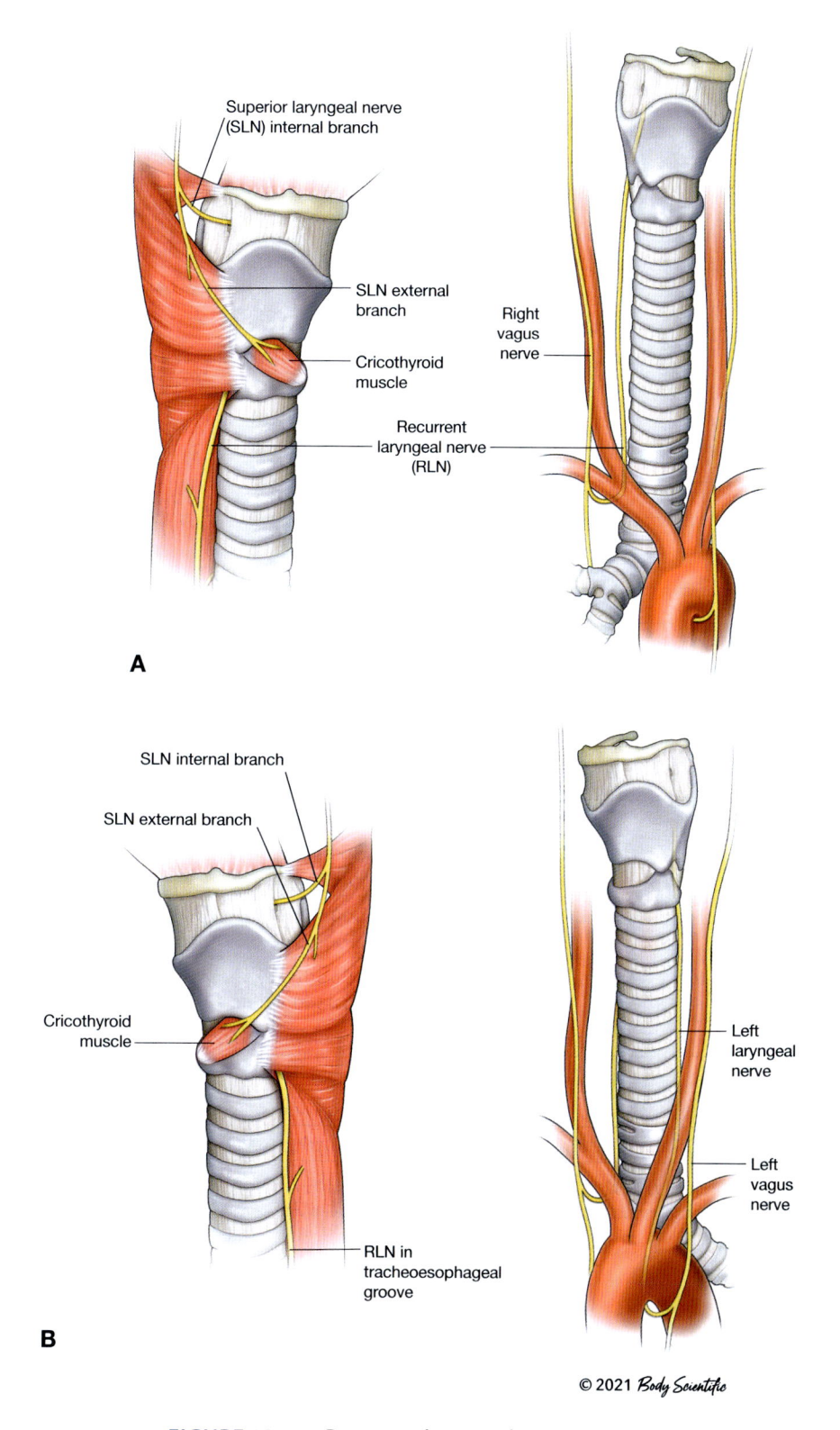

FIGURE 13-15 • Recurrent laryngeal nerve anatomy.

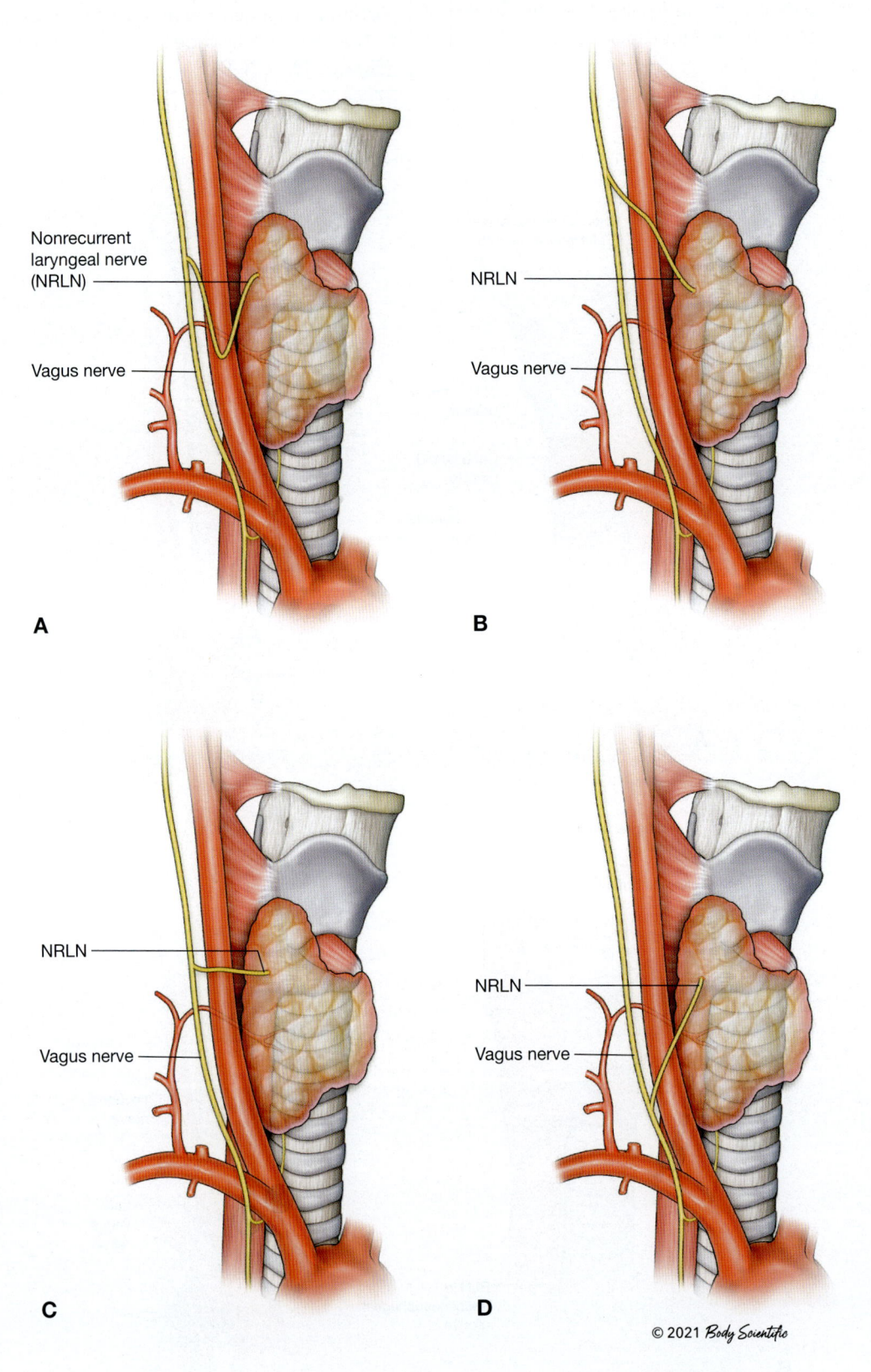

FIGURE 13-16 • Nonrecurrent laryngeal nerve anatomical variations.

Step 7. Dissection of the left recurrent laryngeal nerve and cervical paraesophageal lymph nodes

Adipose tissue bearing station 101R+106recR+105 is detached out of the upper esophagus. The trachea is rolled back carefully and firmly to the right and ventrally, by a grasper holding a small gauze to explore the left aspect of the trachea and the left main bronchus. The left upper mediastinal periesophageal tissue (mesoesophagus) is mobilized on the outermost layer along the left aspect of the trachea and the left bronchus. The outermost layer of the aortic arch, on which left RLN is preserved, is probed, and the adipose tissue bearing the left recurrent nerve nodes (station 106recL) is gently exfoliated on this layer up to the thoracic inlet (**Figures 13-17 A, B**). The upper esophagus is mobilized circumferentially at the level of the aortic arch, and transected using a 45-mm linear stapler. The left upper periesophageal tissue (mesoesophagus) is detached from the left aspect of the upper esophagus in the caudocranial direction up to the top of station 101L marked with the

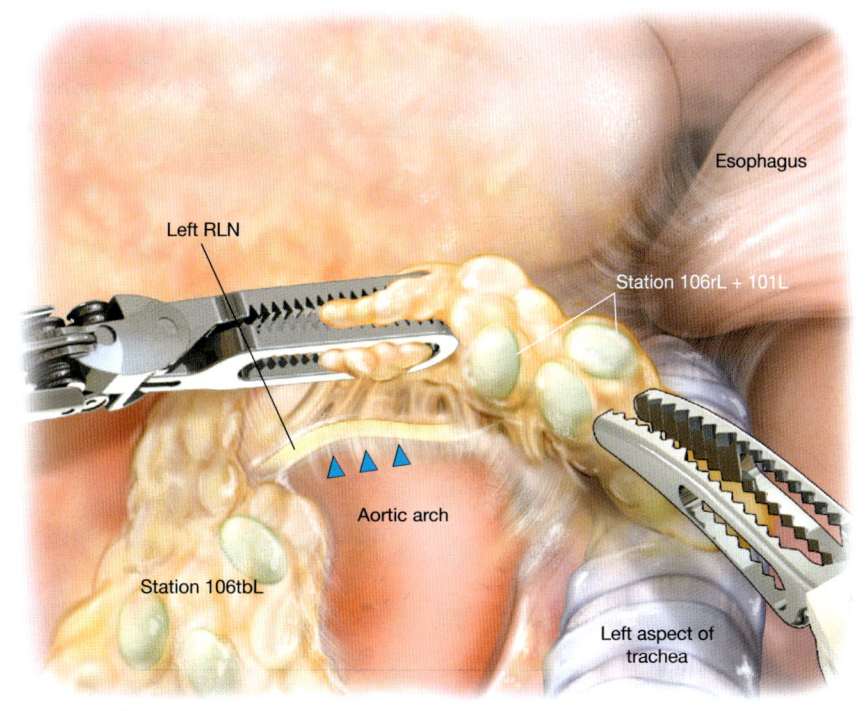

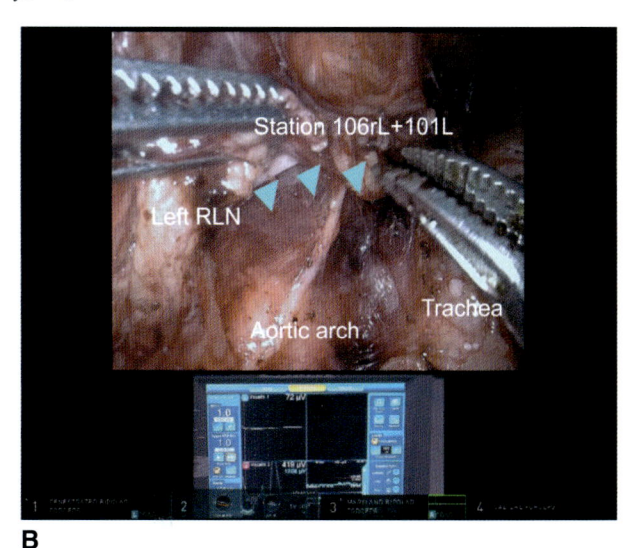

FIGURE 13-17 • Step 7. Dissection of the left recurrent nerve and cervical paraesophageal lymph nodes. *Blue arrowheads:* the outermost layer along the left RLN.

254 The Foundation and Art of Robotic Surgery

C

Esophagus
Left RLN
Station 106rL + 101L
Left aspect of trachea

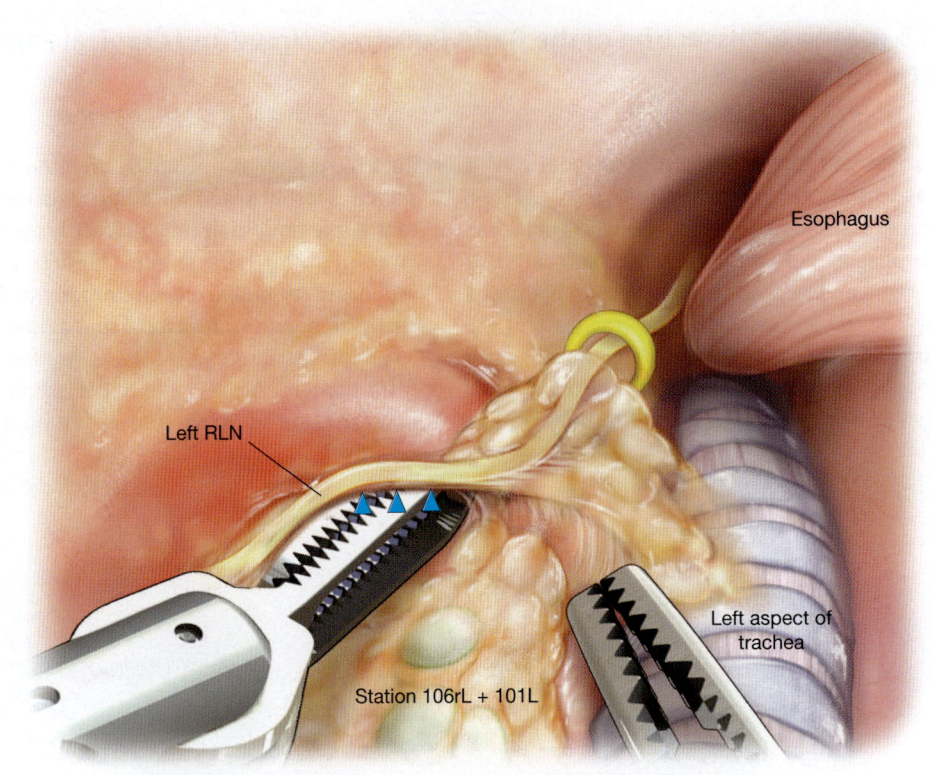

© 2021 Body Scientific

D

Esophagus
Left RLN
Station 106rL+101L
Trachea

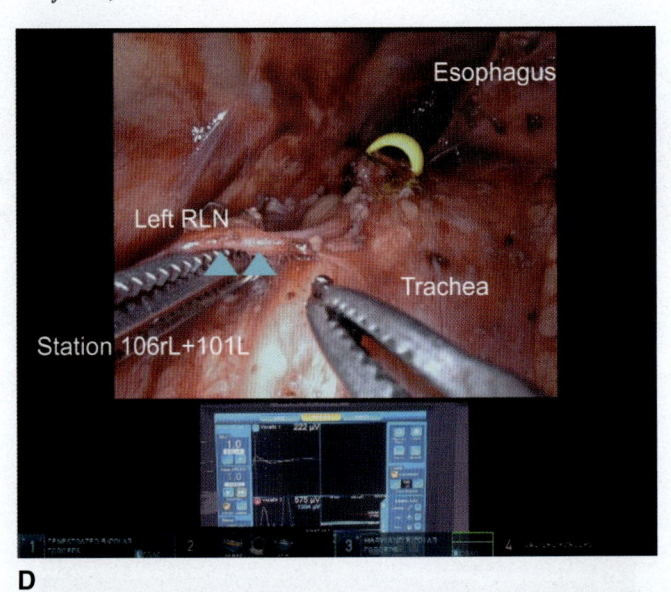

FIGURE 13-17 • *(Continued)*

yellow Vessel Loop, and the esophageal stump is pulled to the back with a stitch. The adipose tissue including the station 106recL+101L nodes is pulled toward the right ventral direction with the R3, and the target tissue is gently exfoliated on the dissectable layer along the left RLN, which is connected to the outermost layer of the aortic arch and the left subclavian artery (**Figures 13-17 C, D**). The esophageal branches of the identified left RLN are divided in turn. The target tissue is mobilized on the outermost layer of the trachea up to the top of station 101L, and the lymphatic connection between station 106recL+101L and the pretracheal nodes (station 106pre) is transected. Finally, the target tissue is flipped up above the left RLN and the ventral aspect of station 106recL+101L is dissected in the craniocaudal direction.

Step 7 average time frame: 40–45 min

▶▶ **TIPS**

Using these surgical maneuvers, the left RLN is preserved including its left ventral aspect, which is covered with a thin membrane-like structure. This membrane may distribute and decrease the tension applied to the nerve during left RLN nodal dissection, possibly leading to reduction in postoperative palsy.

Video 13-5. Step 7. Dissection of the Left Recurrent Nerve and Cervical Paraesophageal Lymph Nodes

Step 8. Dissection of tracheobronchial lymph nodes and posterior mediastinal lymph nodes

The tracheobronchial nodes (station 106tbL) are dissected on the face of the pulmonary artery trunk, preserving the recurrent portion of the left RLN along the outermost layer of the aortic arch (**Figures 13-18 A, B**). At this stage, the left vagus nerve trunk and the left bronchial arteries should be carefully preserved. Then, the caudal side of the divided esophagus is pulled toward the right caudal direction by the assistant surgeon, and the esophageal branches of the left vagus nerve are

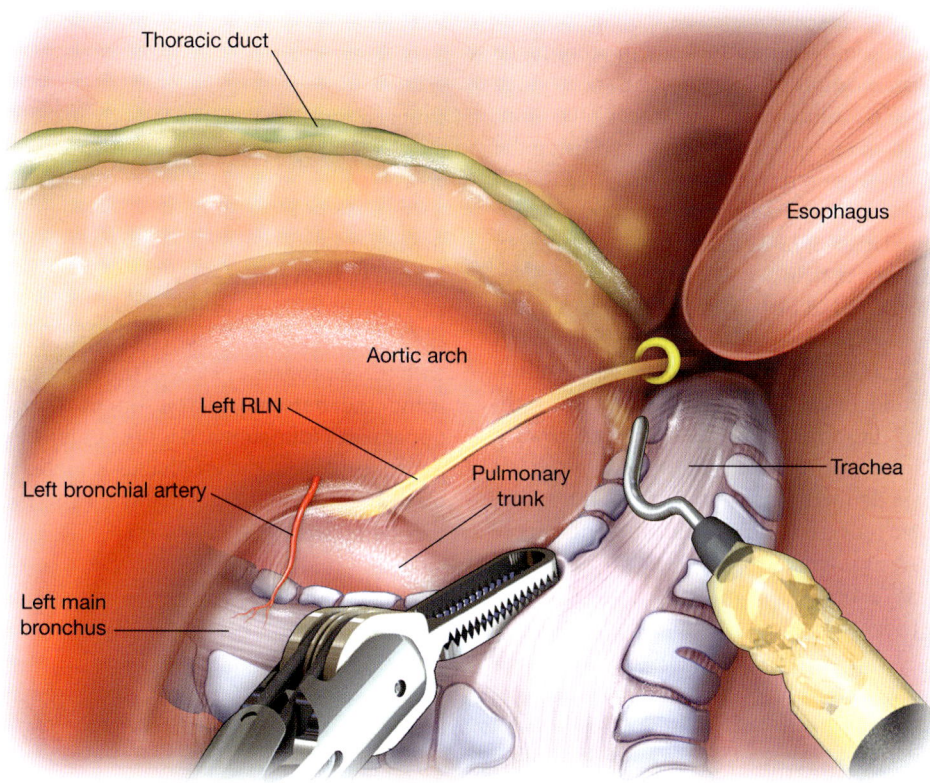

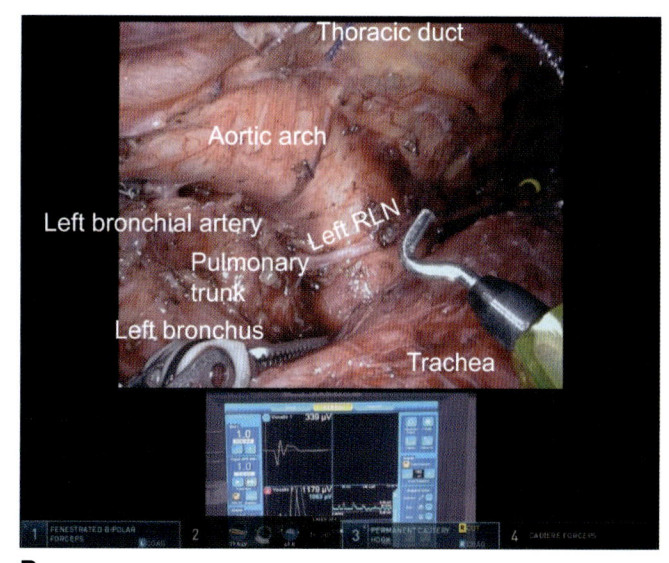

FIGURE 13-18 • Step 8. Dissection of the tracheobronchial lymph nodes and posterior mediastinal lymph nodes.

dissected below the left main bronchus, preserving the left pulmonary branches. Finally, the posterior mediastinal nodes (station 112) are dissected combined with the left mediastinal pleura and the left inferior pulmonary ligament and the thoracic phase of the RE is completed.

Step 8 average time frame: 25–30 min

Stomach Mobilization and Abdominal Lymph Node Dissection

Once the thoracic stage is completed, the patient is turned back to the supine position, and the stomach mobilization is robotically performed. The extent of abdominal lymph node dissection is determined based on the tumor location in accordance with the Japanese Classification of Esophageal Cancer (11th ed., 2015). A 12-mm Kii balloon blunt tip trocar (100 mm, Applied Medical) for the scope is placed on the navel using the Hasson technique. Three 8-mm da Vinci trocars (R1, R2, R3) and a 12-mm assistant port (A1) are placed in the upper abdomen on a straight line (**Figure 13-19**). The distance between each trocar has to be longer than 7 cm. The Nathanson liver retractor (Yufu Itonaga Co. Ltd., Japan) is introduced slightly left caudal to the xiphoid process and the hepatic left lateral segment lifted in a dorsal-to-ventral direction. Kocherization of the duodenum is conducted. Carefully preserving the right gastroepiploic vessels, the omental bursa is opened toward the patient's left, and the root of the gastric branch of the left gastroepiploic artery is divided. The short gastric arteries are divided in turn at their roots, retaining as much blood supply to the greater curvature as possible.

The omental bursa is opened toward the patient's right, the physiological adhesions between the dorsal aspect of the stomach and the pancreatic body are divided, the transverse mesocolon is mobilized along the fusion fascia, and the pancreas is widely exposed. The anastomosis between the right and left gastric arteries along the lesser curvature is divided, and the lesser omentum is opened along the most caudal hepatic branch of the vagus nerve. The dorsal aspect of the stomach is partially mobilized on the subretroperitoneal fascia along the right diaphragmatic crus. The gastropancreatic fold is divided with the appropriate extent of the suprapancreatic lymph nodes using the outermost layer–oriented medial approach. The upper part of the stomach is fully mobilized along the subretroperitoneal fascia, the esophagus is pulled down into the abdomen, and the esophageal hiatus is closed with a nonabsorbable barbed suture.

Average time frame: 90 min

> ▶▶ **TIPS**
>
> In the middle of this step, the left gastrophrenic ligament (composed of loose connective tissue between the upper part of the stomach and the left diaphragmatic crus) is dissected along the posterior aspect of the stomach up to the splenophrenic ligament. Once the splenophrenic ligament is divided, the upper pole of the spleen is exposed, and the most cranial short gastric artery stands upright on the splenic hilum. Using this procedure, the upper pole branch of the splenic artery may easily be preserved.

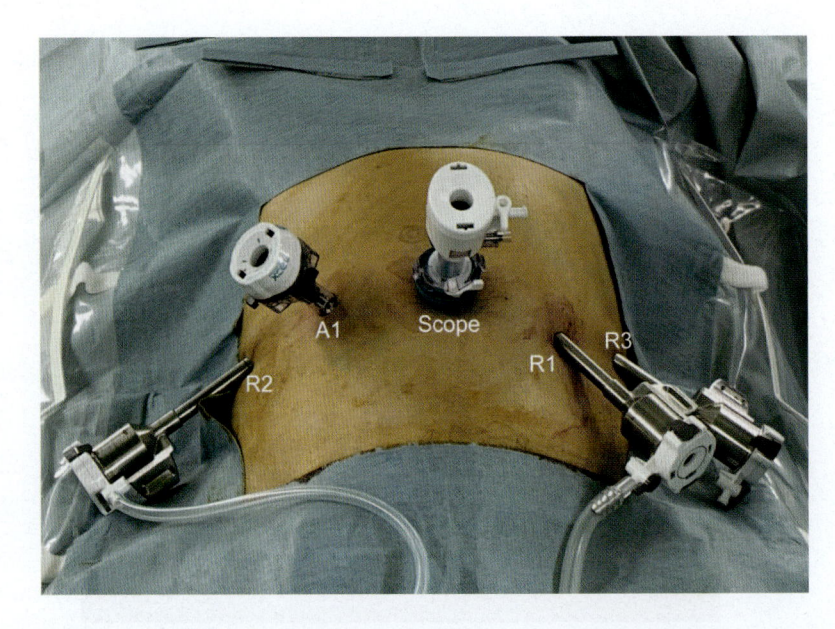

FIGURE 13-19 • Abdominal phase, trocar placement.

▶ **Video 13-6.** Stomach Mobilization and Abdominal Lymph Node Dissection

Specimen Extraction, Extracorporeal Gastric Conduit Creation, Retrosternal Conduit Pull-up, and Cervical Anastomosis

After this phase, a small midline incision is made, a wound protector is placed, the specimen is taken out with the stomach, and a 3.5-cm-wide greater-curvature gastric conduit is created extracorporeally and left cervical esophagogastrostomy is created via the retrosternal route.

▶▶ **TIPS**

End-to-side anastomosis using a circular stapler (25-mm or 21-mm) is performed. When a 21-mm stapler is used, the circumferential stapling line is divided with 1 application of 45-mm linear stapler (Tri-Staple™ purple), to avoid postoperative anastomotic stenosis (so-called keyhole anastomosis).

EDITORIAL COMMENT

Additional description regarding the creation of the gastric conduit can be found in Chapter 12, Ivor-Lewis Esophagectomy.

▶ **Video 13-7.** Esophagectomy Educational Video

Suggested Readings

1. Suda K, Ishida Y, Kawamura Y, et al. Robot-assisted thoracoscopic lymphadenectomy along the left recurrent laryngeal nerve for esophageal squamous cell carcinoma in the prone position: technical report and short-term outcomes. *World J Surg.* 2012;36:1608-1616.
2. Suda K, Nakauchi M, Inaba K, Ishida Y, Uyama I. Robotic surgery for upper GI cancer: current status and future perspectives. *Dig Endosc.* 2016;28:701-713.
3. Suda K, Man-I M, Ishida Y, Kawamura Y, Satoh S, Uyama I. Potential advantages of robotic radical gastrectomy for gastric adenocarcinoma in comparison with conventional laparoscopic approach: a single institutional retrospective comparative cohort study. *Surg Endosc.* 2015;29:673-685.
4. Uyama I, Kanaya S, Ishida Y, Inaba K, Suda K, Satoh S. Novel integrated robotic approach for suprapancreatic D2 nodal dissection for treating gastric cancer: technique and initial experience. *World J Surg.* 2012;36:331-337.
5. Shibasaki S, Suda K, Nakauchi M, et al. Outermost layer-oriented medial approach for infrapyloric nodal dissection in laparoscopic distal gastrectomy. *Surg Endosc.* 2018;32:2137-2148.
6. Cuesta MA, Weijs TJ, Bleys RL, et al. A new concept of the anatomy of the thoracic oesophagus: the meso-oesophagus. Observational study during thoracoscopic esophagectomy. *Surg Endosc.* 2015;29:2576-2582.
7. Nakamura K, Suda K, Akamatsu H, et al. Impact of the Kocher maneuver on anastomotic leak after esophagogastrostomy in combined thoracoscopic-laparoscopic esophagectomy. *Fujita Med J.* 2019; 5:36-44.
8. Japan Esophageal Society. Japanese Classification of Esophageal Cancer, 11th Edition: part I. *Esophagus.* 2017;14(1):1-36. doi: 10.1007/s10388-016-0551-7
9. Giulianotti PC, Coratti A, Angelini M, et al. Robotics in general surgery: personal experience in a large community hospital. *Arch Surg.* 2003;138(7):777-784. doi: 10.1001/archsurg.138.7.777

"The esophageal hiatus may sometimes require diminishing in size in the hopes that this maneuver will help to prevent a recurrence of the hernia; the esophagogastric angle should be reconstituted by fixing the cardia below the diaphragm and so allowing the fundus of the stomach to ballon up under the dome."

—Norman Barrett (1903–1979)

Paraesophageal Hernia Repair

Gabriela Aguiluz • Mario Alberto Masrur • Pier Cristoforo Giulianotti

INTRODUCTION

Hiatal hernias are prevalent gastrointestinal pathology that all physicians will encounter in their practice. The classification of the hiatal hernia consists of 4 types. Type I are sliding hernias, where the gastroesophageal junction migrates above the diaphragm. Type II are pure paraesophageal hernias (PEH), where the gastroesophageal junction remains in its position, but a portion of the fundus herniates through the hiatus parallel to the esophagus. Type III are a combination of the previous 2 types. Type IV includes the presence of a structure other than the stomach, such as the omentum, colon, or small bowel within the hernia sac (**Figure 14-1**). Paraesophageal hernias involve type II-III-IV hiatal hernias (see suggested reading #1). The optimal operative approach varies between institutions; nonetheless, in the last few years, the minimally invasive approach accounts for >90% of elective hernia repairs (see suggested reading #2). The laparoscopic approach requires advanced skills, because the dissection of these hernias can be challenging, especially during the mediastinal portion and mesh fixation. The robotic platform allows for precise hernia sac dissection, esophageal mobilization, accurate reconstruction, and mesh placement, reducing complications such as vagal nerve injuries or esophageal perforations. This chapter will focus on the steps required for a paraesophageal hernia repair.

Indications and Relative Contraindications to the Robotic Approach

The indication for surgical repair is all symptomatic paraesophageal hernias. Relative contraindications for the robotic approach are specific type IV hernias where multiple organs, such as the tail of the pancreas, the spleen, and the colon, in addition to the stomach, herniate through the diaphragm. In those scenarios, a conventional open approach should be considered when planning surgery.

INSTRUMENT REQUIREMENTS

The suggested main robotic instruments/tools can be listed as follows:
- 30° and 0° scope
- Permanent cautery monopolar hook
- Cadière forceps
- Fenestrated bipolar forceps
- 2 needle drivers
- Vessel sealer (in specific cases)

The suggested main laparoscopic instruments/tools can be listed as follows:
- 5-mm scope
- Needle driver
- Graspers
- Scissors
- Clip applier
- Suction-irrigation device

Supplemental materials:
- Gauze sponges
- Penrose drain
- Medium–large clips
- Tailored mesh
- Sutures: Prolene™ 2-0 and 3-0
- Polytetrafluoroethylene (PTFE) pledgets

Photo reproduced with permission from Lord RV. Norman Barrett, "doyen of esophageal surgery." Ann Surg. 1999;229(3):428-439.

Quote reproduced with permission from Stylopoulos N, Rattner DW. The history of hiatal hernia surgery: from Bowditch to laparoscopy. Ann Surg. 2005;241(1):185-193.

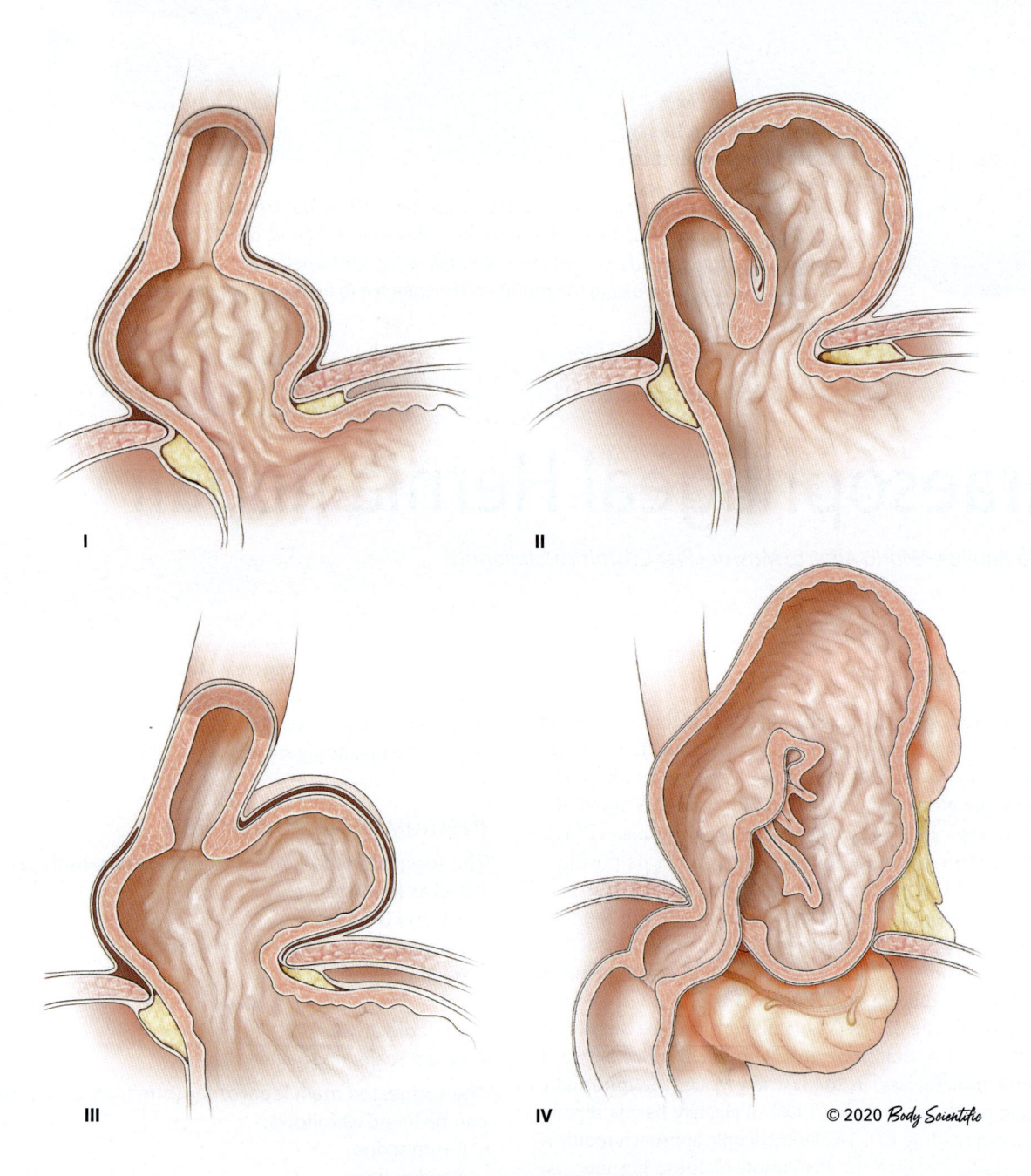

FIGURE 14-1 • Types of hiatal hernia.

Patient Positioning, OR Setup, and Port Setting

After general anesthesia is achieved, the patient's bed is positioned in a 30–45° reversed Trendelenburg, with a 10–15° tilt toward the right side. The patient's legs are parted and protected with intermittent compression devices (**Figure 14-2**). The OR setup is depicted in **Figure 14-3**.

Once pneumoperitoneum is achieved, a 5-mm trocar is placed in the left lateral quadrant, and using a 5-mm laparoscopic camera, initial assessment of the abdominal cavity is performed. Robotic ports are placed along a straight line, 5 cm above the transverse umbilical line, with the scope positioned at the intersection with the left mammary line (**Figure 14-4A**). In obese patients, where the position of the umbilicus is an unreliable landmark, the ports are aligned in a straight line under the costal margins, across the abdomen (**Figure 14-4B**). Additionally, 2 assistant ports (10 and 5 mm) are placed on both sides of the scope. The robotic cart is docked from the patient's right side, and the bedside assistant is positioned between the patient's legs (**Figure 14-3**).

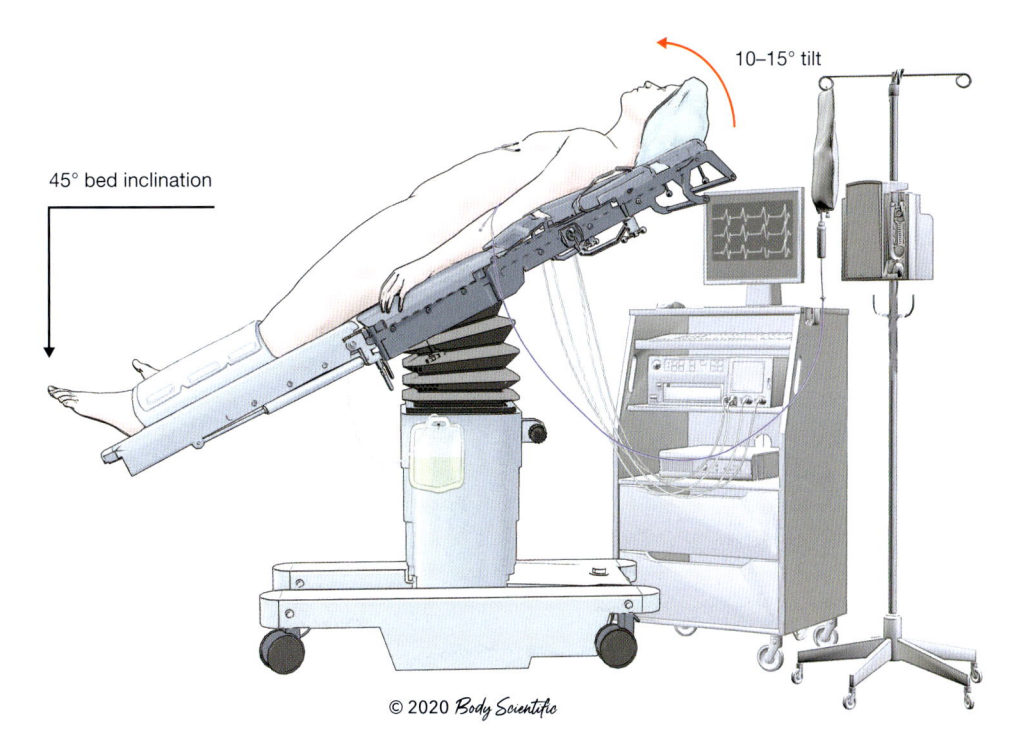

FIGURE 14-2 • Patient positioning.

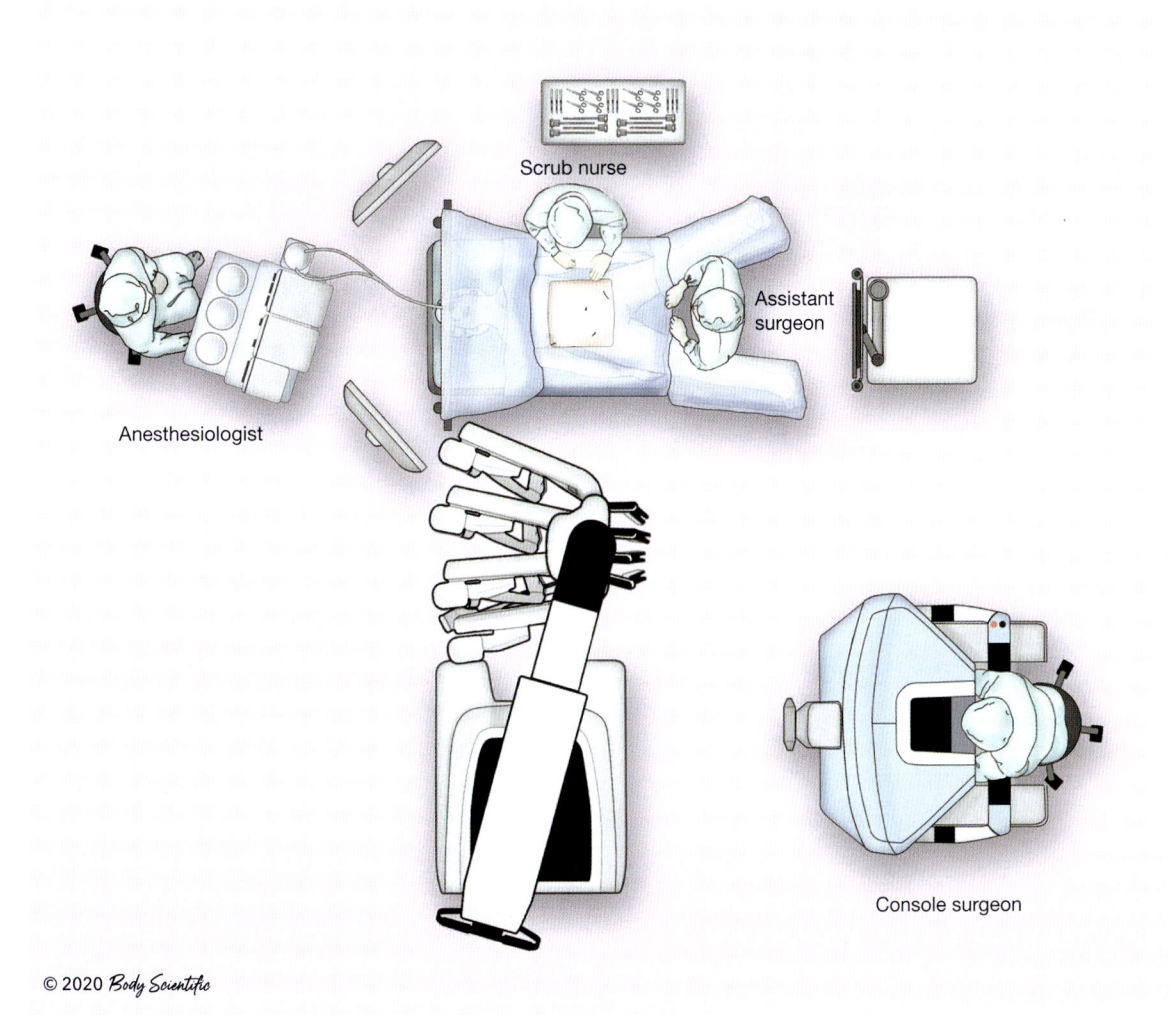

FIGURE 14-3 • OR setup.

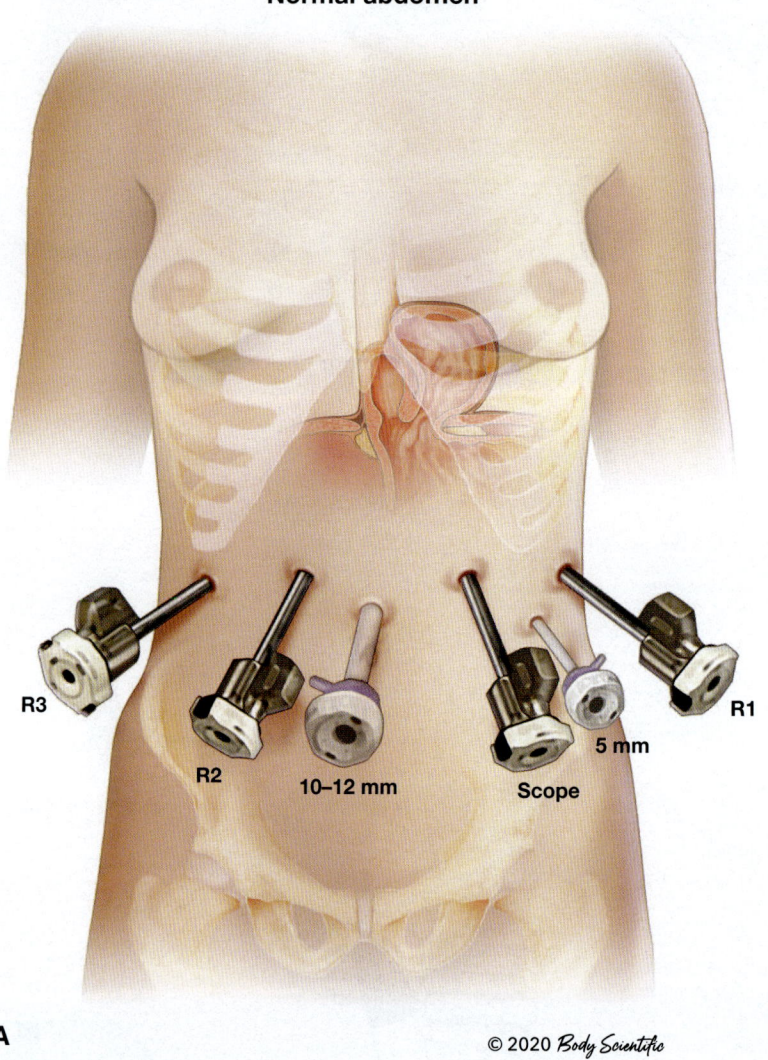

FIGURE 14-4 • Port setting. **A.** Normal abdomen.

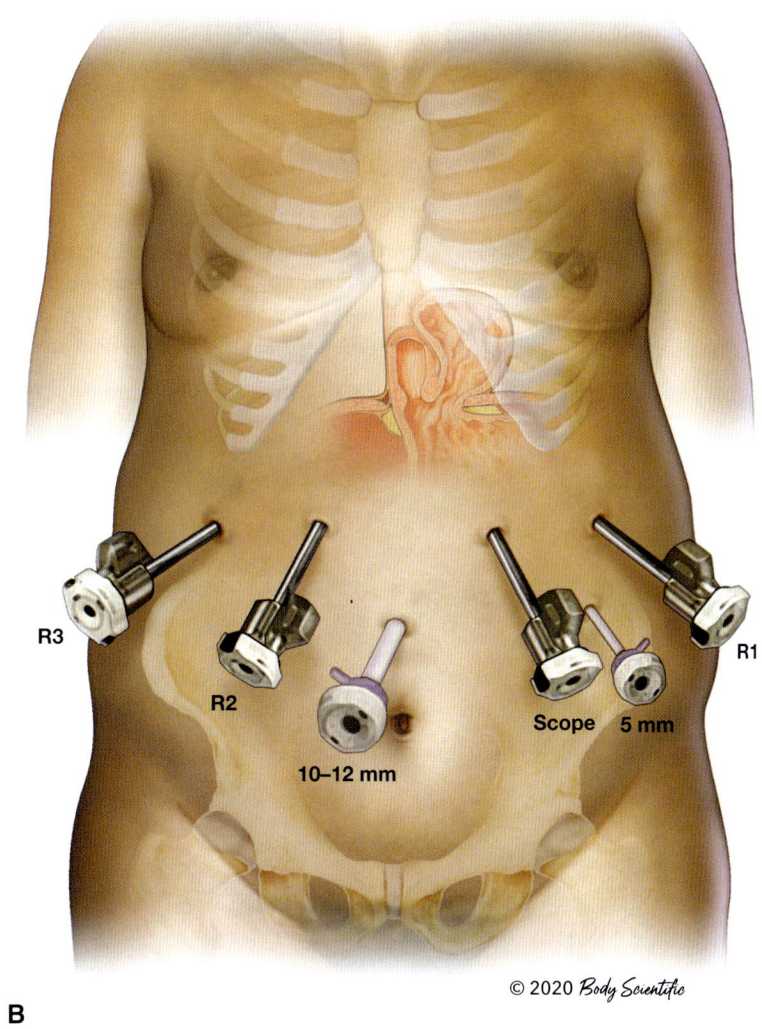

FIGURE 14-4 • (*Continued*) **B.** Wide abdomen.

Surgical Technique

Dissection

▶ **Video 14-1.** Paraesophageal Hernia Dissection Steps

Step 1. Left crus dissection

Once the robot is docked in place, a robotic Cadière forceps protected with a gauze is used through the third arm (R3) to medially retract the left lobe of the liver. Meanwhile, the bedside assistant applies firm traction to the body of the stomach, using 2 atraumatic laparoscopic graspers, and taking good bites of the gastric wall (**Figures 14-5 A, B**). This maneuver allows a partial reduction of the hernia, bringing the stomach back into the abdominal cavity as much as possible.

> ▶▶ **TIPS**
>
> On certain occasions (e.g., bulky segments 2 and 3 of the liver), the hepatic triangular ligament might need to be detached from the diaphragm to allow better exposure of the hiatus.

> ⚠ **PITFALLS**
>
> During this maneuver of retraction, the assistant should be careful not to stretch the omentum or the short gastric vessels, preventing breakage of the capsule of the spleen. The assistant has to grab the stomach, not the omentum.

Dissection continues along the left pillar of the diaphragm using the monopolar hook and the bipolar forceps. The peritoneal sac is incised safely just over the left pillar, and progressively taking down the gastrophrenic ligaments, completely exposing the left crus (**Figures 14-6 A, B**). The scope is advanced into the mediastinum as the next step continues.

Step 1 average time frame: 5–10 min

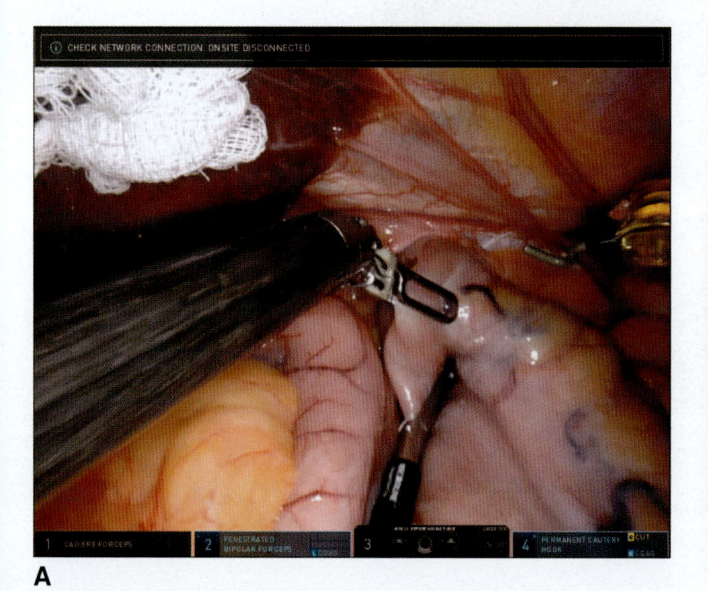

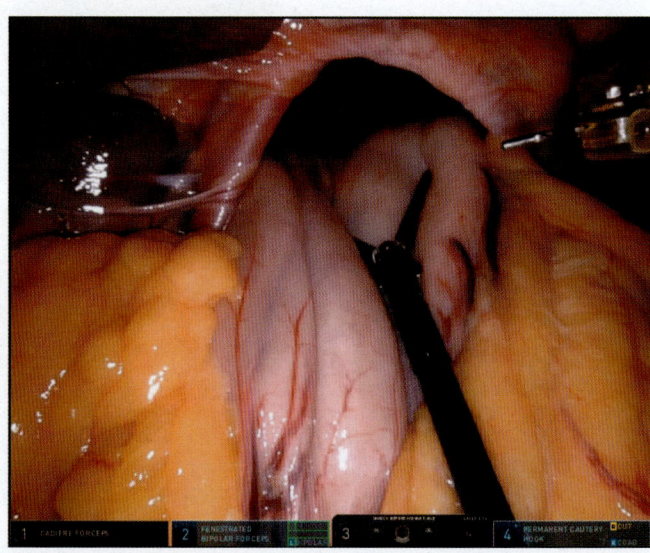

FIGURE 14-5 • Adequate exposure. **A.** In the third arm, a Cadière forceps holding a sponge is used to retract the liver. **B.** Bedside assistant is partially retracting the stomach using an atraumatic grasper.

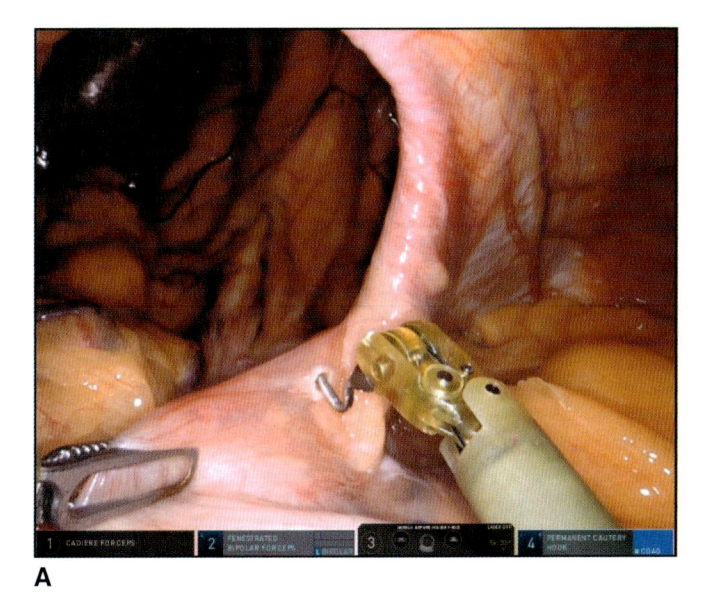

FIGURE 14-6 • Step 1. Left crus dissection. **A.** Peritoneal sac is incised on top of the left pillar, using the tip of the monopolar hook. **B.** Dissection of the peritoneal sac using the back of the instrument.

Step 2. Mediastinal dissection: left side

The dissection progresses inside the mediastinum with the division of the lateral reflection of the hernia sac from the left side of the esophagus, at the 3 o' clock position, and continues to follow a counterclockwise direction (**Figures 14-7 A, B**). The hernia sac's incision is prolonged upward, parallel to the left side of the esophagus.

A combination of blunt and sharp maneuvers is used, following an avascular plane, and paying attention not to injure the left vagal trunk (**Figure 14-8A**). The dissection proceeds posteriorly over the preaortic area (**Figure 14-8B**), until the anterior aspect of the aorta is exposed (**Figures 14-8 B, C**).

Step 2 average time frame: 15–20 min

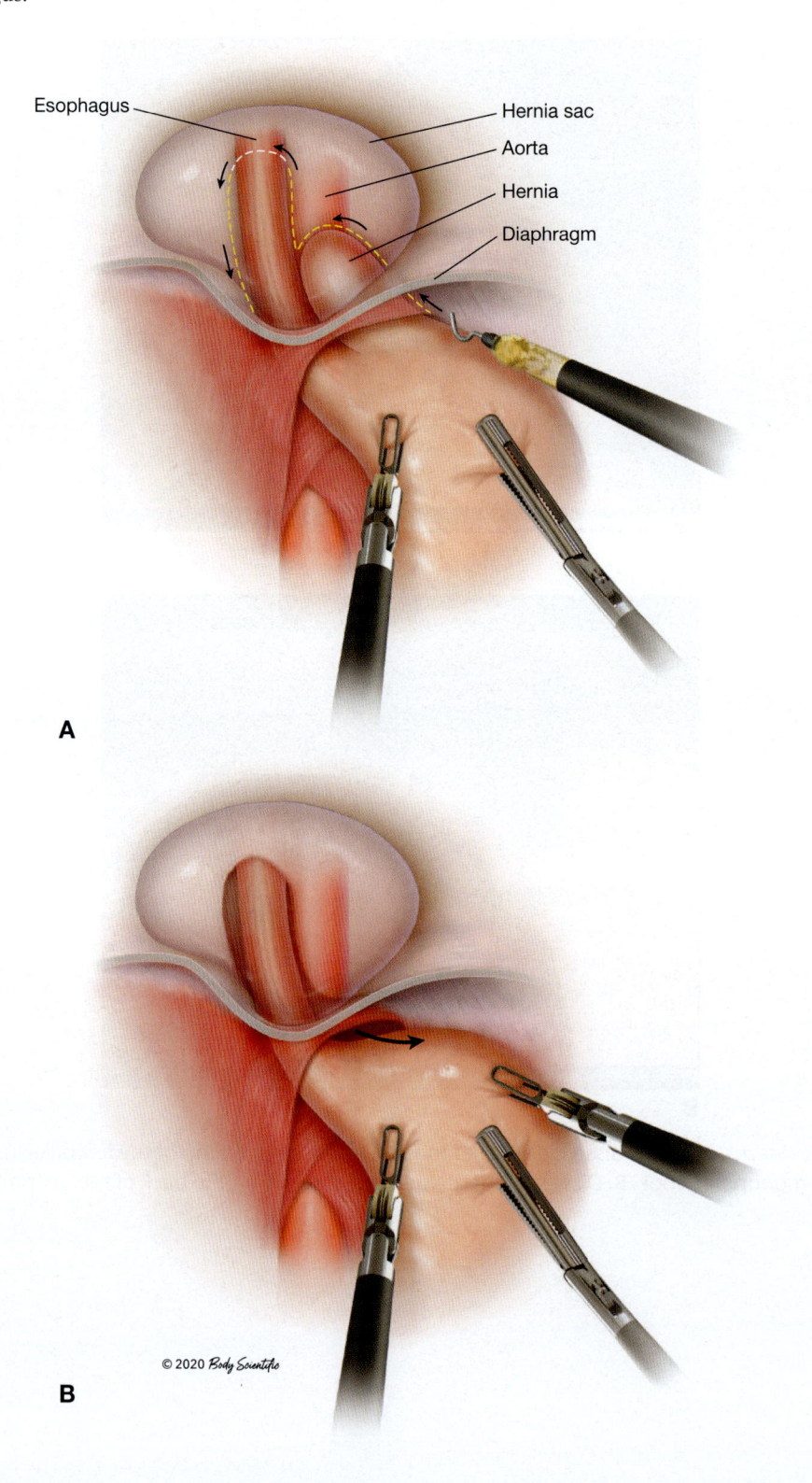

FIGURE 14-7 • Detachment technique of distal esophagus and gastroesophageal junction from the hernia sac. This line of dissection allows a selective separation from the hernia sac, without resecting it in its entirety.

Paraesophageal Hernia Repair 267

▶▶ **TIPS**

Identification of the left vagal trunk should always be attempted to prevent its injury.

▶▶ **TIPS**

In large hernias, the scope might be changed to a 0° angle to allow good visualization and advance the dissection cephalad.

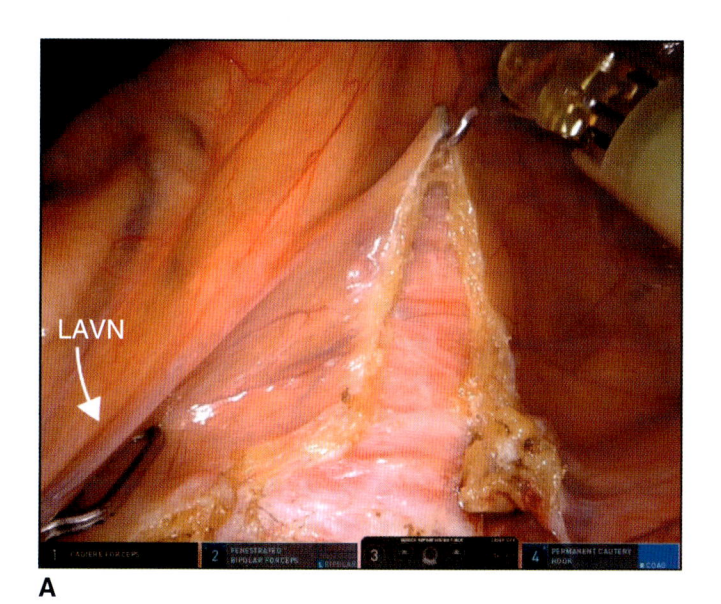

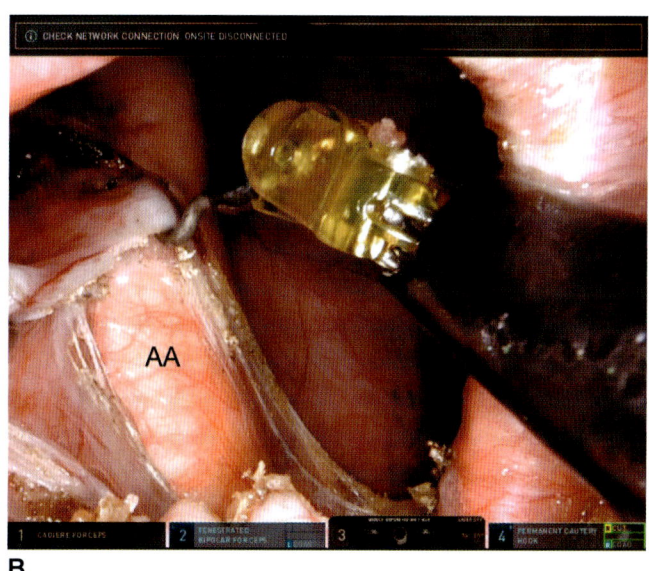

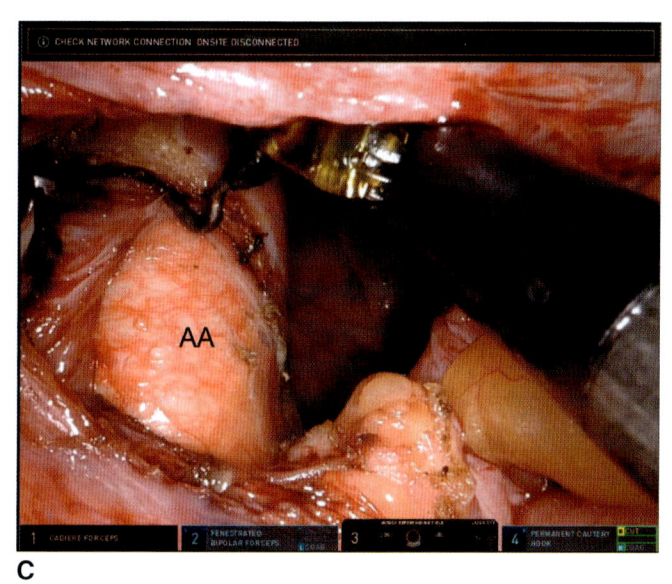

FIGURE 14-8 • Step 2. Mediastinal dissection: left side. Dissection is performed staying preaortic in a plane distant from the position of the left anterior vagal nerve (LAVN). AA, abdominal aorta.

Step 3. Mediastinal dissection: right side, distal esophagus preparation, and Penrose placement

Dissection continues along the right side of the distal esophagus and posteriorly until a retroesophageal window is created (**Figures 14-9 A, B**), joining planes with the left-side dissection anteriorly to the aorta. Dissection should be carried out away from the esophagus to avoid injuring the posterior vagal nerves.

> ▶▶ **TIPS**
>
> A gauze can sometimes be used to facilitate dissection or exposure or to help control small bleeders from the sac mobilization.

Once a proper window is created posteriorly to the esophagus, a Penrose drain is passed around the esophagus, with both ends clipped together. The assistant will be able to apply an effective and safe retraction of the esophagus by pulling the Penrose drain downward (**Figures 14-10 A, B**). This maneuver facilitates the dissection of the right pillar and the mobilization and exposure of the gastroesophageal junction and the posterior part of the distal esophagus (**Figures 14-10 C, D**). On occasions, a lipoma can be found in the posterior aspect of the gastroesophageal junction, consisting of perigastric fat tissue. The excision of this lipoma is required to perform a proper repair.

Step 3 average time frame: 15–20 min

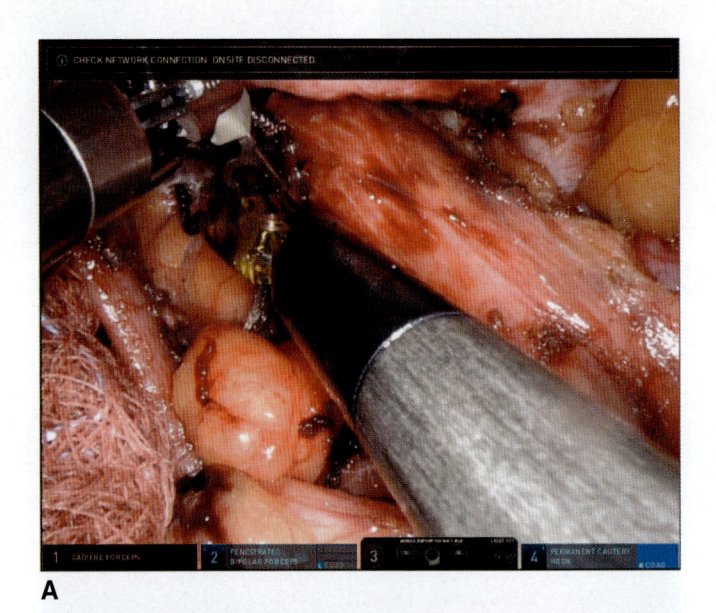

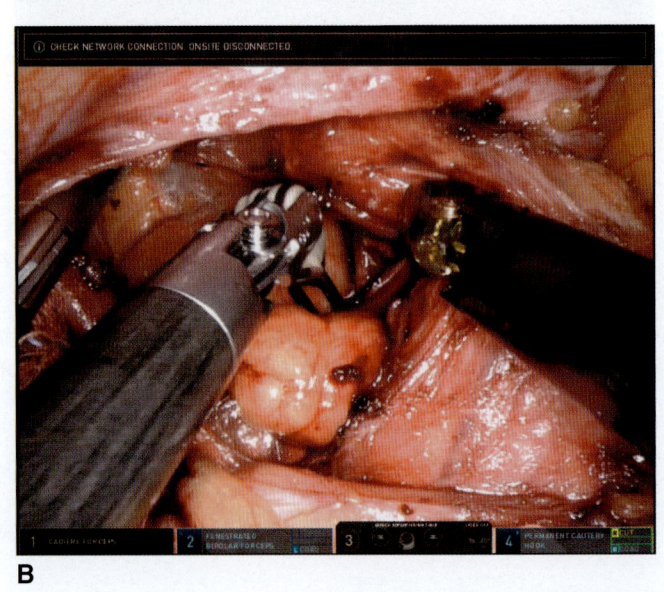

FIGURE 14-9 • Step 3. Mediastinal dissection: right side. **A.** Dissection on the right side of the esophagus. **B.** A retroesophageal window is created to allow the passage of a Penrose drain.

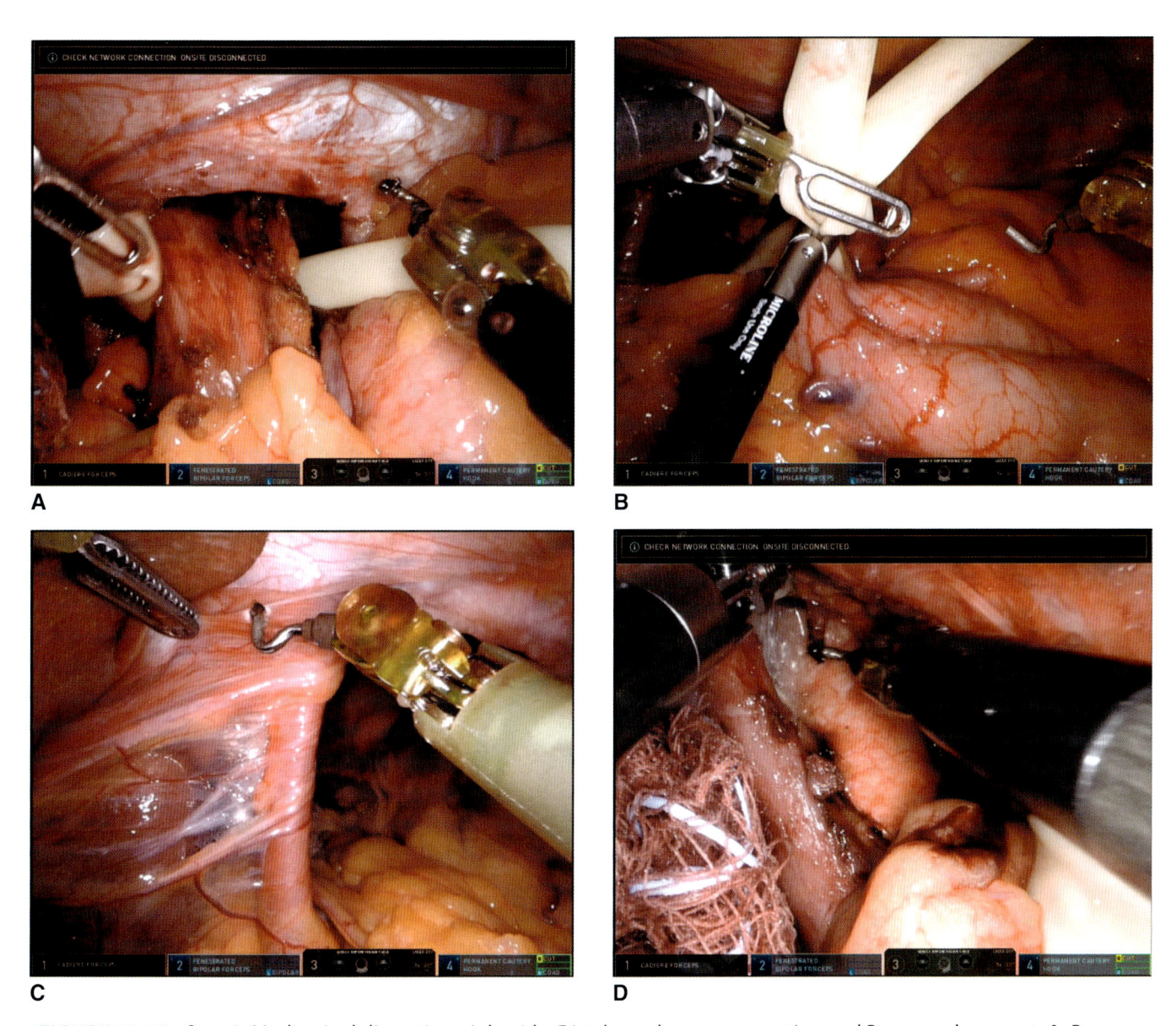

FIGURE 14-10 • Step 3. Mediastinal dissection: right side. Distal esophagus preparation and Penrose placement. **A.** Passage of Penrose drain behind the esophagus. **B.** Penrose is grabbed by the assistant to apply retraction. **C.** Dissection of the right pillar of the diaphragm avoiding vagal fibers in the gastrohepatic ligament. **D.** Preaortic dissection facilitated by the retraction of the esophagus by the assistant.

Step 4. Right crus dissection and completion of esophagogastric mobilization

The procedure continues by approaching the right pillar of the diaphragm. The gastrohepatic ligament is stretched inside the mediastinum making this a complicated step. It is essential to identify and preserve the vascular and neural structures in the lesser curvature of the stomach to prevent the denervation of the stomach and gallbladder that can lead to complications such as gastroparesis or dyspeptic syndromes. Occasionally, an accessory left hepatic artery can be encountered, potentially interfering with the dissection; it should be assessed and, when possible, spared.

The gastrohepatic ligament should be opened in the higher portion of the right pillar, away from the vagal fibers stretched down the ligament (**Figure 14-10C**). After opening the gastrohepatic ligament, it is easier to retract the rest of the ligament downward without unnecessarily dividing neural structures.

The assistant should be able to provide a proper retraction of the stomach to reduce the gastrohepatic ligament into the abdominal cavity. The dissection proceeds by entering the mediastinum until joining the dissection line previously created on the right side of the esophagus.

Step 4 average time frame: 20–30 min

> ▶▶ **TIPS**
>
> When the esophagus is displaced transversally to the right chest, it will be challenging to dissect along the right side of the esophagus, requiring an inversion of Steps 3 and 4. The right pillar should be prepared before addressing the right side of the mediastinum, allowing to stretch the esophagus-gastric junction down, and to complete the dissection on the right side of the esophagus.

> ⚠ **PITFALLS**
>
> The parietal pleura can sometimes be accidentally opened during the mediastinal dissection, leading to an ipsilateral or even bilateral pneumothorax. This event, when identified, should be communicated to the anesthesia team to allow for proper respiratory volume adjustments when necessary. This complication does not typically require extra surgical maneuvers, and it is usually managed conservatively, decreasing the abdominal pressure. On rare occasions, with the worsening of pulmonary parameters, a chest tube drainage placement will be necessary.

> ▶▶ **TIPS**
>
> Attempting the complete excision of the hernia sac in gigantic herniation represents a difficult task. This can lead to unnecessary risks, such as intrathoracic bleeding and vagal injuries, and generate redundant tissue around the gastroesophageal junction, which could hinder the fundoplication. The primary surgical goal is to complete a circumferential detachment of the distal esophagus, the gastroesophageal junction, and the stomach from the hernia sac. This will allow restoring the anatomy into the intra-abdominal cavity.

Reconstruction

▶ **Video 14-2. Paraesophageal Hernia Repair Reconstruction Steps**

Step 5. Cruroplasty

Once the adequate esophageal length is accomplished and both pillars are fully exposed, the cruroplasty is performed. With 2 robotic needle drivers, the hiatus reconstruction is carried out approximating the pillars with 3 to 4 interrupted figure 8 non-absorbable sutures of Prolene® 2-0 (**Figure 14-11A**). In the case of increased tension on the pillars, nonabsorbable stitches reinforced with polytetrafluoroethylene (PTFE) pledgets can be used to decrease the risk of a crural tear (**Figures 14-11 B, C**). The role of the assistant during this step is to retract the esophagus laterally to allow a good exposure of the right and left crus.

Step 5 average time frame: 10–15 min

> ▶▶ **TIPS**
>
> Cruroplasty is typically performed by placing sutures posteriorly. A particular effort should be made to avoid anterior stitches, because they might be the cause of compression on the esophagus, leading to refractory dysphagia. If anterior stitches are required, they should be kept at the minimum with particular attention to avoid stricture and compression.

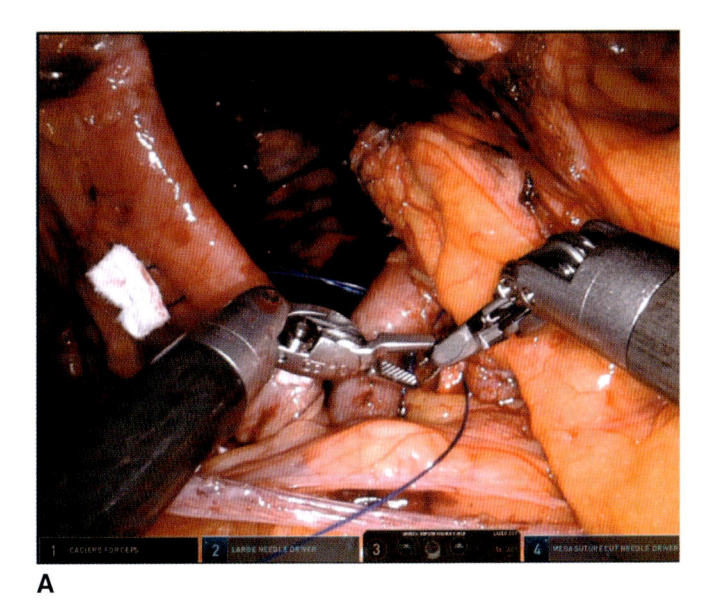

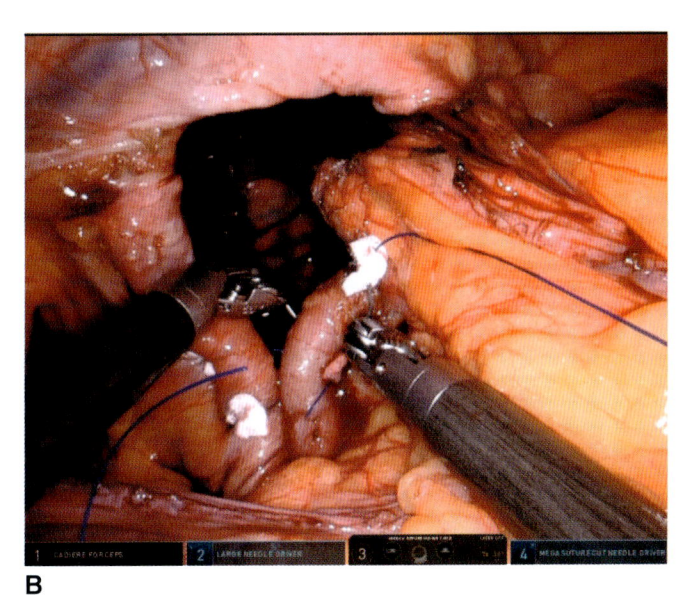

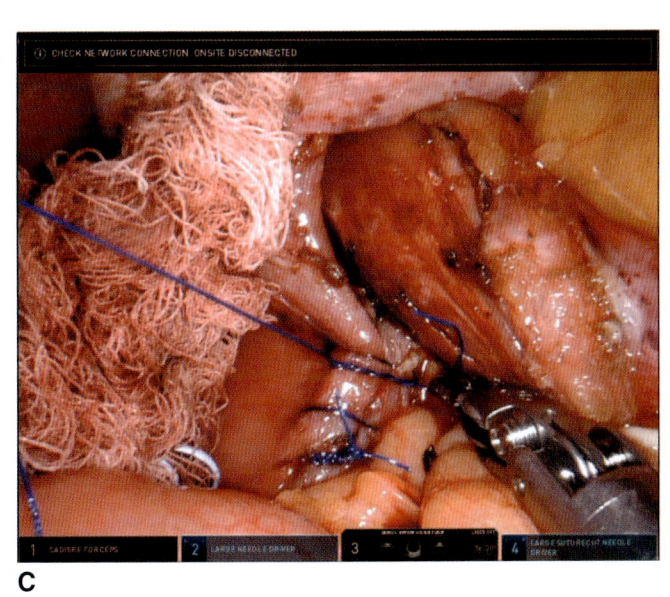

FIGURE 14-11 • Step 5. Cruroplasty. **A, B.** Approximation of pillars reinforced with PTFE pledgets. **C.** Approximation of pillars with nonabsorbable sutures.

Step 6. Mesh reinforcement

Mesh reinforcement is recommended based on short-term outcomes studies. There are different types of mesh, including nonabsorbable and absorbable material. Although absorbable material is associated with fewer complications like esophageal erosions, a higher recurrence rate has been described (see suggested reading #3). A dual-surface polytetrafluoroethylene (ePTFE) material is the suggested mesh option to reinforce the hiatus offering a strong repair with a low complication risk. The mesh is tailored in a U shape to the hiatus (**Figure 14-12**); it is introduced through the 12-mm assistant port and placed adequately around the hiatus. The mesh is fixated with multiple interrupted stitches of Prolene® 3-0 around the pillars, laterally and posteriorly (**Figures 14-13 A–C**).

Step 6 average time frame: 20–30 min

> ▶▶ **TIPS**
>
> Mesh placement is intended to reinforce the pillars of the hiatus. It is essential to avoid contact of the mesh edges with the esophagus because this could result in an esophageal erosion.

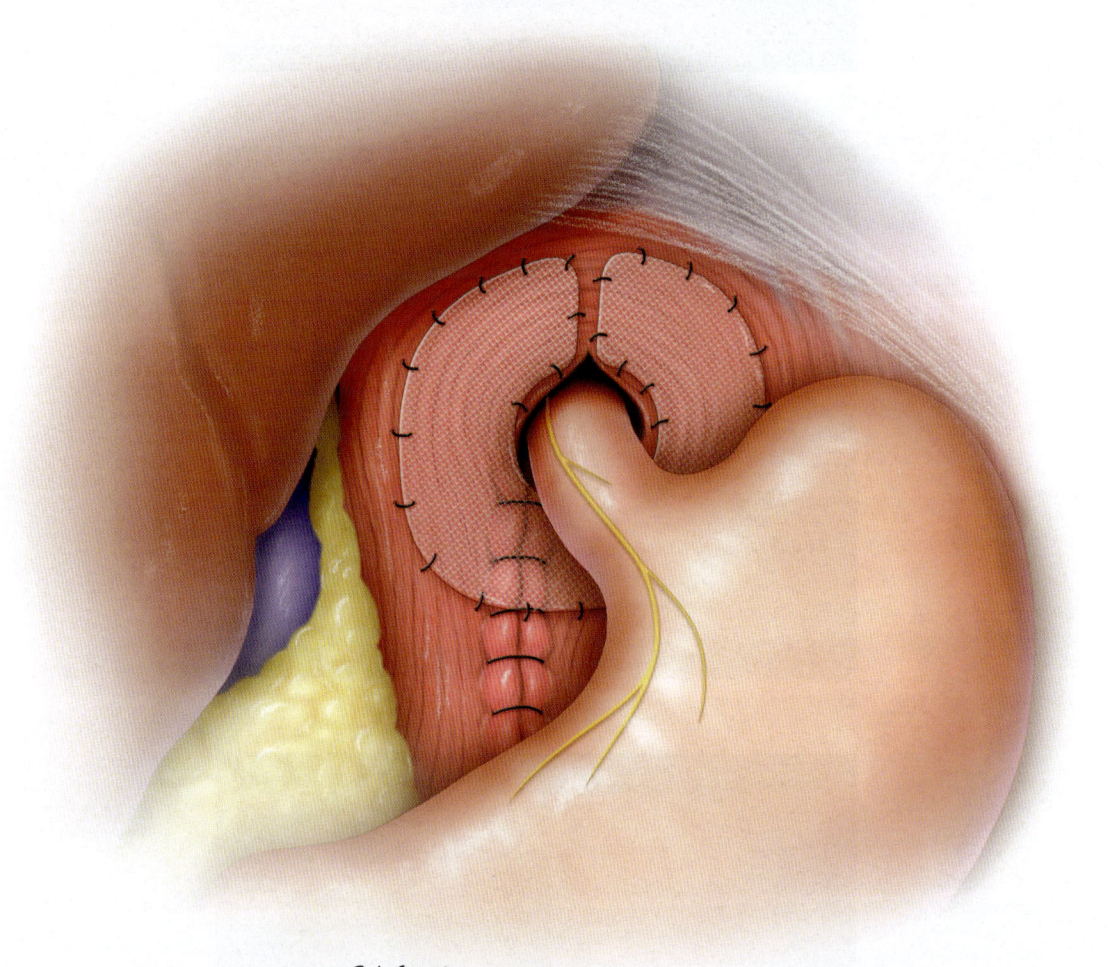

FIGURE 14-12 • Step 6. Mesh reinforcement. Mesh is tailored in a U shape.

Paraesophageal Hernia Repair 273

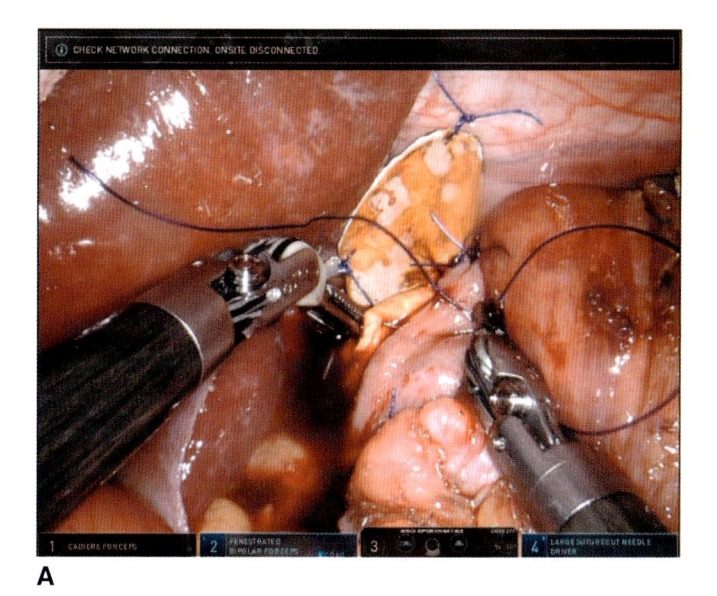

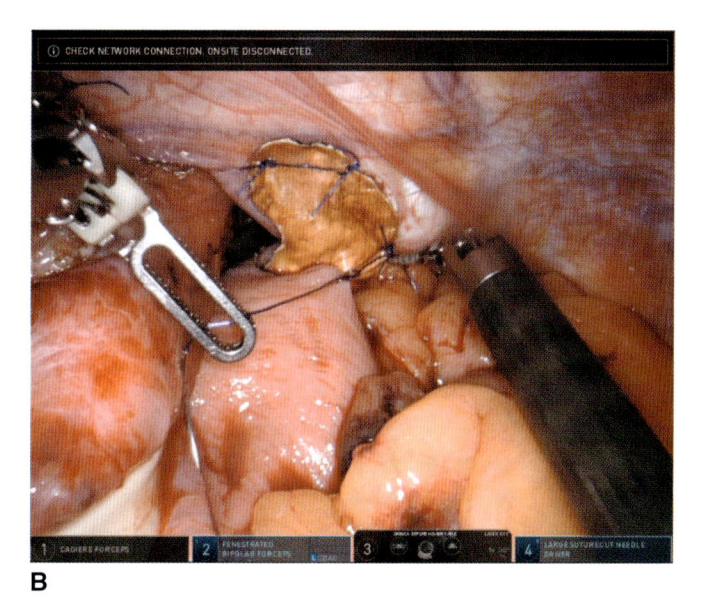

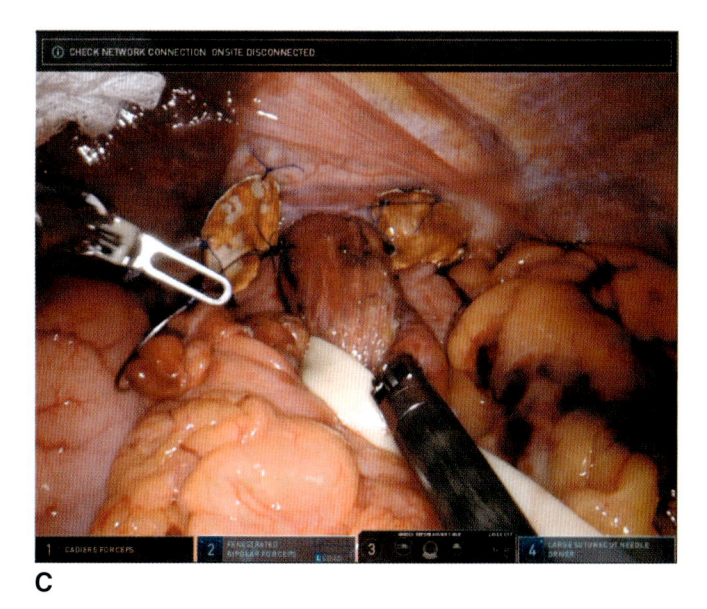

FIGURE 14-13 • Step 6. Mesh reinforcement.

Step 7. Fundoplication

If the patient has symptoms of reflux and/or endoscopic evidence of gastroesophageal reflux disease (GERD), the operation is completed with the construction of an antireflux wrap, usually a Toupet-type (180–270°) fundoplication (**Figure 14-14B**). This represents a posterior partial fundoplication, where part of the gastric fundus is pulled posteriorly behind the gastroesophageal junction. It is fixated with interrupted stitches of Prolene™ 3-0, to the right and left diaphragmatic pillars including the mesh. The placement of sutures on the esophagus should be avoided to prevent damage of vagal fibers.

Nissen fundoplication (360°) can also be considered (**Figure 14-14C**), although a higher incidence of postoperative dysphagia can be observed in this setting.

In patients with dysphagia as the main symptom, restoring the anatomy with at least 2 cm of the intraabdominal esophagus without tension is the preferred surgical treatment. Fundoplication surgical techniques for the management of GERD are described in Chapter 15, Selective Nissen Fundoplication.

Step 7 average time frame: 5–10 min

> ▶▶ **TIPS**
>
> Patients with a surgical indication for giant paraesophageal hernia repair might present a different array of symptoms, GERD refractory to medical therapy, dysphagia, early satiety, postprandial chest or abdominal pain, anemia, or vomiting. When planning the repair, a Nissen-type fundoplication should be performed preferably for patients with refractory GERD symptoms. For the rest of the patients presenting symptoms related to the stomach's physical displacement but not GERD, a Toupet fundoplication is a better option. It avoids the unnecessary risks of postsurgical dysphagia and bloating sometimes associated with the Nissen fundoplication (see suggested reading #6).

> ▶▶ **TIPS**
>
> In selected cases of "super gigantic" hernias where there is a higher risk of early recurrences and there is a need for enhanced stabilization of the reconstruction, supplementary techniques can be used. A gastropexy, applying stitches fixating the fundus to the diaphragm and abdominal wall, may be considered. Rarely, a temporary percutaneous endoscopic gastrostomy fixating the stomach to the abdominal wall, and therefore preventing its migration to the chest, will be needed as an option.

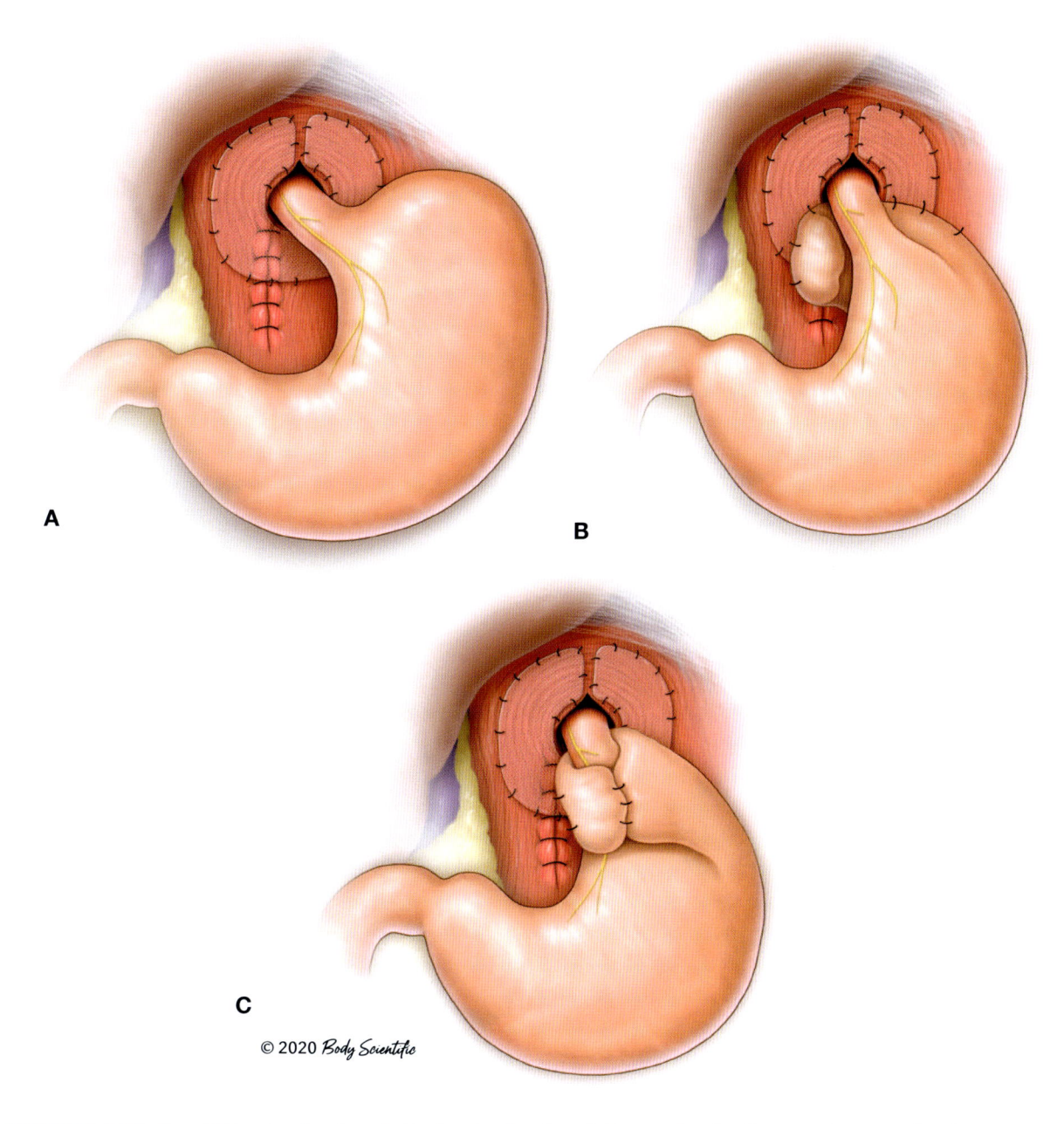

FIGURE 14-14 • Step 7. Fundoplication. **A.** No fundoplication. **B.** Toupet fundoplication. **C.** Nissen fundoplication.

Suggested Readings

1. Kohn GP, Price RR, DeMeester SR, et al. Guidelines for the management of hiatal hernia. *Surg Endosc.* 2013;27(12):4409-4428. doi: 10.1007/s00464-013-3173-3
2. Schlosser KA, Maloney SR, Prasad T, Augenstein VA, Heniford BT, Colavita PD. Mesh reinforcement of paraesophageal hernia repair: trends and outcomes from a national database. *Surgery.* 2019;166(5):879-885. doi: 10.1016/j.surg.2019.05.014
3. Targarona EM, Bendahan G, Balague C, Garriga J, Trias M. Mesh in the hiatus: a controversial issue. *Arch Surg.* 2004;139(12):1286-1296. doi: 10.1001/archsurg.139.12.1286
4. Toupet A. Technique d'oesophago-gastroplastie avec phrenogastropexie appliquee dans la cure radicale des hernies hiatales et comme complement de l'operation de Heller dans les cardiospasmes. *Mem Acad Chir.* 1963;89:394-399.
5. Nissen R. [The relationship between hiatus hernia and reflux esophagits]. *Munchener medizinische Wochenschrift (1950).* 1960;102:1472-1474.
6. Schwameis K, Zehetner J, Rona K, et al. Post-Nissen dysphagia and bloating syndrome: outcomes after conversion to Toupet fundoplication. *J Gastrointest Surg.* 2017;21(3):441-445. doi: 10.1007/s11605-016-3320-y
7. Mertens AC, Tolboom RC, Zavrtanik H, Draaisma WA, Broeders I. Morbidity and mortality in complex robot-assisted hiatal hernia surgery: 7-year experience in a high-volume center. *Surg Endosc.* 2019;33(7):2152-2161. doi: 10.1007/s00464-018-6494-4
8. Giulianotti PC, Coratti A, Angelini M, et al. Robotics in general surgery: personal experience in a large community hospital. *Arch Surg.* 2003;138(7):777-784. doi: 10.1001/archsurg.138.7.777

"One who commits to surgery must, from the first day of training, be made aware not only of the joys, but also the burdens of responsibility."

—Rudolph Nissen (1896–1981)

Selective Nissen Fundoplication

Gabriela Aguiluz • Alberto Mangano • Pier Cristoforo Giulianotti

INTRODUCTION

In the literature, there is a high level of evidence regarding the effectiveness of the surgical approach in treating gastroesophageal reflux disease (GERD). Surgery can present equal or even superior outcomes compared to medical treatment, with reported curative results in up to 93% of patients (see suggested reading #1).

Surgical management addresses the mechanical, anatomical and functional components of GERD, and it can achieve high standards in terms of patient satisfaction. Surgery can also help prevent or revert Barrett's metaplasia.

The Nissen fundoplication was first described in the mid-1950s by Rudolph Nissen. Afterward, the operation gained increasing popularity, and as described by Donahue et al., it has been the antireflux approach of choice for GERD. Over several decades, this approach has been increasingly and extensively performed worldwide, first with the traditional open approach, and subsequently with minimally invasive surgery (MIS) techniques. Currently, there is a vast *corpus* of evidence supporting that the MIS strategy should be the favored approach over traditional open surgery. MIS fundoplication provides better short-term outcomes with no significant differences in long-term failure rate.

Even though the laparoscopic Nissen effectively controls GERD, it is not immune from side effects and complications, such as dysphagia, bloating, and general dyspeptic postprandial symptoms. One of the main reasons for dysphagia is a tight wrap. To avoid this complication, the laparoscopic technique includes an extensive mobilization of the gastric curvature with the division of all short gastric vessels and a complete opening of the gastrohepatic ligament. Such extensive dissection may often create problems such as increased risk of sliding Nissen or vagal disruption of the gallbladder function.

The endowristed capabilities of the robotic approach may allow a very selective dissection around the hiatus with mobilization of the posterior, extraperitoneal part of the gastric fundus. In doing so, the division of the short gastric vessels and the gastrohepatic ligament opening is minimized. A floppy wrap may be obtained without the extensive dissection usually necessary with the laparoscopic approach.

For these reasons, the robotic technique described in this chapter is a new variant of the traditional Nissen, and it is called "selective robotic Nissen fundoplication."

INSTRUMENT REQUIREMENTS

The suggested main robotic instruments/tools can be listed as follows:
- 30° and 0° scope
- Permanent cautery monopolar hook
- Cadière forceps
- Fenestrated bipolar forceps
- 2 large needle drivers
- Vessel sealer (in specific cases)

The suggested main laparoscopic instruments/tools can be listed as follows:
- 5-mm scope
- Needle driver
- Graspers
- Scissors
- Clip applier
- Suction-irrigation device

Supplemental materials:
- Gauze, sponges
- Penrose drains
- Medium–large clips
- Sutures: Prolene™ 2-0 and 3-0

Photo and quote reproduced with permission from Fults DW, Taussky P. The life of Rudolf Nissen: advancing surgery through science and principle. World J Surg. 2011;35(6):1402-1408.

Indications and Relative Contraindications to the Robotic Approach

Currently, the guidelines about the treatment of GERD are evolving. There is still disagreement among different authors, as the available data have low level of evidence, high risk of biases, and most recommendations are therefore conditional/not strong.

However, with a confirmed diagnosis of GERD, the surgical approach should be considered in the following 4 main categories:

1. As an alternative to a lifelong medical treatment in responders who are not complaint, or if there are significant side effects.
2. Early Barret Esophagus (because the operation may reverse the metaplasia).
3. Extraesophageal symptoms (e.g., aspiration, chest pain, cough, asthma).
4. Anatomical hernias.

For more information, see suggested readings #1, 8, 9, 11.

There are no absolute contraindications to the robotic approach for the Nissen fundoplication. A relative contraindication might be the presence of tenacious and extensive adhesions due to a history of multiple open abdominal surgeries. However, the operation can still be conducted in an MIS way depending on the surgical expertise. Patient selection is fundamental, and it should be framed into the specific skills of the surgical team.

Patient Positioning, OR Setup, and Port Setting

After general anesthesia is achieved, the operating table is positioned 30–45° in reverse Trendelenburg, with a 10–15° tilt toward the right side. The patient's legs are parted and protected with intermittent compression devices. The anesthesiologist must place an orogastric tube to decompress the stomach (**Figure 15-1**). The OR setup is depicted in **Figure 15-2**.

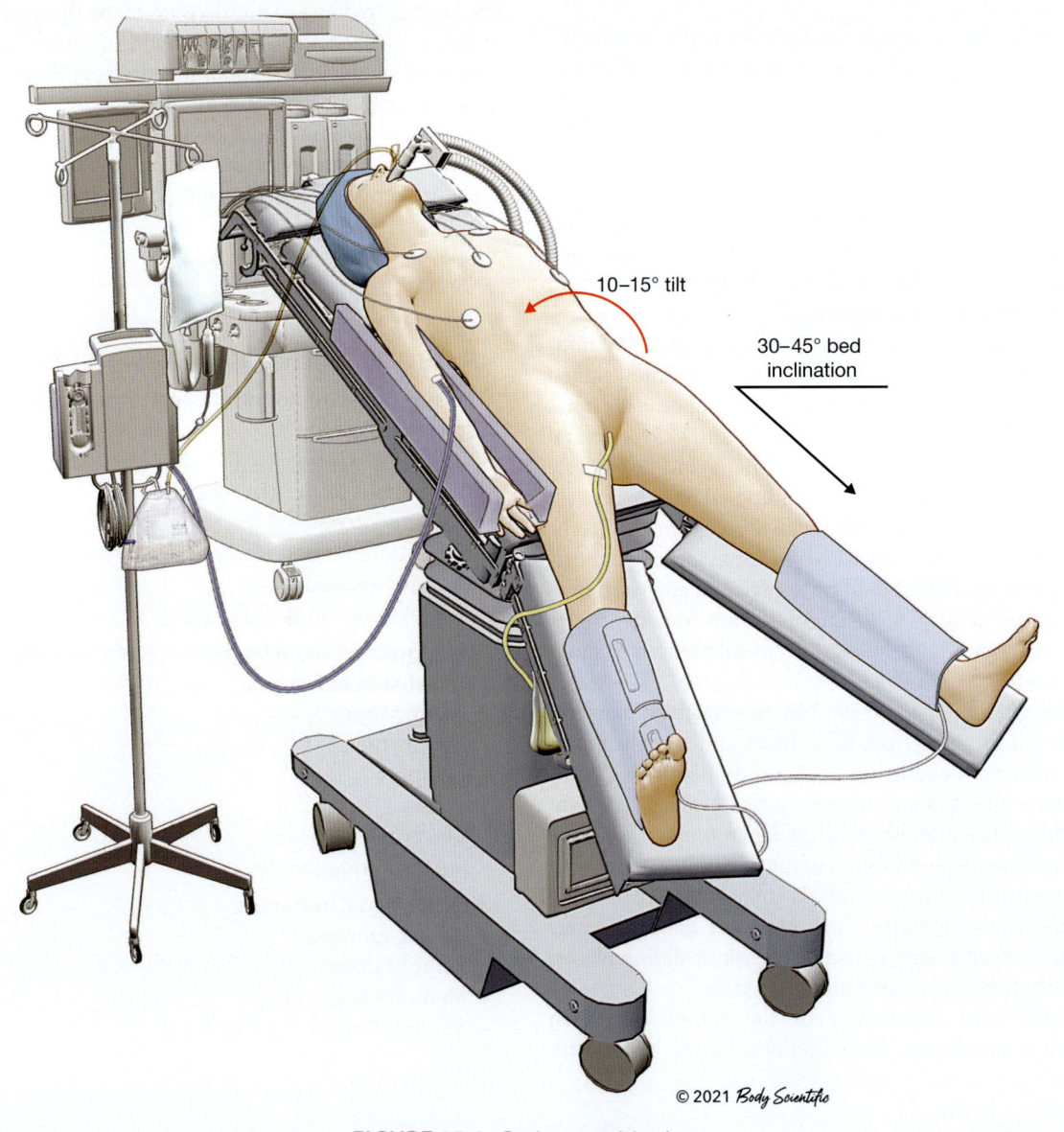

FIGURE 15-1 • Patient positioning.

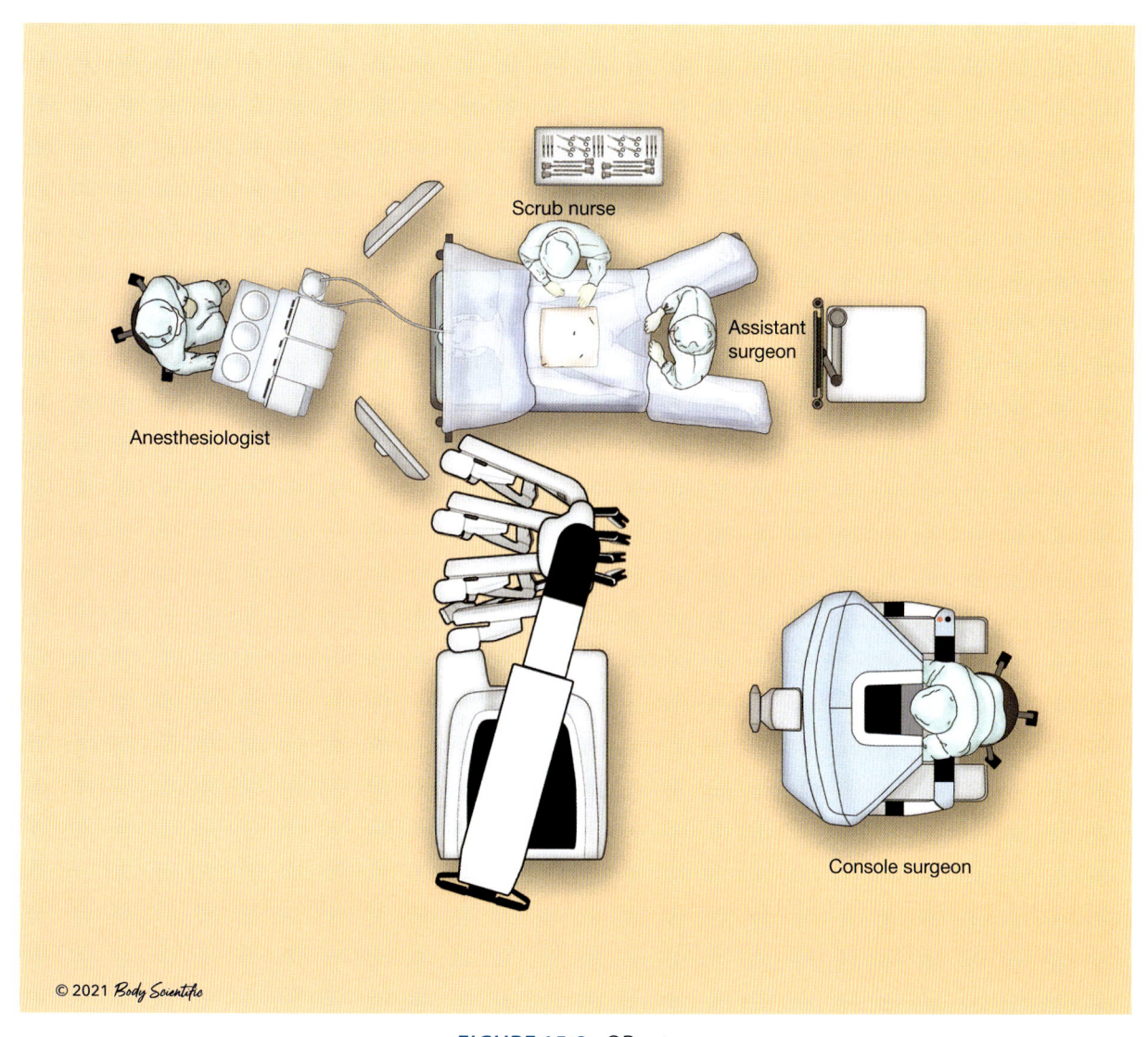

FIGURE 15-2 • OR setup.

Once the pneumoperitoneum is achieved, a 5-mm trocar is placed in the left lateral quadrant, and using a 5-mm laparoscopic camera, an initial assessment of the abdominal cavity is performed. The robotic ports are placed along a straight line, 5 cm above the transverse umbilical line. The scope is positioned at the intersection with the left mammary line (**Figure 15-3A**). In patients with obesity or a wide abdomen, the position of the umbilicus is an unreliable landmark. Hence, the ports are aligned in a straight line under the costal margins, across the abdomen (**Figure 15-3B**). In addition, 2 assistant ports (10 and 5 mm) are placed on both sides of the scope. The robotic cart is docked from the patient's right side, orientating the robotic arms toward the target anatomy, and the bedside assistant is positioned between the patient's legs (**Figure 15-2**).

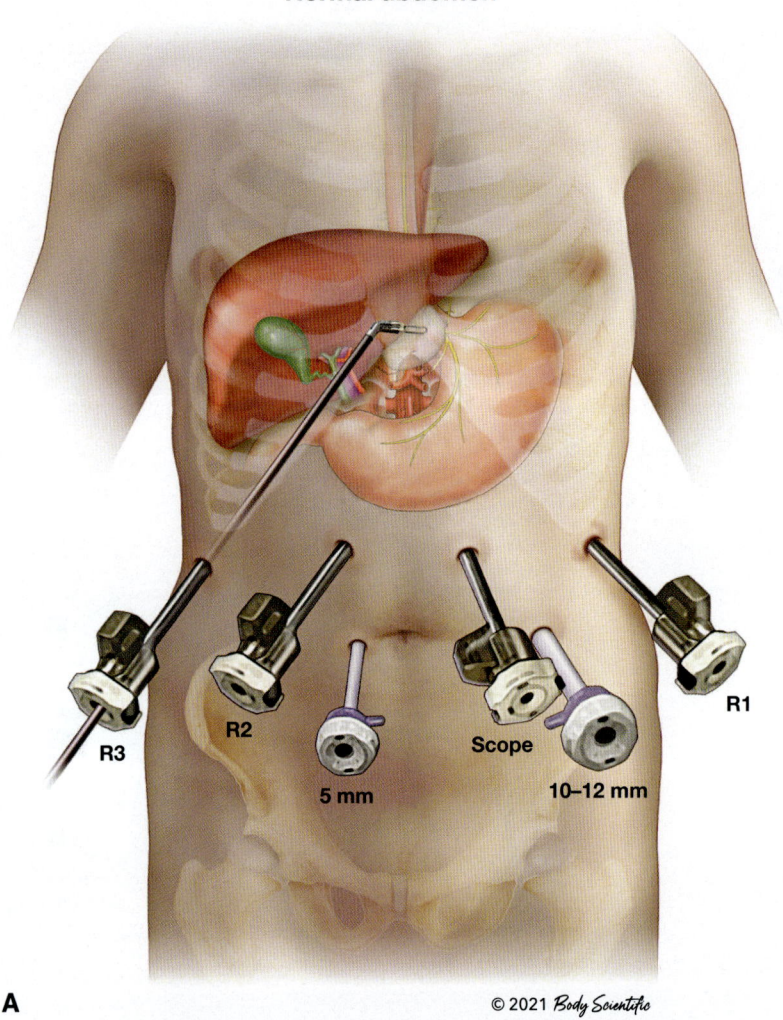

FIGURE 15-3 • Port setting. **A.** Normal abdomen.

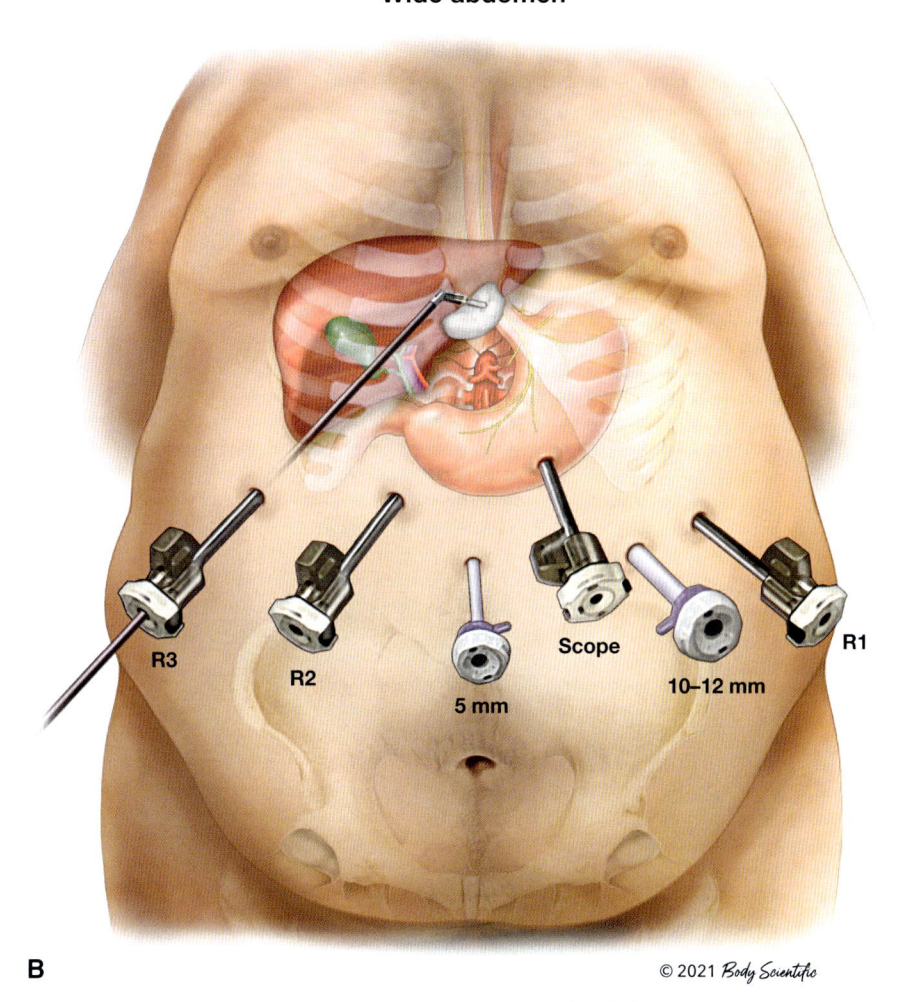

FIGURE 15-3 • (*Continued*) **B.** Wide abdomen.

Surgical Technique

Dissection

▶ Video 15-1. Selective Nissen Fundoplication: Dissection Steps

Step 1. Retraction of the liver and exposure of the hiatus
The surgery starts with adequate exposure of the diaphragmatic hiatus and the gastroesophageal (GE) junction, providing full operational control of an optimal surgical field. Proper exposure is achieved by the R3, positioned in the abdomen's right upper quadrant and the dynamic retraction provided by the beside assistant. A Cadière forceps, protected with a gauze, retracts medially segments 2 and 3 of the liver. Simultaneously, the bedside assistant pulls the gastric fundus downward by holding the gastric wall firmly with laparoscopic graspers and dynamically adjusting retraction throughout the procedure to maintain proper exposure at all times (**Figure 15-4**).

Step 1 average time frame: 3–5 min

▶▶ **TIPS**

In some conditions (e.g., bulky segments 2 and 3 of the liver), the hepatic triangular ligament might need to be detached from the diaphragm to allow proper retraction and better exposure of the hiatus.

⚠ **PITFALLS**

Excessive traction on the omentum may stretch splenic adhesions and cause bleeding. The assistant preferably has to grab the gastric wall and be very careful in retracting the omentum.

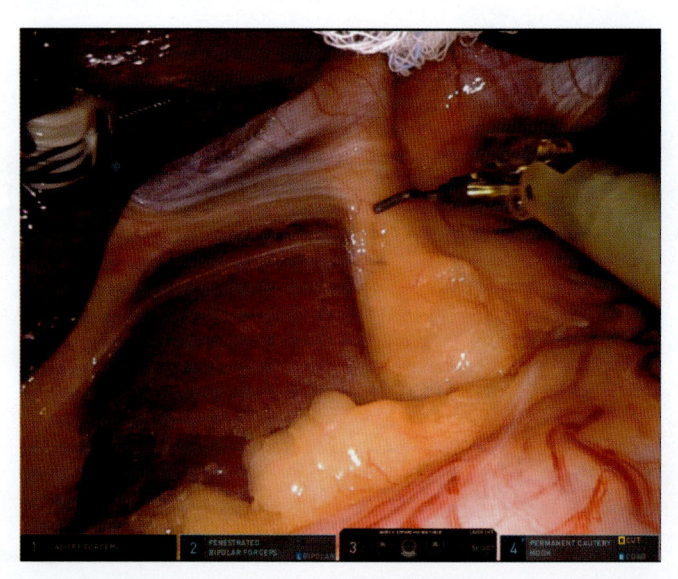

FIGURE 15-4 • Step 1. Retraction of the liver and exposure of the hiatus.

Step 2. Gastrohepatic ligament opening and right crus dissection
The upper portion of the gastrohepatic ligament is selectively opened, staying close to the liver and following a completely avascular surgical plane while avoiding any damage to the vagal fibers or to accessory hepatic arteries (**Figures 15-5 A, B**). The dissection proceeds toward the right pillar. The esophagus is separated from the right crus with a combination of blunt and sharp maneuvers using the monopolar hook, avoiding injuries to the posterior vagus nerve (**Figures 15-6 A, B**).

Step 2 average time frame: 5–10 min

⚠ **PITFALLS**

The monopolar energy should be used cautiously, since the thermal lateral spread might damage the posterior vagus nerve (**Figures 15-7 A–D**).

Selective Nissen Fundoplication 283

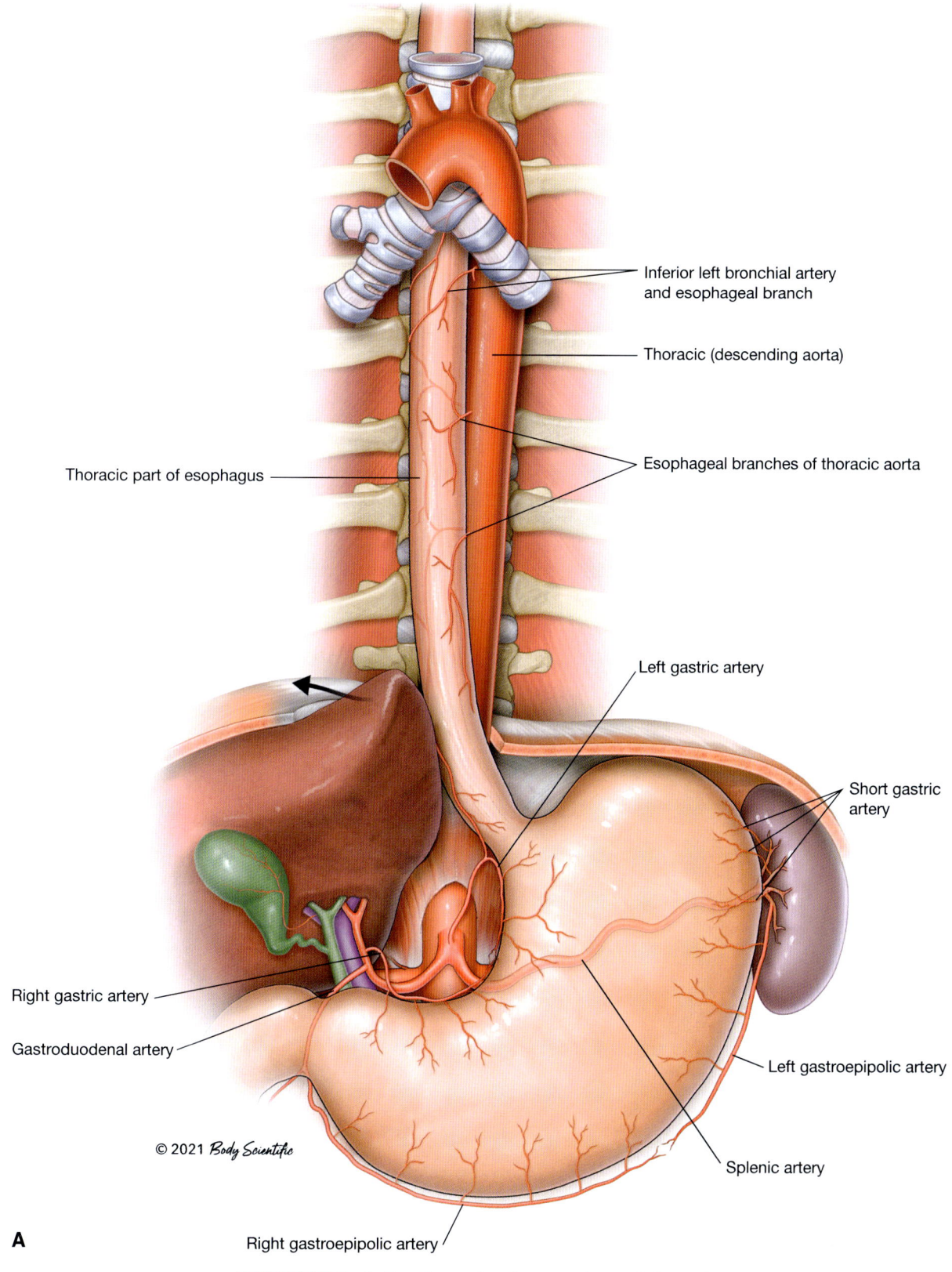

FIGURE 15-5 • **A.** Esophageal and stomach arterial supply.

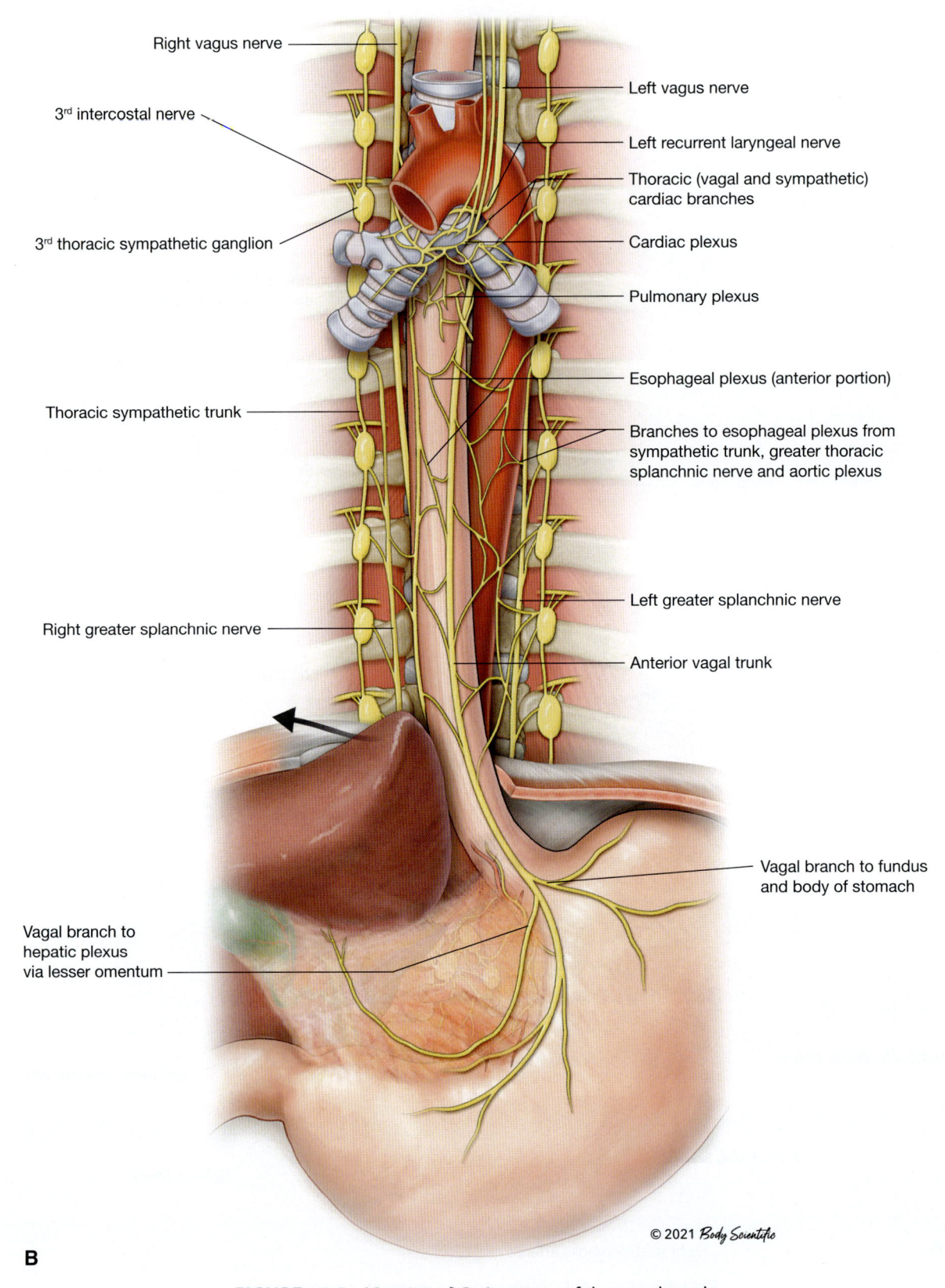

FIGURE 15-5 • (*Continued*) **B.** Anatomy of the vagal trunk.

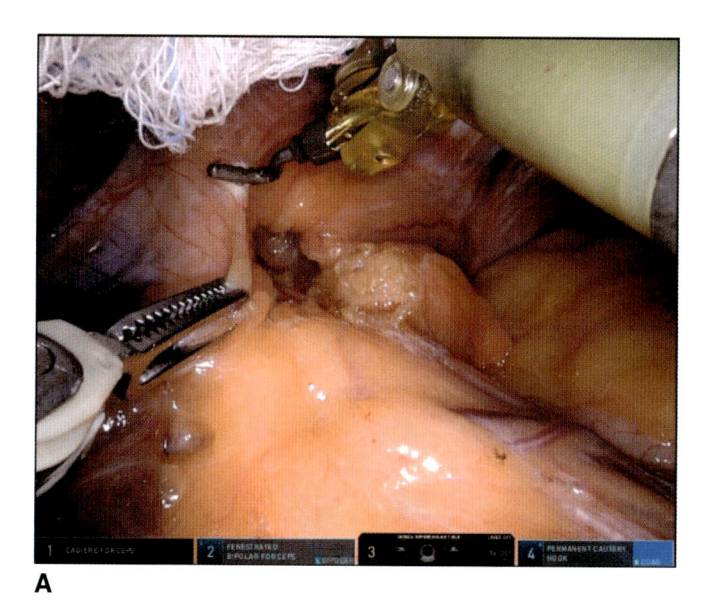

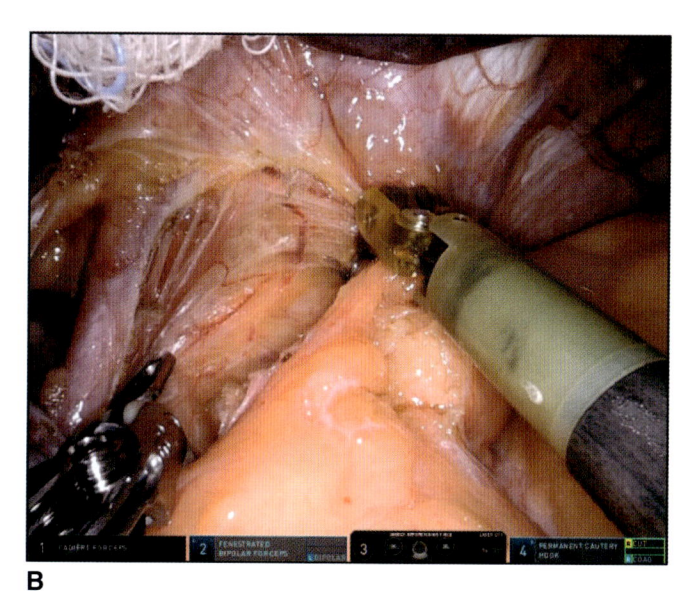

FIGURE 15-6 • Step 2. Gastrohepatic ligament opening and right crus dissection. **A.** Gastohepatic ligament opening using the monopolar hook. **B.** Dissection along the right crus.

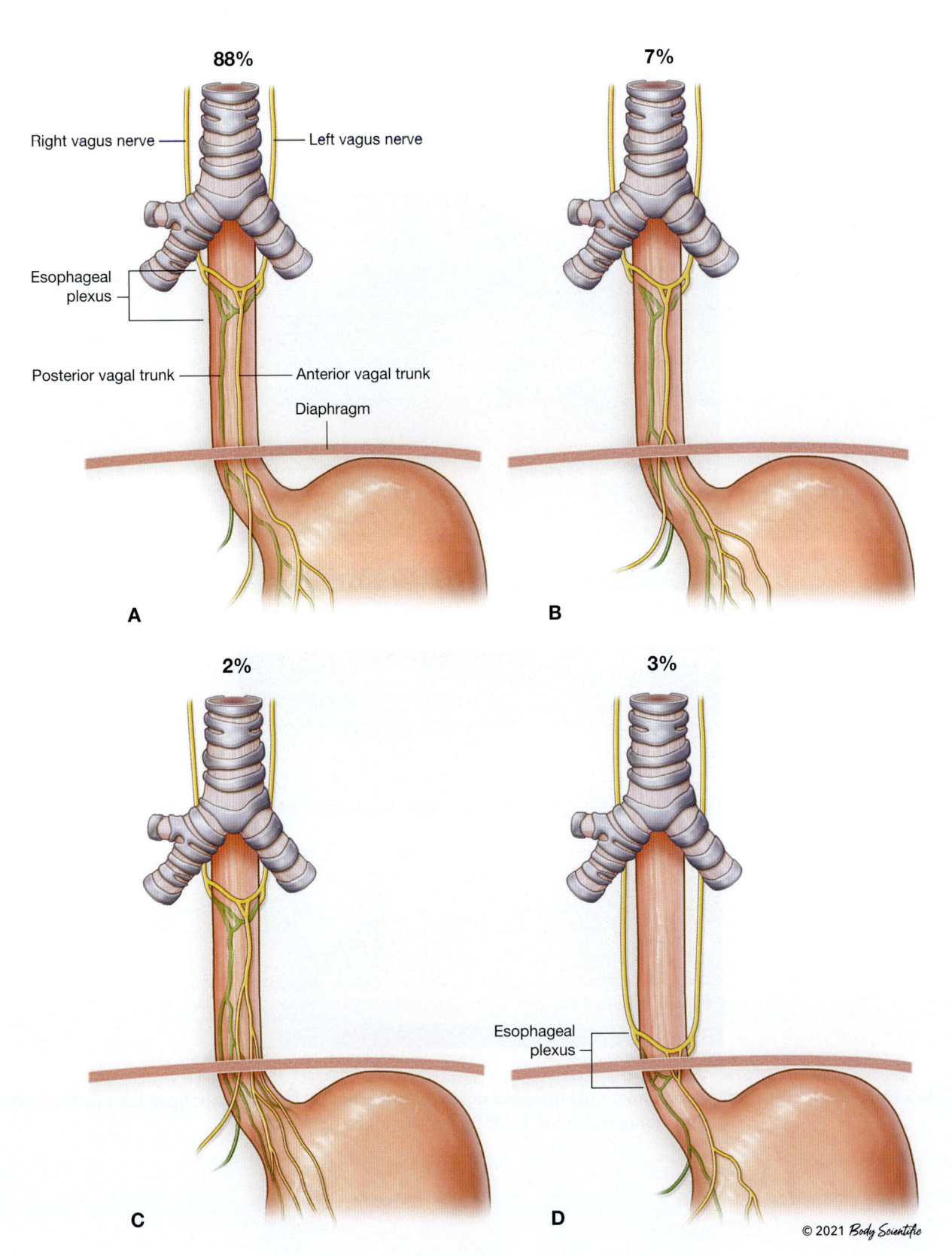

FIGURE 15-7 • Anatomic variations of the vagus nerve.

Step 3. Left crus dissection

The dissection continues, using the monopolar hook and bipolar forceps, progressively taking down the gastrophrenic ligaments and exposing the left crus. In this step, the bedside assistant dynamically exerts proper tension by pulling the stomach downward (while avoiding excessive traction that may damage the short gastric vessels/spleen). While the surgeon continues with the dissection from the esophageal wall, the assistant, through the additional laparoscopic port, can retract laterally the left pillar to provide adequate exposure and field vision (**Figure 15-8**).

Step 3 average time frame: 5–10 min

>> **TIPS**

The best way to prevent injuries of the left anterior vagal trunk is to visualize it.

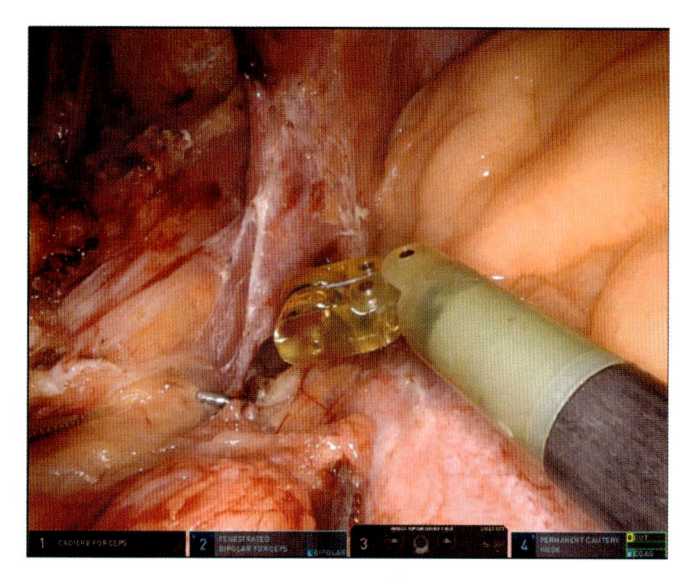

FIGURE 15-8 • Step 3. Left crus dissection.

Step 4. Creation of the retroesophageal window and Penrose placement

The dissection continues around the esophagus, gently separating the pillars from the esophageal wall by blunt dissection, taking precaution not to injure the posterior vagus nerve. A retroesophageal window is created and tailored to allow a floppy wrap (this window cannot be too narrow or too large) (**Figures 15-9 A–D**). A Penrose drain is passed behind the esophagogastric junction, and adequate mobilization of the distal esophagus is carried out to secure a proper segment's length to be placed in the abdomen (**Figures 15-10 A–D**).

Step 4 average time frame: 5 min

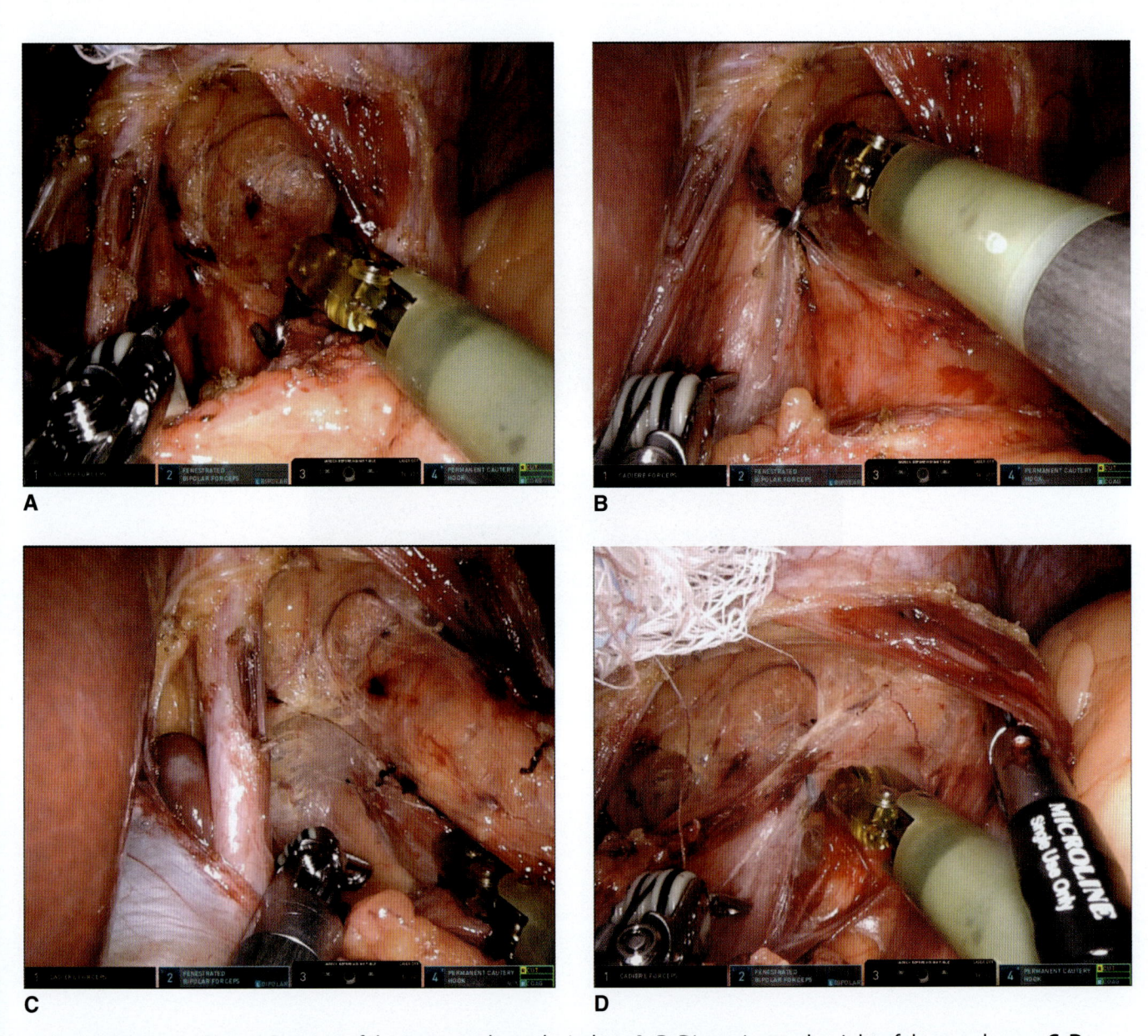

FIGURE 15-9 • Step 4. Creation of the retroesophageal window. **A, B.** Dissection to the right of the esophagus. **C, D.** Dissection to the left of the esophagus.

Selective Nissen Fundoplication 289

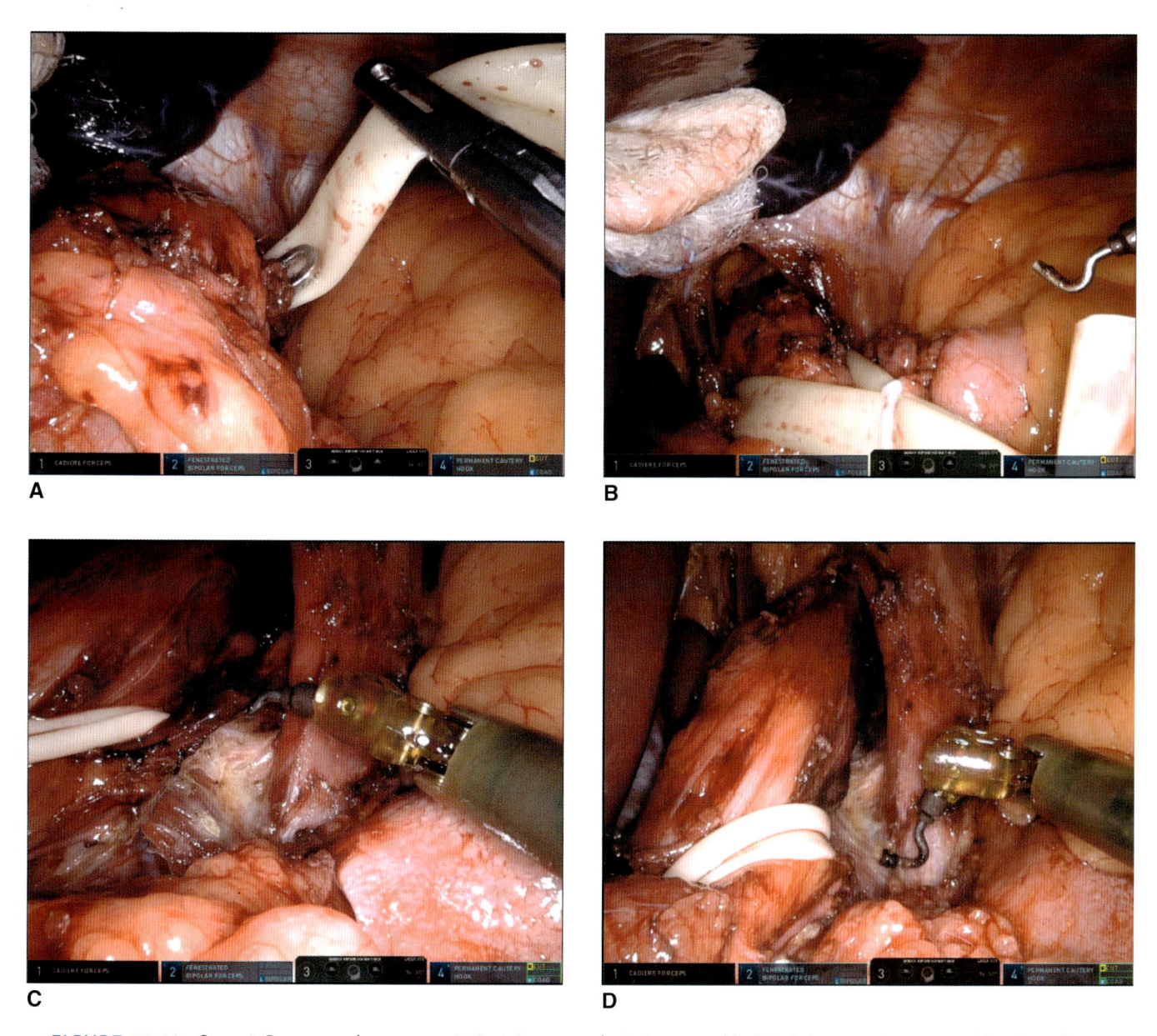

FIGURE 15-10 • Step 4. Penrose placement. **A, B.** A Penrose drain is passed behind the esophagus, and both ends are clipped together with a Hem-o-lok® clip. **C, D.** The assistant provides retraction by pulling from the Penrose and opening up the dissection area.

Step 5. Dissection of the posterior gastric fundus

This step entails a selective mobilization of the posterior aspect of the gastric fundus, targeting the posterior area of the stomach that is not covered by the peritoneum. The gastrosplenic ligament is dissected superiorly, and the connective tissue is divided in order to gain access to the posterior part of the stomach and dissect its attachments, being mindful of the presence of a posterior gastric vessel and its different anatomical variants (**Figures 15-11** and **15-12 A–C**). The lower landmarks of the dissection are the splenic artery and the edge of the pancreatic body.

Step 5 average time frame: 5–20 min

> ▶▶ **TIPS**
>
> In most cases, the fundus's posterior part is large enough, and a floppy Nissen fundoplication can be performed without dissecting the short gastric vessels. However, in some patients, this posterior part of the gastric fundus (not covered by peritoneum) is too short. In these cases, to allow the creation of a floppy Nissen, a very selective division (using the vessel sealer or in between sutures) of 1–2 proximal short gastric vessels might be required.

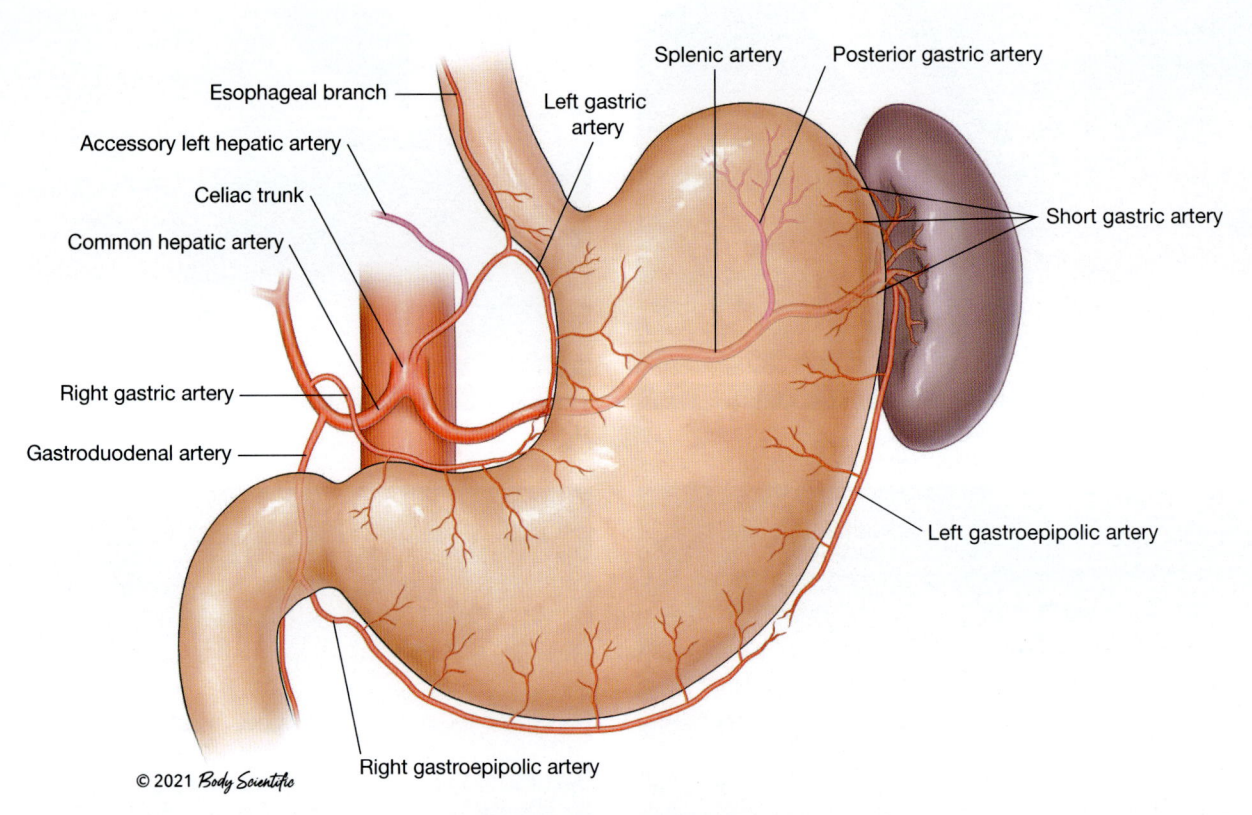

FIGURE 15-11 • Gastric arterial supply.

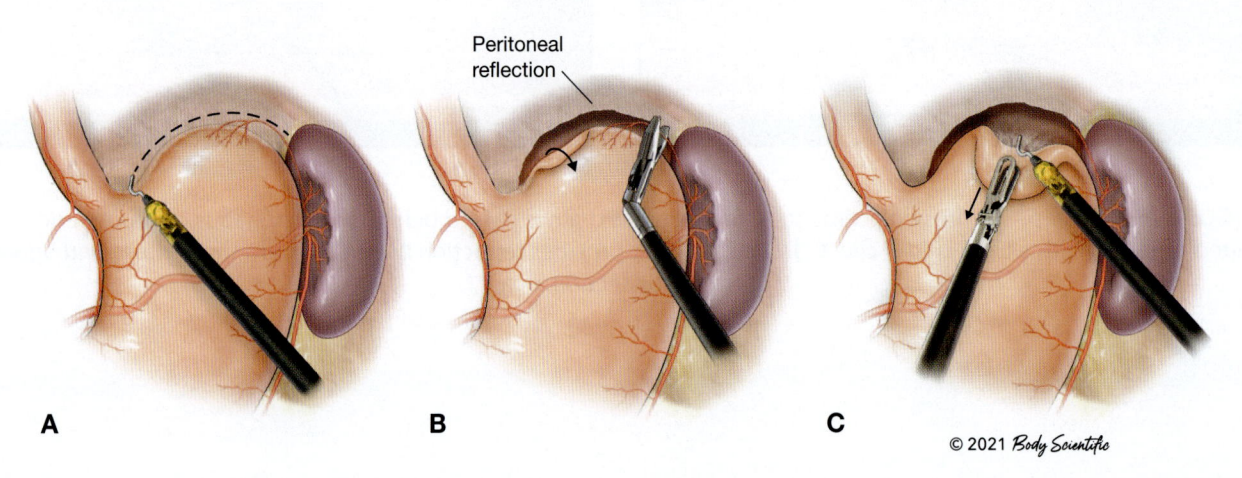

FIGURE 15-12 • Step 5. Dissection of the posterior aspect of the gastric fundus. **A.** Line of dissection in the peritoneal reflection. **B.** One distal short gastric artery is divided with a vessel sealer. **C.** Gastric fundus posterior attachments are dissected using the monopolar hook.

Step 6. Testing of the wrap

Once the gastric fundus has been mobilized, its posterior portion is gently pulled behind the esophagus in a left-to-right direction, using the Cadière forceps.

Once the fundus reaches the right side, it is wrapped around the esophagus, and it is tested for "floppiness." The forceps releases the fundus, and if the wrap stays in place, this is an indication that there is no tension. Conversely, if the wrap shifts behind the esophagus, returning to the left side, this means that tension is present, and more dissection is required (**Figures 15-13 A, B**).

Step 6 average time frame: 5 min

> ⚠️ **PITFALLS**
>
> To use the anterior part of the gastric fundus when transposing it behind the esophagus is wrong. This maneuver can create a "sling effect," increasing the risk of postoperative dysphagia (see **Figures 15-15 A, B**).

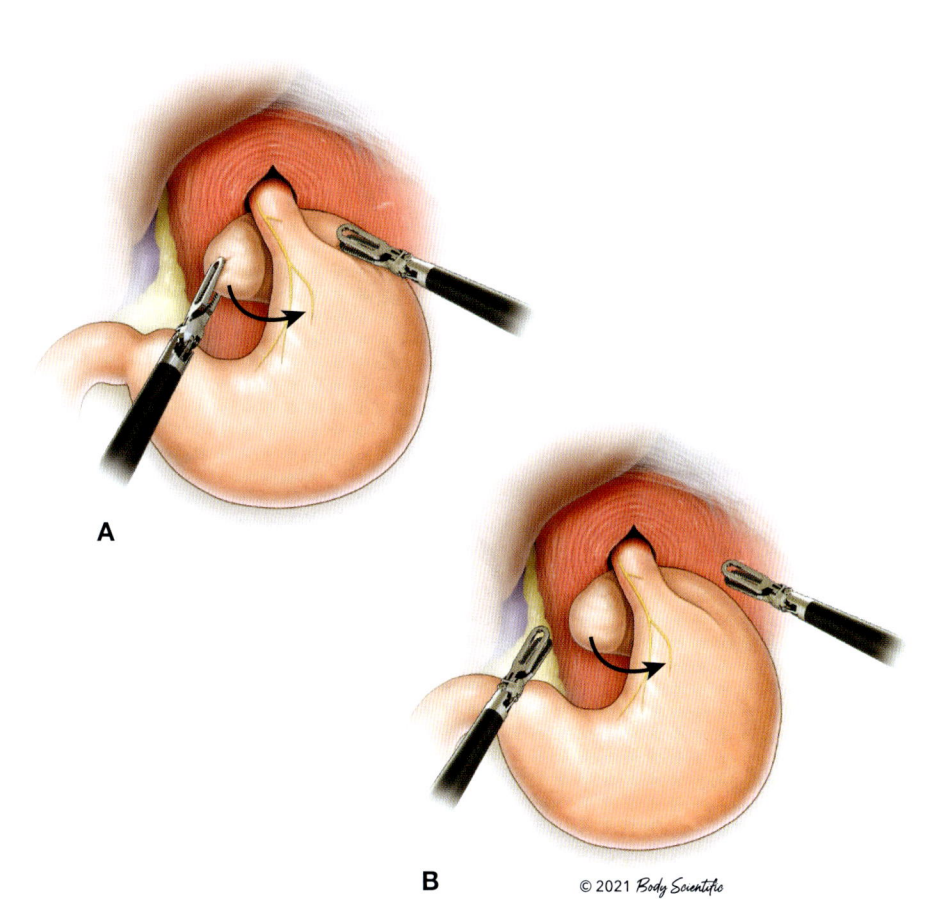

FIGURE 15-13 • Step 6. Testing the wrap. **A.** The fundus is pulled behind the esophagus. **B.** The graspers release the stomach, and the fundus stays in place, indicating that the wrap is not under tension.

Construction

▶ **Video 15-2. Selective Nissen Fundoplication: Construction Steps**

Step 7. Cruroplasty

Occasionally, if the hiatus anatomy is narrow, no hiatoplasty is required. However, in most cases, it is good practice to place 1–2 stitches to calibrate the hiatus. This serves as reinforcement after the esophagus has been dissected from the diaphragm, preventing the risk of a sliding hernia. The pillars are approximated distally with Prolene™ 2-0 single stitches (**Figure 15-14**).

Step 7 average time frame: 10–15 min

> ▶▶ **TIPS**
>
> With experience, it becomes easy to evaluate the adequate closure of the hiatoplasty. At the beginning of the learning curve, it may be prudent to use an endoscopic calibrating bougie size 50–56 Fr to test the tightness of the hiatoplasty and the wrap.

> ⚠ **PITFALLS**
>
> A cruroplasty that is too tight is an important cause of refractory postoperative dysphagia.

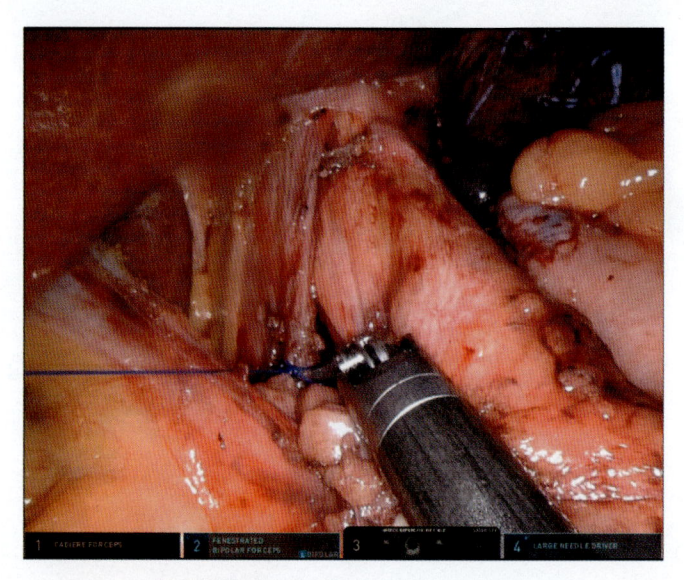

FIGURE 15-14 • Step 7. Cruroplasty.

Step 8. Fundoplication

A short-length Nissen fundoplication is advisable, approximately 1–2 cm, with 3 stitches maximum creating a short bridge connecting the right and left side of the wrap. Using 2 large needle drivers, a Prolene™ 3-0 suture is used to form the plication, taking half-thickness bites of the stomach from each side of the wrap to be sure not to trespass the mucosa. No sutures are placed in the esophageal wall (some surgeons recommend it; if this is done, it is paramount not to include vagal fibers) (**Figures 15-15 A, B** and **15-16 A–C**). In a minority of cases, additional stitches may be required to fix the wrap to the pillar. The most common anatomical patterns of Nissen failures are shown in **Figures 15-17 A–E**.

Step 8 average time frame: 5–10 min

> ▶▶ **TIPS**
>
> It is preferable not to include the esophageal wall when stitching the wrap to avoid the risk of including vagal branches. The reason for anchoring the wrap to the esophagus is to prevent sliding. With the selective mobilization of the robotic Nissen, such a risk is minimal.

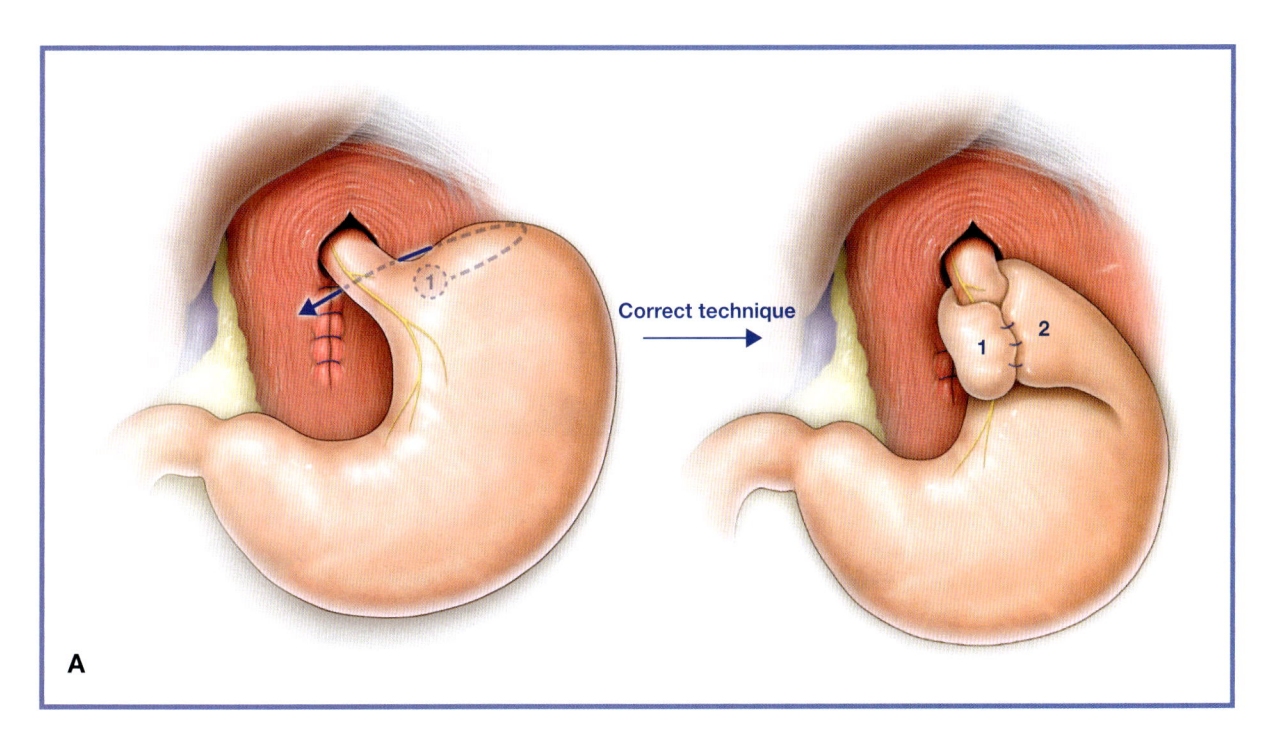

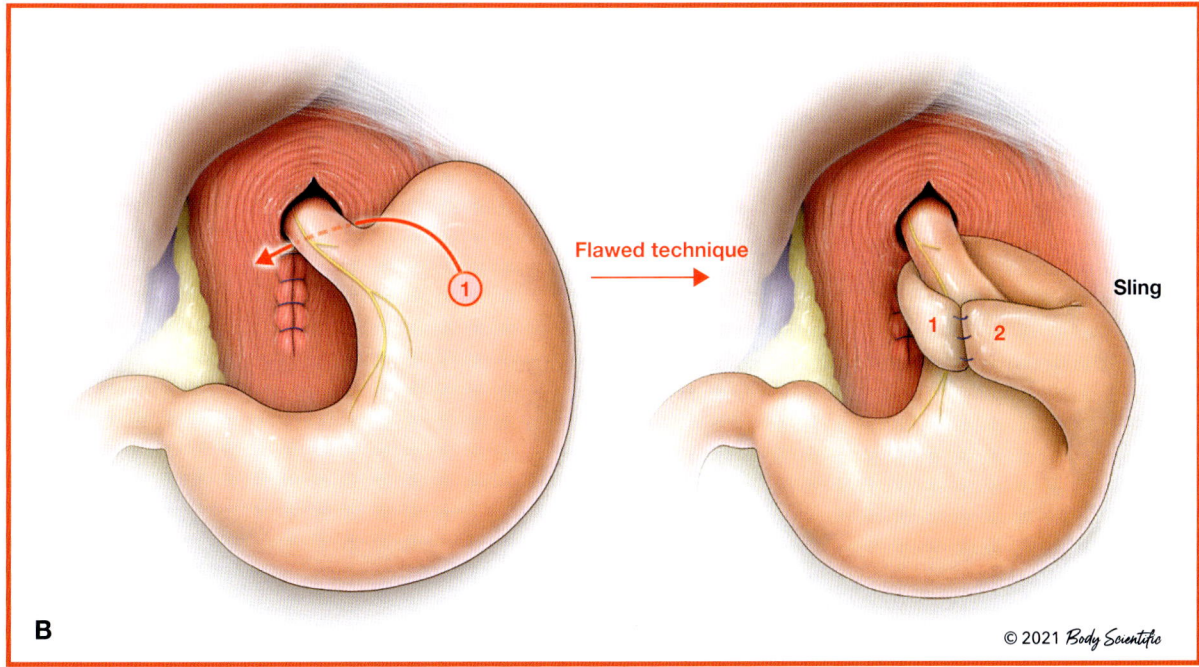

FIGURE 15-15 • Correct (**A**) and flawed (**B**) fundoplication operative technique.

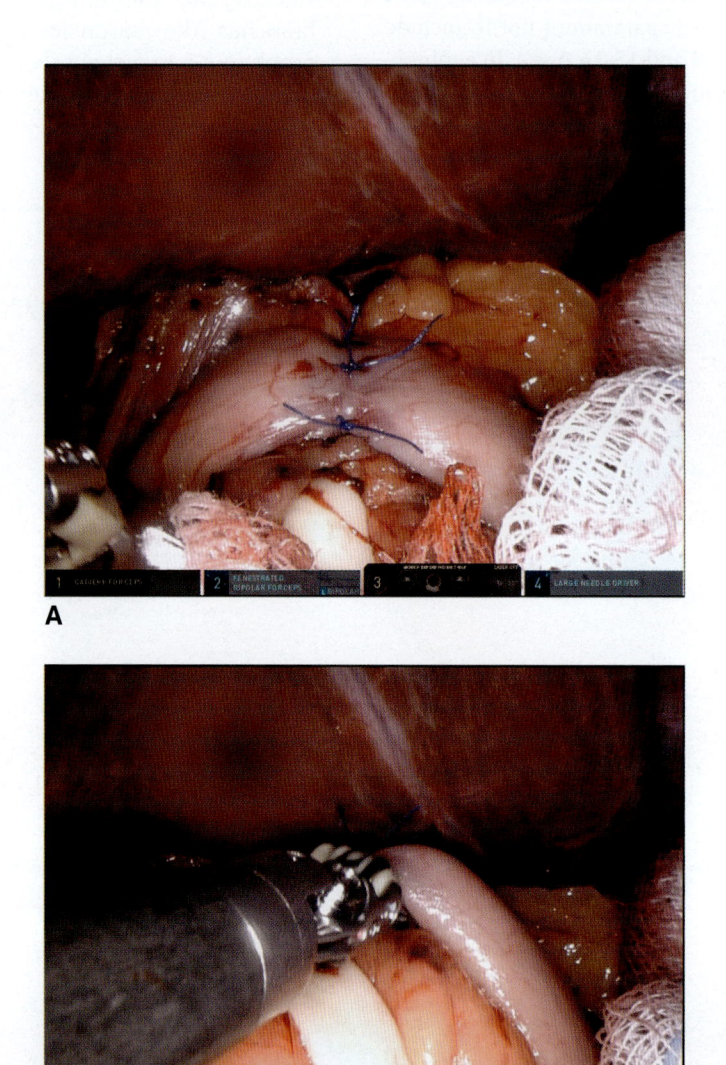

FIGURE 15-16 • Step 8. **Nissen fundoplication. A.** Short bridge with 3 stitches. **B.** The forceps slides underneath the wrap, verifying it is not too tight.

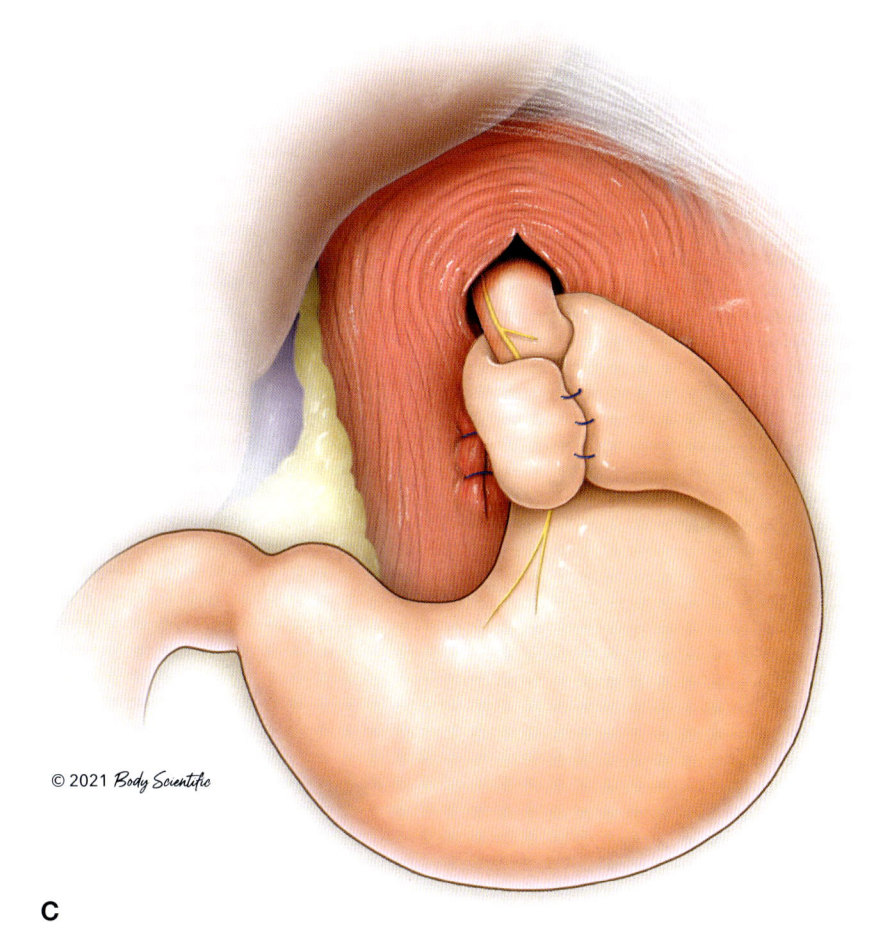

FIGURE 15-16 • (*Continued*) **C.** Final construction.

296　The Foundation and Art of Robotic Surgery

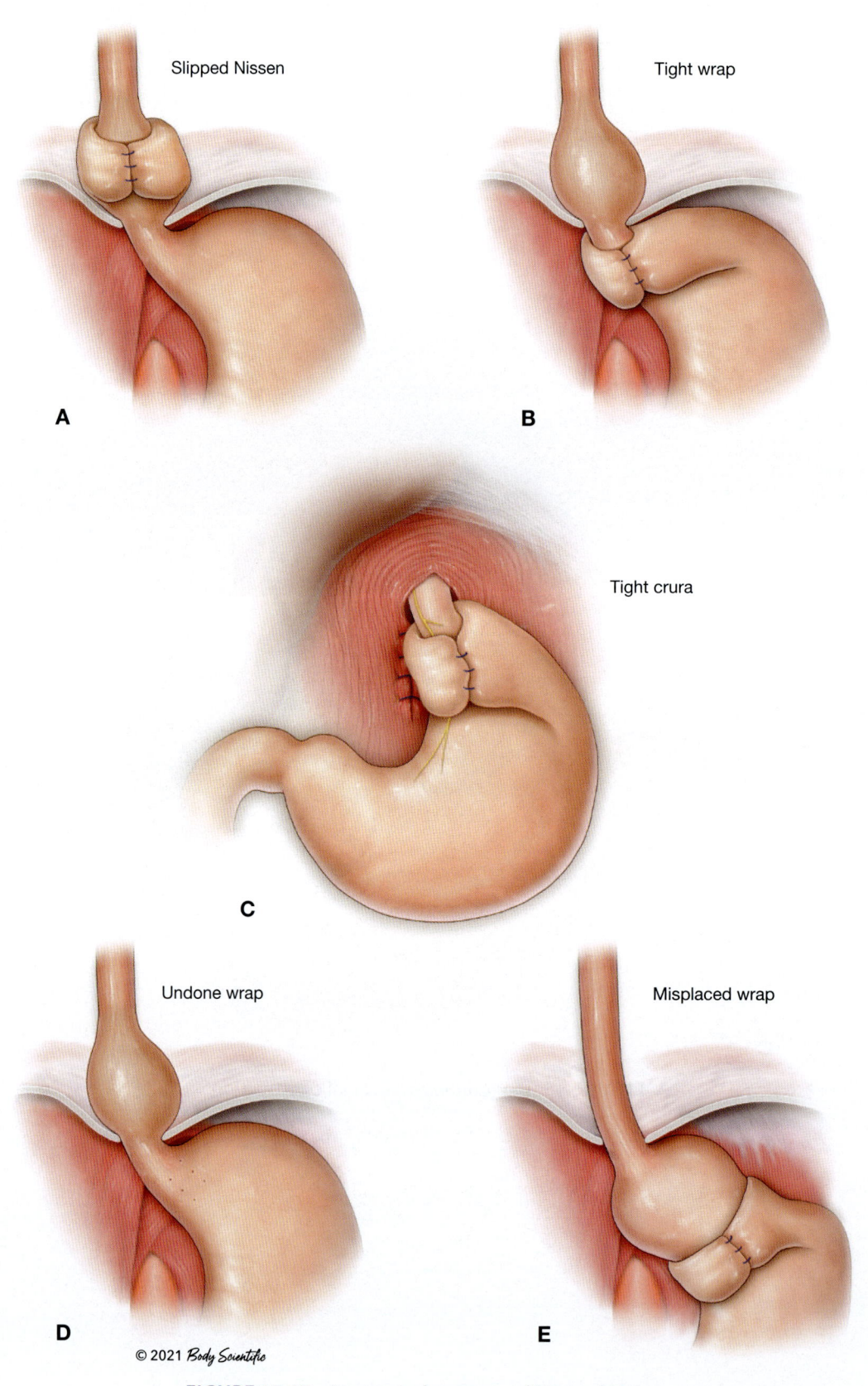

A　Slipped Nissen

B　Tight wrap

C　Tight crura

D　Undone wrap

E　Misplaced wrap

FIGURE 15-17 • Anatomical patterns of Nissen failures.

Video 15-3. Selective Nissen Fundoplication – Full Procedure

Suggested Readings

1. Wykypiel H, Wetscher GJ, Klingler P, Glaser K. The Nissen fundoplication: indication, technical aspects and postoperative outcome. *Langenbecks Arch Surg*. 2005;390(6):495-502. doi: 10.1007/s00423-004-0494-7
2. Hinder RA, Filipi CJ, Wetscher G, Neary P, DeMeester TR, Perdikis G. Laparoscopic Nissen fundoplication is an effective treatment for gastroesophageal reflux disease. *Ann Surg*. 1994;220(4):472-481; discussion 481-483. doi: 10.1097/00000658-199410000-00006
3. Wetscher GJ, Glaser K, Wieschemeyer T, Gadenstaetter M, Prommegger R, Profanter C. Tailored antireflux surgery for gastroesophageal reflux disease: effectiveness and risk of postoperative dysphagia. *World J Surg*. 1997;21(6):605-10. doi: 10.1007/s002689900280
4. Stein HJ, Kauer WK, Feussner H, Siewert JR. Bile reflux in benign and malignant Barrett's esophagus: effect of medical acid suppression and nissen fundoplication. *J Gastrointest Surg*. 1998;2(4):333-341. doi: 10.1016/s1091-255x(98)80072-3
5. Gurski RR, Peters JH, Hagen JA, et al. Barrett's esophagus can and does regress after antireflux surgery: a study of prevalence and predictive features. *J Am Coll Surg*. 2003;196(5):706-712; discussion 712-713. doi: 10.1016/s1072-7515(03)00147-9
6. Nissen R. Eine einfache Operation zur Beeinflussung der Refluxoesophagitis [A simple operation for control of reflux esophagitis]. *Schweiz Med Wochenschr*. 1956;86(Suppl 20):590-592.
7. Donahue PE, Samelson S, Nyhus LM, Bombeck CT. The floppy Nissen fundoplication. Effective long-term control of pathologic reflux. *Arch Surg*. 1985;120(6):663-68. doi: 10.1001/archsurg.1985.01390300013002
8. Lagergren J, Bergström R, Lindgren A, Nyrén O. Symptomatic gastroesophageal reflux as a risk factor for esophageal adenocarcinoma. *N Engl J Med*. 1999;340(11):825-831. doi: 10.1056/nejm199903183401101
9. Oelschlager BK, Eubanks TR, Oleynikov D, Pope C, Pellegrini CA. Symptomatic and physiologic outcomes after operative treatment for extraesophageal reflux. *Surg Endosc*. 2002;16(7):1032-1036. doi: 10.1007/s00464-001-8252-1
10. Giulianotti PC, Coratti A, Angelini M, et al. Robotics in general surgery: personal experience in a large community hospital. *Arch Surg*. 2003;138(7):777-784. doi: 10.1001/archsurg.138.7.777
11. McKinley SK, Dirks RC, Walsh D, et al. Surgical treatment of GERD: systematic review and meta-analysis. *Surg Endosc*. 2021;35(8):4095-4123. doi: 10.1007/s00464-021-08358-5

"Apart from exposing the operative field, the essential problem in extramucosal myotomy is to completely sever the musculature without injuring the mucosa. That this can be done safely only under open operative conditions with direct visual control needs no further justification."

—Ernst Heller (1877–1964)

Heller Myotomy with Modified Dor Fundoplication

Nicolas Hellmuth Dreifuss • Gabriela Aguiluz • Pier Cristoforo Giulianotti

INTRODUCTION

Achalasia is a primary esophageal motility disorder characterized by the absence of relaxation of the inferior esophageal sphincter and lack of esophageal peristalsis in response to swallowing. Preoperative evaluation of these patients must include a high-resolution manometry, barium esophagogram, computed tomography scan, and upper endoscopy. High-resolution manometry confirms the diagnosis of achalasia and defines its subtype according to the Chicago classification (see suggested reading #1). Minimally invasive Heller myotomy and pneumatic dilatation are the best treatment modalities for Chicago type I and II achalasia, while per-oral endoscopic myotomy (POEM) has shown higher success rates in Chicago type III achalasia. POEM is associated with a high incidence of postoperative gastroesophageal reflux. Laparoscopic Heller myotomy has been the preferred surgical approach for decades. This procedure is associated with high clinical success rates (up to 91%) and a low incidence of postoperative reflux (see suggested reading #2). More recently, robotic-assisted Heller myotomy (RHM) proved to be a safe and effective alternative.

As mentioned in Chapters 1 and 2, the robotic platform offers multiple advantages. For this specific procedure, the increased instrument dexterity allows an easier dissection in narrow spaces (mediastinum) and a safer myotomy with lower rates of esophageal mucosal injury when compared with the laparoscopic approach (see suggested reading #3).

In this chapter, the technical aspects of the RHM will be described.

Indications and Relative Contraindications to the Robotic Approach

There are no absolute contraindications to the robotic approach of the Heller myotomy operation. A relative contraindication might be the presence of adhesions due to a history of multiple open abdominal surgeries. Nevertheless, patient selection should be based on the expertise of the surgical team.

Patient Positioning, OR Setup, and Port Setting

After the endotracheal intubation, the patient is positioned supine on a beanbag with arms tucked, and the lower limbs parted in the French position, with a 30° reverse Trendelenburg (**Figure 16-1**). The assistant surgeon is sitting between the patient's legs. The OR setup is explained in **Figure 16-2**.

The pneumoperitoneum is created using the Veress technique. A total of 6 ports (four 8-mm robotic, one 10- to 12-mm

> **INSTRUMENT REQUIREMENTS**
>
> The suggested main robotic instruments/tools can be listed as follows:
> - Needle drivers (round tip or macro)
> - 30°/0° scope
> - Cautery hook/monopolar scissors
> - Bipolar forceps
> - Cadière forceps
>
> The suggested main laparoscopic instruments/tools can be listed as follows:
> - Needle drivers
> - Scissors
> - Graspers
> - Suction-irrigation
>
> Supplemental materials:
> - Gauzes, sponges
> - Sutures: PDS™ 3-0 and 4-0
> - Vessel Loops

Photo reproduced with permission from Haubrich WS. Heller of the Heller myotomy, Clinical-Alimentary Tract Biographical Sketch. Gastroenterology. 2006;130(2):333.
Quote reproduced with permission from Payne WS. Heller's contribution to the surgical treatment of achalasia of the esophagus. 1914. Ann Thorac Surg. 1989;48(6):876-881.

300 The Foundation and Art of Robotic Surgery

assistant port, and one 5-mm assistant port) are used during the procedure. A 5-mm trocar is inserted in the left upper quadrant to perform a diagnostic laparoscopy and for safe placement of the rest of the ports. The four 8-mm cannulas are positioned along a straight line 4–10 cm (depending on the body habitus) above the umbilicus. The camera is introduced in the left paraumbilical trocar, and 2 assistant ports are located on both sides of the scope. Port settings for normal and wide abdomens are explained in **Figures 16-3 A, B**.

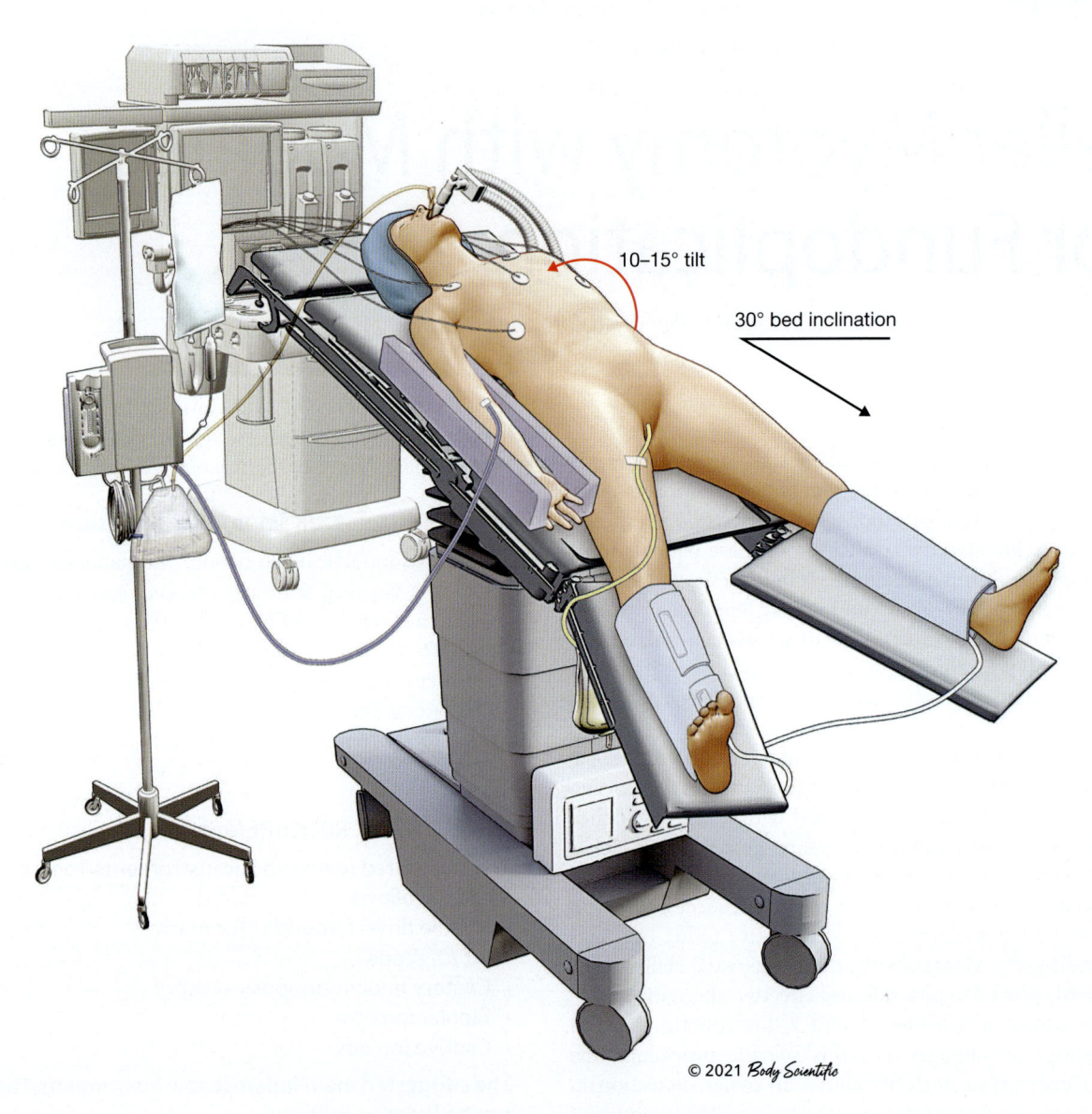

FIGURE 16-1 • Patient positioning.

Heller Myotomy with Modified Dor Fundoplication 301

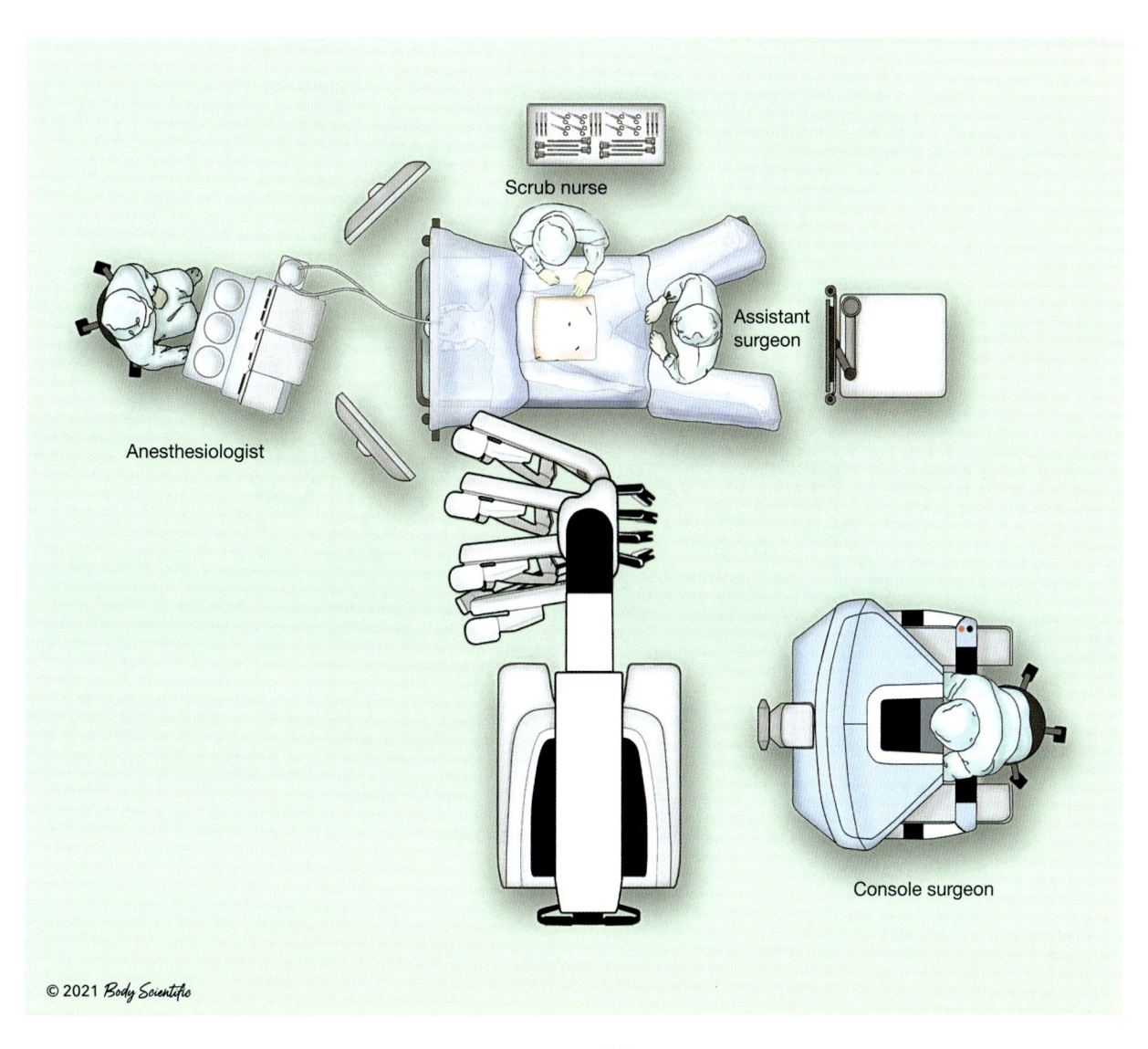

FIGURE 16-2 • OR setup.

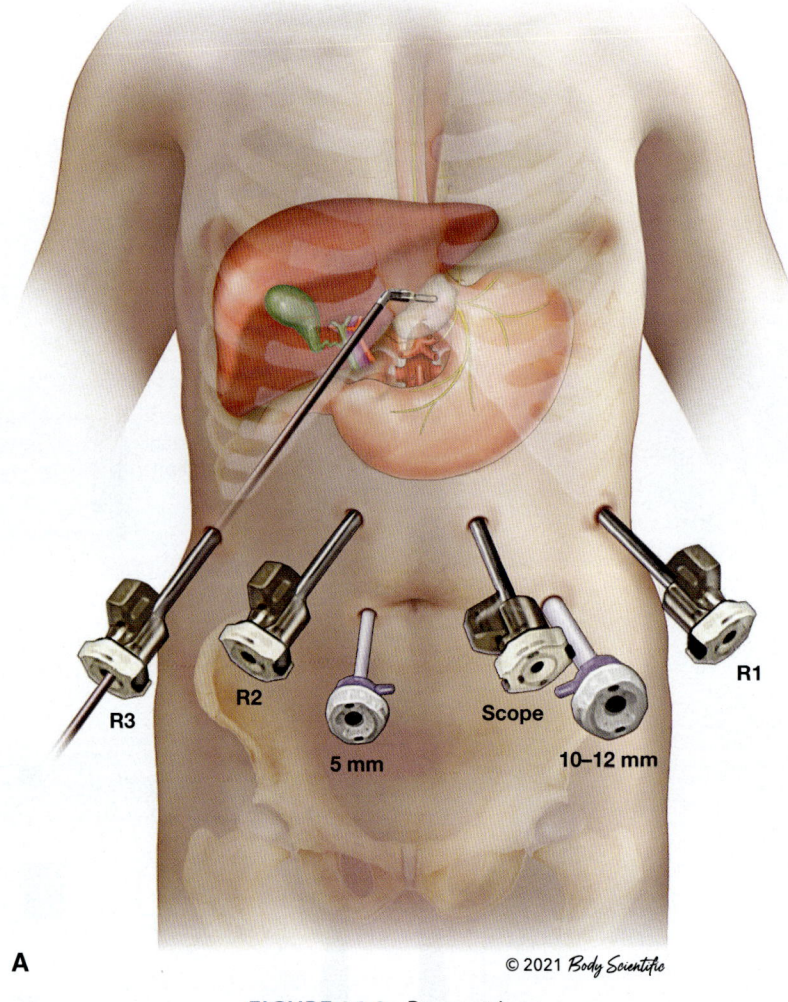

FIGURE 16-3 • Port settings.

Wide abdomen

B

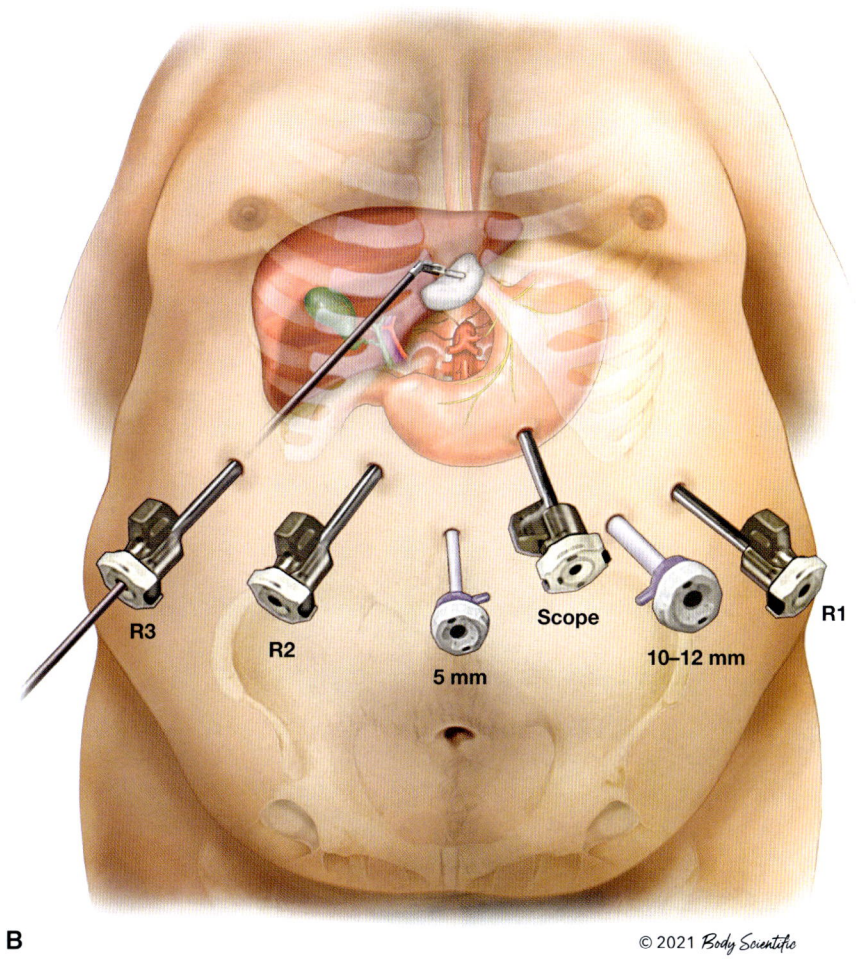

FIGURE 16-3 • *(Continued)*

> ▶▶ **TIPS**
>
> The R3 should not be placed too high and close to the right costal margin, as this will interfere with liver retraction and hiatal exposure.

Surgical Technique

▶ **Video 16-1. Heller Myotomy with Modified Dor Fundoplication**

Step 1. Exposure of the hiatus

After the ports placement, the first step in the operation is to properly expose the diaphragmatic hiatus and the gastroesophageal (GE) junction. Usually, the liver's left lobe is covering the hiatus. A Cadière forceps, protected with a gauze (introduced by the assistant through the 12-mm port), is used through the R3 to retract ventrally and medially segments II and III of the liver. This allows proper visualization of the abdominal esophagus and GE junction and a wider operative field. The assistant surgeon, by retracting the gastric fundus downward with the laparoscopic forceps, helps in maintaining the GE junction exposure (**Figures 16-4 A, B**).

Step 1 average time frame: 3–5 min

> ▶▶ **TIPS**
>
> In some cases, segments II and III of the liver can cover the hiatus and limit the exposure. The division of the left triangular ligament will allow better visualization in this scenario.

A **B**

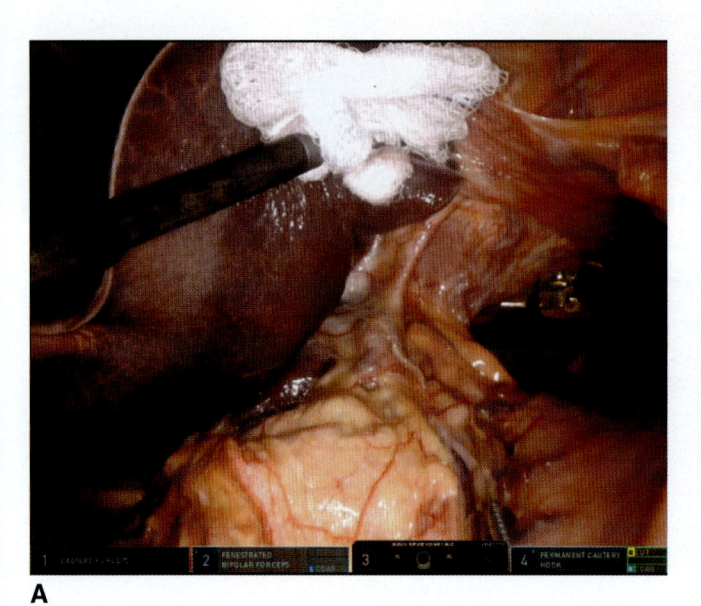

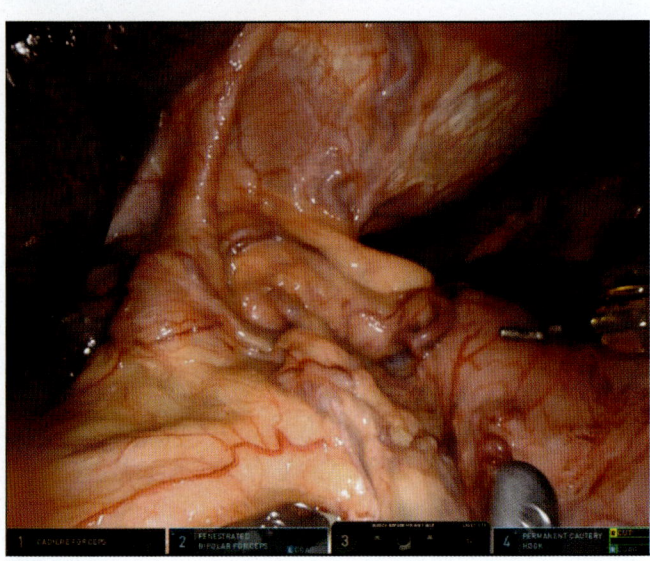

FIGURE 16-4 • Exposure of the hiatus.

> ⚠ **PITFALLS**
>
> Improper retraction with the R3 can cause liver laceration and bleeding.
>
> Insufficient exposure of the hiatus is usually connected to inadequate retraction of the segment II and III of the liver.

Step 2. Division of the anterior phrenoesophageal membrane (Laimer-Bertelli membrane)

The upper portion of the gastrohepatic ligament is minimally opened toward the right diaphragmatic pillar (**Figure 16-5**). Excessive division of the gastrohepatic ligament is unnecessary, as it may cause injury of the vagal fibers going to the liver or an aberrant left hepatic artery. The esophagus is then separated from the right crus with a combination of blunt and sharp dissection using the monopolar hook. When the dissection is near to the right pillar, electrocautery should be used with caution because the thermal lateral spread can damage the posterior vagus nerve. The anterior phrenoesophageal membrane is lifted and then divided with the monopolar hook in a clockwise fashion (**Figures 16-6 A–C**). The left pillar, by blunt dissection, is gently separated from the esophageal wall. To facilitate these maneuvers, the assistant should be able to provide proper retraction of the stomach. As an anterior partial fundoplication will be performed, there is no need for posterior dissection or the creation of a retroesophageal window. This maneuver may cause posterior vagal nerve injury. Moreover, preserving the retroesophageal attachments helps to reduce the risk of postoperative reflux connected to the sliding of the GE junction.

Step 2 average time frame: 5–10 min

> 🔍 **ANATOMICAL HIGHLIGHTS**
>
> Anatomy of the hiatus and esophagogastric junction (**Figure 16-7**).

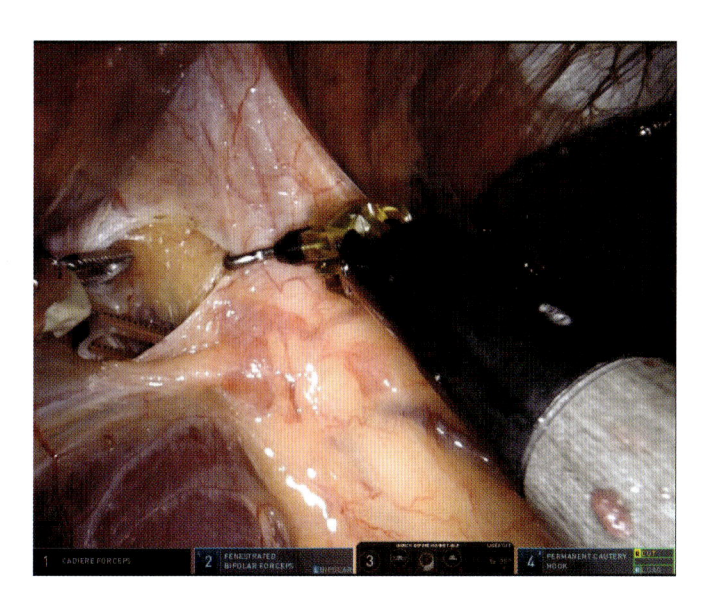

FIGURE 16-5 • Division of the upper portion of the gastrohepatic ligament.

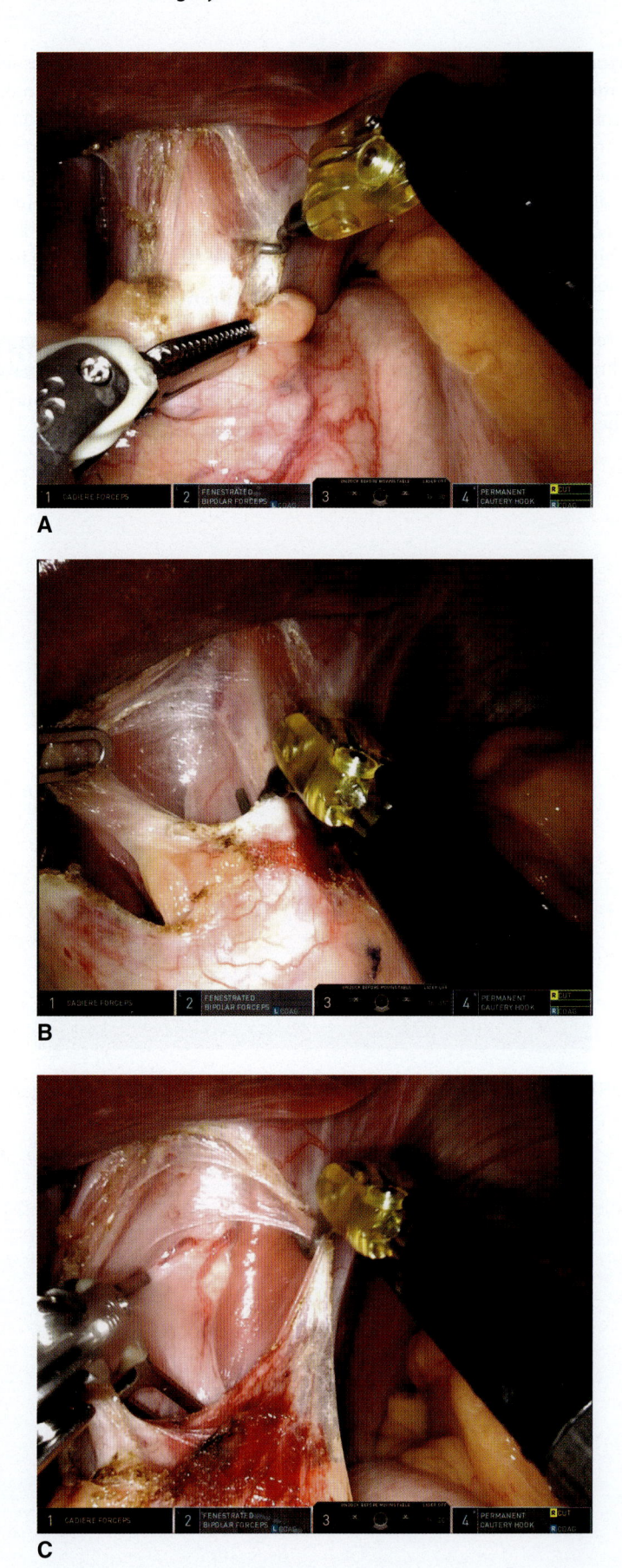

FIGURE 16-6 • Division of the anterior phrenoesophageal membrane.

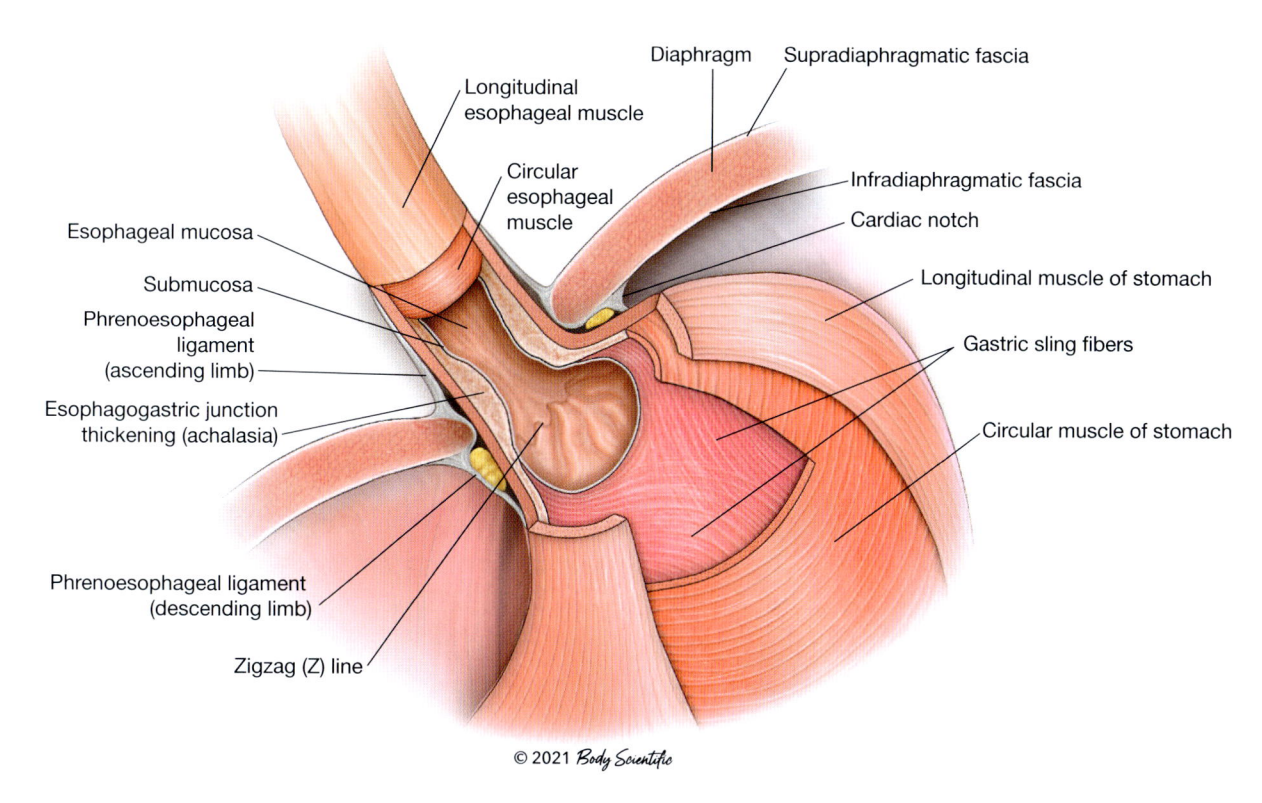

FIGURE 16-7 • Anatomy of the hiatus and esophagogastric junction.

> ⚠ **PITFALLS**
>
> Excessive gastrohepatic ligament division may result in damage to the vagal fibers going to the liver and gallbladder or to an aberrant left hepatic artery.

Step 3. Mediastinal dissection

Dissection of the anterior aspect of the esophagus continues cephalad into the posterior mediastinum. The fundus of the stomach is pulled downward by the assistant surgeon to facilitate distal mobilization of the esophagus. A combination of blunt and sharp dissection with the monopolar hook is performed to expose the esophagus. The anterior surface of the esophagus should be exposed for approximately 10–12 cm. Care must be taken to avoid pleural opening during mediastinal esophagus dissection (**Figures 16-8 A–C**).

Step 3 average time frame: 5–10 min

> ▶▶ **TIPS**
>
> Adequate exposure of the distal esophagus is the key maneuver to perform the subsequent myotomy and fundoplication.

> ⚠ **PITFALLS**
>
> During mediastinal dissection, the parietal pleura might be accidentally opened, leading to a pneumothorax. Usually, this is well tolerated and does not require any intervention. In few cases, it might be necessary to decrease the CO_2 working pressure and/or drain and close the pleural opening with a suture.

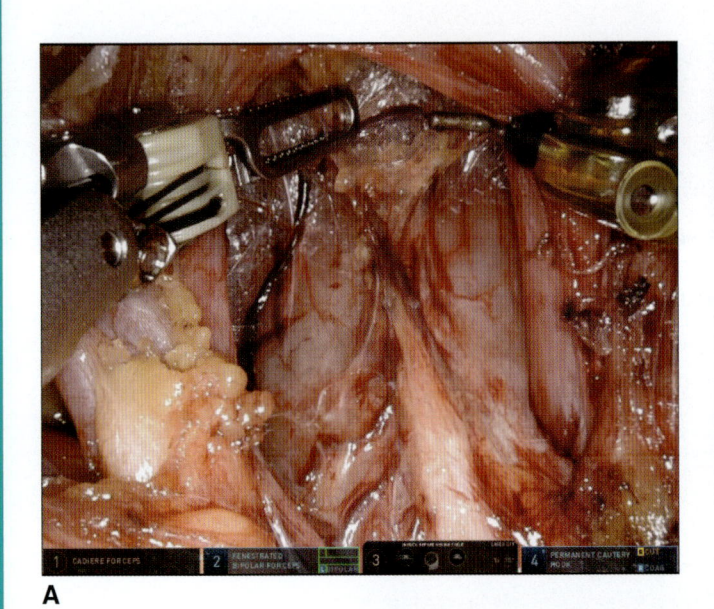

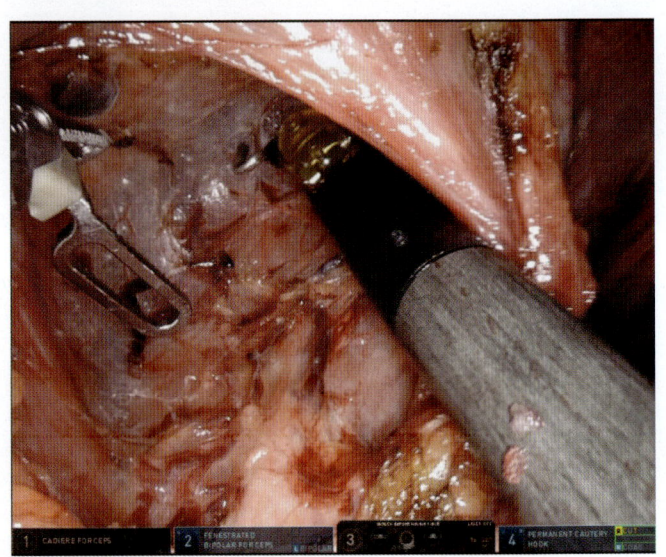

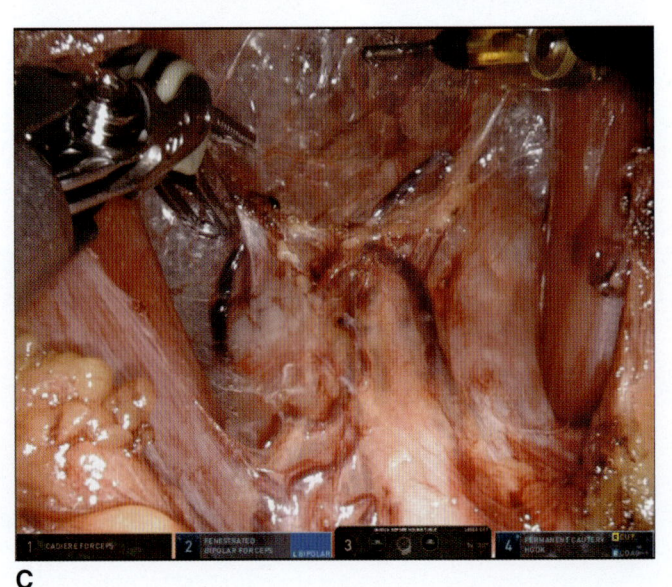

FIGURE 16-8 • Mediastinal dissection.

Step 4. Left vagal trunk identification

Careful identification and handling of the anterior-left vagal trunk is an essential step of the Heller myotomy operation. After the mobilization of the distal esophagus is completed, the anterior-left vagal trunk will be easily identified attached to the esophageal wall. At this level, the left vagal trunk will take an oblique course toward the anterior esophageal wall (crossing the myotomy line) before dividing into its hepatic and gastric branches. Once identified, to avoid thermal injury during the myotomy, the nerve is carefully dissected and gently retracted with a Vessel Loop (**Figures 16-9 A, B**).

Step 4 average time frame: 5–10 min

> ### 🔎 ANATOMICAL HIGHLIGHTS
> Anatomy of the vagal trunk (**Figure 16-10**).
>
> Anatomic variations of the vagus nerve (**Figures 16-11 A–D**).

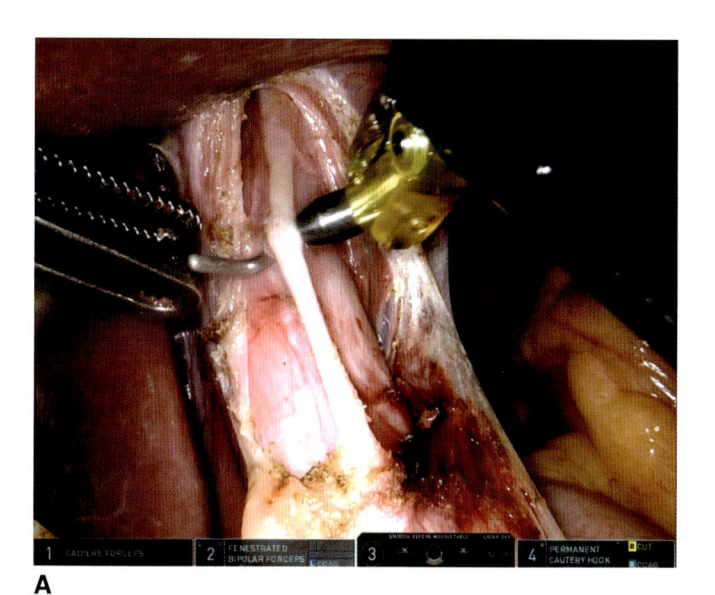

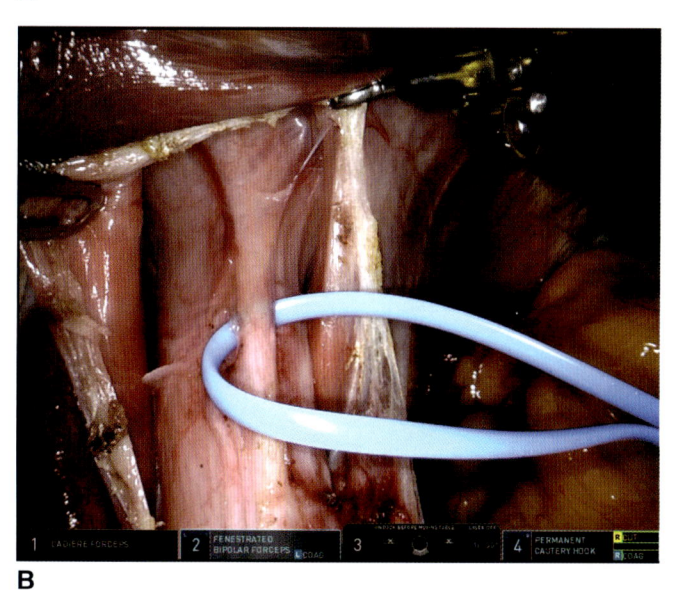

FIGURE 16-9 • Left vagal trunk identification.

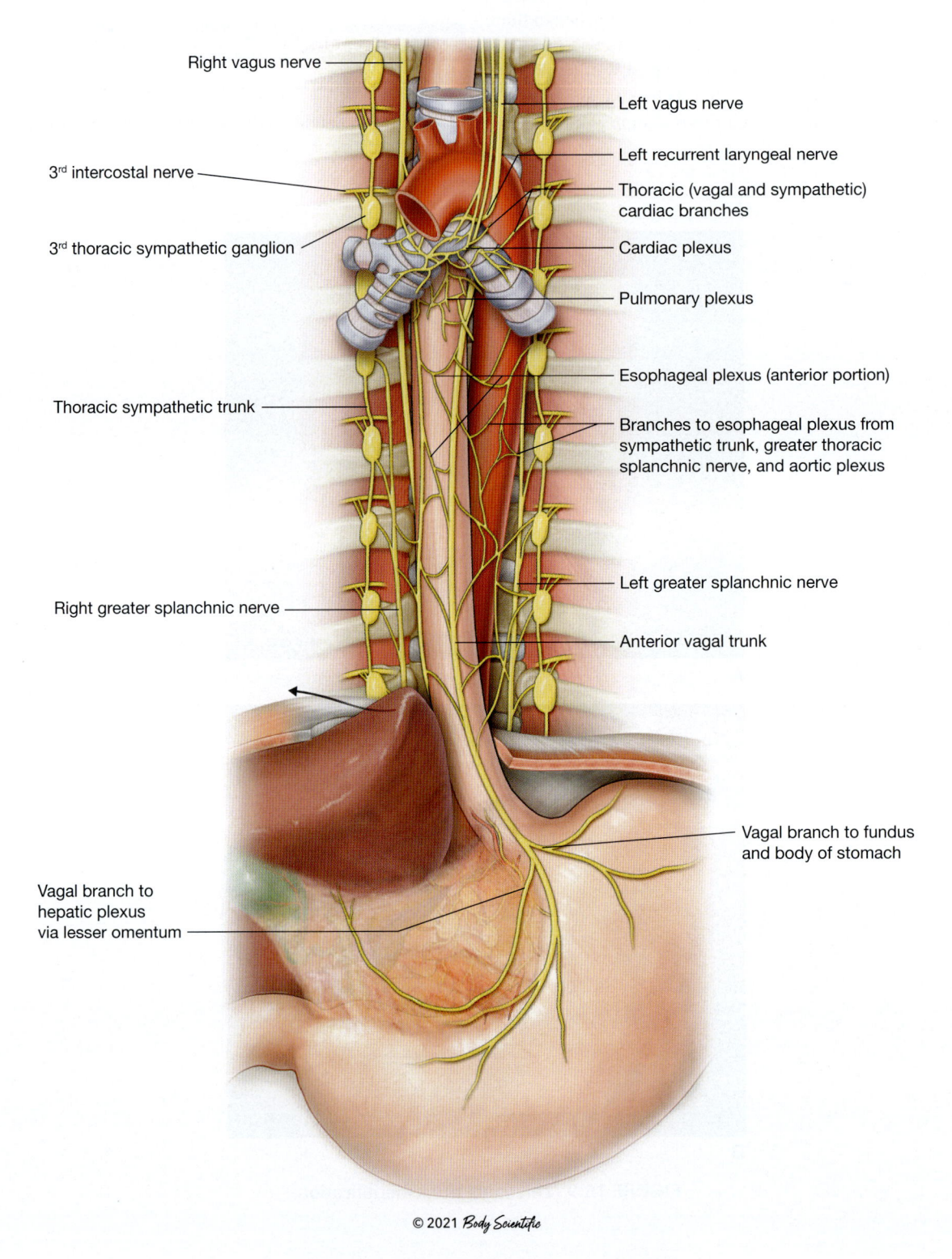

FIGURE 16-10 • Anatomy of the vagal trunk.

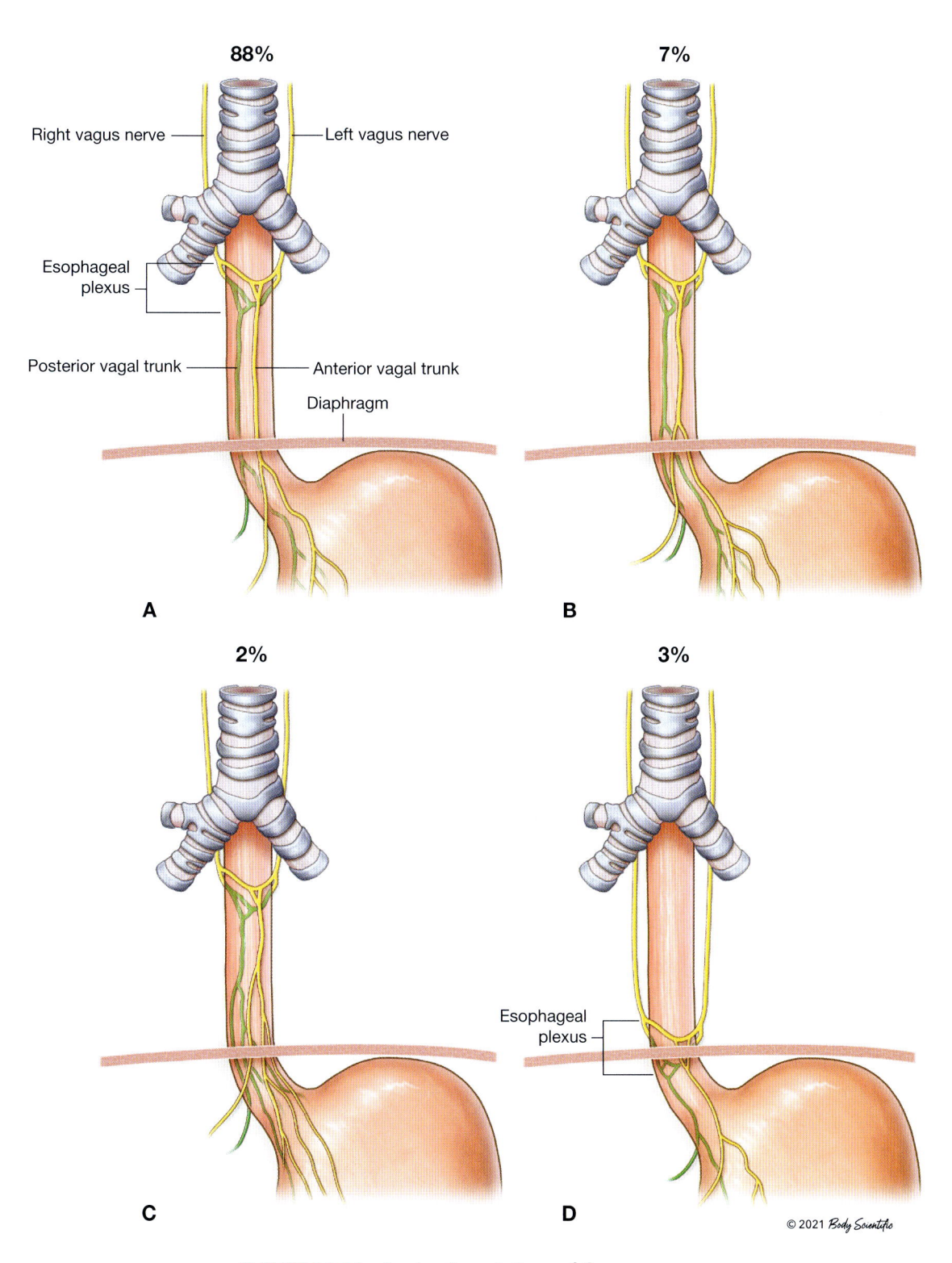

FIGURE 16-11 • Anatomic variations of the vagus nerve.

Step 5. Myotomy

▶ **Video 16-2. Myotomy**

Once the fat pad covering the esophagus and stomach is dissected, and the anterior vagal trunk is retracted, the myotomy is initiated. The esophagogastric junction is pulled downward and leftward by the assistant surgeon. This maneuver provides tension to the longitudinal esophageal muscular fibers facilitating the entering and maintenance of the correct dissection plane. Also, by using the nondominant hand, the surgeon can exert some lateral tension to the circular fibers. The myotomy is started approximately 3 cm above the gastroesophageal junction at the 12 o' clock position. At this level, the submucosal plane is easier to find than the esophagogastric junction, where the layers are not clearly defined. Once the submucosal plane is reached, the longitudinal and circular muscle fibers are divided, using the monopolar hook, until the mucosa is visualized (**Figures 16-12 A–E**). The myotomy is extended proximally for approximately 7–9 cm above the esophagogastric junction and distally for 2–3 cm onto the gastric wall. Fibrosis from previous endoscopic therapies or previous myotomy might increase the difficulty of this step and the risk of perforation.

Step 5 average time frame: 20–25 min

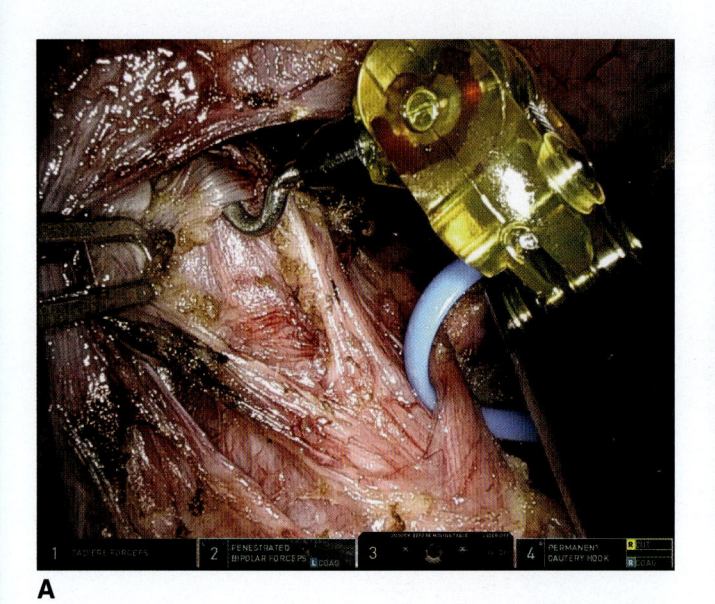

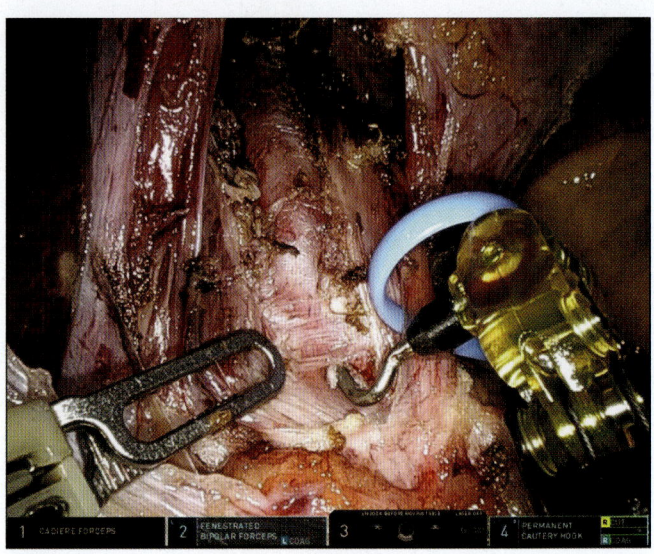

FIGURE 16-12 • Myotomy.

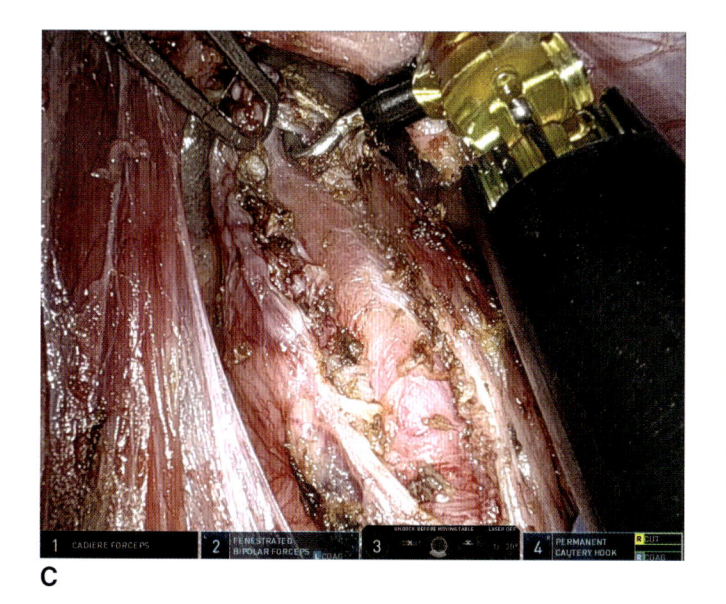

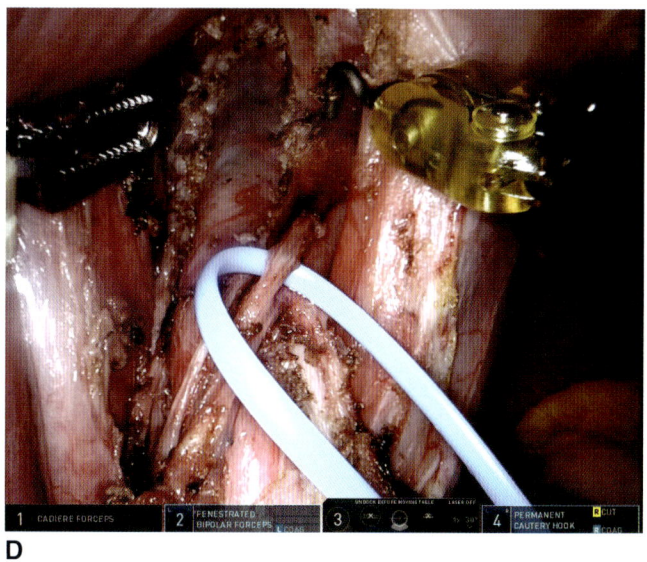

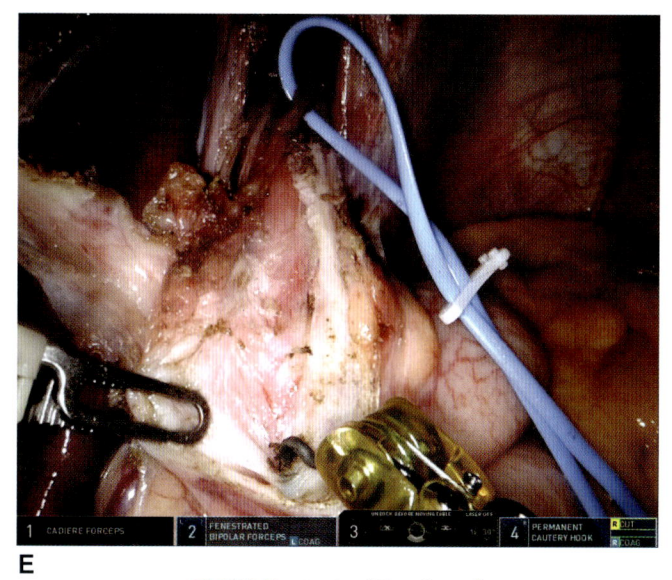

Heller Myotomy with Modified Dor Fundoplication 313

FIGURE 16-12 • (*Continued*)

> 🔍 **ANATOMICAL HIGHLIGHTS**
>
> Layers of the esophageal wall (**Figure 16-13**).

> ▶▶ **TIPS**
>
> The monopolar 90° hook is the perfect tool for performing the myotomy as it allows safe lifting and division of the esophageal circular fibers. To minimize/avert thermal damages, short and intermittent energy applications to divide fiber by fiber are recommended.
>
> The myotomy should not be started at the esophagogastric junction. At this level, the esophageal layers are poorly defined (transition between longitudinal and circular fibers onto the oblique muscular layer), especially if previous endoscopic treatments were performed. The best place to find the plane of dissection is 2–3 cm above the junction, and from there, the myotomy is extended proximally and distally.

314 The Foundation and Art of Robotic Surgery

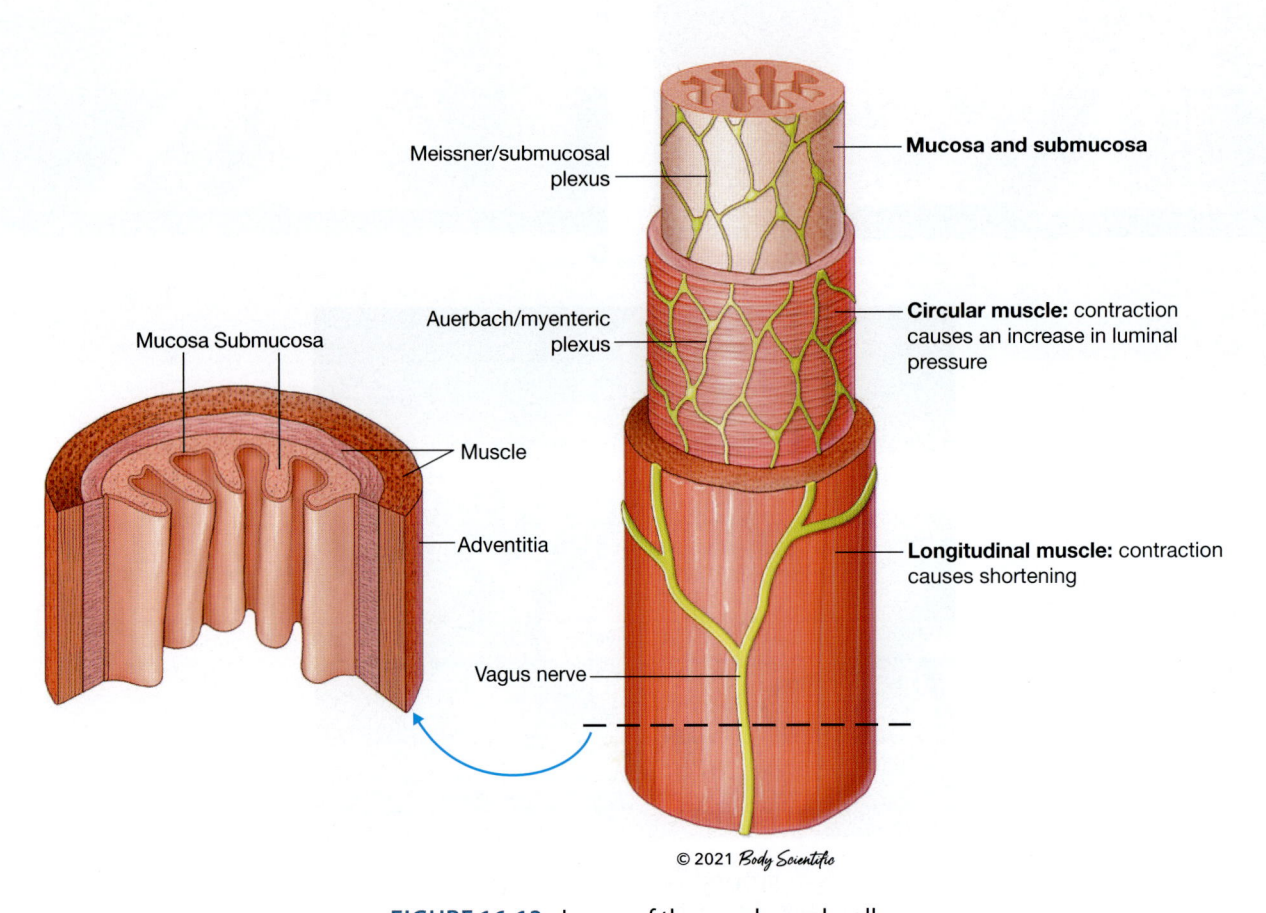

FIGURE 16-13 • Layers of the esophageal wall.

> ⚠ **PITFALLS**
>
> Esophageal perforation. If any perforation occurs during the esophageal myotomy, it should be accurately repaired using interrupted stitches of fine absorbable suture material (PDS™ 4–0).

Step 6. Intraoperative endoscopy

After completing the esophageal myotomy, an intraoperative endoscopy is performed. Careful exploration of the esophagus and the stomach is carried out. The esophageal mucosa is examined for any bleeding, erythema, or evidence of perforation. The myotomy's area is then inspected to assess the completion of the myotomy. An air-leak test could also be performed if a perforation is suspected. Finally, the stomach is decompressed, and the endoscope is pulled out.

Step 6 average time frame: 5–10 min

Step 7. Anterior partial fundoplication

An anterior partial 180° fundoplication (modified Dor) is routinely performed to partially cover the myotomy site and create a valve to prevent postoperative gastroesophageal reflux. At first, the gastric fundus is folded across the exposed esophageal mucosa and fixed to the right pillar of the crus with interrupted stitches of PDS™ 3–0. Then, the superior-anterior aspect of the gastric fundus could also be anchored to the left pillar with 1 or 2 interrupted PDS™ 3-0 stitches. Finally, 1 or 2 additional stitches are placed to fix the superior border of the fundoplication to the anterior rim of the esophageal hiatus (**Figures 16-14 A, B**).

The decision to perform a Dor fundoplication is based on multiple factors:

- Avoidance of posterior mobilization of the esophagus, which increases the chances of sliding of the junction and reason for severe gastroesophageal reflux.
- Less risk of postoperative dysphagia (the Nissen has stronger compression).
- Better coverage of the abdominal portion of the myotomy.

Step 7 average time frame: 10–15 min

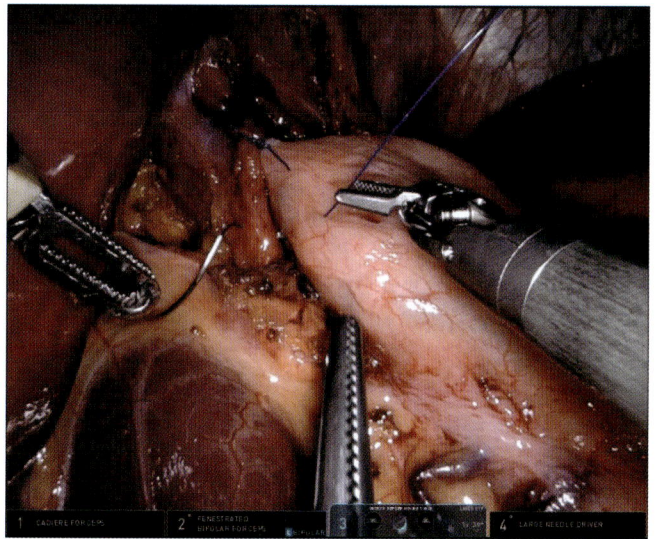

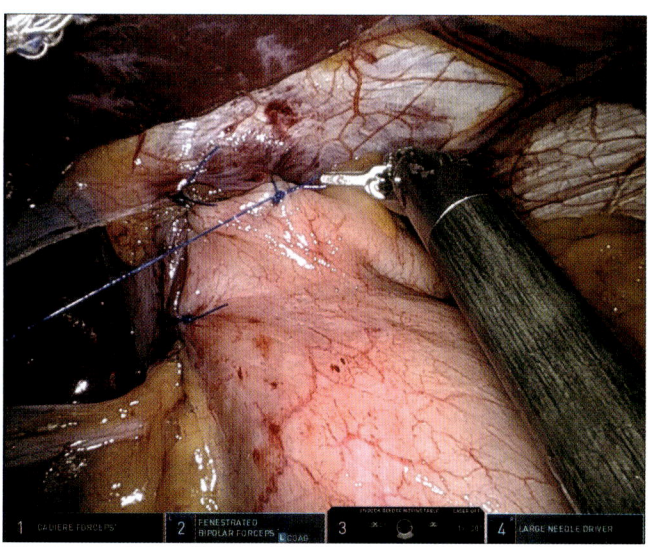

FIGURE 16-14 • Anterior partial fundoplication.

Suggested Readings

1. Kahrilas PJ, Bredenoord AJ, Fox M, et al. The Chicago Classification of esophageal motility disorders, v3.0. *Neurogastroenterol Motil.* 2015;27(2):160-174. doi: 10.1111/nmo.12477
2. Khashab MA, Vela MF, Thosani N, et al. ASGE guideline on the management of achalasia. *Gastrointest Endosc.* 2020;91(2):213-227.e6. doi: 10.1016/j.gie.2019.04.231
3. Milone M, Manigrasso M, Vertaldi S, et al. Robotic versus laparoscopic approach to treat symptomatic achalasia: systematic review with meta-analysis. *Dis Esophagus.* 2019;32(10):1-8. doi: 10.1093/dote/doz062
4. Masrur M, Gonzalez-Ciccarelli LF, Giulianotti PC. Robotic Heller myotomy for achalasia after laparoscopic Roux-en-Y gastric bypass: a case report and literature review. *Surg Obes Relat Dis.* 2016;12(9):1755-1757. doi: 10.1016/j.soard.2016.08.001
5. Zaninotto G, Bennett C, Boeckxstaens G, et al. The 2018 ISDE achalasia guidelines. *Dis Esophagus.* 2018;31(9). doi: 10.1093/dote/doy071
6. Skandalakis JE, Rowe JS Jr, Gray SW, Androulakis JA. Identification of vagal structures at the esophageal hiatus. *Surgery.* 1974;75(2):233-237.
7. Giulianotti PC, Coratti A, Angelini M, et al. Robotics in general surgery: personal experience in a large community hospital. *Arch Surg.* 2003;138(7):777-784. doi: 10.1001/archsurg.138.7.777

"It's not easy to be a pioneer—but oh, it is fascinating!"
—Elizabeth Blackwell (1821–1910)

Lung Lobectomies: General Principles and the Total Port, Transfissure Approach (Fissure First)

Melani Lighter • Gabriela Aguiluz • Fabio Sbrana • Pier Cristoforo Giulianotti

INTRODUCTION

Thoracoscopy was introduced in the early 1990s, a decade after the development of laparoscopic surgery. By 2005, 94% of lobectomies were performed by video-assisted thoracoscopic surgery (VATS), making minimally invasive surgery in anatomical lung resections the standard over the last 20 years. Performing VATS did not change the indications for the operation and has proven to be more advantageous in reducing pain, minimizing complications, decreasing recovery time and hospital stay, and improving overall postoperative quality of life compared to open thoracotomy. More importantly, the short-term mortality, long-term survival rates, and oncologic outcomes are equivalent between VATS and open lobectomy. Despite the progress made with chemotherapy, immunotherapy, and radiotherapy, surgical resection for early stage lung cancer remains the gold standard of cure for these patients, with 5-year recurrence-free survival rates reported to be over 80% for patients with stage I disease.

INSTRUMENT REQUIREMENTS

The suggested main robotic instruments/tools can be listed as follows:
- 30°/0° camera
- Fenestrated bipolar forceps
- Maryland bipolar
- Curved bipolar dissector
- Permanent cautery hook
- Long-tip forceps
- Medium–large clip applier
- Large needle driver
- Monopolar curved scissors
- Tip-up fenestrated grasper
- ProGrasp forceps
- EndoWrist Stapler 45 Curved-Tip
- EndoWrist Stapler 45
- EndoWrist Stapler 30 Curved-Tip

The suggested main thoracoscopic instruments/tools can be listed as follows:
- Nontraumatic forceps
- Needle driver
- Suction device
- Clip applier
- Staplers (optional)

Supplemental materials:
- Roll laparoscopic gauze (cigarette sponges)
- Sutures (Prolene™ 3-0, 4-0, 5-0)
- Vessel loops
- Surgicel®
- Pediatric Foley catheters/Nelaton tubes
- Endo Bag™
- 28-Fr chest tube

Acknowledgement for the photo: The Editors wish to thank the architect Rita Dettori and the photographer/graphic designer Alice Moschin for the drawing they created.
Quote reproduced with permission from Moore W. Elizabeth Blackwell: breaching the barriers for women in medicine. Lancet. 2021;397(10275):662-663.

Robotic-assisted thoracoscopic surgery (RATS) was introduced in the early 2000s. Despite the slow early adoption by thoracic surgeons, there has been an increase in RATS in the second decade since its introduction, from 0.2% to 20%, along with an expansion of indications to more complex cases. Robotic thoracoscopic surgery offers the same advantages as VATS with comparable results and no differences in overall survival or recurrence-free survival. Additionally, the robotic platform provides a shorter learning curve and an improved magnified 3D visualization, allowing a safe, precise dissection around the pulmonary vessels and a delicate lymphadenectomy.

Different techniques of robotic lung resections have been described in the literature. This chapter focuses on the general principles for lung surgery and a step-by-step description of the left upper lobectomy with the transfissure approach.

General Principles for Lung Surgery

1. The anatomy of the lung is complex, and variations are frequent. The vessels and bronchi are designed in a tree-like structure with primary, secondary, and tertiary branches, consequently defining lobes, segments, and subsegments. The functional parenchyma perfectly balances perfusion (inflow/outflow) and ventilation. Surgical anatomical resections should be precise, respecting this balance and preventing mismatching (**Figures 17-1 A–D**).

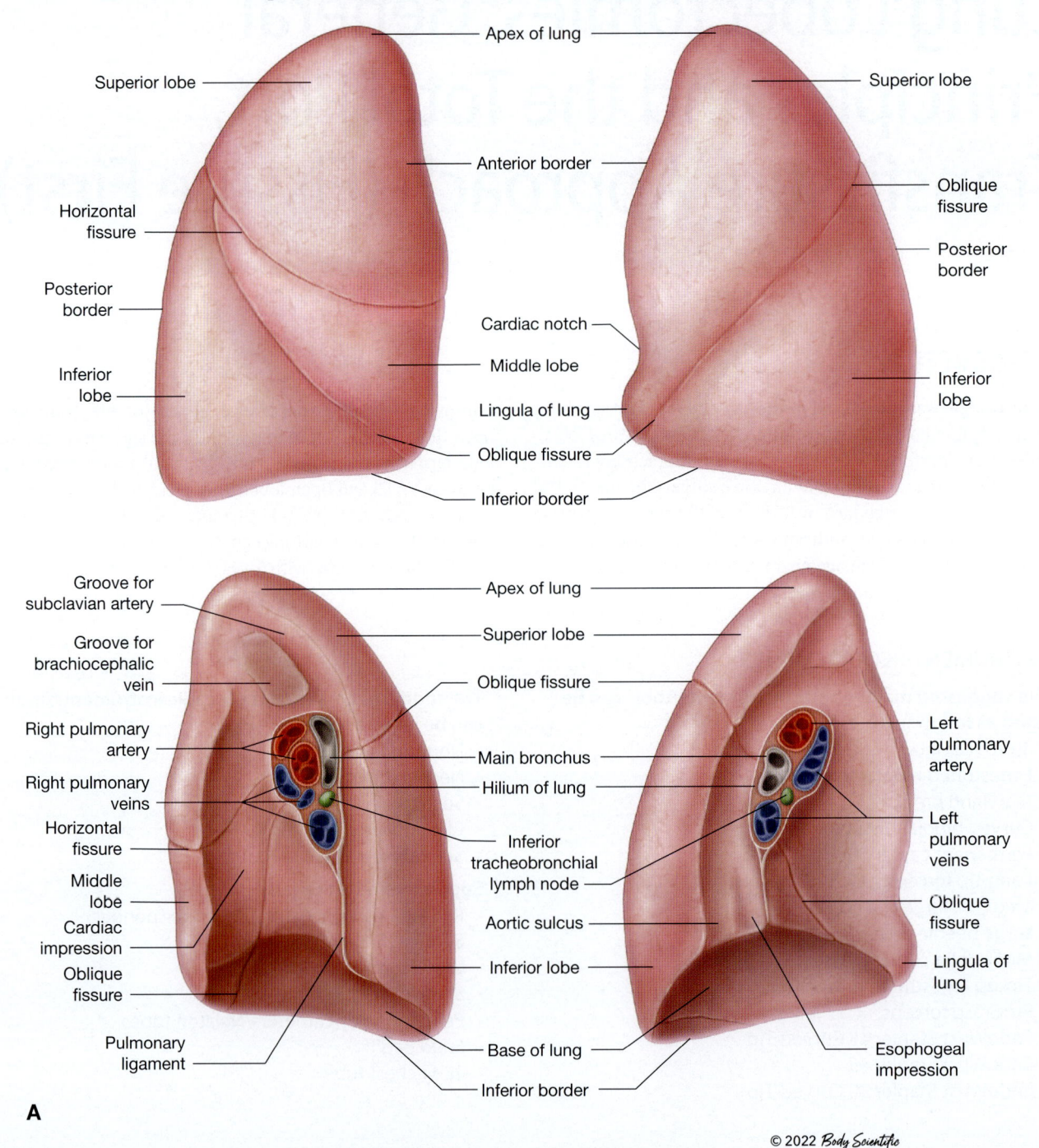

FIGURE 17-1 • A. Right and left lung lobes.

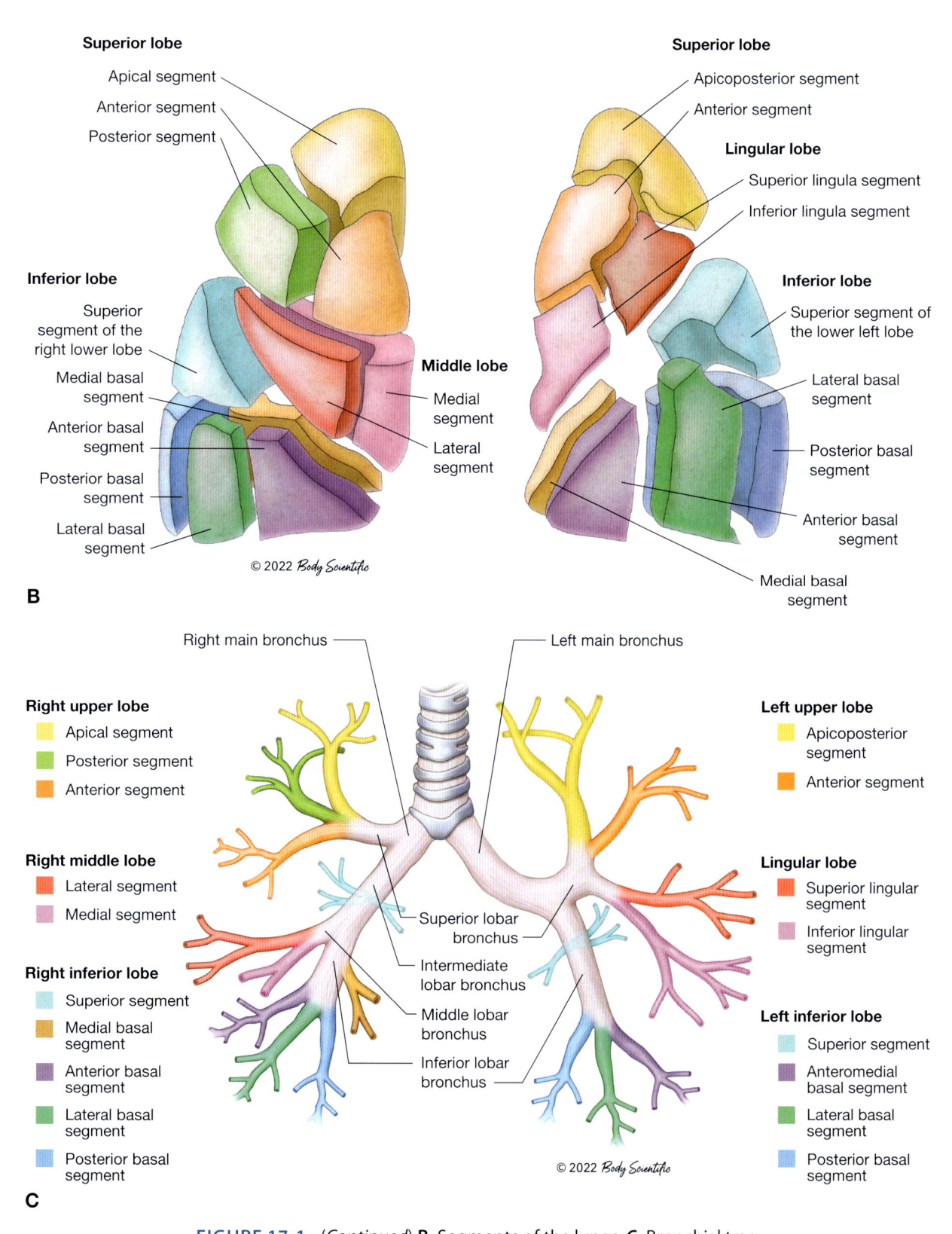

FIGURE 17-1 • (*Continued*) **B.** Segments of the lungs. **C.** Bronchial tree.

320 The Foundation and Art of Robotic Surgery

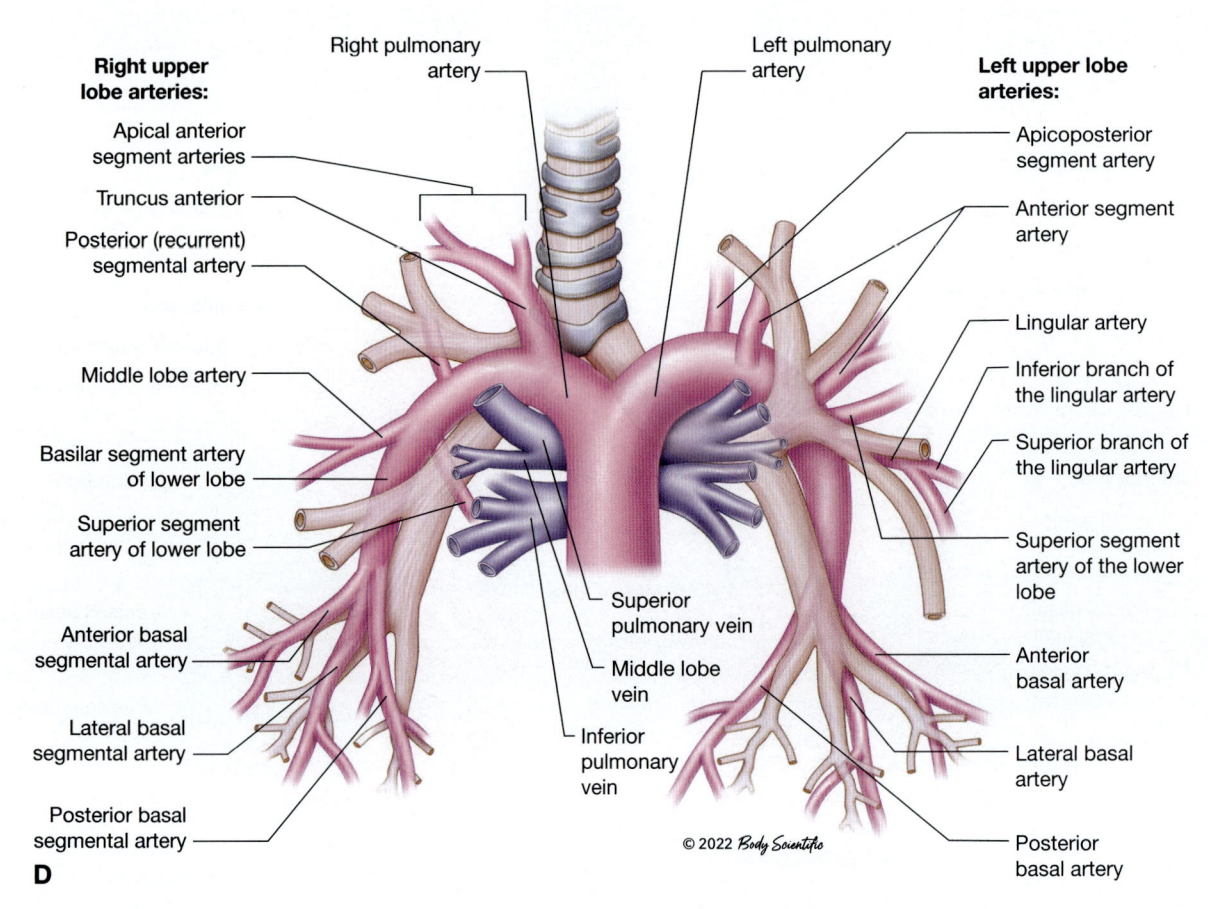

FIGURE 17-1 • *(Continued)* **D.** Pulmonary vasculature.

2. Usually, the main bronchial branches are surrounded by branches of the pulmonary artery and vein (**Figures 17-2 A–C**); this intersectional overlapping makes the preparation of the bronchus during surgery challenging, requiring the division of the vessels first to access the bronchus. The bronchi's structure is more rigid, fragile, and thicker than the vessels and requires a different transection technique. Staplers with wider staples and optional reinforcement should be used.

> ⚠ **PITFALLS**
>
> Fracture of a main lobar bronchus using a vascular stapler with narrow, tight staples.
>
> Air leak from a lobar bronchus is a major complication that may require revisional surgery.

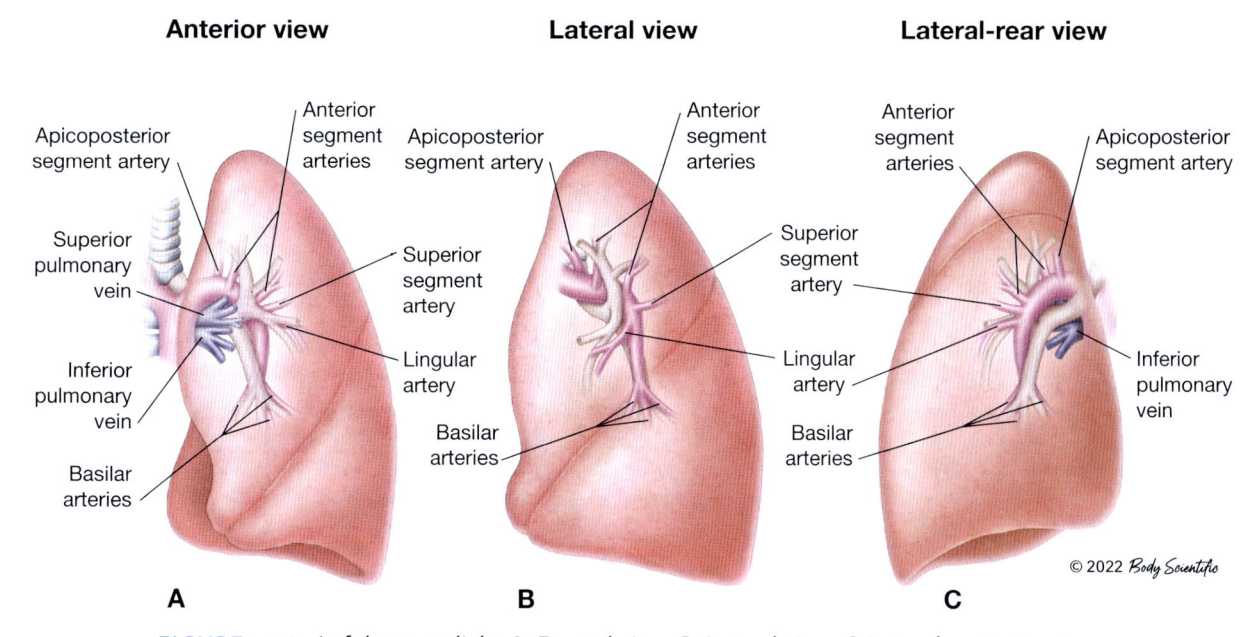

FIGURE 17-2 • Left lung pedicle. **A.** Frontal view. **B.** Lateral view. **C.** Lateral-posterior view.

3. The pulmonary artery is a high-flow but low-pressure system; this vessel differs from the arteries of the systemic circulation. It has thinner walls and is less elastic, making it very fragile and prone to tearing. It must be manipulated very carefully, avoiding direct grasping with surgical instruments, particularly robotic ones, which give only partial force and no tactile feedback (**Figures 17-3 A, B**). Because of the high flow, a tear may result in severe bleeding that is difficult to control.

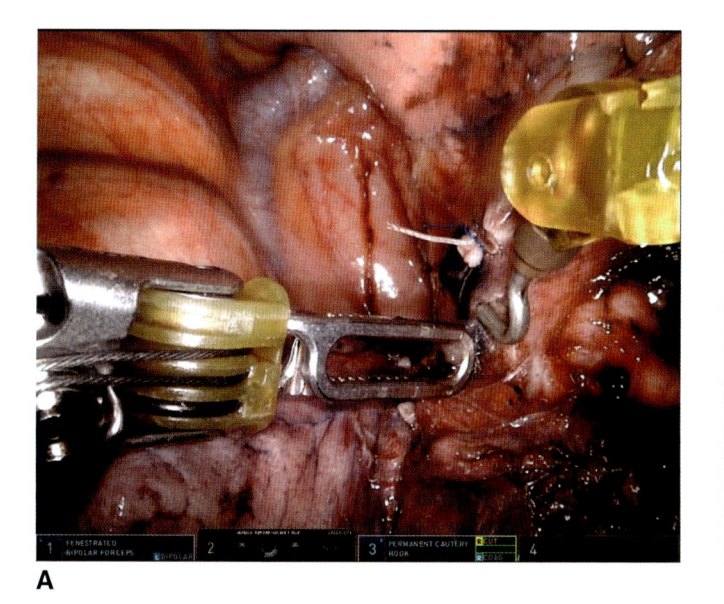

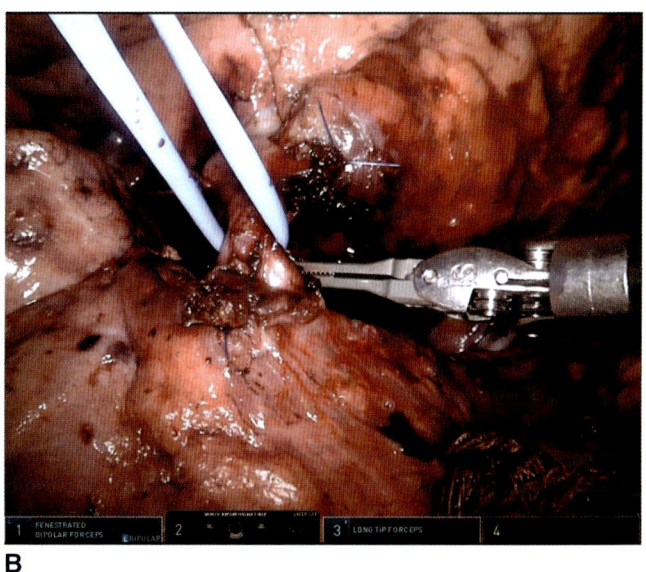

FIGURE 17-3 • The dissection along the arteries should be done delicately, by grasping only the adventitia (**A**) and not the entire vessel itself while manipulating the structures through vessel loops (**B**).

4. The distribution of lymph nodes and lymph nodal stations in the 3 functional compartments of the mediastinum is complex, and their access is hindered by the dense 3D overlapping of vital structures. Intrathoracic lymph nodes locations have been classically divided into 14 stations: stations 1–9 correspond to mediastinal, cephalocaudal and aortic nodes (level 2); while stations 10–14 represent hilar, peripheral and intraparenchymal nodal groups (level 1). A correct lymphadenectomy allows for proper staging of the lung cancer.

5. A precise and accurate lymphadenectomy has a dual value: oncological and technical.

> **ANATOMICAL HIGHLIGHTS**
>
> Lymph nodal sampling for level 2 is made from stations that are more likely involved in cancers originating in a defined lobe according to the original Naruke classification (see **Figure 17-4**):
>
> - **Right upper lobe:** prevascular and retrotracheal N2, N3, 4R, N7
> - **Middle lobe:** N3 and subcarinal N7
> - **Right lower lobe:** N7, N8, N9
>
> See suggested reading #9 for the first lymph nodes map developed by Naruke. See suggested reading #10 for the International Association for the Study of Lung lymph nodes map.

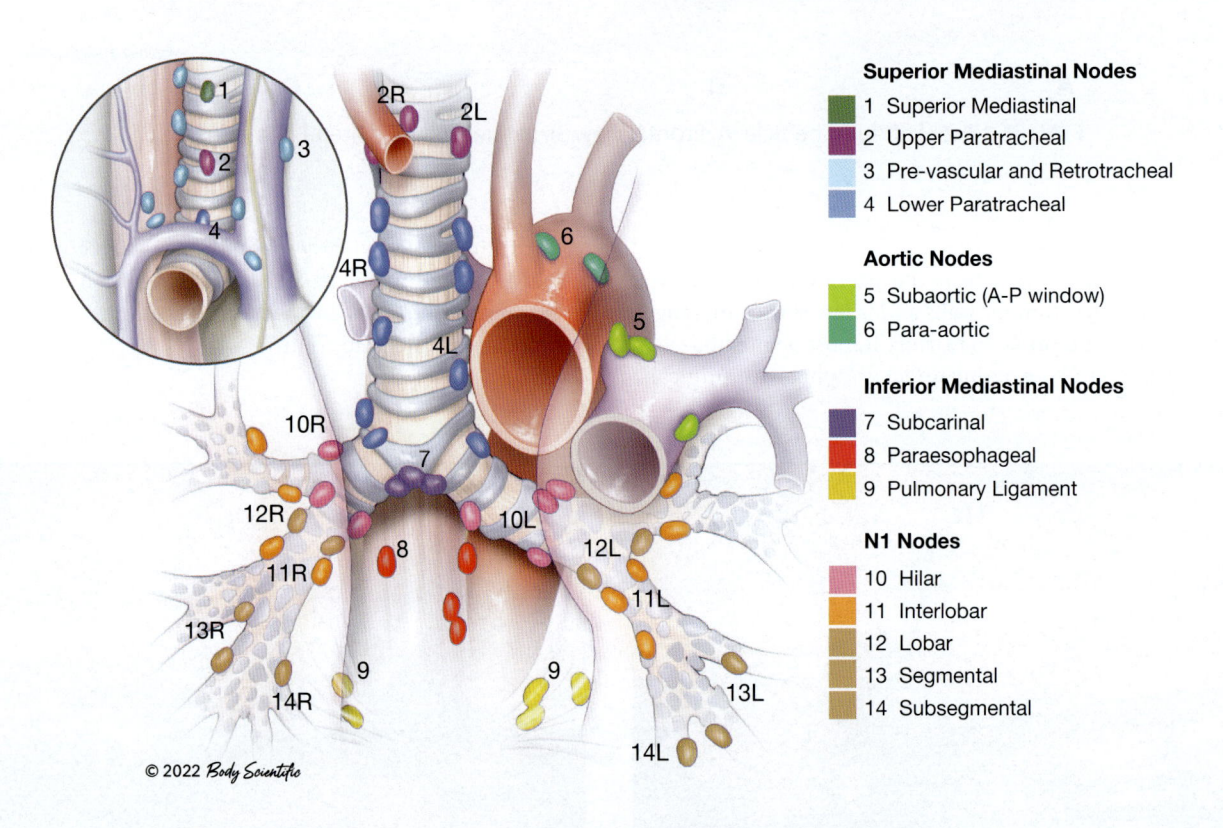

Superior Mediastinal Nodes
1 Superior Mediastinal
2 Upper Paratracheal
3 Pre-vascular and Retrotracheal
4 Lower Paratracheal

Aortic Nodes
5 Subaortic (A-P window)
6 Para-aortic

Inferior Mediastinal Nodes
7 Subcarinal
8 Paraesophageal
9 Pulmonary Ligament

N1 Nodes
10 Hilar
11 Interlobar
12 Lobar
13 Segmental
14 Subsegmental

FIGURE 17-4 • Lymph node classification for lung cancer staging.

It allows a better harvesting of lymph nodal stations. Lymph nodes surround the vascular pedicles and bronchi, and they could be adherent to those structures: clearing them out on the periadventitial plane is the best and safest way to prepare access to the structures that need to be divided.

A complete lymphadenectomy is usually performed in 2 stages. The technical stage is done at the beginning, in preparation or en bloc with the lobectomy (primarily level 1). The oncological stage can be completed/perfected at the end of the procedure (primarily level 2). See **Figure 17-5**.

⚠ PITFALLS

Chronically inflamed lymph nodes (e.g., chronic obstructive pulmonary disease or tuberculosis) may be strongly adherent or fused with the adventitia of the vessels and their dissection carries a risk of vascular injury.

▶▶ TIPS

When feasible, preparation of the vessels should be done simultaneously with the lymphadenectomy of the corresponding station. Stations that are not in the path of the vessel dissection can be addressed at the beginning or at the end of the procedure.

The use of a curved bipolar dissector or Maryland bipolar forceps facilitates the safe removal of intact lymph nodes. Fracturing lymph nodes can theoretically cause cancer cell seeding and immediate bleeding that can be challenging to control, as it is difficult to identify a specific bleeding spot. The best strategy is to apply bipolar coagulation or simply to compress with hemostatic agent (Surgicel®).

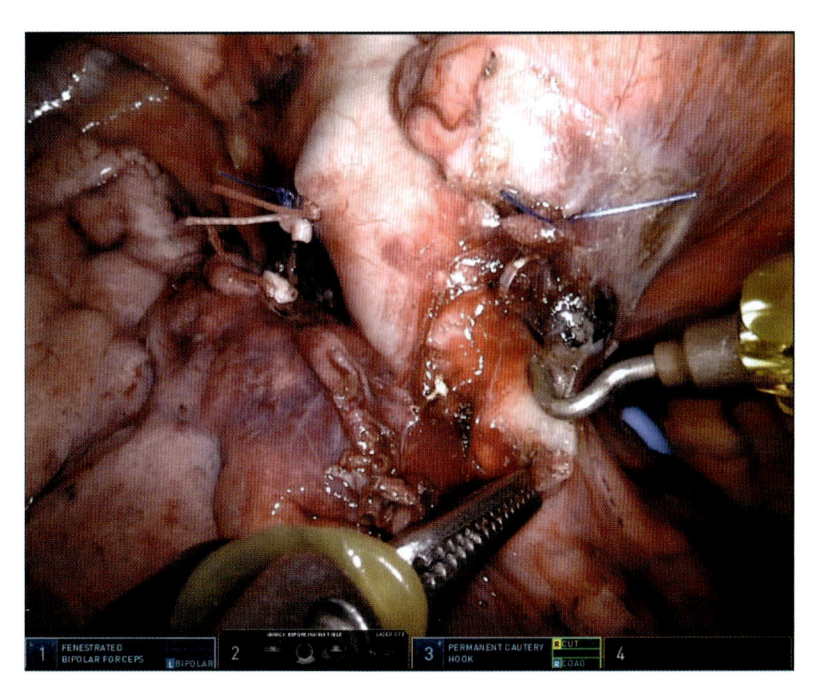

FIGURE 17-5 • Right lower lobectomy, 12R lymph node excision. Underneath, the branches of the basilar trunk have transected between sutures.

6. Robotic port placement must be extremely precise as the trocars become fixed hinges, the intercostal spaces are rigid, and the pleural cavity can be small. If one has suboptimal placement, there is limited room for adjustment (changing the port sites). Incorrect placement can cause poor visualization, restrictions, and collision of operative arms. A good angle of visualization must be kept in mind since the initial planning of the port placement. The port setting should accommodate 3–4 robotic cannulas and 1 or 2 assistant trocars (**Figure 17-6**). Based on the patient's chest anatomy, the main robotic ports are placed in line along the 6th, 7th, or 8th intercostal space, and the assistant's trocars 1 or 2 spaces below. The port setting for upper or lower lobectomies does not differ much because the dissection in the hilum and the main fissure is in the same location, and it might require adjusting only 1 intercostal space higher or lower.

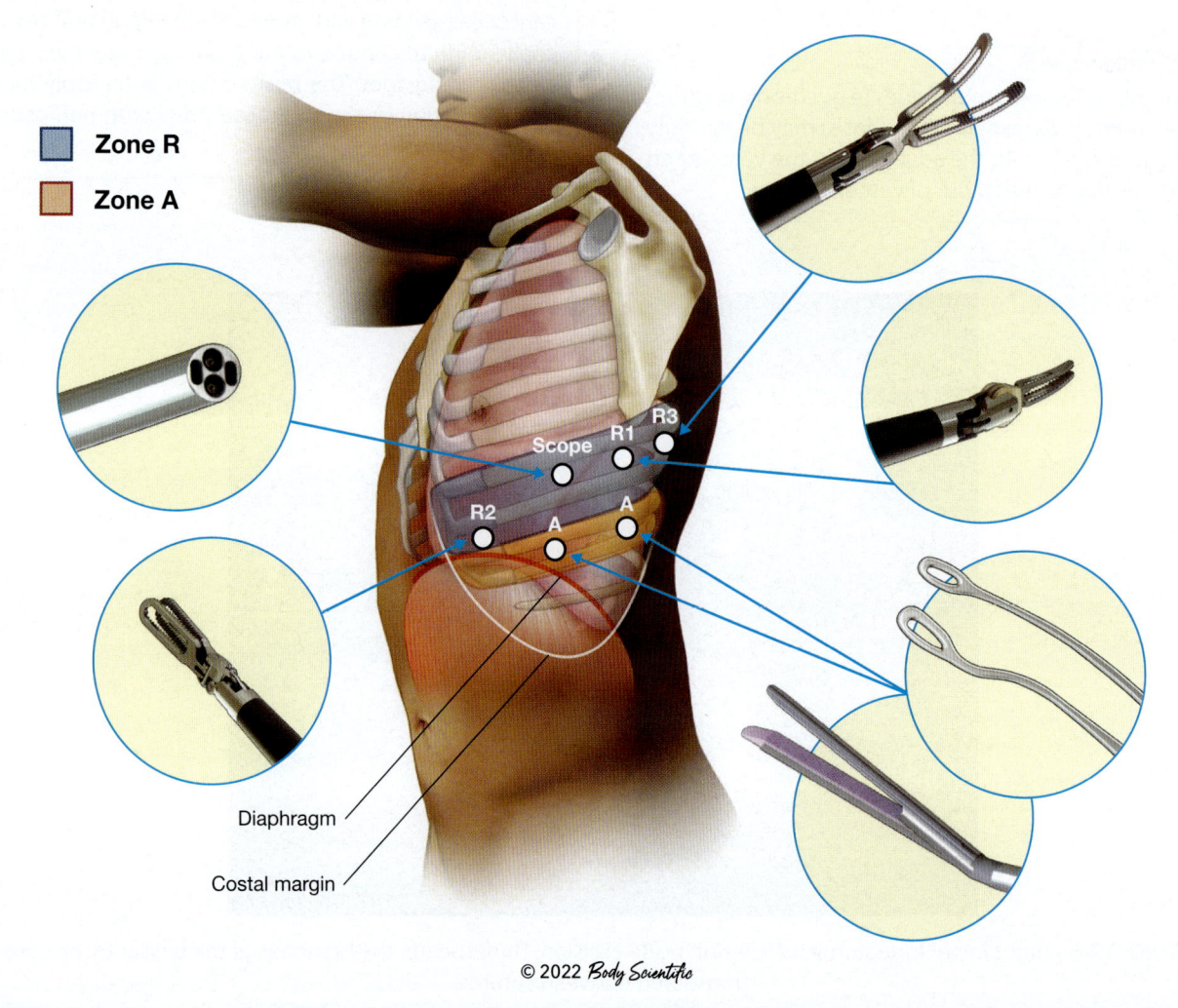

FIGURE 17-6 • Port setting for left lung lobectomy. Zone R is dedicated for robotic ports and Zone A for the assistant's trocars.

7. Pleural adhesions should be taken down completely in the entire lung to have better anatomical control, and to allow for expansion of the remaining lung parenchyma after the lobectomy (filling all the available space since the thoracic wall is rigid and cannot shrink [**Figure 17-7**]). The pleurolysis is better done robotically with the endowristed scissors. The visceral pleura can be plastered to the parietal pleura, making the surgical plane thin and challenging to dissect without making tears of the visceral side (reason for postop air leaks). In the hostile chest (previous surgery/radiation), the first trocar can be difficult to place and must be inserted carefully to avoid entering into the parenchyma. Once some space is created with blunt maneuvers (e.g., the tip of the scope), a couple of robotic trocars are enough to start the dissection.

> ⚠️ **PITFALLS**
>
> Even small parenchymal tears can cause significant and prolonged postoperative air leaks.

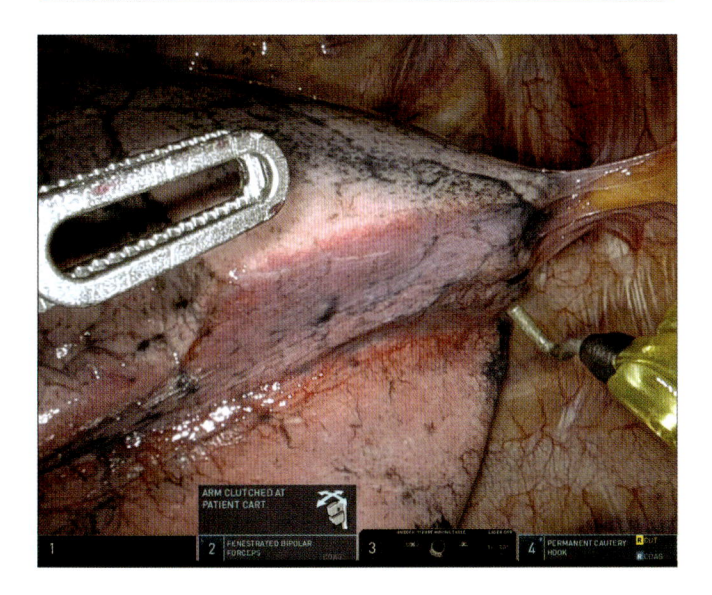

FIGURE 17-7 • Adhesions of the lung to the chest wall, to be divided with monopolar energy.

8. Blood in the chest, even minor bleeds, makes the vision from the camera very dark. Maintaining a clean field with precise dissection and perfect hemostasis (mainly bipolar) minimizes blood loss and allows a superior 3D visualization with recognition of the anatomical details. Usage of white sponges can brighten the operative field, absorbing blood and reflecting white light (**Figure 17-8**).

> ▶▶ **TIPS**
>
> Frequent suctioning and the insertion of an absorbing roll laparoscopic gauze (cigarette sponges) are very helpful in maintaining a dry and clean operative field.

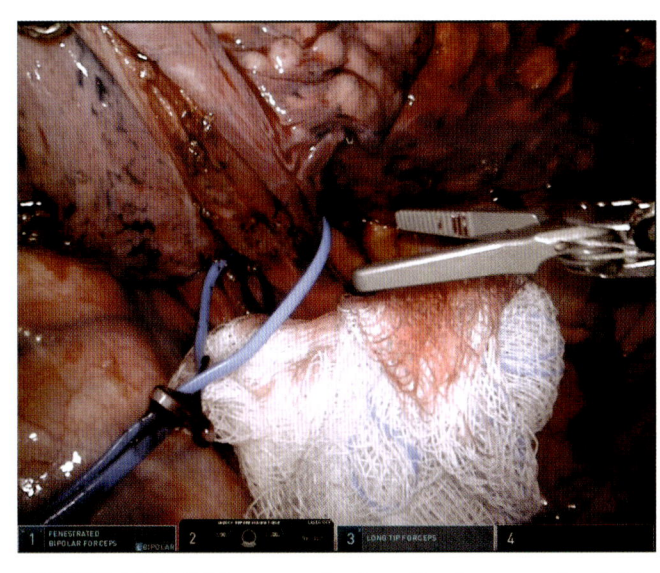

FIGURE 17-8 • White gauze is placed in the operative field, allowing for light reflection and brightening the operative area.

9. It is always better to avoid parenchymal congestion and back bleeding when feasible. Pulmonary artery branches (inflow) should be preferentially divided first before taking down the pulmonary vein (outflow) (**Figure 17-9**).

> **EDITORIAL COMMENT**
>
> It is often difficult or impossible to take down all arterial branches before the pulmonary vein. In many cases, the posterior transfissure approach needs to use a mixed technique. Some arterial branches are easily divided at the beginning, whereas others are taken down after the vein, because the position of the pulmonary vein might have been completely obscuring the access to the artery.

Artery → Vein → Bronchi

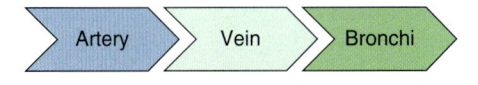

FIGURE 17-9 • Ideal sequence.

10. There are 2 main approaches for the robotic lobectomies:
    a. **Robotic VATS-like** approach with immediate service, anterior, minithoracotomy: there is no possibility of CO_2 insufflation. Through the mini-access, the assistant's instruments, such as staplers, can be introduced, and the incision works also as an extraction site.
    b. **Full robotic (total port)** approach: there is no minithoracotomy, and the chest is closed allowing CO_2 insufflation.

       See **Figure 17-10**.

EDITORIAL COMMENT

	Robotic VATS-like	Full Robotic (Total Port)
Emergency conversion	easy	time-consuming (risky)
Manual lung palpation	possible	not possible
Lung collapse	+	+++
Working space	+	+++
Bleeding (oozing)	+++	+
Cosmesis	suboptimal	good
R3 assistance	not easy	easy
Diaphragmatic injury	possible	infrequent
Improved visualization	good	optimal
Lung exposure to external air	yes	no
Assistant interaction/stapling	easy	more difficult
Postoperative pain	+++	++
Specimen extraction	easy	needs enlarging a trocar site

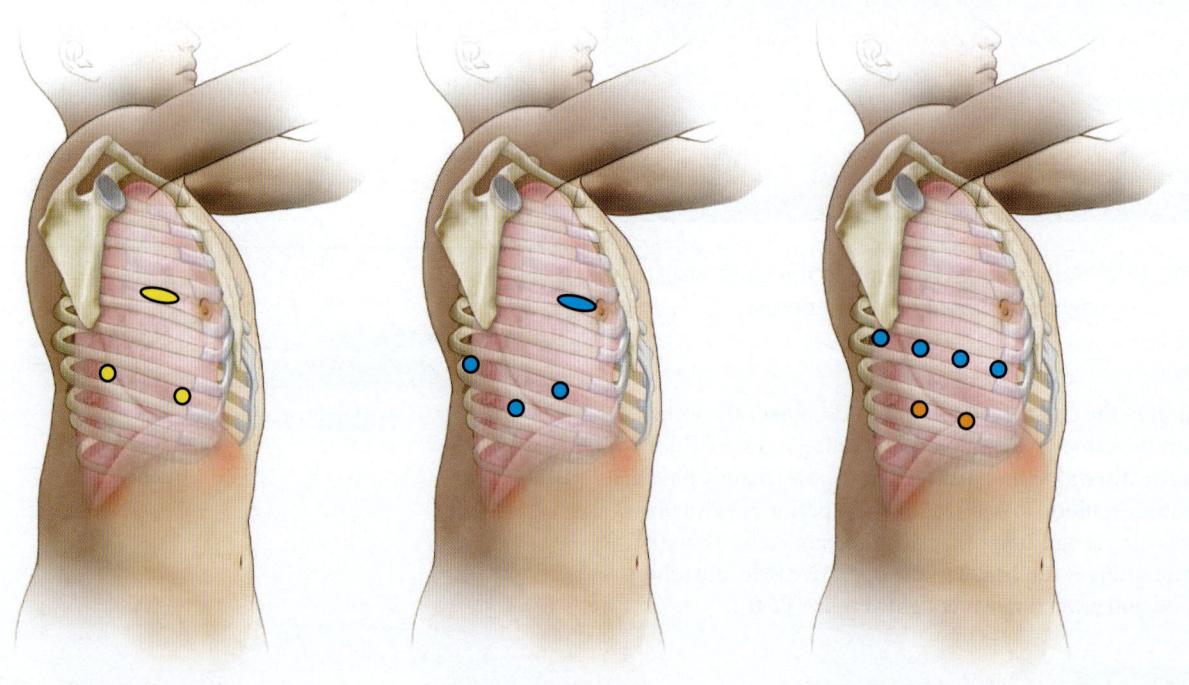

Thoracoscopic approach (VATS) incisions

Robotic VATS-like incisions

Full robotic incisions

© 2022 Body Scientific

FIGURE 17-10 • Different approaches to minimally invasive surgery lung lobectomies.

11. There are 2 main approaches to the vascular dissection necessary for anatomical lobectomy:
    a. The **transfissure approach**, with the goal of addressing the pulmonary artery branches first before the pulmonary vein, is an elegant strategic dissection with less congestion and back bleeding of the parenchyma.
    b. The **anterior approach**, dividing the pulmonary vein first (similarly to many VATS techniques), is more often indicated when the fissure is incomplete or does not exist.
12. There are 2 main techniques for the preparation of pulmonary vessels:
    a. Picking and peeling the peri-adventitia tissue (and lymph nodes) with a curved bipolar dissector or Maryland bipolar forceps (**Figures 17-11 A, B**).
    b. Going around the smaller branches with the monopolar hook used as a right-angle dissector, larger vessels may require a longer, blunt instrument (tip-up forceps or long-tip forceps) (**Figures 17-11 C, D**).

> **EDITORIAL COMMENT**
>
> Both techniques should be practiced and mastered in a simulation lab. The picking and peeling technique is easier and safer and works very well for the main branches of the pulmonary artery, vein, and bronchus.
>
> The hook is a perfect right angle for smaller vessels, but it is more difficult to control the direction of the spread of the monopolar energy. This technique requires a more sophisticated skill set.

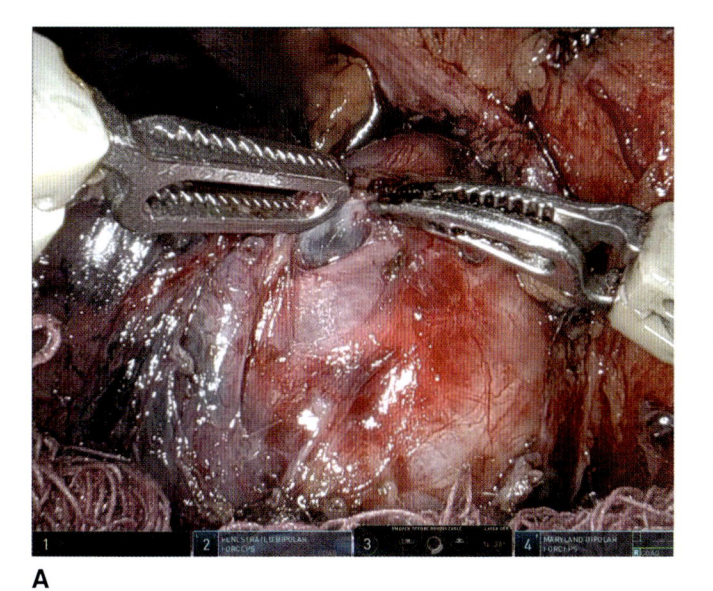

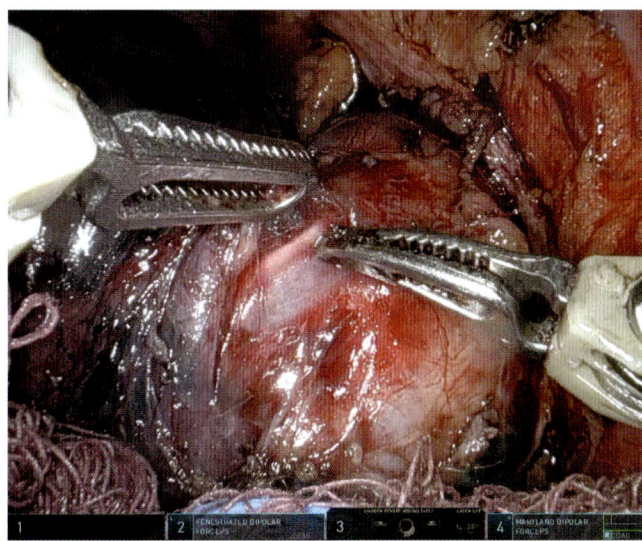

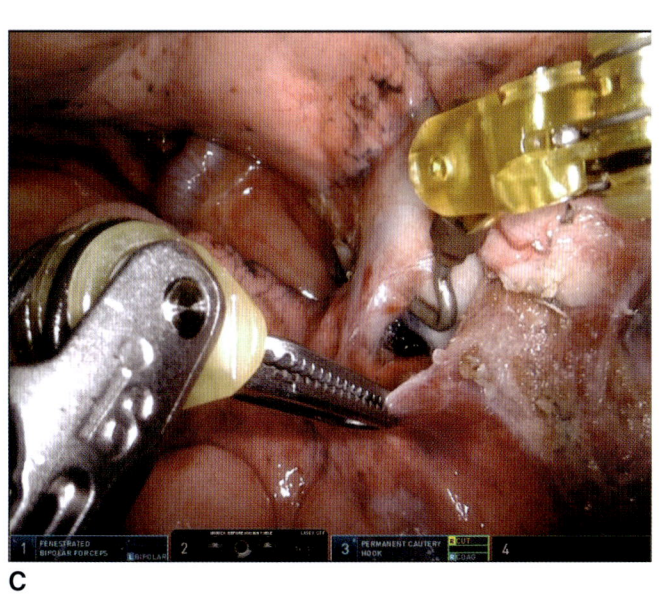

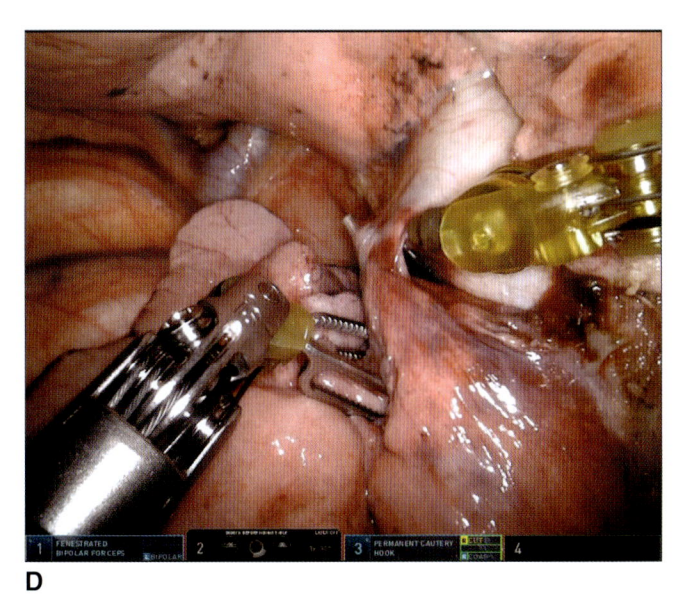

FIGURE 17-11 • **A, B.** Left upper lobectomy, lymph nodal station 7 is being dissected from the vascular structures using the picking and peeling technique. **C, D.** Right lower lobectomy, basilar branches being skeletonized using the monopolar hook.

13. Stapling is the safest and fastest way to control the vascular pedicles and branches. However, the insertion of the staple jaws might be challenging (unfavorable angles, limited space, fixed hinges, presence of other vessels, and structures that can be injured are all limiting factors). A guided stapling technique can be used in some cases (**Figures 17-12 A–C**). Having 2 possible entrance ports for the stapler, 1 more anterior and 1 more posterior, may allow more options for the specific pedicle to be divided. Besides the stapling technique, the surgeon should master all techniques for vascular control, including fine suturing, tying, and application of clips.

> ▶▶ **TIPS**
>
> Using vessel loops or small Nelaton rubber tubes may guide the tip of the stapler in the proper space.
>
> The round, curved tip of the cartridge also facilitates the correct passage of the stapler jaws, decreasing the risk of including other structures.

EDITORIAL COMMENT

The stapler can be thoracoscopic and manually guided by the assistant or full robotic and controlled by the console surgeon.

	Robotic Stapler	Thoracoscopic Stapler	
Width	12 mm	8 mm	12 mm
Staple lines	2	2	3
Controlled	Console surgeon	Assistant	

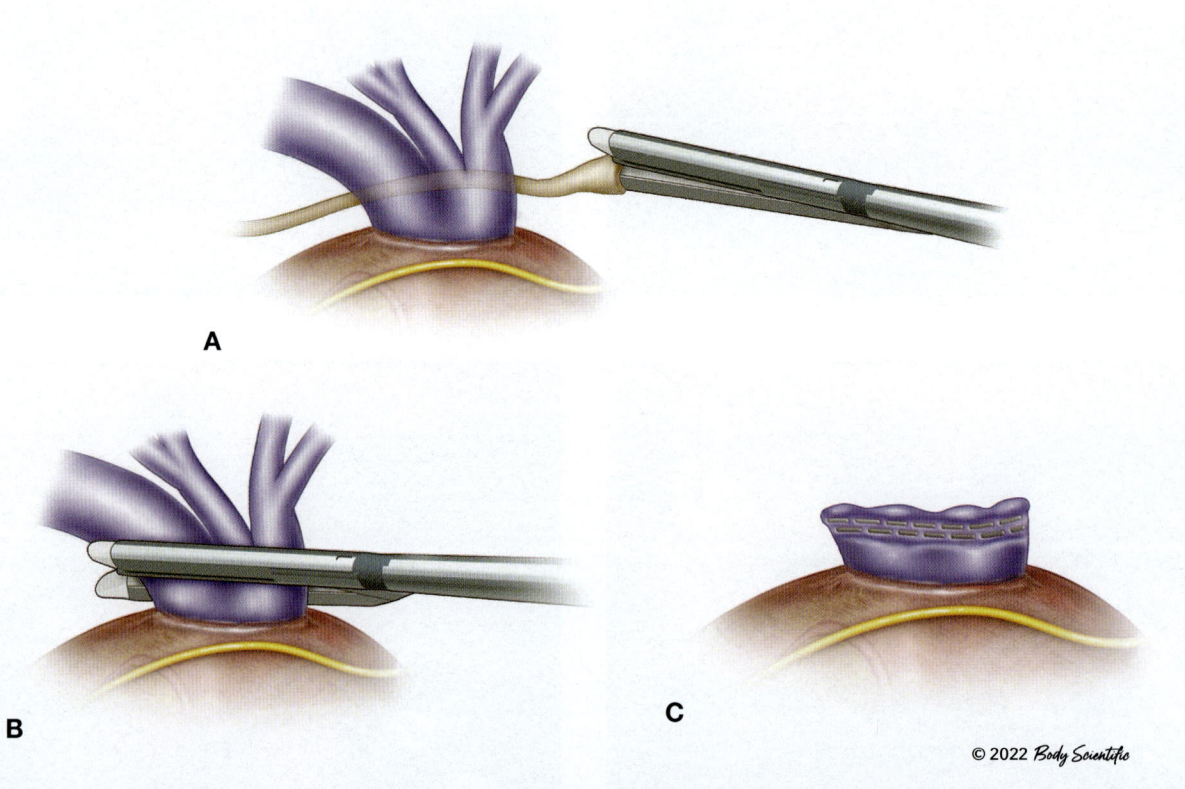

FIGURE 17-12 • Guided stapling vessel technique. **A.** Stapler is being guided by a pediatric Nelaton catheter. **B.** Jaws are closed. **C.** Transected vessels.

14. Before stapling and dividing a bronchus near a bifurcation, it is always prudent to do a clamping ventilation test to ensure there is no side pinching or narrowing of the remaining airways (**Figures 17-13 A–C**).

> ▶▶ **TIPS**
>
> While performing the ventilation test, there is expansion of the remaining lung with loss of working space and vision. It can be time-consuming to exclude the ventilation again and drain the entrapped air in the ventilated parenchyma. Another option can be performing a bronchoscopy to identify the correct placement of the stapler before firing it and transecting the bronchus.

15. The role of the R3 in retraction and exposure during the lobectomy is controversial. It depends on multiple factors, like the size of the working space, ideal port setting, absence of collisions, and presence of an expert assistant at the patient's bedside. A stable exposure generally allows better visualization and facilitates microsurgical dissection.

> ▶▶ **TIPS**
>
> The presence of the R3 increases the chances of collisions and movement restrictions. It is usually set very posteriorly, close to the spine. In some steps of the operation, the R3 can be temporarily undocked when it is not needed. If the lung is collapsed and well deflated of air, the necessary exposure is easily achieved with the surgeon's nondominant hand grasper and the assistant's help.

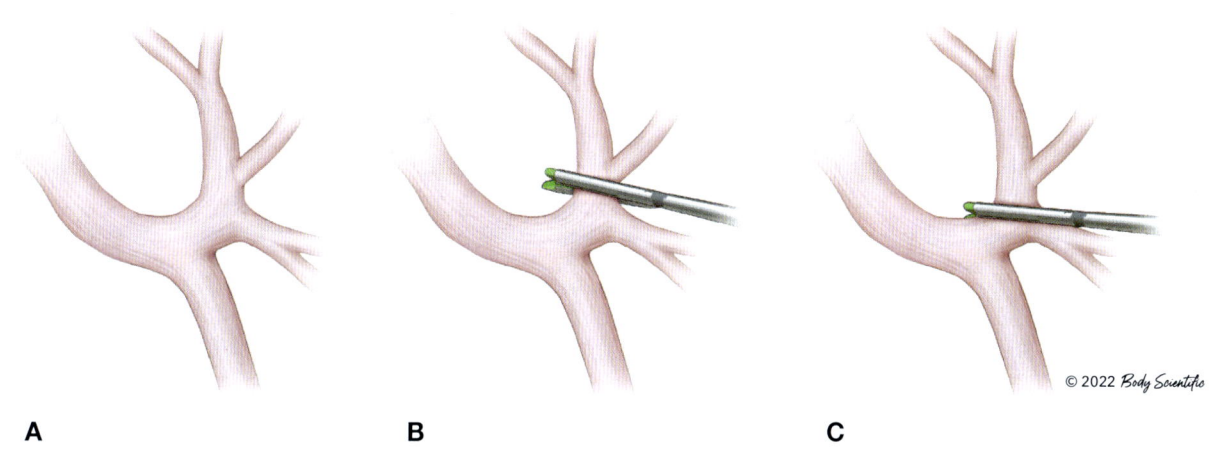

A **B** **C**

FIGURE 17-13 • Technique for adequate placement of stapler for bronchial division. **A.** Left bronchial tree. **B.** Correct placement of the stapler for division of the apicoposterior bronchi, sparing the lingula bronchus. **C.** Incorrect placement of the stapler. Stapler includes a portion of the lingula bronchus, causing pinching and restricting air flow to the lingula.

16. Localization of small nodules in the lung can be challenging, depending on their location and depth inside the parenchyma. If the nodule is superficial, it can be detected by touching the visceral pleura with the tip of the thoracoscopic instruments (indirect tactile feedback). In robotics, the change in texture is recognized by the modification of the reactive pressure lines of the tissue (virtual tactile feedback). For deeper lesions, different techniques have been developed to increase the localization accuracy during thoracoscopies, such as percutaneous metallic wire placement, injection of dye, intraoperative ultrasound scan, magnetic navigation, fluorescent staining, and intraoperative CT in hybrid ORs. The latest technologies, the ION bronchoscopy (Intuitive) or Auris Monarch (J&J), may allow a computerized "robotic" bronchoscopy with the injection of ICG fluorescence into the nodule (**Figures 17-14 A–F**). The patient can undergo robotic lung resection immediately after the robotic bronchoscopy. The ION technique may also be utilized to visualize "sentinel nodes" and perform lymph nodal mapping.

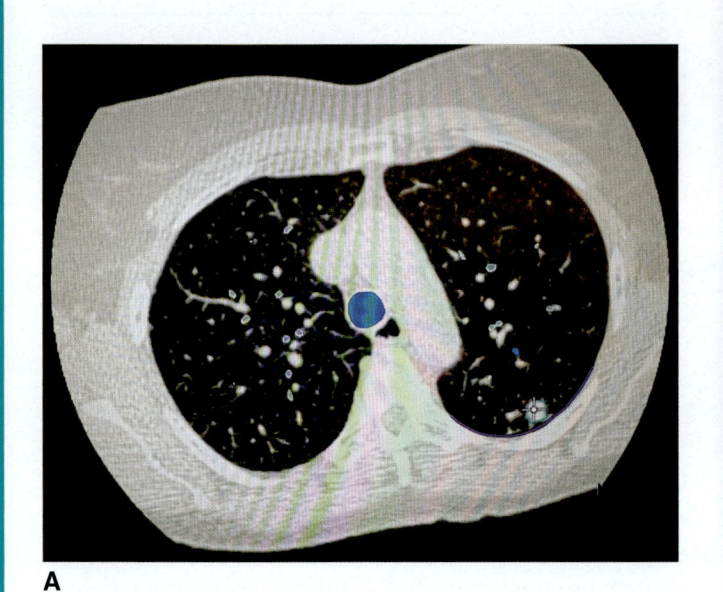

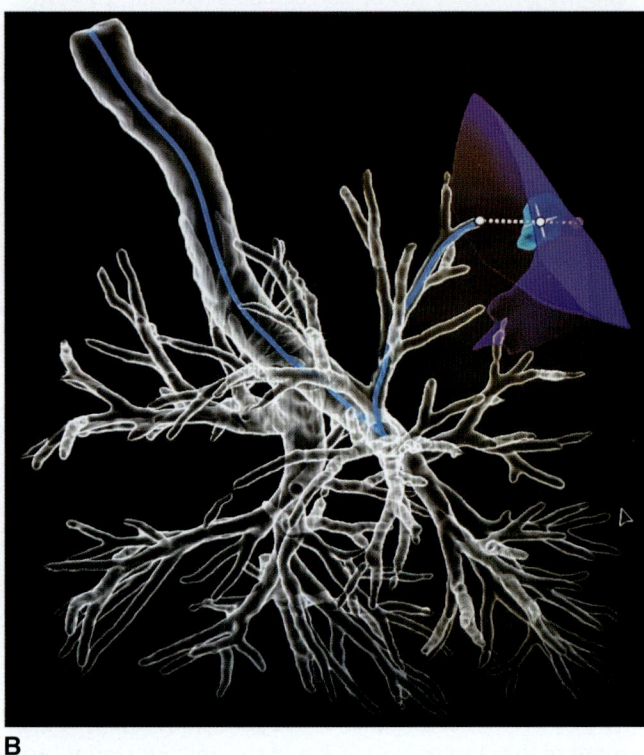

FIGURE 17-14 A, B • Robotic bronchoscopy. The nodule in this case was a peripheral left upper lobe nodule. The robotic bronchoscope is able to reach peripheral nodules given its small-caliber camera and catheter and can also identify and biopsy nodules as small as ~10 mm. Robotic bronchoscopy was used in this case to mark the nodule with ICG and methylene blue in order to identify it intraoperatively with the surgical robot. **A.** ION bronchoscopy CT chest in cross-sectional view. Left upper lobe nodule seen in the posterior left chest marked by navigational program with an X and encircled with a light blue line. The pleural border marker posterior to the nodule is marked in purple. The main airways are marked in blue. **B.** ION bronchoscopy navigational program image of the trachea and bronchial tree. The path to the lesion is noted in blue. The nodule is noted in blue and the pleural boarder in purple. The path created to the nodule will be followed by the robotic bronchoscope to find the lesion for biopsy or marking.

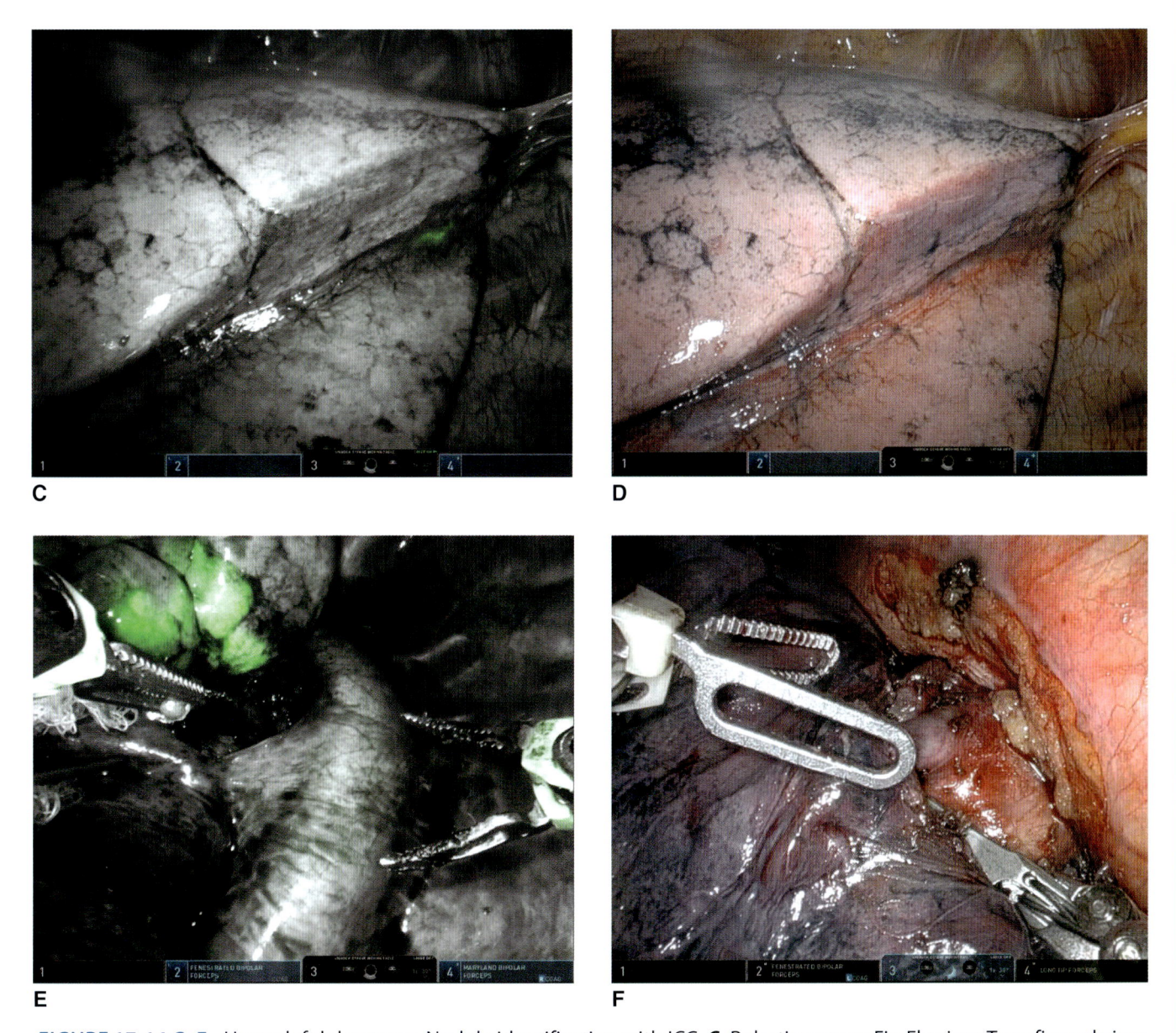

FIGURE 17-14 C–F • Upper left lobectomy. Nodule identification with ICG. **C.** Robotic camera FireFly view: Transfissural view of the left lung with ICG previously injected into the left upper lobe (LUL) nodule seen in the posterior portion of the left upper lobe. **D.** Robotic camera view: Transfissural view without ICG. **E.** Robotic camera FireFly view: Posterior view of the left lung with ICG previously injected into the LUL nodule seen in the posterior portion of the left upper lobe. **F.** Robotic camera view: Posterior view of the left lung without ICG.

TOTAL PORT LEFT UPPER LOBECTOMY WITH THE TRANSFISSURE APPROACH (FISSURE FIRST)

Indications and Relative Contraindications to the Robotic Approach

Multiple aspects should be considered when selecting patients for robotic thoracic surgery, including but not limited to the following: patient's body mass index (BMI), thoracic configuration, anatomical location of the primary lesion, lymph nodal status, the lymph node's relation to vascular structures, presence of adhesions related to prior surgery, infections, chronic lung disease, age, and general comorbidities.

There are no absolute contraindications for the robotic approach, but bulky infiltrative lesions and hostile chest with possible severe adhesions can increase the complexity and length of the operation. Personal judgment should be implemented, taking into consideration the experience and learning curve of the surgeon.

Patient Positioning, OR Setup, and Port Setting

Once the patient is intubated with a double-lumen endotracheal tube and placed on single-lung ventilation, is positioned in the right lateral decubitus. The right arm is extended anteriorly and cranially, and the left arm is positioned anteriorly and toward the head to gain access to the intercostal spaces (**Figure 17-15**). The table's lower section is flexed down and bent to create more space between the hip and the lower border of the rib cage, opening the intercostal spaces. Intermittent compression devices are placed on the lower limbs to decrease the risk of deep vein thrombosis. The robotic cart is placed in front of the patient, and the assistants stand facing the patient's back with easy access to the assistant ports (**Figure 17-16**). Port placement is divided into Zone R for the robotic trocars and Zone A for the assistant's ports. The robotic ports are placed along the 6th, 7th, and 8th intercostal spaces (ICS). Considering the narrowing of the spaces posteriorly, the anterior port might need to be placed 1 ICS below the rest to maintain a straight line. Three robotic trocars are placed along the anterior (R2), middle (S), and posterior (R1)

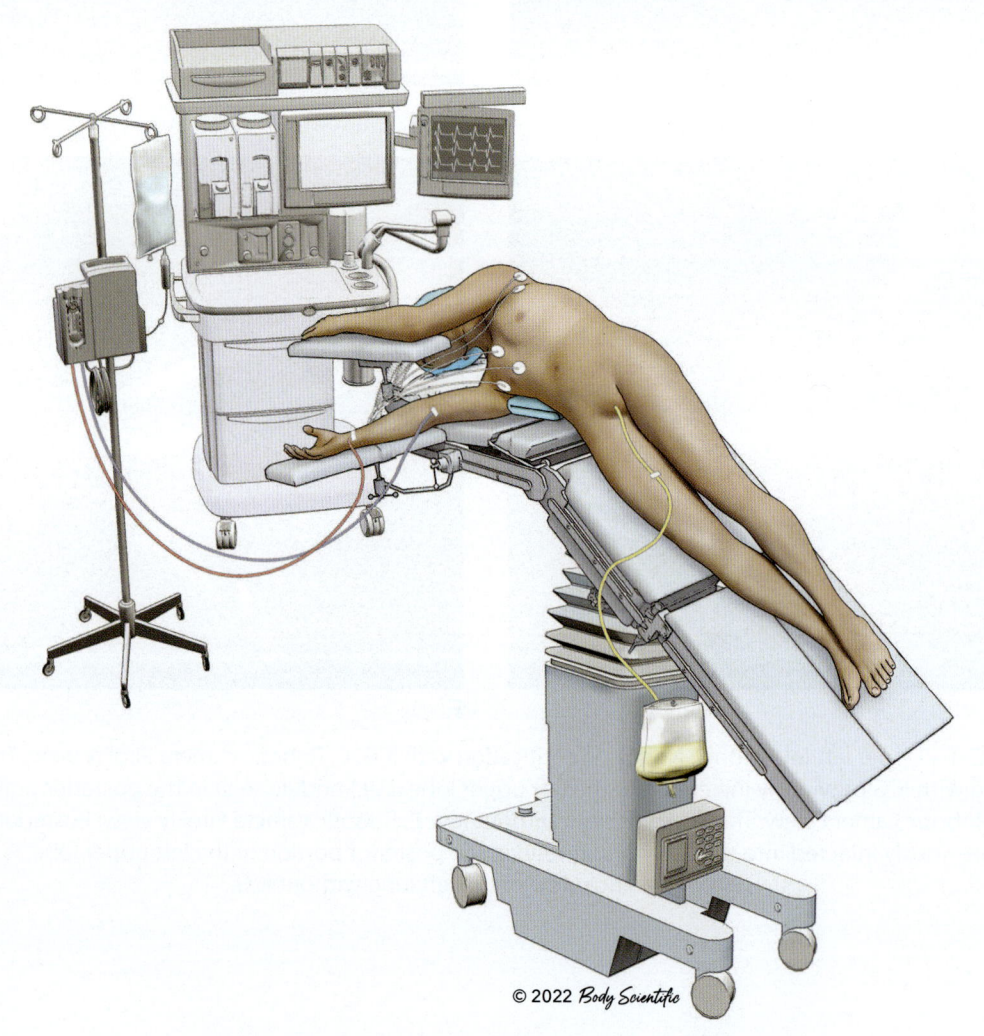

FIGURE 17-15 • Patient positioning for left lung lobectomy.

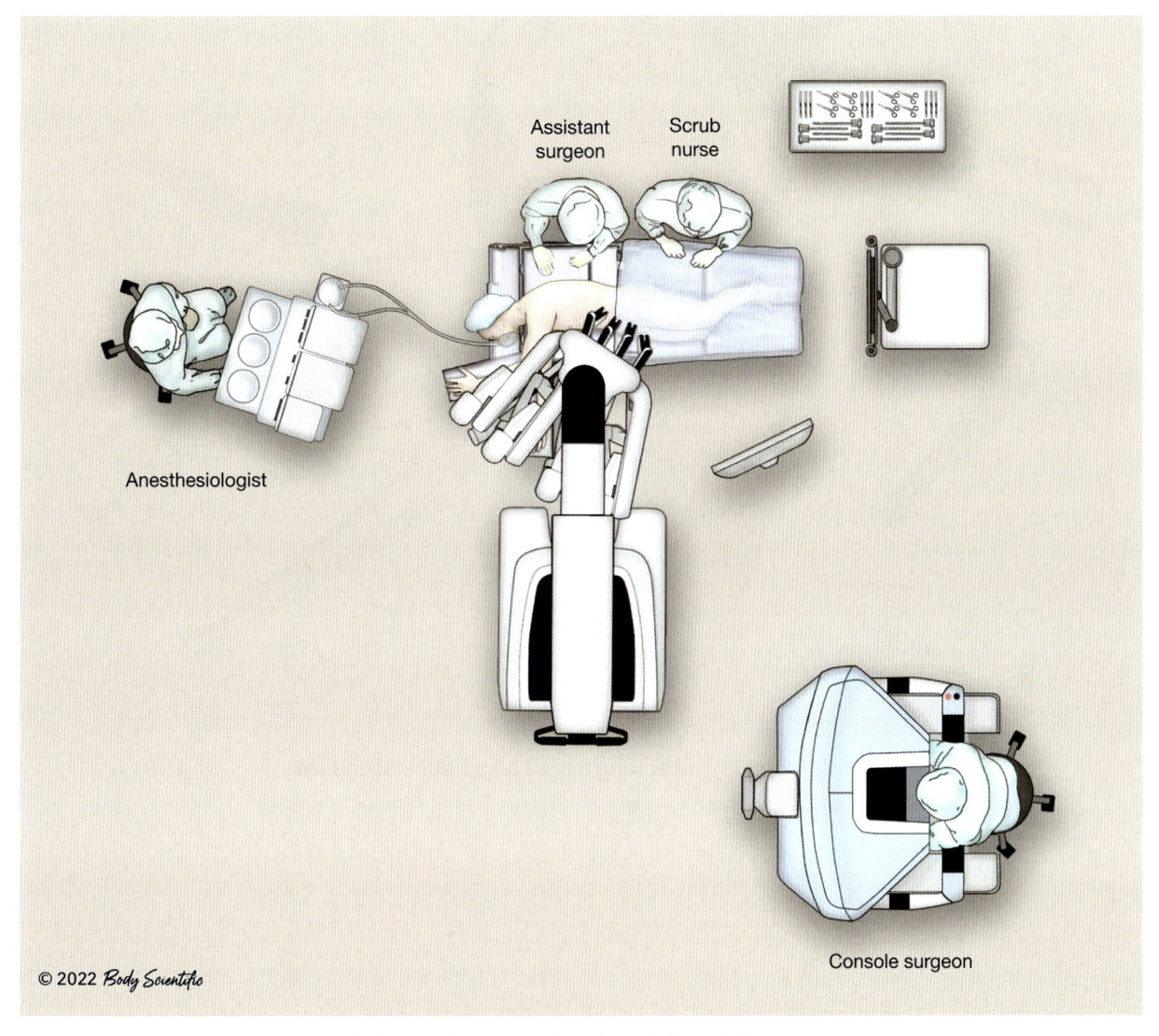

Lung Lobectomies: General Principles and the Total Port, Transfissure Approach (Fissure First) 333

FIGURE 17-16 • OR setup for left lung lobectomy.

axillary lines. When needed, an additional robotic port (R3) can be placed more posteriorly, and it can be undocked when no longer required. Two 12-mm assistant ports are placed 1 or 2 ICS below; both can be used for multiple assistant maneuvers, including thoracoscopic stapling (**Figure 17-17**). If robotic stapling is utilized, some of the operative ports (R1 or R2) should be upgraded to 12-mm size.

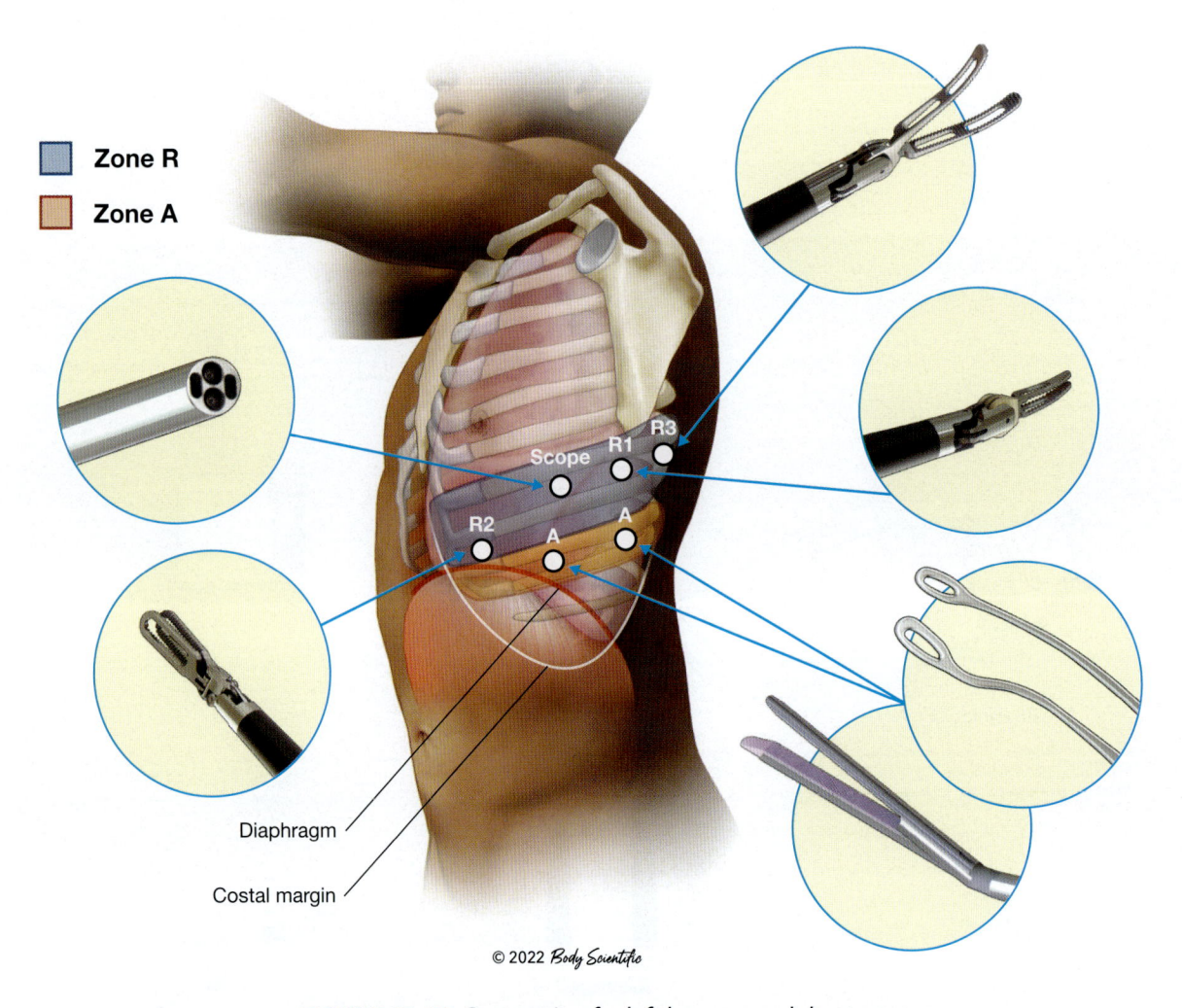

FIGURE 17-17 • Port setting for left lung upper lobectomy.

Surgical Technique

▶ **Video 17-1. Left Upper Lobectomy: Steps 1–4**

Step 1. Inferior pulmonary ligament dissection with station 8–9 lymphadenectomy

If adhesions are present between the lung and the chest wall, they are divided. The lower lobe, posterior and adjacent to the diaphragm, is retracted cephalad in order to gain access to the inferior pulmonary ligament. The left phrenic nerve should be recognized early on. The ligament is carefully divided using monopolar or bipolar cautery. Station 9 lymph nodes are found in this area, which are dissected out and sent for pathology (**Figures 17-18 A, B**). Care is taken to identify and therefore not injure the inferior pulmonary vein, which comes into view as the ligament is dissected toward the hilum. Station 8 lymph nodes are located adjacent to the esophagus; if identified during dissection, these are sent to pathology as well. The dissection proceeds until the inferior pulmonary vein is reached.

Step 1 average time frame: 5–15 min

▶▶ **TIPS**

While making the dissection of the inferior pulmonary ligament, the R3, if utilized, may help retracting cephalad the lower lobe in a very stable way.

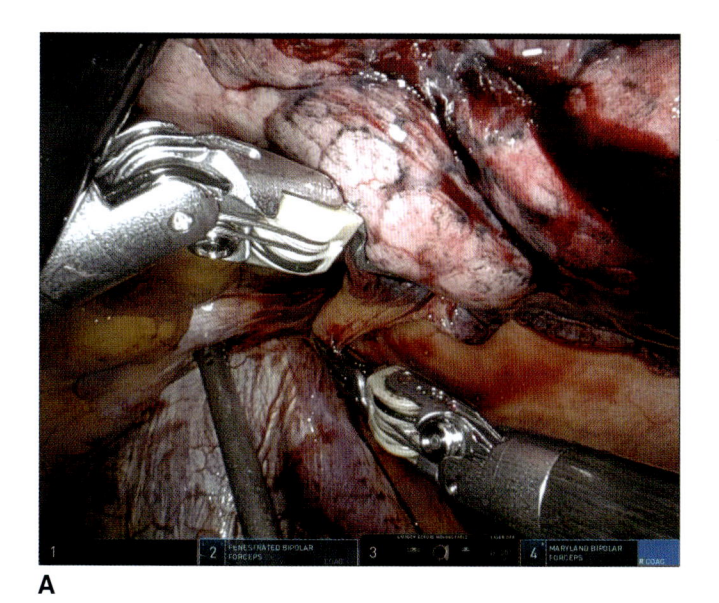

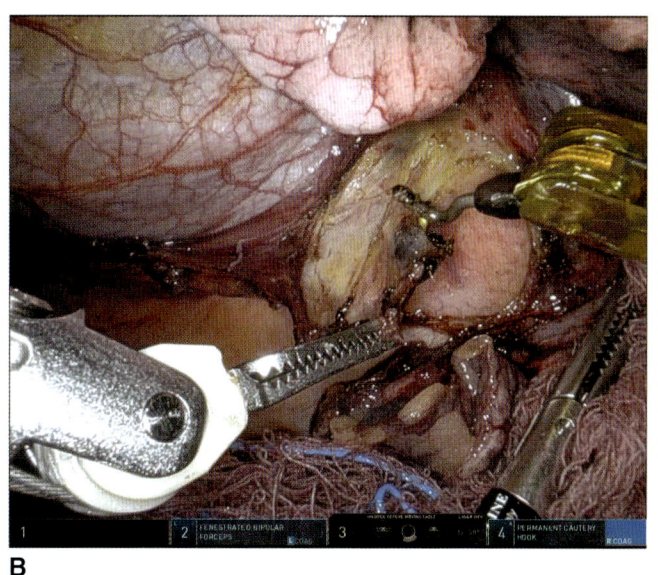

FIGURE 17-18 • Step 1. Inferior pulmonary ligament is divided with station 8–9 lymphadenectomy. **A.** Division of the inferior pulmonary ligament. **B.** Station 9 lymph nodes are removed.

Step 2. Opening of the anterior pleural reflection at the hilum

After dividing the inferior pulmonary ligament, the dissection continues anteriorly with the division of the anterior pleural reflection (**Figures 17-19 A–D**). At this stage, the anatomy of the pulmonary vein must be identified. It is also important to understand the drainage of the lingula into the superior pulmonary vein. If there are enlarged lymph nodes of the station 10L, they should be removed.

Step 2 average time frame: 5–15 min

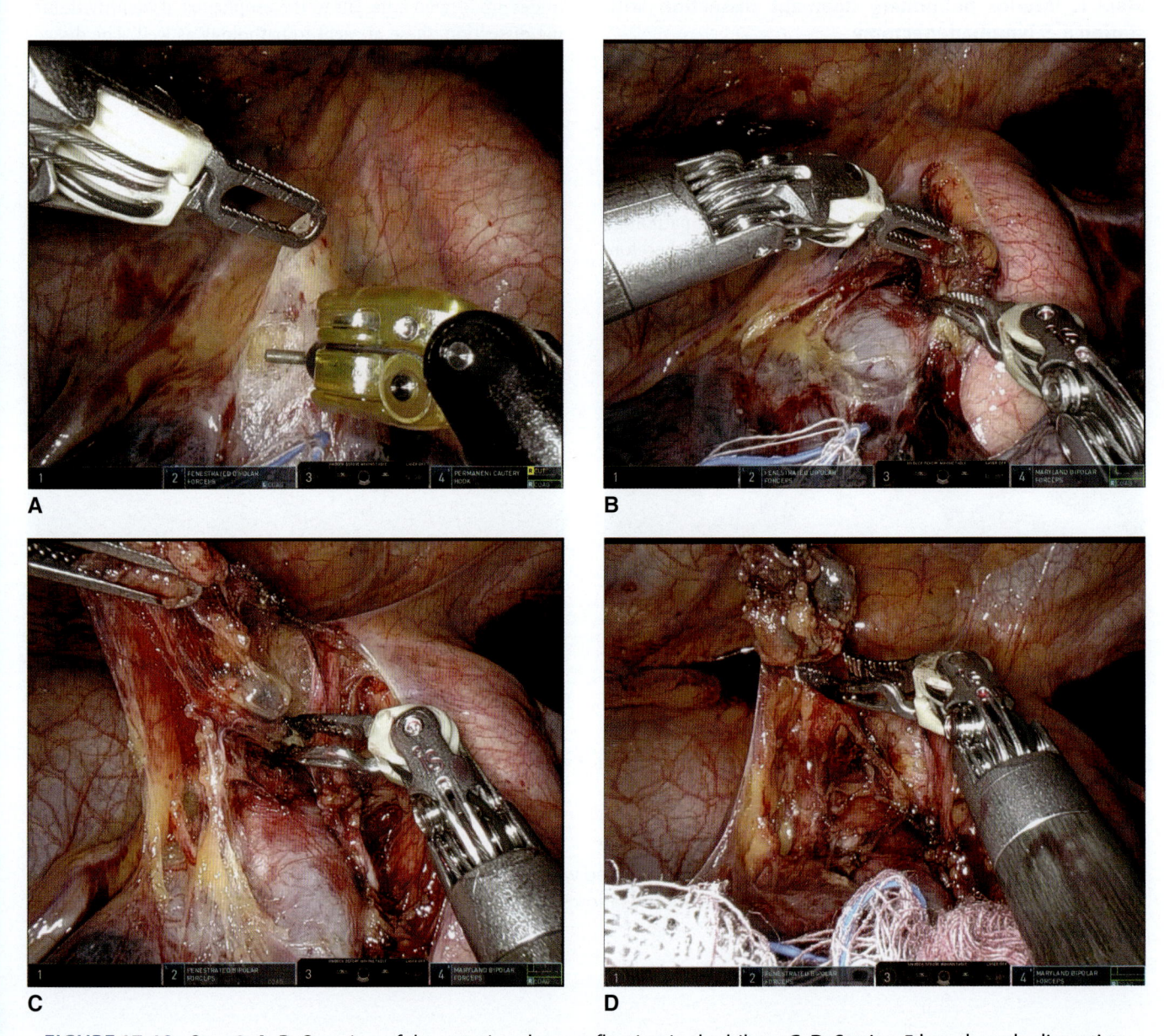

FIGURE 17-19 • Step 2. **A, B.** Opening of the anterior pleura reflection in the hilum. **C, D.** Station 5 lymph node dissection.

Step 3. Opening of the posterior pleural reflection at the hilum

The posterior pleura reflection of the hilum is opened (**Figures 17-20 A–C**). This action gives access to the carina and the station 7 lymph nodes. Those lymph nodes should be removed carefully because they can be adherent to the tracheal bifurcation. The dissection moves cranially, exposing the posterior aspect of the pulmonary artery and reaching the aortopulmonary window (lymph node station 5). Exposing the posterolateral aspect of the pulmonary artery provides an important landmark for the next steps.

Step 3 average time frame: 15–20 min

> ▶▶ **TIPS**
> Bipolar coagulation is the most effective and safest way of removing lymph nodes, avoiding bleeding and inadvertent damage to the vagal nerve (recurrent nerve).

> ⚠ **PITFALLS**
> Damage of the recurrent laryngeal nerve while dissecting lymph nodes from station 5.

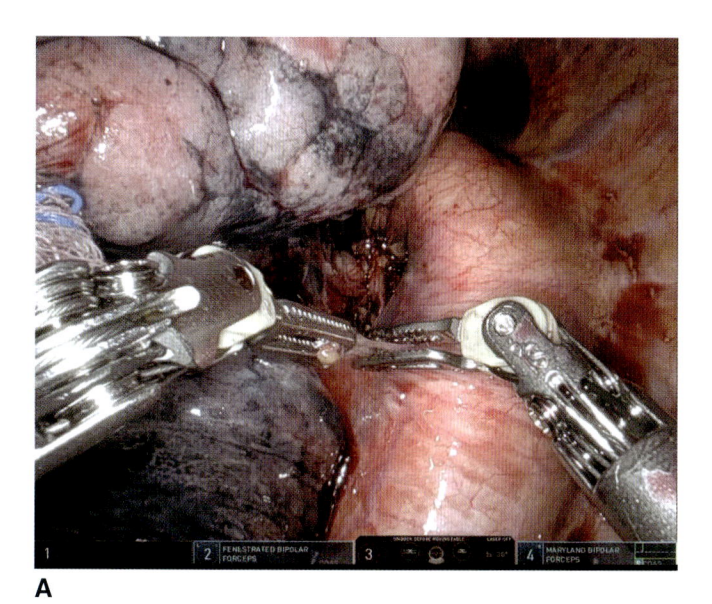

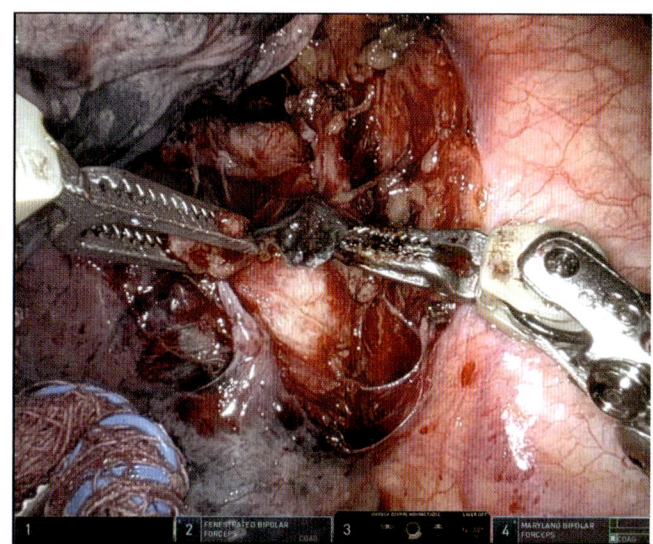

FIGURE 17-20 • Step 3. Opening of the posterior pleural reflection.

Step 4. Dissection of the fissure, preparation of the pulmonary artery, and transection of the posterior pulmonary artery branches

The great oblique fissure has a variable thickness and length. The dissection starts in the middle segment of the fissure and proceeds initially toward the posterolateral aspect (**Figures 17-21 A, B**). If present, a small posterior bridge of the parenchyma might be divided with a stapler at this stage or as described in Step 5. The more the pulmonary artery is exposed, the easier the posterior branches to the upper lobe are recognized and divided with a stapler. The number of the posterior branches varies, from 1 big trunk (A 2–3) to multiple ones (**Figures 17-22 A–F**).

If the procedure includes the lingula resection, 1 or 2 branches for the lingula should be taken down at this stage. Lymph nodes of stations 11 and 12 are removed during this dissection.

Step 4 average time frame: 20–30 min

▶▶ **TIPS**

The stapler could be too cumbersome for some tiny pulmonary artery branches. In this case, they should be divided in between Prolene™ 5-0 sutures.

▶▶ **TIPS**

There is high variability regarding the presence of incomplete fissures. The surgeon should be able to modify their techniques based on the specific anatomy. An incomplete fissure might require an anterior approach to the hilum with take down of the pulmonary vein first, as described in Chapter 18.

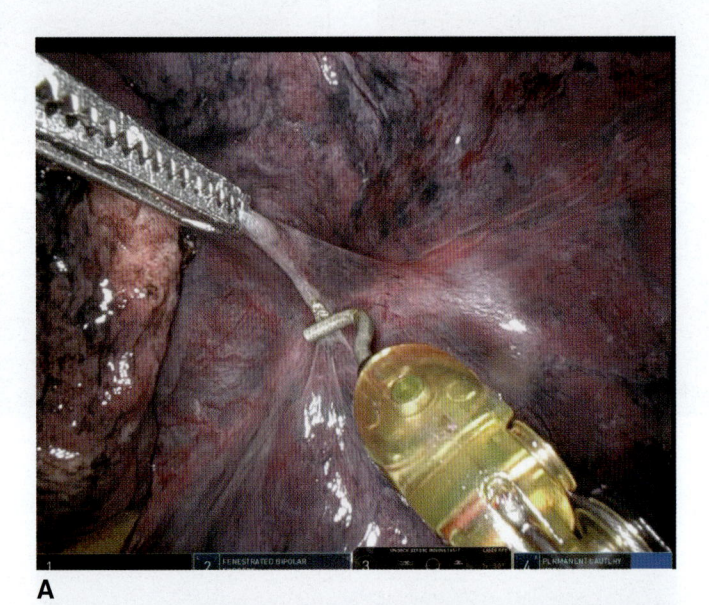

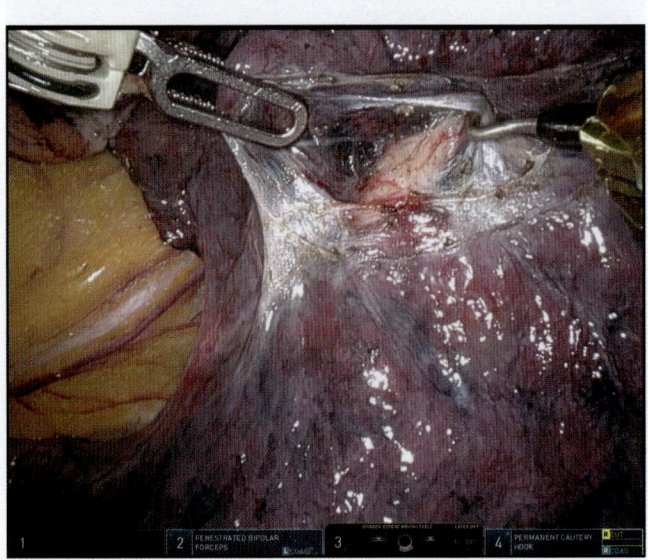

FIGURE 17-21 • Step 4. Division of the fissure.

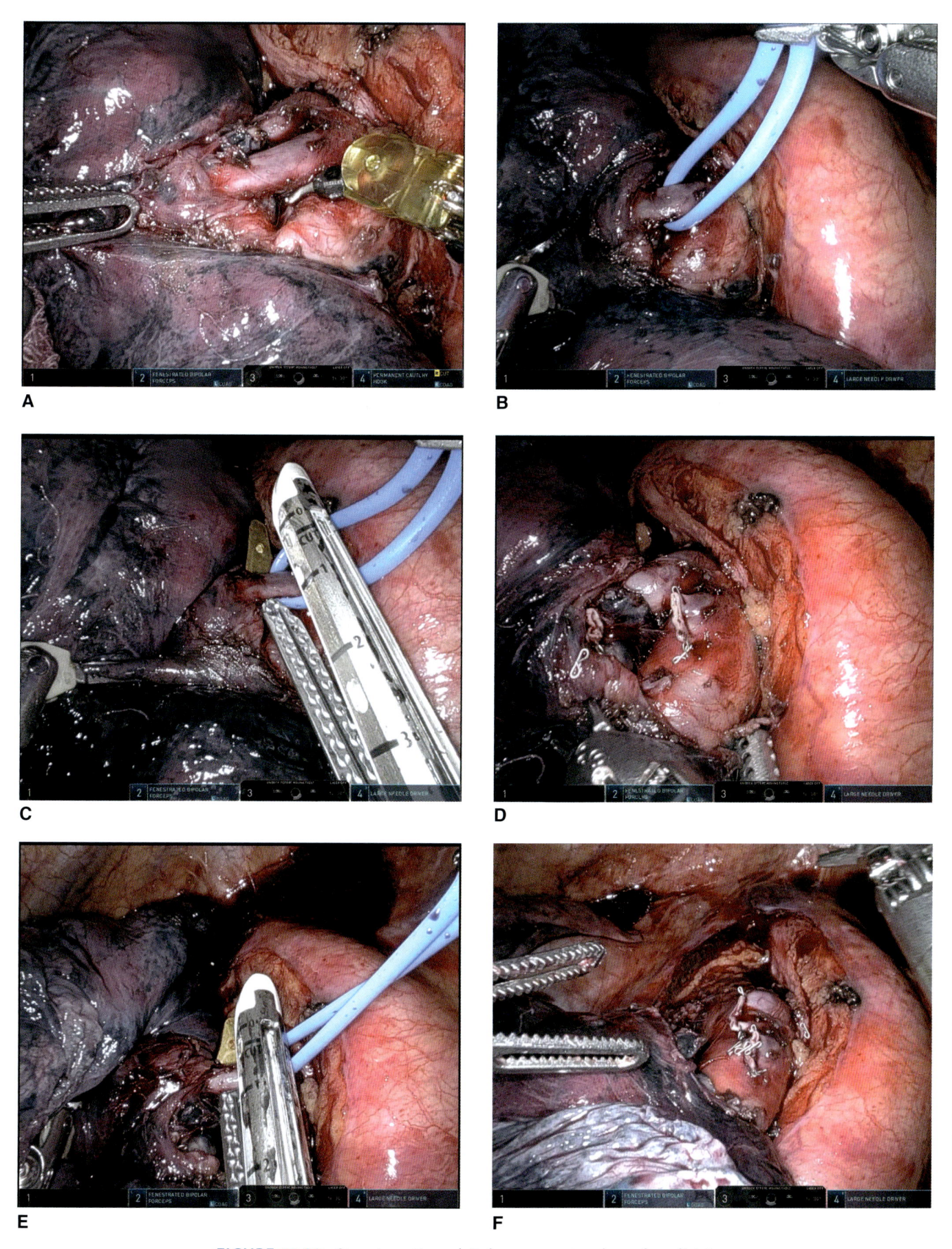

FIGURE 17-22 • Step 4 continued. Pulmonary artery branches division.

Video 17-2. Left Upper Lobectomy: Steps 5–9

Step 5. Transection of the anteromedial and posterolateral parenchymal bridges

Using a stapler, the anteromedial and posterolateral parenchymal bridges between the upper and lower lobes are taken down (**Figures 17-23 A, B**). The anteromedial and posterolateral bridges can be variable, from very thick to nonexistent. (1) The posterolateral bridge is lateral to the main trunk of the pulmonary artery, and when the artery is well exposed, it is quite easy to position the stapler for the transection. (2) The anteromedial bridge is between the 2 pulmonary veins (upper and lower) and the interlobar segment of the pulmonary artery. The preparation of the pulmonary artery, taking down the branches for the lingula, and the anterior dissection of the hilum done in Step 2 give the safe landmarks for the transection of this bridge.

Step 5 average time frame: 10–15 min

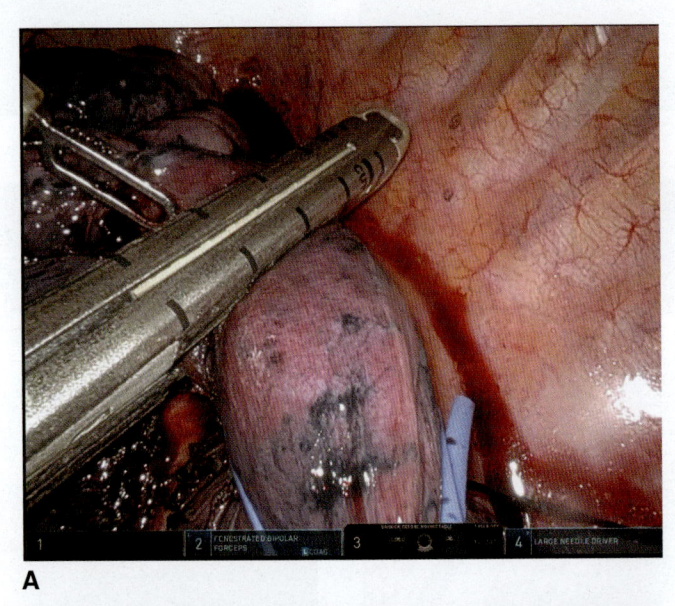

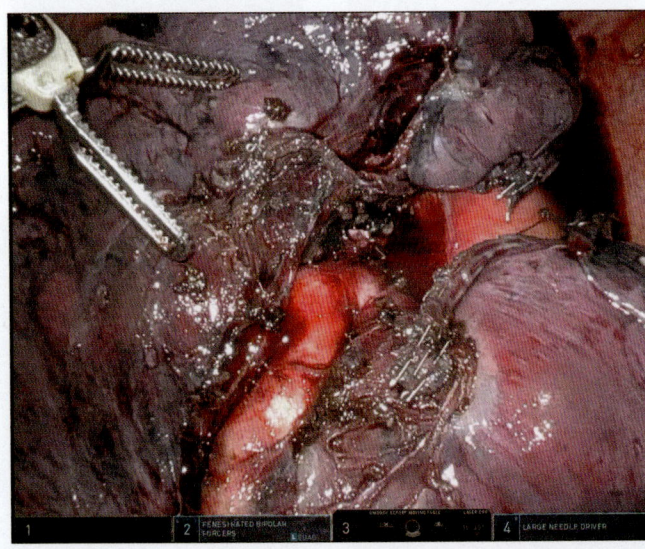

FIGURE 17-23 • Step 5. Transection of posterolateral parenchymal bridge.

Step 6. Preparation and division of the upper pulmonary vein

The upper pulmonary vein should be prepared on a vessel loop. If the segments of the lingula are preserved, the venous drainage should be maintained, and the division of the upper pulmonary vein should be planned accordingly proximal to that drainage (**Figures 17-24 A–D**). The stapling of the vein can be facilitated using a vessel loop or a Nelaton as a guide for the curved tip of the stapler (see **Figures 17-12 A–C**).

Step 6 average time frame: 5–10 min

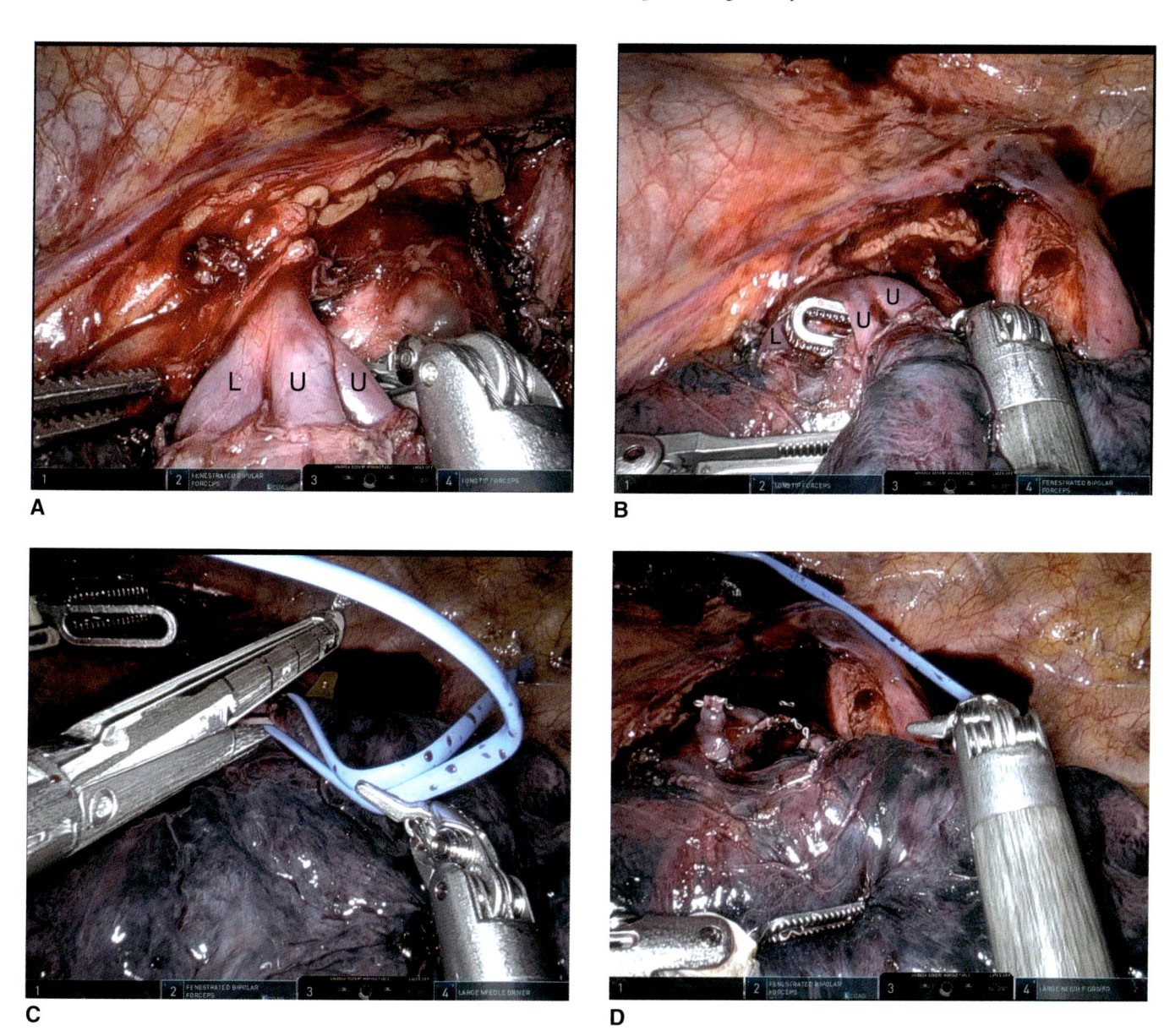

FIGURE 17-24 • Step 6. Preparation and division of the superior pulmonary vein. **A.** Lingula drainage (L) of segments 4 and 5 is preserved. **B.** Drainage (UU) for the upper segments (1, 2, 3) of the upper lobe is prepared and encircled with a vessel loop. **C.** Veins are divided with a vascular stapler. **D.** Vessel's stumps are shown.

Step 7. Transection of the anterior apical pulmonary artery branches

Usually, there are 1 or 2 anterior branches of the pulmonary artery located between the upper pulmonary vein and the bronchus (**Figure 17-25**). After the transection of the vein and the posterolateral preparation of the pulmonary artery, it becomes easier to divide these last branches. Attention should be paid in this step if there are adhesions to the bronchus (chronically inflamed station 11 lymph nodes, like in old tuberculosis). Bipolar dissection and blunt curved instruments might facilitate the separation of the adventitia of the vascular wall from the bronchus. An 8-mm curved-tip stapler usually fits better in the tiny space.

Step 7 average time frame: 15–30 min

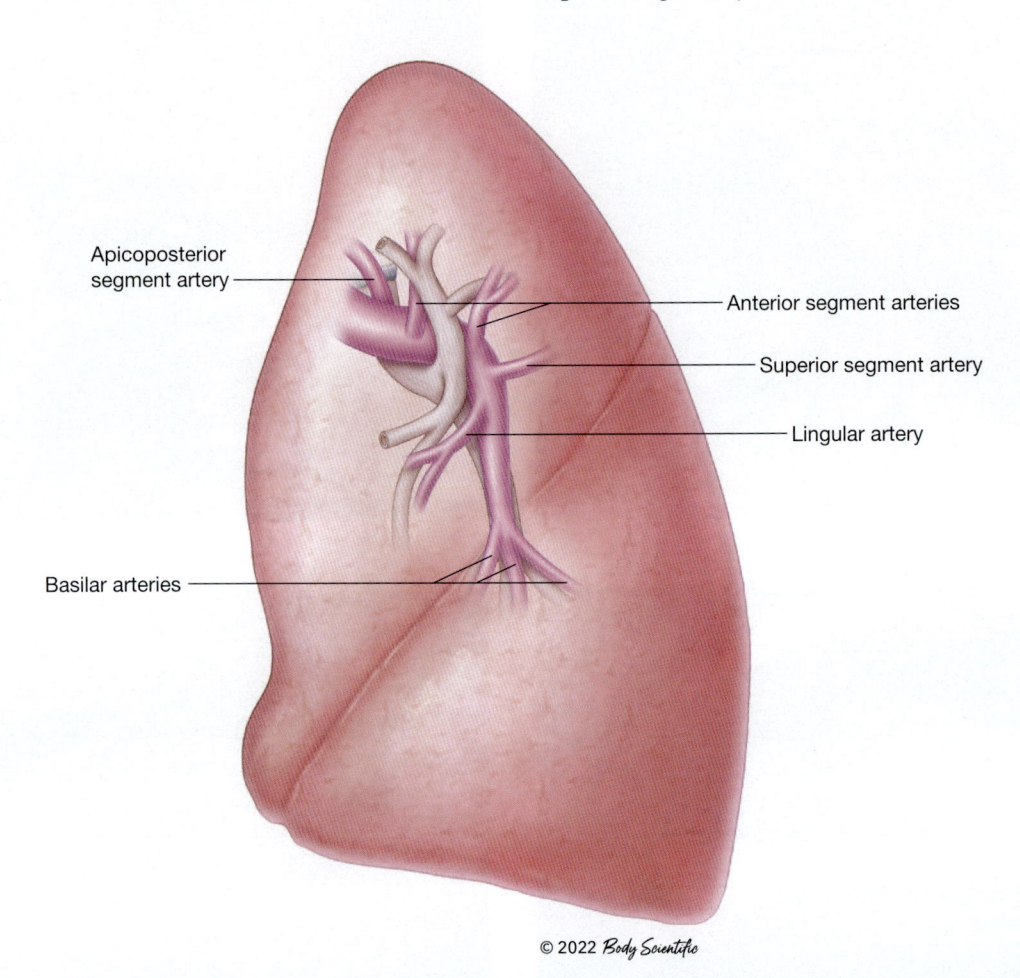

FIGURE 17-25 • Apicoposterior segment artery can be anterior or posterior to the apicoposterior bronchi. When anterior, it is more easily transected after the division of the superior pulmonary vein. When posterior, it is more easily transected after the opening of the posterior reflection of the hilum and the division of the fissure.

Step 8. Division of the bronchus

At this point, the bronchus for the upper lobe is completely accessible and can be transected with a proper application of the stapler with larger staples (green) (**Figures 17-26 A–D**). A robotic or thoracoscopic stapler can be used, selecting the best entry port to achieve a favorable angle. If there are doubts about the anatomy and/or preservation of the lingula segments, an inflation test could be advisable before transecting the bronchus. Reinforcement of the staple line is optional.

Step 8 average time frame: 3–5 min

EDITORIAL COMMENT

If the lingula is preserved, the parenchymal bridge between the lingula and the other segments of the upper lobe is transected after step 8, and verification that the upper bronchus transection didn't compromise the normal ventilation of the lingula (**Figure 17-27**).

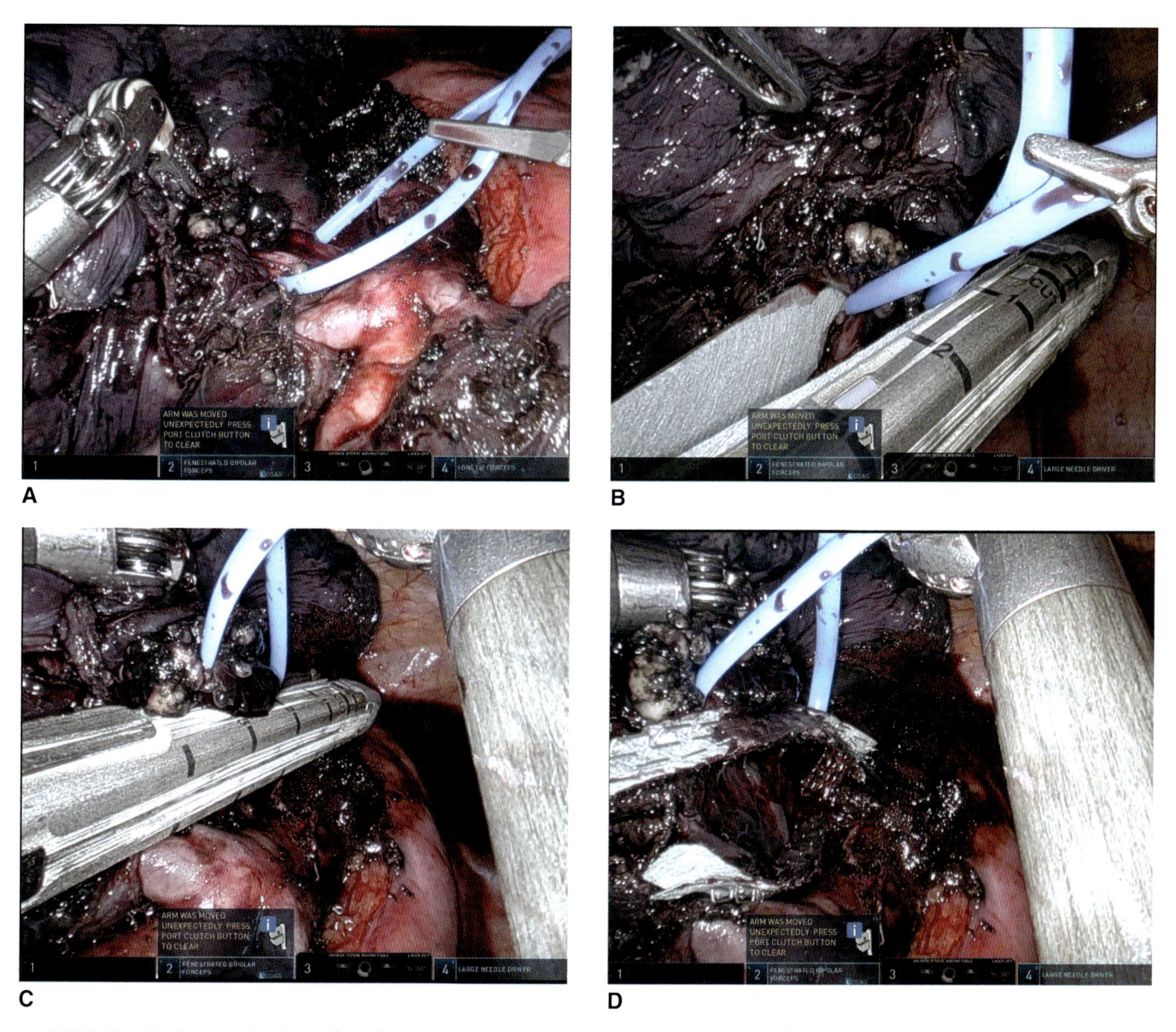

Lung Lobectomies: General Principles and the Total Port, Transfissure Approach (Fissure First) 343

FIGURE 17-26 • Step 8. Division of the bronchus. **A.** Bronchus is encircled by a vessel loop. **B, C.** A staple with reinforcement is used to divide the bronchus. **D.** Bronchial stump is seen after transection.

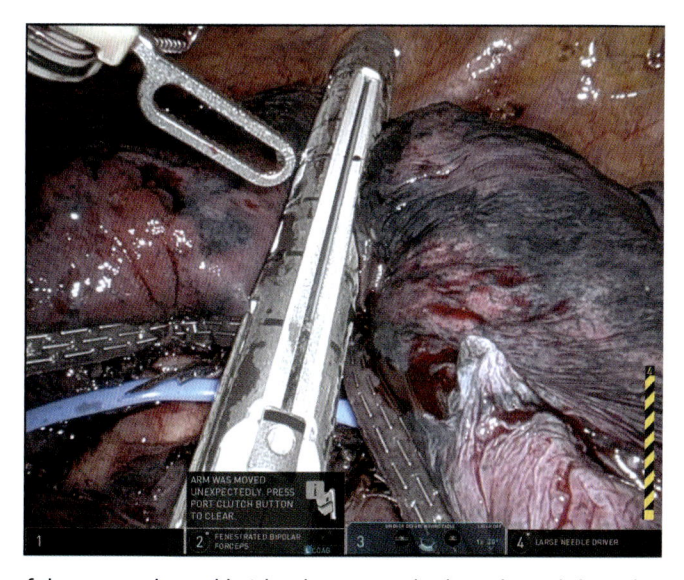

FIGURE 17-27 • Transection of the parenchymal bridge between the lingula and the other segments of the upper lobe.

Step 9. Completion of the lymphadenectomy

If the lymphadenectomy of stations 5–6 was not accomplished or completed earlier during Step 3, it should be done once the lobe is detached. The technique follows the same principles already described.

Step 9 average time frame: 10–20 min

Step 10. Specimen extraction

The specimen is placed in a strong Endobag and retrieved enlarging 1 of the assistant ports without rib spreading (**Figure 17-28**). The operation is completed, leaving 1 or 2 chest tubes and checking thoracoscopically the complete expansion of the lower lobe.

Step 10 average time frame: 10–15 min

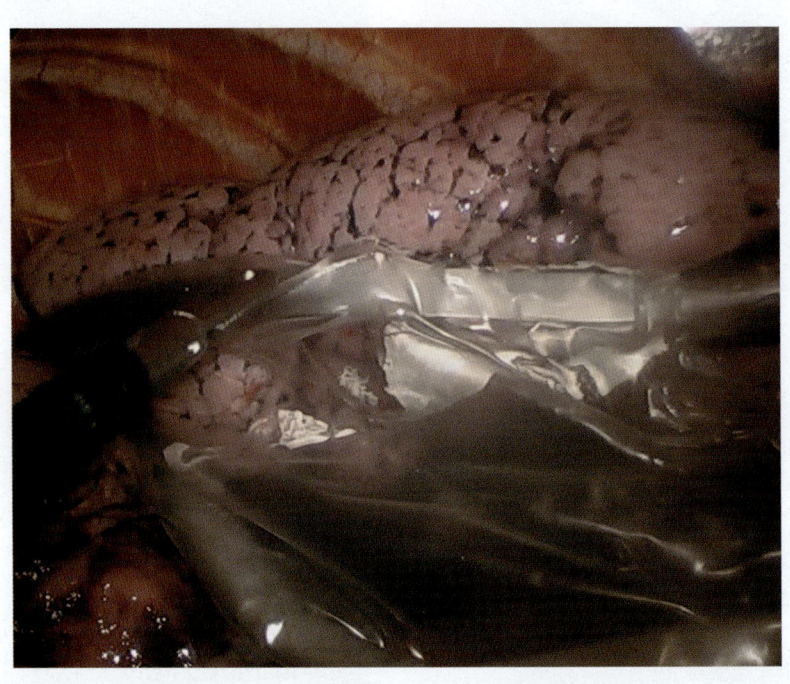

FIGURE 17-28 • Step 10. Specimen extraction.

Video 17-3. Left Upper Lobectomy – Full Procedure

Suggested Readings

1. Sihoe AD. The evolution of minimally invasive thoracic surgery: implications for the practice of uniportal thoracoscopic surgery. *J Thorac Dis.* 2014;6(Suppl 6):S604-6017. doi: 10.3978/j.issn.2072-1439.2014.08.52
2. Khaitan PG, D'Amico TA. Milestones in thoracic surgery. *J Thorac Cardiovasc Surg.* 2018;155(6):2779-2789. doi: 10.1016/j.jtcvs.2017.12.149
3. Detterbeck F, Antonicelli A, Okada M. Results of video-assisted techniques for resection of lung cancer. In: Pass H, Ball D, Scagliotti G. eds. *Thoracic Oncology: The IASLC Multidisciplinary Approach* (2nd ed.). IASLC; 2018.
4. McKenna RJ. Video-assisted thoracoscopic surgery. In: Michael IL, Robert MJ, Jeremy AF, George EC, eds. *Medical Management of the Thoracic Surgery Patient.* Elsevier, Inc.; 2010:75-85:chap 6.
5. Trevis J, Chilvers N, Freystaetter K, Dunning J. Surgeon-powered robotics in thoracic surgery; an era of surgical innovation and its benefits for the patient and beyond. *Front Surg.* 2020;7:589565. doi: 10.3389/fsurg.2020.589565
6. Sihoe ADL. Video-assisted thoracoscopic surgery as the gold standard for lung cancer surgery. *Respirology.* 2020;25 Suppl 2: 49-60. doi: 10.1111/resp.13920
7. Agzarian J, Fahim C, Shargall Y, Yasufuku K, Waddell TK, Hanna WC. The use of robotic-assisted thoracic surgery for lung resection: a comprehensive systematic review. *Semin Thorac Cardiovasc Surg.* 28(1):182-192. doi: 10.1053/j.semtcvs.2016.01.004
8. Kneuertz PJ, D'Souza DM, Richardson M, Abdel-Rasoul M, Moffatt-Bruce SD, Merritt RE. Long-term oncologic outcomes after robotic lobectomy for early-stage non-small-cell lung cancer versus video-assisted thoracoscopic and open thoracotomy approach. *Clin Lung Cancer.* 2020;21(3):214-224.e2. doi: 10.1016/j.cllc.2019.10.004
9. Naruke T, Suemasu K, Ishikawa S. Lymph node mapping and curability at various levels of metastasis in resected lung cancer. *J Thorac Cardiovasc Surg.* 1978;76(6):832-839.
10. Rusch VW, Asamura H, Watanabe H, et al. The IASLC lung cancer staging project: a proposal for a new international lymph node map in the forthcoming seventh edition of the TNM classification for lung cancer. *J Thorac Oncol.* 2009;4(5):568-577. doi: 10.1097/JTO.0b013e3181a0d82e
11. Giulianotti PC, Buchs NC, Caravaglios G, Bianco FM. Robot-assisted lung resection: outcomes and technical details. *Interact Cardiovasc Thorac Surg.* 2010;11(4):388-392. doi: 10.1510/icvts.2010.239541
12. Giulianotti PC, Coratti A, Angelini M, et al. Robotics in general surgery: personal experience in a large community hospital. *Arch Surg.* 2003;138(7):777-784. doi: 10.1001/archsurg.138.7.777

18A

"These are not machines we are treating. ... They are real live human beings."
—Frank H. Netter (1906–1991)

Lung Upper Lobectomies

Giulia Veronesi • Pierluigi Novellis • Piergiorgio Muriana • Gabriela Aguiluz • Francesca Rossetti

INTRODUCTION

The anterior approach with utility incision might have some advantages in robotic lung lobectomy since it allows lung palpation and specimen removal through the same incision. Moreover, in case of bleeding, the utility incision facilitates its rapid control and, if required, conversion to thoracotomy. It can be used by the assistant surgeon to insert additional instruments, such as suction devices, swabs, and sponges, avoiding a fifth trocar incision. On the other side, robotic-assisted lobectomy (RAL), with a utility incision does not allow CO_2 insufflation, that in some situations could be advantageous: obesity, a thick chest wall, diaphragm relaxation, incomplete lung exclusion due to air trapping in chronic obstructive pulmonary disease (COPD), or in case of problems with the orotracheal tube, leading to suboptimal exclusion.

Indications and Relative Contraindications to the Robotic Approach

The elements that have to be considered during the patient selection for robotic thoracic surgery are as follows: body mass index (BMI), anatomical location of the primary lesion and positive (or suspicious) lymph nodes and their relation with vascular structures, history of pleural infections with related effusion or empyema, or previous thoracic surgery (high risk of firm adhesions).

Obesity and adhesions are not absolute contraindications, but they may increase the complexity and duration of surgery. Adhesions are sometimes easier to deal with robotically than with thoracotomy, causing less damage to the visceral pleura, therefore, there is a lower risk of persistent air leak.

Limitations are more related to the surgeon's judgment and personal level of the learning curve. Less experienced surgeons should start with simple lobectomies (absence of pleural adhesions, well-defined fissure, healthy lung parenchyma) and then move on to increasingly complex interventions such as

INSTRUMENT REQUIREMENTS

The suggested main robotic instruments/tools can be listed as follows:
- 30°/0° camera
- Long bipolar grasper
- Fenestrated bipolar forceps
- Tip-up fenestrated grasper
- Medium–large clip applier

Optional instruments:
- Monopolar curved scissors
- Large needle driver
- ProGrasp™ forceps
- Permanent monopolar cautery hook
- EndoWrist® Stapler 45 Curved-Tip
- EndoWrist® Stapler 45
- EndoWrist® Stapler 30 Curved-Tip
- EndoWrist® Stapler 60

The suggested main thoracoscopic instruments/tools can be listed as follows:
- Nontraumatic forceps
- Needle driver
- Suction device
- Staplers
- Clip applier

Supplemental materials:
- Kittner roll laparoscopic gauze (cigarette sponges)
- Sutures (Prolene™ 3-0, 4-0, 5-0,)
- Vessel loops
- Nelaton tubes
- Skin retractor
- Gelport® (optional)
- Hem-o-lok® clips
- Reabsorbable hemostatic material
- EndoBag™
- 28-Fr chest tube

Photo from Dr. Frank H. Netter, MD. The National Library of Medicine.
Quote reproduced with permission from Netter FM, Friedlaender GE. Frank H. Netter MD and a brief history of medical illustration. Clin Orthop Relat Res. 2014;472(3):812-819.

locally advanced N2-positive tumors and complex anatomical resections (anatomical segmentectomies, sleeve bronchial resections). Robotic surgery, although minimally invasive, is closer to traditional open surgery thanks to the maneuverability of the instruments. Therefore, almost every tumor could be approached robotically. Complex intrapericardial pneumonectomies, big masses (more than 10 cm), and lesions requiring vascular sleeve resection and reconstruction are not absolute contraindications to the robotic approach but should be performed only by extremely experienced surgeons.

> ▶▶ **TIPS**
>
> Hilar lymph nodes must always be evaluated on preoperative imaging: calcific lymph nodes, an expression of previous tuberculosis, could make vascular dissection very difficult and risky.

> ▶▶ **TIPS**
>
> To decrease costs, the instruments involved in the dissection can be contained. The main tools are the long bipolar grasper, the tip-up fenestrated grasper, and fenestrated bipolar forceps. The long bipolar grasper is able to make a fine dissection of the periadventitial tissue, removing the lymph nodes around the main vascular structures without injuring the vessels.

> ▶▶ **TIPS**
>
> The assistant surgeon should be well skilled, and all the team must be well-integrated: this is of paramount importance for both the performance of the standard procedure but especially in the event of a vascular accident and emergency conversion.

Right Upper Lobectomy

Patient Positioning, OR Setup, and Port Setting

The patient is positioned in left lateral decubitus, and then forelimbs are extended frontally and secured over supports to allow access to all intercostal spaces. The operating table is flexed down at the level of the fifth intercostal space to lower the hips; alternatively, a roll can be placed under the chest. The patient is intubated with a double-lumen endotracheal tube that ensures single-lung ventilation (**Figures 18A-1** and **18A-2**).

After exclusion of the lung involved in the operation, a 2.5-cm utility incision (Incision R1) is performed anteriorly at the fourth intercostal space, and a skin retractor (Alexis™, Applied Medical, Rancho Santa Margarita, CA) is positioned. Under direct vision with the camera inserted in the utility incision, the thoracic cavity is explored to exclude pleural carcinomatosis or adhesions. An 8-mm port is placed along the anterior axillary line at the seventh intercostal space (Scope-S). This is

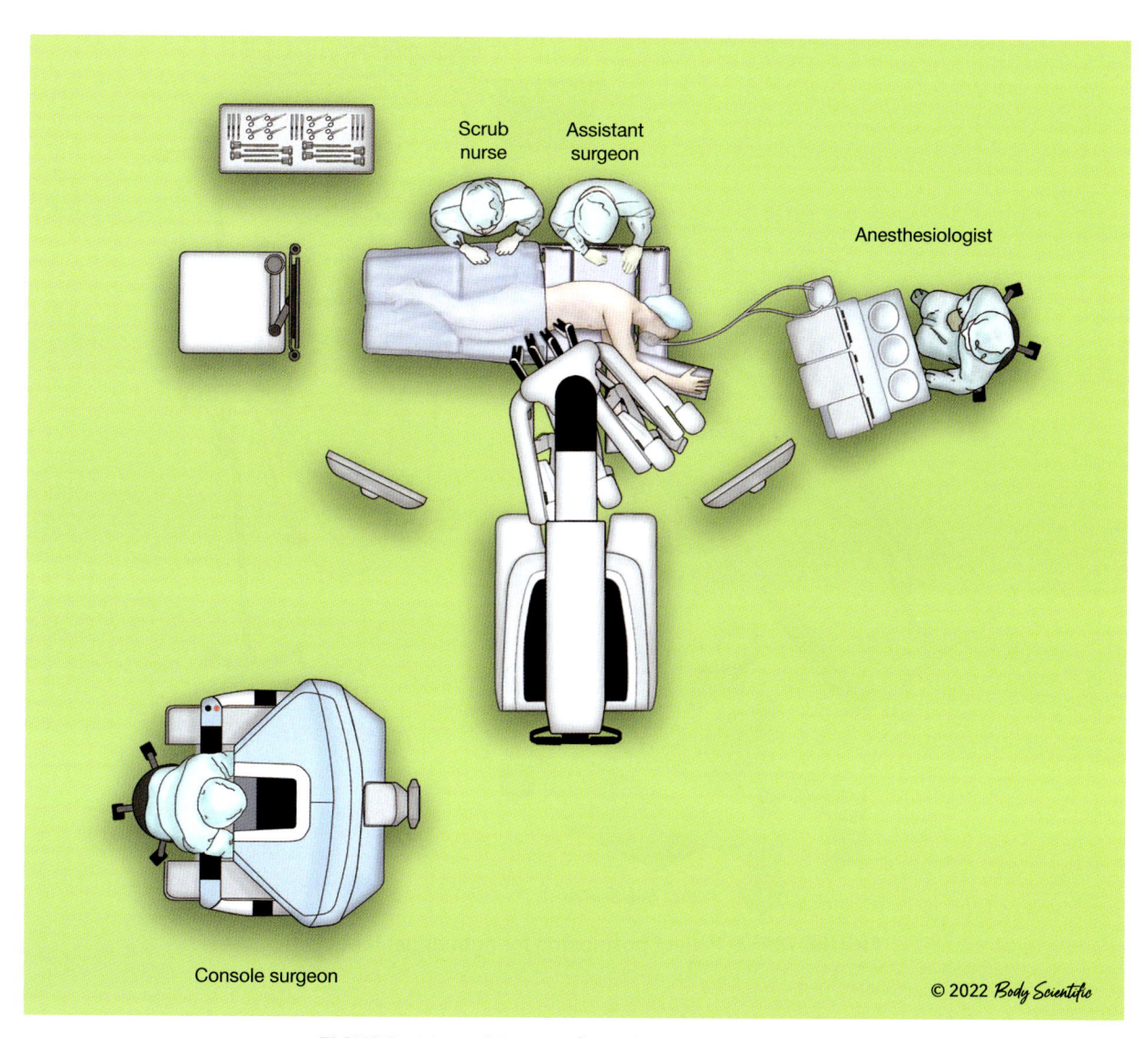

FIGURE 18A-1 • OR setup for right upper lobectomy.

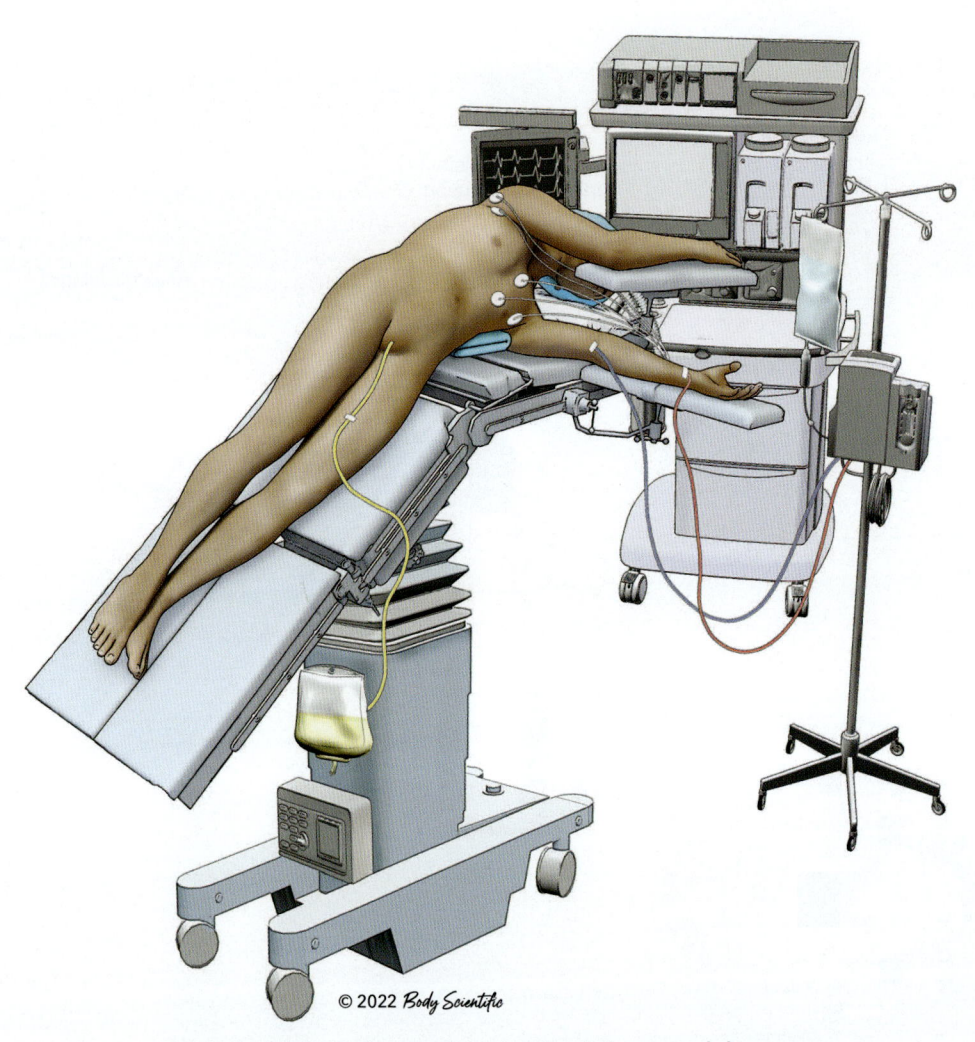

FIGURE 18A-2 • Patient positioning for right upper lobectomy.

Lung Upper Lobectomies

the incision through which the camera is inserted. Afterward, 2 other trocar incisions are performed, an 8- or 12-mm incision on the line of the tip of the scapula at the 8th intercostal space (Port R2) for stapler insertion, and an 8-mm incision in the triangle of auscultation at the seventh intercostal space (Port R3) (**Figure 18A-3**).

The robot is docked in a position that does not interfere with the team's work. The use of the Da Vinci Xi makes docking simpler thanks to the laser centering system (set on port S). Once centered, the robotic arms are connected to the trocars. The dissection instrument, the long bipolar grasper, is positioned in the utility incision (R1), the camera in port S, the fenestrated bipolar forceps in port R2, and the tip-up fenestrated grasper in port R3.

▶▶ **TIPS**

From the utility incision, the assistant surgeon inserts swabs, which can clean the operating field and compress small bleeds.

▶▶ **TIPS**

For a proper port placement, it is necessary to evaluate the following elements: (1) position of the diaphragm: in case of a very high diaphragm (e.g., obese patients), the port incisions should be moved upward, in the 6th or 7th intercostal space, to avoid entering into the abdomen and/or prevent the diaphragm from obscuring the vision, if it is too close to the trocar; (2) presence of cardiomegaly: in this case, if a left lobectomy is performed, it may be necessary to make the incisions more laterally; (3) previous cardiac surgery for "CABG (coronary artery bypass graft)" with the mammary artery: in such cases, preoperative workup is useful to know the bypass course and find out whether the graft is still patent to avoid its inadvertent injury.

▶▶ **TIPS**

The "shape" of the patient's chest and the position of the diaphragm may require adapting the position of the trocar sites. For the lower lobectomies, it is preferable to place all the incisions one space lower to achieve an optimal configuration of the working ports.

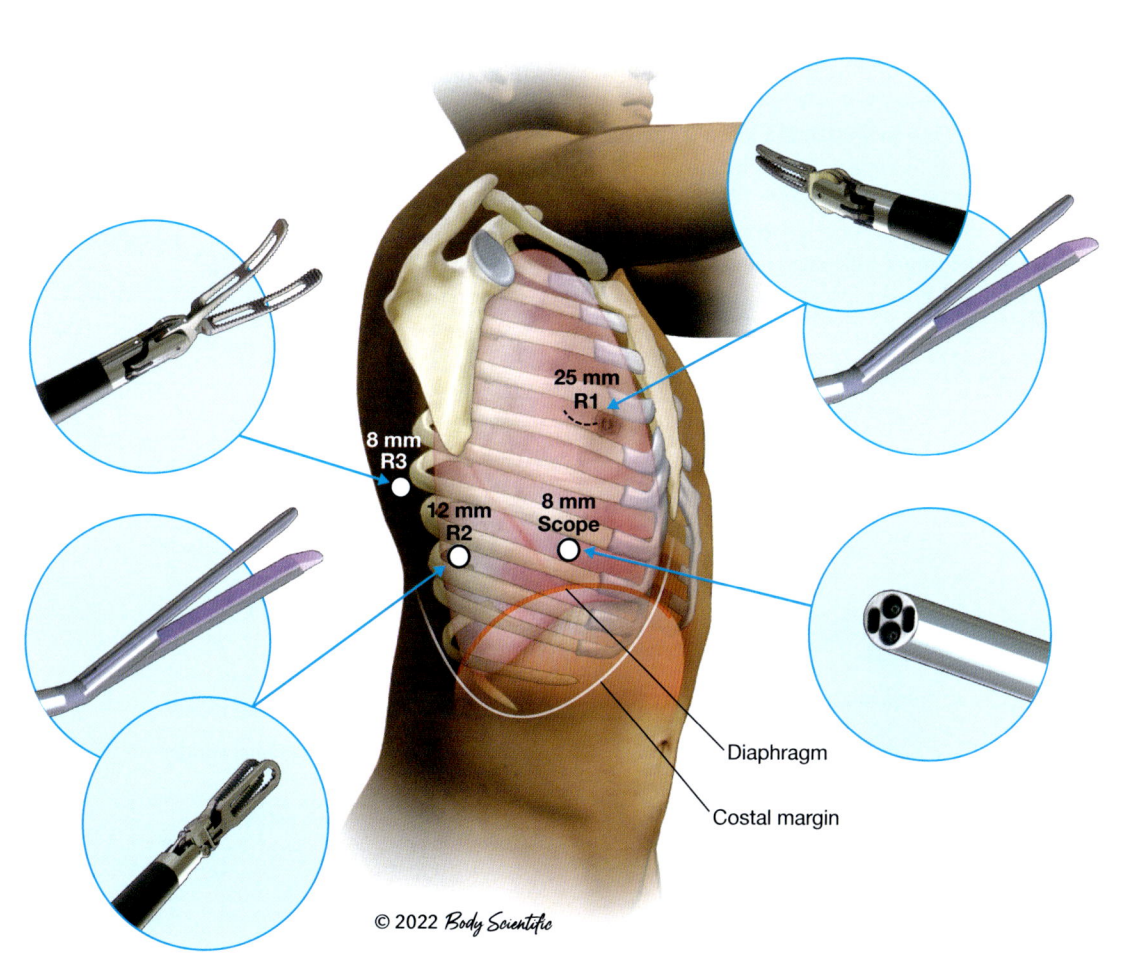

FIGURE 18A-3 • Port setting for right upper lobectomy.

Surgical Technique

▶ **Video 18A-1.** Operative Technique of a Robotic Right Upper Lobectomy. Five Steps Standardized Technique

Step 1. Inspection of the pleural cavity, isolation and division of the right upper pulmonary vein

The thoracic cavity is inspected to exclude the presence of pleural carcinomatosis. When present, adhesions between the visceral and parietal pleura are dissected to achieve a full mobilization of the pulmonary parenchyma. In the absence of a preoperative pathologic diagnosis and a lesion located in the outer third of the lung, not too deep, a wedge resection can be performed with staplers and sent for a frozen section to confirm malignancy.

An anterior "fissureless" approach to hilar structures is used in this technique, with the division of fissures between the right upper lobe and middle and lower lobes being left as the final step of the procedure. Lymphonodal dissection can be performed at the end of the operation in case of stage I tumors. On the contrary, for more advanced cancers, lymphadenectomy should preferably be performed at the beginning to exclude the presence of multistation involvement and to facilitate the dissection of the hilar elements that may be hindered by the presence of bulky lymph nodes.

The lung is gently retracted backward with a sponge held by the tip-up grasper, installed on R3, to visualize the anterior mediastinum. The first step of the right upper lobectomy is isolating the right upper pulmonary vein, which is the most anteriorly located element. The mediastinal pleura is incised parallel to the phrenic nerve to expose the right upper vein. Sharp and blunt dissection is conducted with the long bipolar grasper to identify the confluence between the middle lobe venous branch and the upper lobe stem. The vein is better surrounded by the fenestrated bipolar forceps because of their atraumatic beveled tip and encircled with a vessel loop (**Figures 18A-4 A, B**). The bedside assistant introduces an endoscopic stapler with a 30-mm vascular cartridge through the incision R2 for the vein division.

Step 1 average time frame: 10–15 min

> **EDITORIAL COMMENT**
>
> Careful removal of the lymph nodes around the vascular and bronchial structures is not only an essential onco-logical part of the operation but may facilitate the safe preparation of the pedicles and their division.

> ⚠ **PITFALLS**
>
> Anatomical variants of the pulmonary veins are not uncommon: the presence of a common trunk between upper and inferior veins should always be excluded. A middle lobe branch may merge into the inferior pulmonary vein; therefore, attention should be paid not to confuse it with one of the upper lobe segmental branches (**Figures 18A-5 A–D**).

> ▶▶ **TIPS**
>
> The use of curved tip staplers and a gentle retraction of the vessel loop may help in the safe introduction of the stapler and division of the vein.

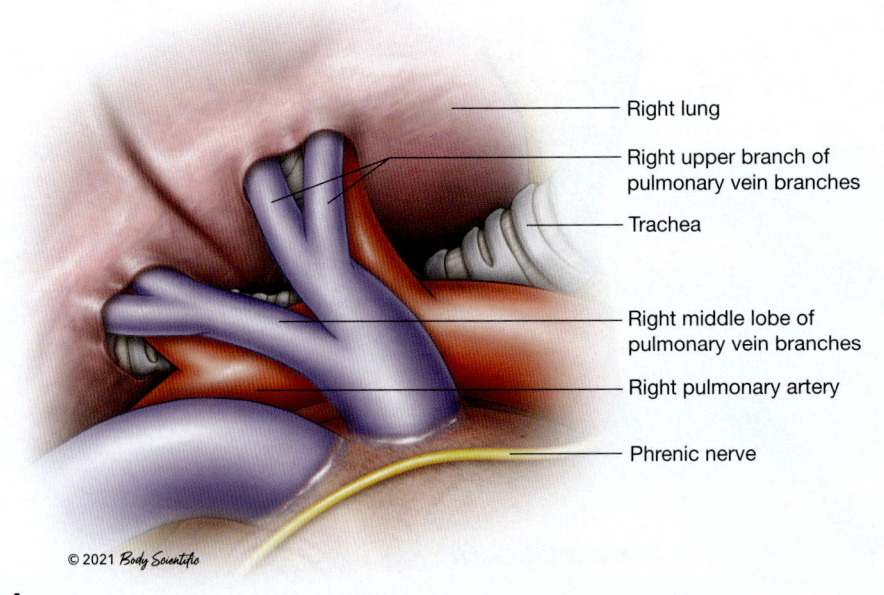

A

FIGURE 18A-4 • **A.** Right pulmonary vein anatomy.

Lung Upper Lobectomies   351

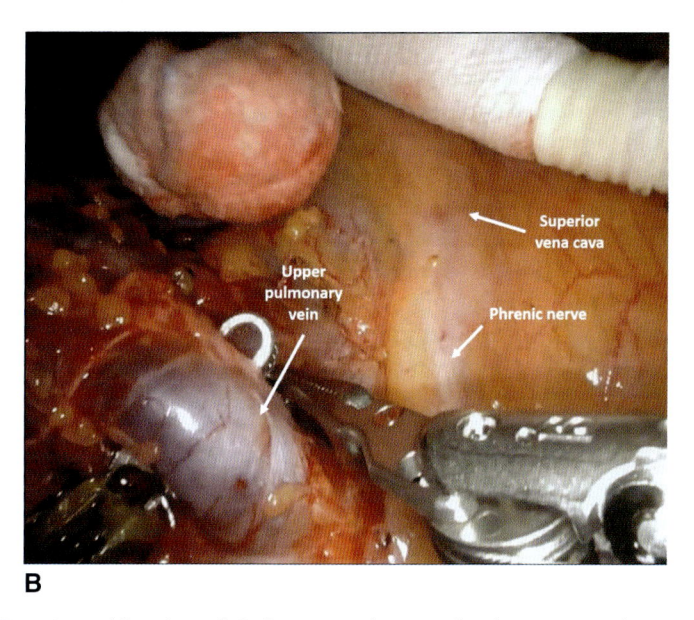

FIGURE 18A-4 • (*Continued*) **B.** Step 1. Isolation of right upper pulmonary vein.

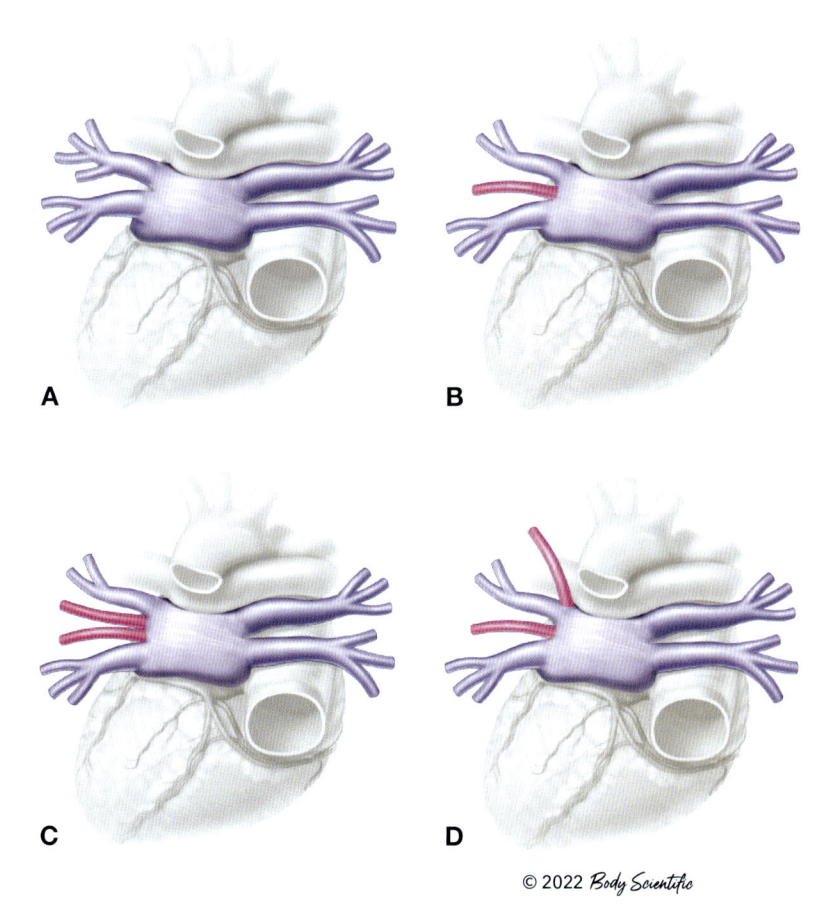

FIGURE 18A-5 • Normal right pulmonary vein anatomy and its variations. **A.** Normal anatomy. **B.** Right middle pulmonary vein. **C.** Two right middle pulmonary veins. **D.** Right middle pulmonary vein and right upper pulmonary vein.

Step 2. Isolation and division of the pulmonary artery branches

After dividing the pulmonary vein and retracting the upper lobe inferiorly, the pulmonary artery branches for the upper lobe are approached. Usually, the upper lobe is supplied by 2 main vessels: the anterior branch (Boyden's trunk) located cranially to the right upper vein, and the posterior ascending artery originating within the fissure. The connective tissue between the vein and the anterior artery, and between the upper border of the artery and the inferior edge of the azygos vein, is dissected and stations 11R and 10R are removed. The anterior artery branch is isolated with the long bipolar grasper, encircled with a vessel loop, and finally divided with a 30-mm vascular reload of the Endostapler, as previously described.

The dissection proceeds on the top of the interlobar artery to identify the ascending branch for the dorsal segment of the right upper lobe. Depending on the diameter of the vessel, either staplers or, in case of small-sized vessels, division between 2 Hemo-lok® clips can be used to section it (**Figures 18A-6 A–C**).

Step 2 average time frame: 20–25 min

> #### 🔍 ANATOMICAL HIGHLIGHTS
> The vascularization of the right upper lobe dorsal segment is variable: usually there are from 1 up to 3 posterior segmental ascending arteries; however, sometimes it is absent, and no branch is found in the fissure (**Figures 18A-7** and **18A-8 A–C**).

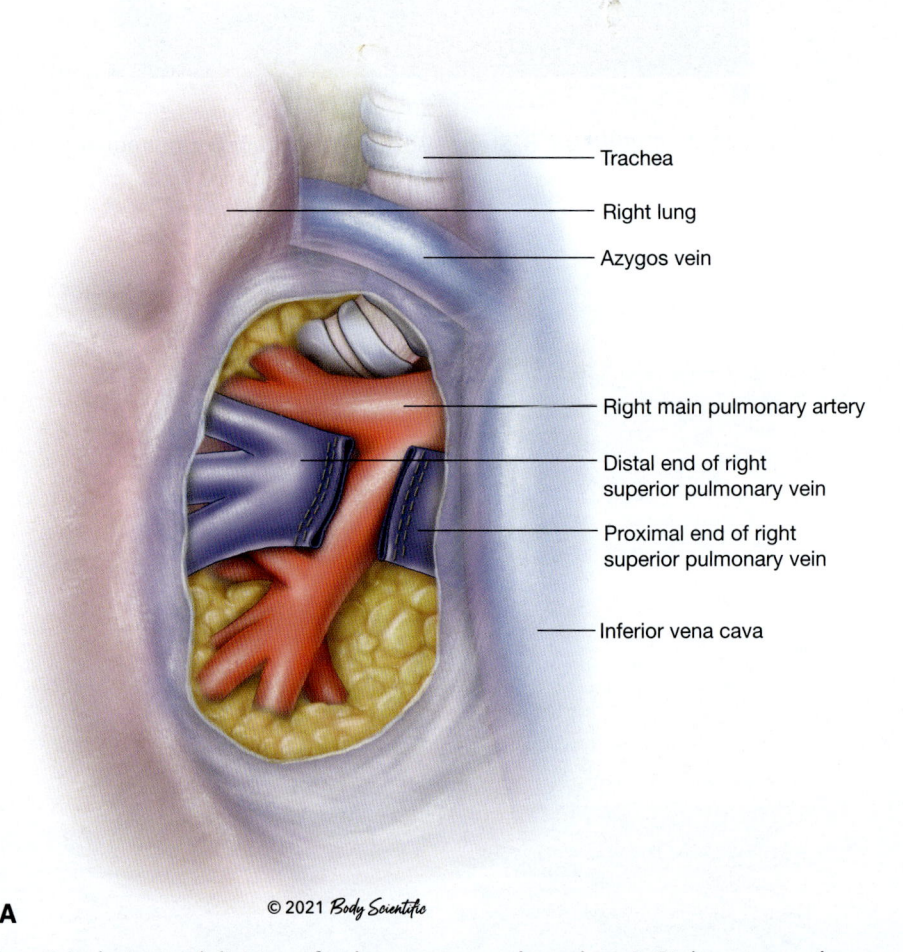

FIGURE 18A-6 • Step 2. Isolation and division of pulmonary artery branches. **A.** Right upper pulmonary vein divided.

Lung Upper Lobectomies   353

B

C

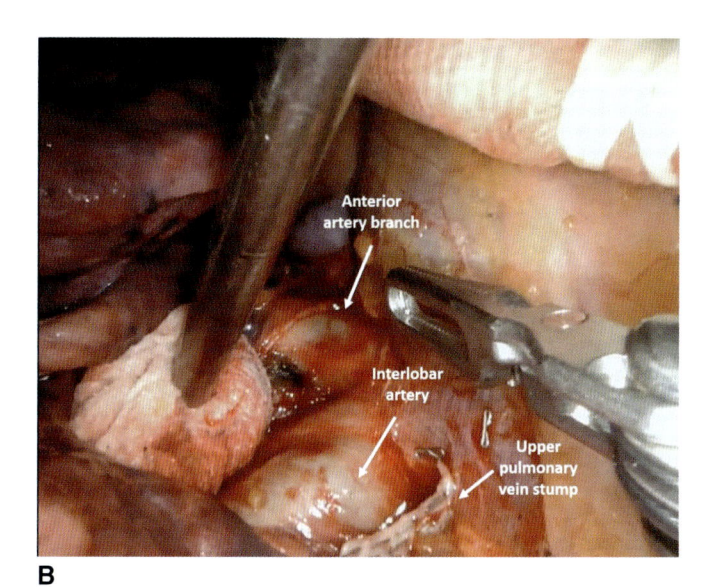

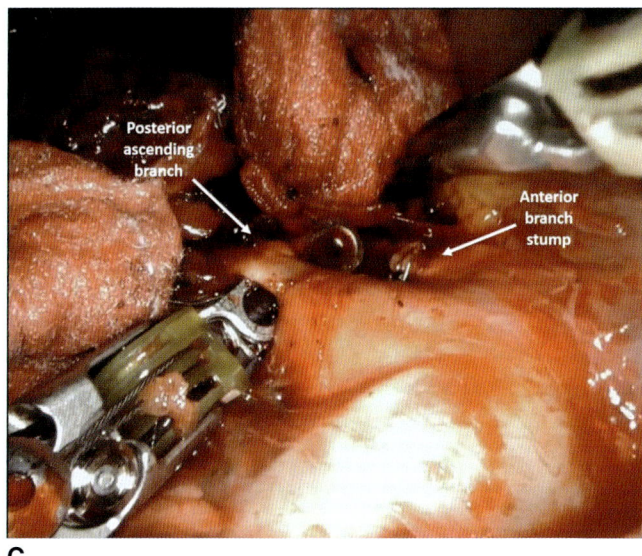

FIGURE 18A-6 • *(Continued)* **B.** Following division of right upper pulmonary vein, the anterior artery branch (Boyden's trunk) is prepared and sectioned. **C.** Posterior ascending arterial branch for right upper dorsal segment (S2).

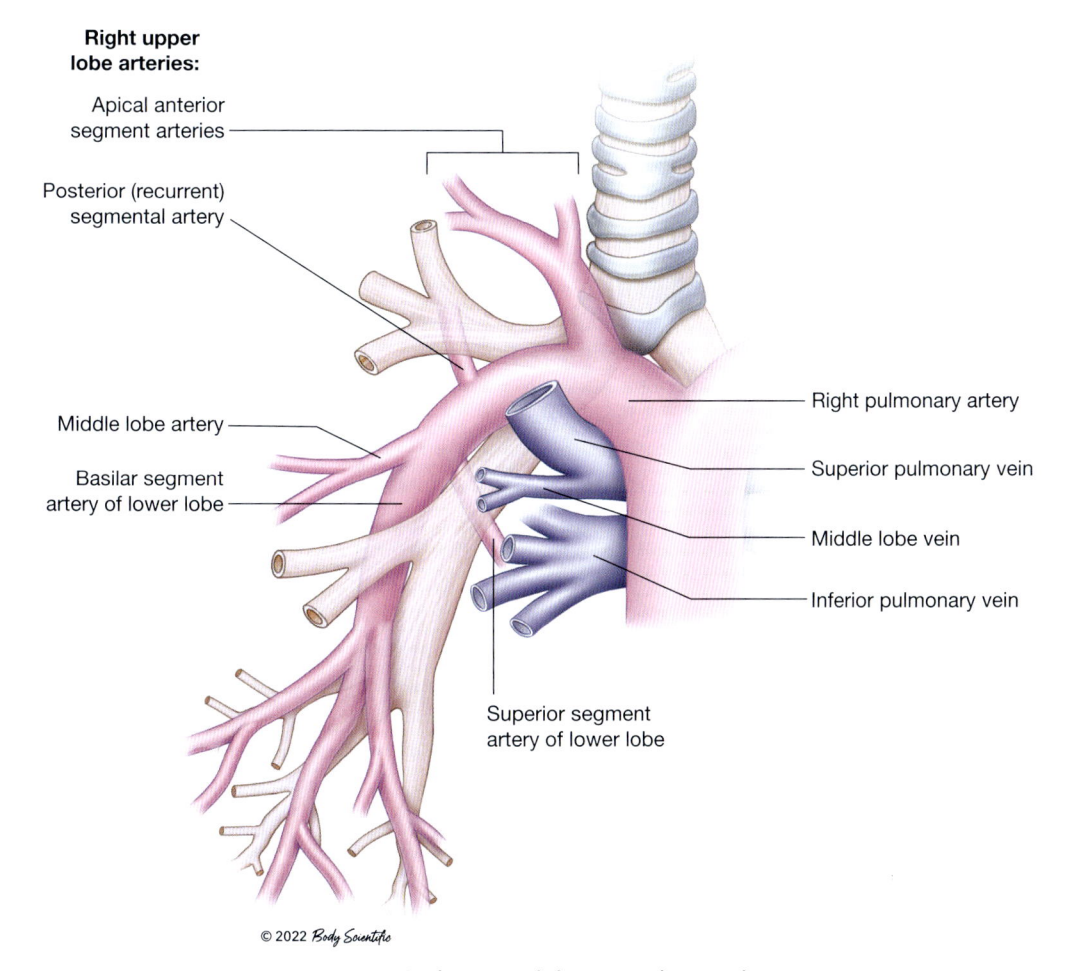

FIGURE 18A-7 • Right upper lobe arterial normal anatomy.

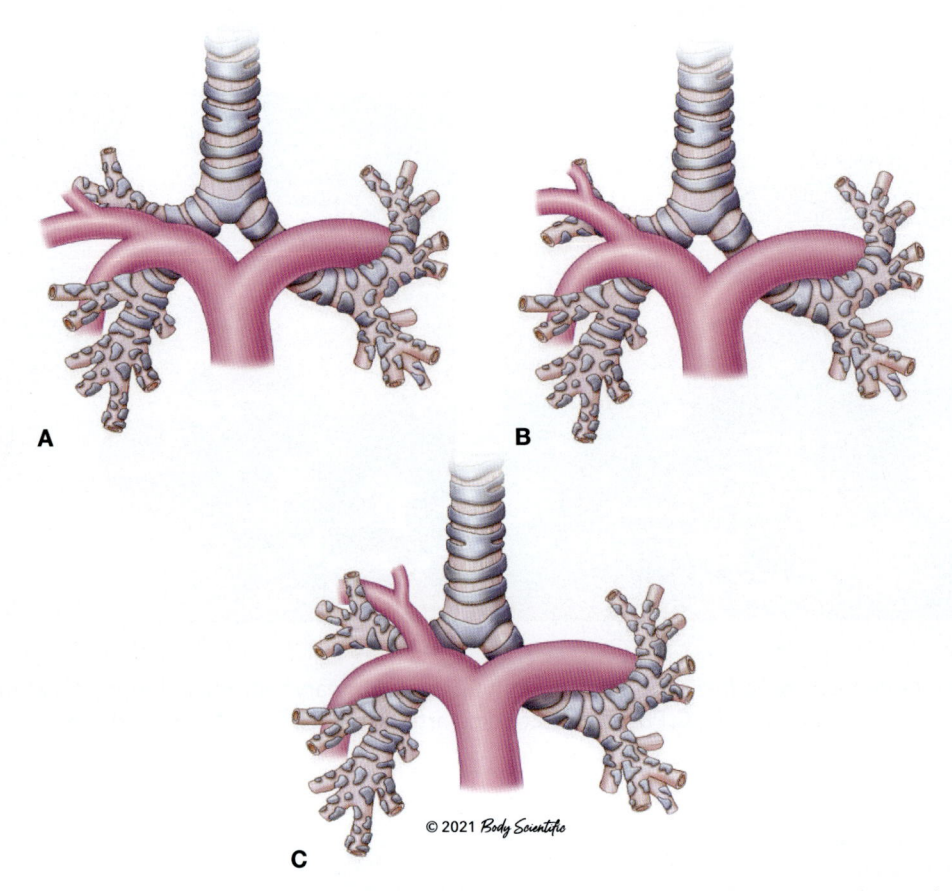

FIGURE 18A-8 • Variations in the relation of bronchi and the right pulmonary arteries. **A.** Artery lower than the bronchus. **B.** Artery on same level with the upper bronchus. **C.** Artery above the level of the upper bronchus.

Step 3. Isolation and division of the right upper lobe bronchus and peribronchial lymph nodes dissection

The lobe is retracted with the tip-up grasper to expose the bronchus. The posterior mediastinal pleura should be widely opened to ease the entry of the stapler. The section line must be cleared from the presence of any peribronchial lymph node (stations 10R and 11R). Cauterization with the long bipolar grasper avoids excessive devascularization and might decrease the risk of postoperative bronchopleural fistulas. After removal of the hilar lymph nodes, always located between the stump of the superior vein and the origin of the bronchus, the bronchus is encircled with a loop (**Figures 18A-9 A, B**) and transected with an Endostapler (Medtronic® purple or black reload) introduced by the bedside assistant through port R2 or the utility incision (R1) (**Figure 18A-3**) depending on the most favorable entry angle. Before firing the stapler, the surgeon might ask the anesthesiologist to ventilate the right lung to check the reexpansion of the remaining lobes to avoid misplacements of the stapler and possible stricture of the middle and lower lobe bronchus.

Step 3 average time frame: 10–15 min

▶▶ **TIPS**

In the case of advanced tumors, a transfissure approach to isolate the ascending artery is preferable because the presence of multiple lymphadenopathies may hinder the anterior approach.

▶▶ **TIPS**

The removal of the hilar lymph nodes between the vein's distal stump and the origin of the bronchus facilitates its preparation. Sometimes, the bronchus should be divided before the ascending artery to ease its isolation.

▶▶ **TIPS**

In patients who have undergone induction chemoradiotherapy, it is advisable to cover the bronchial stump with vital flaps to decrease the risk of bronchial fistulas. Mediastinal fat and pleura can be used for this purpose.

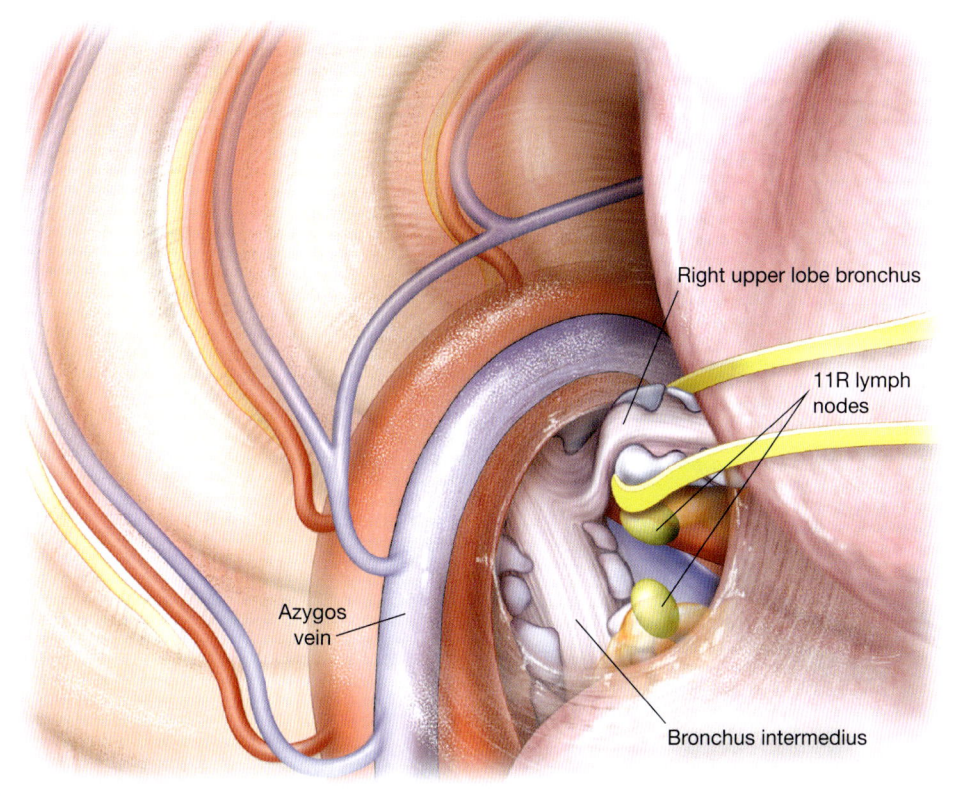

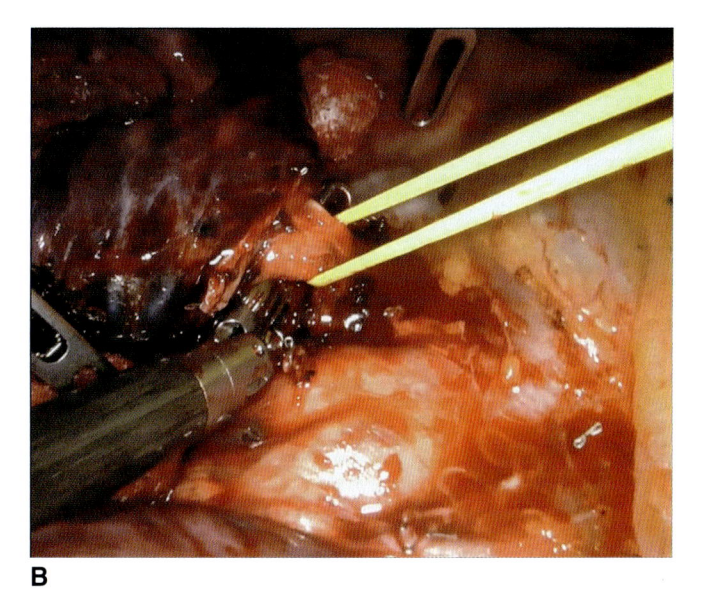

FIGURE 18A-9 • Step 3. Isolation and division of the right upper lobe bronchus and peribronchial lymph node dissection. Right upper bronchus surrounded with a vessel loop.

Step 4. Division of the fissures and specimen extraction

Once the vascular and bronchial elements have been divided, the final step of the procedure consists of the transection of the fissures with multiple 45- or 60-mm parenchymal Endostapler reloads (**Figures 18A-10** and **18A-11**). The location of the vein stump can be used as a landmark to identify the correct plane in case of a fused thick fissure. On the contrary, cauterization can be used if the fissure is represented by a thin pleural flap without the risk of significant postoperative air leak. The lobe is introduced in a retrieval specimen bag and pulled out of the chest through the utility incision.

Step 4 average time frame: 5–10 min

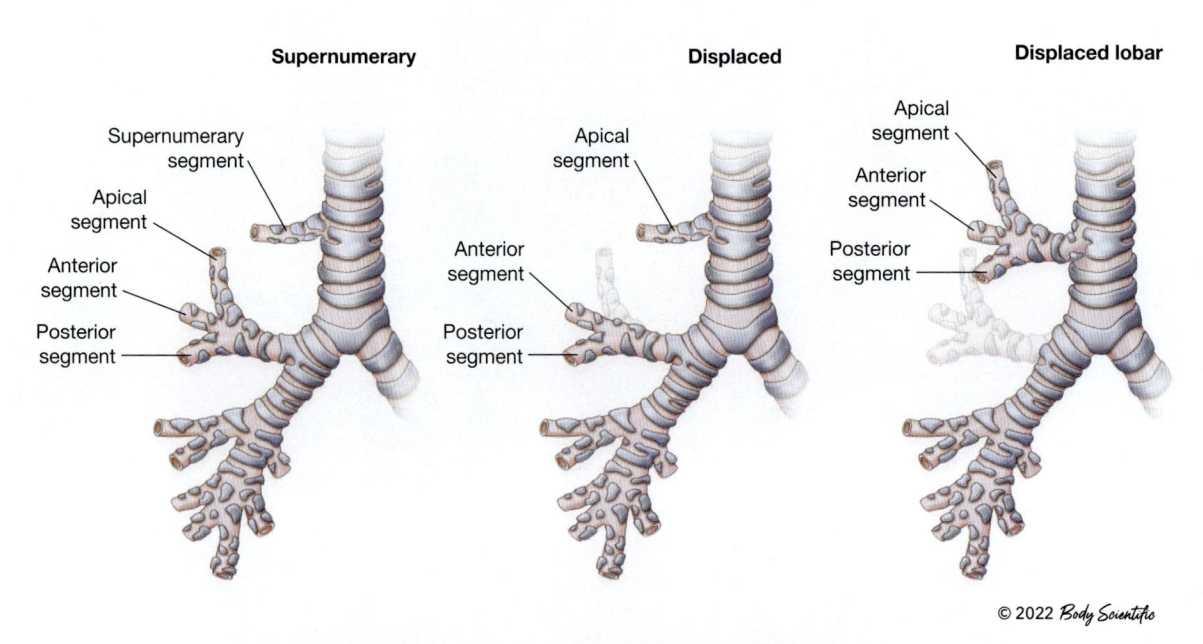

FIGURE 18A-10 • Variations of the bronchi.

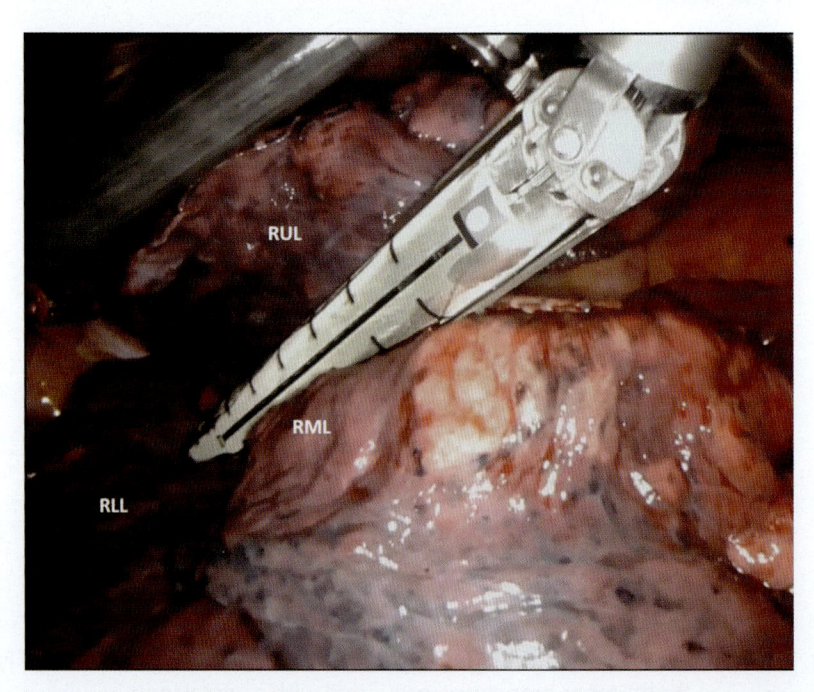

FIGURE 18A-11 • Step 4. Fissure division. RUL, right upper lobe; RML, right middle lobe; RLL, right lower lobe.

Step 5. Mediastinal lymph nodes dissection

The mediastinal pleura is opened from the confluence between the azygos vein and the superior vena cava, proceeding cranially along the lateral side of the vena cava and posteriorly along the course of the vagus nerve. Station 4R and 2R lymph nodes are removed en bloc along with paratracheal fatty tissue (**Figures 18A-12 A, B**).

The lung is then retracted anteriorly-superiorly to expose the subcarinal area. The mediastinal pleura is opened, and station 7 lymph nodes and mediastinal fat are dissected paying attention to avoid lesions to the vagus nerve and/or the esophageal wall. The lymphadenectomy fields are carefully checked to exclude bleeding or lymphatic leakage and filled with an absorbable hemostatic agent.

A 28-Fr chest tube with an accessory hole at 10 cm is inserted in incision S, and the right lung is expanded under endoscopic control.

> ▶▶ **TIPS**
>
> A complete dissection of subcarinal nodes, at the beginning of the operation, with a wide opening of the posterior mediastinal pleura, can facilitate the preparation of the bronchus. Moreover, stapler division of a bridge of the posterior fissure may be required for a better control of the bronchus.

> ⚠ **PITFALLS**
>
> Middle lobe torsion might happen at the reexpansion of the lung, mainly when there is an incomplete fissure. It is important to check this occurrence at the end of the procedure. In this case, the middle lobe should be secured to the upper edge of the inferior lobe.

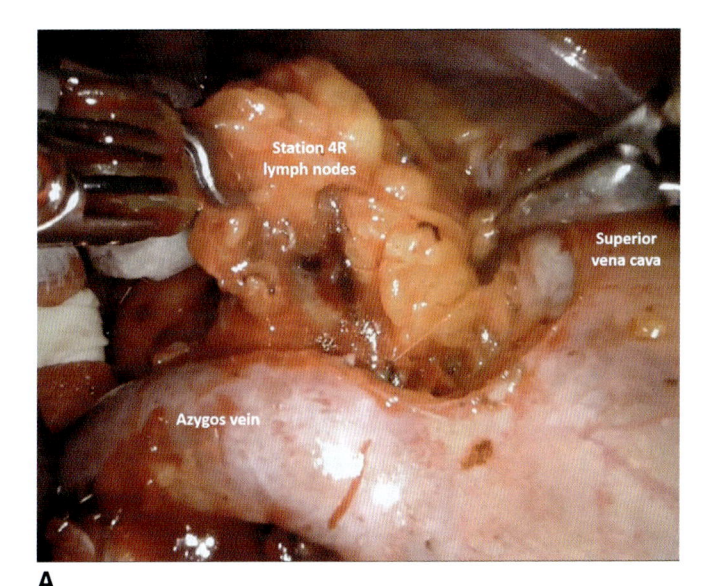

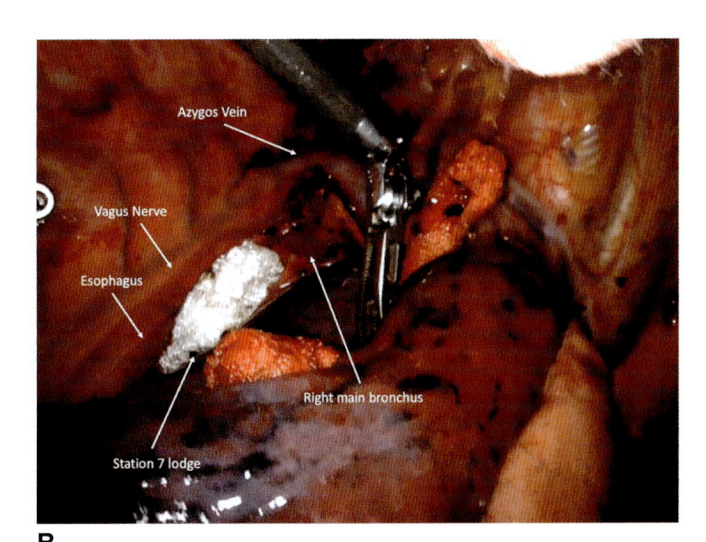

FIGURE 18A-12 • **A.** Barety's lodge lymph node dissection (station 4R). **B.** Lymphadenectomy of subcarinal station.

Left Upper Lobectomy

Patient Positioning, OR Setup, and Port Setting

The patient is positioned in right lateral decubitus, and then the forelimbs are extended frontally and secured over supports to allow access to all the intercostal spaces. The operating table is flexed down at the level of the fifth intercostal space to lower the hips; alternatively, a roll can be placed under the chest. The patient is intubated with a double-lumen endotracheal tube that ensures single-lung ventilation (**Figure 18A-13**).

After the exclusion of the lung involved in the operation, a 2.5-cm utility incision (Incision 2) is performed anteriorly at

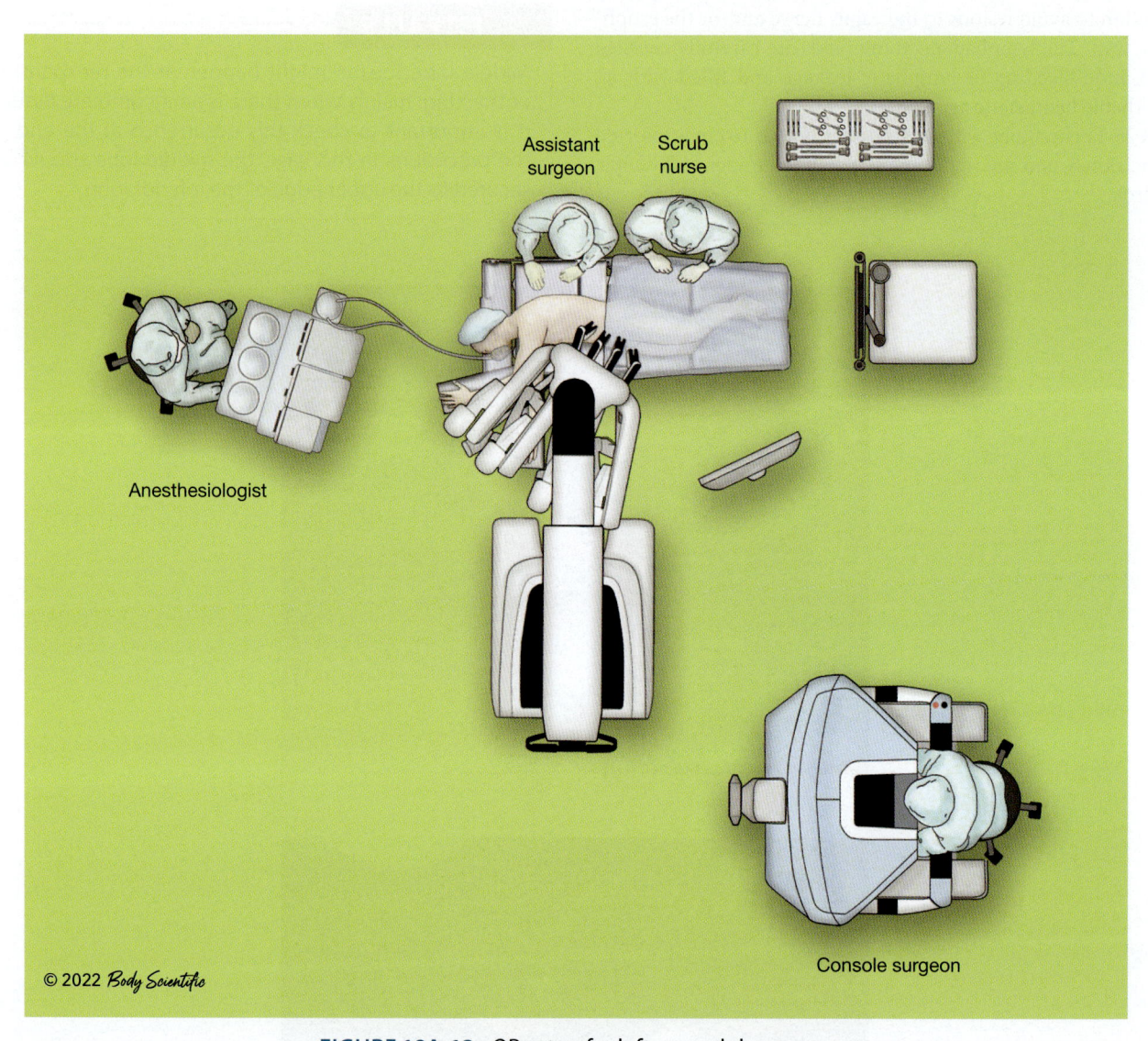

FIGURE 18A-13 • OR setup for left upper lobectomy.

the fourth intercostal space, and a skin retractor (Alexis-Applied Medical, Rancho Santa Margarita, CA) is positioned. Under direct vision with the camera inserted in the utility incision, the thoracic cavity is explored to exclude pleural carcinomatosis or adhesions. An 8-mm port is placed along the anterior axillary line at the seventh intercostal space (S). This is the incision through which the camera is inserted. Afterward, 2 other trocar incisions are performed, an 8- or 12-mm incision on the line of the tip of the scapula at the 8th intercostal space (Port R1) for stapler insertion and an 8-mm incision in the triangle of auscultation at the seventh intercostal space (Port R3) (**Figure 18A-14**).

The robot is docked in a position that does not interfere with the team's work. Once centered, the robotic arms are connected to the trocars. The dissection instrument, a long bipolar grasper, is positioned in the utility incision (R2), the camera in the port (Scope), the fenestrated bipolar forceps in port R1, and the tip-up fenestrated grasper in port R3.

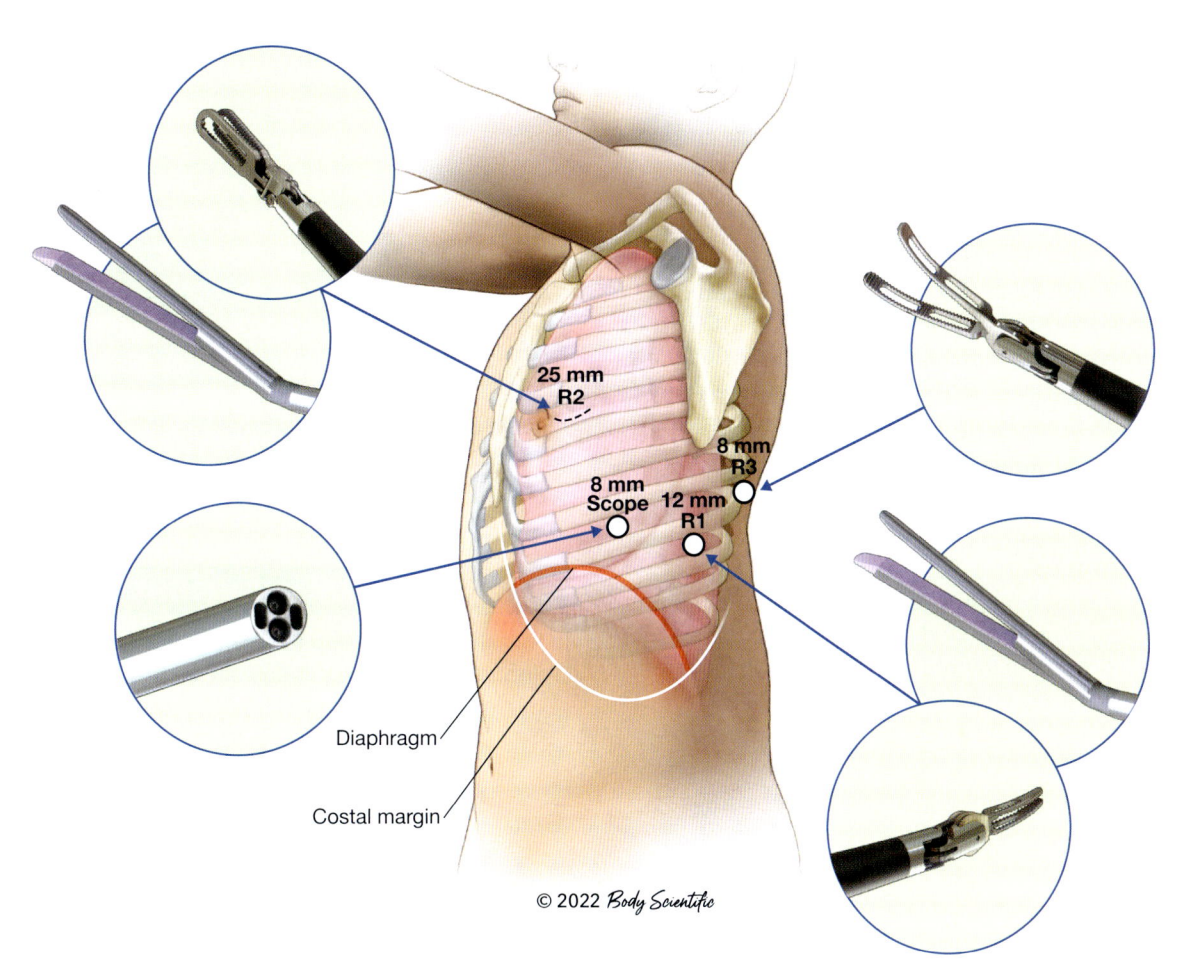

FIGURE 18A-14 • Port setting for left upper lobectomy.

Surgical Technique

▶ **Video 18A-2. Operative Technique of a Robotic Left Upper Lobectomy. Six Steps Standardized Technique**

Step 1. Station 5 lymph nodes dissection and preparation of left upper pulmonary vein

The first step is station 5 (aortopulmonary window) lymph nodes dissection and preparation of the left upper pulmonary vein preparation. The tip-up grasper is used for retracting the upper lobe posteriorly and exposing the hilum. The mediastinal pleura over the vein is opened. The lymph nodes of station 5 can be identified and removed, and the pulmonary artery is exposed. The bifurcation between the upper and lower vein must be identified and dissected: this maneuver helps in the isolation of the vein from the inferior edge of the lobe (**Figures 18A-15** and **18A-16 A–C**). The lingula vein is identified. The tissue surrounding the vein should be carefully dissected with both blunt and sharp dissection to expose the vessel and safely surround it. The use of a vessel loop to encircle the structure is recommended: it may help if the articulation of the stapler is not adequate, and its tip collides against the main pulmonary artery. The stapler is introduced from the port R1.

Step 1 average time frame: 20 min

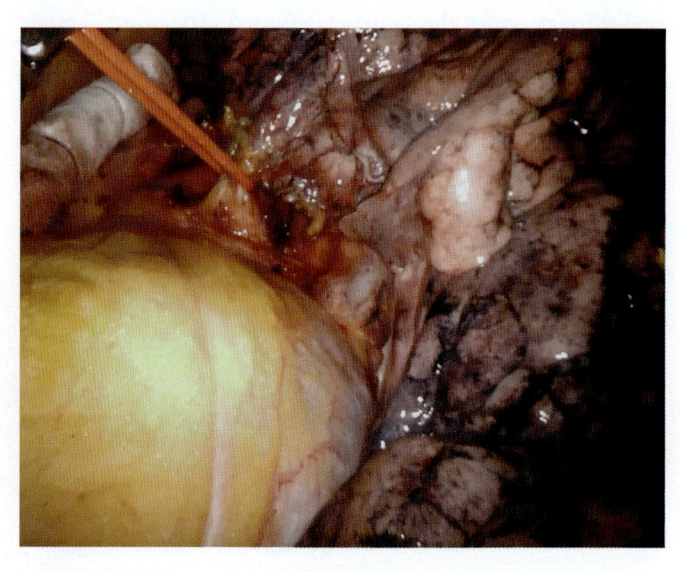

FIGURE 18A-15 • Preparation of the left upper pulmonary vein.

⚠ **PITFALLS**

Particular attention must be paid during the preparation of the posterior portion of the vein because the artery runs just below it. An imprudent maneuver could cause the rupture of the artery.

🔍 **ANATOMICAL HIGHLIGHTS**

It is always necessary to identify the confluence of the lingula vein into the main vein, as it rarely merges into the lower lobe vein.

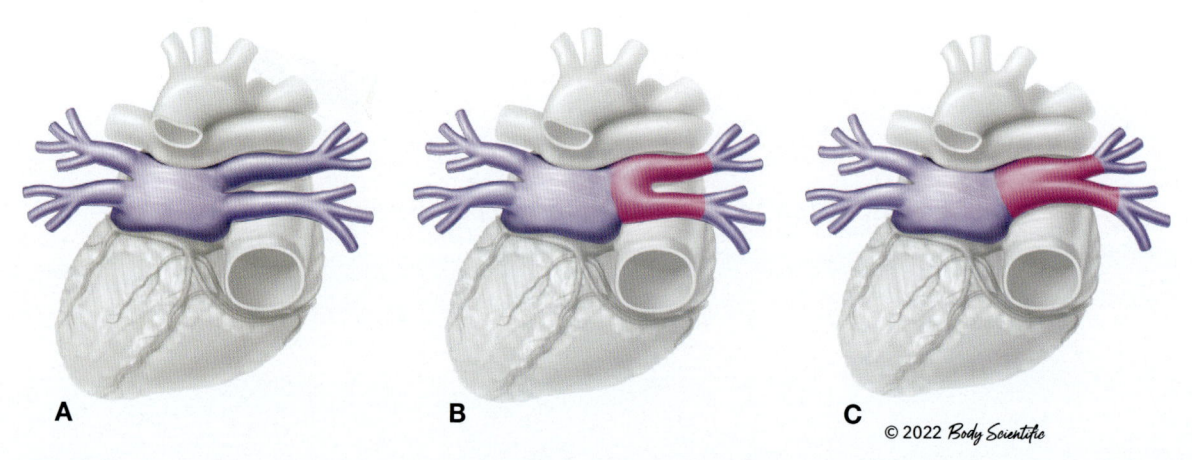

FIGURE 18A-16 • Normal left pulmonary vein anatomy and its variations. **A.** Normal. **B.** Short common left trunk. **C.** Long common left trunk.

Step 2. Preparation and section of the left upper pulmonary artery first branch

The branches of the pulmonary artery (PA) for the left upper lobe are extremely variable both in number and course. There are usually 3 to 5 arterial tributaries to the left upper lobe. Once the vein is divided, usually the PA anterior trunk becomes easily identifiable. Its division as the first step facilitates the isolation and transection of the upper lobe bronchus. The lobe is retracted posteriorly. In some cases, after sectioning the vein, the first branch becomes visible. The PA truncus is dissected using a sharp and blunt dissection; often the removal of hilar lymph nodes, located at the arterial origin, facilitates its isolation and preparation on a vessel loop (**Figure 18A-17**). The instruments inserted in incision R1 and incision R2 can be swapped to use the fenestrated bipolar forceps with a better angle that is less traumatic than the dissection instruments. The division of the arterial branches is performed with a vascular stapler (30 cartridge) introduced through incision R1 (**Figure 18A-18**).

Step 2 average time frame: 10–15 min

> ⚠️ **PITFALLS**
>
> Traction on the vascular stapled suture lines should be avoided because it can cause bleeding.

> 💬 **EDITORIAL COMMENT**
>
> Some of the branches of the pulmonary artery for the upper lobe can be very thin and short, and the introduction of the stapler can be difficult or risky for avulsion, causing major bleeding. In this situation, the safest technique is a classical suture ligation of the branches with Prolene™ 4-0/5-0 and their division with scissors in between sutures.

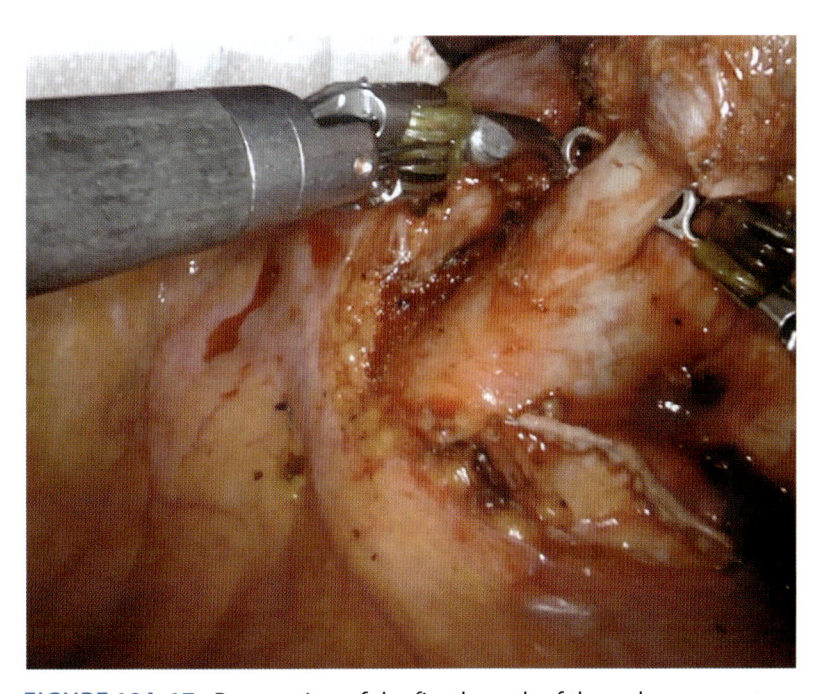

FIGURE 18A-17 • Preparation of the first branch of the pulmonary artery.

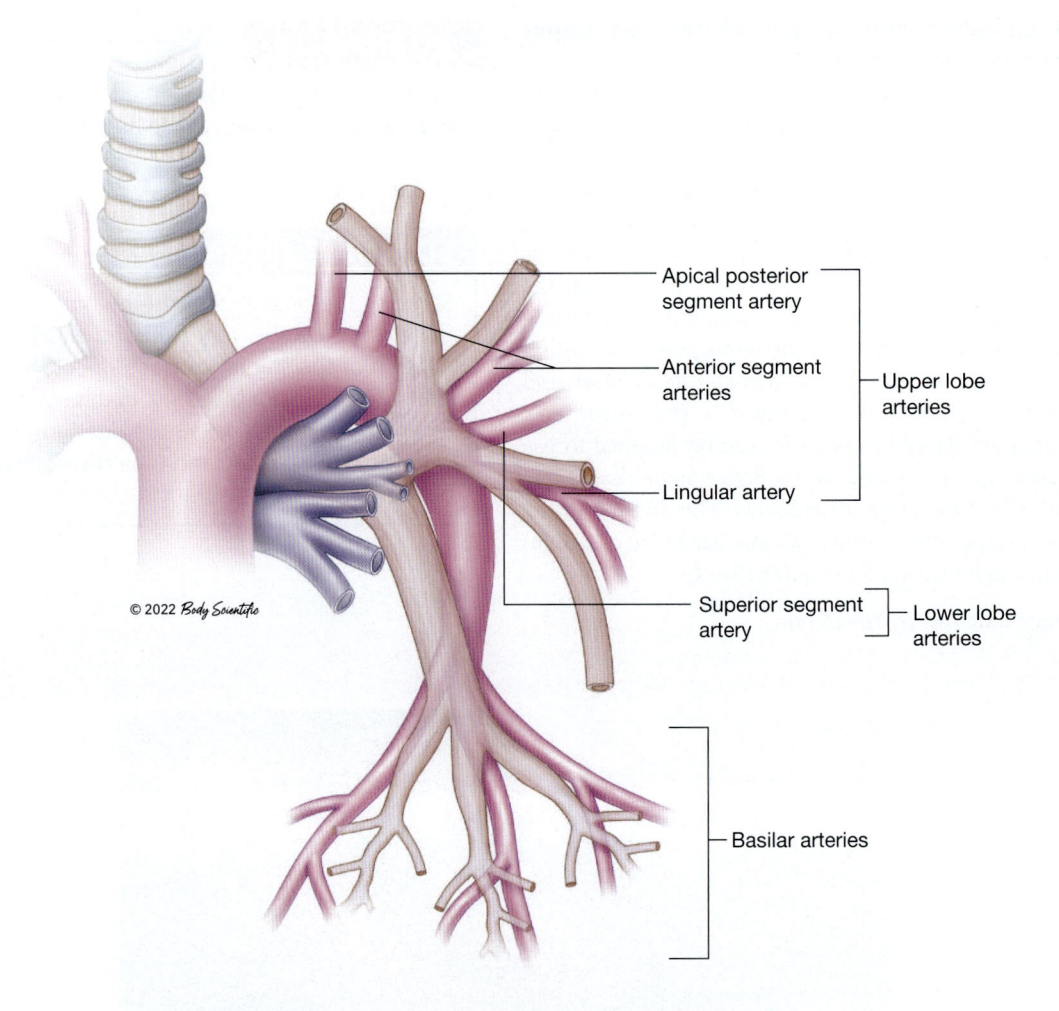

FIGURE 18A-18 • Left upper lobe pulmonary arteries.

Step 3. Preparation and section of the left upper pulmonary bronchus

Once the pulmonary artery anterior trunk is divided, the lobe is retracted upward to facilitate the identification of the upper lobar bronchus that arises vertically from the main bronchus (**Figure 18A-19**). The preparation of the bronchus usually starts from the inferior edge. As for the vein, the lymph nodes that lie between the bronchus and the artery should be removed leaving space for the robotic instruments. Isolation of the left upper bronchus must be performed with extreme caution. As described in Step 2, the instruments inserted in incision R1 and incision R2 can be swapped to use the fenestrated bipolar forceps in contact with the back wall of the bronchus to avoid injuries to the interlobar pulmonary artery. The stapler (usually a 45 curved tip) is again introduced from port R1 (**Figure 18A-20**).

Step 3 average time frame: 10–15 min

▶▶ **TIPS**

Before sectioning the bronchus, an inflation test of the remaining lung can be performed to avoid misplacement of the stapler.

EDITORIAL COMMENT

Inflation test should be done when there are doubts on the correct placement of the stapler. Inflating the lingula and the lower lobe may decrease the working space and suctioning the entrapped* air inside the lung after that might not be easy and it is time consuming.

▶▶ **TIPS**

The peribronchial lymph nodes at this level should always be removed. This allows the creation of a safe dissection plane, reducing the risk of damaging the artery.

⚠ **PITFALLS**

Before stapling the bronchus, it is important to verify that there are no anesthesia catheters or tubes erroneously inserted inside the upper lobe.

Lung Upper Lobectomies 363

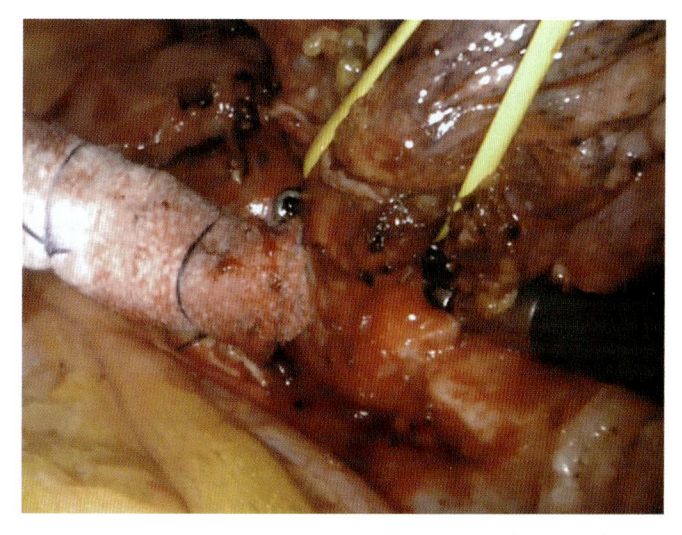

FIGURE 18A-19 • Preparation of the left upper pulmonary bronchus.

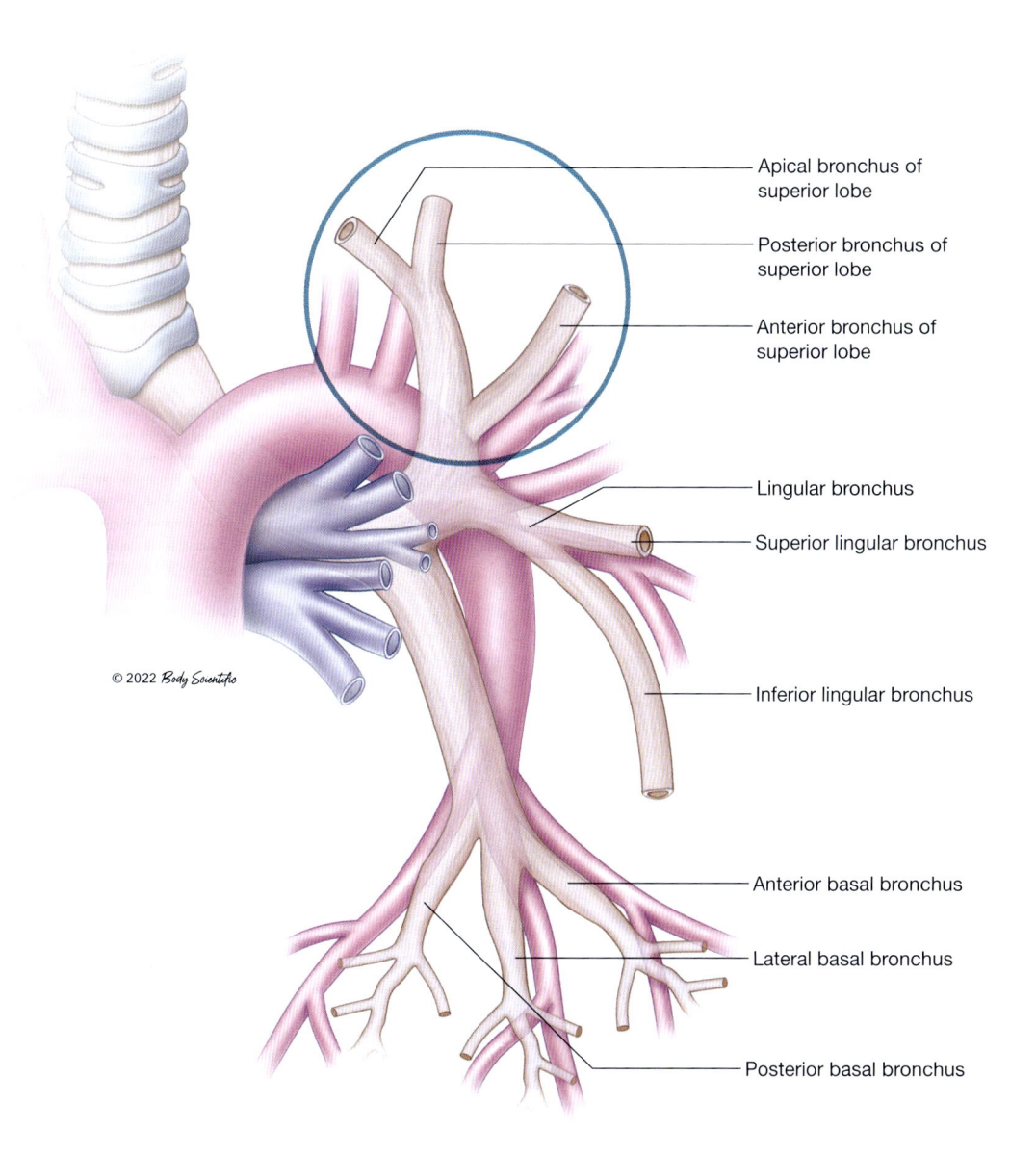

FIGURE 18A-20 • Left upper bronchus.

Step 4. Preparation and section of the remaining left upper pulmonary arteries branches

The lobe is retracted posteriorly. The lingula artery and the posterior ascending branches are isolated and dissected using sharp and blunt maneuvers. The lingula artery is usually resected first, after its identification at the fissure level. The posterior branches are approached afterward (**Figures 18A-21 A–C**). At this stage, the vascular elements of the lobectomy are completed.

Step 4 average time frame: 20–25 min

>> **TIPS**

For small-size vascular branches, depending on the surgeon's preference, a Hem-o-lok® clip can also be used using the medium–large robotic clip applier.

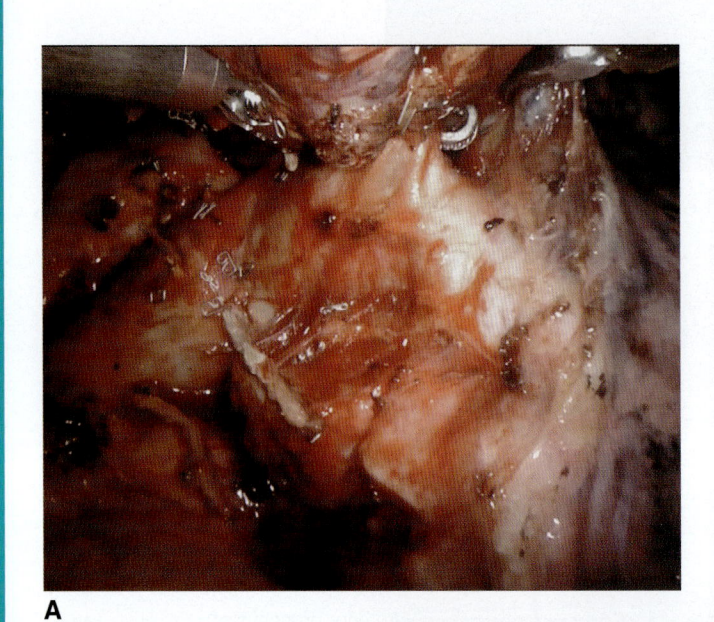

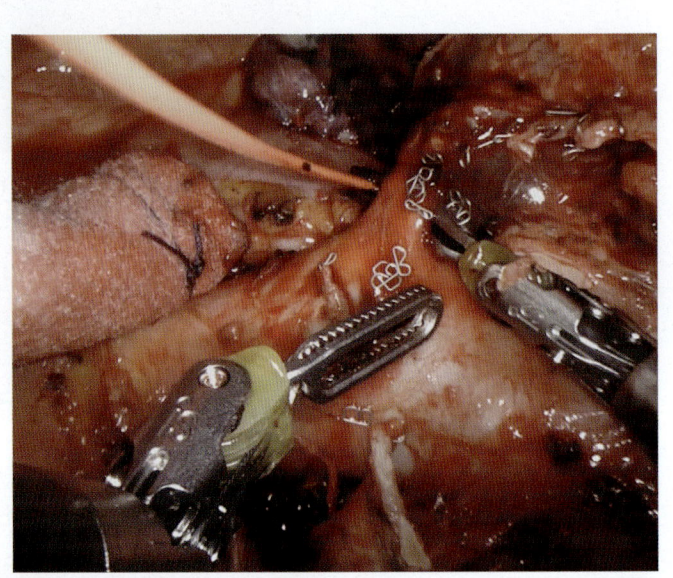

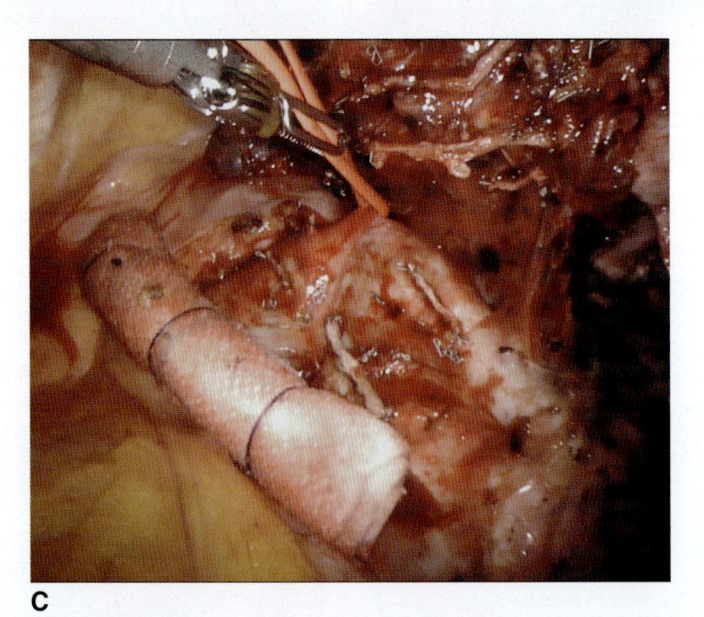

FIGURE 18A-21 • **A.** Preparation of the left lingular artery branch. **B.** Preparation of the 1st posterior left artery branch. **C.** Preparation of the 2nd posterior left artery branch.

Step 5. Preparation and section of the fissure

In accordance with the fissure-less or fissure-last technique, the fissure is sectioned as the last step of the lobectomy. It is necessary to evaluate its characteristics: if it is composed of a thin pleural flap only, it can be dissected by using an energy device; otherwise, in the case of incomplete fissures with pulmonary parenchyma, the use of a stapler is the best option (45 or 60 cartridges depending on the length) (**Figure 18A-22**).

Step 5 average time frame: <10 min

> ⚠ **PITFALLS**
>
> Dividing the lung parenchyma at the fissure with energy instruments is always a potential pitfall and a risk for postoperative air leak. Staplers should be used preferentially.

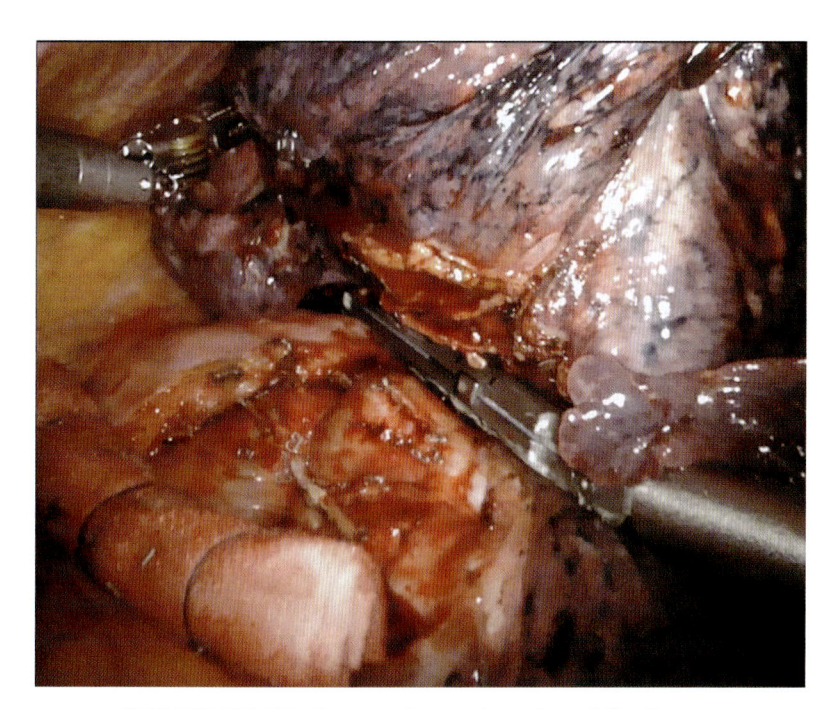

FIGURE 18A-22 • Preparation and section of the fissure.

Step 6. Lymph nodes dissection and specimen extraction

For all cases of malignancy, systematic radical lymph nodes dissection is mandatory. For any left-sided robotic lobectomy, stations 5, 6, and 7 should be removed. L8 and L9 are retrieved mainly in the case of a lower lobectomy when the pulmonary ligament is dissected. Stations 5 and 6 are dissected by opening the mediastinal pleura and proceeding upward along the phrenic nerve to expose the aortic arch. In some cases, the lymphadenectomy of station 5 is performed at the time of preparation of the pulmonary vein, as described in this chapter.

The subcarinal area is approached, retracting the remaining lower lobe anteriorly with the tip-up using a sponge and avoiding direct grasping of the parenchyma. The mediastinal pleura is dissected from the superior edge of the lower lobe vein all the way up along the course of the vagus nerve. Extensive dissection of the posterior mediastinal pleura provides a clear vision of the esophagus and the left main bronchus. The station 7 lymph nodes are removed. The resected lobe is positioned inside a big Endobag and retrieved out of the utility incision (**Figures 18A-23 A, B**). A 28-Fr drainage with an accessory hole at 10 cm is positioned in incision S with the tip located 2 cm lower and away from the apex to avoid postoperative chest and shoulder pain.

Step 6 average time frame: 20–30 min

> ⚠ **PITFALLS**
>
> For the extraction of the specimen, it is always recommended to use an Endobag to avoid the contamination of the extraction site by neoplastic cells.

> ▶▶ **TIPS**
>
> In the subcarinal area, it is recommended to place hemostatic agents to reduce the risk of postsurgical bleeding and lymphatic leakage.

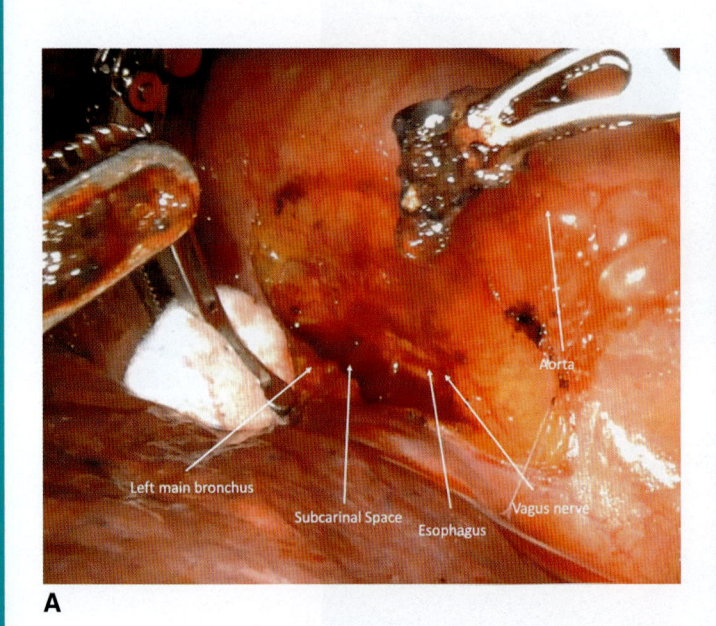

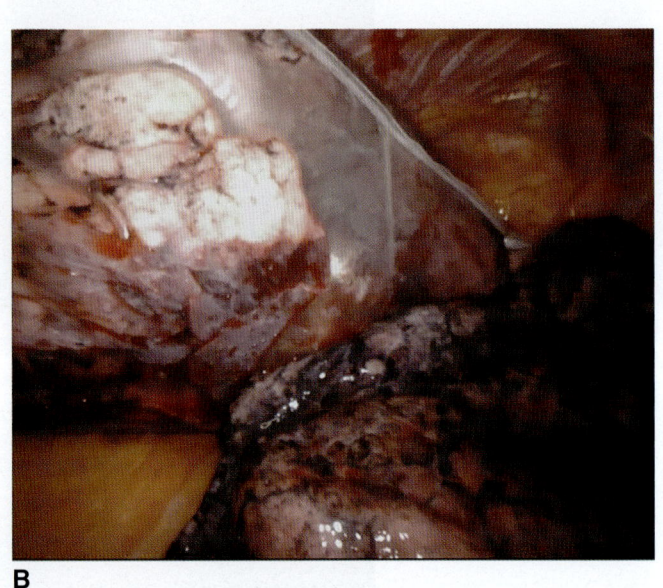

FIGURE 18A-23 • **A.** Station 7 lymph node dissection. **B.** Specimen extraction.

Suggested Readings

1. Veronesi G, Novellis P, Voulaz E, Alloisio M. Robot-assisted surgery for lung cancer: state of the art and perspectives. *Lung Cancer.* 2016;101:28-34. doi: 10.1016/j.lungcan.2016.09.004
2. Novellis P, Alloisio M, Cariboni U, Veronesi G. Different techniques in robotic lung resection. *J Thorac Dis.* 2017;9(11):4315-4318. doi: 10.21037/jtd.2017.10.69
3. Cerfolio RJ, Ghanim AF, Dylewski M, et al. The long-term survival of robotic lobectomy for non-small cell lung cancer: a multi-institutional study. *J Thorac Cardiovasc Surg.* 2018;155(2):778-786. doi: 10.1016/j.jtcvs.2017.09.016
4. Park BJ, Melfi F, Mussi A, et al. Robotic lobectomy for non-small cell lung cancer (NSCLC): long-term oncologic results. *J Thorac Cardiovasc Surg.* 2012;143(2):383-9. doi: 10.1016/j.jtcvs.2011.10.055
5. Oh DS, Reddy RM, Gorrepati ML, Mehendale S, Reed MF. Robotic-assisted, video-assisted thoracoscopic and open lobectomy: propensity-matched analysis of recent premier data. *Ann Thorac Surg.* 2017;104(5):1733-1740. doi: 10.1016/j.athoracsur.2017.06.020
6. Gondé H, Laurent M, Gillibert A, et al. The affordability of minimally invasive procedures in major lung resection: a prospective study. *Interact Cardiovasc Thorac Surg.* 2017;25(3):469-475. doi: 10.1093/icvts/ivx149
7. Bendixen M, Jørgensen OD, Kronborg C, Andersen C, Licht PB. Postoperative pain and quality of life after lobectomy via video-assisted thoracoscopic surgery or anterolateral thoracotomy for early stage lung cancer: a randomised controlled trial. *Lancet Oncol.* 2016;17(6):83-844. doi: 10.1016/S1470-2045(16)00173-X
8. Giulianotti PC, Coratti A, Angelini M, et al. Robotics in general surgery: personal experience in a large community hospital. *Arch Surg.* 2003;138(7):777-784. doi: 10.1001/archsurg.138.7.777

18B

"It will work."
—Nina Starr Braunwald (1928–1992)

Lung Lower Lobectomies

Giulia Veronesi • Pierluigi Novellis • Piergiorgio Muriana • Gabriela Aguiluz • Francesca Rossetti

Right Lower and Middle Lobectomy

Patient Positioning, OR Setup, and Port Setting

In the right lower lobectomies, patient positioning, OR setup, and port setting remain the same when compared to the right upper lobectomies previously described in Chapter 18A (**Figure 18B-1**).

When needed, all incisions can be placed 1 intercostal space lower; in particular, the utility incision might need to be placed at the 5th intercostal space instead of the 4th (**Figure 18B-2**).

> ▶▶ **TIPS**
>
> In lower lobectomies, the stapler is inserted through the utility incision. For the upper and right middle lobectomies, the stapler is usually inserted through the posterior port (incision R2), using a 12-mm trocar, both for the robotic and thoracoscopic stapler.

INSTRUMENT REQUIREMENTS

The suggested main robotic instruments/tools can be listed as follows:
- 30°/0° camera
- Long bipolar grasper
- Fenestrated bipolar forceps
- Tip-up fenestrated grasper
- Medium–large clip applier
- Monopolar curved scissors (optional)
- Large needle driver (optional)
- ProGrasp forceps (optional)
- Permanent monopolar cautery hook (optional)
- EndoWrist® Stapler 45 Curved-Tip (optional)
- EndoWrist® Stapler 45 (optional)
- EndoWrist® Stapler 30 Curved-Tip

The suggested main thoracoscopic instruments/tools can be listed as follows:
- Nontraumatic forceps
- Needle driver
- Suction device
- Staplers
- Clip applier

Supplemental materials:
- Kittner roll laparoscopic gauze (cigarette sponges)
- Sutures: Prolene™ 3-0, 4-0, 5-0
- Vessel loops
- Nelaton tubes
- Skin retractor
- Gelport® (optional)
- Hem-o-lok® clips
- Reabsorbable hemostatic material
- EndoBag™
- 28-Fr chest tube

Photo reproduced with permission from Braunwald E. Nina Starr Braunwald: some reflections on the first woman heart surgeon. Ann Thorac Surg. 2001;71(2 Suppl):S6-S7.
Quote reproduced with permission from Singh S, DiGiacomo JC, Angus LDG. "It Will Work": The Story of Nina Starr Braunwald and the First Successful Mitral Valve Replacement. Ann Thorac Surg. 2021;112(3):1023-1028.

368 The Foundation and Art of Robotic Surgery

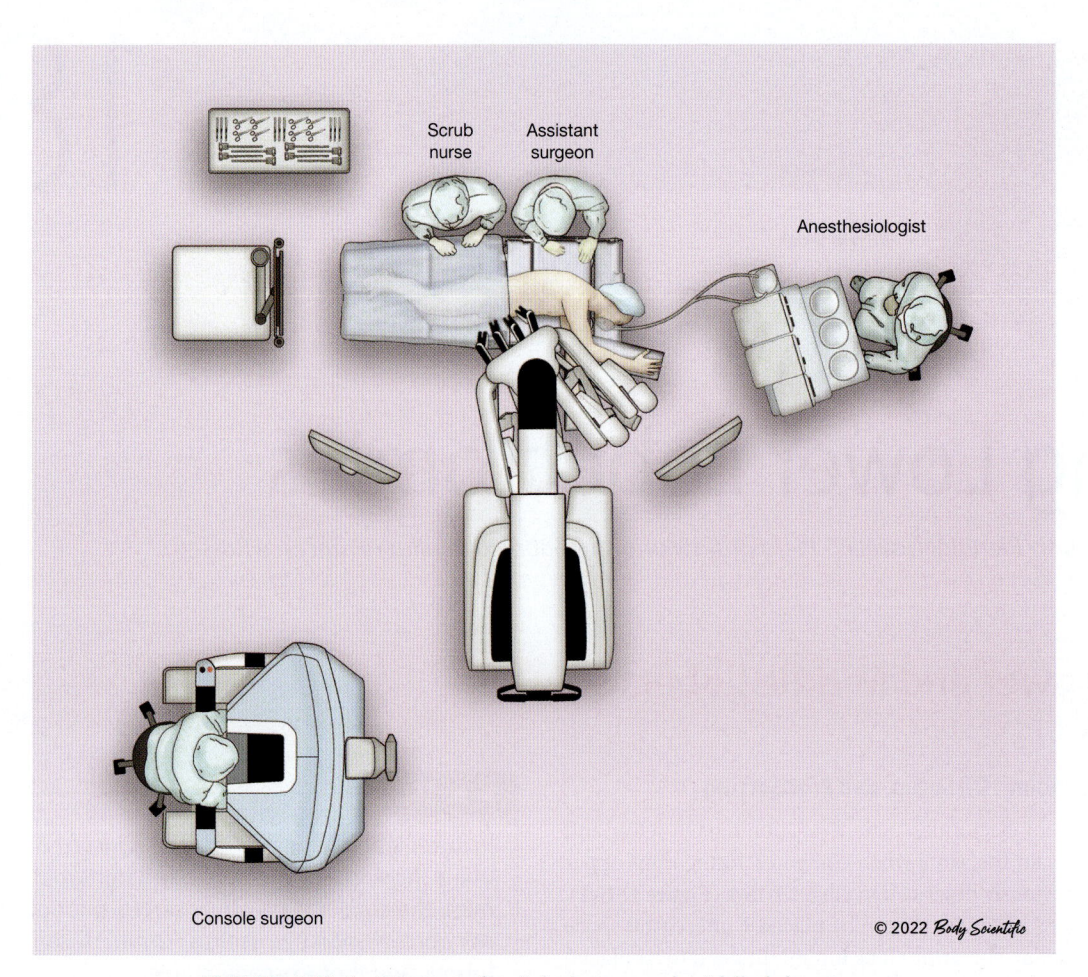

FIGURE 18B-1 • OR setup for right lower and middle lobectomy.

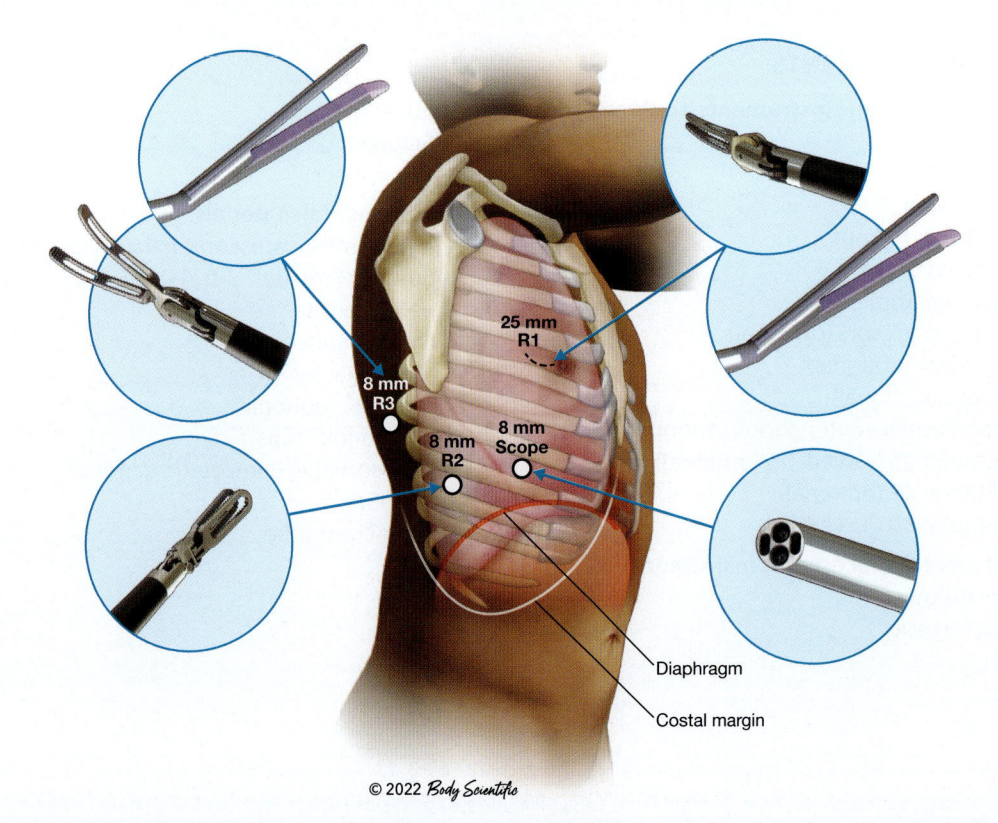

FIGURE 18B-2 • Port setting for right lower and middle lobectomy. Incisions can be placed one intercostal space lower for lower lobectomies.

Right Lower Lobectomy Surgical Technique

▶ **Video 18B-1.** Operative Technique of a Robotic Right Lower Lobectomy. Four Steps Standardized Technique

Step 1. Preparation of the pulmonary ligament and right lower lobe vein isolation

The lung is retracted upward with the tip-up forceps. Dissection proceeds with the long bipolar grasper in the dominant hand and the fenestrated bipolar forceps on the other side. The pulmonary ligament is divided, and the lymphadenectomy of stations 8R and 9R is performed. The lower lobe is kept in traction toward the apex, exposing the inferior pulmonary ligament. In the case of a high diaphragm, it can be retracted down with a grasper holding a sponge by the bedside assistant through the utility incision. In case of patients with obesity, CO_2 insufflation might help in pushing down the diaphragm (see Chapter 17, Lung Lobectomies: General Principles and the Total Port, Transfissure Approach (Fissure First)).

Once the inferior pulmonary vein is visualized, the anterior mediastinal pleura is dissected to expose and identify the middle and upper lobe veins and rule out the presence of abnormal venous anatomy. The posterior pleura is then sectioned to isolate the lower vein. Once prepared, the vein is surrounded by a vessel loop (**Figure 18B-3**). For a smoother maneuver, the instruments connected to R1 and R2 can be inverted to use the less traumatic fenestrated bipolar grasper to go around the vessel. The inferior pulmonary vein is isolated and then divided with a 30-mm vascular stapler through the utility incision.

Step 1 average time frame: 10–15 min

> **EDITORIAL COMMENT**
> CO_2 insufflation works in a closed chest. If there is a utility incision, it should be closed with a sealing device (GelPort®).

> **EDITORIAL COMMENT**
> If the fissure is not too thick, it is convenient to start the dissection from the basilar trunk of the pulmonary artery, which can be easily found at the intersection between the greater and lesser fissures.

> **⚠ PITFALLS**
> Injury of the apical segment venous branch while surrounding the inferior pulmonary vein.

> **▶▶ TIPS**
> The pleura on the backside of the vein should always be opened, allowing a safer separation of the vein from the bronchus.

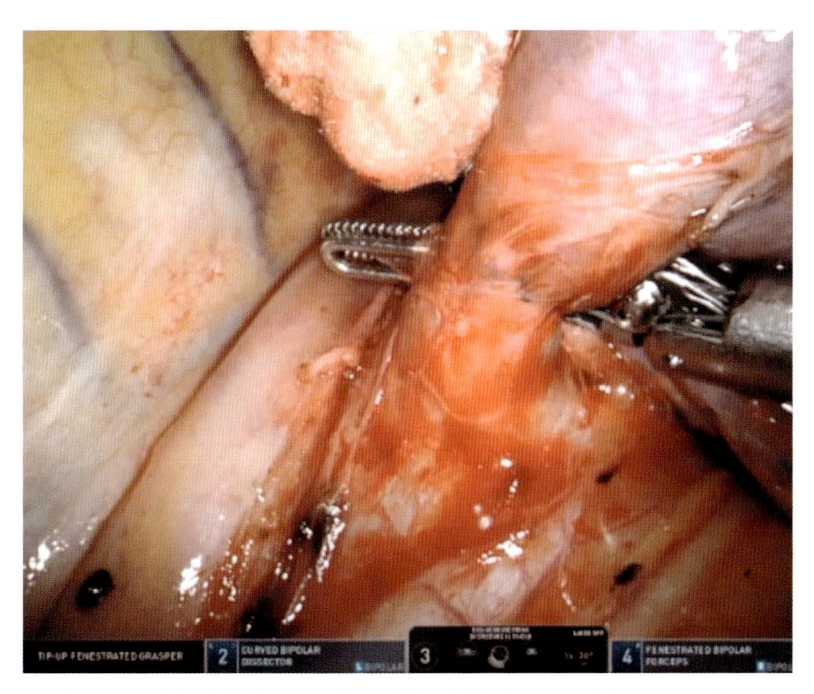

FIGURE 18B-3 • Preparation of the right lower pulmonary vein.

Step 2. Isolation and section of the right lower pulmonary artery

The oblique fissure between the right lower lobe and the middle lobe is divided to expose the pulmonary artery at the fissure level; the vessel is then isolated, proceeding with sharp and blunt dissection. The pulmonary artery is encircled with a vessel loop and divided with a 30-mm vascular stapler introduced from the utility incision. If the origin of the superior segment branch is located far from the basal trunk and it is technically challenging to isolate both branches in a single step, then they should be divided singularly into 2 separate steps (**Figures 18B-4, 18B-5 A, B,** and **18B-6**).

Step 2 average time frame: 20–25 min

> ⚠ **PITFALLS**
> Damage to the visceral pleura of the middle lobe during the preparation of the fissure. This might be the reason for air leak in the postoperative period.

> ▶▶ **TIPS**
> Staplers in the lower lobectomy are better inserted through the anterior utility incision.

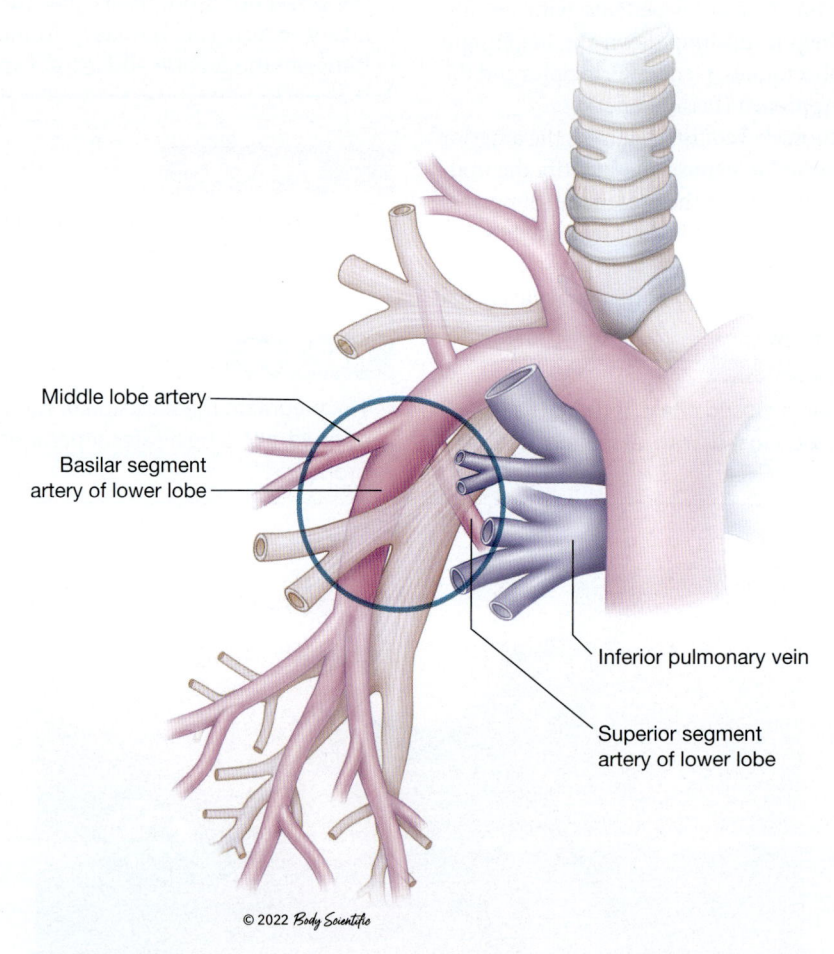

FIGURE 18B-4 • Right pulmonary basilar segment artery of the lower lobe.

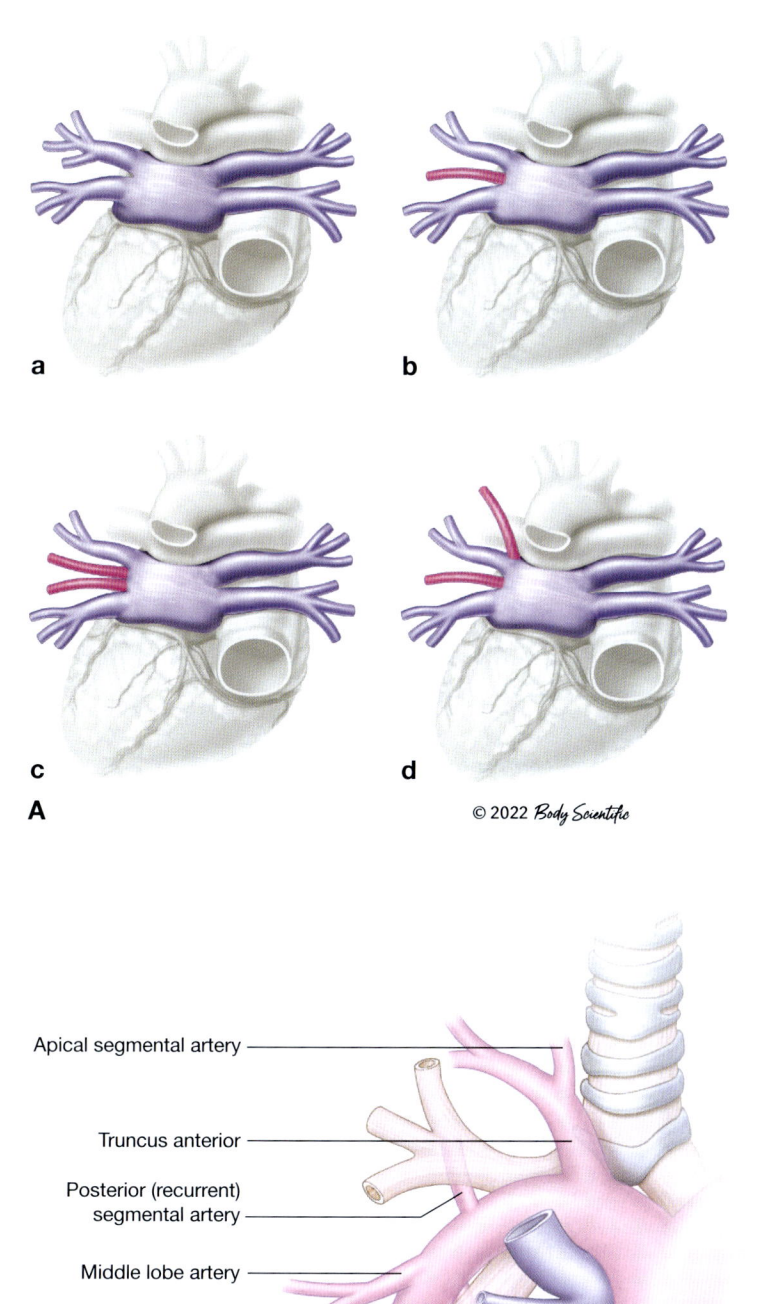

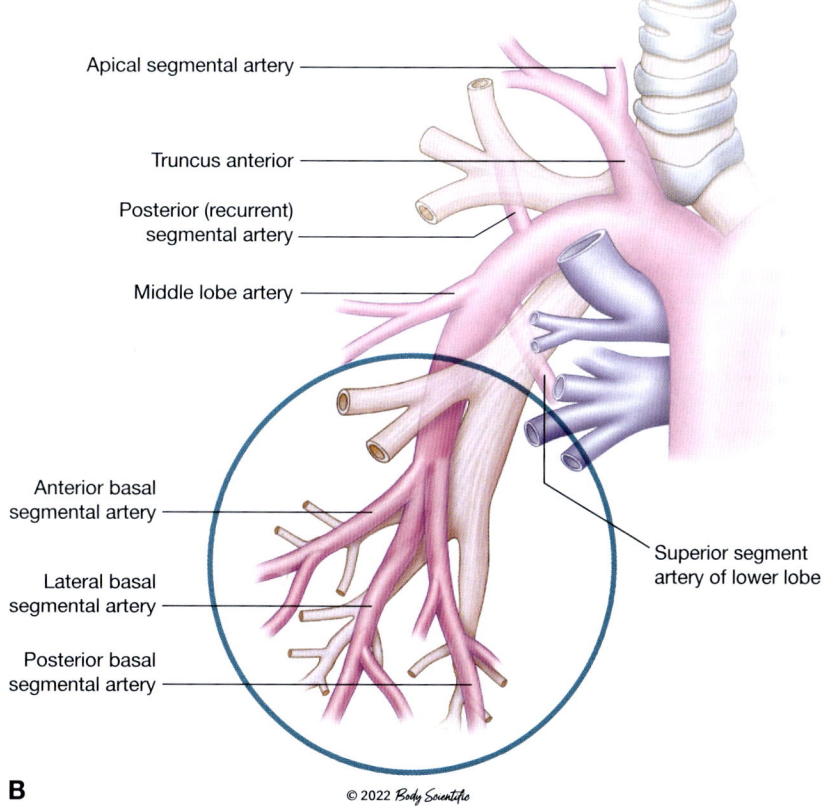

FIGURE 18B-5 • **A.** Normal right pulmonary veins and their variations. Normal anatomy (a). Right middle pulmonary vein (b). Two right middle pulmonary veins (c). Right middle pulmonary vein and right upper pulmonary vein (d). **B.** Right pulmonary basal segmental arteries.

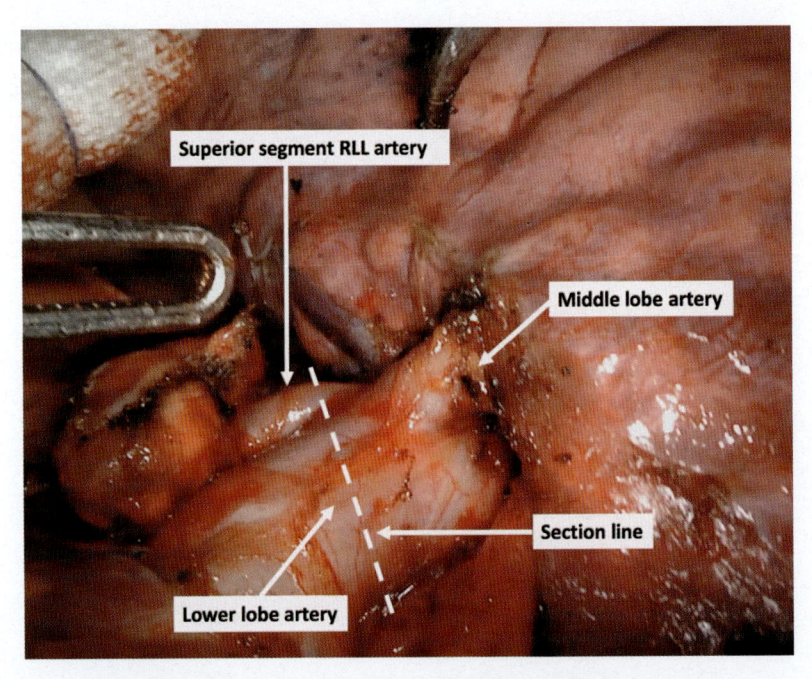

FIGURE 18B-6 • Preparation of right lower pulmonary artery.

Step 3. Isolation and section of the right lower pulmonary bronchus and completion of the fissure

The posterior mediastinal pleura is dissected. All hilar lymph nodes are removed. The fissure can be dissected before or after the bronchus. The fissure is usually sectioned first, using a parenchymal stapler introduced through the utility incision.

Finally, the bronchus is divided with a 45-mm parenchymal curved-tip stapler introduced through the utility incision (**Figures 18B-7 A, B**). The resected lobe is placed inside a specimen bag and retrieved from the mini-thoracotomy.

Step 3 average time frame: 15–20 min

⚠ PITFALLS

Incomplete removal of the peribronchial lymph nodes. They can be erroneously included in the staple line of the bronchial stump.

▶▶ TIPS

Before sectioning the bronchus, proper ventilation of the middle lobe should be confirmed to prevent middle lobe exclusion/persistent atelectasis (ventilation test).

EDITORIAL COMMENT

Inflation test should be done when there are doubts on the correct placement of the stapler. Inflating the lung may decrease the working space and suctioning the entrapped air inside the parenchyma, after that might not be easy and it is time consuming.

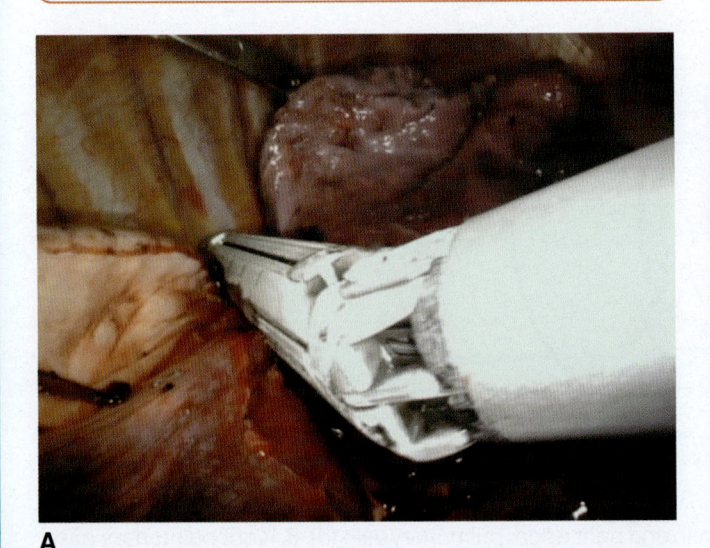

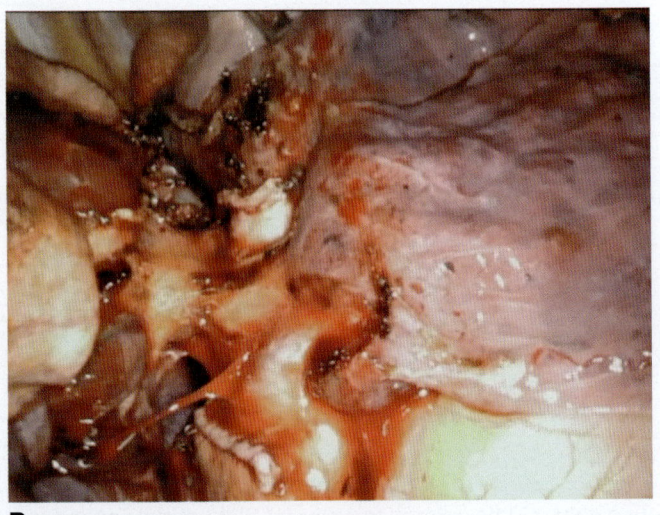

FIGURE 18B-7 • **A.** Fissure section. **B.** Right lower bronchus isolation.

Step 4. Mediastinal lymphadenectomy

If the lobectomy is performed for cancer, it is necessary to complete the surgical procedure with radical lymphadenectomy. In case of advanced tumors or suspicious lymph nodes, performing the lymph nodal dissection before the lobectomy is advisable. The removed mediastinal lymph node stations in the right lobectomies are 2R, 4R, 7, 8R, and 9R. The last 2 are usually removed at the beginning, during the division of the pulmonary ligament, as described in Step 1.

The subcarinal area is approached: to have better exposure of the target area, the remaining lung is retracted cephalad. The mediastinal pleura is opened from the superior edge of the lower lobe vein all the way up along the course of the vagus nerve. The subcarinal lymph nodes are thus radically removed (**Figures 18B-8 A, B**). During paratracheal lymphadenectomy, the azygos-cava confluence is visualized, and the pleura is incised laterally to the cava and above the azygos vein. Therefore, the high (2R) and low (4R) paratracheal lymph nodal tissues are exposed and removed. At the end of the procedure, a chest tube with an accessory hole at 10 cm is inserted through the incision S.

Step 4 average time frame: 15–20 min

> ▶▶ **TIPS**
>
> It is recommended to place a swab of reabsorbable hemostatic material in the subcarinal and paratracheal space to reduce the risk of postoperative lymphatic leakage and bleeding.

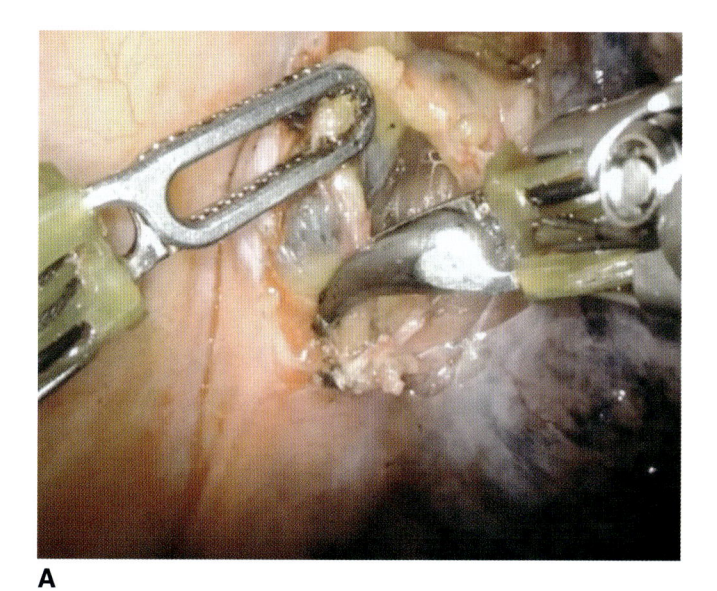

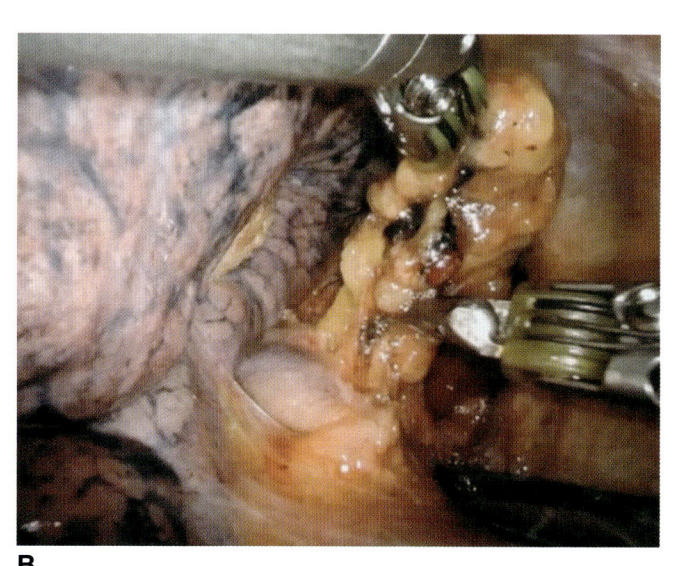

FIGURE 18B-8 • **A.** Lymphadenectomy of the subcarinal station. **B.** Lymphadenectomy of the paratracheal station.

Right Middle Lobectomy Surgical Technique

▶ Video 18B-2. Operative Technique of a Robotic Right Middle Lobectomy. Four Steps Standardized Technique

Step 1. Preparation and division of the middle lobe pulmonary vein

For the right middle lobectomy, an anterior approach is adopted, as for the right upper lobectomy. The surgeon's dominant hand controls the long bipolar grasper for fine dissection introduced through the utility incision. Alternatively, the other hand controls the fenestrated bipolar forceps (R2), or the tip-up grasper with a mounted sponge (R3). The lung is retracted posteriorly with the tip-up grasper. The anterior mediastinal pleura is widely opened parallel and posterior to the course of the phrenic nerve in front of the pulmonary veins. The middle lobe vein, which commonly represents the caudal branch of the right upper pulmonary vein, is identified and encircled with a vessel loop. Depending on the diameter of the vessel and the entry angle, stapling or Hem-o-Lok® clips can be used to divide the vein (**Figures 18B-9 A, B** and **18B-10**).

Step 1 average time frame: 10–15 min

> ⚠ **PITFALLS**
> Injury of the pulmonary artery while isolating the middle pulmonary vein. The pulmonary artery lies right underneath the vein.

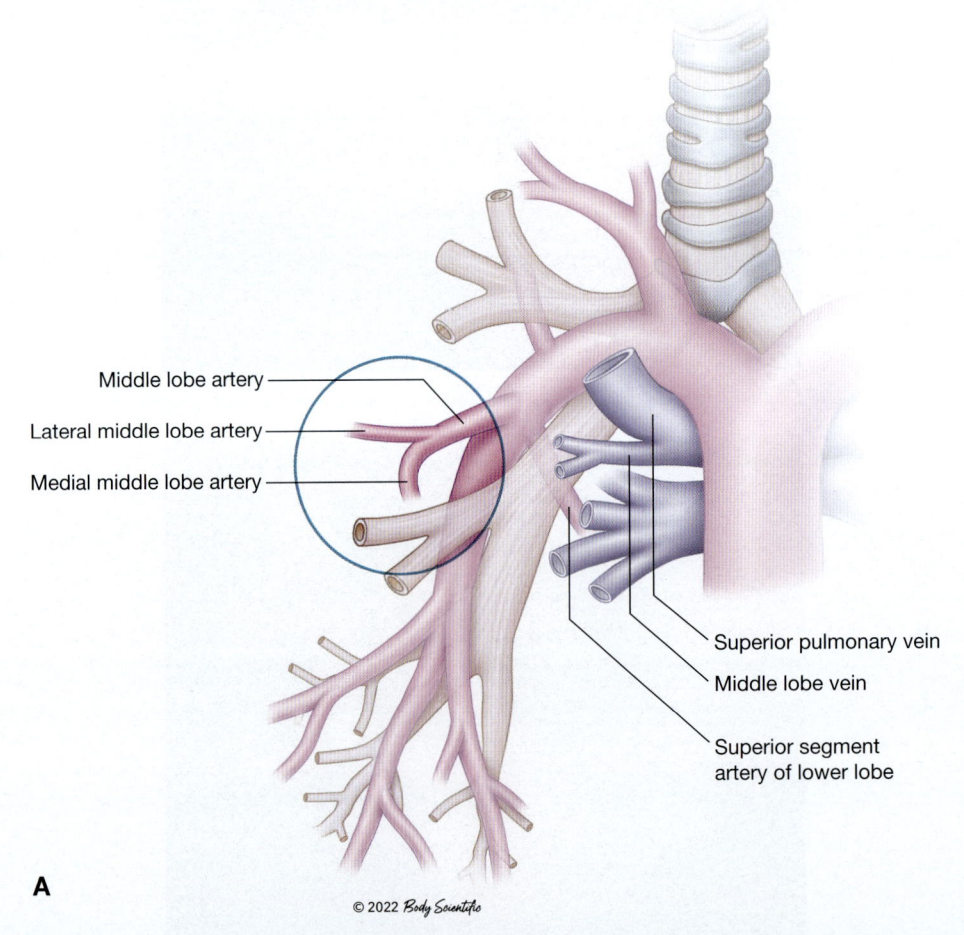

FIGURE 18B-9 • Right pulmonary veins and right middle lobe artery. **A.** Lateral and medial middle lobe branches originate from the middle lobe artery.

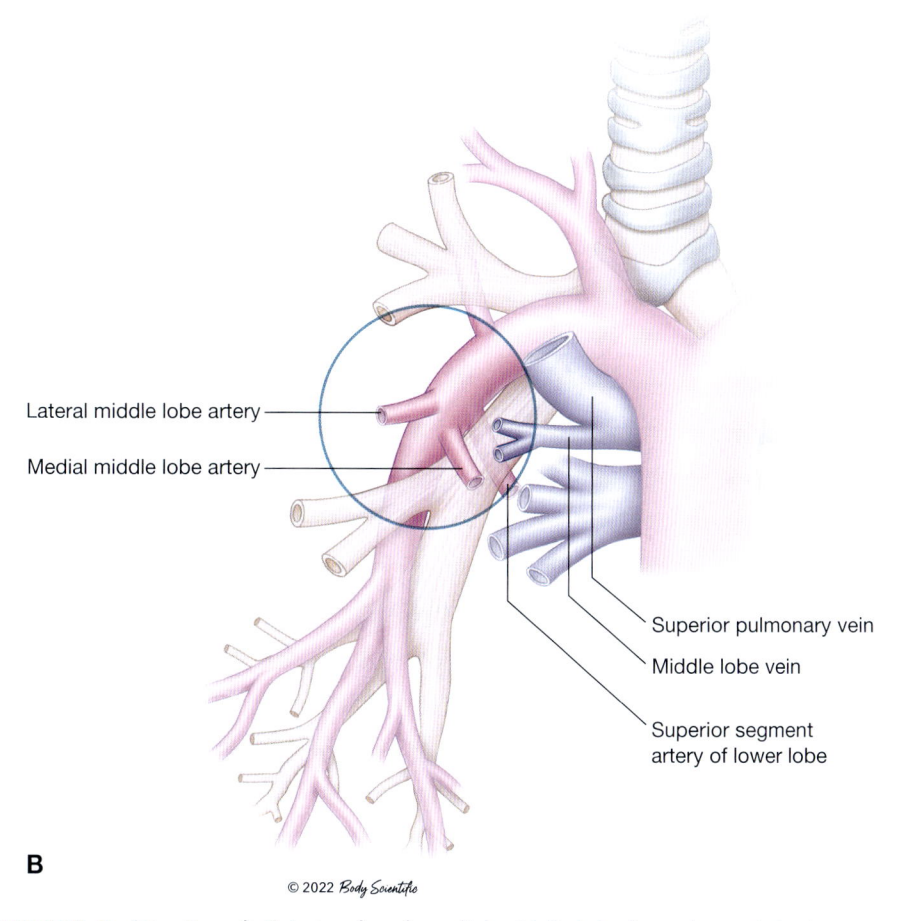

FIGURE 18B-9 • *(Continued)* **B.** Lateral and medial middle lobe branches originate separately.

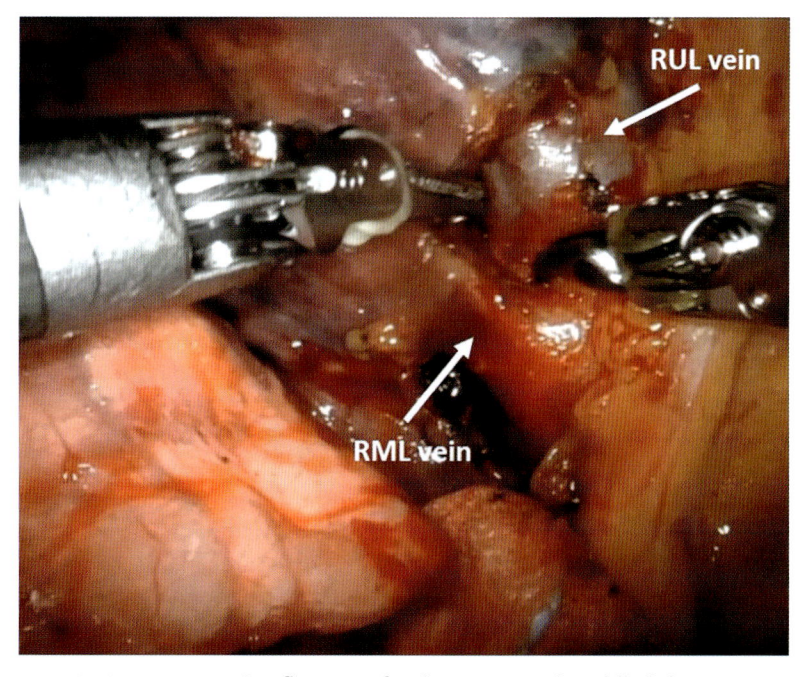

FIGURE 18B-10 • Confluence of right upper and middle lobe veins.

Step 2. Isolation and division of the right middle lobe bronchus

The division of the vein gives access to the bronchus and the arterial branches of the right middle lobe. Usually, the second step of the operation consists in isolating the middle lobe bronchus. Bipolar coagulation and blunt dissection are conducted with the long bipolar grasper. The peribronchial lymph nodes are removed in this phase. Attention must be paid to prevent accidental injury to the arterial branches lying close to the bronchus. The bedside assistant introduces a curved-tip 30-mm Endostapler (black or purple cartridge) through port R2 after momentarily undocking the robotic arm to allow the division of the airway (**Figure 18B-11**).

Step 2 average time frame: 15–20 min

> ⚠️ **PITFALLS**
>
> Injury of the small arterial branches of the middle lobe during the bronchial dissection.

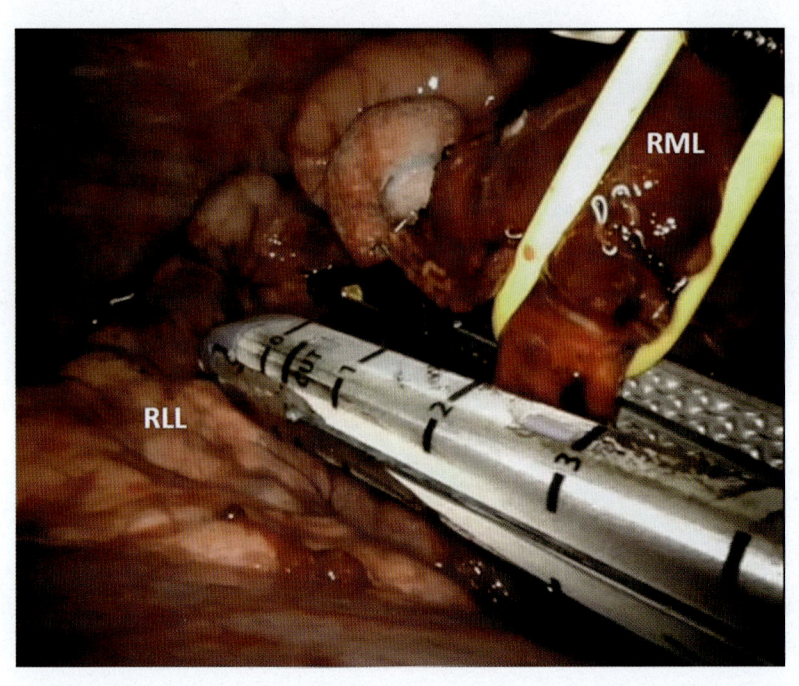

FIGURE 18B-11 • Trasection of the right middle bronchus. RML, right middle lobe; RLL, right lower lobe.

Step 3. Isolation and division of the arterial branch(es)

Once the bronchus is divided, 1 or 2 small arterial branches for the middle lobe are usually identified (**Figure 18B-12**). The vessels are dissected from the pulmonary parenchyma and lymphatic tissue and divided with staplers or between clips, depending on vessel size.

Step 3 average time frame: 15–20 min

> **EDITORIAL COMMENT**
>
> Microsuturing is always the best and safest way to deal with small, fragile branches of the pulmonary artery.

> 🔍 **ANATOMICAL HIGHLIGHTS**
>
> Arterial vascularization of the middle lobe usually includes 2 branches: the medial segmental and the lateral segmental arteries. These vessels can originate separately from the intermediate artery within the fissure or a common trunk arising in front of the ascending posterior branch of the right upper lobe (**Figure 18B-9**).

> ▶▶ **TIPS**
>
> Because the bronchus may lie in a groove surrounded by the 2 segmental arteries, it could sometimes be better to approach the lateral segmental branch at the junction of the transverse and oblique fissures.

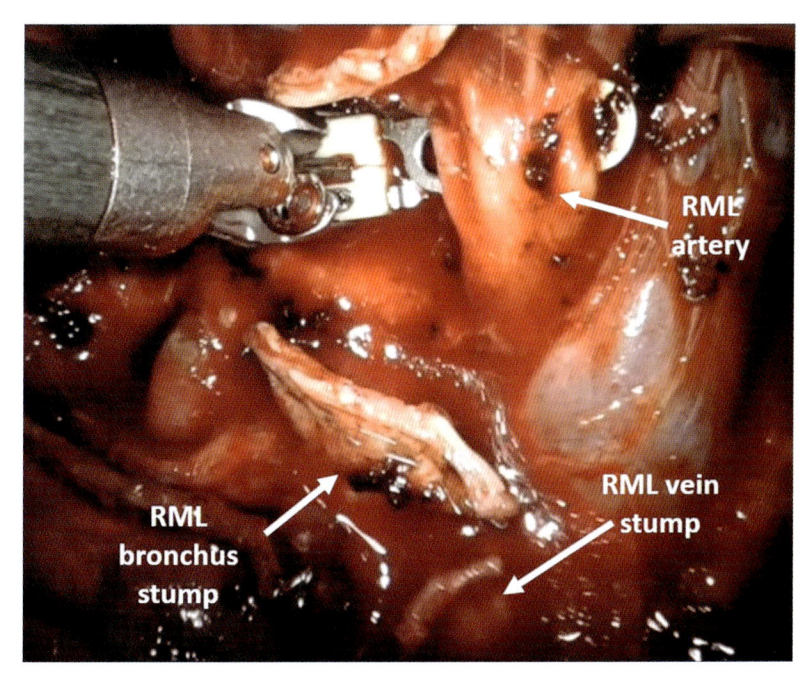

FIGURE 18B-12 • After bronchus division, the middle lobe artery branch is identifiable. RML, right middle lobe.

Step 4. Fissure division

The fissure between the upper and lower lobe is divided by the bedside assistant with multiple cartridges of an Endostapler (usually 45-mm purple reloads), introduced through the utility incision (**Figure 18B-13**). The surgeon at the console retracts the parenchyma to favor the staplers' correct positioning, mainly in case of fused fissures. The specimen is placed inside an Endobag™ and removed through the utility incision. The dissection of 7, 4R, and 2R lymph node stations proceeds as previously described in the right upper lobectomy surgical technique description.

Step 4 average time frame: 10–15 min

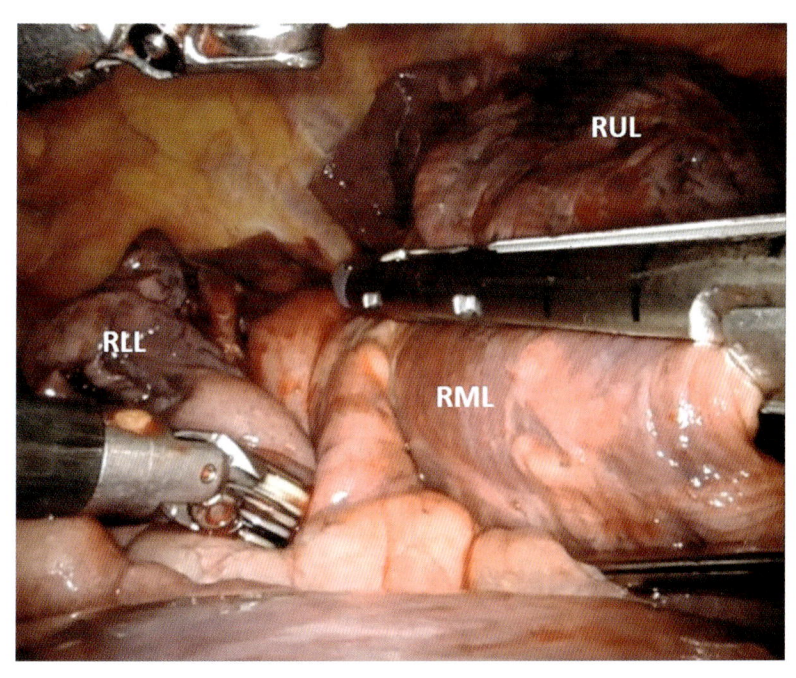

FIGURE 18B-13 • Division of the fissure between the right upper and middle lobes. RUL, right upper lobe; RML, right middle lobe; RLL, right lower lobe.

Left Lower Lobectomy

Patient Positioning, OR Setup, and Port Setting

In left lower lobectomies, patient positioning, OR setup, and port setting remain unchanged when compared to the left upper lobectomies previously described in Chapter 18A (**Figures 18B-14** and **18B-15**).

If necessary, all incisions can be placed 1 intercostal space lower when compared with the upper lobectomy; in particular, the utility incision should be made at the 5th intercostal space instead of the 4th.

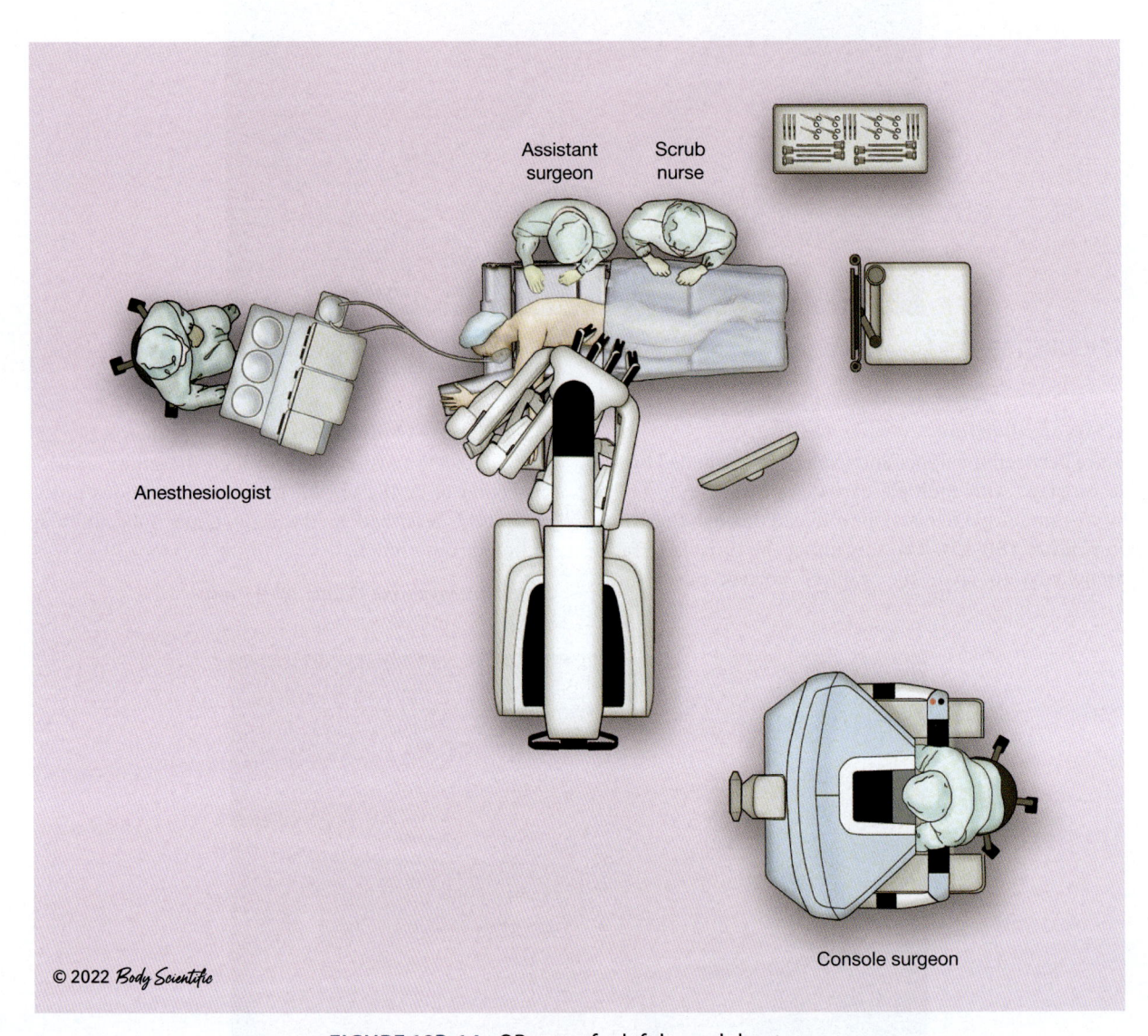

FIGURE 18B-14 • OR setup for left lower lobectomy.

Lung Lower Lobectomies 379

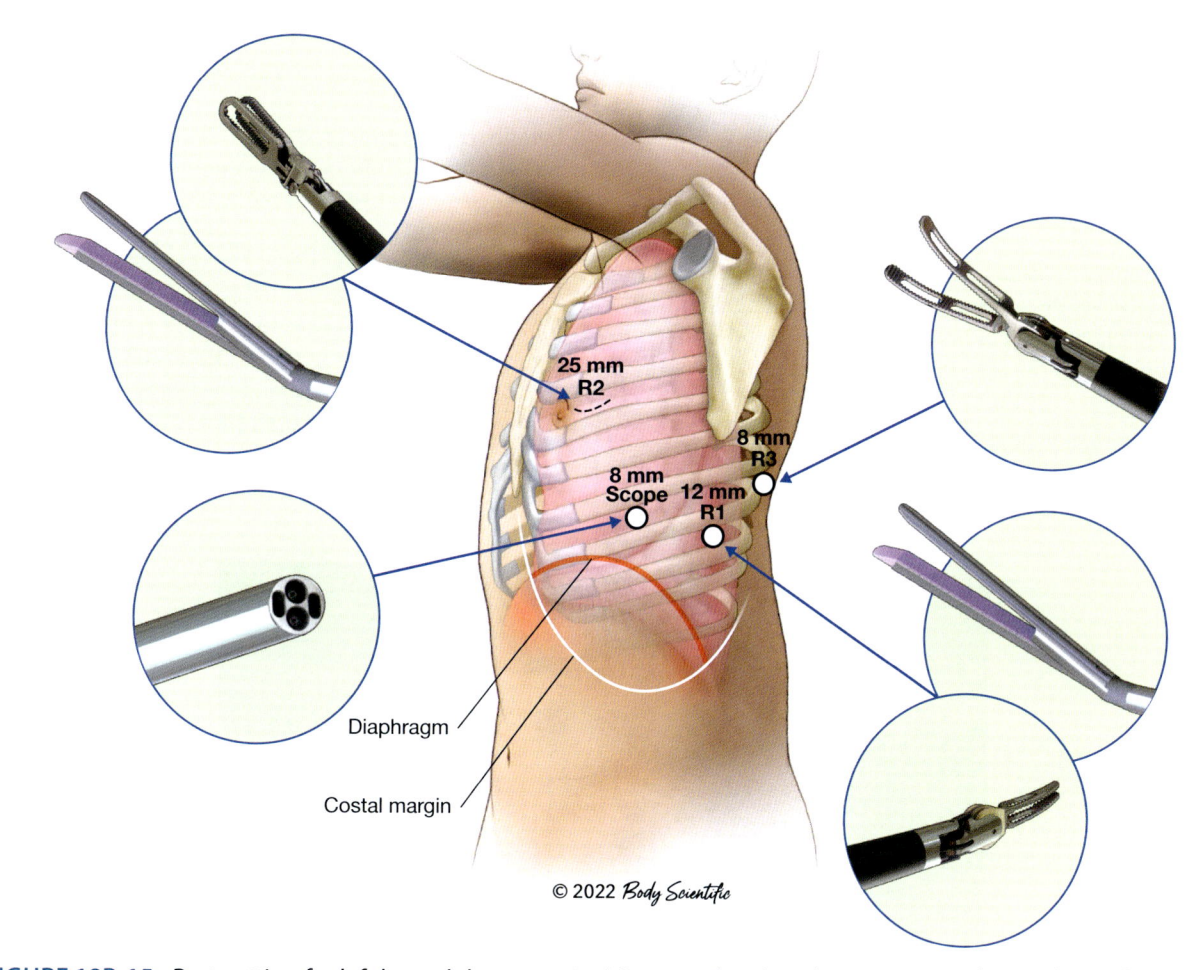

FIGURE 18B-15 • Port setting for left lower lobectomy. Incisions can be placed one intercostal space lower for lower lobectomies.

Left Lower Lobectomy Surgical Technique

Video 18B-3. Operative Technique of a Robotic Left Lower Lobectomy. Four Steps Standardized Technique

Step 1. Dissection of the pulmonary ligament, isolation, and section of the left inferior pulmonary vein

The dissection starts with the takedown of the pulmonary ligament. The lung is retracted upward with the tip-up forceps, while the assistant surgeon retracts the diaphragm downward using a swab inserted through the utility incision, achieving optimal exposure.

The ligament is incised with the long bipolar grasper (a hook or a curved bipolar dissector can also be used) all the way up to the inferior edge of the lower lobe vein.

Once the inferior pulmonary vein is visualized, the hilum is dissected anteriorly to expose and identify the lingula and upper lobe veins and detect the presence of anatomical variations. Once the vein is prepared anteriorly, the lung is moved anteriorly and upward to continue the dissection of the adventitia posteriorly (**Figures 18B-16** and **18B-17 A, B**).

The inferior vein is then isolated, encircled with a vessel loop, and then divided with a 30-mm vascular stapler introduced through the utility incision.

Step 1 average time frame: 15–20 min

> ▶▶ **TIPS**
>
> Lymphadenectomy of stations 8l and 9l is usually performed during pulmonary ligament preparation.

> ▶▶ **TIPS**
>
> The posterior pleura is incised during this step, and station 7 lymphadenectomy can be performed at the beginning of the lobectomy. Sometimes, in early-stage tumors, the station 7 lymphadenectomy can also be performed at the end of the operation, after lobe extraction.

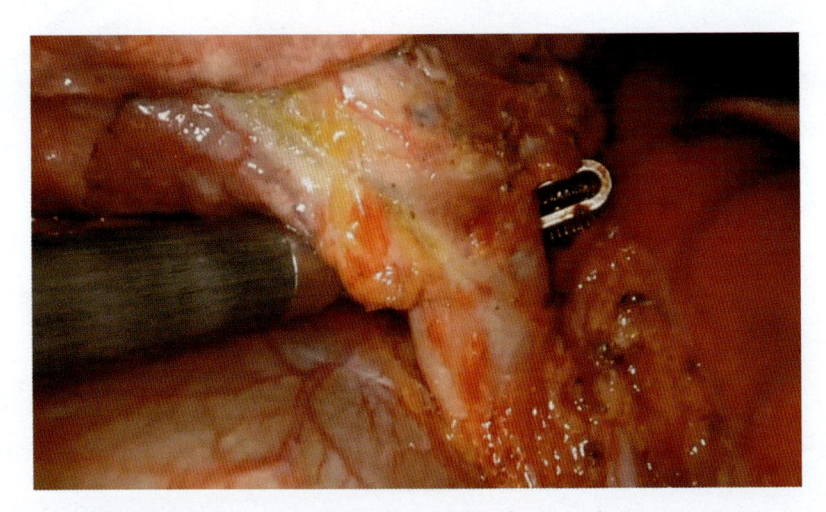

FIGURE 18B-16 • Isolation of the left inferior pulmonary vein.

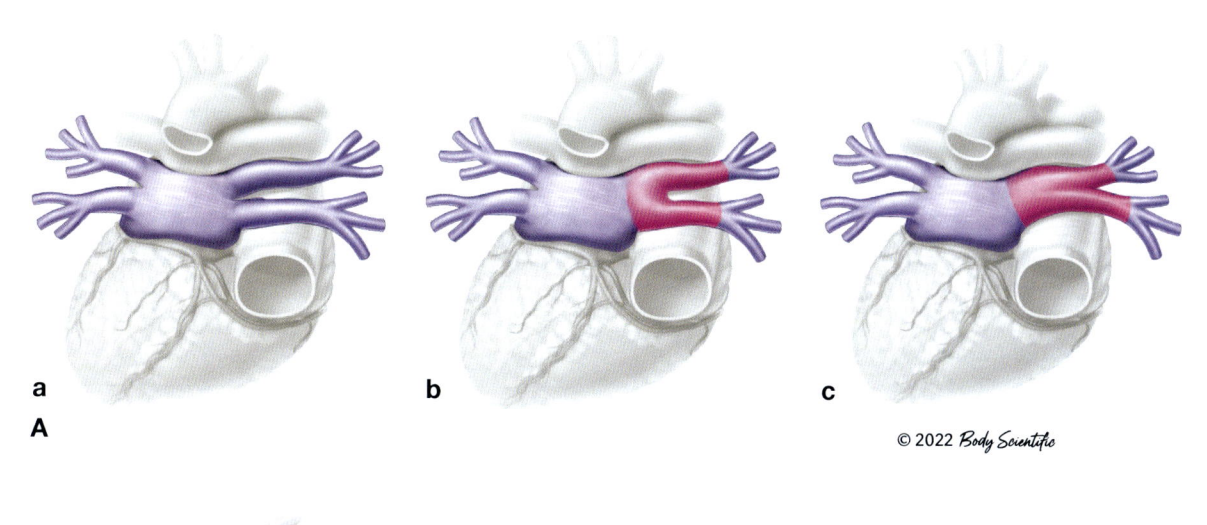

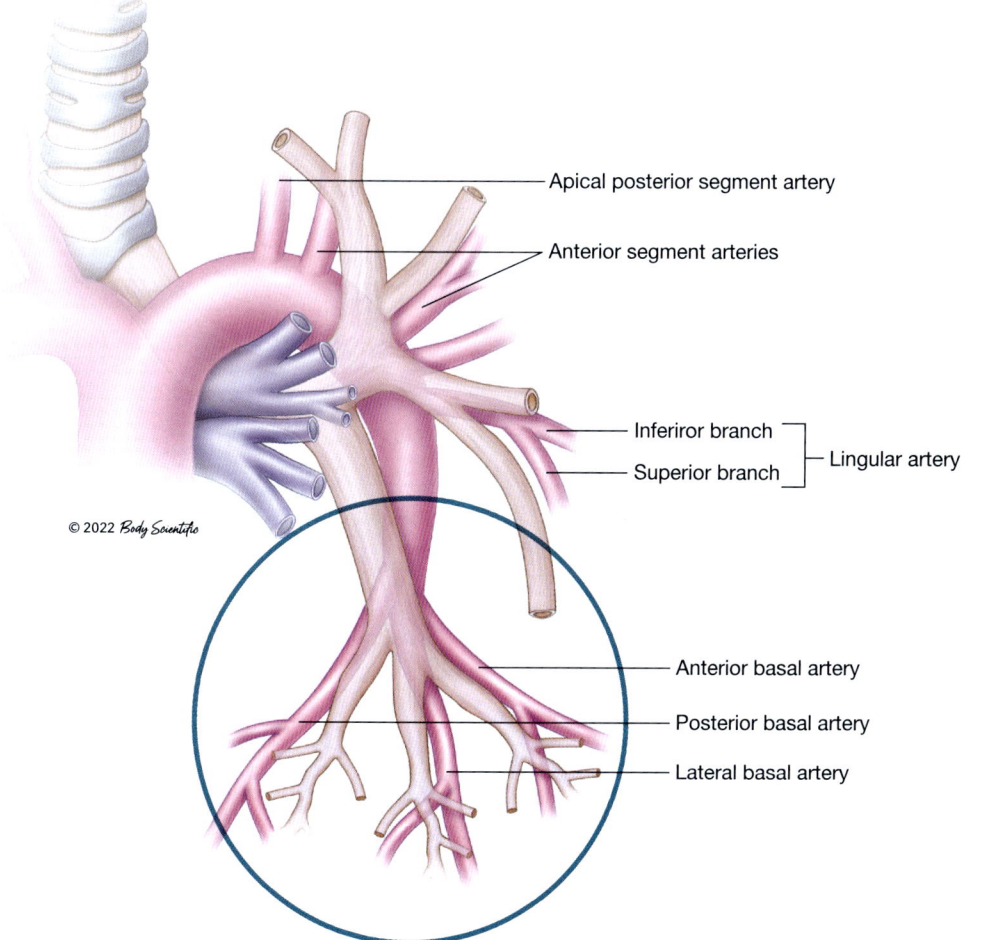

FIGURE 18B-17 • **A.** Normal pulmonary veins and their variation. Normal (a). Short common left trunk (b). Long common left trunk (c). **B.** Left pulmonary arteries.

Step 2. Fissure division and left inferior pulmonary artery isolation

The fissure is now dissected to identify the pulmonary artery (**Figure 18B-18**). Once the artery is visualized, the anterior portion of the oblique fissure is divided. If it consists only of a pleural flap, the long bipolar grasper is used. If lung tissue is present, a parenchymal stapler needs to be used. The interlobar lymph nodes are dissected and removed. This maneuver allows the proper identification of the anterior edge of the basilar trunk. Blunt dissection of the subadventitial plane is then completed to expose the pulmonary artery branch for the upper segment of the lower lobe (segment S6). Both arterial basilar trunk and S6 segmental artery are finally isolated and divided with a 30-mm vascular stapler. This maneuver can also be performed in 2 steps, sectioning the branches individually.

The stapler is usually introduced through the utility incision. Once the artery is divided, it is easy to complete the posterior part of the oblique fissure, in an anterior-to-posterior direction, with a stapler inserted through the utility incision.

Step 2 average time frame: 20–25 min

▶▶ **TIPS**

It is advisable to perform a good interlobar lymphadenectomy to allow better visualization of the artery and bronchus and to avoid leaving residual lymph nodal tissue in the suture line.

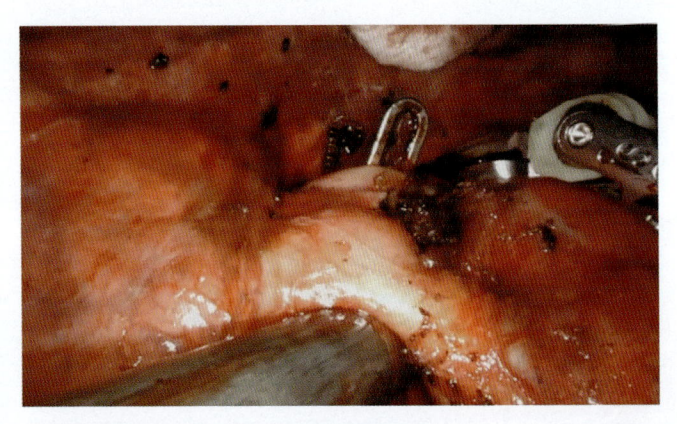

FIGURE 18B-18 • Isolation of the left inferior pulmonary artery.

Step 3. Left lower lobe bronchus isolation and section

The lobe is retracted down and posteriorly with the R3 (tip-up). The bronchus is then divided with a 45-mm curved-tip stapler that should be inserted through the utility incision (**Figure 18B-19**).

The lobe is finally retrieved through the utility incision with an Endobag™.

Step 3 average time frame: 10–15 min

▶▶ **TIPS**

Before dividing the bronchus, while keeping it clamped with the stapler, a ventilation test must be performed to evaluate the correct reexpansion of the upper lobe, especially of the lingula segment.

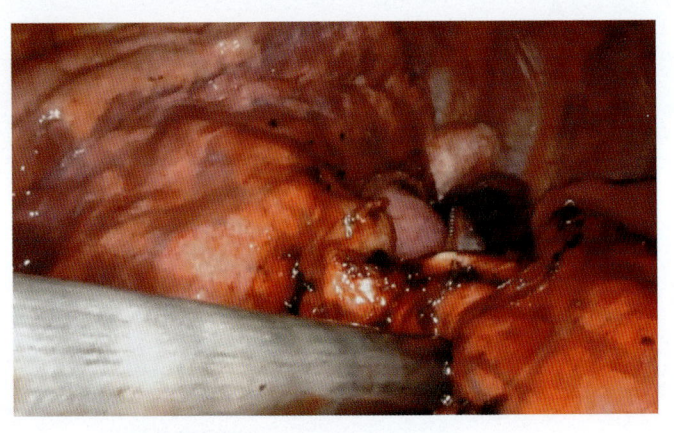

FIGURE 18B-19 • Left lower lobe isolation.

Step 4. Lymph nodal dissection

For left lobectomies, mediastinal lymph nodal stations no. 5, 6, 7, 8L, and 9L are usually removed. Station 5 lymph nodes are removed by retracting the upper lobe inferiorly and posteriorly with the tip-up (R3) to achieve a good exposure of the mediastinum and lung hilum (**Figure 18B-20**). The mediastinal pleura is opened with the long bipolar grasper (R2), and lymph nodes are dissected. For dissection of station 6, the upper lobe is retracted inferiorly and anteriorly with the tip-up (R3).

Stations 8 and 9 are usually removed during the preparation of the pulmonary ligament and dissection of the inferior vein, as previously described (Step 1).

Removing subcarinal lymph nodes (station 7) requires lung retraction anteriorly and superiorly. The posterior pleura is opened from the lower lobe vein stump upward along the course of the vagus nerve to expose the main pulmonary artery. This maneuver facilitates the identification of the target area and allows a correct visualization of the esophagus.

As previously described for other lobectomies, a chest drainage tube with an accessory hole at 10 cm is positioned in incision S.

Step 4 average time frame: 15–30 min

> ⚠ **PITFALLS**
>
> Damage of the left recurrent nerve by improper cauterization during dissection of station 5. The nerve runs in the area, and its damage might cause postoperative dysphonia.

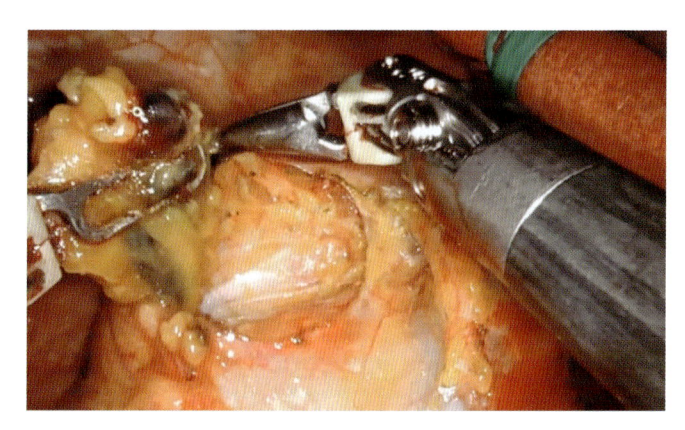

FIGURE 18B-20 • Lymph nodal (station 5) dissection.

Suggested Readings

1. Veronesi G, Novellis P, Voulaz E, Alloisio M. Robot-assisted surgery for lung cancer: state of the art and perspectives. *Lung Cancer.* 2016;101:28-34. doi: 10.1016/j.lungcan.2016.09.004
2. Novellis P, Alloisio M, Cariboni U, Veronesi G. Different techniques in robotic lung resection. *J Thorac Dis.* 2017;9(11):4315-4318. doi: 10.21037/jtd.2017.10.69
3. Cerfolio RJ, Ghanim AF, Dylewski M, et al. The long-term survival of robotic lobectomy for non-small cell lung cancer: a multi-institutional study. *J Thorac Cardiovasc Surg.* 2018;155(2):778-786. doi: 10.1016/j.jtcvs.2017.09.016
4. Park BJ, Melfi F, Mussi A, et al. Robotic lobectomy for non-small cell lung cancer (NSCLC): long-term oncologic results. *J Thorac Cardiovasc Surg.* 2012;143(2):383-389. doi: 10.1016/j.jtcvs.2011.10.055
5. Oh DS, Reddy RM, Gorrepati ML, Mehendale S, Reed MF. Robotic-assisted, video-assisted thoracoscopic and open lobectomy: propensity-matched analysis of recent premier data. *Ann Thorac Surg.* 2017;104(5):1733-1740. doi: 10.1016/j.athoracsur.2017.06.020
6. Gondé H, Laurent M, Gillibert A, et al. The affordability of minimally invasive procedures in major lung resection: a prospective study. *Interact Cardiovasc Thorac Surg.* 2017;25(3):469-475. doi: 10.1093/icvts/ivx149
7. Bendixen M, Jørgensen OD, Kronborg C, Andersen C, Licht PB. Postoperative pain and quality of life after lobectomy via video-assisted thoracoscopic surgery or anterolateral thoracotomy for early stage lung cancer: a randomised controlled trial. *Lancet Oncol.* 2016;17(6):836-844. doi: 10.1016/S1470-2045(16)00173-X
8. Giulianotti PC, Coratti A, Angelini M, et al. Robotics in general surgery: personal experience in a large community hospital. *Arch Surg.* 2003;138(7):777-784. doi: 10.1001/archsurg.138.7.777

SECTION IV

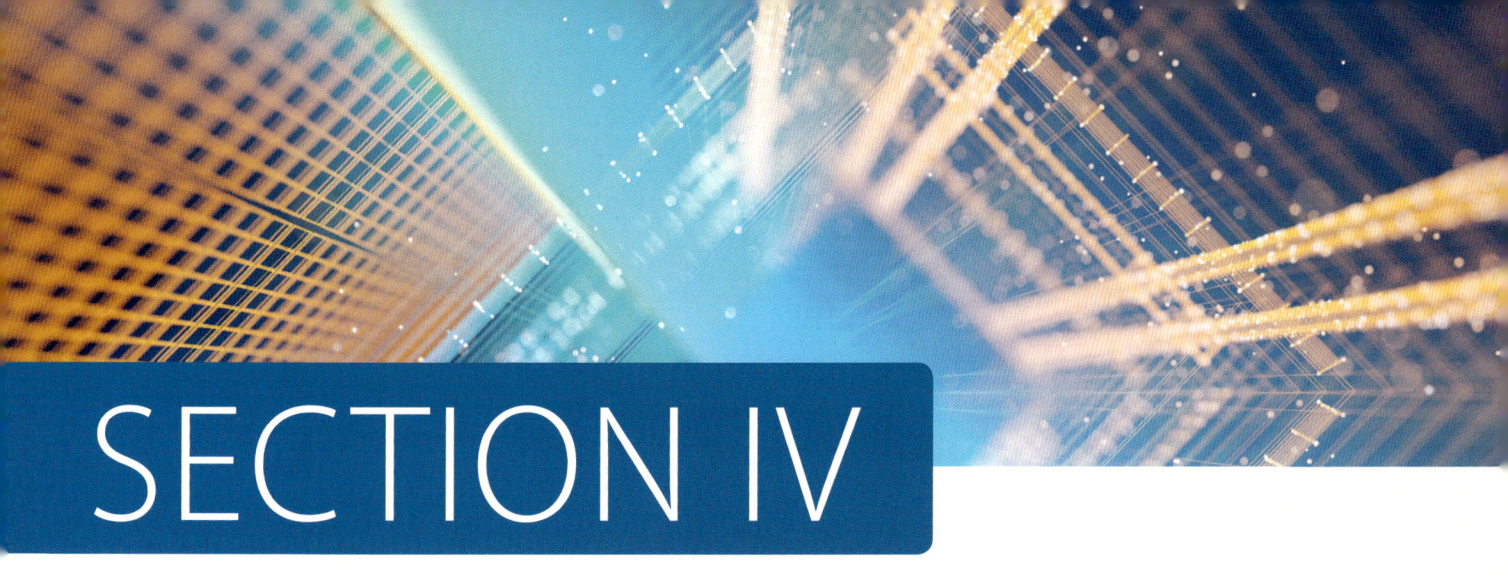

Gastric and Bariatric Surgery

Chapter 19 • D2 Total Gastrectomy 387
Joong Ho Lee • Woo Jin Hyung

Chapter 20 • Sleeve Gastrectomy 407
Chandra Hassan • Alberto Mangano • Yevhen Pavelko

Chapter 21 • Roux-en-Y Gastric Bypass..421
Nicolas Hellmuth Dreifuss • Roberto Bustos • Mario Alberto Masrur

SECTION IV

Gastric and Bariatric Surgery

"Concerning gastric cancer, the MIS, as exeresis surgical tool ... is such a definite and oncological approach as the traditional approach, and superior to this as far as quality of life is concerned."

—Juan Santiago Azagra (1955)

D2 Total Gastrectomy

Joong Ho Lee • Woo Jin Hyung

INTRODUCTION

Because the indications of minimally invasive surgery for gastric cancer are extended, D2 lymph node (LN) dissection is essential for oncologically sound procedures. Robotic total gastrectomy with D2 LN dissection is indicated for advanced gastric cancer of the upper body of the stomach. D2 LN dissection for proximal tumors requires the retrieval of soft tissues around the distal part of splenic vessels and splenic hilum, which contain LNs at stations 11d and 10. Splenic hilar dissection without injury to the spleen is a highly demanding procedure. Nonetheless, the use of magnified 3D views from the robotic system and articulated movements of the robotic arms allow for this complex and challenging procedure to be more easily performed than the laparoscopic approach. Although evidence of the proper indication of robotic surgery is lacking, some experienced surgeons in large-volume centers have shown the feasibility of D2 LN dissection during radical total gastrectomy.

Indications and Relative Contraindications to the Robotic Approach

The indications for robotic gastrectomy for gastric cancer are equivalent to those for laparoscopic surgery. Robotic gastrectomy with limited LN dissection (D1 or D1+) is indicated for cT1N0 cancers that do not meet the criteria for endoscopic procedures. Extended LN dissection (D2) is indicated for the clinically deep submucosal layer, proper muscular infiltration, or deeper invading tumors and for any tumor with a nodal-positive stage. Generally, serosa-involved (cT4a) and more advanced gastric cancers are not appropriate for this type of procedure, but its indication is currently under investigation and the guidelines may change (see **Table 19-1**).

Patient Positioning, OR Setup, and Port Setting

The patient is placed in the supine position with the arms adducted and tucked (unless specific need for anesthesia), and in 30° reverse Trendelenburg (**Figure 19-1**). The assistant

INSTRUMENT REQUIREMENTS

The suggested main robotic instruments/tools can be listed as follows:
- 30° and 0° scope
- Cadière forceps
- Maryland bipolar forceps
- Bipolar forceps
- Permanent cautery monopolar hook/monopolar curved scissors
- Needle drivers (round tip or macro)
- Harmonic shears/vessel sealer
- Clip applier
- Robotic linear stapler and 45-mm loads (optional)

The suggested main laparoscopic instruments/tools can be listed as follows:
- Atraumatic graspers
- Scissors
- Needle drivers
- Suction-irrigation
- Laparoscopic linear stapler and 45-mm loads

Supplemental materials:
- Gauzes, sponges
- Sutures: PDS™ 3-0, 4-0 and Prolene™ 3-0, 4-0
- Hem-o-lok™ clips
- Endobag™

Photo reproduced with permission from Dr. Juan Santiago Azagra.

Quote reproduced with permission from Azagra JS, Goergen M, Lens V, et al. Present state of the mini-invasive surgery (MIS) in esophageal and gastric cancer. Clin Transl Oncol. 2006;8(3):173-177.

The Foundation and Art of Robotic Surgery

TABLE 19-1 • Indications and Contraindications for Robotic Gastrectomy
Indications for robotic gastrectomy requiring D2 LN dissection
T1N1M0, cT2N0/N1M0, cT3N0/N1/N2M0
Expanded indication for robotic gastrectomy requiring D2 LN dissection
Equivocal serosa-positive tumors
Contraindications to robotic gastrectomy
Extensive lymphadenopathy
Definitive serosa-positive tumors
cT4b or distant metastasis

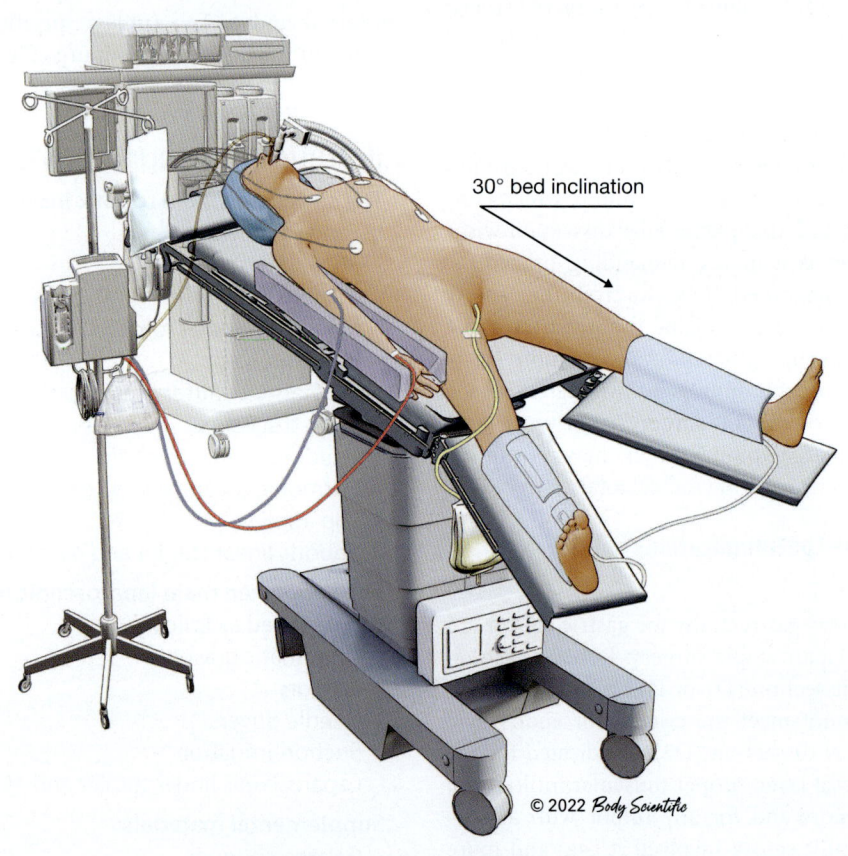

FIGURE 19-1 • Patient positioning.

stands between the patient's legs and the surgical cart is located on the patient's left shoulder (**Figure 19-2**).

> **EDITORIAL COMMENT**
>
> This position is mandatory for the da Vinci® Si™ system. With the Xi™ system, the cart can be set from different directions.

Five ports, including the assistant's port, are used in standard robotic gastrectomy. An 8-mm port is used for camera installation just below the umbilicus with an open technique. After a CO_2 pneumoperitoneum of 12 mm Hg is achieved, the operating table is placed in the 30° reverse Trendelenburg position to lower the transverse colon and small intestine by gravity. After determining the optimal location of the port sites, 4 additional ports are inserted using camera visualization

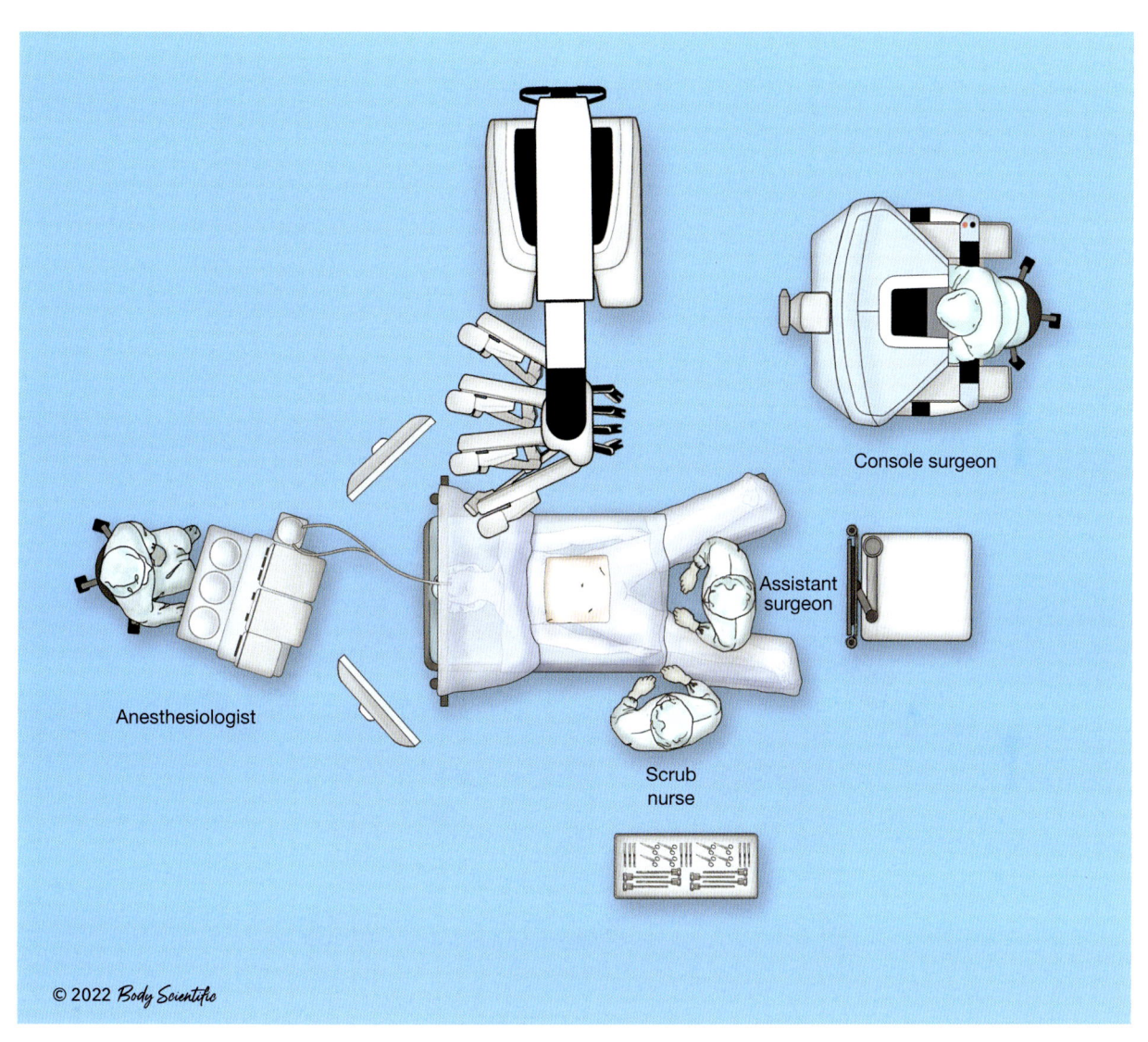

FIGURE 19-2 • OR setup.

(**Figures 19-3 A, B**). Specifically, two 8-mm ports for both lateral robotic arms are placed approximately 1 cm below the costal angle, bilaterally as far laterally as possible. The last 8-mm port for the right second arm is inserted 2–4 cm above an imaginary line intersecting the middle of the camera port and right subcostal port. This step allows easier access to the pancreatic head and duodenum and facilitates a proper angle to use the ultrasonic shears. Next, a 12-mm assistant trocar is placed 1–2 cm below an imaginary line drawn from the insertion site of the left lateral arm to the umbilical port.

> **EDITORIAL COMMENT**
>
> The port setting should be adapted taking into consideration the body habitus. In Western countries, where the overweight population is prevailing, the umbilicus is not a good site to achieve a perfect visualization of the pericardial and perisplenic areas. The port line is usually moved a few centimeters above the transverse umbilical line.

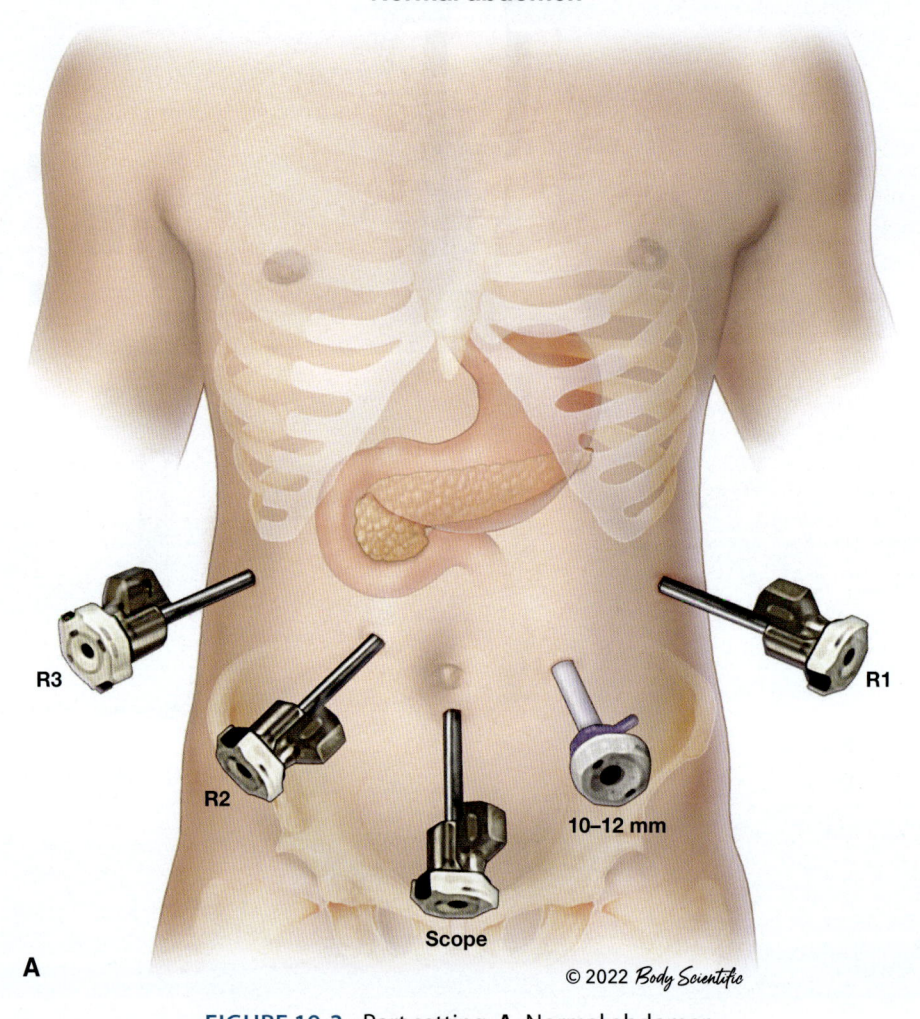

FIGURE 19-3 • Port setting. **A.** Normal abdomen.

Wide abdomen

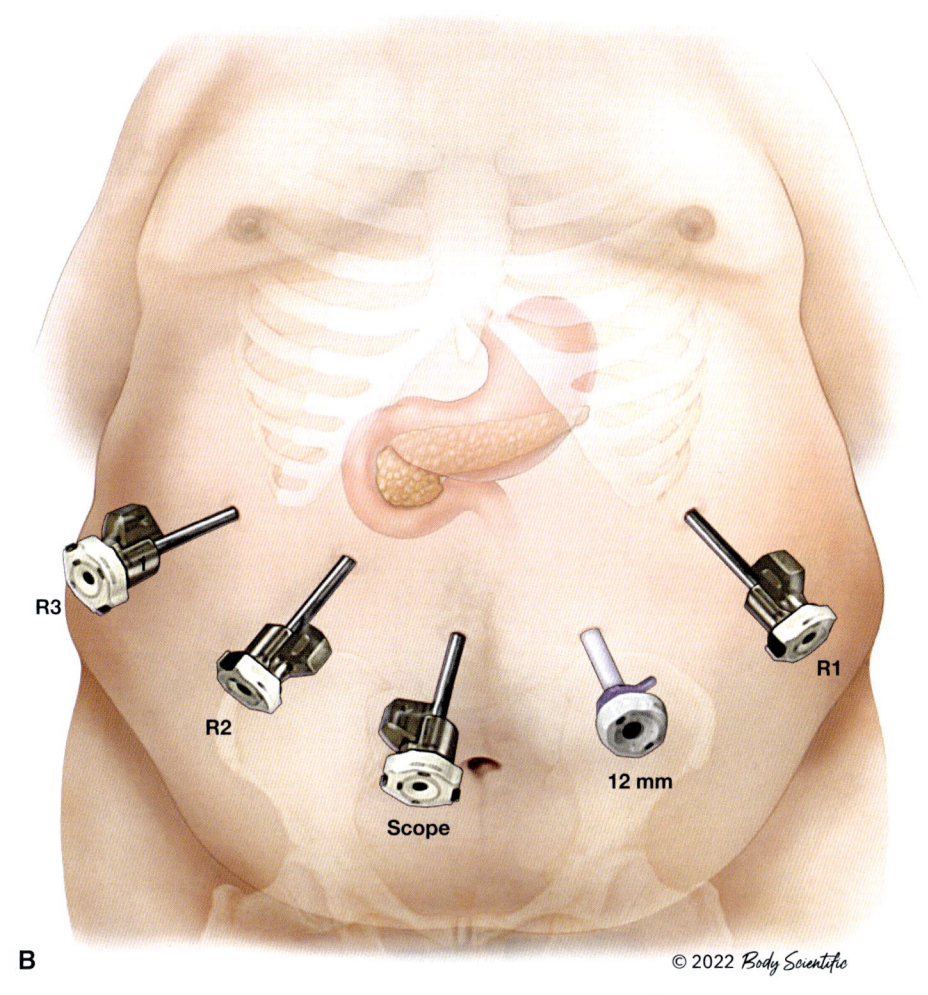

FIGURE 19-3 • (*Continued*) **B.** Wide abdomen.

After completing insertion of the ports, the surgical cart is brought to the operating table to dock the robotic arms. The R1 arm mainly holds Maryland bipolar forceps. The Cadière forceps, whose main function is traction, is inserted through the R3. The R2 interchangeably holds energy devices (ultrasonic shears or monopolar scissors) and Cadière forceps (**Figure 19-4**).

> ▶▶ **TIPS**
>
> When deciding the best location of the ports, the surgical bed should be preliminarily adjusted into the 30° reverse Trendelenburg position in order to make a correct evaluation of the distances.

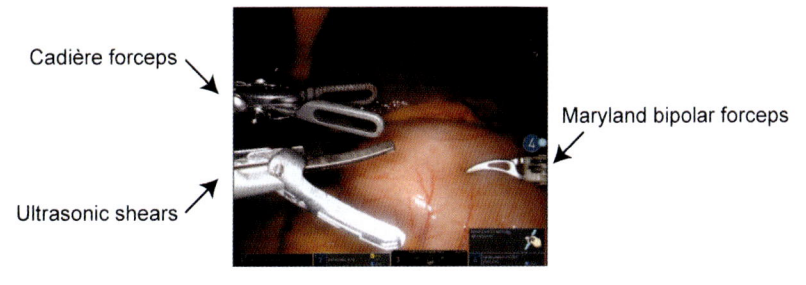

FIGURE 19-4 • Console view of the instruments.

Surgical Technique

▶ **Video 19-1. D2 Total Gastrectomy**

Step 1. General laparoscopic exploration and liver retraction
After completing a comprehensive exploration of the peritoneal cavity, the operation begins with the liver retraction, utilizing a suture and a gauze pad as a "sling." Pushing the liver upward with a Cadière forceps in the right robotic arm exposes the hepatogastric ligament. The *pars flaccida* is divided up to the right side of the esophageal hiatus using an ultrasonic shear in R2. Puncture of the abdominal wall on both sides of the falciform ligament and subcostal margin is performed using a straight needle with thread. The midportion of the thread is anchored to the *pars condensa* with 2 Hem-o-lok™ clips. The V-shaped thread effectively retracts the liver upward (**Figures 19-5 A, B**).

Step 1 average time frame: 3–5 min

> **EDITORIAL COMMENT**
>
> There are other ways to retract the liver effectively and safely. Mainly in obese patients, the liver could be bulky and fatty obscuring the hiatus. The R3 positioned in the lateral right side can be very effective not only to retract the stomach in some steps but also the liver, generally holding a sponge. Another effective way, very common in bariatric surgery, is to use a Nathanson device.

A   **B**

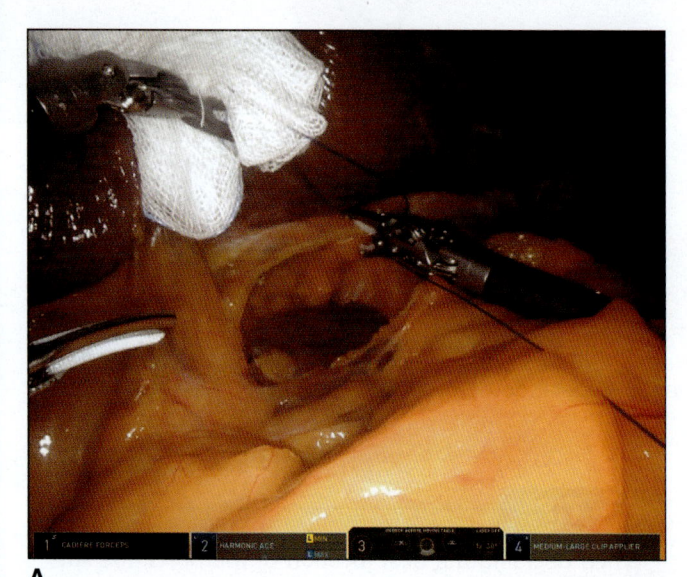

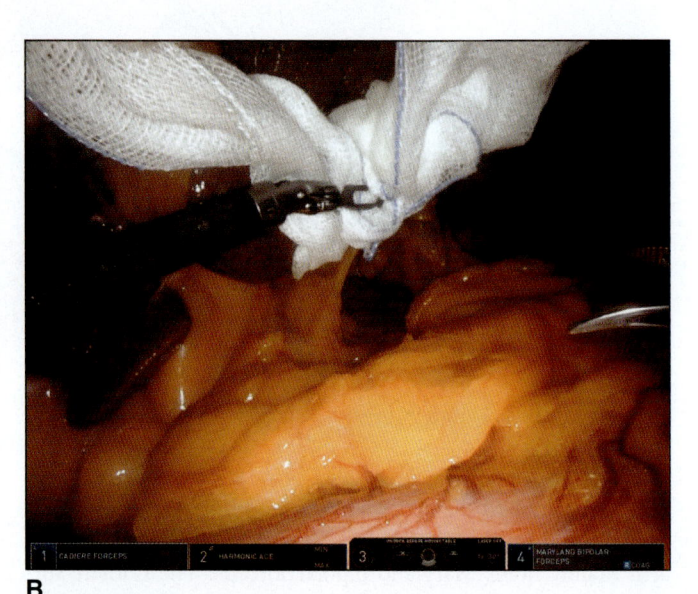

FIGURE 19-5 • Liver retraction.

Step 2. Omentectomy

D2 dissection with total omentectomy is a mandatory procedure for advanced gastric cancers, although the oncological role of total omentectomy remains uncertain for serosa-negative advanced gastric cancers. Robotic total omentectomy is performed using the same procedure as that for open and laparoscopic gastrectomy. Cadière forceps grasp the soft tissues along the greater curvature of the midbody of the stomach and pull them to the anterior abdominal wall. The assistant grasps the transverse colon using an atraumatic grasper to ensure a secure dissection plane. Division of the greater omentum from the transverse colon along the avascular plane using ultrasonic shears is initiated from the midportion of the transverse colon.

The greater omentum is further divided toward the lower pole of the spleen (**Figures 19-7 A, B**). To facilitate the best exposure of the lesser sac, proper repositioning of the omentum by Maryland and Cadière forceps and countertraction of the transverse colon by grasping in the assistant port are essential. The left gastroepiploic vessels are carefully identified and isolated at their roots and ligated using clips to clear LN number 4sb. Next, soft tissue along the surface of the spleen is cleared and short gastric vessels are ligated, which contain LN number 4sb and part of 4sa.

Step 2 average time frame: 15–25 min

> **ANATOMICAL HIGHLIGHTS**
> Anatomy of the omentum (**Figure 19-6**).

> **TIPS**
> When the omentectomy is difficult for adhesions, one trick is to open the gastrocolic ligament. The assistant, using a sponge with the laparoscopic forceps, can enter into the lesser sac and push down the mesentery of the colon applying some tension to it. These divergent actions help in maintaining the correct plane of dissection.

> **PITFALLS**
> While doing the left side omentectomy, there is risk of entering into a wrong plane of the transverse colon mesentery. This risk is higher when there are adhesions between the omentum, the transverse mesocolon, and the pancreatic body and tail.

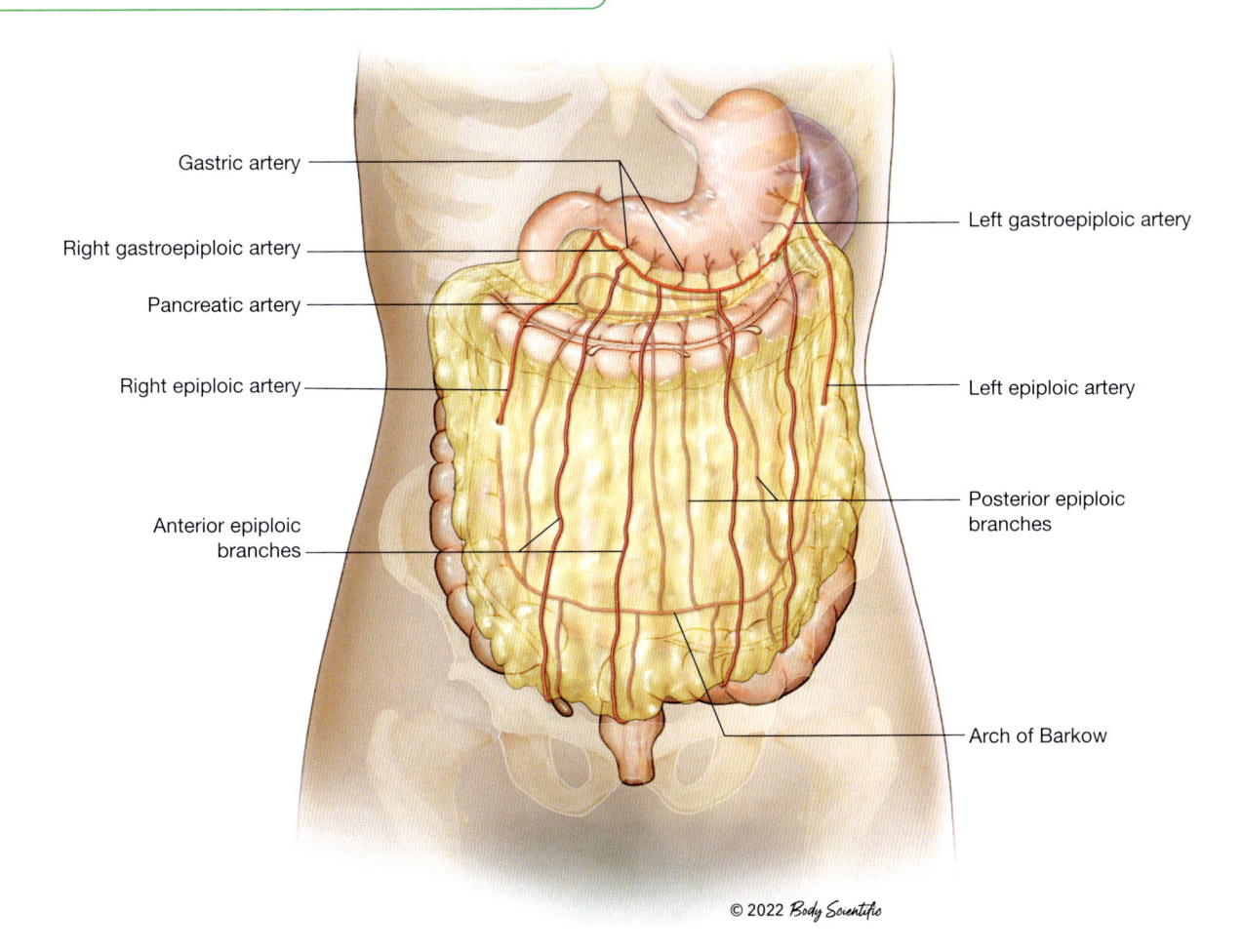

FIGURE 19-6 • Anatomy of the omentum.

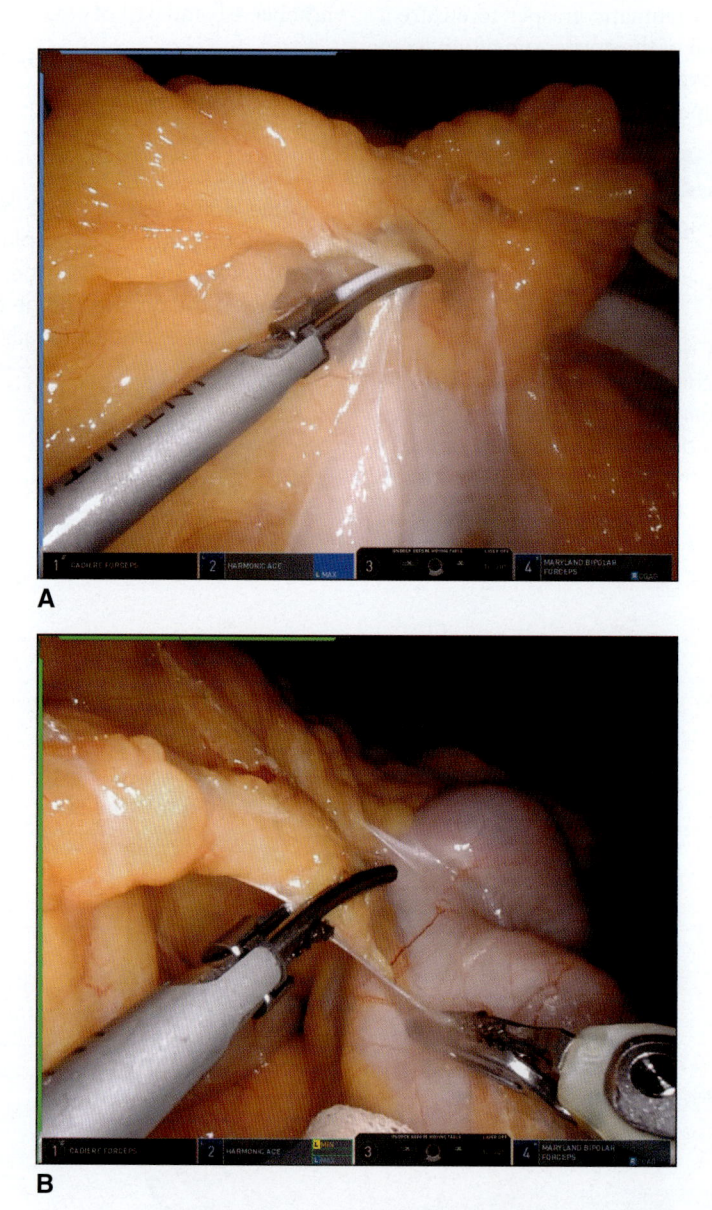

FIGURE 19-7 • Total omentectomy.

Step 3. Dissection of the gastrosplenic ligament with division of the short gastric vessels (LN 4sa) and retrieval of the left paracardial lymph nodes (LN 2)

After division of the left gastroepiploic vessels at their roots, the gastrosplenic ligament is separated by dividing the short gastric vessels along the surface of the spleen. Dissection of the gastrosplenic ligament should be initiated from the adhesions between the lower pole of the spleen and omentum to prevent potential bleeding due to tearing of the splenic capsule. Cadière forceps in the right robotic arm are used to grasp the soft tissues along the greater curvature of the fundus and pull them the cephalad, toward the anterior abdominal wall, to expose the gastrosplenic ligament.

After division of the short gastric vessels at their roots, the esophagophrenic ligament is divided to mobilize the esophagus (**Figure 19-11**). Retroperitoneal attachment of the posterior wall of the upper stomach is detached up to the diaphragmatic crura. The branches of the left subphrenic vessels are identified and ligated (**Figure 19-12**). During this process, injury of the upper pole of the spleen should be avoided, being very careful in dissecting the adhesions of the posterior peritoneum, which is difficult to visualize.

Step 3 average time frame: 10–12 min

> **ANATOMICAL HIGHLIGHTS**
> Gastric arterial supply (**Figure 19-8**)
> Gastric venous drainage (**Figure 19-9**)
> Lymph node stations (**Figures 19-10 A–C**) (see suggested reading #14)

> ▶▶ **TIPS**
> The adhesions between the posterior stomach and the anterior surface of the pancreas should all be released to enhance exposure of the surgical planes around the gastrosplenic ligament.

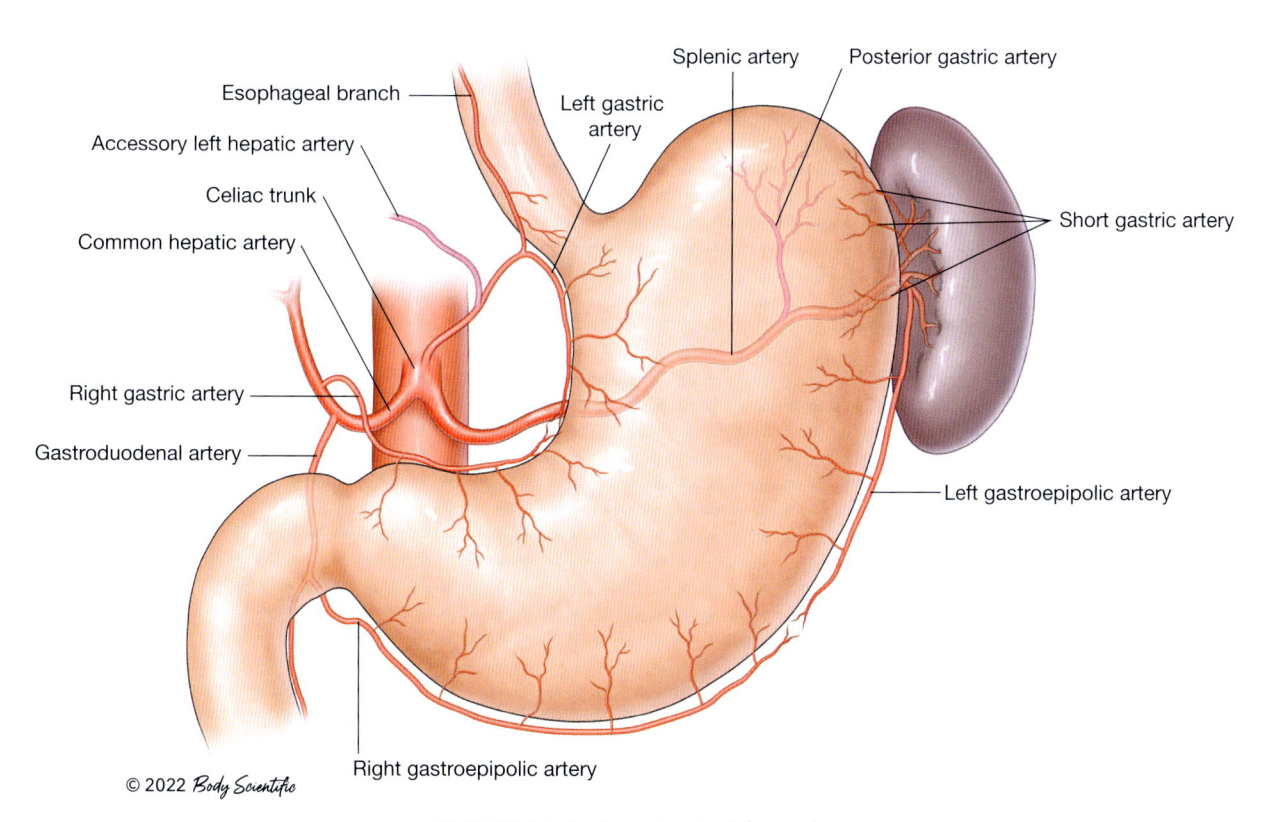

FIGURE 19-8 • Gastric arterial supply.

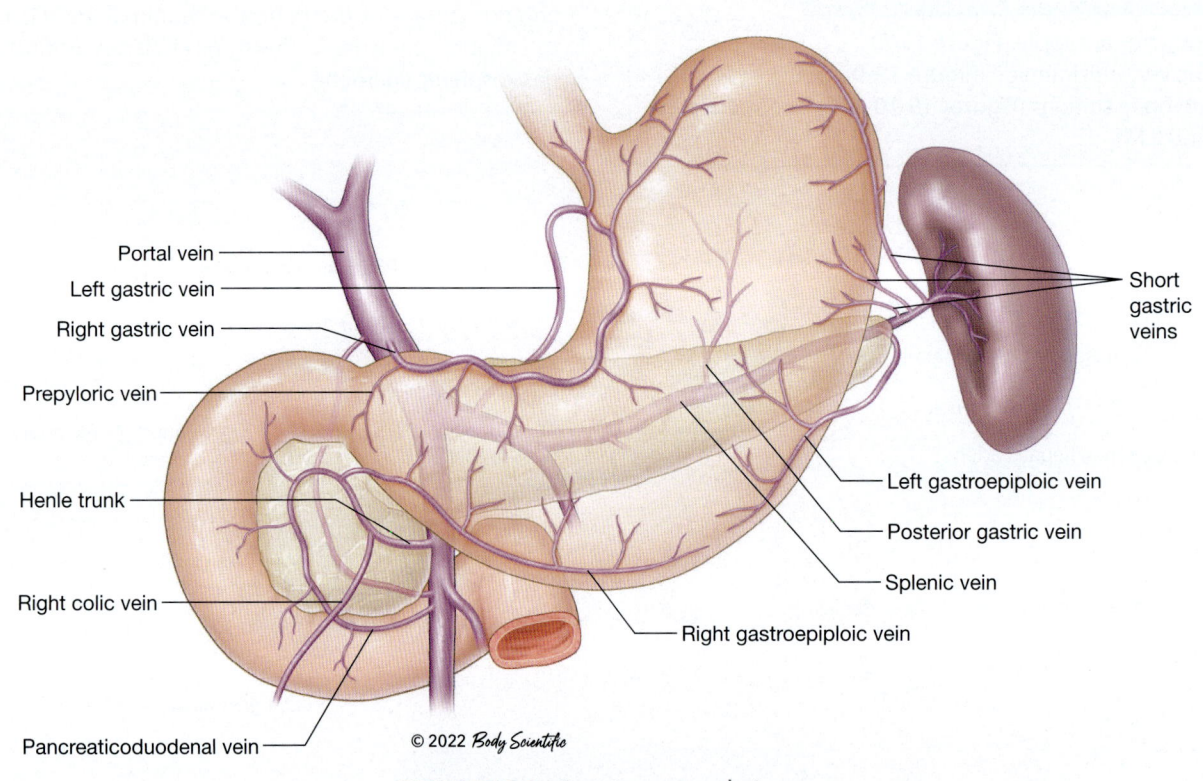

FIGURE 19-9 • Gastric venous drainage.

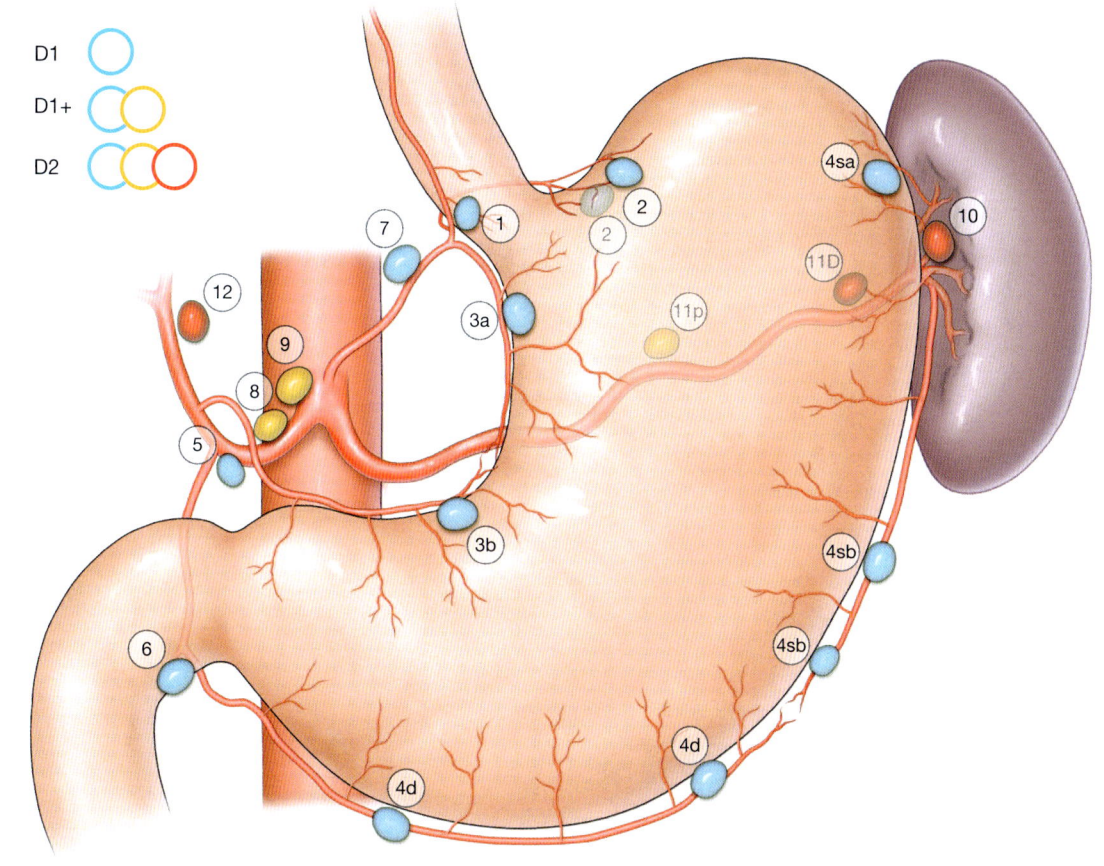

D2 Total Gastrectomy   397

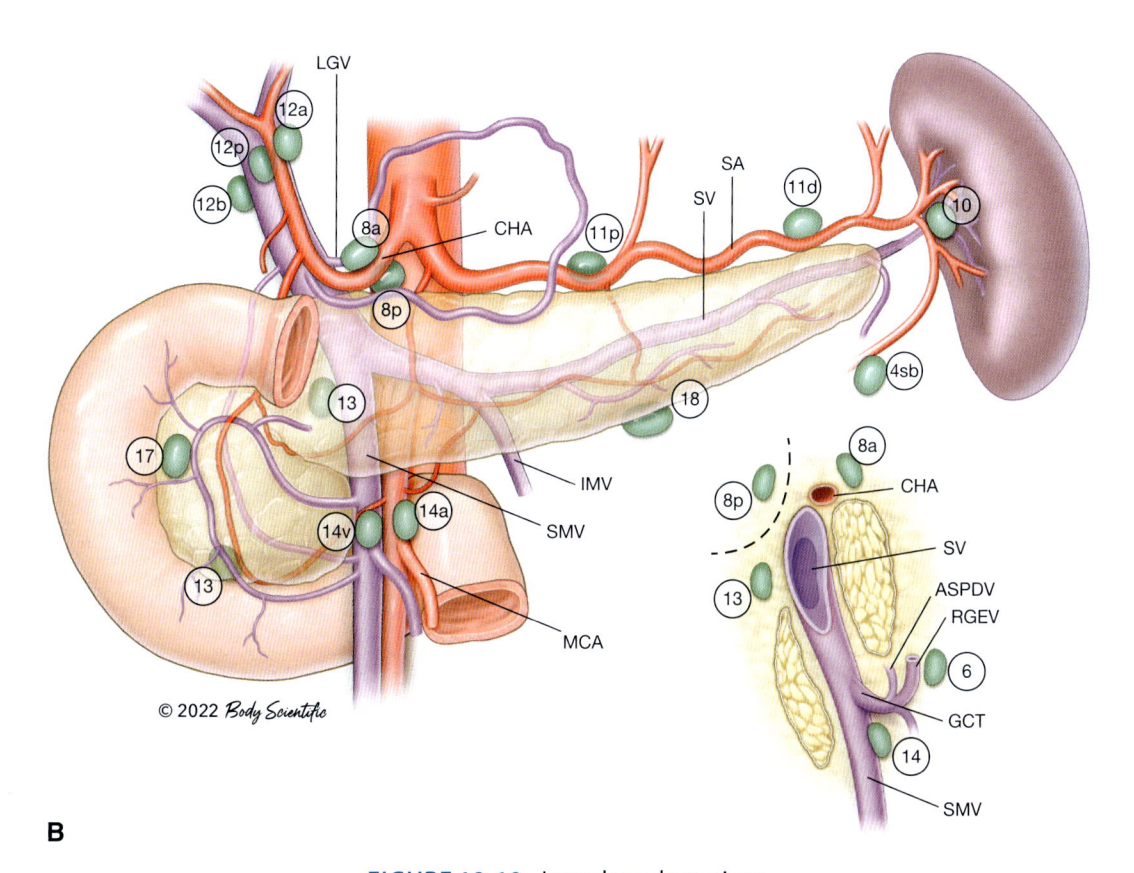

FIGURE 19-10 • Lymph node stations.

398 The Foundation and Art of Robotic Surgery

Left inferior phrenic artery

C

© 2022 Body Scientific

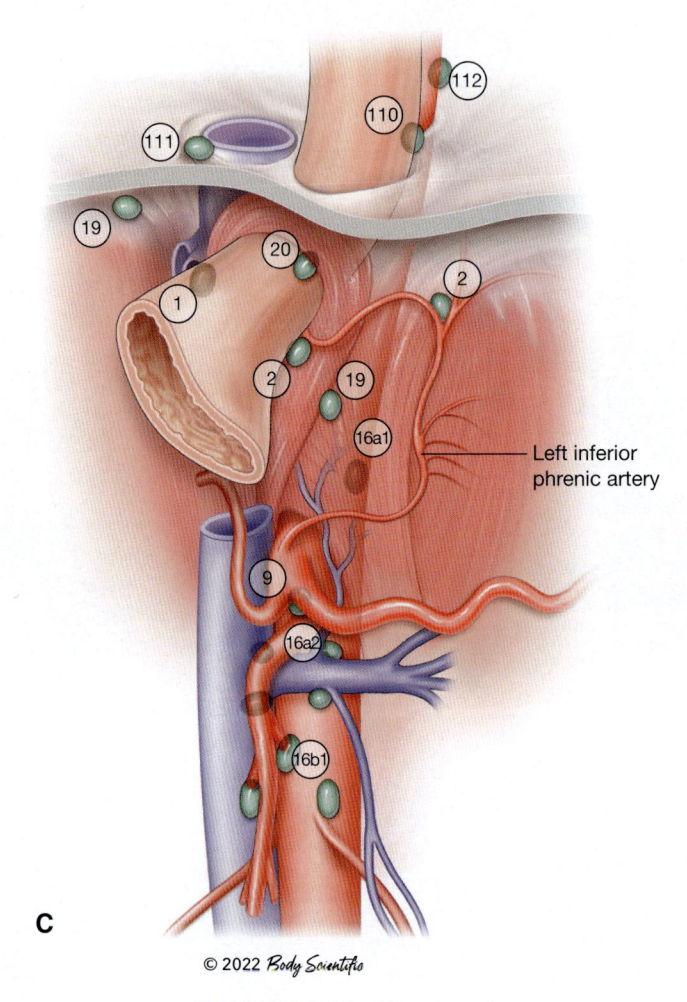

FIGURE 19-10 • (Continued)

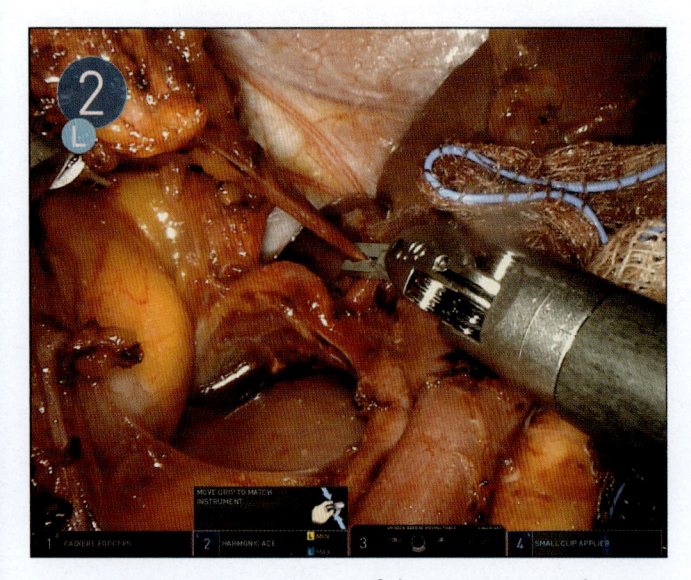

FIGURE 19-11 • Ligation of short gastric vessels.

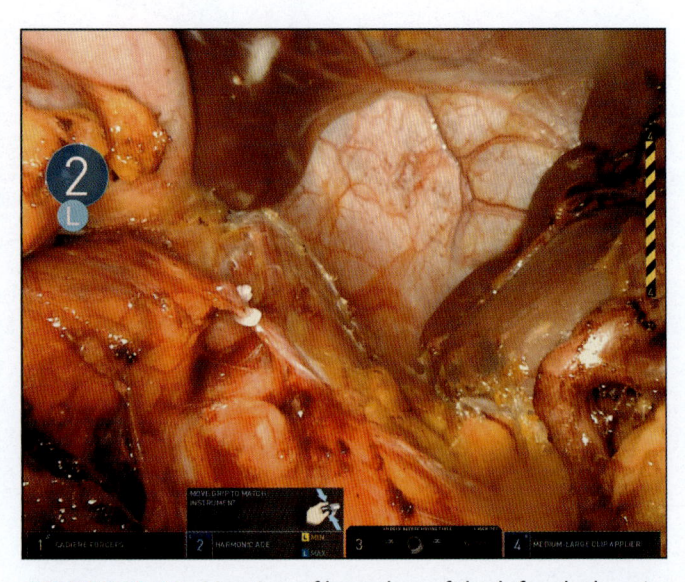

FIGURE 19-12 • Ligation of branches of the left subphrenic vessels.

▶ **Video 19-2. Splenic Hilum–Near infra-red (NIR)**

Step 4. Dissection of the splenic hilum (LN 10)

Splenic hilar lymphadenectomy is necessary for curative total gastrectomy in proximal gastric cancer, especially for advanced tumors. Currently, splenectomy is not recommended for total gastrectomy with D2 lymphadenectomy to prevent additional morbidity. Spleen-preserving splenic hilum lymph node dissection is a highly demanding and time-consuming procedure. The robotic approach could make the performance of splenic hilum lymphadenectomy easier, when compared to laparoscopy.

When dissecting the splenic hilum, there is no need to mobilize the spleen. This maneuver paradoxically can make the exposure of the hilum more difficult because the natural gravitational countertraction is lost. To fully expose the splenic hilar area to remove the LNs at numbers 10 and 11d, the posterior wall of the upper stomach is retracted cephalad using a Cadière forceps in R3. The tail of the pancreas is retracted caudally by the assistant using an atraumatic grasper with gentle pressure.

The proximal splenic vessels are exposed and dissection of suprapancreatic soft tissues continues to the splenic hilum with removal of the LN station 11d. During dissection, soft tissues at the surface of the terminal branches of the splenic vessels are gently lifted ventrally using Maryland bipolar forceps, while the ultrasonic shears are used to dissect the tissues around the terminal branches of the splenic vessels. When dissecting soft tissues behind the splenic vessels, Maryland bipolar forceps are first used to create proper angles in front of the Gerota's fascia, prior to dissecting with ultrasonic shears. Sometimes, nerve fibers around the arteries are gently grasped and retracted to rotate and expose the dorsal side of the vessels. All vessels in the splenic hilum are saved to preserve the spleen.

Step 4 average time frame: 30–40 min

> ▶▶ **TIPS**
>
> To increase the safety of the procedure, surgeons should carefully preoperatively evaluate the splenic vascular anatomy.

▶ **Video 19-3. Infrapyloric Dissection–NIR**

Step 5. Infrapyloric dissection and ligation of the right gastroepiploic vessels (LN 6)

After completing dissection on the left side of the stomach, division of the greater omentum is continued distally toward the pylorus. The distal stomach is retracted ventrally using Cadière forceps. The right side of the omentum is divided along the transverse colon toward the hepatic flexure. The physiological adhesions between the transverse colon and the descending part of duodenum should also be released.

After right side omentectomy, ligation of the right gastroepiploic artery and completion of infrapyloric dissection (LN 6) are performed. To complete the infrapyloric dissection, mobilization of the gastroepiploic pedicle ventrally from the head of the pancreas is facilitated using Cadière forceps. Soft tissues around the right gastroepiploic vessels, as well as soft tissues anterior to the pancreas head, should be dissected using ultrasonic shears and Maryland bipolar forceps until the pancreatic parenchyma is exposed. The right gastroepiploic artery can be identified at the end of the gastroduodenal artery (GDA) and ligated at the root with dissected soft tissues containing LN number 6. Continued dissection will facilitate identification of the infrapyloric artery in most cases, which should be isolated and ligated. The attachment between the posterior wall of the duodenum and the pancreas can be cleared up to the root of the GDA.

Step 5 average time frame: 25–35 min

> ▶▶ **TIPS**
>
> Before performing infrapyloric dissection, physiological adhesions between the posterior wall of the stomach and pancreas should be fully dissected to expose the inferior pancreatic border, which is very helpful in identifying and correctly maintaining the dissection planes.

▶ Video 19-4. Suprapyloric Dissection

Step 6. Suprapyloric dissection and duodenal transection
The duodenum is mobilized from the pancreas along the GDA to prepare for duodenal transection. At this time, the assistant surgeon could retract the distal stomach downward to facilitate better exposure. Soft tissues and supraduodenal vessels are divided by ultrasonic shears just above the pylorus to the bulb of duodenum to make a path for a stapler. Then, the duodenum is stapled and divided about 1–2 cm distal to the pylorus using a 45-mm endoscopic linear stapler through the assistant port, before ligation of the right gastric artery.

Step 6 average time frame: 3–5 min

> ▶▶ **TIPS**
>
> To prevent undesired injury to the common hepatic artery or pancreatic parenchyma during suprapyloric dissection, a gauze should be inserted in the space between the posterior duodenum and the head of the pancreas.

▶ Video 19-5. Right Gastric Artery

Step 7. Ligation of the right gastric artery (LN 5, 12a)
After dividing the duodenum, the stomach is retracted to the patient's left side to identify the right gastric vessels. The right gastric vessels are retracted to the patient's left side using a Cadière forceps in R3 to generate proper tension on the vessels. Dissection is continued along the proper hepatic artery (PHA) until the right gastric vessels are exposed. The right gastric vessels are divided at the root, and LN number 5 is dissected. By dissecting anteriorly and medially to the PHA, LN number 12a is cleared. Complete dissection of LN number 12a is ensured by exposing the portal vein. At this time, the assistant surgeon can retract the common hepatic artery (CHA) inferiorly through a vessel loop, or the PHA toward the patient's right to facilitate better exposure.

Step 7 average time frame: 5–10 min

▶ Video 19-6. Ligation of the Left Gastric Artery and Dissection of the Proximal Splenic Artery

Step 8. Suprapancreatic dissection
After ligation of the right gastric artery, soft tissues around the CHA, which contain LN number 8a, are cleared. The left gastric vessel pedicle is retracted ventrally using Cadière forceps in R3 to expose the lesser curvature and the left gastric vein. The left gastric vein should be identified and securely ligated at the point where it drains into the portal or splenic vein. To continue the retroperitoneal dissection, soft tissues along the left gastric artery, celiac axis, and splenic vessels are removed, which are designated as LN numbers 7, 9, and 11p, respectively. Continued dissection of soft tissues toward the celiac trunk facilitates retrieval of LN number 9. Once the midpoint of the splenic or posterior gastric vessels is reached, the dissection of LN number 11p is complete.

Step 8 average time frame: 12–15 min

Video 19-7. Dissection of the Distal Portion of the Splenic Artery (LN 11d)

Step 9. Dissection of the distal portion of the splenic artery (LN 11d)

After ligation of the left gastric artery and retroperitoneal dissection around the upper body of the stomach, the distal portions of the splenic artery and splenic hilum are well-exposed. After moving the stomach to the left upper quadrant using Cadière forceps in R3, the anterior and superior surfaces of the splenic artery are skeletonized. As the soft tissue is lifted away from the artery, superior dissection helps with exposing the anterior surface of the splenic vein.

Step 9 average time frame: 2–3 min

> ### ▶▶ TIPS
>
> **NIR fluorescent imaging for gastric cancer surgery (see Chapter 7, Fluorescence Imaging: Basics and Clinical Applications):**
>
> NIR fluorescent imaging after peritumoral injection of indocyanine green (ICG) has enabled surgeons to effectively visualize lymphatic anatomy. Fluorescent lymphography using NIR imaging is useful in identifying and retrieving LNs for more thorough intraoperative lymphadenectomy. The peritumoral injection of ICG at the appropriate time before surgery enables visualization of every draining LN from the primary tumor imaged by NIR imaging (**Figures 19-13 A–D**).
>
> The ICG solution is prepared at a concentration of 1.25 mg/mL. One day before surgery, 0.6 mL of the ICG solution is injected into the submucosal layer in 4 points around the primary tumor. The total amount of injected ICG solution is 2.4 mL (3 mg). NIR fluorescent imaging before LN dissection can distinguish between lymphatics and normal tissue, thus avoiding normal tissue injury. NIR imaging after lymphadenectomy can help evaluate the completeness of LN dissection in real time, thus enabling improved surgical quality of the D2 lymphadenectomy.

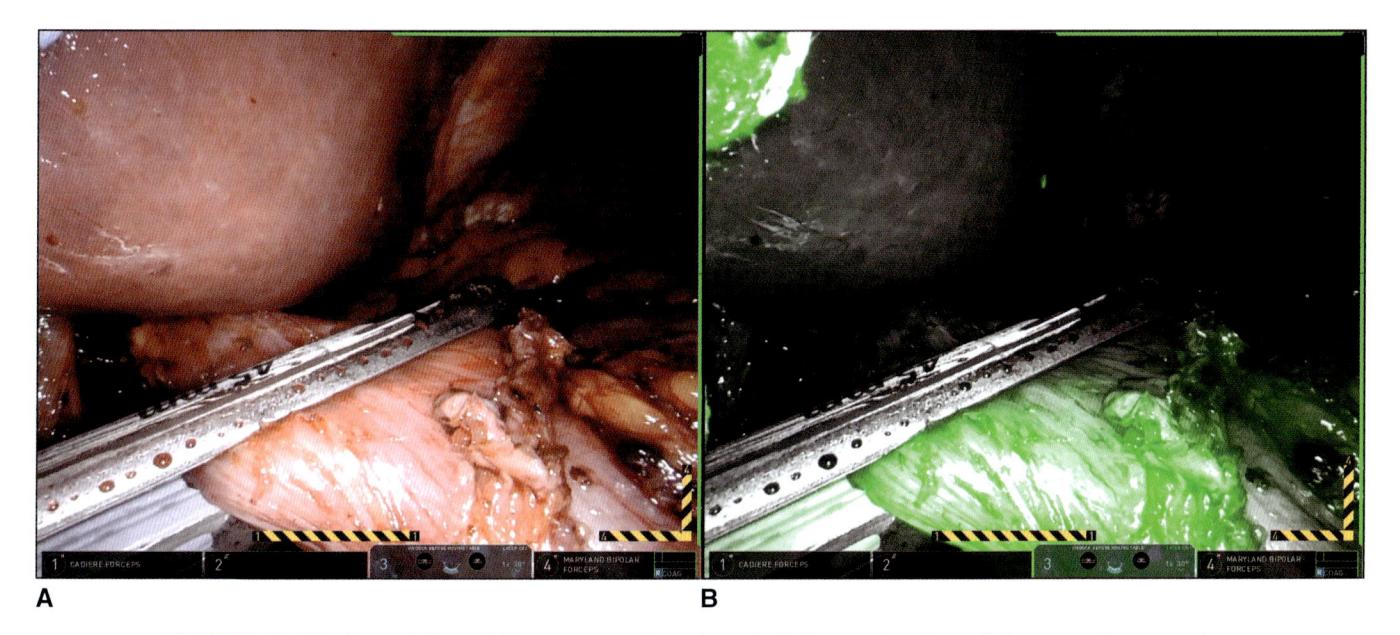

FIGURE 19-13 • Near-infrared fluorescence imaging. A, B. Determination of the resection margin.

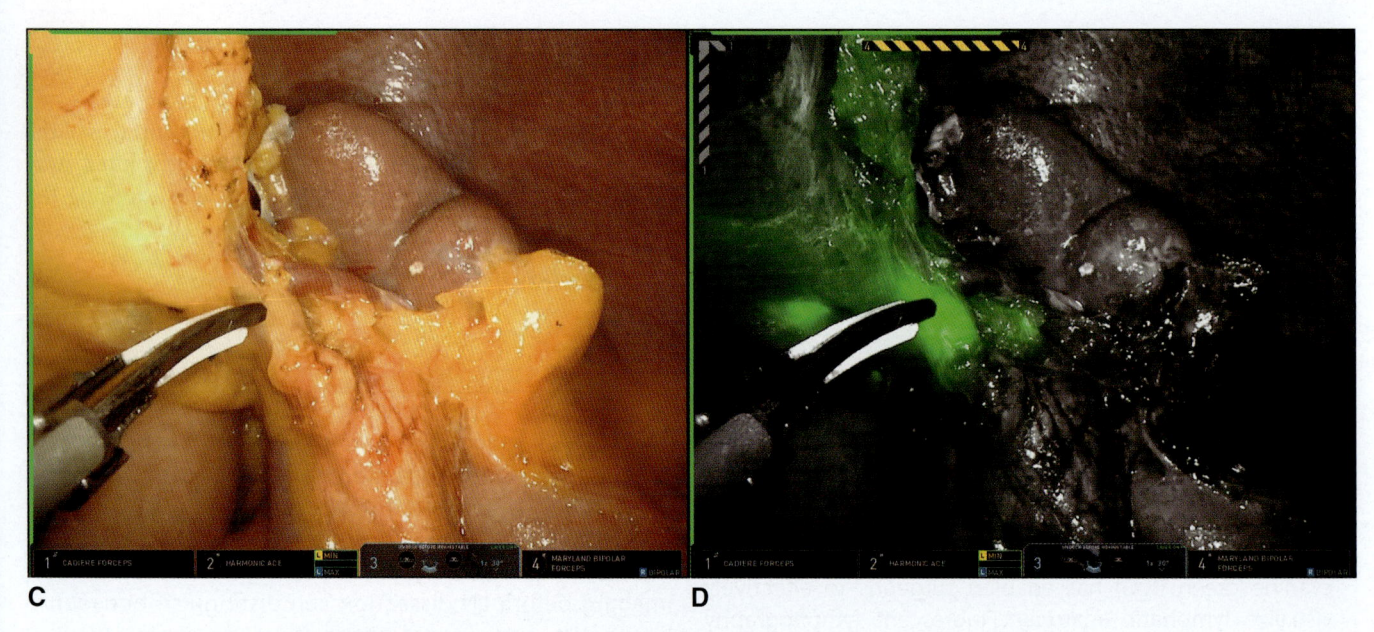

FIGURE 19-13 • (Continued) C, D. Identification of lymphatic anatomy.

Video 19-8. Transection of the Distal Esophagus

Step 10. Transection of the distal esophagus
To be able to use the robotic linear stapler, the 8-mm port of the R2 should be undocked and replaced with a 12-mm trocar. After the stomach is fully mobilized, the distal abdominal esophagus is transected with a 45-mm linear stapler to ensure a sufficient proximal margin. For Roux-en-Y esophagojejunostomy, the abdominal esophagus is transected from the ventral to the dorsal direction by rotating the esophagus counterclockwise. An entry hole of the distal esophagus is made at the dorsal edge of the resection line. Transection of the distal esophagus completes the procedure of robotic D2 lymphadenectomy for total gastrectomy.

Step 10 average time frame: 5–8 min

Video 19-9. Intracorporeal Roux-en-Y Esophagojejunostomy

Step 11. Reconstruction

Intracorporeal antecolic Roux-en-Y esophagojejunostomy using linear staplers is routinely performed after robotic total gastrectomy. After the jejunum is brought up to the transected distal esophagus in a loop fashion, an entry hole is created in the antimesenteric border of the expected anastomosis point of the jejunum. This point is 15–20 cm distal to the Treitz ligament, where no tension is present. A 45-mm linear stapler can then be inserted into the holes using the R2 to create a side-to-side esophagojejunostomy. The common entry hole is subsequently closed with a 45-mm stapler or by suturing. The afferent loop of the jejunum is then transected using a linear stapler. A jejunojejunostomy is finally created 45–60 cm distal to the esophagojejunostomy using a linear stapler. The entry hole is also closed by two 45-mm linear staples (**Figures 19-14 A–C**). The mesenteric defect is closed with running sutures using a robotic handsewn technique. Stapling is performed through the R2 12-mm port when transecting the esophagus, creating the anastomosis, and closing the common entry enterotomy.

Step 11 average time frame: 20–25 min

> **EDITORIAL COMMENT**
>
> There are several techniques for the construction of the esophagojejunostomy. An option is the end-to-side anastomosis using the transoral introduction of the anvil of the circular stapler. The shaft of the stapler is introduced on the left side of the patient entering into the stump of the previously constructed alimentary limb of the Roux-en-Y.

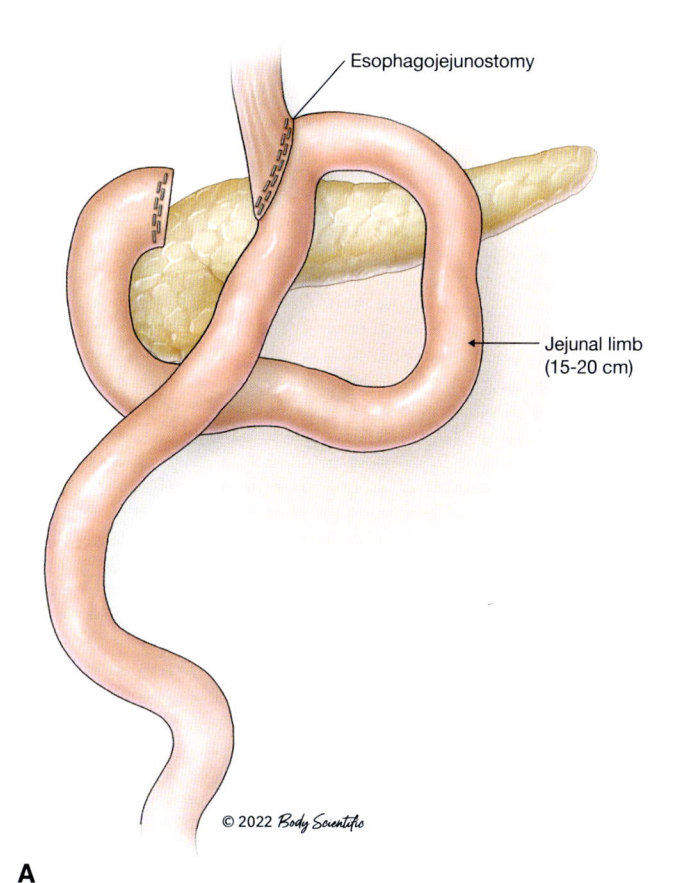

FIGURE 19-14 • Esophagojejunostomy construction. **A.** Step A.

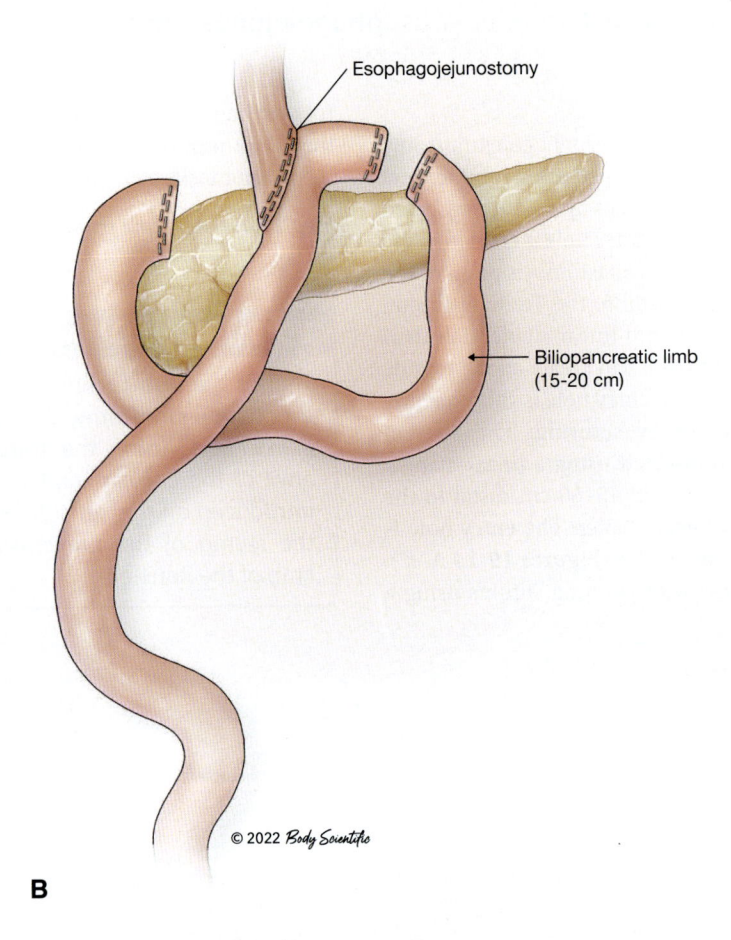

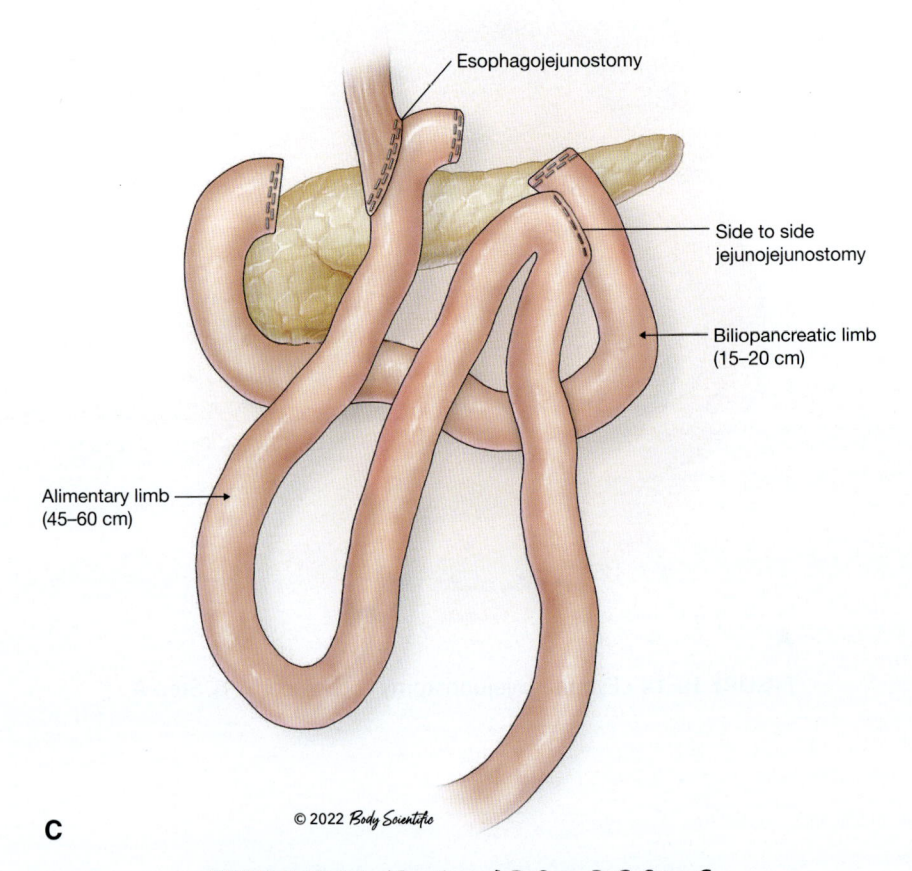

FIGURE 19-14 • (*Continued*) **B.** Step B. **C.** Step C.

Step 12. Specimen extraction
Finally, the specimen is retrieved in an Endobag™ through a 3–4 cm minilaparotomy that is performed by extending the infraumbilical camera port incision. The fascia and skin are then closed in a standard-fashion.

Step 12 average time frame: 10–15 min

> **EDITORIAL COMMENT**
>
> A Pfannenstiel incision may be more indicated for bulky specimens.

Suggested Readings

1. Yang K, Cho M, Roh CK, et al. Robotic spleen-preserving splenic hilar lymph node dissection during total gastrectomy for gastric cancer. *Surg Endosc* 2019;33(7):2357-2363. doi: 10.1007/s00464-019-06772-4
2. Guideline Committee of the Korean Gastric Cancer Association (KGCA), Development Working Group & Review Panel. Korean Practice Guideline for Gastric Cancer 2018: an Evidence-based, Multi-disciplinary Approach [published correction appears in *J Gastric Cancer*. 2019;19(3):372-373]. *J Gastric Cancer*. 2019; 19(1):1-48. doi: 10.5230/jgc.2019.19.e8
3. Japanese Gastric Cancer Association. Japanese gastric cancer treatment guidelines 2018 (5th edition). *Gastric Cancer*. 2021;24(1): 1-21. doi: 10.1007/s10120-020-01042-y
4. Song J, Oh SJ, Kang WH, et al. Robot-assisted gastrectomy with lymph node dissection for gastric cancer: lessons learned from an initial 100 consecutive procedures. *Ann Surg*. 2009;249(6):927-932. doi: 10.1097/01.sla.0000351688.64999.73
5. Woo Y, Hyung WJ, Kim HI, et al. Minimizing hepatic trauma with a novel liver retraction method: a simple liver suspension using gauze suture. *Surg Endosc*. 2011;25(12):3939-3945. doi: 10.1007/s00464-011-1788-9
6. Ri M, Nunobe S, Honda M, et al. Gastrectomy with or without omentectomy for cT3-4 gastric cancer: a multicentre cohort study. *Br J Surg*. 2020;107(12):1640-1647. doi: 10.1002/bjs.11702
7. Kim DJ, Lee JH, Kim W. A comparison of total versus partial omentectomy for advanced gastric cancer in laparoscopic gastrectomy. *World J Surg Oncol*. 2014;12:64. doi: 10.1186/1477-7819-12-64
8. Yu W, Choi GS, Chung HY. Randomized clinical trial of splenectomy versus splenic preservation in patients with proximal gastric cancer. *Br J Surg*. 2006;93(5):559-63. doi: 10.1002/bjs.5353
9. Son T, Lee JH, Kim YM, Kim HI, Noh SH, Hyung WJ. Robotic spleen-preserving total gastrectomy for gastric cancer: comparison with conventional laparoscopic procedure. *Surg Endosc*. 2014;28(9):2606-2615. doi: 10.1007/s00464-014-3511-0
10. Vahrmeijer AL, Hutteman M, van der Vorst JR, et al. Image-guided cancer surgery using near-infrared fluorescence. *Nat Rev Clin Oncol* 2013;10(9):507-518. doi: 10.1038/nrclinonc.2013.123
11. Herrera-Almario G, Patane M, Sarkaria I, Strong VE. Initial report of near-infrared fluorescence imaging as an intraoperative adjunct for lymph node harvesting during robot-assisted laparoscopic gastrectomy. *J Surg Oncol*. 2016;113(7):768-770. doi: 10.1002/jso.24226
12. Kwon IG, Son T, Kim HI, Hyung WJ. Fluorescent lymphography-guided lymphadenectomy during robotic radical gastrectomy for gastric cancer. *JAMA Surg*. 2019;154(2):150-158. doi: 10.1001/jamasurg.2018.4267
13. Giulianotti PC, Coratti A, Angelini M, et al. Robotics in general surgery: personal experience in a large community hospital. *Arch Surg*. 2003;138(7):777-784. doi: 10.1001/archsurg.138.7.777
14. Japanese Gastric Cancer Association. Japanese classification of gastric carcinoma: 3rd English edition. *Gastric Cancer* 14, 101-112 (2011). doi: 10.1007/s10120-011-0041-5
15. Giulianotti PC, Angelini M, Coratti A et al. Technique de la gastrectomie subtotale robotique. *Le Journal de Coelio Chirurgie*. N 43- September 2002.

"I believe the future of sleeve gastrectomy is bright and it will probably become the primary procedure in >75% of patients seeking weight-loss surgery and/or type 2 diabetes surgery."

—Michel Gagner (1960)

Sleeve Gastrectomy

Chandra Hassan • Alberto Mangano • Yevhen Pavelko

INTRODUCTION

The utilization of laparoscopic techniques remains challenging in morbidly obese patients due to the rigidity of the instruments and poor ergonomics. The current robotic system along with its advanced instrumentations, like the vessel sealer and SureForm™ staplers with SmartClamp technology, makes the learning of the surgery potentially easier. Acquiring skills to control the stapling from the console may benefit residents and fellows when introducing them to any of the other complex upper gastrointestinal (GI) robotic surgeries. An increasing number of bariatric patients require revision surgeries for a wide range of reasons including weight recidivism, insufficient weight loss, and complications from the primary bariatric procedure. A considerable number of gastric bands are removed and/or revised to gut anatomy–altering bariatric procedures. This has led to overwhelming numbers of laparoscopic sleeve gastrectomies (SG) followed by Roux-en-Y Gastric Bypass (RYGB) and other newer procedures. Despite advancements in medical weight loss modalities, surgery is the main option to achieve long-term significant results. Laparoscopy remains the most common minimally invasive approach, but an increasing number of bariatric surgeries are performed robotically. The higher level of technical complexities associated with revision surgeries and initial bariatric procedures in higher body mass index (BMI) populations is offset by the advanced technical sophistication of the robotic platform. With a short learning curve for robotic SG and the exponential increase in robotic bariatric surgery in recent years, it is important to learn more about it.

Indications and Relative Contraindications to the Robotic Approach

Patients who qualify for SG under current guidelines of BMI 35 and above should be considered for the robotic approach. More so, the following categories of patients benefit from the robotic technique: super morbid obese and higher BMI, central obesity, double pannus, and revision surgeries.

A history of open abdominal surgeries and possible adhesions are not absolute contraindications.

INSTRUMENT REQUIREMENTS

The suggested main robotic instruments/tools can be listed as follows:
- 30° scope
- Cautery hook/monopolar curved scissors
- Bipolar forceps
- Vessel sealer
- Robotic linear staplers (with different loads)
- Cadiere/ProGrasp forceps
- Needle driver
- Clip applier

The suggested main laparoscopic instruments/tools can be listed as follows:
- 5-mm scope
- Scissors
- Needle driver
- Graspers
- Suction-irrigation

Supplemental materials:
- Sponges
- Sutures (Prolene™ 3-0/4-0)
- Large clips
- ViSiGi®
- Bougie >36 Fr
- Extra-long Veress needle
- Nathanson liver retractor
- Endo-Bag™

Photo reproduced with permission from Michel Gagner, M.D.
Quote reproduced with permission from Gagner M. The future of sleeve gastrectomy. Eur Endocrinol. 2016;12(1):37-38.

Patient Positioning, OR Setup, and Port Setting

The patient is placed supine with the air transfer mattress (deflated) underneath and the firm sponge wedge under the chest to aid anesthesia. Both arms are extended in abducted position resting on surgical arm boards, strapped gently in a comfortable position. Thicker cushioning or extra blankets on the arm board are necessary to prevent pressure damage. A bariatric footrest is attached to the operating table's side rail to provide support when the patient is positioned in reverse Trendelenburg. The stomach is usually decompressed by placing a nasogastric or orogastric tube. A Foley catheter is usually placed for urinary output measurement (**Figures 20-1 A, B**).

An alternative patient position is split leg with knee restraint strap to prevent the patient from sliding during surgery in reverse Trendelenburg. Some surgeons prefer supine on beanbag with lower limbs parted in the French position. It is important to use bariatric reverse Trendelenburg straps to keep the inner thighs in place. Every position has some pros and cons. The final choice is based on the surgeon's preference and patient body *habitus*. For more complex and longer operations, the French position might be preferable, because it gives the assistant surgeon more comfortable control of the instruments in both upper quadrants and at the same time easy access to all robotic arms.

Bariatric table extenders may be necessary to increase the width as well as the length of the table. Sequential compression devices (SCDs) are always applied to the patient's calves.

30° bed inclination

A

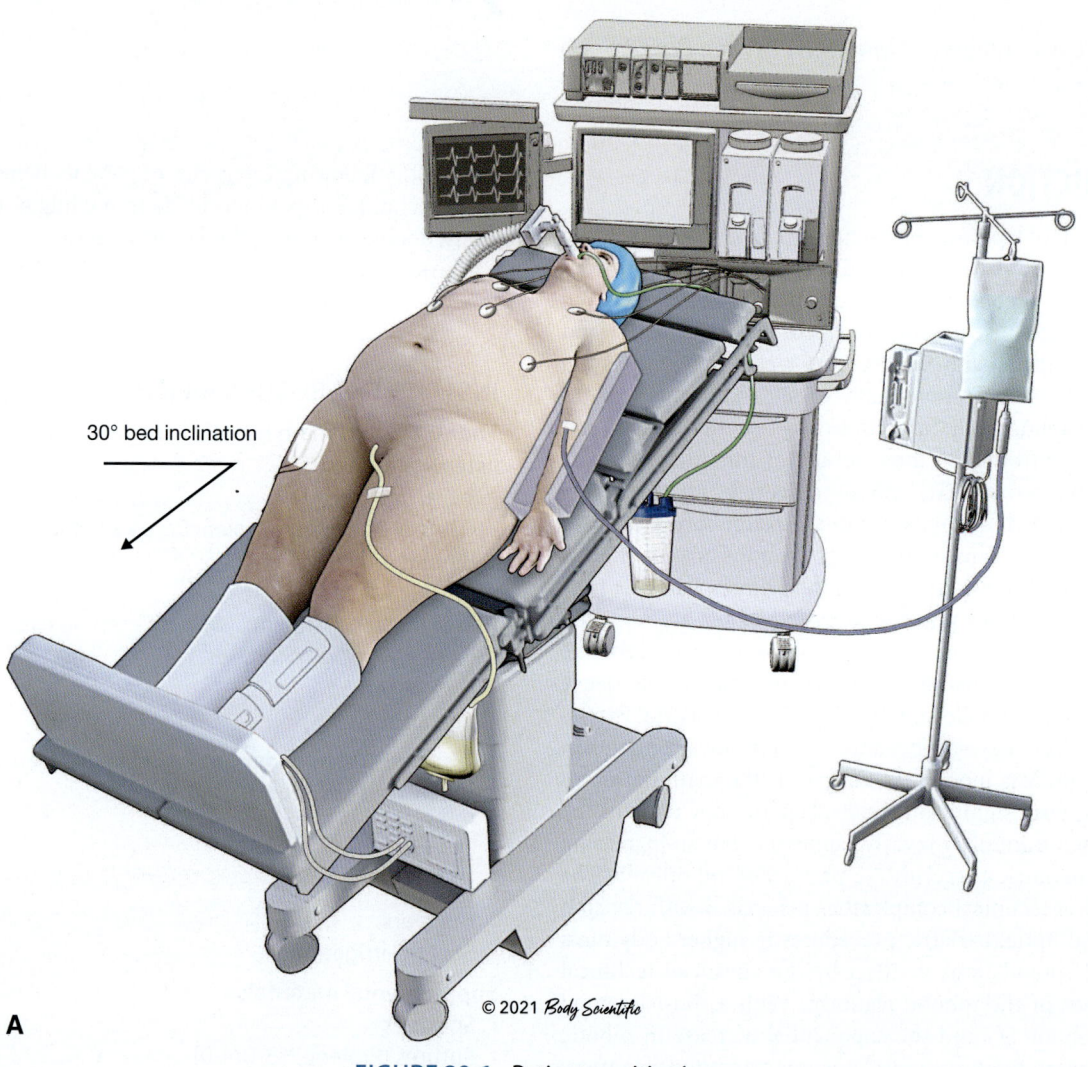

FIGURE 20-1 • Patient positioning.

30° bed inclination

B

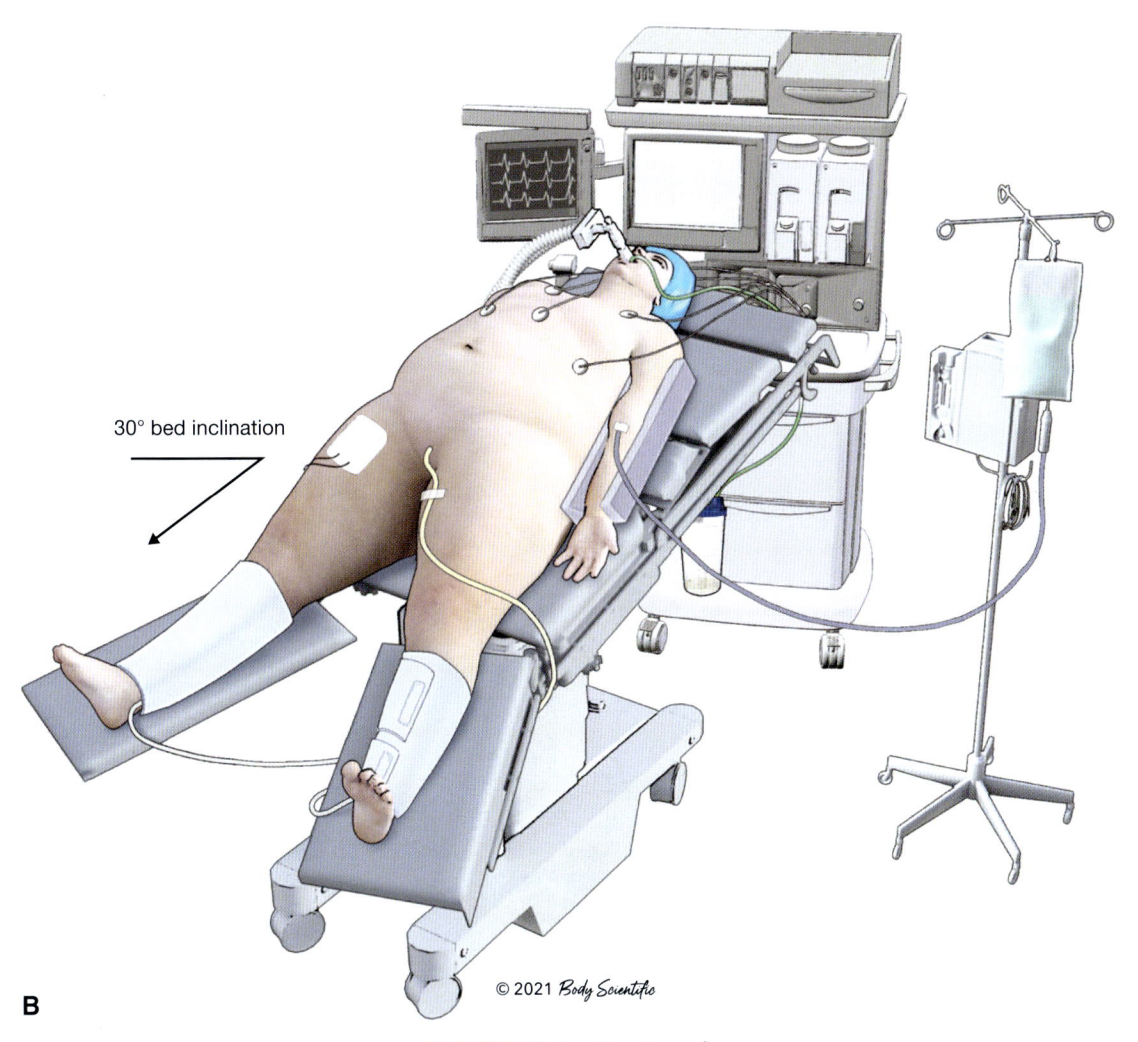

FIGURE 20-1 • *(Continued)*

The assistant's position depends on the patient's position. In the French position, the assistant sits in between the patient's legs; the assistant stands on the right side of the standard supine patient. The pneumoperitoneum is achieved preferably with the Veress needle technique in the left subcostal margin, but in case of failure, there are other options. (See Chapter 2, The Basic Principles of Clinical Applications, for more details.)

The OR setup is described in **Figures 20-2 A, B**.

It is important to be meticulous while creating the pneumoperitoneum to prevent iatrogenic injuries at the beginning of the surgery. Very rarely there is a genuine necessity to use an extra-long Veress needle or extra-long optical trocars for this step, even in patients with central obesity and in BMI above 90. In difficult cases, after few failed attempts with the Veress needle, it is advisable to use other options. If an attempt is made with a 5-mm optical trocar under direct visualization, it should be done in the left lateral upper quadrant where the risk of injuries is less. A quick diagnostic laparoscopy is carefully carried out. This step is performed in order to identify bleeding or iatrogenic bowel injuries or any other conditions that might change the surgical plan. The remaining ports are inserted under direct visualization using a safe track technique.

It is important to recognize that the position of the umbilicus could be much lower than normal, secondary to the pannus. For this reason, creation of the pneumoperitoneum by open methods, including Hasson technique, might be difficult. Whenever a nonrobotic stapler is used, it is preferable to position the 12-mm assistant trocar closer to the midline and on a lower site in relation to the line of the robotic ports. By doing so, a more convenient angle allowing the instrument to

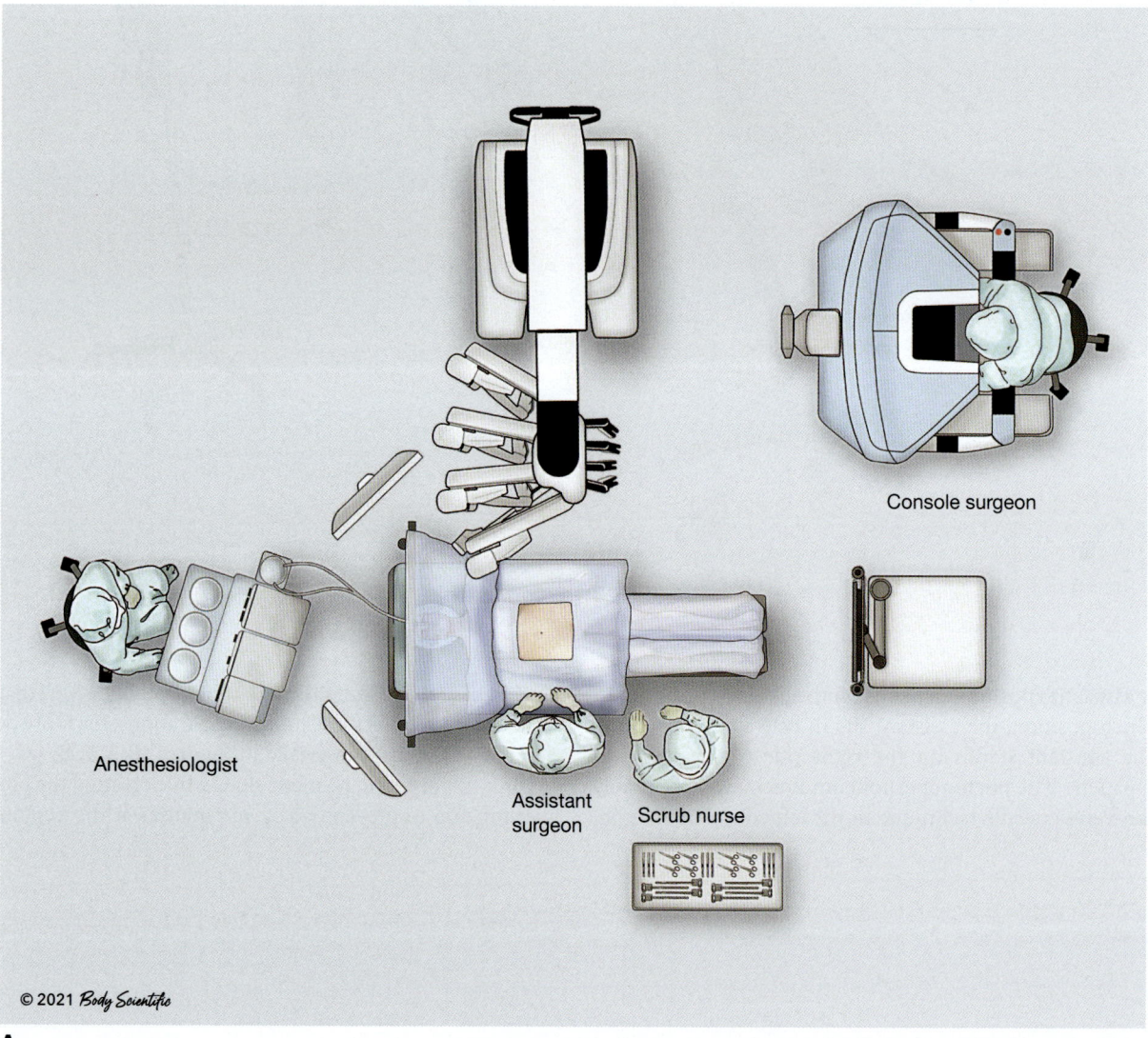

FIGURE 20-2 • OR setup.

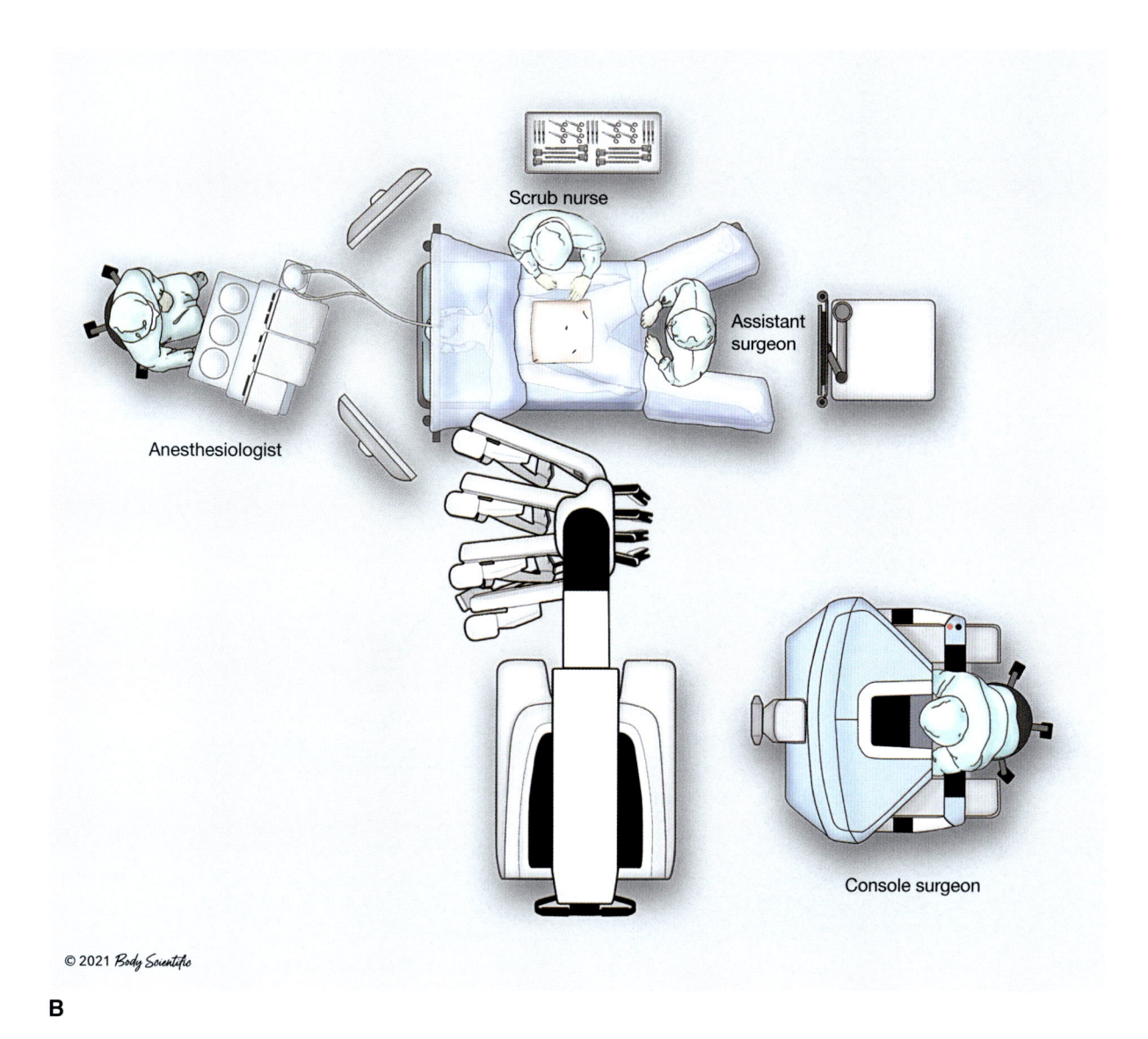

FIGURE 20-2 • (Continued)

be parallel to the greater curvature of the stomach, is achieved. This alignment makes firing with the stapler easier. It is important to keep in mind that the stapler has a long shaft and can easily reach as proximal as the angle of His without extra effort.

It is essential to avoid placement of trocars in the pannus fold at the midabdomen. The lower pannus will greatly compromise the range of movements of the robotic arms. In addition, these incisions are prone to higher incidence of wound infection.

The camera is placed in the patient's left paramedian port for the best visual control of the short gastric vessels while mobilizing the posterior fundus of the stomach from the pancreas and the spleen. The other two 8-mm robotic cannulas and one 12-mm robotic cannula (stapler) are positioned along a horizontal straight line about 20–25 cm from the xiphoid with the camera port at the intersection with the anterior mammillary line (**Figure 20-3**). The body *habitus* and old scars of open surgery may suggest an adaptation of the port placements. All the adhesions in the upper quadrant should be taken down to have secure working space, allowing to safely place all 4 trocars. The adhesions can be taken down laparoscopically or robotically in a 2-step approach (see Chapter 2). In difficult scenarios, an extra 5-mm laparoscopic port can be placed in the lower left quadrant allowing for better assistant interaction.

Wide abdomen

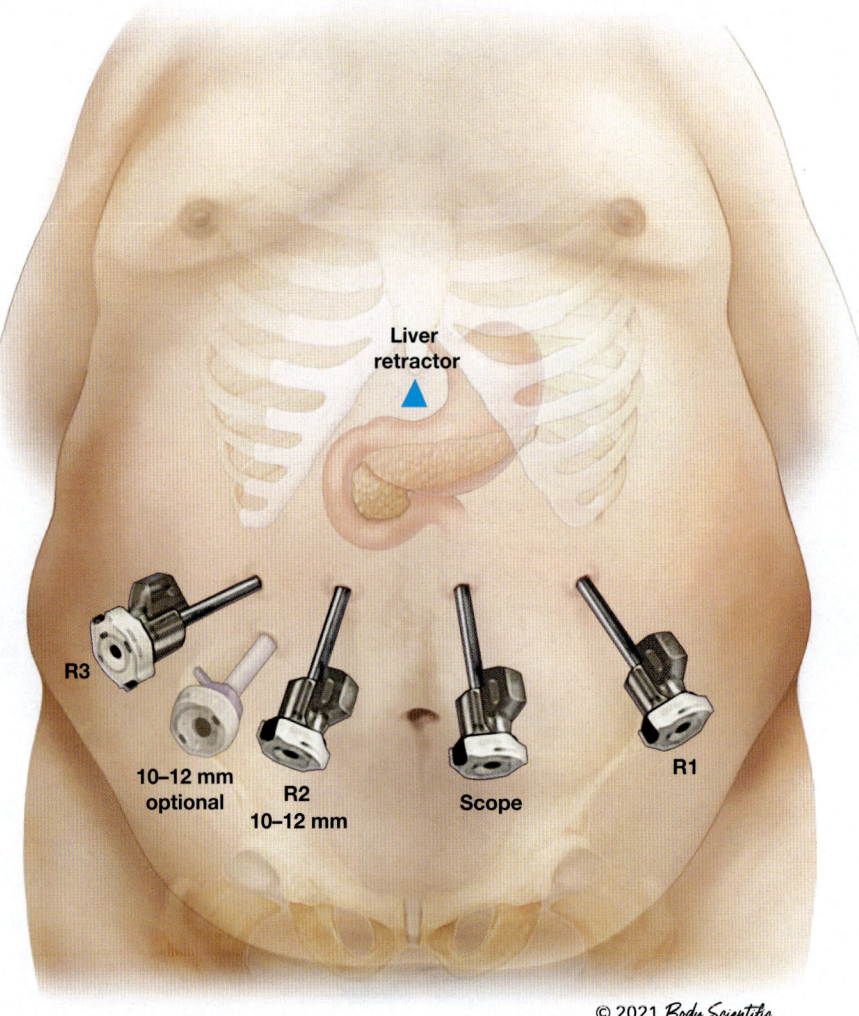

FIGURE 20-3 • Trocars setting wide abdomen.

> ▶▶ **TIPS**
> Patients could still slide down the operating table in reverse Trendelenburg position, even with all these precautions. It is advisable to test steep positions before draping in order to verify, under direct vision, the safety of the setup.

> ⚠ **PITFALLS**
> Extra-long Veress needles are at high risk for iatrogenic injuries of intra- and retroperitoneal organs. A standard-length Veress needle is usually sufficient to create pneumoperitoneum even in patients with central obesity and those who are super morbid obese.

Surgical Technique

▶ **Video 20-1. Sleeve Gastrectomy – Full Procedure**

Step 1. Placement of the Liver Retractor

Before starting the dissection, the size of the left lobe of the liver, the amount of space available in the left upper quadrant, and the size of the spleen are evaluated. A 5-mm epigastric incision is made just below the xiphoid and a track is created by introducing a 5-mm trocar to facilitate the insertion of the Nathanson liver retractor (**Figure 20-4**). The anesthesiologist can gently pass the ViSiGi® bougie 36 F or the preferred size. Any orogastric tube placed for decompression after intubation must be removed because there have been case reports of stapling across the orogastric tube. The operating table is then moved to 30° reverse Trendelenburg. The robotic cart is docked (**Figure 20-4**).

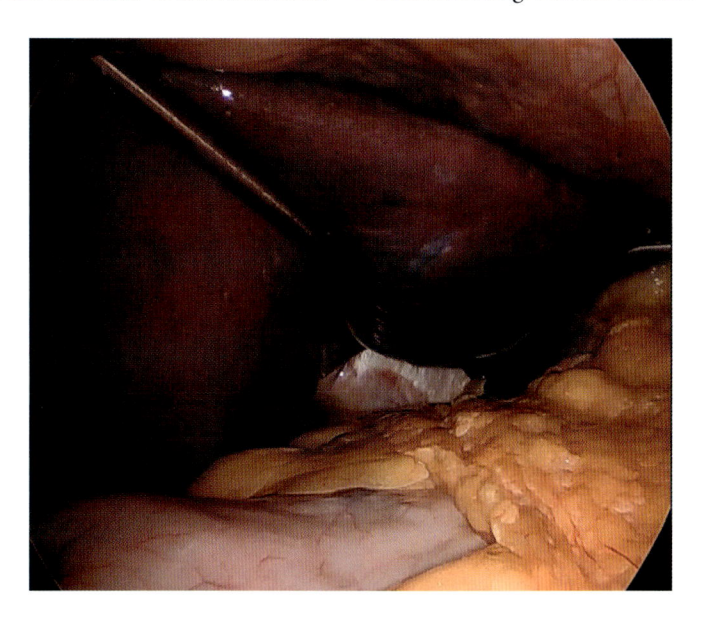

FIGURE 20-4 • Liver retractor placement.

▶ **Video 20-2. Step 1. Liver Retractor Placement**

▶▶ TIPS

It is of paramount importance to coordinate with the anesthesia team the final fixation of the Nathanson liver retractor to the Iron Intern or Martin's Arm to the patient bed. This could compress against the heart and, combined with the pneumoperitoneum and reverse Trendelenburg position, could cause sudden changes in rhythm and vital signs.

⚠ PITFALLS

- Excessive force applied while lifting the left lateral segment of the liver anteriorly could cause liver injury and avoidable hemorrhage. It is well documented that postoperative transient liver dysfunction (POTLD) is a result of liver retractor use during SG.
- Care has to be taken while positioning the retractor to expose the hiatal opening because the free end of the Nathanson retractor could cause damages to the anterior abdominal wall or even to the pericardium in patients with enlarged left lobe of the liver and limited space.

EDITORIAL COMMENT

Instead of the Nathanson retractor, the R3 with a grasper over the sponge is a good tool for exposure, to avoid static force on the liver caused by fixed retractors. The R3 port site should be properly placed on the right side of the patient. During the operation, the grasper hold by the site may also retract the stomach when necessary.

Step1 average time frame: 10–15 min

Step 2. Gastrocolic ligament division

Using the R3, the body of the stomach is lifted upward along the greater curvature with a grasper. The Bouchet transparent zone is identified by putting the gastrocolic ligament under proper tension. This area is opened with the vessel sealer. This maneuver allows the entrance into the lesser sac. The dissection proceeds toward the right side reaching the distance of 5–6 cm from the pylorus, where the staple line will start later on. The arterial branches to the distal stomach and antrum should be addressed while sparing the first branch of the right gastroepiploic artery. Then, the dissection moves toward the left, dividing the branches of the left gastroepiploic artery, always close to the greater curvature of the stomach (**Figures 20-5 A, B**).

▶ **Video 20-3. Step 2. Gastrocolic Ligament Division**

▶▶ **TIPS**

Embryological attachments vary widely, hence precise dissection and clear identification may avoid injuries to structures posterior to the stomach.

⚠ **PITFALLS**

- Staying more lateral, far away from the gastric wall, might injure the transverse colon, the mesentery, the pancreas, and the origin of the left gastroepiploic artery, mainly when there are adhesions with overlapping surgical planes.
- Excessive posterior mobilization of the attachments along the lesser curve, particularly at the incisura, increases the chance of twisting of the newly constructed sleeve.

Step 2 average time frame: 15–20 min

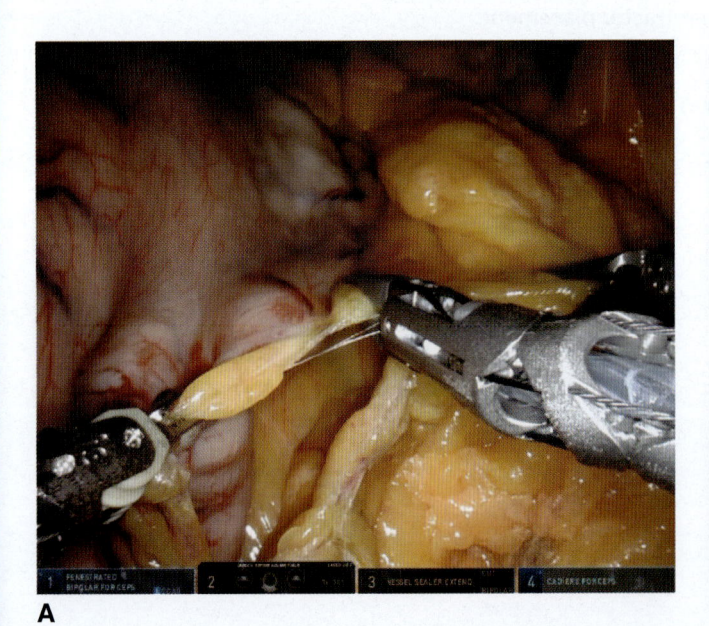

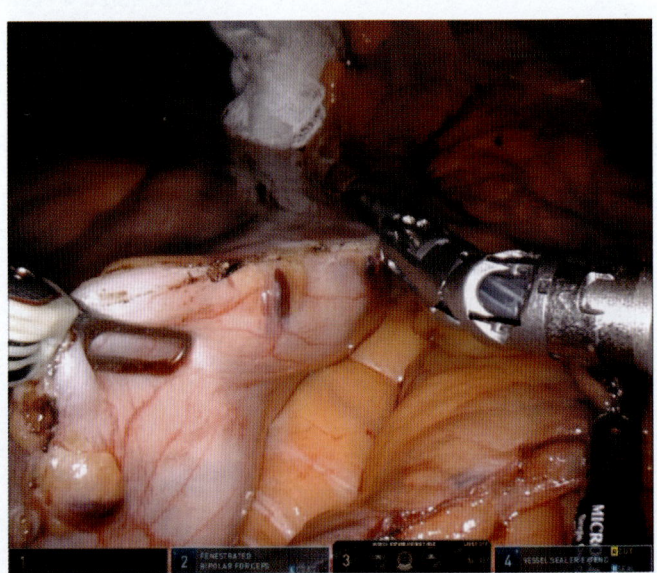

FIGURE 20-5 • Gastrocolic ligament division.

Step 3. Gastrosplenic ligament and short gastric vessels division

The gastrocolic ligament division is continued to include the short gastric vessels in the gastrosplenic ligament. It is important to have precise landmarks to avoid any injury. The short gastric vessels are safely taken down staying close to the gastric fundus reaching up to the left pillar of the diaphragm (**Figures 20-6 A, B**).

Staying closer to the stomach enhances maintenance of the correct dissection plane, thus avoiding inadvertent bleeding or ischemia to a part of the spleen, injury of the splenic vessels, or polar splenic artery. Some types of these injuries can cause portomesenteric vein thrombosis (PMVT <0.3–1.8%), which is a rare but severe complication potentially leading to intestinal infarction, extrahepatic portal hypertension, and even mortality. (For more information, see suggested readings #11, 17.)

> ▶▶ **TIPS**
> The R3 is very important for retraction of the stomach when mobilizing the gastrocolic ligament. To facilitate exposure, the stomach can be retracted by grabbing its posterior wall and putting it under proper tension.

> ⚠ **PITFALLS**
> During this step, retraction needs to be done very carefully. Excessive force applied on some perisplenic omental adhesions can cause lacerations of the splenic capsule and subsequent bleeding.

> **EDITORIAL COMMENT**
> Mainly in patients with congested short gastric vessels or tendency to bleed, dual-coagulation technique with the vessel sealer is advisable; that is, coagulating the distal segment of the vessel first without cutting, then coagulating the proximal segment of the vessel closer to the stomach once, and then cutting.

Step 3 average time frame: 20–30 min

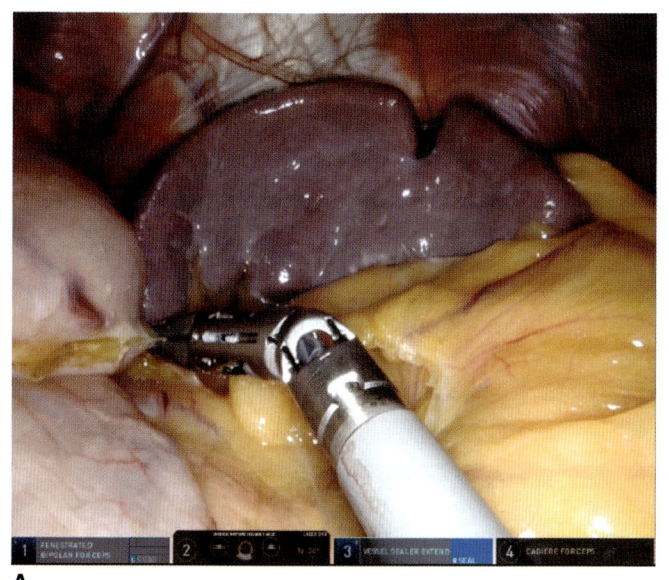

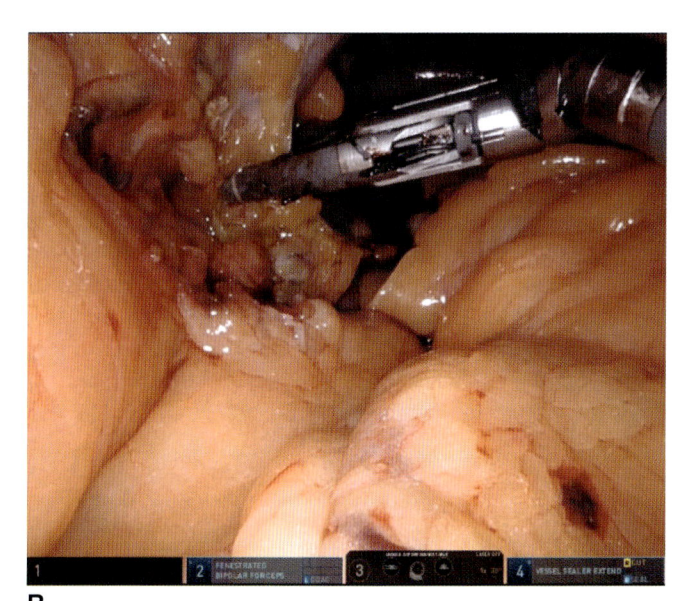

FIGURE 20-6 • Division of short gastric vessels.

Step 4. Mobilization of the posterior gastric fundus

Careful mobilization of the extraperitoneal gastric fundus in proximity to the left pillar of the diaphragm should be performed (**Figure 20-7**).

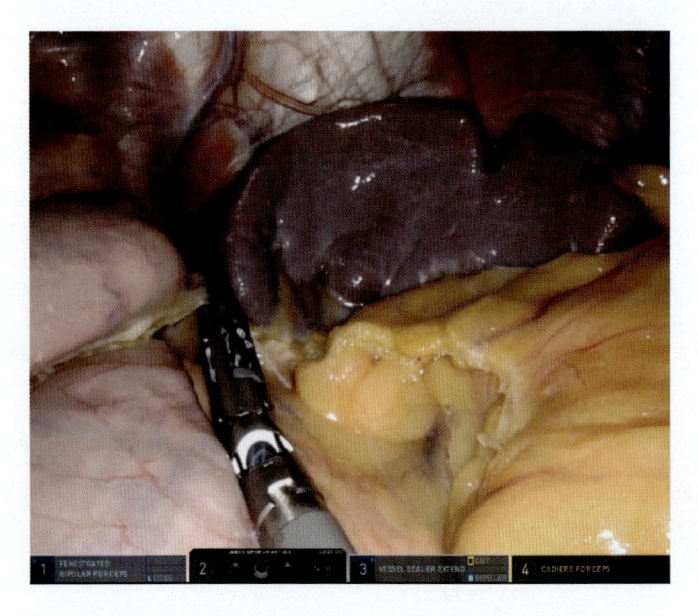

FIGURE 20-7 • Mobilization of the posterior fundus.

Video 20-4. Step 4. Mobilization of the Posterior Fundus

The importance of this step is to avoid the persistence of a large gastric pouch below the gastroesophageal junction. This redundant pouch would make the construction of the sleeve asymmetrical and/or with duplicated walls with increased risk of leak. Once the gastric fundus is completely mobilized, it is much easier to stretch laterally the greater curvature and to apply the staplers in the proper way.

Step 4 average time frame: 15–20 min

> ⚠ **PITFALLS**
>
> Sometimes the splenogastric and splenopancreatic ligaments can be fused, creating a single plane that might contain the posterior gastric artery. Injury of this structure may cause bleeding or splenic focal ischemia if an accessory polar artery is present (**Figure 20-8**).

> 🔍 **ANATOMICAL HIGHLIGHTS**
>
> Anatomy of the posterior fundus (**Figures 20-9 A, B**).

Sleeve Gastrectomy 417

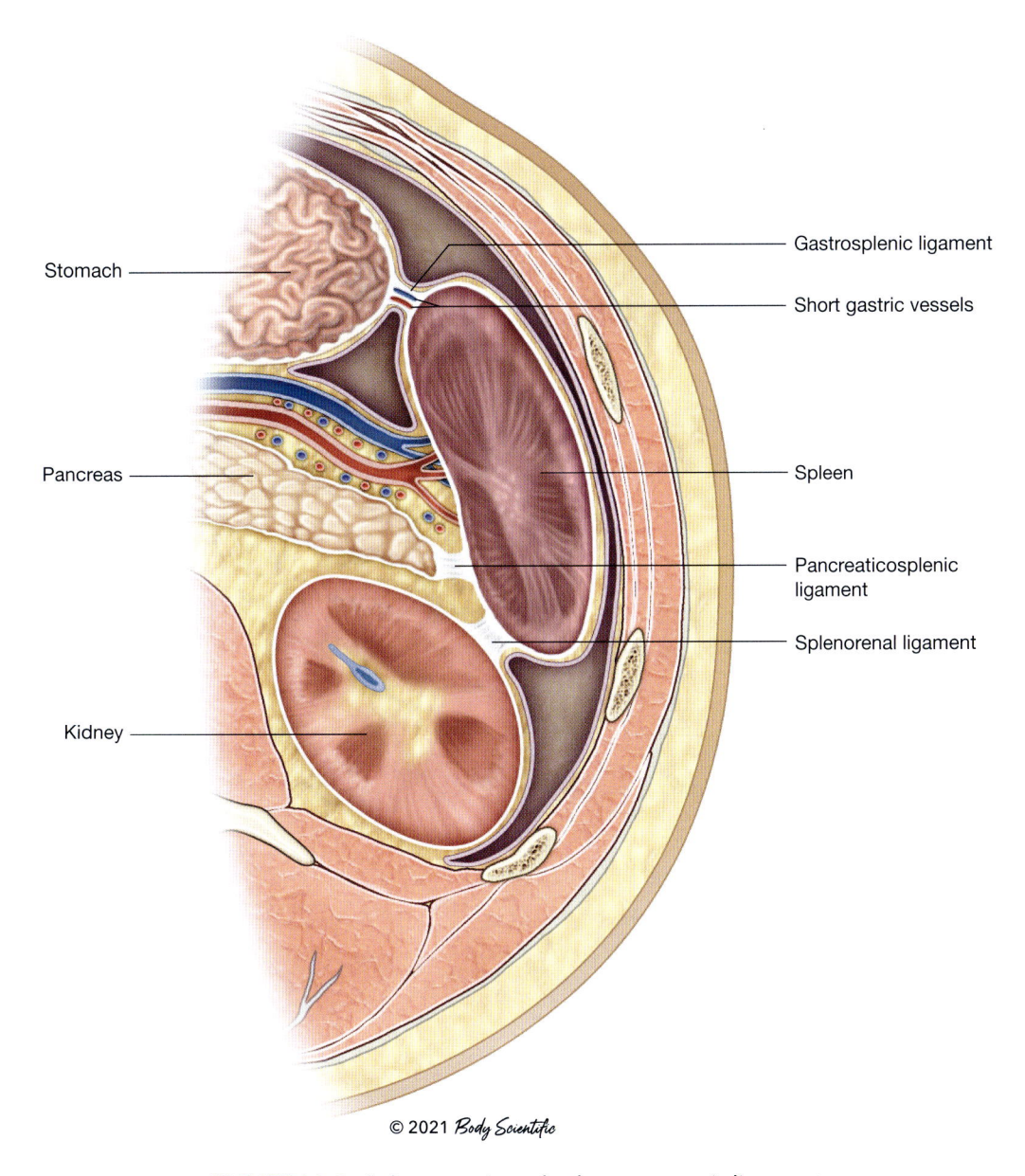

FIGURE 20-8 • Splenogastric and splenopancreatic ligament.

▶▶ TIPS

- Partially withdrawing the bougie above the hiatal opening helps in dissecting along the left crus muscle and mobilization of the posterior fundus of the stomach.
- In difficult cases with limited space or if there is no separation between the planes of the posterior face of the stomach and the spleen, it is better to adopt another strategy. In this situation the gastric wall can be retracted toward the splenic hilum, and the control of the last short gastric vessels could be very challenging with lateral-to-medial direction. Instead, it is safer to dissect along the left diaphragmatic pillar, to divide the peritoneal reflection at the angle of His, between the pillar and the stomach, to complete the mobilization of the extraperitoneal portion of the gastric fundus. Only when this maneuver is completed there is a creation of a window that facilitates taking down the last short gastric vessels with the vessel sealer.

418 The Foundation and Art of Robotic Surgery

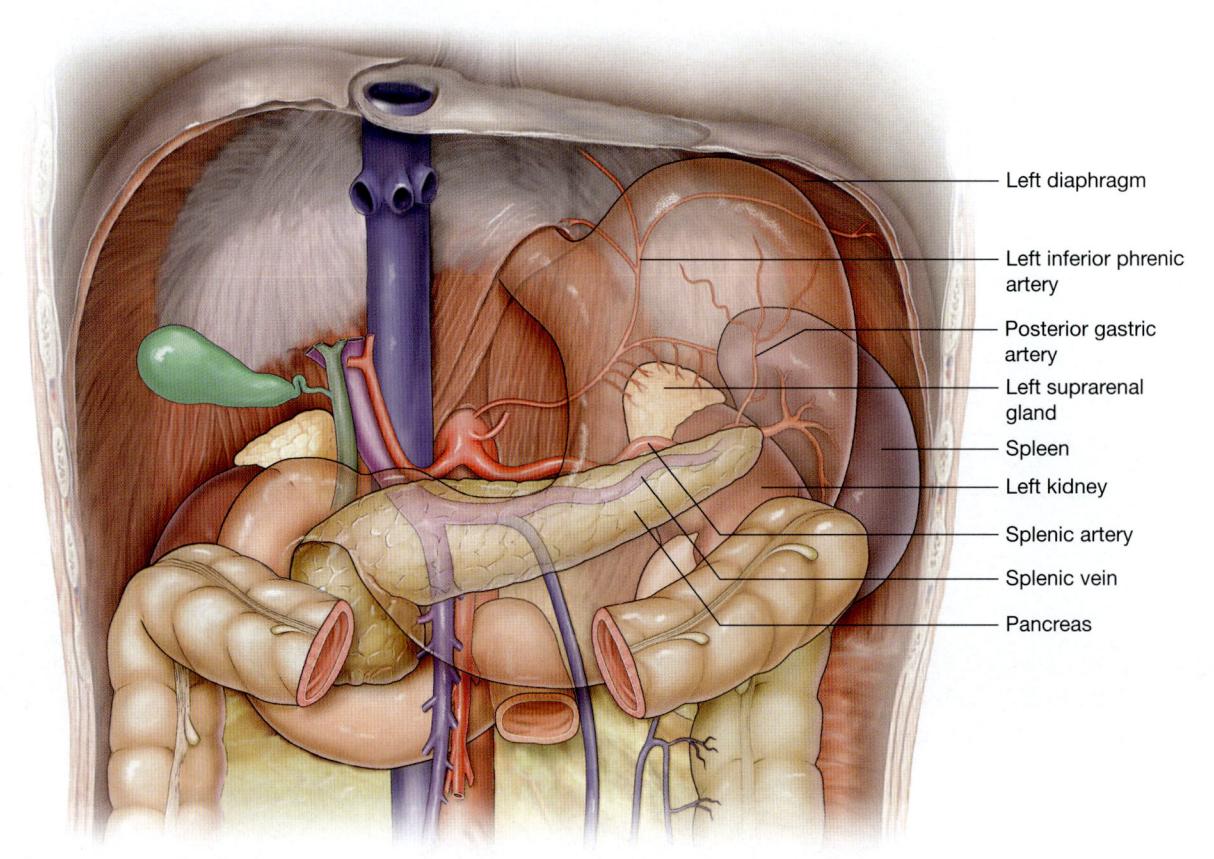

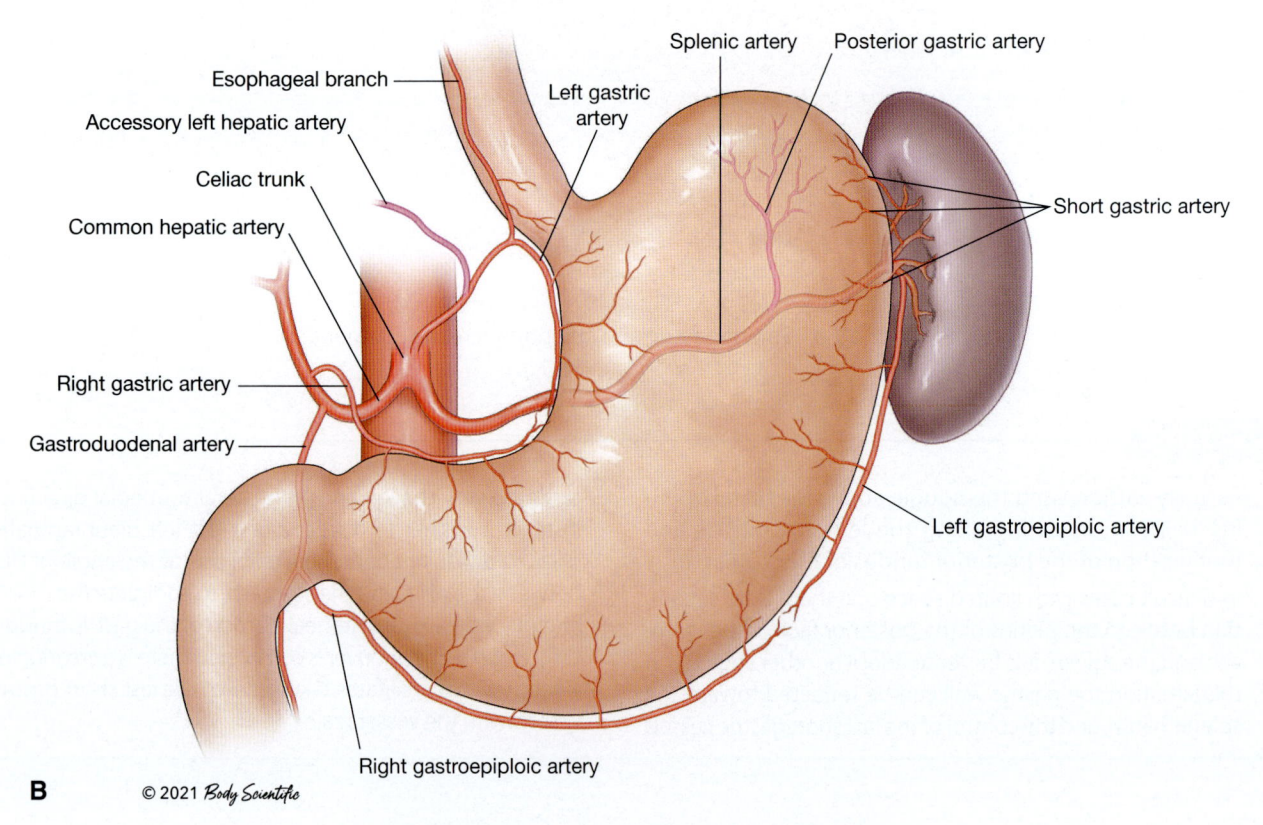

FIGURE 20-9 • Anatomy of the posterior fundus.

Step 5. Stapling and creation of the sleeve gastrectomy

The bougie is advanced and positioned along the lesser curvature of the stomach, with the tip at the pylorus, in preparation for stapling. There is no significant difference between starting the gastric resection at 2 cm or 6 cm proximal to the pylorus. Several stapling devices are available. Endo-GIA™ staplers with black 60-mm linear length for extra-thick tissue with staple line reinforcements are best at the antrum. It is important to avoid stapling tight to the bougie at the incisura. Significant stenosis of SG could happen in this area (**Figures 20-10 A, B**).

> ▶▶ **TIPS**
>
> Before firing the stapler, at the incisura level, the anesthesiologist may be asked to move back and forth the bougie to verify that the stapler jaws, after being closed, are not structuring too much the gastric conduit.

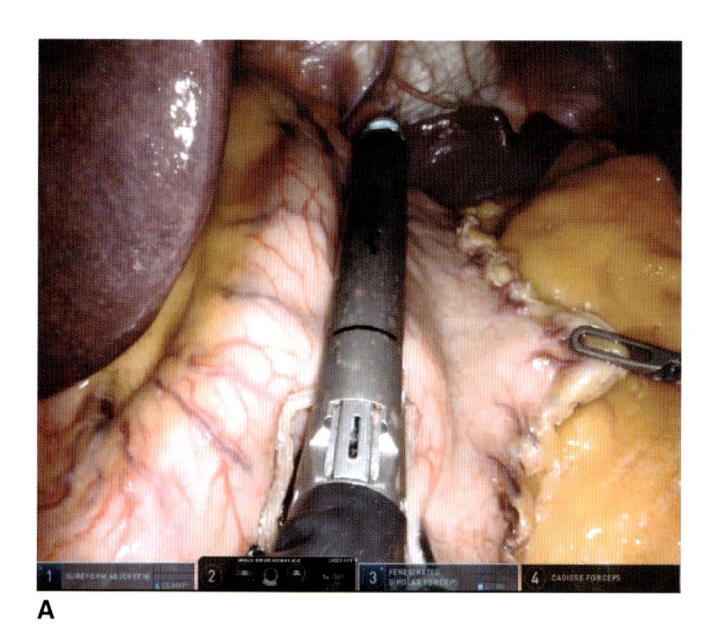

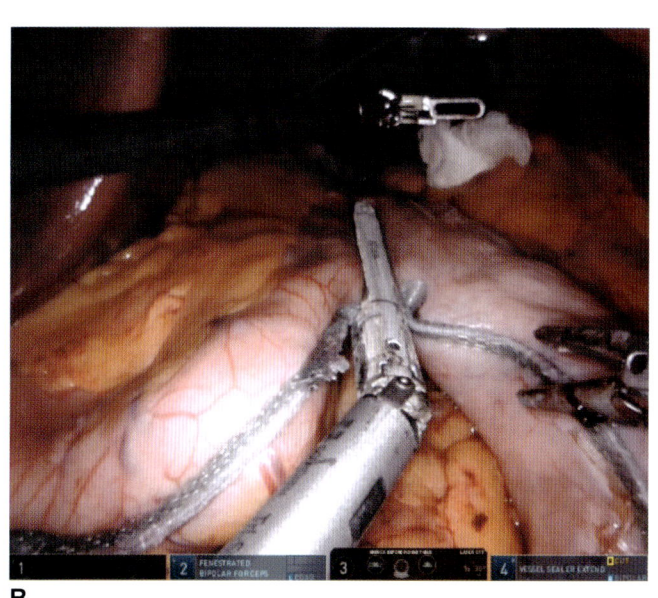

FIGURE 20-10 • **A.** Sleeve gastrectomy robotic stapler. **B.** Sleeve gastrectomy laparoscopic stapler.

▶ Video 20-5. Step 5. Sleeve Gastrectomy

Appropriate closed staple line height to the different tissue thickness from antrum to fundus is essential. The stapler at the angle of His should be angled to the left of the fat pad, which has been shown to lower leak rates. In cases requiring further hemostasis on the staple line, additional sutures may be added. Suturing reinforcement with omentum is left to surgeon discretion. JP drain is not indicated in primary SG. Intraoperative leak tests by methylene blue, ICG, and EGD are available options, even though they have not shown to reduce leaks.

Laparoscopic stapling technique:
The assistant surgeon at the bedside should introduce the stapler using the more right-sided port, which is a 12-mm size. The stapler is positioned 4–6 cm from the pylorus, at an oblique angle, and parallel to the bougie as per the guidance of the console surgeon. It is important to avoid the narrowing at the incisura as already stated. The highest closing height stapler with reinforcement should be used at the antrum. Gradual reduction of the closing height of the stapler to match the thickness of the body and the fundus of the stomach is essential to avoid staple line bleeding and related complications. The console surgeon's role in this step is to help in the exposure of the staple line and to offer proper guidance to the assistant. The mobilized posterior fundus is lifted anteriorly and laterally prior to stapling to avoid formation of neo-fundus. If there is bleeding on the suture line, interrupted stitches of Prolene™ 3-4/0 are applied by the console surgeon.

Robotic stapling technique:
It is necessary to upsize the R1 8-mm port to 12 mm to fit the size of the robotic stapler. Similarly to the laparoscopic technique, the console surgeon starts the stapling at 4–6 cm from the pylorus at an oblique angle and parallel to the bougie. The same advice and precautions described for the laparoscopic technique are also valid for the robotic one.

Step 5 average time frame: 20–30 min

Step 6. Specimen extraction
The gastric specimen is removed via a retrieval bag and sent for pathology. Port-site defects of 10 mm and above are closed with Endoclose™ devices using absorbable sutures. See Chapter 2, The Basic Principles of Clinical Applications, for a comprehensive description of this step and different operative strategies.

Step 6 average time frame: 5–10 min

> **PITFALLS**
> Excessive traction of the gastric wall while firing the stapler can be a reason for coiling of the stomach after removal of the bougie. This is a cause of functional twisting obstruction of the lumen.

> **EDITORIAL COMMENT**
> The laparoscopic technique is a good training model for less experienced surgeons. The staple laparoscopic technique is validated with years of use and thousands of cases, and it results in 3 lines of staples. The robotic technique has similar outcomes, but there are only 2 staple lines. A drawback of the laparoscopic technique is that there is no control of the experienced surgeon over the direct handling of the stapler.

Suggested Readings

1. Pavelko Y, Bustos R, Gruessner S, Hassan C. Acute hiatal hernia with incarcerated proximal half of recent sleeve gastrectomy: super rare complication. *Obes Surg.* 2021;31(1):469-471. doi: 10.1007/s11695-020-05101-2. Epub 2020 Nov 11. PMID: 33179217.
2. Hassan C, Pavelko Y, Gruessner S, et al. Totally robotic sleeve gastrectomy as a training model for residents and fellows. *Clin Endocrinol.* UDK 616.33-089.87-089.819. doi: 10.30978/CEES-2020-4-8
3. Vinzens F, Kilchenmann A, Zumstein V, Slawik M, Gebhart M, Peterli R. Long-term outcome of laparoscopic adjustable gastric banding (LAGB): results of a Swiss single-center study of 405 patients with up to 18 years' follow-up. *Surg Obes Relat Dis.* 2017;13(8):1313-1319.
4. Ramly EP, Alami RS, Tamim H, Kantar R, Elias E, Safadi BY. Concomitant removal of gastric band and sleeve gastrectomy: analysis of outcomes and complications from the ACS-NSQIP database. *Surg Obes Relat Dis.* 2016;12(5):984-988.
5. Chang S, Stoll CRT, Song J, Varela JE, Eagon CJ, Colditz GA. The effectiveness and risks of bariatric surgery: an updated systematic review and meta-analysis, 2003-2012. *JAMA Surg.* 2014;149(3):275-287. doi: 10.1001/jamasurg.2013.3654
6. Mechanick JI, Kushner RF, Sugerman HJ, et al. American Association of Clinical Endocrinologists, The Obesity Society, and American Society for Metabolic & Bariatric Surgery medical guidelines for clinical practice for the perioperative nutritional, metabolic, and nonsurgical support of the bariatric surgery patient. *Obesity (Silver Spring).* 2009;17(suppl 1):S1-S70.
7. Hassan C, Pavelko Y, Gangemi A, et al. Robotic platform represents a good training model for surgical residents in super-morbidly obese patients. 11th CRSA Worldwide Congress; 2019; Durham, NC.
8. Scerbo MH, Alramahi B, Felinski MM, et al. The role of robotics in bariatric surgery. *Curr Surg Rep.* 2020;8(31). doi: 10.1007/s40137-020-00277-z
9. Hiramatsu K, Aoba T, Kamiya T, Mohri K, Kato T. Novel use of the Nathanson liver retractor to prevent postoperative transient liver dysfunction during laparoscopic gastrectomy. *Asian J Endosc Surg.* 2020;13:293-300. doi: 10.1111/ases.12735
10. Perez M, Brunaud L, Kedaifa S, et al. Does anatomy explain the origin of a leak after sleeve gastrectomy? *Obes Surg.* 2014;24(10):1717-1723.
11. Cudworth M, Aguiluz G, Bustos R, et al. A452—Portomesenteric thrombosis (PMVT) after laparoscopic sleeve gastrectomy (LSG). *Surg Obes Relat Dis.* 2018;14(suppl 11):S164-S166.
12. Manos T, Nedelcu M, Cotirlet A, Eddbali I, Gagner M, Noel P. How to treat stenosis after sleeve gastrectomy? *Surg Obes Relat Dis.* 2017;13(2):150-154. doi: 10.1016/j.soard.2016.08.491
13. Silecchia G, Iossa A. Complications of staple line and anastomoses following laparoscopic bariatric surgery. *Ann Gastroenterol.* 2018;31(1):56-64. doi: 10.20524/aog.2017.0201
14. Rosenthal RJ. International sleeve gastrectomy expert panel consensus statement: best practice guidelines based on experience of >12,000 cases. *Surg Obes Relat Dis.* 2012;8(1):8-19.
15. Noel P, Nedelcu M, Gagner M. Impact of the surgical experience on leak rate after laparoscopic sleeve gastrectomy. *Obes Surg.* 2016;26:1782-1787.
16. Villagrán R, Smith G, Rodriguez W, et al. Portomesenteric vein thrombosis after laparoscopic sleeve gastrectomy: incidence, analysis and follow-up in 1236 consecutive cases. *Obes Surg.* 2016;26(11):2555-2561. doi: 10.1007/s11695-016-2183-3
17. Cudworth M, Bustos R, Hassan C, et al. Portomesenteric thrombosis (PMVT) after laparoscopic sleeve gastrectomy (LSG). *Surg Obes Relat Dis.* 2018;14(suppl 11):S164-S166.
18. Giulianotti PC, Coratti A, Angelini M, et al. Robotics in general surgery: personal experience in a large community hospital. *Arch Surg.* 2003;138(7):777-784. doi: 10.1001/archsurg.138.7.777

"An ideal operation for control of obesity should limit ability to overeat and yet should allow normal nutrition."

—Edward E. Mason (1920–2020)

Roux-en-Y Gastric Bypass

Nicolas Hellmuth Dreifuss • Roberto Bustos • Mario Alberto Masrur

INTRODUCTION

Roux-en-Y gastric bypass (RYGB) is one of the most popular procedures for achieving long-term weight loss and resolution of obesity-related comorbidities. This procedure has been modified over several decades to its current version. RYGB has a dual mechanism of action: it restricts the amount of food that the stomach can hold and decreases the absorption of nutrients. Moreover, other proposed mechanisms have been described, such as changes in gut hormones (that reduce appetite and enhance satiety), gut microbiota, bile acids metabolism, and energy expenditure. Minimally invasive RYGB can achieve significant and sustained weight loss with low postoperative morbidity and mortality rates.

The robotic platform might offer several advantages during RYGB. The stability of the platform, along with its articulated instruments, make seamless hand-sewn anastomosis creation much easier. This enhanced suturing capability can also be used for staple line reinforcement, bleeding control, and mesenteric gap closure. Moreover, the robotic platform is especially useful in superobese patients (eliminating the abdominal wall torque effect) and revisional bariatric cases where dense adhesions and altered anatomy are commonly encountered. In this chapter, the technical description of primary robotic RYGB will be detailed.

Indications and Relative Contraindications to the Robotic Approach

Candidates for RYGB should meet the following criteria: BMI ≥40 or BMI ≥35 and two or more obesity-related comorbidities, and inability to achieve sustained weight loss for a significant period with prior weight loss efforts.

Although these indications apply to many different metabolic procedures, the decision for the appropriate operation should consider the patient's characteristics, needs/preference, and surgeon's experience. There are no absolute contraindications for robotic RYGB. The relative contraindications are the same as per the laparoscopic RYGB: severe portal hypertension, dependency on alcohol/drugs, immunosuppression, and intellectual impairment. Special consideration must be taken

INSTRUMENT REQUIREMENTS

The suggested main robotic instruments/tools can be listed as follows:
- 30°/0° scope
- Needle drivers (round tip or macro)
- Permanent cautery monopolar hook/monopolar curved scissors
- Harmonic shears/vessel sealer
- Robotic linear stapler and 60-mm loads
- Bipolar forceps
- Cadière Forceps

The suggested main laparoscopic instruments/tools can be listed as follows:
- Atraumatic graspers
- Scissors
- Needle drivers
- Suction-irrigation
- Laparoscopic linear stapler and 60-mm loads

Supplemental materials:
- Gauzes, sponges
- Sutures: 3-0 PDS™ and 2-0 polyester
- 36 Fr bougie
- Nathanson liver retractor

Photo reproduced with permission from Gupta N, Mason H. Father of bariatric surgery. Indian J Surg. 2021.
Quote reproduced with permission from Mason EE, Ito C. Gastric bypass in obesity. Surg Clin North Am. 1967;47(6):1345-1351.

422 The Foundation and Art of Robotic Surgery

for patients with Crohn's disease, in which the increased risk for complications may outweigh the benefits of the procedure.

Patient Positioning, OR Setup, and Port Setting

After induction of general anesthesia, the patient is positioned supine in 20–25° reverse Trendelenburg and tucked legs with intermittent compression devices (**Figure 21-1**).

The assistant surgeon is located at the patient's right side. The OR setup is explained in **Figure 21-2**.

The pneumoperitoneum is achieved with the Veress needle technique at the modified Palmer's point. A 5-mm optic trocar is inserted in the left upper abdominal quadrant and a diagnostic laparoscopy is carried out. A total of five ports, four 8-mm robotic and one assistant port, are used during the procedure. The scope is placed in the supraumbilical area at the midline. R1 and R2 are placed on the left and right upper quadrant, respectively. The assistant port is inserted between the R2 and the scope. The R3 is placed in the left flank lateral to the R1. Moreover, a 5-mm incision is performed in the epigastrium to introduce the Nathanson's liver retractor (**Figure 21-3**). If stapling will be performed with a laparoscopic device, the assistant port should be 12 mm. If robotic stapling is planned, the R2 port should be upgraded to a 12 mm.

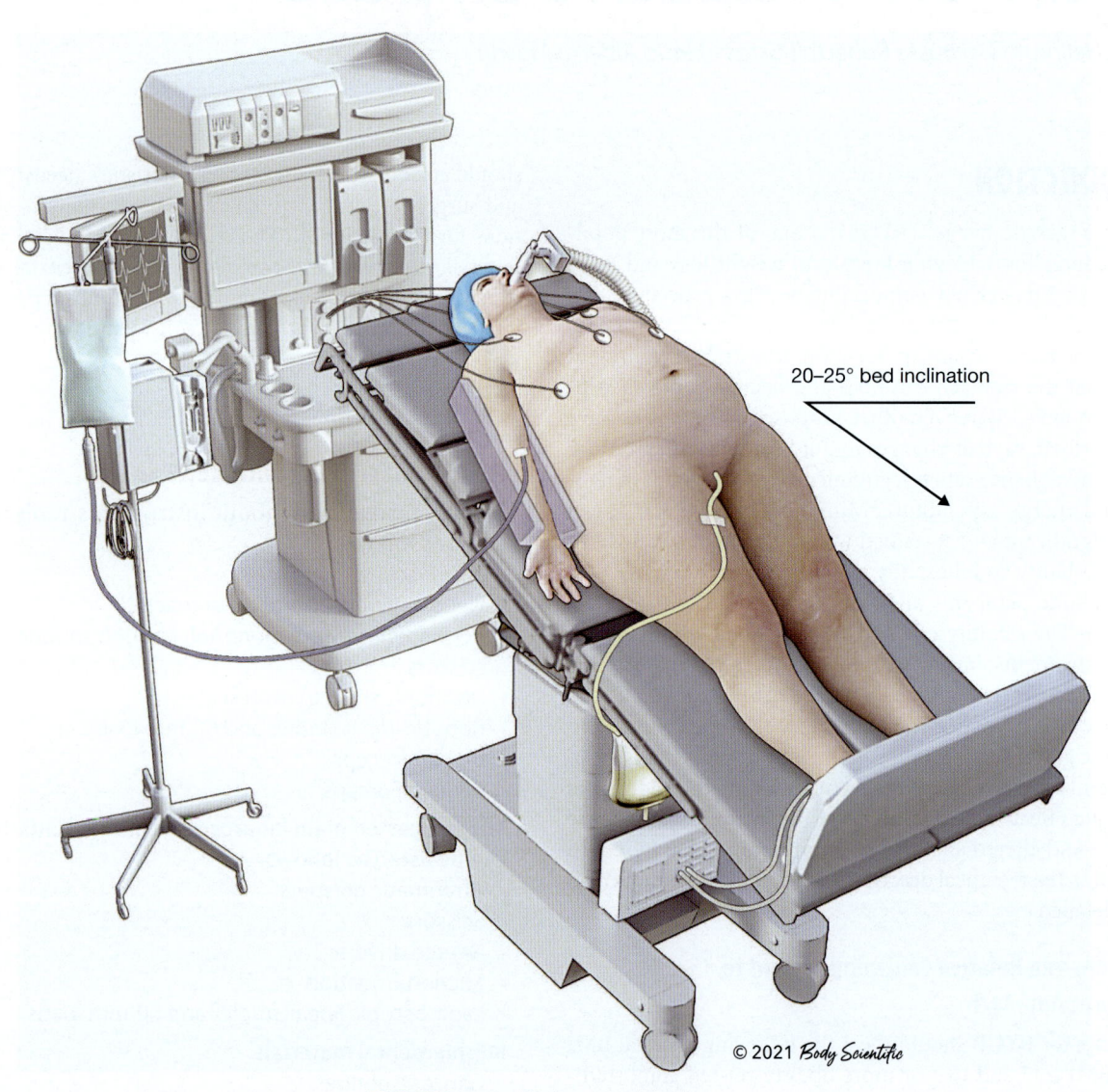

FIGURE 21-1 • Patient positioning.

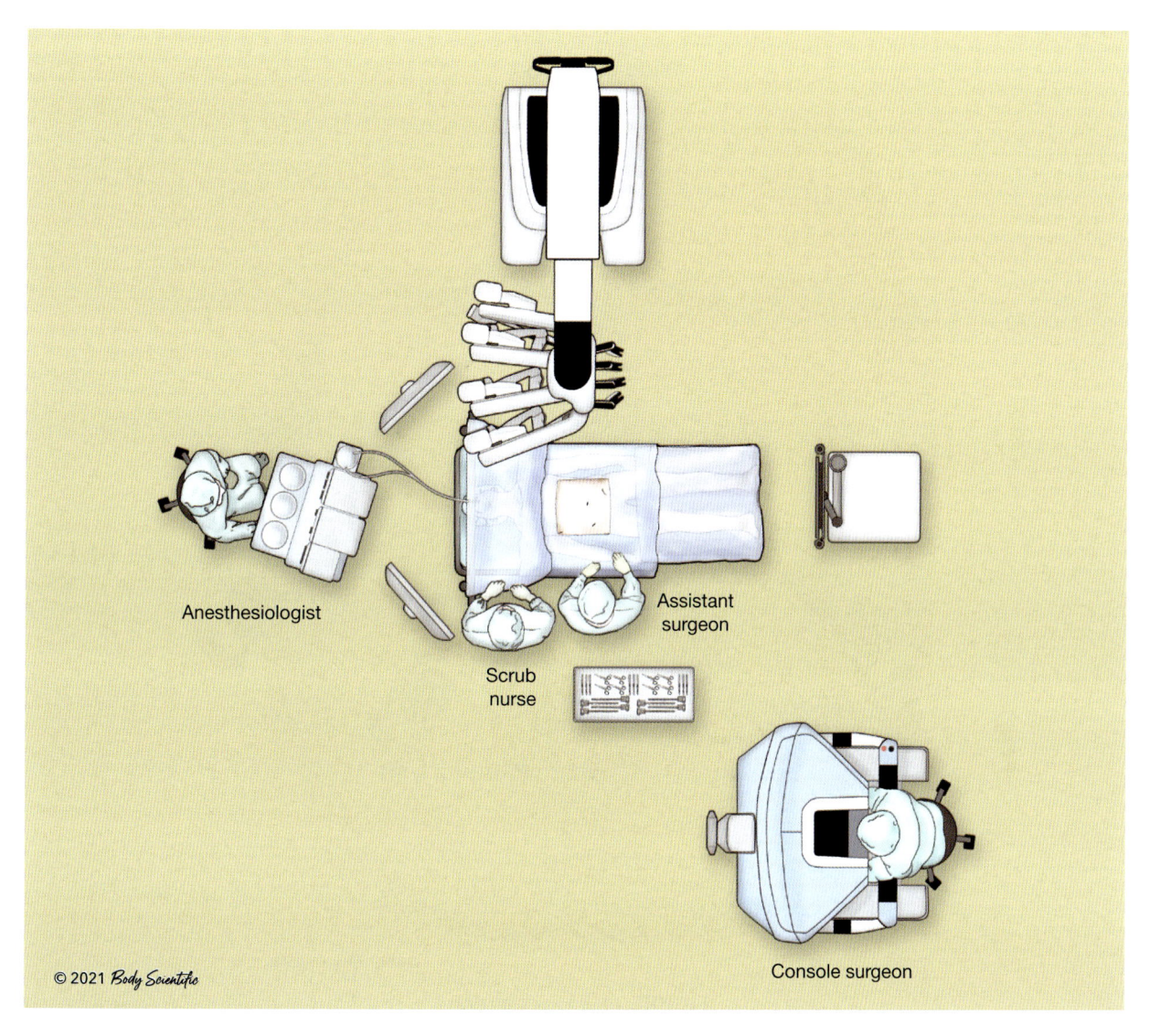

FIGURE 21-2 • OR setup.

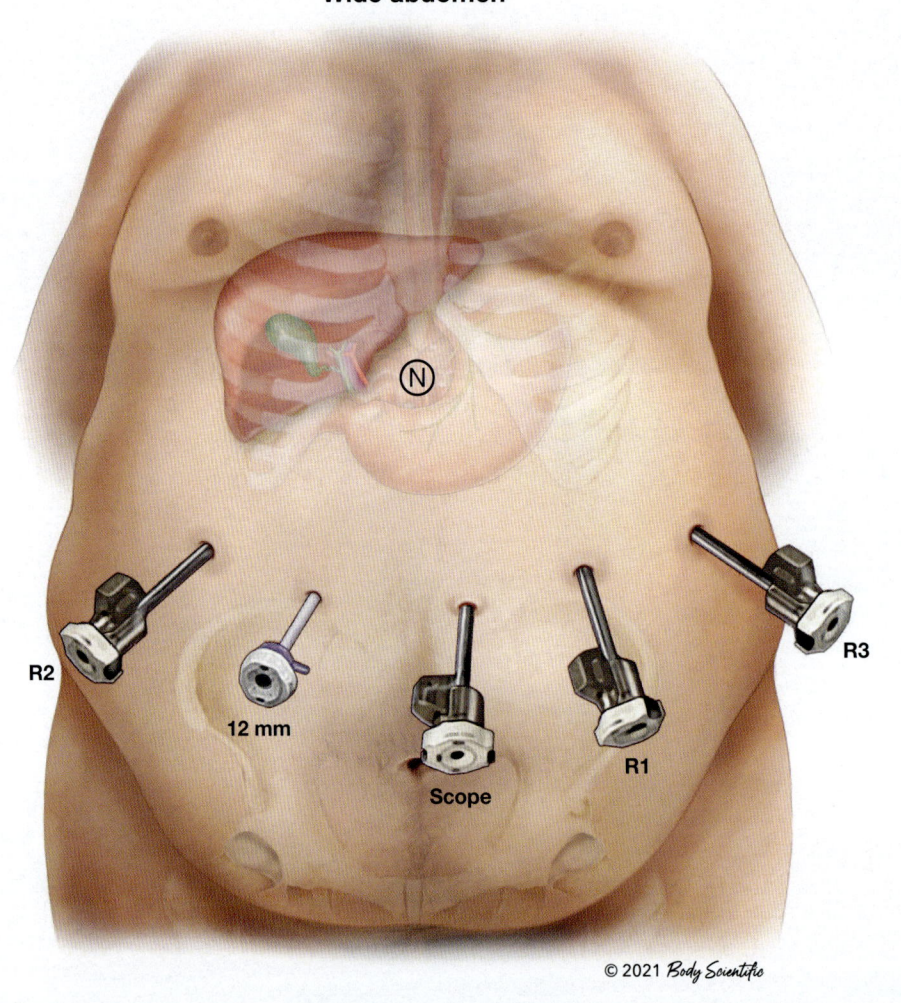

FIGURE 21-3 • Port setting.

Surgical Technique

▶ **Video 21-1** • RYGB Standard Technique

▶ **Video 21-2** • Gastric Pouch Creation

Step 1. Gastric pouch creation

Using the R3, the gastric fundus is retracted downward. The angle of His is exposed and dissected down to the base of the left diaphragmatic pillar using the monopolar hook (**Figures 21-4 A, B**).

Afterward, the gastrohepatic ligament between the second and third branches of the left gastric artery (about 5 cm below the esophagogastric junction) is divided with the vessel sealer to gain entry to the lesser sac. A 50-cc gastric pouch is constructed using reinforced staples. The stapler is introduced through the 12-mm assistant port (laparoscopic stapler) or the R2 (robotic stapler). The first gastric section is performed horizontally. To calibrate the pouch, a 36 Fr bougie is advanced by the anesthesiologist until the horizontal staple line is reached. The Cadière forceps is introduced through the R3 into the lesser sac to lift up the stomach. This maneuver will facilitate the entry of the stapler for the vertical gastric transection. Two or three 60-mm stapler loads are used toward the angle of His to complete the gastric pouch confection (**Figures 21-5 A–E**).

Step 1 average time frame: 10–15 min

> 🔍 **ANATOMICAL HIGHLIGHTS**
> Arterial supply to the stomach (**Figure 21-6**).

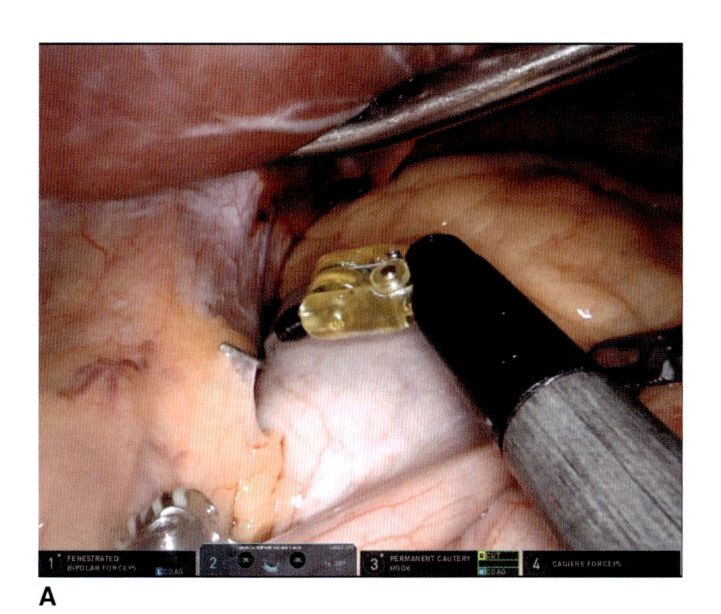

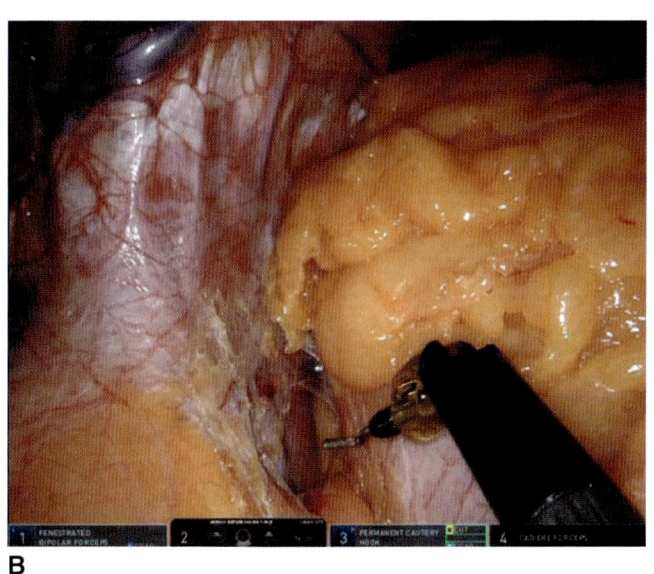

FIGURE 21-4 • Angle of His dissection.

426 The Foundation and Art of Robotic Surgery

A

B

C

D

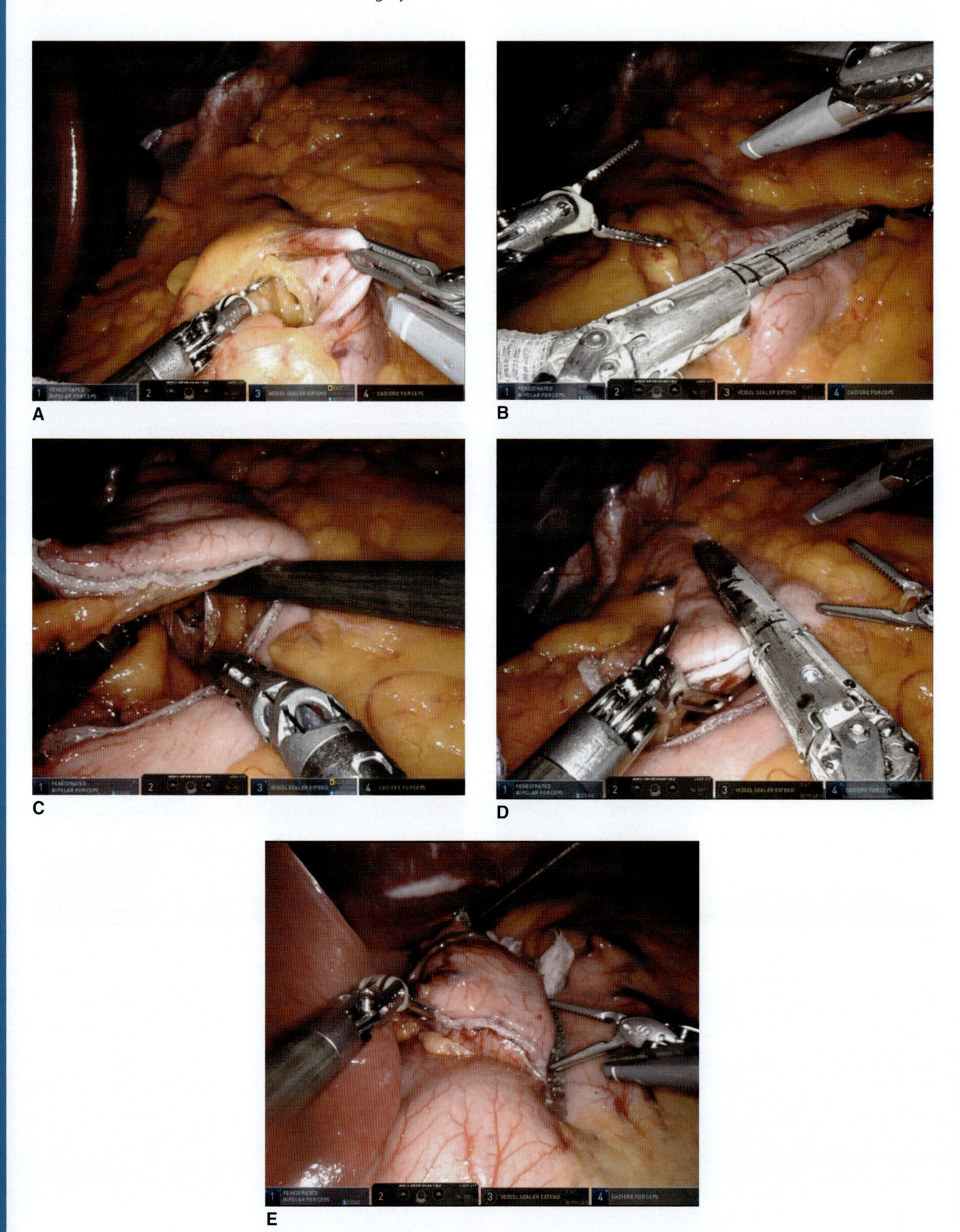

E

FIGURE 21-5 • Gastric pouch creation.

▶▶ TIPS

The ideal length of the gastric pouch should be between 4 and 5 cm. Every additional centimeter of pouch increases the relative risk of marginal ulcers.

It is essential to dissect the gastrophrenic ligament and gastric fundus attachments to the level of the left diaphragmatic pillar to avoid including too much fundus in the pouch. This situation may cause insufficient weight loss as this part of the stomach dilates with time.

⚠ PITFALLS

Care must be taken during the creation of the posterior gastric tunnel to avoid injuries to the pancreas, splenic vessels, or stomach's posterior wall.

The surgeon should verify the complete transection and absence of communication between the gastric pouch and the remnant stomach to avoid gastrogastric fistulas. Additionally, proper hemostasis on the staple line must be carefully checked, because this is one of the main causes of postoperative bariatric hemorrhage.

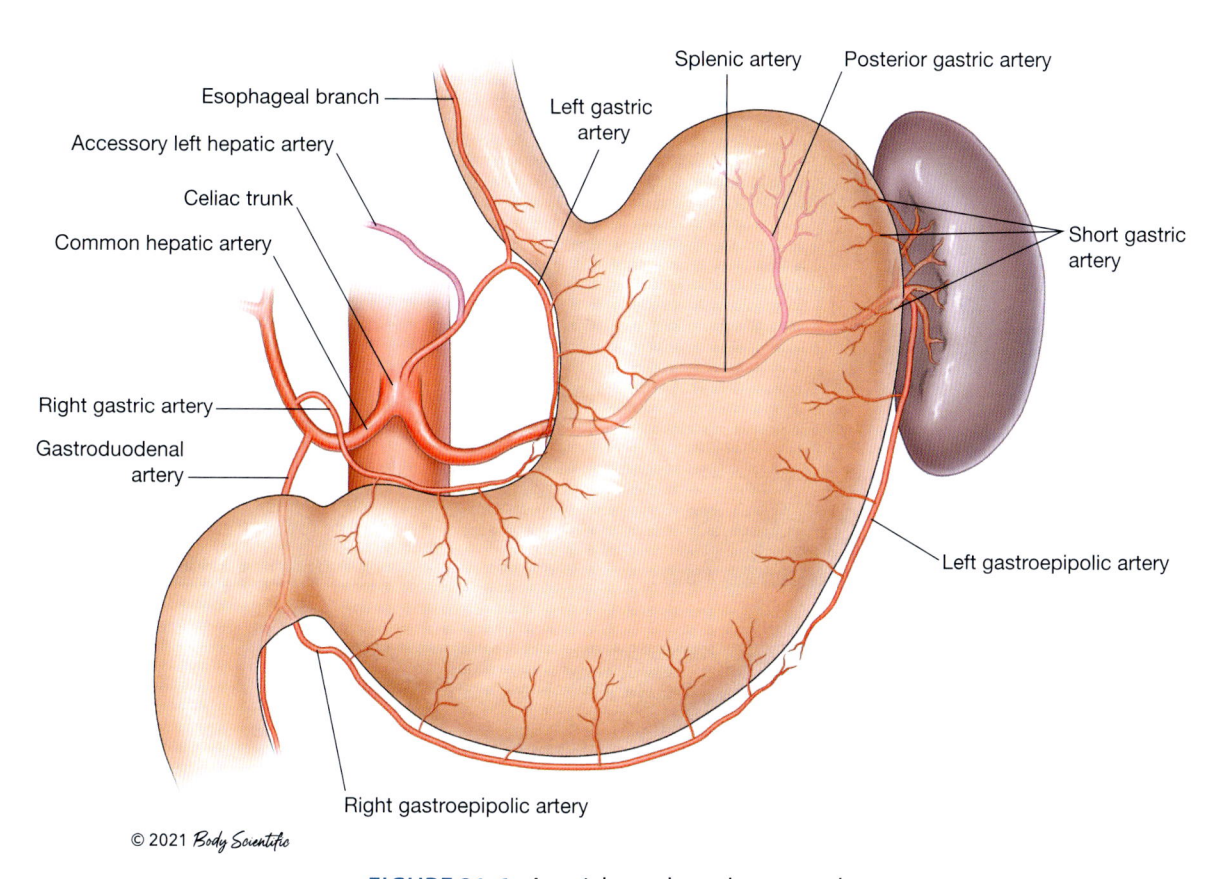

FIGURE 21-6 • Arterial supply to the stomach.

Step 2. Creation of the Roux-en-Y limb

The greater omentum is divided with the vessel sealer around the middle portion of the transverse colon. The transverse colon is retracted cephalad with the R3 to expose the Treitz ligament and the inferior mesenteric vein. After measuring 50 cm of jejunum distal to the Treitz ligament, the jejunal loop is retracted toward the anterior abdominal wall and transected with a linear stapler. The mesentery is further divided 6–8 cm toward the mesentery's root using the linear stapler or vessel sealer. The staple line and the mesentery are inspected for hemostasis. ICG fluorescence is used to assess the small bowel's perfusion prior to the anastomosis construction (**Figures 21-7 A–C**).

Step 2 average time frame: 5–10 min

> ▶▶ **TIPS**
>
> In a standard RYGB, the alimentary limb is around 150 cm and the biliopancreatic limb is around 50 cm. However, this might be tailored according to the patient's BMI and comorbidities. Many studies showed an association between the limb's length and weight loss or obesity-related comorbidities outcomes.

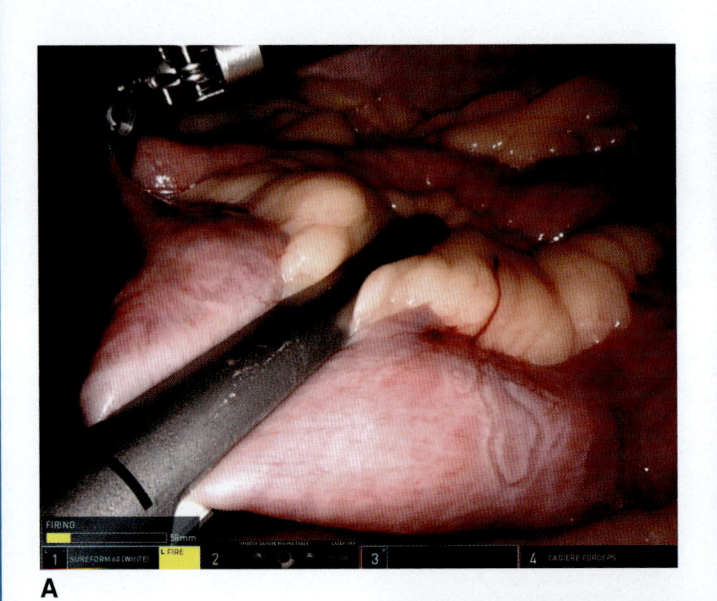

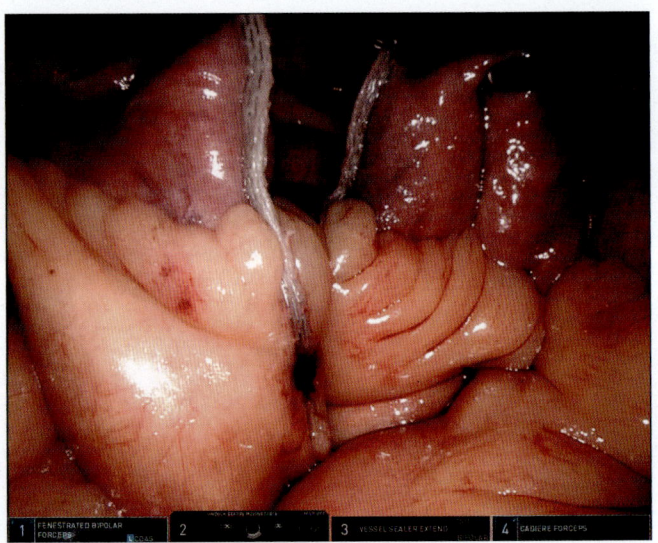

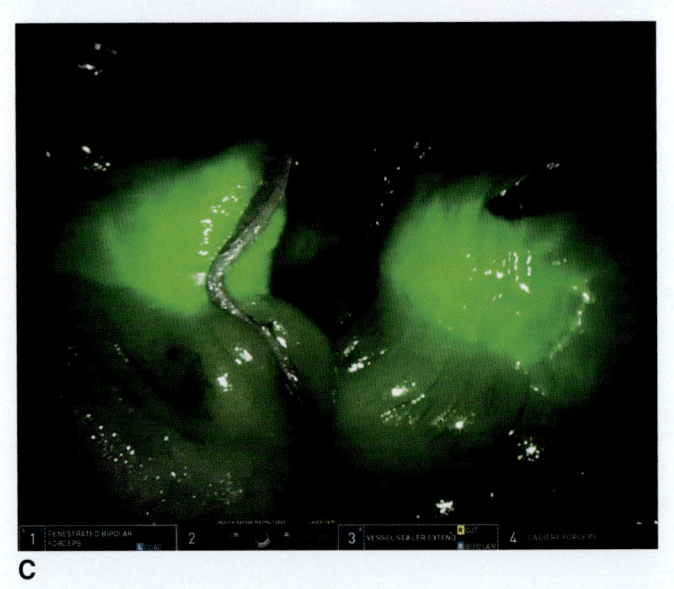

FIGURE 21-7 • Creation of the Roux-en-Y limb.

Step 3. Jejunojejunostomy

A 150-cm Roux limb is measured to determine the site of the jejunojejunostomy. With the help of the R3, the limbs are placed side to side to construct an anisoperistaltic anastomosis. Two small enterotomies are performed in the antimesenteric border of the small bowel using the monopolar hook. A side-to-side jejuno-jejunostomy is created using a 60-mm linear stapler. Afterward, the enterotomy is closed with a two-layered 3-0 PDS™ running suture. Additional 3-0 PDS™ stitches are used to reinforce the biliopancreatic limb staple line (**Figures 21-8 A–D**).

Step 3 average time frame: 15–20 min

> ▶▶ **TIPS**
>
> Proper alignment of the small bowel's mesentery should be checked before firing the linear stapler.

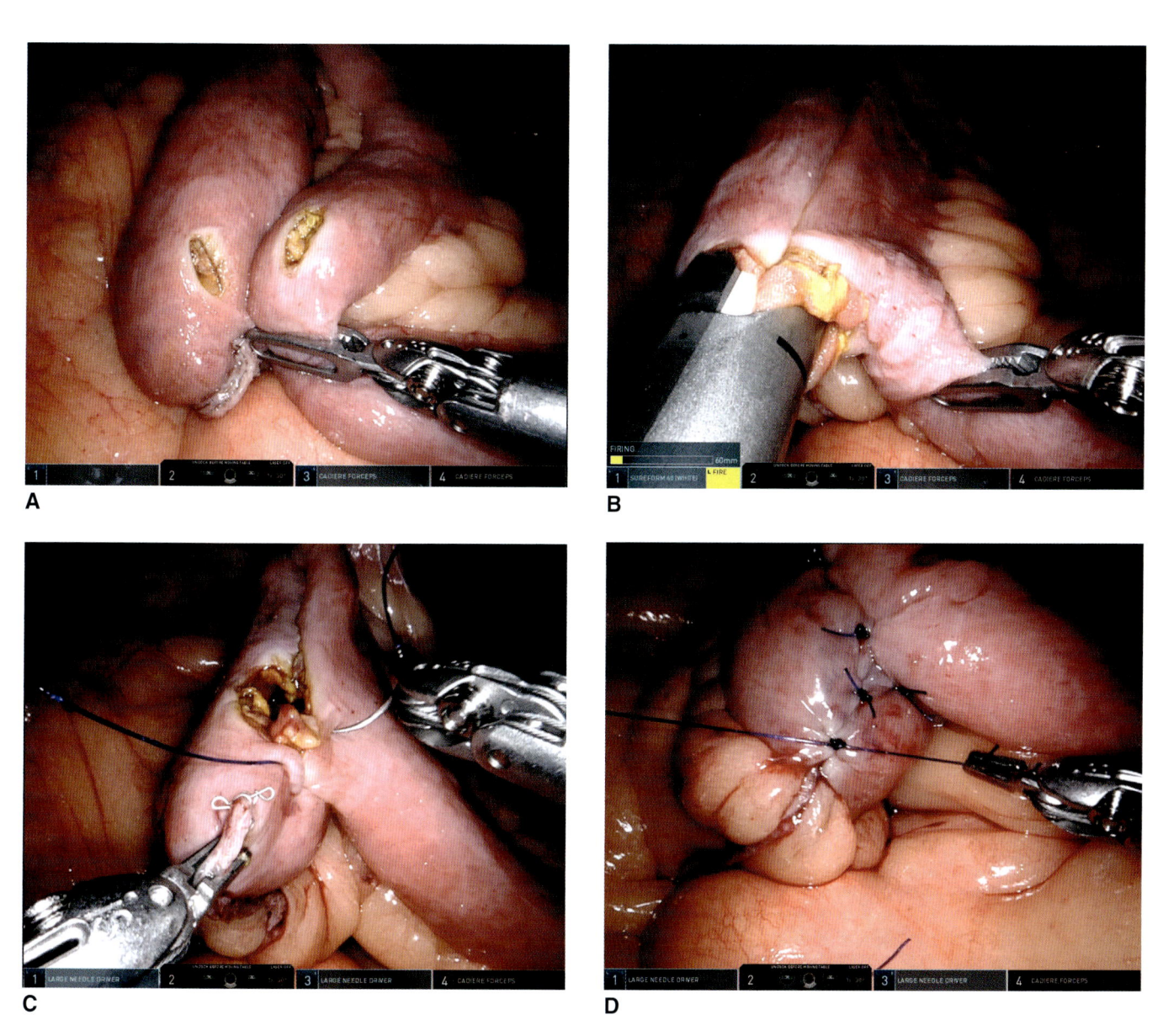

FIGURE 21-8 • Jejunojejunostomy.

Video 21-3 • Gastrojejunostomy

Step 4. Gastrojejunal anastomosis

The alimentary limb is brought antecolic and is held in position with the R3. The stump staple line of the alimentary limb is oriented toward the patient's left side. The end-to-side gastrojejunal anastomosis is performed in two layers. The posterior outer layer is made with a 3-0 PDS™ running suture. A 1.5-cm gastrotomy is performed just above the posterior suture line with the monopolar hook. The enterotomy is made in the antimesenteric border of the alimentary limb. The posterior internal layer is completed with a 3-0 PDS™ running suture. The anterior internal and outer layers are also performed with a 3-0 PDS™ running suture. At last, the alimentary limb's staple line is reinforced with additional PDS™ stitches (Figures 21-9 A–D).

Step 4 average time frame: 15–20 min

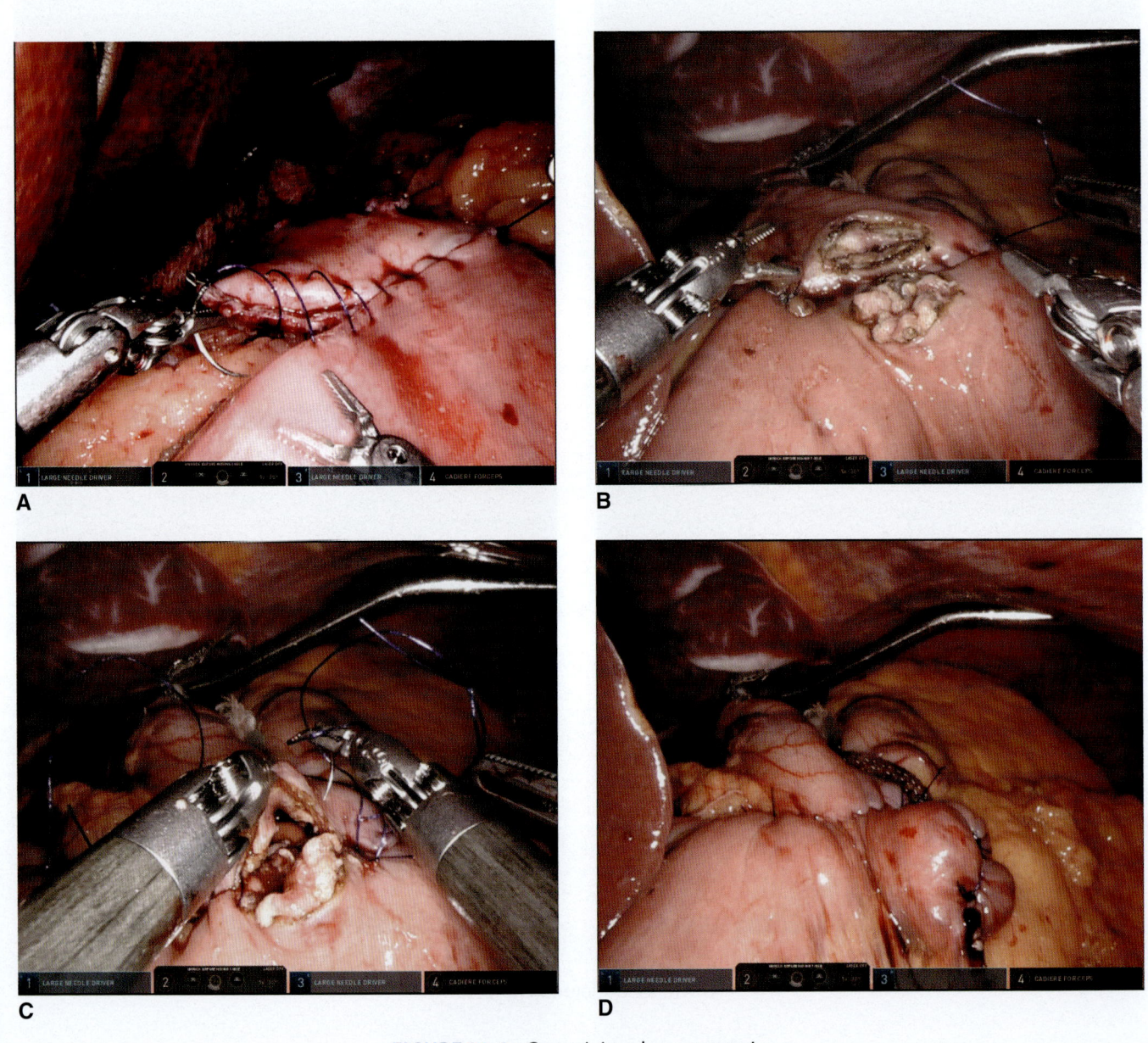

FIGURE 21-9 • Gastrojejunal anastomosis.

🔍 ANATOMICAL HIGHLIGHTS

RYGB anatomy (**Figure 21-10**).

▶▶ TIPS

Recent studies have shown similar outcomes between linear stapled and hand-sewn gastrojejunal anastomosis. However, higher postoperative bleeding and wound infection rates were found with circular staplers.

⚠ PITFALLS

A 36-Fr bougie can be used to calibrate the anastomosis and to avoid including the posterior wall of the pouch/jejunum while performing the anterior suture line.

The key to avoiding anastomotic complications is to create a well-perfused and tension-free gastrojejunal anastomosis. Adequate perfusion may be assessed with ICG fluorescence. Additionally, if the greater omentum is thick (creating tension in the anastomosis), it should be divided with the vessel sealer. If this maneuver fails to guarantee a tension-free anastomosis, a retrocolic or retrogastric transposition of the alimentary limb might be needed.

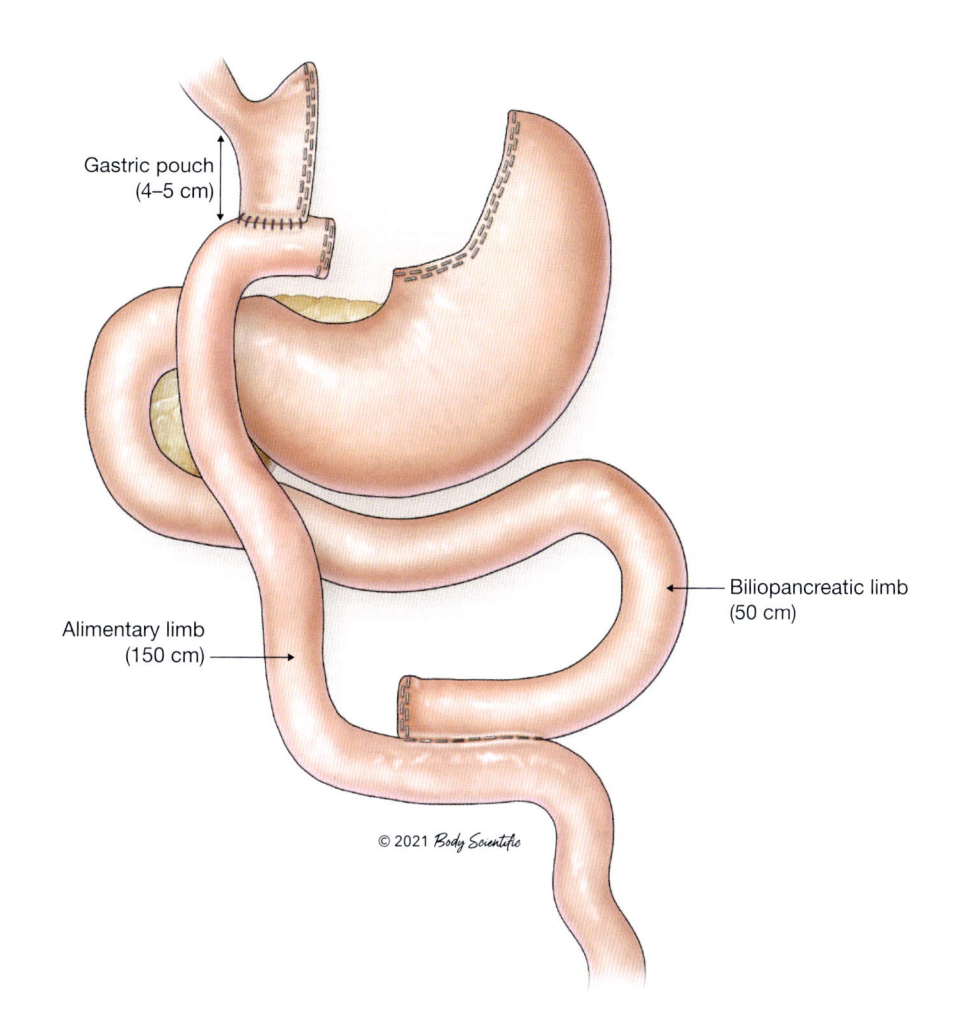

FIGURE 21-10 • RYGB anatomy.

Video 21-4 • Pseudo-Omega Technique

> **EDITORIAL NOTE**
>
> **PSEUDO-OMEGA TECHNIQUE**
>
> The gastrojejunostomy could also be constructed with a different sequence of steps to facilitate the exposure and to speed up the procedure. After measuring 50 cm of jejunum, this pseudo-omega technique consists of bringing up the undivided loop to do the gastrojejunostomy first. Then after measuring a 150-cm alimentary limb, the side-to-side jejunojejunostomy is created. The omega loop at this point is changed into a Roux-en-Y by simply dividing the connection between the gastric pouch and the biliopancreatic limb. See **Figures 21-11 A–C**.

A

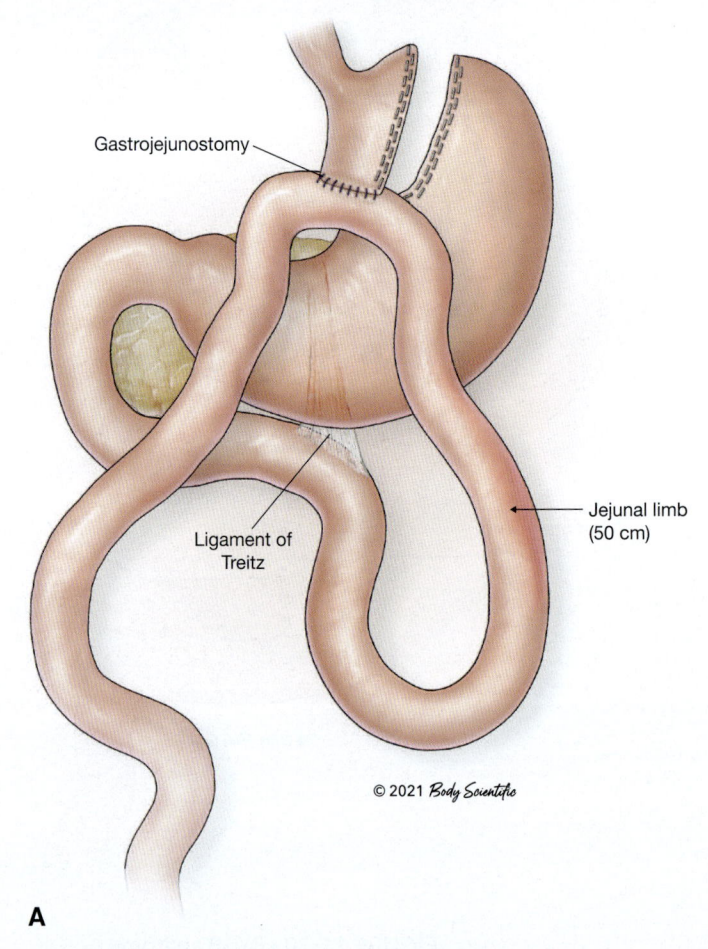

FIGURE 21-11 • Pseudo-omega technique.

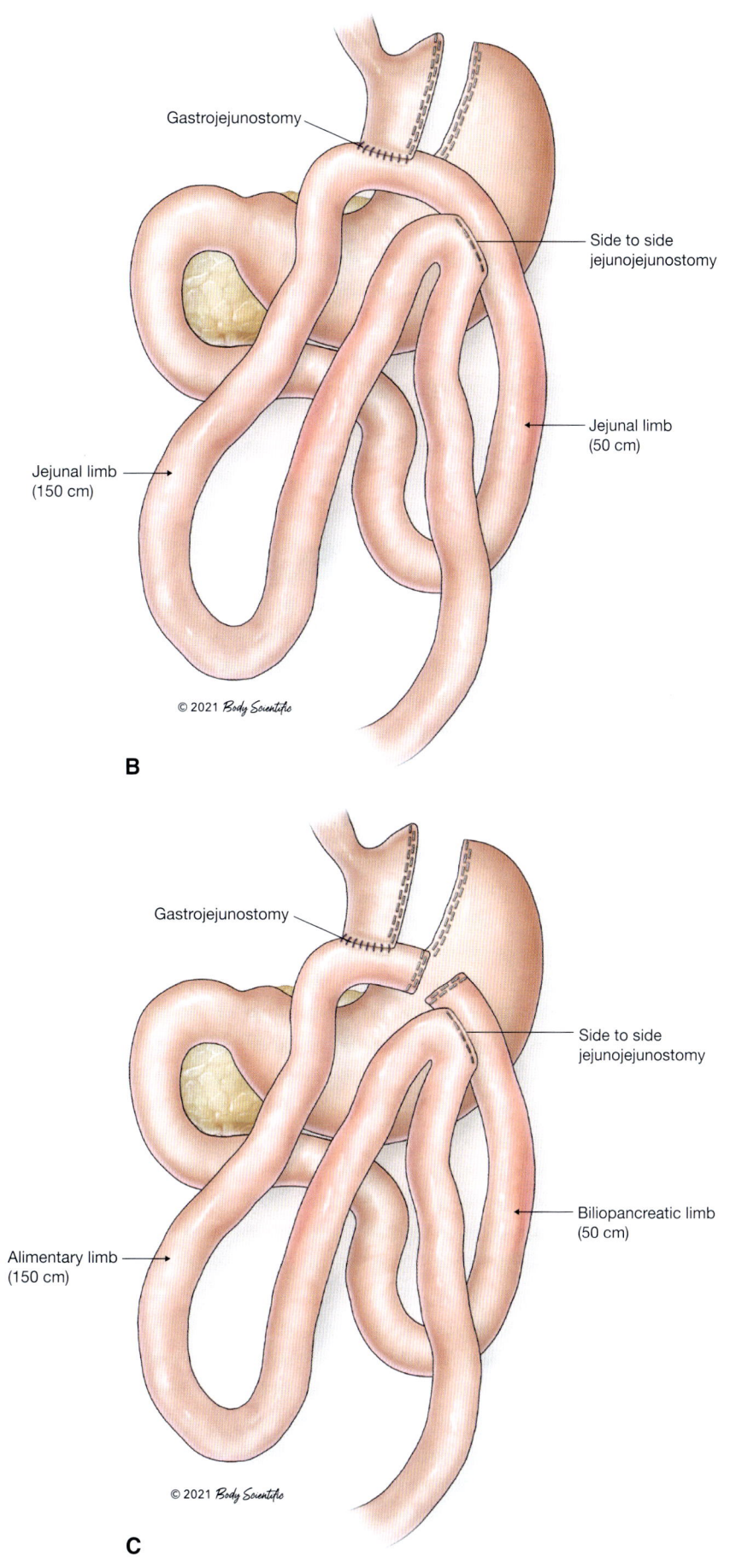

FIGURE 21-11 • *(Continued)*

Step 5. Closure of the mesenteric gap and Petersen space

The mesenteric gap at the jejuno-jejunostomy level is closed with a 2-0 polyester running suture. The space between the alimentary limb and the transverse colon (pseudo-Petersen's defect) is also closed with a 2-0 polyester suture (**Figure 21-12**).

Step 5 average time frame: 5–8 min

> ⚠️ **PITFALLS**
> Special attention should be paid to the stitches' depth to avoid vessel ligation and vascular injury. This might cause anastomotic ischemia or bleeding.

> ▶▶ **TIPS**
> Closure of mesenteric gaps is the key for postoperative internal hernia prevention (a frequent cause of urgent reoperation after RYGB).

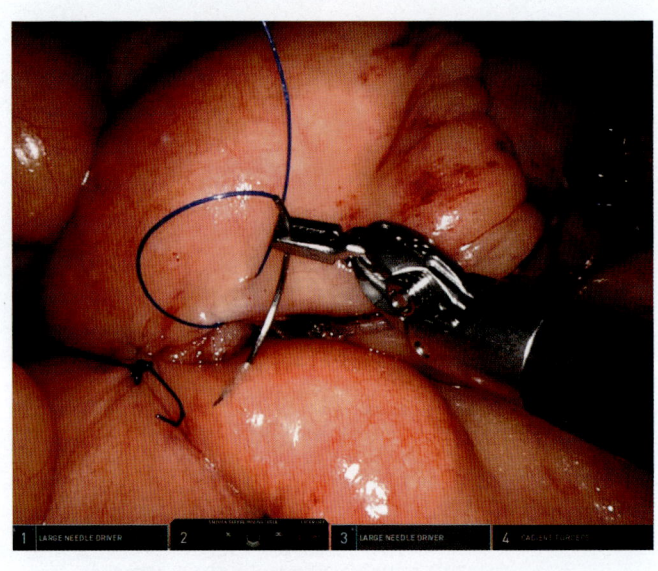

FIGURE 21-12 • Closure of the mesenteric gap.

Video 21-5 • Endoscopy

Step 6. Endoscopic evaluation

The alimentary limb is clamped, and saline is instilled over the anastomosis area. An intraoperative esophagogastroscopy is performed to check the anastomosis for bleeding or leaks. Finally, the pouch is decompressed, and the endoscope is pulled out. At last, all the fluid is aspirated from the abdominal cavity, and the Nathanson liver retractor and trocars are removed under direct vision. Drains are not routinely placed for this operation.

Step 6 average time frame: 5–10 min

Suggested Readings

1. Bindal V, Gonzalez-Heredia R, Masrur M, et al. Technique evolution, learning curve, and outcomes of 200 robot-assisted gastric bypass procedures: a 5-year experience. *Obes Surg.* 2015;25(6): 997-1002. doi: 10.1007/s11695-014-1502-9
2. Dreifuss NH, Mangano A, Hassan C, et al. Robotic revisional bariatric surgery: a high-volume center experience. *Obes Surg.* 2021; doi: 10.1007/s11695-020-05174-z
3. Di Lorenzo N, Antoniou SA, Batterham RL, et al. Clinical practice guidelines of the European Association for Endoscopic Surgery (EAES) on bariatric surgery: update 2020 endorsed by IFSO-EC, EASO, and ESPCOP. *Surg Endosc.* 2020;34(6):2332-2358. doi:10.1007/s00464-020-07555-y
4. Schlottmann F, Galvarini MM, Dreifuss NH, et al. Metabolic effects of bariatric surgery. *J Laparoendosc Adv Surg Tech A.* 2018;28(8): 944-948. doi: 10.1089/lap.2018.0394
5. Gan J, Wang Y, Zhou X. Whether a short or long alimentary limb influences weight loss in gastric bypass: a systematic review and meta-analysis. *Obes Surg.* 2018;28(11):3701-3710. doi: 10.1007/s11695-018-3475-6
6. Jiang HP, Lin LL, Jiang X, et al. Meta-analysis of hand-sewn versus mechanical gastrojejunal anastomosis during laparoscopic Roux-en-Y gastric bypass for morbid obesity. *Int J Surg.* 2016;32:150-157. doi: 10.1016/j.ijsu.2016.04.024
7. Giulianotti PC, Coratti A, Angelini M, et al. Robotics in general surgery: personal experience in a large community hospital. *Arch Surg.* 2003;138(7):777-784. doi: 10.1001/archsurg.138.7.777

SECTION V

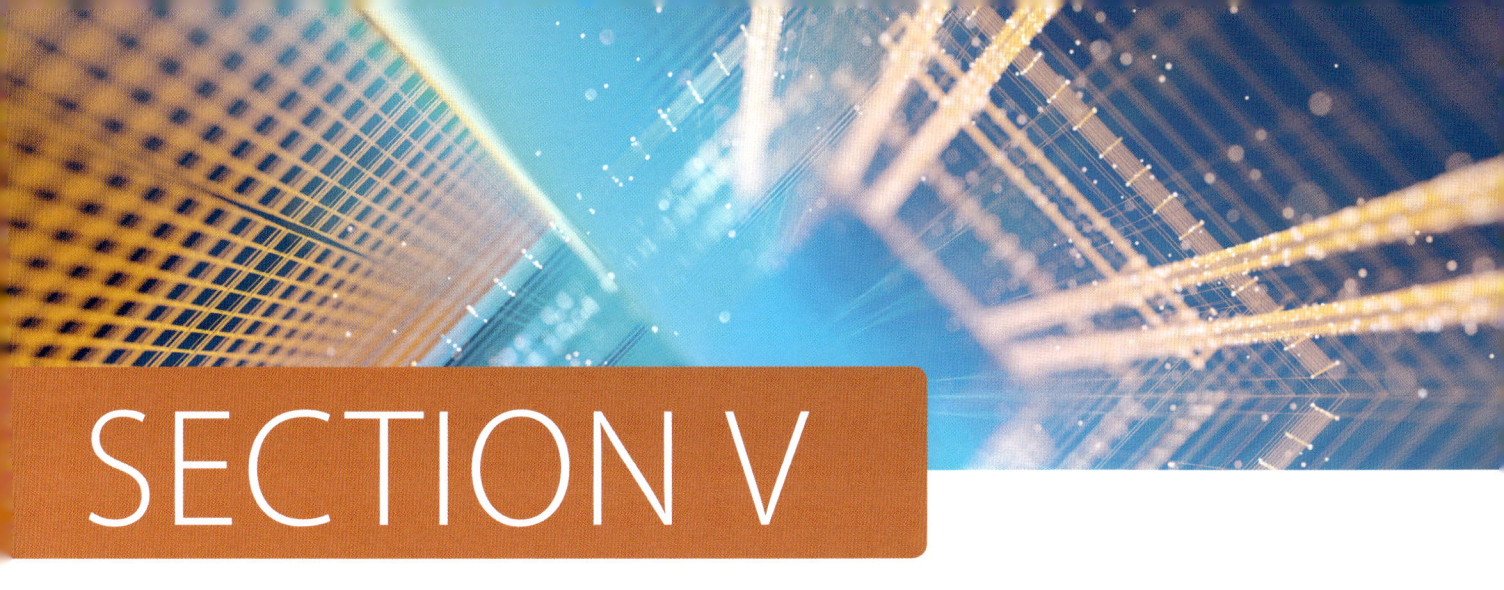

Intestinal Surgery

Chapter 22. Small Bowel Resection 437
Mario Alberto Masrur • Nicolas Hellmuth Dreifuss • Alberto Mangano • Pier Cristoforo Giulianotti

Chapter 23. Radical Right Colectomy with Complete Mesocolic Excision (CME) 455
Alberto Mangano • Valentina Valle • Colton Johnson • Pier Cristoforo Giulianotti

Chapter 24. Left Colectomy 479
Alberto Mangano • Valentina Valle • Pier Cristoforo Giulianotti

Chapter 25. Total Mesorectal Excision for Rectal Cancer 517
Hye Jin Kim • Alberto Mangano • Gyu-Seog Choi

Chapter 26. Abdominoperineal Resection..551
Gerald Gantt • Alberto Mangano • Vivek Chaudhry • Anders F. Mellgren

"… in general, the proper approach to a complete cure is by surgical resection of the diseased segment of the small intestine …"
—Burrill B. Crohn (1884–1983)

Small Bowel Resection

Mario Alberto Masrur • Nicolas Hellmuth Dreifuss • Alberto Mangano • Pier Cristoforo Giulianotti

INTRODUCTION

Small bowel resection (SBR) is one of the most common procedures performed by general surgeons. Frequent indications for this operation include, but are not limited to, partial small bowel obstruction due to adhesions, inflammatory bowel disease, and tumors. Due to the length and mobility of this organ, localization and further treatment of small bowel lesions may be challenging. Historically, SBR has been performed through a traditional open approach because direct palpation of the small bowel lesion was deemed necessary. In the last few decades, laparoscopic surgery, with its known advantages, has gained widespread acceptance in multiple gastrointestinal procedures. In addition, the development of preoperative and intraoperative techniques for small bowel lesion localization (e.g., angiography, video-capsule endoscopy, double-balloon enteroscopy, and laparoscopic sonography) has further increased the applicability of the minimally invasive approach.

Robotic technology has provided several advantages, particularly in case of malignant tumors. While some principles for the resection are universal, certain pathologies may require modifications, such as extension of the resection and associated lymphadenectomy.

This chapter will provide a detailed description of the step-by-step surgical technique for robotic SBR of the jejunum and the ileum.

Indications and Relative Contraindications to the Robotic Approach

There are no absolute contraindications for the robotic approach in the treatment of small bowel disease. Relative contraindications include bulky tumors with vascular invasion, multiple strictures from Crohn's disease, and complete small bowel obstruction with very dilated bowel loops. Previous history of multiple open abdominal operations and high body mass index (BMI) do not represent contraindications. The boundaries of what is feasible and achievable in a robotic way, as well as the patient selection, should be framed into the specific robotic surgical expertise of the console surgeon and of the surgical team. Common indications for SBR include inflammatory bowel disease, ulcers and strictures (Crohn's disease), arteriovenous malformation, tumors (neuroendocrine, gastrointestinal stromal tumors, adenomas, and adenocarcinomas), partial obstruction due to adhesions, and symptomatic diverticula.

INSTRUMENT REQUIREMENTS

The suggested main robotic instruments/tools can be listed as follows:
- 30° scope
- Needle drivers (round tip or macro)
- Cautery hook/monopolar scissors
- Harmonic shears/vessel sealer
- Bipolar forceps
- Cadière forceps
- Robotic linear staplers (with different loads)

The suggested main laparoscopic instruments/tools can be listed as follows:
- Needle drivers
- Scissors
- Graspers
- Suction-irrigation
- Laparoscopic linear staplers (with different loads)

Supplemental materials:
- Gauzes, sponges
- Sutures: PDS™ 2-0, 3-0, and 4-0, Prolene™ 3-0 and 4-0
- Endo Bag™

Patient Positioning, OR Setup, and Port Setting

After induction of general endotracheal anesthesia, the patient is placed supine, with arms tucked. The pneumoperitoneum is achieved with the Veress technique at the modified Palmer's point. The bed is tilted according to the location of the lesion. For lesions in the proximal segments of the small bowel (jejunum), where ports are preferably placed over the right side of the abdomen, a 30° reverse Trendelenburg and a slight right-sided tilting of the table is adopted (**Figure 22-1**). The assistant is located at the patient's right side. A 5-mm trocar is inserted in the right flank of the abdomen at the transverse umbilical line to do the initial laparoscopic assessment (**Figure 22-2**).

For lesions in the distal segments (ileum), where ports are preferably placed over the left side of the abdomen, a 10° Trendelenburg position and a slight left-sided tilting of the table are achieved (**Figure 22-3**). In this setting, the assistant is located at the patient's left side. In order to perform a diagnostic laparoscopy, a 5-mm trocar is inserted in the left flank at the transverse umbilical line (**Figure 22-4**).

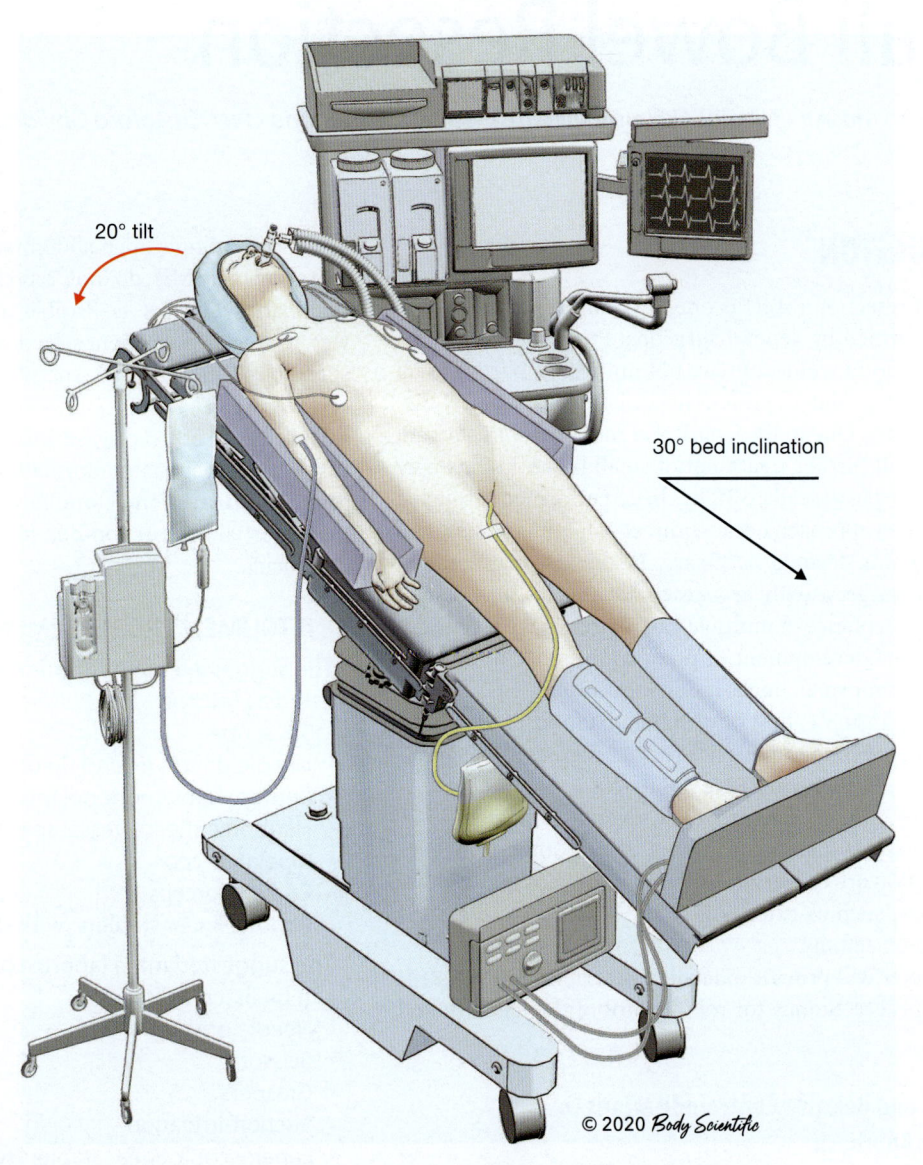

FIGURE 22-1 • Patient positioning in case of proximal small bowel segments.

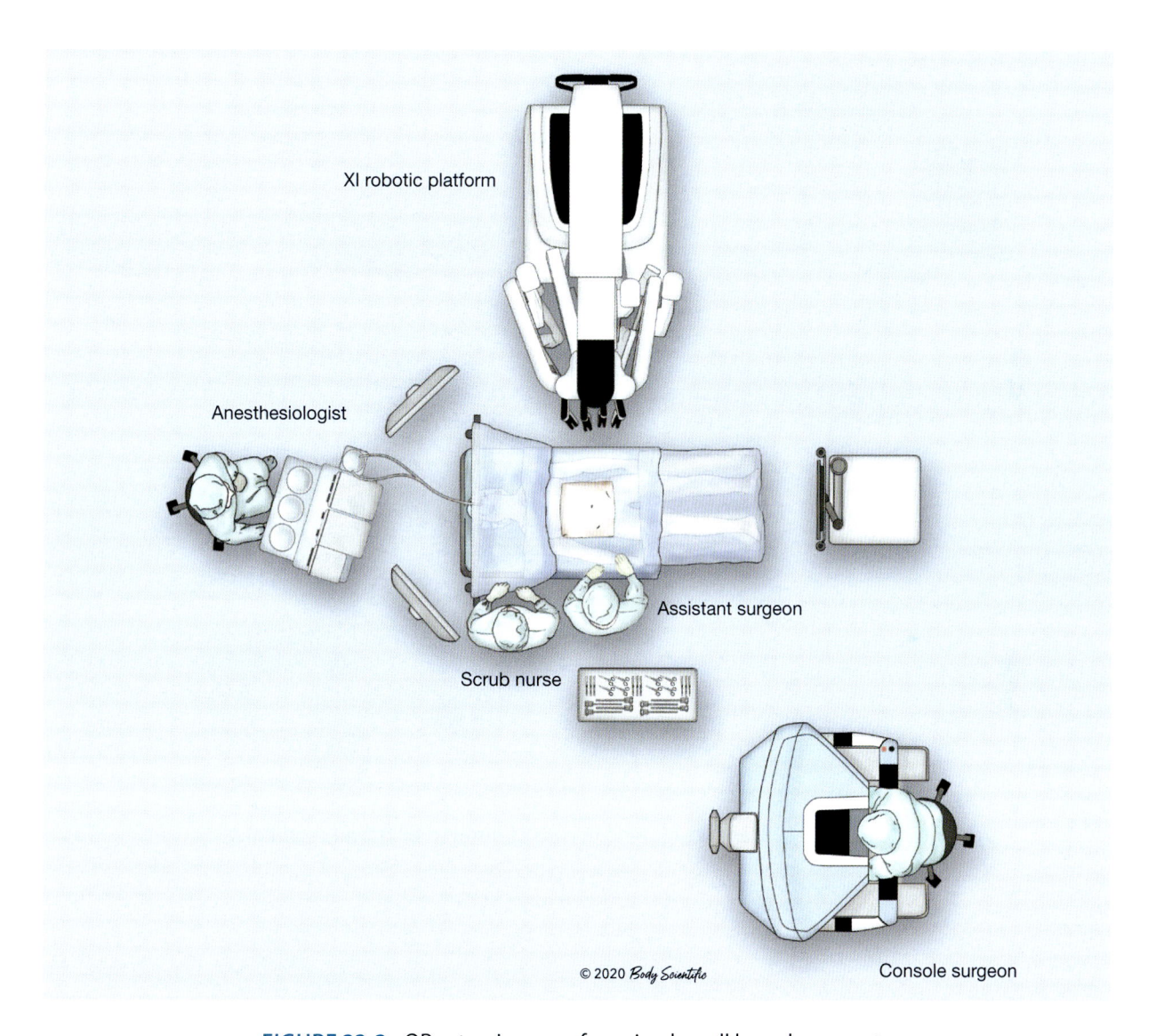

FIGURE 22-2 • OR setup in case of proximal small bowel segments.

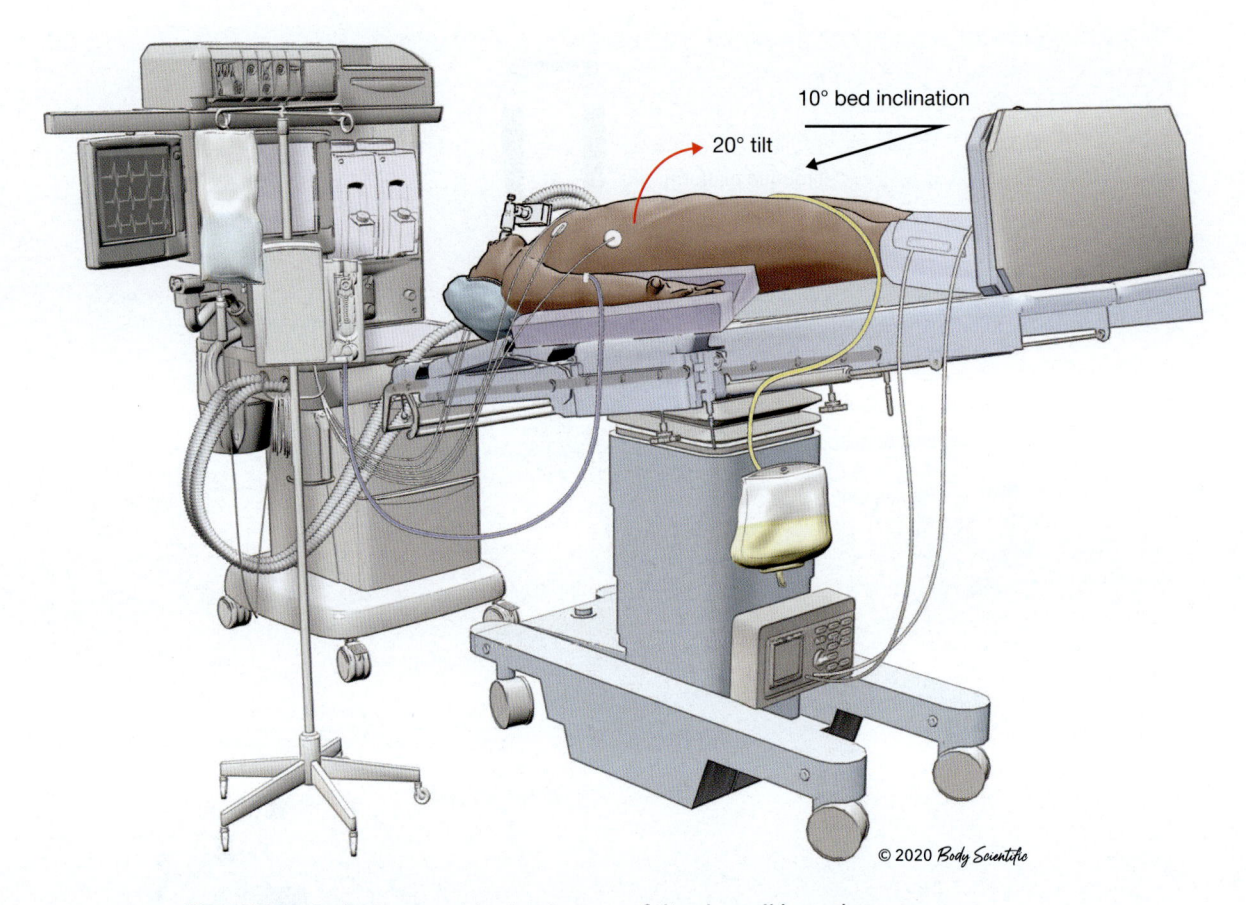

FIGURE 22-3 • Patient positioning in case of distal small bowel segments.

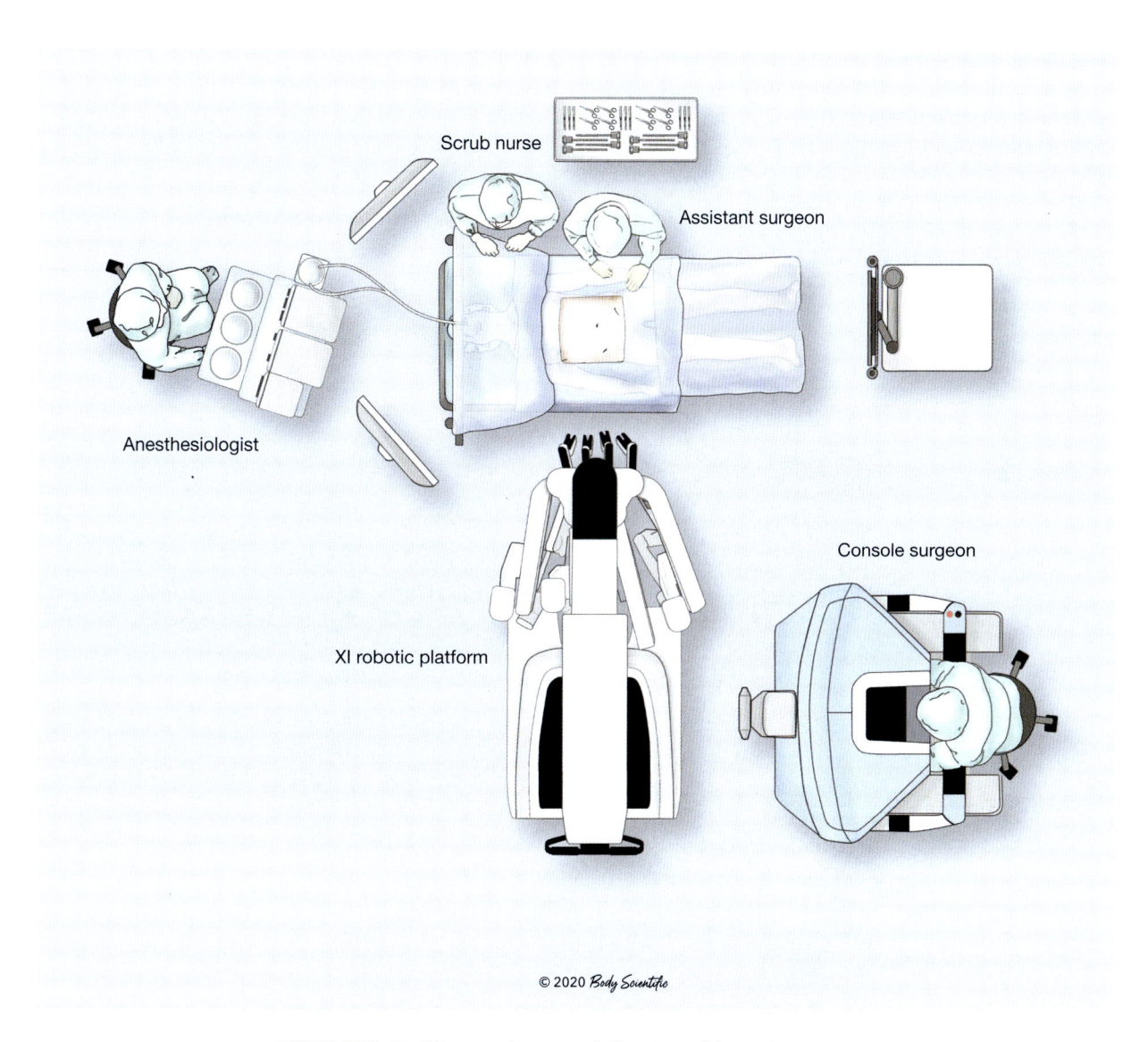

FIGURE 22-4 • OR setup in case of distal small bowel segments.

Surgical Technique

▶ **Video 22-1.** Small Bowel Resection

Step 1. Diagnostic laparoscopy and trocar positioning
During this step, the entire intra-abdominal anatomy is assessed with a 30° 5-mm laparoscopic camera. The small bowel lesion is typically identified, and the peritoneal surfaces evaluated to rule out concurrent pathologies, carcinomatosis, or distant metastasis. For an adequate port placement, the lesion should be properly located, and the small bowel fully inspected. For proximal lesions, two robotic ports (R1 and R2) are placed on the lateral right lower and upper quadrant, respectively. The previously placed 5-mm trocar is then upgraded to an 8-mm robotic camera port, and a 12-mm assistant port is placed between the R1 and camera port. If necessary, an additional 5-mm assistant port could be placed between the R2 and the scope (**Figure 22-5A**). For distal lesions, an 8-mm camera port replaces the trocar of the laparoscopic scope. The first and second robotic arms (R1 and R2) are placed on the lateral upper- and lower-left quadrant, respectively. A 12-mm assistant port is positioned between the R1 and the camera port. Alternatively, if there is not enough space to place a third robotic arm (R3), an additional 5-mm port for the assistant can be used in between the camera port and R2. Finally, if a decision to use the robotic stapler is taken, the R2 can be upgraded to a 12-mm port (**Figure 22-5B**).

Step 1 average time frame: 5–10 min

Normal abdomen

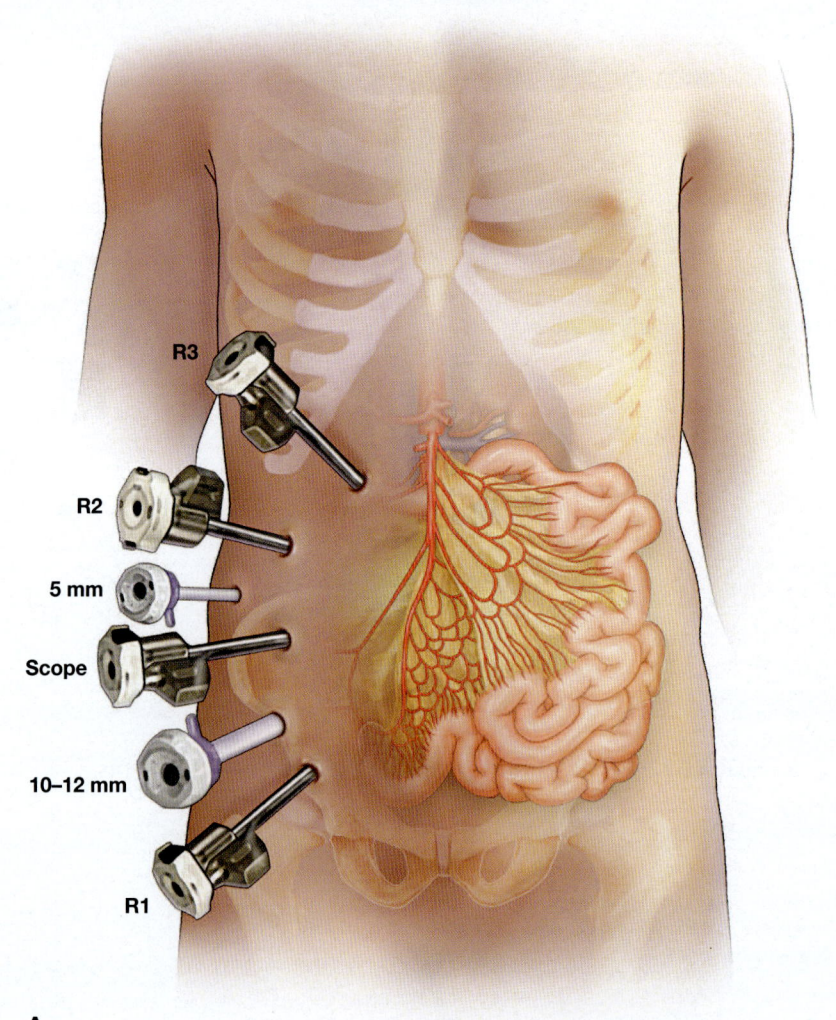

A

FIGURE 22-5 • **A.** Port placement in proximal lesions.

Normal abdomen

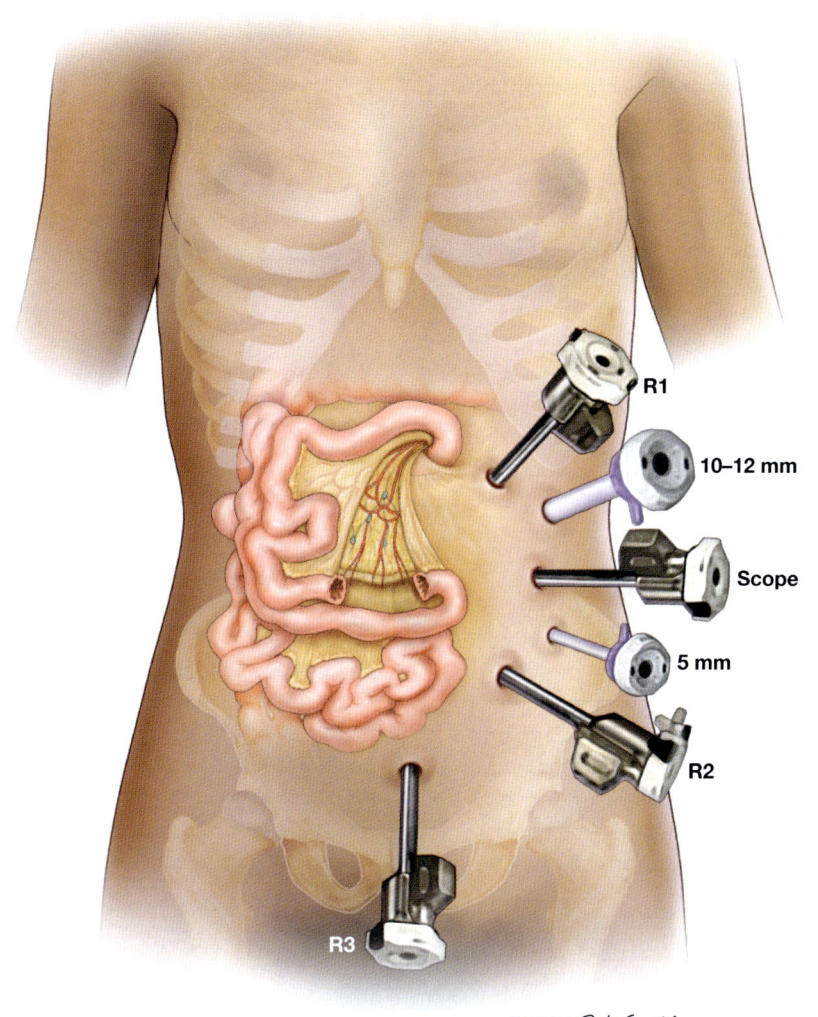

FIGURE 22-5 • (Continued) B. Port placement in distal lesions.

> **▶▶ TIPS**
>
> When the lesion is not visually identified on the initial exploration, a second 5-mm port can be added to allow an assisted exploration using a laparoscopic grasper (indirect palpation).
>
> In right-side settings, the R3 can be placed (if necessary) in the right subcostal area, where more effective retraction of the transverse colon can be achieved.
>
> For left settings, the R3 can be located in the suprapubic area, and it becomes especially useful for lesions in the terminal ileum, allowing a better retraction of the cecum and right colon, as well as facilitating the exposure of the ileocolic vessels.

🎥 Video 22-2. Step 2. Laparoscopic Exploration

Step 2. Laparoscopic evaluation of the entire small bowel
Once the ports are in place, the small bowel is gently run centimeter by centimeter using laparoscopic graspers, and the target segment is properly identified and fully exposed. The mesentery should be assessed: indirect palpation with graspers allows the identification of mesenteric masses or metastatic lymph nodes. An exploration of all abdominal quadrants is mandatory to detect concurrent or distant lesions. After the small bowel lesion is identified, the target segment and mesentery should be left exposed to allow its quick recognition once the robot is docked.

Step 2 average time frame: 15–20 min

> ⚠️ **PITFALLS**
>
> **Small bowel injury:** Adhesiolysis should be performed with sharp scissors and blunt laparoscopic instruments without energy because thermal lateral spread may cause bowel injury. Special care must be taken, while manipulating the dilated bowel loops in case of obstruction or severe inflammation to prevent small bowel perforation.
>
> **Tumor rupture:** In the presence of small bowel tumors, the surgeon should avoid manipulation of the lesion to avoid rupture or peritoneal seeding.

> ▶▶ **TIPS**
>
> When the adhesions are not firm, they can be taken down using laparoscopic instruments. In some cases, accessory ports may be needed to allow a better exposure. Once enough space has been created for the robotic trocar placement, the robot is docked, and adhesiolysis can be continued robotically. More challenging or dense adhesions in narrow spaces, among bowel loops, or involving a previous mesh are better addressed using robotic instruments (see Chapter 2, The Basic Principles of Clinical Applications).

Step 3. Docking time and patient positioning
The robotic cart is then brought from the side and hooked to the robotic trocars. A 30° robotic camera is preferred for this procedure. The patient's position is subsequently modified to a 30° reverse Trendelenburg and a right-side tilting in proximal lesions, whereas a 10° Trendelenburg and left-side tilting position is used for distal lesions. The initial setup is as follows: bipolar forceps in the R2 and monopolar hook in the R1. If the R3 is being utilized, Cadière forceps is the preferred instrument for retraction and exposure.

Step 3 average time frame: 3–5 min

🎥 Video 22-3. Step 4. Mesenteric Dissection

Step 4. Mesenteric dissection and lymphadenectomy
The extent of mesenteric dissection needed depends on the nature of the lesion. In case of benign disease, a minimal mesenteric resection is sufficient to the level of the straight terminal intestinal arteries. This territory can be easily controlled with a vessel sealer. On the contrary, when malignancy is suspected, an associated en bloc lymphadenectomy should be performed with a wider mesenteric dissection. To that end, the larger intestinal arteries involved in the resection require suture ligation, Hem-o-lok™ placement, or stapling. Understanding the small bowel's arterial anatomy (**Figure 22-6A**), its variations (**Figure 22-6B**), venous anatomy (**Figure 22-6C**), and lymphatic drainage is paramount for an adequate oncological resection (**Figure 22-7**). For additional information regarding small bowel arterial anatomy variations, see suggested readings #5, 6.

The area of the resection is established following oncological principles of about 5–10 cm proximally and distally. Free margins, and an average of 8–10 lymph nodes, should be included in the specimen (see suggested reading #7). The mesentery is then marked with a monopolar hook in a triangular wedge shape going from the small bowel to the root of the mesentery. The primary intestinal vessels supplying the affected segment are dissected circumferentially, and then divided at the origin from the superior mesenteric artery, using a stapler, Hem-o-loks™, or suture ligation (**Figures 22-8 A–E**). The adjacent vascular arcades should also be controlled, using suture ligation or a vessel sealer. If the hemostatic effect of the energy device is insufficient, bleeding from the retracted remaining mesentery can occur. In these situations, additional hemostatic sutures can be applied as needed. The mesentery is then fully resected, using a vessel sealer and suture ligation, in a wedge shape until reaching the bowel. During this step, minimal traction on the small bowel should be exerted to avoid tension in the tissue and to prevent ineffective hemostasis (in particular when utilizing the vessel sealer).

Step 4 average time frame: 15–30 min

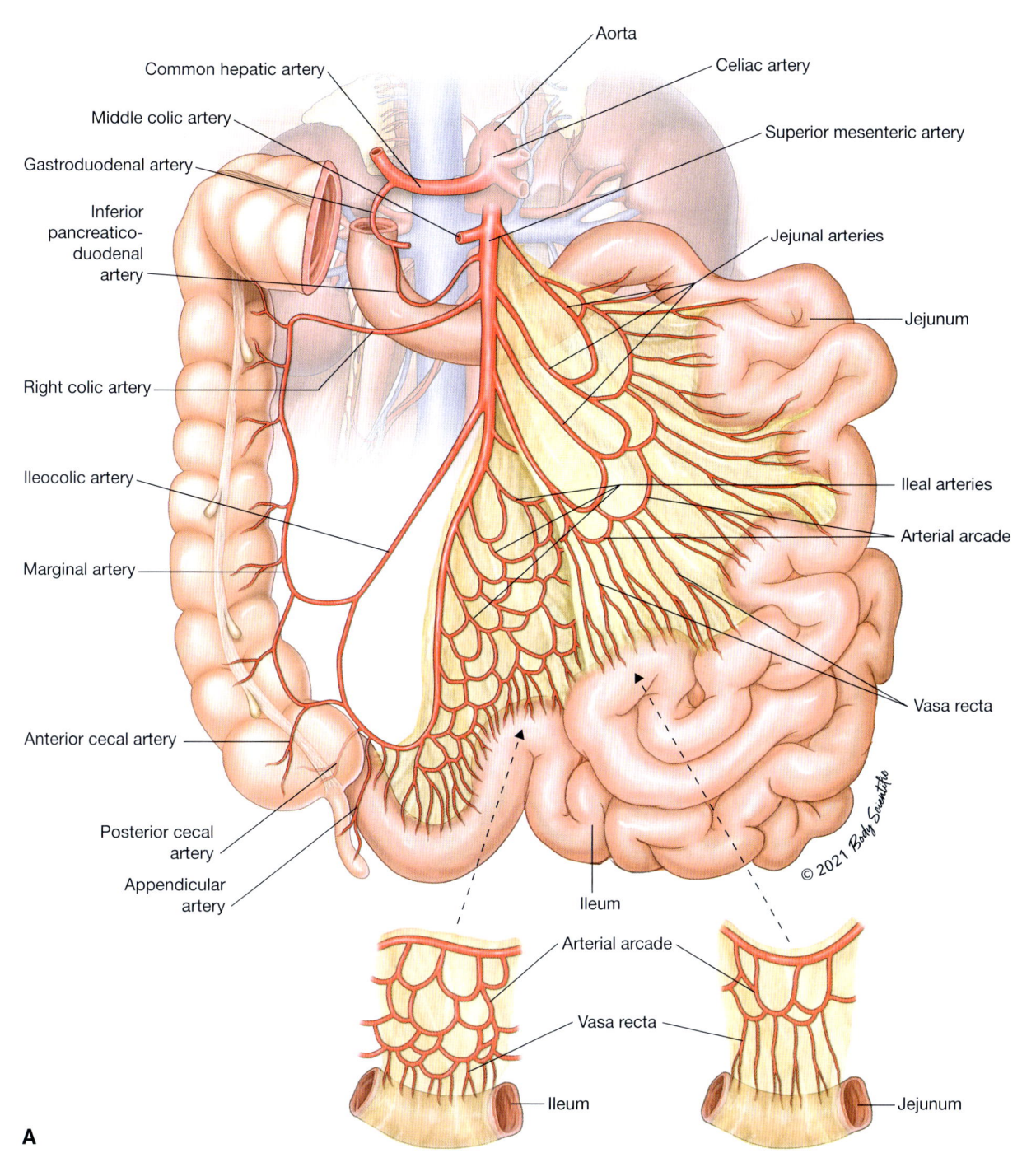

FIGURE 22-6 • **A.** Small bowel arterial anatomy.

446 The Foundation and Art of Robotic Surgery

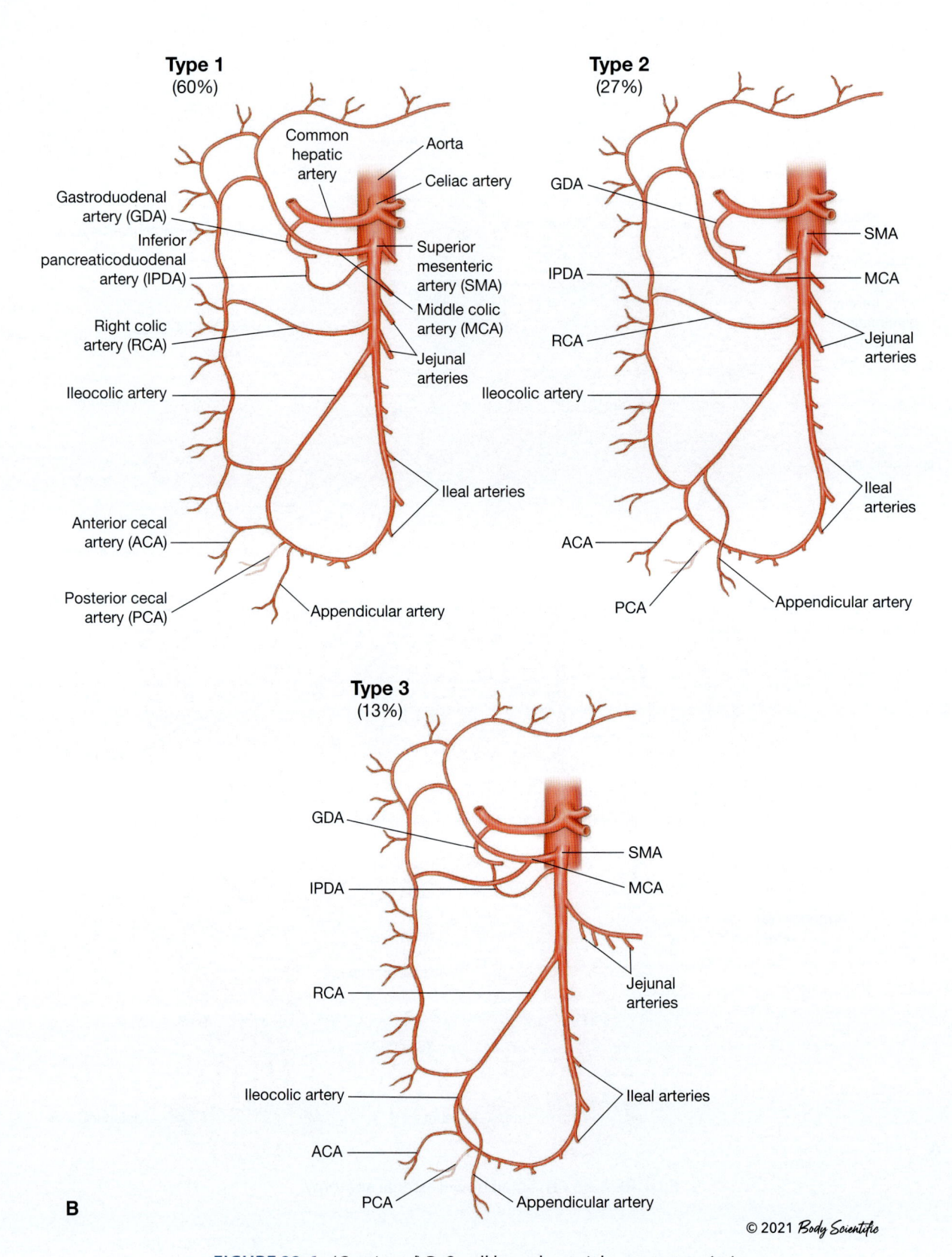

FIGURE 22-6 • (*Continued*) **B.** Small bowel arterial anatomy variations.

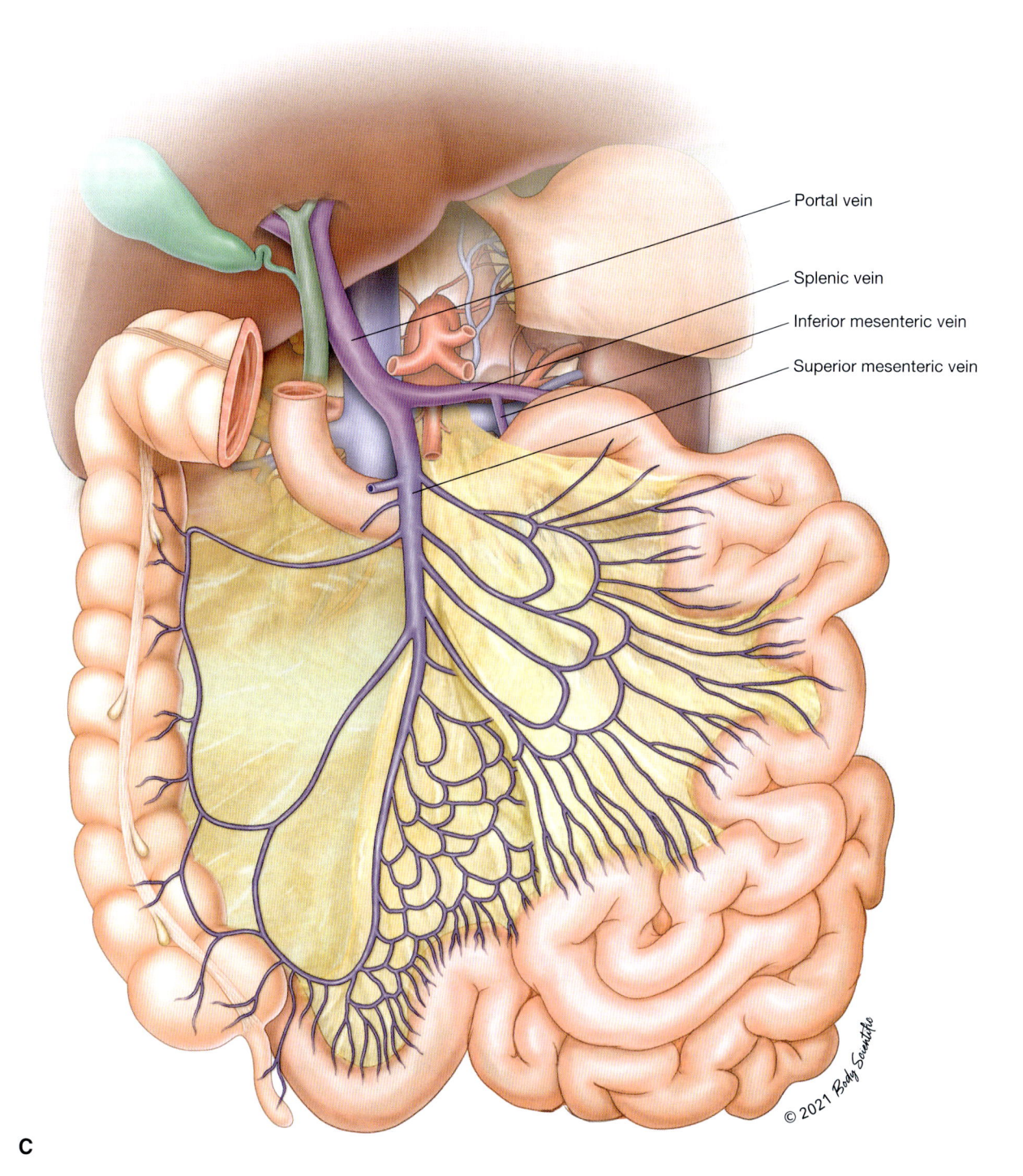

FIGURE 22-6 • *(Continued)* C. Small bowel venous anatomy.

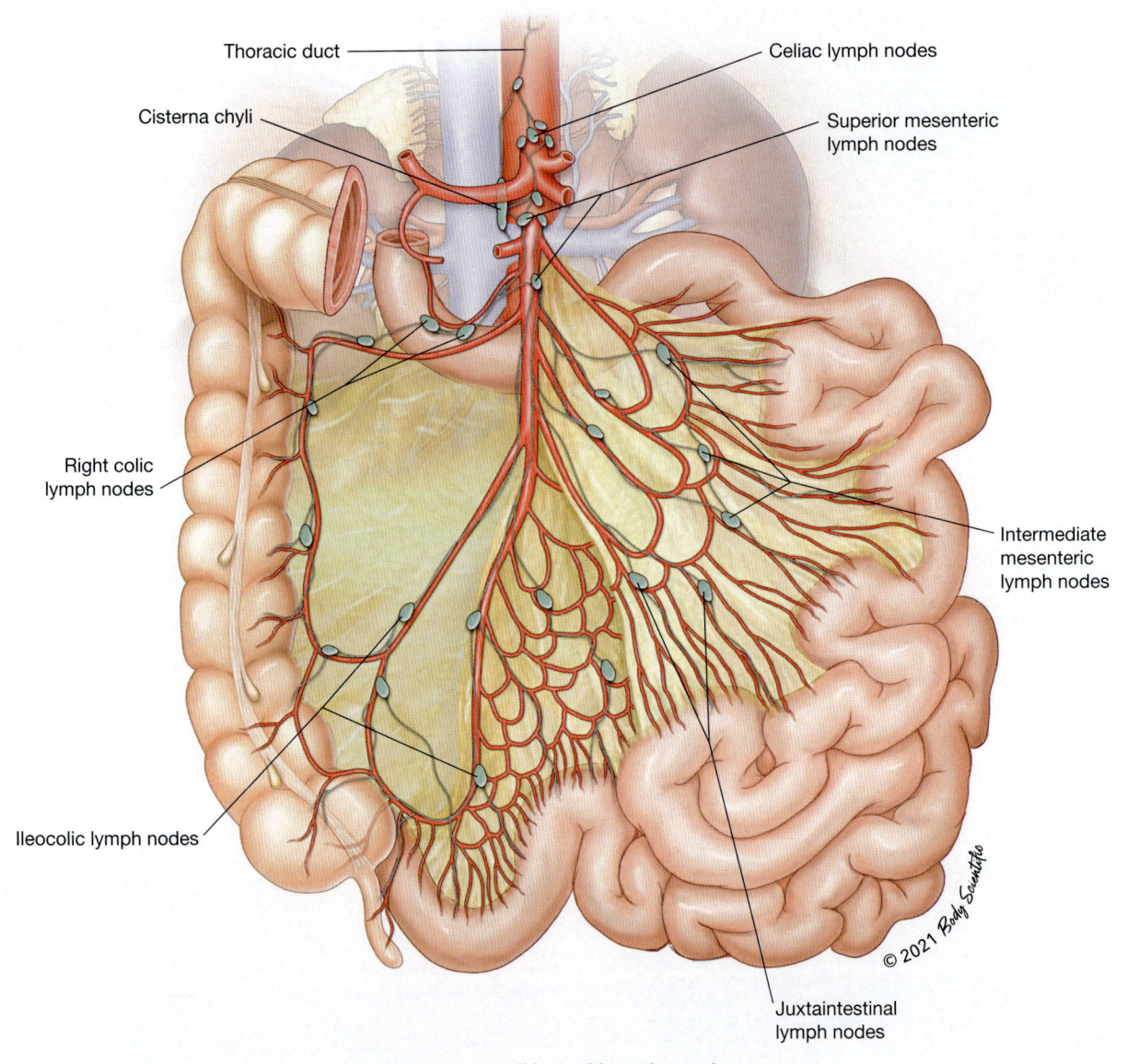

FIGURE 22-7 • Small bowel lymphatic drainage.

Small Bowel Resection 449

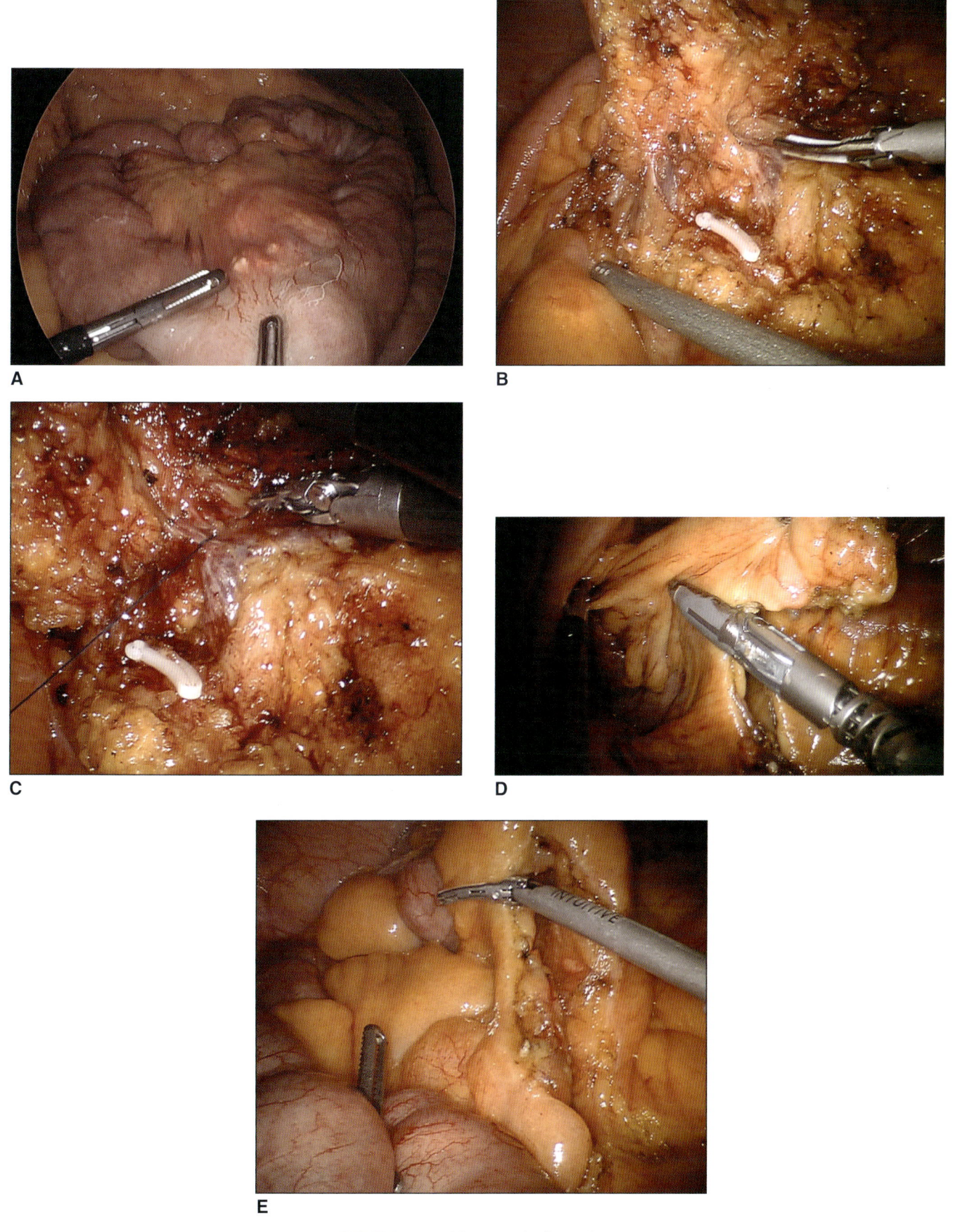

FIGURE 22-8 • Mesenteric dissection.

450 The Foundation and Art of Robotic Surgery

> **ANATOMICAL HIGHLIGHTS**
>
> Small bowel arterial anatomy (**Figure 22-6A**), arterial anatomy variations (**Figure 22-6B**), venous anatomy (**Figure 22-6C**), and lymphatic drainage (**Figure 22-7**).
>
> Structure of the mesentery (**Figures 22-9 A–C**).

A

Labels: Jejunum, Fat, Duodenum, Inferior duodenal fossa, Duodenomesocolic fold, Inferior mesenteric vein, Arterial arcade, Peritoneum, Vasa recta, Ileum

B

Labels: Duodenum, Transverse mesocolon, Root of mesentery, Gastrocolic ligament (greater omentum)

C

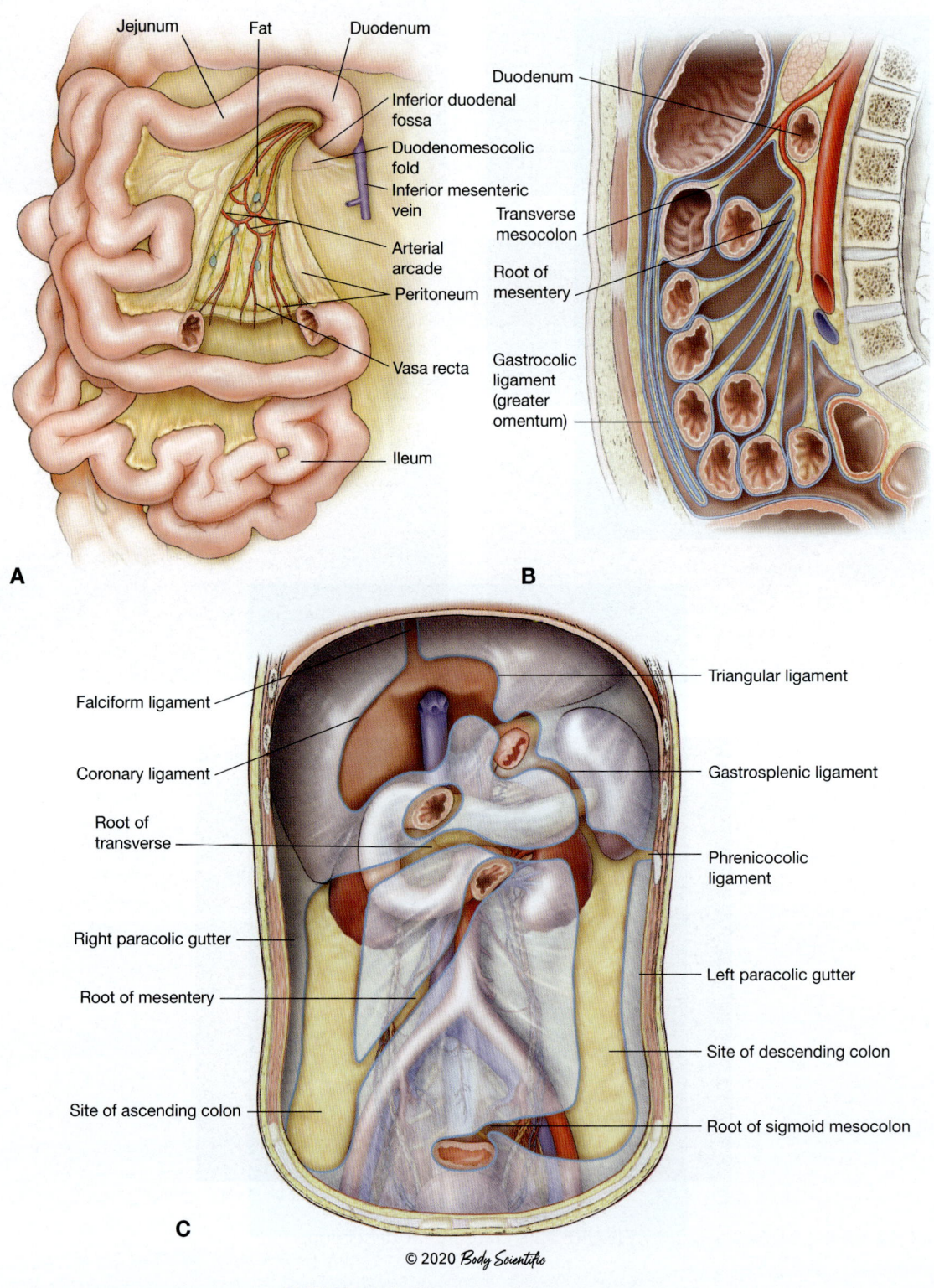

Labels: Falciform ligament, Coronary ligament, Root of transverse, Right paracolic gutter, Root of mesentery, Site of ascending colon, Triangular ligament, Gastrosplenic ligament, Phrenicocolic ligament, Left paracolic gutter, Site of descending colon, Root of sigmoid mesocolon

© 2020 Body Scientific

FIGURE 22-9 • Structure of the mesentery.

►► TIPS

In the case of terminal ileum tumors, an ileocecal resection may be required to achieve good oncological margins and adequate lymph node harvest.

Oncological resections on a proximal segment can be riskier, because in extended resections, the main trunk of the superior mesenteric artery could be compromised. On the contrary, a distal segment tends to be safer: although the terminal branch of the superior mesenteric artery can be compromised, the ileocolic or right colic artery can supply the remaining ileum, cecum, and right colon. The use of indocyanine green (ICG) fluorescence can be useful during this step.

Step 5. Perfusion assessment and transection

Once the mesenteric window has been created, ICG fluorescence is used for perfusion assessment prior to the transection of the small bowel. This represents an additional layer of security that helps with directing the location of the transection line. The division of the bowel is then performed using a linear stapler. The robotic stapler is introduced via a 12-mm port and stapling is controlled by the surgeon. Alternatively, this step can be performed by the bedside assistant using a laparoscopic stapling device (**Figures 22-10 A–C**). If there are doubts about the proper perfusion of the small bowel stumps, the ICG fluorescence assessment can be repeated (**Figures 22-11 A–D**).

Step 5 average time frame: 5–10 min

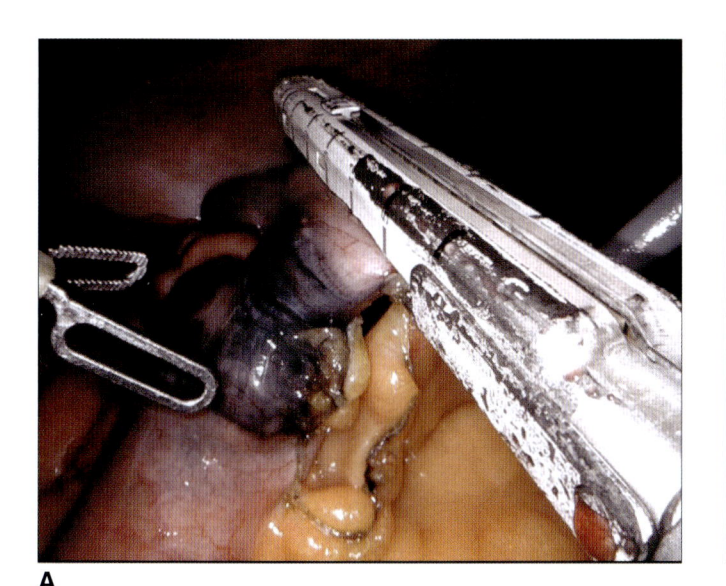

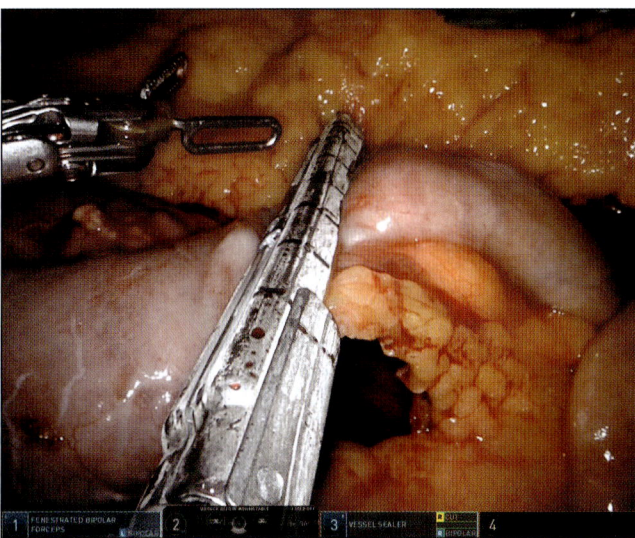

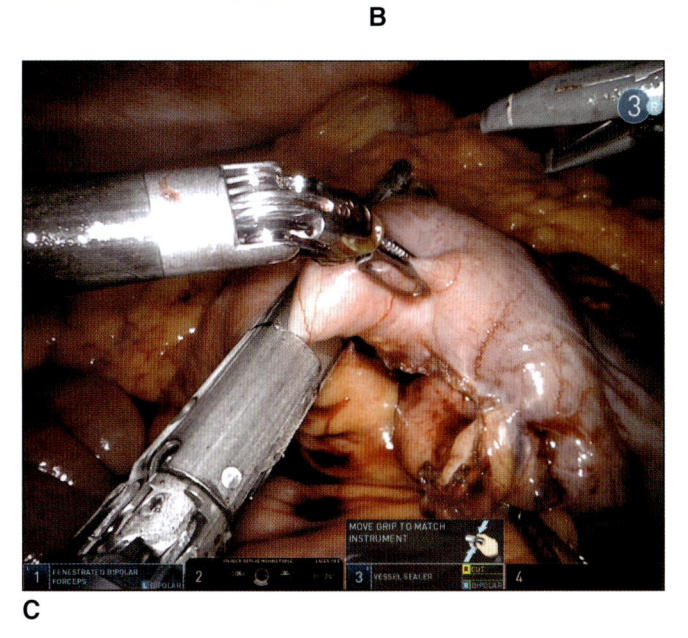

FIGURE 22-10 • Small bowel transection.

452 The Foundation and Art of Robotic Surgery

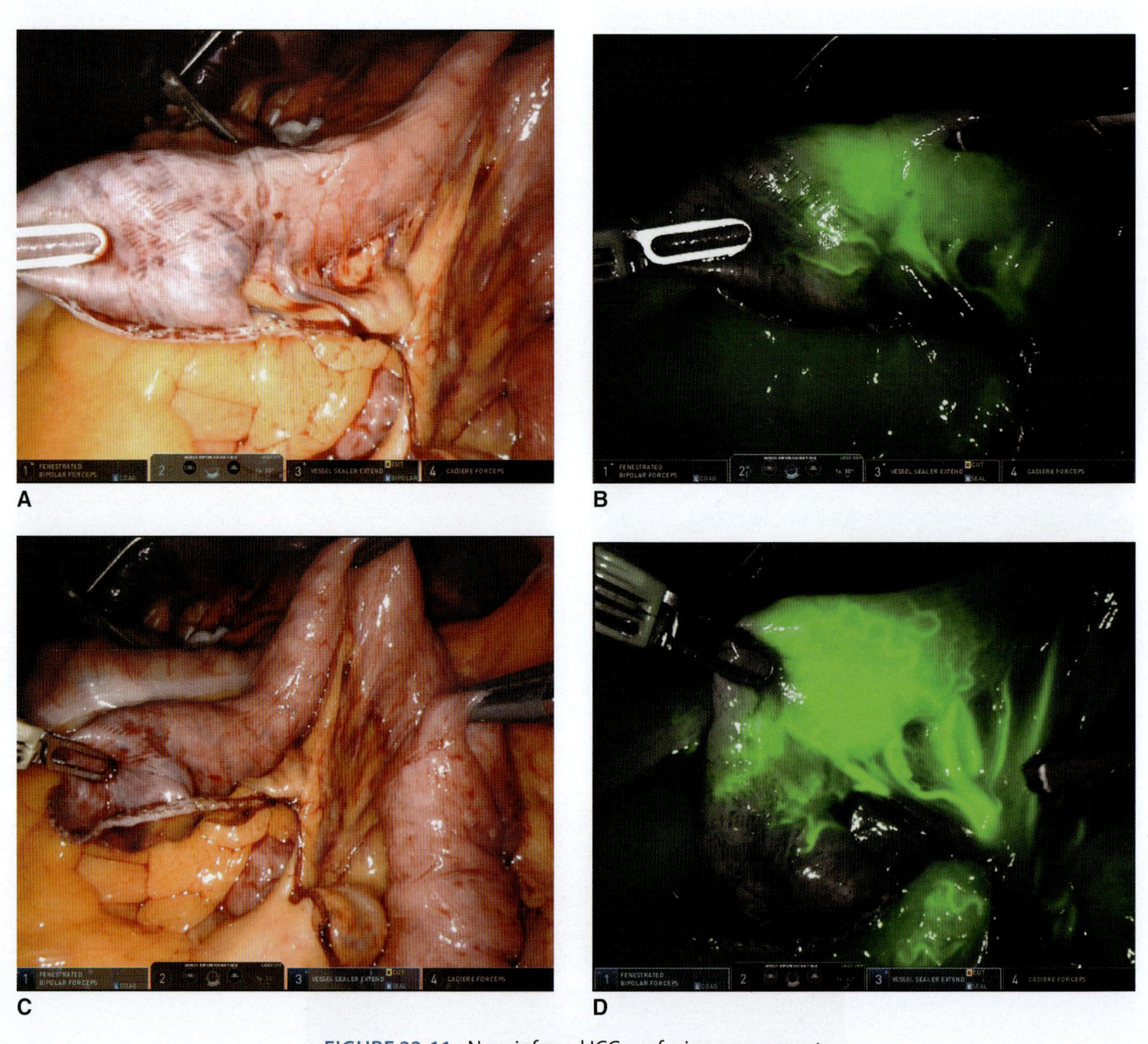

FIGURE 22-11 • Near infrared ICG perfusion assessment.

Small Bowel Resection   453

▶ **Video 22-4. Step 6. Side-to-Side Small Bowel Anastomosis**

Step 6. Reconstruction
Restoring the intestinal continuity after SBR can be performed in several ways, including intra- *versus* extracorporeal anastomosis, side-to-side *versus* end-to-end reconstruction, stapling versus hand-sewn technique, and iso- *versus* antiperistaltic anastomosis. The preferred reconstruction is intracorporeal, side-to-side, isoperistaltic anastomosis performed using a linear stapler.

The bowel stumps are laid overlapping side by side, using an atraumatic grasper. A stay suture is placed to keep the bowel in place with the correct orientation. Small enterotomies are performed at the antimesenteric border of each stump using the monopolar hook. A linear stapler is gently introduced into the small bowel, then the bowel is carefully manipulated with atraumatic robotic forceps and properly positioned onto the stapler. After the stapler is closed, proper inspection is performed to ensure that no other structure is inadvertently caught in between. Finally, the stapler is fired creating a side-to-side anastomosis. The enterotomies are then closed using a running 3-0 PDS with a handsewing robotic technique (**Figures 22-12 A–D**). Reinforcement Prolene™ 4-0 stitches can be placed over the anastomosis and staple lines.

Step 6 average time frame: 15–20 min

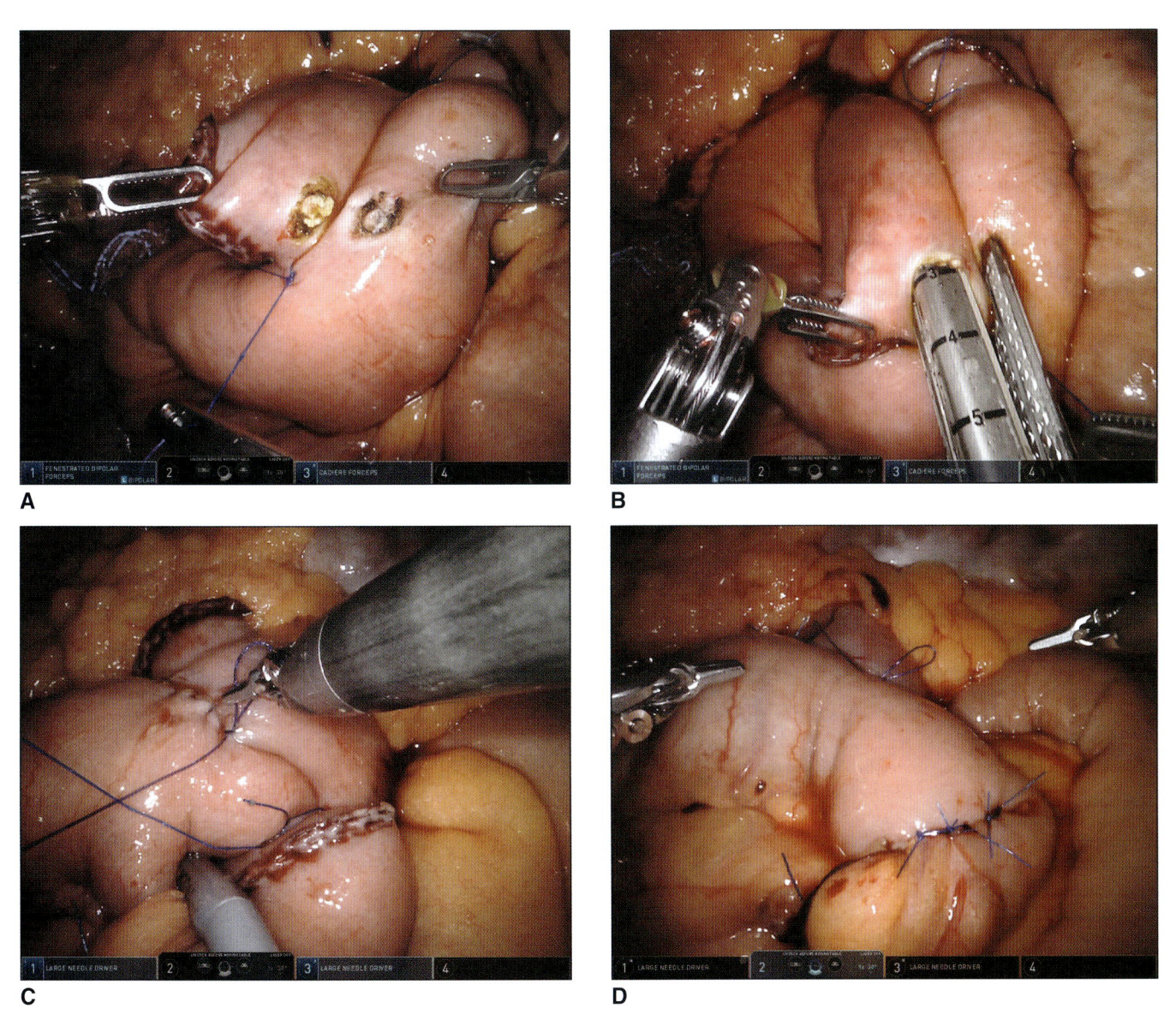

FIGURE 22-12 • Side-to-side small bowel anastomosis.

Step 7. Closure of the mesenteric gap

To avoid potential internal hernia formation, the mesenteric gap is always closed using Prolene™ 3-0 interrupted stiches. The stiches should be carefully placed at the correct depth to avoid mesenteric vessel ligation and vascular injury (**Figure 22-13**).

Step 7 average time frame: 5–10 min

> ⚠️ **PITFALLS**
>
> Hematoma of the mesentery while suturing the mesenteric gap. This condition could end up with compression and relative ischemia of the related bowel. Removing the suture can make the situation worst. In this case it is better to add an additional stitch to stop the intra-mesenteric bleeding, but checking there is no impact on the normal microperfussion of the bowel loop. If necessary, an ICG test can be repeated. Rarely, when ischemia is detected, the bowel loop should be resected again and the anastomosis re-done.

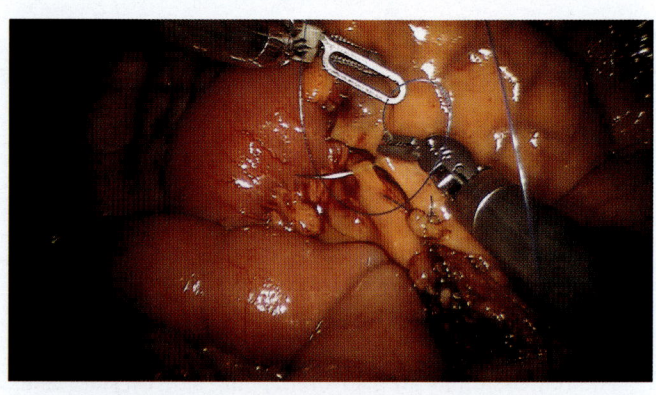

FIGURE 22-13 • Closure of the mesenteric gap.

Step 8. Specimen extraction

The specimen is placed in an Endo bag™ and extracted through a small Pfannenstiel incision or by enlarging a port site incision. Other extraction sites may be considered in the case of previous abdominal surgeries and related scars, in order to achieve better cosmetic results. Suction drain placement is usually not necessary. After controlling for hemostasis, the 12-mm ports fascia and extraction wound are closed with absorbable sutures. Additional detailed information about the closure techniques is provided in Chapter 2, The Basic Principles of Clinical Applications.

Step 8 average time frame: 10–15 min

Suggested Readings

1. Masrur MA, Daskalaki D, Vannucchi A, et al. Minimally invasive treatment of difficult bleeding lesions of the small bowel. *Minerva Chir.* 2016;71(5):293-299.
2. Dasari BVM, McKay D, Gardiner K. Laparoscopic versus open surgery for small bowel Crohn's disease. *Cochrane Database Syst Rev.* 2011;1:CD006956. doi: 10.1002/14651858.CD006956.pub2
3. Patel R, Borad NP, Merchant AM. Comparison of outcomes following laparoscopic and open treatment of emergent small bowel obstructions: an 11-year analysis of ACS NSQIP. *Surg Endosc.* 2018;32(12):4900-4911. doi: 10.1007/s00464-018-6249-2
4. Chen K, Zhang B, Liang YL, et al. Laparoscopic versus open resection of small bowel gastrointestinal stromal tumors: systematic review and meta-analysis. *Chin Med J.* 2017;130(13):1595-1603. doi: 10.4103/0366-6999.208249
5. Igiri AO, Ekong MB, Egemba GO, et al. The pattern of arrangements and distribution of the superior mesenteric artery in a Nigerian population. *Int J Morphol.* 2010;28(1):33-36. doi: 10.4067/S0717-95022010000100005
6. Conley D, Hurst PR, Stringer MD. An investigation on human jejunal and ileal arteries. *Anat Sci Int.* 2010;85(1):23-30. doi: 10.1007/s12565-009-0047-9
7. Benson AB, Venook AP, Al-Hawary MM, et al. Small Bowel Adenocarcinoma, Version 1.2020, NCCN Clinical Practice Guidelines in Oncology. *J Natl Compr Canc Netw.* 2019;17:1109-1133. doi: 10.6004/jnccn.2019.0043
8. Giulianotti PC, Coratti A, Angelini M, et al. Robotics in general surgery: personal experience in a large community hospital. *Arch Surg.* 2003;138(7):777-784. doi: 10.1001/archsurg.138.7.777

23

"All diseases begin in the gut."
—Hippocrates (c. 460 BC–c. 370 BC)

Radical Right Colectomy with Complete Mesocolic Excision (CME)

Alberto Mangano • Valentina Valle • Colton Johnson • Pier Cristoforo Giulianotti

INTRODUCTION

The right colectomy is a procedure that can often be performed, in a relatively easy way, with a laparoscopic approach; and by some authors, it is considered a good model to acquire skills for more complex surgeries. This operation does not require changes in patient positioning, and it may allow hybrid techniques. Extraction mini-laparotomies are sometimes performed to exteriorize the colon, to complete the resection, and to accomplish the anastomosis. In reality, to carry out a right colectomy with a well-conducted complete mesocolic excision (CME) along the main vascular pedicles may be a difficult task that entails a long learning curve. It is during these surgical maneuvers that the robotic approach can make the difference in comparison with traditional laparoscopy.

CME has been a topic of increasing scientific interest in the literature. Growing data in open surgery indicate that it is safe and feasible: it has a similar morbidity profile compared to conventional technique, and it can present advantages in terms of staging (higher number of lymph nodes harvested), it can provide a good specimen quality, and it may have disease-free survival benefits.

The validity of CME has also been confirmed in minimally invasive surgery, offering the same advantages of the open operation. However, the dissection at the mesenteric root, around the superior mesenteric vessels, becomes challenging in laparoscopy, and it may increase the risk of vascular injuries. This technique may require sophisticated skills, experience, and a standardized approach. This is why the robotic platform offers clear advantages over laparoscopy.

In particular, there are three main aspects that play an important role in favor of robotics:

1. The stability of the exposure without need of changing patient positioning.
2. The role of the third arm in improving the retraction and allowing a lateral to medial approach during the mobilization of the right colon mesentery.
3. The EndoWrist™ that allows better and safer dissection of the superior mesenteric vessel pedicles.

INSTRUMENT REQUIREMENTS

The suggested main robotic instruments/tools can be listed as follows:

- 30° scope
- Cautery hook/monopolar scissors
- Vessel sealer
- Needle drivers (round tip or macro)
- Robotic linear staplers (with different loads)
- Multiple Hem-o-lok™ clips
- Medium/large clip-applier
- Bipolar forceps
- Cadière forceps

The suggested main laparoscopic instruments/tools can be listed as follows:

- Needle holders
- Scissors
- Graspers
- Staplers (with different loads)
- Suction-irrigation

Supplemental materials:

- Gauzes, sponges
- Vessel loops (rarely)
- Endo Bag™
- Medium–large clips
- Sutures: PDS™ 3/0–4/0; Prolene™ 3/0–4/0

Photo from Wynnter / Getty Images.

Quote reproduced with permission from Tebala GD. History of colorectal surgery: a comprehensive historical review from the ancient Egyptians to the surgical robot. Int J Colorectal Dis. 2015;30(6):723-748.

Indications and Relative Contraindications to the Robotic Approach

The indications are similar to the ones for open and laparoscopic surgery: malignancies, benign tumors, inflammatory bowel disease, and, more rarely, recurring episodes of diverticulitis.

There are no absolute contraindications to the robotic approach. Extensive and tenacious adhesions, very high body max index (BMI), or bulky cancers in proximity to the duodenum can represent challenging scenarios for laparoscopy. Instead, for an expert robotic surgeon, these situations are not contraindications *a priori* (even though they may increase the surgical time and the technical complexity).

In any case, the limits of what is achievable in a minimally invasive way should always be assessed within the framework of the local surgical expertise. With that in mind, the first phase of the learning curve should consist of smaller lesions, with a safe and stepwise increase of the technical difficulty over time.

Patient Positioning, OR Setup, and Port Setting

The patient is placed in a light Trendelenburg position (10–15°), and the table is tilted 20° toward the left side (to favor small bowel retraction) (**Figure 23-1**). The pneumoperitoneum is achieved with a Veress needle positioned just below the left costal margin (in the modified Palmer's point). The ports are placed as described in **Figure 23-2** for the normal abdomen and as depicted in **Figure 23-3** for the wide abdomen configuration.

A 5-mm VisiPort™ is positioned in the left upper quadrant, and it is used for the initial intra-abdominal assessment (e.g., position of the cecum, possible peritoneal implants, or adhesions). This 5-mm port will be upsized to 10–12 mm and used for one of the assistant ports.

The robotic chart is docked from the patient's right side, and the OR setup is shown in **Figure 23-4**.

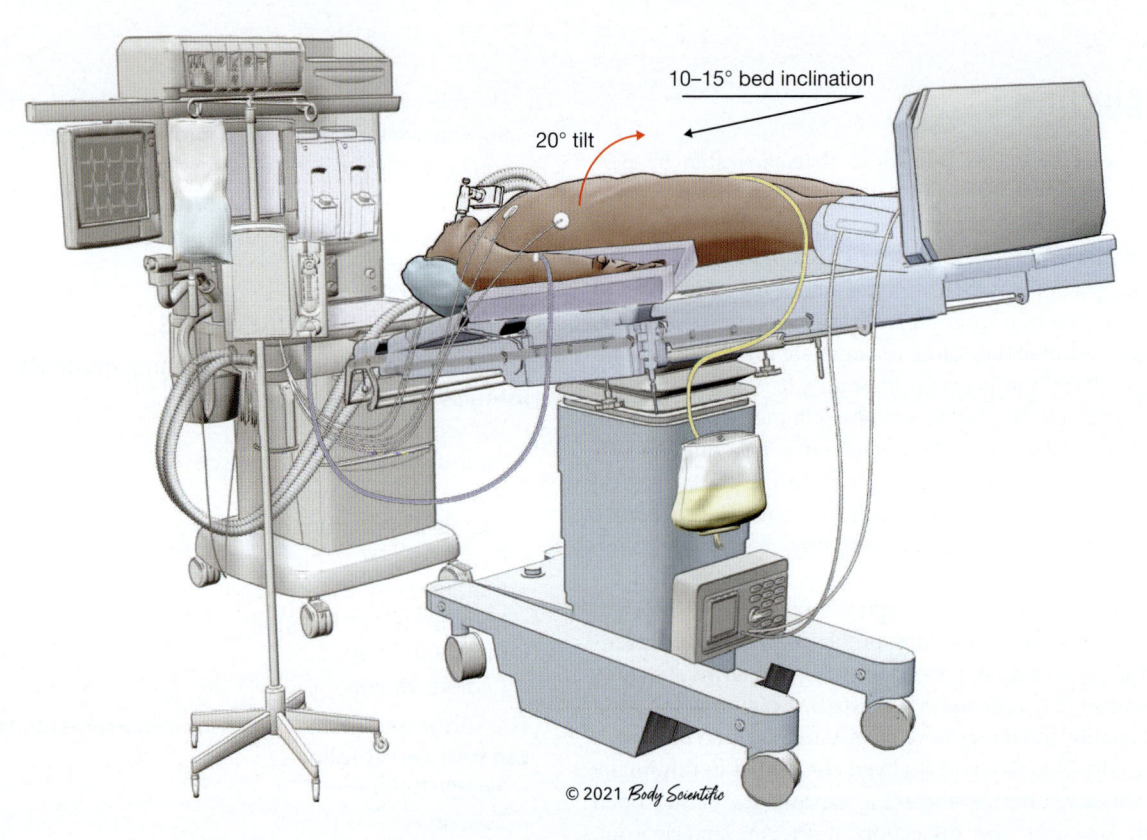

FIGURE 23-1 • Patient positioning.

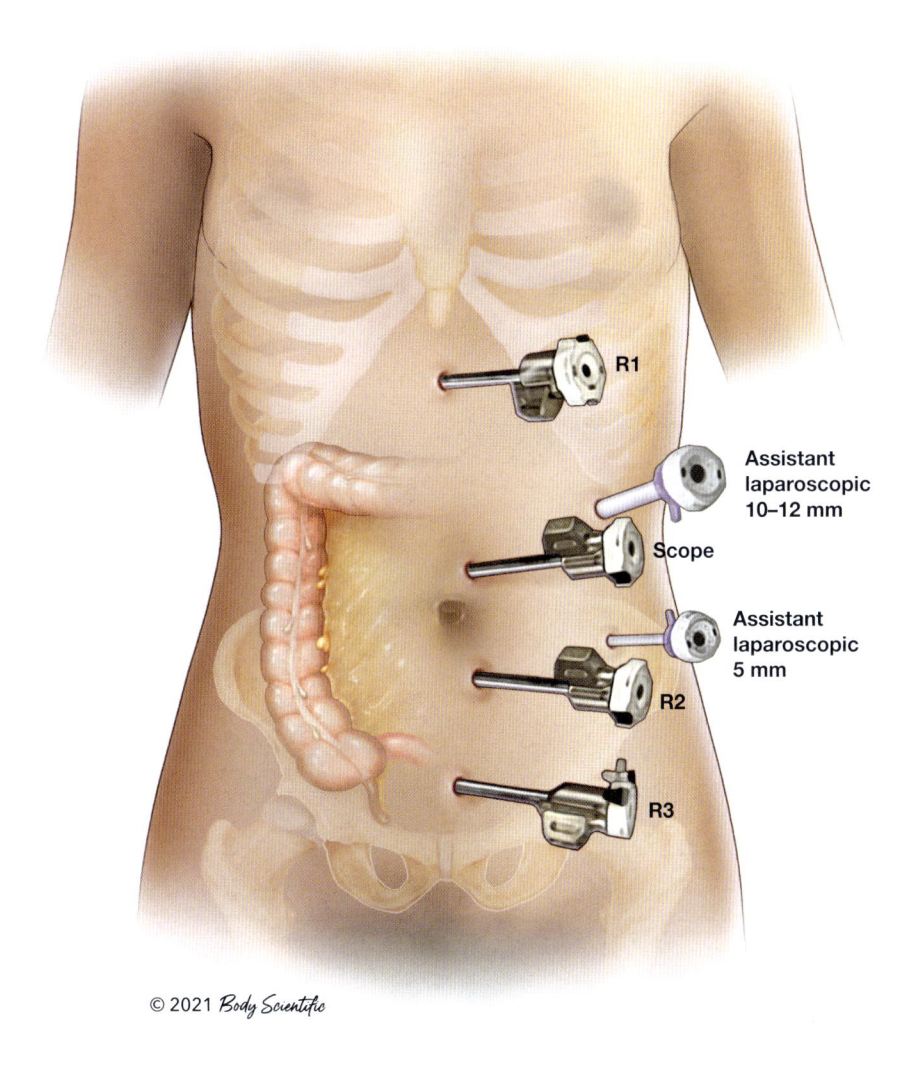

FIGURE 23-2 • Normal abdomen: trocar placement during robotic right colectomy.

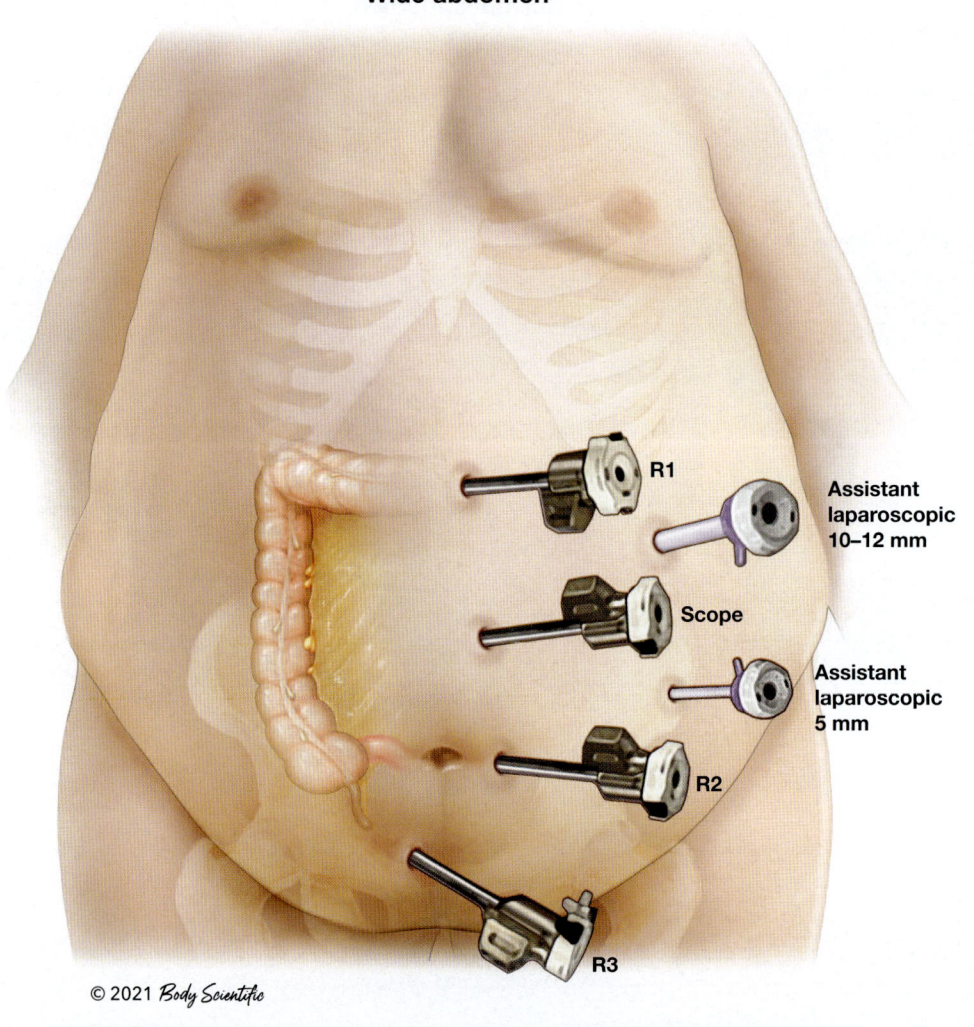

FIGURE 23-3 • Wide abdomen: trocar placement during robotic right colectomy.

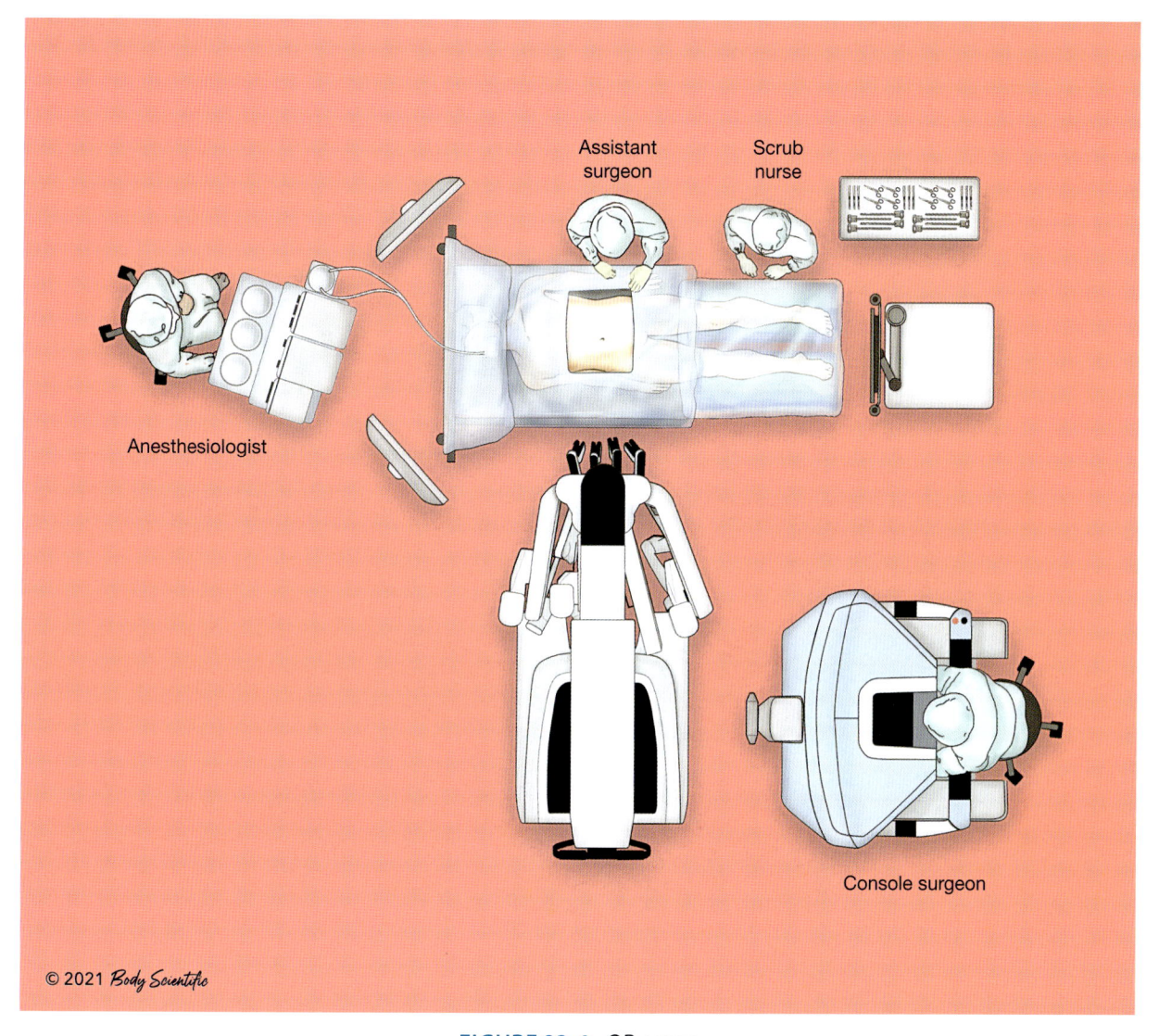

FIGURE 23-4 • OR setup.

Surgical Technique

Step 1. Division of the right side of the omentum

Removing *en bloc* the right side of the omentum is part of the oncological procedure. This maneuver is important because, during the detachment of the omentum, the full understanding of the anatomy of the right colonic flexure can be achieved (e.g., presence of double-folded flexure, adhesions between the ascending colon and the transverse colon). During this step, the lesser sac is entered, and while detaching the omentum, part of the gastrocolic ligament is also removed, staying lateral to the gastroepiploic arcade.

The dissection is started by retracting laterally the right side of the omentum, and its division is started at the level of the middle portion of the transverse colon. The omentum is detached from the colon insertion (**Figure 23-5**).

For these surgical maneuvers, the best tools are the monopolar hook (detachment of the omentum from the colon insertion) and the vessel sealer (division of the omentum itself).

Step 1 average time frame: 15–20 min

> ⚠ **PITFALLS**
>
> Even if they are more common in the left colon, some diverticula may also be present in the right side. During the detachment of the omentum, caution must be taken to avoid their damage.

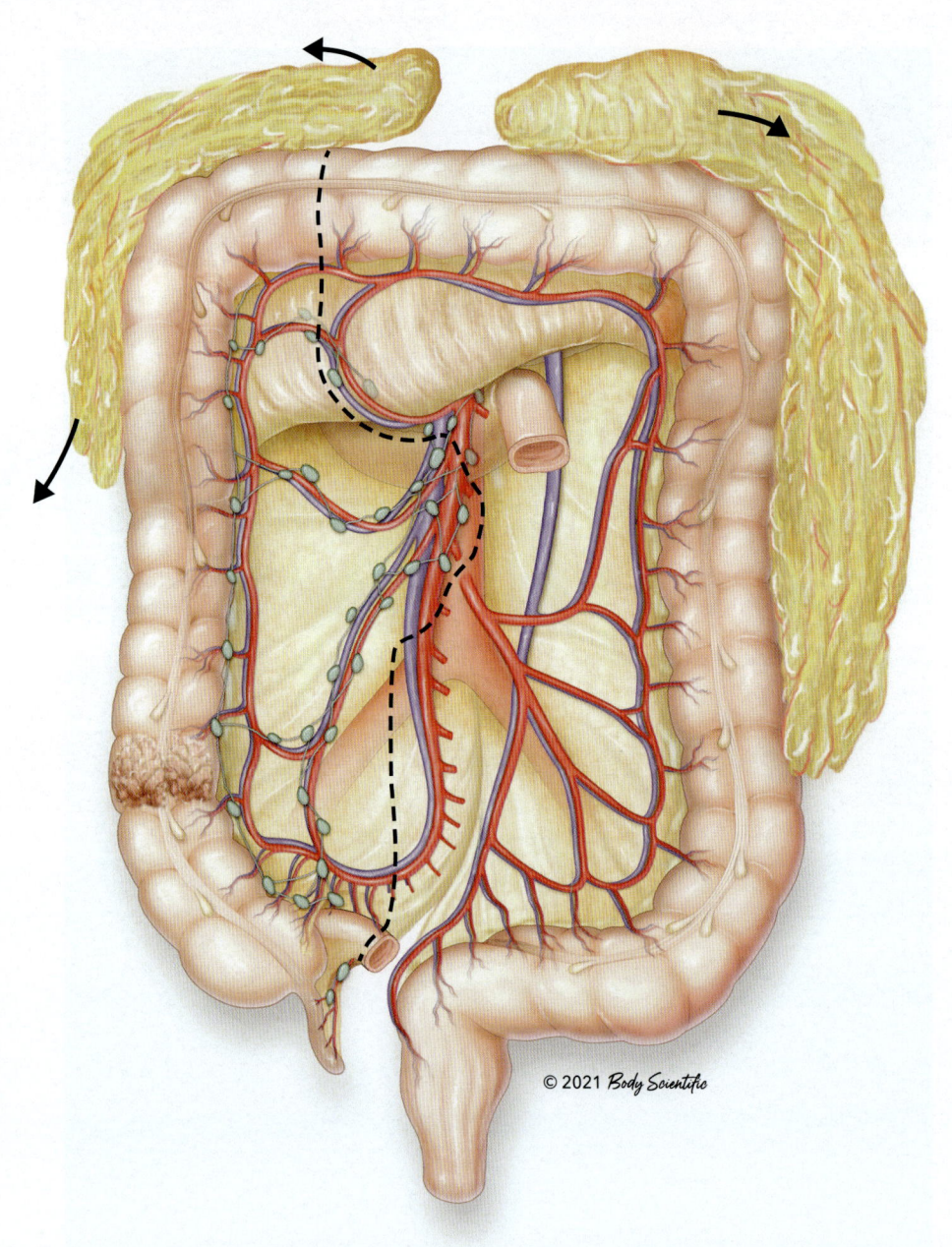

FIGURE 23-5 • Complete mesocolic excision.

Video 23-1. Step 2. Mobilization of the Cecum and Ascending Colon

Step 2. Mobilization of the cecum and ascending colon
In laparoscopy, most authors adopt a strictly medial-to-lateral dissection. An early hepatic flexure mobilization can interfere with a proper exposure. The mobilized colon tends to fold down, obstructing the surgical view and requiring additional maneuvers by the assistant to maintain the exposure.

Using the robotic approach, the R3 can dynamically lift the cecum/ascending colon, allowing an optimal vision of the surgical field. This makes possible an "open-like" technique: the dissection is usually started with the mobilization of the mesentery (see **Figure 23-6** for mesentery anatomy). The detachment of the mesentery of the right colon from the retroperitoneum facilitates, even in thick/obese patients, the identification of the vascular pedicles and of the main superior mesenteric trunks. Also, the dissection becomes safer, decreasing the risk of injury of the retroperitoneal elements such as the ureter and the gonadal vessels. The dissection starts at the cecal base, moving cranially up to the right flexure, while the R3 is counter-retracting the colon medially.

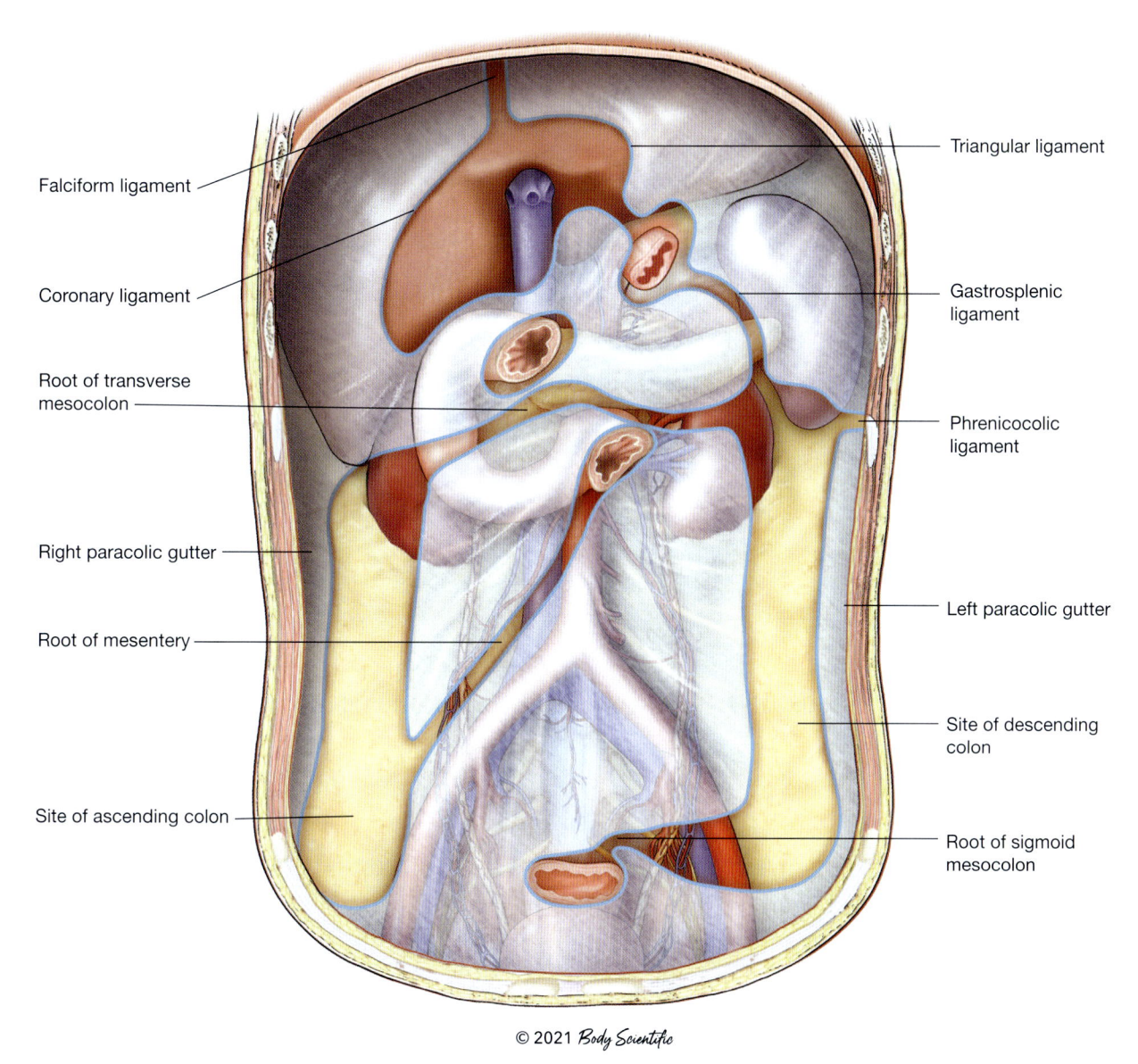

FIGURE 23-6 • Mesentery structure. General anatomy.

The peritoneal reflection of the paracolic gutter is dissected, the retroperitoneal plane is entered staying in front of the Toldt's fascia (see **Figure 23-7** for Toldt's and Gerota's surgical planes), and then the dissection is continued in a bottom-up and lateral-to-medial direction up to duodenal portion (D) II identification.

The aim of this step is to detach the mesentery of the ascending colon, and the flexure from the retroperitoneum. While making this dissection, the surgical landmarks and limits that have to be identified are as follows: gonadic vessels, ureter, vena cava (VC), DII, and DIII. Medially, the attachment of the mesentery of the terminal ileum should also be mobilized, and the iliac vessels should be identified.

All those structures should be exposed before starting Step 3. The dissection proceeds toward the flexure on top of the Toldt's fascia, which is more evident at this level than at the level of the cecum. The hook is the preferred tool for this step.

Step 2 average time frame: 15–20 min

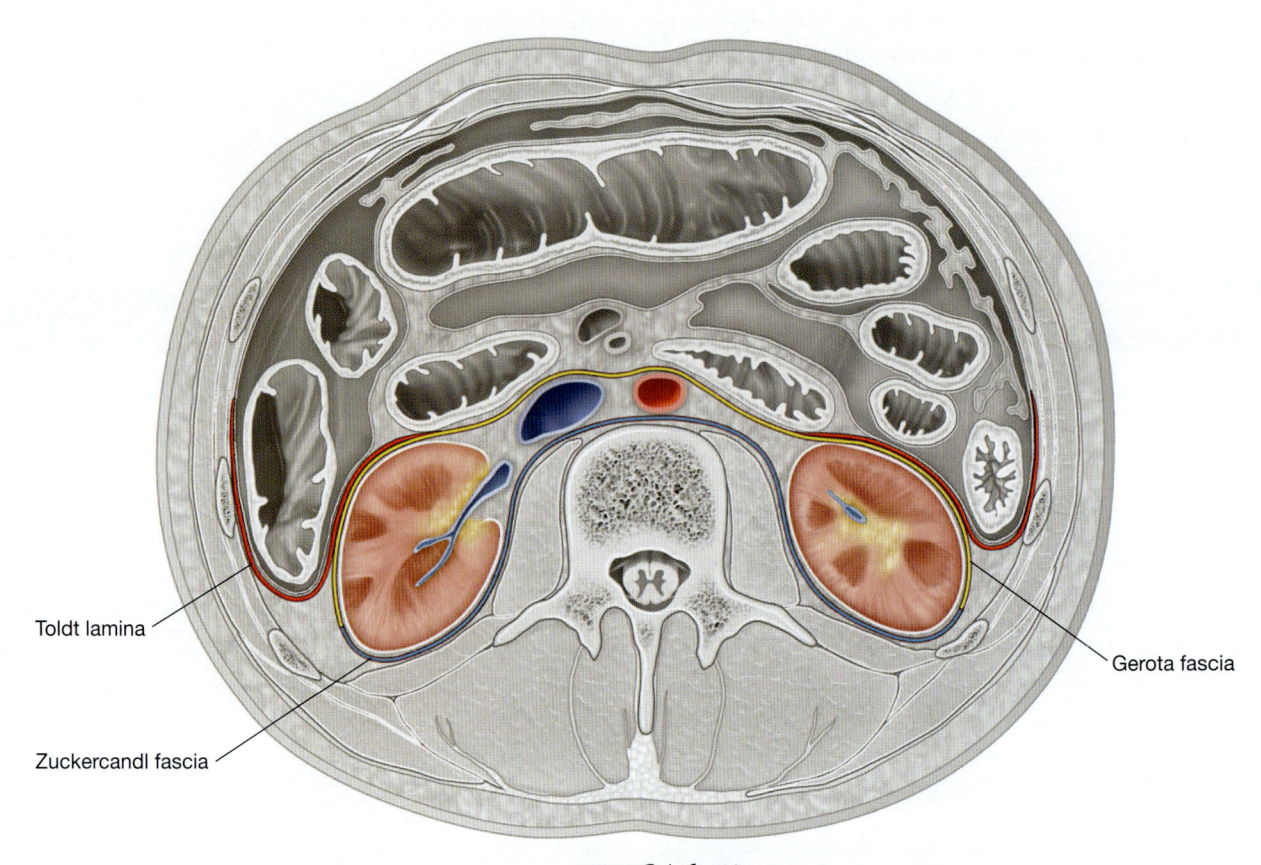

FIGURE 23-7 • Laminae and fasciae of surgical relevance.

▶▶ TIPS

The role of the assistant in this step is to improve the retraction of the right colon toward the midline. In fact, R3 is often colliding with the operative arms, at this stage, and its efficacy may be limited.

⚠ PITFALLS

When mobilizing the mesentery of the right colon, the gonadic vessels or the ureter may be lifted along with the mesentery, and in doing so, there is an increased risk of injuring those structures (see **Figure 23-8** for the standard anatomy). To avoid damages, these anatomical elements must be pushed down while lifting up the mesentery of the colon.

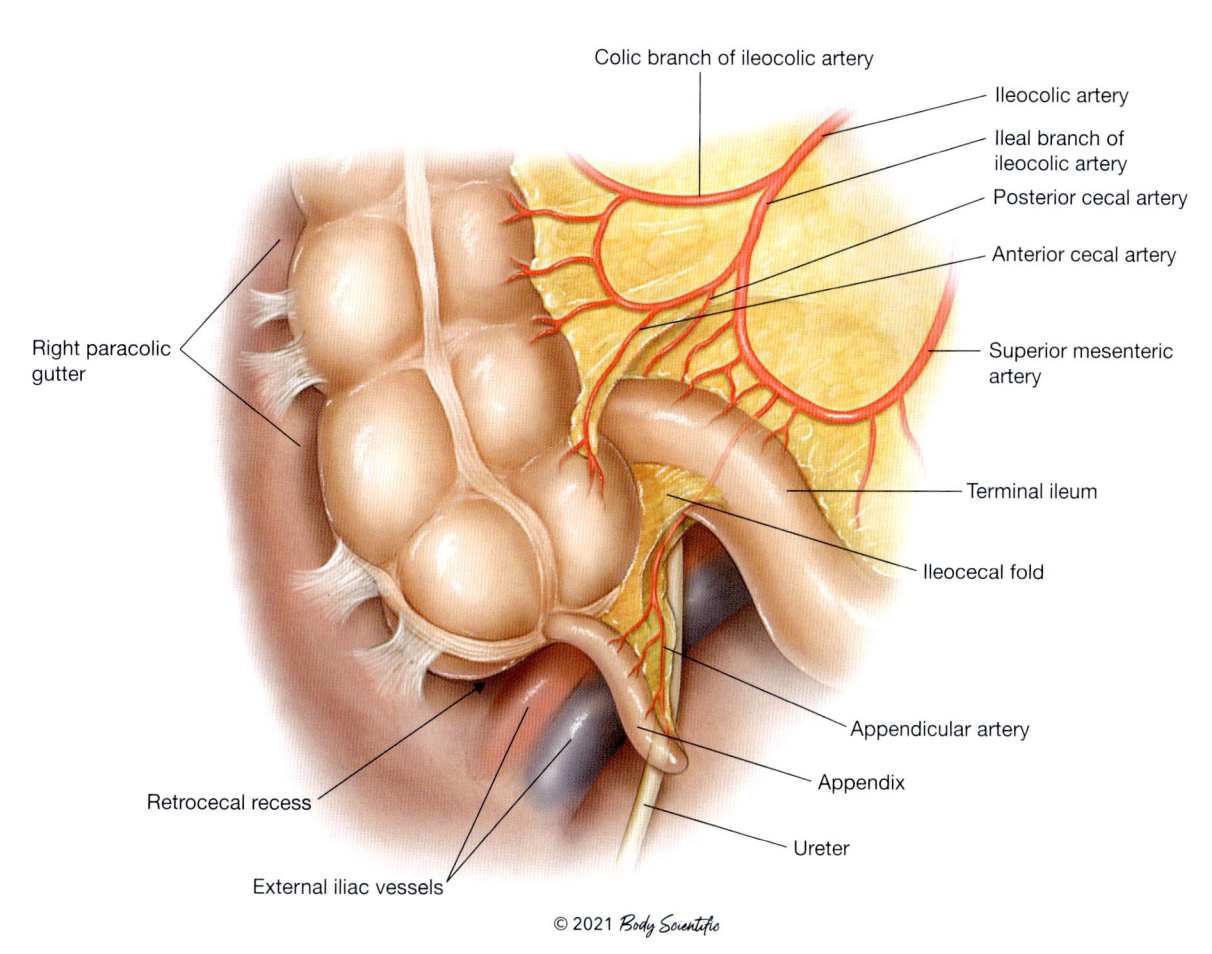

FIGURE 23-8 • Ileocecal region anatomy.

Video 23-2. Step 3. Mobilization of the Right Colonic Flexure

Step 3. Mobilization of the right colonic flexure
This step requires different concerted actions and surgical maneuvers (**Figures 23-9 A–C** and **23-10**). The assistant and the nondominant hand of the console surgeon pull down the flexure, creating some tension on the peritoneal reflection/layer between the colonic flexure and the renal capsule. This area is the reflection of the parietal peritoneum into the visceral peritoneum. This is described by some authors as the hepatocolic ligament or renocolic ligament, and it is the area where the dissection is started. The space in front of the Toldt's fascia is opened up, the dissection is continued downward, DII is recognized, and the head of the pancreas is progressively exposed.

The mesentery of the right colon is separated from DIII reaching the confluence of the right colonic venous drainage into the superior mesenteric vein (SMV). The mobilization of the flexure is also carried out in a cranial to caudal fashion, reaching the previously dissected surgical field (i.e., the mobilization of the ascending colon).

The landmarks for this step are as follows: the VC, DII, DIII, and the right venous discharge into the SMV. If these structures are not properly seen, it means that the mobilization is not completed (see **Figure 23-11** for the venous anatomy of the right colon).

Step 3 average time frame: 15–20 min

> ▶▶ **TIPS**
>
> A complete mobilization of the right colonic flexure requires a good exposure of the pancreatic head.
>
> The access to the lesser sac, obtained in Step 1, facilitates a better understanding of the relation with the pancreas and the anatomy of the vascular connections with the SMV system.

> ▶▶ **TIPS**
>
> If there are bulky liver and/or high flexure and/or adhesions, a specific and more stable hepatic retraction may be needed and the position of R3 may be temporarily changed from the lower to the left lateral upper quadrant. Placing the R3 in the higher port requires resetting the function of all the other cannulas (including the scope which becomes in a more caudal position). (See **Figures 23-2** and **23-3**.)

> ⚠ **PITFALLS**
>
> The traction maneuvers should be performed with caution. The more extensive the mobilization, the more fragile the connections of right colonic veins into the SMV will become. There is a risk of laceration of these venous confluences, with possible major bleeding that is difficult to control. In addition to the traction exerted by the console surgeon, the traction of the assistant should also be considered.

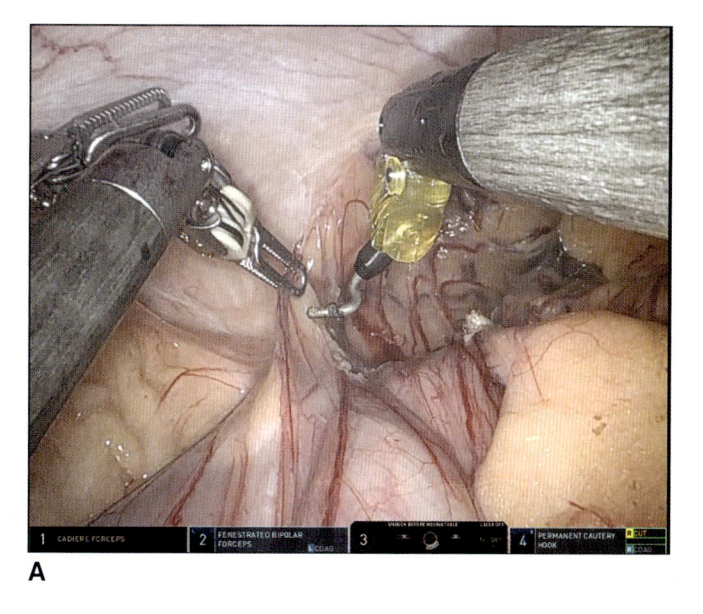

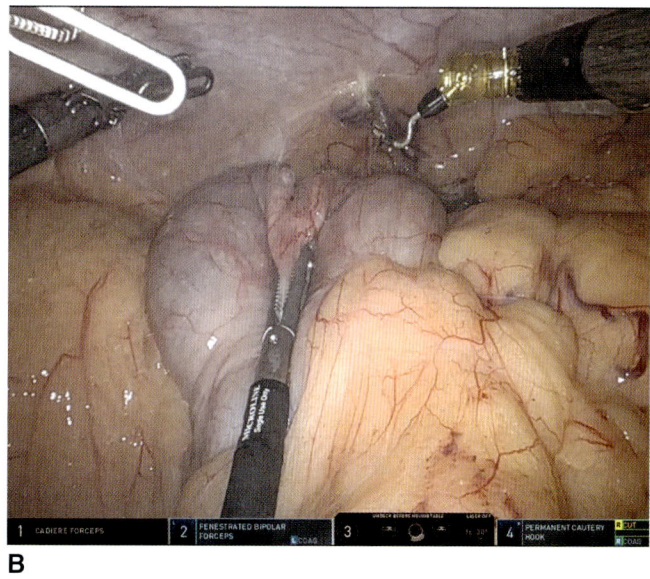

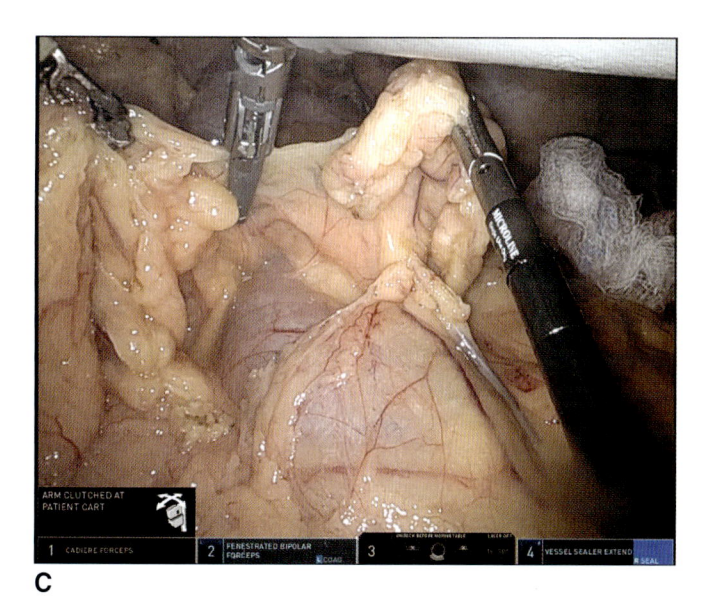

FIGURE 23-9 • Step 3. Mobilization of the right colonic flexure.

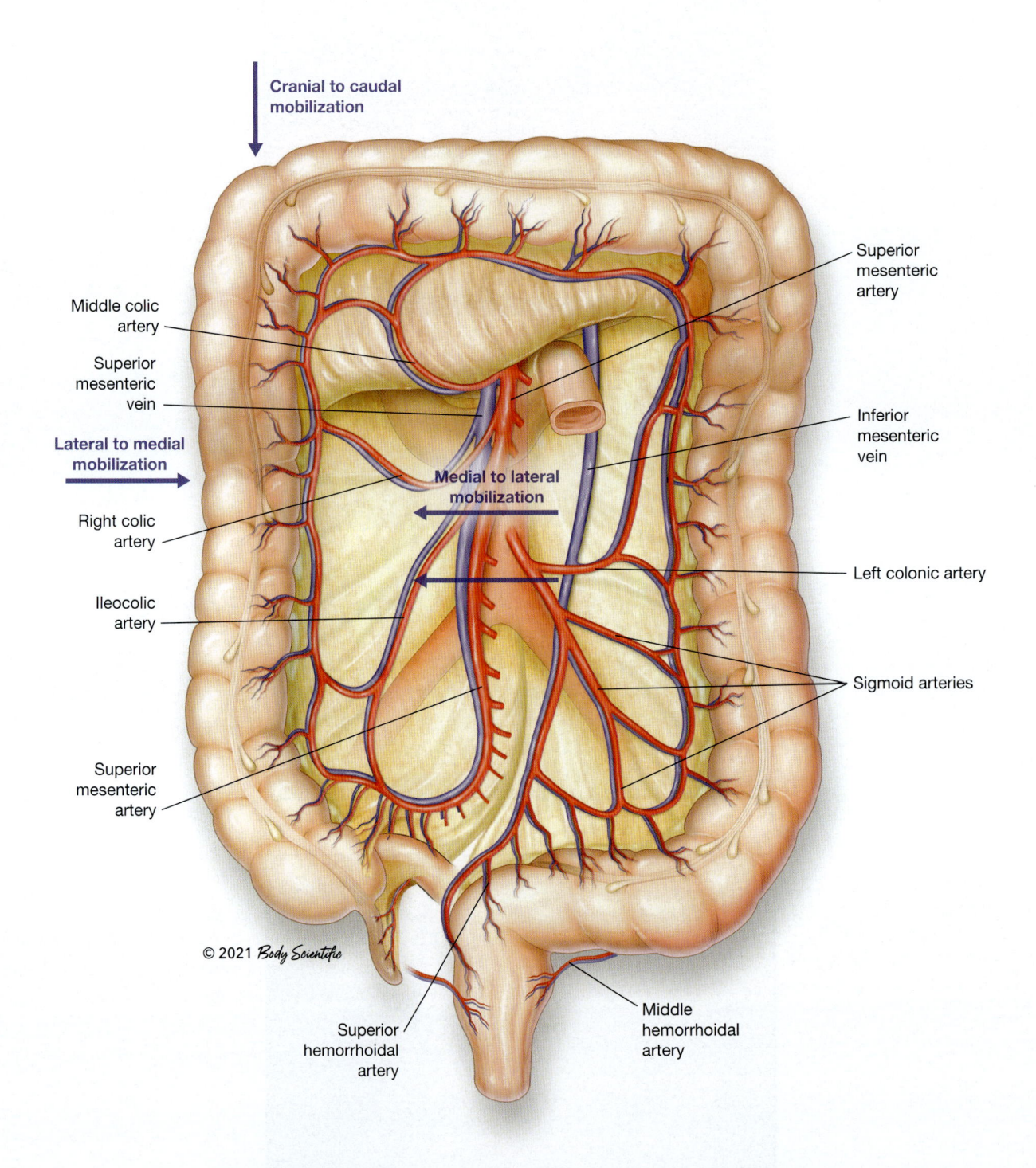

FIGURE 23-10 • Different pathways of right colonic flexure mobilization.

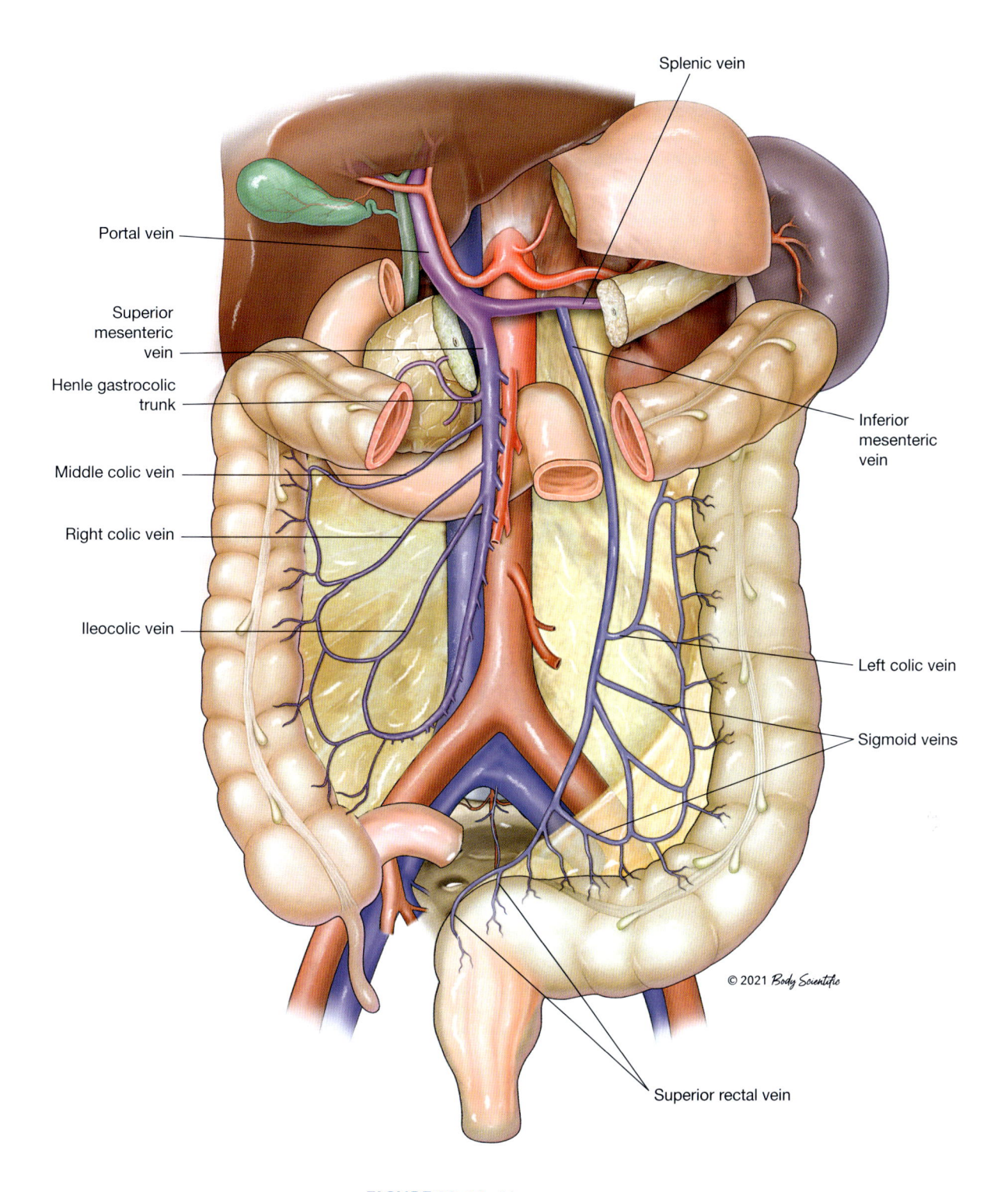

Radical Right Colectomy with Complete Mesocolic Excision (CME)   467

FIGURE 23-11 • Venous anatomy.

Video 23-3. Step 4. Medial-to-Lateral Dissection with CME and Division of the Ileocolic Vessels

Step 4. Medial-to-lateral dissection with CME and division of the ileocolic vessels

At this point, there is a change in retraction: the R3 is lifting the ascending colon. The mesentery of the mobilized ascending colon is stretched up. An avascular triangle is delimited by the branches of the ileocolic vessels (or by the right colic vessels depending on the anatomy) and DIII (see **Figure 23-12** for standard anatomy and **Figures 23-13 A–I** for variations in the colic arteries). By entering into this avascular plane, a communication is created with the dissection previously performed on the other side during the right colonic flexure mobilization.

While pulling up the mobilized colonic mesentery, tension is exerted on the tissue, the profile of the trunk of the SMV is also lifted, and it can be more easily identified (even in patients with a high BMI).

The hook is used to start the dissection on the left side of the SMV. The CME is carried out: the lymph nodes around the SMV and around the confluence of the ileocolic vein into the SMV are removed. This extended lymphadenectomy is called "complete" because the lymph nodes on top and around the SMV, and the lymph nodes around the confluence of the ileocolic vessels into the SMV, are all removed *en bloc* with the vascular pedicles (**Figures 23-5** and **23-14**).

This maneuver is facilitated by the previous mobilization that makes it easier to separate the ileocolic vein and artery. The superior mesenteric artery should not be routinely exposed, unless there are visible and enlarged lymph nodes. However, the dissection should include the anterior part of the tissue between artery and vein. The ileocolic vessels are then divided in between clips, or sutures, or alternatively utilizing a vascular stapler if proper skeletonization was performed.

Step 4 average time frame: 20–30 min

▶▶ TIPS

Instead of going straight down on top of the SMV, it is easier to follow the structure of the ileocolic pedicle and approach the right side of the vein first, where the position of the main trunk is recognized (even in high BMI patients); then, the anterior aspect of the artery is followed as well, and the lymphadenectomy around the trunk can be performed.

⚠ PITFALLS

Bleeding from lacerations of the veins are potential pitfalls. This can occur mainly when enlarged metastatic lymph nodes are present. Careful suturing may be required, because energy-based devices or clips are not effective and may even be dangerous in this situation.

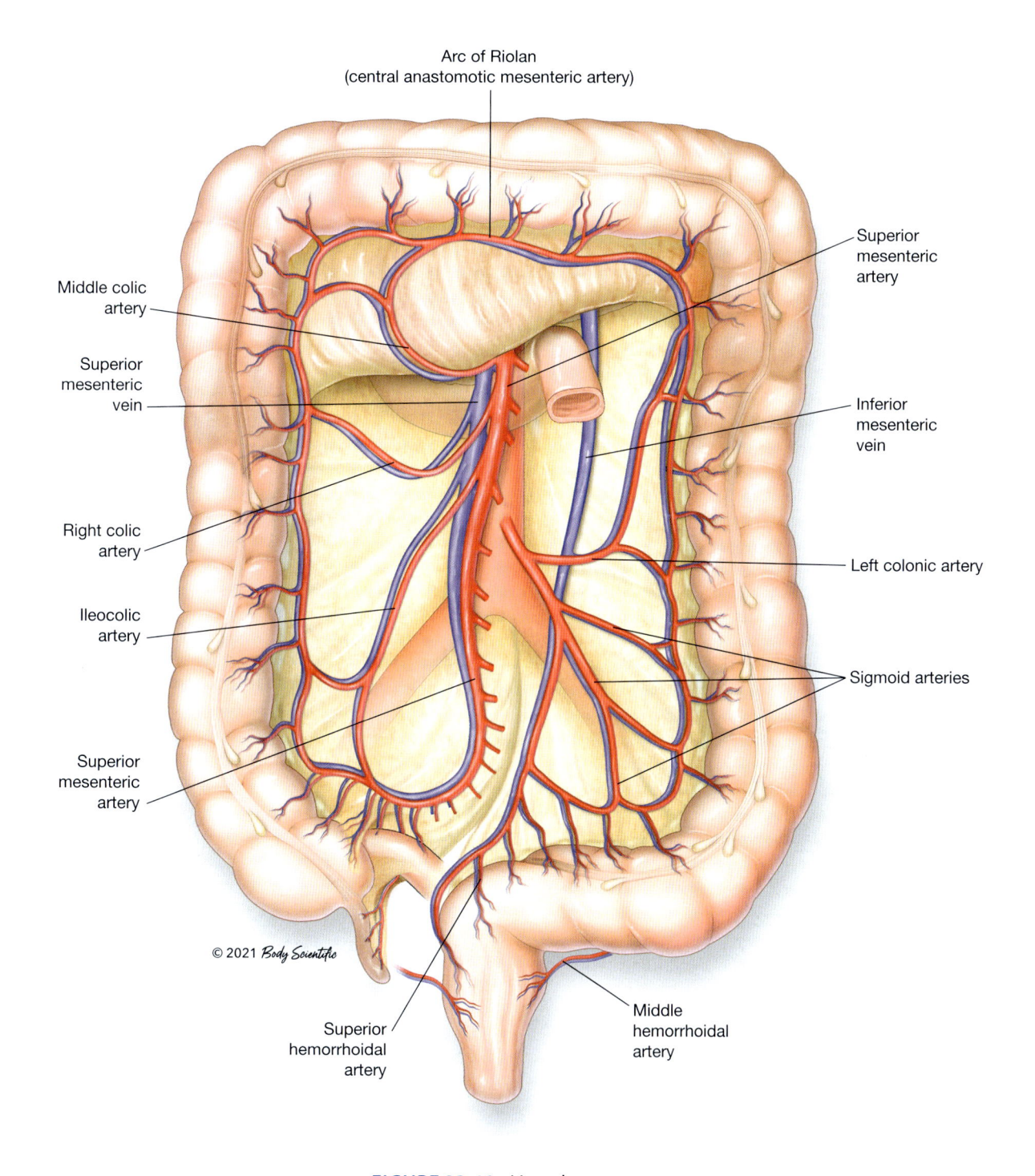

FIGURE 23-12 • Vascular anatomy.

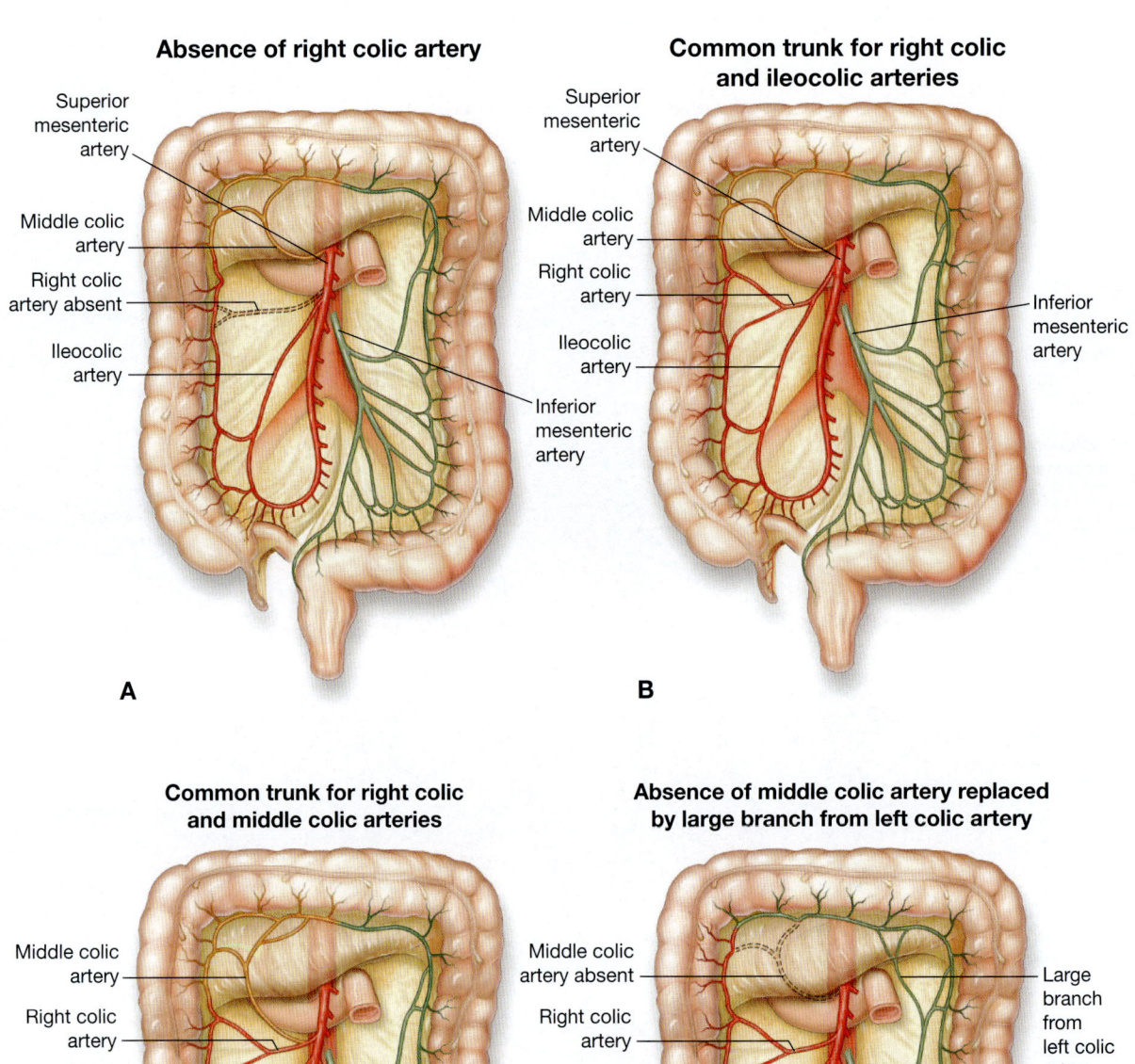

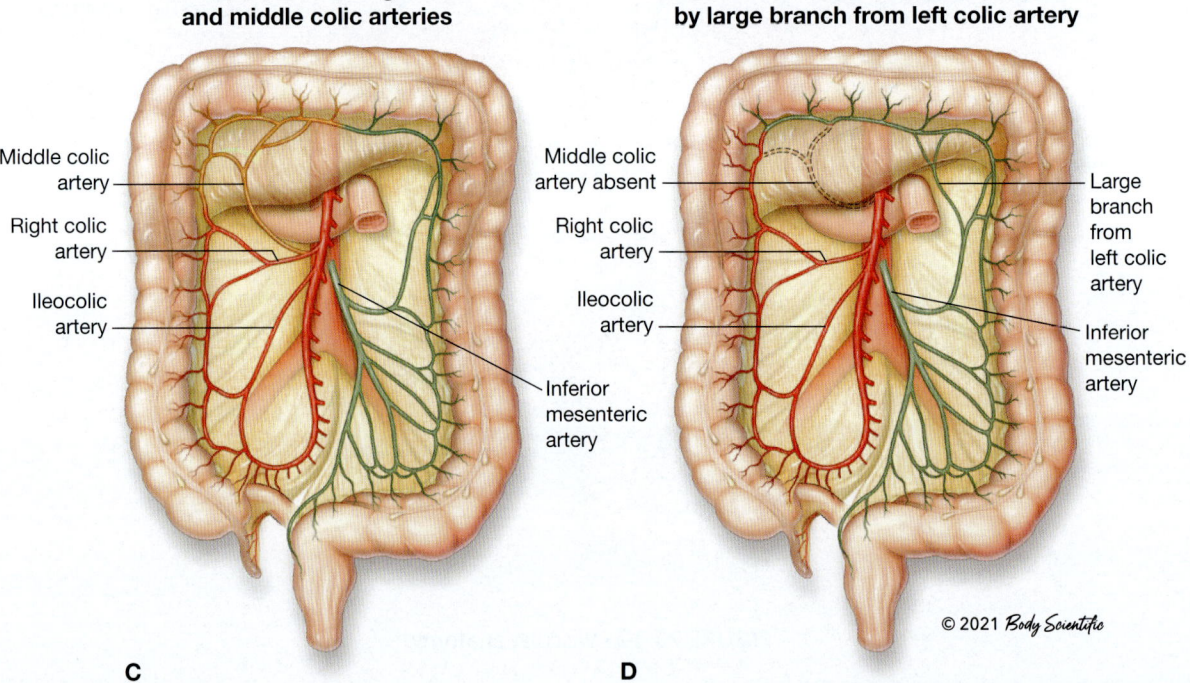

FIGURE 23-13 • Anatomical variations of the colonic arteries that may be encountered during right colectomy.

Discontinuity of marginal artery (between right colic and ileocolic arteries)

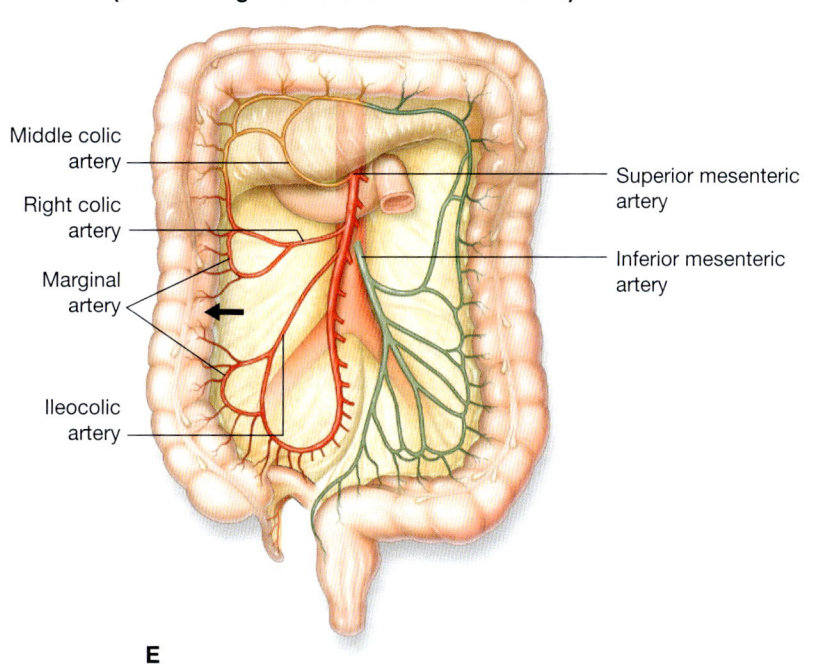

E

Middle colic artery originates from dorsal pancreatic artery

F

Middle colic artery originates from celiac trunk via dorsal pancreatic artery

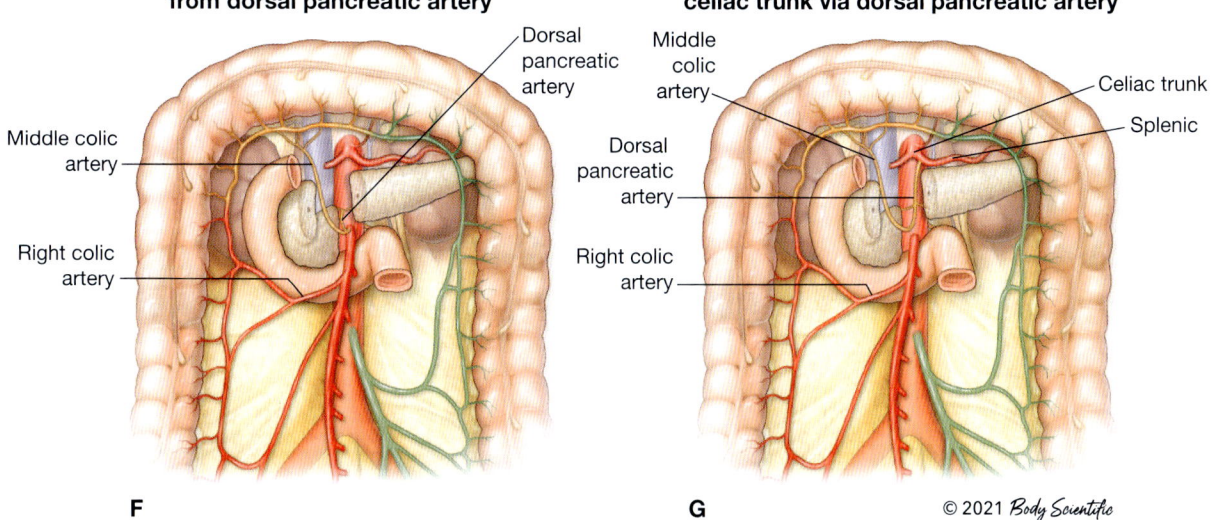

G

FIGURE 23-13 • *(Continued)*

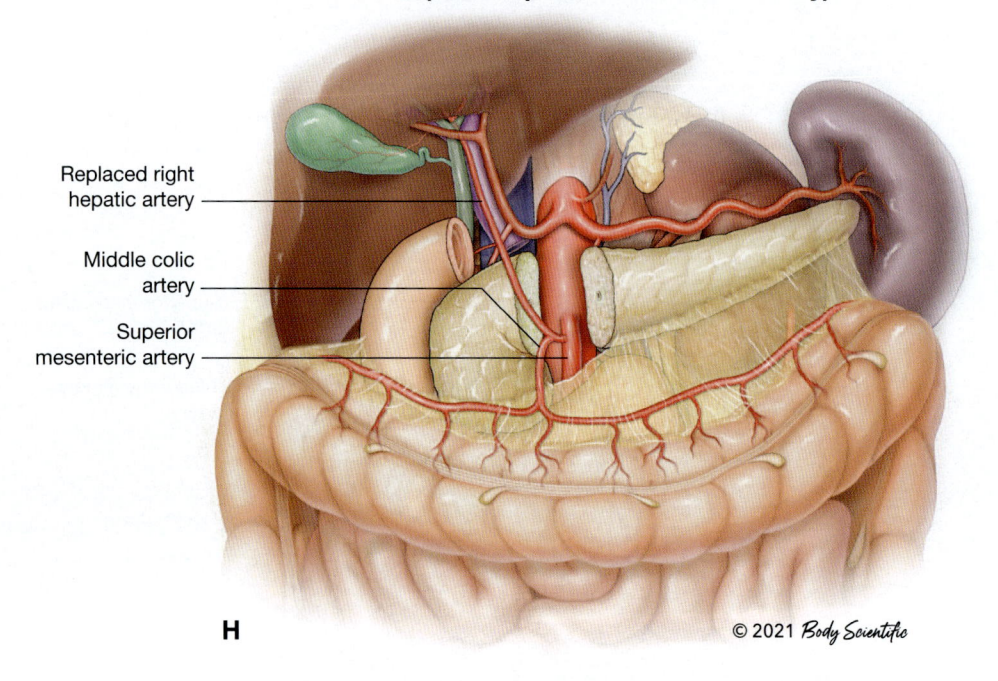

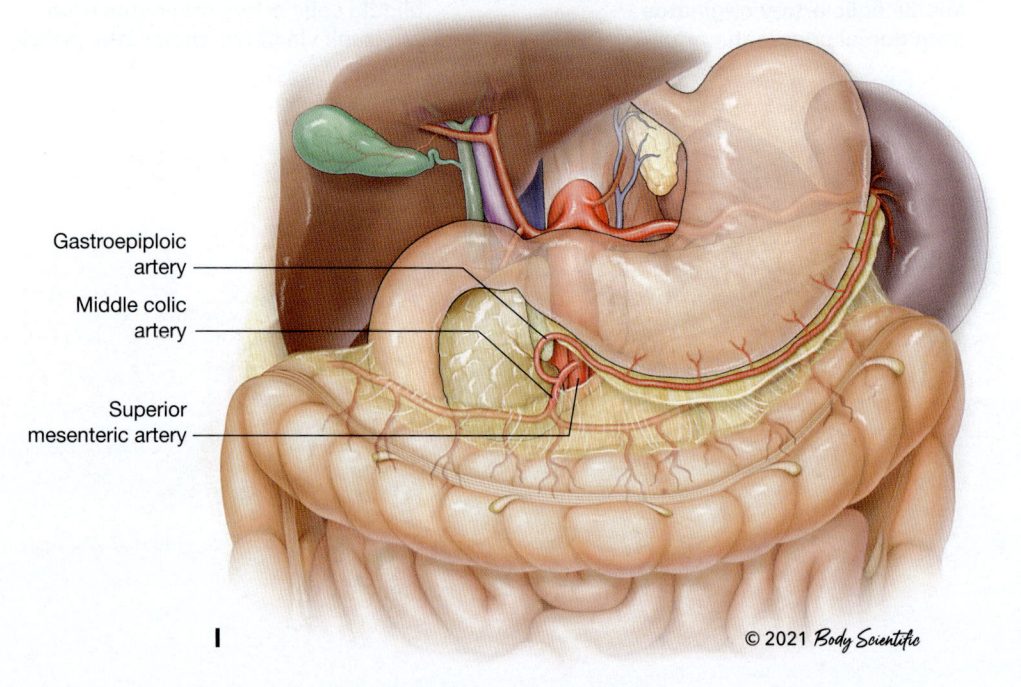

Middle colic artery originates from replaced right hepatic artery (from superior mesenteric artery)

- Replaced right hepatic artery
- Middle colic artery
- Superior mesenteric artery

H

The superior mesenteric artery gives origin to the right gastroepiploic artery and to the middle colic artery

- Gastroepiploic artery
- Middle colic artery
- Superior mesenteric artery

I

FIGURE 23-13 • *(Continued)*

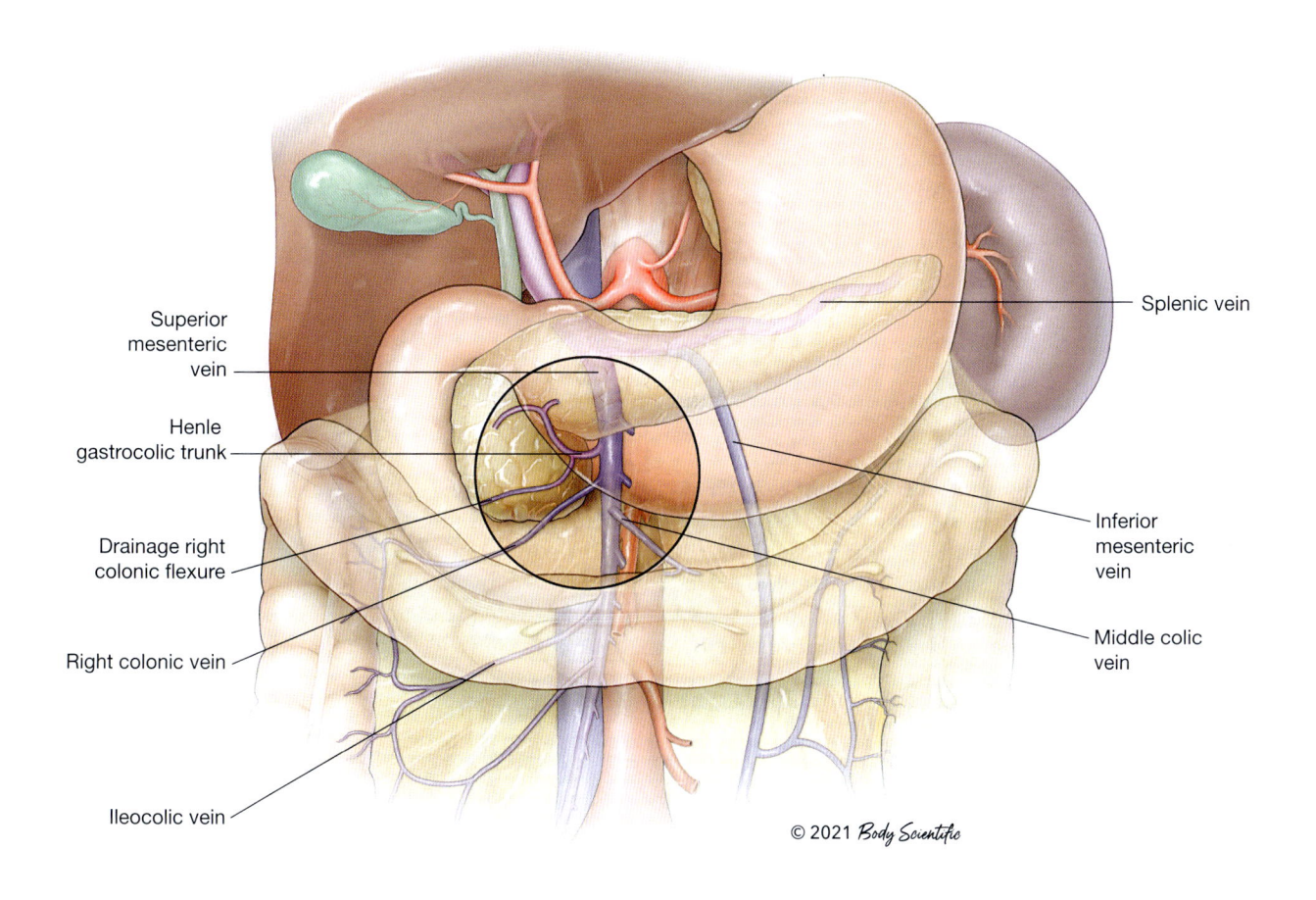

FIGURE 23-14 • Complete mesocolic excision: anatomy.

▶ Video 23-4. Step 5. Division of the Mesentery of the Terminal Ileum

Step 5. Division of the mesentery of the terminal ileum
Once the ileocolic vessels are divided, using a vessel sealer, it is easier to divide the mesentery of the terminal ileum because the cecum was previously fully mobilized. The double coagulation technique is recommended, and, if there is a thick mesentery, a vascular stapler is a better option. Additional Prolene™ 3-0 stitches can be added on the mesenteric edge to perfect the hemostasis and decrease the risk of delayed bleeding and hematomas.

Step 5 average time frame: 5–10 min

▶ Video 23-5. Step 6. Division of the Terminal Ileum

Step 6. Transection of the terminal ileum
This maneuver is performed with a linear stapler either laparoscopic or robotic. A near-infrared indocyanine green (ICG) perfusion test may be used to check the blood supply of the segments selected for the anastomosis.

Step 6 average time frame: 5–10 min

> ⚠ **PITFALLS**
>
> If the mesentery of the terminal ileum was not completely detached from the retroperitoneum, this maneuver can be difficult or dangerous. Before dividing the terminal ileum, confirmation should be obtained that the mesentery is completely detached.

▶ Video 23-6. Step 7. Transverse Colon Division

Step 7. Transverse colon division with the right branch of the middle colic artery
The sequence of Steps 7 and 8 can be interchangeable: which step is performed first depends on the difficulty of the detachment of the venous drainage of the right colon into the SMV. If it is difficult, the transverse colon should be divided first. By doing so, a portion of the resected mesentery can be retracted toward the right side. This maneuver, combined with the lateral to medial dissection that was previously performed, is giving a better exposure of the "focal point," which is the merging of the right colonic drainage into the SMV or Henle's trunk. This extended lymphadenectomy (removing lymph nodes draining toward Henle's trunk, the gastroepiploic arcades, and the SMV) is part of the CME (see **Figure 23-15** for lymph nodes standard anatomy), and it is particularly important when the location of the cancer is higher: in the ascending colon or in the flexure.

If the detachment of the venous drainage of the right colon into the SMV is easy, due to favorable connections (e.g., right colonic drainage going directly into the SMV and a good exposure is present), then these structures can be divided before transecting the transverse colon.

The transection of the transverse colon, for the hemicolectomy procedure, is usually close to the midline. The transverse colon is divided with a stapler. Then, starting from the point where the colon was divided, the dissection of the mesentery proceeds caudally, with the vessel sealer, toward the root of the mesentery, including the right branch of the middle colic artery. In doing so, two dissection planes are joined together: the one from below and the one from above.

If the tumor is distal to the right colonic flexure, it may be necessary to extend the lymphadenectomy to the origin of the middle colic vessels, with their sacrifice. For ascending colon or proximal tumors of the right colon, this extended lymphadenectomy is not necessary because it may increase the risk of ischemia of the distal colonic stump.

Step 7 average time frame: 15–20 min

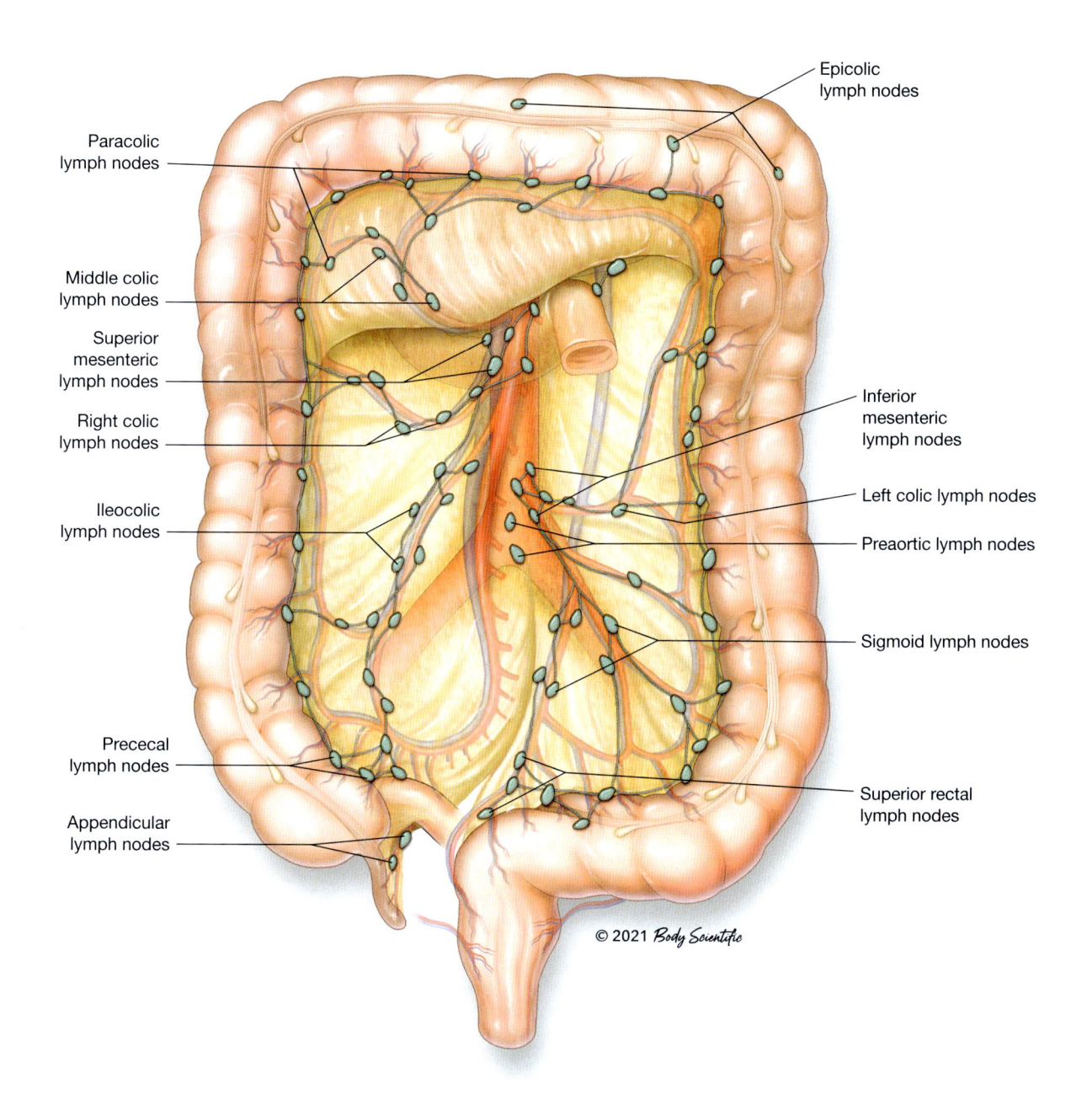

FIGURE 23-15 • Lymph node anatomy.

Video 23-7. Step 8. Downward Division of the Transverse Colon Mesentery with Anatomical Control

Step 8. Downward division of the transverse colon mesentery with anatomical control of the colonic flexure venous drainage into the mesenteric system

This is the trickiest step, and a full understanding of the specific anatomy is essential. The most critical area is around the SMV. In this region, the right colonic vein is merging with the SMV with very heterogenous anatomical variations and pathways. In Chapter 28, Pancreaticoduodenectomy, it is described how, at times, the right colonic vein is merging independently into the SMV, or in other cases, it drains into the right gastroepiploic, into Henle's trunk, or into the middle colic veins (see **Figures 23-16 A–E** for variations of Henle's trunk).

At this point of the procedure, the mesentery of the colon is attached only with venous connections. If required, a combination of top-down and bottom-up dissection is carried out until reaching the origin of these vessels. The lymphadenectomy is carried out around the confluence of the gastroepiploic, Henle's trunk, and the middle colic, and the lymphatic tissue is removed *en bloc*. These veins can be divided at their merging in between clips, sutures, or rarely with a stapler. To avoid the risk of local recurrence, a radical lymphadenectomy has to be performed correctly and accurately without leaving unwanted lymphatic tissue behind.

Sometimes, during the downward dissection toward the root of the mesentery, after having already detached the ileocolic, the right branch of the middle colic, and the venous attachments of the right flexure, there may be still an independent arterial branch: the right colonic artery. This it is not a branch of the ileocolic, but it is a vessel having origin independently from the segment of the SMA between the middle colic and the ileocolic. This structure should be divided independently in between sutures or clips.

Step 8 average time frame: 20–30 min

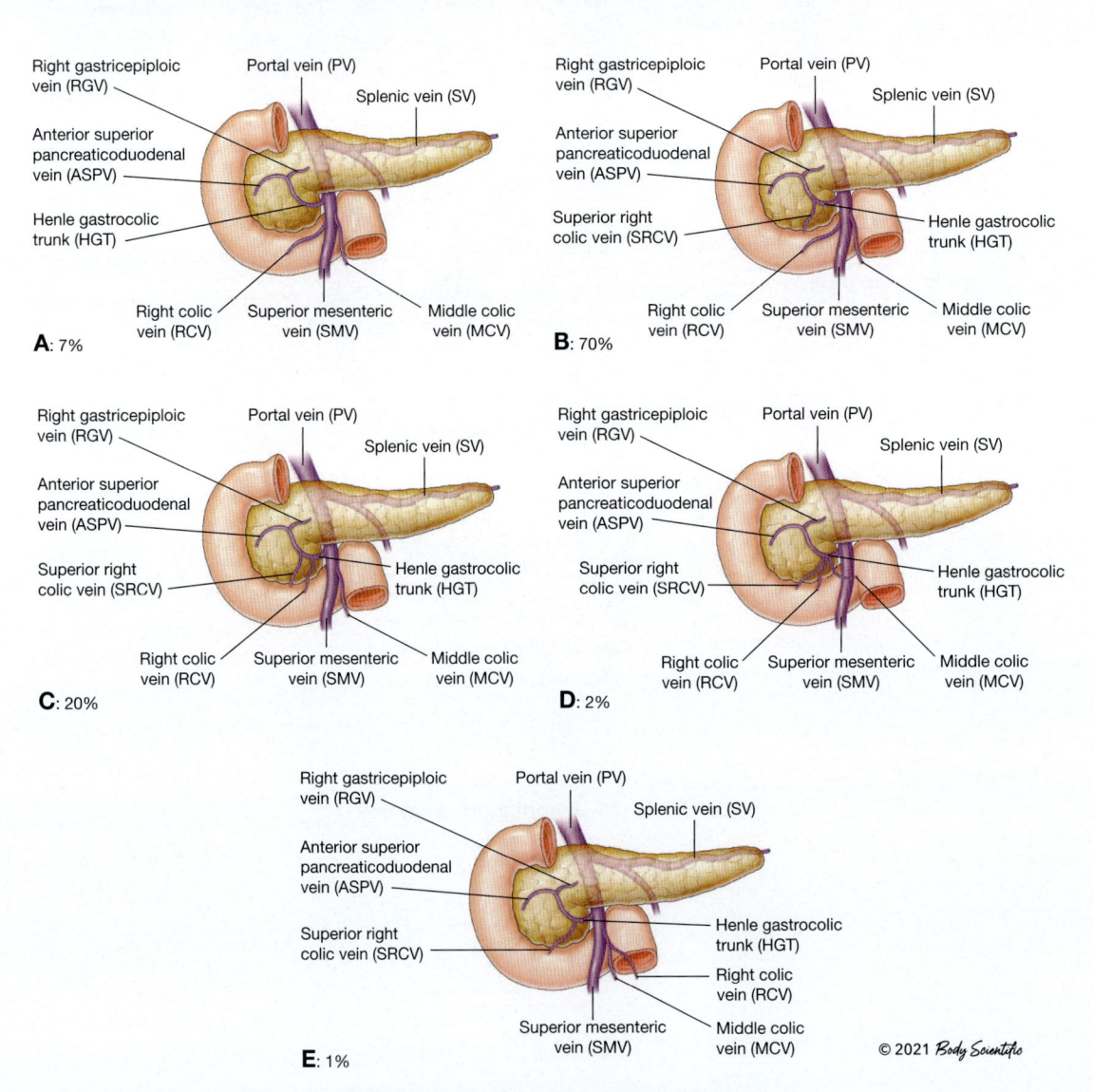

FIGURE 23-16 • Variations of Henle's trunk.

Reconstruction

Video 23-8. Step 9. Reconstruction Ileocolic Isoperistaltic Anastomosis

Step 9. Reconstruction
The specimen is momentarily left inside the abdomen, in a position not interfering with the completion of the operation, usually between the diaphragm and the right lobe of the liver, or in the pelvis.

It is important to check that that there is the proper amount of mobilization of the terminal ileum, making sure that it is reaching the transverse colon without tension. If not, further mobilization will be carried out. Also, ICG should be used to check that the ileal and transverse stumps are well perfused.

The reconstruction is routinely performed in an intracorporeal way, with an isoperistaltic side-to-side anastomosis (**Figures 23-17 A, B**). A stay suture is applied to approximate the terminal ileum and the transverse colon, while R3 helps in getting and maintaining the proper position of the bowel segments with an ideal angle for the stapler. Unless the colon is distended, the hook diathermy is usually used to perform the enterotomies (see the following Pitfalls box). The anastomosis can be fashioned either by the assistant using laparoscopic staplers or with a robotic stapling technique. The enterotomies are closed with running PDS™ 3-0. Sometimes, interrupted Prolene™ 3-0 or 4-0 stitches are placed to strengthen or to control possible bleeding on the suture line and on the two blind ends of the bowel. Usually, to prevent potential internal hernias, it is advisable to close the mesenteric defect with PDS™ 3-0 interrupted stitches, being careful during the maneuver not to damage the vessels close to the edges of the mesentery, to avoid ischemia on the anastomosis. Another ICG perfusion check may be repeated at this time (**Figures 23-18 A, B**).

Step 9 average time frame: 15–20 min

> ⚠ **PITFALLS**
>
> If the colon is very distended by gas (with possible presence of methane), the monopolar cautery may be dangerous because it may cause explosion of the colon. In this case, the colon should be opened using cold scissors or harmonic. This risk is less important for the ileum.

Step 10. Specimen extraction
The extraction of the specimen is usually carried out through a small Pfannenstiel (using a wound protector). See Chapter 2, The Basic Principles of Clinical Applications, for more details.

Step 10 average time frame: 15–20 min

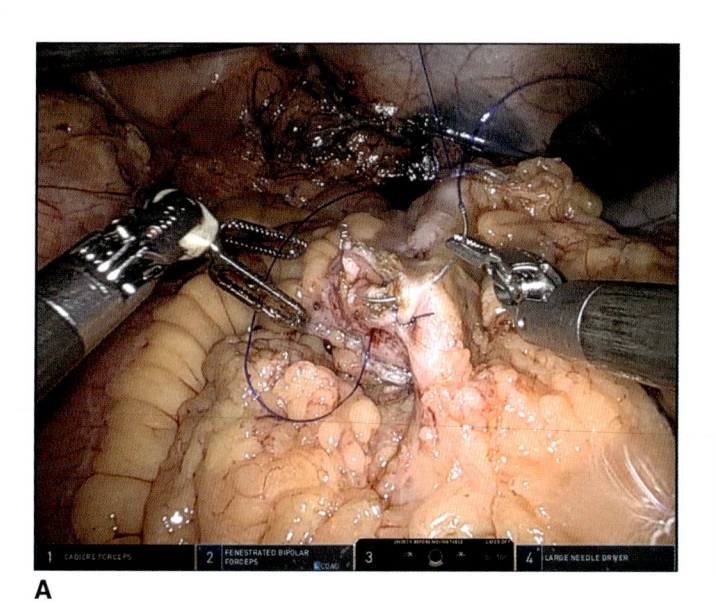

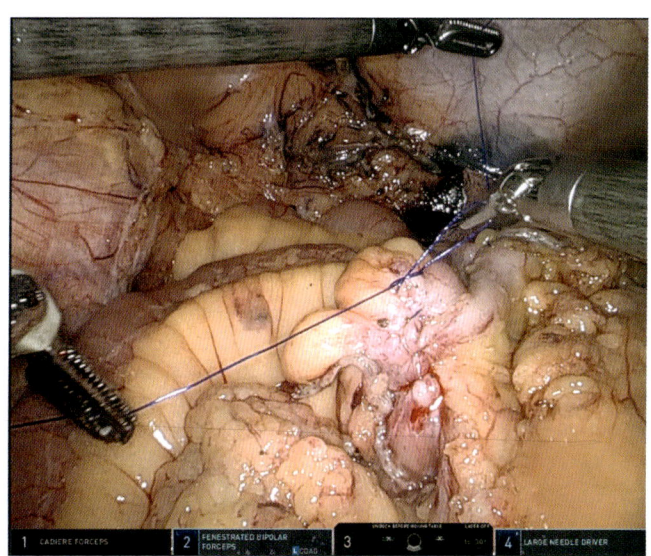

FIGURE 23-17 • Step 9. Reconstruction: ileocolic isoperistaltic anastomosis.

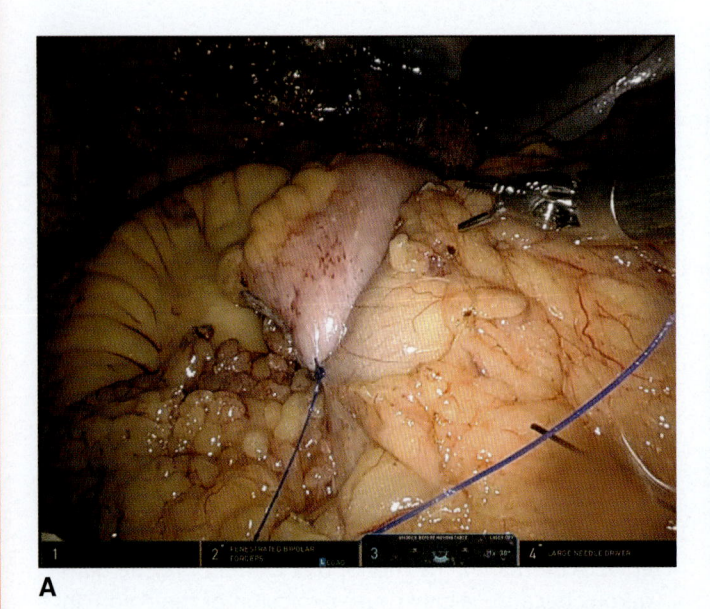

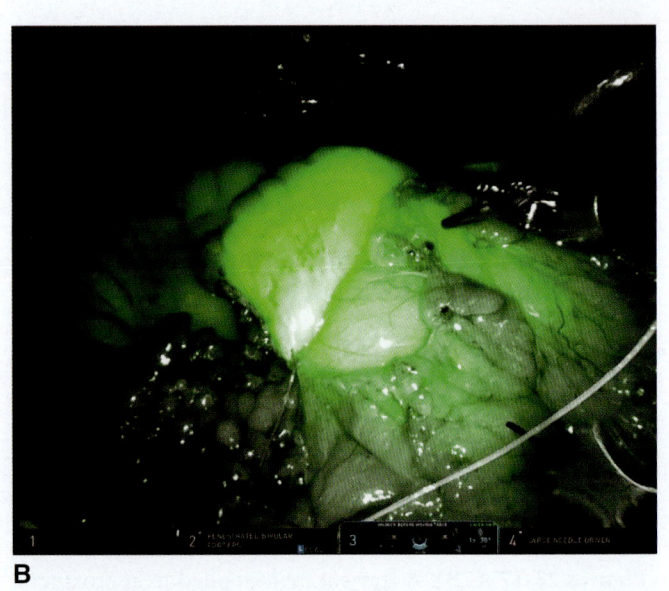

FIGURE 23-18 • Step 9. Reconstruction: ICG test.

Video 23-9. Radical Right Colectomy with Complete Mesocolic Excision (CME) – Full Procedure

Suggested Readings

1. Khan JS, Ahmad A, Odermatt M, et al. Robotic complete mesocolic excision with central vascular ligation for right colonic tumours a propensity score-matching study comparing with standard laparoscopy. *BJS Open*. 2021;5(2):zrab016. doi: 10.1093/bjsopen/zrab016
2. Larach JT, Flynn J, Wright T, et al. Robotic complete mesocolic excision versus conventional robotic right colectomy for right-sided colon cancer: a comparative study of perioperative outcomes. *Surg Endosc*. 2022;36(3):2113-2120. doi: 10.1007/s00464-021-08498-8
3. Athanasiou CD, Markides GA, Kotb A, Jia X, Gonsalves S, Miskovic D. Open compared with laparoscopic complete mesocolic excision with central lymphadenectomy for colon cancer: a systematic review and meta-analysis. *Colorectal Dis*. 2016;18(7):O224-O235. doi: 10.1111/codi.13385
4. Ferri V, Vicente E, Quijano Y, et al. Right-side colectomy with complete mesocolic excision vs conventional right-side colectomy in the treatment of colon cancer: a systematic review and meta-analysis. *Int J Colorectal Dis*. 2021;36(9):1885-1904. doi: 10.1007/s00384-021-03951-5
5. Mazzarella G, Muttillo EM, Picardi B, Rossi S, Muttillo IA. Complete mesocolic excision and D3 lymphadenectomy with central vascular ligation in right-sided colon cancer: a systematic review of postoperative outcomes, tumor recurrence and overall survival. *Surg Endosc*. 2021;35(9):4945-4955. doi: 10.1007/s00464-021-08529-4
6. Xu L, Su X, He Z, et al. RELARC Study Group Collaborators, Short-term outcomes of complete mesocolic excision versus D2 dissection in patients undergoing laparoscopic colectomy for right colon cancer (RELARC): a randomised, controlled, phase 3, superiority trial. *Lancet Oncol*. 2021;22(3):391-401. doi: 10.1016/S1470-2045(20)30685-9
7. Mangano A, Gheza F, Bustos R, et al. Robotic right colonic resection. Is the robotic third arm a game-changer? *Minerva Chir*. 2020;75(1):1-10. doi: 10.23736/S0026-4733.18.07814-8
8. Mangano A, Bustos R, Fernandes E, et al. Surgical technique in robotic right colonic resection. *Minerva Chir*. 2020;75(1):43-50. doi: 10.23736/S0026-4733.18.07815-X
9. Nelson H, Sargent DJ, Wieand HS, et al. A comparison of laparoscopically assisted and open colectomy for colon cancer. *N Engl J Med*. 2004;350(20):2050-2059.
10. Guillou PJ, Quirke P, Thorpe H, et al. Short-term endpoints of conventional versus laparoscopic-assisted surgery in patients with colorectal cancer (MRC CLASICC trial): multicentre, randomised controlled trial. *Lancet (London, England)*. 2005;365(9472):1718-1726.
11. Lacy AM, Delgado S, Castells A, et al. The long-term results of a randomized clinical trial of laparoscopy-assisted versus open surgery for colon cancer. *Ann Surg*. 2008;248(1):1-7.
12. Papanikolaou IG. Robotic surgery for colorectal cancer: systematic review of the literature. *Surg Laparosc Endosc Percutan Tech*. 2014;24(6):478-483.
13. Zhang X, Wei Z, Bie M, Peng X, Chen C. Robot-assisted versus laparoscopic-assisted surgery for colorectal cancer: a meta-analysis. *Surg Endosc*. 2016;30(12):5601-5614.
14. Cheng CL, Rezac C. The role of robotics in colorectal surgery. *BMJ (Clinical Research ed.)*. 2018;360:j5304.
15. Park JS, Choi GS, Park SY, Kim HJ, Ryuk JP. Randomized clinical trial of robot-assisted versus standard laparoscopic right colectomy. *Br J Surg*. 2012;99(9):1219-1226.
16. Giulianotti PC, Coratti A, Angelini M, et al. Robotics in general surgery: personal experience in a large community hospital. *Arch Surg*. 2003;138(7):777-784. doi: 10.1001/archsurg.138.7.777

24

"It is current practice to remove cancers of the terminal pelvic colon by way of a very major operation, namely an abdominal-perineal resection of the rectum. For two patients with colostomies following obstruction, I decided, upon reflection, to confine my excision to the segment of colon, with its accompanying ganglionic territory, proximal to the anus and rectum. Then I closed the superior part of the rectum and left it in the peritoneum without disturbing the perineal floor. The practicalities of the operation itself in the two cases were as straightforward as removing a non-inflamed appendix. Leaving a rectal dead end did not present any inconveniences, and my patients are still very well, now 9- and 10-months post-operation respectively."

—Henri Albert Hartmann (1860–1952)

Left Colectomy

Alberto Mangano • Valentina Valle • Pier Cristoforo Giulianotti

INTRODUCTION

The left colectomy and the low anterior resections (LARs) are important procedures in abdominal surgery and essential models for developing and refining surgical skills. They are multiquadrant procedures, where the minimally invasive approach may be challenging for a variety of reasons. Also, between left colectomy and LARs, there are other types of left-sided colon resections, which share common aspects (sigmoidectomy, Hartmann, etc.):

1. The exposure of the surgical target can be hindered by small bowel distension, adhesions, anatomical anomalies of the mesentery, inflammation, diverticulitis, bulky lesions, or narrow pelvis.
2. Gravitational retraction, sometimes adopting an extreme patient positioning, is necessary to favor proper exposure.
3. Left colectomy and LAR are both following avascular embryological planes for mobilization, dissection, control of the vascular pedicles, and lymphadenectomy.

INSTRUMENT REQUIREMENTS

The suggested main robotic instruments/tools can be listed as follows:
- 30° and 0° scope
- Cautery hook/monopolar scissors
- Vessel sealer
- Robotic linear staplers (with different loads)
- Needle drivers (round tip or macro)
- Multiple Hem-o-lok™ clips
- Medium–large clip applier
- Bipolar forceps
- Cadière forceps/tip-up fenestrated grasper

The suggested main laparoscopic instruments/tools can be listed as follows:
- Graspers
- Scissors
- Staplers (linear and circular)
- Needle drivers
- Suction-irrigation
- Fan retractor

Supplemental materials:
- Gauzes, sponges
- Vessel loops
- Alexis™ wound protector/retractor
- Endobags™
- Medium–large clips
- Sutures: Prolene™ 3-0 and PDS™ 3-0

Photo reproduced with permission from Université de Paris.
Quote reproduced with permission from Hartman MH. New procedure for the removal of cancers of the terminal part of the pelvic colon. Paris. Thirtieth Congress of Surgery, Strasbourg; 1921.

4. Four distinct dissection surgical phases are in common:
   a. Proximal colon mobilization.
   b. Central lymphadenectomy, and during the LAR, also total mesorectal excision.
   c. Specimen extraction with or without proximal anastomotic stump preparation.
   d. Colorectal anastomosis.
5. A crucial technical point is the mobilization of the splenic flexure. This maneuver should be performed in all cases independently from the sigmoid redundancy:
   a. It provides a well-perfused, longer, proximal colonic segment, which allows a floppy anastomosis.
   b. If the mobilization of the splenic flexure is not performed preventively, and the proximal colon becomes too short, going back for further mobilization of the flexure can be very difficult (mainly if the anastomosis was already done), and the blood flow of the marginal arcade can be compromised.
   c. It permits a wider oncological dissection with easier lymphadenectomy.
   d. It allows the mastering of a surgical maneuver that, similarly to the Kocher maneuver in hepato-pancreato-biliary surgery, can be used in other/different operations (e.g., distal pancreatectomy, splenectomy). Some authors claim potential drawbacks connected to the routine splenic flexure mobilization, such as (1) risk of splenic injuries and (2) extended operative time. However, in expert hands, such occurrences are rare.
6. If the splenic flexure mobilization is done systematically, both the left colectomy and the LAR become multiquadrant operations characterized by 4 distinct phases and 2 different surgical fields. The first surgical field is the left upper quadrant for the mobilization of the left colonic flexure. The second one is the lower quadrants for the aorto-pelvic phase. These double surgical fields require to achieve an optimal control, 2 different patient positionings, 2 potentially distinct port settings, and 2 separate robotic cart dockings.
7. Since minimally invasive surgery (MIS) penetrance in left colonic resections is still relatively low, robotics can be of value by making the operation easier, with a shorter learning curve, and decreasing the risk of conversion.

> **EDITORIAL COMMENT**
>
> The single docking approach for left colectomies and LAR is popular in Asia, where the majority of patients have a very favorable body conformation and/or the splenic mobilization is achieved with hybrid techniques (laparoscopy). In Western countries, with higher body mass index (BMI) patients, this approach may result in poor visualization and limited instrument control.

In this chapter, a standardized approach to robotic left colonic resections, with routine splenic flexure mobilization, is presented. This technique can be defined as the "triple two" procedure because it is composed of 2 patient positionings, 2 different port settings, and 2 dockings.

Indications and Relative Contraindications to the Robotic Approach

The indications are similar to the ones for open and laparoscopic surgery: malignancies, benign tumors, inflammatory bowel disease, and recurrent diverticulitis.

Extensive and/or tenacious adhesions, morbid obesity, and bulky cancers may increase the difficulty of the procedure, but they are not absolute contraindications.

The boundaries of what is achievable with a robotic MIS should always be assessed according to the local surgical expertise. With that in mind, the first part of the colorectal learning curve should consist of easy cases with smaller lesions, adopting a safe and stepwise progressive increase of the technical difficulty.

Patient Positioning, OR Setup, and Port Setting

The specific patient positioning, OR setup, and port setting are depicted in the illustrations at the beginning of each of the 4 phases.

As far as possible, the goal should be to use/reuse the same trocars, with a different direction of work characteristic of the specific phase. To facilitate the accomplishment of this goal, the trocar placement should be planned keeping in mind the different phases, and with the construction of 2 different triangles of work, each of which is characterized by 2 distinct target anatomies.

The first triangle for Phase A is centered around the central/left upper quadrants (for the mobilization of the left colonic flexure and inferior mesenteric vein [IMV] division). The other triangle of work is for the following phases, and it is directed toward the aortopelvic region.

The position of the scope is the first priority during the port placement. It is placed on the right side of the umbilicus (in normal size patients) to give more room for R3, which is useful during the retraction of the sigmoid colon and rectum. The scope, while pointing at different directions, will stay in the same location during the entire procedure. The other trocars are placed in a way to be able to construct 2 triangles of work. The first triangle is facing the splenic flexure, and the second one downward toward the pelvis. The complete port setting is done at the beginning of the procedure, but some of the ports are working as robotic ports, and others as assistant ports, and *vice versa* in the different phases of the operation.

Surgical Technique

Intrabdominal Exploration and Anatomical Understanding

This step is important to take the proper technical decisions, to establish what is safe, and to acquire any information relevant for the strategy of the entire operation.

If the surgical indication is cancer, it is essential to complete a staging assessment with potential changes in treatment plans (e.g., peritoneal carcinomatosis).

Also, the presence of adhesions and/or concomitant pathologies that can modify the strategy of access to the abdominal cavity must be ruled out. The specific anatomy of the left colonic flexure should be also evaluated: e.g., the presence of diverticula, omental adhesions, or double-folded flexure (i.e., when the distal transverse and the descending colon are tightly attached with a shape resembling a "double barrel shotgun"), or when the flexure is in an unusually cranial position (going beyond the splenic hilum).

After the specific anatomical assessment, the best tailored approach can be decided, adapting the trocar sites and choosing the most appropriate combination of the different left colonic mobilization strategies (see TIPS box).

Video 24-1. Left Colectomy – Full Pocedure

Phase A

The OR setting, the patient positioning, and the port placement for Phase A are depicted in **Figures 24-1**, **24-2**, and **24-3**.

The exact sequence of some of the surgical steps can be variable according to the specific anatomy and surgical case. The most frequent order for Phase A is as follows: left omentum-colic detachment, splenocolic ligament dissection, lateral-to-medial mobilization, transverse colon mesenteric root detachment from the pancreatic body, and then medial-to-lateral dissection with IMV division. However, in some situations (see TIPS box), it is preferable to start with medial to lateral or with gastrocolic access.

Landmarks of Phase A are: lower edge of the pancreatic body, Toldt's fascia, inferior mesenteric vein (IMV), Treitz, and lower pole of the spleen.

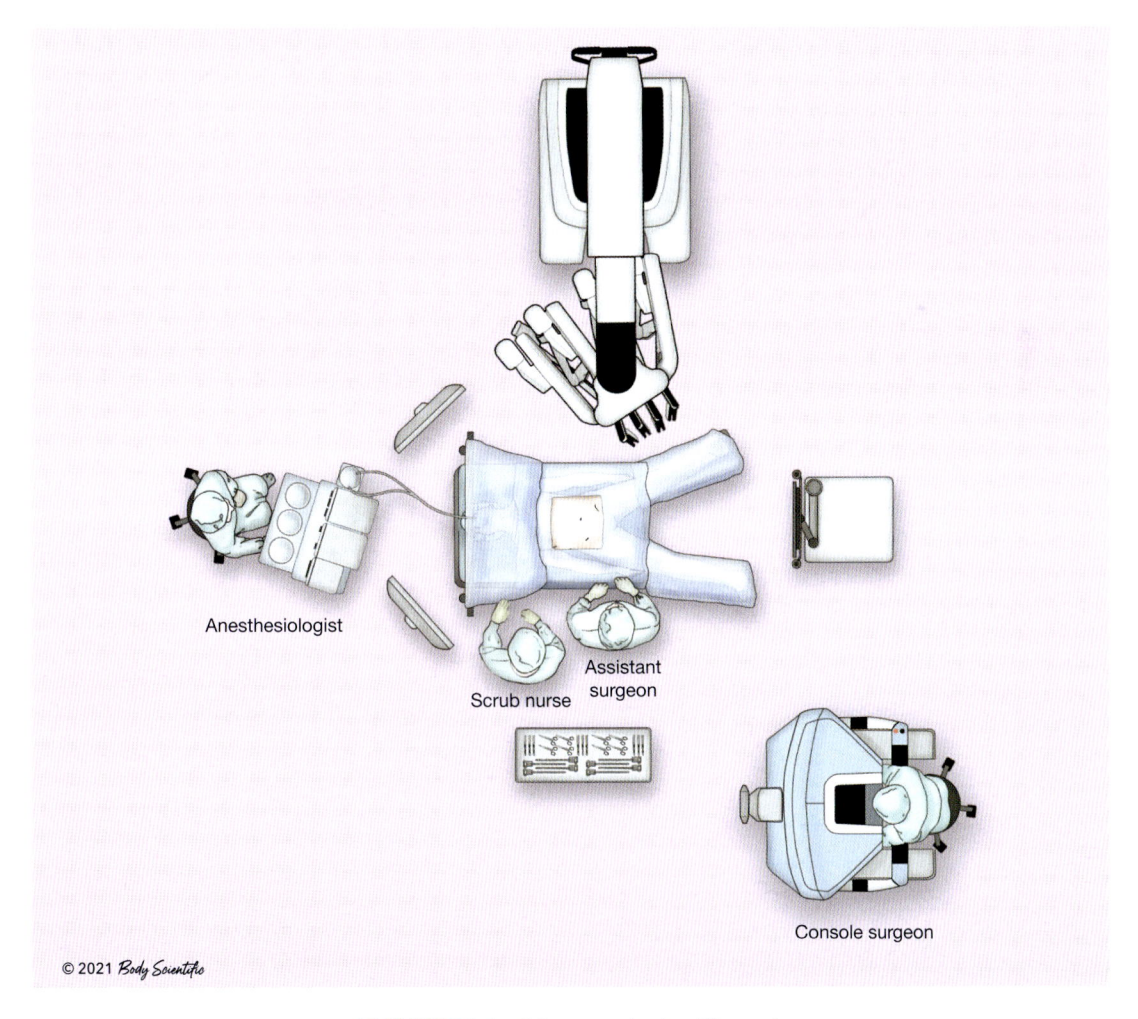

FIGURE 24-1 • OR setup during Phase A.

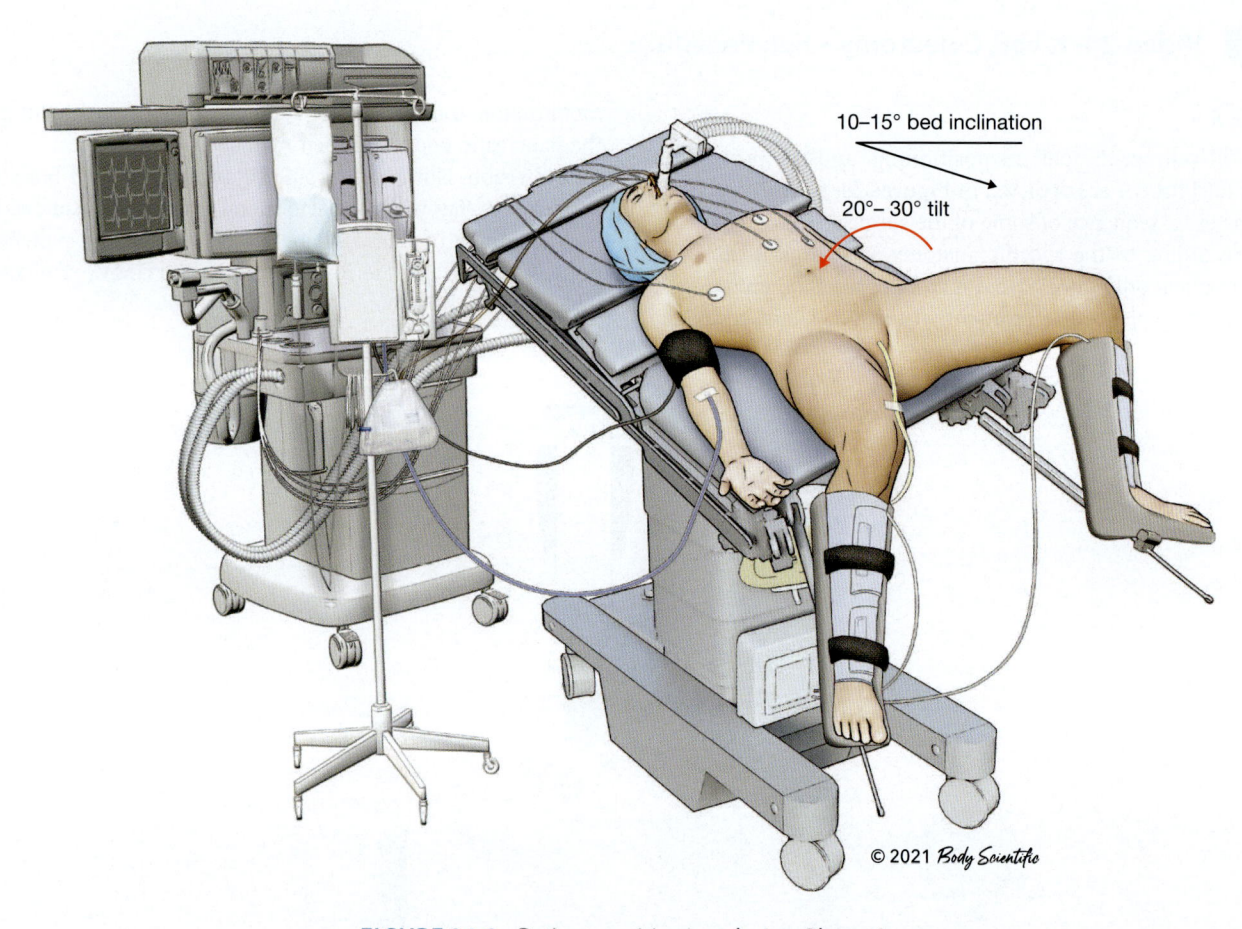

FIGURE 24-2 • Patient positioning during Phase A.

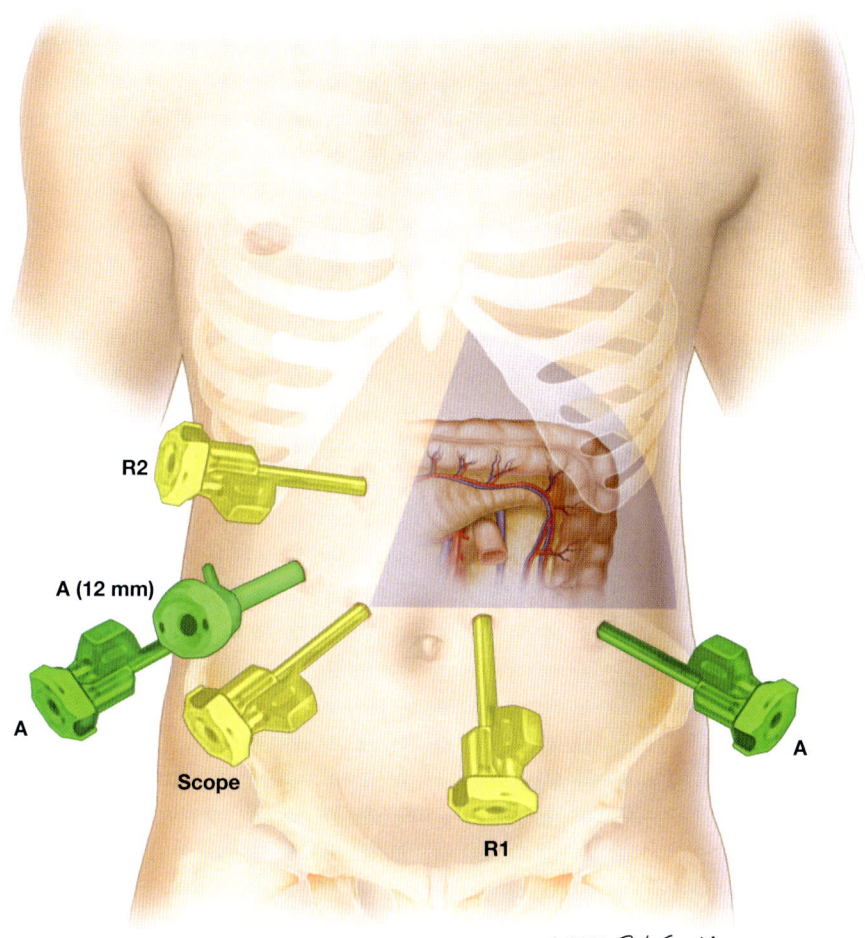

Left Colectomy 483

FIGURE 24-3 • Port setting during Phase A. The robotic ports in this phase are depicted in yellow. The ports that may be used by the Assistant are depicted in green.

> ▶▶ **TIPS**

There are 4 different possible dissection pathways that must be mastered for the left colonic flexure mobilization. Usually, this maneuver is carried out by adopting a variable combination of at least 2 or 3 of these 4 pathways which are used with a different sequence/order according to the specific clinical case and anatomy.

The 4 pathways are:

1. Lateral-to-medial dissection (**Figure 24-4**).
2. Medial-to-lateral dissection (**Figure 24-5**).
3. Top-down dissection with omental-colonic detachment (**Figure 24-6**).
4. Top-down approach with opening of the gastrocolic ligament (transgastrocolic access) (**Figure 24-7**). If there are adhesions, diverticulitis, or the presence of many diverticula, the omental detachment can be dangerous. In this case, the omentum may be left attached to the colon, and the gastrocolic ligament is divided with an omental flap adherent to the flexure. In this approach, the left colonic flexure is taken down with the omentum attached.

In this chapter, the most typical combination and sequence of these approaches will be described for the left colonic resection.

> ▶▶ **TIPS**

The classical sequence of splenic flexure mobilization is: medial-to-lateral and then lateral-to-medial dissection. However, the order of the steps can be changed when there is an anatomical situation that suggests that one of the pathways is easier:

1. If the small bowel is distended, going medial-to-lateral is troublesome: there are dilated bowel loops, and it's possible to make injuries with the instruments while trying to visualize the base of the mesentery and the IMV. In this situation, it is better to give priority to lateral-to-medial approach, being careful not to open the mesentery. The mesentery becomes like an "apron" that can be mobilized/lifted while, at the same time, retracting the small bowel.
2. In skinny patients with no bowel distension, it is easier to start with the medial-to-lateral dissection. After preparing the Toldt's fascia, using a medial-to-lateral approach, the dissection may be completed with top-down detachment of the insertion to the edge of the pancreas.
3. A perfect mobilization requires the knowledge of all 4 pathways of the left colonic flexure takedown. In any case, every pathway is convergent to the Toldt's fascia. Also, dissecting along the correct plane from one side allows the subsequent dissection to be carried out along the other directions.

> ▶▶ **TIPS**

The assistant has to exert the proper amount of tension on the colon and on the mesentery of the transverse colon. This maneuver allows a better understanding and the separation of different anatomical planes/structures: the omentum, the gastrocolic ligament, and the mesentery. If the specific anatomy is well understood, the risk of injury to the blood supply is reduced.

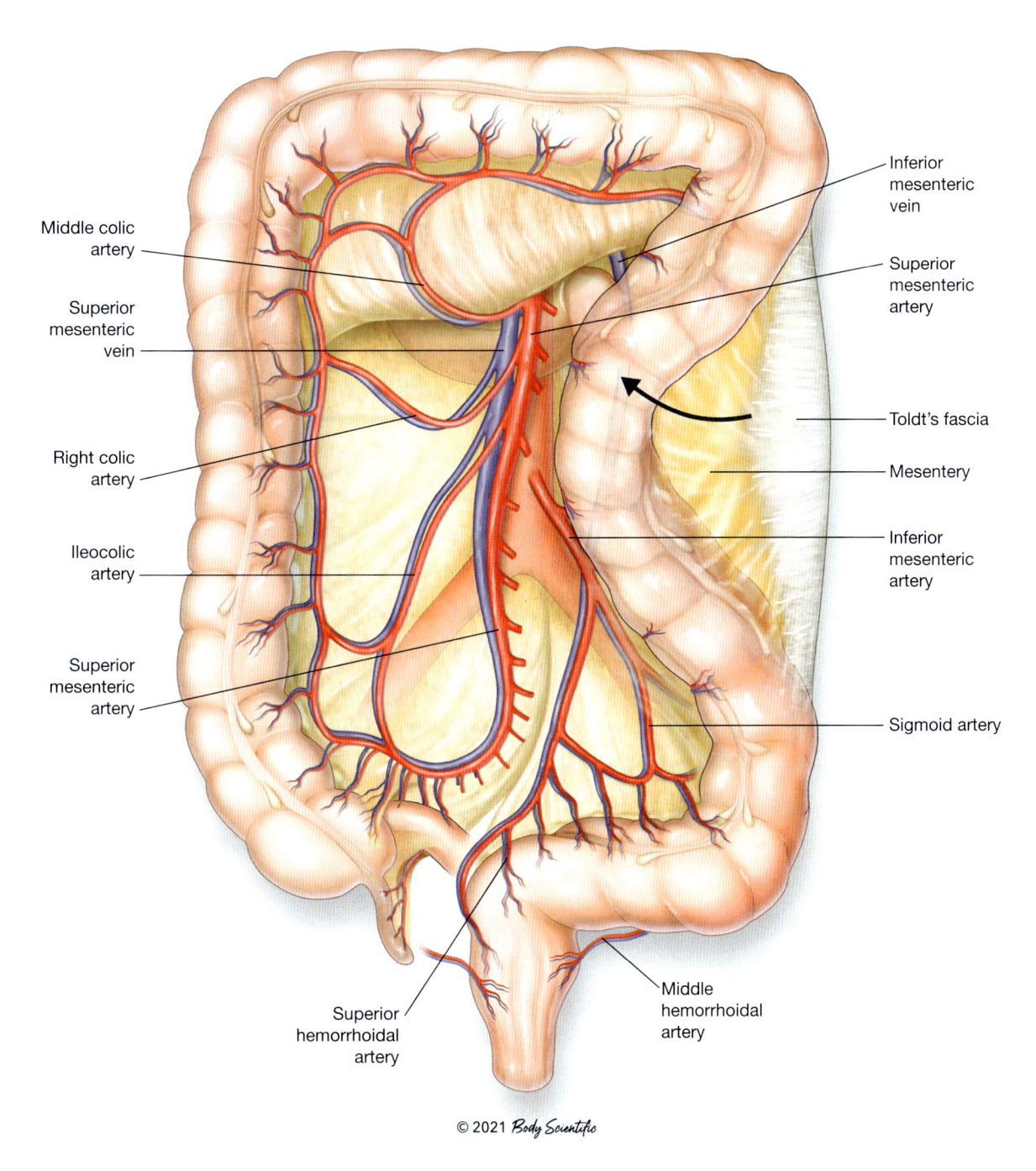

FIGURE 24-4 • Lateral-to-medial mobilization.

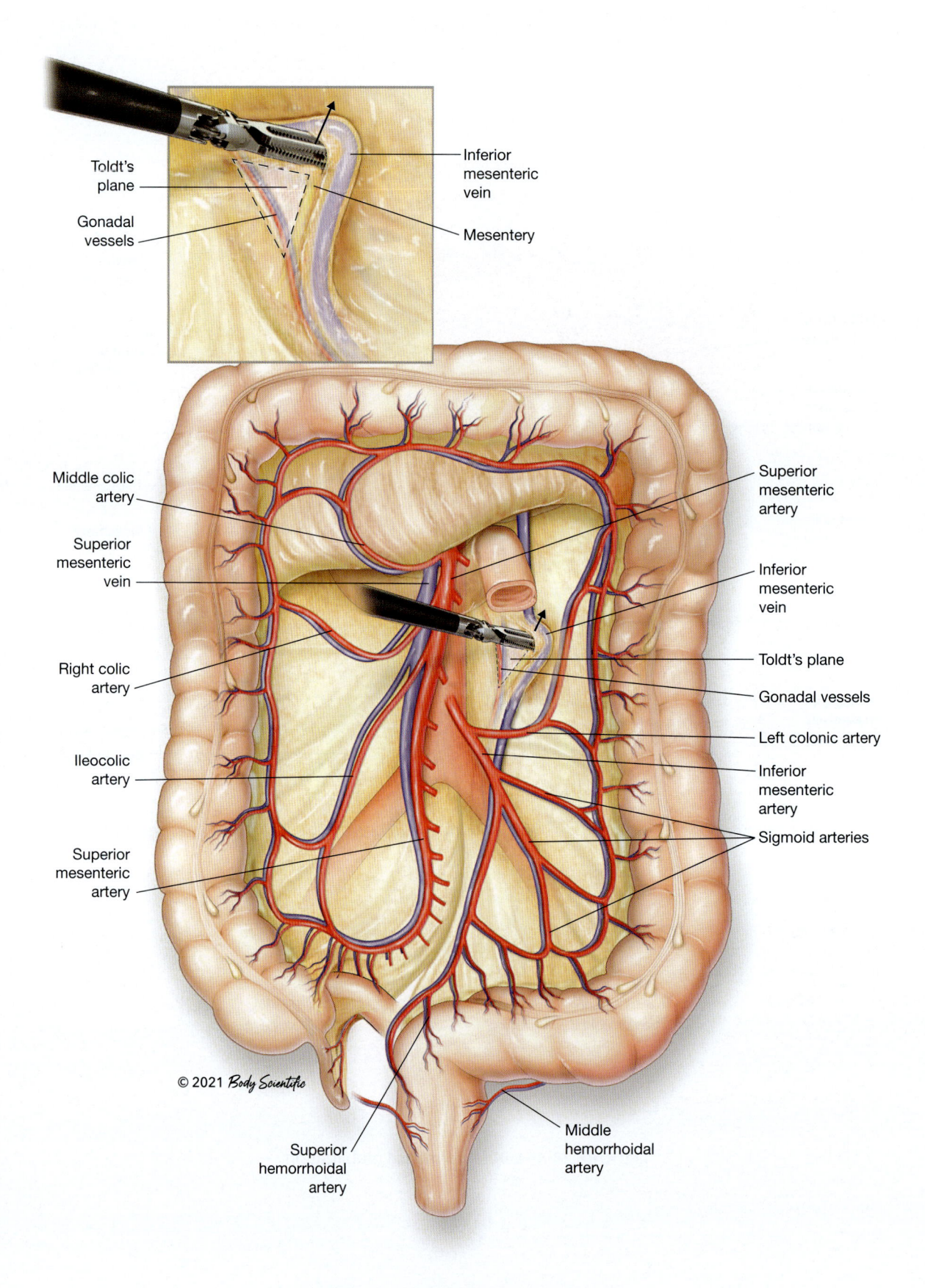

FIGURE 24-5 • Medial-to-lateral dissection.

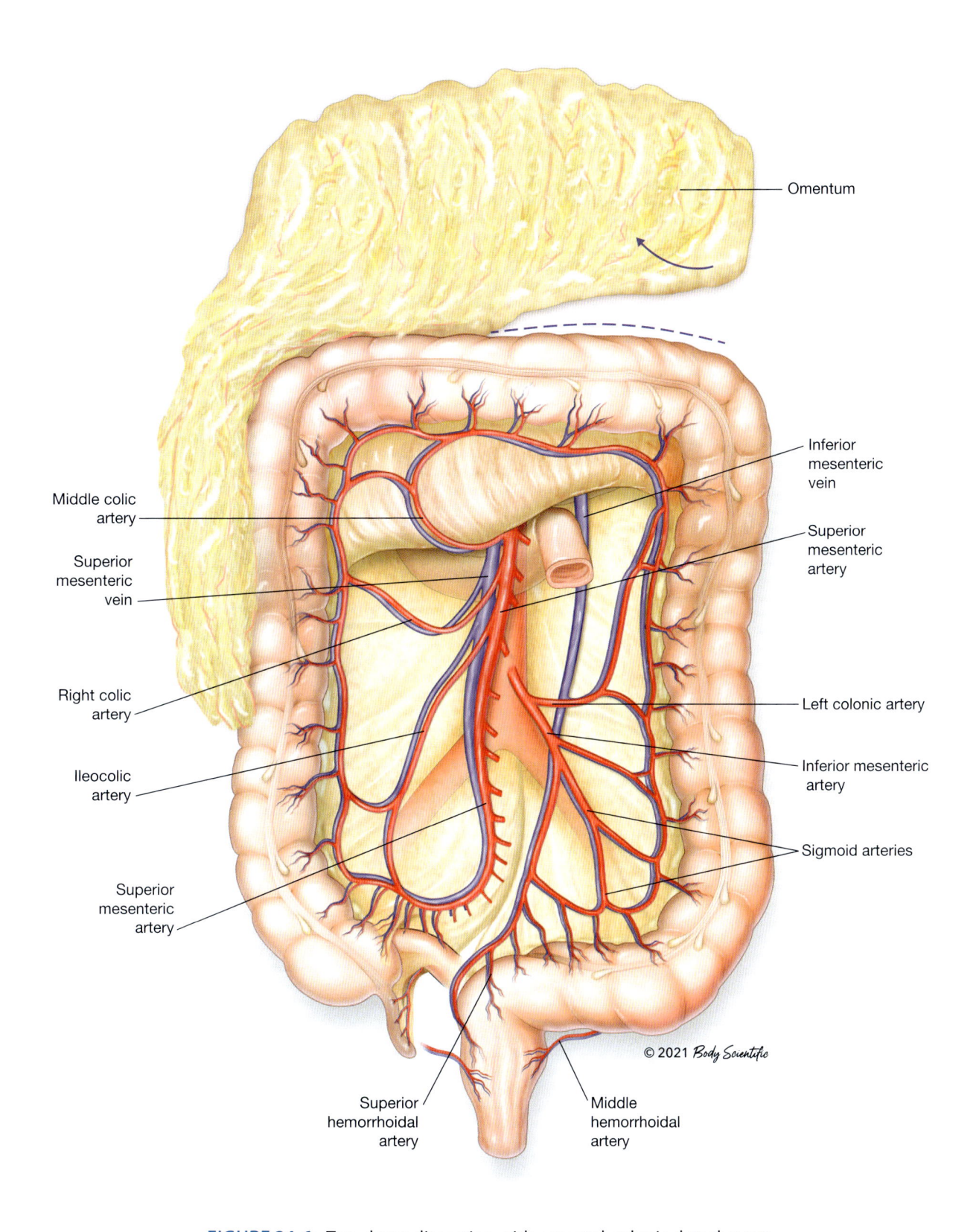

FIGURE 24-6 • Top-down dissection with omental-colonic detachment.

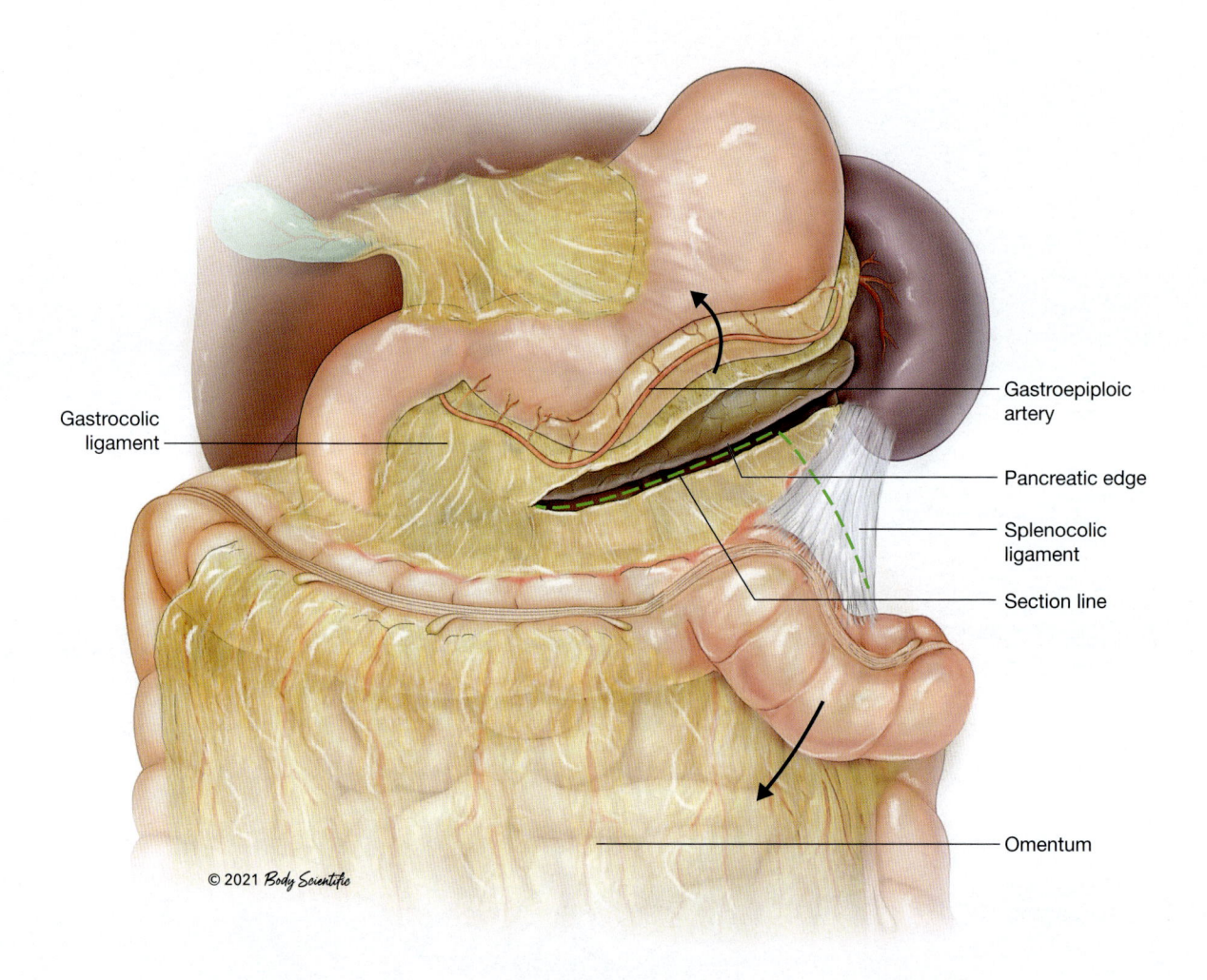

FIGURE 24-7 • Top-down approach with opening of the gastrocolic ligament.

Step 1. Left omentum-colic detachment

In the classical and most common situation, the omental detachment from the insertion of transverse colon should be performed first. If the flexure is very high, it may not be possible to complete all the detachment. However, if the specific situation allows it, the left side of the omentum is divided from the transverse colon attachment, being careful not to damage possible diverticula. During this step, the gastrocolic ligament can be detached and the lesser sac can be entered. This maneuver gives the surgeon control of the insertion of the mesentery of the transverse colon. This detachment proceeds medial to lateral, but it may be difficult to complete it with one approach only and, at some point, the lateral-to-medial pathway will be adopted.

Step 1 average time frame: 10–15 min

> **▶▶ TIPS**
>
> For this step, the best instrument is the monopolar hook or the scissors because they are forcing the surgeon to stay in the correct avascular plane. The vessel sealer may be useful for thick or hypervascular omentum as in cirrhotic patients with portal hypertension.

> **⚠ PITFALLS**
>
> If the surgical planes are not clearly defined, it is possible to mistakenly enter into the mesentery of the transverse colon, injuring the blood supply (e.g., the marginal arcade) of the flexure.

Step 2. Splenocolic ligament dissection

The splenocolic ligament is carefully dissected staying close to the colonic wall ("onion peeling technique"). Particular attention should be paid not to injure the pancreatic tail.

The in-depth knowledge of the anatomy of this region and its different ligaments is essential (**Figure 24-8**).

Step 2 average time frame: 5–10 min

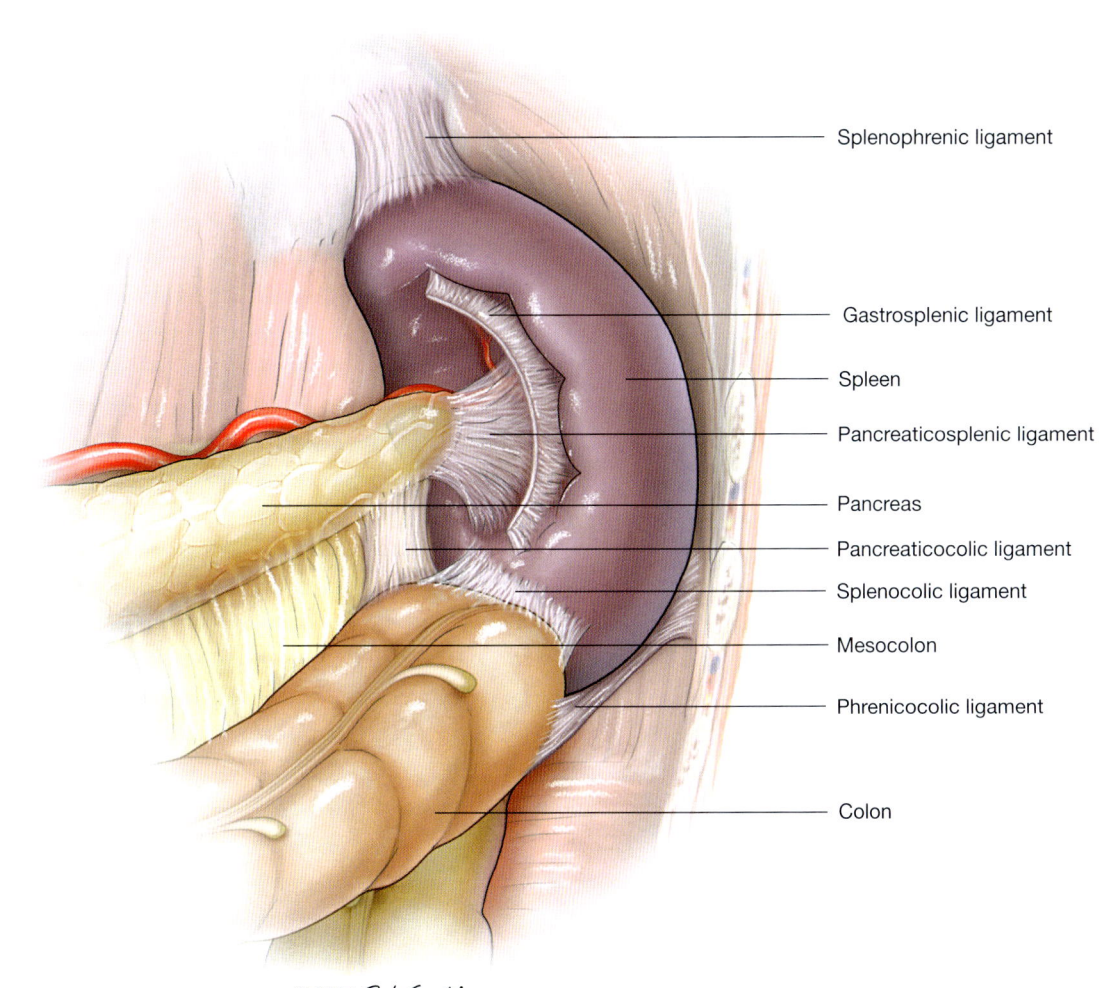

FIGURE 24-8 • Ligaments of the spleen.

Step 3. Lateral-to-medial dissection

The mobilization of the descending colon is started. The most favorable point to start the lateral-to-medial dissection is 5–6 cm below the left colonic flexure. This area is where the reflection of the lateral peritoneum on the Gerota's capsule is more evident. The correct plane can be recognized by proper exposure: the assistant is retracting medially the descending colon, possibly with 2 laparoscopic forceps. The main surgeon is adding a finer, precise traction on the peritoneal reflection and it becomes easy to enter into the proper avascular plane in front of the Toldt's fascia (see **Figures 24-9 A, B** for Toldt's fascia anatomy).

The dissection can join the plane that was previously prepared, and the detachment of the splenocolic ligament can be completed achieving the entire takedown of the flexure.

Step 3 average time frame: 5–10 min

▶ **Video 24-2. Step 3. Lateral-to-Medial Dissection**

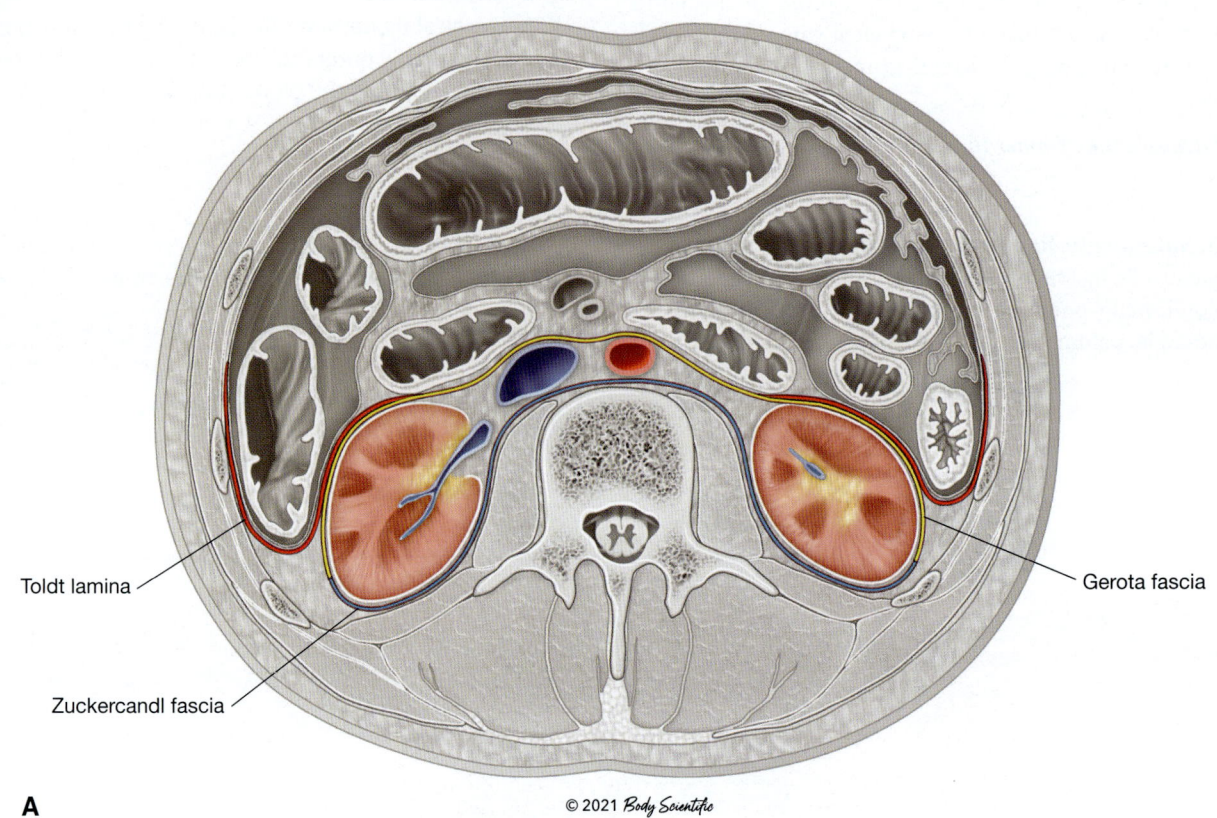

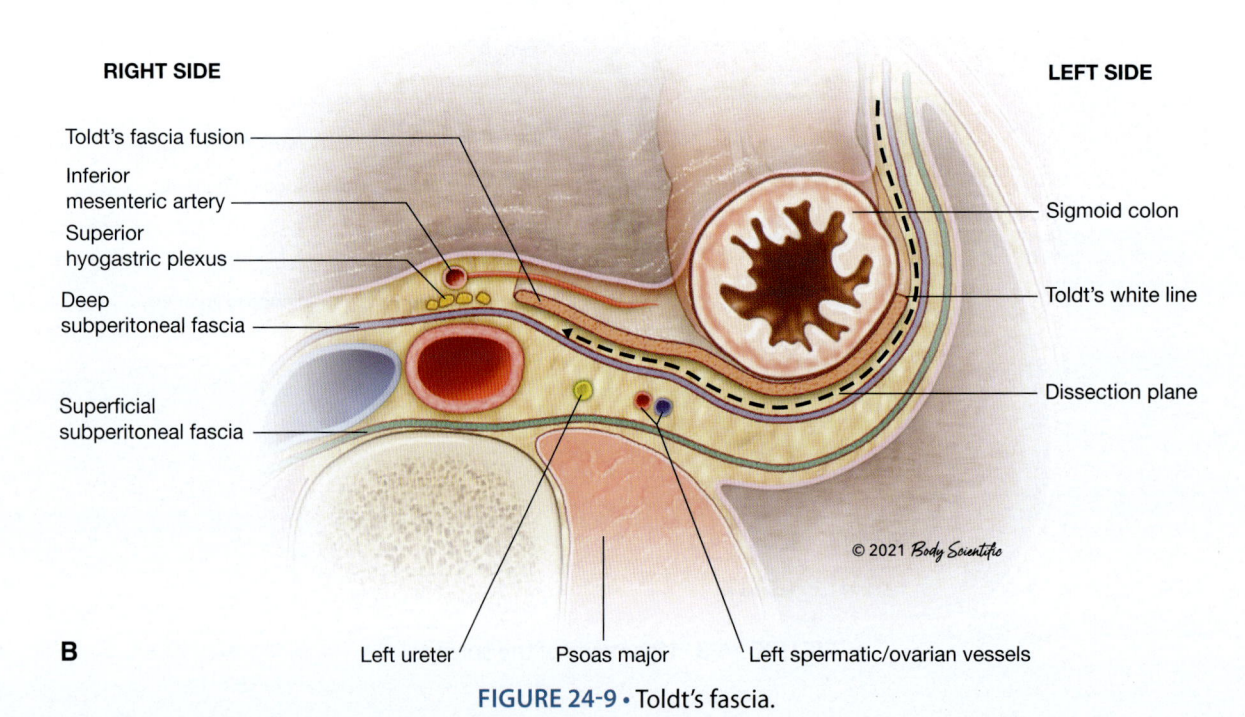

FIGURE 24-9 • Toldt's fascia.

Step 4. Transverse colon mesenteric root detachment from the pancreatic body

The transverse colon mesenteric root (**Figure 24-10**) is carefully detached from the edge of the pancreatic body. The dissection starts with a medial-to-lateral direction following the lower edge of the pancreatic body, and attention should be paid not to injure the pancreatic parenchyma. The dissection plane is usually totally avascular, with some exceptions like cirrhotic patients, and going down on top of the Toldt's fascia. The most difficult points are close to the pancreatic tail and the splenic colonic flexure where the anatomical relationships between the tail of the pancreas and the colon could be variable.

Step 4 average time frame: 3–5 min

> ⚠️ **PITFALLS**
>
> Lesions of the pancreatic parenchyma can occur during the detachment of the mesenteric root of the transverse colon. When the pancreas is inadvertently injured, usually there is a bleeding that cannot be controlled with bipolar coagulation but it requires application of stitches. Bleeding should be, in this step, a warning sign of a wrong plane with risk of pancreatic injury.

▶ **Video 24-3.** Step 4. Transverse Colon Mesenteric Root Detachment from the Pancreatic Body

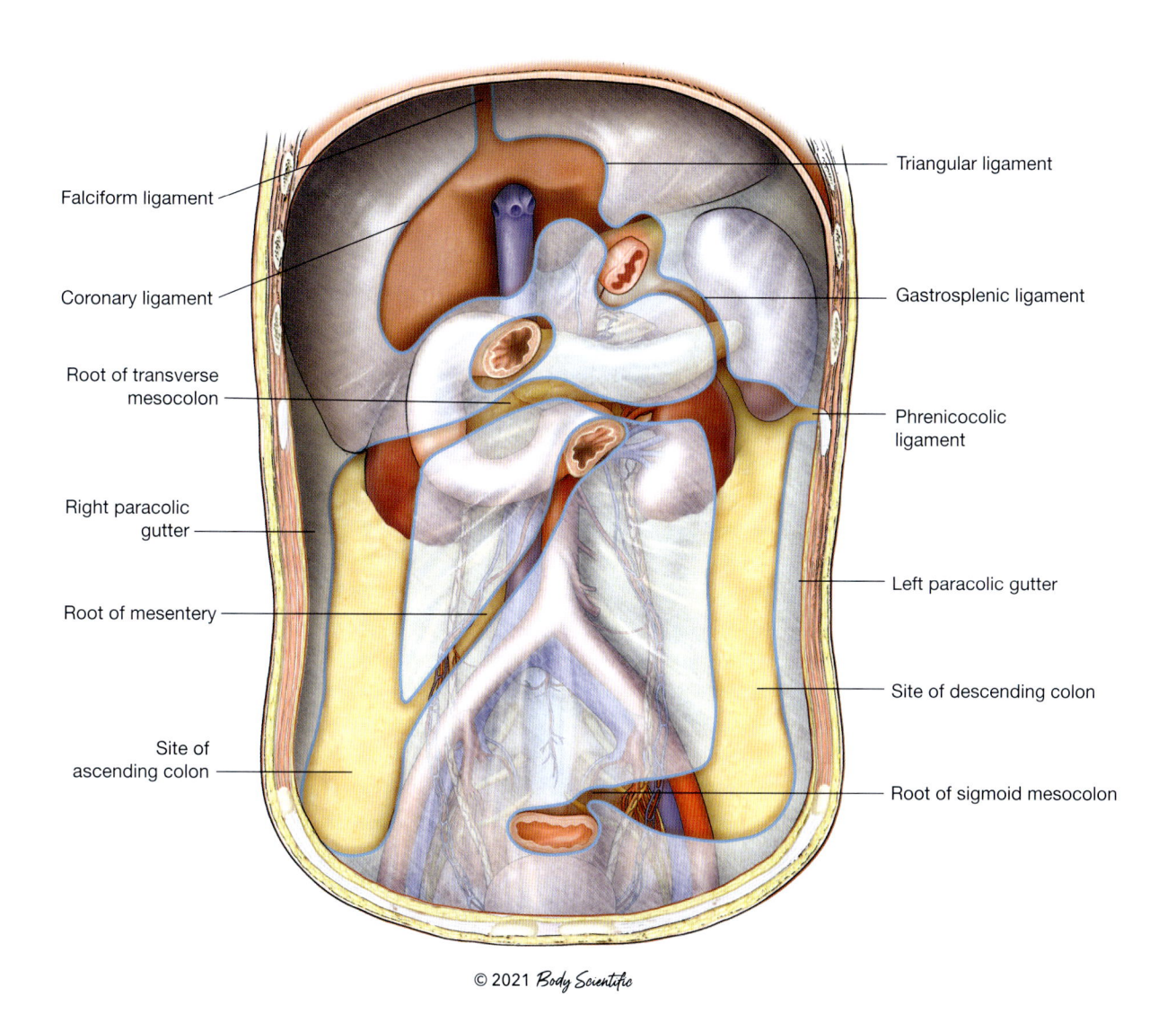

FIGURE 24-10 • Structure of the mesentery.

Step 5. Medial-to-lateral dissection and IMV division

At this time, the exposure is changing. The assistant pulls up the mesentery of the transverse colon, using 1 laparoscopic forceps, while with another laparoscopic forceps, the proximal jejunal loops are retracted medially. In doing so, the IMV is exposed. The venous anatomy is depicted in **Figure 24-11**.

The Treitz is very lateral sometimes, and in such cases, it has to be partially mobilized and retracted medially. If the proximal jejunal loops are too lateral, they may go underneath the mesentery of the descending colon after the reconstruction. This can cause postoperative partial obstruction due to internal herniation.

The reflection of the peritoneum underneath the IMV is identified. This peritoneal layer should be opened in a parallel fashion very close to the lower margin of the IMV.

At this point, the IMV is lifted and the dissection planes that were previously created are joined together.

The division of the IMV can be performed with clips, or preferably with the stapler. If the latter is chosen, the ascending branch of the left colonic artery can be included in the dissection. This maneuver opens up the vascular arcade and the mesentery allowing an elongation of the descending colon.

At this stage, Phase A of the procedure is completed.

Step 5 average time frame: 5–10 min

▶▶ **TIPS**

What are the limits of the mobilization of the flexure at this stage?

Once the IMV is transected, the mesentery of the descending colon can be lifted and retracted downward, staying on the correct plane as much as it is technically feasible and easy. At some point, the instruments will be perpendicular or in reverse position, and the surgeon will be restricted during the surgical maneuvers. At least, the IMV should be divided, and if possible, the origin of the inferior mesenteric artery (IMA) should be reached. In doing so, Phase B will be facilitated.

The IMA should not be controlled during Phase A. The reason for this advice is, at this point, the surgeon is working with the instruments at the limits of the surgical field. Also, the exposure is not optimal because the small bowel is in front of the aorta due to the reverse Trendelenburg position.

At this stage, the tip of the flap of the descending colonic mesentery has been created (the tip of this flap is the stump of the IMV). Then, the origin of the IMA is reached, and when the instruments start having some restrictions, the mobilization should be stopped. Usually, at this point, the left colonic flexure is completely detached and mobilized.

Left Colectomy 493

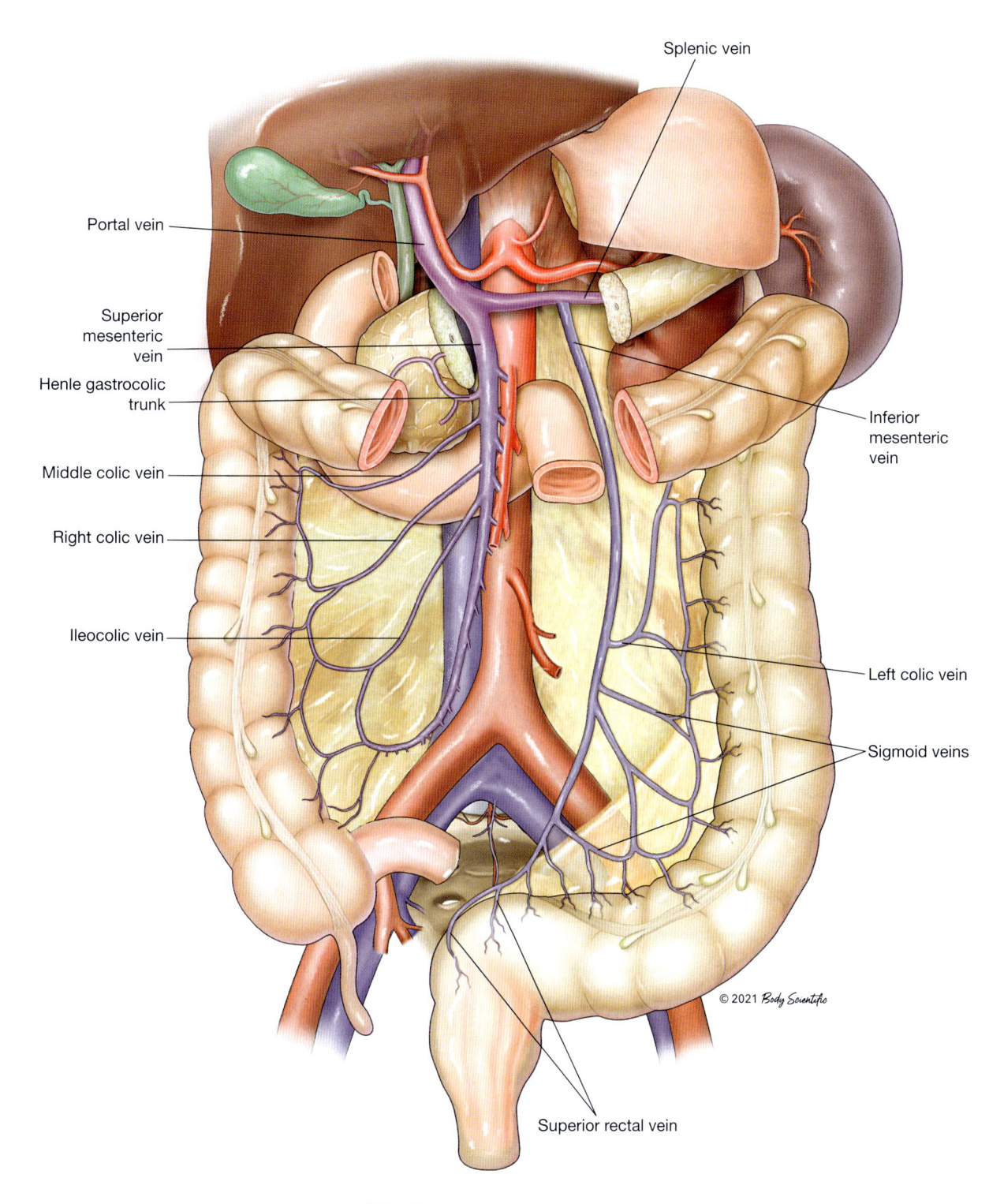

FIGURE 24-11 • Venous anatomy.

▶ Video 24-4. Step 5. Medial-to-Lateral Dissection

> ⚠️ **PITFALLS**
>
> Entering into the wrong surgical plane with the intention to divide the IMV is not too infrequent. A deeper plane includes the gonadal vessels. The IMV is on a more superficial level. Especially in skinny patients, it is easy to go too deep and below the gonadal vessels, with potential injury of them and/or of the ureter.

> ⚠️ **PITFALLS**
>
> - Direct lesions of the spleen are possible, but rare. More commonly, indirect lesions may occur when there are adhesions between the omentum and the splenic capsule. Traction must be exerted carefully, considering the sum of the surgeon's traction forces plus the assistant's ones and the gravitational forces.
> - Putting the stapler in the wrong way and reaching the marginal arcade while dividing the IMV. If the colon has a folded or short anatomical configuration, it is possible to reach the marginal arcade with just one stapler application. If the marginal arcade is damaged, there may be a risk of segmental colonic ischemia (which may not be diagnosed intraoperatively).

Phase B

The OR setting, the patient positioning, and the ports setting for Phase B are depicted in **Figures 24-12**, **24-13**, and **24-14**.

The robot is temporarily undocked. The position of the patient is changed from a reverse Trendelenburg to a steep Trendelenburg. The goal is to remove the bowel loops from the pelvis and to expose the aorta to visualize the IMA origin. The degree of surgical table tilting should be the minimum necessary to achieve these goals, reducing the hemodynamic consequences of the Trendelenburg position. Also, the assistant may help with exposure by using laparoscopic retraction. However, the ideal situation is to reach the perfect exposure just by gravitation. After changing the position, before redocking the robotic cart, a laparoscopic check may be performed to make sure that those exposure goals are correctly achieved.

The scope stays in the same place at the right side of the umbilicus for the entire operation.

Left Colectomy 495

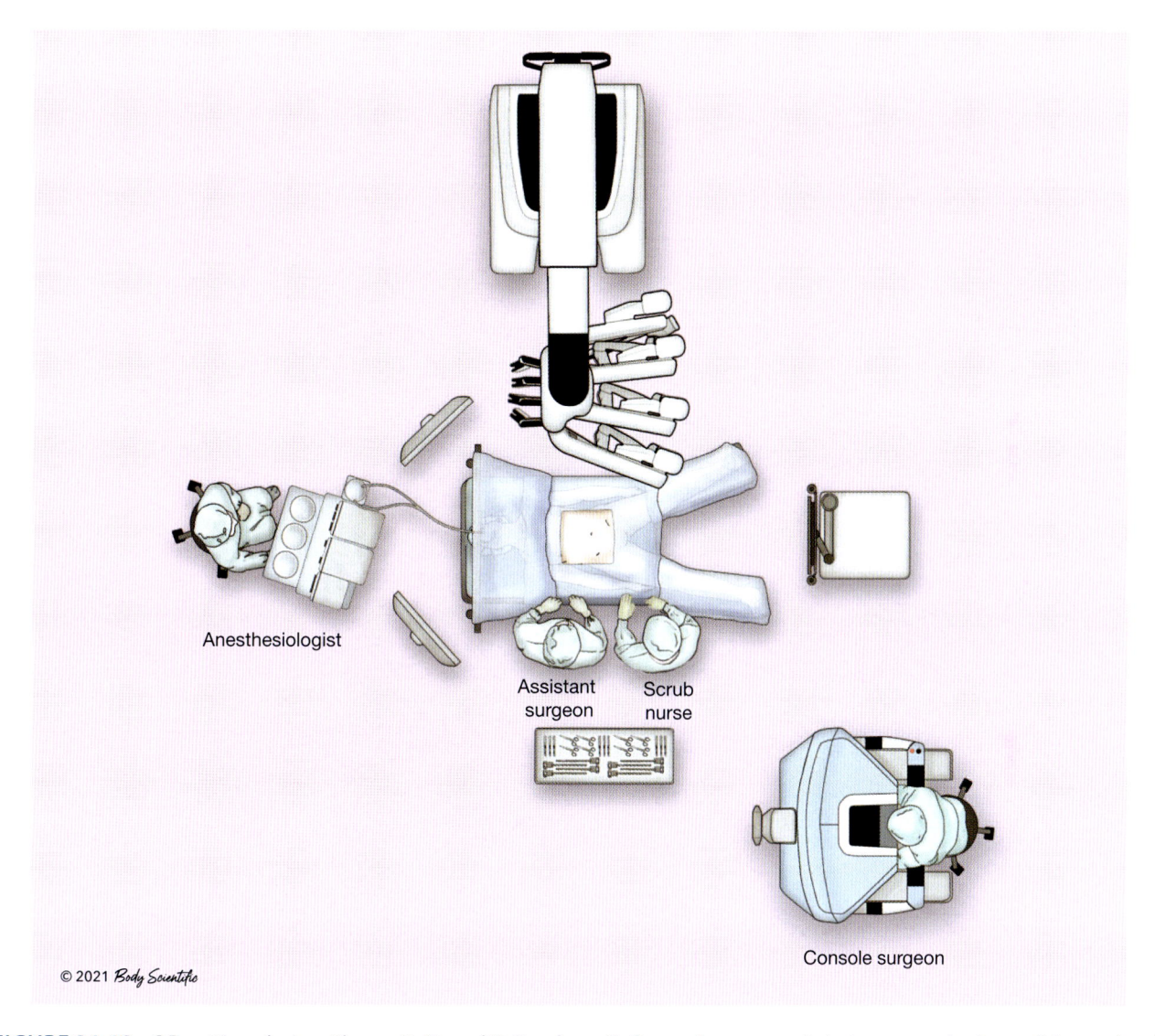

FIGURE 24-12 • OR setting during Phases B, C, and D (in phase D the main surgeon is in between the legs of the patient).

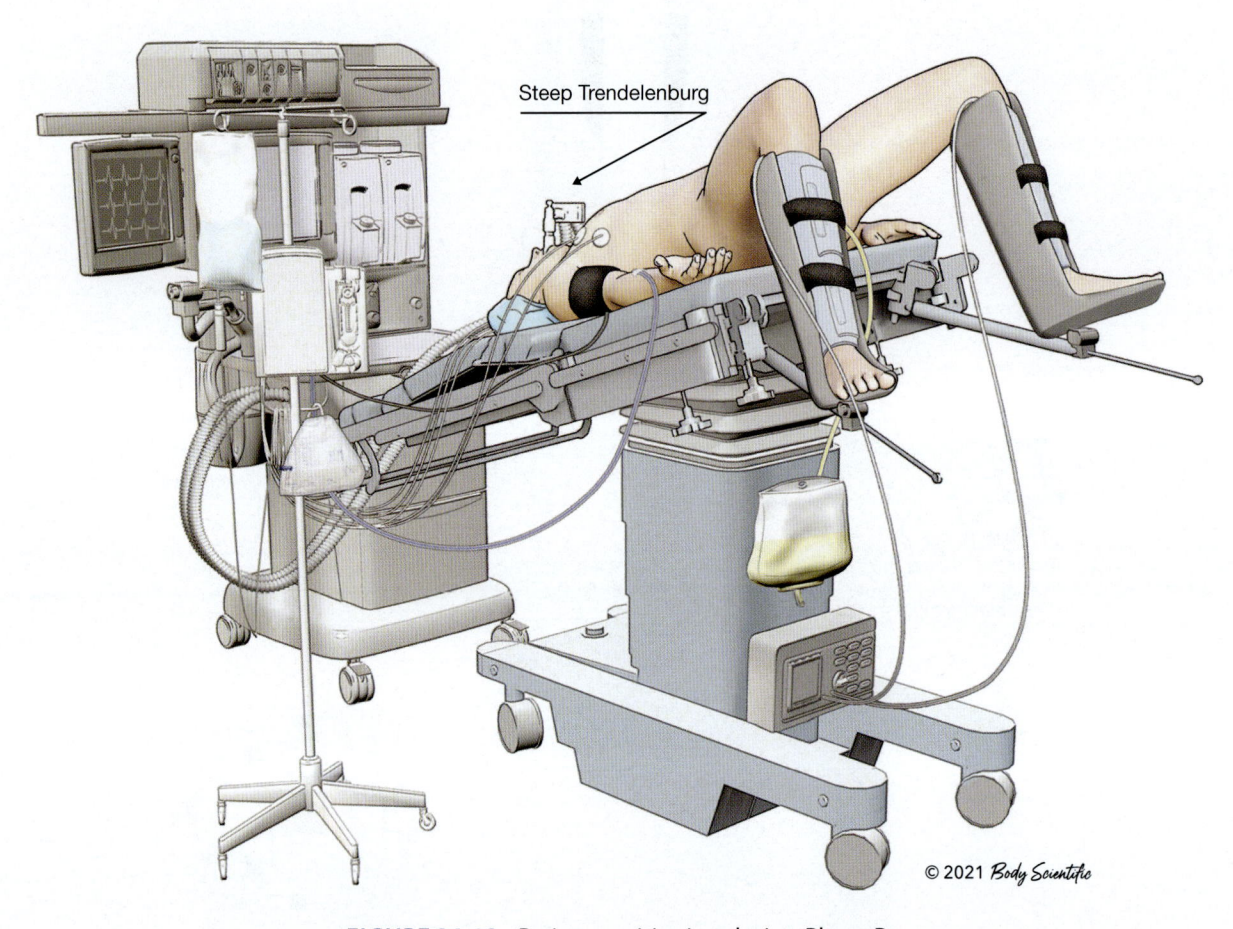

FIGURE 24-13 • Patient positioning during Phase B.

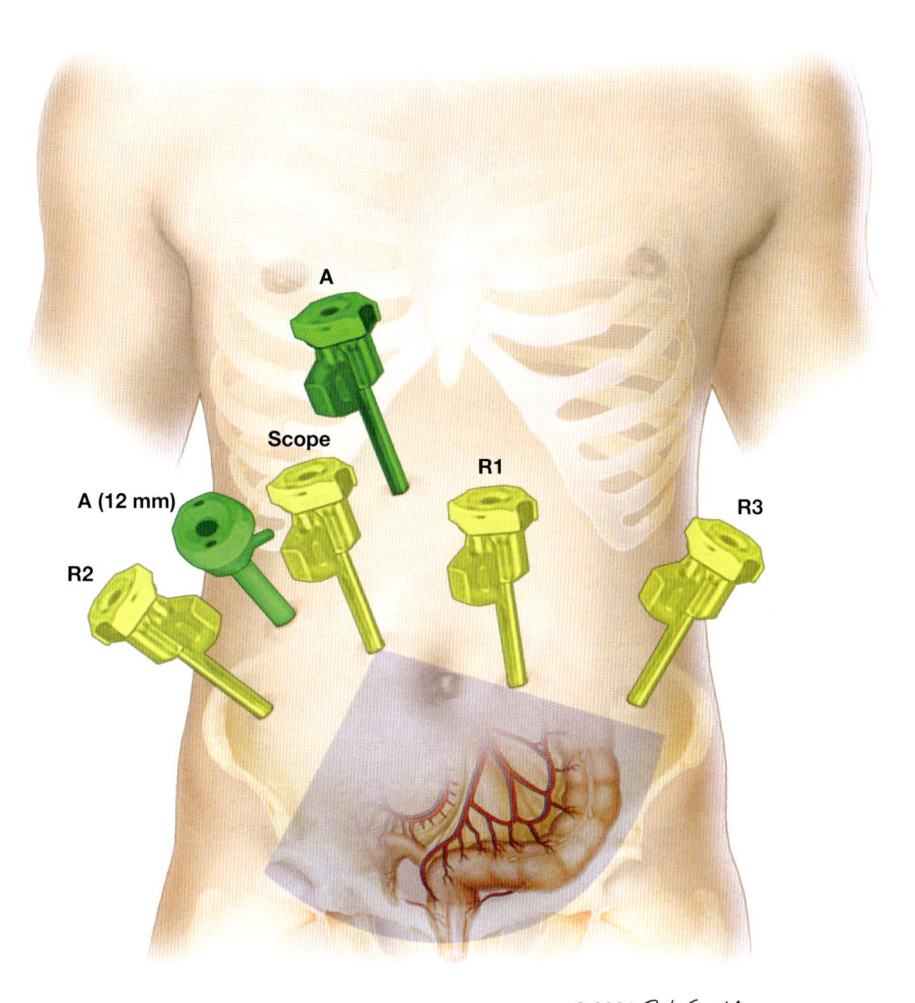

Left Colectomy

FIGURE 24-14 • Port setting during Phase B. The robotic ports in this phase are depicted in yellow. The ports that may be used by the Assistant are depicted in green.

Step 6. Localization of the promontory, lifting the mesentery of the sigmoid colon, retrograde preaortic dissection, and left ureter identification

The promontory is localized by visual, or sometimes, "virtual" tactile feedback. The safest point to start the dissection is at the root of the insertion of the mesentery of the sigmoid colon (on the right side of the sigmoid colon mesentery). The promontory may be less or more prominent depending on the anatomy of the spine and the bifurcation of the aorta and the vena cava.

To facilitate the maneuver, the mesentery of the sigmoid colon must be lifted with R3, putting in tension the insertion of the mesentery. In doing so, at the promontory, it is easier to perform the longitudinal opening at the base of the mesentery along the lateral reflection of the peritoneum. This is the area, in front of the promontory, where the mesentery of the sigmoid colon is encountering the mesorectum. The CO_2 usually spreads in the retroperitoneum, facilitating a "natural" dissection along the proper plane. This allows a retrograde dissection, which is carried out in front of the aortic bifurcation, almost up to the origin of the IMA.

It is advisable first to go down to some extent (without going too far/deep) while staying in front of the promontory and entering into the 2 layers of the mesorectal fascia. This dissection provides a better working area, with more clear landmarks, and a superior visualization of the anatomy of the hypogastric plexus and nerves (see **Figures 24-15 A–C**). During this step, it is essential to clearly recognize the anatomy, specifically, the ureters and the hypogastric neural plexus.

> ▶▶ **TIPS**
>
> Lifting the mesentery of the sigmoid colon by R3 puts some tension on the string of the sigmoidorectal artery, which is lifted as well, creating a V-shape of the space in front of the aorta. The lower edge of this vascular string naturally brings to the origin of the IMA. The neural plexus is bluntly lowered down toward the aorta.

Such maneuvers will be useful to join, at a later stage, the rectosigmoidal junction for the resection. Once the space is achieved, a retrograde dissection is started. Here, the trick is to lift the string of the rectal artery and the IMA. In this region, a triangle can be defined: the upper edge is the string of the rectal artery and the IMA, while the lower edge is the aorta. By following the 2 sides of the triangle, the surgeon reaches the point where the 2 lines are merging together (insertion of the IMA). In this process, care must be taken to avoid staying too close to the aorta, not because of the risk of injury to this vessel (since this is a very strong structure), but mainly because of possible neural damage to the preaortic plexus. During the retrograde dissection, the left ureter should be identified, and it is usually located deeper to the correct dissection plane (which is in front of Toldt's fascia—**Figures 24-9 A, B**). The Toldt's fascia, in its lower portion, is frequently less anatomically defined and represented. So, it is easier to mistakenly go deeper with the dissection (which is why it is important to visualize the ureter).

Step 6 average time frame: 15–20 min

Left Colectomy 499

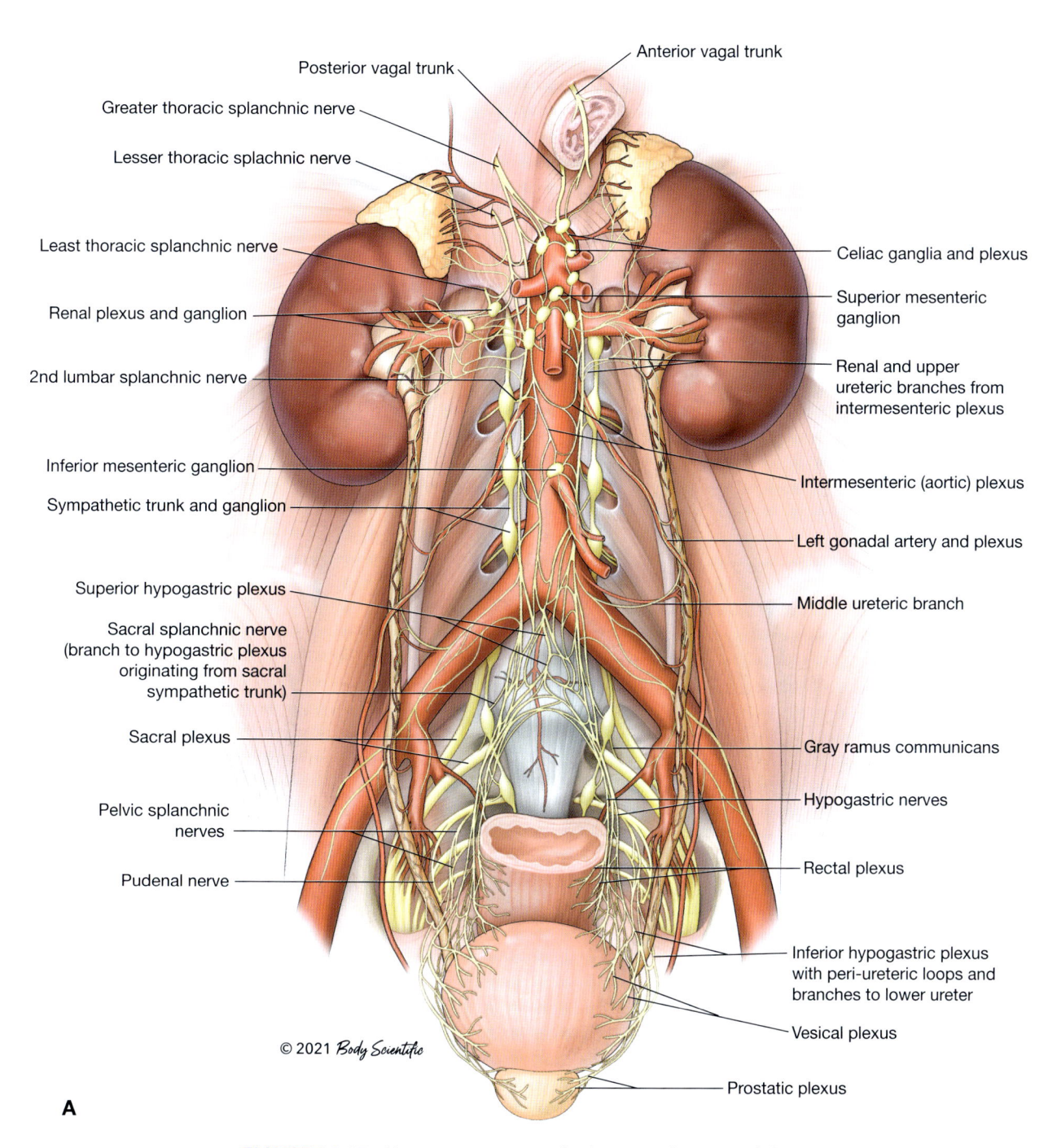

FIGURE 24-15 • Nerve structures and relation with origin of the IMA.

A

500 The Foundation and Art of Robotic Surgery

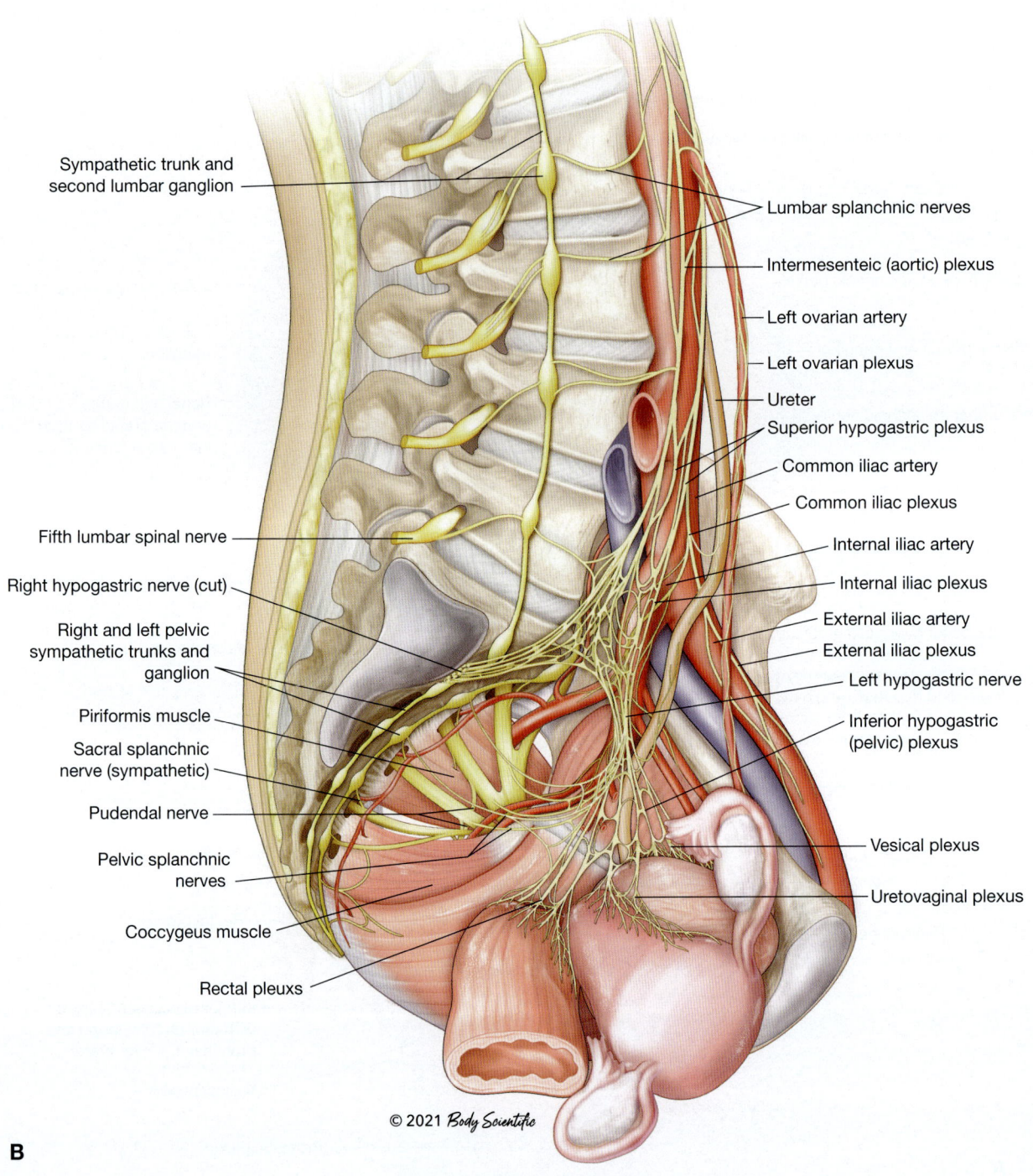

FIGURE 24-15 • *(Continued)*

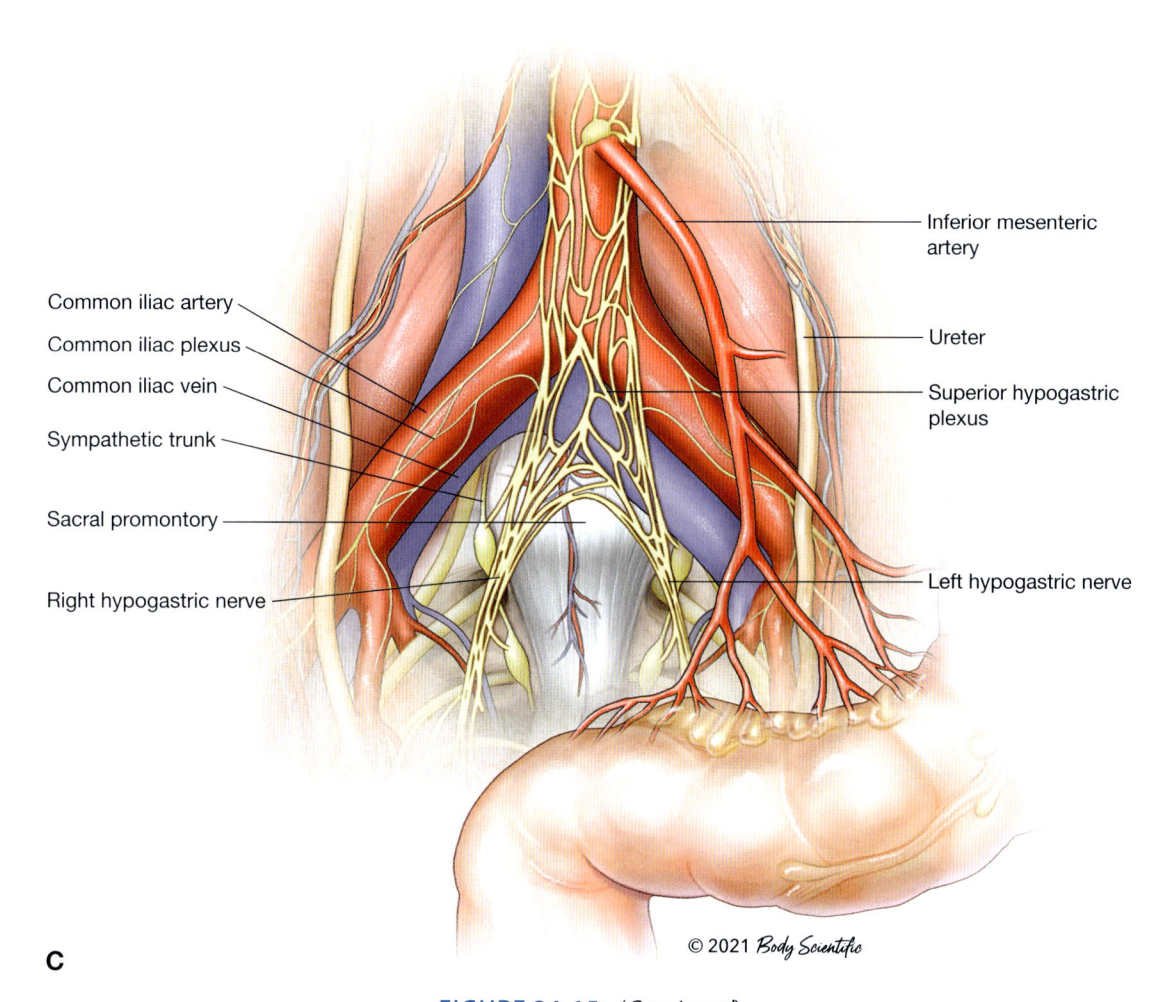

FIGURE 24-15 • *(Continued)*

Step 7. Sigmoid colon mobilization (by lateral-to-medial dissection)

The mobilization of the sigmoid colon with the remaining part of the attachment of the descending colon (which was partly previously mobilized) is carried out. The dissection is performed staying in front of the retroperitoneal structures (left iliac vessels, left ureter, left hypogastric plexus). The lateral-to-medial dissection is continued until reaching the periaortic area.

Step 7 average time frame: 10–15 min

▶ Video 24-5. Step 7. Sigmoid Colon Mobilization

Step 8. Control and division of the IMA

At this point, due to the dissections previously performed in front of the aorta, and the lateral-to-medial approach, the mesentery is attached to the IMA only.

The IMA is divided (**Figures 24-16 A, B**) using the stapler or clips. Staplers seem the safest option and are the preferred instrument. It is important not to divide the IMA too close to the aorta for the following reasons: (1) to avoid damage to the hypogastric plexus (situated on a plane in front of the aorta); and (2) if bleeding occurs from the aorta, this is difficult to control.

After dividing the IMA, it is easy to identify the 2 vascular landmarks for the central lymphadenectomy: the stumps of IMV and of the IMA.

Those are the anatomical landmarks for the lymphadenectomy, and they guide how to divide the mesentery of the descending colon.

Knowledge of the standard vascular anatomy and its variations is key (**Figures 24-17** and **24-18 A–I**) (see also suggested reading #5).

Step 8 average time frame: 3–5 min

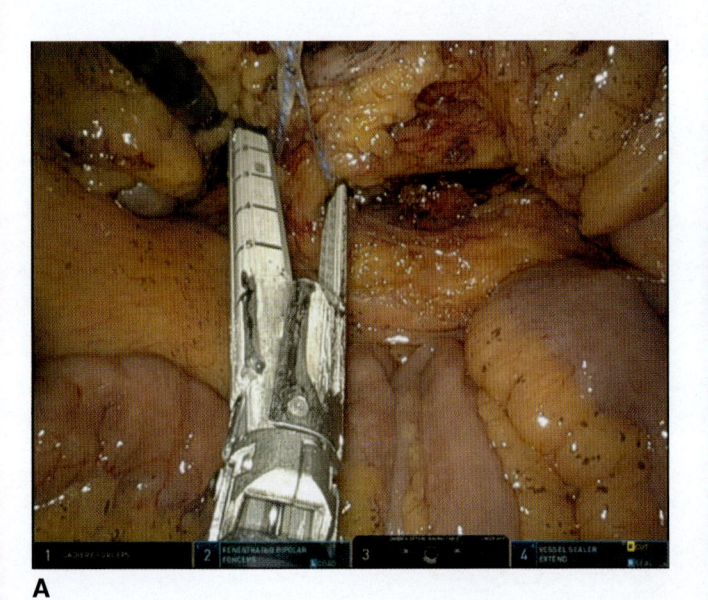

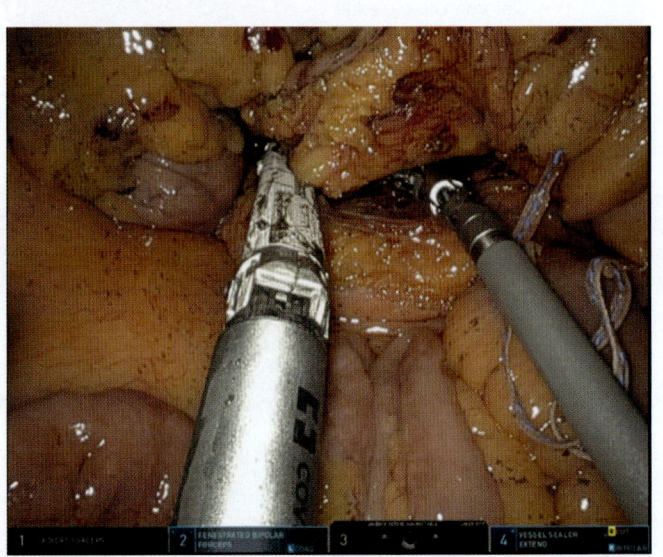

FIGURE 24-16 • Control and division of the IMA.

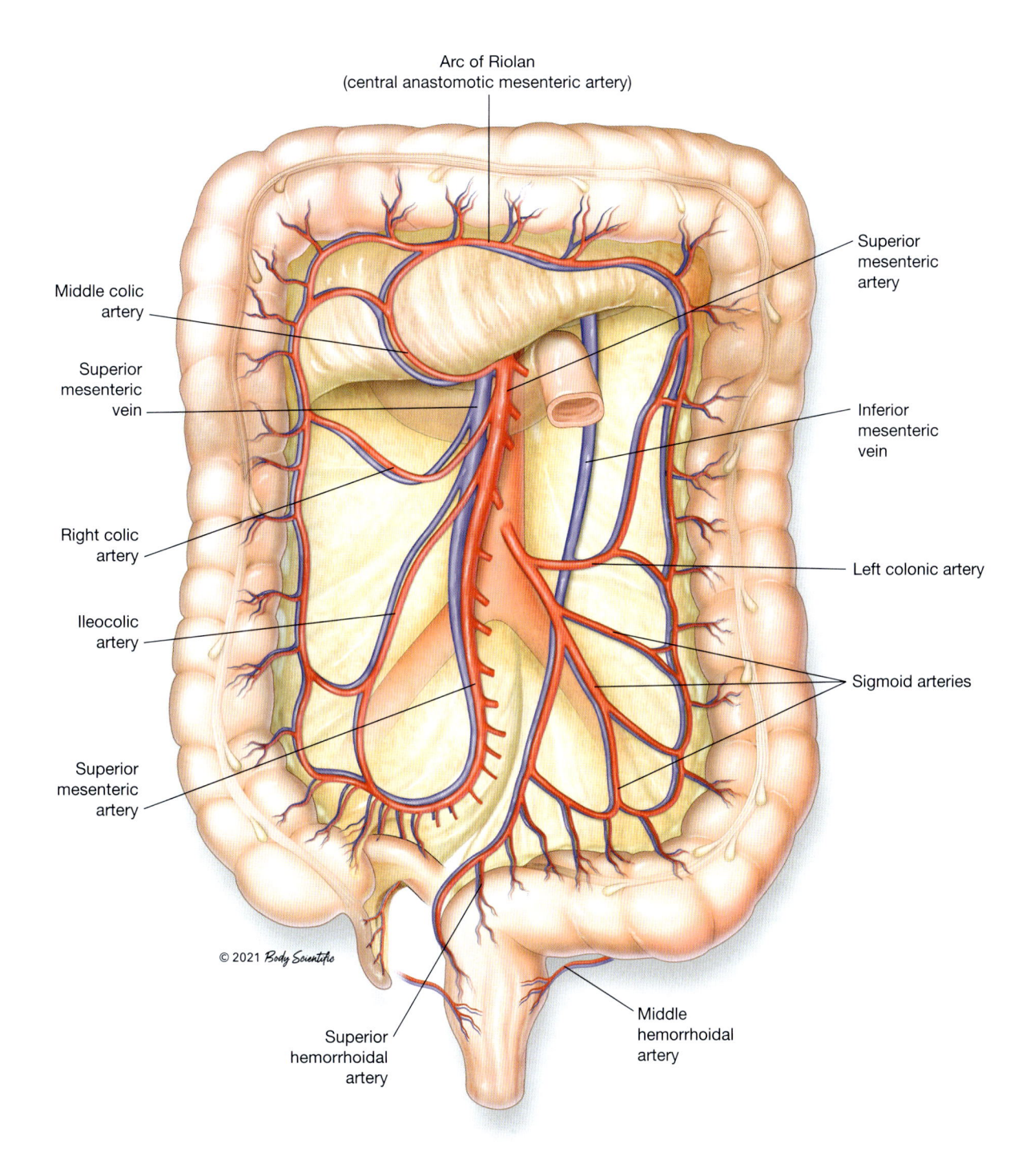

FIGURE 24-17 • Standard vascular anatomy.

504 The Foundation and Art of Robotic Surgery

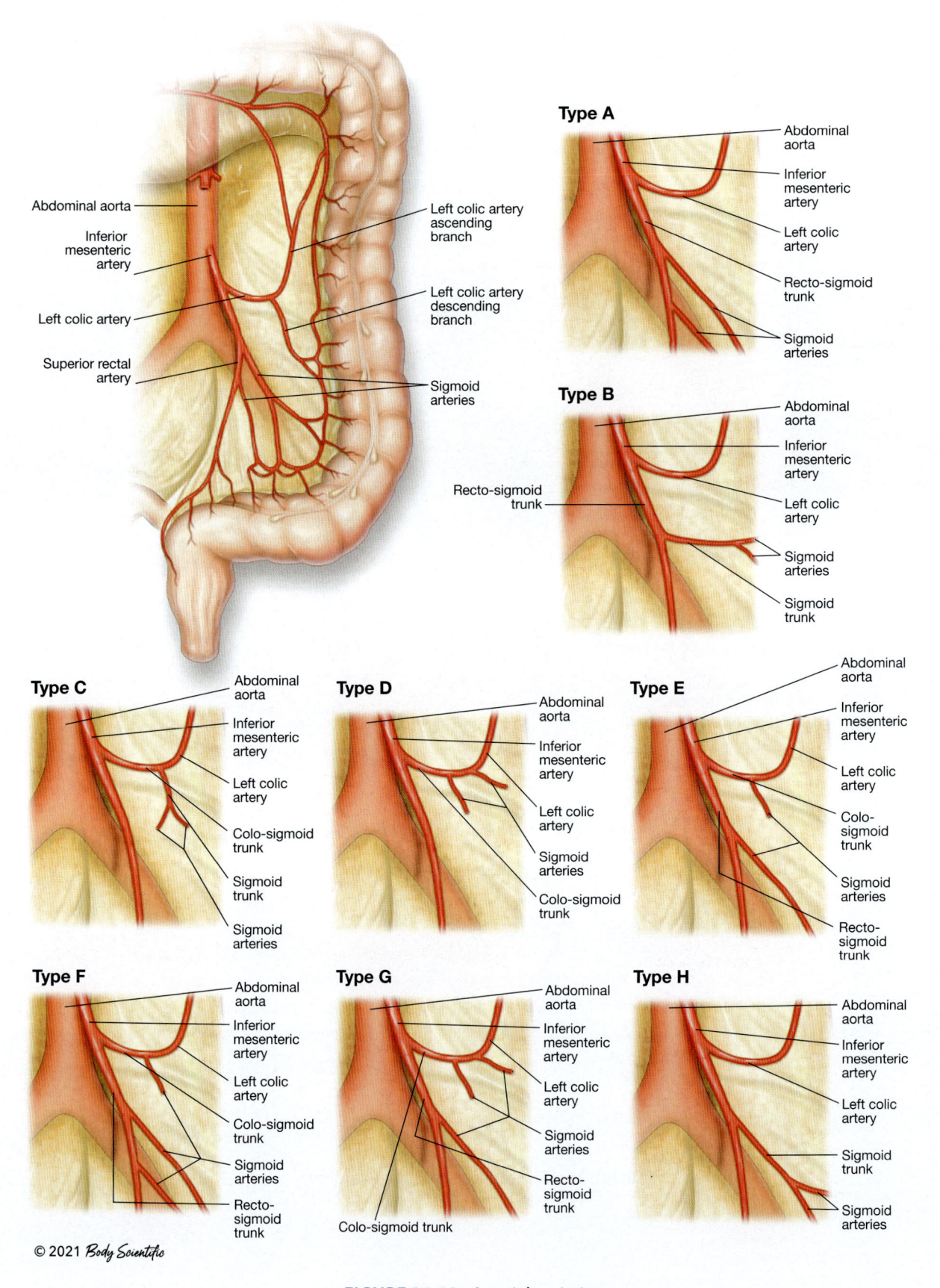

FIGURE 24-18 • Arterial variations.

Arch of Riolan between middle colic and left colic arteries

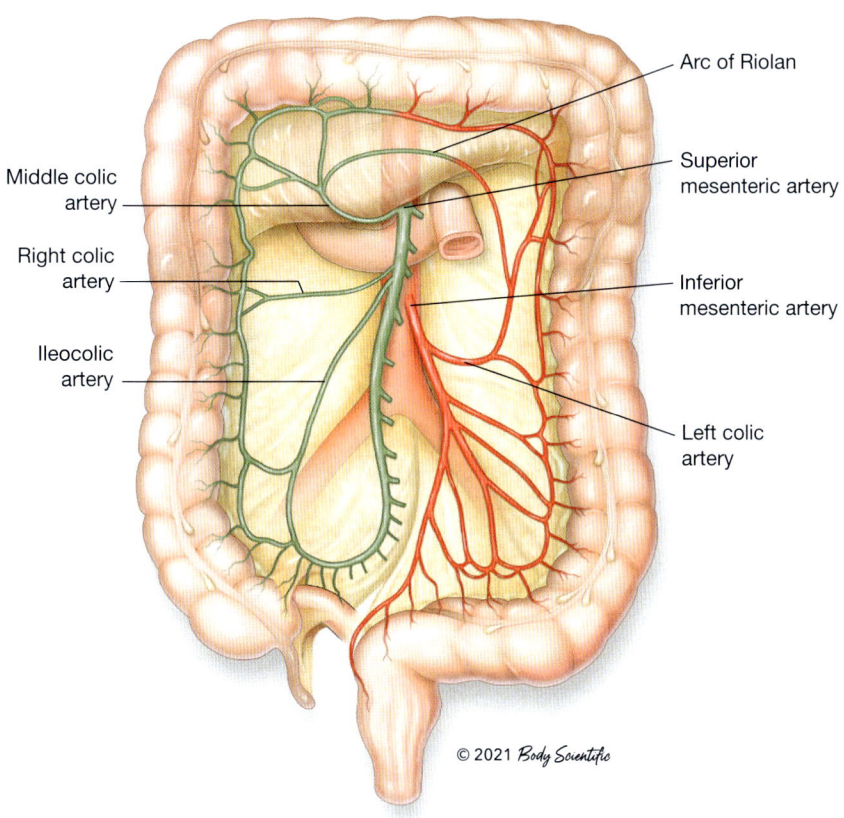

I

FIGURE 24-18 • (Continued)

Step 9. Sigmoidal-rectal transection

The mesentery is divided, using the vessel sealer, at the rectosigmoid junction and including the rectal artery (**Figures 24-19 A, B**). The hemostasis of the distal rectal artery stump may be reinforced with Prolene™ 3-0 stitches.

The rectum is divided (**Figures 24-20 A, B**), using a stapler with medium-sized load, at the junction between the intraperitoneal portion of the rectum with the sigmoid colon

Step 9 average time frame: 10–15 min

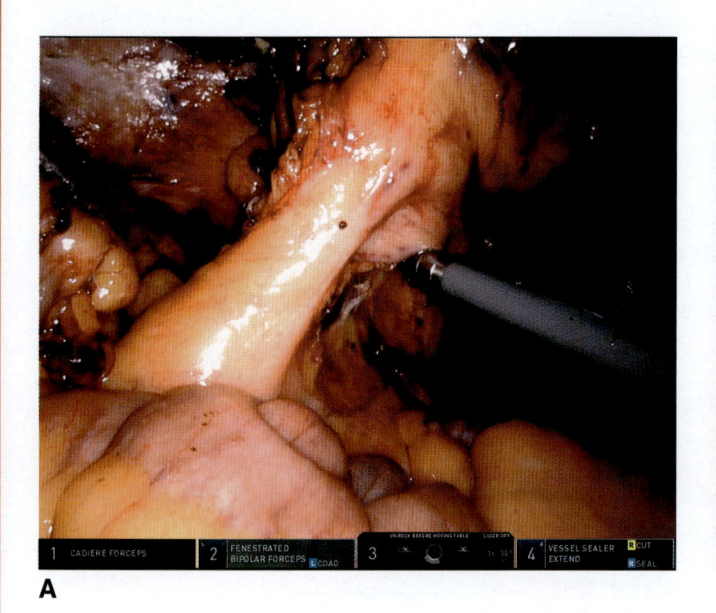

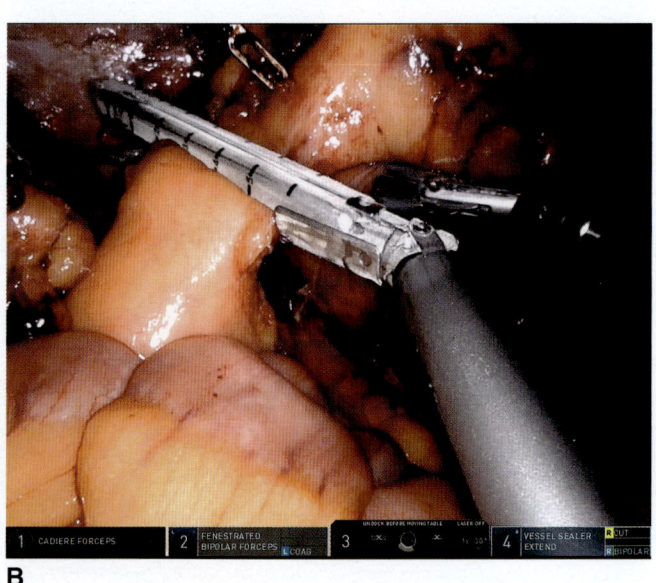

FIGURE 24-19 • Division of the mesentery with the rectal artery.

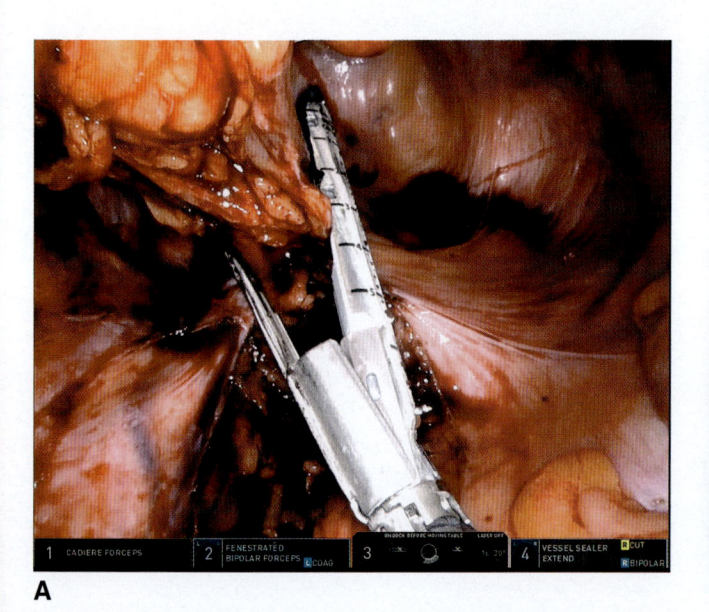

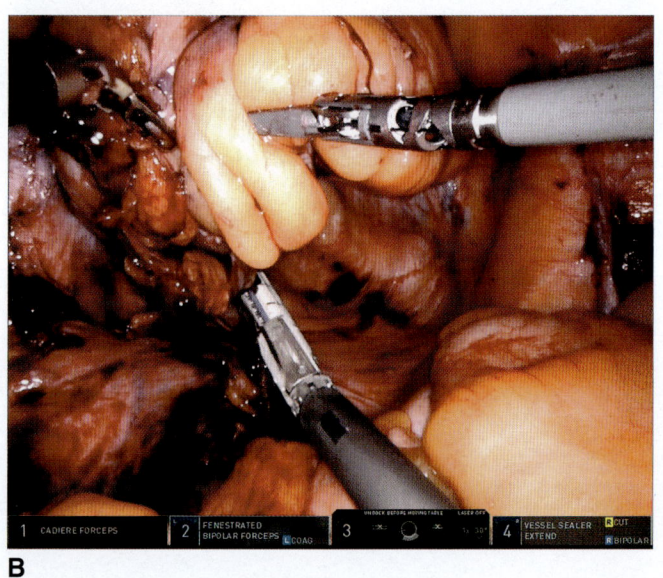

FIGURE 24-20 • Division of the rectum.

Step 10. Identification of the principal lymph nodes (LNs) pedicle and division of the descending colon mesentery

The lines of dissection in the mesentery of the descending colon must be identified. Starting from the IMA and IMV stumps, the length of the descending colon and the distance of the planned area for the anastomosis must be carefully assessed. A flap of mesentery is created (**Figures 24-21 A, B**) with the vessel sealer, containing all the LNs that should be removed, together with the specimen. The division of the marginal arcade (**Figure 24-22**) interrupts the blood supply distal to the transection line. The width and position of the flap are conditioned by the location of the tumor. The planned resection line of the colon is assessed for microcirculation by a near-infrared ICG perfusion test. If the perfusion is not optimal, a more proximal colonic segment is selected. ICG allows evaluation of the perfusion of the stumps in a totally intra-abdominal way. The LNs' anatomy is depicted in **Figures 24-23 A, B**.

Step 10 average time frame: 10–15 min

EDITORIAL COMMENT

An alternative way to complete the lymphadenectomy and to prepare the proximal colonic stump is to exteriorize the specimen with the proximal colon through the extraction site (usually a Pfannenstiel). Once the recto-sigmoidal junction is divided, the tip of the specimen is grabbed with a laparoscopic forceps and exteriorized through the wound protector. The marginal arcade is divided extracorporeally, the specimen is resected, and the proximal colon stump is checked for blood supply and length. The anvil of the stapler is inserted into the stump and fixed with a purse string of Prolene™ 2-0.

▶▶ TIPS

The vessel sealer should be used in the division of the mesentery with the double-coagulation technique.

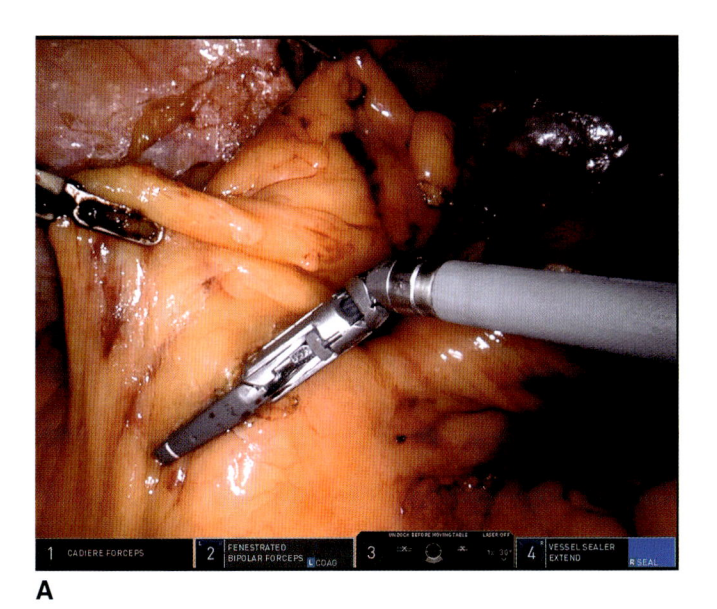

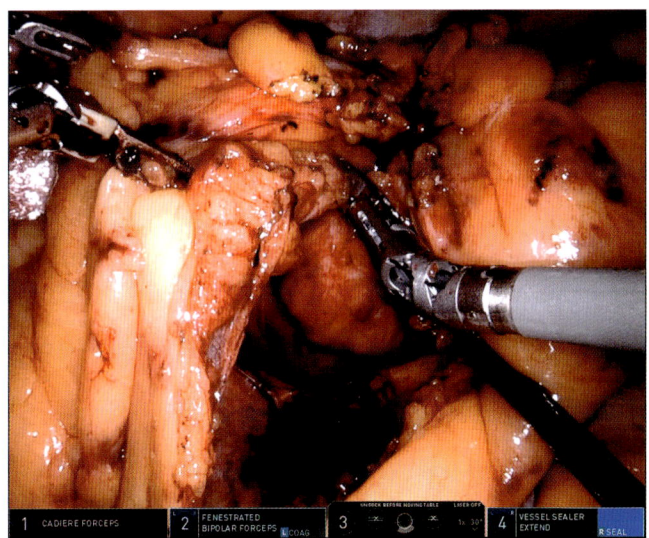

FIGURE 24-21 • Division of the mesentery.

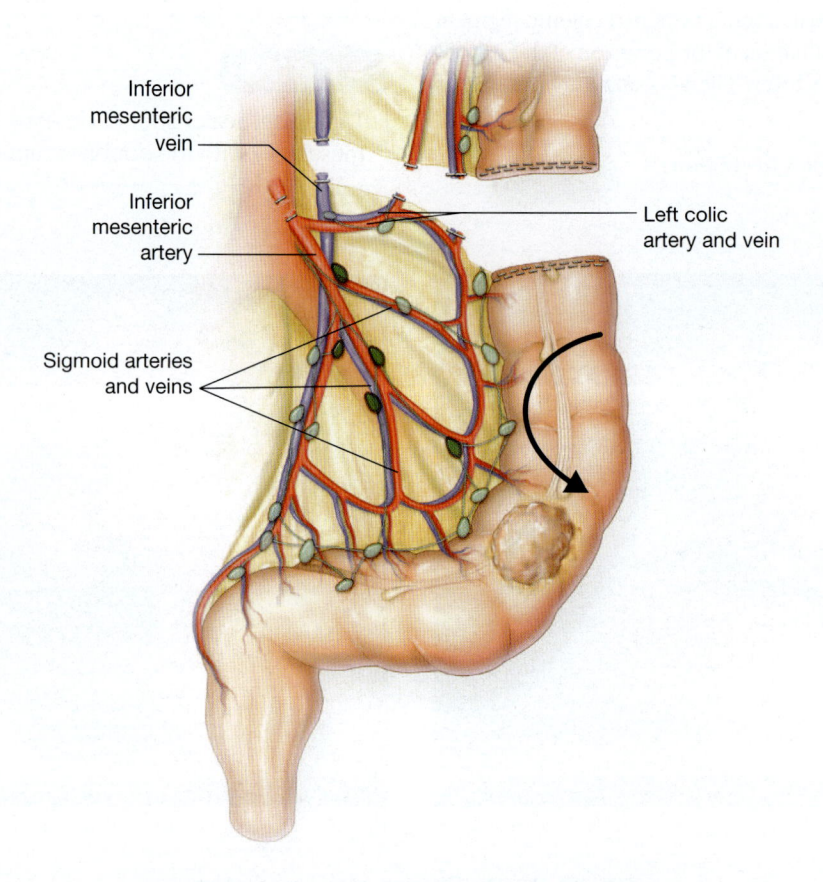

FIGURE 24-22 • Vessels and proximal stump divided.

Left Colectomy

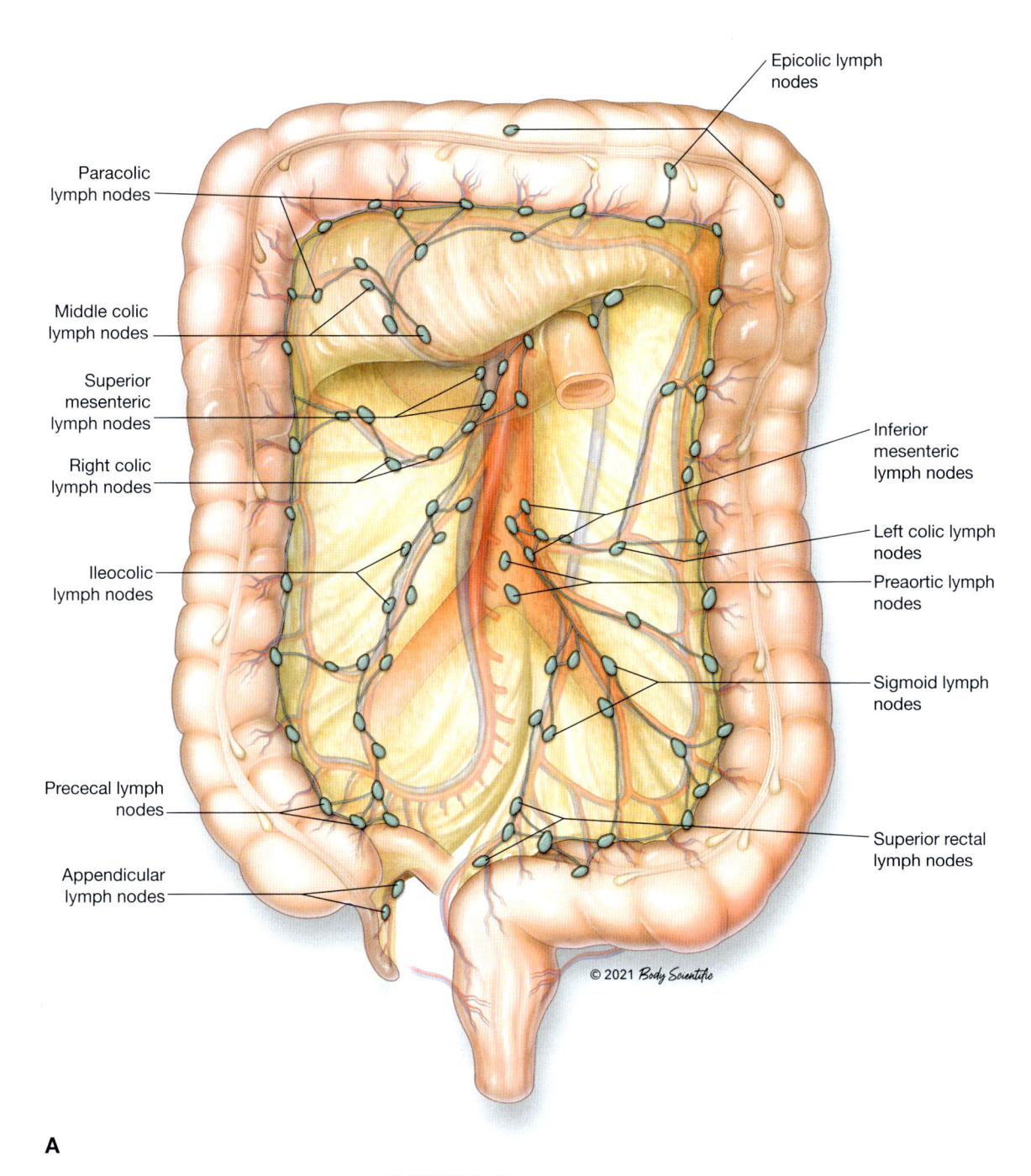

FIGURE 24-23 • LNs anatomy.

510 The Foundation and Art of Robotic Surgery

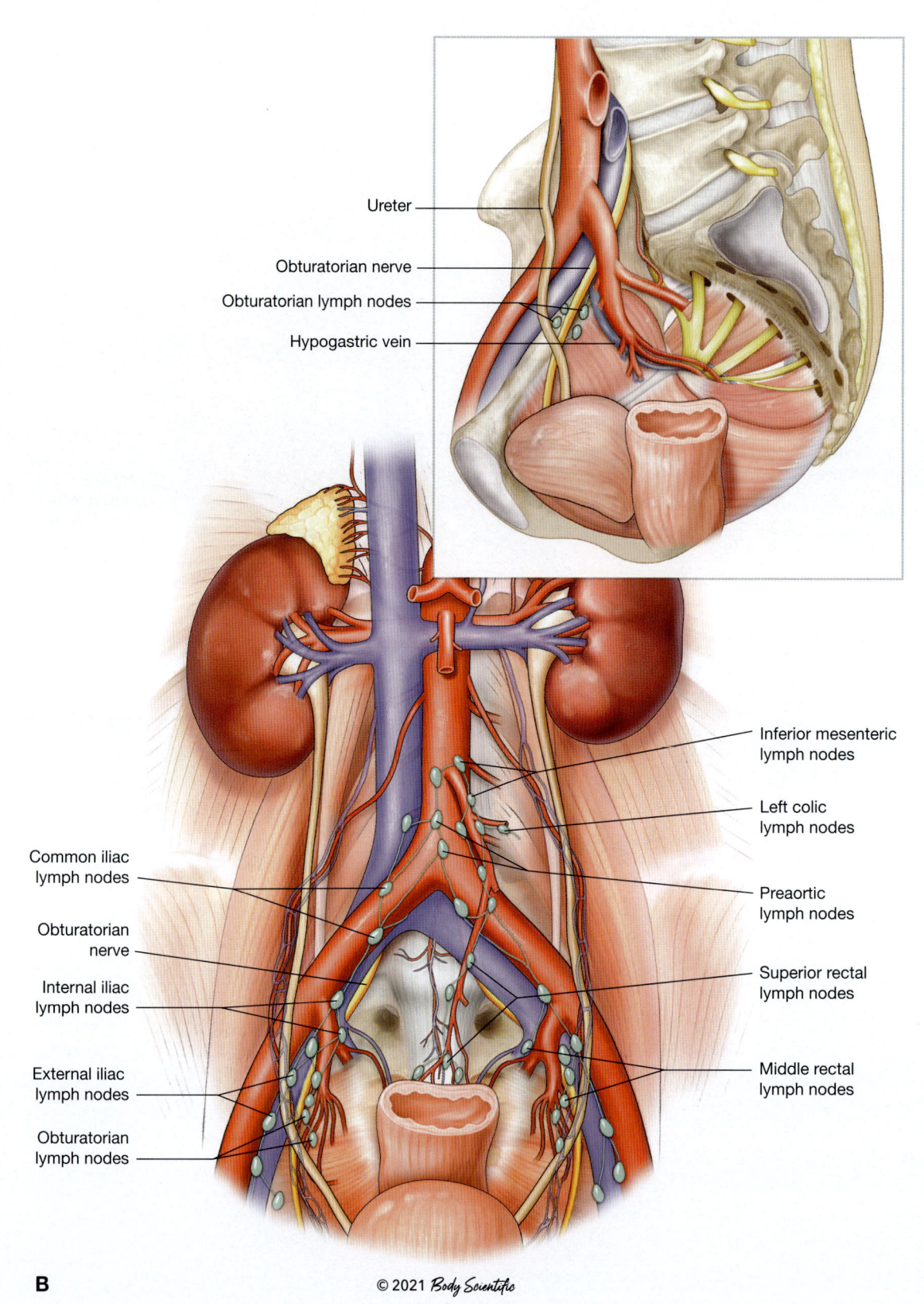

FIGURE 24-23 • (Continued)

Step 11. ICG perfusion check and proximal colon transection

After carrying out the division of the marginal arcade, an ICG test must be performed: if the perfusion is not optimal, another more proximal segment should be chosen.

The descending colon is finally divided with a stapler (**Figures 24-24 A, B**).

Step 11 average time frame: 5–10 min

Phase C

The OR setting is similar to the one already depicted in **Figure 24-12**. Patient positioning and port setting for Phase C are represented in **Figures 24-25** and **24-26**, respectively.

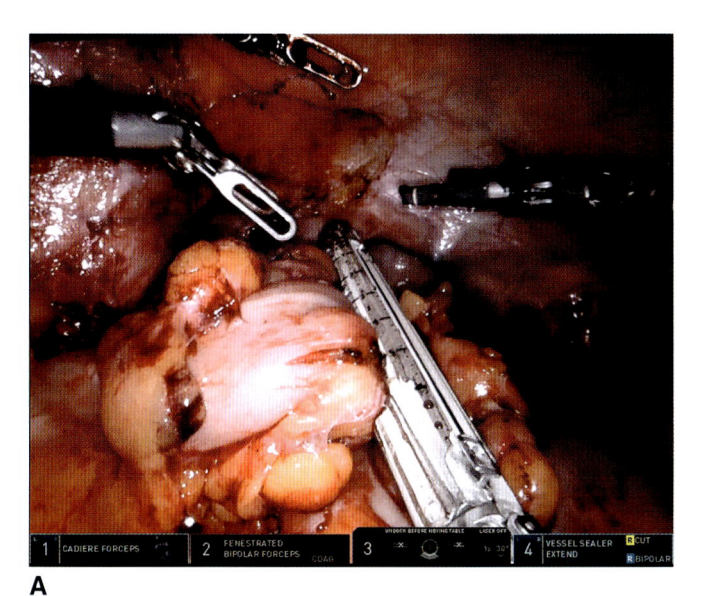

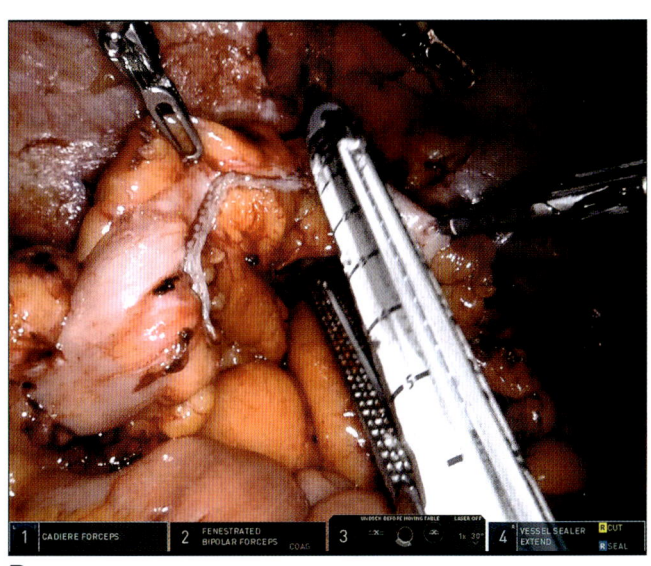

FIGURE 24-24 • Division of the colon.

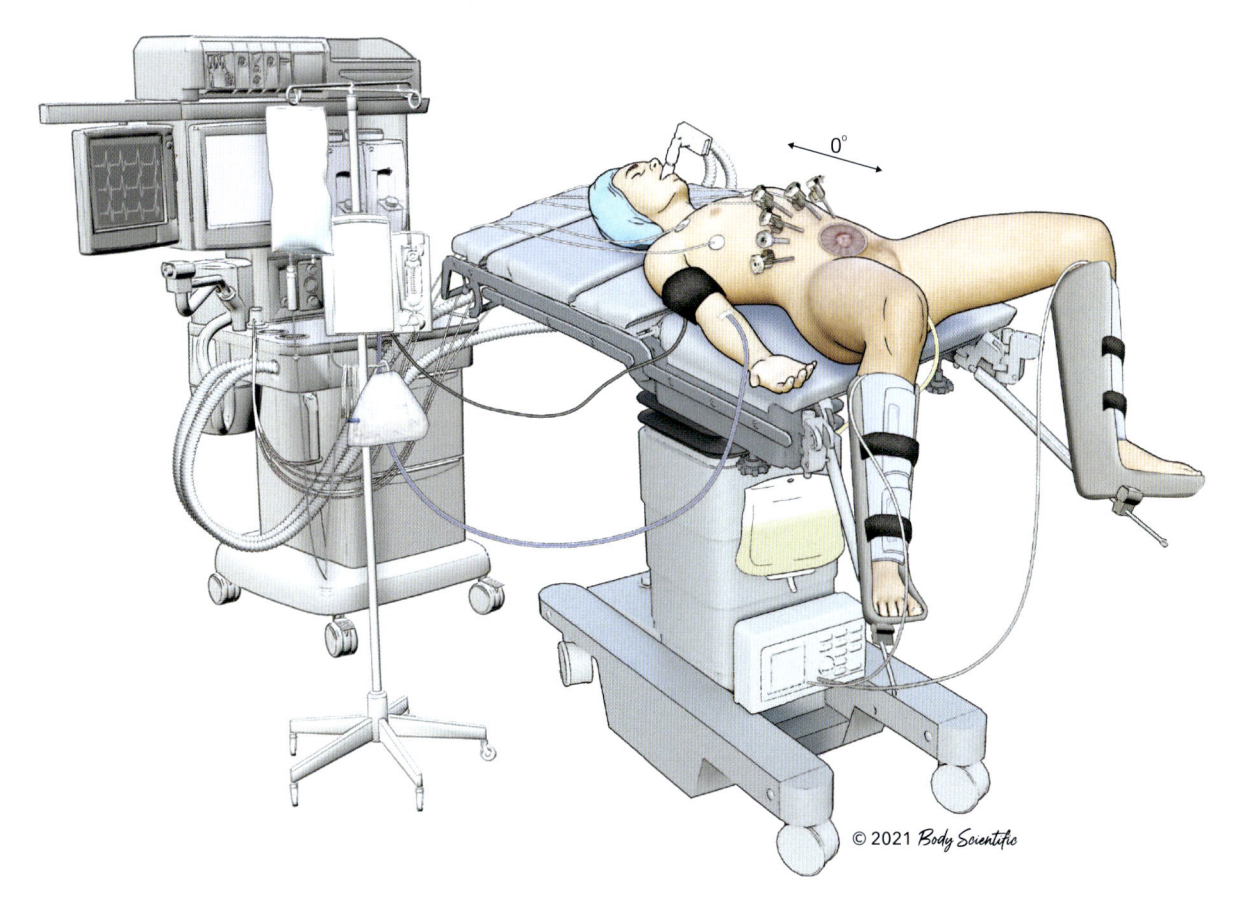

FIGURE 24-25 • Patient positioning during Phase C.

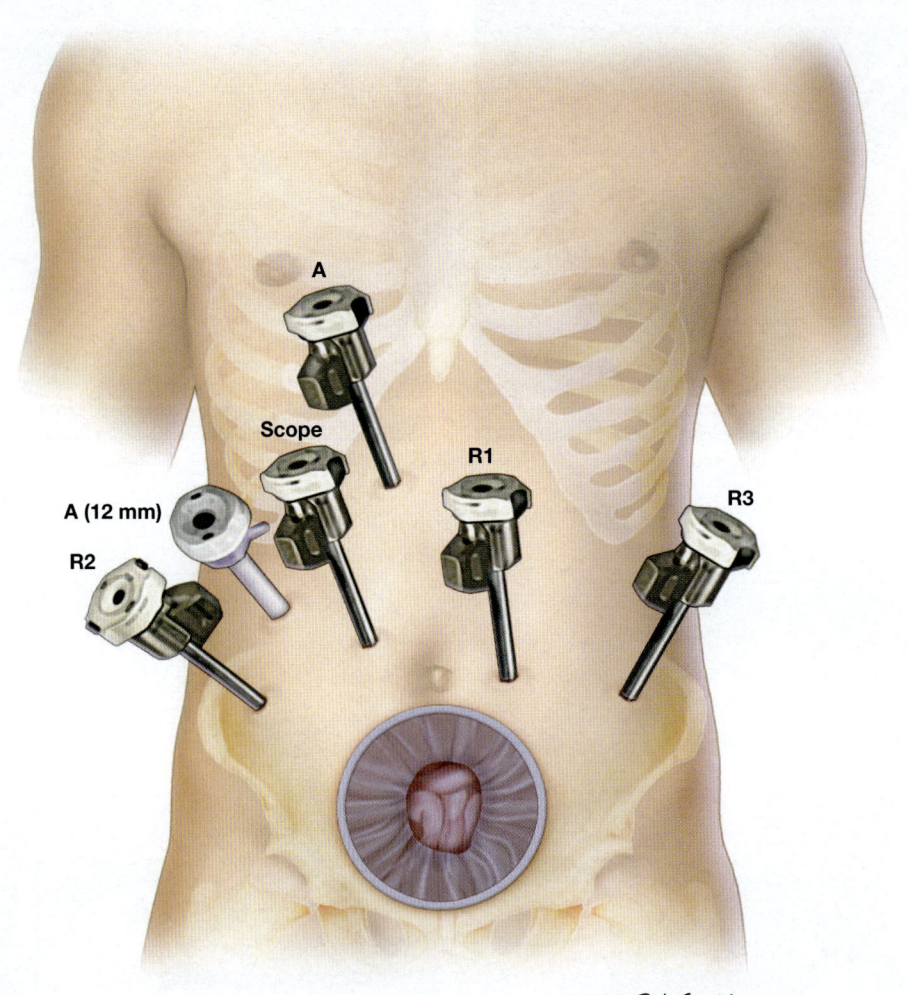

FIGURE 24-26 • Port setting during Phase C (the ports are not colored because are not used at this time).

Step 12. Specimen extraction, proximal colon exteriorization, and anvil placement

At this point, the specimen is completely detached inside the abdomen. The robot is momentarily undocked. The operating table is adjusted in a neutral position (patient supine). A Pfannenstiel incision is usually performed (unless there are previous surgical scars that may be used as an access). A wound protector is applied (Alexis™). The specimen is extracted. The proximal colon is exteriorized. The anvil of the stapler is better placed extra-abdominally by a purse string in the proximal stump (this maneuver is also possible intra-abdominally, but there may be a higher risk of contamination). At this time, an additional verification of the length of the proximal colon is carried out.

Step 12 average time frame: 20–25 min

Phase D

The OR setting is similar to the one already depicted in **Figure 24-12** (but the main surgeon is in between the patient's legs). The patient positioning and port setting for Phase D are represented in **Figures 24-27** and **24-28**, respectively.

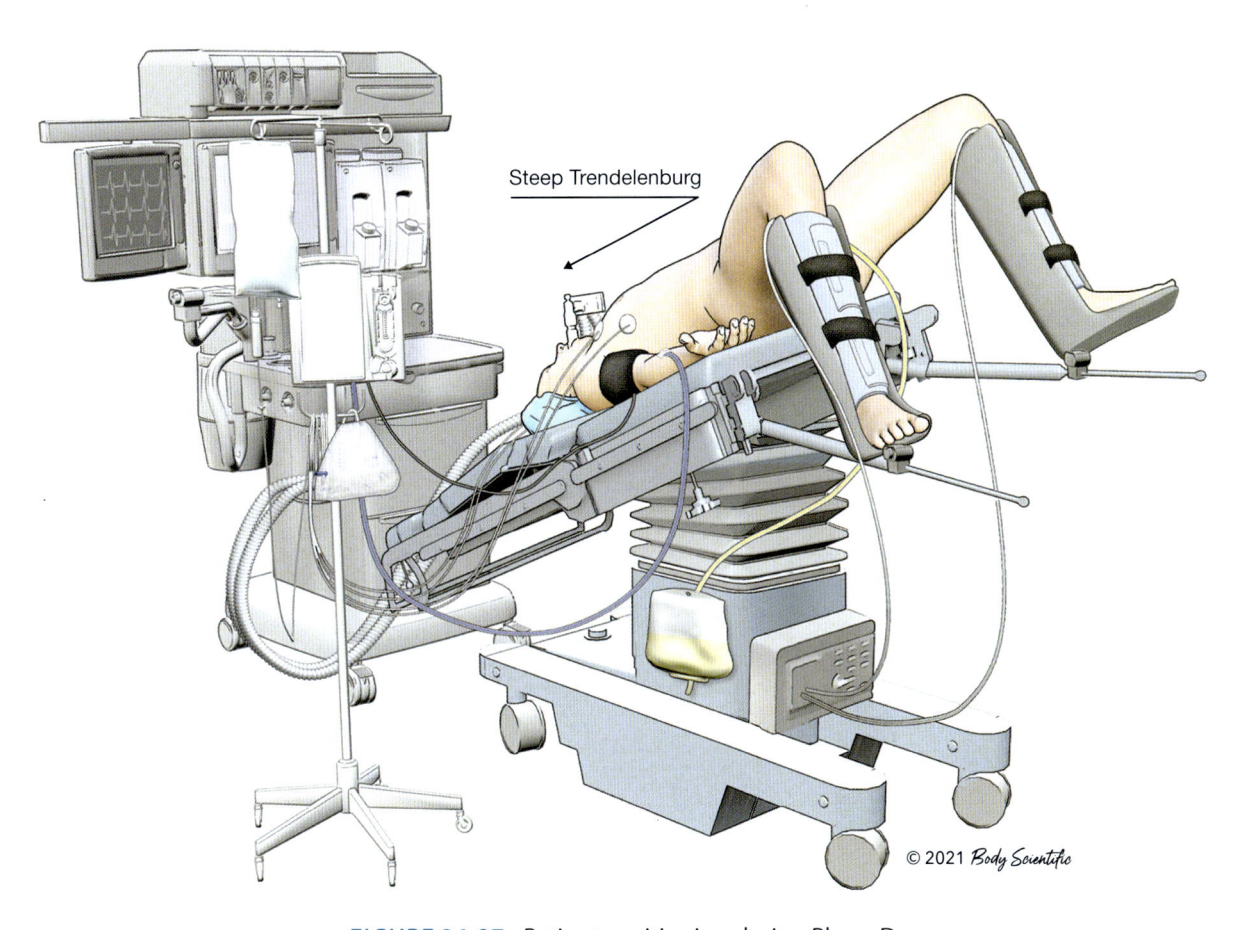

FIGURE 24-27 • Patient positioning during Phase D.

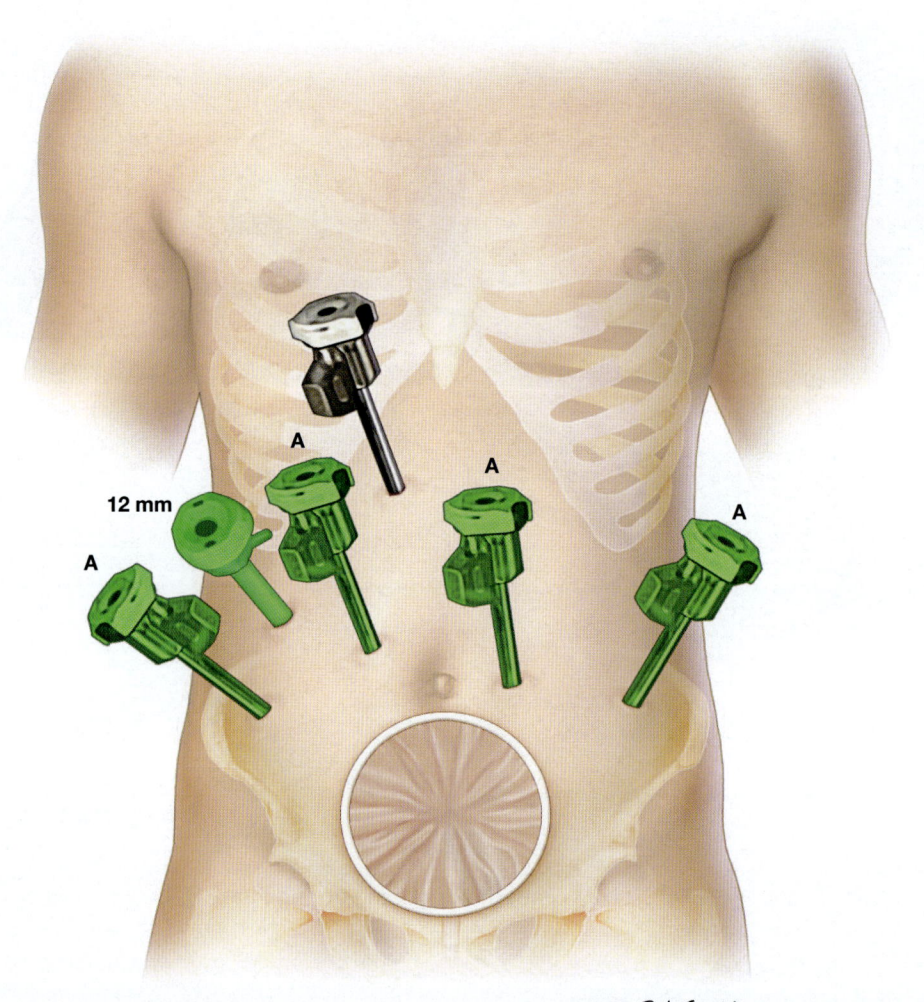

FIGURE 24-28 • Port setting during Phase D. The ports in green may be used by the assistant.

Step 13. End-to-end transanal stapled anastomosis

The wound protector is temporarily closed. The pneumoperitoneum is reestablished. The surgical table is adjusted to a lesser degree of Trendelenburg. The senior surgeon is using the transanal stapler controlling the perfect alignment of the stump, while the assistant (laparoscopically) favors the engagement of the stapler shaft with the anvil. The stapler is fired and an end-to-end transanal anastomosis is carried out. The anastomotic rings, extracted from the stapler, are routinely checked to confirm that they are intact.

Step 13 average time frame: 5–10 min

Video 24-6. Step 13. ICG Check of the Anastomosis

> **TIPS**
> The anastomosis at the level of the intraperitoneal rectum is usually strong. If there are any doubts, or if bleeding is suspected, it may be necessary to assess the anastomosis endoscopically. Some additional stitches (PDS™ 3-0) may be placed to reinforce the anastomosis should the need arise.

> **PITFALLS**
> Poor perfusion of the proximal segment, due to incorrect division of the mesentery or insufficient mobilization. This may lead to leaks or strictures.

Suggested Readings

1. Giulianotti PC, Coratti A, Angelini M, et al. Robotics in general surgery: personal experience in a large community hospital. *Arch Surg.* 2003;138(7):777-784. doi: 10.1001/archsurg.138.7.777
2. Mangano A, Valle V, Fernandes E, Bustos R, Gheza F, Giulianotti PC. Operative technique in robotic left colonic resection. *Minerva Chir.* 2019;74(5):431-437. doi: 10.23736/S0026-4733.18.07807-0
3. Mangano A, Gheza F, Giulianotti PC. Iatrogenic spleen injury during minimally invasive left colonic flexure mobilization: the quest for evidence-based results. *Minerva Chir.* 2018;73(5):512-519. doi: 10.23736/S0026-4733.18.07737-4
4. Mangano A, Gheza F, Chen LL, Minerva EM, Giulianotti PC. Indocyanine green (ICG)-enhanced fluorescence for intraoperative assessment of bowel microperfusion during laparoscopic and robotic colorectal surgery: the quest for evidence-based results. *Surg Technol Int.* 2018;32:101-104.
5. McSweeney W, Kotakadeniya R, Dissabandara L. A comprehensive review of the anatomy of the inferior mesenteric artery: branching patterns, variant anatomy and clinical significance. *SN Compr Clin Med.* 2020;2:2349-2359. doi:10.1007/s42399-020-00541-4
6. Gass JM, Daume D, Schneider R, et al. Laparoscopic versus robotic-assisted, left-sided colectomies: intra- and postoperative outcomes of 683 patients. *Surg Endosc.* 2022. doi:10.1007/s00464-021-09003-x

25

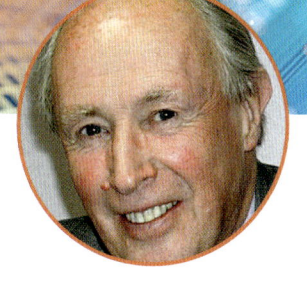

"The tumor is more apt to spread initially along the field of active lymphatic and venous flow. In my view the fascia itself is 'impenetrable' only in the sense of being an avascular interface between viscus and soma—it is indeed the 'Holy Plane.'"

—Bill Heald (1936)

Total Mesorectal Excision for Rectal Cancer

Hye Jin Kim • Alberto Mangano • Gyu-Seog Choi

INTRODUCTION

Laparoscopic total mesorectal resection (TME) for rectal cancer is widely accepted as a standard treatment since several randomized clinical trials have reported better short-term outcomes and noninferior oncological results in comparison to open surgery.

Meanwhile, robotic surgery has been gaining popularity and is expected to improve the quality of minimally invasive surgery due to the mechanical and visualization superiority compared to laparoscopy. This chapter describes the basic techniques of robotic TME using da Vinci Xi–Si and SP surgical systems.

Indications and Relative Contraindications to the Robotic Approach

The indications for the robotic approach are the same as for laparoscopy. However, robotic surgery is generally recommended in complex middle or lower rectal cancers, where laparoscopy has more challenges. Robotic surgery for rectal cancer is associated with a reduced conversion rate to open compared to the laparoscopic approach. There is a shorter learning curve, and there are probably better functional results at least in the short term. The oncological outcomes seem to be equivalent.

Locally advanced cancers (T3–T4) after neoadjuvant treatment and history of previous abdominopelvic surgery increase the complexity of the operation and require an expert team, however these are not absolute contraindications to the robotic approach.

INSTRUMENT REQUIREMENTS

The suggested main robotic instruments/tools can be listed as follows:
- 30°, 0° scope
- Single port access device
- Monopolar scissors/cautery hook
- Vessel sealer
- Robotic linear staplers (with different loads)
- Needle drivers (round tip or macro)
- Multiple Hem-o-lok™ clips
- Medium–large clip applier
- Bipolar forceps
- Cadière forceps/tip-up fenestrated grasper

The suggested main laparoscopic instruments/tools can be listed as follows:
- Needle drivers
- Scissors
- Graspers
- Staplers (linear and circular)
- Suction-irrigation
- Fan retractor (optional)

Supplemental materials:
- Gauzes, sponges
- Vessel loops
- Endobag™
- Wound protector/retractor
- Medium–large clips
- Sutures: Prolene™ 3-0, 4-0, and PDS™ 3-0

Photo reproduced with permission from Editorial Board of the British Journal of Surgery. Br J Surg. 1993;80(4):409.
Quote reproduced with permission from Heald RJ. The 'Holy Plane' of rectal surgery. J R Soc Med. 1988;81(9):503-508.

The preoperative assessment for pathologically diagnosed rectal cancer consists of pelvic magnetic resonance imaging (MRI), abdominopelvic and chest computed tomography (CT) with or without positron emission tomography (PET) as well as routine laboratory tests.

Endoscopic ultrasound (EUS) increases the accuracy of preoperative staging, mainly in early lesions. EUS-guided fine-needle aspiration may be useful in patients with early T-stage and suspicious pelvic lymph nodes.

Routine mechanical bowel preparation is done accordingly to surgeon's preference, and it is not different from open and laparoscopic surgery. The majority of surgeons do not do any bowel preparation.

Antithromboembolic stockings and sequential compression devices are applied to prevent deep venous thromboses. A Foley catheter is inserted after induction of anesthesia. Intravenous antibiotics are administered just before the beginning of the procedure. A nasogastric tube is mostly omitted.

> **EDITORIAL COMMENT**
>
> An orogastric tube may be indicated to decompress the stomach that sometimes is distended after the induction of the anesthesia. The decompression of the stomach makes the retraction of the bowel easier, mainly during the mobilization of the splenic flexure.

Patient Positioning and OR Setup

The patient is placed in the lithotomy position and tilted toward the right side (10–15°) down with thighs below the flat level and knees slightly flexed. Both arms are tucked to the body to prevent shoulder injuries and to maximize the working space for the surgical staff (**Figure 25-1**).

Ports Setting and Docking Using S or Si Systems

Understanding the unique concept of "camera cone" in robotic surgery is crucial for proper port setup, mainly using the S or Si system. It means that the entire surgical field should be included in the area of visualization (cone) obtained with a single docking (**Figure 25-2A**). Ideally, a port for the camera for the low anterior resection (LAR) procedure should be placed near the umbilicus in the middle and at the top of the camera cone. The remaining 3 ports are placed along the curvilinear line connecting both anterior superior iliac spines and the camera port, with evenly spacing, approximately 8 cm apart from each other, after full pneumoperitoneum. For hybrid laparoscopy–robotic approaches, an additional two 5-mm ports for the assistant on the upper midline and right upper quadrant of the abdomen are needed (**Figure 25-2A**). In case a diverting ileostomy is planned, that incision can be anticipated and a single port access device (**Figure 25-2B**) can be placed in that location (right lower quadrant). This access is utilized for 1 robotic port, and also for a laparoscopic assistant instrument (e.g., stapler). With this strategy, the upper midline 5-mm assistant port can be avoided (**Figure 25-2B**).

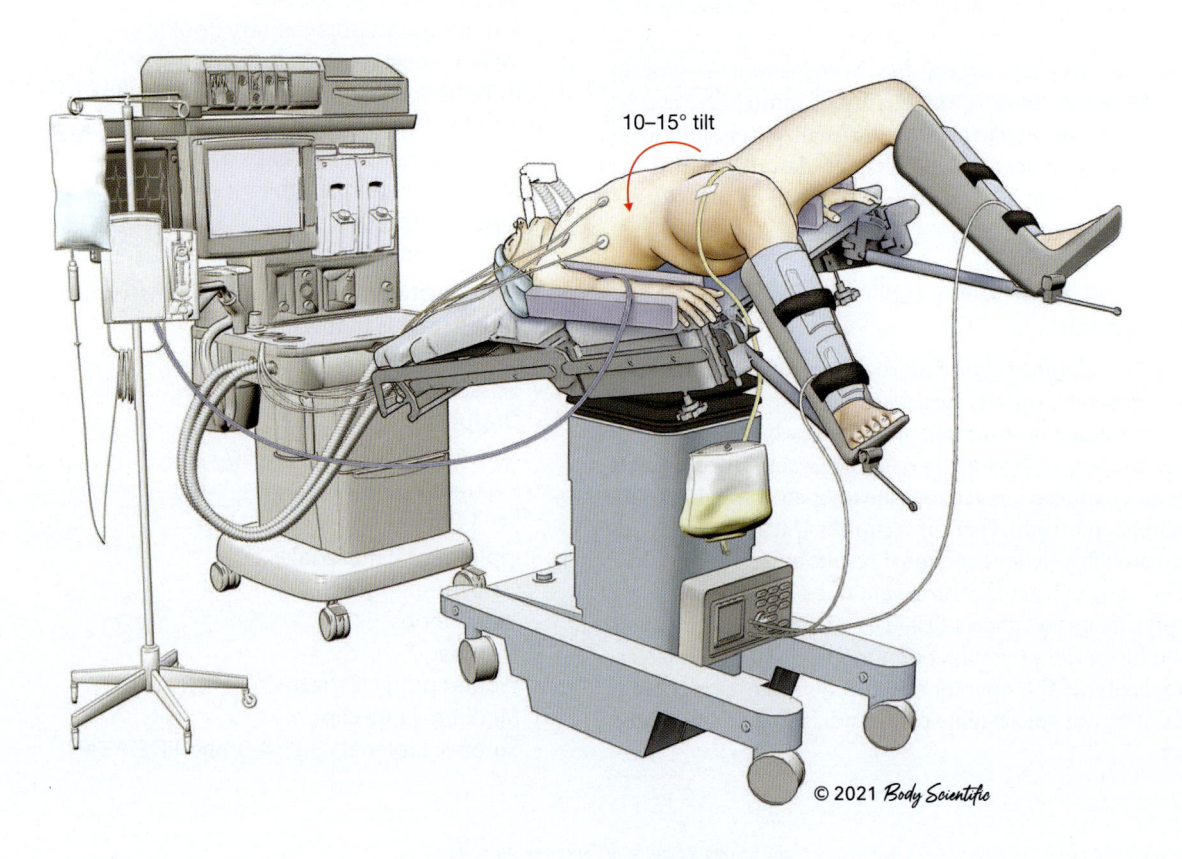

FIGURE 25-1 • Patient position.

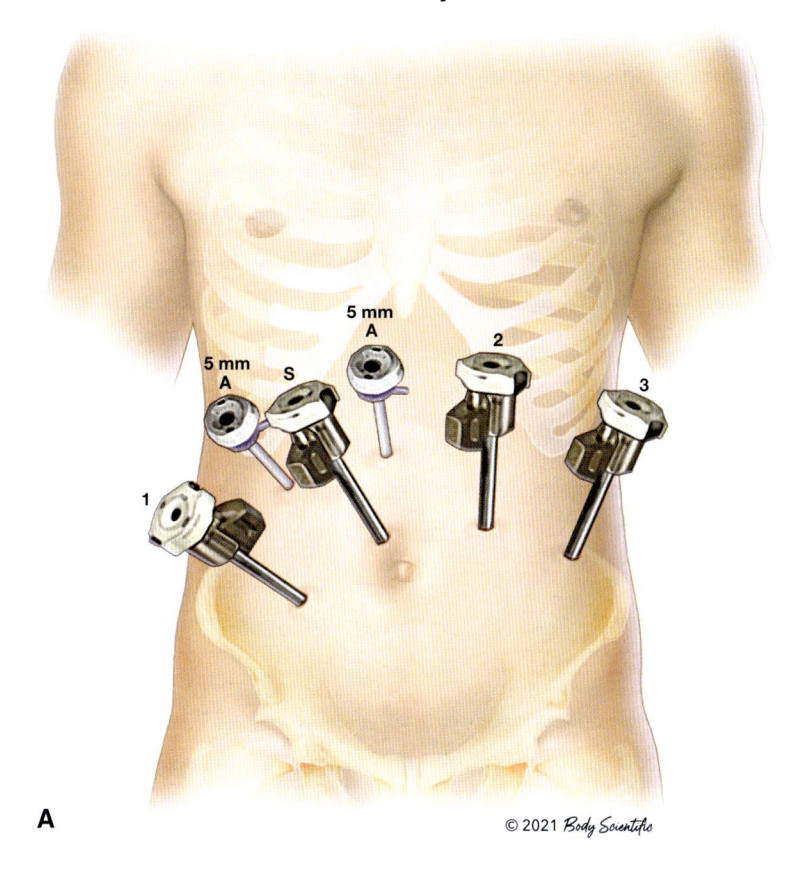

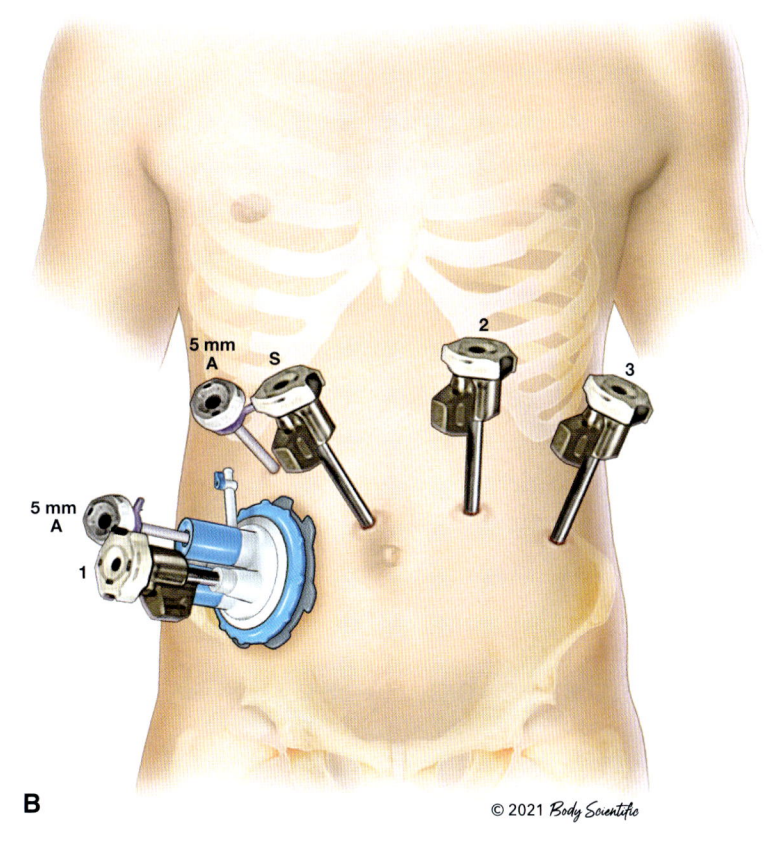

FIGURE 25-2 • Port setup in S or Si system. **A.** In case of using a single port access device. **B.** Uniport.

The patient should then be positioned as described. Before docking the robotic cart, a careful laparoscopic check is necessary to be sure that all the small bowels loops are swept to the right upper abdomen out of surgical field, since changing position of the patient is not allowed when the robot is docked in (unless there is a synchronized table).

In the hybrid approach, after laparoscopic inferior mesenteric artery (IMA) and inferior mesenteric vein (IMV) ligation and left colon mobilization, the robotic cart can be placed between the patient's legs for the pelvic dissection (TME). In the full robotic approach, where the takedown of the IMA and the colon mobilization are done robotically, it is more convenient to place the robotic cart parallel to the left thigh of the patient. This compromised position of the cart allows better movement of the instruments in the periaortic area (**Figures 25-3 A, B**), reducing arm collision during IMA ligation and sigmoid colon mobilization and, at the same time, allowing pelvic dissection. One of the advantages of this docking is maintaining free access to the perineum for rectal examination or transanal stapling without interfering with the procedure.

Ports Setting and Docking Using the Xi System

The current da Vinci Xi system has improved range of motion by top-mounted rotatable boom arms with additional joints, which enables the surgeon to make an easier mobilization of the left colon, including the splenic flexure, and, at the same time, a complete TME with a single docking. Ports setup is simplified by placing all trocars on a straight line from left subcostal margin to the right lower quadrant, at an even distance of 6–8 cm of each other. An additional 12-mm laparoscopic port is placed in the right upper abdomen similarly to the previous version (**Figures 25-4 A, B**). Usually, docking from the left side of the patient is recommended since the assistance is preferably working from the right side (**Figure 25-5**). This setup can be modified according to the local space availability in each OR. **Figure 25-6** shows, after docking, a picture of the trocar positioning with Xi.

> ### EDITORIAL COMMENT
>
> The low anterior resection of the rectum with TME is a multiquadrant operation, involving at least 3 quadrants. The mobilization of the left colonic flexure is always necessary. This step is done at the beginning of the procedure and can be performed laparoscopically with a hybrid technique before carrying out the robotic pelvic dissection, or with a full robotic approach (preferred). This latter technique may require a compromised port setting and docking. In Western populations, with higher BMI, it may be difficult to achieve both the splenic flexure mobilization and the pelvic work with the same patient positioning, port setting, and docking (see Chapter 24, Left Colectomy).
>
> Also, with the oblique straight line of the port setting, the highest port in the left upper quadrant may have problems in reaching down the pelvis in a narrow/deep anatomy, limiting the action of the supported instruments.

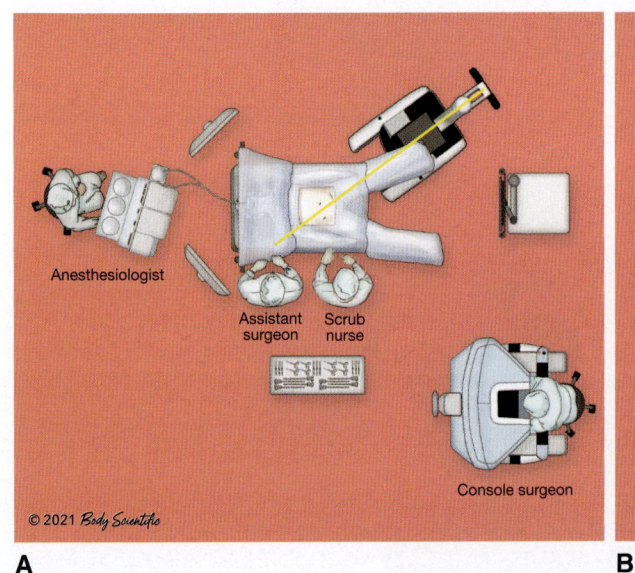

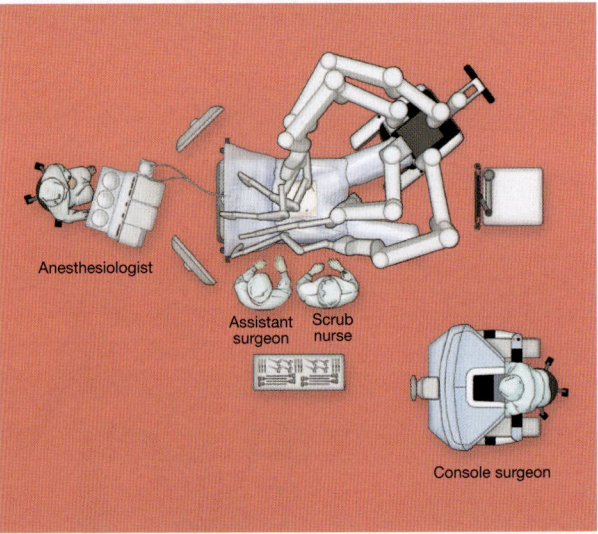

FIGURE 25-3 • OR setup with S or Si system.

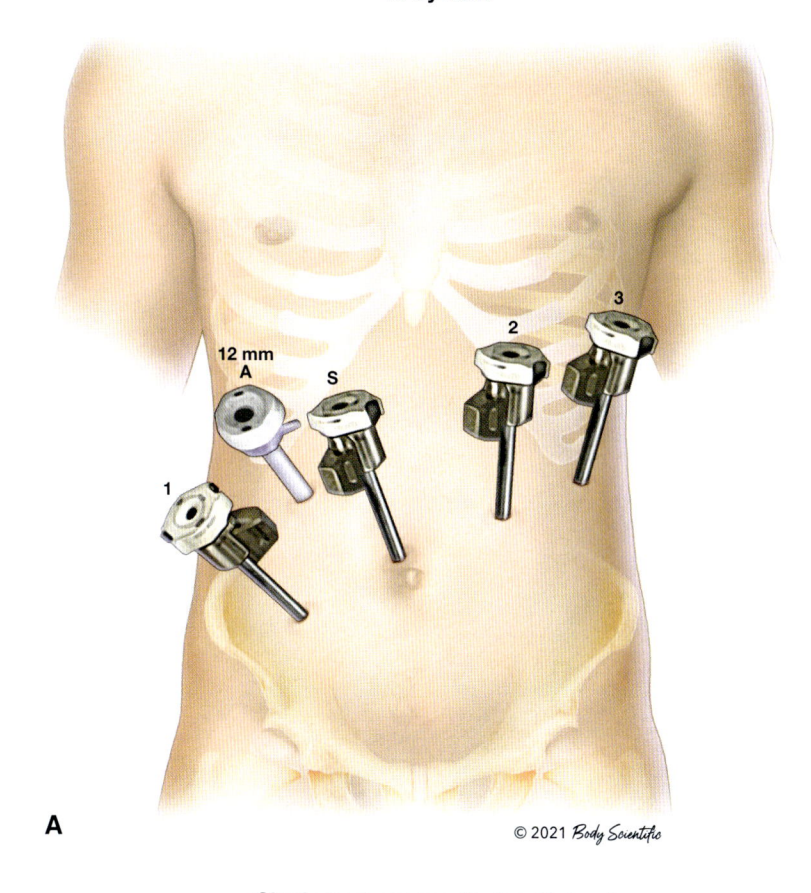

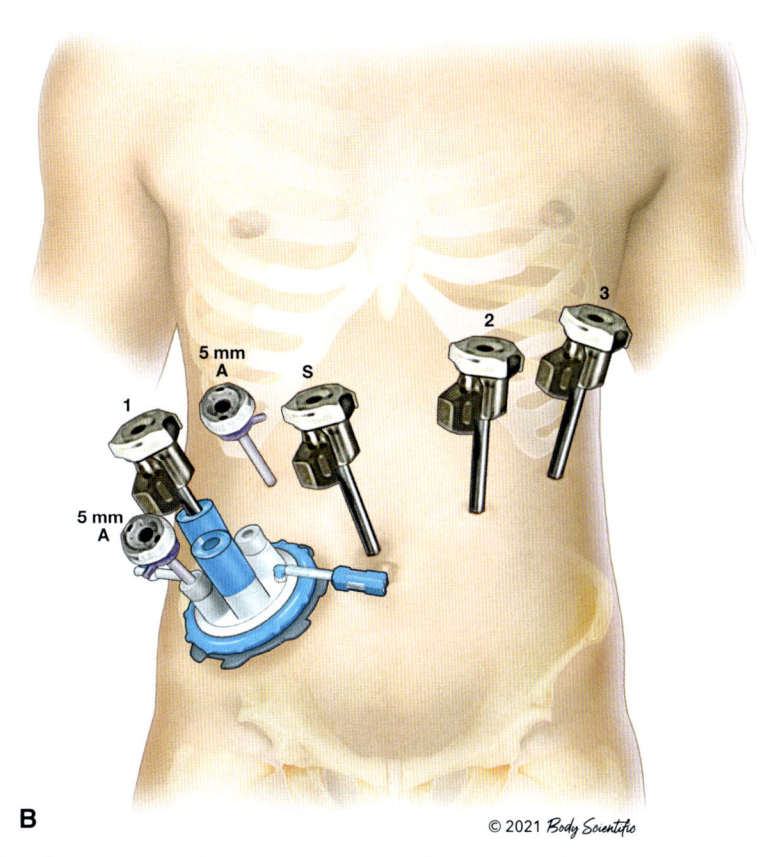

FIGURE 25-4 • Port setup in Xi system. **A.** In case of using a single port access device. **B.** Uniport.

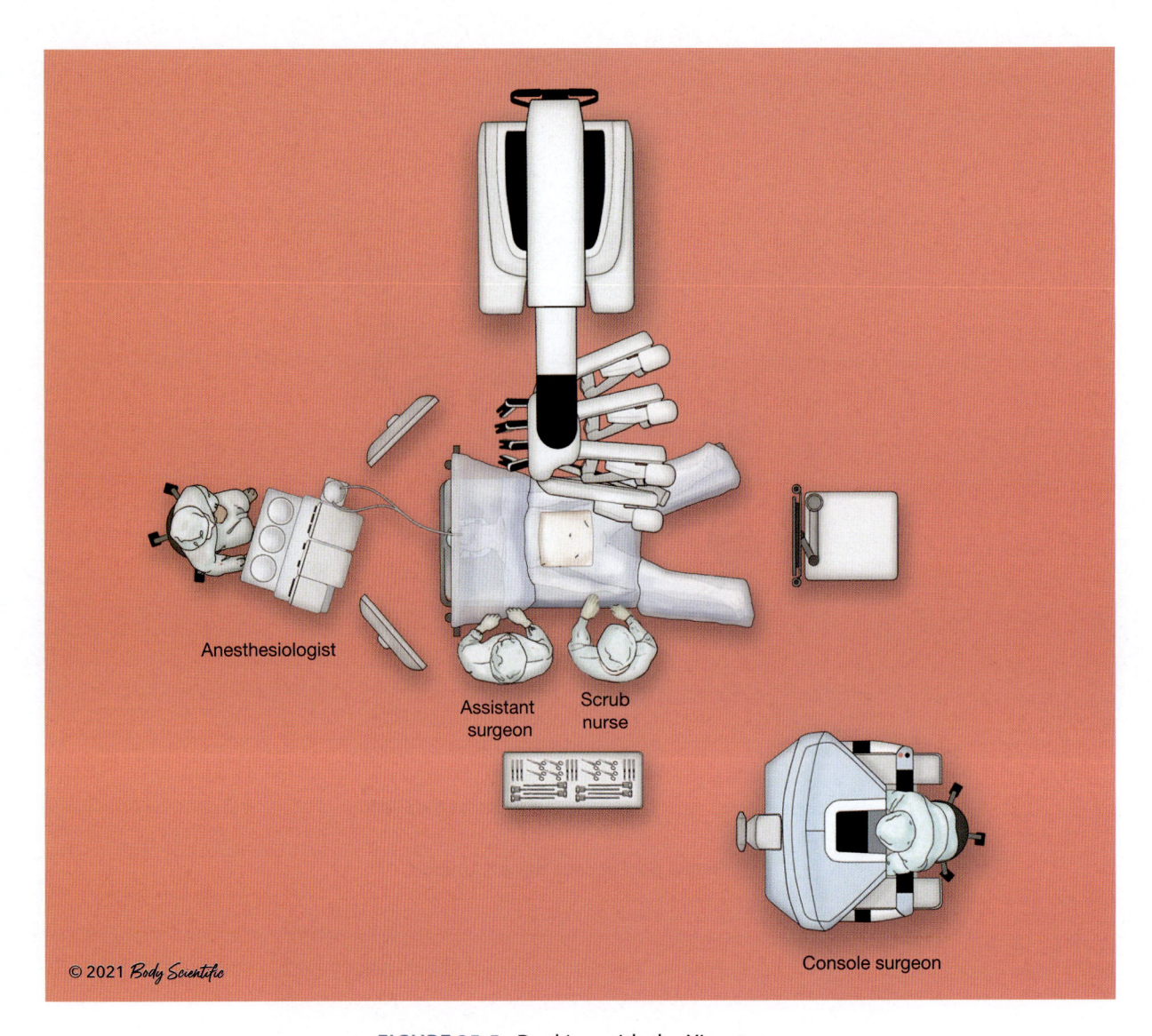

FIGURE 25-5 • Docking with the Xi system.

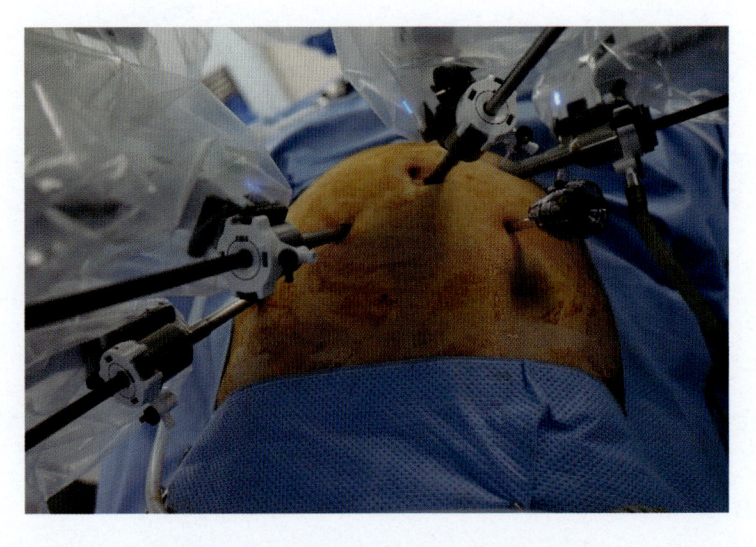

FIGURE 25-6 • After docking with Xi system.

Surgical Techniques

Hybrid Laparoscopic–Robotic Approach

In the laparoscopic phase of the takedown of the splenic flexure, the surgeon uses 2 trocars on the right side of the patient, and the assistant works with the remaining ones. Briefly, the dissection starts with IMA and IMV division, and a full mobilization of the left colon is performed in a medial to lateral fashion. Once this preliminary phase of the operation is completed, the robotic cart is docked in to perform the TME.

Full Robotic Approach

After docking the robotic arms to the trocars, a tip-up fenestrated grasper, bipolar Cadiére forceps, hot-shears, and camera are installed in R1, R2, R3, and S, respectively.

The procedure starts by entering the avascular interfascial space near the sacral promontory, or in a higher position below the inferior mesenteric vein where this space is well developed. The assistant stretches up the mesentery of the sigmoid colon lifting the arcade of the inferior mesenteric artery/sigmoidorectal artery, and the surgeon carefully incises the peritoneal sulcus of the rectosigmoid by monopolar cautery held in the dominant hand coordinated with gentle countertraction by the Cadière forceps in the nondominant hand (**Figures 25-7 A, B**).

Then, the dissection plane is extended cephalad by sweeping the hypogastric plexus down until the origin of the IMA is identified (**Figure 25-8A**). The assistant grabs the IMV so that the surgeon may find the proper plane underneath the vein. At this point, special care must be taken to secure the autonomic nerves because those fibers of the preaortic plexus on the right side of IMA can be easily seen, but on the left side is often hidden behind the IMA. Cautious division of the nerve branch, at

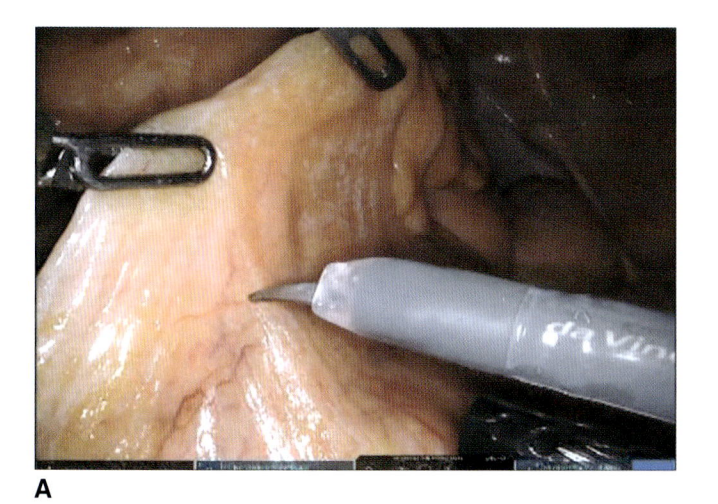

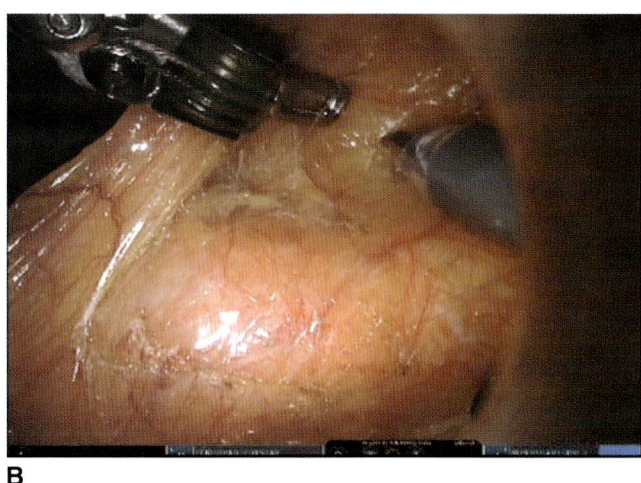

FIGURE 25-7 • **A.** Traction method to incise the peritoneum. **B.** Countertraction by Cadière forceps.

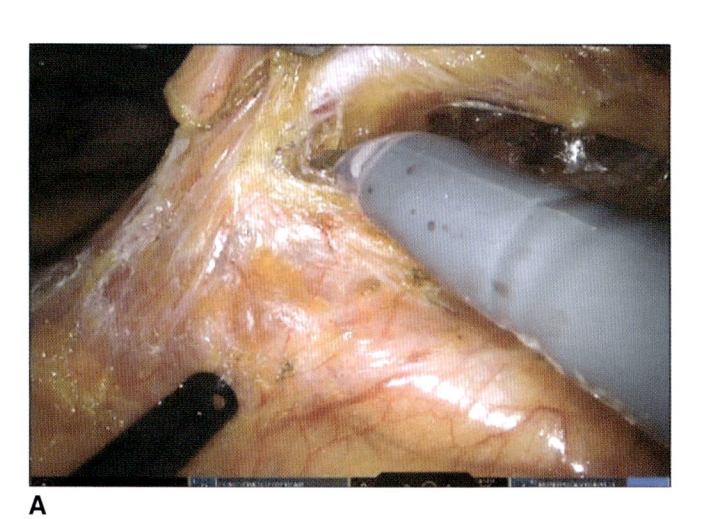

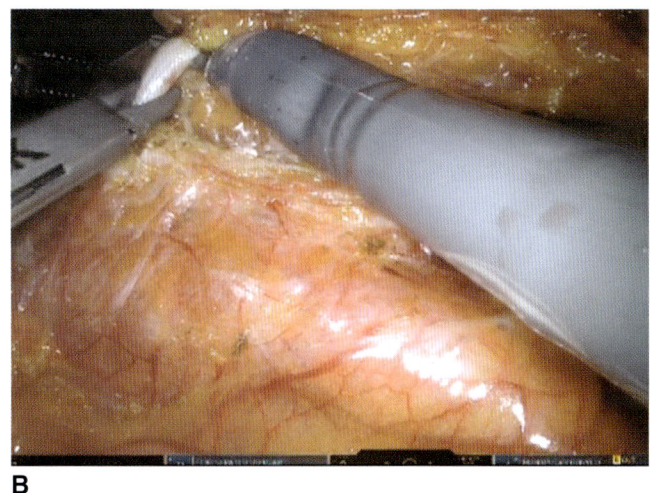

FIGURE 25-8 • IMA ligation. **A.** Identification of right branches of preaortic plexus. **B.** IMA ligation.

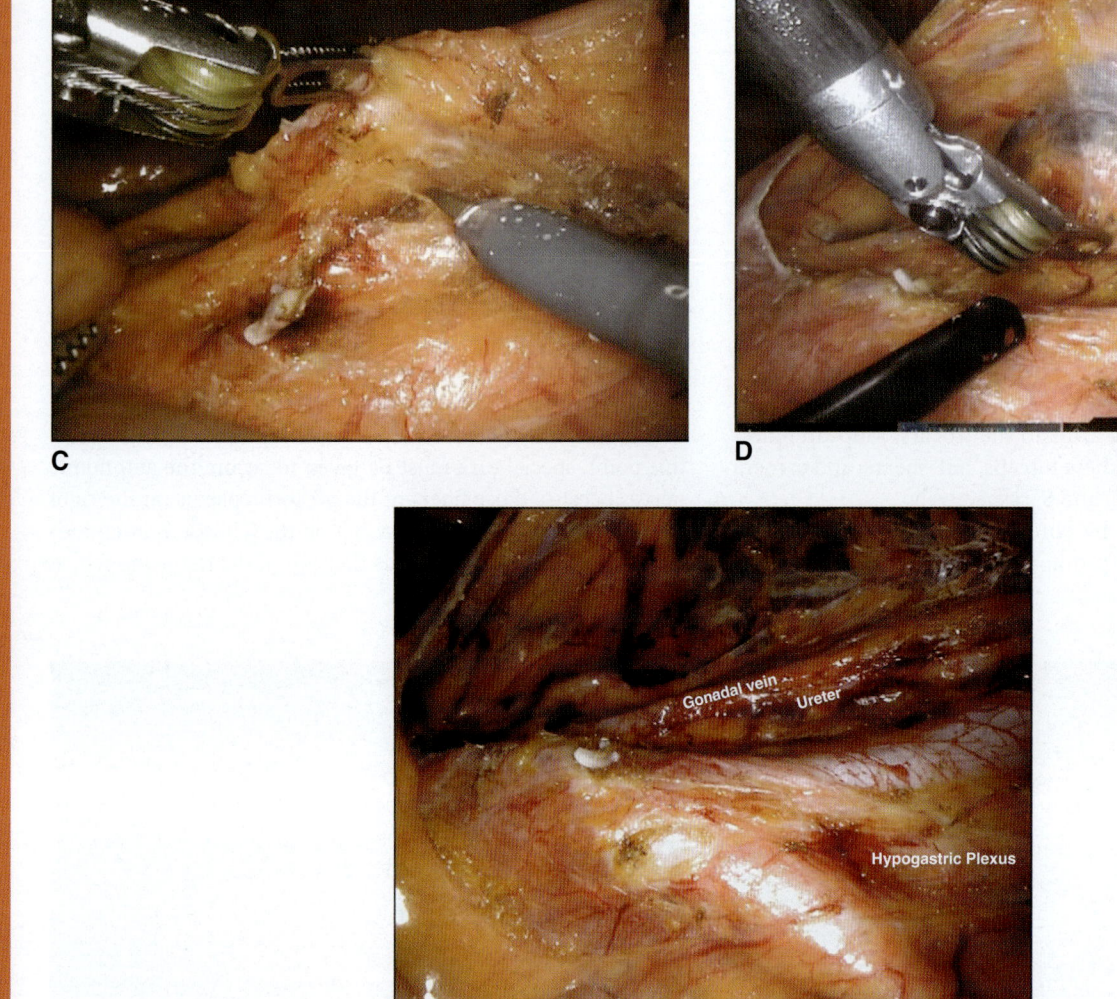

FIGURE 25-8 • (Continued) **C.** Preservation of the left branches of the preaortic plexus. **D.** Medial-to-lateral dissection. **E.** After IMA ligation.

the right front side of the artery, unveils the origin of the IMA. The artery is divided in between clips (Hem-o-lok™) or using a vascular stapler (**Figure 25-8B**). After that, the simple lifting up of the IMA stump enables the surgeon to identify the left side branches of preaortic plexus (**Figure 25-8C**).

The remaining part of the medial-to-lateral dissection is relatively straightforward, because the separation of the mesentery from the Toldt's fascia can be easily carried out by detaching the mesocolon from the ureter and the gonadal vessels, while the tip-up fenestrated grasper is holding the mesocolon ventrally (**Figures 25-8 D, E**).

The IMV is cut just below the lower border of the pancreas (**Figure 25-9A**). The medial-to-lateral dissection ends when the pancreas on the top (cephalad), the descending paracolic gutter on the side (laterally), and the ureter (passing over the left iliac vessels) are identified (**Figures 25-9 B, C**).

Subsequently, once an incision is made in the paracolic gutter, the peritoneal attachment along the left colon is released.

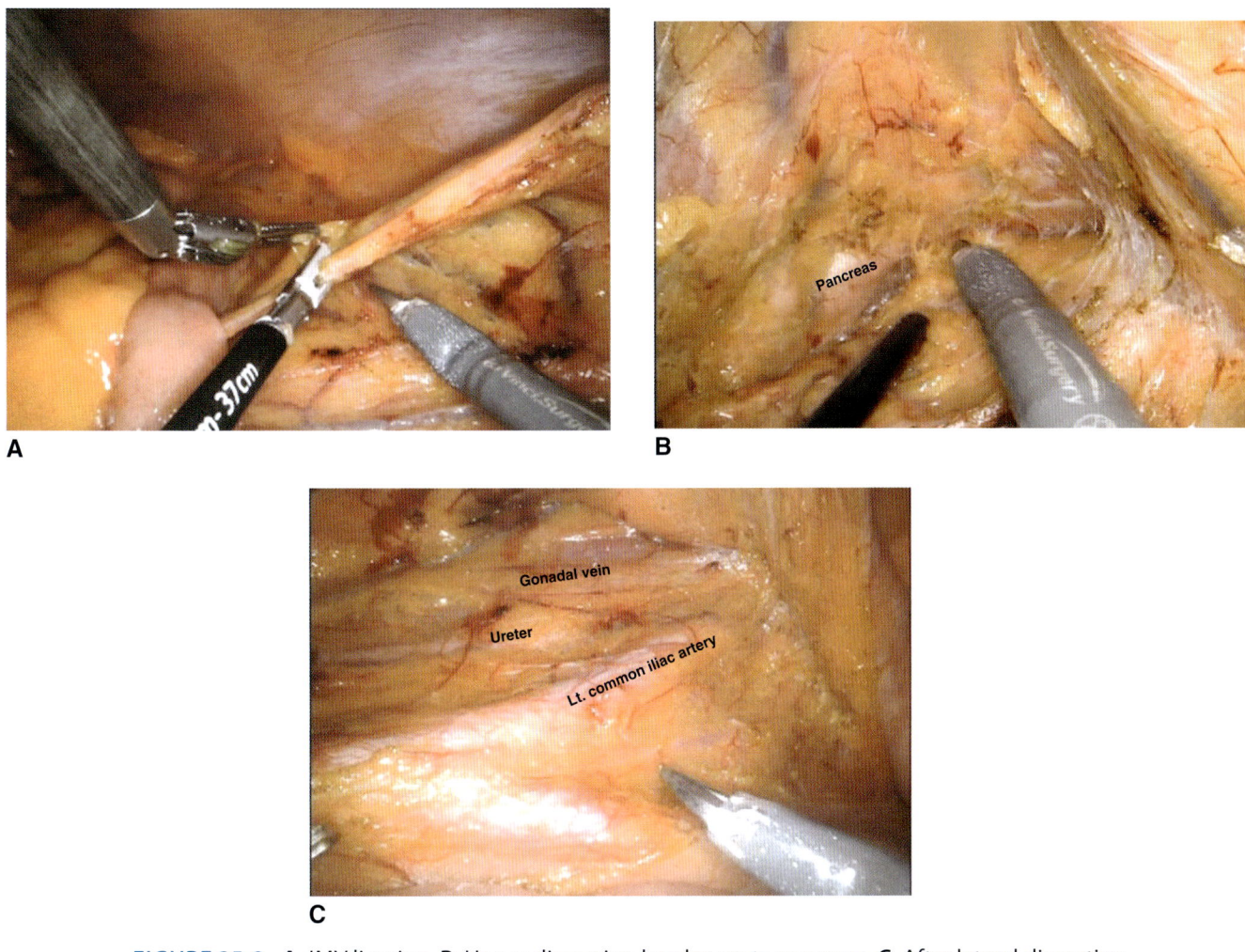

FIGURE 25-9 • **A.** IMV ligation. **B.** Upper dissection border, up to pancreas. **C.** After lateral dissection.

The assistant facilitates the maneuver straightening and pulling the colon medially together with the robotic grasper in R3. The dissection proceeds in a bottom-up direction, reaching the splenic flexure (**Figures 25-10 A–C**).

There are several methods for the takedown of the splenic flexure (see Chapter 24 for more details). First, if the pancreas is easily visible during medial-to-lateral mesocolon mobilization, the simplest way is to enter the lesser sac by cutting the pancreatocolic ligament (insertion of the mesentery of the transverse colon) from below (**Figure 25-11A**).

If this is not easy, a lateral dissection of the splenocolic ligament is suggested to separate the greater omentum from the colon. At this point, a useful tip is pulling the omentum while another grasper is holding the colon to put in tension the dissection plane (**Figure 25-11B**). The most efficient way to get enough length of proximal colon is to perform a complete mobilization of the left colonic flexure, including the insertion of the left side of the mesentery of the transverse colon to the lower edge of the pancreas (**Figure 25-11C**).

> **EDITORIAL COMMENT**
>
> More details on the splenic flexure mobilization are described in Chapter 24.

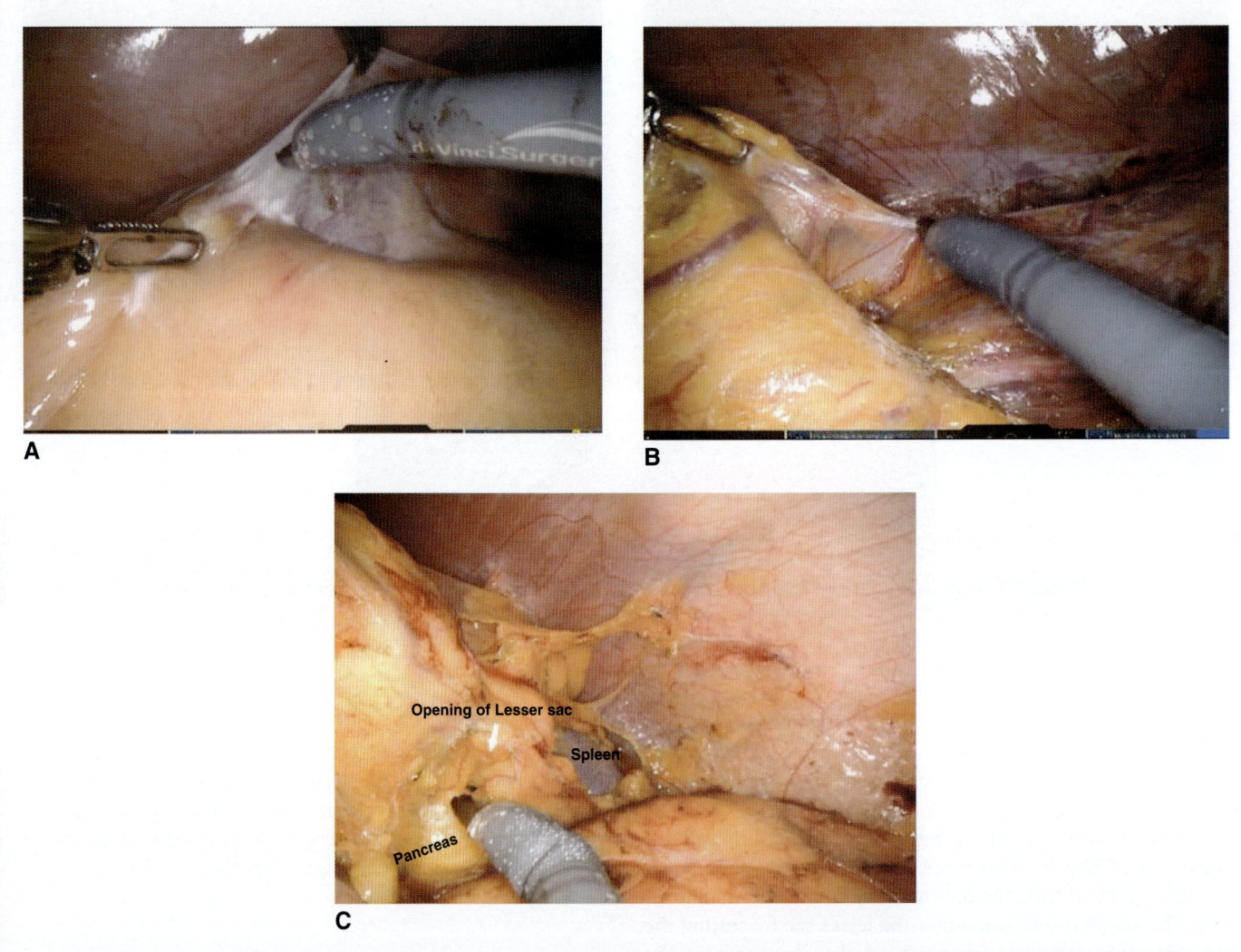

FIGURE 25-10 • Lateral dissection. **A.** Incision in paracolic gutter and releasing the left colon (**B**) up to the spleen (**C**).

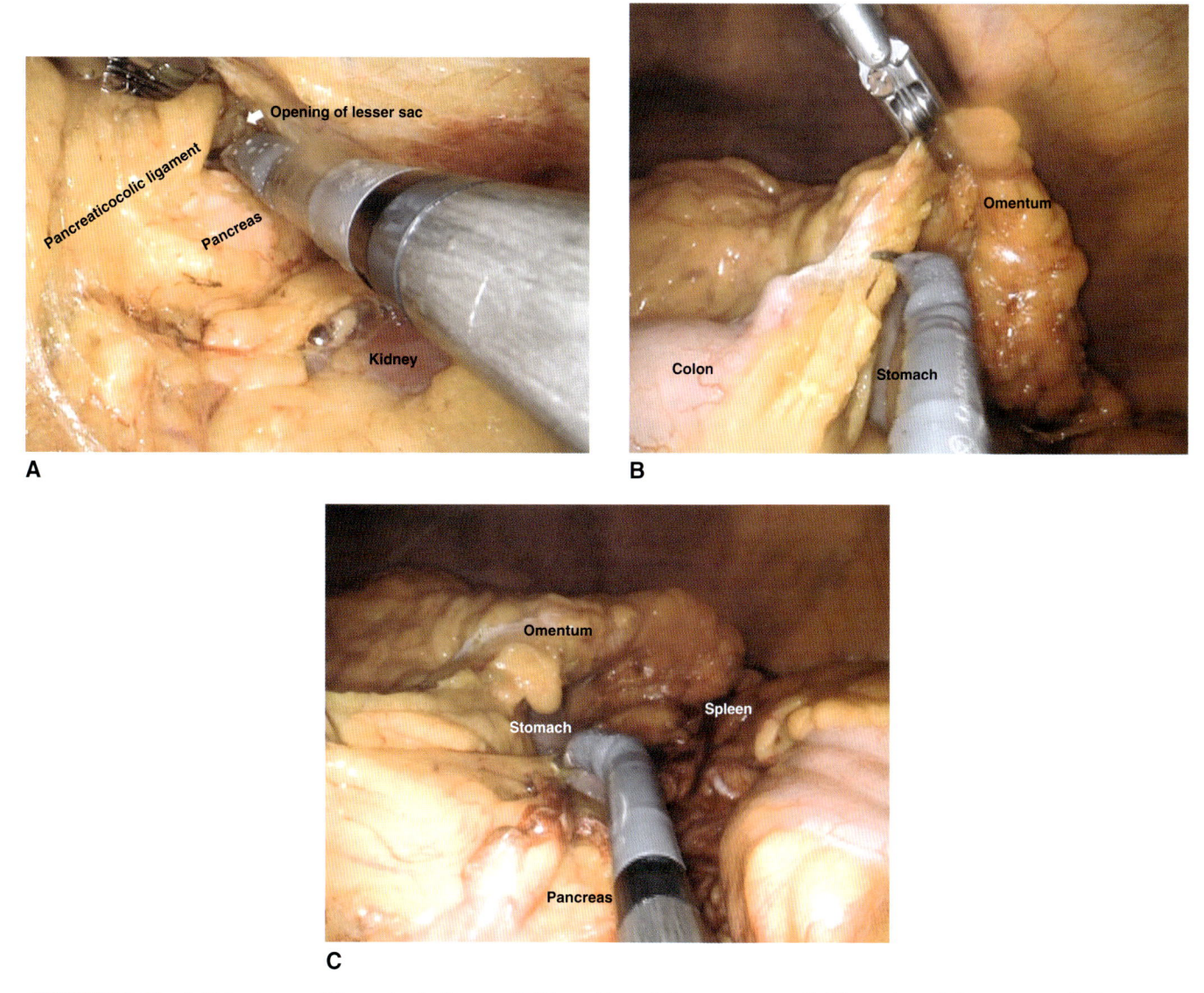

FIGURE 25-11 • **A.** Takedown of the splenic flexure. **B.** Dissection of the omentum. **C.** Dissection of the gastrocolic ligament.

TME

Essential Considerations for Rectal Cancer Surgery

Anatomy Based on Embryology

The rectum is embryologically developed in a tube-like organ with a lumen. Nutrition of this tube is supplied mainly by the IMA and partly by branches of the internal iliac artery (medium hemorrhoidal artery). The draining veins and lymphatics run reversely along with the arteries, with the exception of the IMV that directly drains into the splenic vein. This lymphovascular network is well organized and maintained within the fatty cushion of the mesorectum. All these structures are covered by a thin membrane of peritoneum (visceral mesorectal fascia) that finally fuses and attaches to the lining of retroperitoneum (parietal mesorectal fascia) and a part of genitourinary organs during the embryologic development.

Hence, one of the basic principles in rectal cancer surgery is to separate these fascial adhesions back to the earlier embryonic stages and to remove the tumor-bearing segment within a package of visceral mesorectal fascia.

Fasciae and Autonomic Nerves

As described, the peritoneal membrane covers not only the rectum, but also most of the pelvic organs, so it develops into a "fascia" of various names through a complex fusion process. A good understanding of the relationship of these fasciae helps to facilitate surgery, to reduce bleeding, to maintain physiological functions, and to secure oncological radicality (see **Figures 25-12, 25-13 A, B,** and **25-14**).

The pelvic autonomic nerves also emerge from the spine and intertwine in front of the aorta to form the preaortic nerve plexus, which leads to the superior hypogastric nerve plexus, which diverts into both sides and becomes the left and right hypogastric nerves, which are responsible for the sympathetic innervation. The sympathetic ganglion chains, on both sides of the aorta, run down and are connected with some fibers of sacral nerves (parasympathetic) bilaterally in front of the sacrum to form the pelvic splanchnic nerves and merge with the hypogastric nerves to develop the pelvic plexus, which attributes mixed sympathetic and parasympathetic innervation (**Figure 25-15**). This part is less evident, since the S2-S4 sacral nerves proper are rather located in a deeper space and are mostly unseen in normal rectal surgery and merge with the lumbar trunk to become the femoral nerve descending to the leg.

Different Levels of Retraction

In the TIPS box, different levels of retraction are described. These maneuvers will be useful during the procedure described in this chapter.

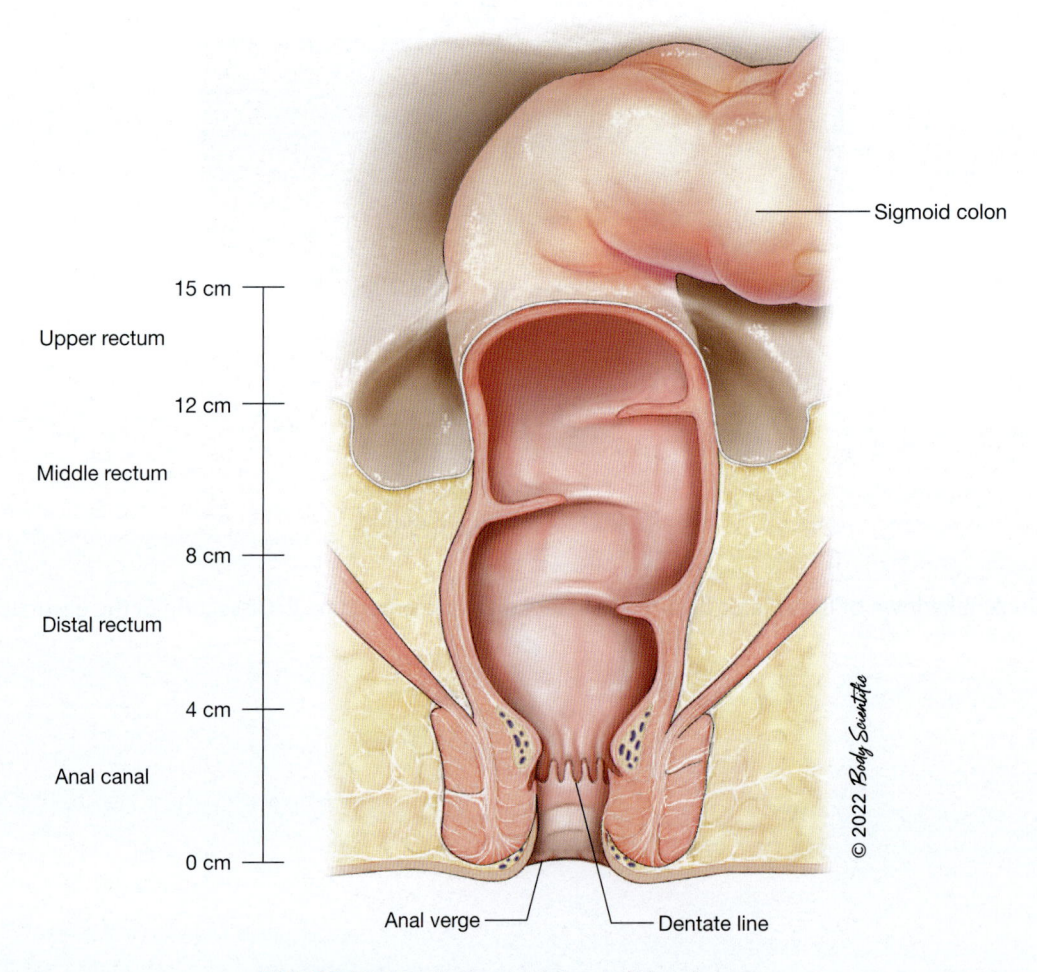

FIGURE 25-12 • Upper, middle, and distal rectum.

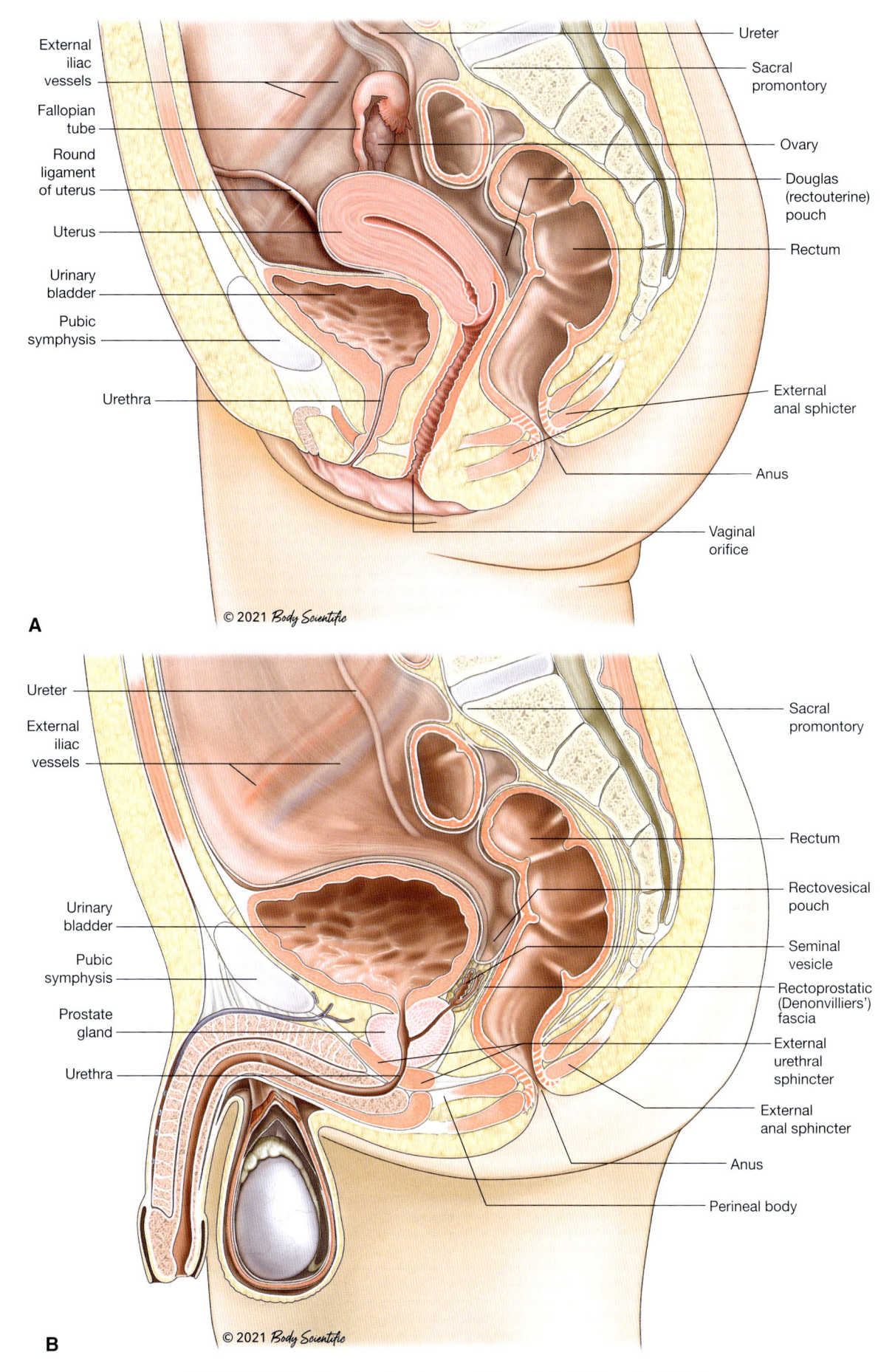

FIGURE 25-13 • Standard anatomy of the pelvis: **A.** Female. **B.** Male.

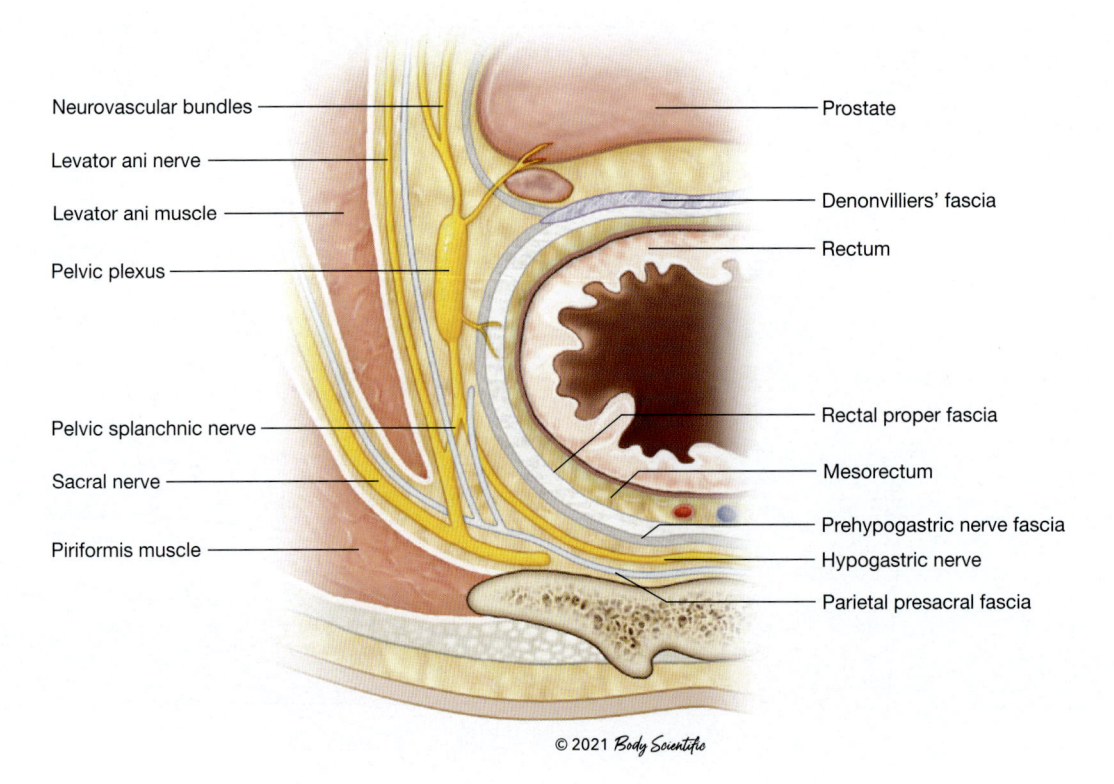

FIGURE 25-14 • Pelvic fasciae and autonomic nerves.

Superior view

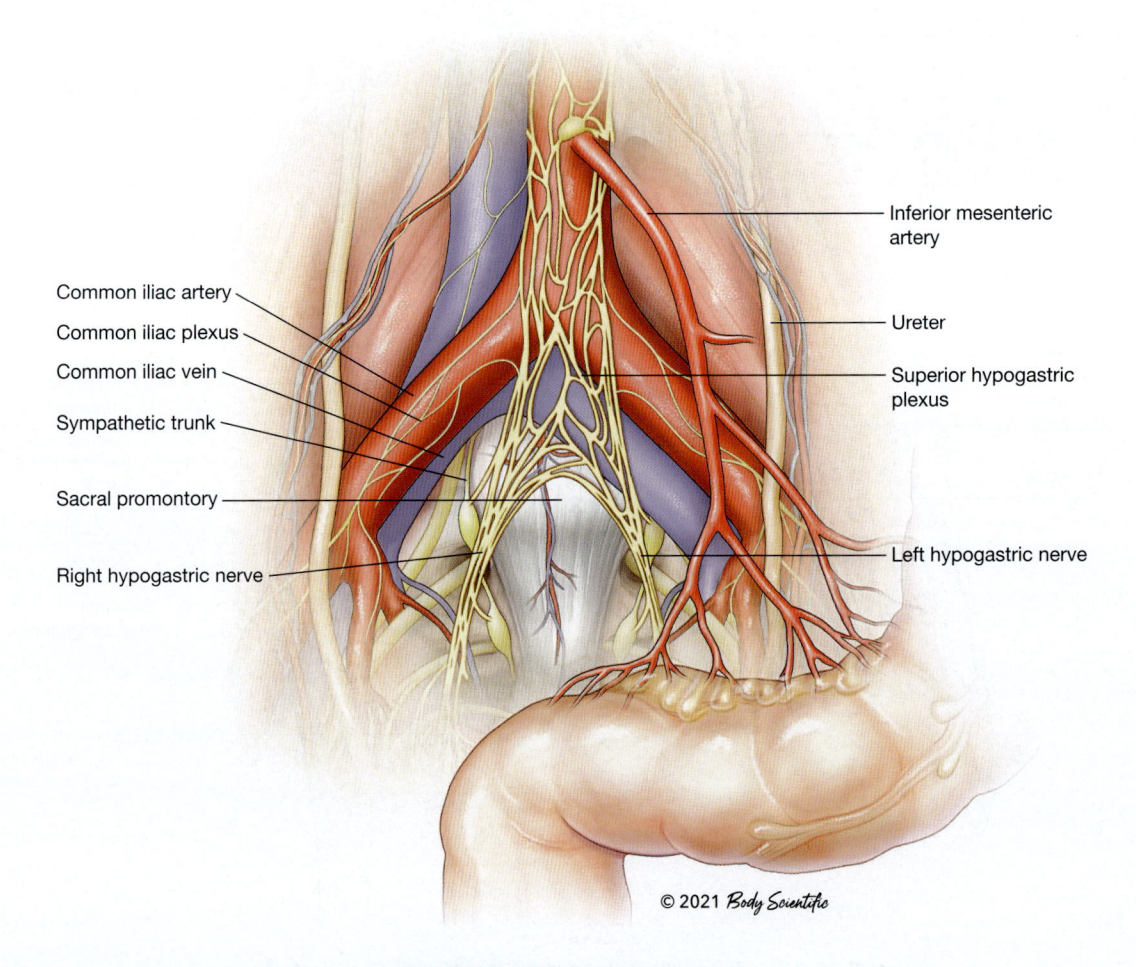

FIGURE 25-15 • Neural anatomy.

►► TIPS

Different levels of retraction (**Figures 25-16 A–D**)

1. Major retraction is maintained by the assistant keeping the rectum in appropriate tension to visualize the target area clearly.
2. Counter-retraction is handled by a tip-up fenestrated grasper held in the R3 to create a wide surgical field while it is lifting, pushing the pelvic wall or the rectum.
3. Minor traction is achieved with the surgeon's non-dominant hand with bipolar Cadière forceps to adjust the dissection plane.
4. Finally, the dissection itself is carried out by the surgeon's dominant hand with a hot-shears or hook.

EDITORIAL COMMENT

For more information on the different levels of retraction, see Chapter 2, The Basic Principles of Clinical Applications. The R3 has a fundamental role in maintaining stable/constant exposure during the dissection. Its role changes in different steps of the TME. During the posterior dissection, the R3 does the main retraction, lifting, and pushing the rectum anteriorly; while during the anterior dissection, it is retracting the prostate, the bladder, or the uterus, and the assistant is handling the sigmoid and the rectum. The assistant and the R3 are doing complementary actions, and their roles swap depending on the required exposure.

A

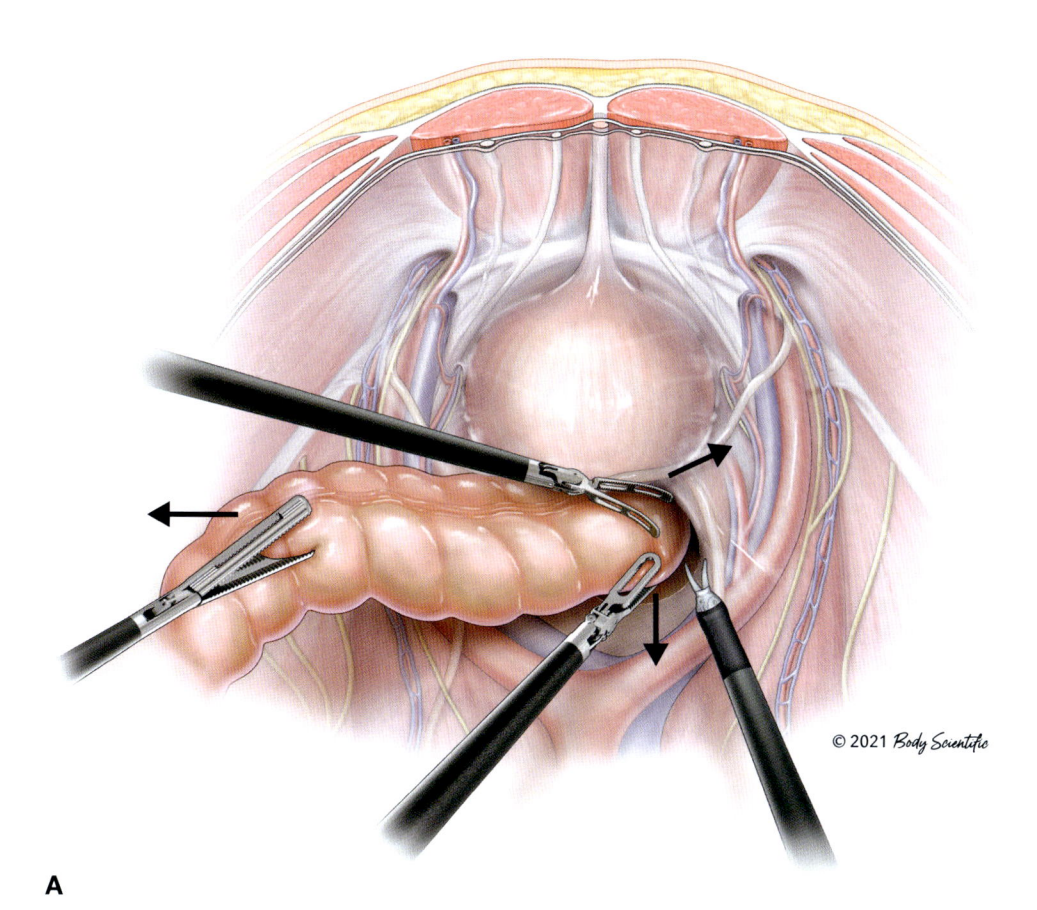

FIGURE 25-16 • Main techniques of tractions during: **A.** Right side.

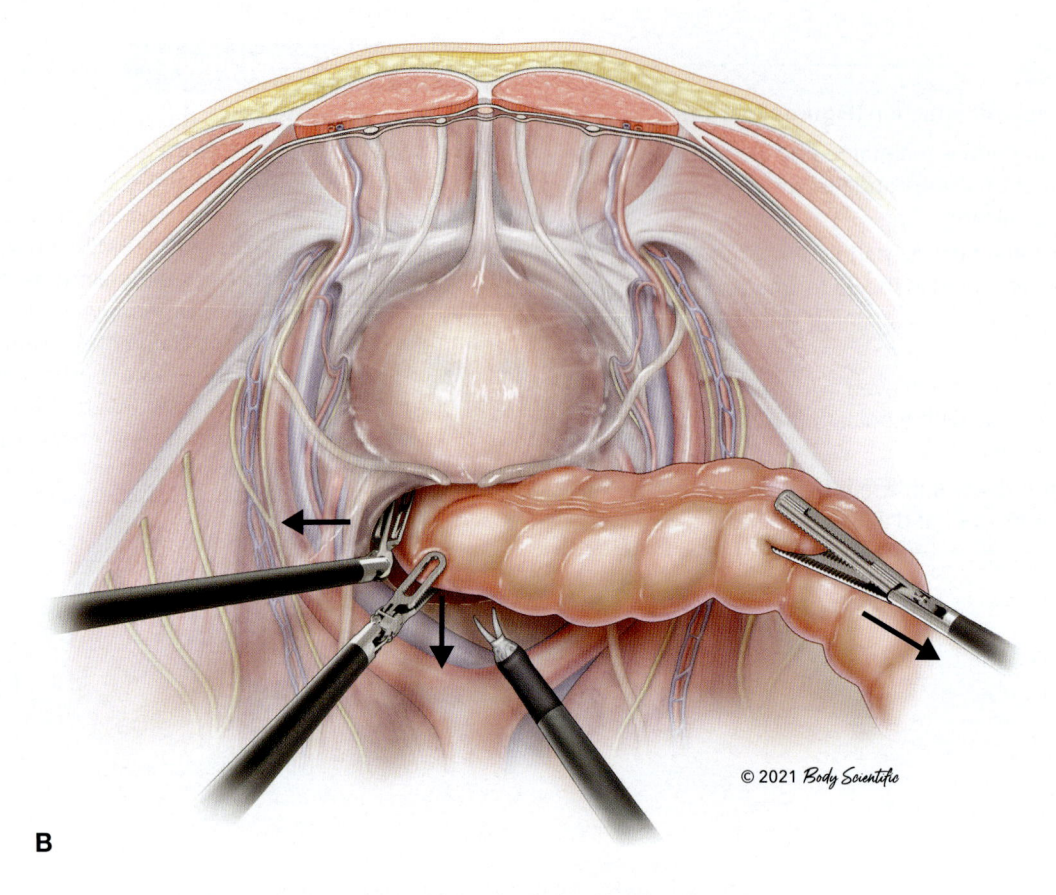

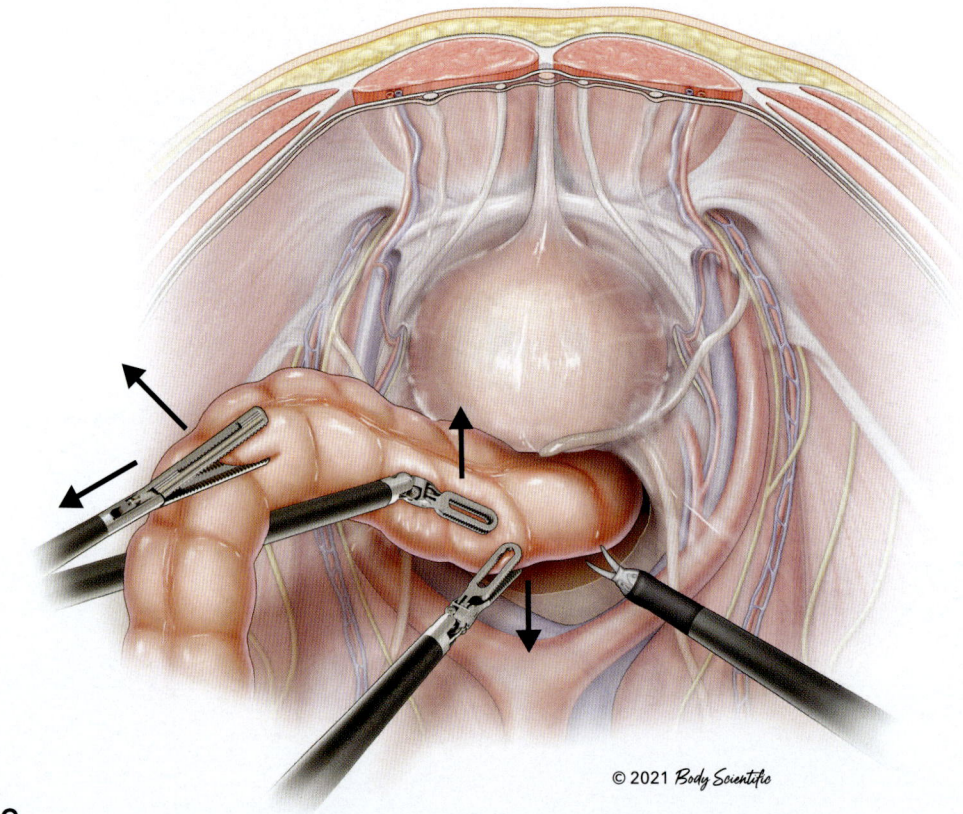

FIGURE 25-16 • *(Continued)* **B.** Left side. **C.** Posterior side.

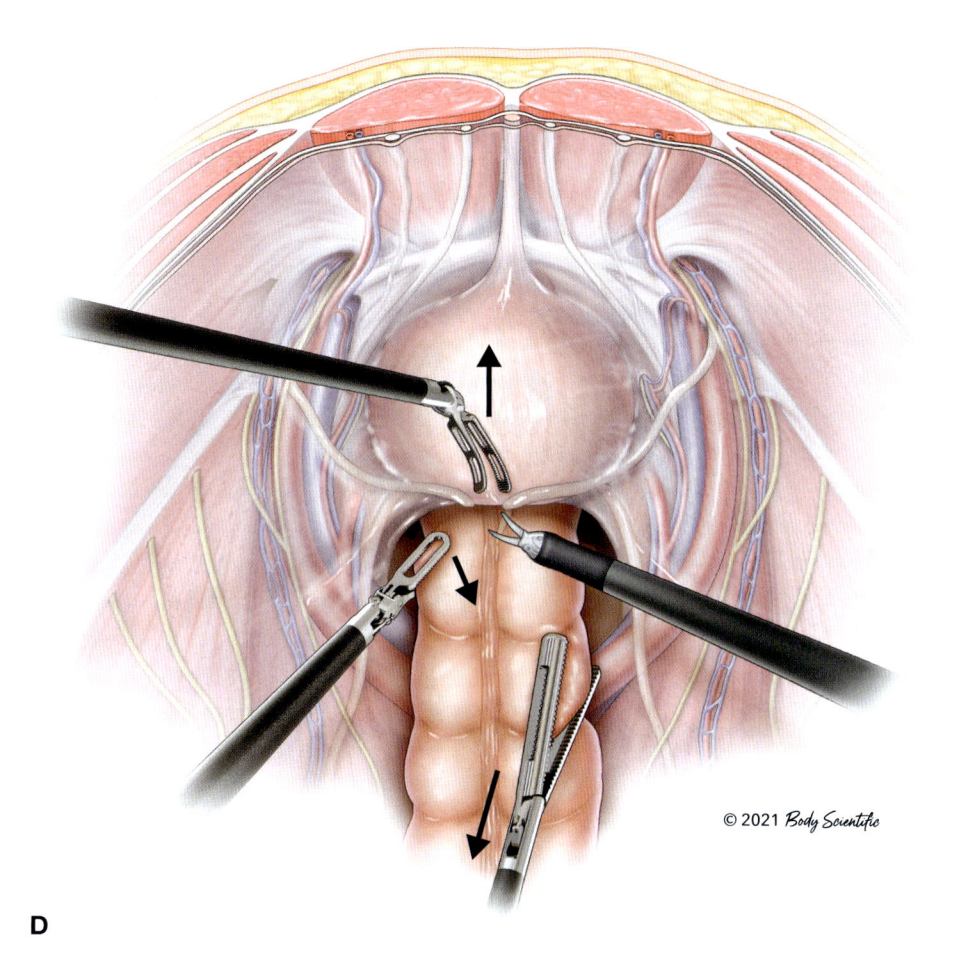

FIGURE 25-16 • (*Continued*) **D.** Anterior side dissection.

TME: Technical Steps

Step 1. Posterior dissection

The mobilization of the rectum begins in front of the promontory, with the dissection already created in the previous phase and extending the avascular planes already developed. The assistant holds the cut edge of mesocolon to lift it up; also, a grasper through the R3 grabs the upper rectum for better exposure (**Figures 25-17 A, B**). The CO_2 helps in opening up the "holy plane", down between the 2 layers of the mesorectal fascia. This is a totally avascular plane. It is worth noting that the avascular planes posterior to the mesorectum are 2 narrow spaces defined by 3 layers of the mesorectal fascia proper (or visceral endopelvic fascia), prehypogastric nerve fascia, and parietal endopelvic fascia (**Figure 25-17C**). As Heald emphasizes "intra-fascial TME" or "yellow side of the white," meticulous dissection between the first 2 fasciae can achieve both autonomic nerve preservation and oncologic TME. Hence, superior hypogastric plexus and hypogastric nerves can be relatively easily identified and preserved, as long as this interfascial dissection is maintained. However, excessive traction or thermal injury should be avoided.

The dissection should proceed downward and vertically in the midline as much as possible, reaching the thickenings of the fascia (which are called sacrorectal ligaments). When these ligaments are divided, the rectum and mesorectum change their shape from an L-shape to a straight one, allowing the formation of a larger working space, creating some mobility of the mesorectum.

The anatomy of the mesorectum is represented in **Figure 25-18**.

Step 1 average time frame: 10–15 min

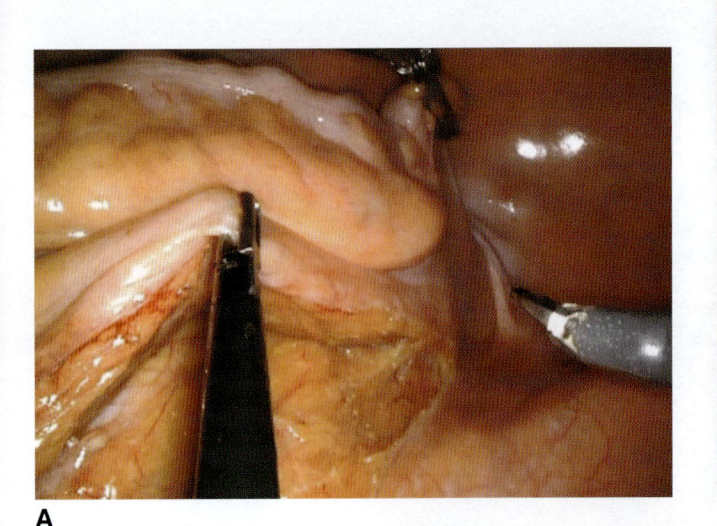

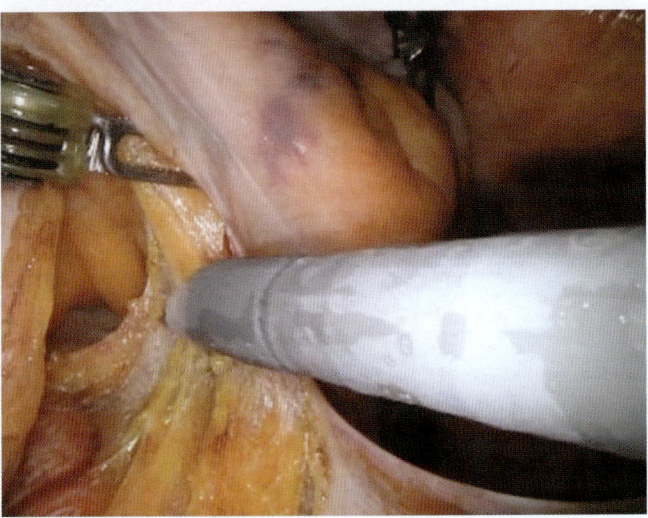

FIGURE 25-17 • Pelvic dissection. **A.** Traction method. **B.** Dissection of the posterior side of the rectum at sacral promontory. **C.** Pelvic cavity.

> **⚠ PITFALLS**
>
> Entering into a deeper space, below the endopelvic fascia, and damaging the presacral veins. These veins can bleed massively and be difficult to control. Compression with a sponge and hemostatic agent is the first measure to adopt in such event. Bipolar coagulation may be ineffective or cause more bleeding, and suturing with Dacron® pledgets on the periostium is challenging.

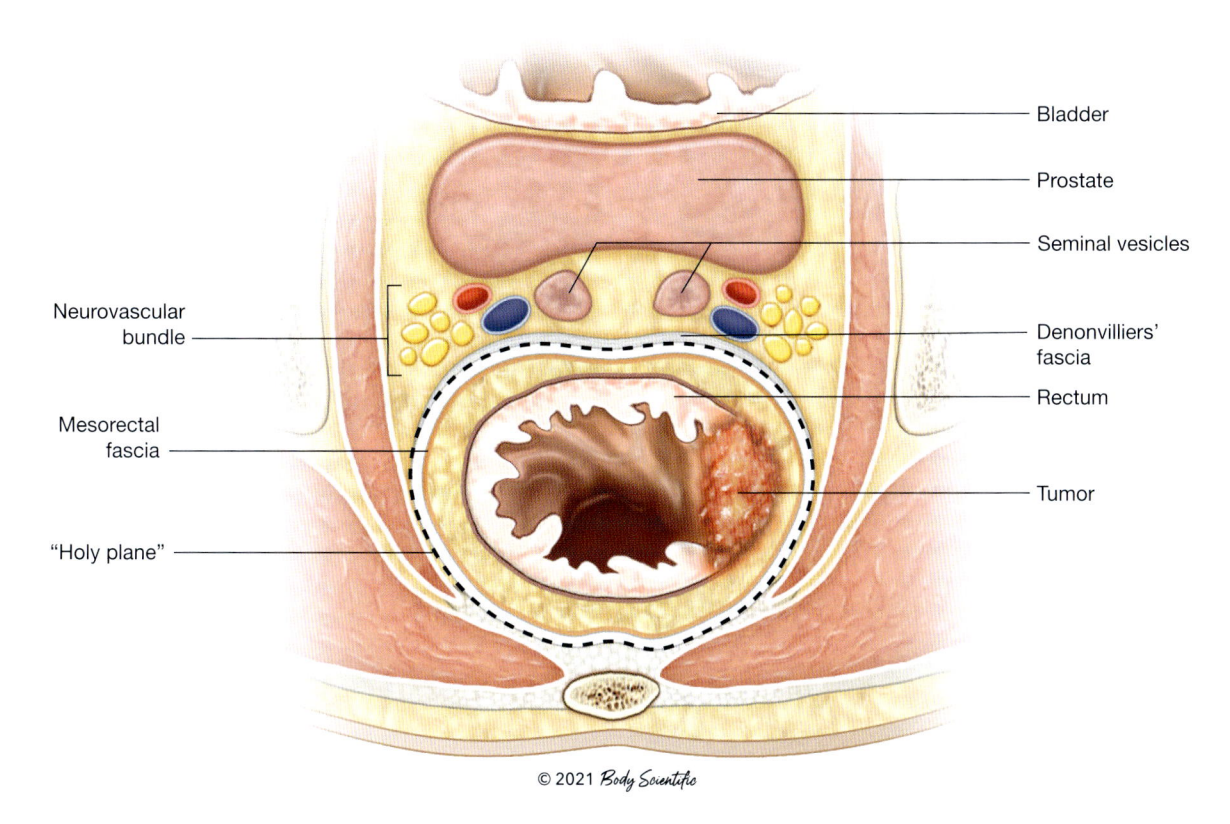

FIGURE 25-18 • Mesorectum.

Step 2. Postero-bilateral dissection

The lateral dissection, on both sides, is made easier when there is a good posterior plane already done. During this lateral dissection phase, the anatomy of the hypogastric nerves needs to be recognized. This anatomy can be variable because the bifurcation of the plexus (nerve formation) is inconstant: higher (close to the aorta) or lower (promontory). Here, the anatomy must be assessed, and the dissection should be kept medial to the nerves. Great care must be taken to keep pelvic splanchnic nerves (parasympathetic predominant) intact, which are running perpendicularly and merging with hypogastric nerves (sympathetic predominant) to form pelvic plexus (mixed autonomic). Laterally, the fascia is less evident than posteriorly. A trick to maintain the proper dissection plane is to push the mesorectum towards the counter-lateral side. Some of the fibers of the plexus entering into the mesorectum are lifting the bundle, and by pulling toward the contralateral side, the homolateral nerves can be stretched and visualized. This dissection has to include the middle hemorrhoidal vessels, which sometimes may not be recognized (they may be small and be coagulated). These structures, anatomically, are not represented in 100% of cases. The lateral dissection should proceed downward/vertically to avoid to go too much lateral. Here, laterally, some clinically relevant damage may occur (in men, ejaculation or erection can be affected).

This posterolateral dissection should proceed from the easiest side to the counter lateral part, and it may require some back and forth to be symmetrical on both sides.

As the mobilization proceeds, the assistant grabs the cut edge of the mesorectum more distally and pulls it ventrally and toward the counter lateral side, and then a tip-up fenestrated grasper, with its jaws opened (R3), makes countertraction, and the surgeon's left hand gently pushes the mesorectum medially to continue the mesorectal dissection through the Holy Plane (**Figures 25-19 A, B** and **25-20 A, B**).

Step 2 average time frame: 20–30 min

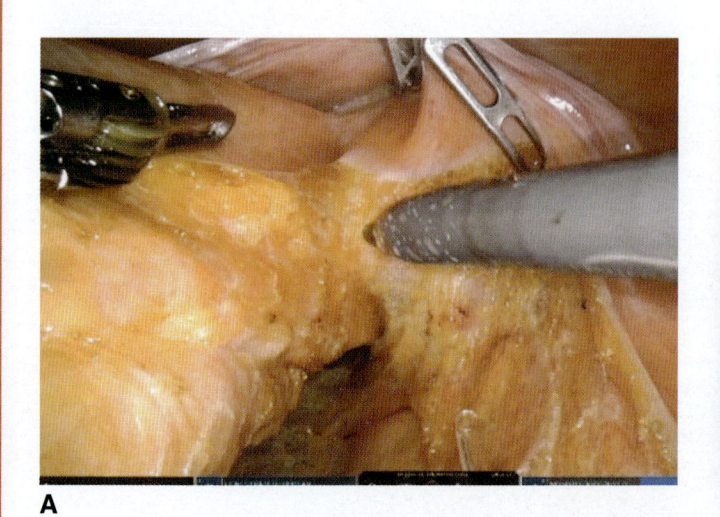

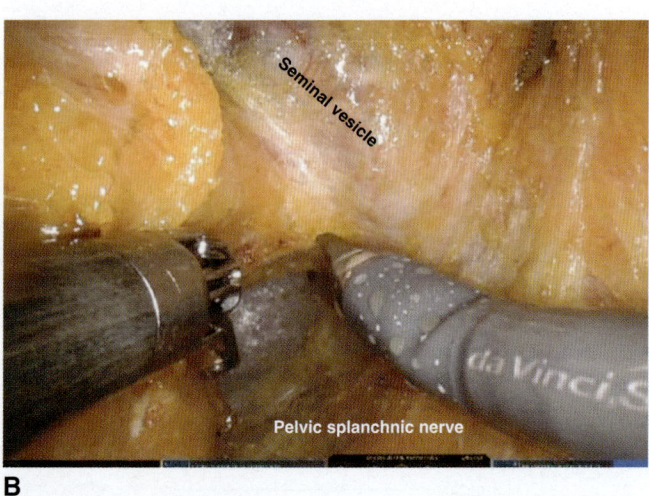

FIGURE 25-19 • Right side dissection of the rectum. **A.** Traction method. **B.** Preservation of the pelvic nerves.

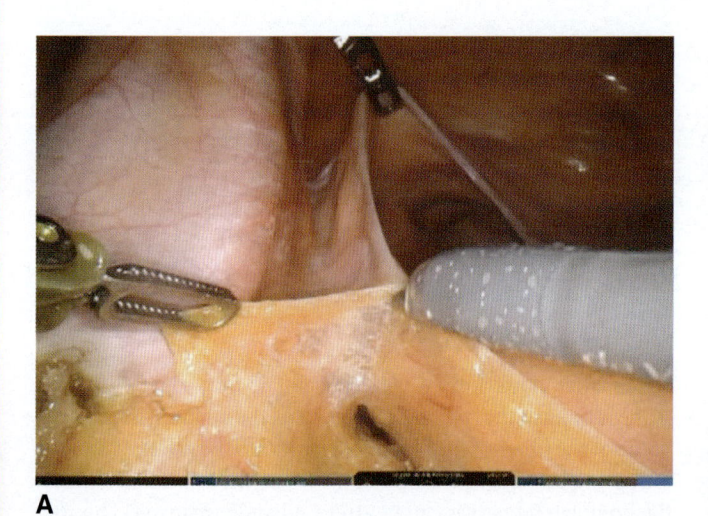

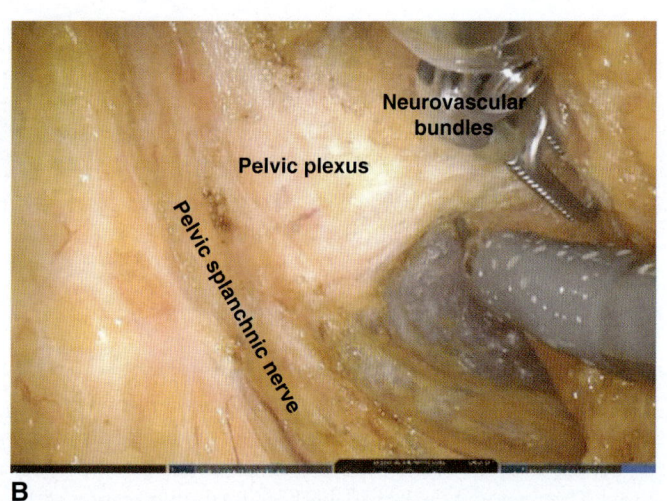

FIGURE 25-20 • Right side dissection of the rectum. **A.** Traction method. **B.** Preservation of the pelvic nerves.

🔍 ANATOMICAL HIGHLIGHTS

Vascular, lymph nodal, and neural anatomy are described in **Figures 25-21, 25-22,** and **25-23.**

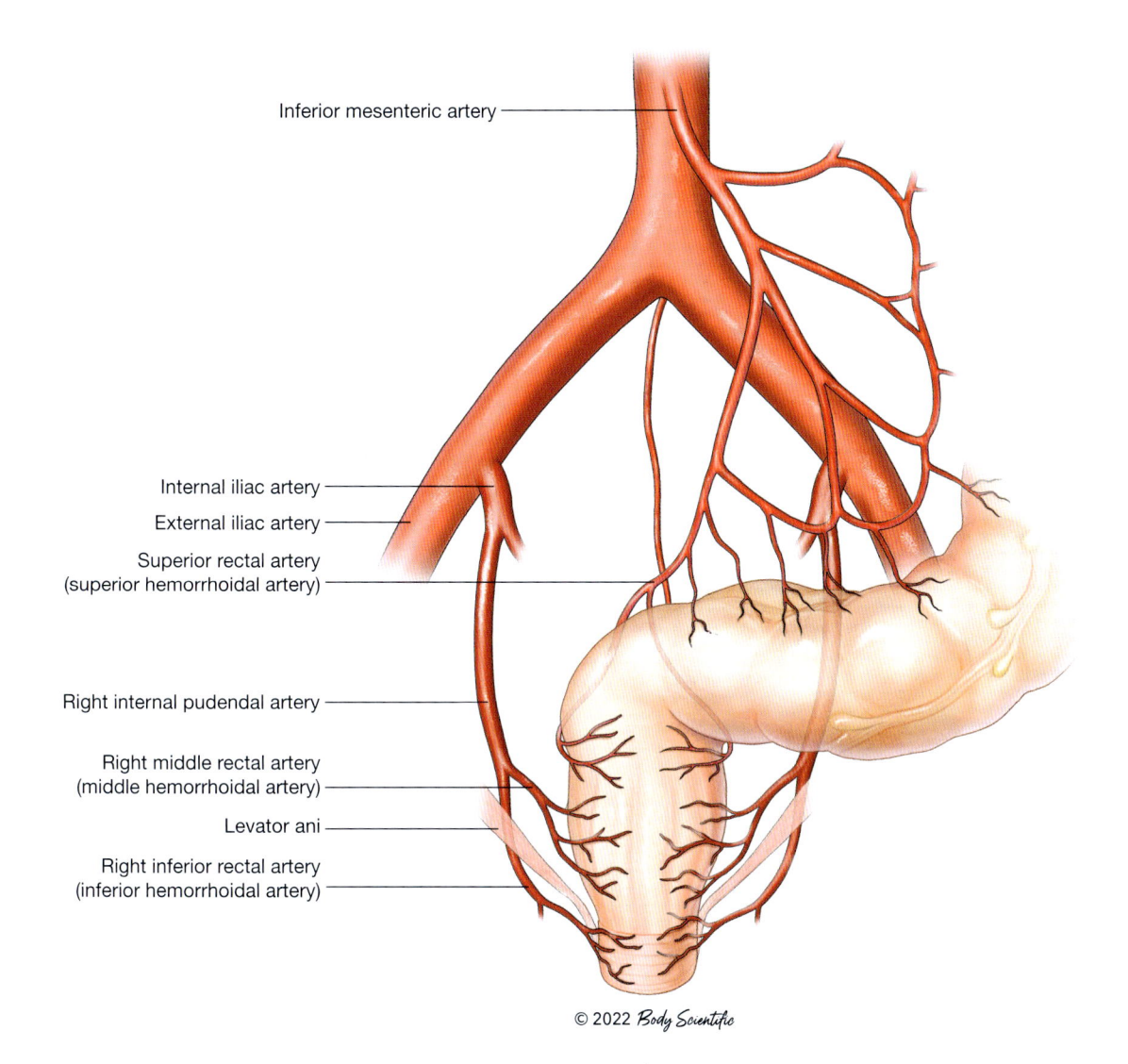

FIGURE 25-21 • Arterial anatomy.

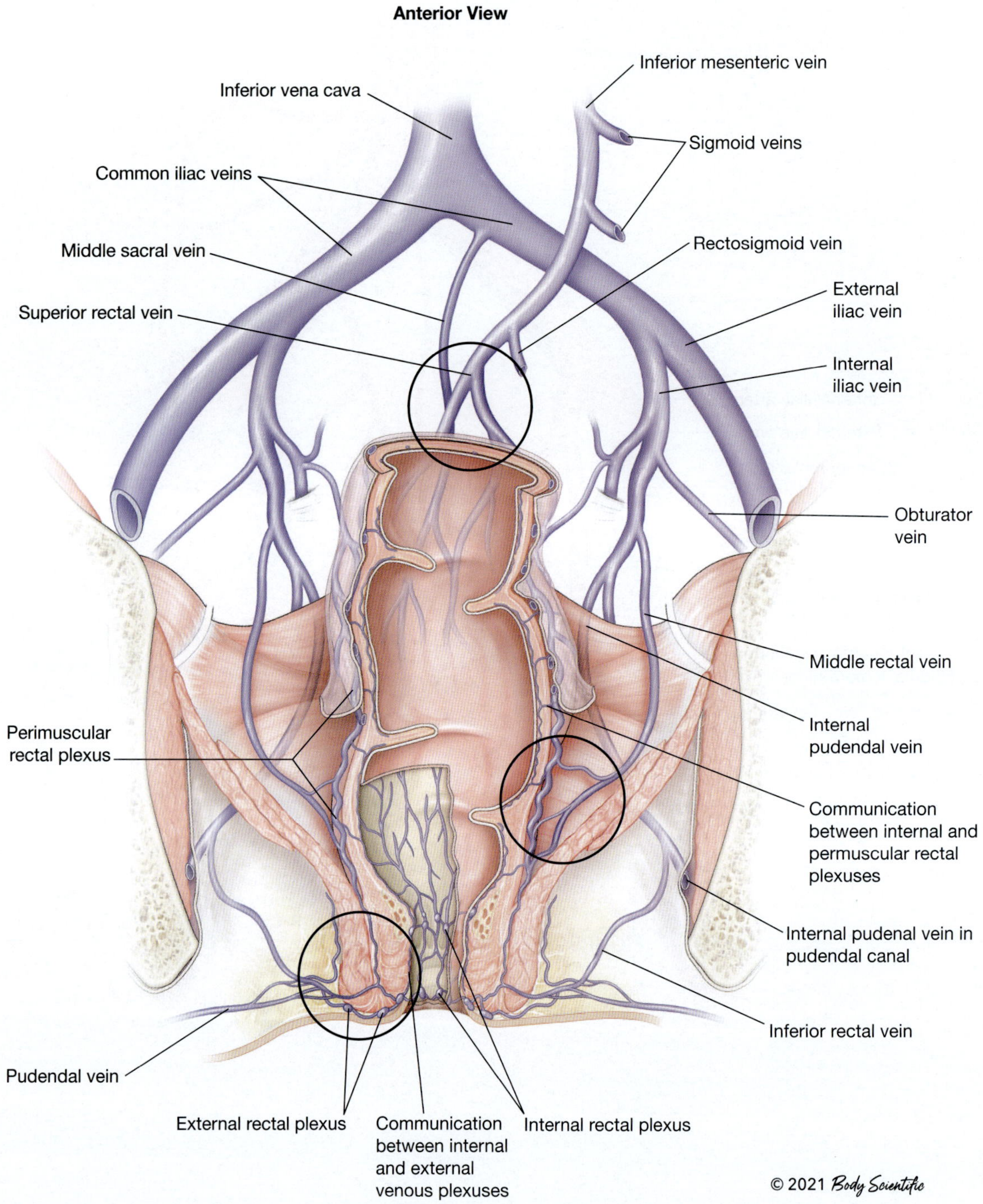

FIGURE 25-22 • Venous anatomy.

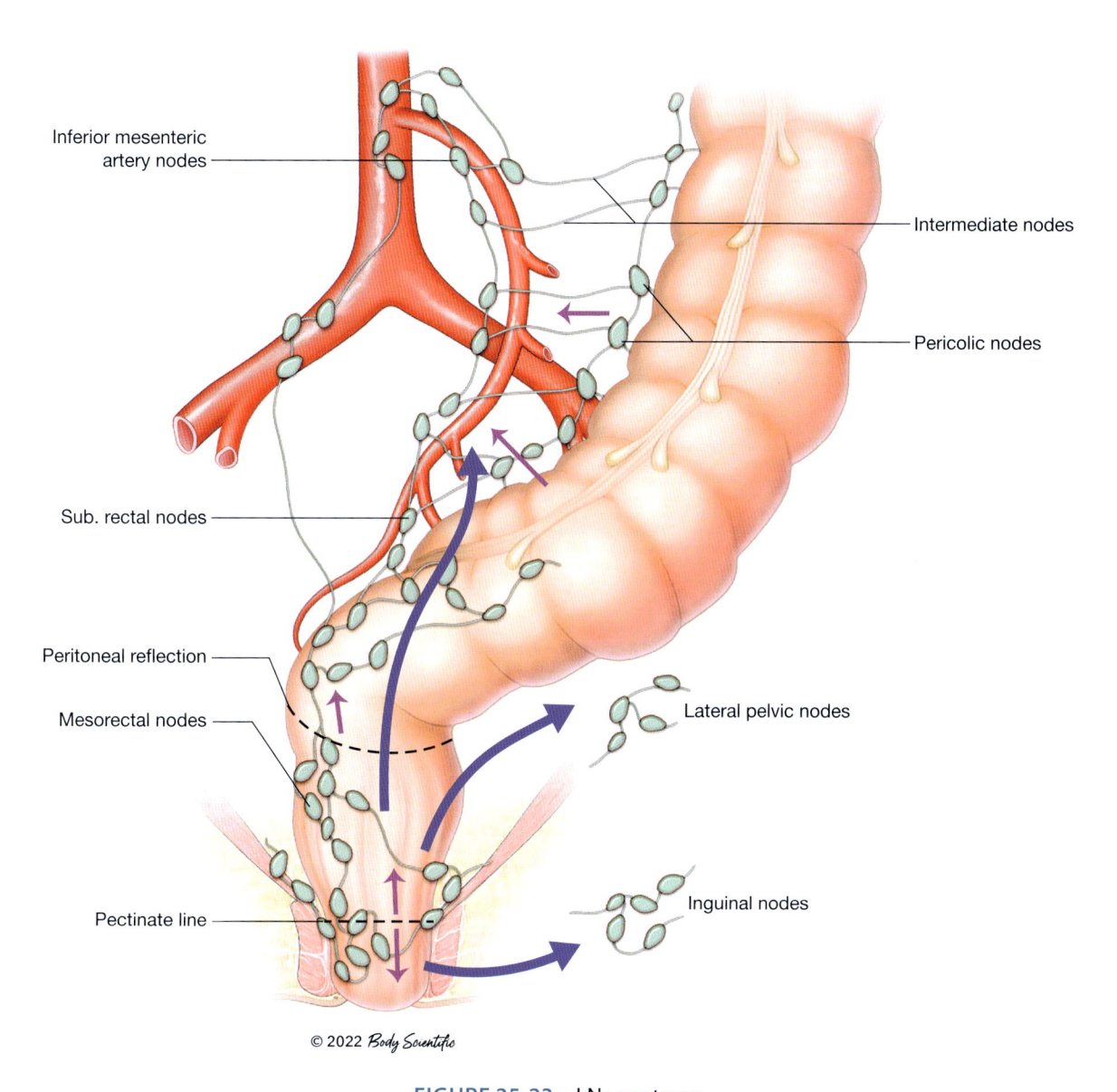

Total Mesorectal Excision for Rectal Cancer 539

FIGURE 25-23 • LNs anatomy.

Step 3. Anterior and anterolateral dissection

The anterior dissection changes if the patient is female or male. The reflection of the Douglas (recto-uterine pouch), in women, or the recto-vesical pouch, in men, has to be incised. In men, the dissection proceeds entering below the prostate: the Denonvilliers' fascia (recto-prostatic fascia) (**Figure 25-24**) is usually left untouched (anteriorly); only in anterior/advanced cancers does it have to be removed for a better oncological radicality. This plane in front of the Denonvilliers' fascia is more difficult and vascularized; also, it is riskier for neurological damage. In the majority of cases, the Denonvilliers' fascia is left intact.

The main trick of the step is to put in tension the dissection plane: in females, by retracting with R3 the uterus and by stretching the vaginal–rectum septum; whereas, in males, by pushing the prostate up and forward with the R3.

The surgeon's left hand with a Cadière/bipolar forceps is making downward countertraction of the rectum.

This traction (R3) and countertraction (surgeon's nondominant hand) are opening the space for the dissection.

The first few centimeters are not difficult. The peritoneum is incised, then with R3 by lifting up the anterior prostate or the vaginal–rectum septum, and subsequently going distally toward the pelvic floor.

After a clear exposure of the seminal vesicles in their medial portion, the dissection proceeds laterally. The lateral corner of the seminal vesicles is the most dangerous area for neural injuries: as this area is reached, the dissection has to change direction going downward/more vertically (because laterally there are autonomic branches for sexual innervation) (**Figures 25-25 A, B**).

If the posterior and posterolateral dissection areas have been well prepared in the earlier steps, then the 2 planes will be joined easily.

Step 3 average time frame: 20–30 min

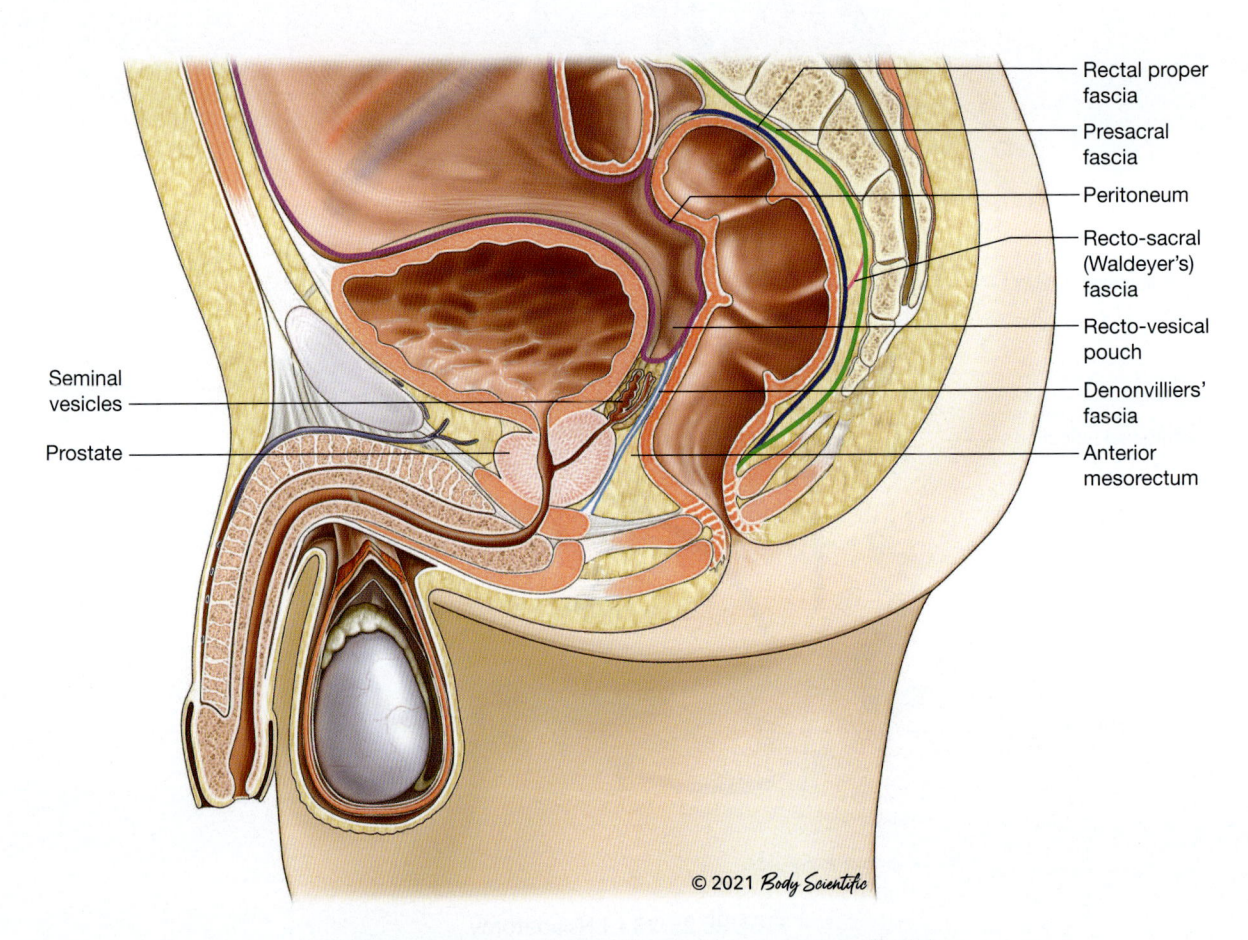

FIGURE 25-24 • Denonvilliers' fascia (recto-prostatic fascia).

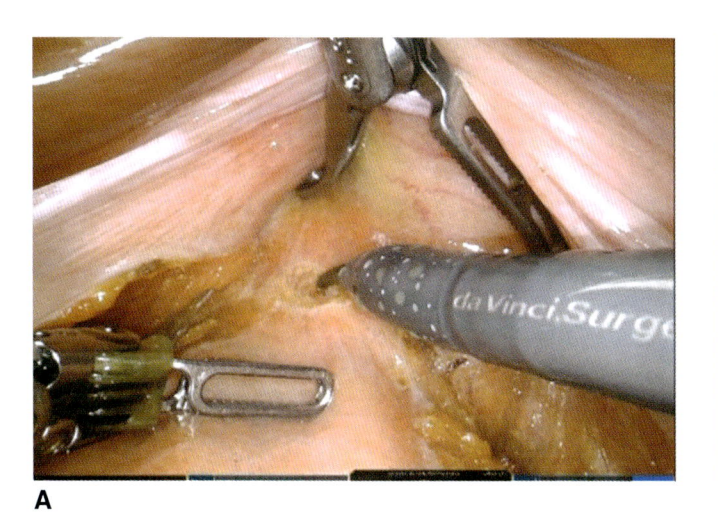

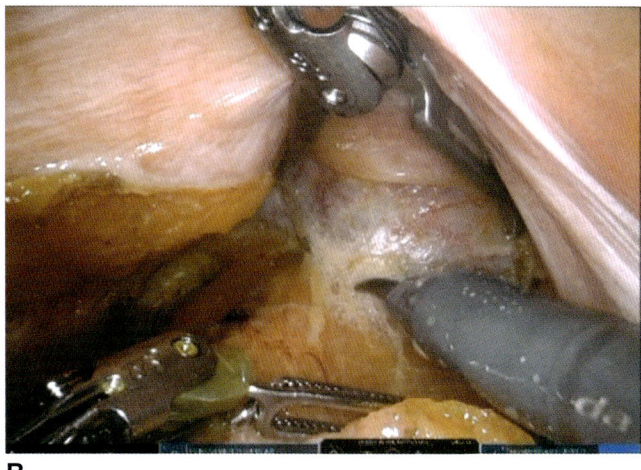

Total Mesorectal Excision for Rectal Cancer   541

FIGURE 25-25 • Anterior side dissection of rectum. **A.** Traction method. **B.** Preservation of neurovascular bundles.

Step 4. Circular concentric dissection (cylinder) of the distal mesorectum

After passing the seminal vesicles and the middle hemorrhoidal vessels, with the posterior dissection already performed, the rectum and the mesorectum become vertical. This is a concentric/circular dissection, while keeping the cylinder of the mesorectum intact, until the pelvic floor. No portion of the mesorectum should be left behind, despite the narrowing of the surgical space. The fascia, distally, is not so well represented as in the upper mesorectum. Hence, it is easier to get confused. The more dissection is carried out posteriorly, the easier the verticalization of rectum and mesorectum will be. Depending on the cancer location, the dissection has to be performed up to the anal canal, or the internal sphincter may be detached from pelvic floor muscles (**Figure 25-26**) for the intersphincteric resection.

Step 4 average time frame: 15–30 min

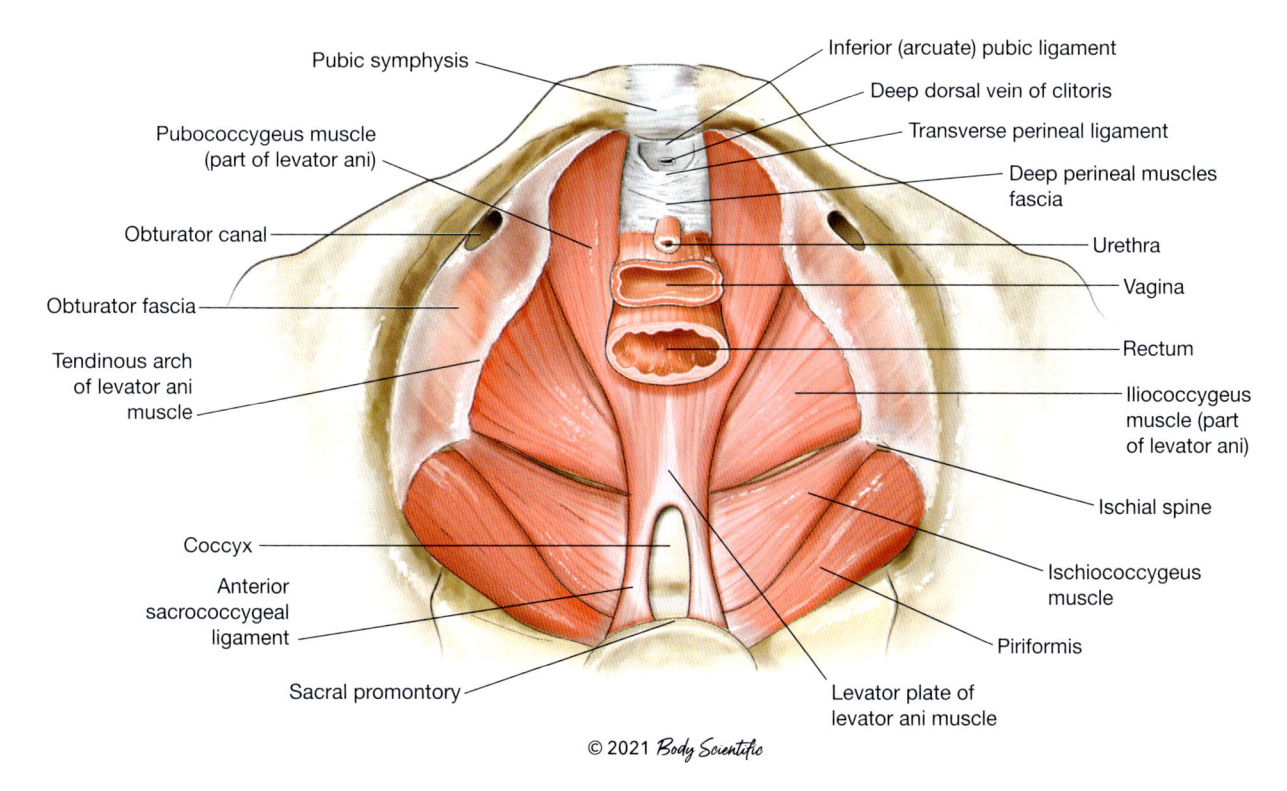

FIGURE 25-26 • Pelvic floor muscles.

⚠ PITFALLS

During the distal mesorectal dissection, getting too close to the rectal wall (mainly lateral and posteriorly) and compromising the radicality of the TME. Instead of a cylinder, the dissection takes the shape of a cone.

▸▸ TIPS

A very useful technique developed by Kyungpook National University for deep posterior dissection of the rectum is to use a tip-up fenestrated grasper in R3 to lift up the mesorectum and to provide clear surgical field between the rectum and sacrum (**Figure 25-27**). This maneuver enables the surgeon to use both hands to facilitate fine dissection around the last part of the rectum, even to be able to enter into the intersphincteric space (**Figures 25-28 A, B**).

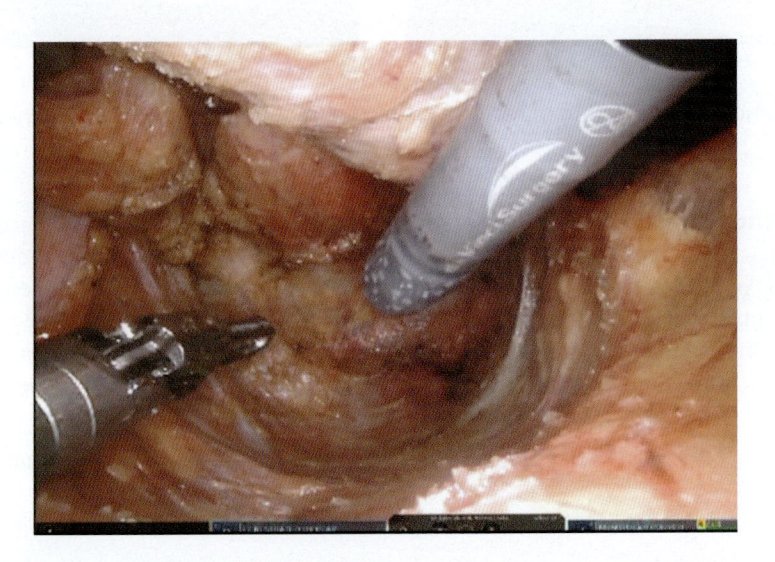

FIGURE 25-27 • Use of a tip-up fenestrated gasper for deep posterior dissection.

A

B

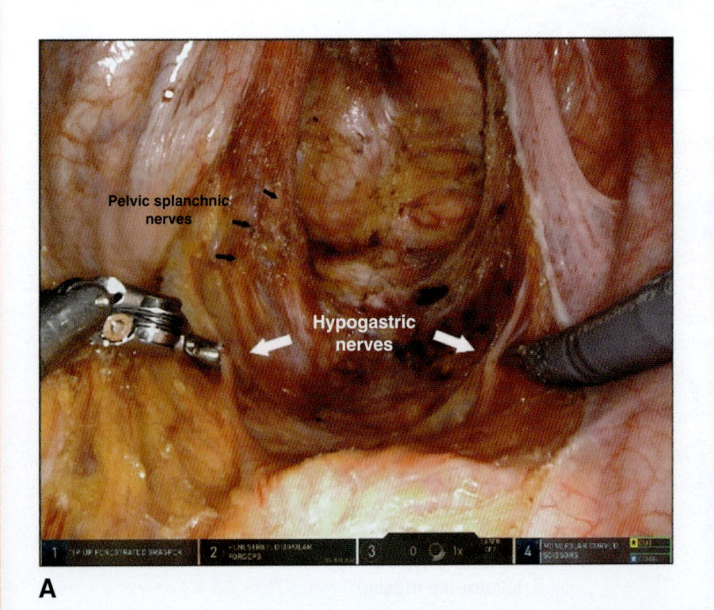

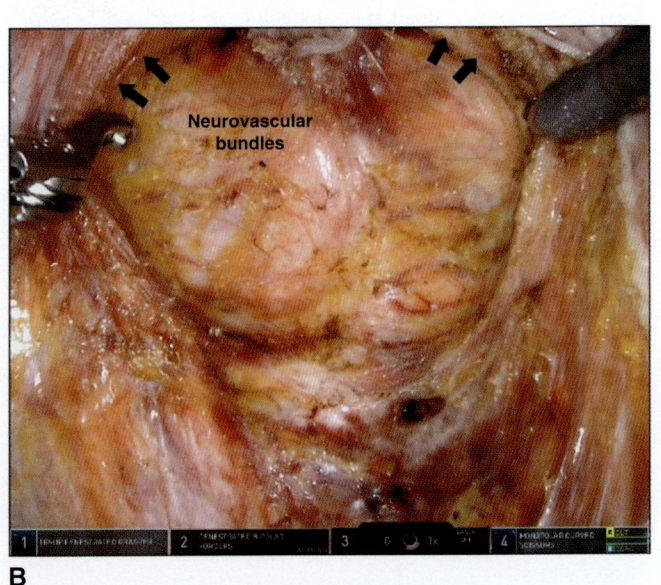

FIGURE 25-28 • Pelvic view after completion of TME. **A.** Whole pelvis. **B.** Lower pelvis.

Step 5. Division of the distal rectum

Improved technology in robotic stapling has made it easier to cut and anastomose the lower rectum. However, the double stapling technique, developed by Griffin and Knight decades ago, has not basically changed. When the rectum is sufficiently mobilized below the tumor and clamped distally to the tumor with a detachable clamp or tip-up fenestrated grasper, the distal rectal stump can be washed out with betadine solution through the anus (**Figure 25-29A**). A robotic linear stapler, engaged in R1, is introduced through the right lower quadrant trocar to divide the rectum (**Figure 25-29B**). In most cases, a stapler of 60 mm is sufficient, but sometimes, when additional cartridges are needed, cutting only two-thirds of the rectum might be an option, so that with the next stapling becomes easier to complete a perpendicular transection, and this allows a "crossing point" of staple lines positioned at the center of the rectal stump, which will be taken out by the final circular stapler (**Figure 25-29 C**).

Step 5 average time frame: 10–15 min

> ⚠️ **PITFALLS**
>
> Creating too many overlapping staple lines. Ideally 1–2 loads should be used to divide the lower rectum (because distally, it is smaller in diameter).

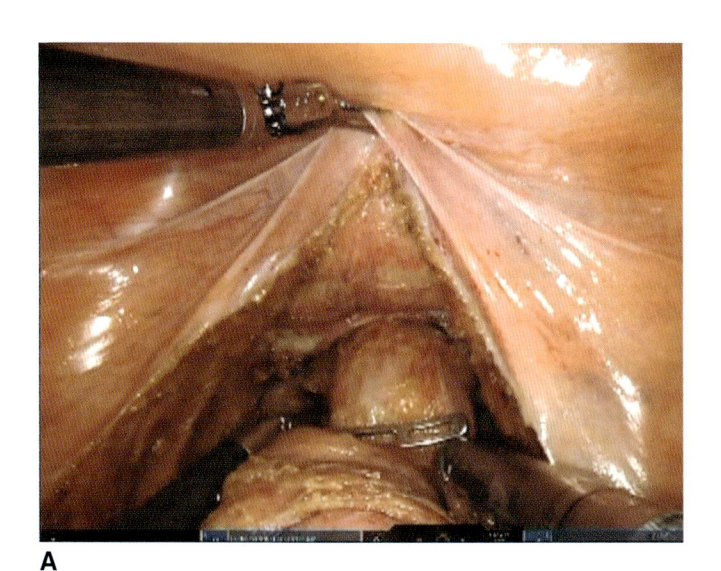

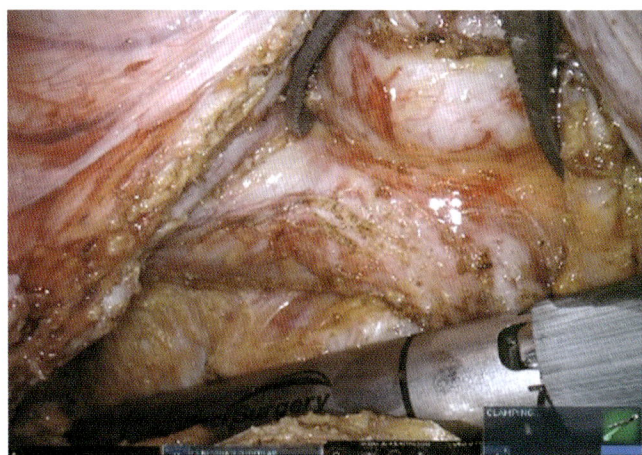

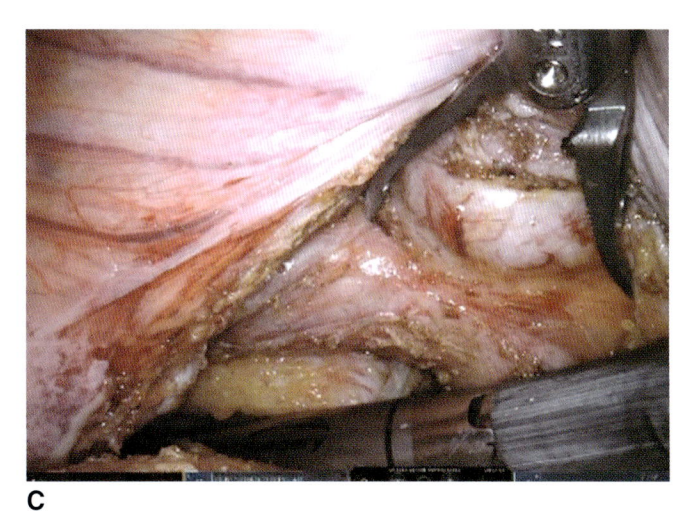

FIGURE 25-29 • **A.** Rectal washing. Introducing the first (**B**) and the second robotic linear staplers (**C**).

Step 6. Proximal colon preparation

Once the distal rectum is divided, the preparation of the proximal colon transection line starts.

Some surgeons perform this step exteriorizing the specimen and the proximal colon through the extraction wound, but it is better done inside the abdomen under direct robotic visualization.

In this way, there is a better evaluation of the lymphatic pedicles (part of the oncological dissection) and a superior understanding of the proper length of the proximal colon. Also, ICG microperfusion is assessed before dividing the colon to be sure that the blood supply is optimal (see Chapter 24).

The stump of the IMA is retracted down and medially, and the mesentery of the distal descending colon is divided with the vessel sealer (or stapler) staying lateral to the IMA stump and being sure to maintain a good mesenteric lymph nodal flap on the specimen side.

The colon, at the selected transection site, is then divided with a stapler.

Step 6 average time frame: 15–20 min

Step 7. Specimen extraction

The extraction site is usually a small incision in the right lower quadrant, especially if a diverting ileostomy is planned or a single access device was already placed in that location.

A wound protector is applied into the incision. The specimen is retrieved and the proximal colon is exteriorized.

The anvil of the circular stapler is inserted into the proximal colon stump (see Chapter 24 for more details), and the colon is then placed again inside the abdominal cavity. The pneumoperitoneum is restored closing the wound protector.

Step 7 average time frame: 15–20 min

> **EDITORIAL COMMENT**
>
> If there is no plan for ileostomy or other reason to place the extraction site in the right lower quadrant, the Pfannenstiel incision is a good alternative. The robotic cart could be partially undocked to make the access. The incidence of incisional hernias here is much lower.

Step 8. Colorectal/coloanal anastomosis

The robot is not undocked until the colorectal anastomosis is completed. It may be useful to have a correct evaluation of the tension and orientation of the proximal colon mesentery. In selected cases, with favorable pelvic anatomy, some reinforcing stitches can also be applied to the anastomotic corner of the Knight Griffin. The shaft of the stapler is carefully inserted transanally after gentle anal dilation. The correct position of the hinge is verified before going through the rectal stump, engaging the anvil, and firing the staples. The integrity of the anastomotic rings should be verified, and a final check should be performed with an air leak test or colonoscopy. In patients with very low tumors after an intersphincteric resection, a handsewn side-to-end coloanal external anastomosis is performed. A diverting ileostomy is created or omitted on an individual basis (local and general conditions/surgeon preference). A pelvic drainage is usually omitted.

Step 8 average time frame: 10–20 min

> **⚠ PITFALLS**
>
> Incorrect positioning and centering of the hinge of the circular stapler increases the risk of leaks.

SP Robotic Rectal Cancer (Off-Label Indication)

Port Placement and Robotic Docking

A 4-cm transverse incision is made in the right lower quadrant, and a Uniport™ (Dalim, Korea) containing a 25-mm multichannel SP trocar, a 12-mm assistant port, and two 5-mm assistant ports are introduced. An additional 5-mm assistant port is placed in the right upper quadrant (**Figure 25-30**).

The robotic system approaches from the left side of the patient (**Figure 25-31A**). The camera is placed in the down-up mode, and da Vinci SP monopolar curved scissors, SP fenestrated bipolar forceps, and an SP round tooth retractor are engaged into SP trocar in counterclockwise order. To deploy the robotic instruments in the working space, the tip of the cannula of the SP system should be suspended in the air (floating docking) (**Figure 25-31B**). Therefore, the tip of the cannula, and the abdominal incision, must be taped to seal the abdominal cavity and allow insufflation of CO_2 gas via the plastic wound retractor using a Uniport. The assistant is positioned on the right side of the patient, and 2 ports are used for suctioning and for additional retraction.

Because the SP system does not have a vessel sealer, the assistant has to insert Hem-o-lok™ clips and/or control vessels using a laparoscopic vessel sealer (**Figure 25-32**). Full mobilization of the left colon and splenic flexure is performed robotically (**Figure 25-33**). Thereafter, the surgeon uses the relocate pedal to move the 3 instruments and the camera, as a single unit, toward the pelvis.

SP system

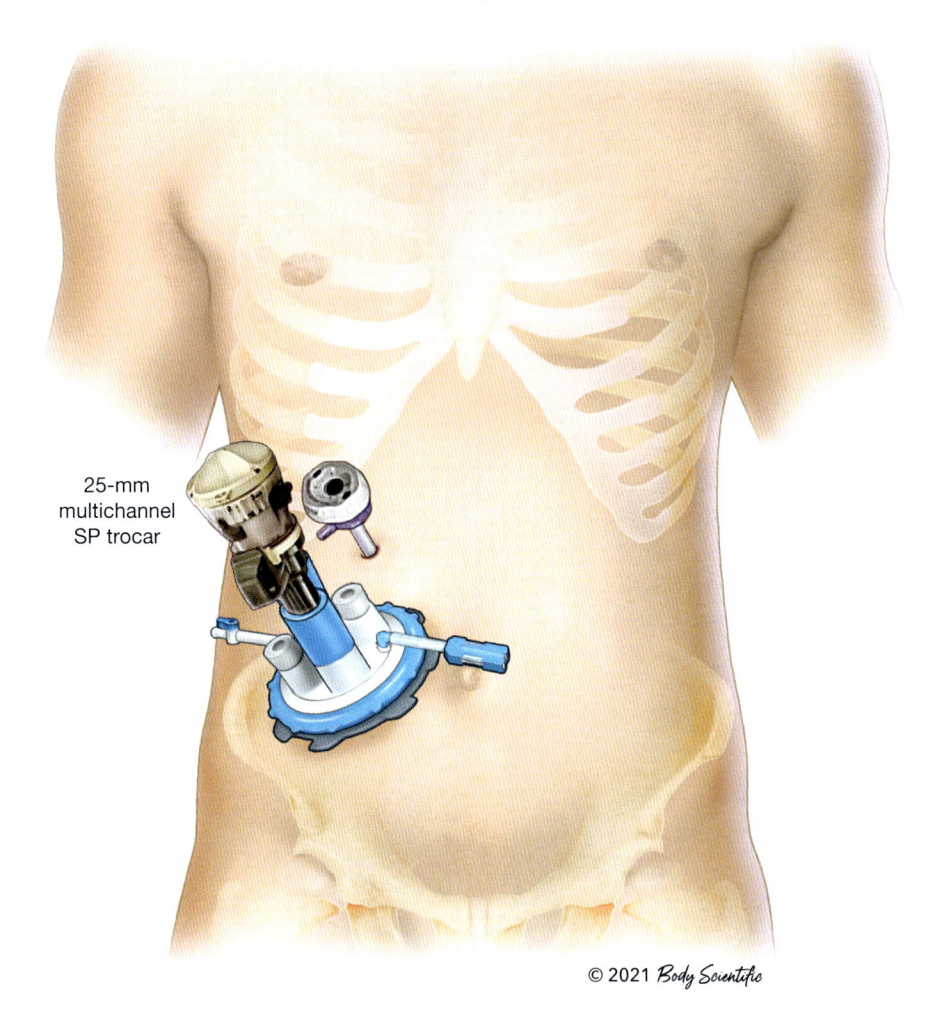

FIGURE 25-30 • Port setup in SP system.

546 The Foundation and Art of Robotic Surgery

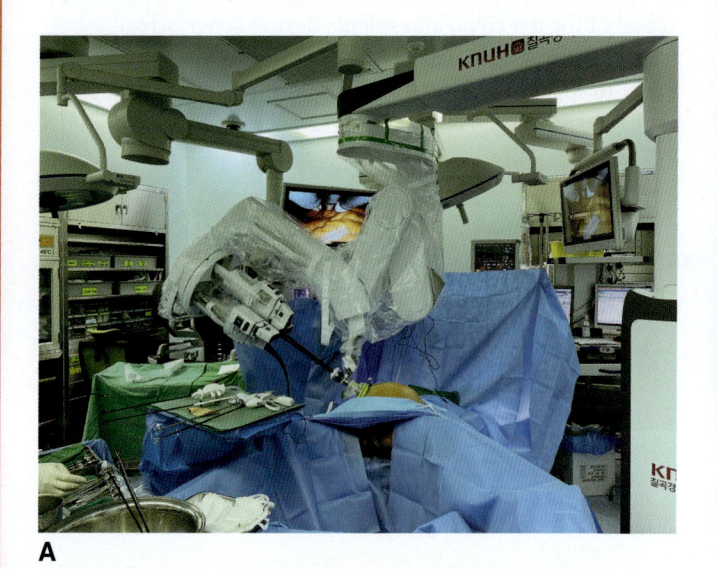

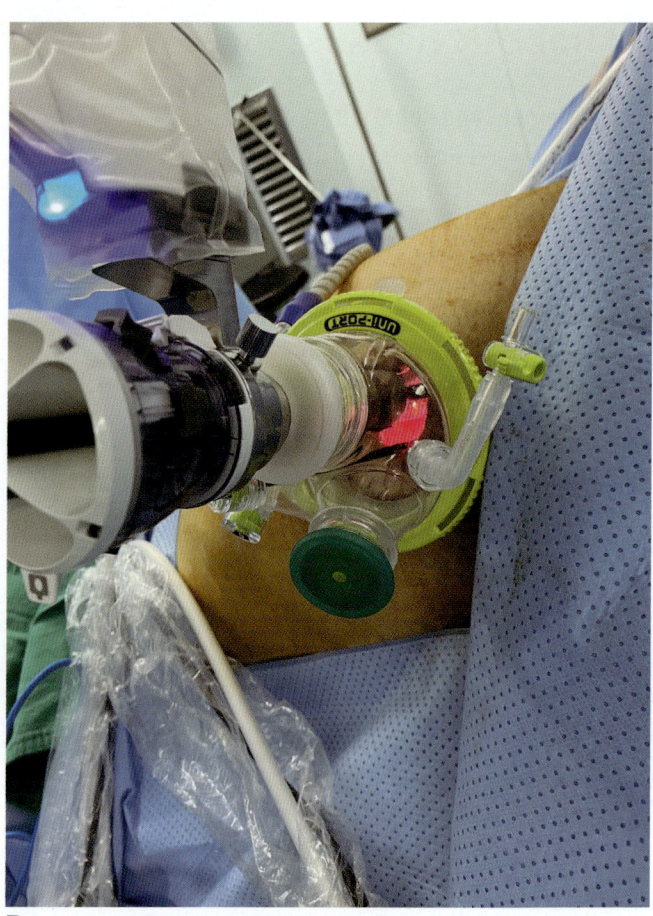

FIGURE 25-31 • SP robotic system docking. **A.** Location of the SP cannula. **B.** Ligation of the inferior mesenteric vessels and mobilization of the left colon.

Total Mesorectal Excision and Anastomosis

The rectum is mobilized using the monopolar cautery scissors by dissecting through the avascular plane between the endopelvic fascia to preserve the autonomic nerves (**Figure 25-34A**). SP monopolar curved scissors and fenestrated bipolar forceps are used for fine dissection and retraction, respectively. Additionally, an SP round tooth retractor is used for suspension of the rectum, simultaneously pushing the pelvic structures in different directions. It is particularly useful for retracting the prostate or the vagina, when dissecting the anterior side

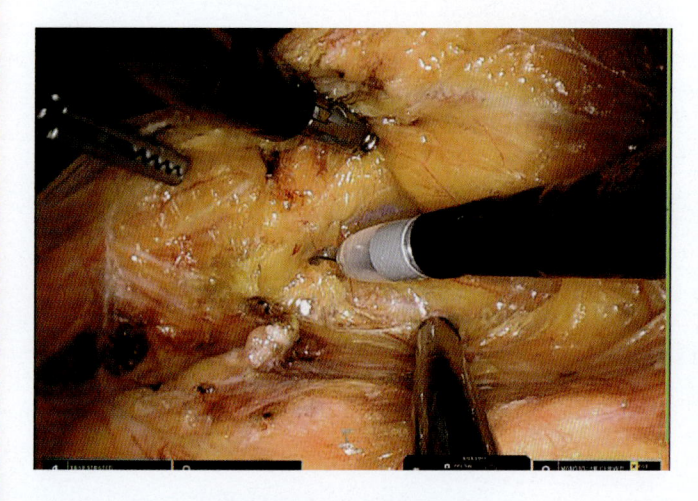

FIGURE 25-32 • IMA ligation.

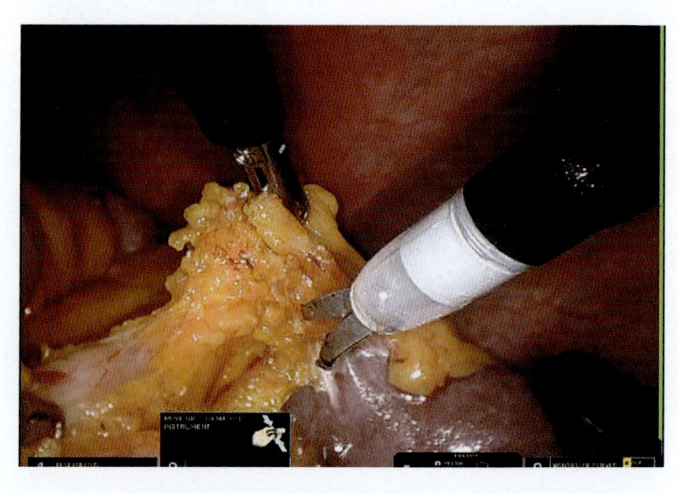

FIGURE 25-33 • Splenic flexure mobilization.

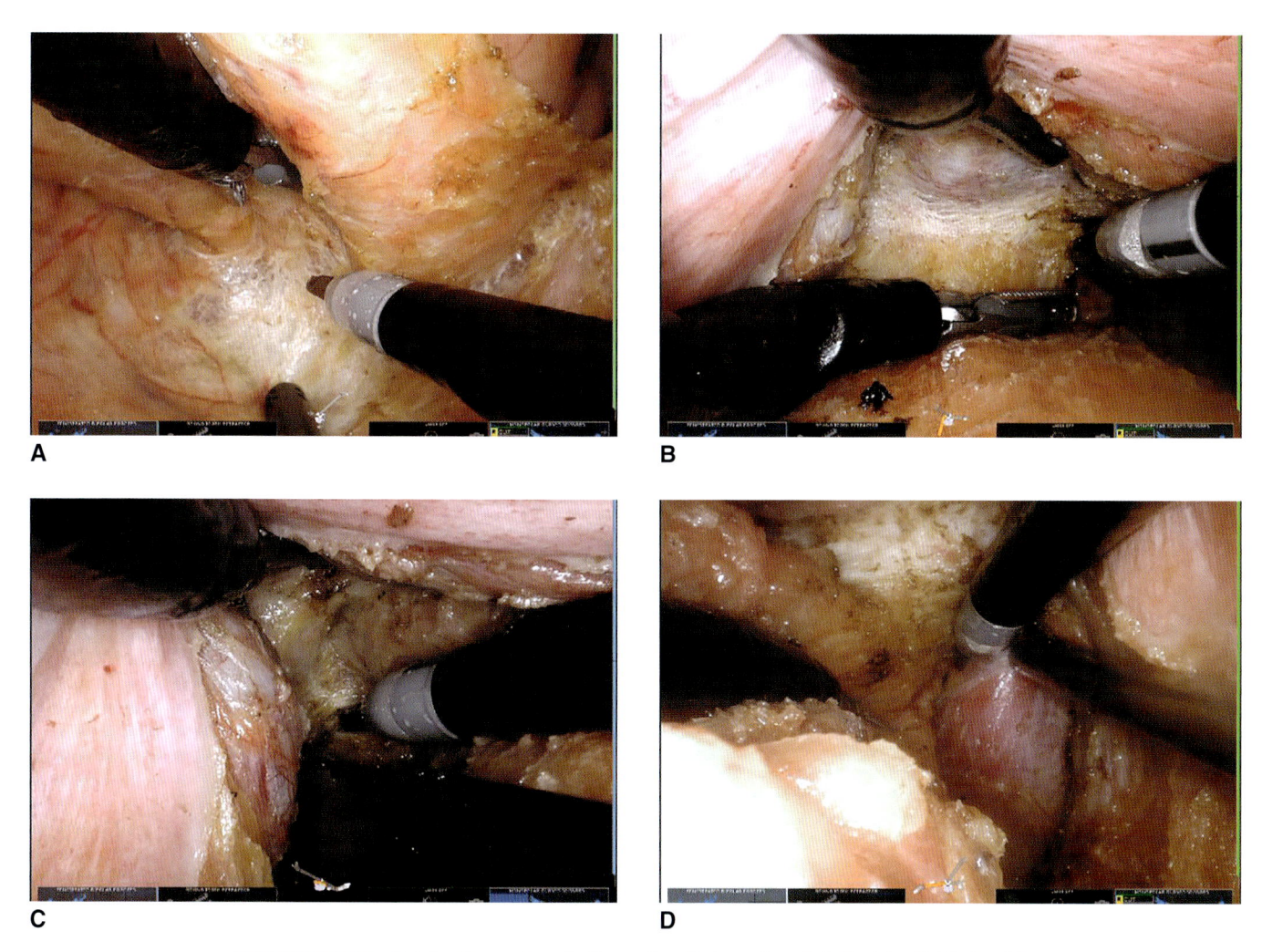

FIGURE 25-34 • Pelvic dissection. **A.** Posterior. **B.** Anterior. **C.** Left side. **D.** Right side.

of the rectum (**Figure 25-34B**). An assistant retracts the entire rectum using the right upper quadrant laparoscopic port and performs suction using the 5-mm port of the Uniport while sharing the SP port. After complete dissection of the mesorectum (**Figures 25-34 C, D**), the rectum is transected using a laparoscopic Endo-linear stapler through a 12-mm port inserted into the Uniport™ access.

The specimen is extracted through the 4-cm minilaparotomy, used for the SP trocar insertion. An intracorporeal end-to-end anastomosis is created using a circular stapler. In patients with very low tumors, intersphincteric resection and handsewn side-to-end coloanal anastomosis are performed. A pelvic drain is occasionally placed, and a protective ileostomy is created in the right lower quadrant, with the same incision, as per the surgeon's discretion (**Figure 25-35**).

EDITORIAL COMMENT

In the standard Western population with larger BMI and narrow/deep pelvis, the anterior retraction of the mesorectum and prostate or vagina could be very challenging with the Sp system. The situation may require a multiport assistance.

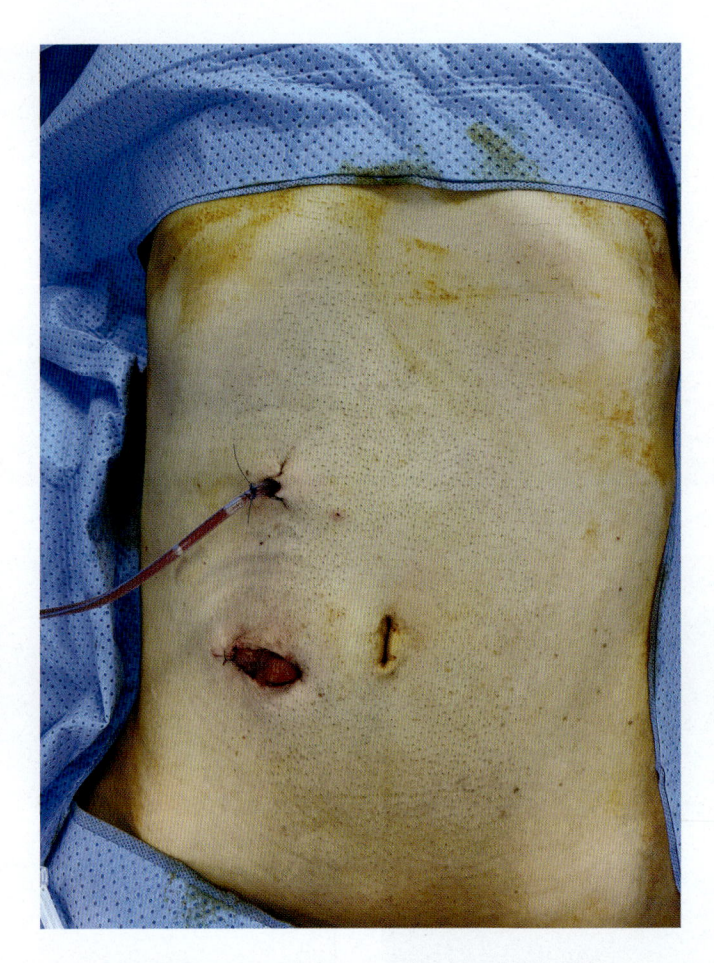

FIGURE 25-35 • Abdomen after SP robotic TME.

Suggested Readings

1. Park JS, Choi GS, Lim KH, Jang YS, Jun SH. Robotic-assisted versus laparoscopic surgery for low rectal cancer: case-matched analysis of short-term outcomes. *Ann Surg Oncol.* 2010;17(12):3195-3202.
2. Park JS, Choi GS, Lim KH, Jang YS, Jun SH. S052: A comparison of robot-assisted, laparoscopic, and open surgery in the treatment of rectal cancer. *Surg Endosc.* 2011;25(1):240-248.
3. Kim HJ, Choi GS, Park JS, Park SY. Multidimensional analysis of the learning curve for robotic total mesorectal excision for rectal cancer: lessons from a single surgeon's experience. *Dis Colon Rectum* 2014;57(9):1066-1074.
4. Park SY, Choi GS, Park JS, Kim HJ, Ryuk JP. Short-term clinical outcome of robot-assisted intersphincteric resection for low rectal cancer: a retrospective comparison with conventional laparoscopy. *Surg Endosc.* 2013;27(1):48-55.
5. Kim JY, Kim NK, Lee KY, Hur H, Min BS, Kim JH. A comparative study of voiding and sexual function after total mesorectal excision with autonomic nerve preservation for rectal cancer: laparoscopic versus robotic surgery. *Ann Surg Oncol.* 2012;19(8):2485-2493.
6. Park EJ, Kim CW, Cho MS, et al. Multidimensional analyses of the learning curve of robotic low anterior resection for rectal cancer: 3-phase learning process comparison. *Surg Endosc.* 2014;28(10):2821-2831.
7. Hellan M, Anderson C, Ellenhorn JD, Paz B, Pigazzi A. Short-term outcomes after robotic-assisted total mesorectal excision for rectal cancer. *Ann Surg Oncol.* 2007;14(11):3168-3173.
8. Pigazzi A, Luca F, Patriti A, et al. Multicentric study on robotic tumor-specific mesorectal excision for the treatment of rectal cancer. *Ann Surg Oncol.* 2010;17(6):1614-1620.
9. deSouza AL, Prasad LM, Marecik SJ, et al. Total mesorectal excision for rectal cancer: the potential advantage of robotic assistance. *Dis Colon Rectum* 2010;53(12):1611-1617.
10. Kang J, Min BS, Park YA, et al. Risk factor analysis of postoperative complications after robotic rectal cancer surgery. *World J Surg.* 2011;35(11):2555-2562.
11. Yang Y, Wang F, Zhang P, et al. Robot-assisted versus conventional laparoscopic surgery for colorectal disease, focusing on rectal cancer: a meta-analysis. *Ann Surg Oncol.* 2012;19(12):3727-2736.
12. Trastulli S, Farinella E, Cirocchi R, et al. Robotic resection compared with laparoscopic rectal resection for cancer: systematic review and meta-analysis of short-term outcome. *Colorectal Dis.* 2012;14(4):e134-156.
13. Mak TW, Lee JF, Futaba K, Hon SS, Ngo DK, Ng SS. Robotic surgery for rectal cancer: a systematic review of current practice. *World J Gastrointest Oncol.* 2014;6(6):184-193.
14. Memon S, Heriot AG, Murphy DG, Bressel M, Lynch AC. Robotic versus laparoscopic proctectomy for rectal cancer: a meta-analysis. *Ann Surg Oncol.* 2012;19(7):2095-2101.

15. Luca F, Valvo M, Ghezzi TL, et al. Impact of robotic surgery on sexual and urinary functions after fully robotic nerve-sparing total mesorectal excision for rectal cancer. *Ann Surg*. 2013;257(4):672-678.
16. Baik SH, Kim NK, Lim DR, Hur H, Min BS, Lee KY. Oncologic outcomes and perioperative clinicopathologic results after robot-assisted tumor-specific mesorectal excision for rectal cancer. *Ann Surg Oncol*. 2013;20(8):2625-2632.
17. Kim HJ, Choi GS, Park JS, Park SY, Yang CS, Lee HJ. The impact of robotic surgery on quality of life, urinary and sexual function following total mesorectal excision for rectal cancer: a propensity score-matched analysis with laparoscopic surgery. *Colorectal Dis*. 2018;20(5):O103-O113. doi: 10.1111/codi.14051
18. Jayne D, Pigazzi A, Marshall H, et al. Effect of robotic-assisted vs conventional laparoscopic surgery on risk of conversion to open laparotomy among patients undergoing resection for rectal cancer: the ROLARR randomized clinical trial. *JAMA*. 2017;318(16):1569-1580. doi: 10.1001/jama.2017.7219
19. Kim J, Baek SJ, Kang DW, et al. Robotic resection is a good prognostic factor in rectal cancer compared with laparoscopic resection: Long-term survival analysis using propensity score matching. *Dis Colon Rectum*. 2017;60(3):266-273. doi: 10.1097/DCR.0000000000000770
20. Kim HJ, Choi GS. Robot-assisted multiport tme with low colorectal anastomosis. In: Dapri G, Marks J (eds). *Surgical Techniques in Rectal Cancer*. Tokyo: Springer; 2018. doi: 10.1007/978-4-431-55579-7_13
21. Mangano A, Valle V, Fernandes E, Bustos R, Gheza F, Giulianotti PC. Operative technique in robotic rectal resection. *Minerva Chir*. 2019;74(6):501-508. doi: 10.23736/S0026-4733.18.07808-2
22. Mangano A, Gheza F, Chen LL, Minerva EM, Giulianotti PC. Indocyanine green (ICG)-enhanced fluorescence for intraoperative assessment of bowel microperfusion during laparoscopic and robotic colorectal surgery: the quest for evidence-based results. *Surg Technol Int*. 2018;32:101-104.
23. Giulianotti PC, Coratti A, Angelini M, et al. Robotics in general surgery: personal experience in a large community hospital. *Arch Surg*. 2003;138(7):777-784. doi: 10.1001/archsurg.138.7.777
24. Kim HJ, Choi GS, Song SH, et al. An initial experience with a novel technique of single-port robotic resection for rectal cancer. *Tech Coloproctol*. 2021;25(7):857-864. doi: 10.1007/s10151-021-02457-0

"Never cut what you cannot see ... always know what you are going to do next."
— William Ernest Miles (1869–1947)

Abdominoperineal Resection

Gerald Gantt • Alberto Mangano • Vivek Chaudhry • Anders F. Mellgren

INTRODUCTION

The management of rectal carcinoma has considerably evolved over time. It shifted from a defunctioning colostomy strategy (for palliation) during the 18th century to the current minimally invasive surgery (MIS) radical operations.

In 1908, Sir W.E. Miles, well aware of the issue of local relapse, paved the way for the existing rectal cancer surgery, publishing the abdominoperineal resection (APR) technique. After that, for a long time, the APR has been the gold standard for most cancers of the rectum. Later, much evidence has shown that, from a pathological standpoint, the lymphatic spreading occurs mostly cranially. This made possible the development of the "sphincter-sparing paradigm," which does not worsen the oncologic outcomes.

Over the last few decades, the indications for APR have become less and less frequent. This is partly due to the increasingly more numerous therapeutic options available, including sphincter preservation techniques, total mesorectal excision (TME), low anterior resections (LARs), neoadjuvant and multimodal therapies, and the advancements in MIS.

For low rectal cancers, the distal resection margin (DRM) required for curative intent is constantly decreasing: the previous dogmatic DRM of 5 cm has shifted to 1 cm or less (in the TME context with multimodal therapy). The neoadjuvant therapies have allowed better locoregional control, as well as downstaging/downsizing. Currently, the sphincter-preserving strategy is possible in most cases. Moreover, the evolution of

INSTRUMENT REQUIREMENTS (INTRABDOMINAL PHASE)

The suggested main robotic instruments/tools can be listed as follows:
- 30°, 0° scope
- Monopolar scissors/cautery hook
- Vessel sealer
- Robotic linear staplers (with different loads)
- Needle drivers (round tip or macro)
- Multiple Hem-o-lok™/clips
- Medium/large clip applier
- Bipolar forceps
- Cadière Forceps/tip-up fenestrated grasper

The suggested main laparoscopic instruments/tools can be listed as follows:
- Needle drivers
- Scissors
- Graspers
- Staplers (linear)
- Suction-irrigation
- Fan retractor (optional)

Supplemental materials:
- Gauzes, sponges
- Vessel loops
- Medium–large clips
- Sutures: Prolene™ 2-0, 3-0, 4-0, and PDS™ 3-0

Photo reproduced with permission from Campos FG. The life and legacy of William Ernest Miles (1869-1947): a tribute to an admirable surgeon. Rev Assoc Med Bras (1992). 2013;59(2):181-185.

Quote reproduced with permission from Campos FG. The life and legacy of William Ernest Miles (1869-1947): a tribute to an admirable surgeon. Rev Assoc Med Bras (1992). 2013;59(2):181-185.

the stapling devices, the TME, and MIS have further reduced how often the APR is performed.

The overall survival outcomes for the APR are worse than for the anterior rectal resections. Moreover, the local recurrence rate is higher (see suggested readings #1–4): there are multiple factors, including biases, that have an impact on these paradoxical outcomes.

Multiple approaches for APR have been described. An in-depth discussion of all the technical variations of the abdominoperineal excision goes beyond the aim of this chapter (for more information, see suggested reading #5).

Despite the aforementioned advancements in neoadjuvant/multimodal therapy and the evolution of the surgical technology, a radical resection is still the main therapeutic goal. When the sparing of the sphincter is oncologically and technically impossible, the APR may still be the best option for the cancer treatment. There are 2 distinct phases for the APR procedure:

1. **The intrabdominal phase.** This, traditionally, has been done open. The goals are the abdominal lymphadenectomy, the TME, the pelvic dissection, and the colostomy fashioning. Currently, this part of the procedure is done laparoscopically/robotically in most centers.
2. **The abdominoperineal phase**. The dissection of the pelvic floor is completed from the outside, the specimen is removed, and the defect is closed (sometimes the closure is very complex, and it may require the help of plastic surgeons).

In the past, the classical version of the APR was completely (i.e., both phases) performed in an open way. In the attempt to minimize the trauma of this invasive operation, the abdominal part is currently done in an MIS way. This hybrid approach, composed of laparoscopic (for the intra-abdominal phase) plus open (for the perineal phase) techniques, has become the standard of care.

More recently, the abdominal phase of the APR has been further facilitated and perfected by the adoption, in some centers, of the robotic technique, which has all its well-known advantages in comparison to the classical laparoscopy. However, the procedure still remains hybrid—robotic plus open—and the steps are similar to the traditional laparoscopic approach.

The robotic benefits are particularly evident in the case of a narrow anatomical field (e.g., a narrow pelvis), or when severe adhesions are present. Also, the robotic technique may have a role in helping to achieve a precise surgery, with a faster/safer learning curve and potentially lower conversion rates.

In laparoscopy, some authors prefer the 2-team operative technique, which is performing the perineal phase at the same time as the intra-abdominal steps. In robotics, depending on the type of the robotic platform (Si vs. Xi), the one-team approach, due to the space limitations, is usually the preferred strategy.

Promising data are growing about the robotic approach, and adopting a standardized operative procedure is key in this evidence-based validation process. In this chapter, a standardized dual-phase, hybrid (robotic plus open) technique for APR will be described.

Indications and Relative Contraindications to the Robotic Approach

APR is indicated in the following situations:

1. For rectal cancers involving the sphincteric complex or that cannot be excised with an adequate distal resection margin without compromising the sphincter
2. For anal cancers that are refractory to conservative treatment (e.g., radiation) or are recurrent
3. If there are concerns for fecal incontinence in patients who otherwise could undergo a low colorectal anastomosis
4. In some old/fragile patients, when the lesion cannot be removed even with a Hartmann procedure, and the construction of the coloanal anastomosis, after an intersphincteric resection, may prolong the operation and increase the overall perioperative risk
5. In patients with Crohn's disease with extensive recalcitrant perianal disease

If there is a correct indication for performing an APR, there are no absolute technical contraindications regarding the adoption of the robotic procedure (for the abdominal part). However, the boundaries of what is feasible in a robotic way have to be framed according to the local operative expertise of the surgeons and the surgical team.

Abdominal Phase

Intra-abdominal Phase Surgical Technique

The surgical technique, for the intra-abdominal portion of the APR, is basically similar to the one previously described (see Chapter 25, Total Mesorectal Excision for Rectal Cancer). The important points that should be underlined are:

1. There is no need of splenic flexure mobilization (indeed, if performed, it may increase the risk of prolapse of the colostomy). The APR requires fewer access ports (for the lymphadenectomy and the TME) and only 1 patient positioning for the abdominal phase, and it is faster.
2. The colostomy is permanent; hence, it should be carefully located, with preoperative marking, to allow the construction of a stoma, which must be comfortable for the patient in their everyday activities. The predesigned colostomy site can be used for one of the laparoscopic/robotic ports. There are different techniques to construct a permanent colostomy, but the preparation of an extraperitoneal tunnel may decrease the long-term complications of the stoma.
3. The central lymphadenectomy is similar to lower anterior resection (LAR), with a high ligation of the inferior mesenteric artery, but the left colonic artery is usually spared, and the level of transection of the bowel is at the end of the descending colon.
4. The TME follows the same steps described for the LAR, with particular attention for the more distal portion, to avoid compromising the cylindrical shape of the specimen in order to maintain an adequate distance from the area of the invasive cancer.
5. In a difficult narrow pelvis with bulky distal lesions, the decision when to stop the pelvic dissection of the abdominal phase may be challenging.

> ▶▶ **TIPS**
>
> There are important landmarks that need to be reached before ending the abdominal phase and starting the perineal one:
>
> 1. In males, the **prostate.** This is the landmark for the anterior dissection. The more progress that is made posteriorly to the prostate, in the Denonvilliers septum, the easier it will be to join the 2 surgical lines from the perineal and abdominal side, decreasing the risk of false planes and injuries to the urethra. Once the prostate is overcome, the perineal phase can be started.
>
> In females, the **rectovaginal septum** should be followed as much as possible, if there is no invasion of the vagina and the need of its partial resection.
>
> 2. The **coccyx.** This is the landmark for the posterior dissection both in male and female patients. Once the vertical component of the TME is completed, it is not too difficult to understand where the horizontal muscles of the pelvic floor start. The abdominal dissection, after reaching the coccyx, may be stopped, and the perineal part can be started. In fact, the coccyx is also a very important landmark during the perineal phase.

The patient positioning, trocar placement, and OR setup for the intrabdominal phase of the procedure are described in **Figures 26-1**, **26-2**, and **26-3**, respectively.

A few reminders of the anatomical key points are described in **Figures 26-4 A, B** and **26-5**.

> **EDITORIAL COMMENT**
>
> The lymphatic spread of low rectal cancer is following the same pathways described in the LAR chapter (see Chapter 25, Total Mesorectal Excision for Rectal Cancer), but it is important to remember that, in some tumors, like the squamocellular carcinomas of the anus, the inguinal nodes are a possible site of metastatic spread.

554   The Foundation and Art of Robotic Surgery

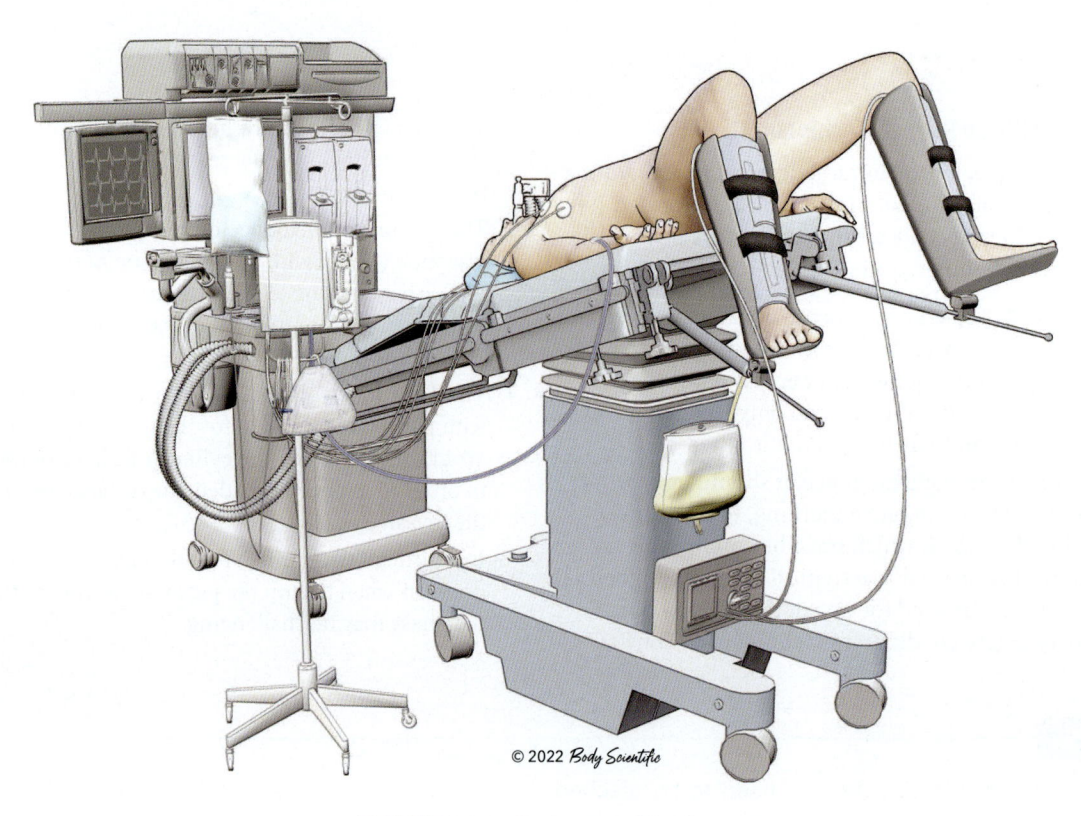

FIGURE 26-1 • Patient positioning.

Normal abdomen

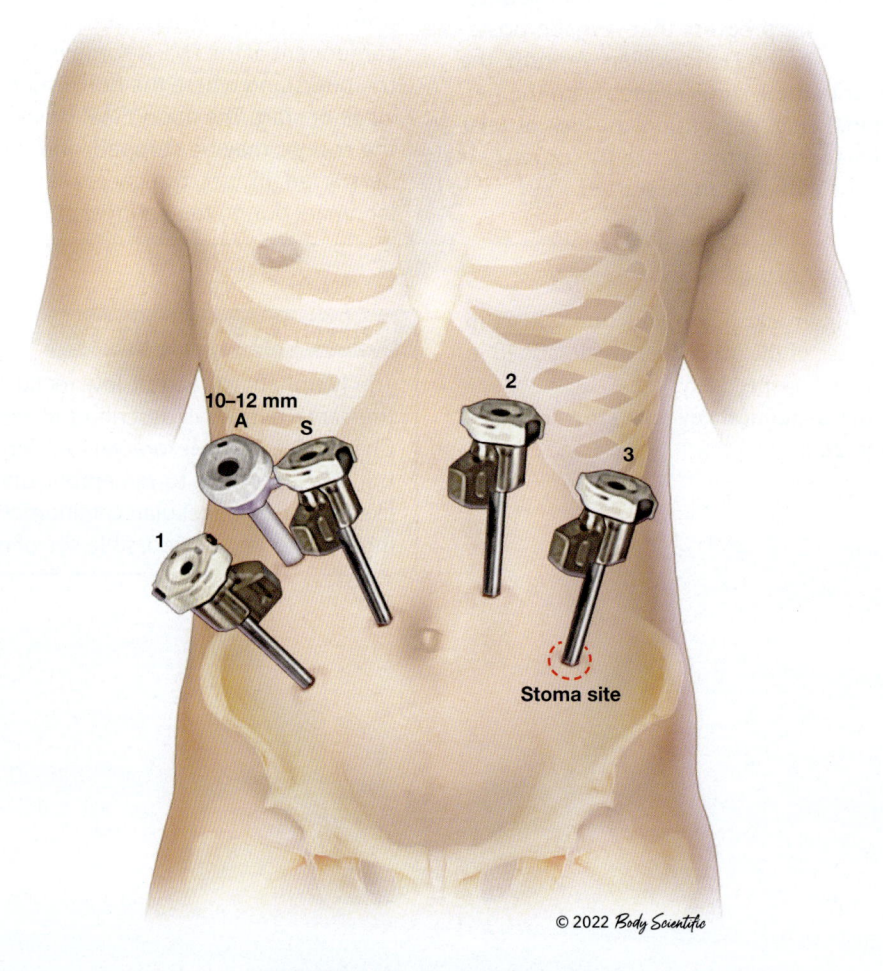

FIGURE 26-2 • Trocar placement.

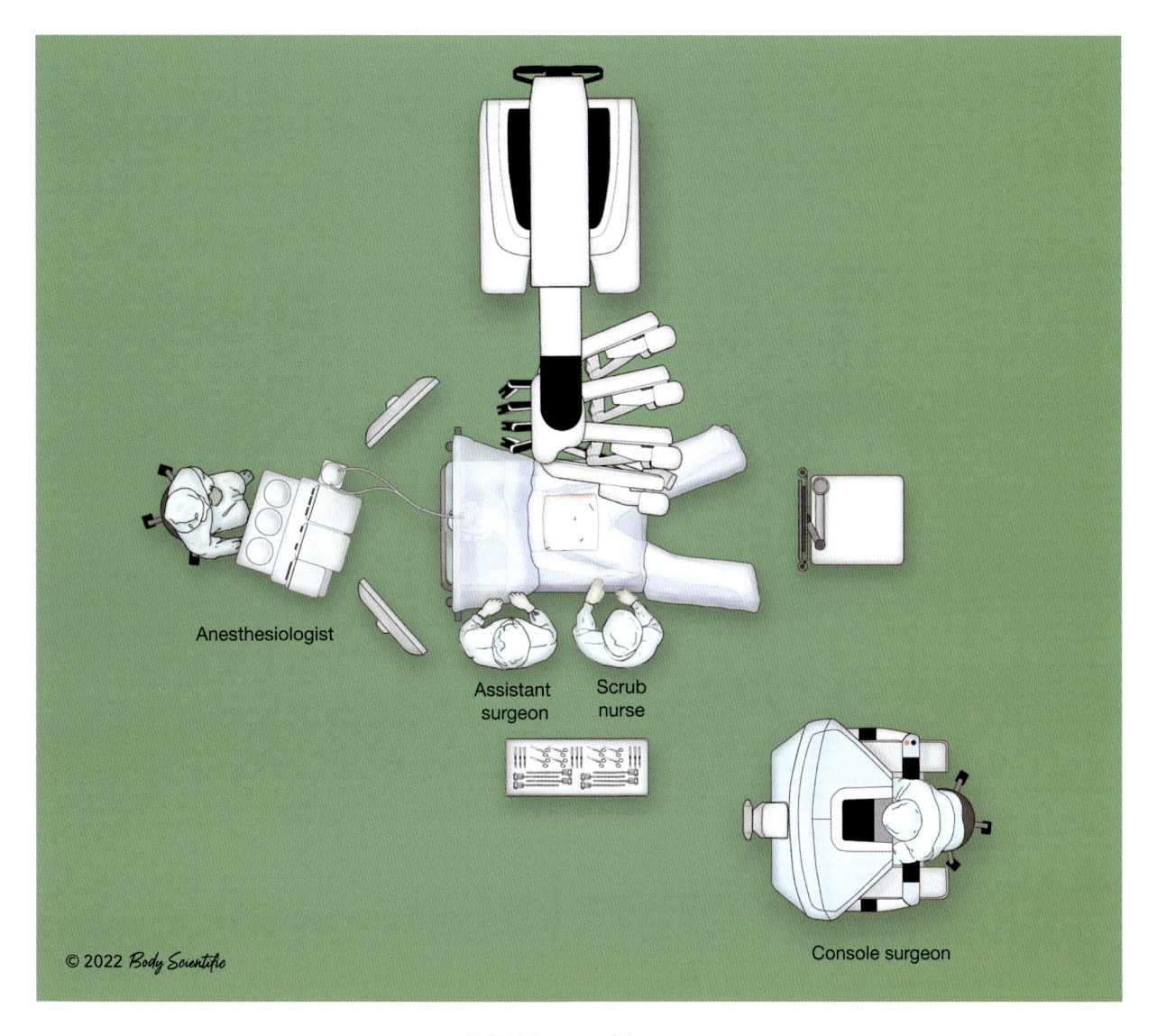

FIGURE 26-3 • OR setup.

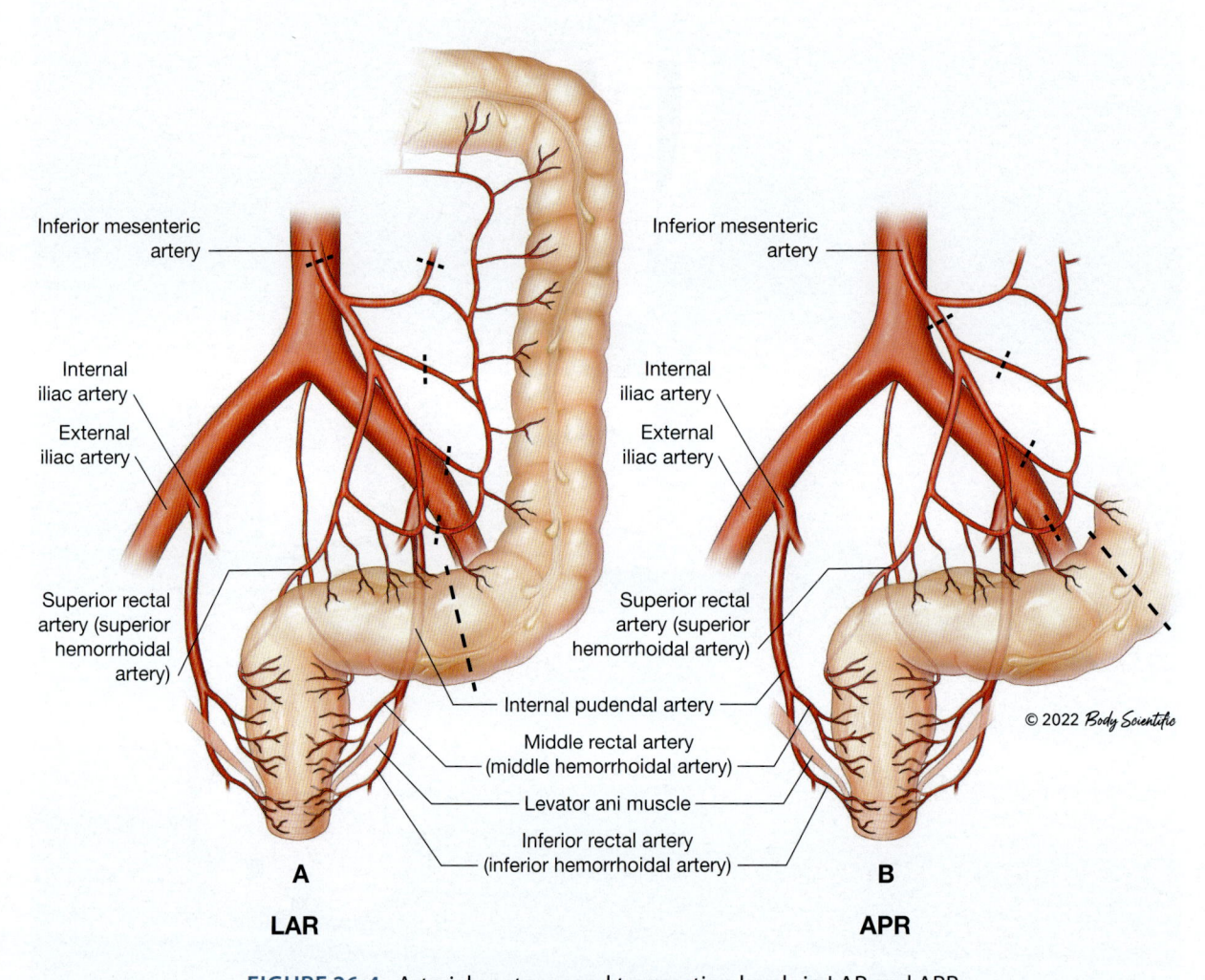

FIGURE 26-4 • Arterial anatomy and transection levels in LAR and APR.

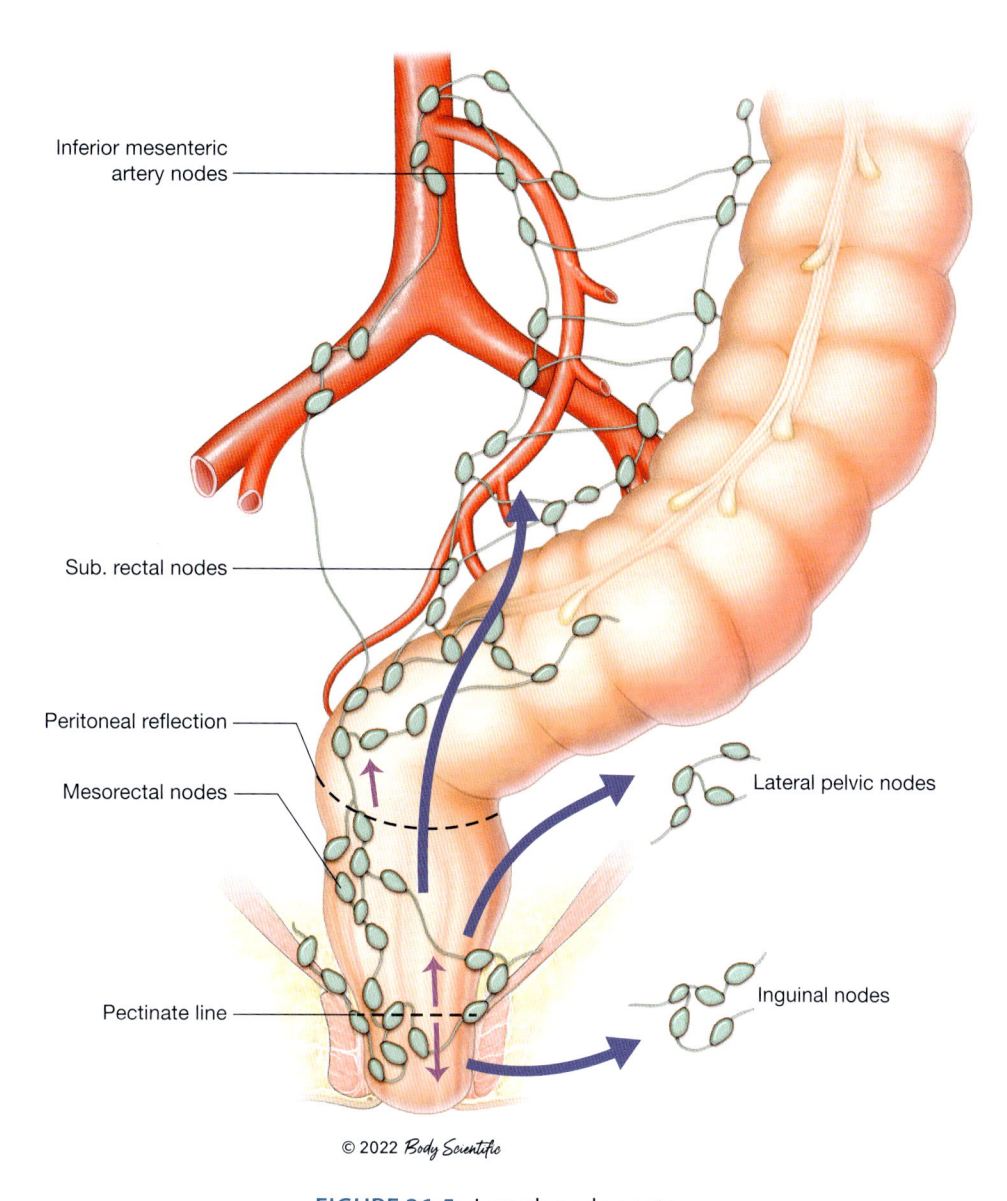

FIGURE 26-5 • Lymph node anatomy.

Perineal Phase Surgical Technique

Depending on the extension of the lesion, on the type of cancer, and on the patient conditions, the surgical dissection of the perineal phase can be performed in different ways:

Extrasphincteric APR

This is the most frequent option; it entails less dissection of the pelvic floor in comparison to the extralevator approach (which is described next). The incision should be kept at around 2.5 cm from the anal canal. The subcutaneous tissue and the pelvic floor are opened from the perineal side. The dissection is conducted laterally to the external sphincter, which is removed with the anal canal. Hence, the defect will be easy to close. The extrasphincteric APR is the main technique described in this chapter (see below) (**Figure 26-6**).

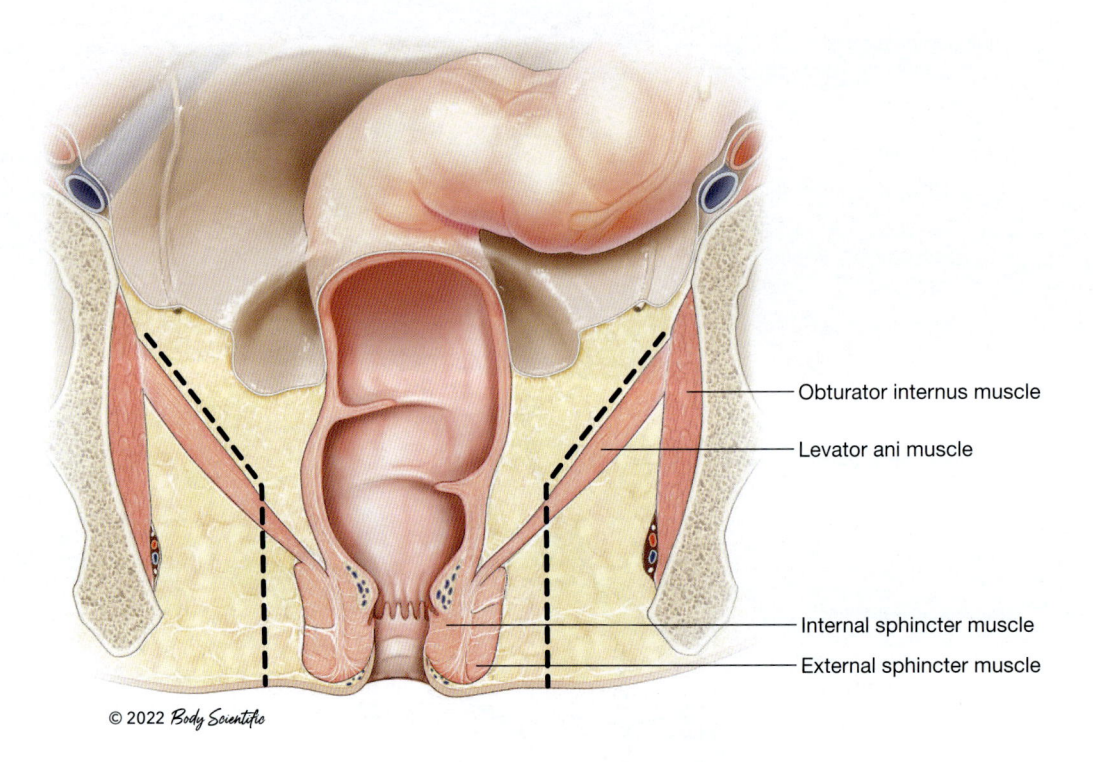

Extrasphincteric dissection

FIGURE 26-6 • Extrasphincteric dissection.

The Extralevator Abdominoperineal Excision

This technique entails a more extensive lateral dissection, including part of the pelvic floor, and the assistance of a plastic surgeon may be required to close the defect (**Figure 26-7**).

The Intersphincteric APR

This option is performed very rarely and requires a minimal dissection of the pelvic floor. An intersphincteric plane is followed with excision of the submucosa, mucosa, and *muscularis*, sparing the external sphincter. Usually, this dissection is concluded with a coloanal transperineal anastomosis. In particular patients not candidate for a pouch reconstruction, the small defect is primarily closed and then a permanent colostomy is performed. Therefore, it is classified as a type of abdominoperineal resection (**Figure 26-8**).

INSTRUMENT REQUIREMENTS (PERINEAL PHASE)

The suggested main instruments/tools can be listed as follows:
- Monopolar cautery
- LigaSure™
- Lonestar retractor
- Right-angle retractors
- St. Marks perineal retractors
- Needle drivers
- Forceps (DeBakey)
- Scissors

Supplemental materials:
- Gauzes, sponges
- Suction/irrigation
- Close suction drains
- Sutures: Prolene™ 2-0, 3-0, 4-0; PDS™ 1-0; Vycril™ 2/0, 0; Nylon 2/0; Silk 2/0

Extralevator dissection

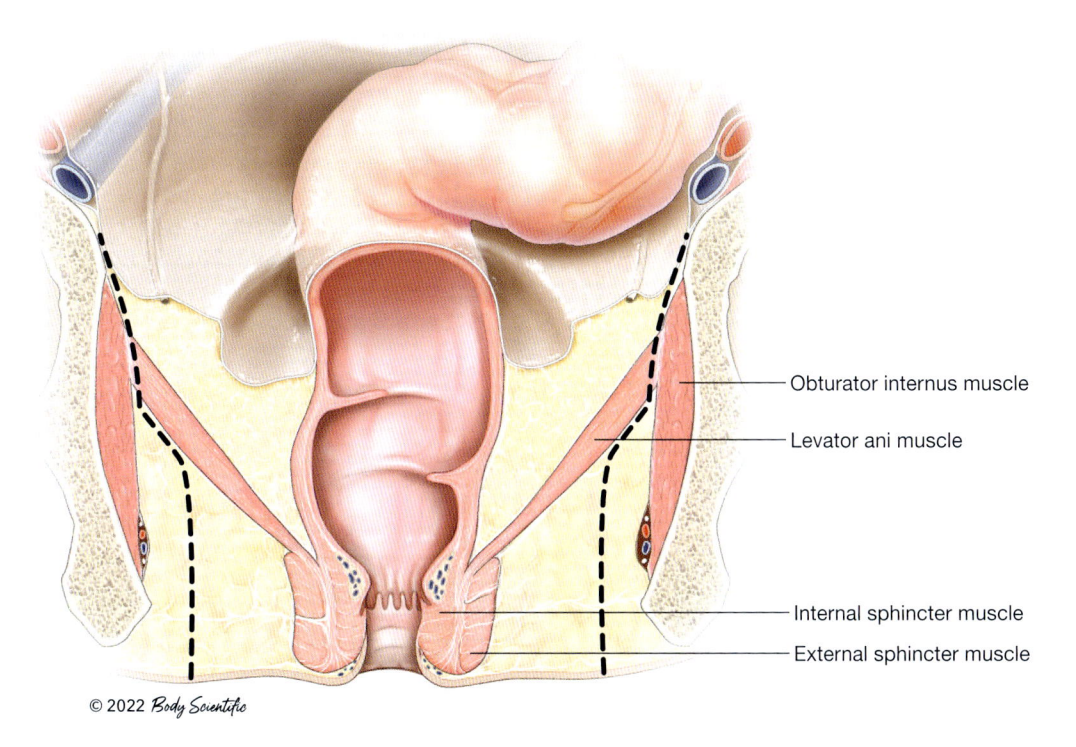

FIGURE 26-7 • Extralevator dissection.

Intersphincteric dissection

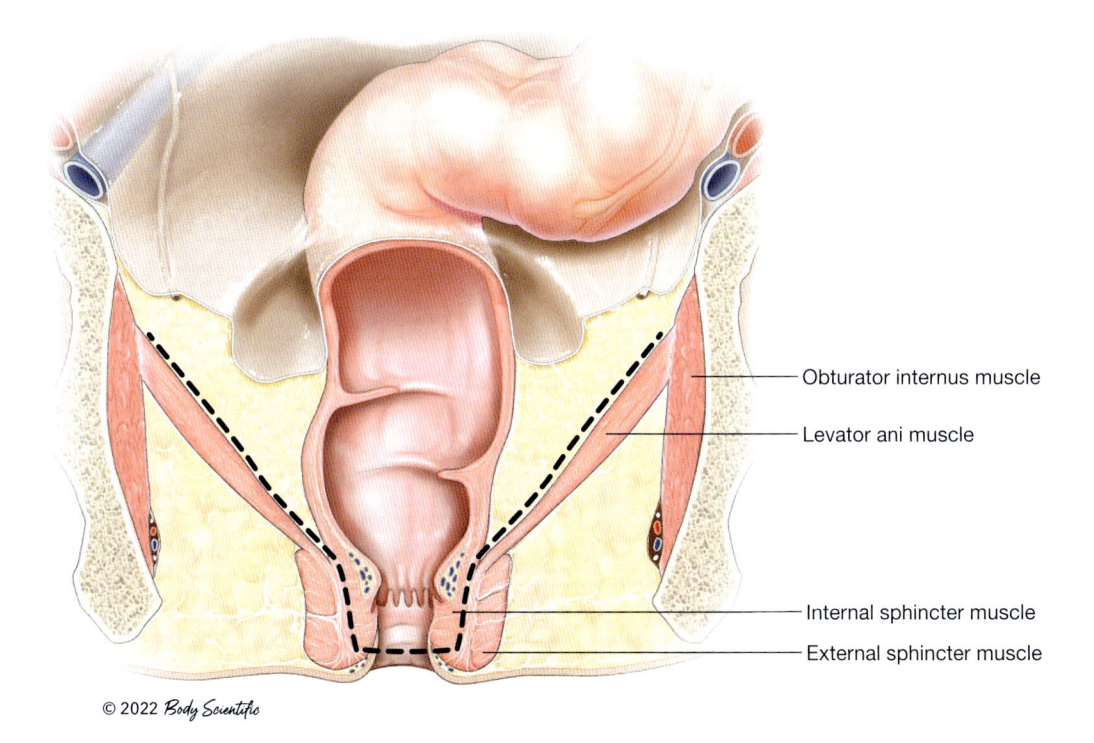

FIGURE 26-8 • Intersphincteric dissection.

Patient Positioning and OR Setup

The perineal portion of the APR may be performed either in lithotomy (preferred position) or in prone jackknife. The latter requires repositioning of the patient. The OR setup is explained in **Figure 26-9**.

> **EDITORIAL COMMENT**
>
> The advantage of the lithotomy position is that the perineal step can be started with the abdomen still open, and it allows the simultaneous work of 2 teams. The procedure is therefore less time consuming, and it may allow combined maneuvers. The disadvantage is represented by a more limited vision and access, particularly in the anterior part of the pelvic floor (prostate area).

Lithotomy

The patient is placed in high lithotomy position (**Figures 26-10 A, B**), with the buttocks within the break of the OR bed, which should be assured at the beginning of the case. Care should be taken to avoid injuries to the common peroneal and posterior tibial nerves. A 3/4 surgical drape, with or without a Mayo stand, may be used to extend the sterile field. The patient is placed in the Trendelenburg position at an appropriate height, so that the perineal portion can be carried out from a seated position. The surgeon and the assistant are both sitting between the patient's legs. A separate surgical tray and scrub nurse can facilitate this portion of the procedure.

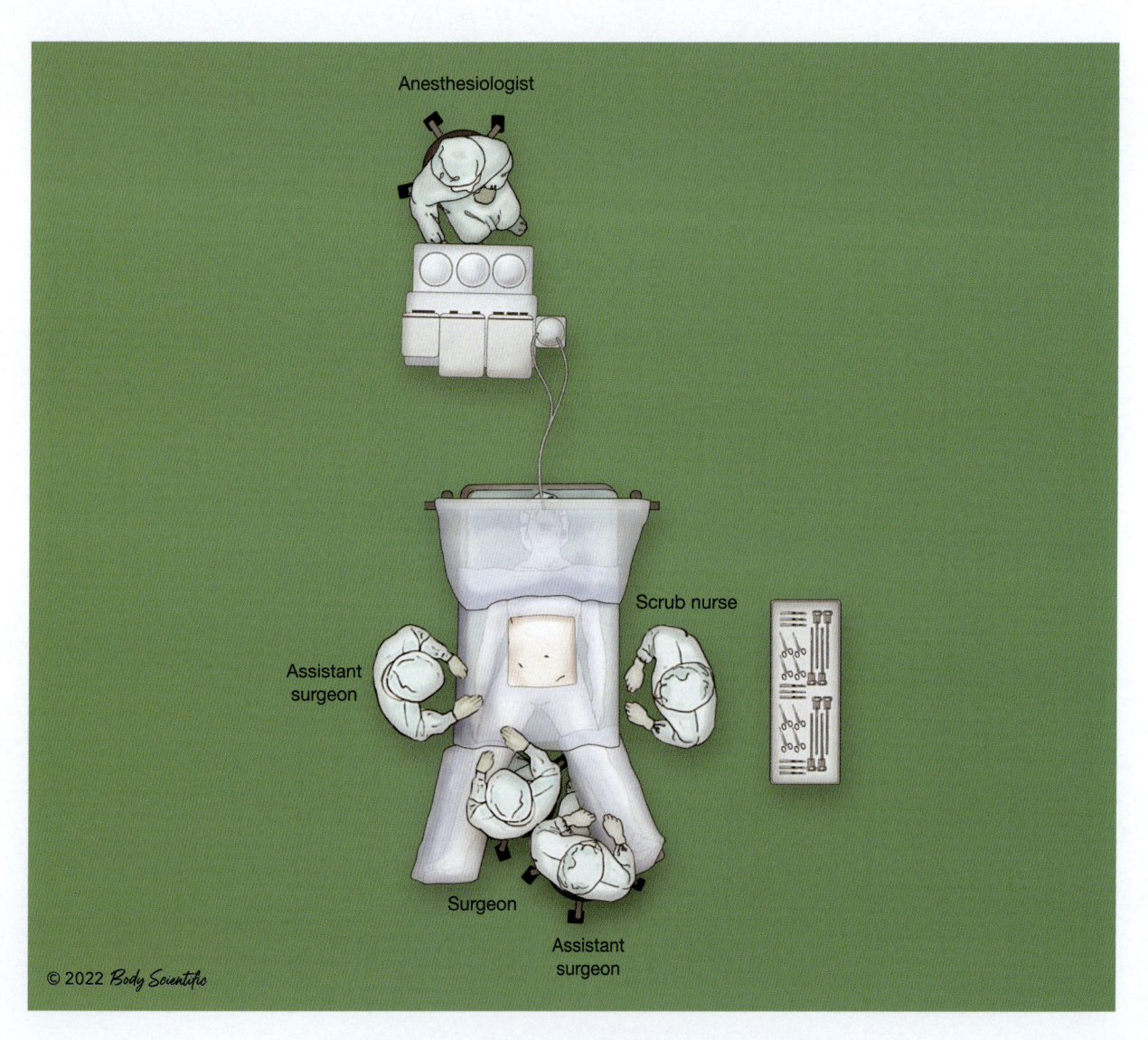

FIGURE 26-9 • OR setup (perineal portion of APR).

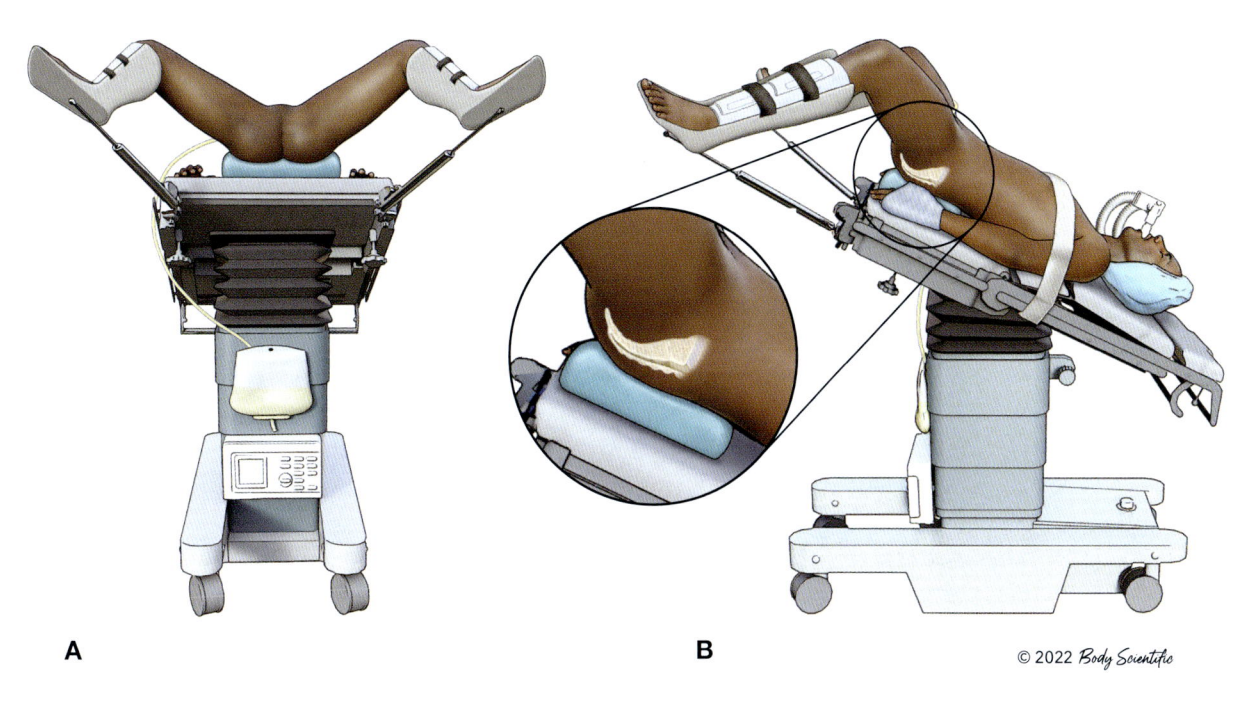

FIGURE 26-10 • Lithotomy position.

Prone Jackknife

The prone jackknife position (**Figures 26-11 A, B**) may facilitate the visualization of some steps of the perineal dissection, particularly anteriorly; or for extended resection involving the sacrum and coccyx. The abdomen should be closed and the colostomy matured prior to placing the patient in prone position. A second OR bed is brought into the room, and the patient is flipped into the prone position with the face placed in a foam prone-cutout pillow or face rest. A gel roll is placed under the anterior superior iliac spines at the break of the table, which is then flexed and the patient is placed in the Trendelenburg position.

> **EDITORIAL COMMENT**
>
> The main drawback of the jackknife prone position is that all the incisions, for the intrabdominal phase, must be closed prior to changing the decubitus of the patient. Any simultaneous, combined intra-abdominal/perineal maneuver is precluded. Also, the final laparoscopic verification is not doable or may require another patient position change and reopening of the port sites.

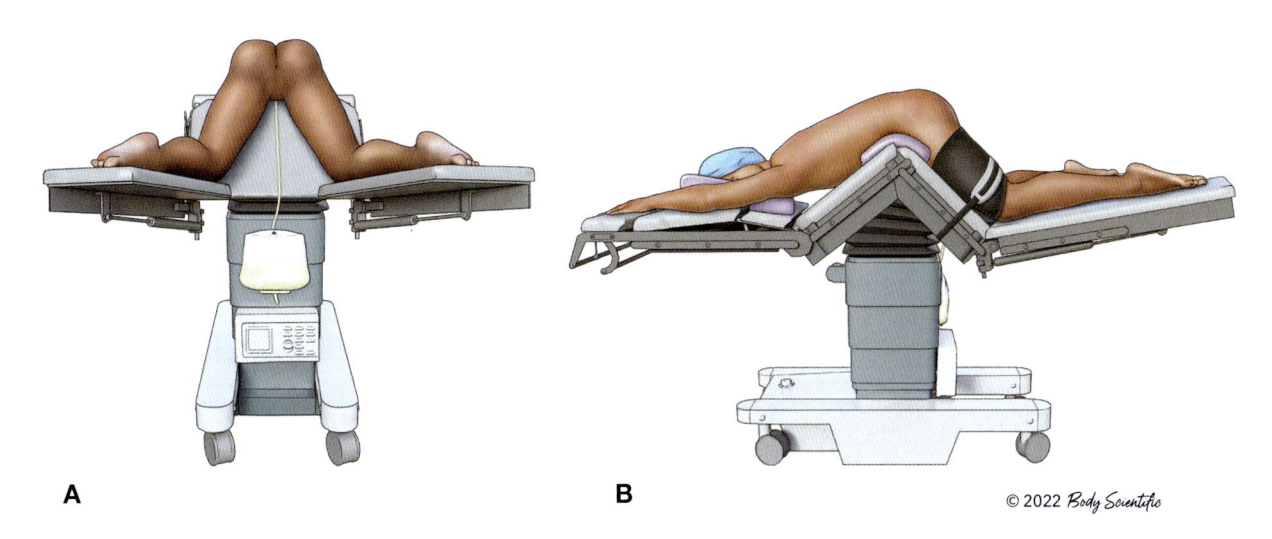

FIGURE 26-11 • Jackknife prone position.

In **Figures 26-12 A, B**, **26-13**, **26-14**, and **26-15**, some anatomical reminders are depicted.

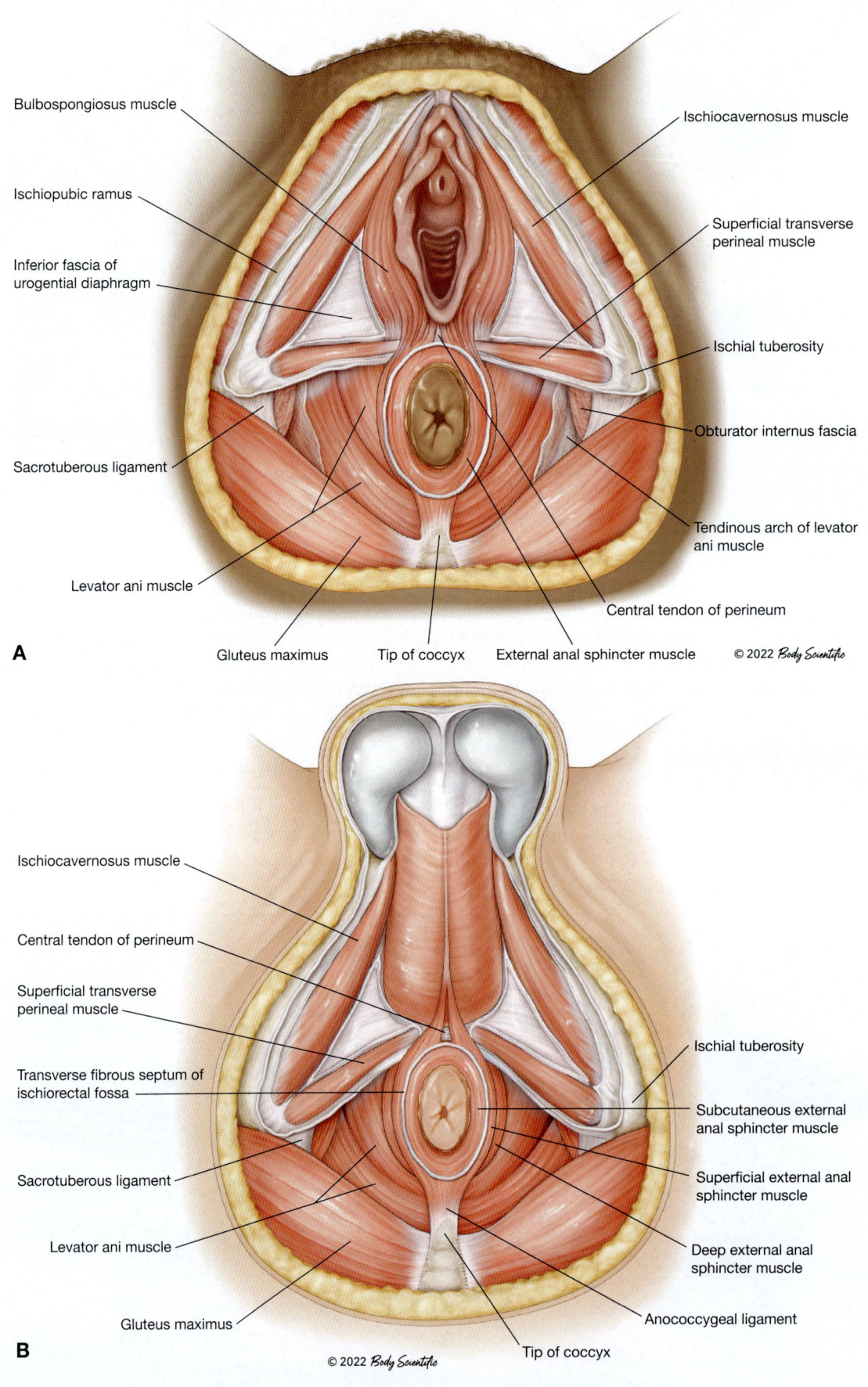

FIGURE 26-12 • Perineal anatomy. **A.** Female. **B.** Male.

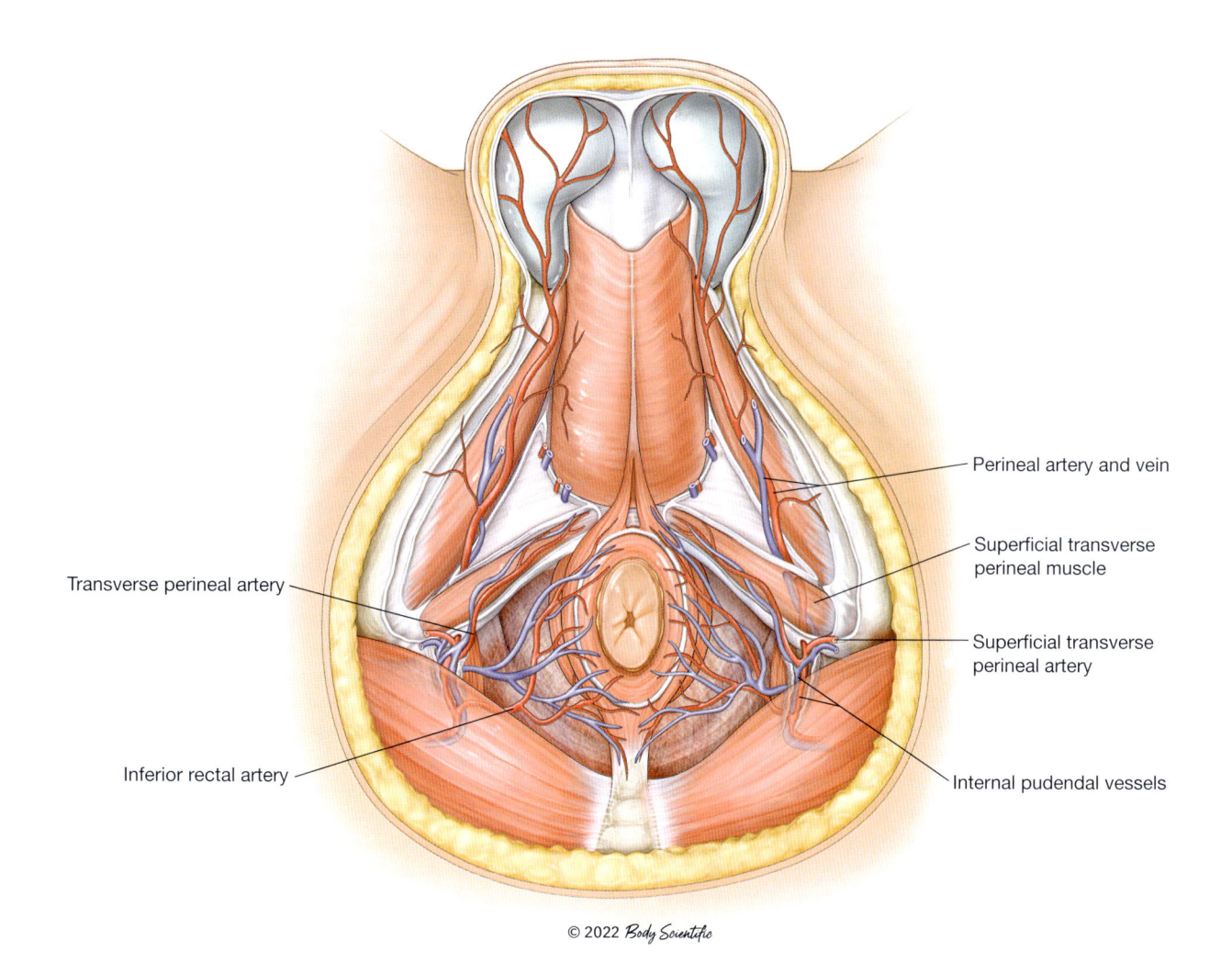

FIGURE 26-13 • Vascular anatomy.

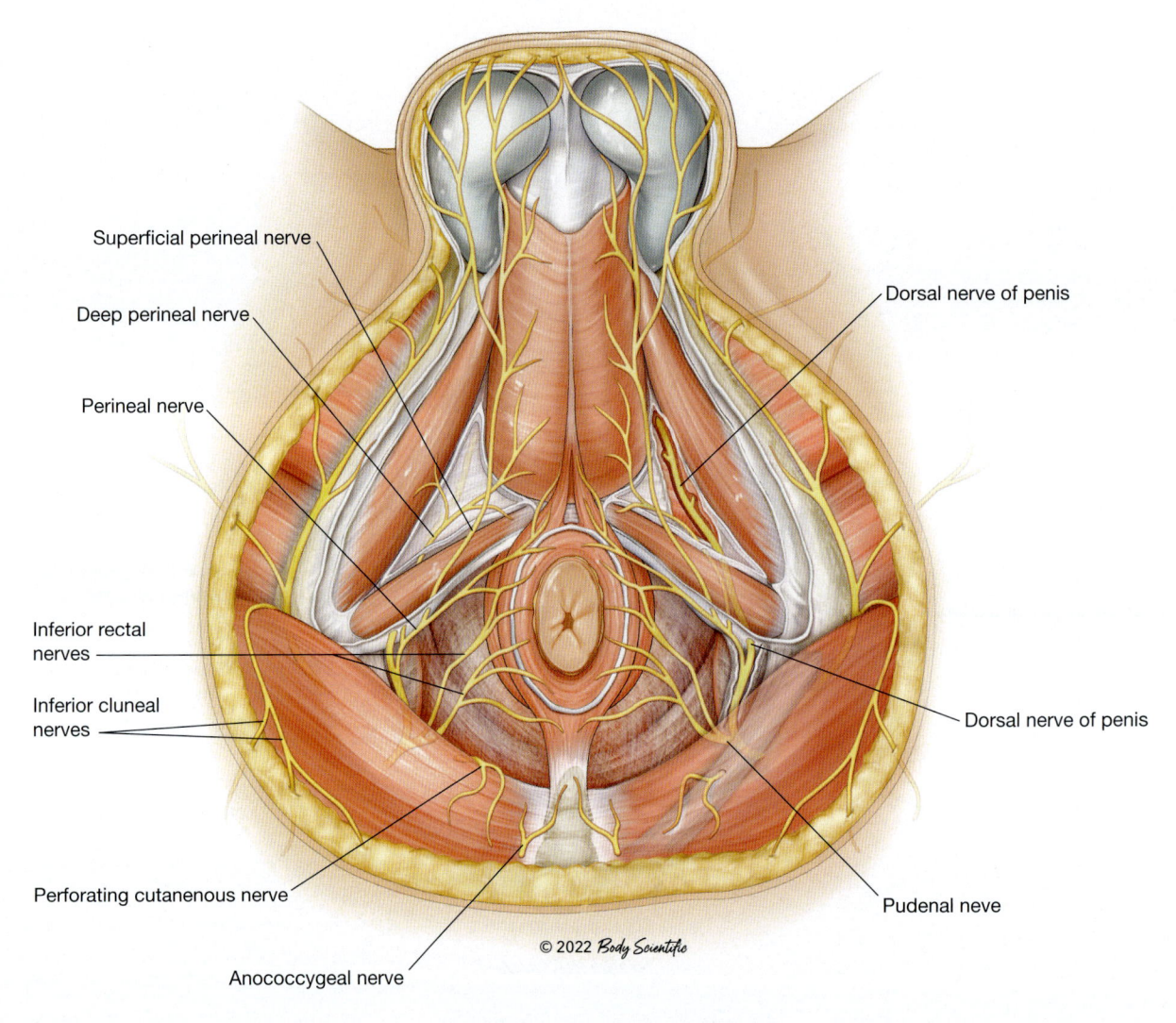

FIGURE 26-14 • Nerves (male).

Abdominoperineal Resection 565

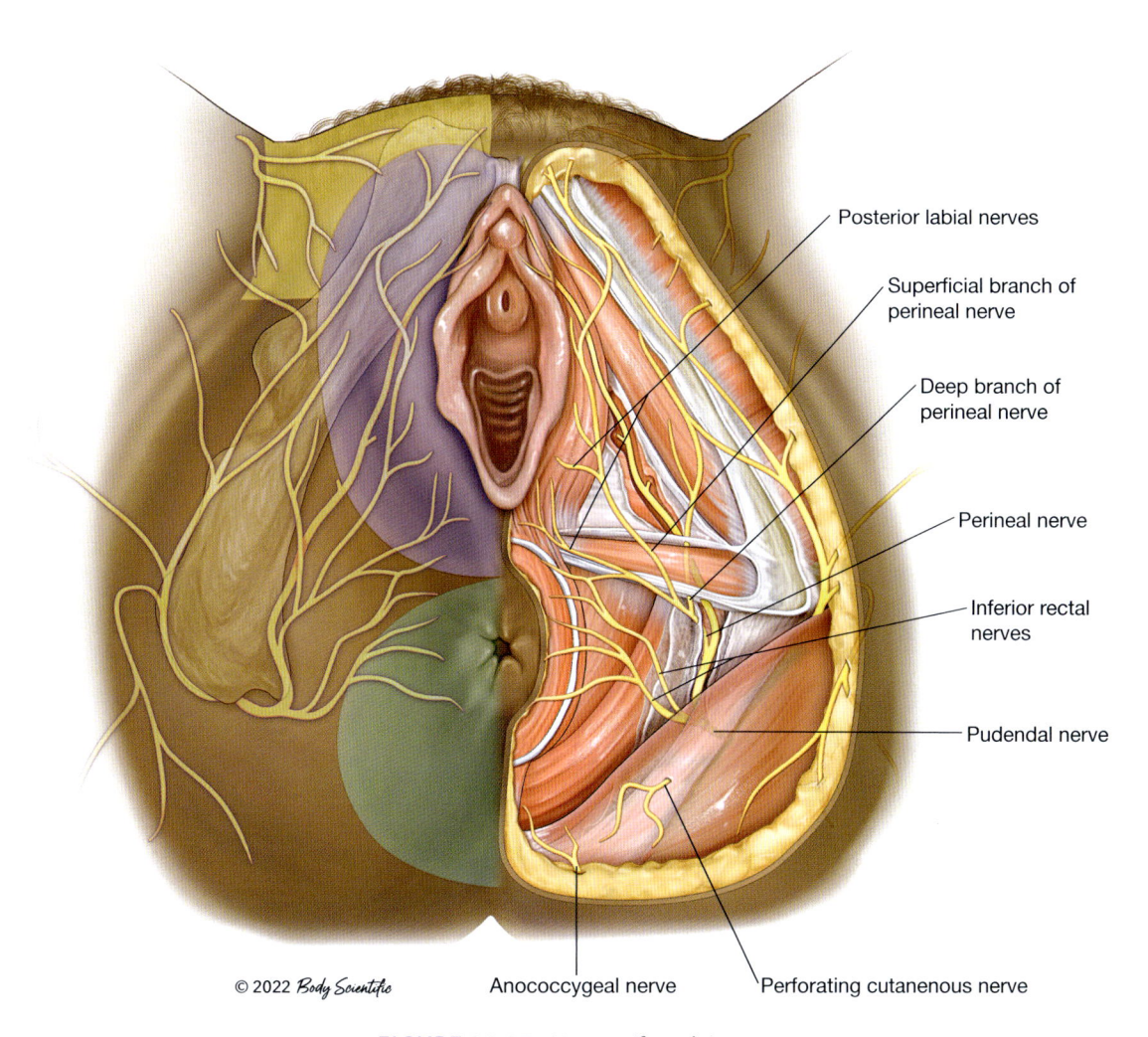

FIGURE 26-15 • Nerves (female).

Step 1. Perianal incision

An incision is made around the sphincter complex (**Figures 26-16 A, B**). After the skin incision, the anus is sutured closed with a silk 2-0 to prevent contamination. The suture is left long and it can be used to make longitudinal traction and countertraction on the specimen. The incision should be halfway between the anal verge and the coccyx, perineal body, and bilateral ischia for most dissections.

If the malignancy extends onto the perianus, the incision should be enlarged to ensure an appropriate margin. In selected cases of an *en bloc* vaginectomy, the anterior part of the incision will extend onto the vaginal fourchette or labia or encompass the urethra in cases of pelvic exenteration. After making the initial incision, the dermis is then divided with electrocautery. A Lonestar™ retractor (**Figure 26-17**) can be used to facilitate a deeper exposure. In the prone position, the incision can also be extended over the sacrum when necessary (**Figure 26-18**).

Step 1 average time frame: 10–15 min

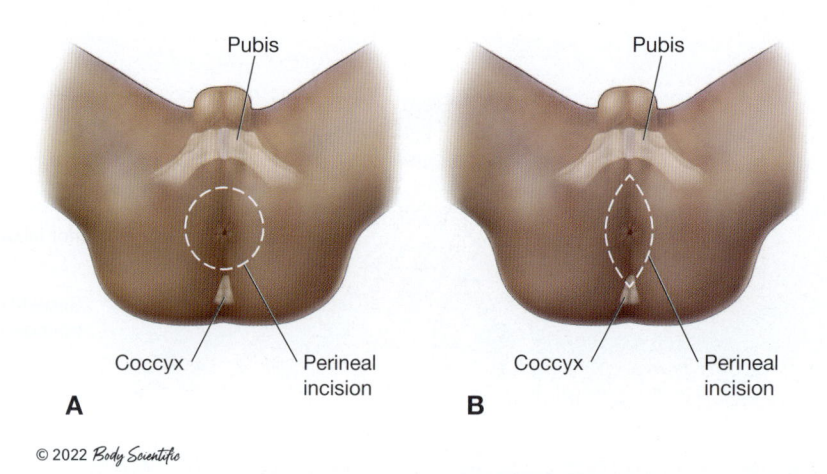

FIGURE 26-16 • Types of perineal incision.

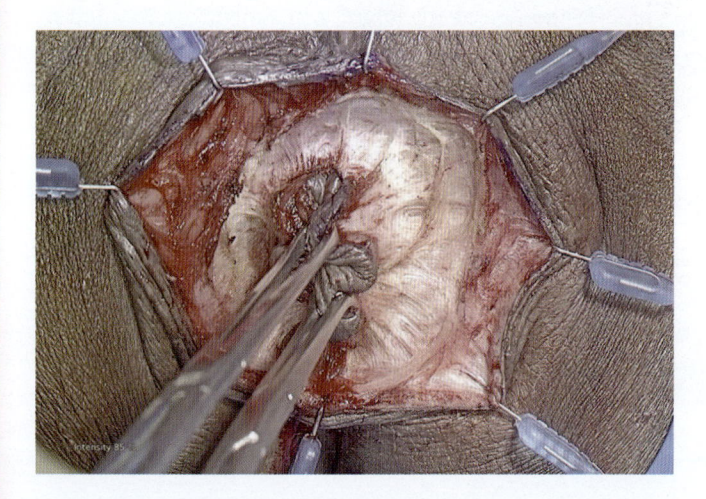

FIGURE 26-17 • Perineal dissection after incising the dermis. (Reproduced with permission from Dr. Gerald Gantt Jr.)

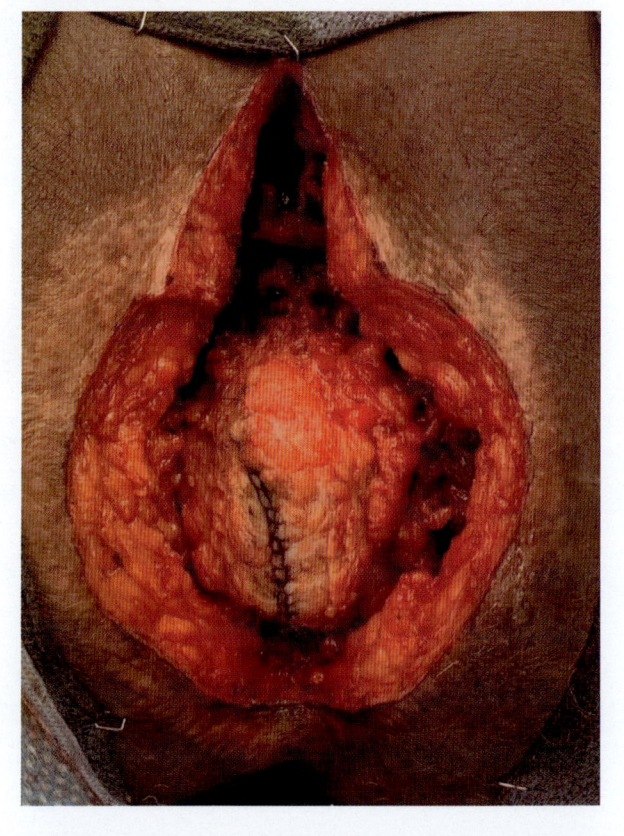

FIGURE 26-18 • "Teardrop" incision extended over the sacrum in the prone position. (Reproduced with permission from Dr. Gerald Gantt Jr.)

Step 2. Ischiorectal dissection: Extrasphincteric approach

The traditional extrasphincteric approach is carried out by dividing the ischiorectal fat outside of the sphincter complex with electrocautery. As the incision is deepened, a perineal St. Marks retractor or right-angle retractors are used by the assistant to pull the ischorectal fat laterally, anteriorly, and posteriorly. The rectum is manipulated by placing Allis clamps on the closed specimen, or pulling on the strong suture closing the anus. The superficial branches of the internal pudendal artery and vein are cauterized or ligated as they are encountered. As the dissection plane deepens, a long-tipped electrocautery device is used. This dissection is carried to the levator ani muscles circumferentially.

Step 2 average time frame: 10–15 min

Step 3. Entrance into the pelvis and detachment of the rectum from the pelvic floor

Once the levator ani muscles are reached, the abdomen can be entered by dividing these muscles with a *rendezvous* with the abdominal dissection already created from above. The initial entry into the abdomen is done posteriorly where the coccyx provides a safe landmark. The pelvis is then reached, in front of the coccyx, by dividing the recto-sacral fascia of Waldeyer. After entering the pelvis, the opening is enlarged enough to allow the exteriorization of the specimen. The proximal stump of the sigmoid rectum is pulled completely outside, and the rectum remains anchored to the pelvic floor only anteriorly and laterally on both sides.

The remaining levator muscles are hooked with an index finger and then divided with electrocautery or a vessel sealer device (**Figure 26-19**). The dissection is usually carried from the posterior midline, bilaterally, and then anteriorly at the end.

Step 3 average time frame: 20–30 min

> ▶▶ **TIPS**
>
> If the perineal portion is being carried out in lithotomy position, then some steps of the dissection may be facilitated by an assistant guiding the maneuvers from the abdomen. This may happen mainly in patients with very thick perineal layers and a deep pelvic floor.

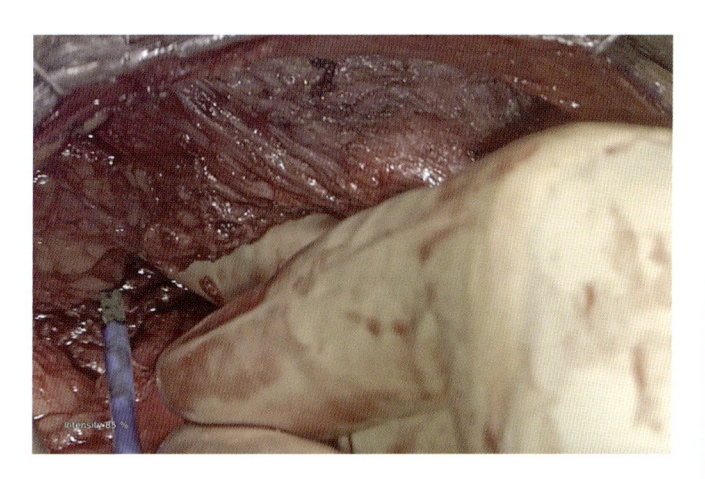

FIGURE 26-19 • Entrance into the pelvis. The levators are divided laterally using manual palpation and electrocautery. (Reproduced with permission from Dr. Gerald Gantt Jr.)

Step 4. Anterior dissection

The specimen is pulled with countertraction to facilitate the anterior dissection.

In women, this dissection may be aided by placing a finger in the vagina to delineate the rectovaginal septum. The posterior wall of the vagina is well vascularized, and bleeding during this step indicates that the dissection plane may be too close to the internal vaginal layers.

In men (**Figure 26-20**), care should be taken to avoid blood loss from the prostate or injury to the membranous urethra. This can be achieved by paying close attention to the position of the Foley catheter.

This portion of the dissection can be difficult, because the anterior rectal wall and the rectovaginal septum are intimately attached to the perineal body. The anterior wall of the rectum is at risk of being violated, mainly if the preparation of the proper surgical plane was not completed during the intra-abdominal phase or in case of advanced cancer involving this area. Using the lateral dissection plane already done, as a guide, is very useful during this step. The anterior dissection is completed with division of the recto-*urethralis* and deep transverse perineal muscles. In case of an anterior rectal cancer, a portion of the posterior vagina or prostate should be taken *en bloc* to ensure negative circumferential resection margins.

Step 4 average time frame: 15–30 min

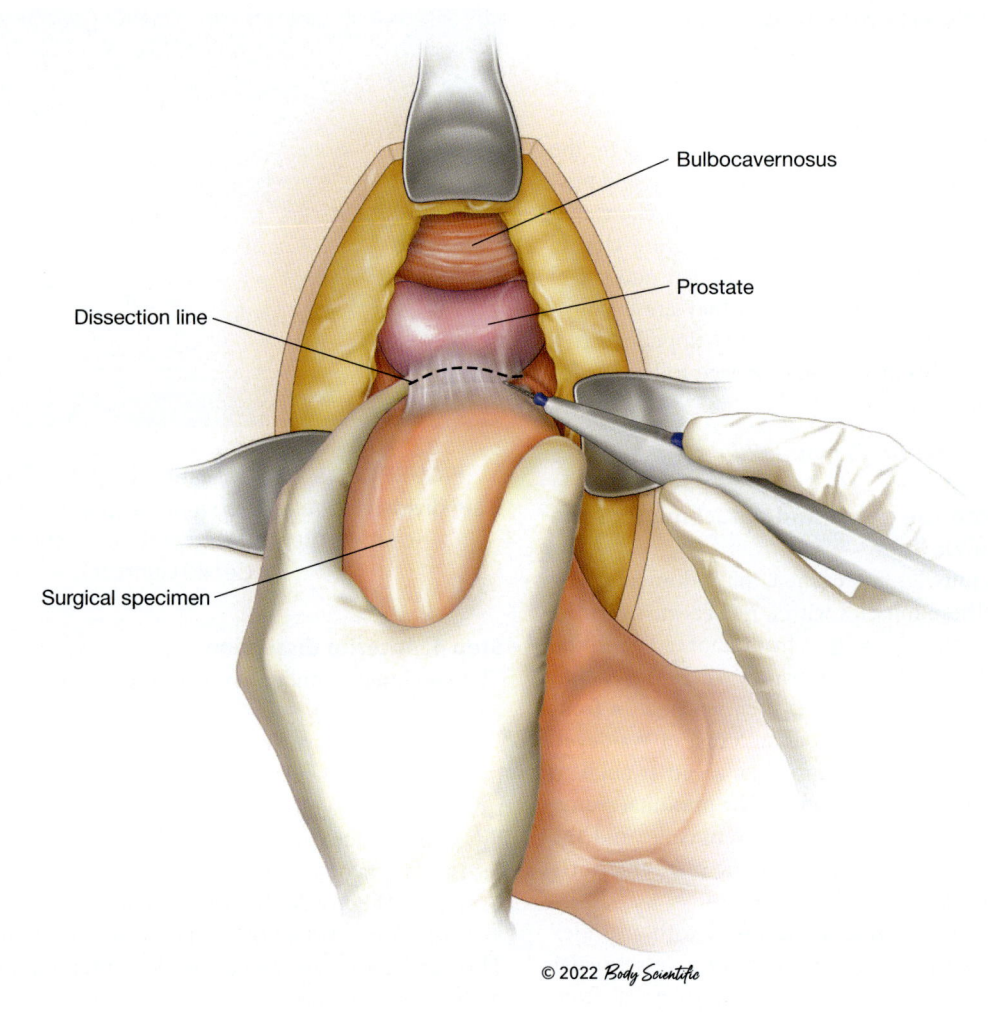

FIGURE 26-20 • Anterior dissection (in male patient).

> **EDITORIAL COMMENT**
>
> The importance of an adequate preparation of the anterior mesorectal space, either periprostatic or rectovaginal septum, during the earlier abdominal steps should not be underestimated. The presence of the right plane between the rectum and the prostate (or the vagina), when the specimen is exteriorized posteriorly during the perineal phase, allows the index of the surgeon to hook the specimen following the right surgical plane and to guide the dissection from the perineal side.

> ⚠ **PITFALLS**
>
> The anterior dissection plane is often difficult to discern. In men, the membranous urethra may be injured. Frequent palpation of the Foley catheter should be used as a reference for the distance. Brisk bleeding from the prostate capsule or posterior wall of the vagina may happen, and it can be controlled with monopolar coagulation or, better, with sutures of Vicryl™ or Prolene™ 2-0 or 3-0. The neurovascular bundles, derived from the inferior hypogastric plexus, course anterolaterally to the rectum and are intimately involved with the rectovaginal/rectovesicular septum. Thus, dissecting too far anteriorly can result in sexual and urinary dysfunction. Conversely, dissecting too far posteriorly can lead to perforation of the anterior rectal wall. Palpation of the rectal tube, manipulation of the posterior vaginal wall, and eversion of the specimen through the perineal defect are all helpful maneuvers to decrease the chances of injuring these structures. Additionally, prone positioning greatly increases the visualization of the anterior structures and should be considered for anterior/advanced tumors.

Step 5. Closure of the perineal wound

The perineal wound may either be closed primarily or with flap reconstruction depending on the size of the defect. Prior to the closure, a closed suction drain can be placed in the pelvis either transabdominally or through the perineal incision. Transabdominal placement of the drain is preferred to avoid wound complications. The primary closure is performed by reapproximating the levators (if still present) and the ischiorectal fat in a series of interrupted single or figure 8 stitches, layer by layer sutures with Vicryl™ 2-0 or 0. The dermis is then approximated with Prolene™ 2-0 or Nylon 2-0 vertical mattress interrupted stitches and removed 2–4 weeks postoperatively. Alternatively, the dermis may be closed with a running subcuticular suture of absorbable material (**Figure 26-21**).

Step 5 average time frame: 15–20 min

> **EDITORIAL COMMENT**
>
> The skin closure of the perineal wound is better done with interrupted stitches. In case of infection, requiring reopening of the wound, only a few stitches can be removed.

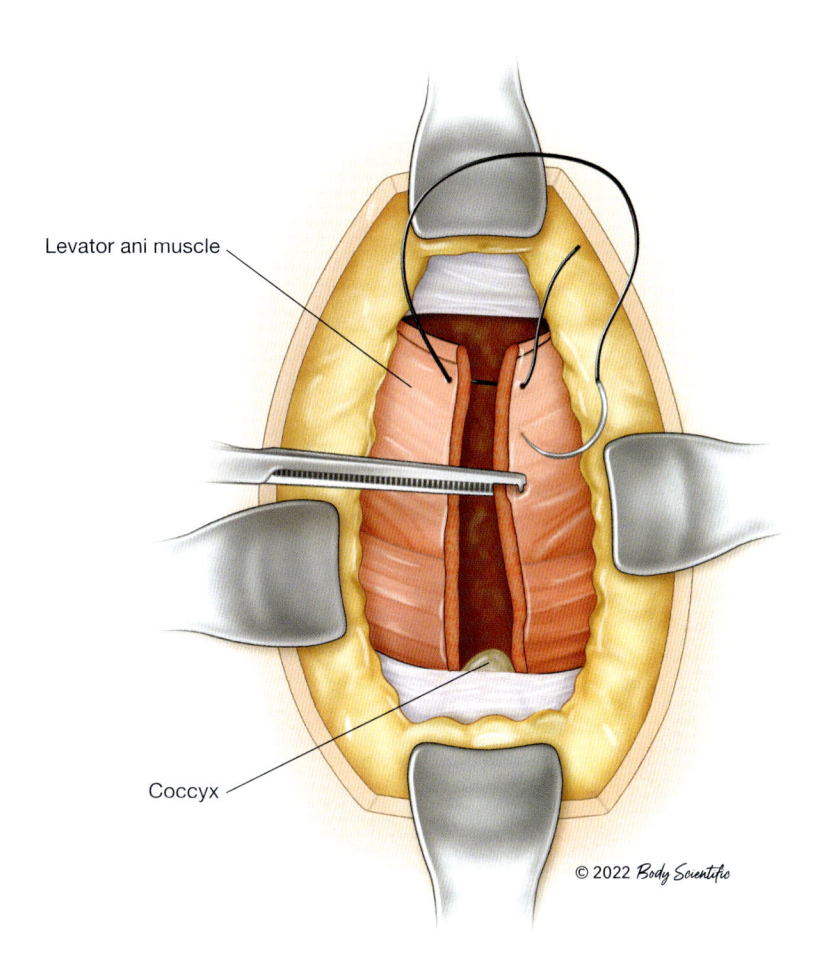

FIGURE 26-21 • Closure of the perineal wound.

Step 6: Left iliac end-colostomy fashioning and intra-abdominal laparoscopic final check

In the majority of cases, the abdominal phase is not completed, with the closure of the accesses and the fashioning of the colostomy, until the end of the perineal phase. This strategy allows the final verification of the hemostasis and the correct positioning of the bowel into the pelvis.

Therefore, the patient is repositioned supine, the laparoscopic ports are reinserted, and a general overview of the abdominal cavity is achieved. A left iliac retroperitoneal tunnel is prepared laparoscopically, in correspondence of the incision where the stoma will be placed (usually utilized for one of the operative robotic trocars).

A round incision is performed in this previously planned area. A small opening in the lateral oblique muscles is made. The proximal descending colon is brought out to perform a left iliac end-colostomy (usually it is halfway in the line between the umbilical scar and the left anterior superior iliac spine). The colon is affixed to the fascia after being "tunnelized" extraperitoneally and then also attached to the skin. A final additional laparoscopic check is usually performed to have a general verification of the correct positioning of the colon and hemostasis. The abdomen is then deflated, and the port sites are closed with interrupted stitches and glue.

Step 6 average time frame: 15–20 min

CONSIDERATIONS ABOUT THE EXTRALEVATOR DISSECTION

An extralevator dissection removes the levator muscles at the pelvic sidewalls resulting in a cylindrical specimen without the "wasting" (hourglass shape) sometimes seen with the traditional, more conservative, extrasphincteric approach. The goal, with this technique, is to minimize the risk of positive circumferential resection margins at the anorectal junction for more advanced lesions.

After incising the perianal skin, the ischiorectal fat is divided along the sphincter complex. The dissection is then carried laterally to reach the insertion of the levator ani muscles in the pelvic sidewall. During this dissection, the terminal branches of the pudendal nerve, leading to the levator ani muscles and peri-anus, will be transected. The genital branches of the pudendal nerve should be preserved. The levator ani muscles are divided, at their origin, using electrocautery.

For tumors extending into the perianal skin or ischiorectal fossa, an ischiorectal resection can be performed. The skin incision is tailored to the tumor to ensure at least a 2-cm margin. After incising the dermis, the dissection is carried laterally to the ischial tuberosities and along the fascia of the *obturator internus* muscle using diathermy or a vessel sealing device. This dissection can be performed either unilaterally or bilaterally, depending on the location of the tumor. The levator ani muscles are then divided as in the standard extralevator approach. For more information, see suggested reading #5.

In essence, several lines of evidence have shown that there are conflicting results about this approach, and more data are needed to validate the claims of the "extralevator superiority" in terms of survival outcomes. At this stage, this approach should be adopted in selected cases, with high intraoperative perforation risk, or clear MRI involvement of the levator muscles (for more information, see suggested readings #1–5, 19).

CONSIDERATIONS ABOUT THE INTERSPHINCTERIC DISSECTION

An intersphincteric dissection may be performed for patients with inflammatory bowel disease who require a proctectomy, but are not candidates for a pouch procedure, or for low rectal cancers that do not involve the sphincter complex. This dissection allows the removal of the rectal tube, leaving the external sphincter behind.

This technique allows a simpler closure of the perineal defect, as the external sphincter can be easily reapproximated, and decreases the risk for wound healing complications. A Lonestar™ retractor is placed with the hooks at the anal verge to expose the dentate line. Local anesthetic with epinephrine is injected in the intersphincteric groove using a 25-g needle to facilitate dissection. An incision is made just proximal to the dentate line circumferentially. The rectum is then sutured closed with a Prolene™ 2-0 in a purse-string fashion. The dissection is then carried cephalad in the intersphincteric space with electrocautery. Once the abdominal dissection plane is encountered, the rectum is dissected circumferentially. The specimen may then be removed from the perineum (for more information, see suggested reading #5).

Suggested Readings

1. Prytz M, Angenete E, Ekelund J, Haglind E. Extralevator abdominoperineal excision (ELAPE) for rectal cancer—short-term results from the Swedish Colorectal Cancer Registry. Selective use of ELAPE warranted. *Int J Colorect Dis.* 2014;29(8):981-987.
2. den Dulk M, Marijnen CA, Putter H, et al. Risk factors for adverse outcome in patients with rectal cancer treated with an abdominoperineal resection in the total mesorectal excision trial. *Ann Surg.* 2007;246(1):83-90.
3. Marr R, Birbeck K, Garvican J, et al. The modern abdominoperineal excision: the next challenge after total mesorectal excision. *Ann Surg.* 2005;242(1):74-82.
4. Nagtegaal ID, van de Velde CJ, Marijnen CA, van Krieken JH, Quirke P. Low rectal cancer: a call for a change of approach in abdominoperineal resection. *J Clin Oncol.* 2005;23(36):9257-9264.
5. Hawkins AT, Albutt K, Wise PE, et al. Abdominoperineal resection for rectal cancer in the twenty-first century: indications, techniques, and outcomes. *J Gastrointest Surg.* 2018;22(8):1477-1487. doi: 10.1007/s11605-018-3750-9
6. Miles WE. A method of performing abdomino-perineal excision for carcinoma of the rectum and of the terminal portion of the pelvic colon (1908). *CA: Cancer J Clin.* 1971;21(6):361-364.
7. Heald RJ, Ryall RD. Recurrence and survival after total mesorectal excision for rectal cancer. *Lancet (London, England).* 1986;1(8496):1479-1482.
8. MacFarlane JK, Ryall RD, Heald RJ. Mesorectal excision for rectal cancer. *Lancet (London, England).* 1993;341(8843):457-460.
9. Quirke P, Durdey P, Dixon MF, Williams NS. Local recurrence of rectal adenocarcinoma due to inadequate surgical resection. Histopathological study of lateral tumour spread and surgical excision. *Lancet (London, England).* 1986;2(8514):996-999.
10. Sauer R, Becker H, Hohenberger W, et al. Preoperative versus postoperative chemoradiotherapy for rectal cancer. *N Engl J Med.* 2004;351(17):1731-1740.
11. Bordeianou L, Maguire LH, Alavi K, Sudan R, Wise PE, Kaiser AM. Sphincter-sparing surgery in patients with low-lying rectal cancer: techniques, oncologic outcomes, and functional results. *J Gastrointest Surg.* 2014;18(7):1358-1372.
12. Mangano A, Valle V, Fernandes E, Bustos R, Gheza F, Giulianotti PC. Operative technique in robotic rectal resection. *Minerva Chir.* 2019;74(6):501-508. doi: 10.23736/S0026- 4733.18.07808-2
13. Giulianotti PC, Coratti A, Angelini M, et al. Robotics in general surgery: personal experience in a large community hospital. *Arch Surg.* 2003;138(7):777-784. doi: 10.1001/archsurg.138.7.777
14. Stelzner S, Holm T, Moran BJ, et al. Deep pelvic anatomy revisited for a description of crucial steps in extralevator abdominoperineal excision for rectal cancer. *Dis Colon Rectum.* 2011;54(8):947-957. doi: 10.1097/DCR.0b013e31821c4bac
15. Liu P, Bao H, Zhang X, et al. Better operative outcomes achieved with the prone jackknife vs. lithotomy position during abdominoperineal resection in patients with low rectal cancer. *World J Surg Onc.* 2015;13:39. doi: 10.1186/s12957-015-0453-5
16. Holm T, Ljung A, Häggmark T, Jurell G, Lagergren J. Extended abdominoperineal resection with gluteus maximus flap reconstruction of the pelvic floor for rectal cancer. *Br J Surg.* 2007;94:232-238. https://doi-org.proxy.cc.uic.edu/10.1002/bjs.5489
17. Perry WB, Connaughton JC. Abdominoperineal resection: how is it done and what are the results? *Clin Colon Rectal Surg.* 2007;20(3):213-220. doi: 10.1055/s-2007-984865
18. Holm T. Controversies in abdominoperineal excision. *Surg Oncol Clin N Am.* 2014;23(1):93-111. doi: 10.1016/j.soc.2013.09.005
19. Negoi I, Hostiuc S, Paun S, Negoi RI, Beuran M. Extralevator vs conventional abdominoperineal resection for rectal cancer–a systematic review and meta-analysis. *Am J Surg.* 2016;212(3):511-526.

SECTION VI

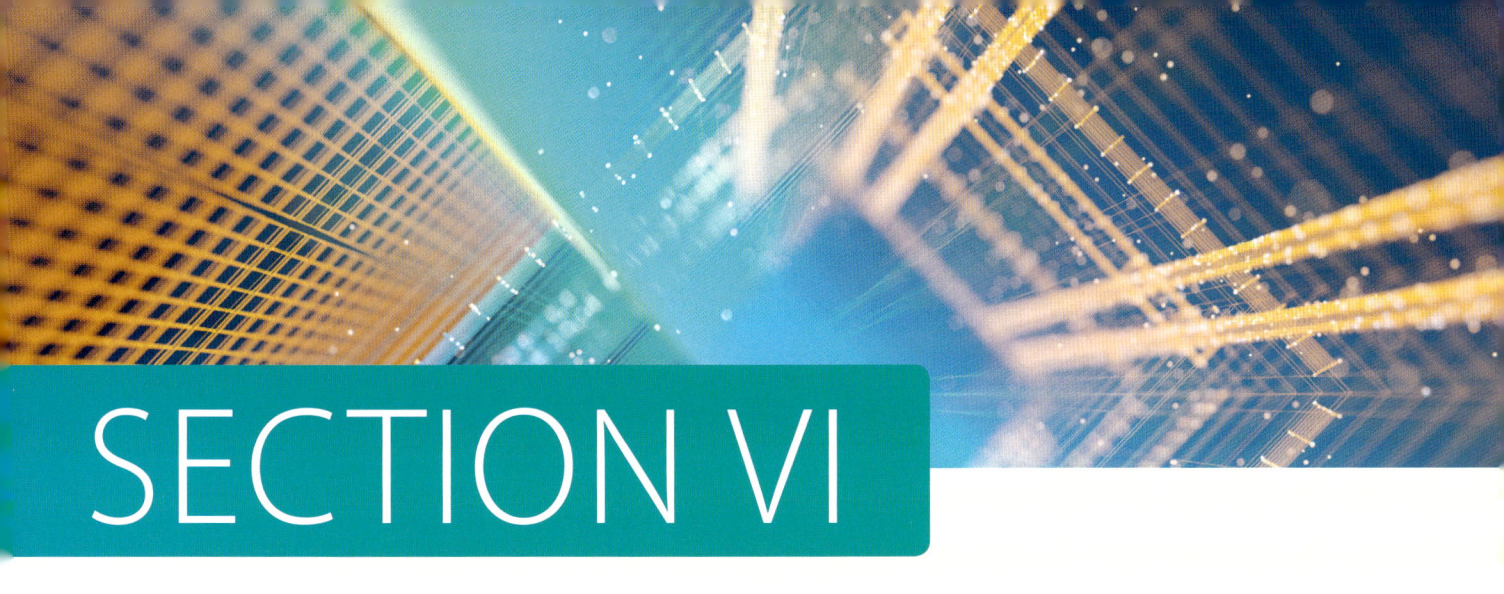

Surgery of the Spleen and Pancreas

Chapter 27 • Splenectomy 575
Valentina Valle • Alberto Mangano • Pier Cristoforo Giulianotti

Chapter 28 • Pancreaticoduodenectomy 599
Pier Cristoforo Giulianotti • Valentina Valle • Roberto Bustos • Alberto Mangano

Chapter 29 • Radical Antegrade Modular Pancreatosplenectomy 635
Rong Liu • Qu Liu

Chapter 30 • Spleen-Preserving Distal Pancreatectomy 653
Valentina Valle • Alberto Mangano • Antonio Cubisino • Pier Cristoforo Giulianotti

Chapter 31 • Central Pancreatectomy 673
Antonio Cubisino • Valentina Valle • Nicolas Hellmuth Dreifuss • Pier Cristoforo Giulianotti

Chapter 32 • Enucleation of Pancreatic Tumors 689
Graziano Pernazza • Antonio Cubisino

"The aim of laparoscopic splenectomy, described in 1991, was achieving results identical to those of open surgery in terms of efficacy and safety but with hope for benefits resulting from the reduced trauma to the abdominal wall, the usually simpler postoperative course, and a shorter duration of hospitalization."

—Bernard Delaitre (1937–)

Splenectomy

Valentina Valle • Alberto Mangano • Pier Cristoforo Giulianotti

INTRODUCTION

Laparoscopic splenectomy was first reported in 1991 by Delaitre and Maignien. After a gradual and progressive adoption, the laparoscopic approach to this operation is now supported by increasing evidence and by surgical societies. According to the literature data from the National (US) Surgical Quality Improvement Program database (NSQIP), laparoscopy is an increasingly chosen strategy for elective splenectomy, being adopted in more than 60% of cases (see suggested reading #1).

The laparoscopic technique is regarded as safe and feasible for most indications, while retaining all the well-established advantages of a minimally invasive surgery (MIS) approach. Even in case of severe splenomegaly, the splenectomy is often feasible, and for benign pathology, the specimen can be morselized for the retrieval.

In the last decade, robot-assisted laparoscopy has been increasingly adopted. It provides several additional technical advantages, mainly during the preparation of the vessels at the hilum, where microdissection capabilities and superior visualization can matter. The technical advancements of the platform allow the inclusion of more complex indications, probably with the reduction of conversion rate and specific morbidity.

According to meta-analytic data from recent literature, the robotic approach represents up to 39% of the MIS splenectomies for nontraumatic indications (see suggested reading #2).

INSTRUMENT REQUIREMENTS

The suggested main robotic instruments/tools can be listed as follows:
- 30° scope
- Permanent cautery monopolar hook
- Cadière forceps
- Fenestrated bipolar forceps
- Vessel sealer
- Needle drivers
- Clip applier
- (SureForm™ Robotic Stapler: white cartridge)

The suggested main laparoscopic instruments can be listed as follows:
- 5-mm scope
- Graspers
- Needle drivers
- Scissors
- Suction-irrigation device
- Laparoscopic 45-mm stapler (vascular load)

Supplemental materials:
- Gauze, sponges
- Penrose drains/vessels loops
- Hem-o-lok™ clips
- Sutures: Prolene™ 3-0, 4-0, and 5-0
- Endo Bag™

Picture provided by Marine Delaitre, the daughter of Dr. Bernard Delaitre.
Quote reproduced with permission from Delaitre B, Blezel E, Samama G, et al. Laparoscopic splenectomy for idiopathic thrombocytopenic purpura. Surg Laparosc Endosc Percutan Tech. 2002;12(6):412-419.

Indications and Relative Contraindications to the Robotic Approach

The indications for splenectomies can be classified into 2 main groups: (1) operations performed to provide a diagnosis; and (2) procedures carried out to treat a disease. In the first case, the splenectomy is mostly done to assess the presence of subdiaphragmatic extension of Hodgkin lymphoma or to analyze the nature of a splenic lesion (e.g., cyst/abscess/benign or malignant tumors).

When splenectomies are performed as treatment of a disease, they are usually carried out to relieve symptomatic splenomegaly, to avoid the risk of splenic rupture (infectious mononucleosis), to treat hypersplenism (hematologic disorders), or to remove a focal pathology. See **Table 27-1** for details.

There are no absolute surgical contraindications to the robotic approach for elective splenectomies.

Relative contraindications may be: large splenomegaly (more than 20 cm), hostile abdomen, portal hypertension, and hemodynamically unstable patients. Multiple parameters should be examined when evaluating the indications: the experience of the team, if the specific disease/indication entails an increased risk of intraperitoneal rupture, and the extraction strategy.

> **EDITORIAL COMMENT**
>
> As it is for all elective splenectomies (open and MIS), the patient should be prophylactically vaccinated to be protected against encapsulated microorganisms (meningococcus, pneumococcus, and *Haemophilus influenzae* spp.), and to decrease the risk of post-splenectomy sepsis.

Patient Positioning, OR Setup, and Port Setting

The patient is positioned supine, with parted legs, and both arms tucked to the side. The stomach is usually decompressed by placing a nasogastric or orogastric tube. A Foley catheter is placed for urinary output control (**Figure 27-1**).

TABLE 27-1 • Diagnosis and Treatment	
Diagnosis	**Treatment**

• **Hodgkin lymphoma**
• **Non-Hodgkin lymphoma**
• **Splenic masses:**
  - Cysts
  - Abscesses
  - Primary/adjacent tumors
  - Metastasis
	• **Hematologic disorders:**
	  - Idiopathic thrombocytopenic purpura
	  - Thrombotic thrombocytopenic purpura
	  - Hereditary hemolytic anemia
	  - Hereditary spherocytosis
	  - Sickle cell disease
	  - Beta thalassemia
	• **Malignancies:**
	  - Lymphoma (Hodgkin/non-Hodgkin)
	  - Lymphoproliferative disorders (acute myeloid leukemia, acute lymphoid leukemia)
	  - Hairy cell leukemia
	  - Myelofibrosis
	• **Risk of rupture/contained rupture:**
	  - Infectious mononucleosis
	• **Others:**
	  - Felty syndrome*
	  - Gaucher disease**
	  - Splenic artery aneurism
	  - Splenic vein thrombosis
	  - AIDS

*Rare disorder defined by the presence of rheumatoid arthritis, splenomegaly, and neutropenia, which causes repeated infections.
**Genetic disorder in which the deficiency of the enzyme glucocerebrosidase leads to accumulation of glucocerebroside in certain organs inducing multiple symptoms (e.g., hepatosplenomegaly).

Splenectomy 577

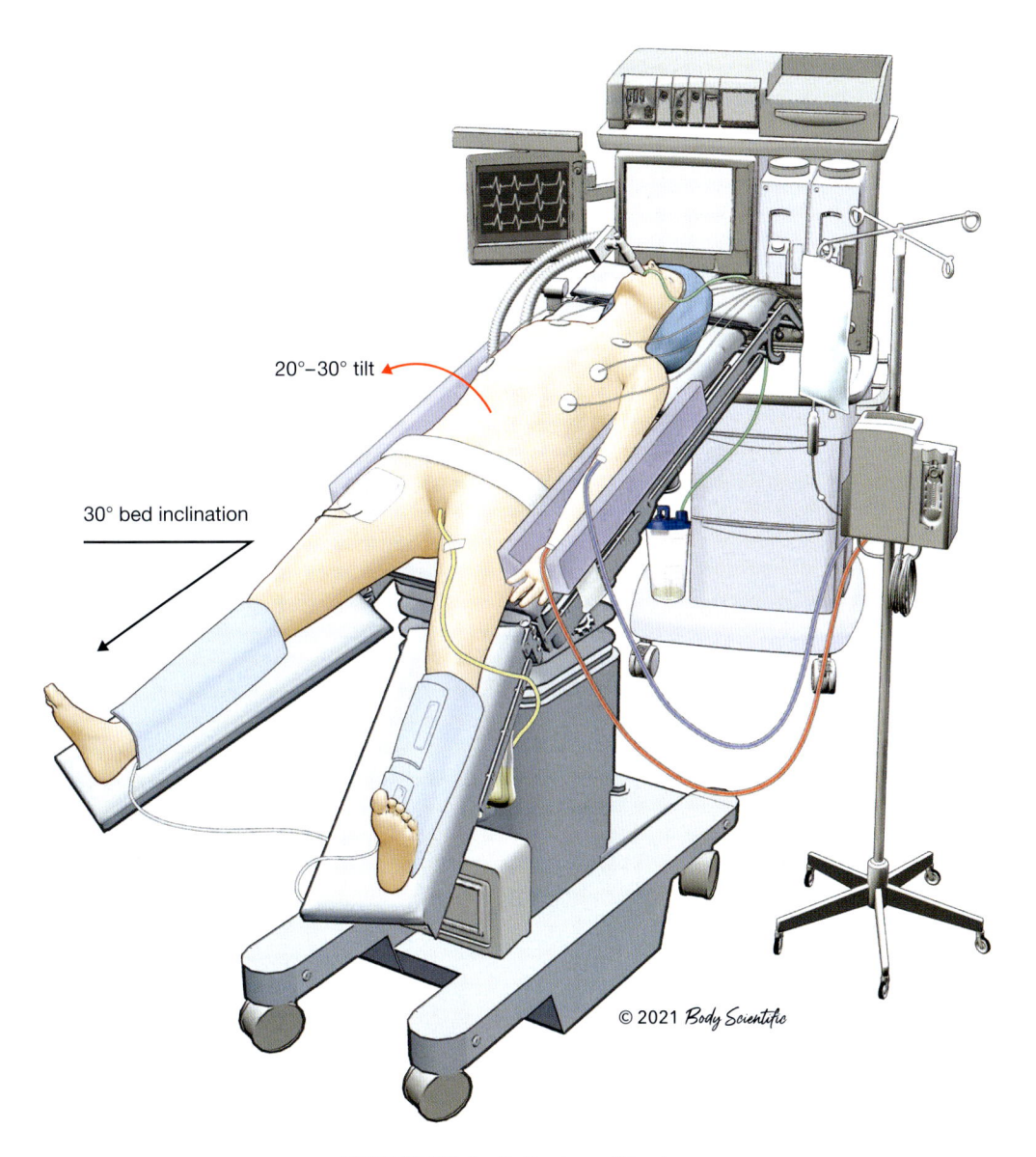

20°–30° tilt

30° bed inclination

© 2021 Body Scientific

FIGURE 27-1 • Patient positioning.

The OR setup is described in **Figure 27-2**. The assistant surgeon is positioned between the patient's legs, and the scrub nurse is on the opposite side of the robotic cart.

Pneumoperitoneum is achieved with the Veress needle technique: in case of splenomegaly, it can be placed below the umbilicus (further details are available in Chapter 2, The Basic Principles of Clinical Applications).

A 5-mm VisiPort™ is placed in the right upper quadrant; this trocar is later replaced by a robotic one. An intra-abdominal exploration is performed to rule out adhesions, to assess the general position and dimensions of the spleen, and to detect any other factors that may affect the operative plan.

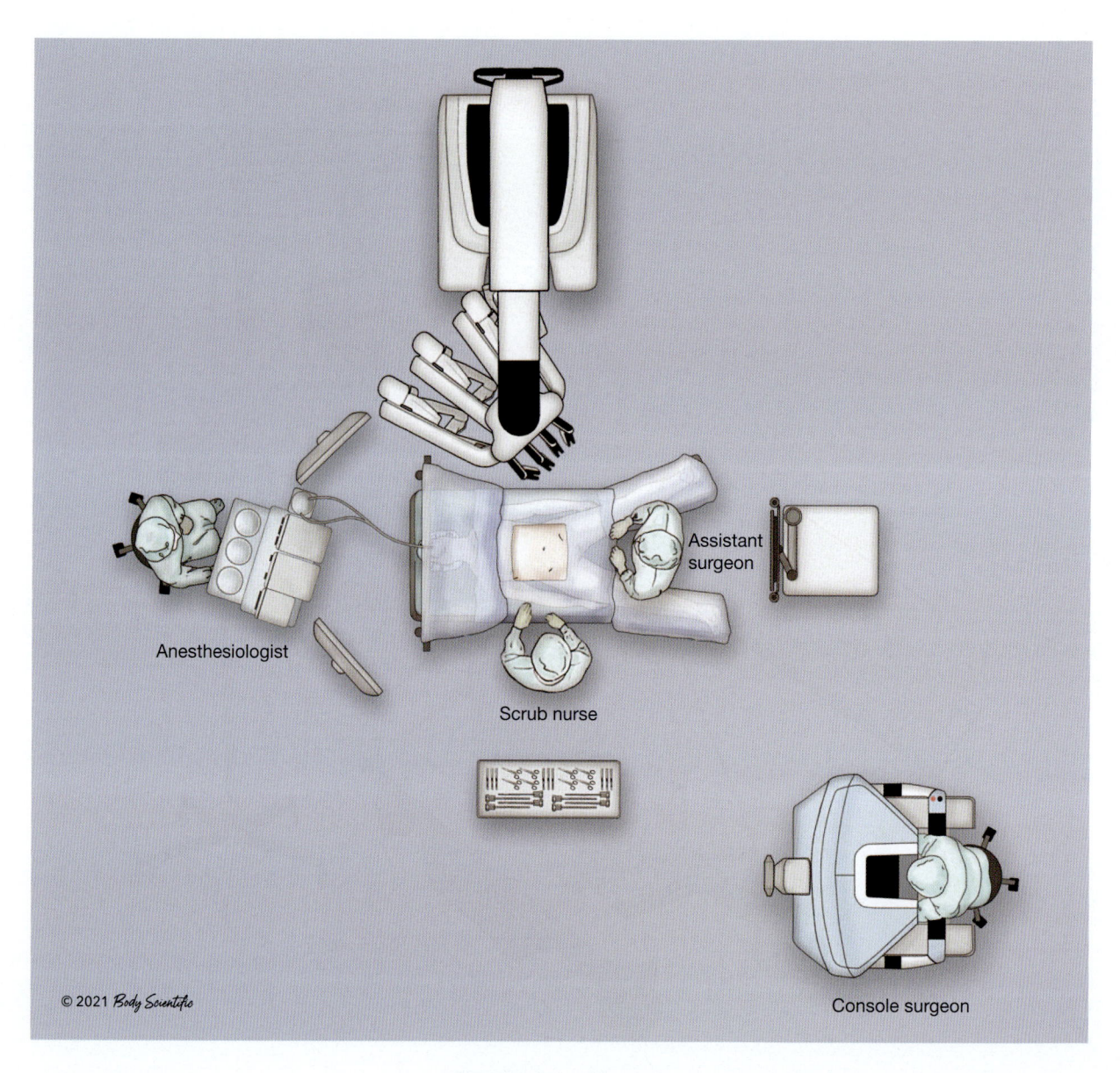

FIGURE 27-2 • OR setup.

Splenectomy **579**

The camera trocar is positioned at the intersection of the left pararectal line with a straight line oriented in an oblique fashion going from the left lower to the right upper quadrant. Once the anatomy is assessed, three 8-mm ports are positioned along this oblique line (**Figures 27-3 A, B**).

Two assistant ports are placed a few centimeter below: one is a 12-mm cannula in between the R1 and the scope, and the other is a 5-mm port positioned in between the scope and the R2 trocar.

The operative table is then adjusted to a 30° reverse Trendelenburg and tilted 20–30° to the right side. The robotic cart is placed preferably on the left of the patient to facilitate the assistant surgeon's work targeting toward the spleen, and to give room to a second assistant or a scrub nurse on the right side.

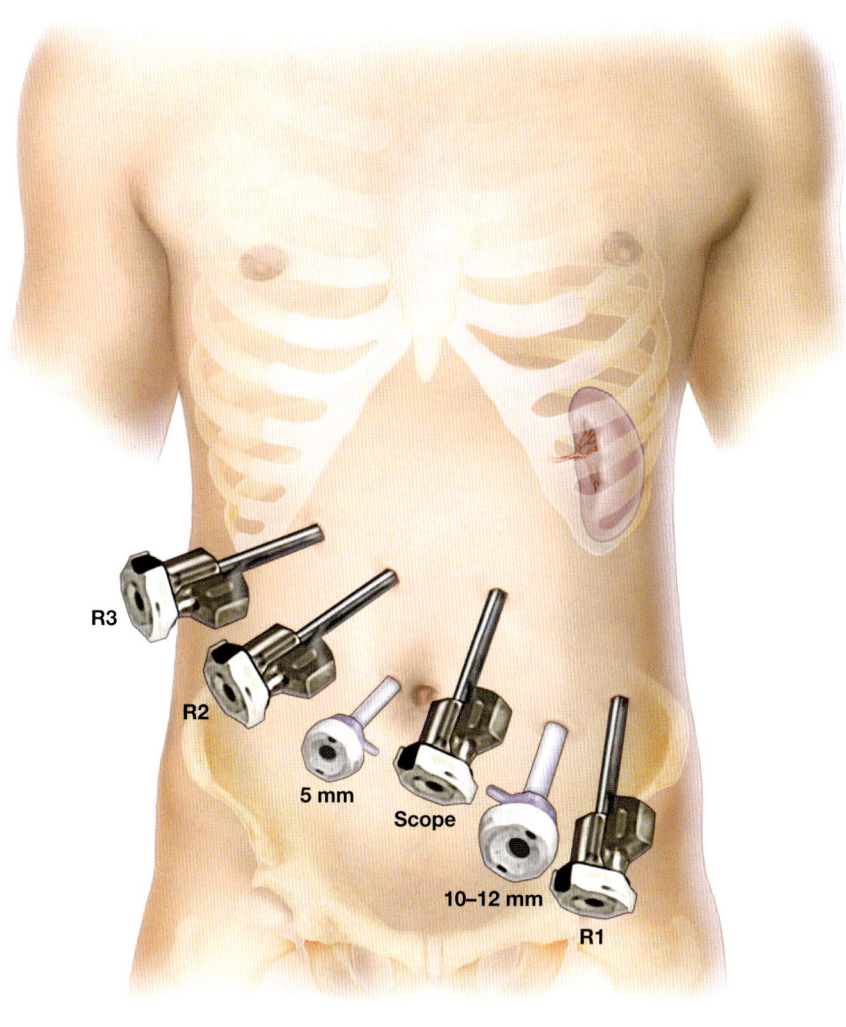

Normal abdomen

FIGURE 27-3 • Port settings. **A.** Normal abdomen.

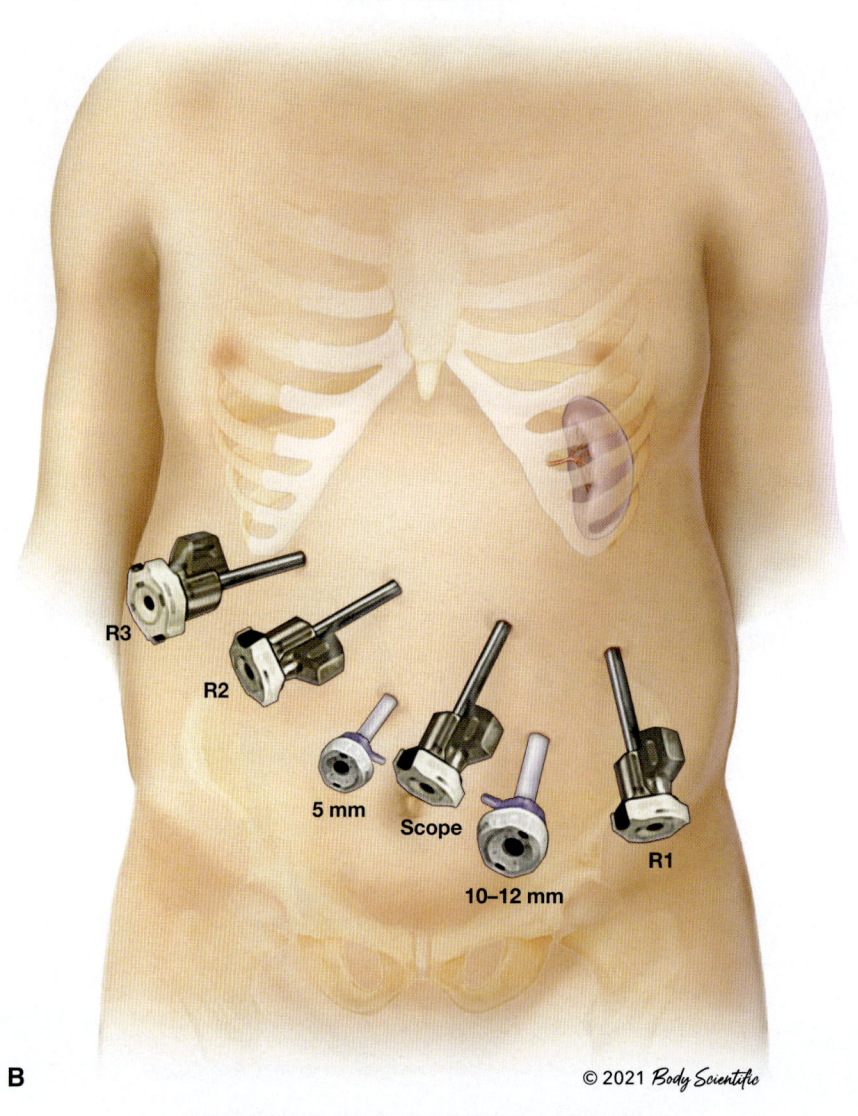

FIGURE 27-3 • (*Continued*) **B.** Wide abdomen.

Surgical Technique

▶ Video 27-1. Splenectomy – Full Procedure

Step 1. Gastrocolic ligament division

The stomach is retracted cephalad and medially using the R3. The Bouchet's transparent zone is identified by putting the gastrocolic ligament under tension. This area is opened using the cautery hook and the vessel sealer, and the access to the lesser sac is achieved. The dissection proceeds toward the short gastric vessels (which, at this point, are not dissected yet) (**Figures 27-4 A–C** and **27-5**). The maneuver guarantees the access to the lesser sac, facilitating the mobilization of the left colonic flexure and the identification of the lower edge of pancreatic body.

Step 1 average time frame: 10–15 min

> ▶▶ **TIPS**
>
> The assistant should maintain gentle tension on the transverse colon to help keep the correct avascular dissection plane and to avoid entering the mesocolon with the risk of damaging the blood supply of the transverse colon.

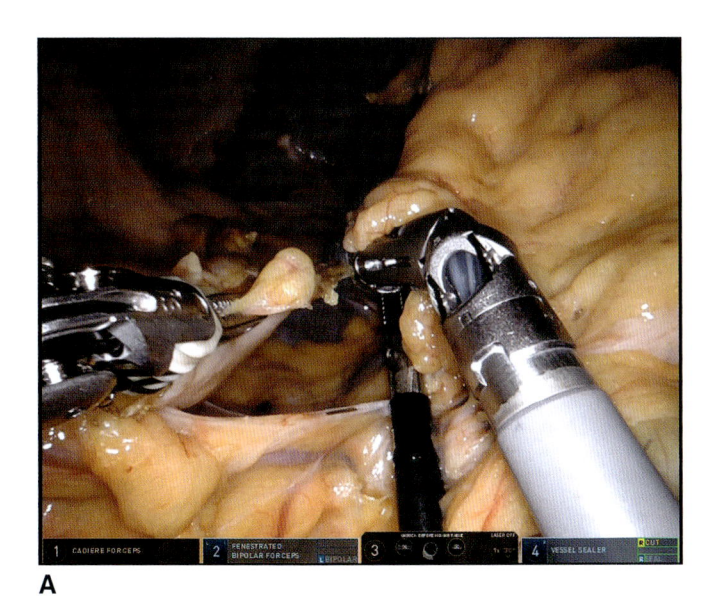

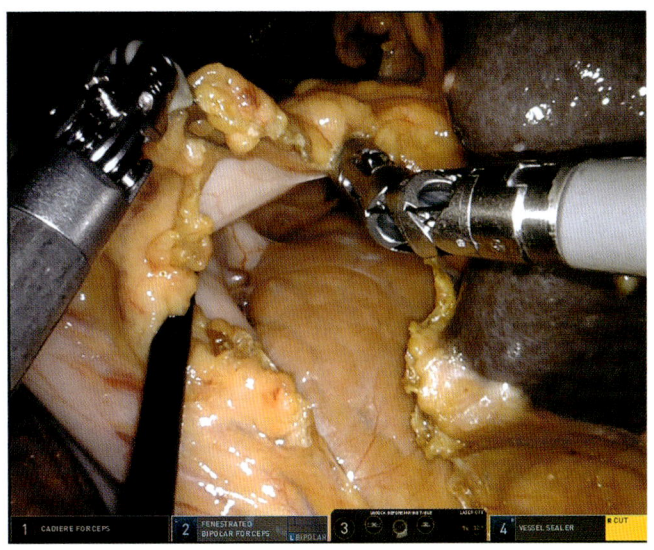

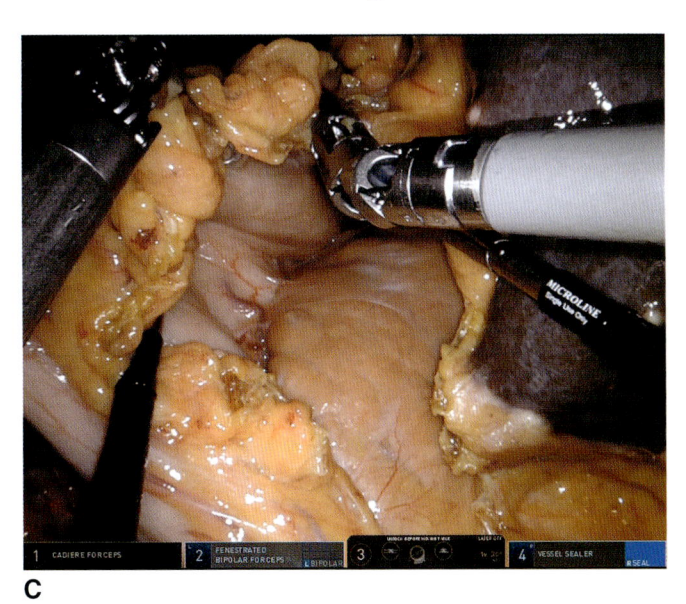

FIGURE 27-4 • Gastrocolic ligament division.

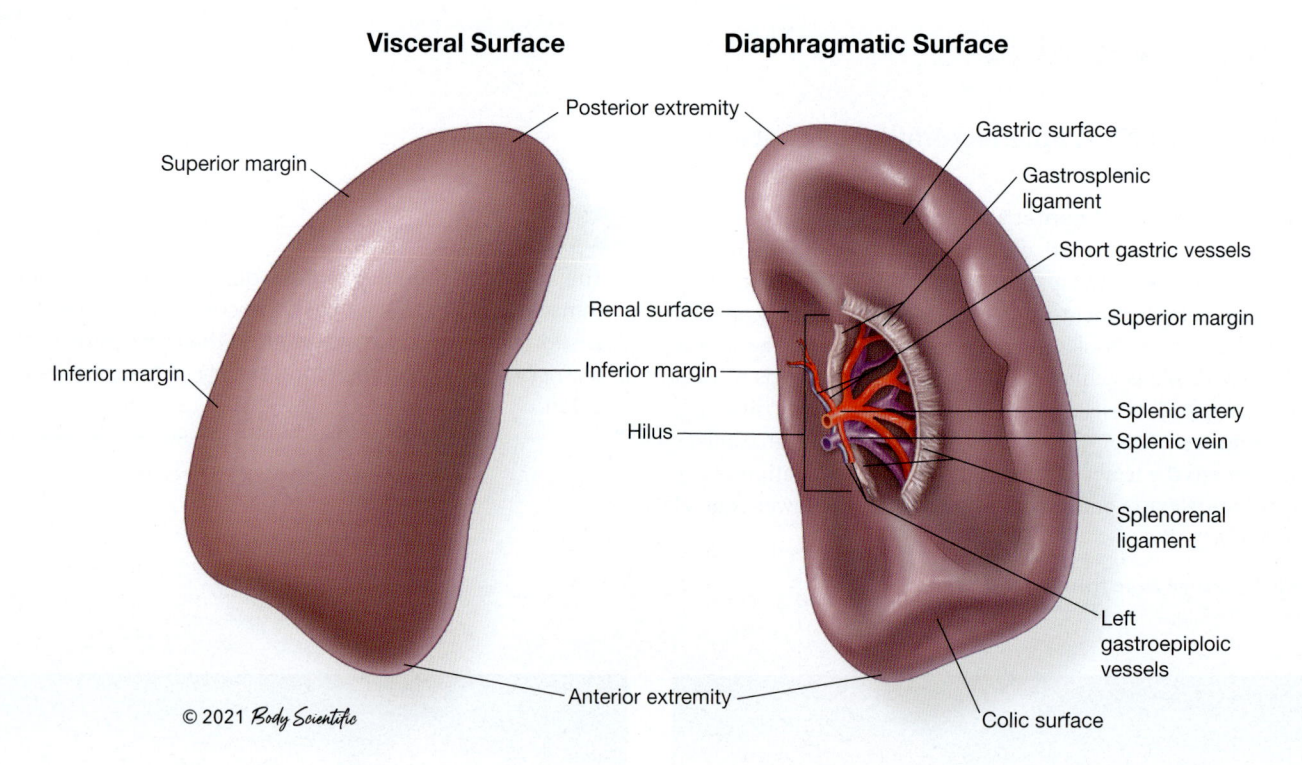

FIGURE 27-5 • Spleen: visceral and diaphragmatic surfaces.

▶ Video 27-2. Step 2. Mobilization of the Left Colonic Flexure

Step 2. Mobilization of the left colonic flexure

Using the monopolar hook and the bipolar forceps, the left colonic flexure and the proximal descending colon are mobilized, with a lateral to medial approach, keeping the dissection plane in front of the Toldt's fascia. The assistant surgeon, using atraumatic graspers, retracts the colon caudally and medially. The splenorenal and splenocolic ligaments are taken down, allowing the separation of the spleen from the colon. The correct plane can be identified and maintained by a precise combination of traction and counter traction on the mesentery of the descending colon and the Toldt's fascia (for more details about the splenic flexure mobilization pathways, see Chapter 24, Left Colectomy). This step is important to expose the inferior edge of the pancreatic body and tail (see **Figures 27-6** and **27-7**).

Step 2 average time frame: 15–20 min

> ⚠ **PITFALLS**
>
> Lacerations of the splenic capsule.
>
> During this step, retraction needs to be exerted very carefully to avoid pulling on possible adhesions between the omentum and the spleen, because this may cause lacerations of the splenic capsule and bleeding.

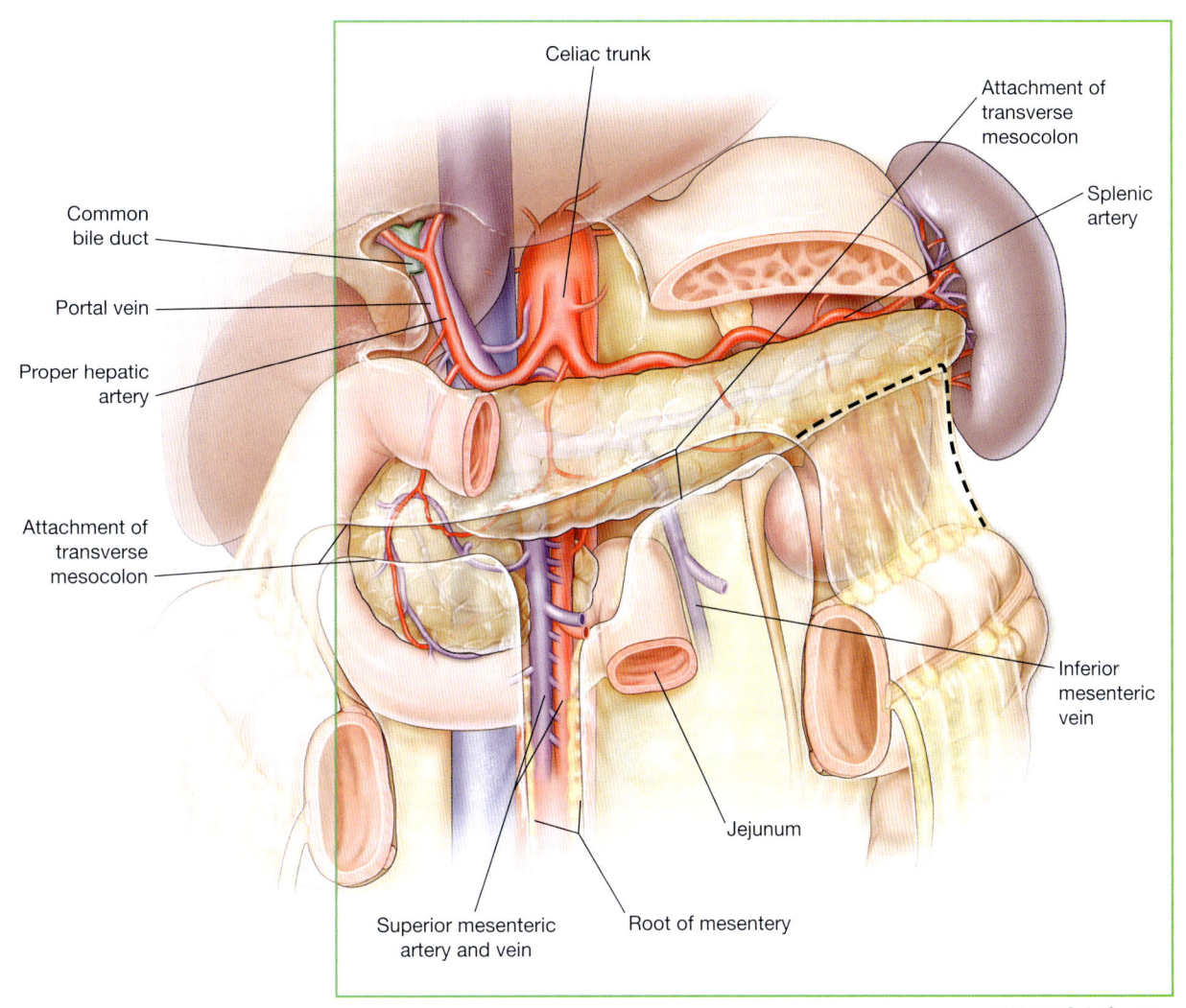

FIGURE 27-6 • General anatomy.

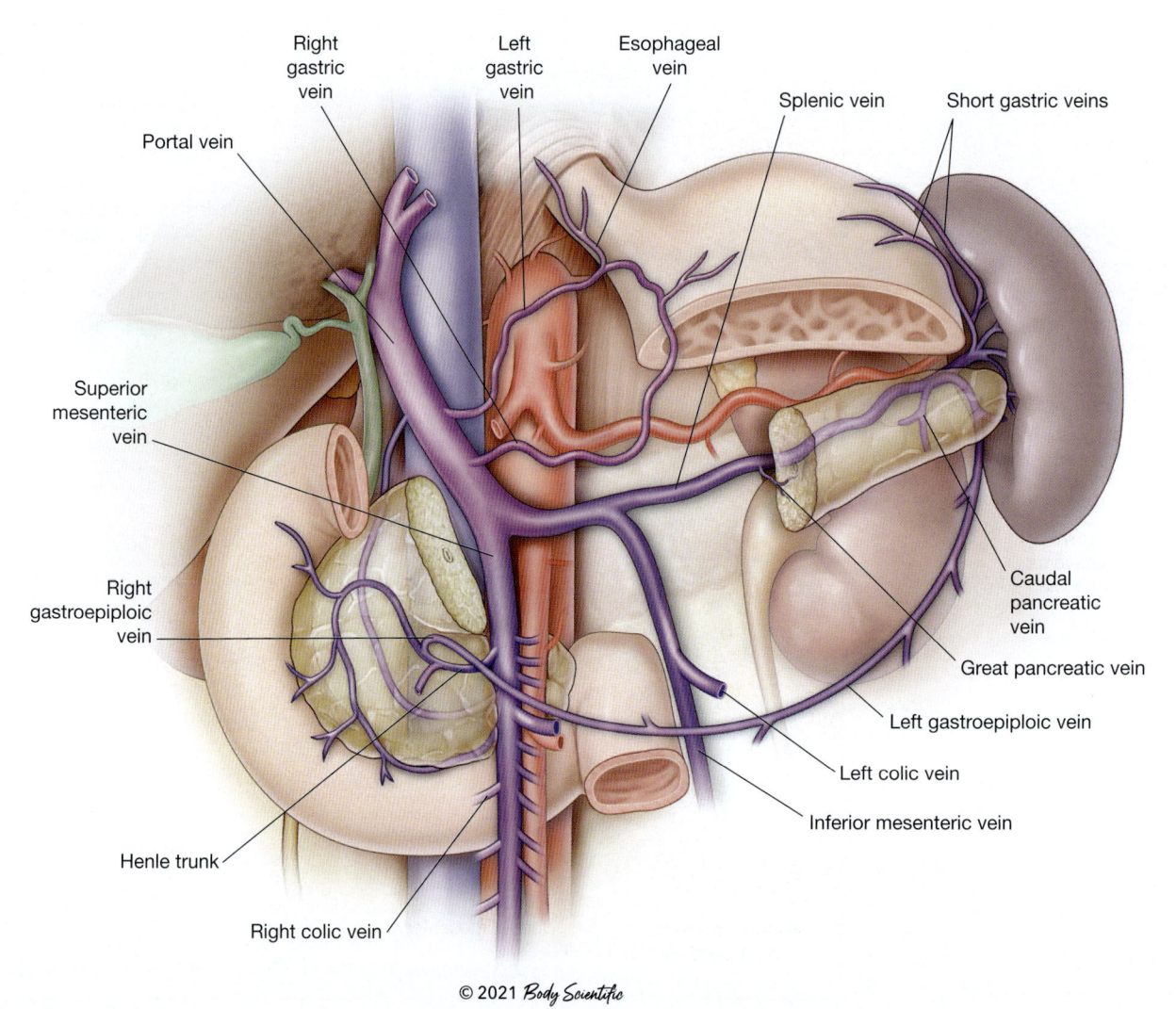

FIGURE 27-7 • Venous general anatomy.

Splenectomy 585

Video 27-3. Step 3. Splenic Artery Control

Step 3. Splenic artery control
At this point, the most distal portion of the splenic artery, that can be easily identified, should be selected for the preliminary control. A careful dissection is performed along the artery using the monopolar hook as a right angle, and a vessel loop is placed around the vessel for a better manipulation, retraction, and possible clamping. The splenic artery often presents multiple kinkings, can be tortuous, and can disappear behind the pancreatic tail (some anatomical reminders are provided in **Figures 27-5** to **27-7**). The artery should be prepared on a loop, where it is easy to do that, and staying as far distal as possible (**Figures 27-8 A–C**).

Step 3 average time frame: 5–15 min

🔍 ANATOMICAL HIGHLIGHTS
The most relevant variations of the splenic artery are described in **Figures 27-9 A, B** (for more information, see suggested reading #7).

⚠ PITFALLS
Damage of the splenic vein during the preparation of the artery.

The splenic vein can be attached to the artery, and it can be inadvertently damaged during the preparation. The bleeding can be difficult to control and may require suturing between the artery and the vein, making the preparation of the artery in that segment impossible.

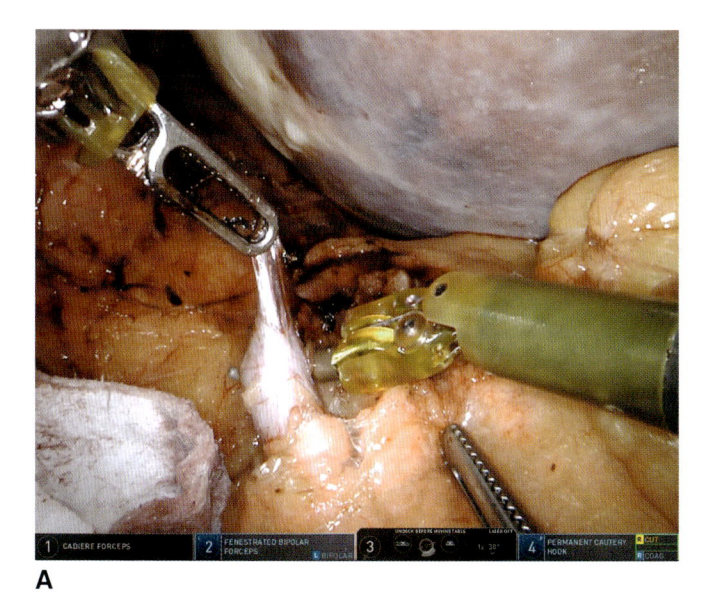

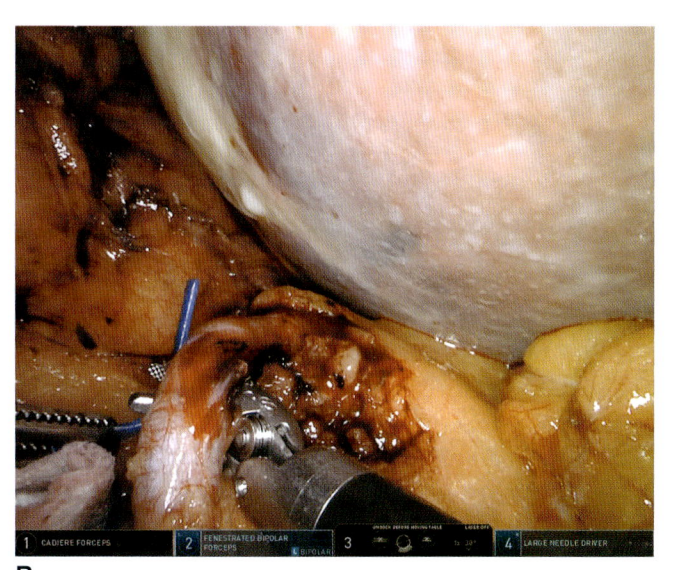

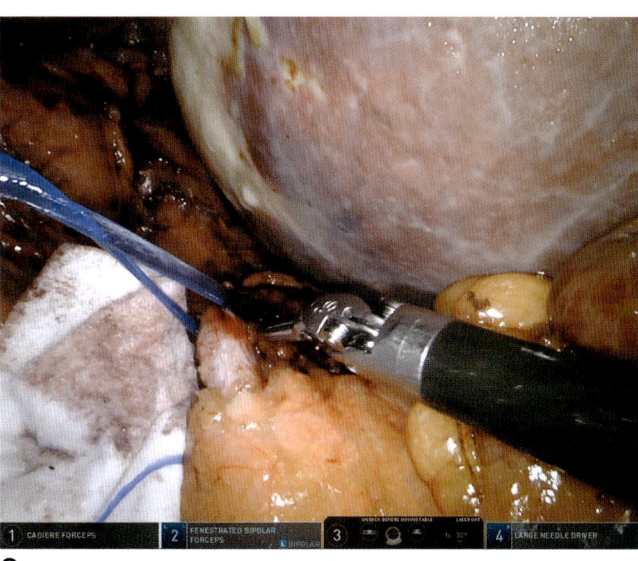

FIGURE 27-8 • Splenic artery control.

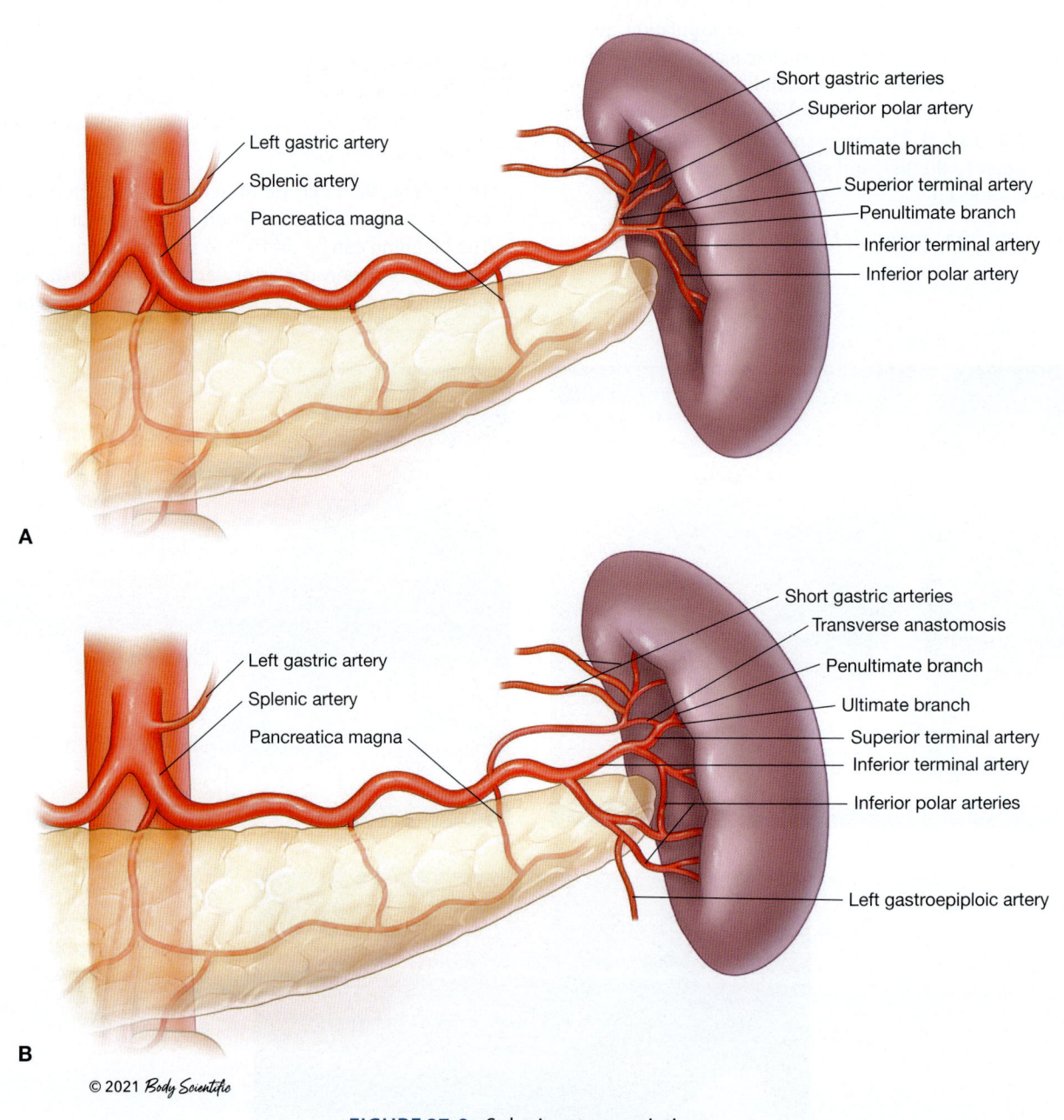

FIGURE 27-9 • Splenic artery variations.

Splenectomy 587

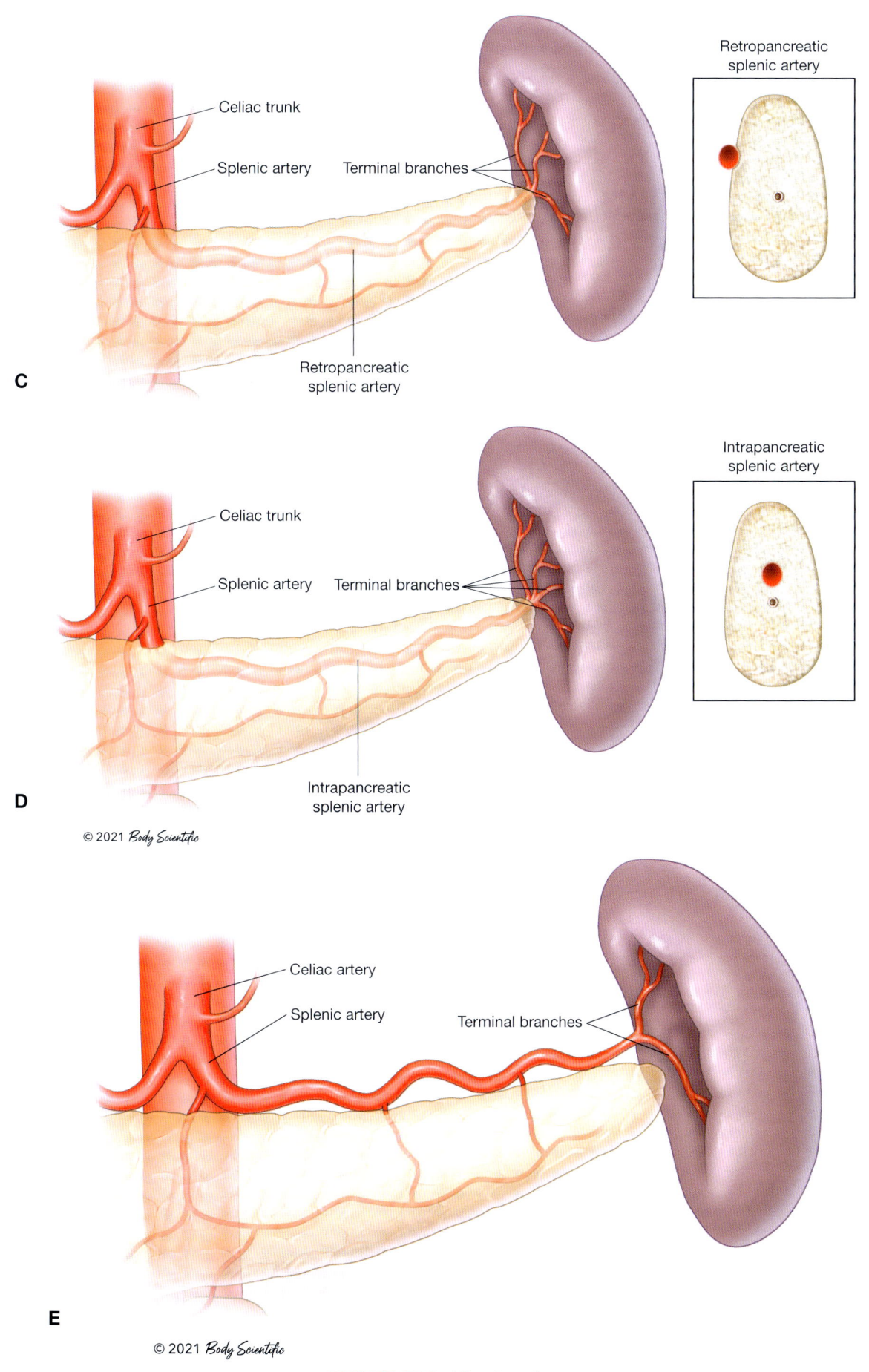

FIGURE 27-9 • *(Continued)*

Step 4. Take-down of the short gastric vessels

This maneuver can be performed using the vessel sealer in R1, the bipolar forceps in R2, and the R3 with a grasper for exposure. The Cadiére in R3 needs to be frequently repositioned to provide an effective traction of the posterior gastric wall and to optimize the visualization.

All short gastric vessels must be divided until reaching the left diaphragmatic pillar, as shown in **Figure 27-10**. To minimize the risk of rebleeding, this step is better achieved with the dual coagulation technique, using the vessel sealer twice on the same vessel, and leaving a longer-occluded stump toward the stomach side.

Step 4 average time frame: 15–20 min

> ▶▶ **TIPS**
>
> In certain cases, the splenic vein can be compressed, or thrombosed, causing left-sided portal hypertension and short gastric vein varices. When such districtual portal hypertension is present, in order to prevent some backflow bleeding, it is better to anticipate the clamping of the splenic artery (SA) before dividing the congested short gastric vessels.

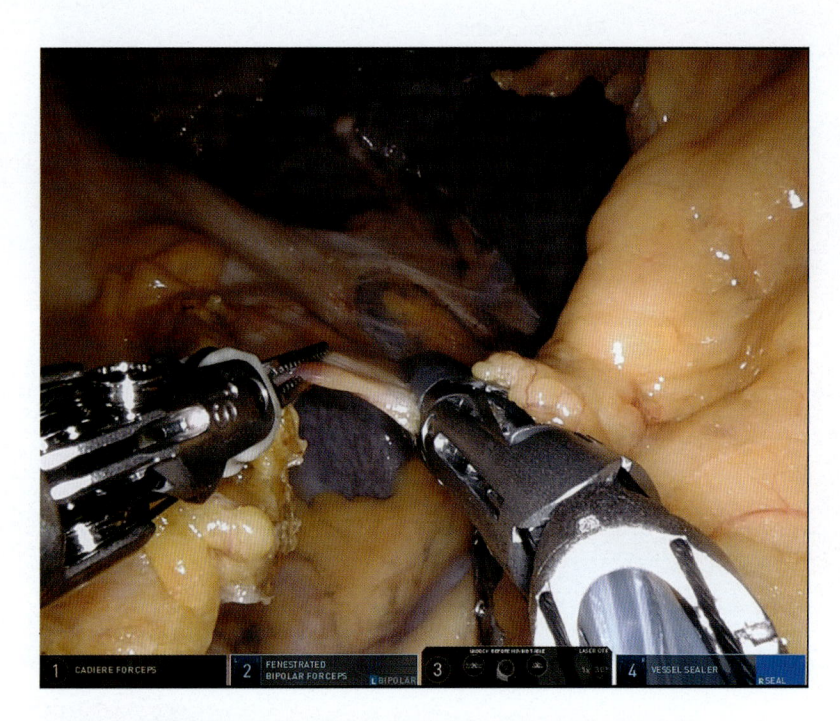

FIGURE 27-10 • Division of the short gastric vessels.

Step 5. Take-down of the phrenogastric and phrenosplenic ligaments with partial mobilization of the spleen

The phrenogastric and the phrenosplenic ligaments (see **Figures 27-11 A, B**) must be divided to achieve a partial mobilization of the spleen (**Figures 27-12 A–C**). This maneuver increases the ability to control the splenic hilum. If major bleeding occurs and the spleen is still fixed and completely attached to retroperitoneum, maneuvers like the insertion of the stapler become difficult and dangerous. The exposure is achieved with R3 retracting the stomach. The phrenosplenic ligaments are better approached from below the spleen, following the avascular plane of Toldt's fascia in front of the left kidney. A grasper with a sponge may be used to gently lift the pancreatic body/tail, and the R1 with the monopolar energy is cutting the ligaments and the posterior attachments of the spleen. For the phrenogastric and the upper portion of the phrenosplenic ligament, the dissection proceeds in the groove between the diaphragm and the upper pole of the spleen. The grasper with the sponge in R2 is gently pushing the spleen downward, opening the space.

The dissection proceeds until it is easily done.

Step 5 average time frame: 10–15 min

> ⚠️ **PITFALLS**
>
> Opening the diaphragm and the left pleura during the mobilization of the spleen.
>
> This complication usually happens with severe perisplenitis, when the capsule of the spleen is fused with the diaphragm.

A

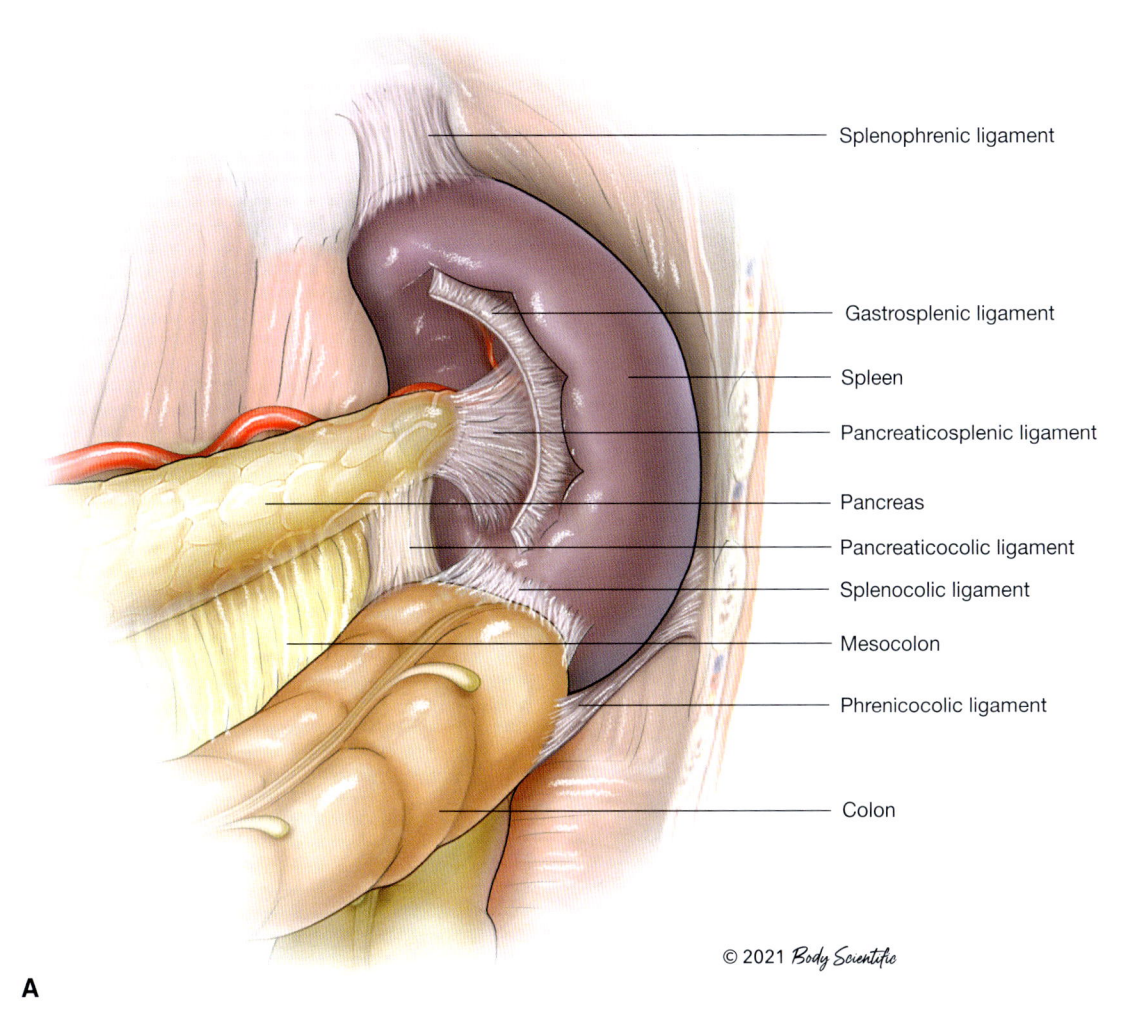

FIGURE 27-11 • Ligaments of the spleen.

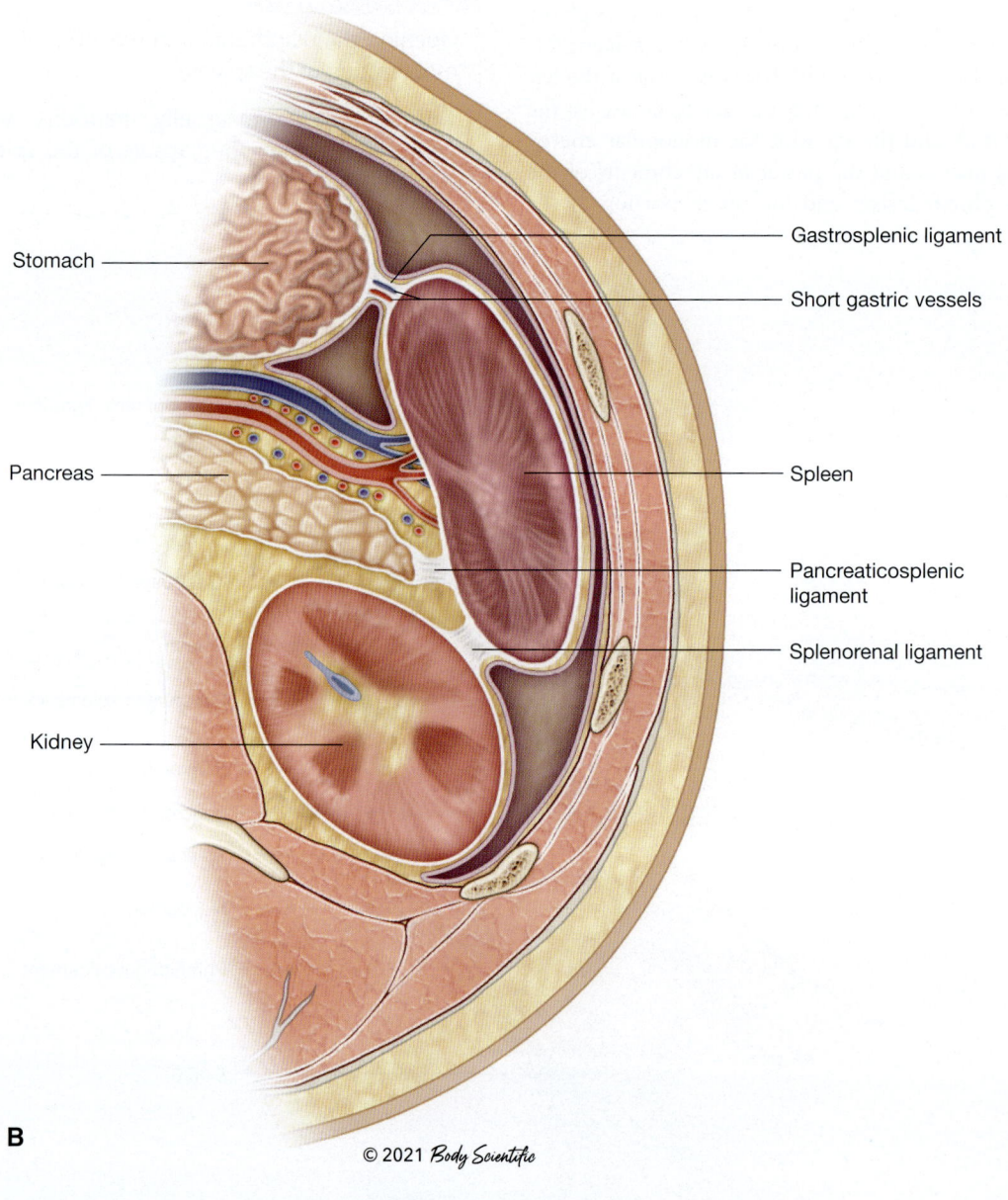

FIGURE 27-11 • (Continued)

Splenectomy 591

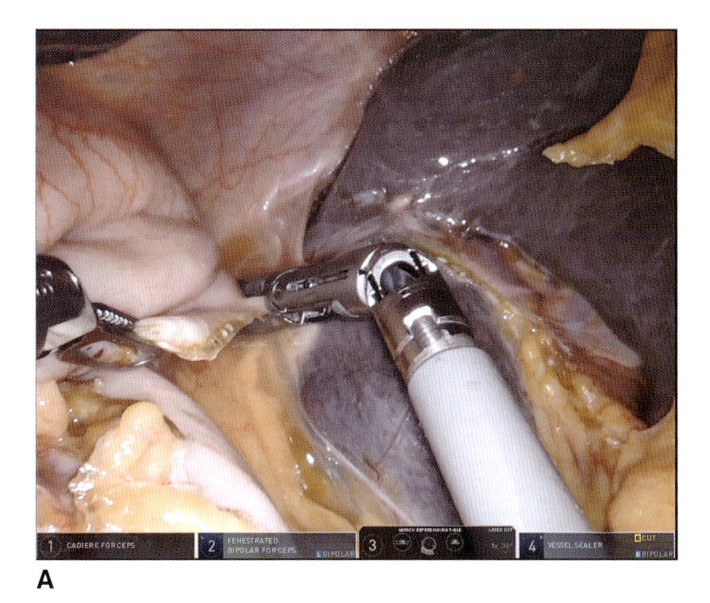

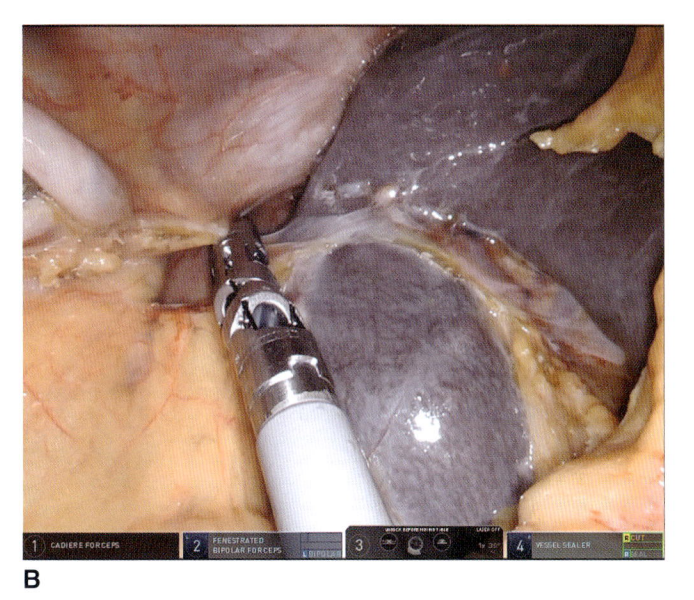

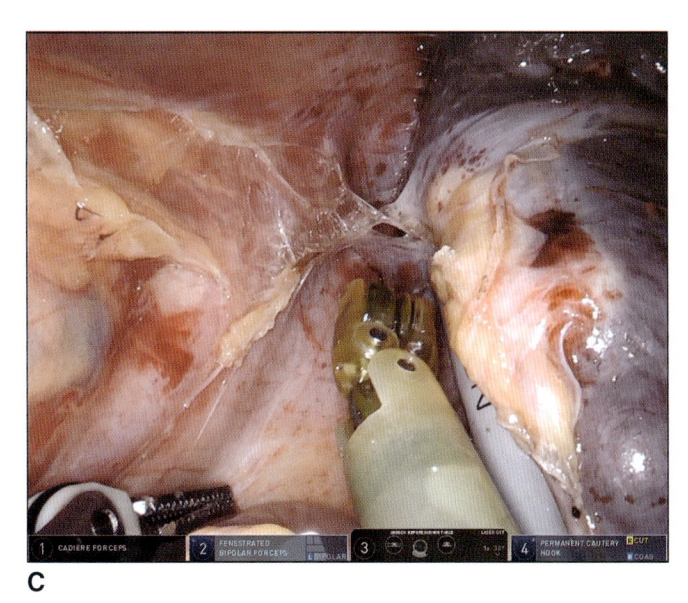

FIGURE 27-12 • Take-down of the phrenogastric and the phrenosplenic ligaments (partial mobilization of the spleen).

Video 27-4. Step 6. Retraction of the Pancreatic Tail

Step 6. Exploration of the splenic hilum and retraction of the pancreatic tail

Understanding the anatomy of the pancreatic tail, including the different morphologies, is very important in order to avoid the crushing transection of the pancreatic parenchyma during the following step. The splenic hilum is prepared for the transection. Usually, the lower and upper pole branches of the artery and vein can be individually ligated and divided (Prolene™ 4-0). Sometimes, an upper pole artery from the posterior gastric artery or the splenic artery is found, and they need to be divided (see **Figures 27-13 A–D**; see suggested reading #8). This maneuver makes the hilum narrower and easier to staple without including pancreatic parenchyma.

Step 6 average time frame: 15–20 min

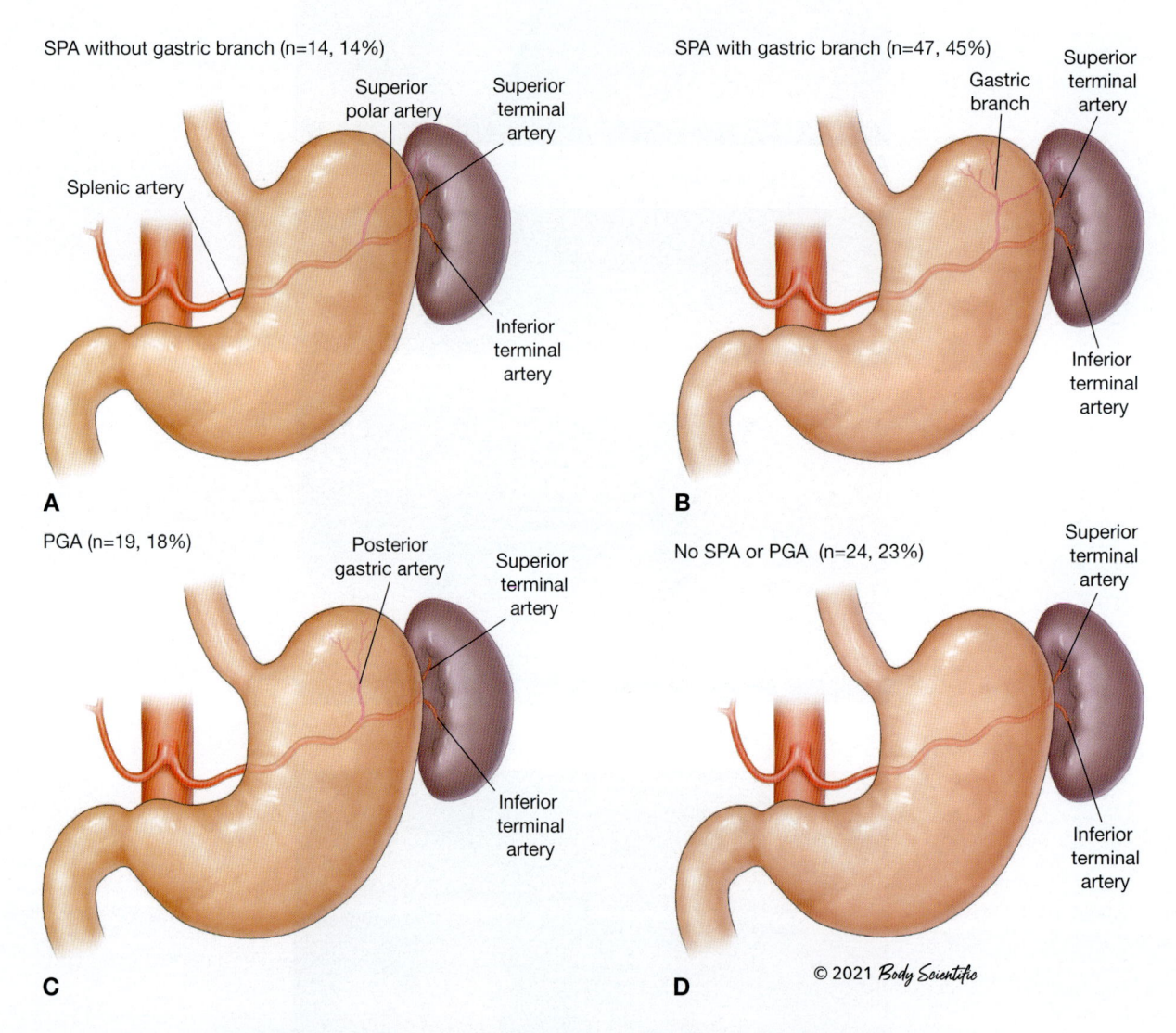

FIGURE 27-13 • Posterior gastric artery and superior polar artery variations.

Splenectomy

▶▶ TIPS

In some difficult splenic hilums, after the preparation of the retroperitoneal plane behind the pancreas, it may be useful to pass an umbilical tape around the pancreatic tail to facilitate the retraction of the gland (**Figures 27-14 A, B**)

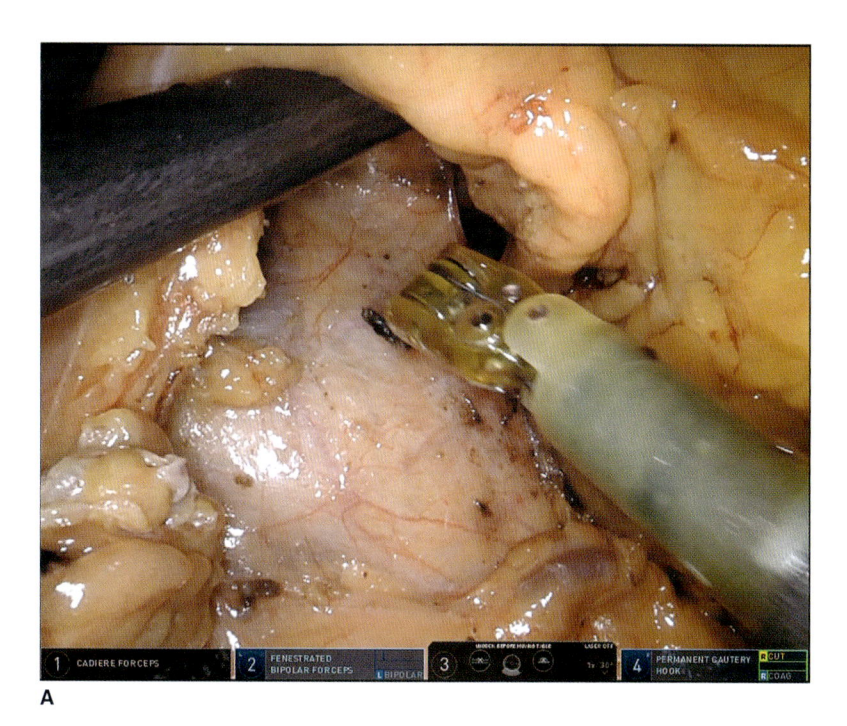

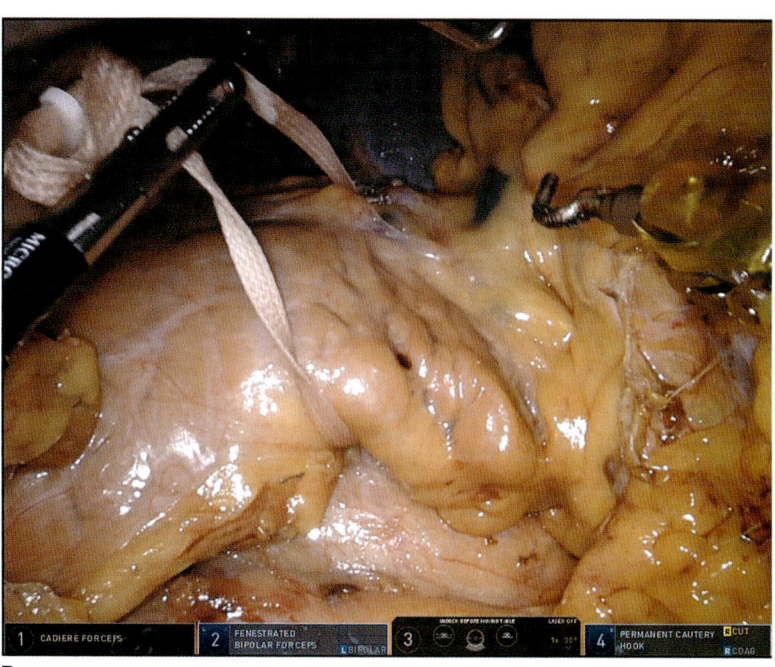

FIGURE 27-14 • Step 6. Retraction of the pancreatic tail.

594 The Foundation and Art of Robotic Surgery

> 🔍 **ANATOMICAL HIGHLIGHTS**
>
> Anatomical variations of the pancreatic body and tail (Figures 27-15 A–E).

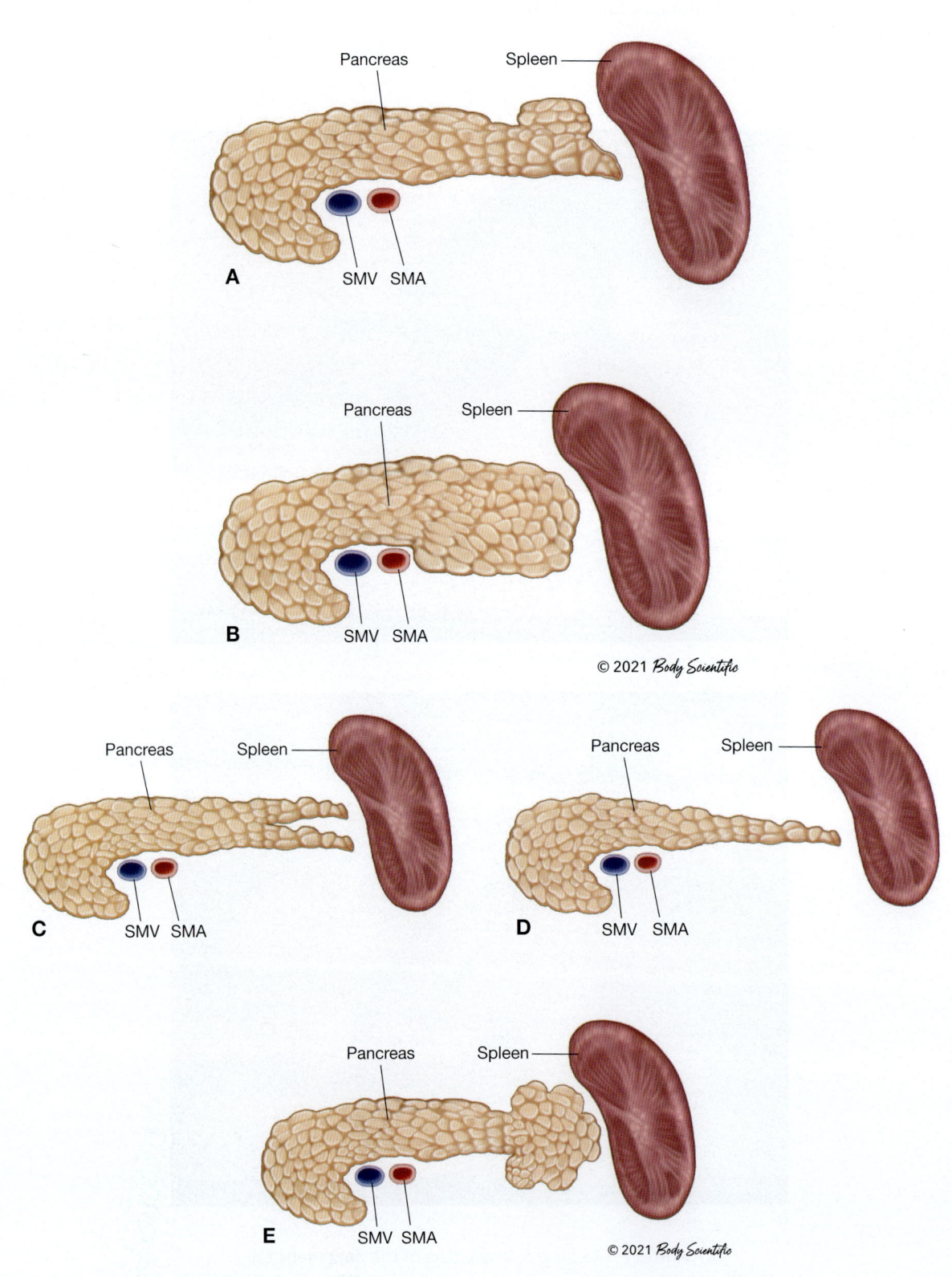

FIGURE 27-15 • Anatomical variations of the pancreatic body and tail.

Step 7. Transection of the splenic vessels

If the preliminary control of the splenic artery was very distal, close to the hilum, the artery could be divided at that level using a vascular stapler; otherwise, if the control was too proximal, a bulldog clamp may be applied without dividing the artery, to have less splenic inflow. At this point, a stapler is inserted toward the splenic side of the hilum: the partial mobilization of the spleen facilitates this maneuver. Both artery and vein are divided, simultaneously, with the stapler (see **Figures 27-16 A–E** for some anatomical reminders; also see **Figure 27-17** for the splenic vessels transection).

Step 7 average time frame: 5–10 min

> ▶▶ **TIPS**
>
> If a bulldog clamp is preliminarily applied to the artery, it is convenient to wait a few minutes before dividing the hilum, allowing the blood pooled in the spleen to be drained into the venous system.

A

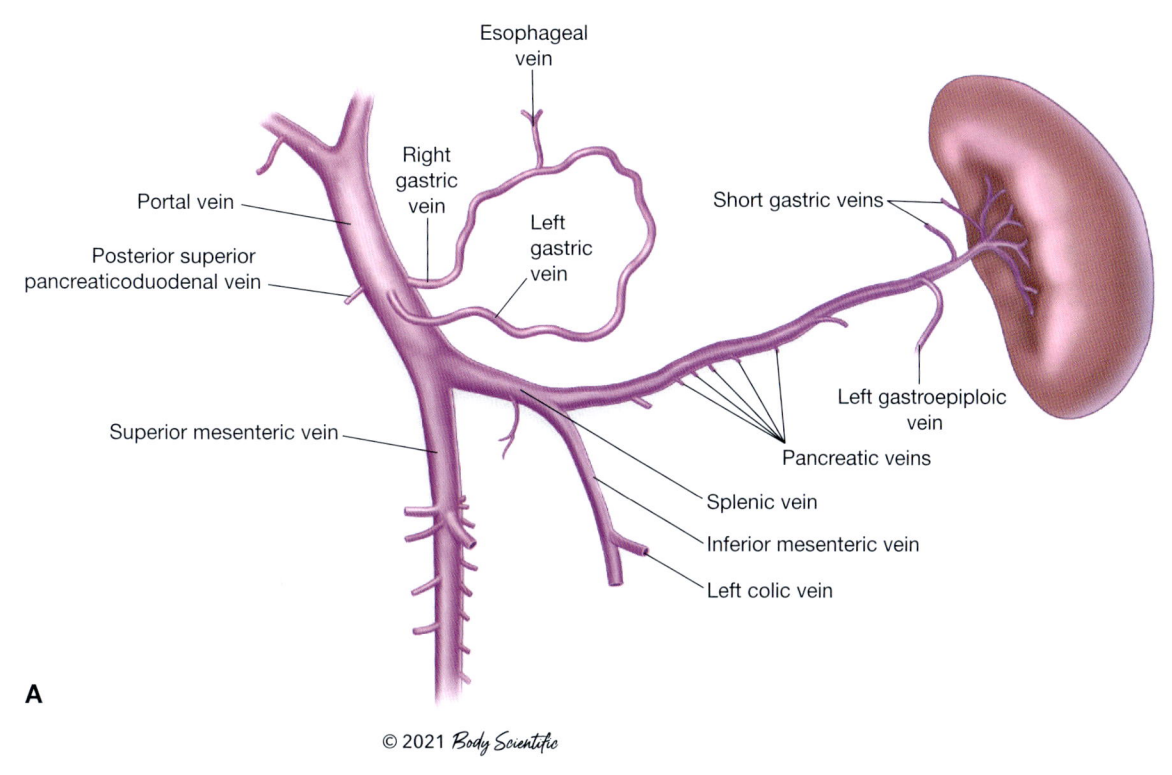

FIGURE 27-16 • Splenic venous anatomy variations.

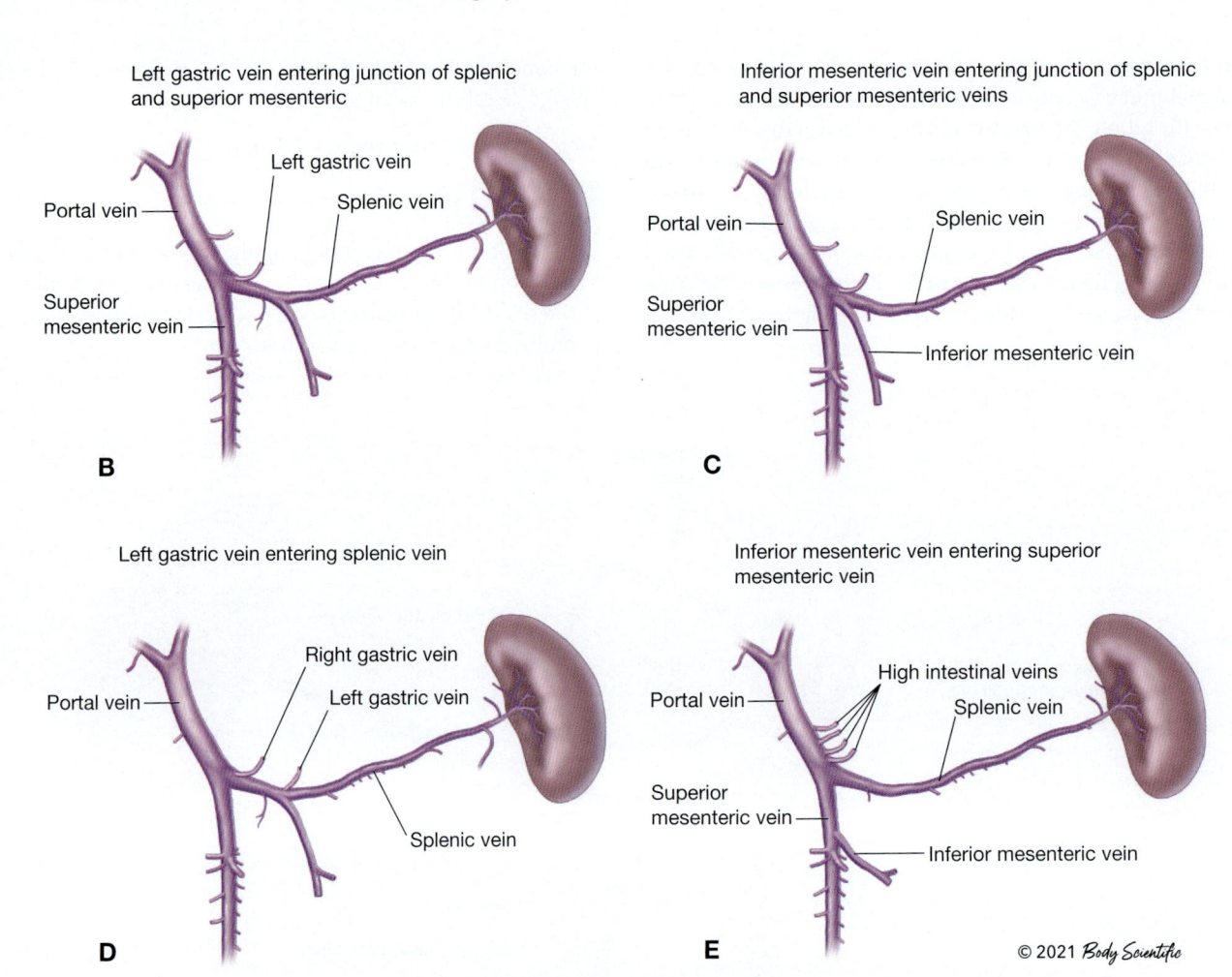

FIGURE 27-16 • *(Continued)*

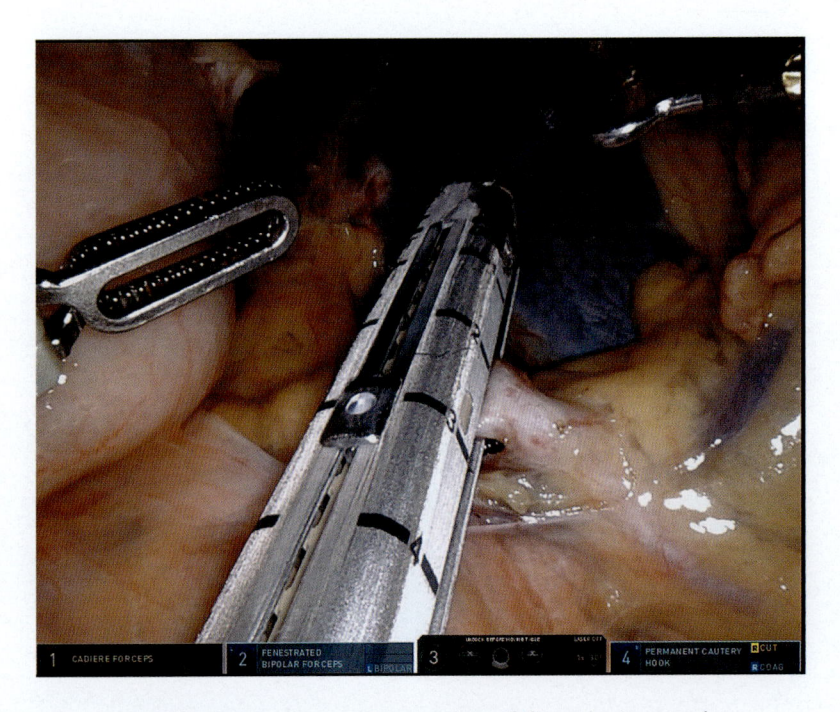

FIGURE 27-17 • Step 7. Transection of the splenic vessels.

Step 8. Completion of the splenic mobilization, specimen extraction, and hemostasis review

At this point, using a monopolar hook and/or a vessel sealer, the spleen is fully detached from the posterior plane and from the lateral retroperitoneal tissue, while paying attention not to break the capsule during the manipulation (**Figure 27-18**; see suggested reading #9).

The specimen is placed in an Endo Bag™, and it is removed by extending a trocar site or making a Pfannenstiel incision (further details are available in Chapter 2, The Basic Principles of Clinical Applications).

According to the specific surgical indications and the size of the spleen, some specimens can be morselized to be more easily retrieved.

During the extraction, the robotic cart is temporarily undocked. After closing the retrieval site, the robot is docked again to perform the final overview.

The surgical field is carefully inspected to perfect the hemostasis. Some additional suture of Prolene™ may be placed in the pedicle of the artery and vein. Also, the diaphragmatic area should be checked. The inspection is completed, evaluating all the possible sites for accessory spleens, to be sure that no splenic tissue is left behind.

In this step, the role of the bedside assistant is to maintain a clean operative field and an optimal exposure with an active, effective suction/irrigation, and proper retraction. Usually, no drains are left in place.

Step 8 average time frame: 15–25 min

⚠ PITFALLS

After a splenectomy, leaving behind some splenic tissue should be avoided, because it can be source of future diagnostic problems, or recurrence of disease/splenosis.

The most frequent reasons are:
1. Severe perisplenitis: splenic tissue can inadvertently be left in place with patches of thick capsule. The remnant tissue can increase in size over time.
2. Breaking the spleen during extraction or morselization.
3. Ignoring the presence of accessory spleens (**Figure 27-19**; see suggested reading #11).

EDITORIAL COMMENT

The dissection of the splenic hilum can also be done in a different way with individual ligation of the vessels. This technique requires more experience, and it is not always feasible. However, it has the advantage of clear visualization of the pancreatic parenchyma with less risk of its damage.

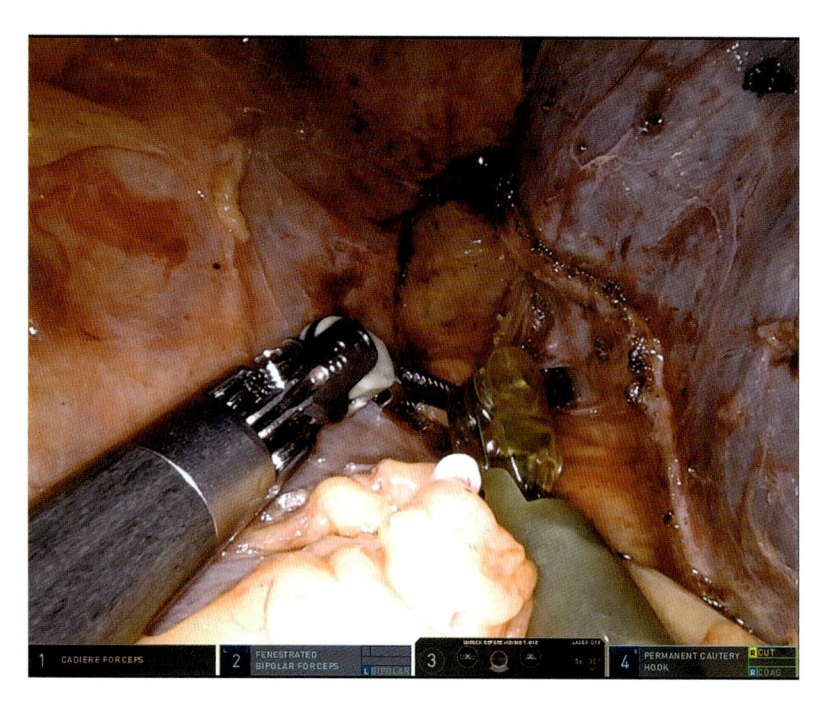

FIGURE 27-18 • Completion of the spleen mobilization.

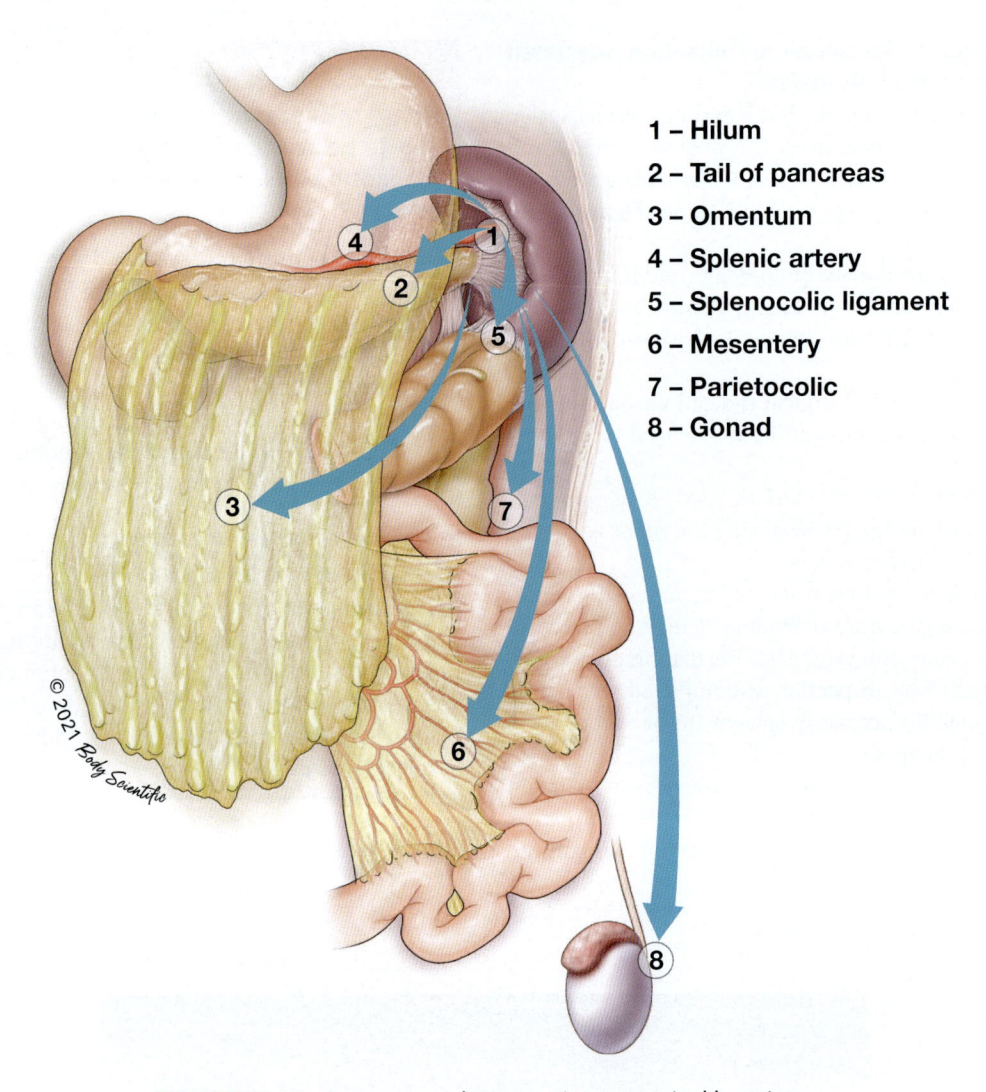

1 – Hilum
2 – Tail of pancreas
3 – Omentum
4 – Splenic artery
5 – Splenocolic ligament
6 – Mesentery
7 – Parietocolic
8 – Gonad

FIGURE 27-19 • Accessory spleens: main anatomical locations.

Suggested Readings

1. Deeb AP, Kim AJ, Fleming FJ, et al. The impact of operative approach in elective splenectomy: a multivariate analysis of outcomes from the NSQIP database. *Surg Laparosc Endosc Percutan Tech.* 2012;22(5):4159. doi: 10.1097/SLE.0b013e31825cba10
2. Bhattacharya P, Phelan L, Fisher S, Hajibandeh S, Hajibandeh S. Management of non-traumatic splenic pathologies: a systematic review and meta-analysis. *Am Surg.* 2022;88(1):38-47. doi: 10.1177/0003134821995057
3. Misiakos EP, Bagias G, Liakakos T, Machairas A. Laparoscopic splenectomy: current concepts. *World J Gastrointest Endosc.* 2017;9(9):428-437. doi: 10.4253/wjge.v9.i9.428
4. Delaitre B, Maignien B. Splenectomy by the laparoscopic approach. Report of a case. *Presse Med.* 1991;20:2263.
5. Society of American Gastrointestinal and Endoscopic Surgeons. Guidelines for the performance of minimally invasive surgery. July 2021. https://www.sages.org/publications/guidelines/guidelines-for-the-performance-of-minimally-invasive-splenectomy
6. Giulianotti PC, Buchs NC, Addeo P, et al. Robot-assisted partial and total splenectomy. *Int J Med Robot.* 2011;7(4):482-488. doi: 10.1002/rcs.409
7. Pandey SK, Bhattacharya S, Mishra RN, Shukla VK. Anatomical variations of the splenic artery and its clinical implications. *Clin Anat.* 2004;17(6):497-502. doi: 10.1002/ca.10220
8. Ishikawa Y, Ehara K, Yamada T, et al. Three-dimensional computed tomography analysis of the vascular anatomy of the splenic hilum for gastric cancer surgery. *Surg Today.* 2018;48(9):841-847. doi: 10.1007/s00595-018-1679-y
9. Omeri AK, Matsumoto S, Kiyonaga M, et al. Contour variations of the body and tail of the pancreas: evaluation with MDCT. *Jpn J Radiol.* 2017;35(6):310-318. doi: 10.1007/s11604-017-0635-x
10. Manatakis DK, Piagkou M, Loukas M, et al. A systematic review of splenic artery variants based on cadaveric studies. *Surg Radiol Anat.* 2021;43(8):1337-1347. doi: 10.1007/s00276-020-02675-5
11. Vikse J, Sanna B, Henry BM, et al. The prevalence and morphometry of an accessory spleen: a meta-analysis and systematic review of 22,487 patients. *Int J Surg.* 2017;45:18e28. doi: 10.1016/j.ijsu.2017.07.045
12. Giulianotti PC, Coratti A, Angelini M, et al. Robotics in general surgery: personal experience in a large community hospital. *Arch Surg.* 2003;138(7):777-784. doi: 10.1001/archsurg.138.7.777

"What should be recognized as a landmark date in the history of pancreatic resection was February 9, 1898 when Alessandro Codivilla of Imola, Italy performed what should be acknowledged as the first pancreatoduodenectomy."

Pancreaticoduodenectomy

Pier Cristoforo Giulianotti • Valentina Valle • Roberto Bustos • Alberto Mangano

INTRODUCTION

Indications for minimally invasive pancreatic surgery have been rapidly increasing. There are a wide range of operative approaches described, ranging from combined multivisceral operations to enucleation or wedge resections. Despite advancements in other therapeutic domains (e.g., chemotherapy/radiotherapy), the surgical approach is still the main option to pursue a curative treatment for cancer. For pancreatic cancer, the resectability rate is less than 20%. Proper lymphadenectomy and obtaining negative resection margins are paramount elements for the improvement of the oncological outcomes. The laparoscopic pancreaticoduodenectomy (LPD) is not a widely used approach given its level of technical sophistication and the significant learning curve. The first worldwide robotic pancreaticoduodenectomy (RPD) was carried out in 2001 (and later published in 2003) by PC Giulianotti. Over 20 years of practice in this area allowed standardization of the technique. The robotic platform provides multiple and well described benefits, especially during the pancreatic uncinate process dissection, the lymphadenectomy, and the reconstructive phase.

Indications and Relative Contraindications to the Robotic Approach

The elements to be considered while selecting the patients are: body mass index (BMI), anatomical location of the lesion and its relation with major vascular/lymphatic structures, and previous intra-abdominal surgeries.

Obesity and tenacious adhesions are not absolute contraindications, but they may increase the surgical time and complexity.

The boundaries of what is feasible should always be carefully evaluated within the framework of the specific expertise. Even in the event of vascular involvement (where open surgery is usually preferred), graft interposition, end-to-end reconstruction, and tangential resections are robotically feasible in the hands of expert surgeons. With that in mind, the first phase of the learning curve should consist of smaller lesions.

INSTRUMENT REQUIREMENTS

The suggested main robotic instruments/tools can be listed as follows:
- 30° scope
- Needle drivers (round tip or macro)
- Cautery hook/monopolar scissors
- Harmonic shears™/vessel sealer
- Robotic linear staplers (with different loads)
- Multiple Hem®-o-lok-clips
- Medium/large clip-applier
- Bipolar forceps
- Cadière forceps

The suggested main laparoscopic instruments/tools can be listed as follows:
- Needle drivers
- Scissors
- Graspers
- Staplers (with different loads)
- Suction-irrigation
- Laparoscopic ultrasound (drop-in probe or handheld)

Supplemental materials:
- Gauzes, sponges
- Penrose drains
- Vessel loops
- Endobags™
- Medium–large clips
- Sutures: Prolene™ 2-0, 3-0, 4-0, and 5-0
- PDS™ 3-0, 4-0, and 5-0

Photo source: Alessandro Codivilla, National Library of Medicine.
Quote reproduced with permission from Schnelldorfer T, Adams DB, Warshaw AL, et al. Forgotten pioneers of pancreatic surgery: beyond the favorite few. Ann Surg. 2008;247(1):191-202.

▶▶ **TIPS**

The best instrument for dissection is the EndoWrist® hook. This tool is very versatile: it can work as right-angle forceps without the energy and divide tissue while coagulating or cutting. The application of energy with the tip can be very sharp, but when using the back of the instrument, the coagulation becomes spray type.

Patient Positioning, OR Setup, and Port Setting

The patient is placed supine on a beanbag, with arms tucked and lower limbs parted in the French position, with a 20–30° reverse Trendelenburg and a slight left-sided tilting of the table (**Figure 28-1**). The assistant surgeon is sitting between the patient's legs. The OR setup is explained in **Figure 28-2**.

The pneumoperitoneum is achieved with the Veress technique in a region very close to the costal margin and more cranial than Palmer's point (modified Palmer's point). A 5-mm trocar is inserted into the left upper abdominal quadrant and a 4-quadrant diagnostic laparoscopy is carefully carried out. This step is performed in order to exclude possible surgical contraindications (e.g., undiagnosed liver metastases or carcinomatosis) and to insert the remaining ports under safe visualization.

Whenever possible for the available space, the third robotic arm (R3) is better positioned on the right side. In doing so, a more effective retraction of the pancreatic head can be achieved during the uncinate process dissection.

In order to exclude hepatic metastatic involvement, an accurate laparoscopic ultrasound is carried out, before docking the robotic cart.

The port setting in the RPD procedure is very important (**Figures 28-3** and **28-4**).

A correct position of the ports allows an optimal visual control of the anatomical target, an unrestricted range of instruments motion, and a better working space for the assistant surgeon with full surgical, bi-handed capabilities. Six cannulas are utilized (4 robotic and 2 assistant ports).

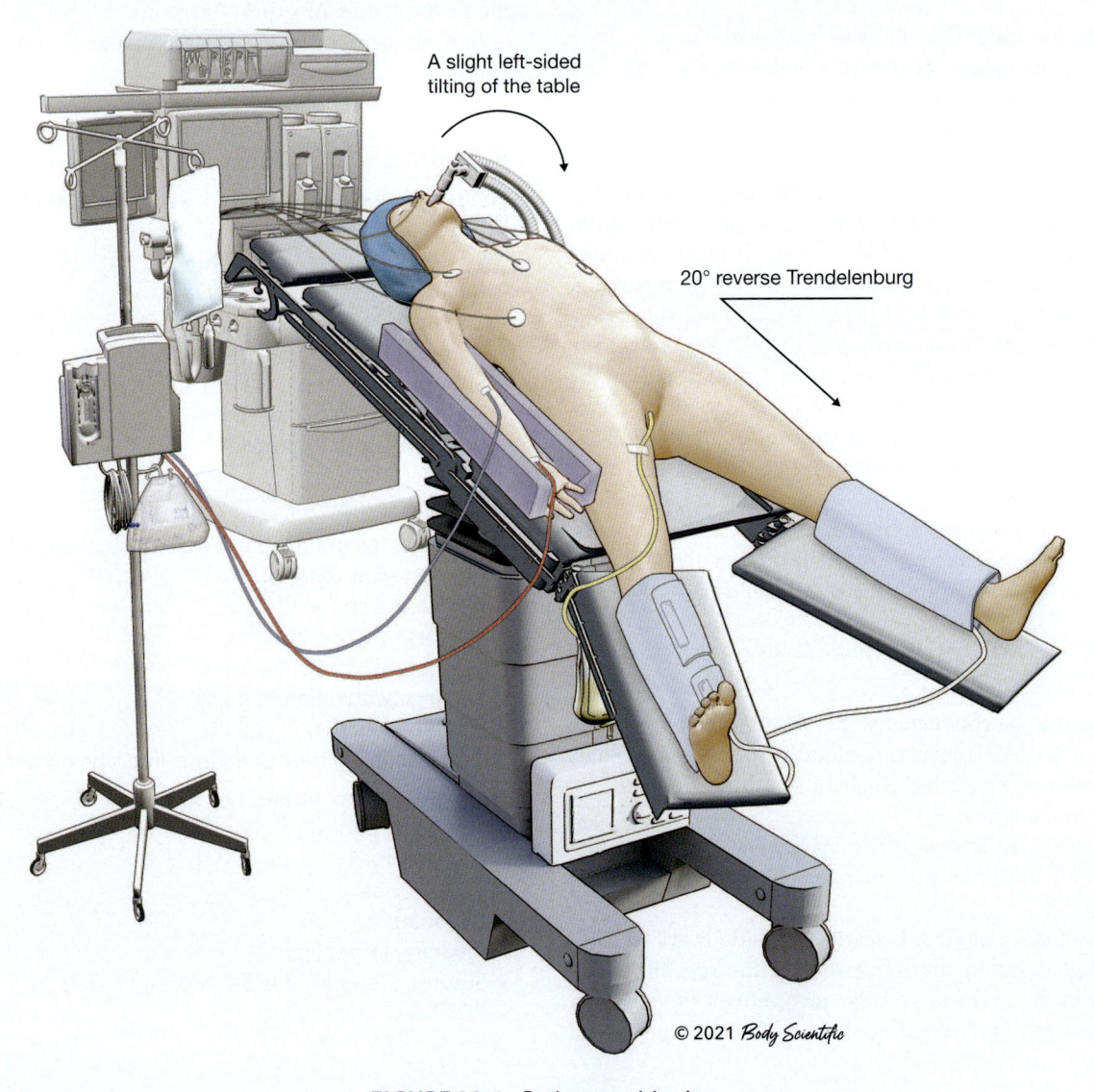

FIGURE 28-1 • Patient positioning.

The four 8-mm robotic cannulas are positioned along a straight line, usually 2 cm above the transverse umbilical line. The scope is placed in the right paraumbilical position, for most part of the case, in order to achieve the best visual control of the superior mesenteric vein (SMV) and the right side of the portal vein.

The advantage of moving the scope to different ports is clear when doing the pancreaticojejunostomy. In this step, the scope is repositioned into the paramedian left port, that is closer to the anastomotic site, allowing a better definition of the technical details.

The two 10–12-mm assistant ports are placed on both sides of the midline, in the lower quadrants, and are conveniently parted from the other ports allowing a good assistant interaction.

However, in a very narrow abdomen, there is not enough space for three ports in the right lateral quadrant, and to avoid mechanical conflicts, the R3 is set in the left lateral position.

> ▶▶ **TIPS**
>
> The body habitus may suggest an adaptation of the port setting, moving the straight line cephalad or caudally according to the distance of the target (pancreatic head) in relation to external landmarks (umbilicus, costal margin). The initial laparoscopic overview helps in defining the proper position of the ports for the operation.

> ▶▶ **TIPS**
>
> The R3 is better placed in the right lateral position, in wide/large abdomens where this setting is feasible without collisions achieving a better retraction of the pancreatic head during the uncinate dissection.

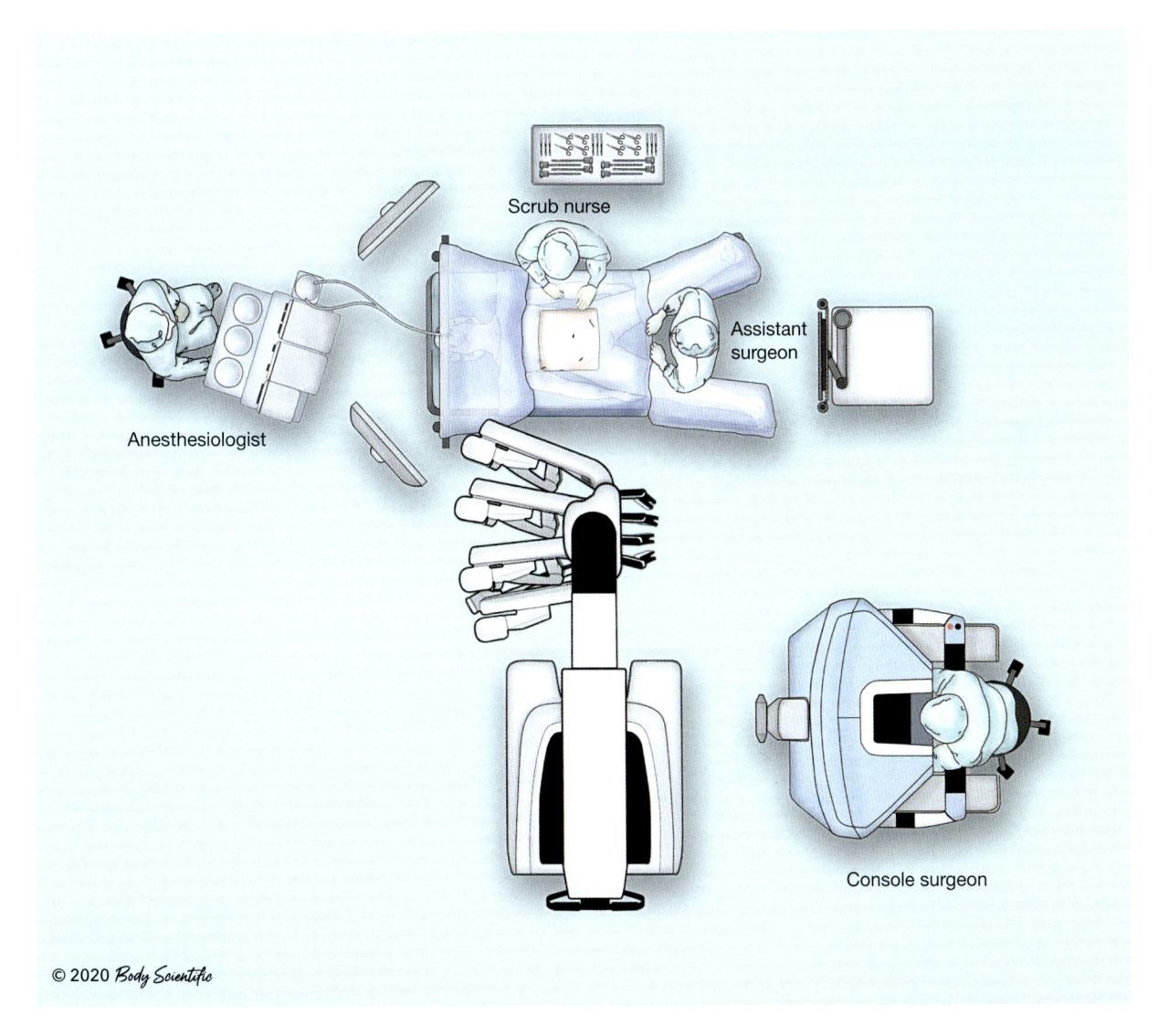

FIGURE 28-2 • OR setting.

FIGURE 28-3 • Port setting normal abdomen.

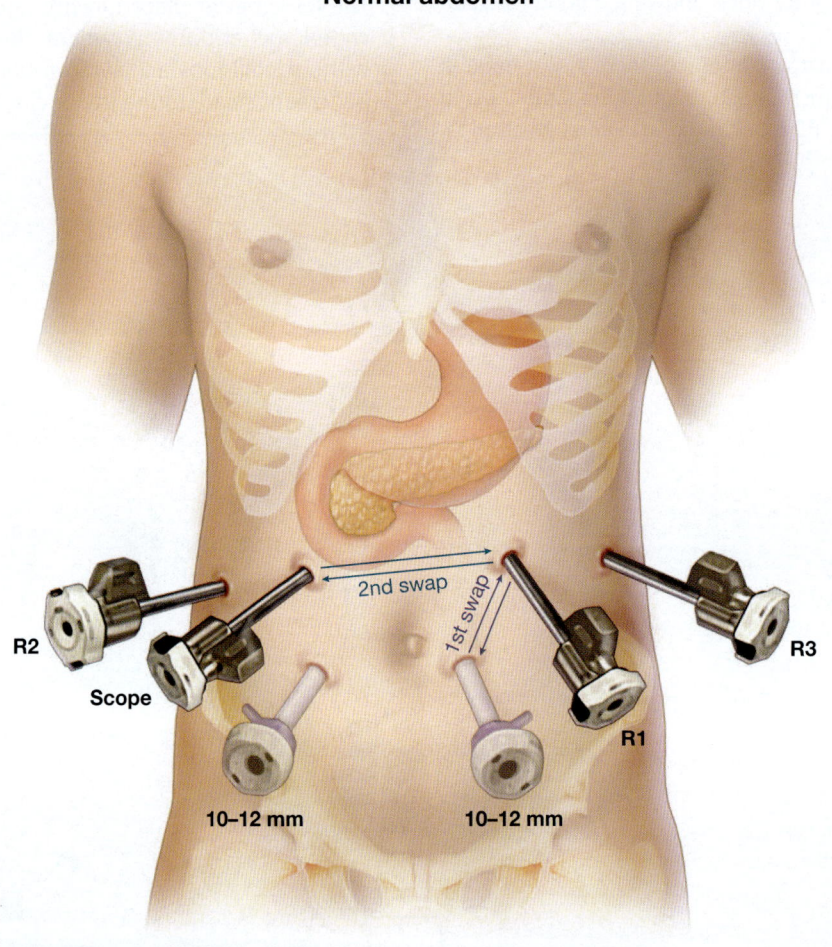

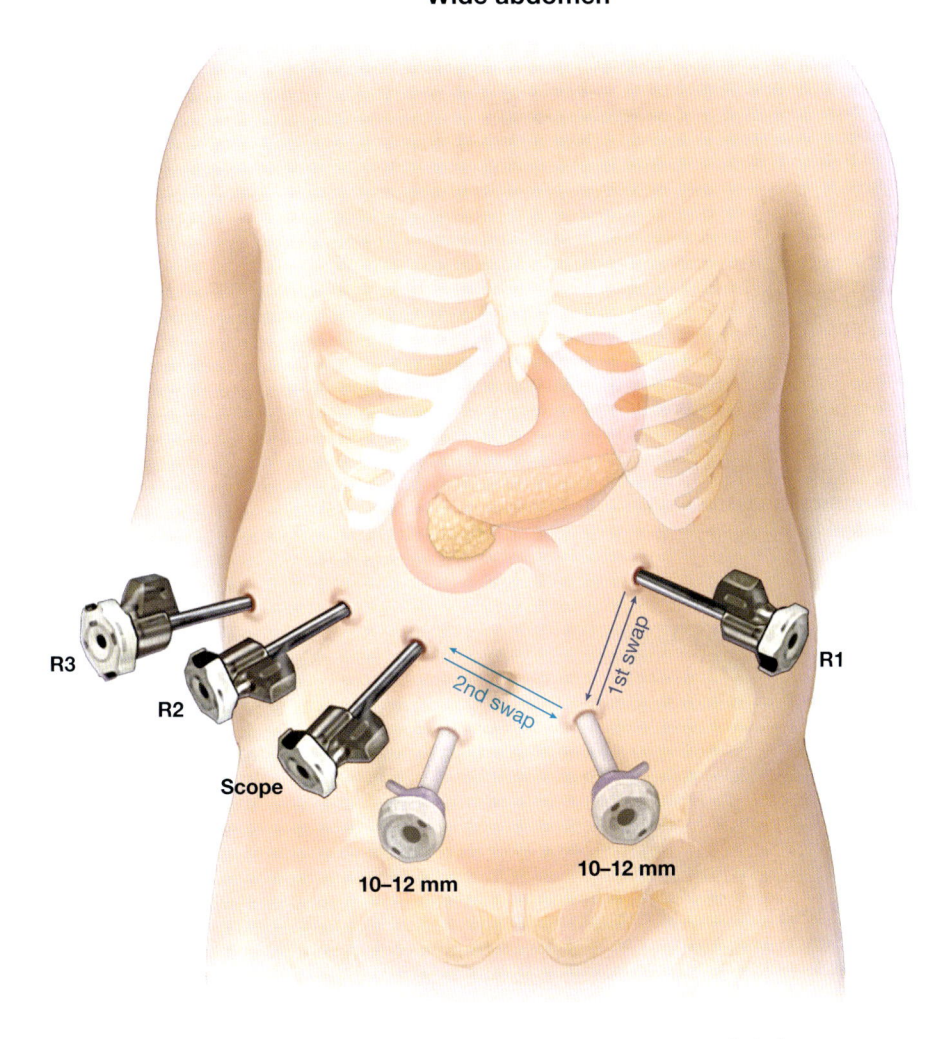

FIGURE 28-4 • Port setting wide abdomen.

Surgical Technique

Video 28-1. Pancreaticoduodenectomy – Full Procedure

> ▶▶ **TIPS**
>
> A hepato-pancreatico-biliary surgeon should be skilled in intraoperative ultrasound (IOUS). Nonetheless, the precise role of IOUS in pancreatic surgery is questionable. While it may help in detecting small nodules, like neuroendocrine tumors, or in scanning the liver for metastatic lesions, it is not very useful in ruling out the resectability of a cancer. There are many artifacts and the interpretations of the images can be very difficult.
>
> The final assessment relays on the surgical dissection of the vascular structures around the tumor: narrowing of a vein, changes in color, and indirect tactile feedback (based on tissue deformation in response to local pressure) are all important elements.

Dissection

Before starting the dissection, a gross inspection with exclusion of any obvious liver and peritoneal metastases are performed. Biopsy of suspected lesions may be necessary.

Step 1. Gastrocolic ligament division

Using the R3, the stomach is lifted upward with a grasper. The Bouchet's transparent zone is identified by putting the gastrocolic ligament under proper tension. This area is opened with the hook, this maneuver allows entrance into the lesser sac to inspect the pancreas (anteriorly) and the stomach (posteriorly) to rule out tumor spread/carcinomatosis.

If a PPPD (pylorus-preserving pancreaticoduodenectomy) is planned, in order to guarantee a proper pyloric blood supply, it is important to spare the right gastroepiploic arcade.

The gastrocolic ligament opening (**Figure 28-5**) is widened before reaching the left gastroepiploic and short gastric vessels (which have to be preserved). The SMV/portal vein confluence (located below the pancreatic neck) is assessed. An essential part of the resectability evaluation also entails assessing the SMV–portal vein confluence.

Step 1 average time frame: 10–15 min

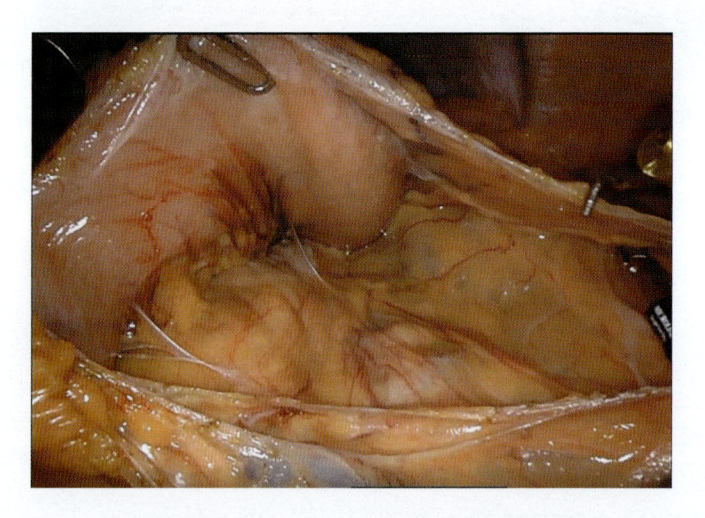

FIGURE 28-5 • Step 1. Gastrocolic opening.

Step 2. Hepatic flexure mobilization

This apparently simple step cannot be understated. A generous detachment of the right colonic flexure and ascending colon is "opening" the surgical field, and is facilitating many other subsequent maneuvers.

The vena cava, the entire second portion of the duodenum, and the head of the pancreas should be exposed.

Depending on the vascular anatomy of the mesentery of the right colon, it may be difficult to open the space to have a complete exposure of the head of the pancreas. This situation may require the division, between clips or ligatures, of the right colonic vein just before its merging into the SMV or middle colic vein. The dissection is easily done with the monopolar energy, staying in front of the prerenal Toldt's fascia, and using the bipolar forceps to perfect the hemostasis. The assistant surgeon helps with the laparoscopic forceps in maintaining the exposure and retracting the colon medially and downward (**Figures 28-6 A–C**). The right colonic vein presents multiple anatomical variations that are important to be aware of (**Figures 28-7 A–E**). (For more information, see suggested readings #11, 12, 13.)

Step 2 average time frame: 10–15 min

> ▶▶ **TIPS**
>
> Asking the assistant to maintain some tension on the mesentery of the flexure helps in keeping the proper avascular dissection plane between the two fascia layers.
>
> The main landmarks of dissection should be checked (head of pancreas, entire second portion of the duodenum).
>
> The monopolar hook or scissors are the best tools to find and maintain the right plane.

> 🔍 **ANATOMICAL HIGHLIGHTS**
>
> The right colonic drainage into the Henle's trunk, the middle colic vein, and the right gastroepiploic vein.

> ⚠ **PITFALLS**
>
> Entering the renal/Gerota's fat pad.
>
> Insufficient, incomplete mobilization.

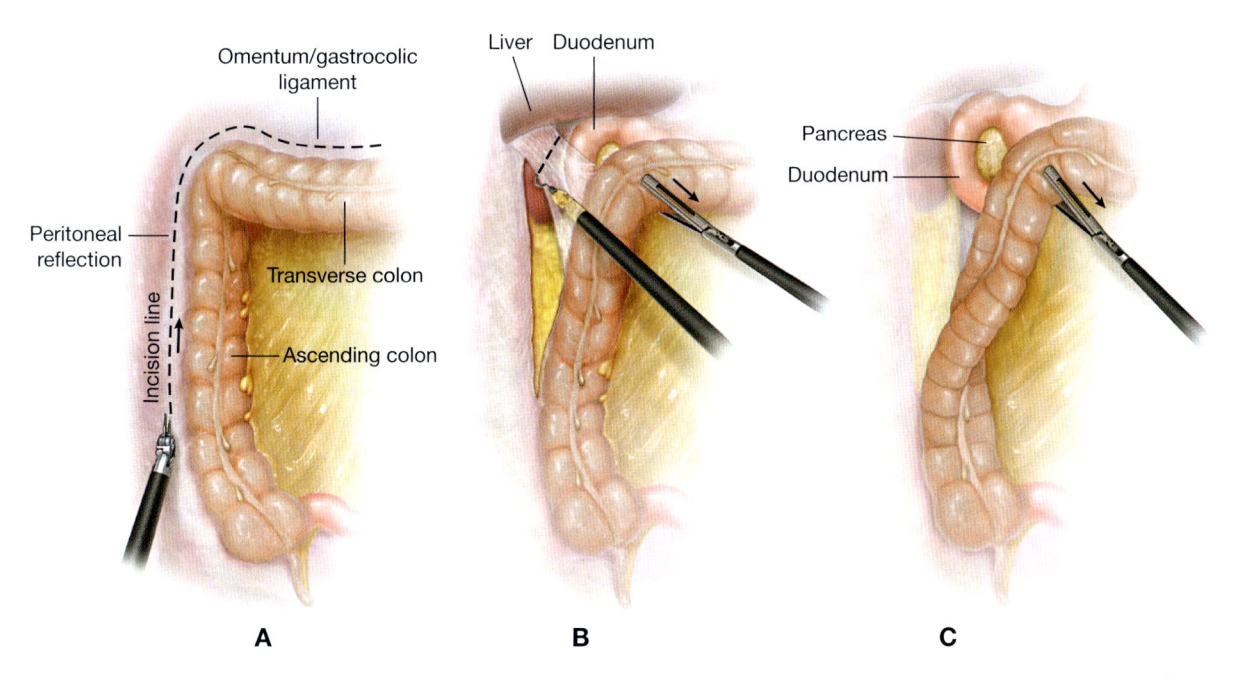

FIGURE 28-6 • Step 2: Hepatic flexure mobilization.

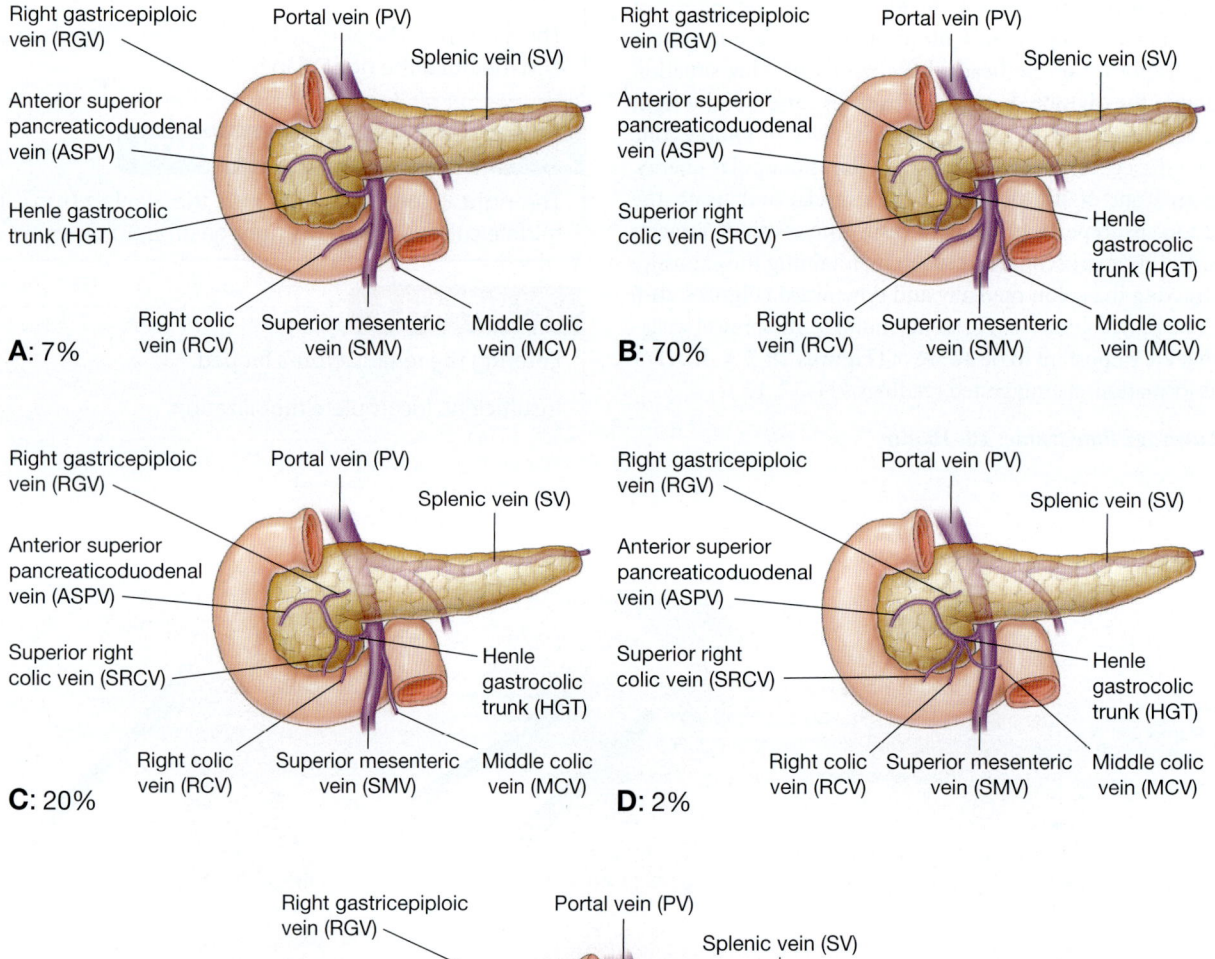

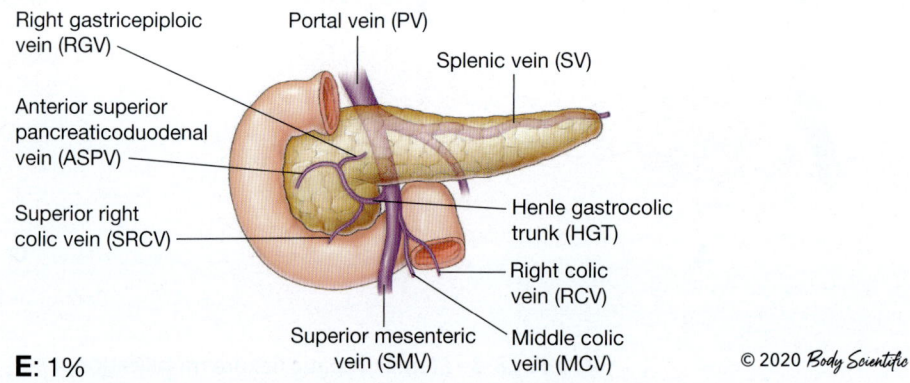

FIGURE 28-7 • Right colonic vein anatomical variations.

Video 28-2. Step 3. Kocher Maneuver

Step 3. Kocher maneuver
This maneuver, named after Emil Theodore Kocher, is one of the most useful ones in general surgery, necessary in many situations and different operations. It entails the complete detachment of the duodenum and the head of the pancreas from the retroperitoneum. In the Whipple procedure, it is fundamental for staging of the pancreatic cancer, anatomical assessment of resectability, and to make the final steps of the dissection, involving the uncinate process, easier and safer.

The peritoneal reflection from the Winslow foramen is incised immediately lateral to the second duodenal portion, and the entire duodenum is mobilized with the pancreatic head. The posterior face of the pancreatic head is completely detached from the retroperitoneum. In the laparoscopic/robotic pancreatoduodenectomy, the Kocher maneuver should be even more extensive than in the open operation, exposing the vena cava, the left side of the aorta, the left renal vein, and the origin of the superior mesenteric artery (SMA) (**Figures 28-8** and **28-9 A–C**).

During this step, enlarged lymph nodes can be retrieved in the preaortic space (station 16 as part of an extended lymphadenectomy).

The R3, if positioned in the left side of the patient, may help in the exposure, holding and progressively retracting the duodenum with an atraumatic grasper.

The assistant is further implementing the exposure, retracting the colon and, if necessary, the duodenum, and retrieving tissues (e.g., lymph nodes) for pathology.

Step 3 average time frame: 20–30 min

▶▶ TIPS

The full, extended Kocher maneuver may be difficult to complete in one step at the beginning. It may require a stepwise dissection and it becomes easier to do while the entire operation progresses. It is anyway important that no attempt at dividing the pancreas is done before the Kocher maneuver is completed. Monopolar energy, with the hook or scissors, is the main tool for this step. The Harmonic shears, or the vessel sealer, may be used to retrieve lymph nodes from the preaortic space.

ANATOMICAL HIGHLIGHTS

Retroaortic left renal vein (rare occurrence). In this case, the left renal vein is not a landmark for the origin of the SMA.

PITFALLS

Incomplete Kocher maneuver.

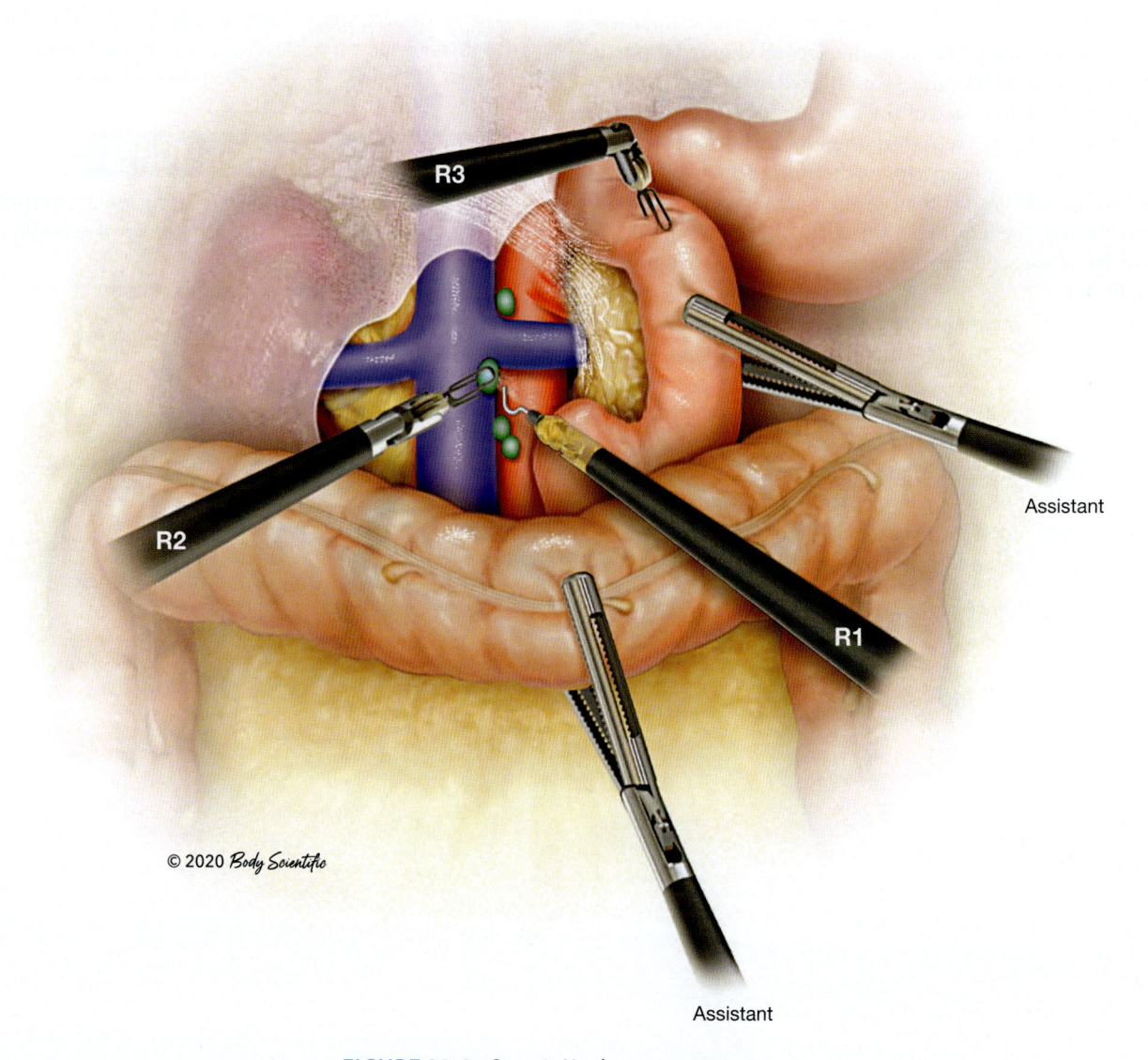

FIGURE 28-8 • Step 3. Kocher maneuver.

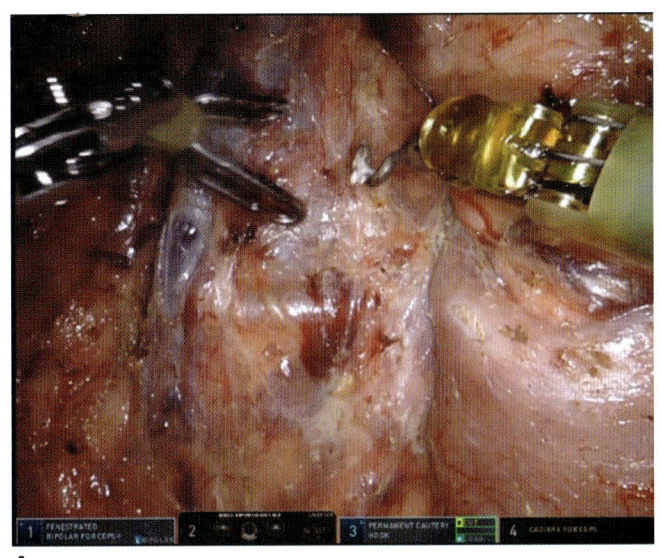

Pancreaticoduodenectomy 609

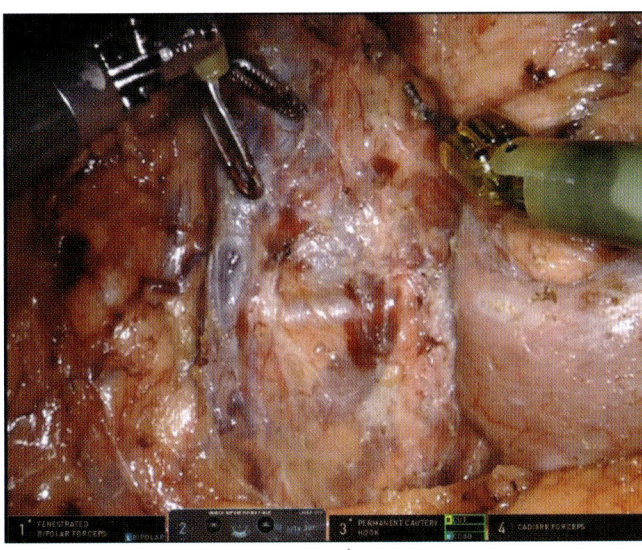

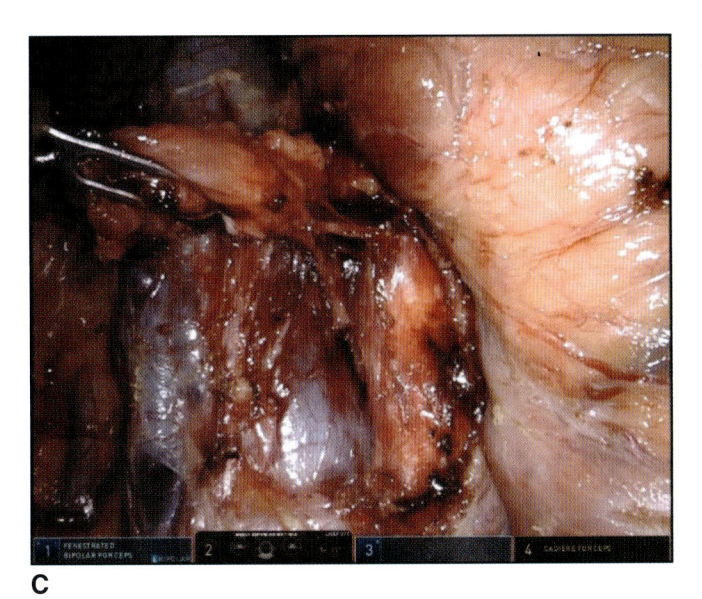

FIGURE 28-9 • Step 3. Kocher maneuver.

Step 4. Hepatic hilum and station 12 lymphadenectomy
The dissection in the liver hilum and hepatoduodenal ligament has 3 goals: oncological assessment for possible carcinomatosis or diffuse lymphatic spread, lymphadenectomy of station 12, and precise vascular anatomy evaluation. A "frozen" hilum is a contraindication to proceed with the resection.

The dissection starts at the hilar plate coming down (**Figure 28-10**). Lymphatic tissue and lymph nodes around the bifurcation of the hepatic artery are gently removed and sent for permanent pathology (**Figures 28-11 A–C**). The understanding of the general anatomy is important (**Figure 28-12**), including the knowledge of the lymph node stations involved in the RPD (**Figures 28-13 A, B**). (For more information, see suggested reading #14.) In particular, an early recognition of the vascular anatomy is mandatory, because it may change the conduction of the operation. Inadvertent injuries of aberrant arteries should be avoided. A totally replaced or accessory right hepatic artery coming from the SMA is present in up to 20% of cases. Depending on its relevance, size, and cancer involvement, preservation or ligation (rarely reimplantation/bypass) is required.

Step 4 average time frame: 15–20 min

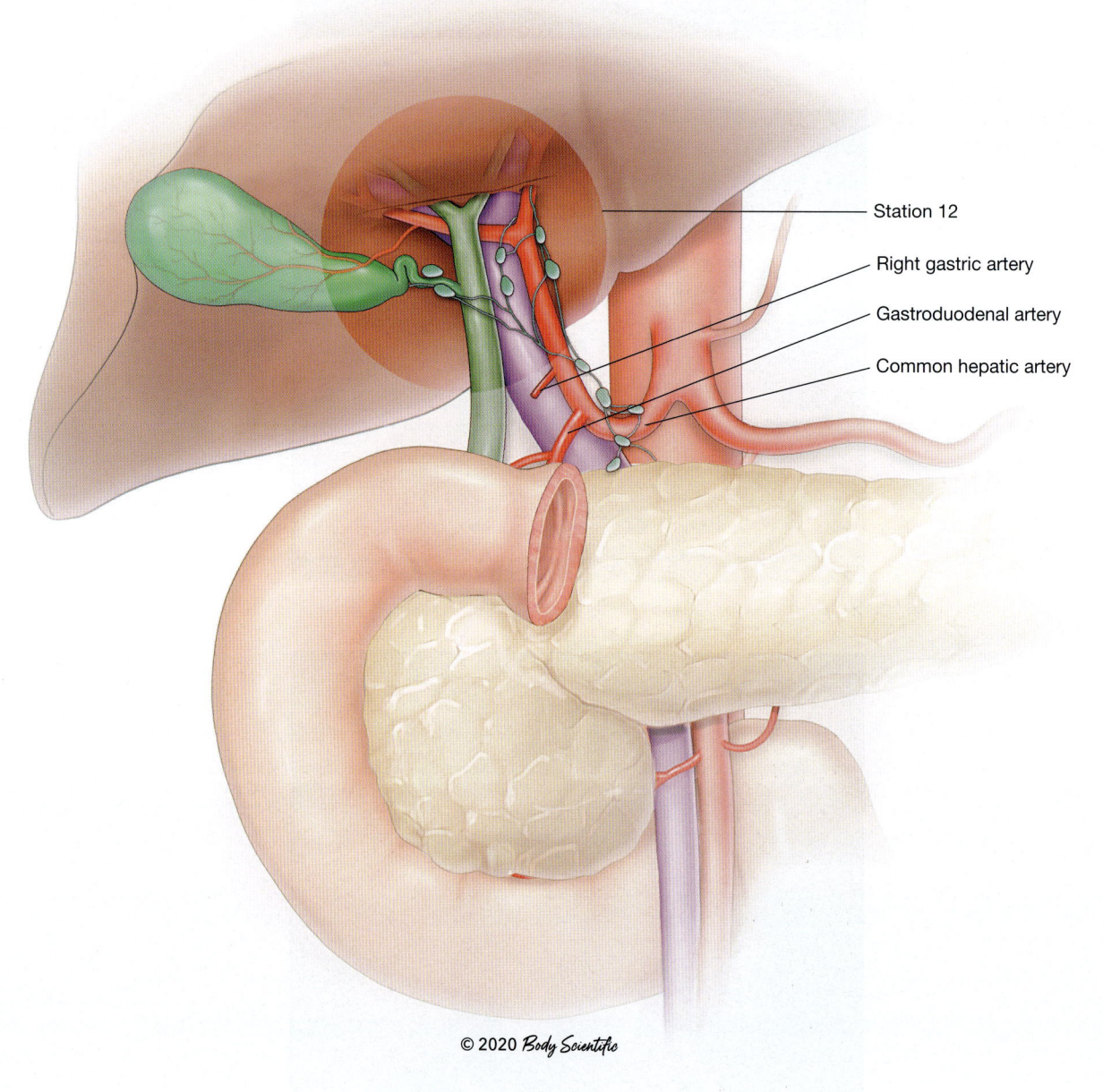

FIGURE 28-10 • Step 4. Hilum exploration.

Pancreaticoduodenectomy

▶▶ TIPS

A correct positioning of a grasper holding a sponge, handled by the third robotic arm, is opening the liver hilum (segment 4b).

The ICG fluorescence may help in defining the biliary anatomy, mainly in cases where the common bile duct is not dilated.

Individual groups of lymph nodes can be easily retrieved through the laparoscopic trocars using a "cheap" home-made Endobag™ (the cut fingers of a glove).

⚠ PITFALLS

Insufficient exposure of the hilum.

Vascular injuries due to poor understanding of the vascular anatomy.

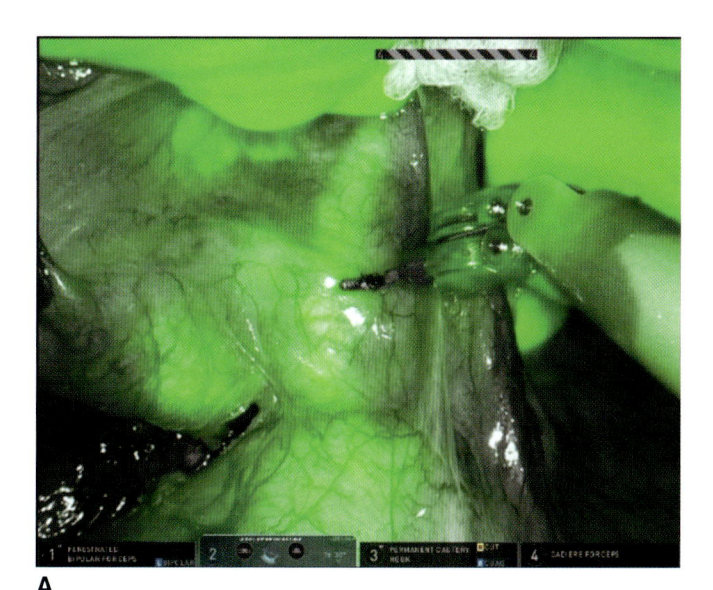

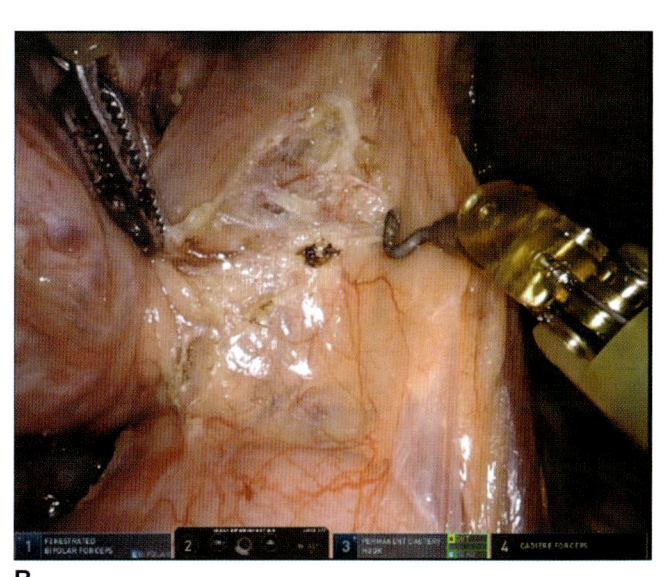

FIGURE 28-11 • Step 4. Hilum exploration.

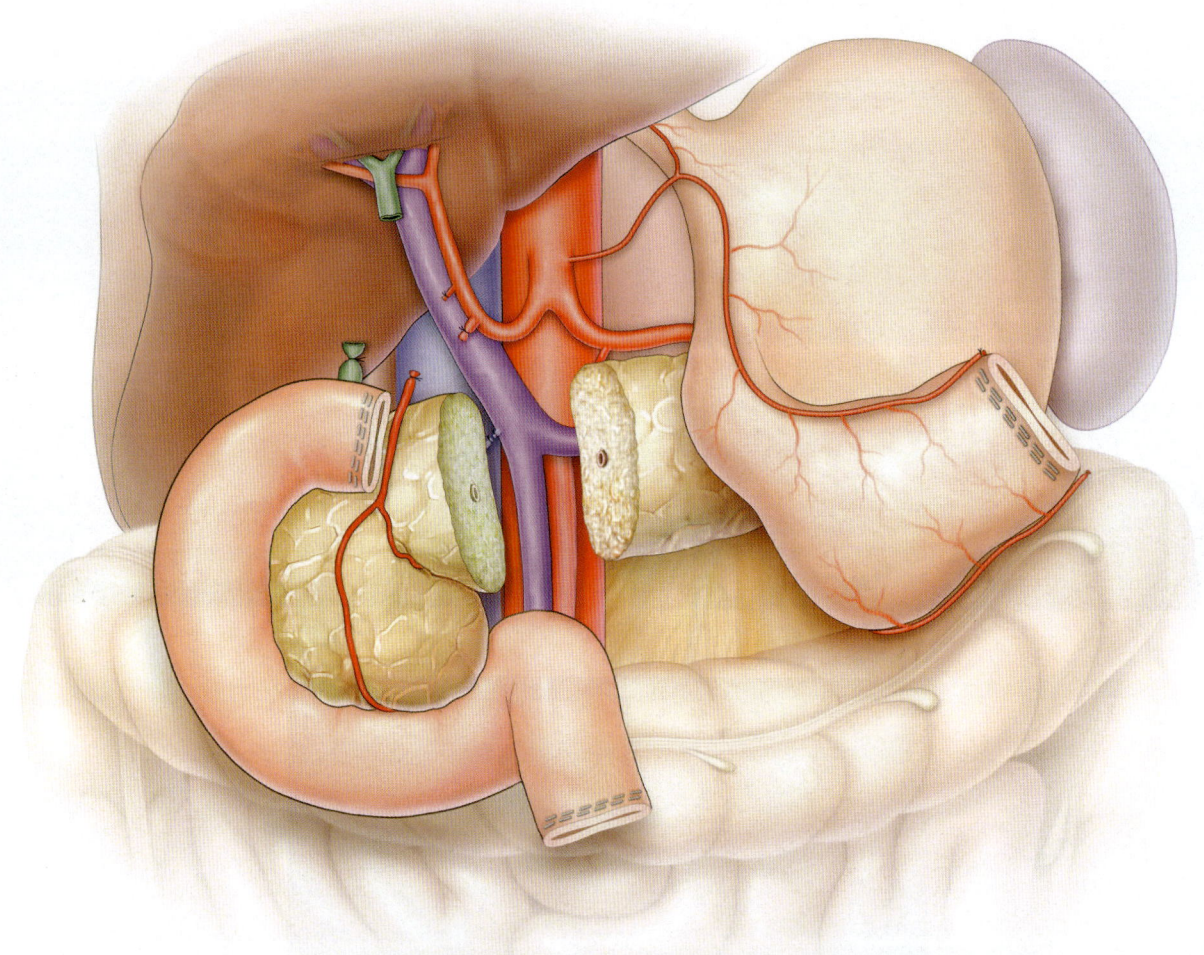

FIGURE 28-12 • General anatomy.

Pancreaticoduodenectomy 613

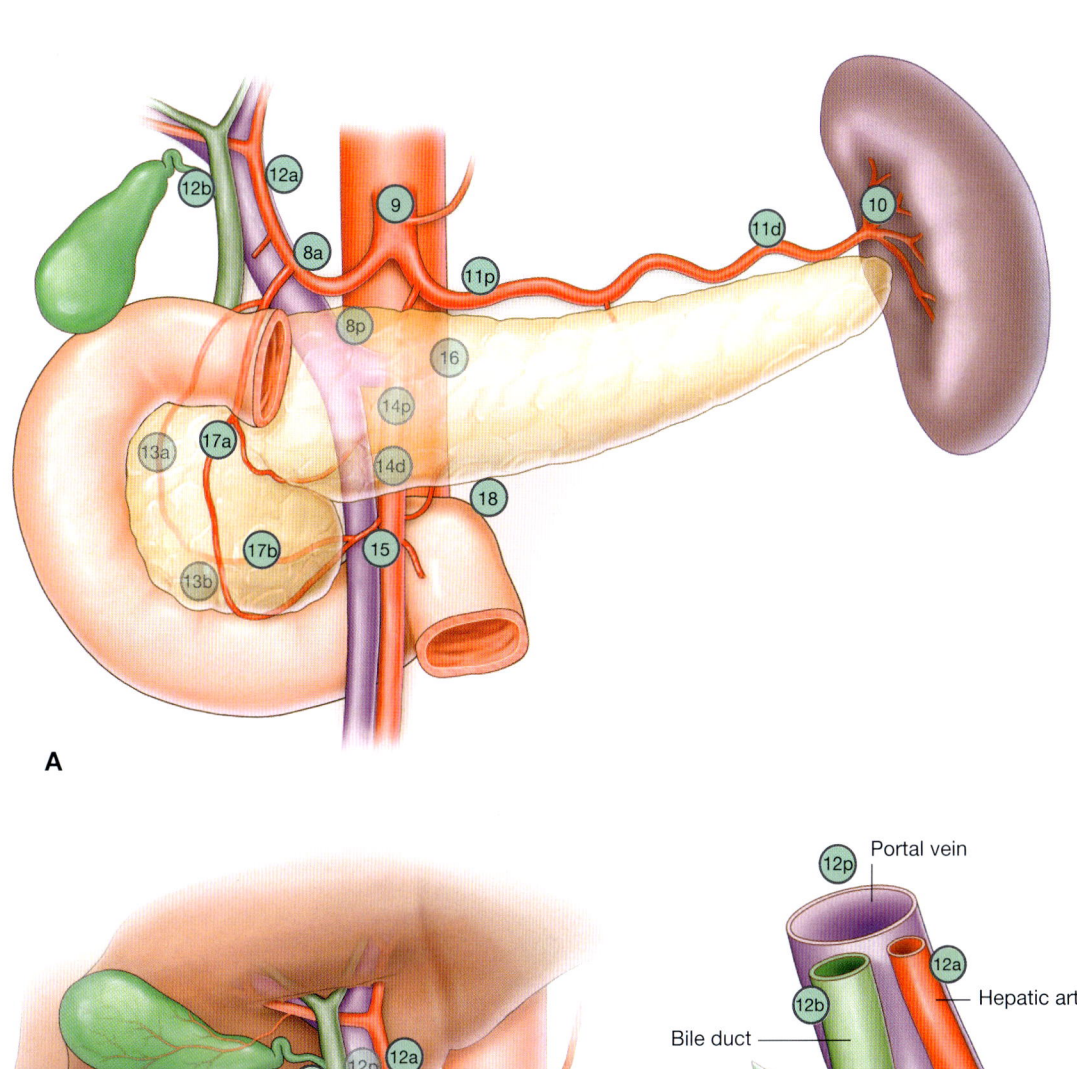

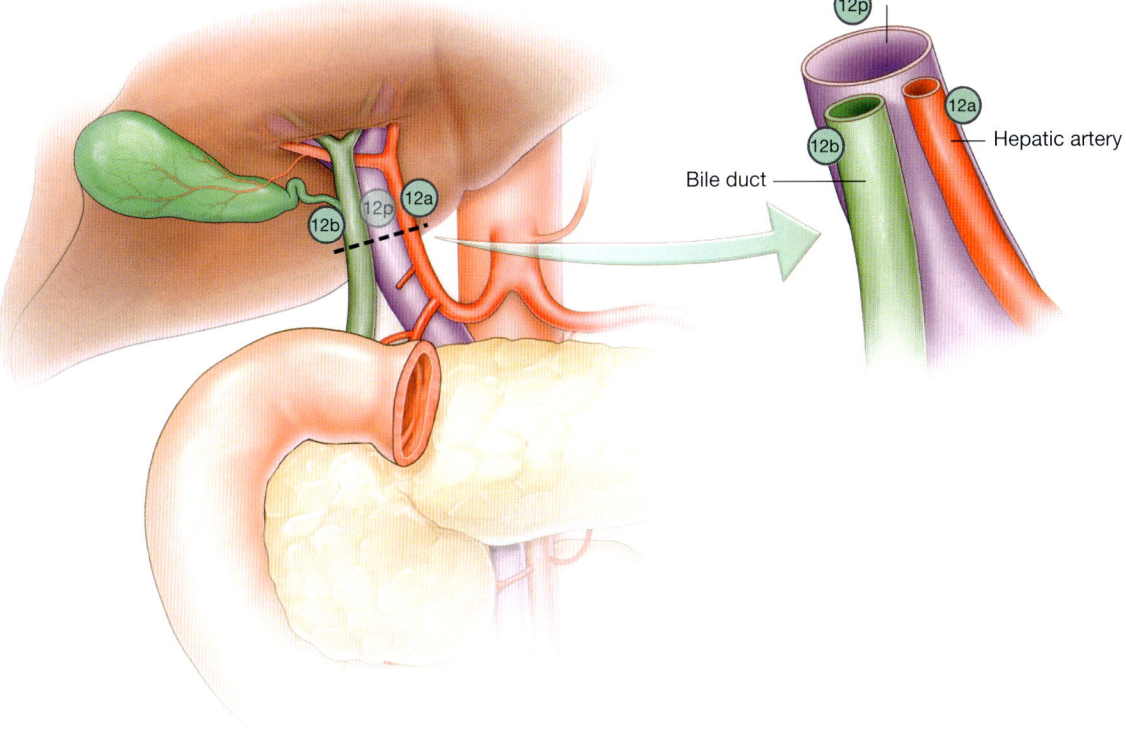

FIGURE 28-13 • Lymph node stations for RPD.

Step 5. Right gastric artery division

The division of the right gastric artery is part of the overall dissection/lymphadenectomy of the hepatoduodenal ligament (suprapyloric lymph nodes, station 5), and it is also necessary to detach the pylorus from its vascular connections (**Figure 28-14**). Suture ligation with Prolene™ 4-0 is preferable to clips or energy-based devices.

The right gastric artery may originate from the proper hepatic artery in more than 50% of patients, from the common hepatic artery in 20%, and less frequently from the left hepatic artery or gastroduodenal artery (GDA).

Step 5 average time frame: 10–15 min

> ▶▶ **TIPS**
>
> A perfect understanding of the vascular anatomy is necessary before dividing the artery. Lifting and retracting the antropyloric region with a grasper may put in evidence the arterial connections. The artery should be divided, at the very origin, and the suprapyloric/periduodenal lymph nodes are removed and sent apart for pathology. It must be kept in mind that the preservation of vagal innervation to the pylorus, in the gastrohepatic ligament, is essential for a proper recovery of the gastric emptying.

> ⚠ **PITFALLS**
>
> 1. Incomplete suprapyloric lymphadenectomy.
> 2. The right gastric artery divided far away from its origin and creating ischemia of the pyloric region.

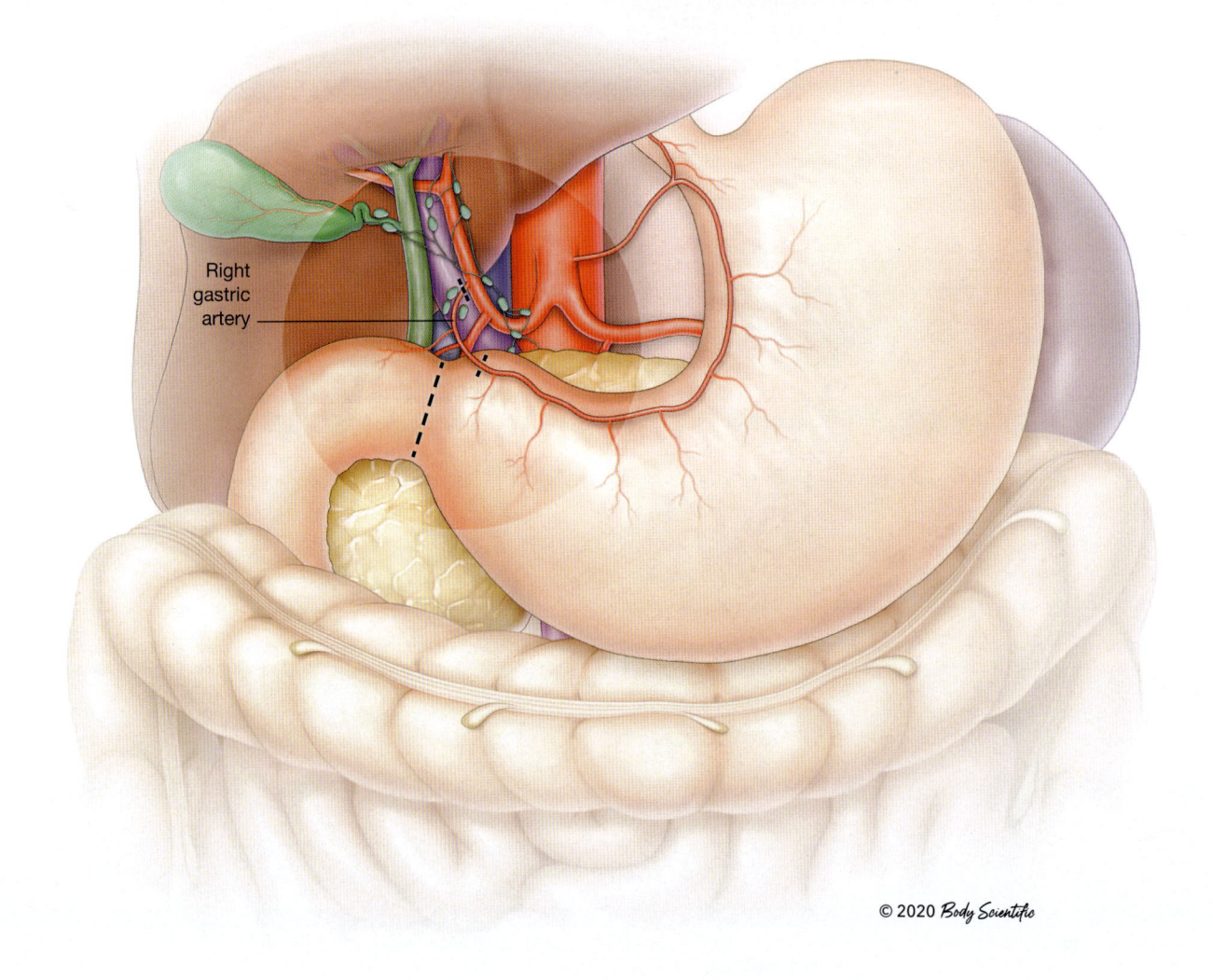

FIGURE 28-14 • Step 5. Right gastric artery division.

Step 6. Right gastroepiploic artery division

This step requires a perfect understanding of the vascular anatomy, performing an adequate lymphadenectomy of the infrapyloric and retropyloric lymph nodes (station 6), and at the same time, maintaining a good blood supply to the pylorus. Station 6 remains attached to the head of the pancreas, and it is part of the "en bloc" lymphadenectomy. The gastroepiploic vein and artery should be divided 2–3 cm from the pancreatic capsule (origin of the right gastroepiploic from the GDA) (**Figure 28**-15). A vascular stapler, or the vessel sealer, can be used for this step. The transection site should, at the same time, respect the integrity of the gastroepiploic vascular arcade supplying the pylorus, and maintain the retropyloric LN attached to the specimen (lymphoadenectomy).

Step 6 average time frame: 10–15 min

> ▶▶ **TIPS**
>
> Lifting the antrum with the third robotic arm puts some tension on the gastroepiploic arcade and helps in clarifying its relation with the duodenal wall and the pyloric region.

> ⚠ **PITFALLS**
>
> The gastroepiploic arcade is divided too far from its origin from the GDA, and its interruption may critically decrease the blood supply to the pylorus.

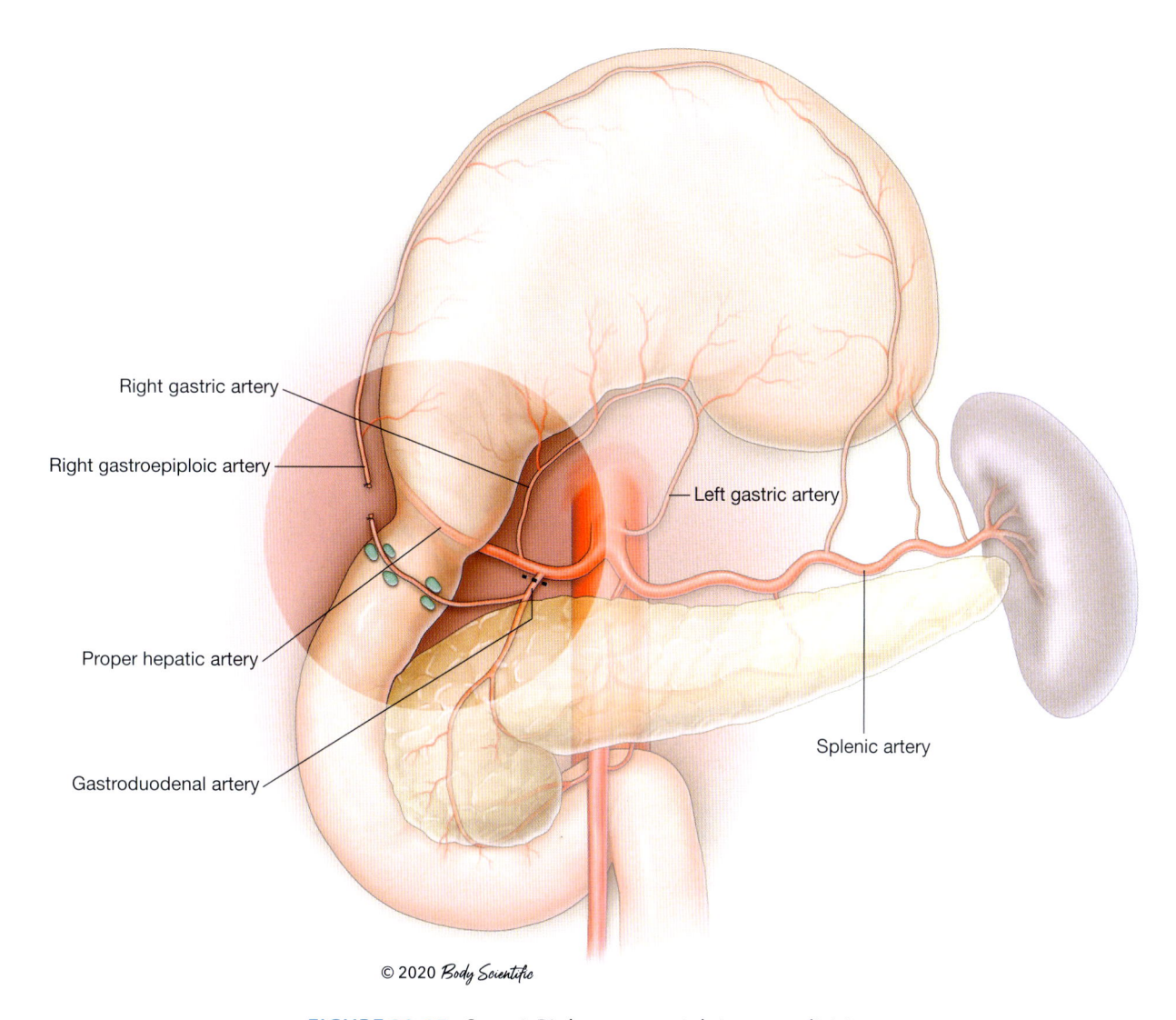

FIGURE 28-15 • Step 6. Right gastroepiploic artery division.

Step 7. Transection of the duodenum

If Steps 5–6 are well done, the transection of the duodenum in the pylorus-preserving technique is fast and simple. A medium range load stapler is applied a couple of centimeters distal to the pyloric canal (**Figure 28-16**). Then, the entire stomach is retracted to the left, opening the surgical field on the pancreatic head.

Step 7 average time frame: 5–10 min

> ▶▶ **TIPS**
>
> Lifting the stomach on a vertical direction gives a favorable approach to the stapler.
>
> Either the robotic stapler, or the assistant-controlled laparoscopic one, is easily applied.

> ⚠ **PITFALLS**
>
> Dividing the duodenum too close to the pylorus or damaging the sphincter.

Step 8. Cholecystectomy

The cholecystectomy (**Figure 28-17**) is a necessary step of the Whipple procedure: preserving the gallbladder with the bilioenteric anastomosis creates conditions for recurrent infections.

Taking down the gallbladder anterogradely, opens the space in the hilum, and facilitates the lymphadenectomy of the hepatoduodenal ligament. The cystic artery is divided in between Prolene™ 4-0 sutures or clips.

The gallbladder, detached from the liver, is momentarily left attached to the common bile duct and the final specimen (en bloc resection). The hepatic duct will be divided later just above the confluence of the cystic duct.

Step 8 average time frame: 15–20 min

> ▶▶ **TIPS**
>
> Emptying a distended gallbladder with the suction device facilitates its detachment. The small hole in the gallbladder fundus is then closed with a stitch. A meticulous bipolar coagulation of the liver bed may avoid continuous oozing.

> ⚠ **PITFALLS**
>
> Prolonged dissection time because of an over-distended gallbladder.

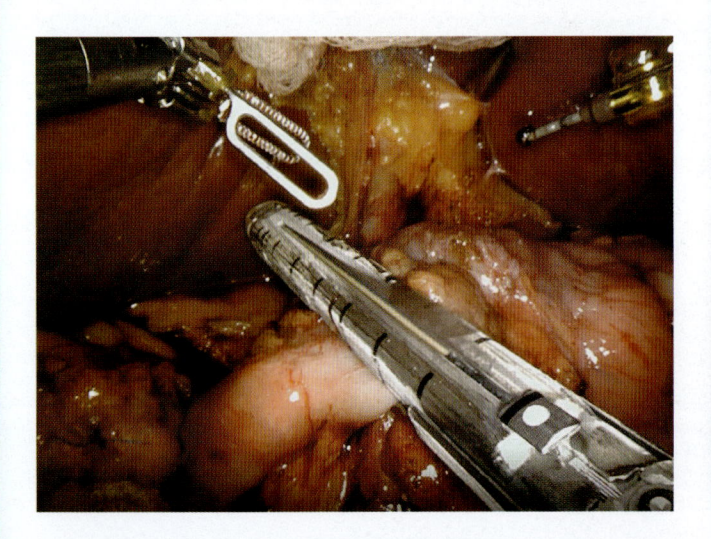

FIGURE 28-16 • Step 7. Transection of the duodenum.

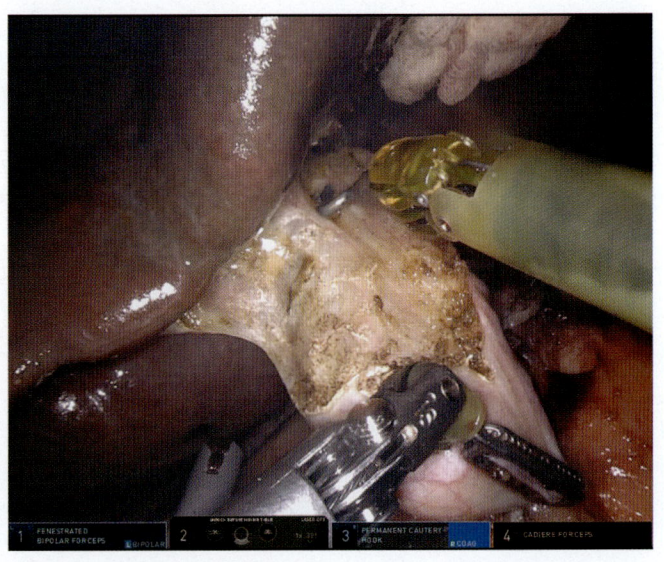

FIGURE 28-17 • Step 8. Cholecystectomy.

▶ **Video 28-3.** Step 9. CBD Transection

Step 9. Common bile duct transection

The division of the hepatic duct (**Figures 28-18 A–C**), just above the confluence of the cystic duct, is an important step. It gives access to the portal vein and allows better control of the GDA.

The proximal stump is clamped, with a soft bulldog, to avoid spillage of bile into the surgical field. A sample of the section line is sent for frozen intraoperative pathology. The distal stump is sutured with a long stay stitch, which avoids retrograde contamination from the specimen side, allowing downward retraction and further exposure of the portal vein.

If the bile duct is thin-walled and not dilated, it is better to be cut with cold scissors to avoid thermal injury; if it is thick and dilated (sometimes previously stented), the monopolar hook can be used.

All the lymph nodes lateral and posterior to the portal vein are detached and removed en bloc with the specimen (station 12p).

Step 9 average time frame: 10–15 min

> ▶▶ **TIPS**
>
> The posterior wall of the hepatic duct should be divided from inside the lumen while lifting the bile duct. This maneuver allows the recognition of the aberrant vascular structures between the bile duct and the portal vein.

> ⚠ **PITFALLS**
>
> Injury of aberrant hepatic arteries on the posterior right side of the common bile duct.

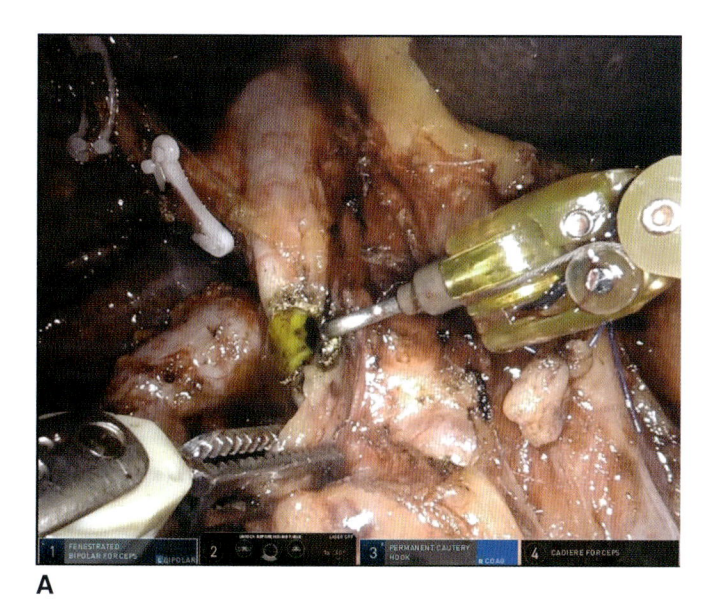

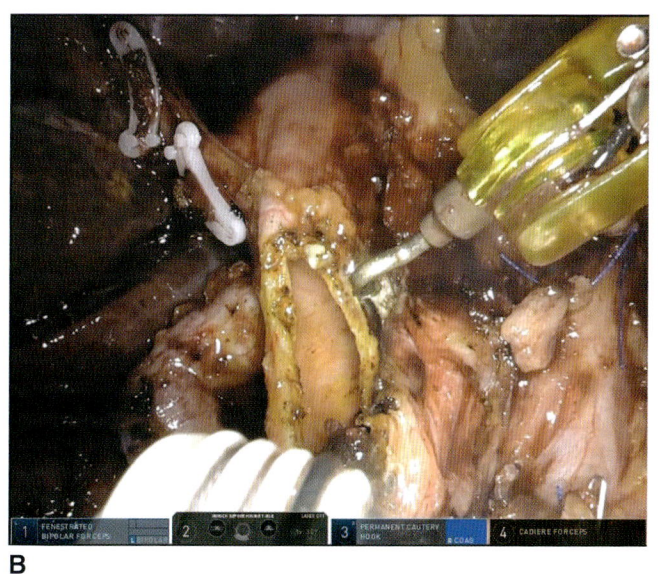

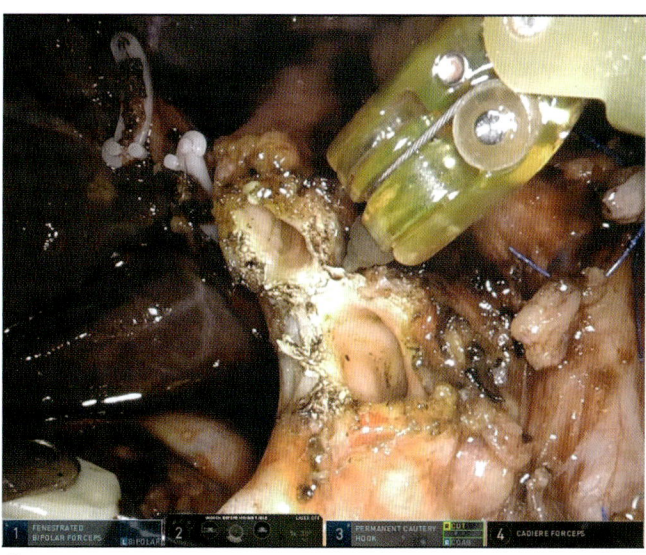

FIGURE 28-18 • Step 9. Transection of common bile duct.

Video 28-4. Step 10. GDA Transection

Step 10. Division of the GDA and completion lymphadenectomy around the hepatic artery and the celiac trunk

The preliminary preparation of the common and proper hepatic arteries on vessel loops allows atraumatic retraction, completion lymphadenectomy reaching the celiac trunk (station 9), and easier insertion of the vascular stapler to divide the GDA. Knowledge of the vascular anatomy, and in particular the anatomical variations of the hepatic artery, is essential (**Figure 28-19**). (Multiple anatomical variants can occur, and these can be classified in different ways. Here, the most clinically significant have been reported. For more information, see suggested readings #16–21.)

The safe division of the GDA (**Figures 28-20 A–C**) is one of the most important vascular steps of the procedure. The stump of the GDA may be the source of intraoperative and postoperative bleeding complications (pseudo-aneurysm). Clips should be avoided if possible; suture ligation with a good cuff or stapling is preferred.

Step 10 average time frame: 15–20 min

Type 1: the right, middle, and left hepatic arteries arise from the common hepatic artery (≈75%)

Type 2: the right hepatic artery arises from the superior mesenteric artery (≈12%)

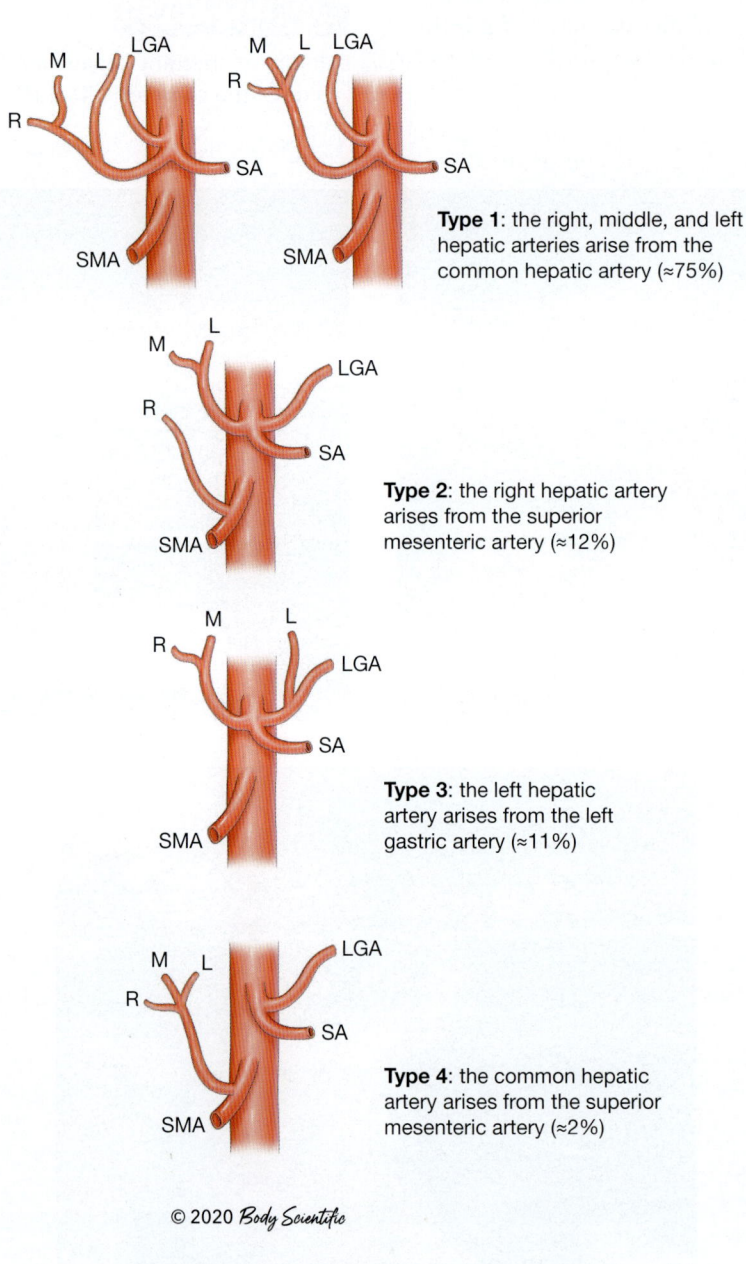

Type 3: the left hepatic artery arises from the left gastric artery (≈11%)

Type 4: the common hepatic artery arises from the superior mesenteric artery (≈2%)

© 2020 Body Scientific

FIGURE 28-19 • Right hepatic artery variants.

ANATOMICAL HIGHLIGHTS

Knowledge of the most common anatomy of the GDA (**Figure 28-21**) and the anatomical variations of its trunk origin is paramount (**Figures 28-22 A–C**). It could be a long segment without collaterals, or a very short one with early branches. A tricky situation is also represented by the presence of a right gastric vein merging into the portal vein, crossing or adjacent to the GDA.

PITFALLS

Inadvertent lesions of collaterals with brisk bleeding. Blind suturing may end up including the anterior wall of the portal vein underneath.

▶▶ TIPS

Careful and precise utilization of the hook (**Figures 28-23 A–E**) at a right angle usually allows a bloodless and clean dissection. Two needle drivers and Prolene™ 4-0, 5-0. Suturing of small branches are very effective.

To avoid venous congestion of the antropyloric region, the left gastric vein should be preserved.

The vascular stapler cartridge with a curved blunt tip is preferred.

Retracting the vessel loops on the common and proper hepatic artery facilitates the insertion of the stapler for the GDA division and avoids the risk of tangential inclusion/stricture of the hepatic artery.

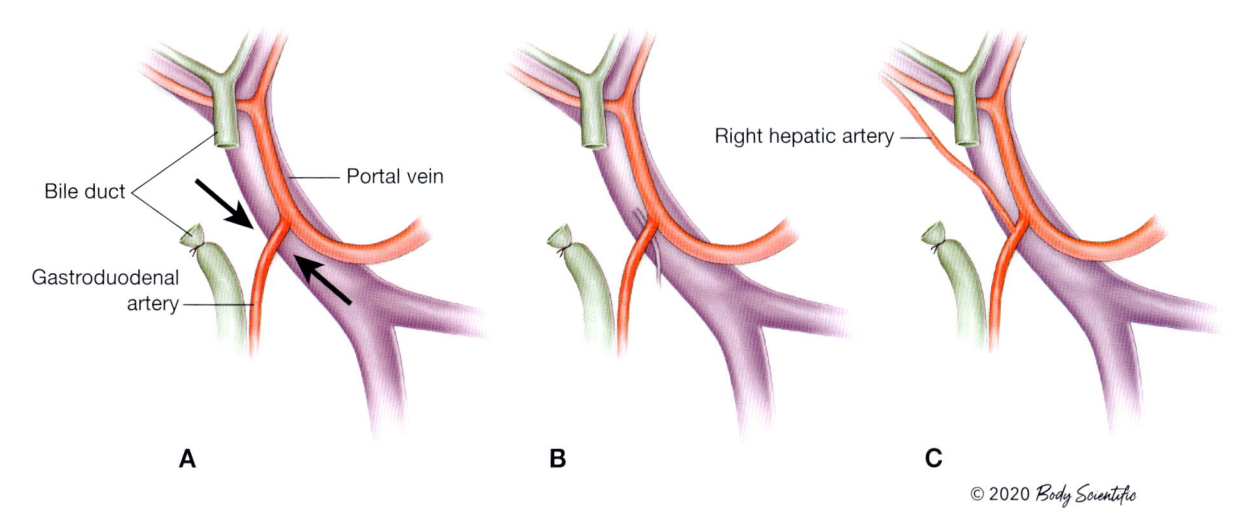

FIGURE 28-20 • Step 10. Gastroduodenal artery transection.

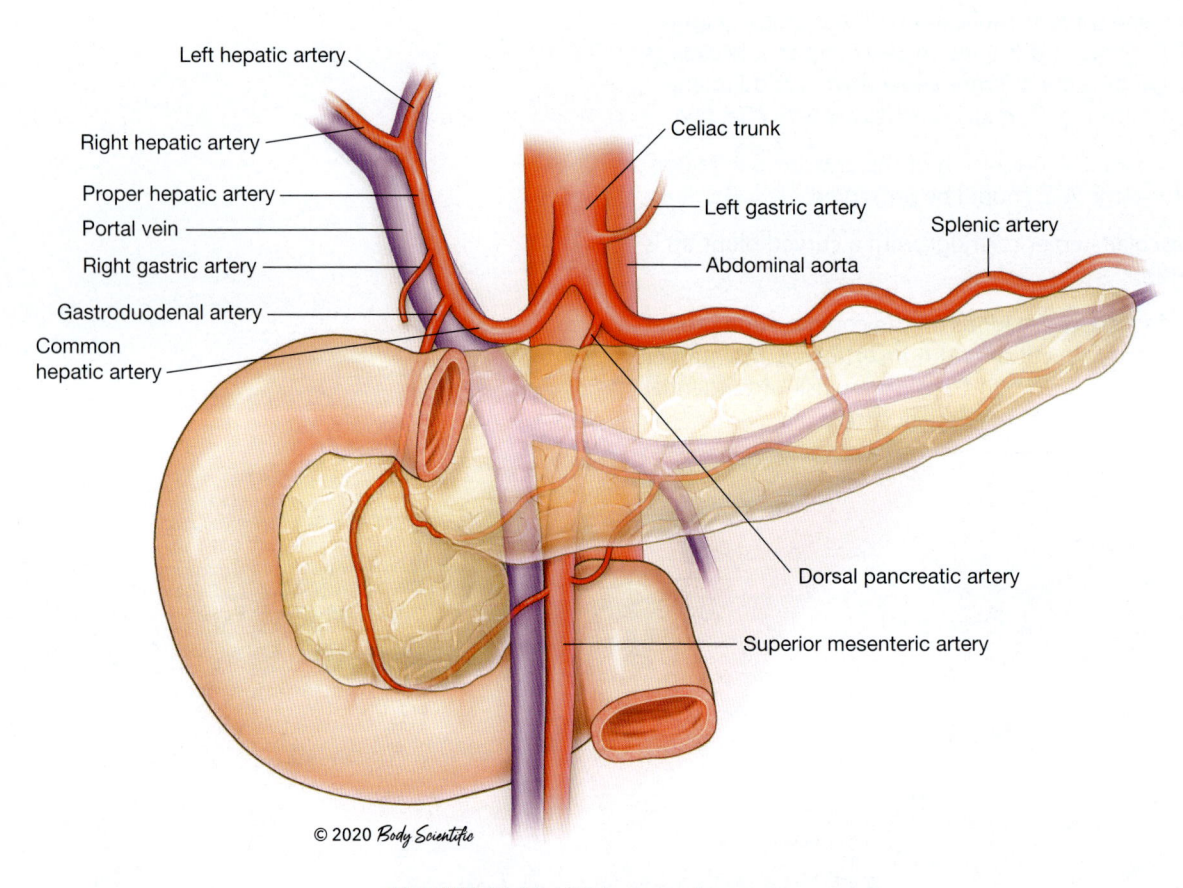

FIGURE 28-21 • GDA general anatomy.

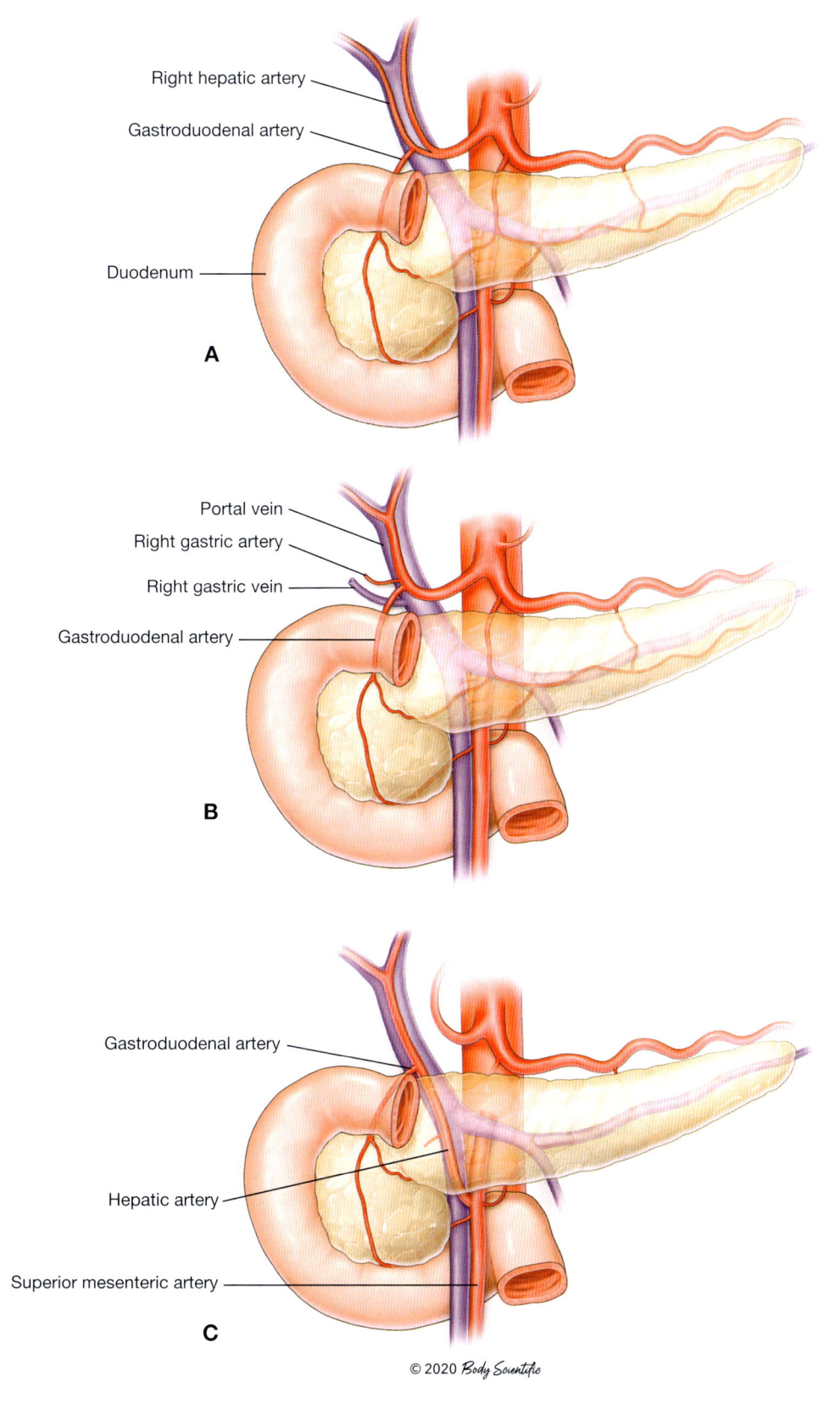

FIGURE 28-22 • Variations of the gastroduodenal artery.

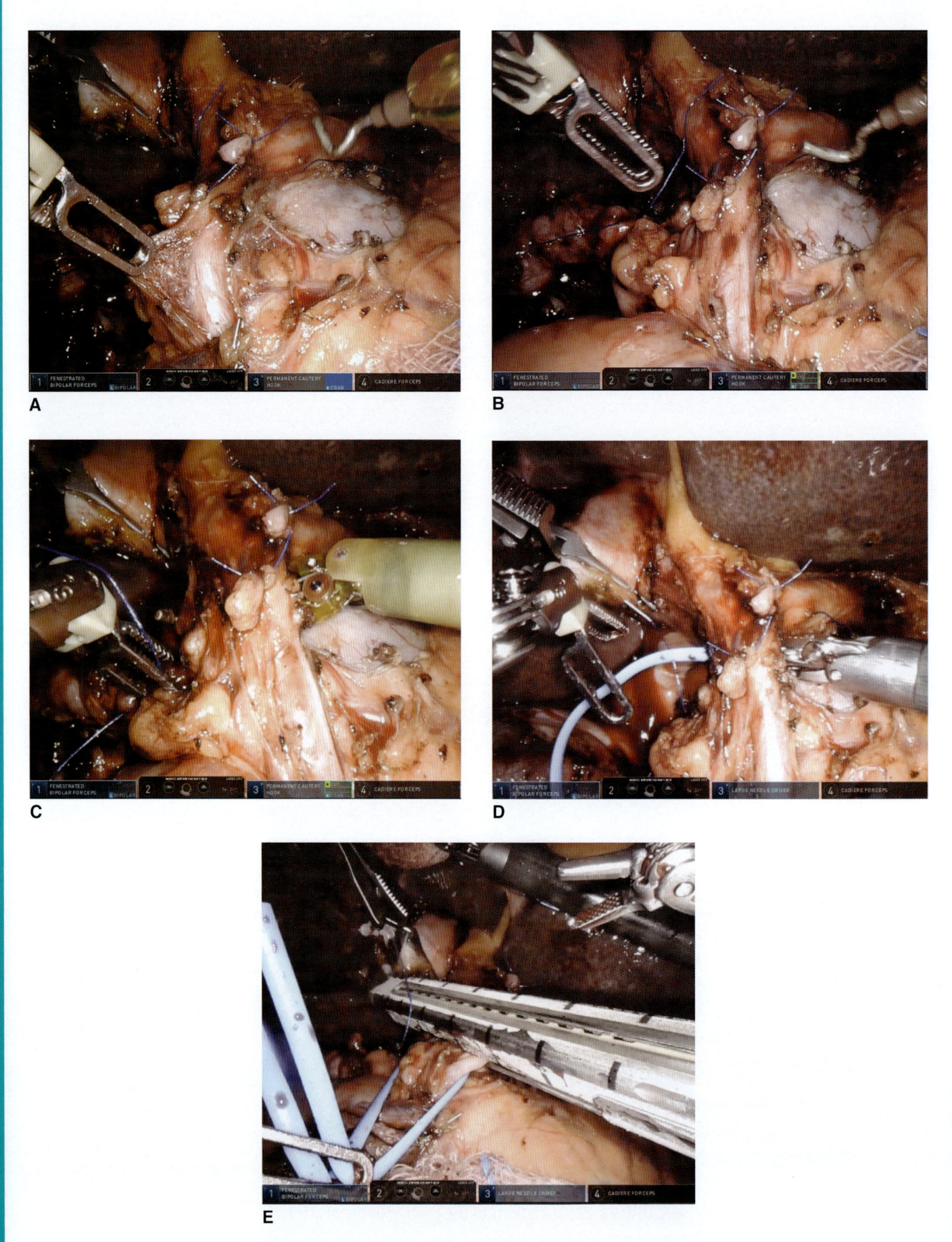

FIGURE 28-23 • Step 10. Gastroduodenal artery transection.

Step 11. Treitz transection and duodenal derotation

Before dividing the pancreas, the duodenojejunal flexure needs to be transected (**Figures 28-24 A–C**). The R3 grasper is positioned to retract cephalad the mesentery of the transverse colon, exposing the ligament of Treitz and the inferior mesenteric vein. The peritoneum is incised medially to the inferior mesenteric vein (if the retroperitoneal window is not already open from previous dissection in Step 3). The first jejunal loop is divided with the stapler. The ligament of Treitz is dissected with the Harmonic shears. The first jejunal branches of the SMA and SMV are divided from the left side, exerting some gentle traction on the duodenal stump. The more dissection is done from the left, the easier the right side derotation of the duodenum becomes. Releasing the retraction of the mesocolon and returning to the right upper quadrant, the fourth duodenal segment and duodenojejunal flexure are completely shifted on the right side of the SMV.

Step 11 average time frame: 15–20 min

> ▶▶ **TIPS**
>
> Meticulous and patient dissection of the ligament of Treitz should be performed. If any bleeding occurs, Prolene™ 3-0 or 4-0 stitches are used to make hemostasis on the mesentery; bipolar coagulation should not be trusted.

> ⚠ **PITFALLS**
>
> Insufficient dissection of the ligament of Treitz with difficult derotation. Bleeding from the posterior mesentery on the left side of the SMA.

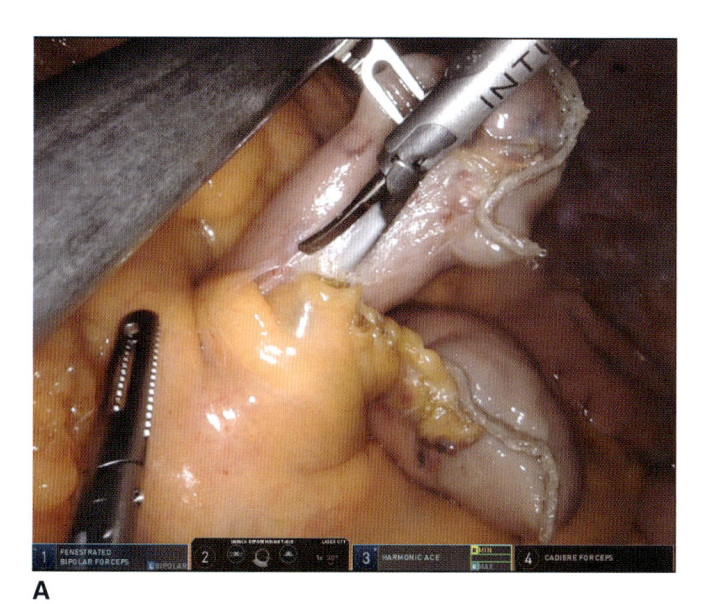

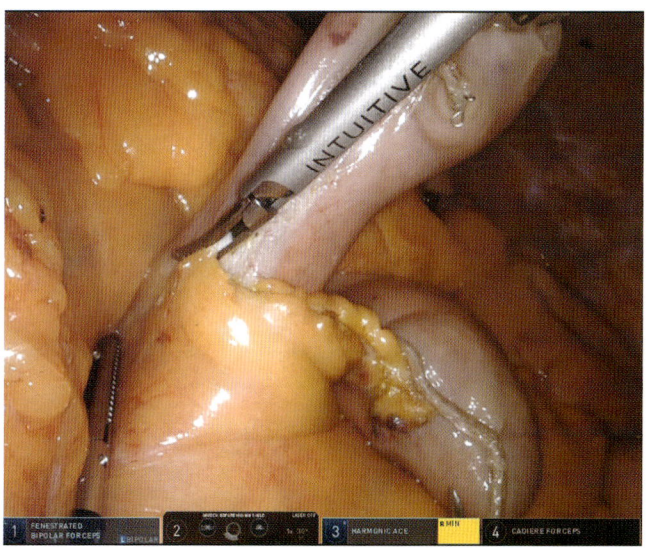

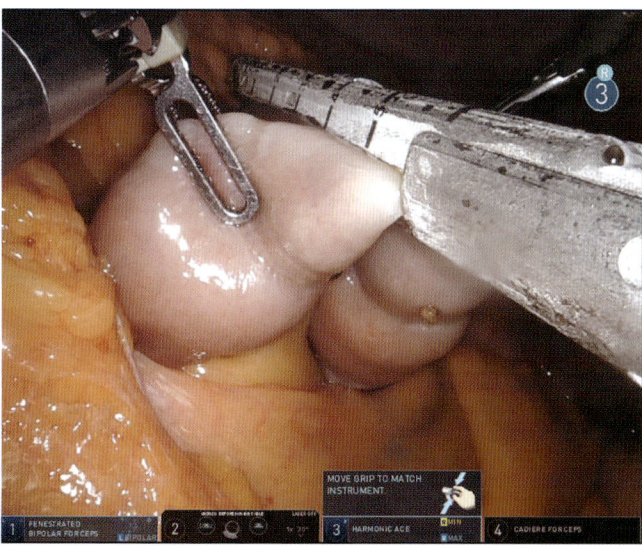

FIGURE 28-24 • Step 11. First jejunal loop transection at the ligament of Treitz.

Video 28-5. Step 12. Parenchyma Transection

Step 12. Transection of the pancreatic neck

The division of the pancreas (**Figures 28-25 A, B**) does not require the creation of a complete tunnel between the portal vein and the posterior aspect of the pancreatic neck, a typical maneuver described in open surgery textbooks. If it is easy, it can be done by passing a vessel loop underneath the neck, lifting the pancreas away from the vein, but this maneuver can be very difficult due to peripancreatic inflammation or if the tumor is adjacent to the vein.

Applying 2 Prolene™ 2-0 stay sutures, on both the lower right and left side of the neck, allows some preventive hemostasis and lifting traction. The plane in front of the portal vein may be gradually dissected while splitting the parenchyma anterogradly. The preferred tool for the pancreatic division is the Harmonic shears, using the inactive blade on the portal side. Usually, the pancreatic duct is recognized, when transected, because clear pancreatic fluid is released.

A complete hemostasis may require some additional interrupted stiches of Prolene™ 4-0, mainly at the upper border. A sample of the pancreatic duct is sent for frozen pathology (section margin). A small stent, with side holes, is placed inside the distal pancreatic duct and secured with a PDS™ 4-0 stich. The proximal section line is further sutured with a long "U" Prolene™ 2-0 stitch that will be used for traction of the specimen.

Step 12 average time frame: 15–20 min

▶▶ TIPS

Using the active blade of the Harmonic shears like a scalpel, when in close proximity to the pancreatic duct, avoids the sealing effect.

If the pancreatic duct is inadvertently closed, once the pancreatic division is completed, the pancreatic margin should be carefully inspected, and the duct immediately reopened.

IV infusion of octreotide 50 mg/h is started by the anesthesiologist before the pancreatic transection.

⚠ PITFALLS

Inadvertent and not recognized.

Sealing/closure of the distal pancreatic duct using the Harmonic shears.

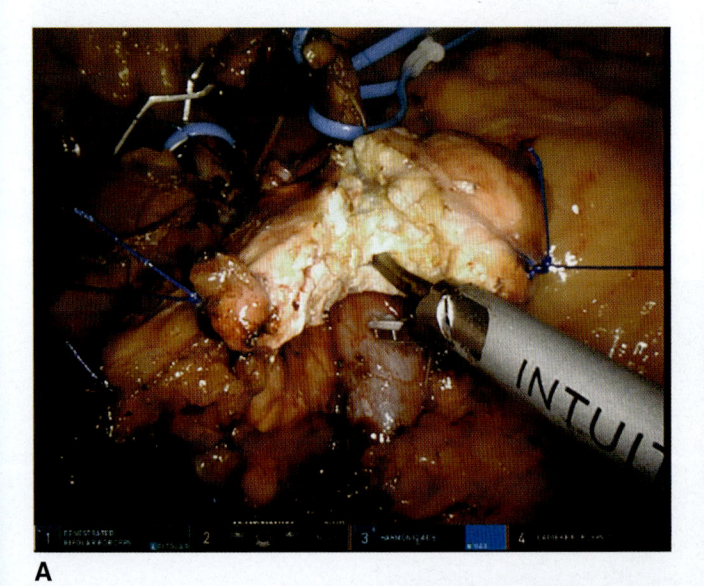

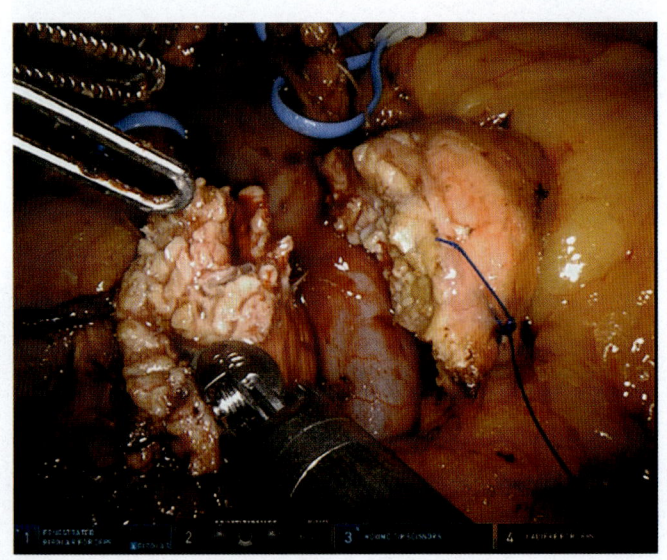

FIGURE 28-25 • Step 12. Transection of the pancreatic neck.

▶ **Video 28-6.** Step 13. Uncinate Process Dissection 1

▶ **Video 28-7.** Step 13. Uncinate Process Dissection 2

▶ **Video 28-8.** Step 13. Uncinate Process Dissection 3

Step 13. Uncinate process dissection
This is the most complex step and where severe intraoperative bleeding complications may happen!

It is also the step where the microsurgical capabilities of the robotic platform play an important role. The dissection has to be conducted meticulously in a kind of bench surgery fashion.

The R3 has an important function; the stable and progressive lateral lifting of the pancreatic head opens the grove between the SMA/SMV and the uncinate process with its vascular connections.

First, the venous Henle's trunk, connecting the right lateral side of the pancreatic neck with the SMV, should be divided in between Prolene™ 4-0 or 5-0 sutures. This detachment is essential because it allows a complete exposure of the uncinate behind the SMV.

The following dissection proceeds from ventral to cephalad. An attempt should be made to expose the anterior, safe aspect of the SMA working on the left side of the SMV (artery first). This maneuver may require suture ligation of some branches of the SMV, including sometimes the middle colic vein. Exposing the SMA gives an important landmark for the dissection. A gentle inspection of the posterior face of the SMV allows the identification of the posterior branches, mainly the pancreaticojejunal trunk.

After precise understanding of the anatomy, by working with the hook as a right-angle instrument, a window is created, and a vessel loop is passed around the SMV (hanging maneuver) (**Figure 28-26**).

Careful traction on the vessel loop by the assistant (**Figures 28-27 A–D**) improves the control of the lower corner of the uncinate process where the pancreaticojejunal trunk is located. Suture ligation of this trunk with Prolene™ 4-0 is usually feasible. Disconnecting the lower corner opens the grove between the uncinate and SMA.

At this point, the dissection in the connective tissue on the right side of the SMA is conducted with small bites of tissue. The lateral traction of the R3 on the pancreatic head is progressively adjusted.

The arterial branches from the SMA to the ventral pancreas can be variable, but the most constant and important vessel is the inferior pancreaticoduodenal artery. This big branch can be suture ligated or clipped and suture ligated. If there are no oncological concerns, the dissection can be also conducted in the connective tissue just lateral to the SMA leaving some tissue on the artery. In this case, the Harmonic shears, or the vessel sealer, may take down the arterial branches included in that tissue. Suture reinforcements are always advisable. The last vessel to be divided (clip or suture) is the superior pancreaticoduodenal vein, in the upper right side of the portal vein.

Step 13 average time frame: 30–40 min

> **▶▶ TIPS**
>
> Before starting the uncinate dissection, it must be checked that the extended Kocher maneuver is complete. If the pancreatic head is completely detached from the retroperitoneum (origin of the SMA), the dissection is faster and safer. In case of bleeding, the detachment of the uncinate can be sped up allowing better control of the situation.
>
> Prevention of bleeding is always recommended; the control of the vascular connection must be meticulous and precise.
>
> If bleeding happens, this situation should not cause panic. The reason of the bleeding must be understood, the anatomical landmarks should be kept in mind, and the communication with the team must be calm, clear, and precise.
>
> Exposure, surgical suctioning, and retraction of the SMV with the "hanging maneuver" may require an expert assistant.
>
> Advanced robotic suturing skills are mandatory.

> **🔍 ANATOMICAL HIGHLIGHTS**
>
> In up to 5% of cases, the SMV can be double.
>
> The inferior mesenteric vein merges into the splenic vein in 56% of cases, into the SMV in 26%, and into the spleno-mesenteric angle in 18%. (For more information, see suggested reading #15.)

> **⚠ PITFALLS**
>
> Incomplete understanding/exposure of the SMA/SMV with unsafe blind dissection.
>
> Bleeding from the posterior aspect of the SMV.
>
> Bleeding from the lateral side of the SMA.
>
> Excessive oozing from the specimen, because of an early ligation of the superior pancreaticoduodenal vein.

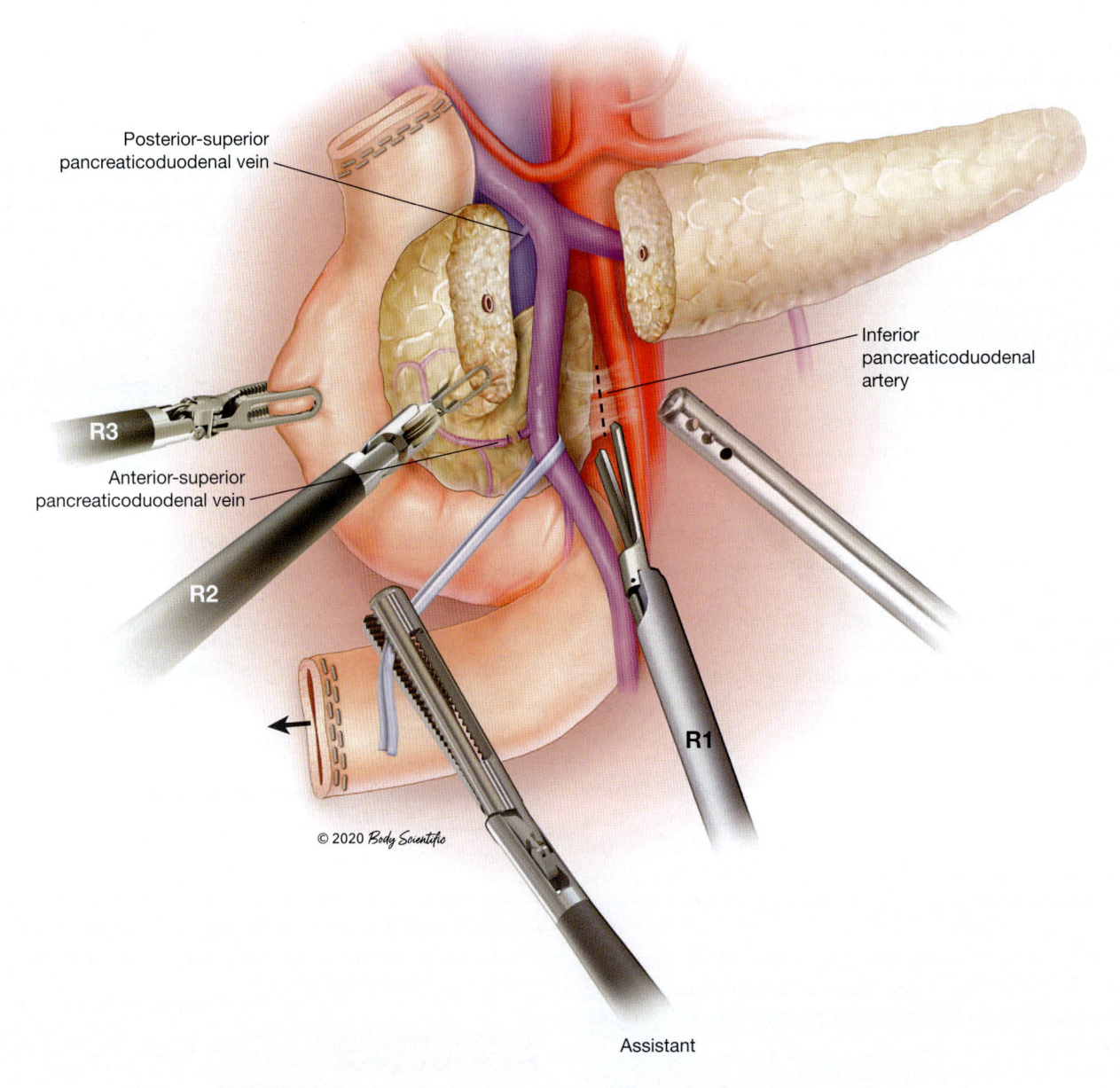

FIGURE 28-26 • Step 13. Uncinate process dissection/hanging maneuver.

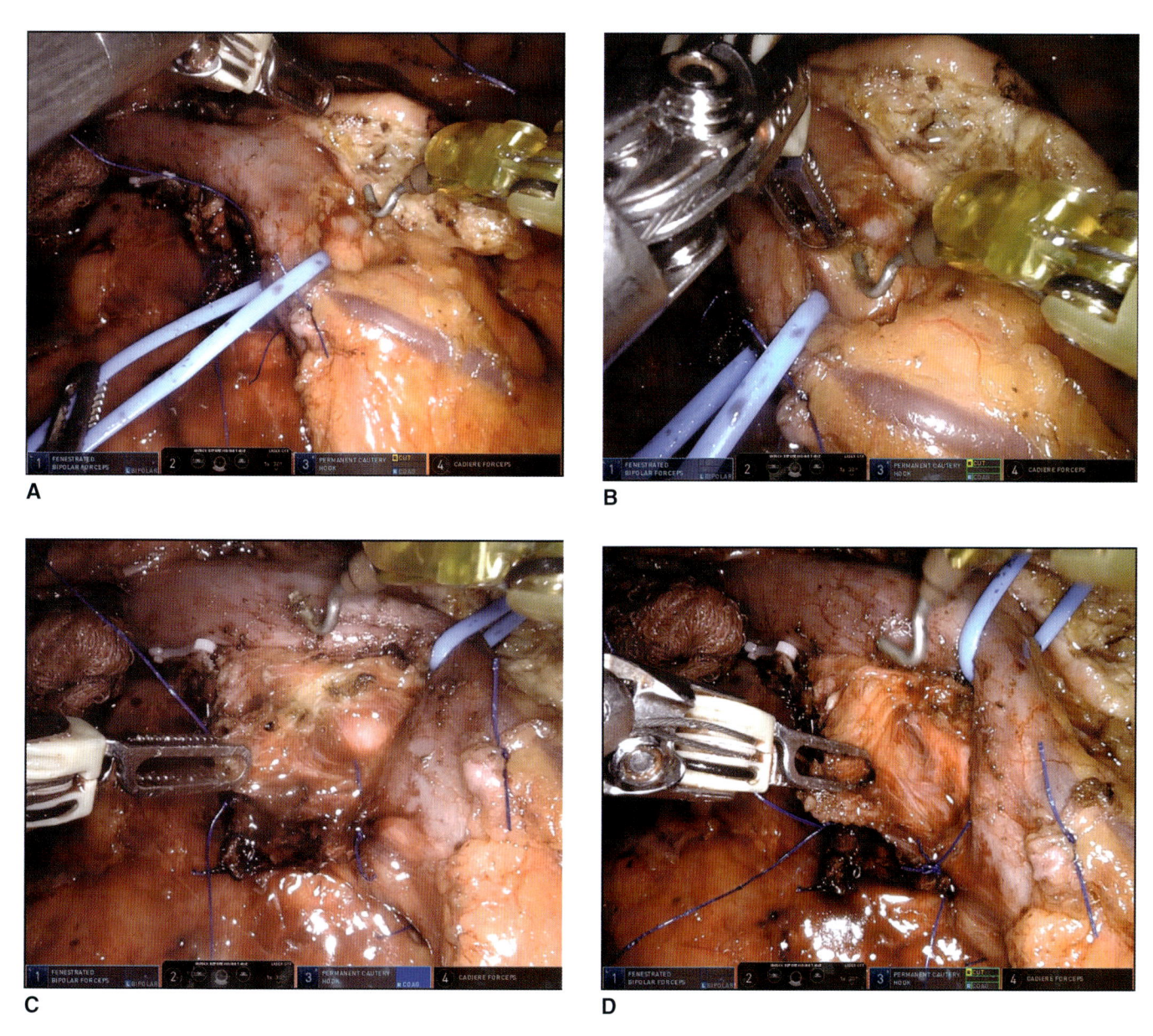

FIGURE 28-27 • Step 13. Uncinate process dissection.

RECONSTRUCTION

Similar to open surgery pancreatoduodenectomy, there are multiple techniques for the pancreatic digestive reconstruction.

Two options are most frequently used: the pancreaticojejunostomy and the pancreaticogastrostomy.

The choice should be based on several parameters, knowing pros and cons of both. The pancreaticojejunostomy has better functional long-term results (endocrine and exocrine), but if the "activated juice" fistula occurs, it is more severe and risky. The pancreaticogastrostomy has a higher rate of long-term anastomotic strictures, and a higher risk of postoperative intragastric bleeding, but the pancreatic fistula is milder and better tolerated (inactive secretions).

The parameters to consider to select the pancreatic anastomosis are: overall risk of fistula, quality of the pancreas, size of the pancreatic duct, age, long-term prognosis, and patient's ability to tolerate severe complications (e.g., leaks).

If a classical Whipple procedure with gastric antrectomy is performed, the pancreaticogastrostomy becomes technically complex with overlapping anastomotic lines, and therefore is not recommendable.

Video 28-9. Step 14-a. End-to-Side Pancreaticojejunostomy

Step 14-a. End-to-side pancreaticojejunostomy
If the quality of the pancreatic tissue is not too friable, and the size of the pancreatic duct is more than 3–4 mm, the mucosa-to-mucosa pancreaticojejunostomy is the best option. It does not require a long mobilization of the pancreatic stump, just 1 cm to allow the posterior anchoring suture. Small collateral vessels (splenic branches) are divided in between Prolene™ 5-0 sutures.

The first jejunal loop is brought to the upper quadrants with the shortest and most favorable route, retromesenterically (duodenal bed). A running suture of Prolene™ 4-0 is performed between the posterior pancreatic capsule and the serosa of the jejunum, being careful not to include the pancreatic duct (previously stented), which may be very close to the posterior surface of the pancreas. A small opening in the jejunum is made in front of the pancreatic duct, and a PDS™ 5-0 running suture makes the posterior row of a mucosa-to-mucosa anastomosis. The proximal tip of the stent is inserted into the jejunal lumen, and the anterior row is completed with interrupted stitches of PDS™ 5-0. All stitches are momentarily individually controlled with clips, and tied at the end, to be able to see the details of the needle's passage (see **Video 28-9**). A final anterior running suture of Prolene™ 4-0 completes the anastomosis. This step is shown in **Figures 28-28 A–D**.

Step 14-a average time frame: 30–40 min

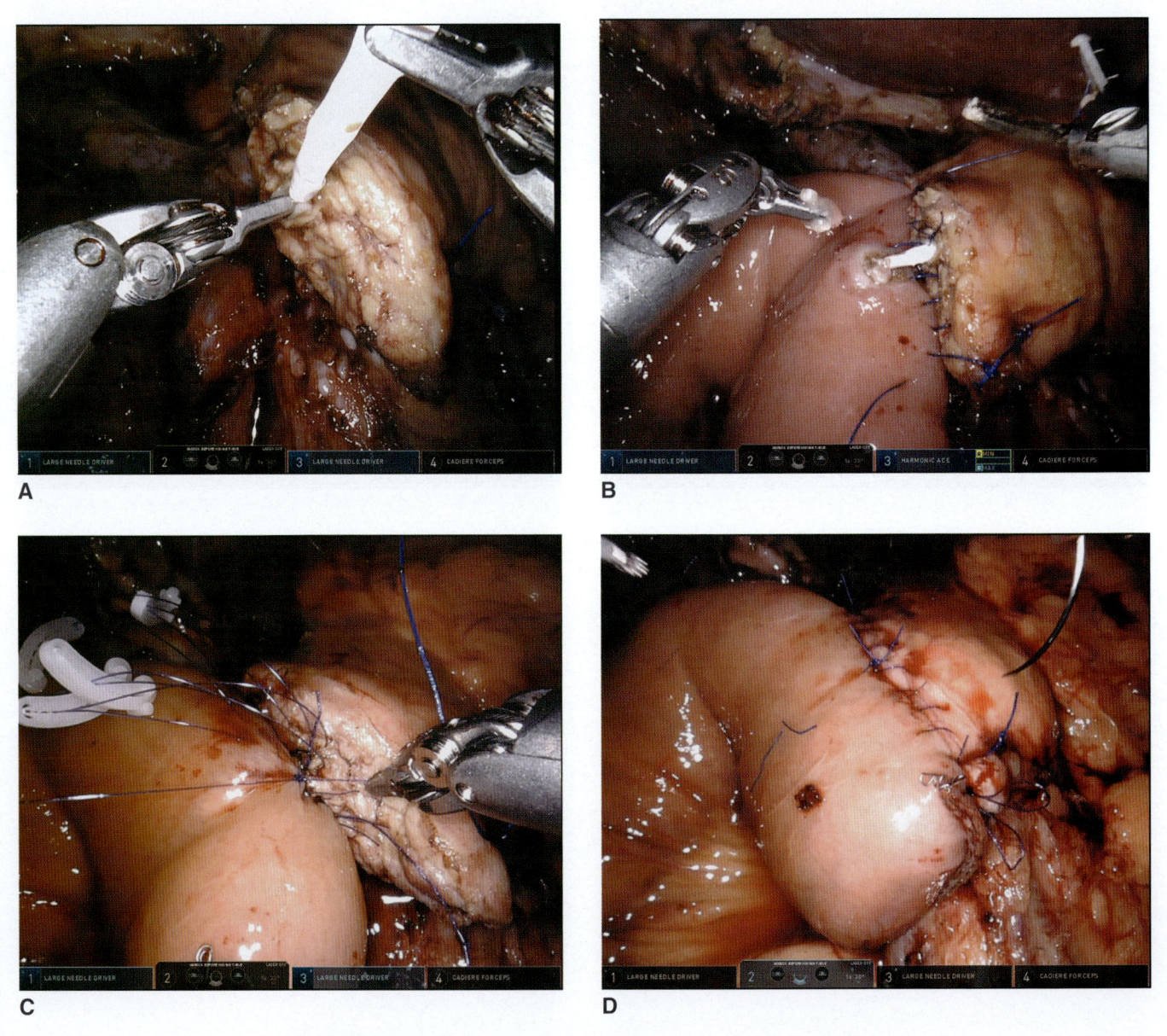

FIGURE 28-28 • Step 14-a. End-to-side pancreaticojejunostomy.

> **▶▶ TIPS**
>
> After the construction of the posterior anchoring suture, it must be checked if the pancreatic juice is naturally flowing out of the stent.
>
> As an alternative for fragile parenchyma, Blumgart-type anchoring stitches may replace the posterior running suture.

> **⚠ PITFALLS**
>
> Inadvertent inclusion of the pancreatic duct in the posterior suture. This can potentially be a reason of severe complications (pancreatitis and leak). A loose posterior running/anchoring suture may lead to side branch pancreatic leak (usually reason for the majority of type A leaks).

▶ Video 28-10. Step 14-b. Pancreaticogastrostomy

Step 14-b. Transgastric pancreaticogastrostomy

The pancreatic stump has to be prepared for deep invagination into the stomach. At least 4–5 cm of the pancreatic body should be skeletonized, taking down (between Prolene™ 5-0 sutures) all the arterial and venous connections with the splenic vessels.

Two stay sutures of Prolene™ 2-0 are applied at the upper and lower margins of the pancreatic stump.

A small opening in the posterior gastric wall is created where the stump is naturally laying without tension.

A longitudinal vertical anterior gastrotomy is performed near the posterior opening, and the pancreas is gently pulled inside the stomach with a complete invagination of the mobilized stump.

Interrupted stiches of PDS™ 4-0 are used from inside the stomach to fix the pancreatic capsule to the gastric wall.

The hemostasis must be perfect, and every minor bleeding should be treated with independent, separate stitches of Prolene™ 4-0.

At this point, the anesthesiologist is asked to adjust the position of the nasogastric tube to be able to effectively drain the stomach in the early postop.

The anterior gastrostomy is then closed with a running suture of PDS™ 3-0.

This step is shown in **Figures 28-29 A, B**.

Step 14-b average time frame: 30–40 min

> **▶▶ TIPS**
>
> A Prolene™ 3-0 purse string, made at the beginning of the creation of the posterior gastric opening, may be tied from inside the stomach after the pancreatic stump is completely introflexed, being sure to avoid stricturing the stump, that could be reason of venous congestion and bleeding.
>
> At the end of the anastomosis, the suture line should be completely dry. Even minor bleeding should be treated with additional hemostatic sutures.
>
> Moving the camera port site temporarily to the left quadrant may facilitate an optimal visual control of the anastomotic details.

> **⚠ PITFALLS**
>
> Incomplete mobilization of the pancreatic stump with difficult and short dunking effect.
>
> A too large posterior gastric opening can be a possible reason for gastric leaks.
>
> Suboptimal hemostasis, with risk of postoperative intragastric bleeding.

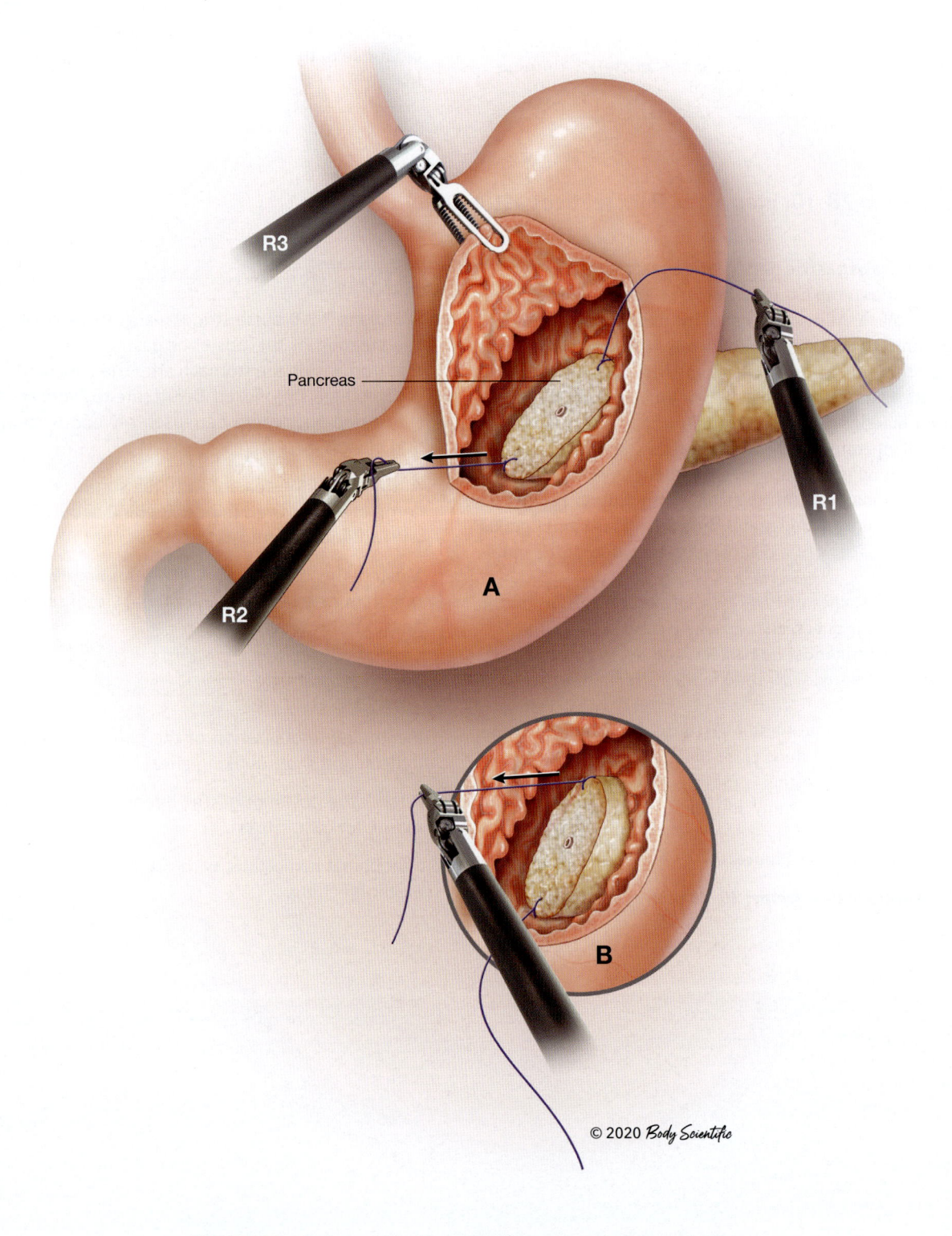

FIGURE 28-29 • Step 14-b: Transgastric pancreaticogastrostomy.

Step 15. Bilio-digestive anastomosis

The hepaticojejunostomy (**Figure 28-30**) is an end-to-side reconstruction, and depending on the size/thickness of the bile duct, it can be of variable complexity.

Very dilated ducts are usually an easy suturing task, which is performed with two half-running PDS™ 4-0 sutures.

The same jejunal loop, 20–30 cm distal to the pancreaticojejunostomy, is the anastomotic site.

If the bile duct is thin (4–5 mm), the technical challenge is more complex.

A posterior short running suture is carried out, and the anterior aspect of the anastomosis is constructed with interrupted PDS™ 4-0 or 5-0 single stitches.

Every suture is mounted on a clip, and all stitches are tied, one by one, at the end. Attention should be paid not to break the tissue while tying. Optimal visual feedback is necessary to adjust the tension of the knots.

Step 15 average time frame: 20–30 min

▶▶ TIPS

Starting the anastomotic row from lateral to medial allows a better open angle of vision than vice versa. The bowel opening needs to be created before making the posterior suture line.

The assistant may decrease the tension, when tying the knots, pushing the jejunal loop up toward the liver with a grasper.

⚠ PITFALLS

Stricture/leaks of the anastomosis due to poor visualization of the anastomotic edges.

Tension on the anastomotic line during the construction and risk of tissue breaks.

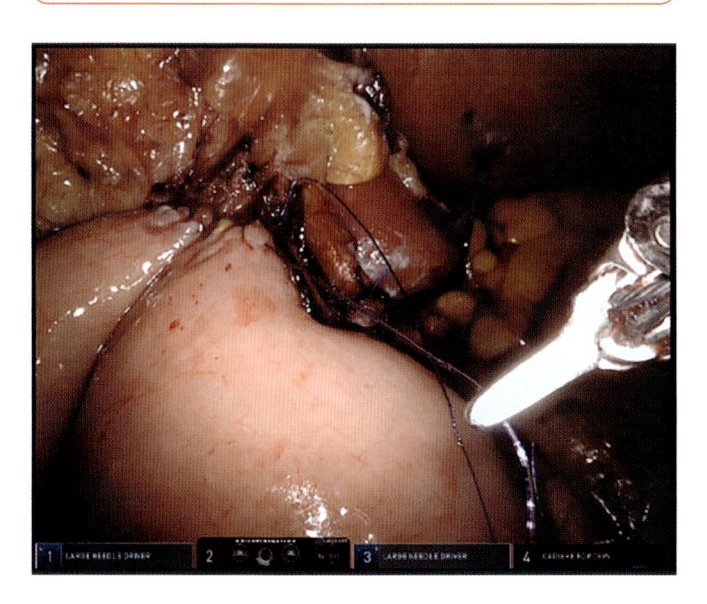

FIGURE 28-30 • Step 15. Hepaticojejunostomy.

Step 16. The digestive reconstruction

When a pylorus-preserving procedure is done, a simple reconstruction 50–60 cm distal to the hepaticojejunostomy and an end-to-side pylorojejunostomy is performed.

Two half-running PDS™ 3-0 sutures are used for the posterior and anterior row.

This step is represented in **Figures 28-31** and **28-32 A–F**.

Step 16 average time frame: 20–30 min

▶▶ TIPS

The microperfusion of the pylorus should be checked with ICG. A very short duodenal stump, distal to the pylorus, is necessary to anchor the suture and respect the integrity of the sphincter.

⚠ PITFALLS

A too long duodenal cuff beyond the pylorus leading to suboptimal perfusion, potentially delayed gastric emptying, and pyloric dysfunction.

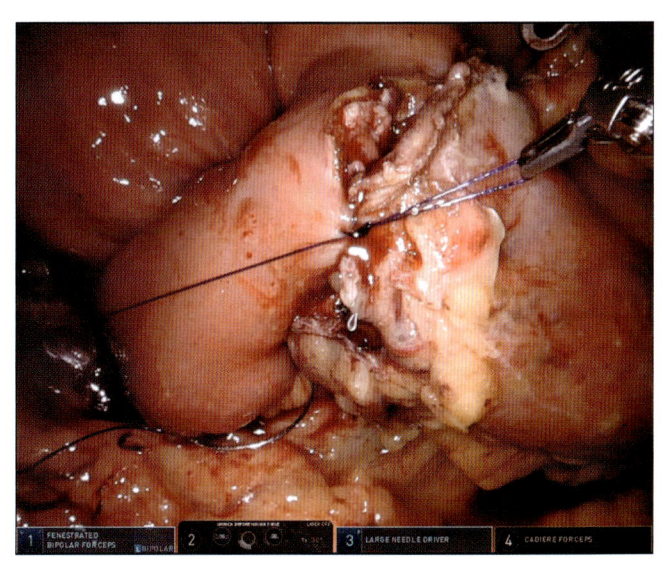

FIGURE 28-31 • Step 16. Gastrojejunostomy.

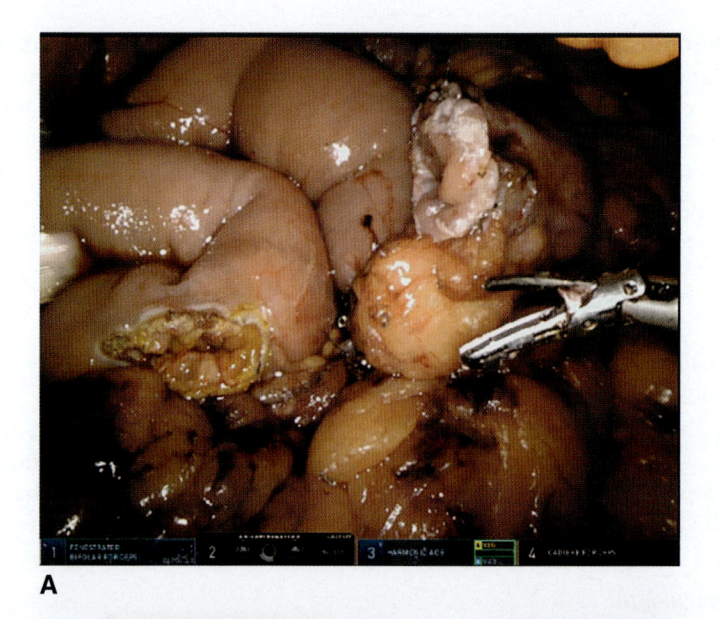

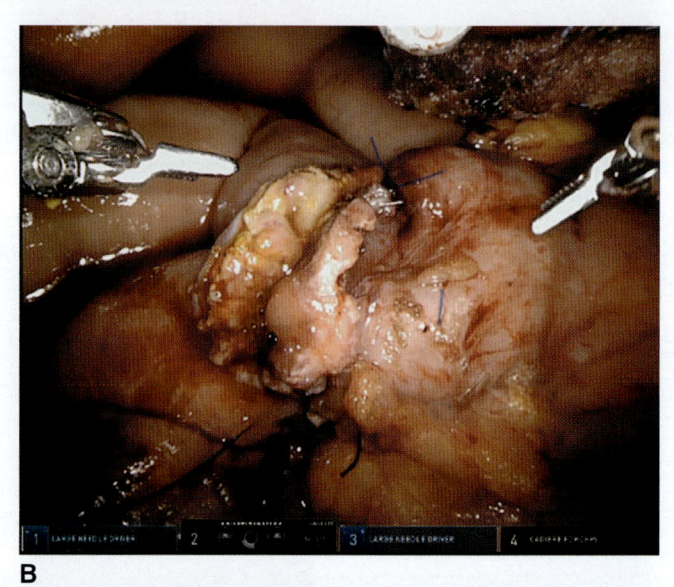

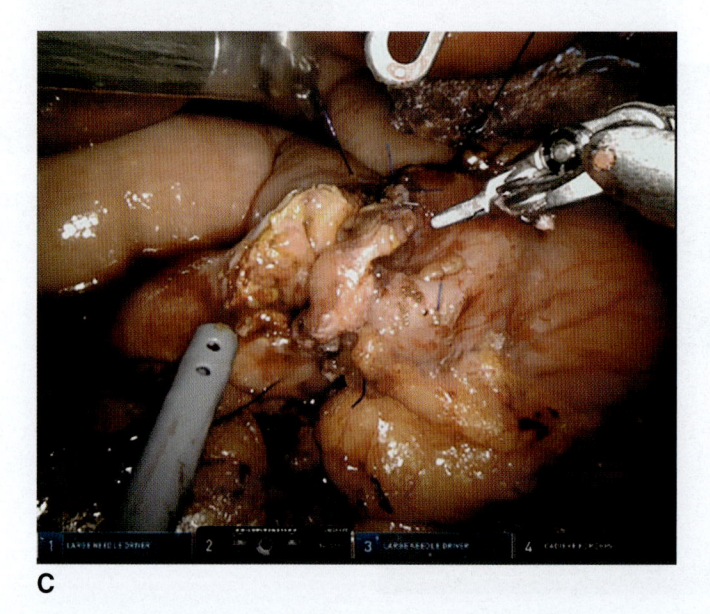

FIGURE 28-32 • Step 16. Pylorojejunostomy.

Pancreaticoduodenectomy 633

D

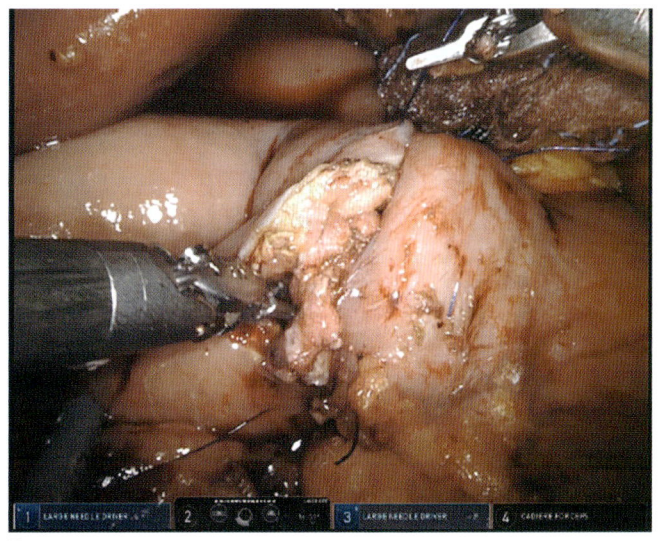

E

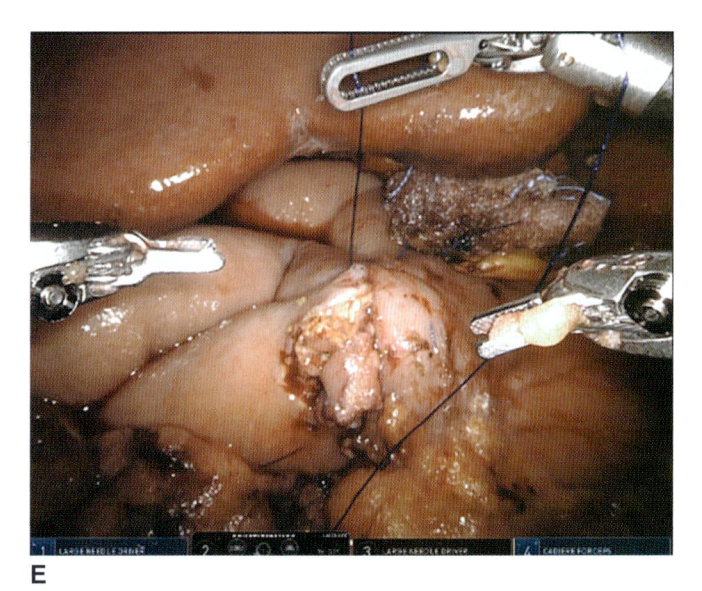

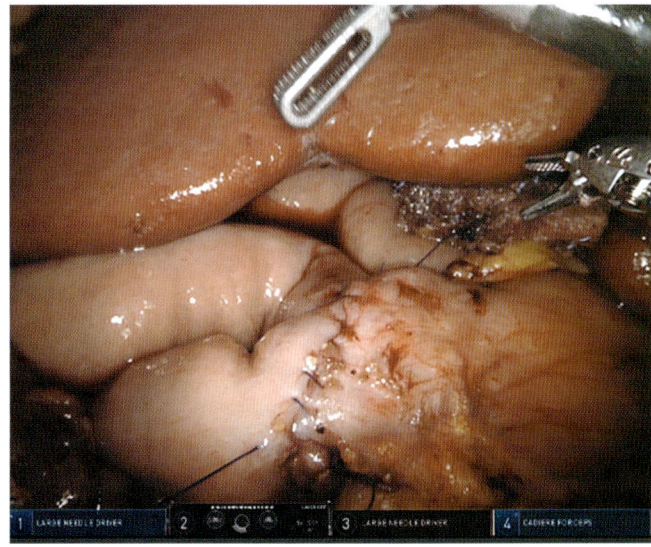

F

FIGURE 28-32 • (*Continued*)

Step 17. Specimen extraction

The specimen is placed into an Endobag™ and retrieved through a Pfannenstiel incision (see Chapter 2, The Basic Principles of Clinical Applications, for additional details). The extraction can be made immediately before the reconstructive phase, temporarily undocking the robot, or at the end of the procedure. If the suprapubic space is not easily available from previous operations in the lower quadrants, other extraction sites can be considered (midline supraumbilical mini-laparotomy).

Two drains are left in the gallbladder fossa and near the pancreatic anastomosis (behind the stomach). The amylase is checked on the first, third, and fifth postop days, and the drains are removed if the test is negative.

Step 17 average time frame: 20–30 min

Suggested Readings

1. Pancreatic Cancer Treatment (Adult) (PDQ®)–Health Professional Version. National Cancer Institute Web site. https://www.cancer.gov/types/pancreatic/hp/pancreatic-treatment-pdq.
2. NCCN Guidelines. Pancreatic Adenocarcinoma. NCCN Evidence Blocks.™ https://www.nccn.org/guidelines/guidelines-detail? category=1&id=1455
3. Giulianotti PC, Mangano A, Bustos RE, et al. Operative technique in robotic pancreaticoduodenectomy (RPD) at University of Illinois at Chicago (UIC): 17 steps standardized technique: Lessons learned since the first worldwide RPD performed in the year 2001. *Surg Endosc* 2018;32(10):4329-4336. doi: 10.1007/s00464-018-6228-7
4. Giulianotti PC, Mangano A, Bustos RE, et al. Educational step-by-step surgical video about operative technique in robotic pancreaticoduodenectomy (RPD) at University of Illinois at Chicago (UIC): 17 steps standardized technique. Lessons learned since the first worldwide RPD performed in the year 2001. *Surg Endosc* 2020;34(6):2758-2762. doi: 10.1007/s00464-020-07383-0
5. Klompmaker S, van Hilst J, Wellner UF, et al. Outcomes after minimally-invasive versus open pancreatoduodenectomy: a Pan-European propensity score matched study. *Ann Surg.* 2020;271(2):356-363. doi: 10.1097/SLA.0000000000002850
6. Giulianotti PC, Coratti A, Angelini M, et al. Robotics in general surgery: personal experience in a large community hospital. *Arch Surg.* 2003;138(7):777-784. doi: 10.1001/archsurg.138.7.777
7. Giulianotti PC, Gheza F. Robotic pancreatoduodenectomy. In: Fong Y, Woo Y, Hyung WJ, Lau C, Strong VE, eds. *The SAGES Atlas of Robotic Surgery*. Springer; 2018:311-318.
8. Kornaropoulos M, Moris D, Beal EW. Total robotic pancreaticoduodenectomy: a systematic review of the literature. *Surg Endosc.* 2017;31(11):4382-4392. doi: 10.1007/s00464-017-5523-z
9. Ricci C, Casadei R, Taffurelli G, et al Minimally invasive pancreaticoduodenectomy: what is the best "choice"? A systematic review and network metanalysis of non-randomized comparative studies. 2018. *World J Surg.* 2018;42(3):788-805. doi: 10.1007/s00268-017-4180-7
10. Yan JF, Pan Y, Chen K, et al. Minimally invasive pancreatoduodenectomy is associated with lower morbidity compared to open pancreatoduodenectomy: an updated meta-analysis of randomized controlled trials and high-quality nonrandomized studies. *Medicine (Baltimore).* 2019;98(32):e16730. doi: 10.1097/MD.0000000000016730
11. Alsabilah J, Kim WR, Kim NK. Vascular structures of the right colon: incidence and variations with their clinical implications. *Scand J Surg.* 2017;106(2):107-115. doi: 10.1177/1457496916650999
12. Alsabilah JF, Razvi SA, Albandar MH, et al. Intraoperative archive of right colonic vascular variability aids central vascular ligation and redefines gastrocolic trunk of Henle variants. *Dis Colon Rectum.* 2017;60(1):22-29. doi: 10.1097/DCR.0000000000000720
13. Murono K, Kawai K, Ishihara S, et al. Evaluation of the vascular anatomy of the right-sided colon using three-dimensional computed tomography angiography: a single-center study of 536 patients and a review of the literature. *Int J Colorectal Dis.* 2016;31(9):1633-1638. doi: 10.1007/s00384-016-2627-1
14. *Japan Society of Pancreatic Cancer Classification of Pancreatic Carcinoma*. Fourth English Edition. Japan Pancreas Society: 2017.
15. Graf O, Boland GW, Kaufman JA, et al. Anatomic variants of mesenteric veins: depiction with helical CT venography. *AJR Am J Roentgenol.* 1997;168(5):1209-1213. doi: 10.2214/ajr.168.5.9129413
16. Anwar AS, Srikala J, Papalkar AS, et al. Study of anatomical variations of hepatic vasculature using multidetector computed tomography angiography. *Surg Radiol Anat.* 2020;42(12):1449-1457. doi: 10.1007/s00276-020-02532-5
17. Yan J, Feng H, Wang H, et al. Hepatic artery classification based on three-dimensional CT. *Br J Surg.* 2020;107(7):906-916. doi: 10.1002/bjs.11458
18. Hiatt J R, Gabbay J, Busettil R W. Surgical anatomy of the hepatic arteries in 1000 cases. *Ann Surg.* 1994;220(1):50-52. doi: 10.1097/00000658-199407000-00008
19. Zhang W, Wang K, Liu S, et al. A single-center clinical study of hepatic artery variations in laparoscopic pancreaticoduodenectomy: a retrospective analysis of data from 218 cases *Medicine (Baltimore).* 2020;99(21):e20403. doi: 10.1097/MD.0000000000020403
20. Noussios G, Dimitriou I, Iosif Chatzis I, et al. The main anatomic variations of the hepatic artery and their importance in surgical practice: review of the literature. *J Clin Med Res.* 2017;9(4):248-252. doi: 10.14740/jocmr2902w
21. Michels NA. Newer anatomy of the liver and its variant blood supply and collateral circulation. *Am J Surg.* 1966;112:337-347. 10.1016/0002-9610(66)90201-7
22. For updates on Robotic Surgery Congresses and thousands of educational surgical videos and presentations please visit the Clinical Robotic Surgery Association Website (CRSA): https://clinicalrobotics.com/
23. Schnelldorfer T, Adams DB, Warshaw AL, Lillemoe KD, Sarr MG. Forgotten pioneers of pancreatic surgery: beyond the favorite few. *Ann Surg.* 2008;247(1):191-202. doi: 10.1097/SLA.0b013e3181559a97
24. Giulianotti PC, Angelini M, Sbrana F, et al. Les Résections Coelioscopiques du Pancréas. *Le Journal de Coelio Chirurgie.* N 54- Decembre 2004.

"Surgery is an art, as well as a science, and requires a delicate balance of knowledge, skill, and creativity."

—Harvey Cushing (1869–1939)

Radical Antegrade Modular Pancreatosplenectomy

Rong Liu • Qu Liu

INTRODUCTION

Conventional distal pancreatectomy with splenectomy for pancreatic cancer of the body and tail have been associated with a high positive margin rate, low lymph nodes retrieval, and poor overall survival. This approach, which proceeds in a left-to-right retrograde fashion, has been suggested to result in limited visualization of the posterior plane of dissection, potential hemorrhage, and inadequate lymphadenectomy, particularly regarding the lymph nodes around the celiac and superior mesenteric arteries.

In 2003, Strasberg et al. (see suggested readings #1, 2) introduced a novel approach for cancers of the body and tail of the pancreas called radical antegrade modular pancreatosplenectomy (RAMPS). The RAMPS proceeds in a right-to-left antegrade fashion with early control of the splenic vessels, celiac artery, superior mesenteric artery (SMA), and improved visualization of the retroperitoneal plane of dissection. It was designed to increase the rate of R0 resection and the extent of lymph nodes dissection. This procedure is modular in that the plane of the posterior dissection can be directed on the left adrenal gland and Gerota's fascia (anterior RAMPS) or can be posterior to the adrenal gland and Gerota's fascia (posterior RAMPS), depending on the extent of penetration of the tumor on the preoperative workup.

Indications and Relative Contraindications to the Robotic Approach

Malignant tumors located in the body and tail of the pancreas are eligible for robotic RAMPS (RRAMPS). Obesity and history of intra-abdominal surgeries are not absolute

INSTRUMENT REQUIREMENTS

The suggested main robotic instruments/tools can be listed as follows:
- 30° scope
- Needle drivers (round tip or macro)
- Cautery hook
- Harmonic shears/vessel sealer
- Scissors
- Cadiére grasper
- Linear staplers
- Medium/large clip applier
- Bipolar forceps

The suggested main laparoscopic instruments/tools can be listed as follows:
- Needle drivers
- Scissors
- Graspers
- Staplers (with different loads)
- Suction-irrigation
- Laparoscopic ultrasound (drop-in probe or handheld)

Supplemental materials:
- Gauzes, sponges
- Penrose drains
- Vessel loops
- Endo Bags™
- Sutures: Prolene™ 2-0, 3-0, 4-0, and 5-0 and PDS™ 3-0, 4-0, and 5-0
- Multiple Hem-o-lok-clips®

Photo reproduced with permission from Doyle NM, Doyle JF, Walter EJ. The life and work of Harvey Cushing 1869-1939: A pioneer of neurosurgery. J Intensive Care Soc. 2017;18(2):157-158.
Quote reproduced with permission from Cushing H. The Life of Sir William Osler. Oxford UK: Oxford University Press; 1925.

contraindications, but they may increase the surgical time and complexity.

Patient Positioning, OR Setup, and Port Setting

The patient is positioned supine with legs parted and arms tucked to the side as described in **Figure 29-1**.

The assistant sits between the legs. The OR setup is shown in **Figure 29-2**.

The pneumoperitoneum is achieved using a Veress needle placed in the left subcostal space. After induction of pneumoperitoneum, a 5-mm port is placed with the Optiview® technique laterally in the left upper quadrant near the anterior axillary line. An initial abdominal exploration, using a 5-mm laparoscope, is mandatory to assess for adhesions or signs of advanced disease that may modify the operative plan.

Five or six trocars are placed under direct visualization as shown in **Figures 29-3 A, B** (four robotic and one or two assistant ports).

The four robotic ports are inserted along a straight line. The camera port is placed slightly above the transverse umbilical line at the intersection with the left pararectal line. The 5-mm trocar that was initially placed for abdominal exploration is replaced by the 8-mm first robotic arm port (R1). The second arm working port is placed at the level above the transverse umbilical line and medial to the right pararectal line (R2). The third arm trocar (R3) is inserted at the level of the right anterior axillary line. In doing so, a more effective retraction of the stomach can be achieved during the dissection and resection of the pancreas. Two 10–12-mm assistant ports are preferred (**Figures 29-4 A, B**). The first one is placed slightly inferior between the first robotic arm and the scope, and the second one is inserted around the umbilicus. All port placements should be slightly adjusted according to the patient's body habitus and tumor location. Following the port placement, the bed is adjusted in a 30° reverse Trendelenburg position and slightly tilted to the right. The robotic cart is docked from the left side of the bed.

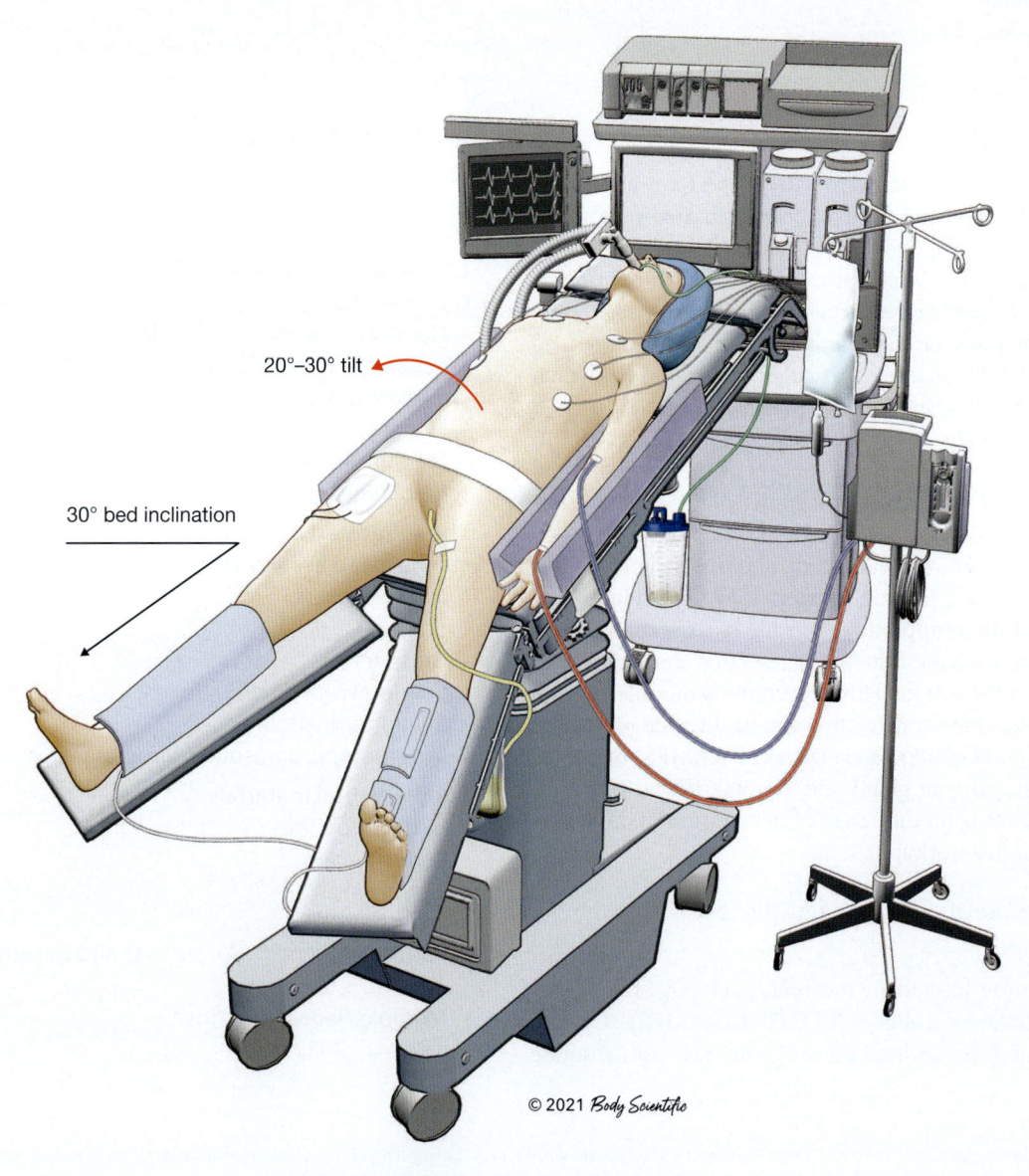

FIGURE 29-1 • Patient positioning.

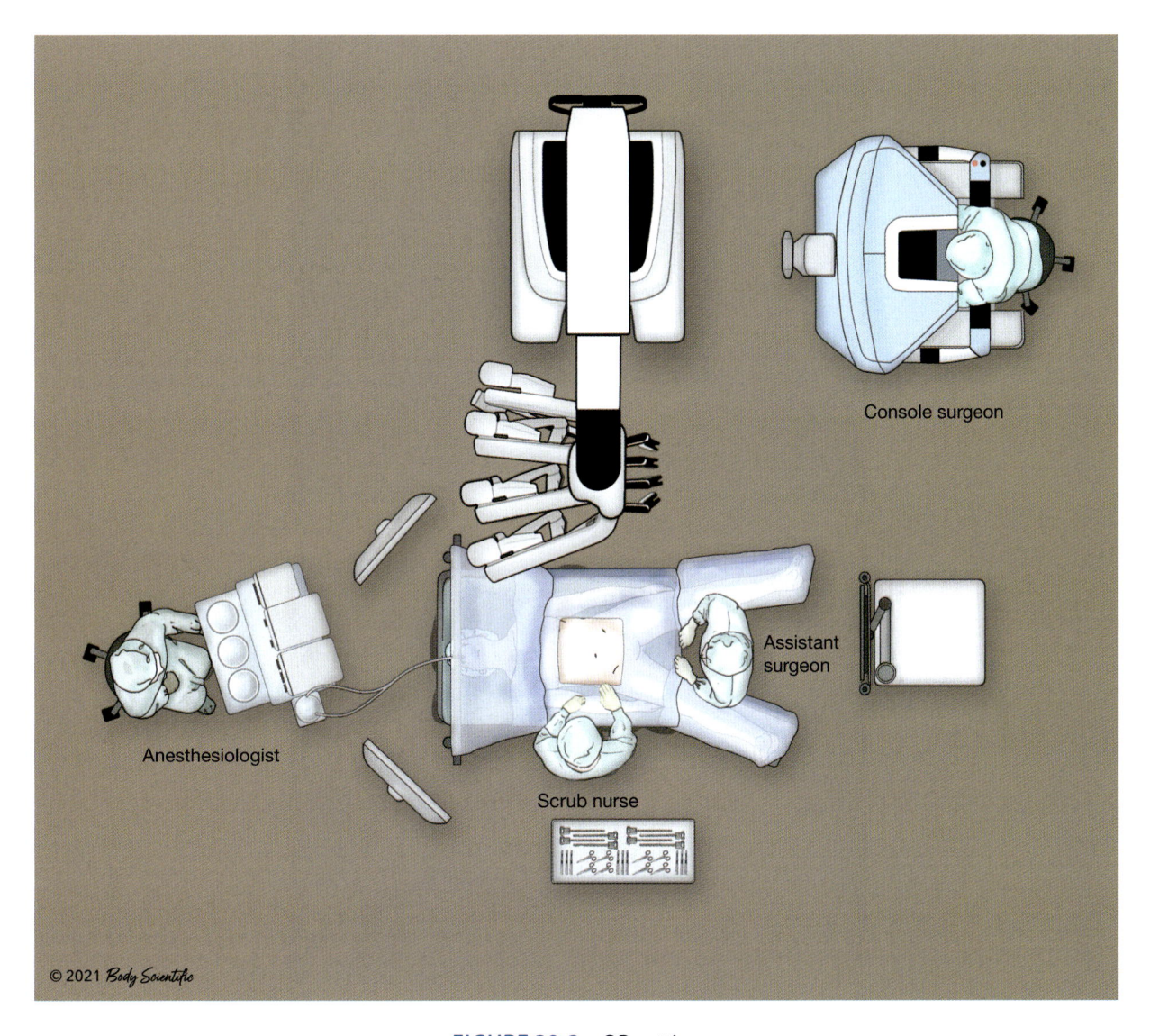

FIGURE 29-2 • OR setting.

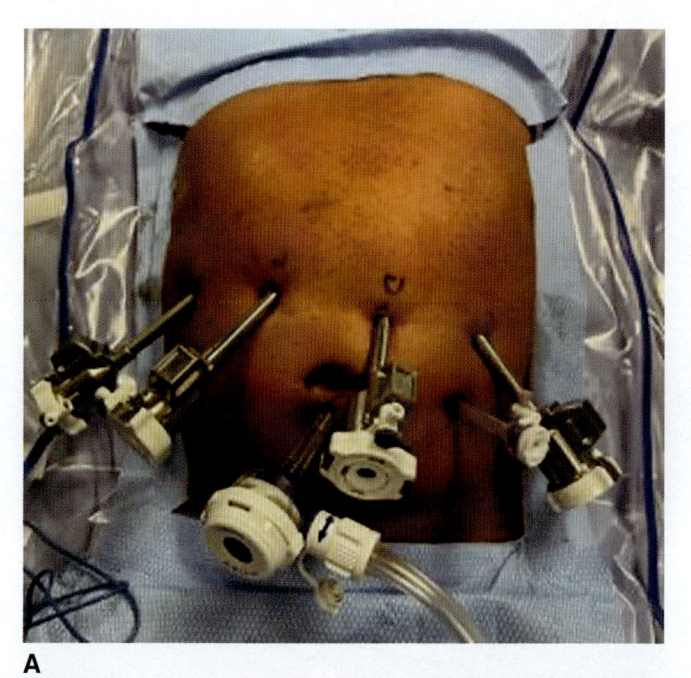

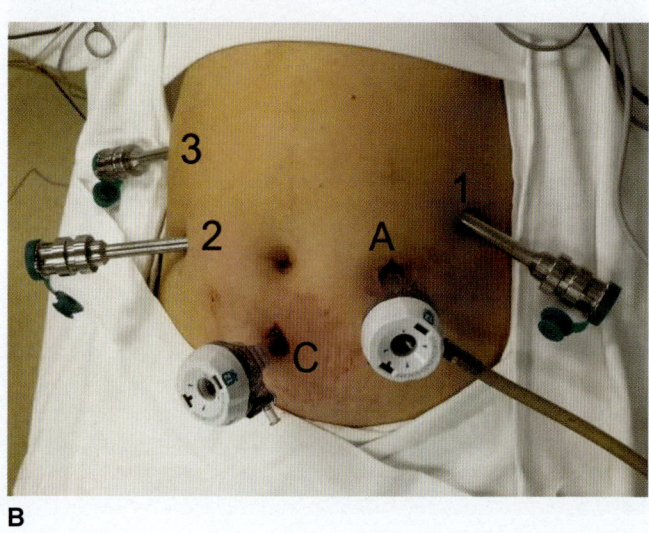

FIGURE 29-3 • **A.** Xi port placement. **B.** Si port placement.

Radical Antegrade Modular Pancreatosplenectomy 639

EDITORIAL COMMENT

In many countries, the Si system is still the most available platform. However, the Xi system is the standard technology in US and Europe and its ports setup is shown in **Figures 29-4 A, B**.

Normal abdomen

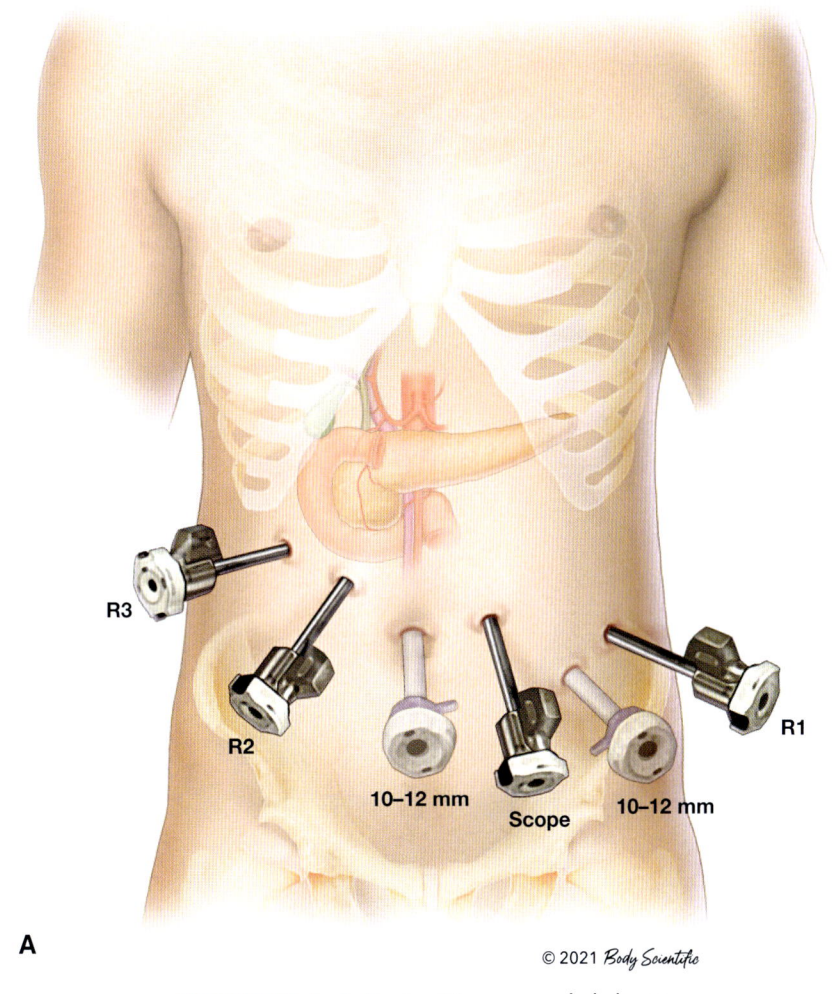

FIGURE 29-4 • **A.** Port setting normal abdomen.

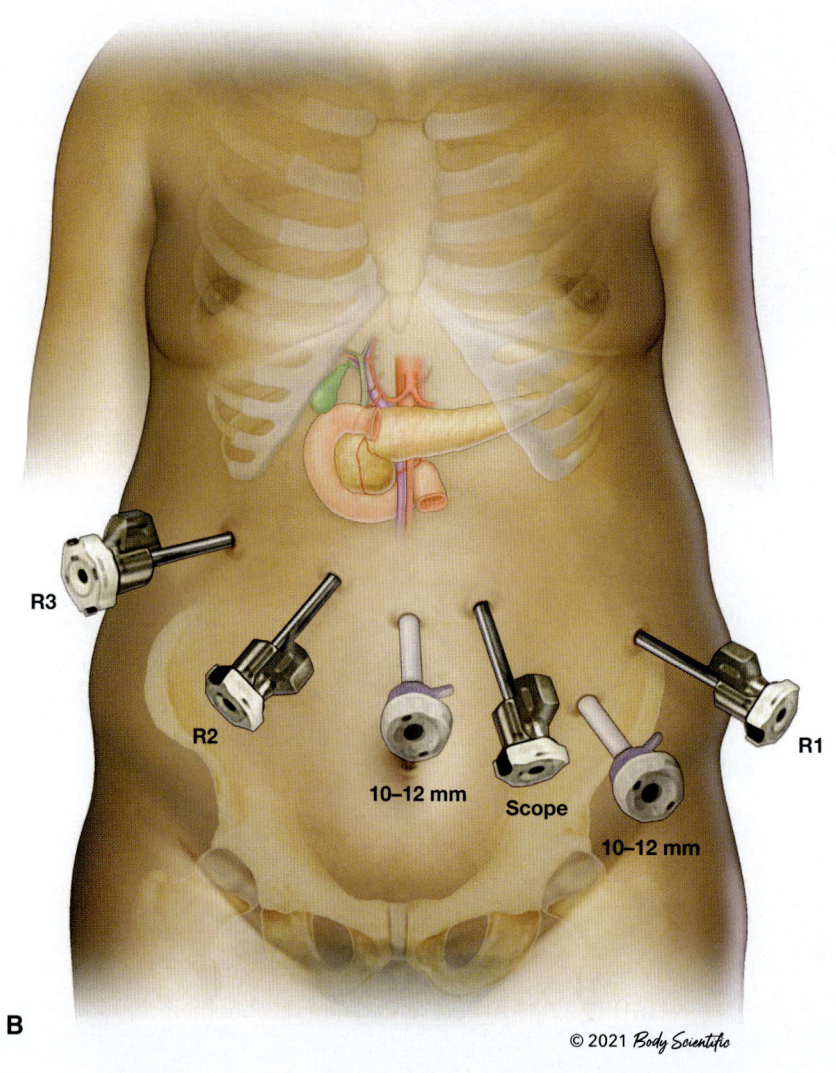

FIGURE 29-4 • (Continued) B. Port setting wide abdomen.

Surgical Technique

▶ **Video 29-1. RRAMPS – Full Procedure**

Step 1. Gastrocolic ligament division

Using the third robotic arm (R3), the stomach is lifted upward with Cadière forceps putting the gastrocolic ligament under proper tension. The gastrocolic ligament is divided using the hook or Harmonic shears/vessel sealer starting in the middle and then moving laterally to the left to expose the tail of the pancreas and hilum of the spleen. The short gastric vessels and the left gastroepiploic vessels are not dissected yet, as shown in **Figure 29-5**.

This maneuver allows the exploration of the lesser sac, which provides initial intraoperative assessment of the cancer staging. Important finding to look for are: local involvement of the serosa, local carcinomatosis, enlarged lymph nodes, and encasement of major vessels. Based on this assessment, the surgeon may need to take a biopsy of the suspicious tissue for frozen pathology.

Step 1 average time frame: 10–15 min

▶▶ **TIPS**

Asking the assistant to maintain gentle tension on the transverse colon helps in keeping the proper avascular dissection plane, avoiding the risk of damaging the blood supply of the transverse colon.

⚠ **PITFALLS**

Incomplete gastrocolic ligament division may not allow a comprehensive examination of the lesser sac. Sometimes, there are adhesions between the posterior wall of the stomach and the pancreas. Those adhesions have to be carefully taken down in order to complete the exploration of the lesser sac and the assessment of the pancreatic body.

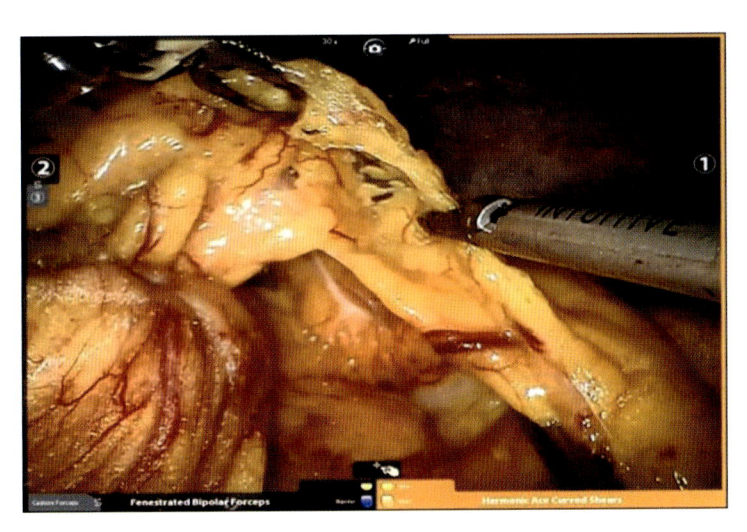

FIGURE 29-5 • Gastrocolic ligament division.

Step 2. Mobilization of the left colonic flexure

The left colonic flexure and descending colon are mobilized along the Toldt's fascia inferiorly and medially, using the monopolar hook and the bipolar forceps, as shown in **Figure 29-6**.

The splenorenal and splenocolic ligaments are taken down, allowing the complete detachment of the spleen from the colon. The mobilization should be generous in order to expose the underlying inferior edge of the pancreas and Gerota's fascia of the left kidney.

Step 2 average time frame: 15–20 min

> ▶▶ **TIPS**
> It is important to use dynamically the R3 during this step to achieve an efficient exposure. The borders of the distal pancreas can be better exposed by retracting the posterior wall of the stomach instead of the anterior one.

> ⚠ **PITFALLS**
> During this step, omental and gastric retraction should be made very carefully in order not to pull on splenic adhesions, with the risk of laceration of the splenic capsule and subsequent bleeding.

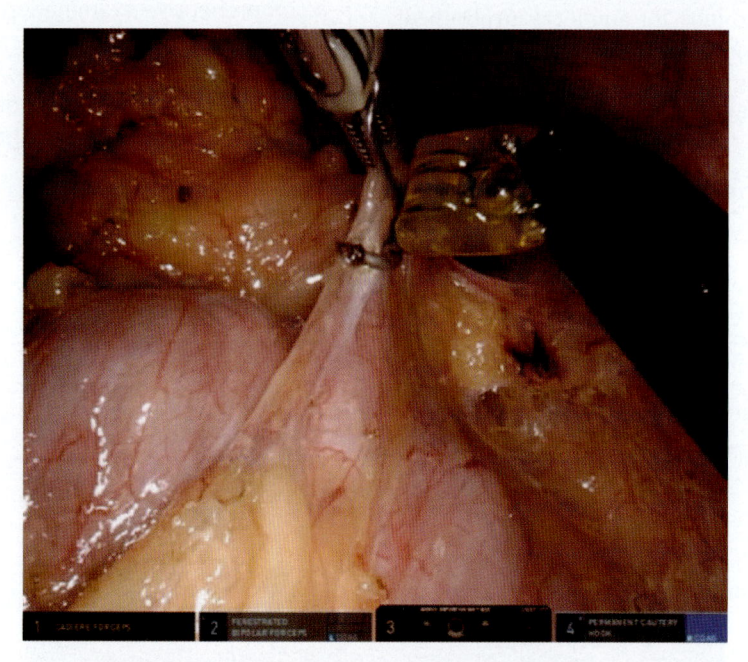

FIGURE 29-6 • Mobilization of the left colonic flexure.

Step 3. Preparation of the neck of the pancreas, assessment of the resectability, and intraoperative ultrasound

The retrogastric adhesions with the pancreas, if present, are dissected while moving toward the posterior wall of the gastric antrum. The assessment of the pancreatic neck is an important step to rule out a possible local infiltration (tangential abutment/encasement) of the superior mesenteric vein (SMV) or the portal axis (see **Figures 29-7 A, B** for detailed description of the pancreas anatomy).

When the anterior wall of the pancreatic isthmus has been exposed, an intraoperative ultrasound scan can be used for more detailed evaluation of the extent of the lesion, to assess its proximity with nearby structures, and to identify suspicious lymphadenopathies or tumor infiltration into the retropancreatic adipose tissue.

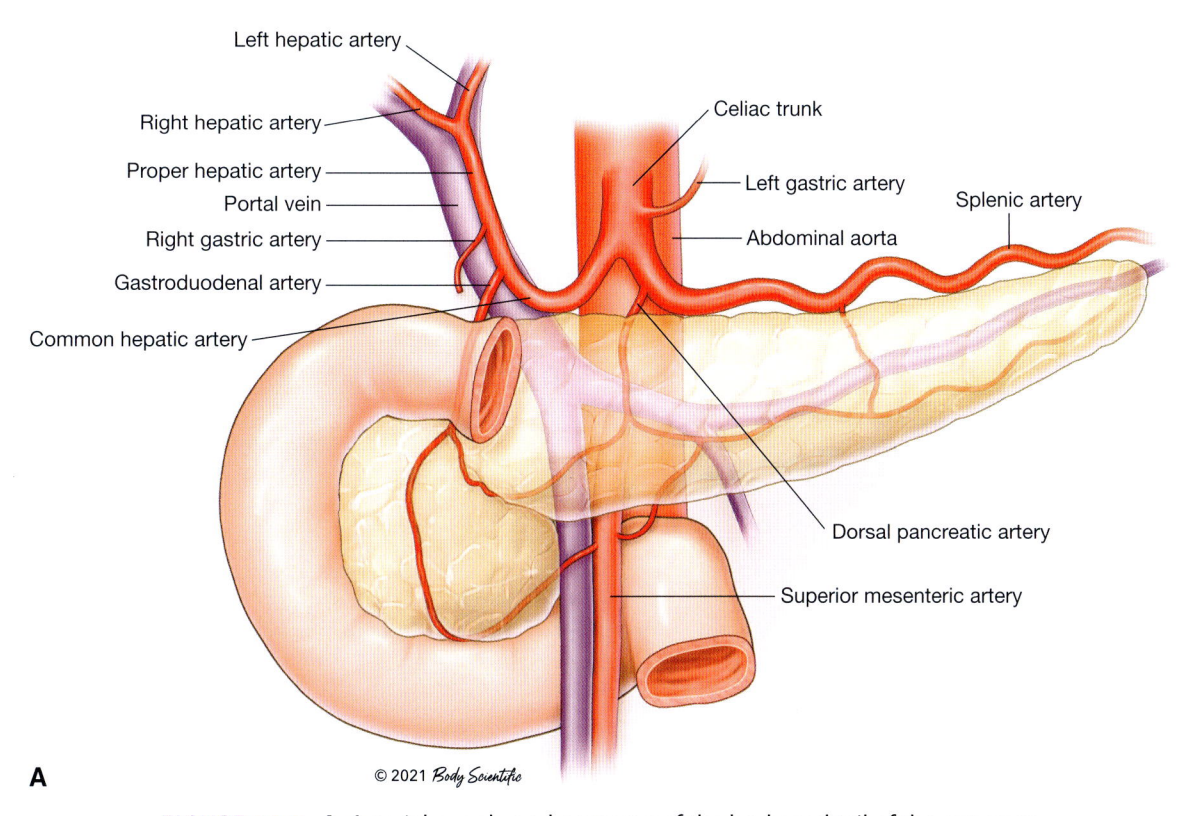

FIGURE 29-7 • **A.** Arterial supply and anatomy of the body and tail of the pancreas.

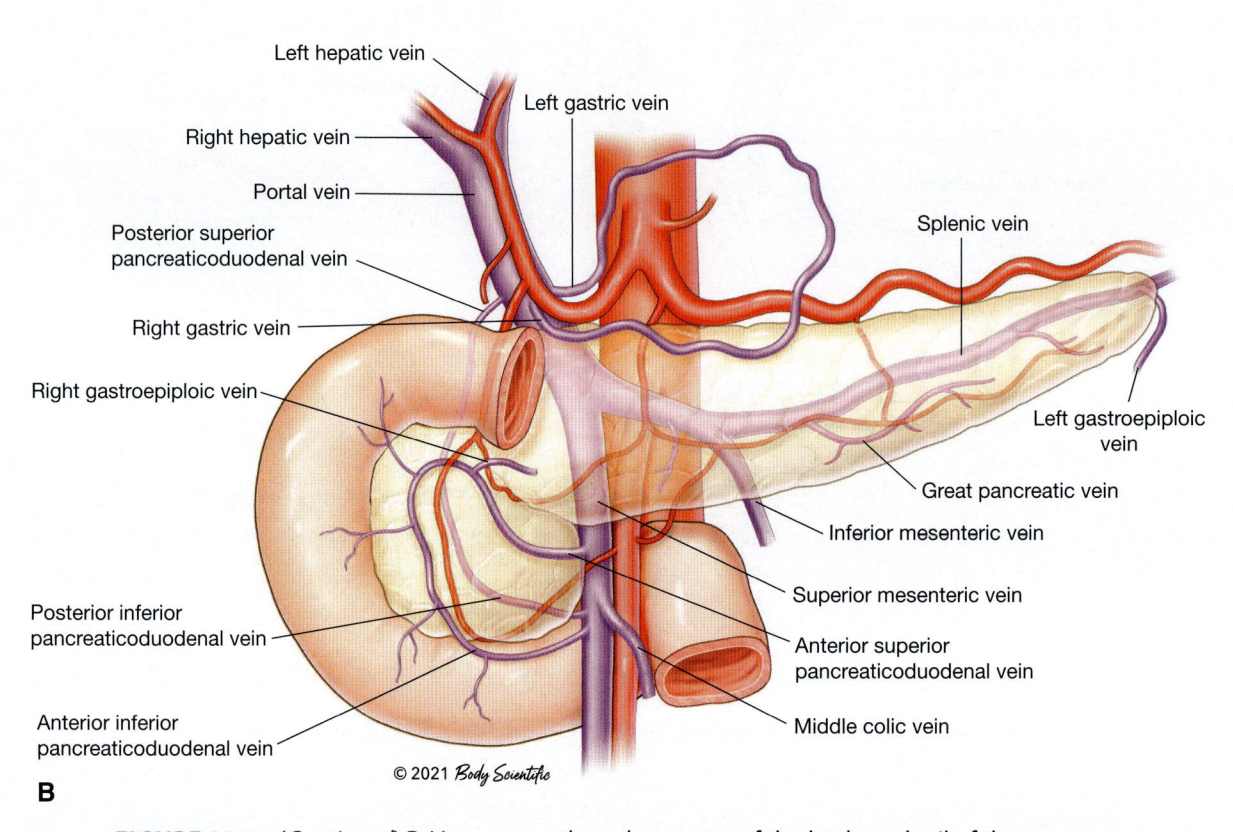

FIGURE 29-7 • (*Continued*) **B.** Venous supply and anatomy of the body and tail of the pancreas.

Final resectability assessment should rely not only on the results of an ultrasound, but also on the surgical dissection of the vascular structures around the tumor.

Before preparing the retropancreatic tunnel, the peritoneal reflection at the junction of the mesocolon and pancreatic neck is carefully dissected, exposing the superior and inferior borders of the isthmus of the pancreas with a monopolar hook alternated to bipolar energy. The partial mobilization of the body and tail of the pancreas from the transverse mesocolic root is necessary to achieve adequate exposure of the inferior mesenteric vein (IMV) that is an important surgical landmark. During this step, it is also important to divide, if present, the small branches of the middle colic vein joining the pancreas (using Prolene™ 5-0). This maneuver allows better access to the confluence of the SMV and portal vein.

Step 3 average time frame: 15–20 min

> ▶▶ **TIPS**
>
> Narrowing of a major vein, changes in color and indirect tactile feedback based on tissue deformation in response to local pressure are all important feedback. The middle colic vein is a useful landmark to localize the confluence of the SMV with the portal vein. In an obese patient with thick mesentery, this is particularly helpful.

▶ **Video 29-2.** Preparation of the Neck of the Pancreas, and Intraoperative Ultrasound

Step 4. Division of the left gastroepiploic artery and short gastric vessels

The dissection of the gastrocolic ligament is continued toward the short gastric vessels, as shown in **Figure 29-8**.

The left gastroepiploic artery and all short gastric vessels have to be divided until reaching the left diaphragmatic pillar. This maneuver can be perfectly executed using a vessel sealer and the R3 in a "dynamic fashion." The R3 has to be frequently repositioned providing traction on the posterior wall of the stomach for optimal exposure. The vessel sealer progressively seals and divides the short gastric vessels and the splenogastric ligament moving toward the fundus.

Step 4 average time frame: 5–10 min

> ▶▶ **TIPS**
>
> In certain cases, a bulky lesion can compress the splenic vein causing left-sided portal hypertension and gastric varices. When left-sided portal hypertension is present, it is better to divide the splenic artery (SA) before ligating the congested short gastric vessels and division of the pancreas decreasing the backflow bleeding. The SA can be controlled using a vascular stapler or Prolene™ 3-0 suture. The short gastric vessels are better divided using the vessel sealer with the so-called "dual application," which means to coagulate twice before cutting in the middle.

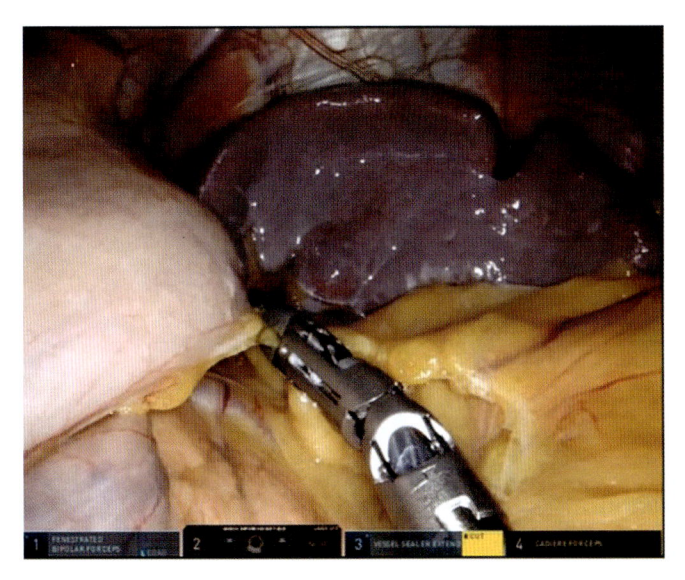

FIGURE 29-8 • Division of the short gastric vessels.

Step 5. Control and division of the splenic artery and celiac lymphadenectomy

A lymphadenectomy with skeletonization of the common hepatic artery, left gastric artery, and celiac trunk is performed. The origin of the splenic artery is exposed (see **Figures 29-9** and **29-10 A–D** for a detailed description of the anatomy and the lymph nodes mapping of the celiac trunk and the pancreas).

The peritoneum is divided at the base of the caudate lobe, and connective tissue, lympho-neural tissue, and lymph nodes are dissected inferiorly off the crus of the diaphragm. The splenic artery is divided, close to its origin, with a vascular stapler as shown in **Figure 29-11**.

Step 5 average time frame: 20–30 min

> ▶▶ **TIPS**
>
> A perfect understanding of the vascular anatomy is necessary before dividing the artery.
>
> For bulky lesions in proximity of the pancreatic neck, it may be necessary to change the steps of the procedure, dividing the pancreas first and controlling the confluence of the splenic vein and origin of the splenic artery after lifting the distal pancreatic stump.

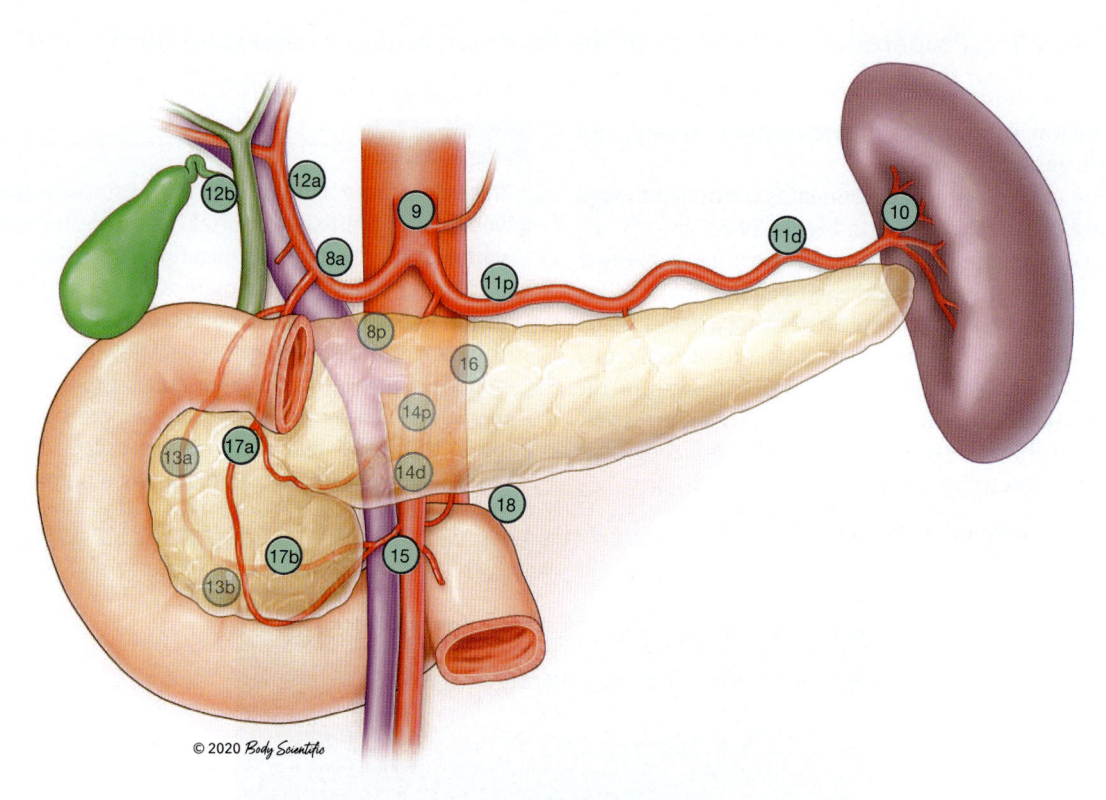

FIGURE 29-9 • Lymph nodes mapping of the pancreas.

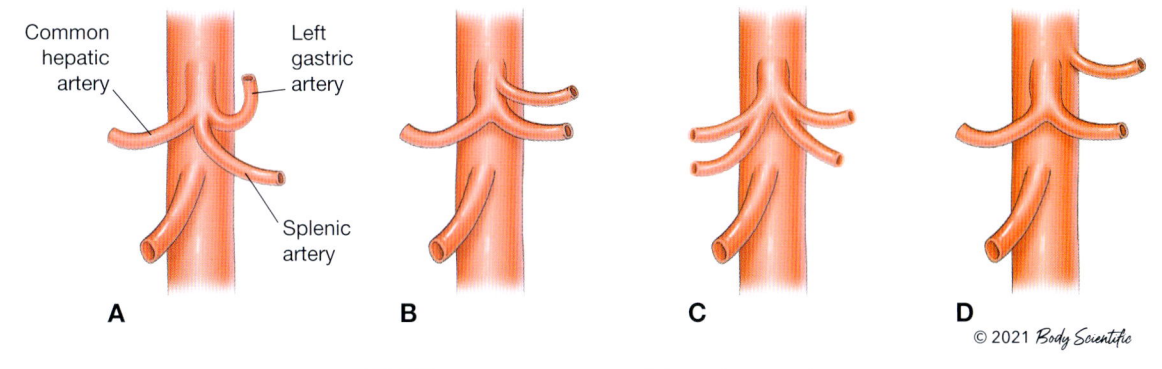

FIGURE 29-10 • Anatomy of the celiac trunk.

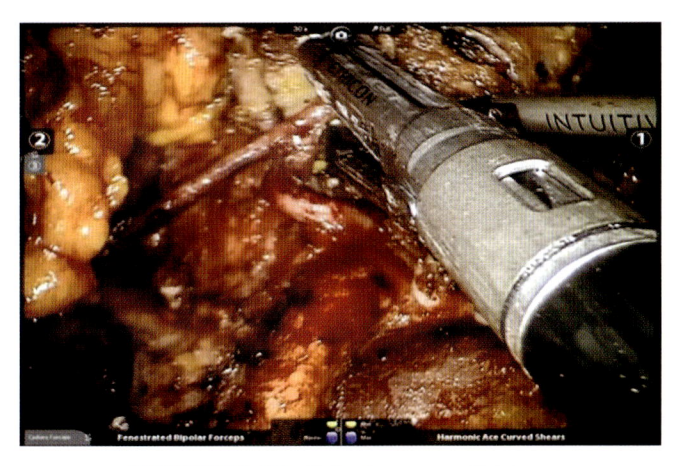

FIGURE 29-11 • Splenic artery division.

▶ **Video 29-3. Step 6. RRAMPS Pancreas Transection**

Step 6. Division of the pancreas
The pancreas is transected either by Harmonic shears or with a triple row stapler as described in **Video 29-3**. The device selection depends on the preference of the surgeon, pancreatic thickness, and parenchymal texture. Sometimes, it is simple to create a complete retropancreatic tunnel underneath the neck for division of the pancreas. In this case, a vessel loop can be passed underneath the neck, lifting the pancreas away from the vein. However, this maneuver can be very difficult if peripancreatic inflammation or a tumor infiltrating the vein are present. Two Prolene™ 2-0 stay sutures are applied on both the inferior right and left side of the neck, allowing some preventive hemostasis and lifting traction. The retropancreatic dissection needs to be created by a gentle blunt technique along the mesenteric-portal axis. The tunnel is necessary if the pancreas is transected by a stapler. In cases where the tunnel is difficult, the pancreas may be gradually divided with the Harmonic shears, while splitting the parenchyma layer by layer in antegrade fashion, using the inactive blade close to the portal vein. The main proximal pancreatic duct needs to be identified by a released clear pancreatic juice and oversewn with a figure 8 Prolene™ 3-0 or 4-0 suture as shown in **Figure 29-12**.

A sample of the distal pancreatic duct is sent for frozen pathology. A strong Prolene™ 2-0 stay suture is used on the distal stump to lift the pancreas and to facilitate the medial to lateral dissection.

Step 6 average time frame: 15–20 min

▶▶ **TIPS**

For thick and delicate pancreas parenchyma, the preferred tool for transection is the harmonic scalpel. For thin and fibrotic parenchyma, a triple raw stapler is generally used.

The surgeon has to be skilled and proficient with suturing technique. Bleeding from the pancreatic stump is a common event either with a stapler or Harmonic scalpel. It can be controlled with some additional interrupted stiches of Prolene™ 4-0, mainly at the upper border of the pancreas.

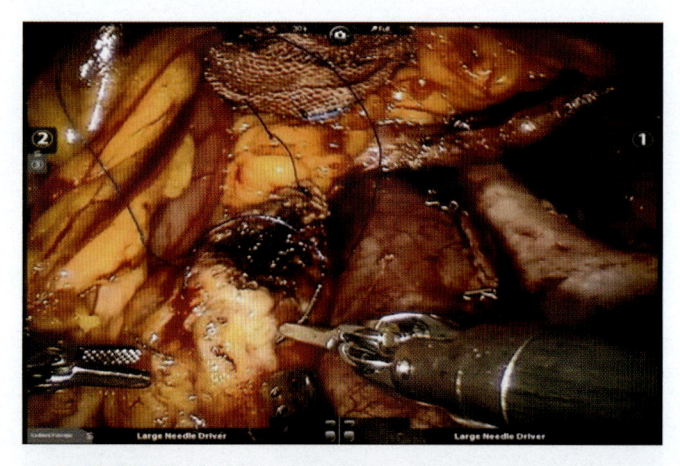

FIGURE 29-12 • Oversewing of the pancreatic stump.

Step 7. Inferior mesenteric vein division

After the transection of the pancreatic neck, it is important to reevaluate the location of the major vessels. The division of the IMV is an important surgical step. Sometimes the vein can be preserved when its confluence is into the portal vein or very close to it. Depending on the anatomy (see **Figures 29-13 A–C** for IMV anatomy), the IMV can be divided between transfixing sutures or stapler.

Step 7 average time frame: 10–15 min

> ▶▶ **TIPS**
>
> For the RRAMPS procedure, the IMV has to be divided in between Prolene™ 4-0 sutures or by vascular stapler if it joins with the splenic vein. It is better not to use clips for the IMV division. Later on when taking down the splenic vein, clips in close proximity to the vessel can be trapped between the jaws of the stapler causing a malfunction.

> 🔎 **ANATOMICAL HIGHLIGHTS**
>
> The IMV can drain into the splenic vein (more commonly) or into the portal vein.

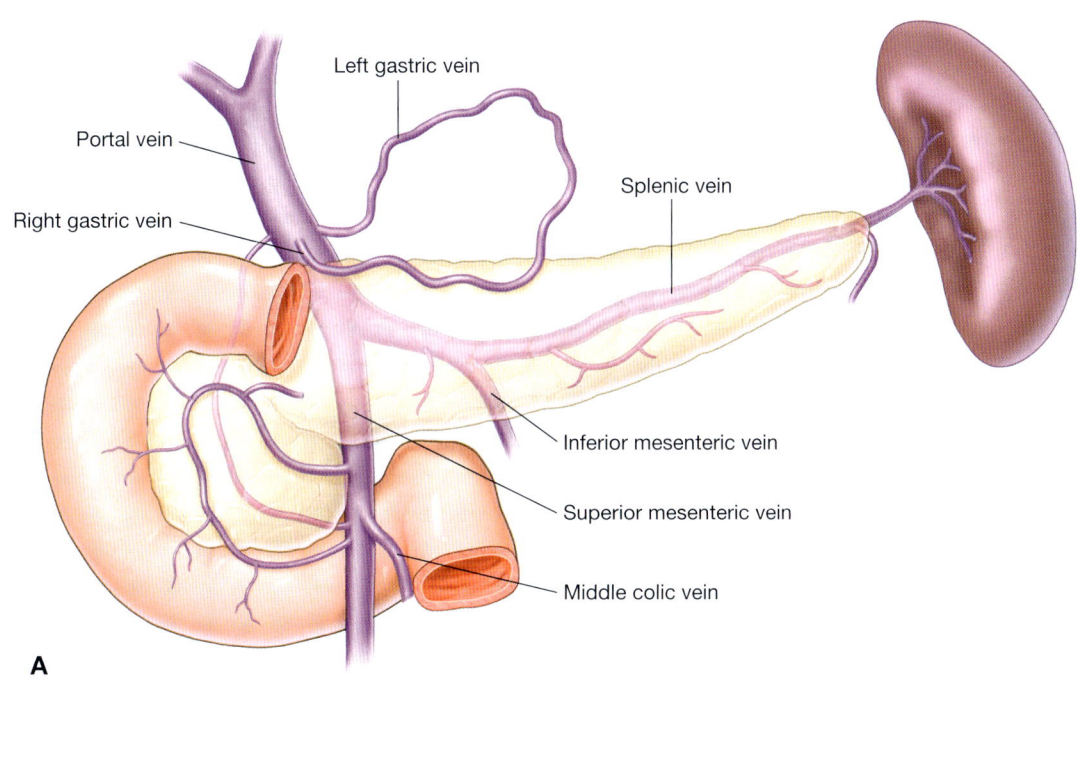

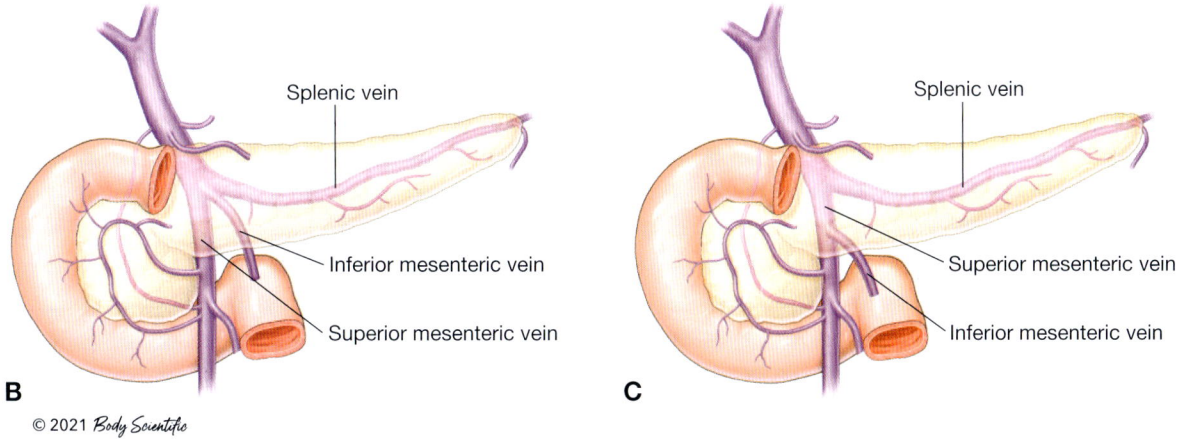

FIGURE 29-13 • Inferior mesenteric vein variations.

Video 29-4. Step 8. Splenic Vein Division

Step 8. The splenic vein division
The splenic vein is isolated at its junction with the SMV and divided with a vascular stapler, as shown in **Figure 29-14**.

This step opens up the retroperitoneal preaortic space while the pancreatic stump is more progressively retracted toward the left side.

Step 8 average time frame: 20–30 min

▶▶ TIPS
If the tumor invades the portal vein, resection and reconstruction of the portal vein may be necessary.

⚠ PITFALLS
Sometimes, the left gastric vein has its insertion into the portal vein, splenic vein, or directly at the confluence of portal and splenic veins. If the anatomy of the left gastric vein is not recognized, trying to dissect around its confluence can cause bleeding difficult to control.

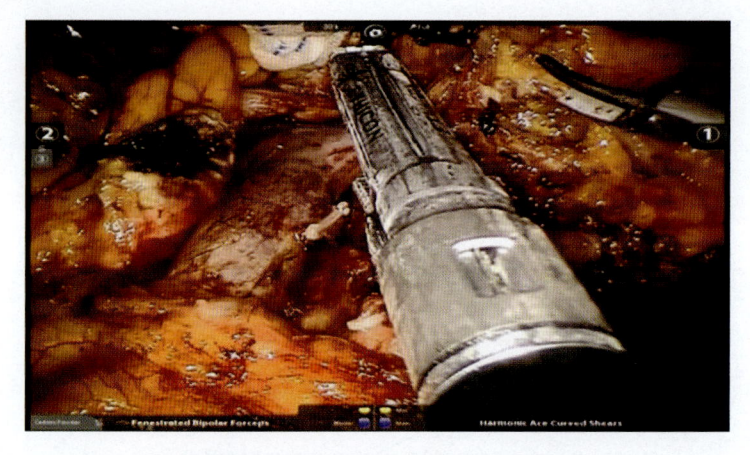

FIGURE 29-14 • Splenic vein division.

Step 9. Dissection of the retroperitoneum and left adrenalectomy

At this point, the lymphadenectomy around the SMA proceeds with a longitudinal dissection from the origin of the middle colic artery up to the origin of the SMA. When the anterior border of the aorta is reached, the plane of dissection proceeds posteriorly in the sagittal plane down both sides of the aorta toward the diaphragm. Then, the fat and fibrous tissue anterior to the aorta, the inferior vena cava, and the left renal vein are divided. The adrenal vein is divided at its junction with the renal vein. The dissection proceeds posterior to the adrenal gland, and then continues laterally behind Gerota's fascia directly onto the surface of the proper kidney capsule. The entire specimen, including the distal pancreas, the adrenal gland, and all the retroperitoneal fat is removed en bloc (see **Figures 29-15 A, B**).

Step 9 average time frame: 40–50 min

▶▶ TIPS

- If the tumor infiltrates the middle colic artery and the transverse mesocolon, the involved part should be removed.
- The left renal vein is the inferior border of the dissection and the diaphragm is the superior border.
- The inferior vena cava and the aorta are fully exposed.
- An interaortocaval lymph nodes dissection is routinely performed.
- Exposure, surgical suctioning, and retraction of the SMA with the hanging maneuver may require an expert assistant.

⚠ PITFALLS

Lesion of the SMA/SMV. Blind dissection, in this area, is risky because the vessels are very close. The periadventitial plane of the artery is the safest way to separate the artery from the perivascular tissue.

Incomplete lymphadenectomy. The main lymph nodal stations, part of the oncological procedure, should be included in the dissection. Some lymph nodes are numbered and sent separately. Some other stations are included en bloc with the specimen.

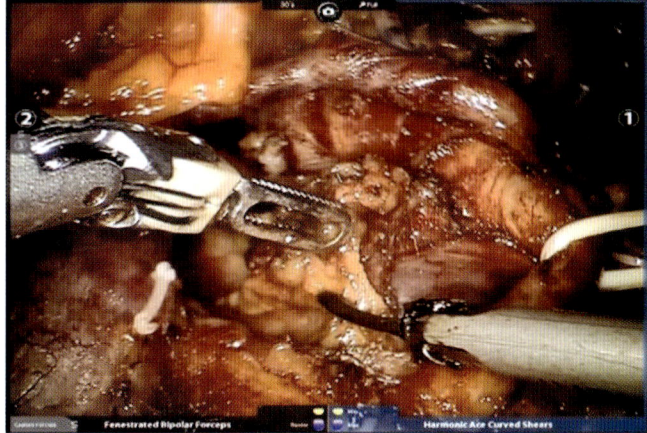

FIGURE 29-15 • **A.** Dissection of the retroperitoneum with left adrenalectomy. **B.** General overview of the surgical field.

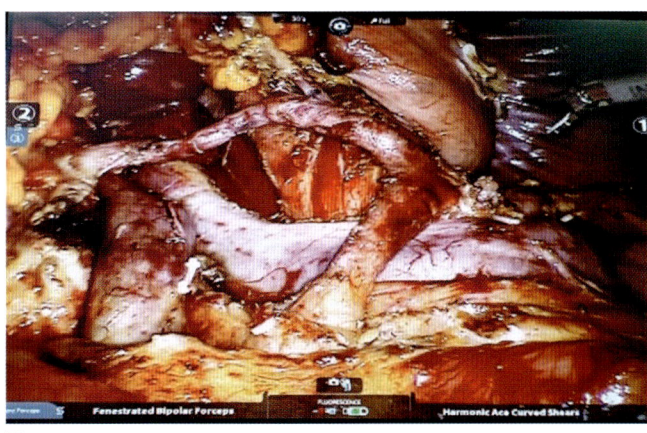

Step 10. Specimen extraction
The specimen is placed into an Endobag™ and removed through a suprapubic Pfannenstiel incision or from an extended trocar incision. Two drains are placed in proximity to the pancreatic stump. The amylase is checked on the first, third, and fifth postop days, and the drains are removed if the test is negative.

Step 10 average time frame: 15–20 min

Suggested Readings

1. Strasberg SM, Linehan DC, Hawkins WG. Radical antegrade modular pancreatosplenectomy procedure for adenocarcinoma of the body and tail of the pancreas: ability to obtain negative tangential margins. *J Am Coll Surg*. 2007;204(2):244-249.
2. Strasberg SM, Drebin JA, Linehan D. Radical antegrade modular pancreatosplenectomy. *Surgery* 2003;133(5):521-527.
3. Choi SH, Kang CM, Lee WJ, Chi HS. Multimedia article. Laparoscopic modified anterior RAMPS in well-selected left-sided pancreatic cancer: technical feasibility and interim results. *Surg Endosc*. 2011;25(7):2360-2361.
4. Mitchem JB, Hamilton N, Gao F, et al. Long-term results of resection of adenocarcinoma of the body and tail of the pancreas using radical antegrade modular pancreatosplenectomy procedure. *J Am Coll Surg*. 2012;214(1):46-52.
5. Kawabata Y, Hayashi H, Takai K, et al. Superior mesenteric artery-first approach in radical antegrade modular pancreatosplenectomy for borderline resectable pancreatic cancer: a technique to obtain negative tangential margins. *J Am Coll Surg*. 2015;220(5):e49-54.
6. Aosasa S, Nishikawa M, Hoshikawa M, et al. Inframesocolic superior mesenteric artery first approach as an introductory procedure of radical antegrade modular pancreatosplenectomy for carcinoma of the pancreatic body and tail. *J Gastrointest Surg*. 2016;20(2):450-454.
7. Grossman JG, Fields RC, Hawkins WG, et al. Single institution results of radical antegrade modular pancreatosplenectomy for adenocarcinoma of the body and tail of pancreas in 78 patients. *J Hepatobiliary Pancreat Sci*. 2016;23(7):432-441.
8. Giulianotti PC, Coratti A, Angelini M, et al. Robotics in general surgery: personal experience in a large community hospital. *Arch Surg*. 2003;138(7):777-784. doi: 10.1001/archsurg.138.7.777

30

"Benign lesions, as well as low-grade malignancy of the body and tail of the pancreas, may be indications for this procedure. Surgeons should know the techniques and significance of spleen-preserving distal pancreatectomy (SpDP) with conservation of the splenic artery and vein, which is a very safe and reliable method."

—Wataru Kimura (1953)

Spleen-Preserving Distal Pancreatectomy

Valentina Valle • Alberto Mangano • Antonio Cubisino • Pier Cristoforo Giulianotti

INTRODUCTION

Over the last 2 decades, there has been increasing evidence supporting the minimally invasive approach as the preferred treatment for benign and low-grade malignant tumors located on the left side of the pancreas. In addition, this notion was further confirmed, in 2020, by the "Miami International Evidence-Based Guidelines on Minimally Invasive Pancreas Resection." For these lesions, given the increasing knowledge about the immunologic splenic functions, a spleen-preserving distal pancreatectomy has been progressively advocated.

There are 2 main techniques to achieve a spleen-preserving distal pancreatectomy: (1) the Kimura technique (with splenic vessel preservation), first described as an open procedure in 1996, and (2) the Warshaw technique (with splenic vessel transection), which was described, as an open approach as well, in 1988.

The Warshaw technique includes the proximal and distal division of the splenic vessels while preserving the short gastric vessels to supply the spleen. However, several studies have shown an increased risk of splenic infarction, and perigastric varices (up to 25% and 20%, respectively), associated with this approach.

The splenic vessel preservation technique (Kimura) is a more challenging procedure because it entails a precise control of multiple small vascular branches.

The laparoscopic approach to spleen-preserving distal pancreatectomy was first described in 1997 by Gagner et al. Despite having the minimally invasive advantages, the laparoscopic spleen-preserving distal pancreatectomy (most notably

INSTRUMENT REQUIREMENTS

The suggested main robotic instruments/tools can be listed as follows:
- 30° scope
- Permanent cautery monopolar hook/monopolar scissors
- Cadière forceps
- Fenestrated bipolar forceps
- Harmonic shears/vessel sealer
- Needle drivers
- Clip applier
- SureForm™ Robotic Stapler: with different loads

The suggested main laparoscopic instruments/tools can be listed as follows:
- 5-mm scope
- Graspers
- Scissors
- Needle drivers
- Staplers (with different loads)
- Suction-irrigation device
- Laparoscopic ultrasound (drop-in probe or handheld)

Supplemental materials:
- Gauzes, sponges
- Penrose drains
- Vessel loops
- Endobags™
- Hem-o-lok™ clips
- Sutures: Prolene™ 2-0, 3-0, 4-0, and 5-0

Photo reproduced with permission from Dr. Wataru Kimura.
Quote reproduced with permission from Kimura W, Yano M, Sugawara S, et al. Spleen-preserving distal pancreatectomy with conservation of the splenic artery and vein: techniques and its significance. J Hepatobiliary Pancreat Sci. 2010;17(6):813-823.

the Kimura) has been adopted in just a few referral centers, due to the complexity of some of the surgical steps.

The robotic spleen-preserving distal pancreatectomy can overcome some of the laparoscopic hurdles and technical limitations. The robotic technique was first performed by PC Giulianotti in 2001. Since then, in comparison to laparoscopy and open techniques, the robotic approach has shown several additional advantages. These benefits are mostly related to microdissection capabilities and improved visualization, which allow spleen preservation in a higher number of cases, a lower conversion rate, and a shorter hospital stay.

Indications and Contraindications to the Robotic Approach

Benign and/or low-grade malignant lesions, located in the body and tail of the pancreas, are eligible for robotic spleen-preserving distal pancreatectomy. Indications are evolving, but at the present time, they can be summarized as follows:

- Well-differentiated (G1-G2) pancreatic neuroendocrine tumors (pNETs) (less than 3–4 cm) not meeting the criteria for enucleation (see Chapter 32, Enucleation of Pancreatic Tumors).
- Mucinous cystadenomas without any sign of malignant transformation (size < 5 cm; absence of thickened, irregular, or calcified walls).
- Noninvasive and symptomatic branch, or segmental main duct intraductal papillary mucinous neoplasms (IPMNs) without high-risk features (main duct ≥10 mm; main duct between 5 and 9 mm associated with thickened walls, and/or intraductal mucin and/or mural nodules).
- Symptomatic serous cystadenomas.
- Selected patients with symptomatic chronic pancreatitis predominantly confined in the body and the tail of the pancreas (refractory pseudocysts after failed drainage).
- Other, less common, benign symptomatic selected lesions/conditions rarely requiring surgical treatment, such as solid pseudopapillary tumors.

In patients with pNETs or IPMNs, a regional lymph nodes sampling should always be performed in order to have a proper staging in case of postoperative cancer confirmation. Distal splenopancreatectomy with formal regional/radical lymphadenectomy is still the gold standard treatment for documented pancreatic adenocarcinoma.

Contraindications to spleen-preserving distal pancreatectomy are:

- Left-sided portal hypertension with compression/thrombosis of the splenic vein.
- Bulky lesions with vessel involvement.
- Documented ductal adenocarcinomas.
- Concomitant splenomegaly and/or hypersplenism.

Relative contraindications of the operation could be history of previous multiple surgeries, including organ-specific procedures, body habitus, and an unexperienced surgical team.

Patient Positioning, OR Setup, and Port Setting

The patient is placed supine on a beanbag, with arms tucked and lower limbs parted in the French position, with a 30° reverse Trendelenburg, and a slight right-sided tilting of the table. The patient's position is secured to avoid slippage. The bedside assistant sits between the patient's legs (**Figure 30-1**).

The robotic cart is placed on the left of the patient to facilitate the assistant's work targeting toward the spleen and giving room to a second assistant, or a scrub nurse on the right side (**Figure 30-2**).

The pneumoperitoneum is achieved with the Veress technique at the modified Palmer's point. A 5-mm trocar is then inserted into the left lateral upper quadrant.

Spleen-Preserving Distal Pancreatectomy 655

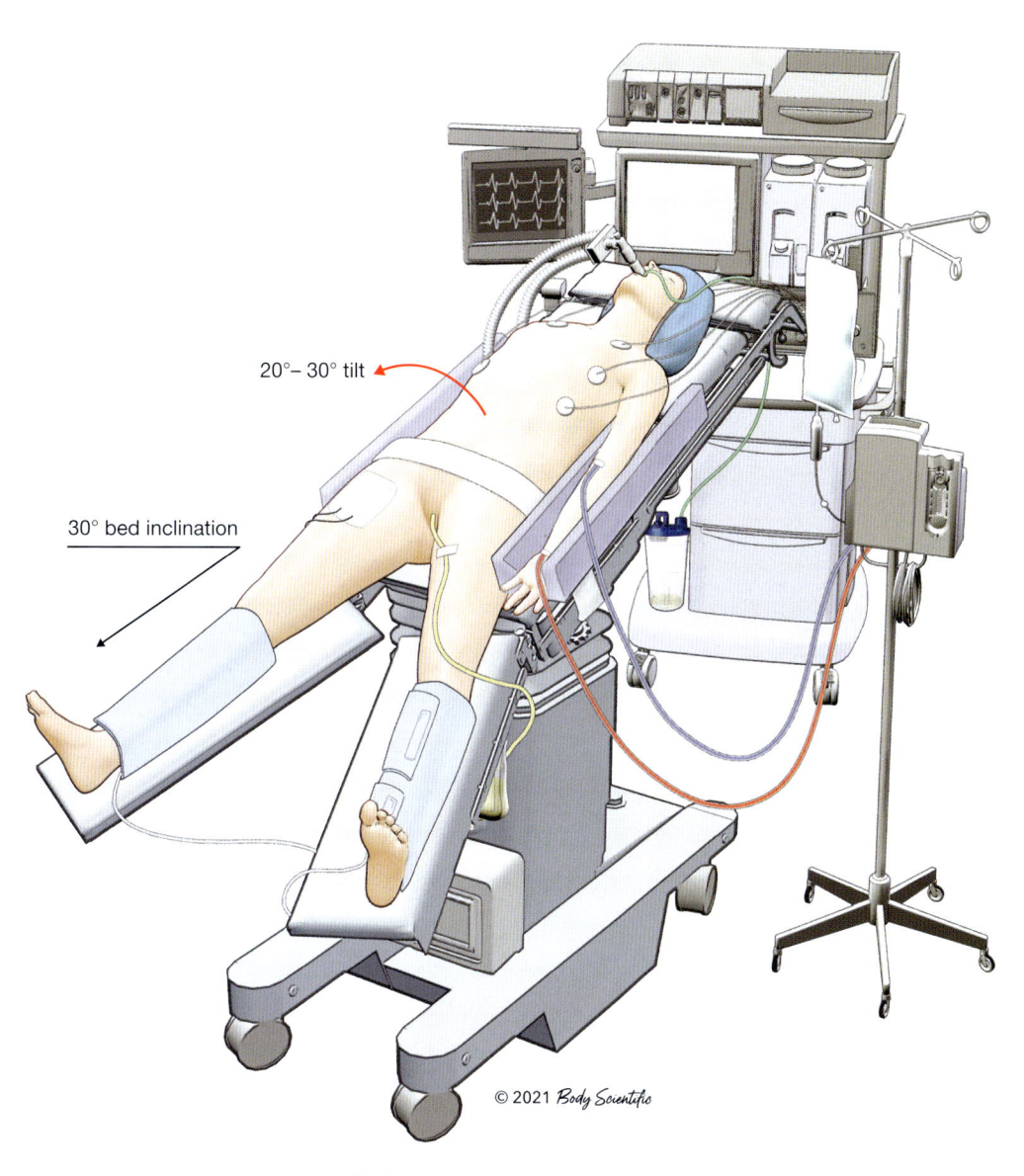

20°– 30° tilt

30° bed inclination

© 2021 Body Scientific

FIGURE 30-1 • Patient positioning.

656 The Foundation and Art of Robotic Surgery

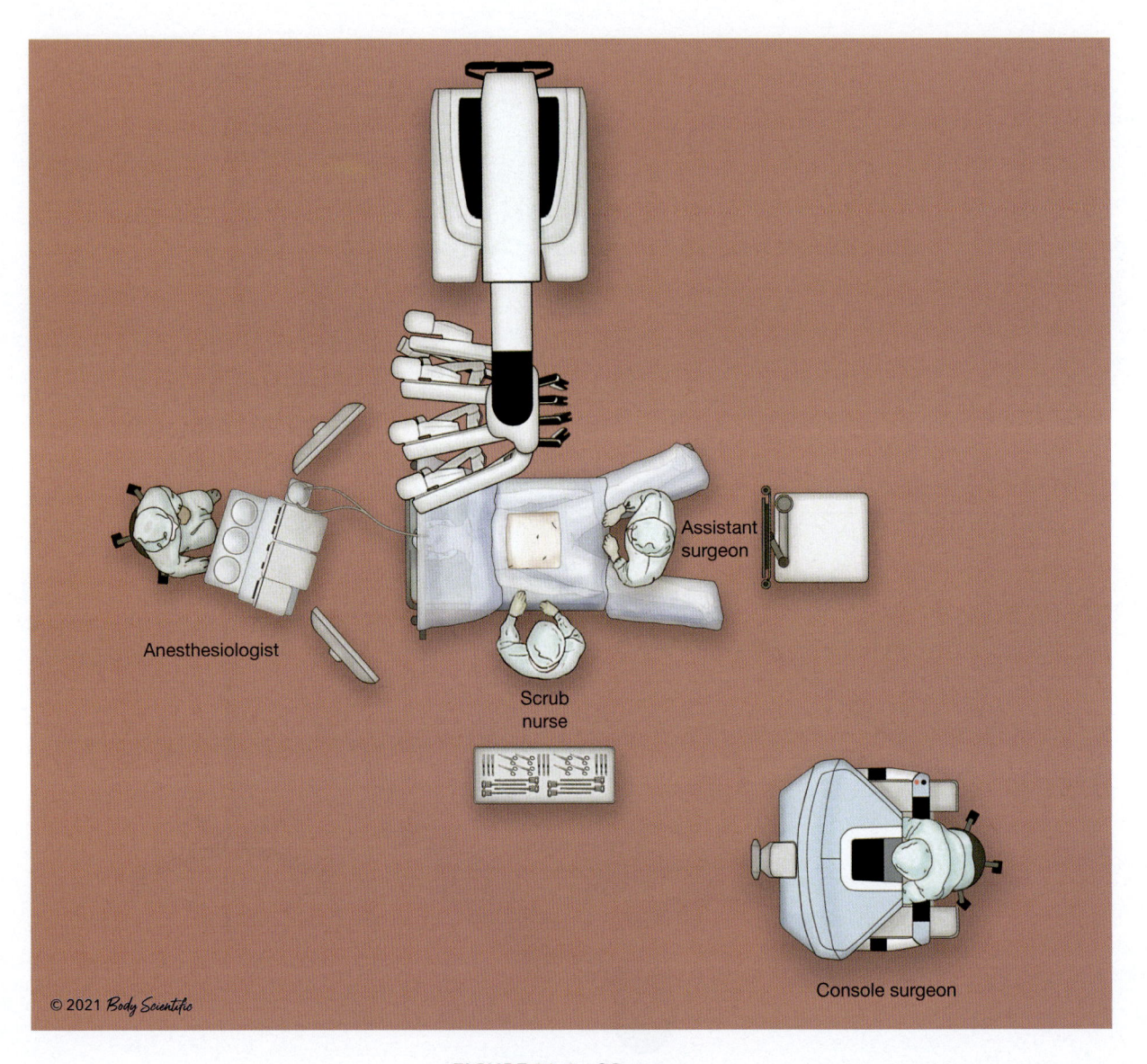

FIGURE 30-2 • OR setup.

A diagnostic-laparoscopy is carried out (this maneuver has multiple goals, which are already detailed in Chapter 2, The Basic Principles of Clinical Applications).

Four 8-mm trocars are arranged along a straight line above the umbilicus. The 5-mm port used for the abdominal exploration is replaced by the R1. The camera port is placed slightly above the transverse umbilical line, at the intersection with the left pararectal line. The R2 is positioned at the same level, medial to the right pararectal line, and the R3 is inserted at the right anterior axillary line.

Two assistant ports are placed, on both sides of the midline, a few centimeters below: one is a 5-mm cannula between R1 and the scope, and the other is a 10–12-mm port positioned between the scope and the R2 trocar as depicted in **Figures 30-3 A, B.**

Normal abdomen

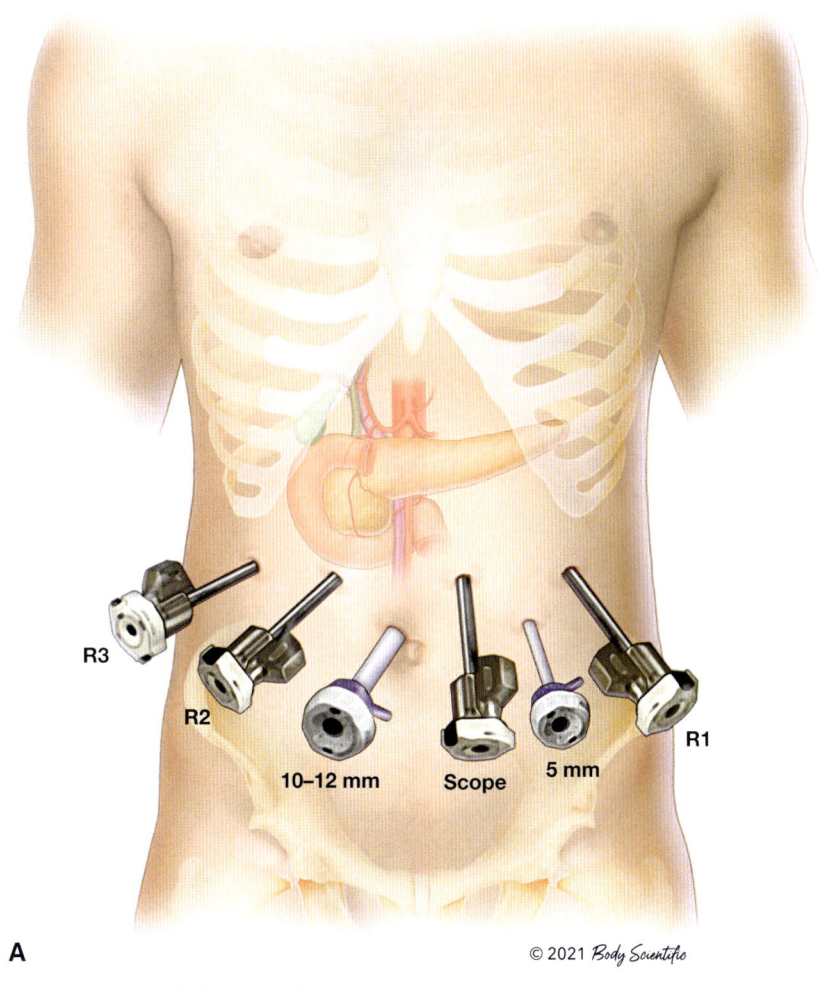

FIGURE 30-3 • **A.** Port setting normal abdomen.

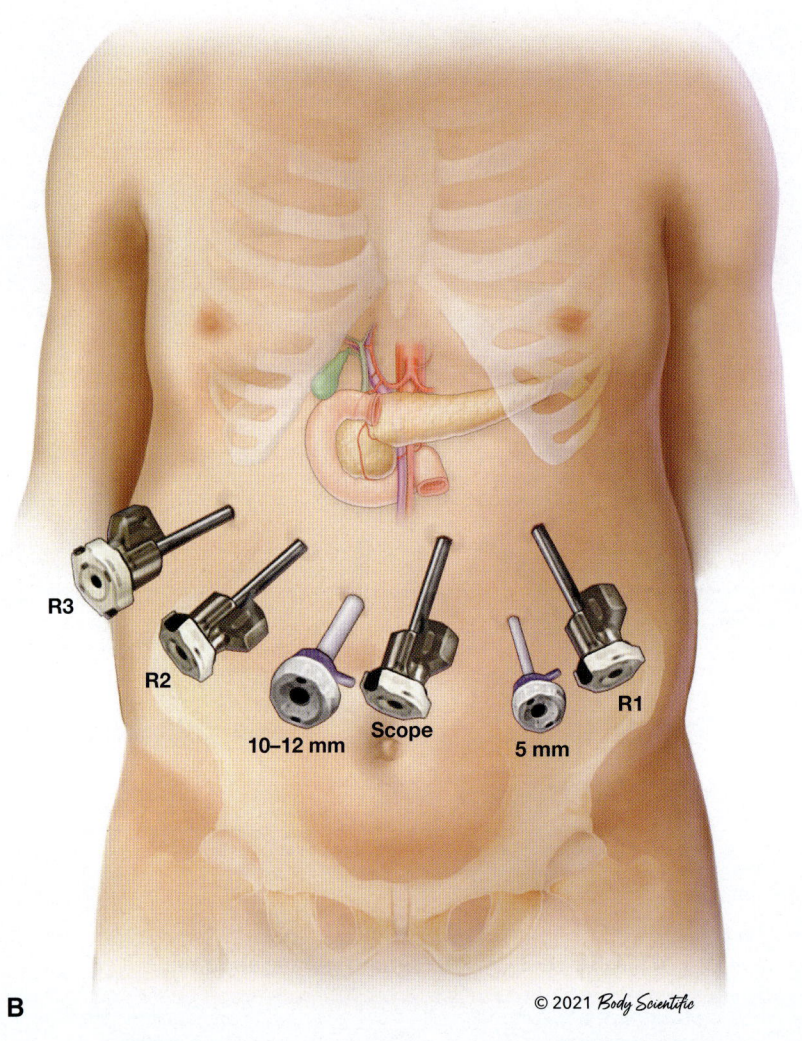

FIGURE 30-3 • (Continued) B. Port setting wide abdomen.

Surgical Technique

▶ **Video 30-1. Spleen-Preserving Distal Pancreatectomy – Full Procedure**

Step 1. Gastrocolic ligament opening

The stomach is retracted upward using a grasper positioned in the R3. After exerting traction on the gastrocolic ligament, by using the hook placed in R1, an incision is performed to open the Bouchet's transparent zone, and access the lesser sac. This maneuver allows the exploration of the lesser sac, the possible confirmation of the lesion, and the evaluation of the pancreatic gland with the identification of the anatomical landmarks.

The gastrocolic ligament opening is widened with the vessel sealer until reaching the left gastroepiploic artery, which is usually divided either with the vessel sealer or in between clips: this maneuver allows a better exposure of the pancreatic tail (**Figures 30-4 A, B**). The short gastric vessels are generally preserved. On the right side, the dissection reaches the origin of the right gastroepiploic vessels that must be preserved.

Step 1 average time frame: 10–20 min

> ▶▶ **TIPS**
>
> The identification of the anatomical landmarks, such as the celiac trunk and the mesenterico-portal confluence, is facilitated by maneuvers such as retracting upward the posterior wall of the stomach and following the vertical fold of the left gastric artery, or looking at the direction of the middle colic vein going toward the neck of the pancreas (some anatomical reminders are depicted in **Figure 30-5**).

> ⚠ **PITFALLS**
>
> When there are adhesions between the gastrocolic ligament, the mesentery of the transverse colon, and the posterior face of the stomach, particular attention should be paid not to enter a wrong plane, because this may increase the risk of damaging the pancreas or the blood supply to the colon.

A

B

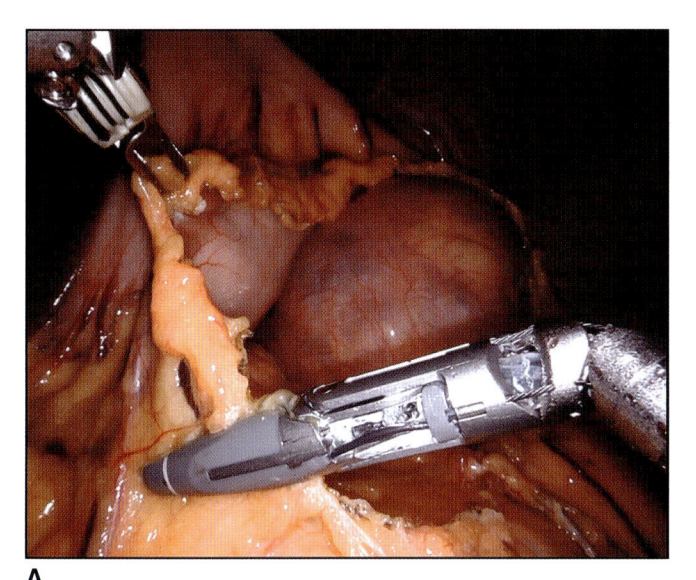

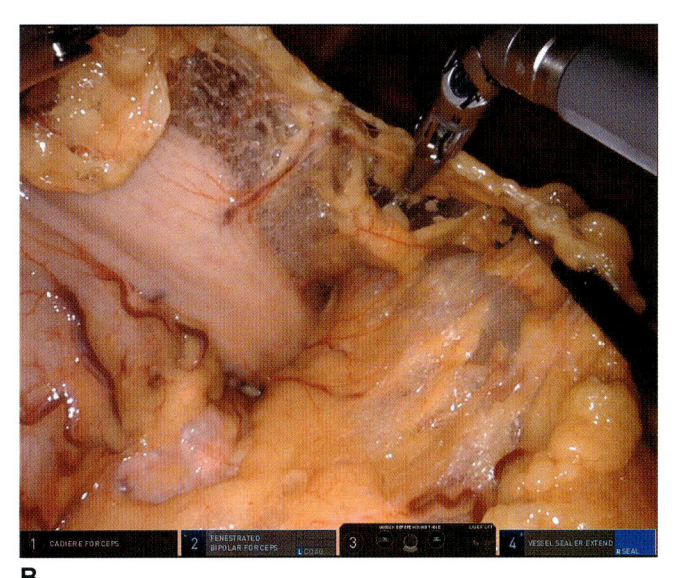

FIGURE 30-4 • Gastrocolic ligament division.

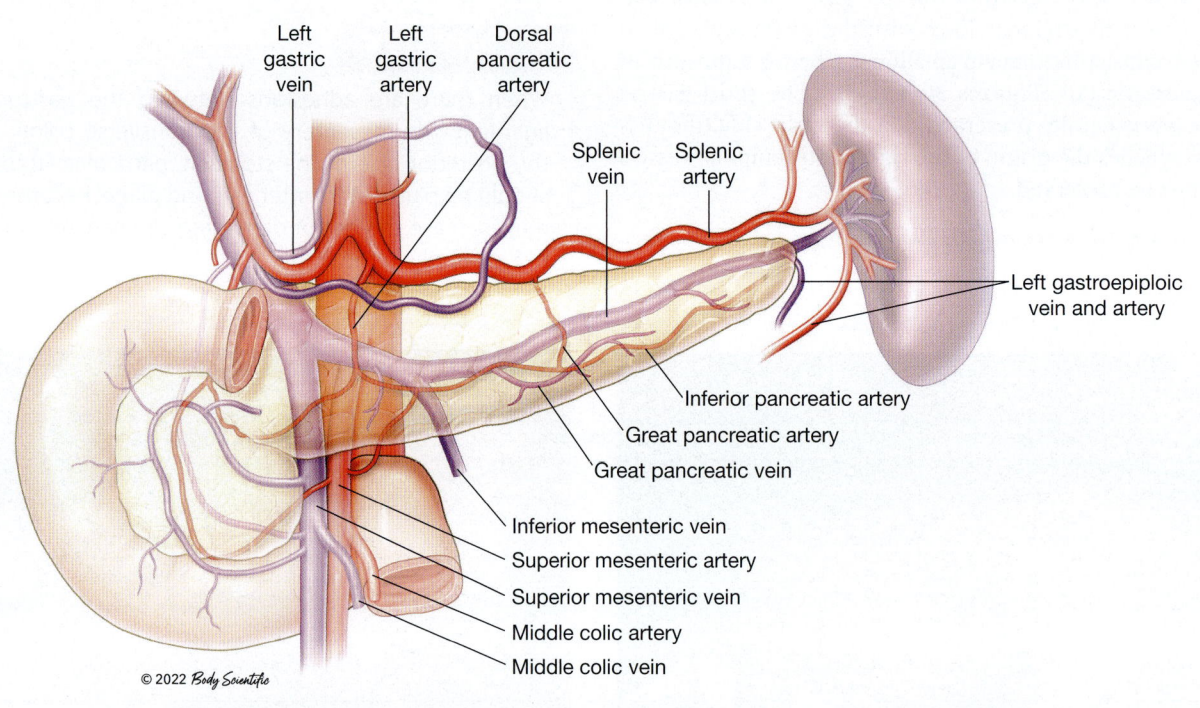

FIGURE 30-5 • Pancreatic body and tail anatomy: Arterial and venous anatomy.

Video 30-2. Step 2. Preparation of the Origin of the Splenic Artery

Step 2. Preparation of the origin of the splenic artery

The splenic artery is carefully dissected at its origin, while paying attention to its small branches. The maneuver is performed using the monopolar hook as a right angle, and a vessel loop is placed around the vessel for better manipulation, retraction, and possible clamping (**Figures 30-6 A–C**). The preparation of the artery on a loop allows the placement of a bulldog clamp in case of bleeding. The clamping of the proximal splenic artery doesn't completely control the bleeding, because the pancreatic body and tail have a powerful collateral circulation (short gastric and intrapancreatic vessels); however, this clamping decreases its amount, facilitating the suture repair of the bleeding spots.

Step 2 average time frame: 5–15 min

> ⚠ **PITFALLS**
>
> Misjudging the origin of the splenic artery with the origin of the common hepatic artery.
>
> This mistake is favored by bulky, redundant retroperitoneal tissue, or intraparenchymal route of the arteries. This kind of error may lead to ineffective clamping in case of bleeding, or even worse, it may cause the transection of the common hepatic artery in case of conversion to splenopancreatectomy. The identification of the celiac trunk, following the left gastric artery, may help in avoiding this pitfall.

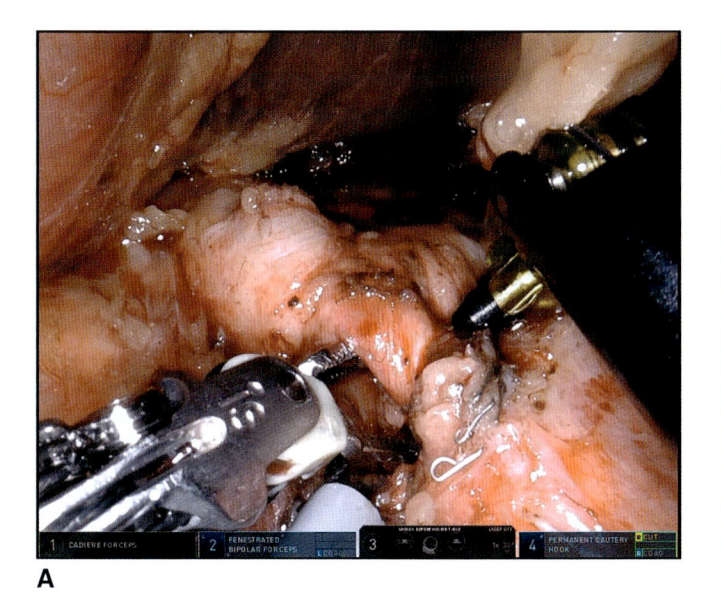

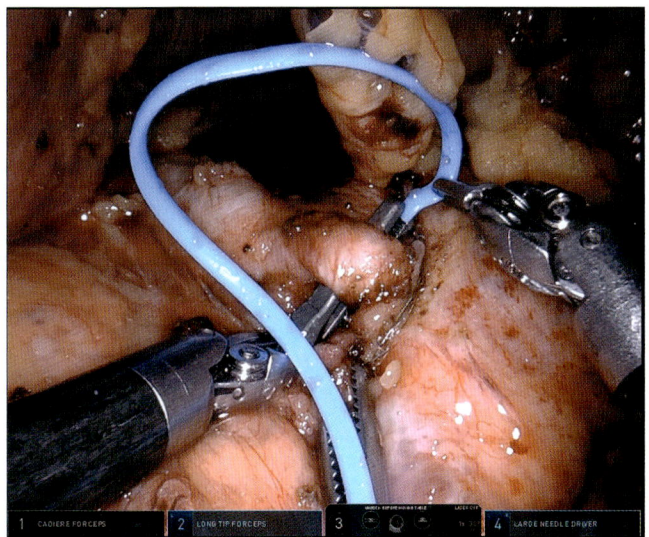

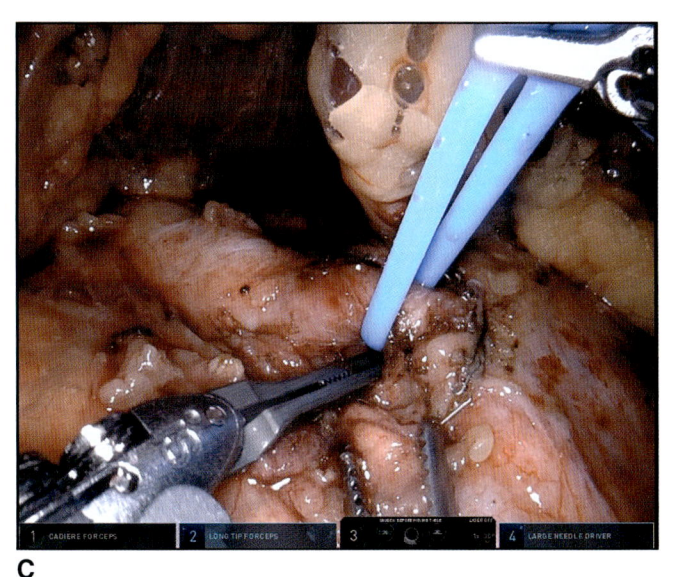

A

B

C

FIGURE 30-6 • Preparation of the origin of the splenic artery.

Video 30-3. Step 3. Left Colonic Flexure Mobilization

Step 3. Left colonic flexure mobilization

This step allows a better access to the retroperitoneum and the visualization of the tail of the pancreas and its inferior aspect. The dissection is more easily done using the monopolar energy, following the surgical plane in front of the Toldt's fascia (**Figure 30-7**). The assistant surgeon helps, with the laparoscopic forceps, in maintaining the exposure and retracting the colon medially and downward (for more details about the splenic flexure mobilization pathways, see Chapter 24, Left Colectomy).

Step 3 average time frame: 15–20 min

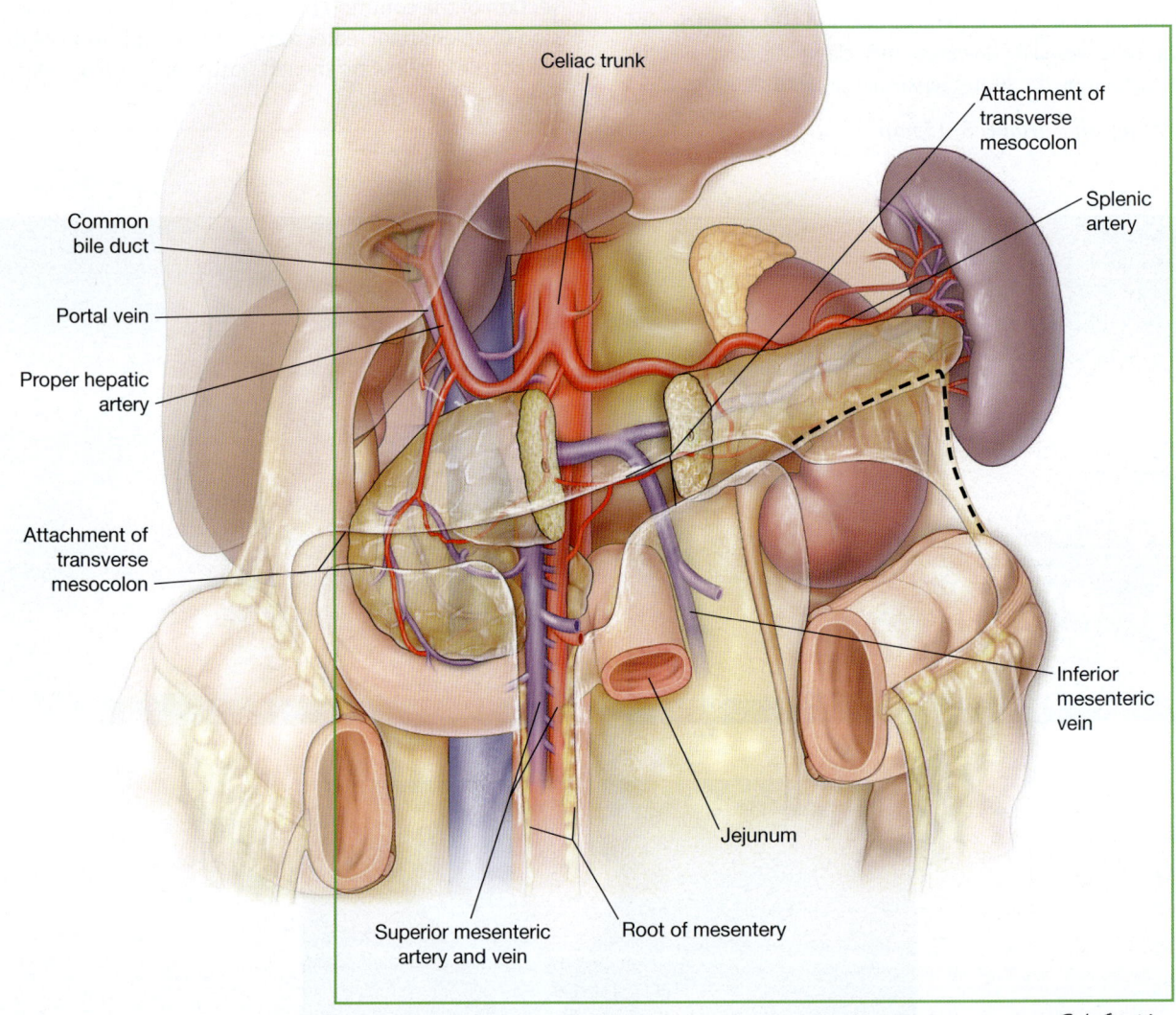

FIGURE 30-7 • Left colonic flexure mobilization.

Step 4. Localization of the lesion and decision of the dissection strategy

At this point, an intraoperative ultrasonography (IOUS) should be carried out mainly when the lesion is not visible at the pancreatic capsule (**Figure 30-8**). The ultrasound may give more details about the nodule localization, its margins, and the anatomical relationship with the main vessels.

Depending on the position of the lesion, the surgical plan may change. For small lesions of the tail, a "parenchymal sparing" lateral-to-medial technique should be preferred; for lesions of the proximal body, the division of the neck with a medial-to-lateral approach should be chosen.

Step 4 average time frame: 5–10 min

> **EDITORIAL COMMENT**
>
> The short gastric vessels are usually spared in the spleen-preserving technique. In selected cases, they need to be sacrificed to increase the exposure of the splenic hilum, or to decrease the risk of bleeding during challenging dissection of the splenic vessels.

> **ANATOMICAL HIGHLIGHTS**
>
> For the anatomical relationships of the splenic artery and vein, see **Figures 30-9 A–C**.

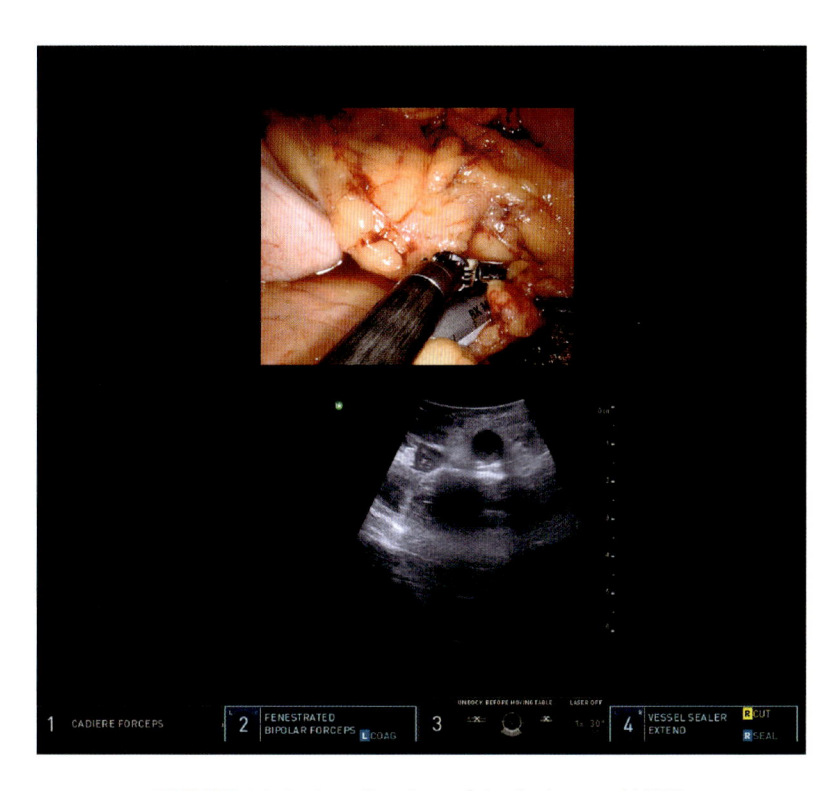

FIGURE 30-8 • Localization of the lesion and IOUS.

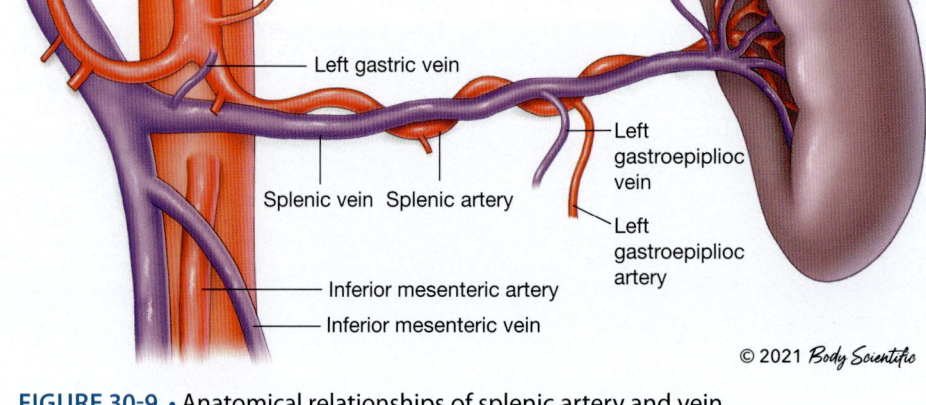

FIGURE 30-9 • Anatomical relationships of splenic artery and vein.

Video 30-4. Step 5. Preparation of the Pancreatic Neck and Retropancreatic Tunnel Creation

Step 5. Preparation of the pancreatic neck and retropancreatic tunnel creation

For proximal lesions, a medial-to-lateral approach is preferred. With the monopolar hook in the R1 and the bipolar forceps in the R2, the dissection is performed at the peritoneal reflection between the mesocolon and the inferior border of the pancreas. This maneuver allows an initial exposure of the pancreatic neck and of the superior mesenteric vein.

A tunnel is created between the confluence of the splenic vein and the superior mesenteric vein with the posterior wall of the pancreas. The pancreatic neck preparation may require a precise microdissection of small venous branches merging into the confluence of the splenic vein with the superior mesenteric vein; those should be divided in between sutures of Prolene™ 5-0 or 6-0.

When it is possible, a vessel loop is placed around the pancreatic neck to lift the pancreas. This pancreatic "hanging" maneuver facilitates the following parenchymal transection (**Figure 30-10**).

However, as described in Chapter 28, Pancreaticoduodenectomy, the creation of the tunnel can sometimes be incomplete. This mostly occurs in cases of severe inflammation, or if the lesion is near to the vessels.

Step 5 average time frame: 25–30 min

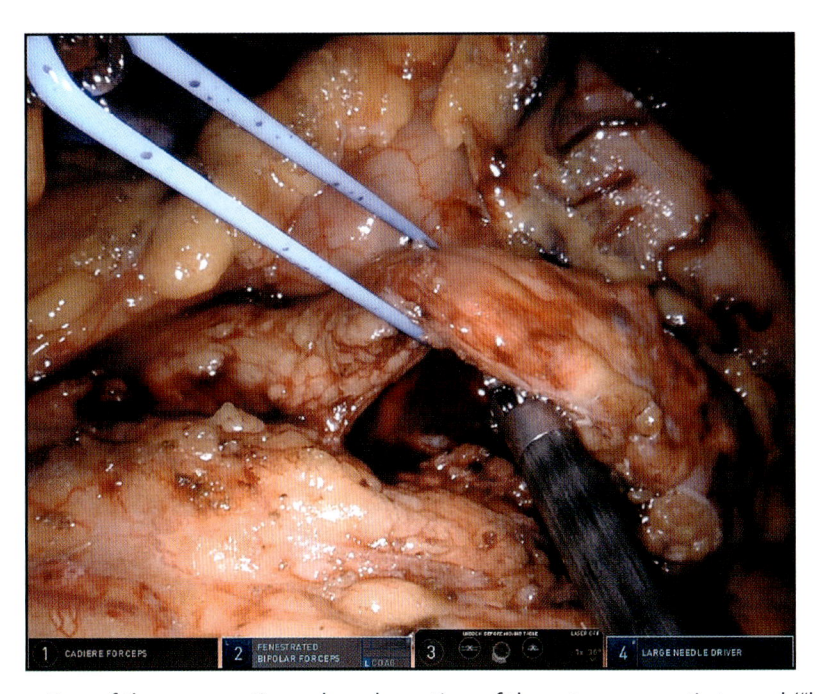

FIGURE 30-10 • Preparation of the pancreatic neck and creation of the retropancreatic tunnel ("hanging" maneuver).

Step 6. Division of the pancreas

Two Prolene™ 2-0 stay sutures are applied on both sides of the lower edge of the pancreatic neck for hemostasis and traction purposes.

Depending on the thickness and size of the neck, a stapler, or the Harmonic shears, or the vessel sealer, can be used to divide the parenchyma (**Figures 30-11 A, B**). The tunnel creation is required for the use of the stapler. When this is not feasible, the pancreas may be divided with the Harmonic shears, while splitting the parenchyma layer by layer. In this case, additional stiches on the proximal suture line are required to seal the proximal pancreatic duct.

A frozen section analysis is performed to obtain confirmation of negative margins.

Step 6 average time frame: 15–20 min

> ▶▶ **TIPS**
>
> If the pancreatic parenchyma is thin and fibrotic, the use of the stapler is preferred. On the contrary, with a thick and soft pancreas, the Harmonic shears are used to avoid the "crushing effect" of the stapler. To complete the hemostasis, stiches of Prolene™ 3-0 can be applied.

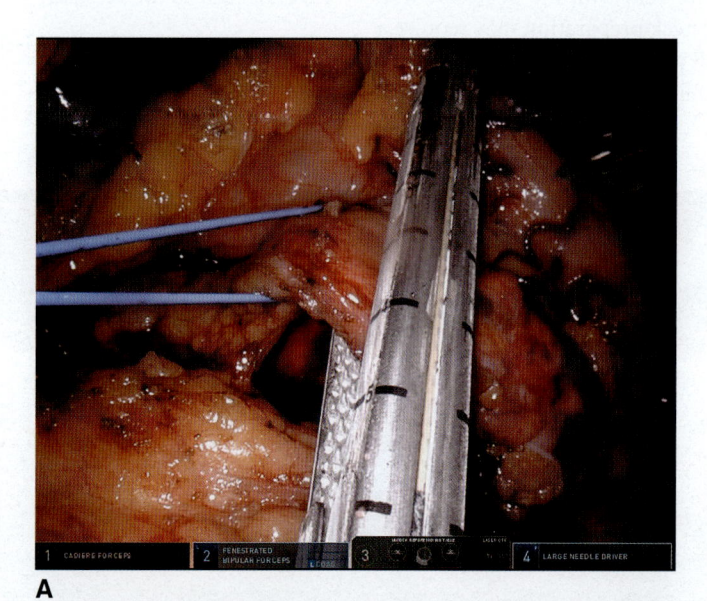

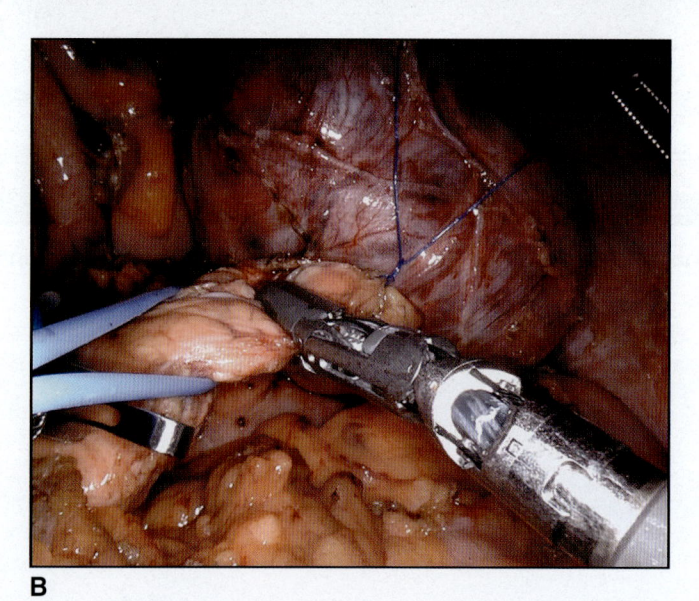

FIGURE 30-11 • Division of the pancreas.

Video 30-5. Step 7. Pancreatic Body and Tail Mobilization

Step 7. Pancreatic body and tail mobilization
On the distal section line of the pancreatic body, 2 Prolene™ 2-0 stitches are applied to be used during the traction of the specimen.

A meticulous dissection is required to separate the pancreas from the splenic vessels. More frequently, the artery may present numerous kinkings; therefore, the angle of the dissection should be changed accordingly. Small branches can be divided in between sutures of Prolene™ 5-0 or 6-0 (**Figures 30-12 A–C**).

Clips are rarely used because their dimensions do not fit the space available and/or they interfere with the dissection maneuvers.

Depending on the specific anatomy, the dissection may continue from above or below the pancreas, and it proceeds until the complete detachment of the pancreas is achieved (**Figure 30-13**).

Step 7 average time frame: 30–60 min

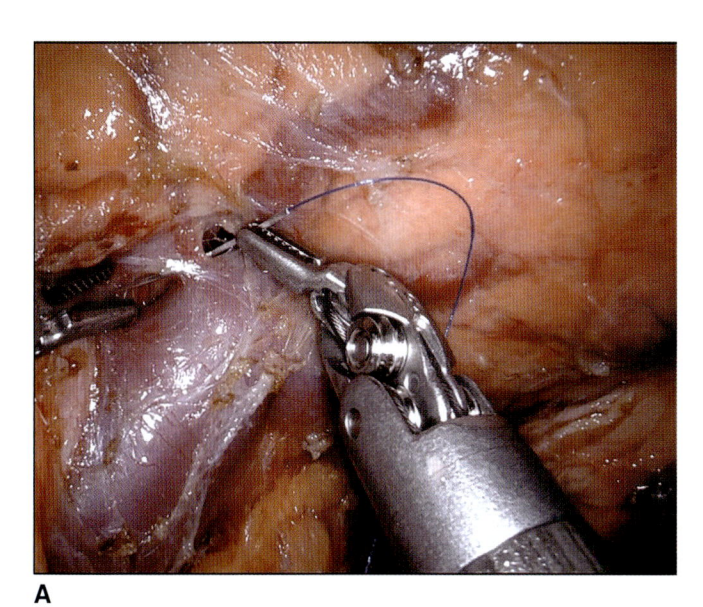

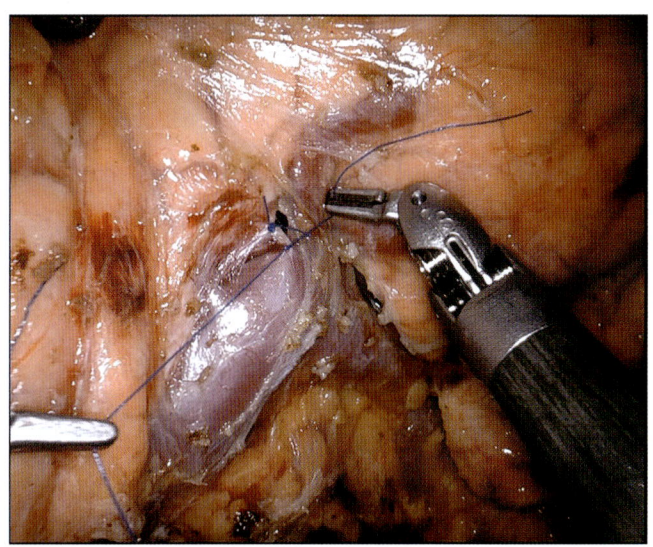

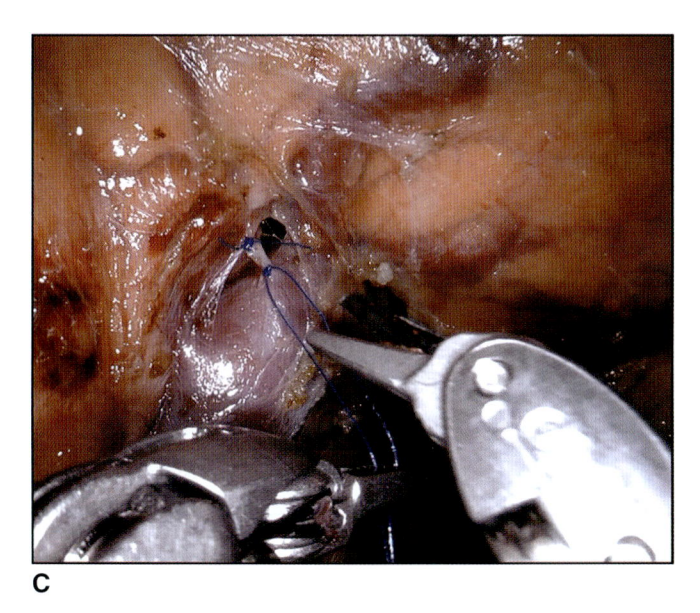

FIGURE 30-12 • Pancreatic body and tail mobilization: Division of short venous branches.

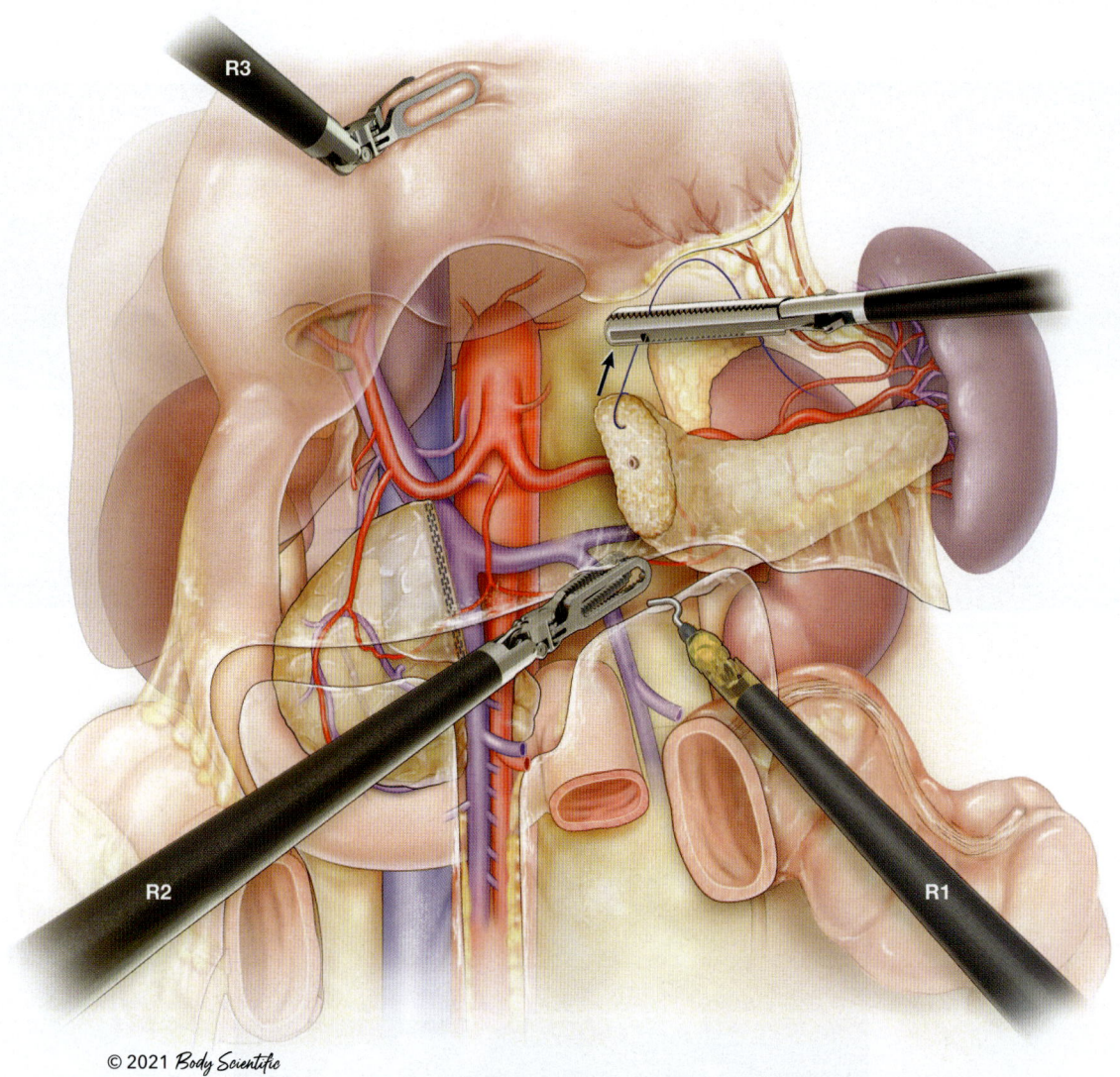

FIGURE 30-13 • Pancreatic body and tail mobilization: Medial-to-lateral dissection.

EDITORIAL COMMENT

For very distal lesions, a lateral-to-medial approach is preferred. This dissection starts from the tail of the pancreas. By placing 2 Prolene™ 2-0 stay sutures, a gentle medial retraction is applied to the tail, while carefully separating the parenchyma from the splenic hilum. The maneuver proceeds opening the retropancreatic plane until a safe resection margin is reached, and the pancreas is completely detached (**Figure 30-14**).

This approach allows more pancreatic parenchyma to be spared. If there are any doubts about the precise tumor location and the resection margins, an IOUS should be repeated.

At this point, the transection of the pancreas is carried out, and a frozen section analysis is performed to confirm negative margins.

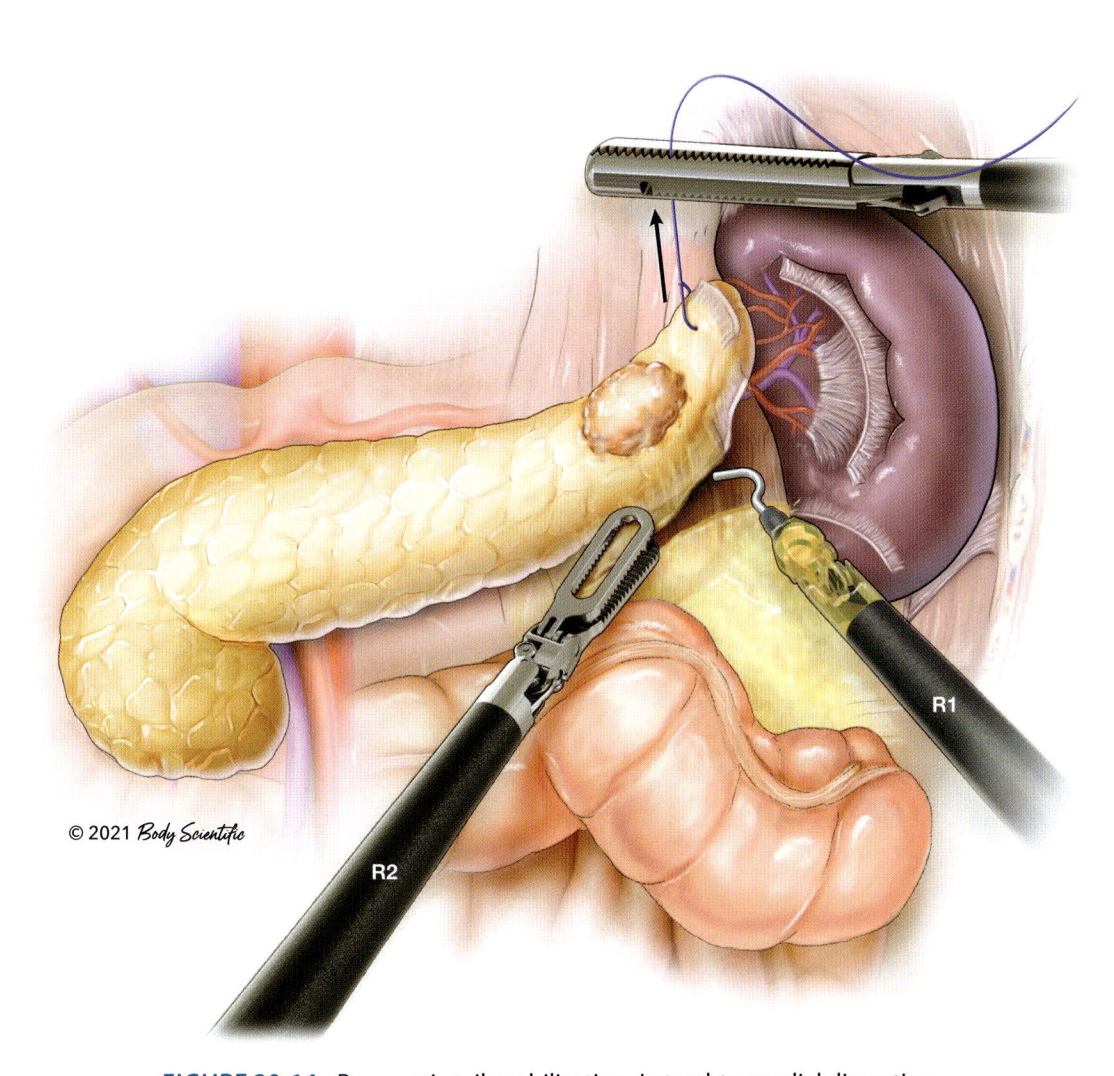

FIGURE 30-14 • Pancreatic tail mobilization: Lateral-to-medial dissection.

ANATOMICAL HIGHLIGHTS

For anatomical variations of the pancreatic body and tail, see **Figures 30-15 A–E**.

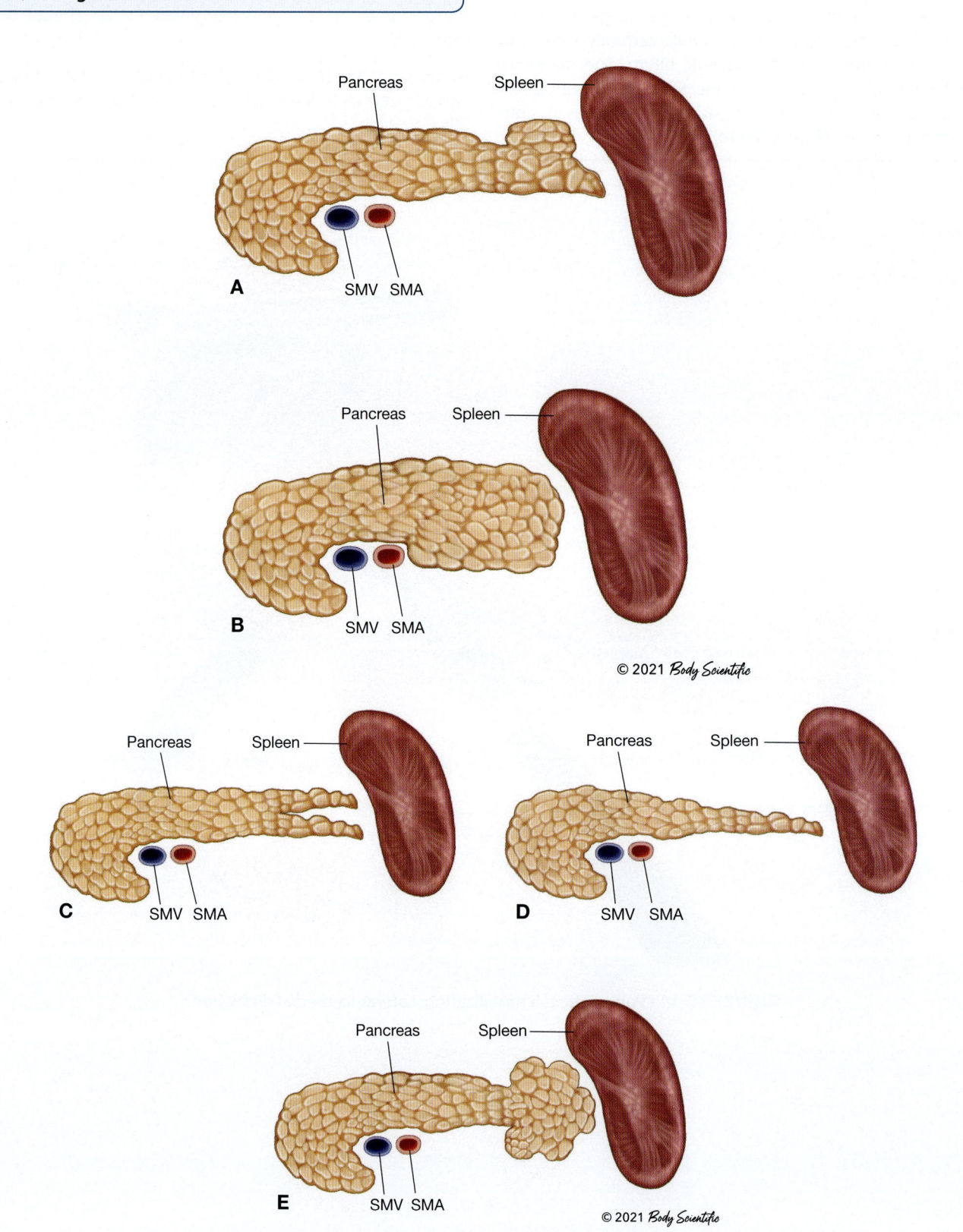

FIGURE 30-15 • Anatomical variations of the pancreatic body and tail.

▶ **Video 30-6. Step 8. ICG Fluorescence Splenic Inflow and Outflow Check**

Step 8. Specimen extraction
The specimen is placed in an Endobag™, and it is retrieved by enlarging one of the port sites, or through a Pfannenstiel incision, depending on the size of the specimen, and on the specific cosmetic requirements of the patient (further details are available in Chapter 2, The Basic Principles of Clinical Applications).

The normal inflow and outflow of the splenic vessels can be verified with ICG fluorescence. Fibrin glue is applied on the section line, and 2 Jackson-Pratt drains are left in place, and positioned close to the pancreatic resection line. The amylase is checked on the 1st, 3rd, and 5th postoperative days, and the drains are removed if the test is negative.

Step 8 average time frame: 10–20 min

Suggested Readings

1. Giulianotti PC, Coratti A, Angelini M, et al. Robotics in general surgery: personal experience in a large community hospital. *Arch Surg.* 2003;138(7):777-784. doi: 10.1001/archsurg.138.7.777
2. Asbun HJ, Moekotte AL, Vissers FL, et al. The Miami International Evidence-Based Guidelines on Minimally Invasive Pancreas Resection. *Ann Surg.* 2020;271(1):1-14. doi: 10.1097/SLA.0000000000003590
3. Gavriilidis P, Roberts KJ, Sutcliffe RP. Comparison of robotic vs laparoscopic vs open distal pancreatectomy. A systematic review and network meta-analysis. *HPB.* 2019;21(10):1268-1276. doi: 10.1016/j.hpb.2019.04.010
4. Warshaw AL. Conservation of the spleen with distal pancreatectomy. *Arch Surg.* 1988;123:550-553.
5. Halfdanarson TR, Strosberg JR, Tang L, et al. The North American Neuroendocrine Tumor Society Consensus Guidelines for Surveillance and Medical Management of Pancreatic Neuroendocrine Tumors. *Pancreas.* 2020;49(7):863-881. doi: 10.1097/MPA.0000000000001597
6. Fernandes E, Giulianotti PC. Robotic-assisted pancreatic surgery. *J Hepato-Biliary-Pancreat Sci.* 2013;20(6):583-589. doi: 10.1007/s00534-013-0615-1
7. Song J, He Z, Ma S, Ma C, Yu T, Li J. Clinical comparison of spleen-preserving distal pancreatectomy with or without splenic vessel preservation: a systematic review and meta-analysis. *J Laparoendosc Adv Surg Tech A.* 2019;29(3):323-332. doi: 10.1089/lap.2018.0135
8. Lü SC, Shi XJ, Wang HG, et al. Follow-up studies for long-term postoperative complications of Warshaw operation. *Zhonghua Yi Xue Za Zhi.* 2013;93(14):1096-1098.
9. Giulianotti PC, Angelini M, Sbrana F, et al. Les Résections Coelioscopiques du Pancréas. *Le Journal de Coelio Chirurgie.* 2004.

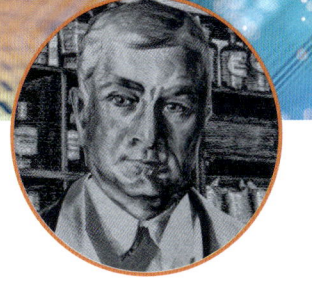

"...partial pancreatic resection with pancreatico-jejunostomy as a technically demanding but safe procedure with all the advantages of minimally invasive surgery will find a firm place in laparoscopic pancreatic surgery."

—Ivo Baca (1947)

Central Pancreatectomy

Antonio Cubisino • Valentina Valle • Nicolas Hellmuth Dreifuss • Pier Cristoforo Giulianotti

INTRODUCTION

Central pancreatectomy (CP) involves a limited resection of the middle segment of the pancreas. As a tissue-sparing procedure, it allows preservation of more functional parenchyma, decreasing the risk of exocrine and/or endocrine insufficiency, and also avoids the unnecessary mutilation of organs such as the spleen as in distal splenopancreatectomies. These features may have a favorable impact on clinical outcomes and quality of life. There are 3 factors that limit a wide adoption of the technique, which was first described in open surgery in 1957 by Guillemin and Bessot with a double anastomosis:

- The technical challenge of the dissection and reconstruction requires microsurgical skills. The neck of the pancreas lays on top of a crossway of important vessels.
- The contained resection and lymphadenectomy do not qualify the procedure as a cancer operation and the indications should be carefully selected.
- The risk of pancreatic fistula seems to be significantly higher than in other more standardized pancreatic resections.

Variations and modifications of the technique have been proposed through the years with constructions of 2 pancreatico-enteric anastomoses or only the distal one with closure of the proximal pancreatic stump. The first laparoscopic CP was described by Baca and Bokan in 2003.

The progressive development of robotics in advanced laparoscopy seems at least to decrease the technical challenges of the procedure. The first robotic CP was performed in 2004 by Dr. PC Giulianotti (and later published in 2010).

In 2018, in China, Rong Liu described a modification of the robotic technique with an end-to-end reconstruction/anastomosis of the 2 pancreatic stumps on a stent.

INSTRUMENT REQUIREMENTS

The suggested main robotic instruments/tools can be listed as follows:
- 30° scope
- Cautery hook/monopolar scissors
- Needle drivers (round tip or macro)
- Bipolar forceps
- Cadière forceps
- Harmonic shears/vessel sealer
- Robotic linear staplers (with different loads)
- Medium/large clip applier
- Round tip scissors

The suggested main laparoscopic instruments/tools can be listed as follows:
- Needle drivers
- Scissors
- Graspers
- Endostapler (with different loads)
- Suction-irrigation
- Laparoscopic ultrasound (drop-in probe or laparoscopic handheld)

Supplemental materials:
- Gauzes, sponges
- Penrose drains
- Vessel loops
- Multiple Hem-o-lok™ clips
- Endobag™
- Medium–large clips
- Sutures: Prolene™ 3-0, 4-0, and 5-0; PDS™ 3-0, 4-0, and 5-0

Acknowledgement for the photo: The Editors wish to thank the architect Rita Dettori and the photographer/graphic designer Alice Moschin for the drawing they created.
Quote reproduced with permission from The Influence of European Surgery on American Practice. St. Paul M J 1914;16:601-605.

Indications and Relative Contraindications to the Robotic Approach

CP can be used to treat benign and/or low-grade malignant lesions located in the neck and proximal body of the pancreas. When one of these lesions is greater than 2 cm and/or located near to the main or accessory pancreatic duct (<3 mm), a formal enucleation is contraindicated. Usually, it is possible to perform a CP for all benign lesions that are located on the left side of the gastroduodenal artery, allowing a long distal pancreatic remnant (**Figure 31-1**). A lymph node sampling is possible with the CP to have a tumor staging assessment, mostly in patients with pancreatic neuroendocrine tumors (pNETs) or intraductal papillary mucinous neoplasms (IPMNs). The presence of worrisome malignant features is a contraindication for a CP. pNETs with enlarged lymph nodes or distant metastasis, IPMNs with a main duct >10 mm or with thickened walls, intraductal mucin, or mural nodules are examples of these contraindications. A comprehensive preoperative workup of these lesions is always crucial to establish the appropriate treatment. The ideal procedure should balance the short- and long-term outcomes with the risk of the procedure and the life expectancy of the patient.

Preserving the pancreatic functions in a young patient with a benign lesion should be considered a priority.

Indications for a CP are as follows:

- Well-differentiated (G1-G2) pNETs not susceptible to enucleation (>2 cm and located <3 mm from the main pancreatic duct)
- Mucinous cystadenomas with no signs of malignant transformation (size >5 cm; thickened or irregular cyst wall; calcification of the cyst wall)
- Noninvasive and symptomatic branch or segmental main duct IPMNs without high-risk features (main duct ≥10 mm; main duct between 5 and 9 mm associated with thickened walls and/or intraductal mucin and/or mural nodules)
- Symptomatic serous cystadenomas
- Other less common benign symptomatic selected lesions/conditions rarely requiring surgical treatment such as solid pseudopapillary tumors

A standard pancreaticoduodenectomy or distal pancreatectomy with regional lymphadenectomy is still recommended for malignant lesions or low-grade malignant tumors with associated lymph node involvement.

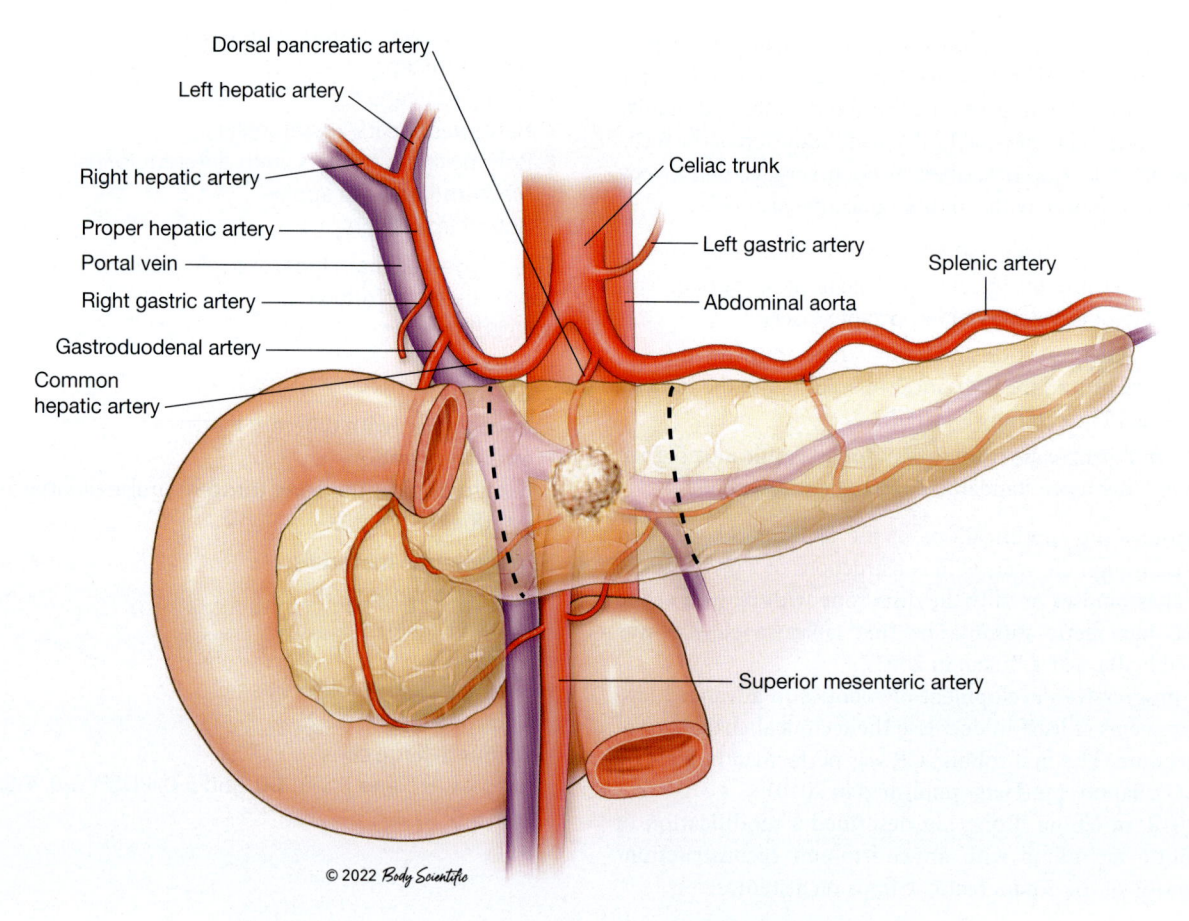

FIGURE 31-1 • Central pancreatic lesion and anatomical landmarks.

Patient Positioning, OR Setup, and Port Setting

The patient is placed supine on a beanbag with both arms tucked and parted legs in the French position, with a 30° reverse Trendelenburg to achieve adequate exposure of the surgical field. The assistant surgeon is sitting between the patient's legs (**Figure 31-2**). The OR setup is explained in **Figure 31-3**.

A total of 6 ports (four 8-mm robotic, one 10–12 mm, and one 5-mm assistant trocars) are used during the procedure. The pneumoperitoneum is induced with the Veress needle at the modified Palmer's point, and a preliminary diagnostic laparoscopy is usually performed with a 30° scope before completing the port setting. This initial exploration has multiple goals: detecting incidental findings, unexpected changes in staging, presence of adhesions or other reasons that may suggest a change in the overall surgical strategy, and a more precise tailoring of the port location. The position of the 2 assistant ports, placed on both sides of the scope, allows the assistant surgeon to have a real active role during the entire procedure (**Figure 31-4**).

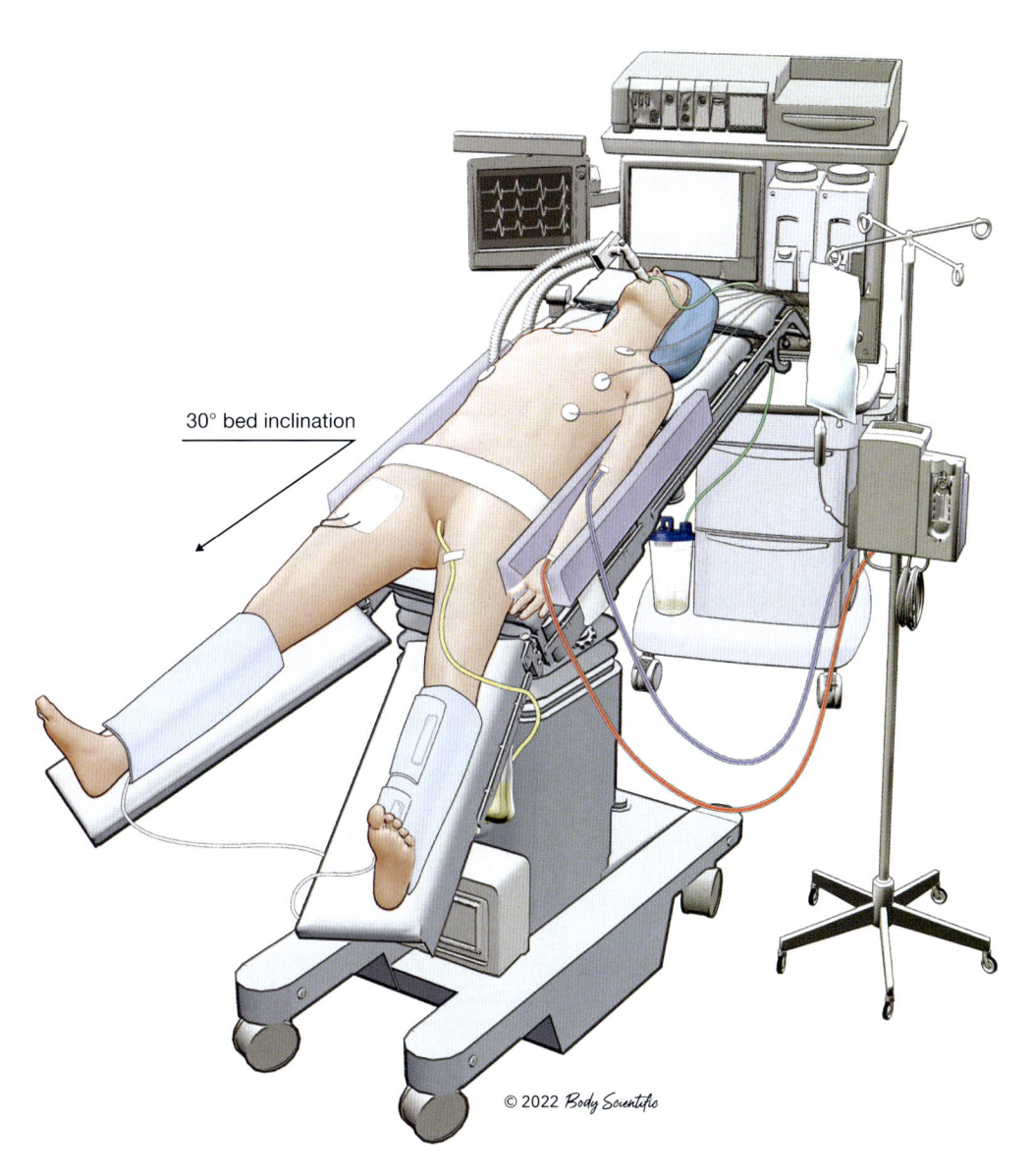

FIGURE 31-2 • Patient positioning.

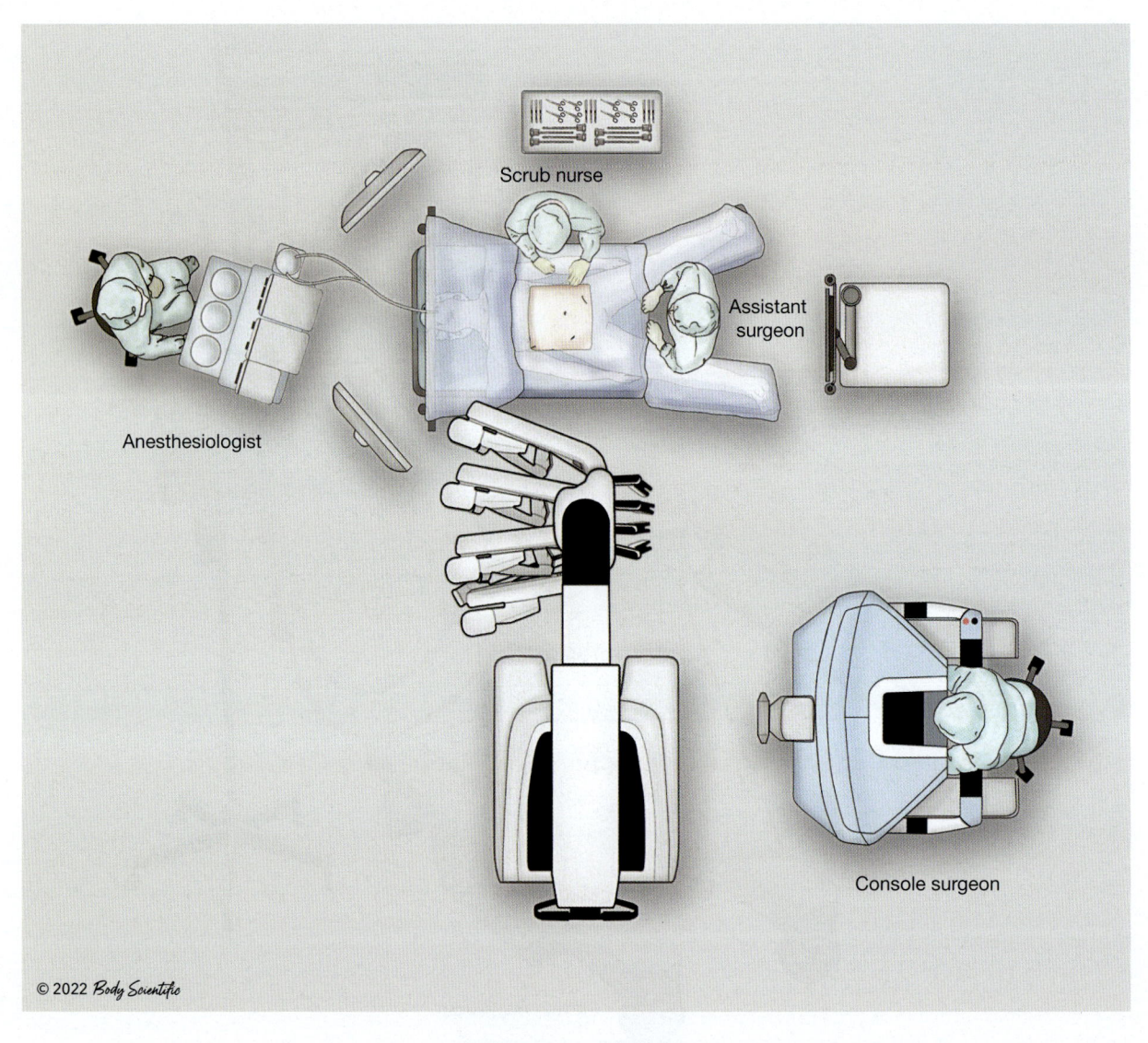

FIGURE 31-3 • OR setup.

Central Pancreatectomy

> ▶▶ **TIPS**
>
> In the usual port setting, the scope is placed in the left paraumbilical position, achieving an adequate visualization on top of the mesenterico-portal confluence. However, in some steps of the procedure, or depending on the local anatomy, moving the scope in the contralateral (right) paraumbilical position allows a better definition of some anatomical details. This dynamic variation of the port setting entails the relocation of the position of the scope, the R3, and the other operative instruments.

Normal abdomen

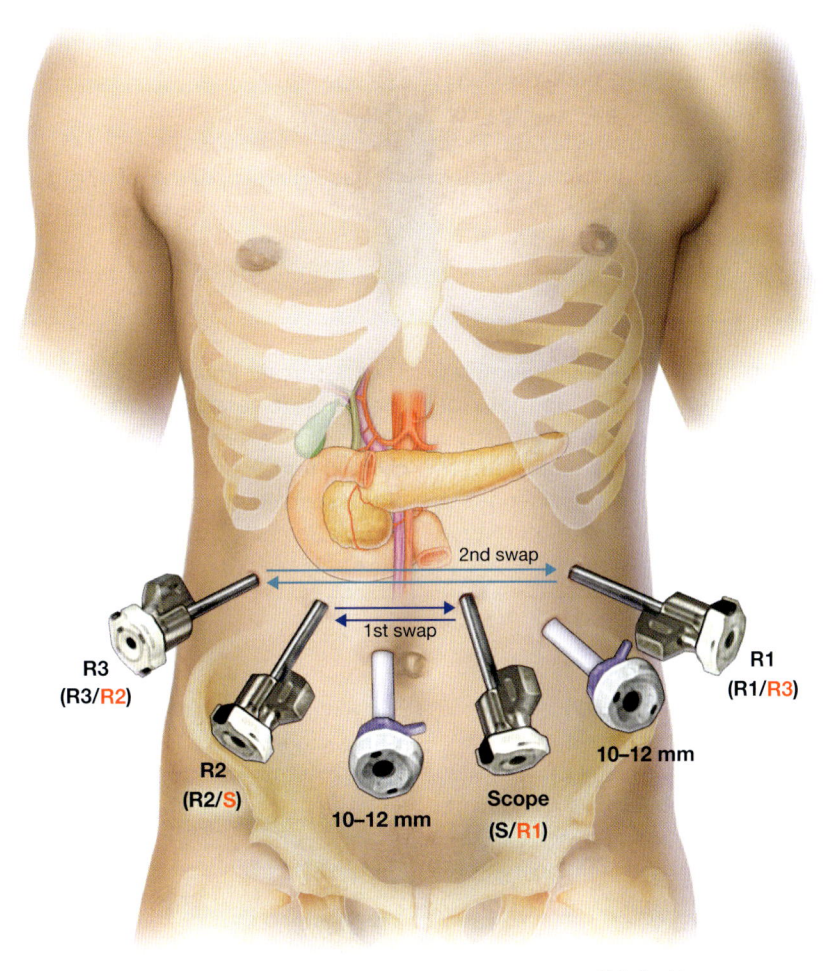

FIGURE 31-4 • Port placement.

Surgical Technique

▶ **Video 31-1.** Central Pancreatectomy – Full Procedure

▶ **Video 31-2.** Step 1. Opening of the Gastrocolic Ligament

DISSECTION

Step 1. Opening of the gastrocolic ligament

By using a grasper in the R3, the stomach is lifted upward, putting the gastrocolic ligament under proper tension. To enter into the lesser sac and expose the pancreas, the gastrocolic ligament is opened at the level of the Bouchet's transparent zone and it is progressively taken down, preserving the gastroepiploic arcade. Possible minor adhesions between the pancreatic capsule and posterior wall of the stomach should be entirely dissected with the monopolar cautery hook. This first step allows a complete exploration of the lesser sac with an initial assessment of the central segments of the pancreas.

Step 1 average time frame: 10–15 min

> ⚠ **PITFALLS**
>
> Inadequate opening of the gastrocolic ligament with uncomplete lesser sac examination.

> ▶▶ **TIPS**
>
> The opening of the gastrocolic ligament usually requires a combination of monopolar energy dissection (hook or scissors) and bipolar coagulation/transection of the larger omental vessels. The monopolar energy is more precise and safer to open up the proper surgical plane when there are adhesions between the ligament and the transverse mesocolon.
>
> The gastrocolic ligament dissection should not include the short gastric vessels and/or the left gastroepiploic artery. Their sacrifice does not increase the exposure of the surgical field for CP and may limit the technical options in case of unexpected injury of the proximal portion of the splenic artery (Warshaw's spleen preserving technique).

Step 2. Intraoperative ultrasonography (IOUS)

To confirm the tumor location and its relationship with vascular structures, an IOUS is usually carried out with a drop-in or laparoscopic handheld probe. Although the final assessment of tumor resectability depends on the surgical dissection, the IOUS remains a powerful tool that provides additional information such as:

- Ruling out other possible concomitant small pancreatic lesions
- Defining anatomical relationships of the tumor (vessels and pancreatic ducts)
- Evaluating the position of potential free margins

Ultrasonographic incidental findings can modify the planned surgical strategy and the extension of the surgical resection. However, the main goal of IOUS remains to assess the adequacy of the surgical margins, allowing maximal parenchyma sparing, while ensuring a complete resection (**Figures 31-5** and **31-6**).

Step 2 average time frame: 5–10 min

> ▶▶ **TIPS**
>
> Depending on the location of the tumor, when the potential proximal margins are extending on the right side of the portal vein, a better exposure of the pancreatic head is needed. This situation may require a mobilization of the right colonic flexure and a Kocher maneuver.

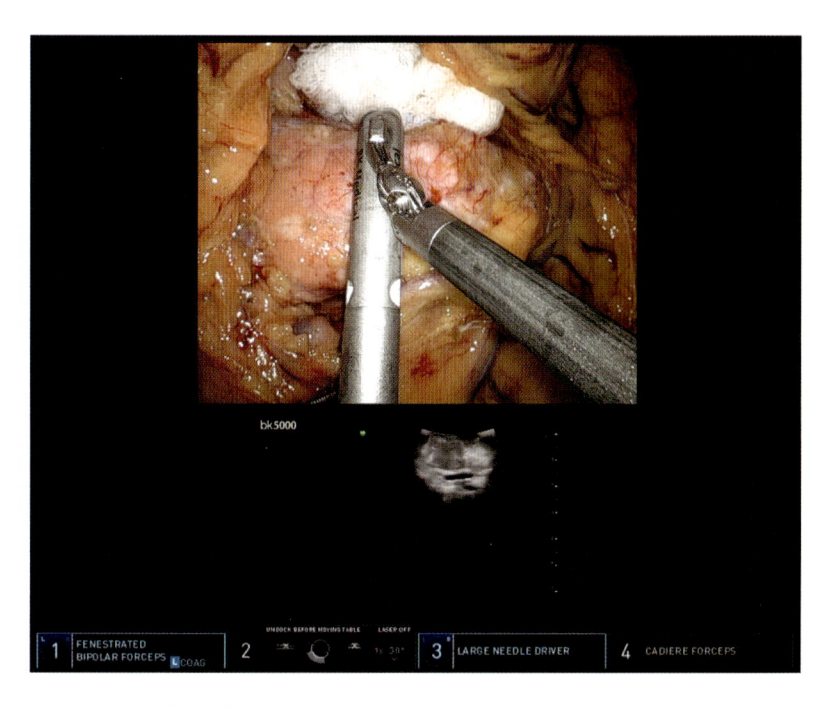

FIGURE 31-5 • Intraoperative ultrasonography.

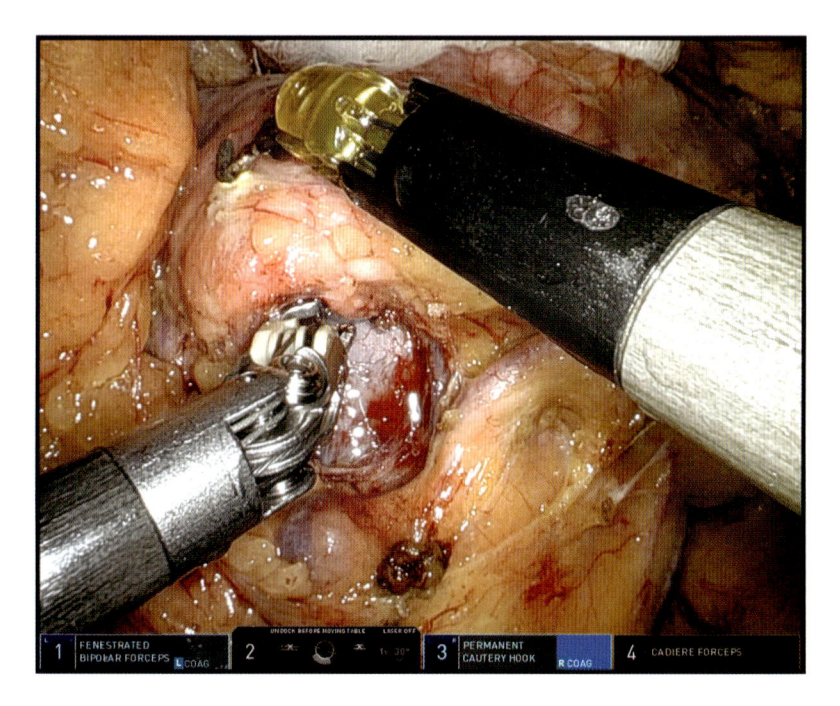

FIGURE 31-6 • Marking the proximal resection margin.

Video 31-3. Step 3. Preparation of the Pancreatic Neck

Step 3. Preparation of the pancreatic neck

Once the ultrasonographic evaluation of the pancreatic gland is completed, the peritoneal reflection between the mesocolon and the inferior border of the pancreas is carefully dissected with the monopolar hook. This maneuver allows an initial exposure of the pancreatic isthmus and of the underlying superior mesenteric vein. In presence of a thick colonic mesentery, following the middle colic vein may facilitate the finding of its merging into the superior mesenteric vein or the mesenterico-portal junction.

An initial, partial retropancreatic tunnel is then created between the inferior edge of the pancreatic neck and the mesenterico-portal axis. The pancreatic neck preparation may require a precise microdissection of tiny venous branches that may hinder the access to the portal vein (**Figure 31-7**).

Usually, those tiny branches are more frequent on the left side of the mesenterico-portal junction. They have to be carefully prepared and divided in between sutures of Prolene™ 5–0 (**Figure 31-8**). The pancreatic mobilization at the level of the portal axis allows a better evaluation of the tumor extension and its resectability.

Step 3 average time frame: 10–25 min

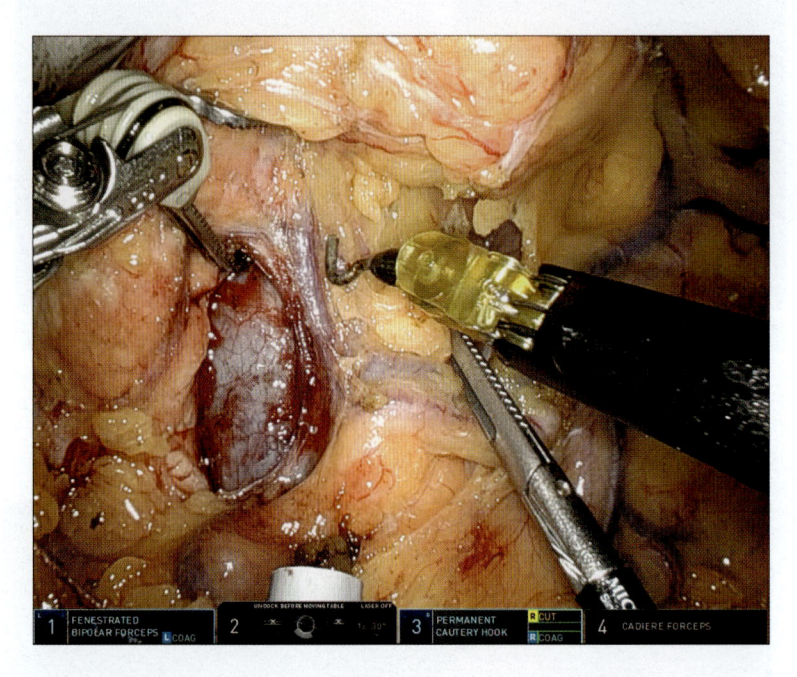

FIGURE 31-7 • Retropancreatic neck dissection.

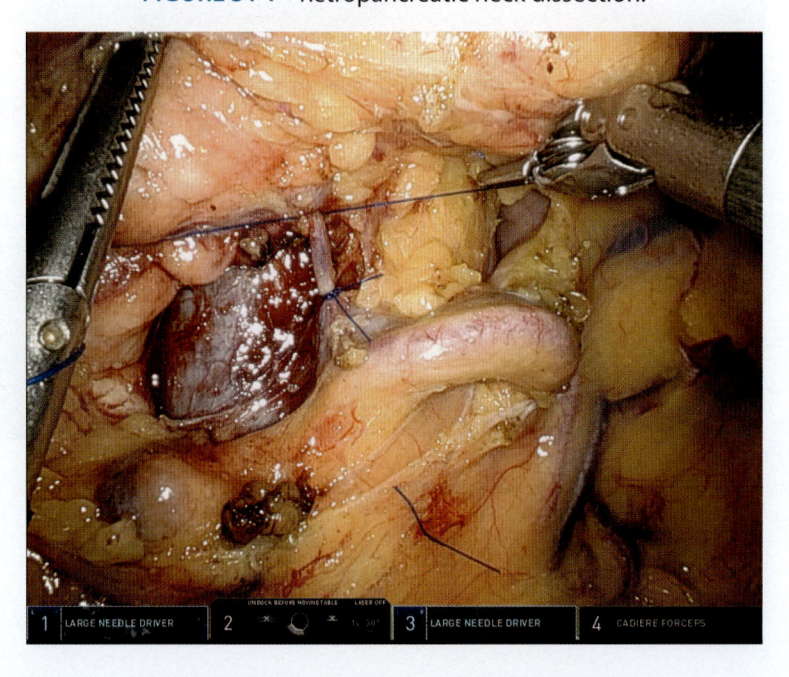

FIGURE 31-8 • Small retropancreatic vein control.

▶ **Video 31-4. Step 4. Preparation of the Pancreatic Arteries and Sample Lymphadenectomy**

Step 4. Preparation of the main peripancreatic arteries and sample lymphadenectomy

A careful dissection is then performed at the superior border of the pancreatic neck exposing the proximal portion of the common hepatic artery. This maneuver is extended along the major vascular axis until reaching the gastroduodenal artery, which represents the proximal pancreatic resection limit.

The progressive mobilization of the superior pancreatic edge may facilitate the identification of the left gastric vein, reducing the risk of its inadvertent injury during the subsequent retropancreatic dissection. The proximal portion of the splenic artery is similarly prepared and encircled with a vessel loop to facilitate its atraumatic retraction and dissection.

The best way to prepare these main peripancreatic vessels is to proceed with a periadventitial vascular dissection detaching the lymph nodes that always go along the main arteries (**Figure 31-9**). This surgical plane allows to skeletonize the vessels and, at the same time, to retrieve the corresponding lymph nodes. This lymph nodal sampling may be important to complete the oncological procedure, mainly in case of low-grade pNETs.

The ultimate goal of the peripancreatic vascular dissection is to allow a less risky parenchymal transection, creating a safe space between the pancreatic gland and the main vessels.

Step 4 average time frame: 20–40 min

> ⚠ **PITFALLS**
>
> Insufficient pancreatic detachment from the main peripancreatic arteries. This situation may increase the risk of vascular injuries during the following steps.

> ▶▶ **TIPS**
>
> The peripancreatic arteries should be manipulated carefully, never touching the vessels directly with the robotic instruments. The lack of tactile feedback and the only partial force feedback may increase the risk of applying excessive forces and damaging the structure of the artery. The application of a vessel loop allows traction and retraction without the risk of injuries.

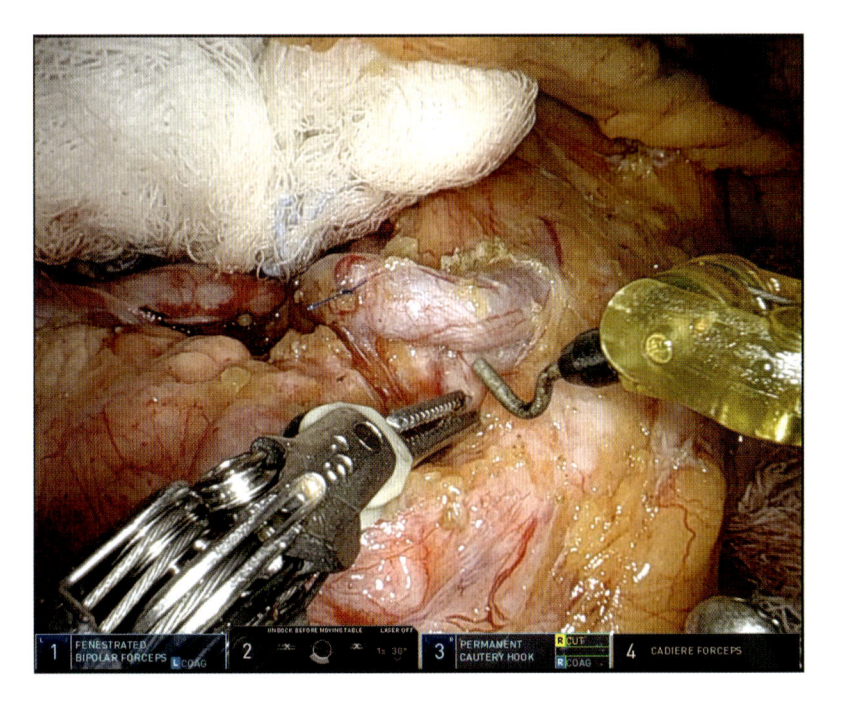

FIGURE 31-9 • Splenic artery dissection.

Video 31-5. Step 5. Completion of the Retropancreatic Tunnel

Step 5. Completion of the retropancreatic tunnel

The retropancreatic tunnel is progressively completed, with a careful blunt technique, between the posterior surface of the pancreas and the mesenteric-portal axis. With the grasper stable in the R3 retracting the stomach, the retropancreatic dissection is usually performed with the monopolar cautery hook in the R1 and the bipolar grasper in the R2.

The posterior mobilization of the neck sometimes requires the detachment of tiny vascular venous branches at the splenoportal confluence. Those delicate structures are meticulously prepared and divided in between sutures of Prolene™ 5-0.

The accomplishment of an adequate posterior dissection of the pancreatic neck allows an easy positioning of a vessel loop, which is then used to lift the pancreas away from the portal vein. This pancreatic "hanging maneuver" facilitates the following parenchymal transection.

Step 5 average time frame: 15–25 min

>> **TIPS**

When there are intense inflammatory adhesions between the pancreatic neck and the portal vein, the blunt dissection of the tunnel may be risky. In this case, there are 2 possible technical options:
- Antegrade dissection of the pancreatic neck, lifted with 2 stay sutures placed at the inferior edge. While the dissection is progressing with the Harmonic shears, more access is achieved on top of the portal vein with better control. The anterior aspect of the portal vein is progressively exposed while the pancreas is split.
- The periadventitial dissection of the anterior aspect of the portal vein is conducted with microsurgical dissection (smoot rounded scissors) (**Figure 31-10**). This technique requires a mature experience because a tear of the portal vein with the pancreas undivided may present a very difficult challenge.

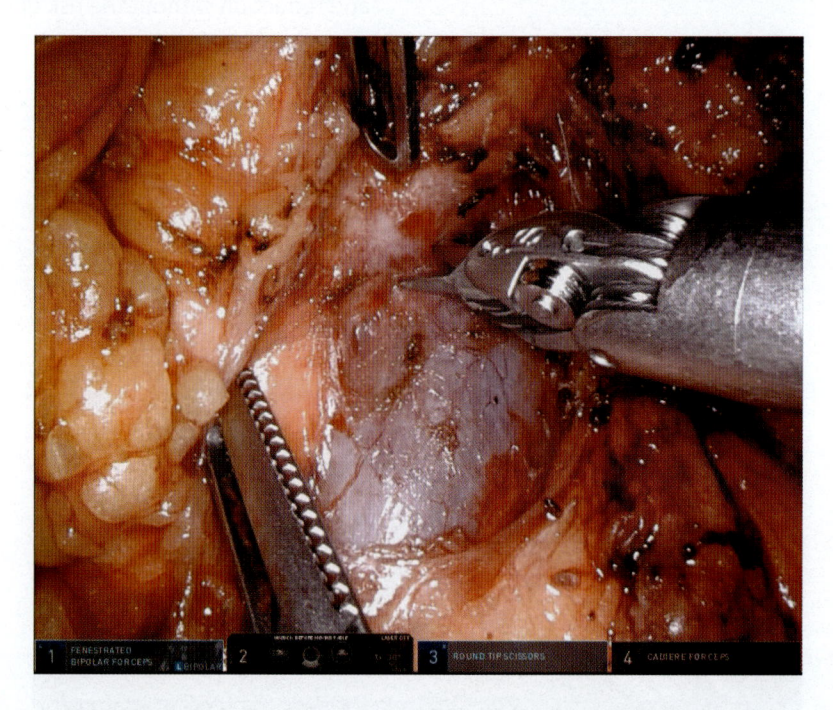

FIGURE 31-10 • Sharp dissection of the retropancreatic portal vein.

Video 31-6. Step 6. Proximal Pancreatic Transection

Step 6. Proximal pancreatic transection

Once the retropancreatic tunnel is completed, 2 stay sutures are applied at the inferior edge of the pancreas to facilitate the glandular transection and to ensure a better preventive hemostasis. The two transection margins were already defined and marked on the pancreatic surface with monopolar electrocautery during the IOUS (tattooed margins).

Depending on tumor location, pancreatic neck size, and texture (soft, intermediate, or hard), a stapler or Harmonic shears should be used for the pancreatic transection (**Figure 31-11**). When the Harmonic device is used, the inactive blade is placed near the portal vein to avoid thermal injuries. The proximal section line is inspected, and the hemostasis is verified and improved with Prolene™ 3-0 or 4-0 stitches. The main proximal pancreatic duct is then identified and oversewn with a Prolene™ 3-0 or 4-0 suture (**Figure 31-12**).

Step 6 average time frame: 15–20 min

> ▶▶ **TIPS**
>
> If there are any doubts about the precise tumor location and the resection margins, the IOUS should be repeated.

> ▶▶ **TIPS**
>
> The proximal and distal pancreatic transection (Steps 6 and 8) can be inverted depending on the location of the tumor. If the lesion is located more toward the pancreatic body, it is simpler to divide the pancreatic neck first and only after then prepare the distal portion. If the tumor is in the neck of the pancreas, it may be easier to divide the pancreatic body first and then to retract the proximal stump to the right side. In order to achieve a proper proximal margin, in some cases, it may also be necessary to prepare the right side of the portal vein.
>
> To achieve the most favorable angle for the proximal pancreatic transection with the Harmonic shears, it is often necessary to swap the instrument control between the 2 hands, having the shears maneuvered with the left hand and coming from the right side of the patient.

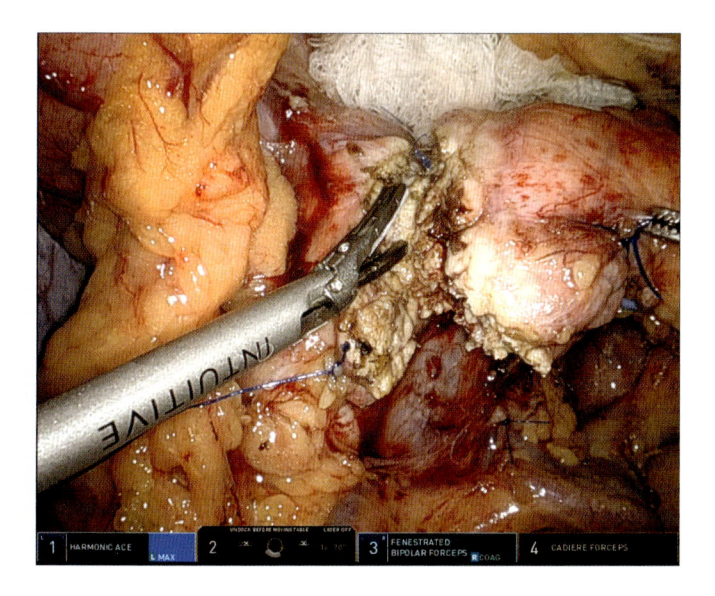

FIGURE 31-11 • Proximal pancreatic transection.

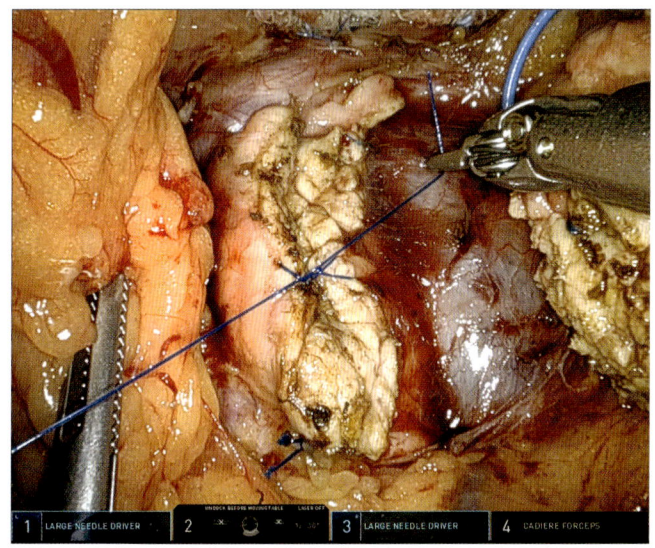

FIGURE 31-12 • Oversewing of the proximal pancreatic duct.

Step 7. Mobilization of the proximal pancreatic body

To reach the distal transection margin, the pancreatic mobilization is extended toward the body.

The vascular dissection should follow the proximal segment of the splenic artery and the splenic vein starting close to the junction with the portal vein and proceeding distally.

A meticulous dissection and control with Prolene™ 5-0 sutures is performed on all small venous and arterial branches connecting the posterior pancreatic surface with the splenic vessels (**Figure 31-13**).

Suturing is always the most secure way to obtain a hemostatic control of these tiny arteries and veins. The use of energy devices to control these small vascular branches should be discouraged to minimize the risk of an unstable hemostasis and delayed bleeding.

The dissection proceeds until the predetermined distal margin on the pancreatic body is reached. At this point, the left pancreas is gently lifted and ready for the transection.

Step 7 average time frame: 15–35 min

> **🔍 ANATOMICAL HIGHLIGHTS**
>
> The left gastric vein can drain into the portal vein, splenic vein, or directly at their confluence. The exact understanding of this vascular anatomy can avoid difficult bleedings during the dissection of the spleno-portal confluence (**Figures 31-14 A–C**).

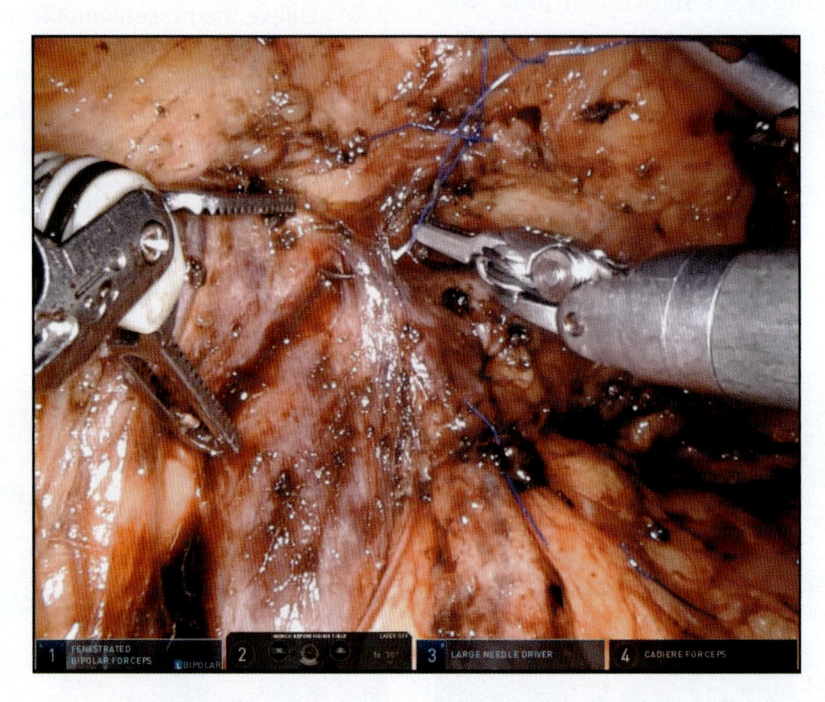

FIGURE 31-13 • Vascular control of small venous branches.

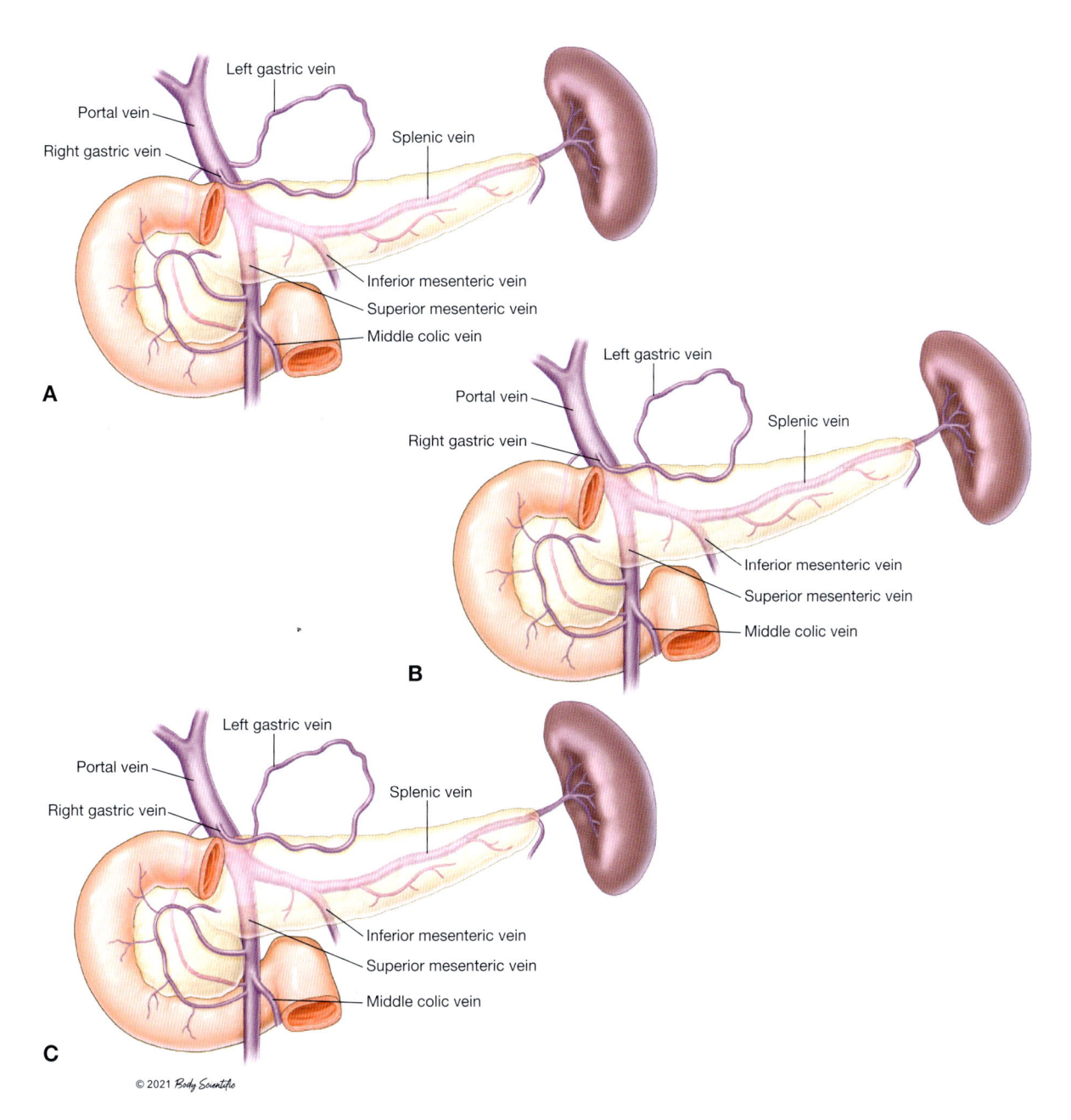

FIGURE 31-14 • Left gastric vein variations.

Step 8. Distal transection of the pancreas

At this point, to confirm the correct position of the distal pancreatic resection margin, a further IOUS may be necessary (**Figure 31-15**).

While lifting and retracting the stay suture with a grasper in the R2, the distal pancreatic margin is progressively transected, thus completing the dissection phase of the procedure (**Figure 31-16**). The Harmonic shears should be used with the open jaws near to the pancreatic duct to avoid the sealing effect. Mainly in the small-size duct, a complete closure may create problems in its identification. The distal duct, if sealed, should be reopened for the anastomosis.

Once the distal transection is completed, the specimen is temporarily placed into an Endobag™ for subsequent extraction and moved in a position where it is not interfering with the completion of the operation, usually above the liver in the right upper quadrant. The hemostasis on the distal pancreatic section line is verified and improved with Prolene™ 4-0 stitches.

Step 8 average time frame: 10–25 min

> ▶▶ **TIPS**
>
> Before starting the reconstruction, an intraoperative frozen section analysis of the proximal and distal margins is always possible and recommended when the lesion is close to a section line.

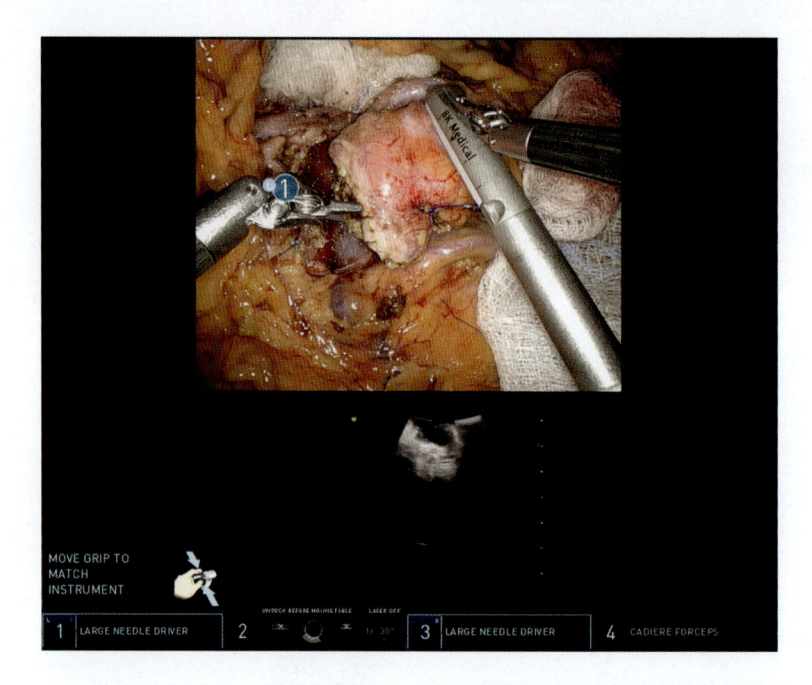

FIGURE 31-15 • IOUS–Distal pancreatic margin assessment.

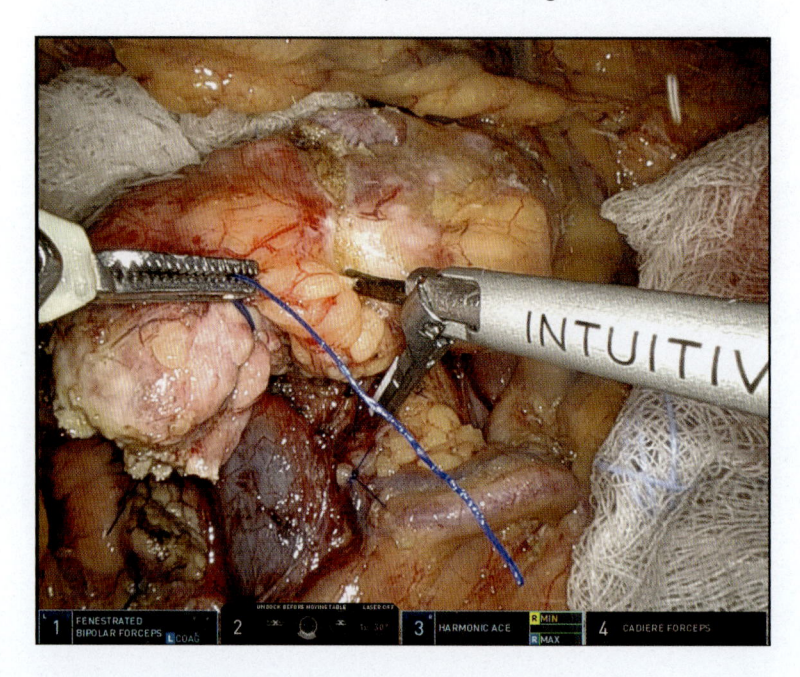

FIGURE 31-16 • Distal pancreatic transection.

RECONSTRUCTION

Similarly to what is described in Chapter 28, Pancreaticoduodenectomy, the main options for the pancreatico-digestive anastomosis are pancreaticojejunostomy and pancreaticogastrostomy (see Chapter 28 for precise indications).

Here, the pancreaticojejunal anastomosis is described.

Step 9. Preparation of a Roux-en-Y jejunal loop

Before starting the reconstructive phase, the distal pancreatic stump is evaluated for the anastomosis. If necessary, it is further mobilized for a couple of centimeters in order to have enough space for the posterior anastomotic layer. Also, the pancreatic duct is explored, and when it is less than 3–4 mm in size, it is stented with a small cannula that is fixed in place with a 4-0 absorbable monofilament suture. To prepare the Roux limb, the second jejunal loop is divided at about 30 cm from the Treitz ligament using a vessel sealer for the mesentery and a linear stapler (**Figure 31-17**). A side-to-side jejunojejunostomy is distally performed to create an isolated loop of about 60 cm. The anastomosis is carried out with a stapling technique (see Chapter 21, Roux-en-Y Gastric Bypass).

The transverse mesocolon is carefully opened with the cautery hook in an avascular area, usually on the right side of the middle colonic vessels, and the Roux limb is transposed into the lesser sac.

Step 9 average time frame: 20–35 min

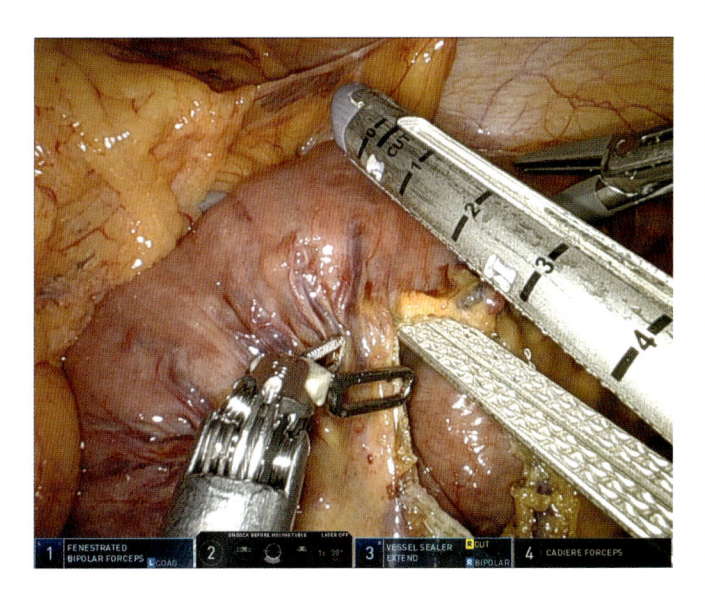

FIGURE 31-17 • Second jejunal loop transection.

Video 31-7. Step 10. Distal Pancreaticojejunostomy

Step 10. Distal pancreaticojejunostomy

A small (pinpoint) enterotomy is performed in the jejunum in a position that will match the location of the pancreatic duct without tension. Then, a posterior Prolene™ 4-0 suture capsule-serosa is performed approximating and stabilizing the 2 openings (pancreatic duct with the stent and the point enterotomy). A mucosa-to-mucosa anastomosis is carried out with interrupted absorbable stitches of PDS™ 4-0 or 5-0. An anterior capsule-serosa layer with Prolene™ 4-0 completes the reconstruction (see Chapter 28 for more details) (**Figure 31-18**).

Step 10 average time frame: 30–40 min

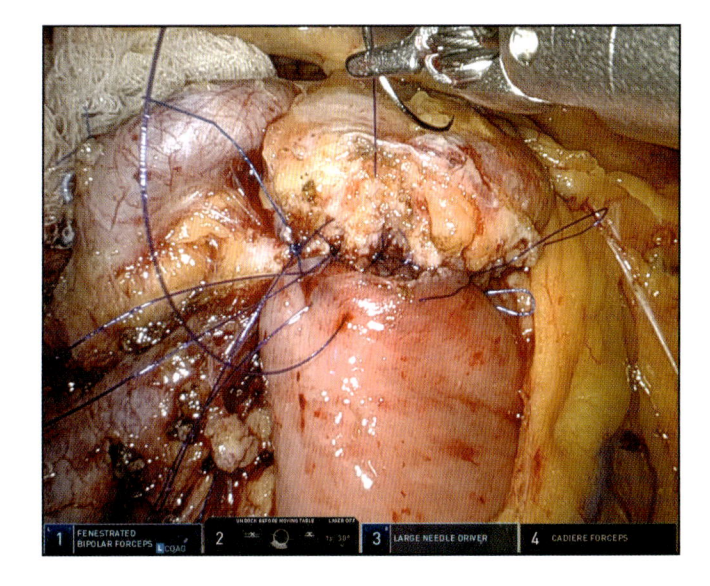

FIGURE 31-18 • Duct-to-mucosa pancreaticojejunostomy.

Step 11. Specimen extraction

Once the reconstructive phase is completed, the hemostasis should be carefully verified and perfected. Fibrin glue is applied on the pancreaticojejunostomy, and 2 Jackson-Pratt drains are then placed near the anastomosis. The robotic arms are undocked and the Endobag™ with the surgical specimen is retrieved through a small Pfannestiel or, more frequently, by enlarging the size of one of the assistant trocars site. The choice is based on the volume of the specimen and the specific anatomical details of the patient (e.g., body mass index, previous scars, etc.).

Step 11 average time frame: 10–20 min

Suggested Readings

1. Giulianotti PC, Sbrana F, Bianco FM, Addeo P, Caravaglios G. Robot-assisted laparoscopic middle pancreatectomy. *J Laparoendosc Adv Surgi Techniq.* 2010;20(2):135-139. doi: 10.1089/lap.2009.0296
2. Dreifuss NH, Cubisino A, Schlottmann F, Giulianotti PC. Robotic-assisted central pancreatectomy: a minimally invasive approach for benign and low-grade lesions. *Surg Oncol.* Published online March 2022:101736. doi: 10.1016/j.suronc.2022.101736
3. Xu SB, Zhu YP, Zhou W, Xie K, Mou YP. Patients get more long-term benefit from central pancreatectomy than distal resection: a meta-analysis. *Eur J Surg Oncol.* 2013;39(6):567-574. doi: 10.1016/j.ejso.2013.02.003
4. Rompianesi G, Montalti R, Giglio MC, Caruso E, Ceresa CDL, Troisi RI. Robotic central pancreatectomy: a systematic review and meta-analysis. *HPB.* 2022;24(2):143-151. doi: 10.1016/j.hpb.2021.09.014
5. Iacono C, Verlato G, Ruzzenente A, et al. Systematic review of central pancreatectomy and meta-analysis of central versus distal pancreatectomy. *Br J Surg.* 2013;100(7):873-885. doi: 10.1002/bjs.9136
6. DiNorcia J, Ahmed L, Lee MK, et al. Better preservation of endocrine function after central versus distal pancreatectomy for midgland lesions. *Surgery.* 2010;148(6):1247-1256. doi: 10.1016/j.surg.2010.09.003
7. Liu R, Wang ZZ, Gao YX, Xu Y. Application of end-to-end anastomosis in robotic central pancreatectomy. *J Vis Exp.* 2018;(136):57495. doi: 10.3791/57495
8. Sauvanet A, Partensky C, Sastre B, et al. Medial pancreatectomy: a multi-institutional retrospective study of 53 patients by the French Pancreas Club. *Surgery.* 2002;132(5):836-843. doi: 10.1067/msy.2002.127552
9. Crippa S, Bassi C, Warshaw AL, et al. Middle pancreatectomy: indications, short- and long-term operative outcomes. *Ann Surg.* 2007;246(1):69-76. doi: 10.1097/01.sla.0000262790.51512.57
10. Shi Y, Jin J, Huo Z, et al. An 8-year single-center study: 170 cases of middle pancreatectomy, including 110 cases of robot-assisted middle pancreatectomy. *Surgery.* 2020;167(2):436-441. doi: 10.1016/j.surg.2019.09.002
11. Goudard Y, Gaujoux S, Dokmak S, et al. Reappraisal of central pancreatectomy: a 12-year single-center experience. *JAMA Surg.* 2014;149(4):356. doi: 10.1001/jamasurg.2013.4146
12. Halfdanarson TR, Strosberg JR, Tang L, et al. The North American Neuroendocrine Tumor Society Consensus Guidelines for Surveillance and Medical Management of Pancreatic Neuroendocrine Tumors. *Pancreas.* 2020;49(7):863-881. doi: 10.1097/MPA.0000000000001597
13. Giulianotti PC, Angelini M, Sbrana F, et al. Les resections coelioscopiques du pancreas. *Le Journal de Coelio Chirurgie.* 2004, 52:19-27.
14. Giulianotti PC, Coratti A, Angelini M, et al. Robotics in general surgery: personal experience in a large community hospital. *Arch Surg.* 2003;138(7):777-784. doi: 10.1001/archsurg.138.7.777.

"Simplicity is the ultimate sophistication."
—Leonardo da Vinci (1452–1519)

Enucleation of Pancreatic Tumors

Graziano Pernazza • Antonio Cubisino

INTRODUCTION

The mainstay treatment for benign and low-grade malignant tumors of the pancreas is still resection, either pancreaticoduodenectomy (PD) or left pancreatectomy (LP). In these procedures, a large amount of normal parenchyma is removed along with the tumor; therefore, there is a high risk of endocrine and/or exocrine insufficiency. Enucleation consists of resection of the mass, sparing the surrounding tissue, as an alternative to major resections. This may allow a shorter operative time and reduced intraoperative blood loss with consequent shorter intensive care unit (ICU) stay and equal or shorter length of hospital stay. When correctly indicated, this procedure has good long-term clinical and oncological outcomes with a lower risk of exocrine and/or endocrine insufficiency.

Mortality, overall complications, reoperation rates, delayed gastric emptying, and overall survival are not significantly different between enucleation and resection. Similar to the standard pancreatic resection, postoperative pancreatic fistula (POPF) remains the main complication of pancreatic enucleation. The POPF incidence is strictly related to the tumor position and its proximity to the pancreatic ducts. The higher-risk zones in developing POPF after enucleation are the ventral head parenchyma and the uncinate process. Even though the rate of clinically significant fistulas (grades B and C) is higher with enucleation, this does not seem to significantly affect morbidity and mortality.

This procedure can be considered for well-differentiated pancreatic neuroendocrine tumors (pNETs) and pancreatic cystic neoplasms (PCNs). These 2 types of tumors include benign lesions and potentially more aggressive ones, with a higher malignant potential.

pNETs represent less than 5% of all pancreatic tumors. Most of them are sporadic, while approximately 10% are associated with multiple endocrine neoplasia type 1 (MEN1), von Hippel-Lindau syndrome (VHL), tuberous sclerosis complex, and neurofibromatosis (NF1).

These patients more frequently have multifocal tumors, with an earlier disease onset, and need a precise preoperative evaluation and an accurate intraoperative ultrasonography (IOUS).

INSTRUMENT REQUIREMENTS

The suggested main robotic instruments/tools can be listed as follows:
- 30° scope
- Cautery hook/monopolar scissors
- Harmonic shears™
- Maryland bipolar forceps
- Cadière forceps
- Vessel sealer (optional)
- Needle drivers (round tip or macro)

The suggested main laparoscopic instruments/tools can be listed as follows:
- Needle drivers
- Scissors
- Graspers
- Suction-irrigation
- Laparoscopic ultrasound (drop-in probe or handheld)

Supplemental materials:
- Gauzes, sponges
- Penrose drains
- Vessel loops
- Endobag™
- Medium–large clips
- Fibrin sealant
- Sutures (Prolene™ 3-0, 4-0, and 5-0)

pNETs are generally nonfunctional tumors—only 10% secrete hormones. Functional pNETs include insulinomas (35–40%), gastrinomas (16–30%), glucagonomas, VIPomas, and somatostatinomas (rare).

The measures of proliferative index (Ki-67 and mitotic index) are used to assign pNETs histologic grade and have significant implications on treatment and prognosis. An ideal indication for enucleation is the presence of a pNET smaller than 2–3 cm, with a Ki-67 <3% (G1), located >3 mm from the main or accessory pancreatic duct.

PCNs comprise intraductal papillary mucinous neoplasms (IPMNs) in 20–50% of cases, mucinous cystic neoplasms (MCNs) in 10–45% of cases, serous cystoadenomas (SCAs) in 32–39% of cases, and solid pseudopapillary neoplasms (SPNs) in less than 10% of cases.

Routine preoperative workup involves triple-phase contrast-enhancement computed tomography (CT), magnetic resonance imaging (MRI), endoscopic ultrasonography (EUS), IOUS, tumor markers (CA19.9, chromogranin A, neuron-specific enolase), and endocrine assessment if indicated on basis of the biopsy. CT makes it possible to evaluate the tumor's characteristics (e.g., localization, size, density, presence of a capsule, vascularization, malignant features), its proximity or involvement of surrounding structures (biliopancreatic ducts, portal vein, superior mesenteric vein, superior mesenteric artery), and potential nodal or distant metastases. An MRI scan can help to identify small lesions that cannot be accurately studied with CT scans. Echo-endoscopy is an extremely specific method for the study of the pancreas. It allows performance of tumor biopsies and fluid analysis in cystic tumors (for more information, see suggested readings #2, 3, 4).

> **EDITORIAL COMMENT**
>
> Endocrine assessment and somatostatin receptor–based imaging play an important role in the suspect of functional pNETs. Gallium-68 (^{68}Ga)-DOTATOC positron emission tomography (PET)-CT is a very useful imaging investigation for diagnosing and staging pNETs. It has proven to have a higher sensitivity and specificity when compared to the previously widely used Octreoscan®.
>
> Another effective functional imaging technique is the use of ^{18}F-fluorodeoxyglucose (^{18}F-FDG) PET/CT for detecting and staging nonfunctional pNETs.

Indications and Relative Contraindications to the Robotic Approach

The risk of malignant transformation/dissemination and the presence of systemic symptoms, due to hormone overproduction or related to local mass compression, represent the most common indications to resect a pNET. The diagnostic and therapeutic approach should depend on specific factors such as functional status, proliferative activity (Ki-67 index and mitotic count), tumor growth rate, and extent of the disease (**Figure 32-1**).

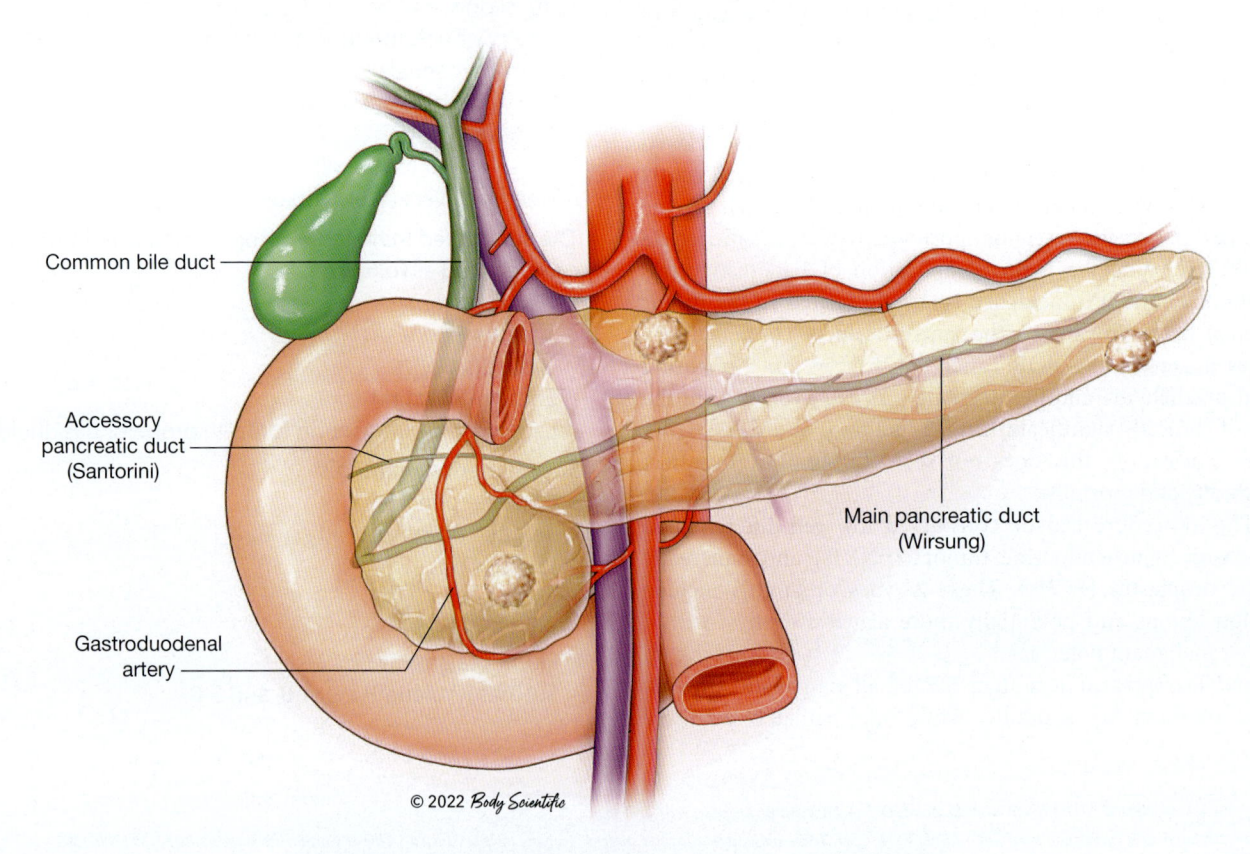

FIGURE 32-1 • Pancreatic nodules and anatomical landmarks.

There is a strong consensus about pancreatic enucleation for small insulinomas and nonfunctional pNETs (<2 cm), located >3 mm from the main or accessory pancreatic duct. Similar to these lesions, the gastrinoma may also be enucleated when <2 cm. However, it is useful to mention that its risk of malignancy remains high (60–90% vs 5–15% of insulinomas).

Other functional pNETs, such as VIPoma, glucagonoma, and somatostatinoma, are typically large and most often metastatic at diagnosis. For these reasons, they should be treated with a standard pancreatectomy.

Some guidelines state that patients with incidentally diagnosed, small low-grade NF-pNETs (<1 cm) could be managed conservatively but a general consensus is still missing. This means that the decision to observe or resect an asymptomatic pNET <1 cm in size should be individualized.

EDITORIAL COMMENT

Indications for pancreatic enucleations can be resumed as follows:
- Small nonfunctional pNETs <2 cm, with a low Ki-67 and that are located >3 mm from the main or accessory pancreatic duct.
- Functional pNETs as insulinoma and gastrinoma <2 cm, with a distance greater than 3 mm from the main or accessory pancreatic duct.
- A standard pancreatectomy with regional lymphadenectomy is still recommended for larger tumors at risk for cancerization, with possible associated lymph nodes involvement.

▶▶ TIPS

Pancreatic nodules may be in any region of the gland. They can be exophytic or immersed in the parenchyma and not visible at the surface.

The use of an ultrasound system with a drop-in or handled probe is mandatory to explore the gland, identify the nodule, and determine its relationship with the vascular structures, the eventual involvement of the duct, and the presence of additional lesions. All these characteristics may influence the final surgical approach and can be useful during the enucleation to dynamically verify the dissection plane excluding any residual disease.

Patient Positioning, OR Setup, and Port Setting

The patient is placed supine, with arms tucked and lower limbs parted in the French position, with a 20° reverse Trendelenburg. If the nodule is located inside the head of the pancreas, a slight left-sided down tilting of the table can be useful. On the contrary, in case of lesions located in the tail, a slight right-sided tilting of the table will be preferred (**Figure 32-2**).

The extreme versatility of the da Vinci® Xi™ system, with its rotating boom-mounted arms, makes single docking easy even for complex multiquadrant procedures. Despite that the robotic cart can be docked from any position around the patient, the ideal cart position should be homolateral to the surgical target. This setting allows a better OR setup with the scrub nurse and/or the second assistant in a more functional and appropriate position (**Figure 32-3**).

The pneumoperitoneum is achieved with the usual technique described in Chapter 2, The Basic Principles of Clinical Applications. A full diagnostic laparoscopy is carefully carried out before confirming the line of port setting. The ports are placed under direct visualization.

The port position is chosen based on the nodule location. If the nodule is located on the proximal part of the gland, port placement will be like the one described for robotic PD (see Chapter 28, Pancreaticoduodenectomy), while in case of distal location, the placement will be like robotic LP (see Chapter 29, Radical Antegrade Modular Pancreatosplenectomy) (**Figure 32-4**).

Correct port position is crucial to have good exposure and unrestricted operative arms. Usually, at least 5 ports are needed (4 robotic and 1 or 2 assistant ports).

▶▶ TIPS

External landmarks may be unreliable to choose the right port placement mainly in obese patients. If the location of the lesion is not completely clear in the preoperative workup the laparoscopic ultrasound scan may be anticipated before completing the entire line of ports.

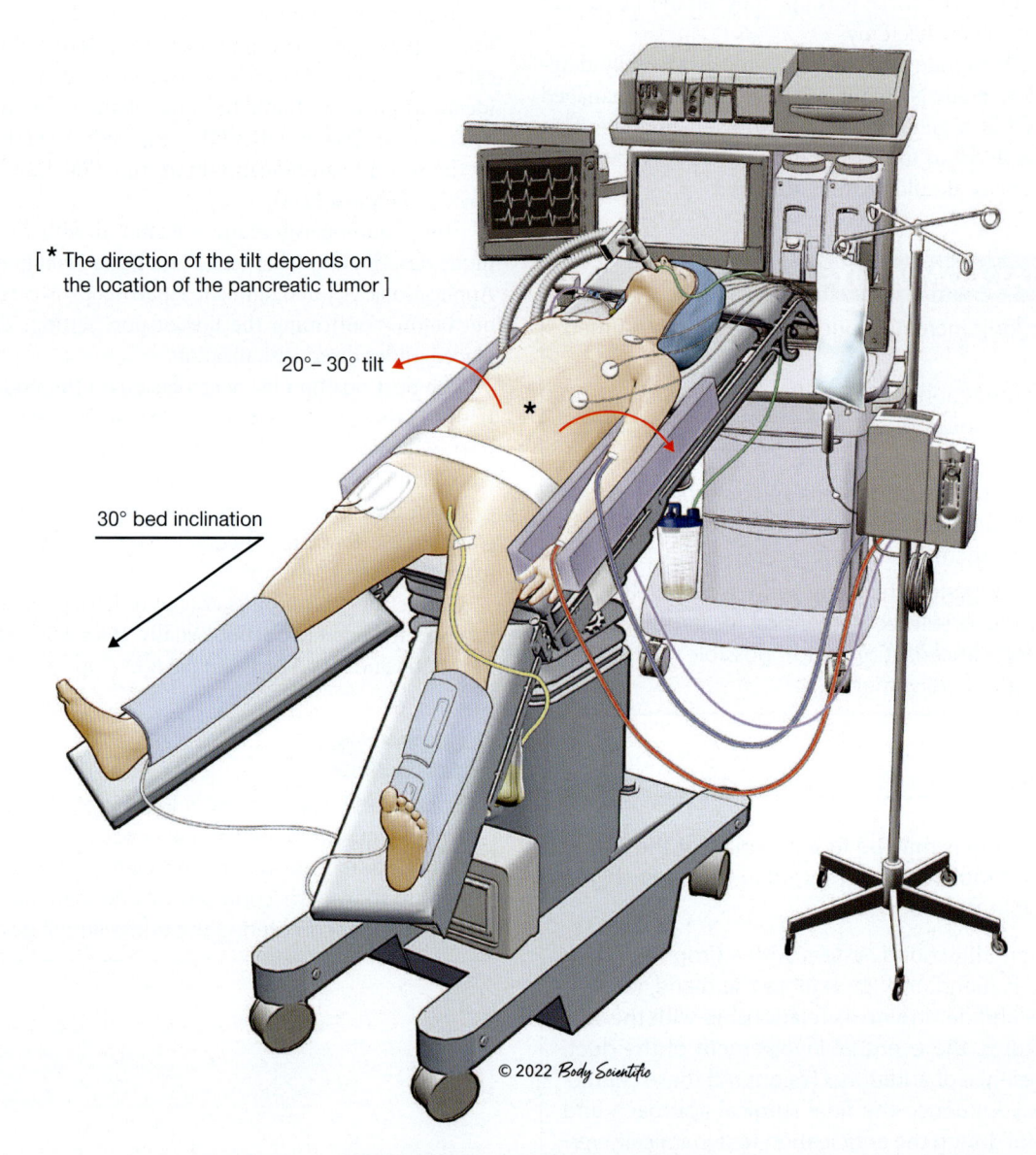

FIGURE 32-2 • Patient positioning.

FIGURE 32-3 • OR setup.

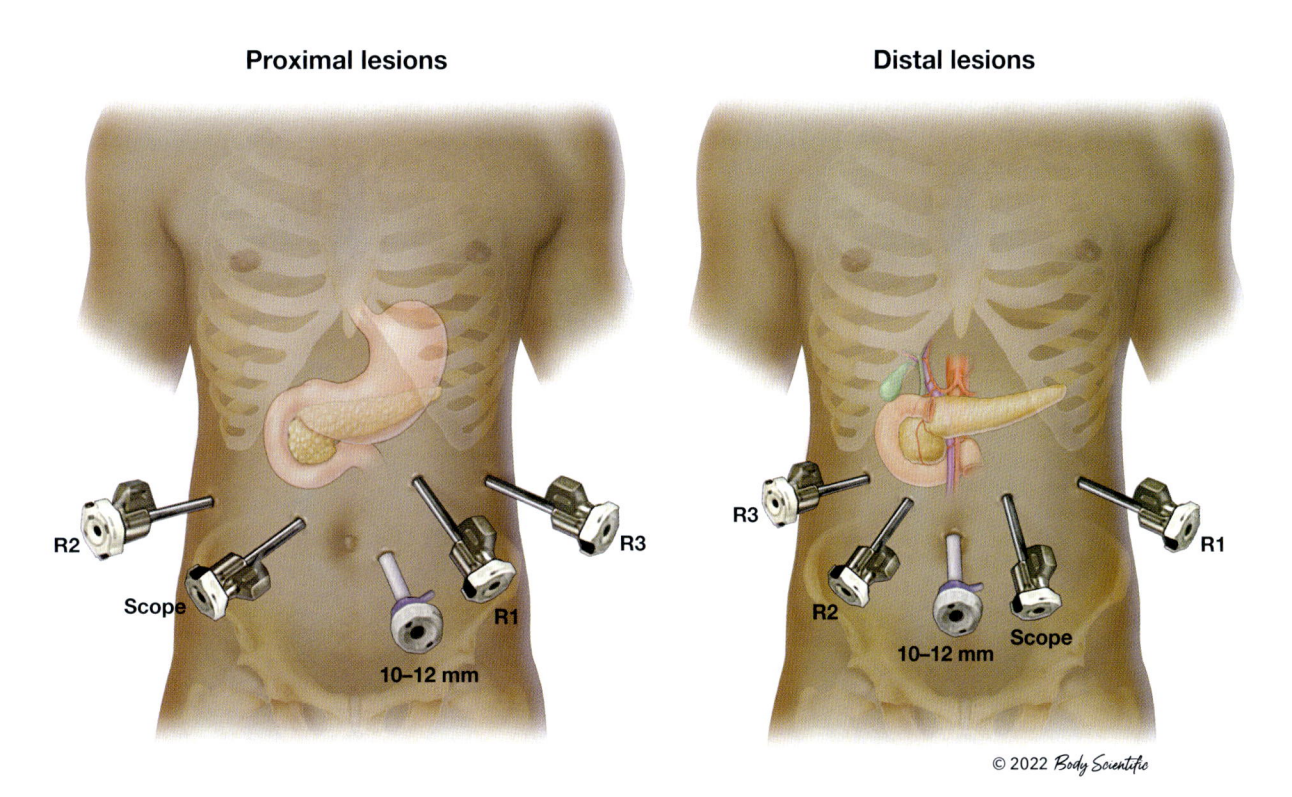

FIGURE 32-4 • Port setting.

Surgical Technique

Step 1. Pancreatic gland exposure

Using the R3, the stomach is lifted upward with a grasper. The Bouchet's transparent zone is identified by putting the gastrocolic ligament under proper tension. This area is opened with the monopolar cautery hook or the scissors, and this maneuver allows entrance into the lesser sac to inspect the pancreas (anteriorly).

The gastrocolic ligament opening is widened until reaching the left and right gastroepiploic vessels on each side and preserving entirely the gastroepiploic arcade. The superior mesenteric vein (SMV)/portal vein confluence (located at the pancreatic neck) should be assessed systematically. The body and tail of the pancreas are completely exposed dividing adhesions between the stomach, pancreas, and omentum, if present.

The right colonic flexure is completely mobilized (see Chapter 28, Pancreaticoduodenectomy).

Step 1 average time frame: 15–20 min

▶ **Video 32-1. Step 2. Ultrasound Exploration**

Step 2. Ultrasound exploration

The pancreatic gland should be entirely scanned with overlapping sweeps in the transverse and sagittal planes to ensure complete coverage of the organ.

It is necessary to allow a close contact between the transducer and the gland. No specific acoustic coupling material is generally necessary. The transducer is lightly applied to the surface of the pancreas, and the moisture of the exposed gland suffices to achieve acoustic coupling. Sometimes, a poor acoustic coupling occurs, due to an irregular glandular surface or location of a lesion immediately adjacent to the surface of the transducer.

When performing a laparoscopic IOUS, it is important to select the most appropriate port site location for insertion of the transducer, because even in case of articulated probes, the port site angle determines which structures can be optimally scanned, and in which planes.

A careful ultrasound examination can help to achieve an adequate surgical margin with maximal preservation of pancreatic parenchyma. One of the main criteria for the resection is the distance between the tumor and the Wirsung duct, which must be assessed. The preoperative study must accurately define this aspect.

Step 2 average time frame: 10–15 min

> ▶▶ **TIPS**
>
> IOUS should assess:
> - echogenic characteristics of the lesion;
> - dimension of the lesion;
> - relationship between the lesion and the other vascular/ductal structures;
> - resection plans and strategy.

> ⚠ **PITFALLS**
>
> Another diagnostic pitfall occurs when direct pressure exerted on the pancreas with the transducer causes vascular or ductal compression, which might be misinterpreted as narrowing or occlusion. In such situations, a sterile saline solution may be helpful to obtain an acoustic offset.

> ▶▶ **TIPS**
>
> In case of lesions in proximity (≤3 mm) of the Wirsung duct, the risk of accidental damage increases and therefore the risk of pancreatic fistula. In these cases, the preoperative insertion of a temporary endoscopic stent should be considered.
>
> Fluorescence imaging using indocyanine green (ICG) may visualize pancreatic lesions, especially in presence of small and superficial pNETs (**Figure 32-5**).

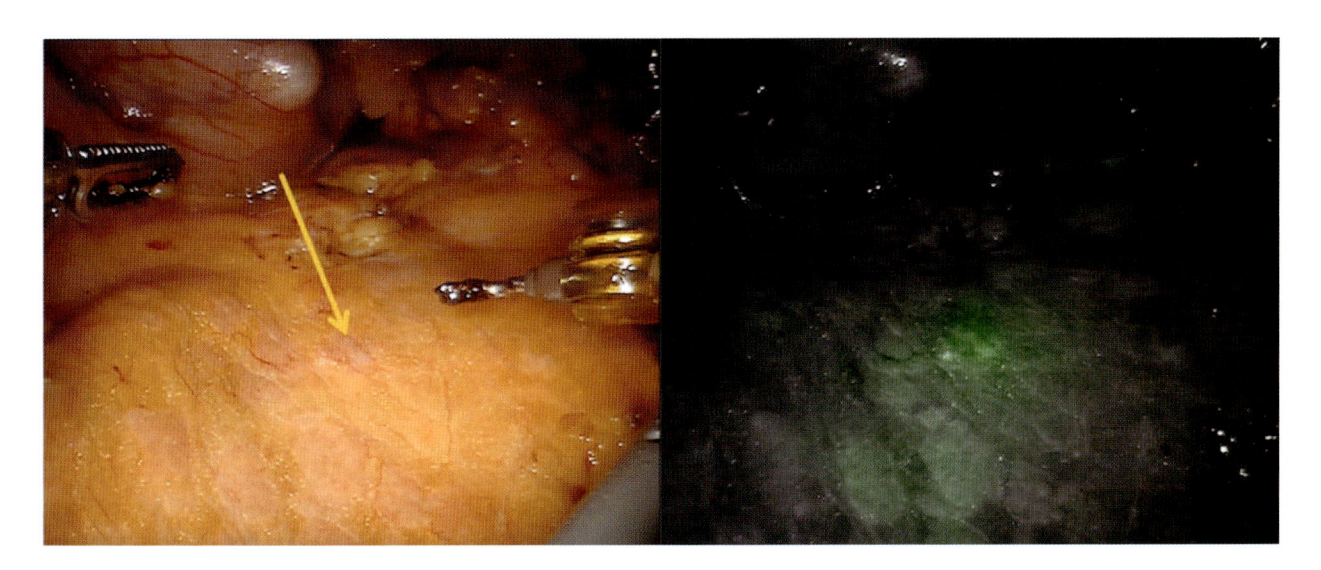

FIGURE 32-5 • ICG fluorescence imaging.

Step 3. Mobilization of the gland

Tumor location is a crucial technical factor. A wider mobilization of the pancreatic gland is not always necessary. In some cases, however, this must be done to allow a safer access and to have an adequate exposure of the tumor. This can occur even in lesions of the isthmus, which may come in contact with the mesenteric-portal (see **Video 32-1**) or splenic venous axis, for lesions located within the uncinate process or immersed in the gland, not emerging to the capsule.

In the presence of proximal lesions posteriorly located, a complete Kocher maneuver may allow a more stable exposure of the proximal retropancreatic surface. In this case, the medial duodenal retraction is carried out with a Cadière forceps in R3, ensuring a better exposure and a more stable operating field.

A complete retropancreatic tunnel between the mesenteric-portal axis and the pancreatic gland is usually needed in case of posterior lesions in the body or tail of the pancreas. An anterior approach to these tumors significantly increases the risk of major vascular lesions and pancreatic duct infractions.

The uncinate process remains the most challenging location for a pancreatic enucleation. When the lesion is located in its posteromedial surface, a wide Kocher maneuver and a careful preparation of the SMV may be requested in order to expose the surgical target avoiding major vascular injuries.

Step 3 average time frame: 10–40 min (extremely variable)

> ▶▶ **TIPS**
>
> Sometimes, it is necessary to use loops around the vessels or around the gland to lift or make tractions on them without directly grasping them. These maneuvers may decrease the risk of inadvertent injuries of major vessels and may favor vascular control in case of bleeding.

> ⚠ **PITFALLS**
>
> Incomplete or inadequate mobilization may lead to intraoperative complications. In particular, when lesions are close to main vessels (hepatic artery, gastroduodenal artery, splenic artery, portal or splenic veins), it is necessary to perform an appropriate mobilization of the gland to detach the plane form the vascular structures and to gain an adequate room for dissection.

▶ **Video 32-2. Step 4. Enucleation**

Step 4. Enucleation

Under direct or ultrasound-guided vision, the pancreatic capsule must be opened. The interruption of the capsule around the lesion generally determines a "decompression" of the nodule from the gland and lesions tends to "emerge." This makes it easier to identify a razor-thin margin between the tumor and pancreas, which has to be reached and followed detaching the tumor without breaking its capsule.

It is useful to use the R3 to get an adequate exposure and keep the operative field stable. The preferred instruments to perform dissection are monopolar (hook or scissors) and bipolar Maryland forceps.

Monopolar energy should be kept as low as possible to avoid any thermal damage to normal pancreatic tissue and to avoid tissue charring or eschar formation.

A gauze must always be available within the operating field to allow a clean vision and to perform a focal and targeted hemostasis.

Focused bipolar energy can be very useful for hemostasis, keeping clear the dissection plane, and dissociating tissues by gentle blunt and sharp dissection and occasionally exploiting the cavitation effect between the branches of the bipolar forceps.

Great attention must be paid to tumor manipulation. The accidental rupture of the capsule should be avoided. It is important not to grab the neoplasm directly; using gentle tractions or pushing with a sponge may favor the luxation of the nodule.

If there is any doubt about the radicality of the primary excision, an intraoperative frozen section represents an excellent way to evaluate the resection margins and at the same time to confirm the diagnosis.

Step 4 average time frame: 20–40 min

> ▶▶ **TIPS**
>
> The nodule may have some patchy areas of normal parenchyma attached to its capsule. This area may be used for a gentle grasping with the Cadière or bipolar forceps without the risk of breaking the tumor capsule, which always has a fragile tension.

Step 5. Specimen extraction, final hemostasis verification, and drain

Once the enucleation is completed, the specimen should be immediately removed from the operative field using a retrieval bag in order to avoid any spillage or cell seeding. It is advisable to extract the specimen through a small incision and not directly through cannulas even for small-sized lesions. Squeezing the nodule through the cannula may accidentally rupture the capsule and not allow a proper pathology examination.

At this point, an IOUS should always be performed to finally confirm the radicality of the resection. Moreover, in case of proximity of the lesion to the Wirsung duct, it is necessary to check its integrity evaluating the residual parenchymal margin.

Hemostasis must be accurate through the entire operation, but it should be always carefully verified at the end of the procedure. Prolene™ 4-0 stitches may be necessary to consolidate the bleeding control.

Clinical evidence on the role of sealants in pancreatic surgery is limited, but the use of sealing material and patches on the dissection area can be helpful in limiting minor leaks from the gland and reducing the spread of pancreatic fluid around the area of enucleation. However, the use of these aids cannot substitute for an accurate dissection technique and perfect control of the hemostasis.

A Penrose drain is left close to the dissection area. Amylase from the secretion retrieved in the drain should be measured on postoperative days 1, 3, and 5 to evaluate the presence of a POPF.

Step 5 average time frame: 10–15 min

> ▶▶ **TIPS**
>
> If there is an unclear damage of the main pancreatic duct and the fistula is doubtful, a way to clarify is to use an intraoperative secretin IV injection test.

> ▶▶ **TIPS**
>
> During the use of bipolar coagulation, a gentle irrigation made by the assistant to keep the dissection area clean and allow the surgeon to identify the source of bleeding is helpful. Moreover, saline solution improves the transmission of bipolar energy between the branches of the bipolar forceps and reduces the lateral thermal focal dispersion.

Suggested Readings

1. Giulianotti PC, Sbrana F, Bianco FM, et al. Robot-assisted laparoscopic pancreatic surgery: single-surgeon experience. *Surg Endosc.* 2010;24(7):1646-1657. doi: 10.1007/s00464-009-0825-4
2. Howe JR, Merchant NB, Conrad C, et al. The North American Neuroendocrine Tumor Society consensus paper on the surgical management of pancreatic neuroendocrine tumors. *Pancreas.* 2020;49(1):1-33. doi: 10.1097/MPA.0000000000001454
3. McKenna LR, Edil BH. Update on pancreatic neuroendocrine tumors. *Gland Surg.* 2014;3:258–275. doi: 10.3978/j.issn.2227-684X.2014.06.03
4. Marini F, Giusti F, Tonelli F, Brandi ML. Pancreatic neuroendocrine neoplasms in multiple endocrine neoplasia type 1. *IJMS* 2021;22:4041. doi: 10.3390/ijms22084041
5. Duconseil P, Marchese U, Ewald J, et al. A pancreatic zone at higher risk of fistula after enucleation. *World J Surg Onc* 2018;16:177. doi: 10.1186/s12957-018-1476-5
6. Cauley CE, Pitt HA, Ziegler KM, et al. Pancreatic enucleation: improved outcomes compared to resection. *J Gastrointest Surg.* 2012;16:1347-1353. doi: 10.1007/s11605-012-1893-7
7. Hackert T, Hinz U, Fritz S, et al. Enucleation in pancreatic surgery: indications, technique, and outcome compared to standard pancreatic resections. *Langenbecks Arch Surg.* 2011;396(8):1197-1203. doi: 10.1007/s00423-011-0801-z
8. Chua TC, Yang TX, Gill AJ, Samra JS. Systematic review and meta-analysis of enucleation versus standardized resection for small pancreatic lesions. *Ann Surg Oncol.* 2016;23(2):592-599. doi: 10.1245/s10434-015-4826-3
9. Ei S, Mihaljevic AL, Kulu Y, et al. Enucleation for benign or borderline tumors of the pancreas: comparing open and minimally invasive surgery. *HPB (Oxford).* 2021;23(6):921-926. doi: 10.1016/j.hpb.2020.10.001
10. Zhou Y, Zhao M, Wu L, Ye F, Si X. Short- and long-term outcomes after enucleation of pancreatic tumors: an evidence-based assessment. *Pancreatology.* 2016;16(6):1092-1098. doi: 10.1016/j.pan.2016.07.006
11. Talamini MA, Moesinger R, Yeo CJ, et al. Cystadenomas of the pancreas: is enucleation an adequate operation? *Ann Surg.* 1998;227(6):896-903. doi: 10.1097/00000658-199806000-00013
12. Jin JB, Qin K, Li H, et al. Robotic enucleation for benign or borderline tumours of the pancreas: a retrospective analysis and comparison from a high-volume centre in Asia. *World J Surg.* 2016;40(12):3009-3020. doi: 10.1007/s00268-016-3655-2
13. Song KB, Kim SC, Hwang DW, et al. Enucleation for benign or low-grade malignant lesions of the pancreas: single-center experience with 65 consecutive patients. *Surgery.* 2015;158(5):1203-1210. doi: 10.1016/j.surg.2014.10.008
14. Crippa S, Bassi C, Salvia R, Falconi M, Butturini G, Pederzoli P. Enucleation of pancreatic neoplasms. *Br J Surg.* 2007;94(10):1254-1259. doi: 10.1002/bjs.5833
15. Kaiser J, Fritz S, Klauss M, et al. A treatment alternative for branch duct intraductal papillary mucinous neoplasms. *Surgery.* 2017;161(3):602-610. doi: 10.1016/j.surg.2016.09.026
16. Kabir T, Tan ZZX, Syn N, Chung AYF, Ooi LLPJ, Goh BKP. Minimally-invasive versus open enucleation for pancreatic tumours: a propensity-score adjusted analysis. *Ann Hepatobiliary Pancreat Surg.* 2019;23(3):258-264. doi: 10.14701/ahbps.2019.23.3.258
17. Ore AS, Klompmaker S, Stackhouse K, et al. Does surgical approach affect outcomes of enucleation for benign and low-grade pancreatic tumors? An ACS-NSQIP evaluation. *HPB (Oxford).* 2019;21(11):1585-1591. doi: 10.1016/j.hpb.2019.03.375
18. Hüttner FJ, Koessler-Ebs J, Hackert T, Ulrich A, Büchler MW, Diener MK. Meta-analysis of surgical outcome after enucleation versus standard resection for pancreatic neoplasms. *Br J Surg.* 2015;102(9):1026-1036. doi: 10.1002/bjs.9819
19. Bartolini I, Bencini L, Bernini M, et al. Robotic enucleations of pancreatic benign or low-grade malignant tumors: preliminary results and comparison with robotic demolitive resections. *Surg Endosc.* 2019;33(9):2834-2842. doi: 10.1007/s00464-018-6576-3
20. Giulianotti PC, Coratti A, Angelini M, et al. Robotics in general surgery: personal experience in a large community hospital. *Arch Surg.* 2003;138(7):777-784. doi: 10.1001/archsurg.138.7.777

SECTION VII

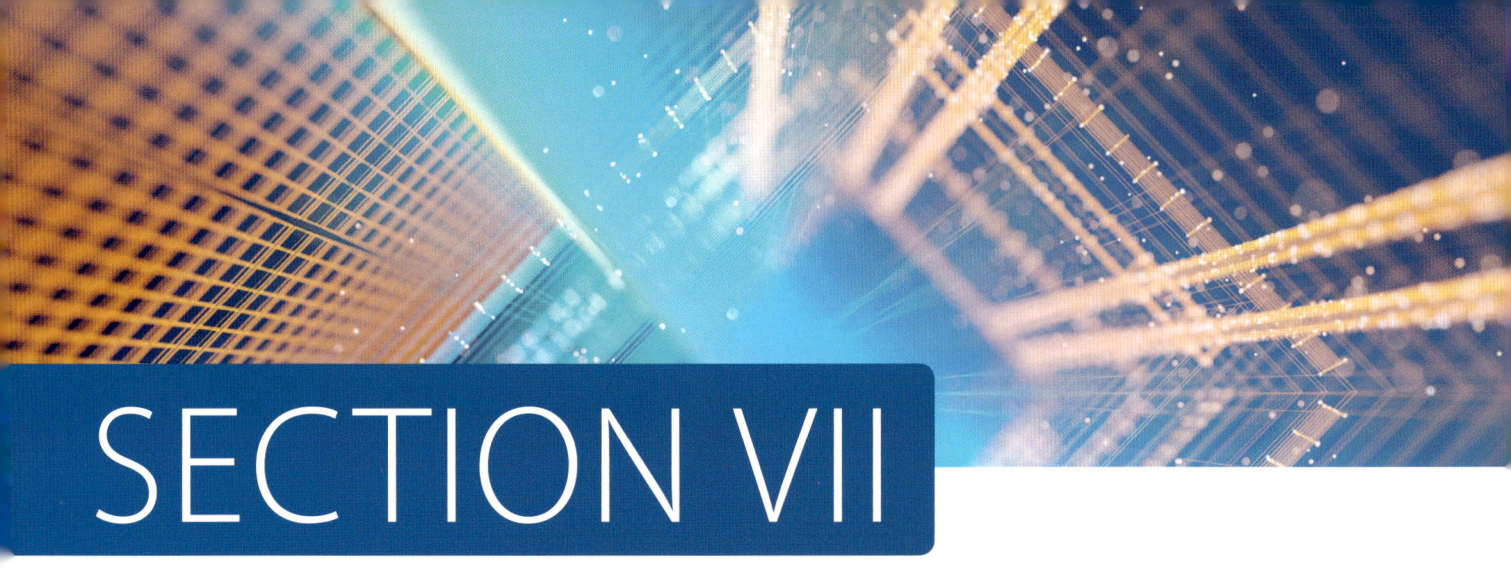

Liver Surgery

Chapter 33 • Right Hepatectomy 701
Eduardo Fernandes • Alberto Mangano • Valentina Valle • Pier Cristoforo Giulianotti

Chapter 34 • Left Hepatectomy 733
Antonio Cubisino • Carolina Baz • Nicolas Hellmuth Dreifuss • Pier Cristoforo Giulianotti

Chapter 35 • Liver Sectionectomies: Left Lateral Sectionectomy 755
Alberto Mangano • Valentina Valle • Pier Cristoforo Giulianotti

Chapter 36 • Segmental and Atypical Liver Resections 769
Francesco Guerra • Carolina Baz • Alberto Patriti

"The benefits of minimally invasive surgery for malignancy are negated if proper oncologic resection is compromised."
—Brice Gayet (1949)

Right Hepatectomy

Eduardo Fernandes • Alberto Mangano • Valentina Valle • Pier Cristoforo Giulianotti

INTRODUCTION

Minimally invasive liver surgery has historically been a niche subspecialty. In the past, the high technical demand and the lack of familiarity of the hepato-pancreato-biliary (HPB) and transplant specialists with minimally invasive techniques have relegated this field to a handful of surgeons. In more recent times, early training opportunities to develop laparoscopic and robotic skills have significantly changed the *status quo*, fostering an increase in popularity of robotic HPB surgery. For the vast majority of liver resections, including right and left hepatectomies, a minimally invasive approach is currently considered the standard of care.

In this section of the book, the basic principles of robotic liver surgery will be illustrated. A detailed description of the most commonly performed liver resections will be provided, and a standardized approach to robotic right hepatectomy will be described.

A fundamental prerequisite to a safe approach to liver surgery is an accurate and in-depth knowledge of liver anatomy (**Figures 33-1** and **33-2**).

INSTRUMENT REQUIREMENTS

The suggested main robotic instruments/tools can be listed as follows:
- 30° scope or 0° scope (the latter in very few cases when the surgical field is very deep. See Chapter 2, The Basic Principles of Clinical Applications.)
- Needle drivers (round tip or macro)
- Cautery hook/monopolar scissors
- Harmonic shears/vessel sealer (subcortical layer parenchyma transection)
- Robotic linear staplers (with different loads, for the core layer of parenchymal transection)
- Multiple Hem-o-lok™ clips
- Medium/large clip-applier
- Bipolar forceps
- Long-tip forceps
- Cadière forceps

The suggested main laparoscopic instruments/tools can be listed as follows:
- Needle drivers
- Scissors
- Graspers
- Staplers (with different loads)
- Suction-irrigation
- Laparoscopic ultrasound (drop-in probe or handheld laparoscopic)

Supplemental materials:
- Gauzes, sponges
- Penrose drains
- Vessel loops
- Endobags™
- Hem-o-lok®
- Sutures: Vicryl™ 3-0, silk 3-0, Prolene™ 2-0, 3-0, 4-0, and 5-0

Photo reproduced with permission from Dr. Brice Gayet.
Quote reproduced with permission from Gayet B, Cavaliere D, Vibert E, et al. Totally laparoscopic right hepatectomy. Am J Surg. 2007;194(5):685-689.

Indications and Relative Contraindications to the Robotic Approach

Like in any surgical procedure, the patient's selection is of paramount importance. There are currently no absolute contraindications to robotic liver resections; rather, the indication to these procedures should be based on a surgeon's skills and experience. Particular attention in weighting risks and benefits of a robotic liver resection should be paid in the following circumstances:

1. Tumor invasion of major vascular structures. These types of resections are possible, but require high levels of skills and should be approached only by very experienced surgeons.
2. Bulky lesions that involve the diaphragm, especially in its posterior portion in proximity to the vena cava.
3. Presence of multiple lesions where hybrid techniques of resection are necessary. In cases where many parenchymal sparing resections, associated with multiple radiofrequency ablations throughout the liver are required, an open procedure is probably more suitable. An exception to these considerations is perhaps represented by large hemangiomas, which feature significant volume reduction after arterial blood supply is interruption.
4. Patients' conditions can also preclude safe performance of robotic liver surgery. Individuals with cardiorespiratory comorbidities, who are unfit for major surgery, should not be offered a robotic procedure either.

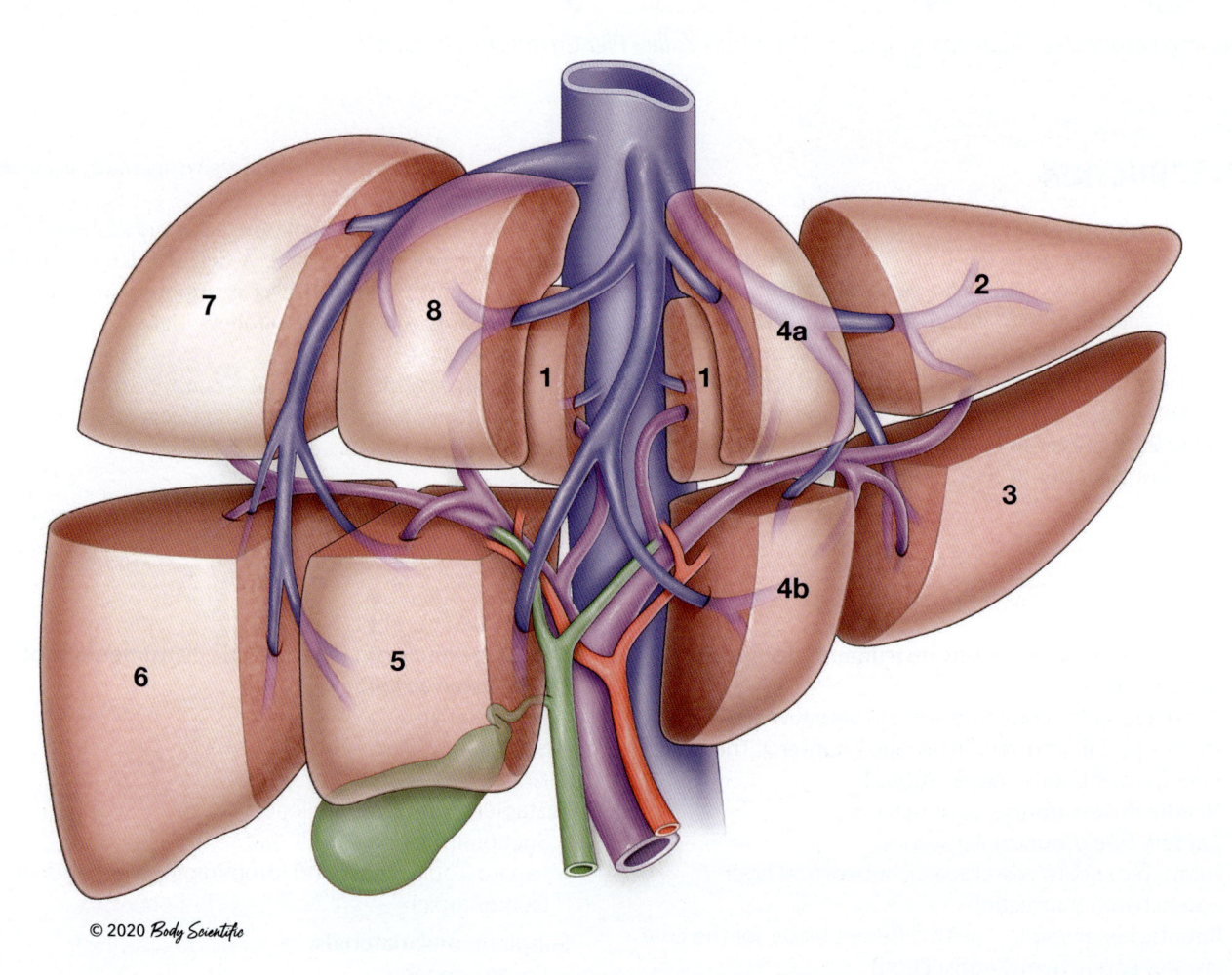

FIGURE 33-1 • Segmental liver anatomy.

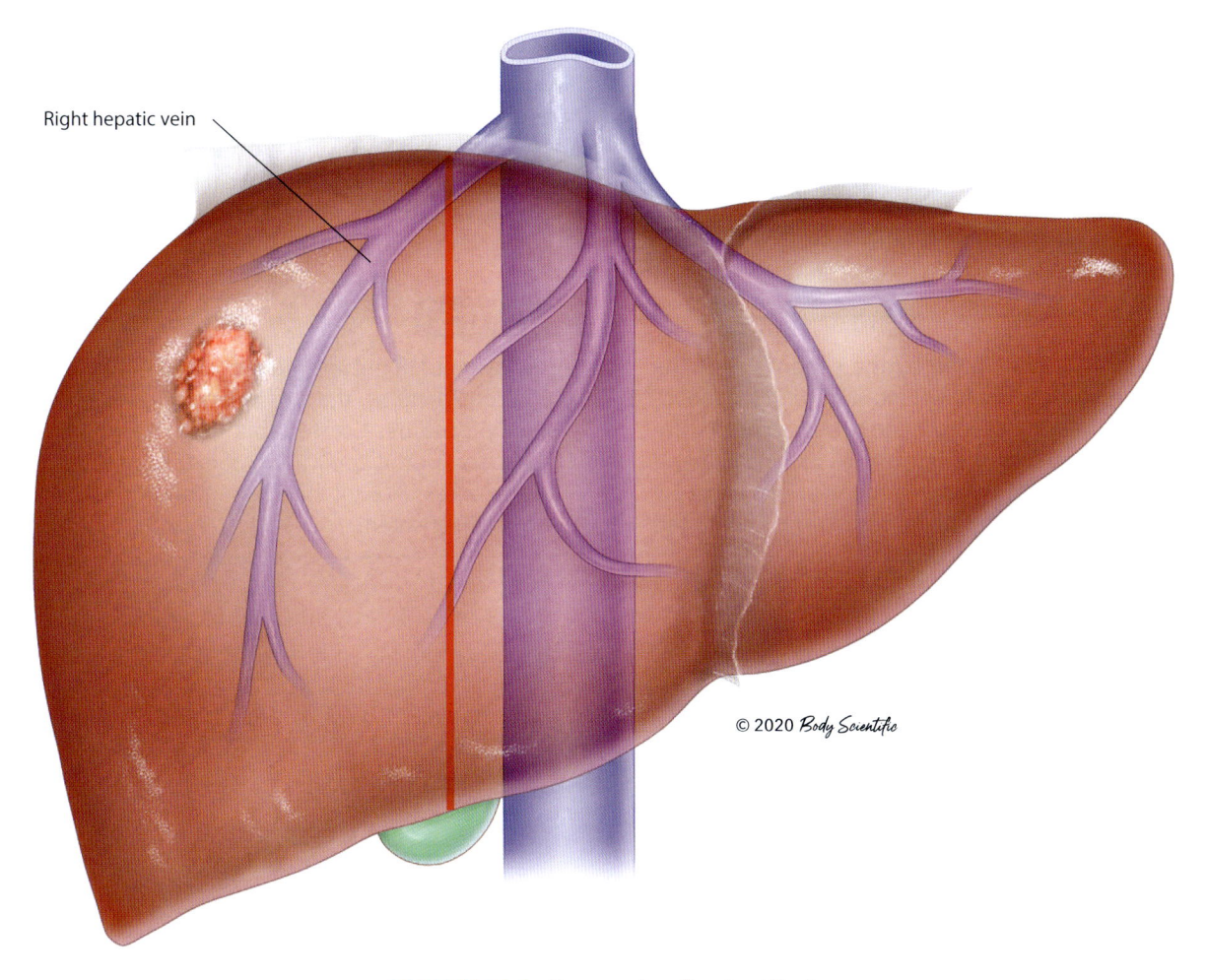

FIGURE 33-2 • Transection line (red line).

Robotic Right Hepatectomy – Surgical Technique

▶ **Video 33-1. Right Hepatectomy – Full Procedure**

Patient Positioning, OR Setup, and Port Setting

The patient positioning (**Figure 33-3**) reflects the one described for all the major foregut robotic procedures. The patient is placed supine, with arms tucked and parted legs. A 30° reverse-Trendelenburg tilt is important to prevent crowding of any hollow organs in the right upper quadrant. The table is tilted slightly toward the left, which provides a more effective retraction of the left lobe as the parenchyma is transected (Step 3). The assistant surgeon is positioned between the patient's legs (**Figure 33-4**).

Pneumoperitoneum is achieved with a Veress needle at the modified Palmer's point. A 5-mm VisiPort™ is placed in the left upper quadrant, which is later upgraded to a robotic trocar. Intra-abdominal exploration is carried out to rule out adhesions and peritoneal tumor extension and to assess the general position of the liver within the right upper quadrant. As per any other robotic procedure, the strategy of trocar placement is important for the success of the operation.

The ports are positioned transversally along a line 5 cm above the transumbilical one (**Figure 33-5**). This setting can and must be adjusted for patients with atypical body habitus.

The camera trocar is positioned on the right midclavicular line along the inferior vena cava axis. The remaining trocar placement is detailed in **Figure 33-5**. A 12-mm assistant port is positioned in between the R1 and the scope. Frequently, this can be hidden around the umbilical scar. The assistant trocar can be utilized for stapling, retraction, suction, and irrigation. An additional 5-mm assistant port (upgradable to a 12 mm if needed) is also placed in between the scope and the R2 (**Figure 33-5**).

▶▶ **TIPS**

The vision cart is positioned by the patient's feet. The wires/suction tubes should not interfere with the movements of the bedside assistant and the scrub nurse. The latter is positioned to the left of the patient to hand instruments onto the bedside surgeon's right hand. By doing so, it is natural that the robotic cart is positioned on the patient's right (**Figure 33-4**).

▶▶ **TIPS**

The overall OR setup (**Figure 33-4**) should also take into consideration the possibility of conversion to an open procedure. Comfortable robotic cart maneuvering, space for the application of external retractors, and ease of access to all of the open surgery armamentarium should be ensured.

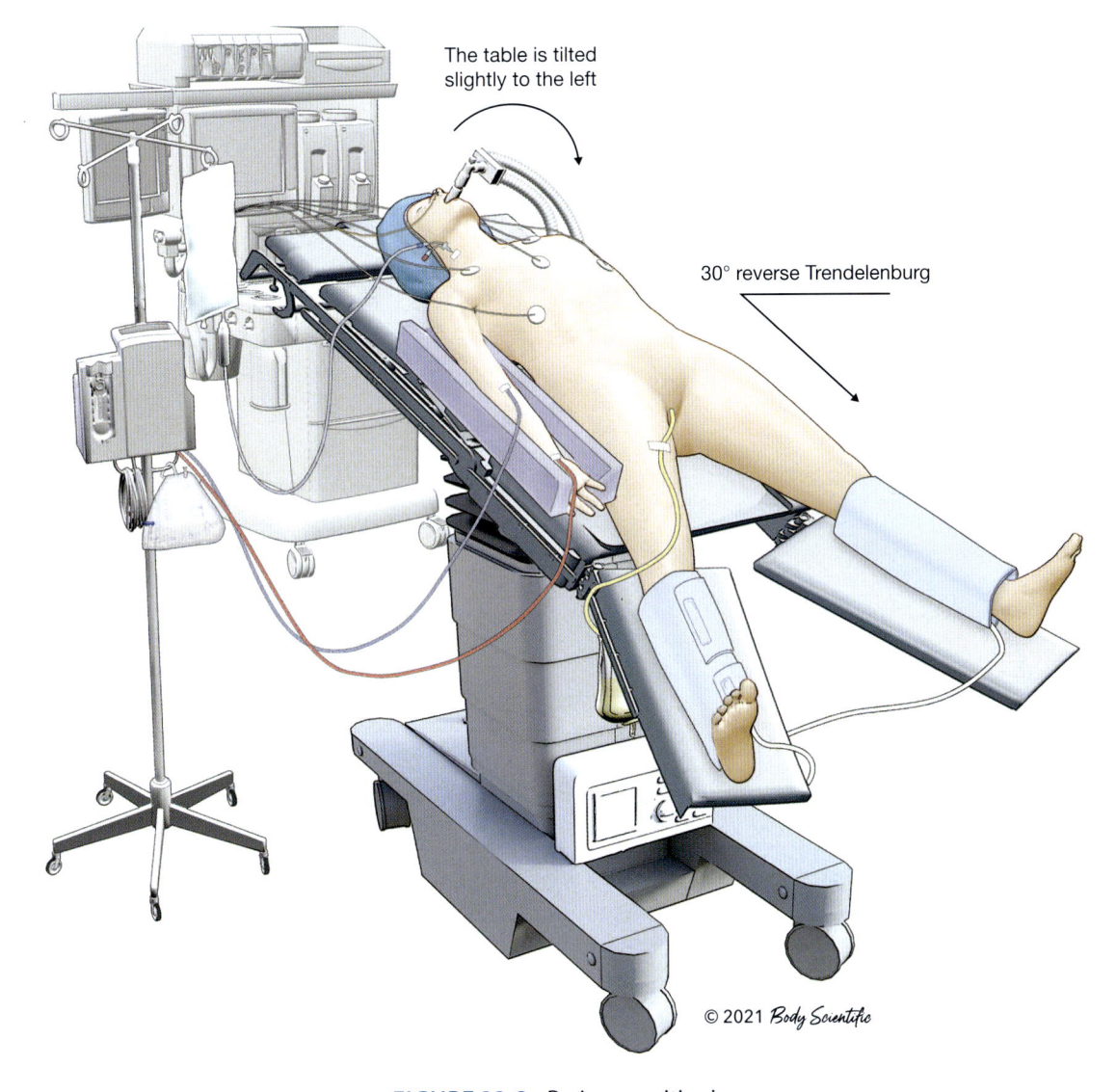

FIGURE 33-3 • Patient positioning.

706 The Foundation and Art of Robotic Surgery

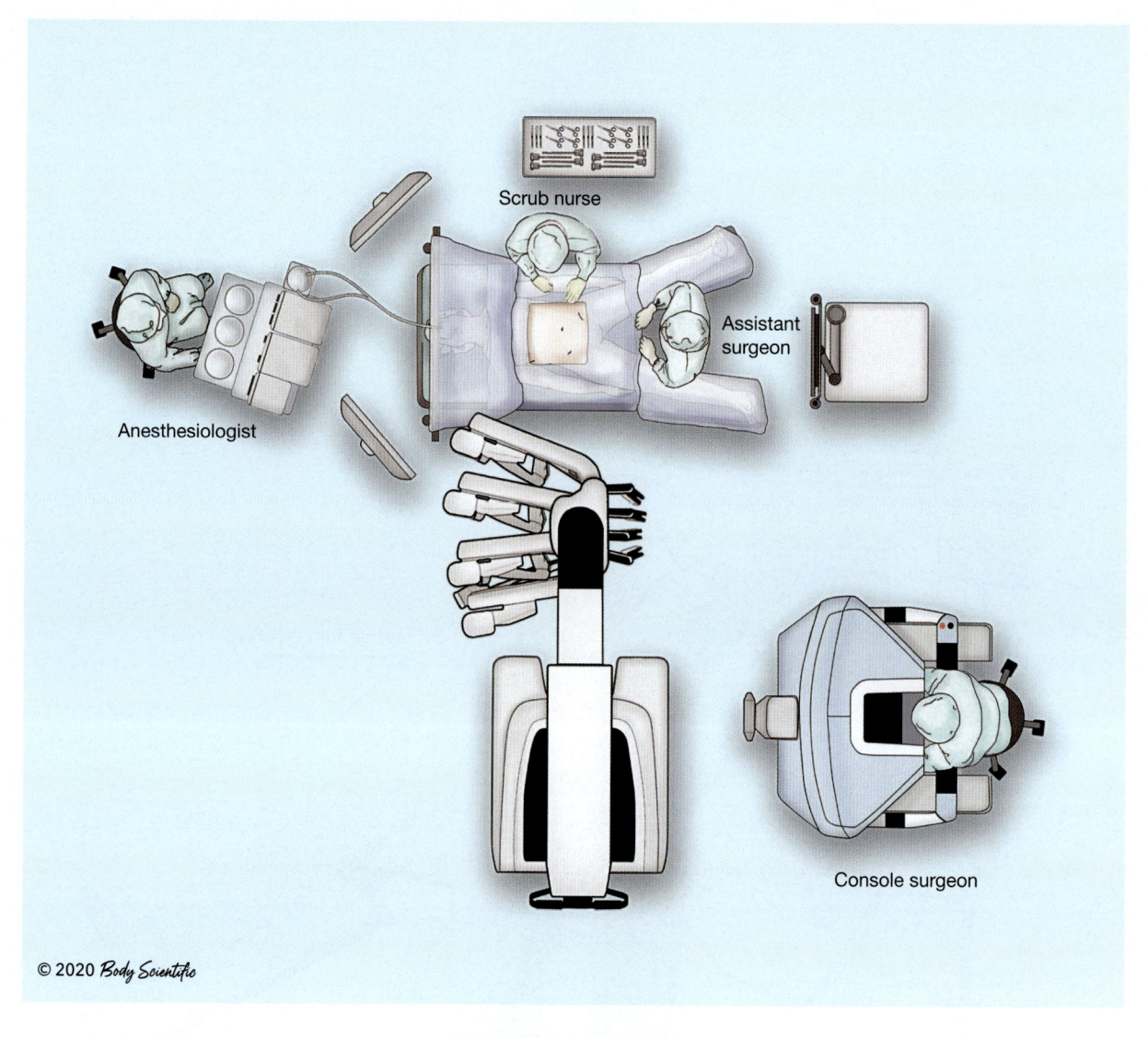

FIGURE 33-4 • OR setup.

▶▶ TIPS

The position of the camera trocar is very important. The best strategy to achieve both a perfect vision and control of the surgical field is a 45° angle between the shaft of the camera/instruments and the target anatomy. Greater angles (90°/perpendicular) would cause loss of perception of the field depth, while smaller angles (30°) would create an excessive tangential view (see Chapter 2, The Basic Principles of Clinical Applications, for additional details).

R3 has important retracting functions during hilar dissection, liver mobilization, and parenchymal transection. It should not be placed too parallel to the lower edge of the liver, because this setting would cause difficulties when retracting the right lobe during the hepatocaval dissection. It should be a compromise according to the step. R3 positioning too high or too low should be avoided.

When dissecting the coronary ligament, the R3 can be used to gently press down the dome of the liver and facilitate the dissection of the paracaval portion of the ligament. This allows to divide the reflection of the peritoneum between the vena cava and the liver.

🔍 ANATOMICAL HIGHLIGHTS

Certain patients, especially the ones with an "hourglass body" habitus (**Figure 33-6**), present a "low" costal margin that lies low over the inferior edge of the liver. When that is the case, there is limited space between the liver and the chest wall upon induction of the pneumoperitoneum (the rib cage is rigid and doesn't expand). The end result of this situation is a very difficult anterior retraction of the liver making its mobilization difficult. This occurrence must be recognized, and may sometimes require to adapt the position of the trocars, decrease the pneumoperitoneum, or even an early open conversion.

Normal abdomen

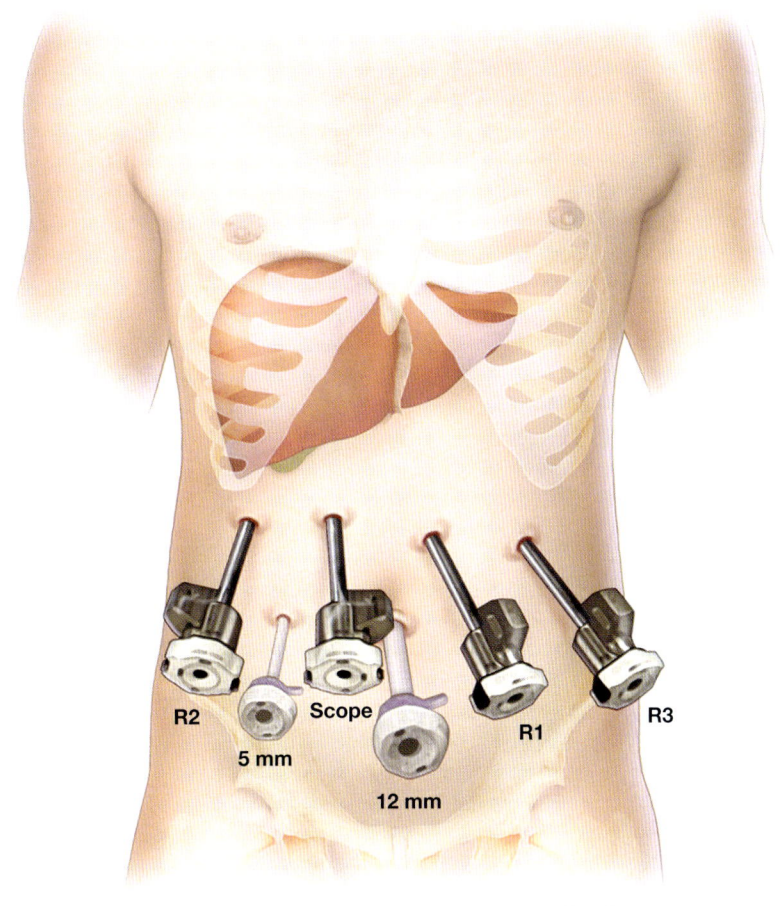

FIGURE 33-5 • Trocar positioning.

Step 1. Dissection of the falciform ligament and intraoperative ultrasound

The initial steps of the procedure should aim to evaluate the feasibility of the operation and to make an adequate surgical plan. In case of malignancy, peritoneal extension of the disease would have been determined at the initial laparoscopy. To facilitate the process, the falciform ligament is usually divided (**Figure 33-7**) and the intraoperative ultrasound (IOU) is carried out (**Figure 33-8**). Although it is beyond the scope of this chapter to describe in details IOU techniques, it is well known that it is important to learn the anatomical relationship of the target lesion with any of the segmental pedicles, the portal vein, hepatic artery, hepatic vein, and the major communicating branches.

The minimally invasive surgery (MIS) ultrasound technique is more difficult to master than the open one. In particular, interventional procedures involving three-dimensional targeting, such as laparoscopic biopsies or radiofrequency ablations, are more challenging in MIS compared to open surgery.

When performing these procedures in MIS, two types of IOU devices are available:

1. "Drop in" robotic probes. These are small probes with a flexible cable that can be controlled by the surgeon at the console.
2. Handheld laparoscopic probes. These devices have a rigid shaft with a flexible head and are generally maneuvered by the assistant surgeon.

It is far preferable to use the console surgeon-driven IOU probes, because they allow the ultrasound to be performed directly by the operating (and likely more expert) surgeon, who can map, with the assistance of the "tile pro" function, the target anatomy and plan the resection appropriately.

Step 1 average time frame: 5–10 min

708   The Foundation and Art of Robotic Surgery

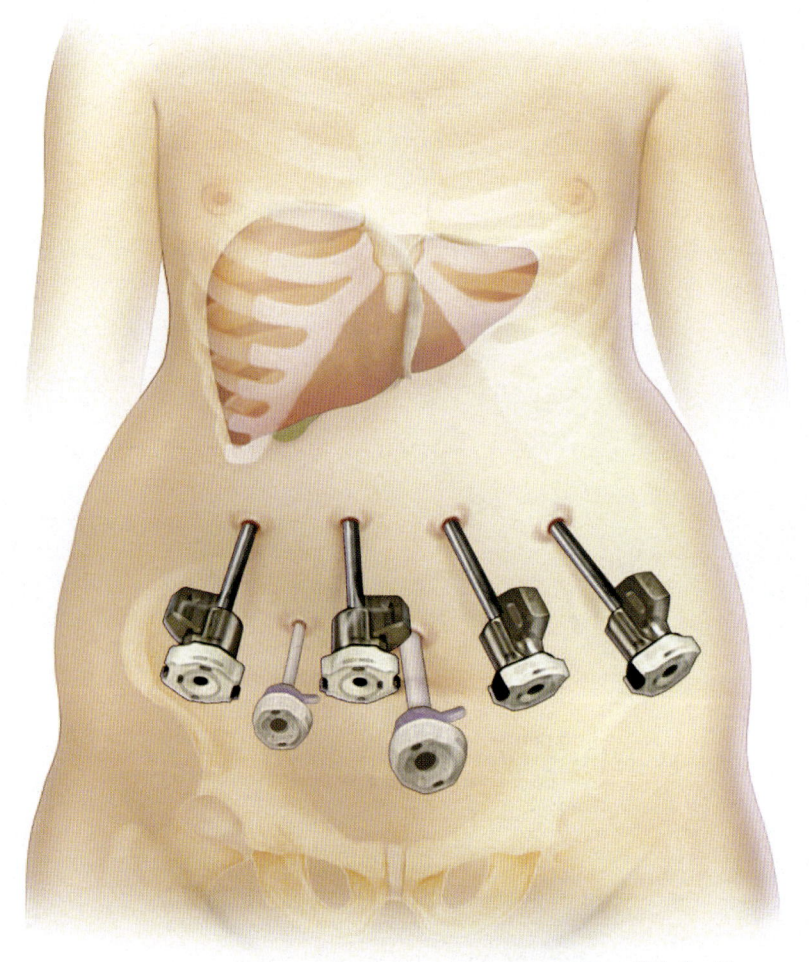

FIGURE 33-6 • Hourglass body habitus.

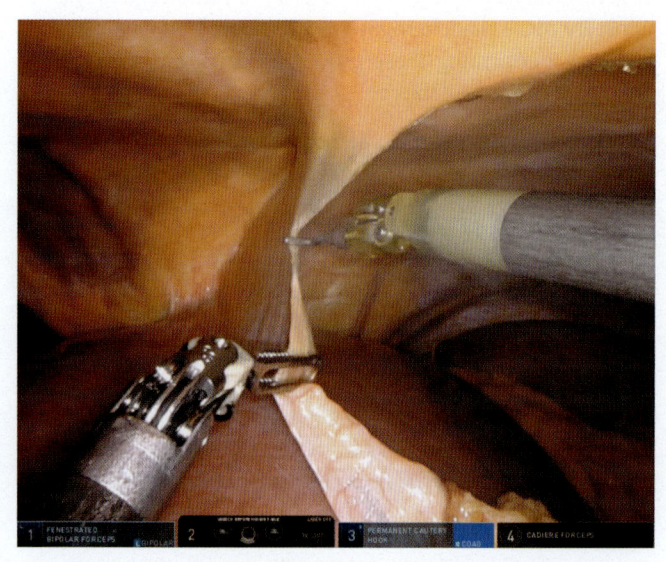

FIGURE 33-7 • Dissection of the falciform ligament.

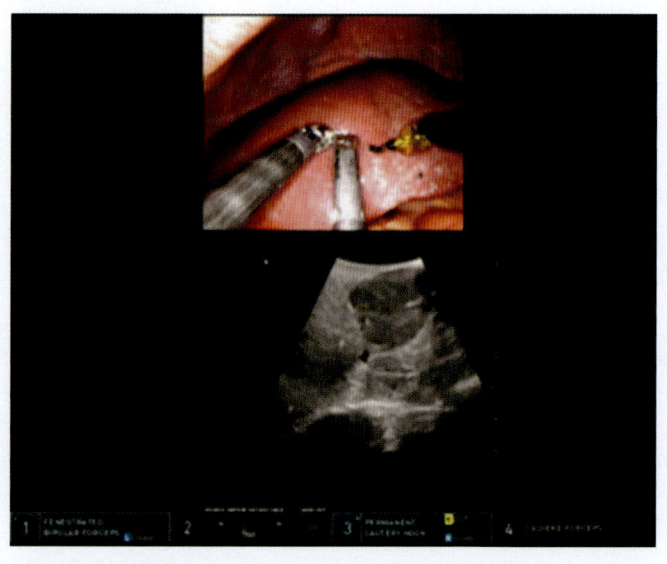

FIGURE 33-8 • Intraoperative ultrasound.

Steps of Hepatic Hilum Dissection

Step 2. Liver hilum exposure/evaluation and cholecystectomy

Exposure of the hilum (**Figure 33-9**) is obtained with the upward traction of segment 4b by the R3 over a sponge. An indocyanine green (ICG) cholangiogram may be helpful, at this point, for exploring the hilum (**Figures 33-10 A, B**) and in identifying anatomical biliary variations. The ICG iv injection is made at least 1 hour in advance before starting the operation in order to maximize the visualization of the bile ducts (see Chapter 7, Fluorescence Imaging: Basics and Clinical Applications, for more information).

A cholecystectomy is carried out. The cystic duct is ligated with Vicryl™ 3-0 ties and divided. The stump is kept long to facilitate traction (by the assistant surgeon or the R3) (**Figure 33-11**) and exposure of the more posterior hilar structures (portal vein, retroportal lymph nodes). The dissection proceeds with extreme care with the monopolar hook, which is the best instrument for this step (see Chapter 1, What Robotic Surgery Is, and Chapter 2, The Basic Principles of Clinical Applications), and also the bipolar cautery when necessary. The lower edge of segment 4b is dissected off the higher portion of the hilum exposing the bile duct bifurcation (lowering of the plate).

Step 2 average time frame: 10–15 min

▶ **Video 33-2. Step 2. Retraction of the Cystic Duct**

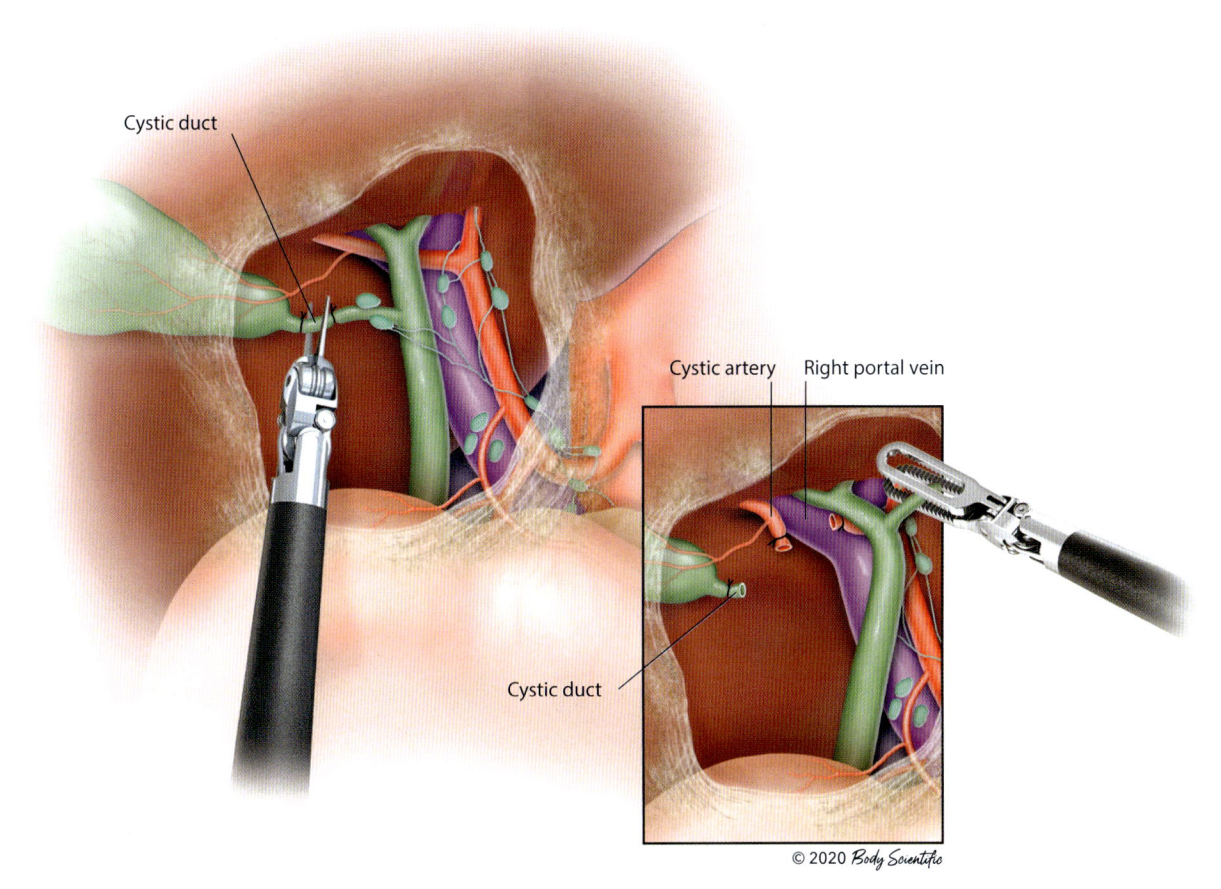

FIGURE 33-9 • Hilum exposure.

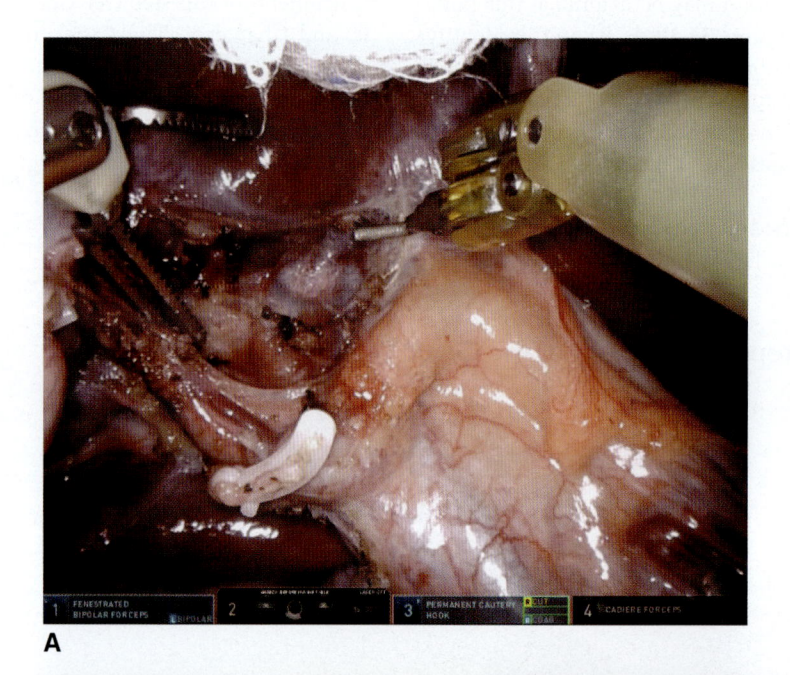

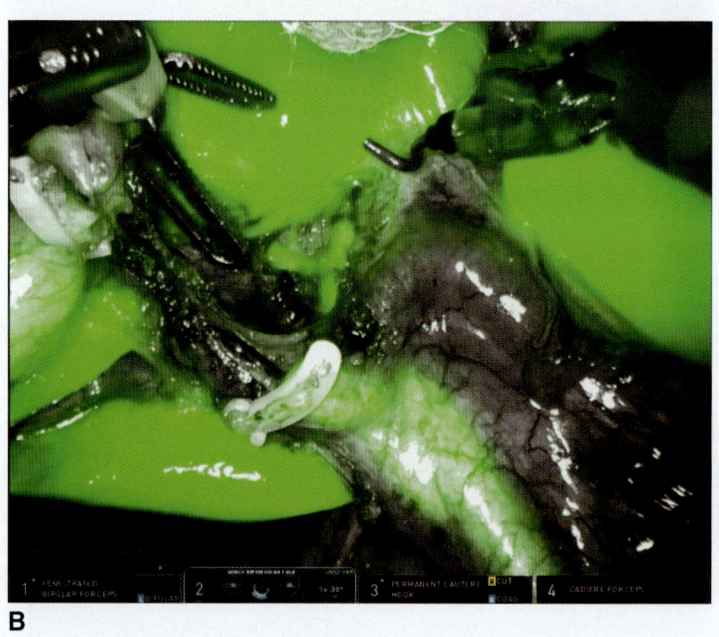

FIGURE 33-10 • ICG during hilum exploration.

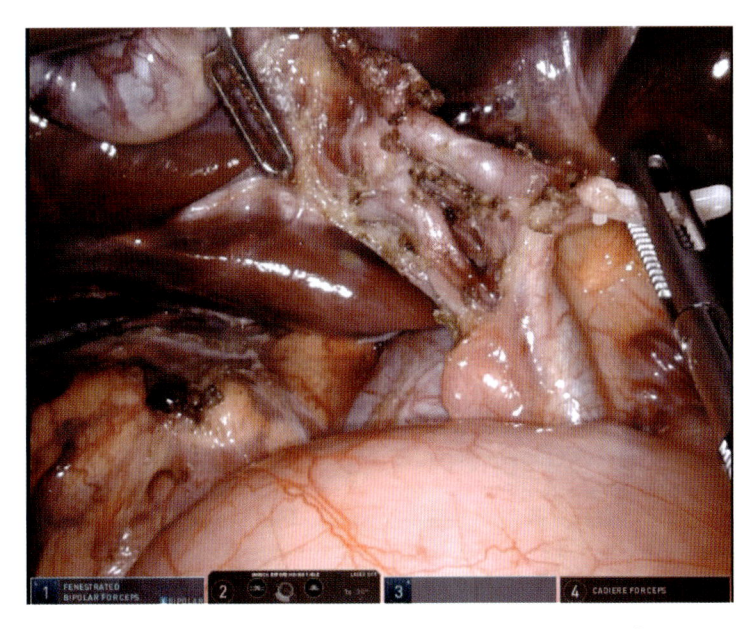

FIGURE 33-11 • Retraction maneuver on the cystic duct.

▶▶ **TIPS**

The right colonic flexure is mobilized if adhesions with the liver are encountered. Moreover, if the anatomy of the flexure is interfering with a proper visualization, the vena cava must be exposed, and a partial Kocher maneuver may be necessary.

The common bile duct should not be manipulated with traumatic robotic instruments, because they can cause significant damage.

In case of redo hilar dissection (e.g., following cholecystectomy), when the cystic duct stump is not identifiable or too short, a good strategy is to pass a vessel loop around the common bile duct and use it for retraction.

▶▶ **TIPS**

The robotic hook is the ideal instrument for the hilar dissection. Its many degrees of freedom make it versatile in the dissection of delicate hilar structures. Application of energy while lifting the tissue prevents unwanted heat spread to lateral and deeper structures. It is safer than other instruments, also due to the small amount of tissue that can be handled at any one time (for more details, see Chapter 2, The Basic Principles of Clinical Applications).

▶▶ **TIPS**

Leaving the cystic duct stump long has a twofold advantage: (1) when retracted medially, it allows excellent exposure of the hilar deeper structures; and (2) it provides an easy point of access to the biliary tree when the cholangiography is needed.

ICG can be used to identify the biliary anatomy. When used in the "arterial phase," it is also useful in identifying arterial anatomy (for more details, see Chapter 7, Fluorescence Imaging: Basics and Clinical Applications).

Step 3. Hepatic artery

Multiple arterial anatomical variations can occur, and these should be borne in mind and recognized in good time (**Figure 33-12** and see the Anatomical Highlights box of this step. For additional information, see suggested readings #11, 14–16.)

The right hepatic artery (RHA) is dissected and skeletonized (**Figures 33-13 A–E**).

If the operation is performed for some malignant disease such as cholangiocarcinoma, the dissection around the proper and common hepatic artery is part of the procedure. On the contrary, it may not be required if the procedure is conducted for other diseases and the anatomy of the RHA is very clear. If the anatomy is unclear, the hepatic artery lymph nodes can be lifted off and removed, and the course of the common hepatic artery can be followed up to the bifurcation. Safe dissection of the artery takes place via the identification of a safe spot where it is possible to encircle the vessel with a soft vessel loop. The RHA is ligated with Prolene™ 3-0 or 4-0 and the transfixing technique is the preferred one. If the RHA is long enough, a vascular stapler (in particular, the 8-mm staplers with curved tip occupy less space) can be used (energy based devices [EBD] or clips should be avoided). Prior to the RHA ligation, the artery is clamped with a bulldog, and the Doppler signal on the left hepatic artery (LHA) is evaluated to ensure that good pulsatile flow is confirmed.

The presence of an accessory RHA arising from the superior mesenteric artery should be known preoperatively and its control must be achieved at this time. To this purpose, medial retraction on the cystic duct stump is exerted, and lymphatic tissue to the right of the bile duct is dissected until the artery is identified. It should also be kept in mind that additional anomalies may occur. These concerns the distribution of the RHA, which may supply segment 4b, or the fact that the RHA may be disproportionately larger than the LHA; the LHA may lie very lateral, or the hepatic artery bifurcation be very high. If there are any doubts, it is essential to dissect the vessel further and evaluate with the bulldog test the expected demarcation line. Notably, the demarcation line following arterial clamping takes several minutes to become evident, and it is more subtle than the demarcation line obtained following portal vein clamping. In case of doubt, IOU may clarify the anatomy.

Step 3 average time frame: 10–15 min

▶ **Video 33-3. Step 3. Right Hepatic Artery**

▶▶ TIPS

Artery manipulation (lifting/retraction) should always occur in an indirect fashion with a soft vessel loop. Grabbing the vessel directly with any robotic instruments may potentially result in formation of wall hematomas, dissection, or even rupture.

The use of clips, during hilar dissection, should be minimized for two reasons: (1) instability: metal/titanium clips are not stable enough to halt pressure on large arterial vessels, and they can easily slide off venous structures; and (2) need for stapling.

When stapling is used, especially in a semiemergency situation, previous clips may be caught in between the jaws of the stapler and cause misfiring.

🔍 ANATOMICAL HIGHLIGHTS

An accessory RHA must be promptly identified. With the cystic and common bile duct retracted medially, the lymphatic tissue to the right of the bile duct is carefully dissected, and the accessory artery identified. Several other arterial variations can occur, and multiple heterogenous classifications are available in the literature. (For additional information, see suggested readings #11, 14–16.)

In **Figure 33-12**, the most surgically relevant variations are reported. These should be remembered and recognized in good time.

Right Hepatectomy   713

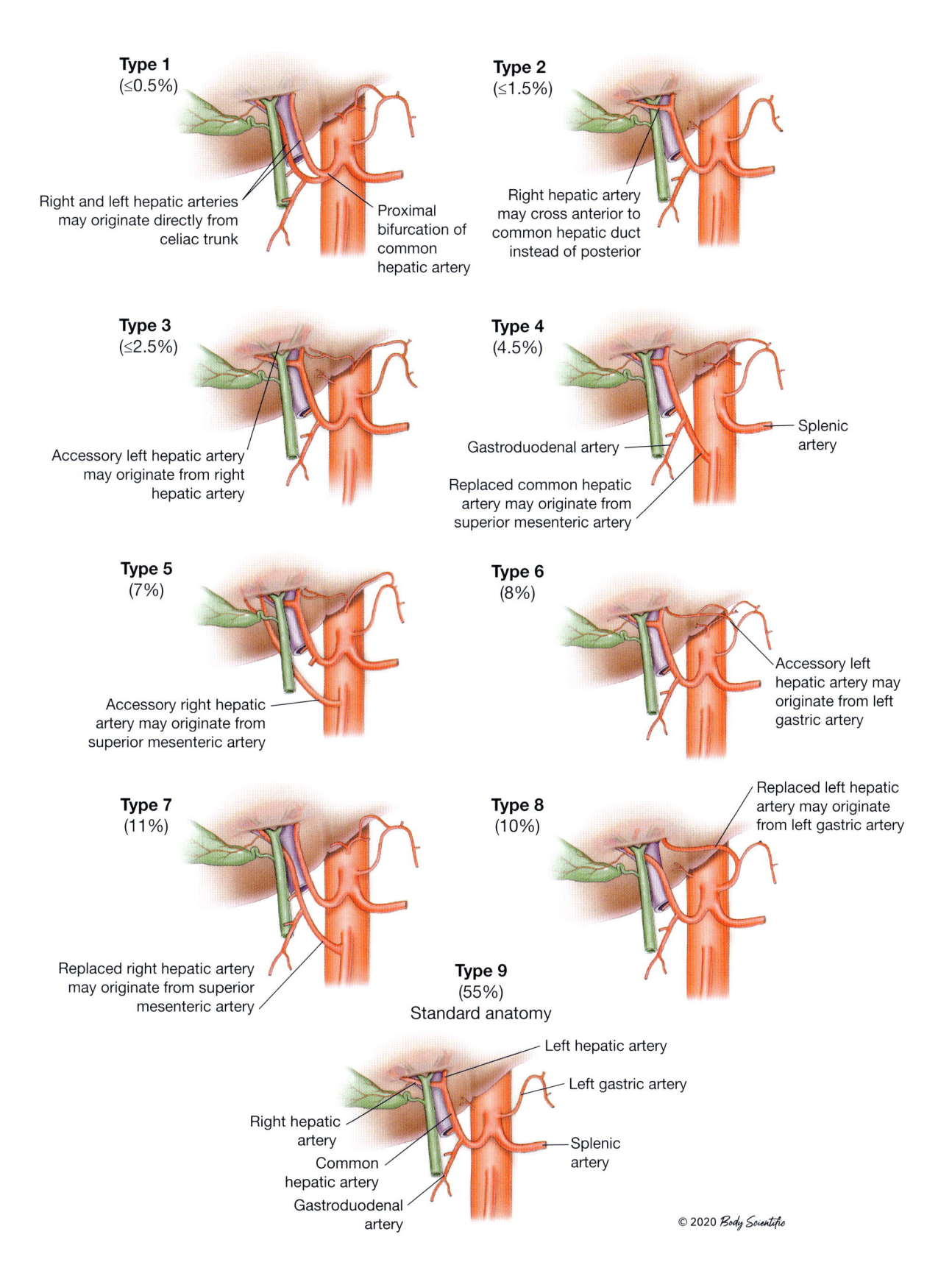

Type 1 (≤0.5%)
Right and left hepatic arteries may originate directly from celiac trunk
Proximal bifurcation of common hepatic artery

Type 2 (≤1.5%)
Right hepatic artery may cross anterior to common hepatic duct instead of posterior

Type 3 (≤2.5%)
Accessory left hepatic artery may originate from right hepatic artery

Type 4 (4.5%)
Gastroduodenal artery
Splenic artery
Replaced common hepatic artery may originate from superior mesenteric artery

Type 5 (7%)
Accessory right hepatic artery may originate from superior mesenteric artery

Type 6 (8%)
Accessory left hepatic artery may originate from left gastric artery

Type 7 (11%)
Replaced right hepatic artery may originate from superior mesenteric artery

Type 8 (10%)
Replaced left hepatic artery may originate from left gastric artery

Type 9 (55%)
Standard anatomy
Left hepatic artery
Left gastric artery
Right hepatic artery
Splenic artery
Common hepatic artery
Gastroduodenal artery

© 2020 Body Scientific

FIGURE 33-12 • Hepatic artery variations (**Types 1–9**).

714 The Foundation and Art of Robotic Surgery

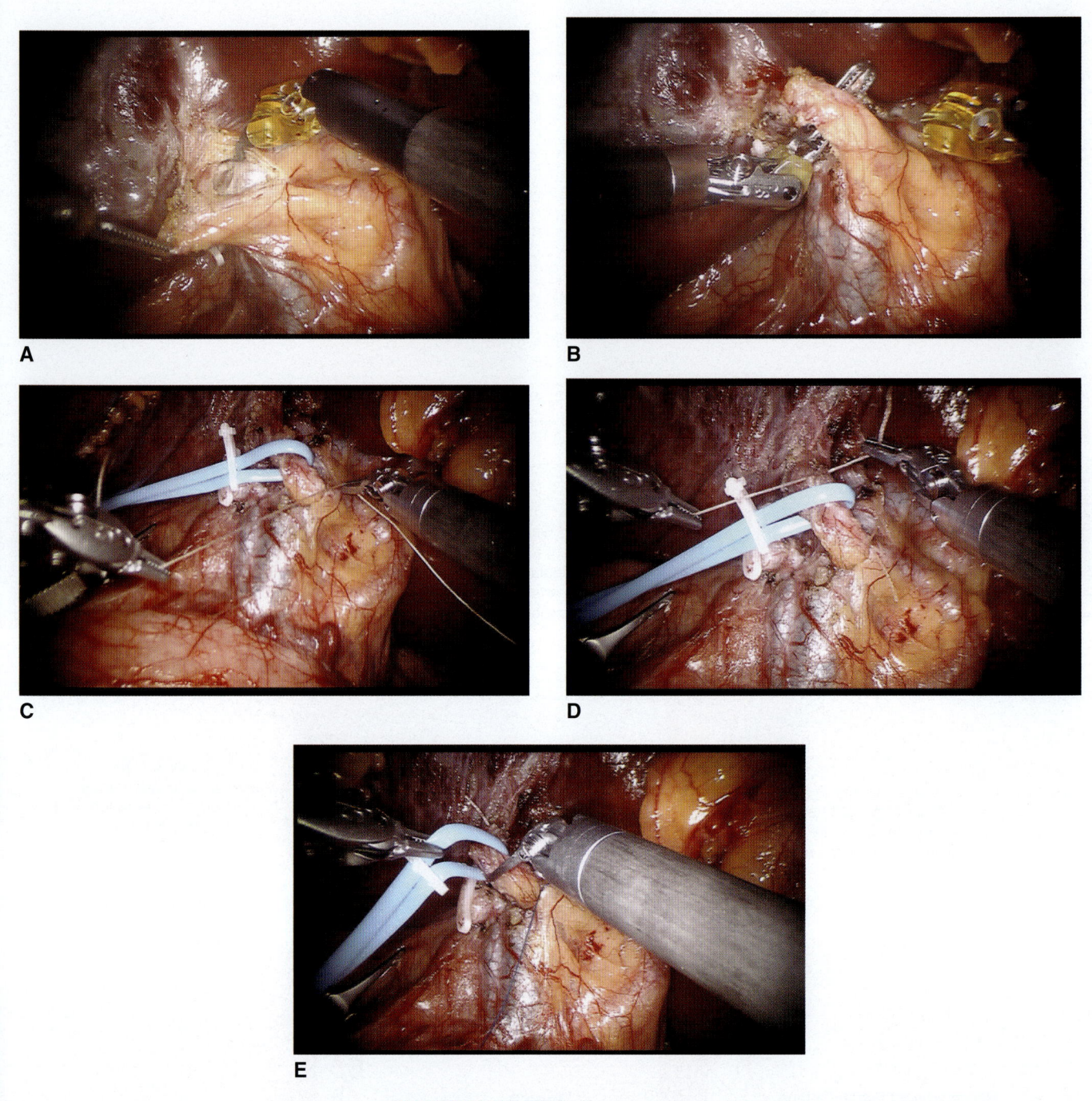

FIGURE 33-13 • Right hepatic artery.

Step 4. Portal vein

After the RHA has been ligated, traction on the cystic duct is applied medially to expose the portal vein and its bifurcation. Some degree of periportal lymph node dissection is required to expose the portal vein. This structure can have several anatomical variations with multiple heterogenous classifications available in the literature. The knowledge of these scenarios is essential. (For additional information, see suggested readings #17, 18.) In **Figure 33-14**, the most surgically relevant variations are reported.

The portal vein (**Figures 33-15 A–D**) is more resilient to robotic instrument manipulation; however, it still must be handled with extreme care, because damages, at this stage, result in bleeding that is potentially difficult to control. The portal vein is surrounded by areolar-lymphatic tissue. With prudent use of the hook and bipolar forceps, the periadventitial plane must be identified. After the correct plane is entered, additional dissection will allow the identification of the bifurcation and circumferential control of the right portal vein. This is encircled with a vessel loop. A long-tip forceps, that has longer jaws and a blunt smooth tip, is the ideal instrument to pass behind and around the right portal vein. This maneuver must be executed with extreme care in order to avoid damages to small portal branches, supplying segment 1 of the liver (**Figure 33-16**), which arise

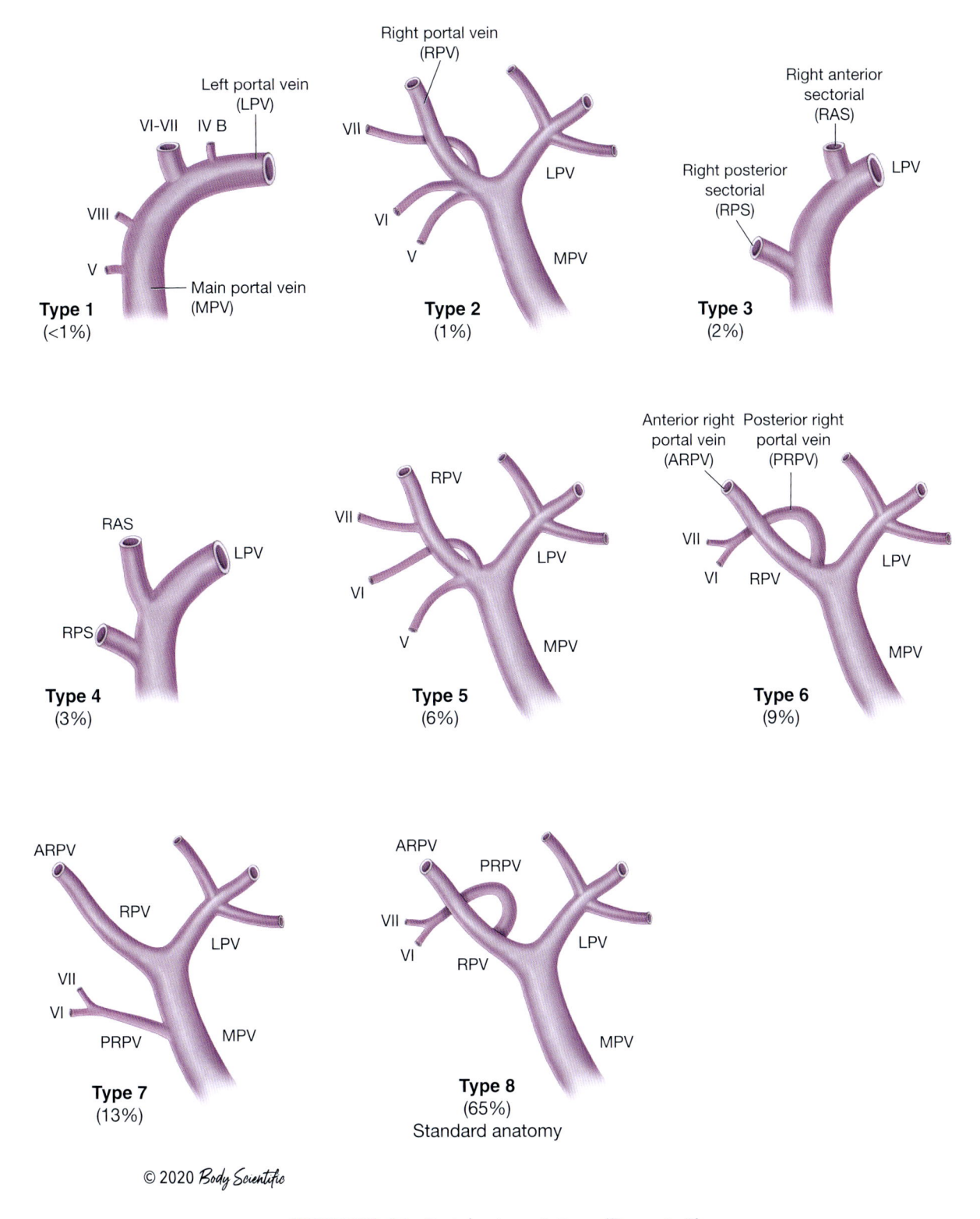

FIGURE 33-14 • Portal vein variations (Types 1–8).

from the posterior aspect of the right portal vein. Prior to the right portal vein ligation, it is necessary to gain additional length for a safe application of staple or sutures. In order to achieve this, it is often needed to divide one or two minor branches supplying the caudate lobe. Failure to do so may result in their avulsion and bleeding. The short length of these small vessels can make their control difficult. The best strategy is to start ligating these branches on the portal vein side. If additional space allows, the liver parenchymal end of the vessel can be ligated. If double ligation is not possible, the vessels can be divided without distal ligation. This will result in minimal bleeding from the parenchyma, which can be controlled with bipolar forceps. After these vessels are divided, additional sutures with Prolene™ 4-0 or 5-0 can be applied to the stump on the portal vein side for additional safety.

716 The Foundation and Art of Robotic Surgery

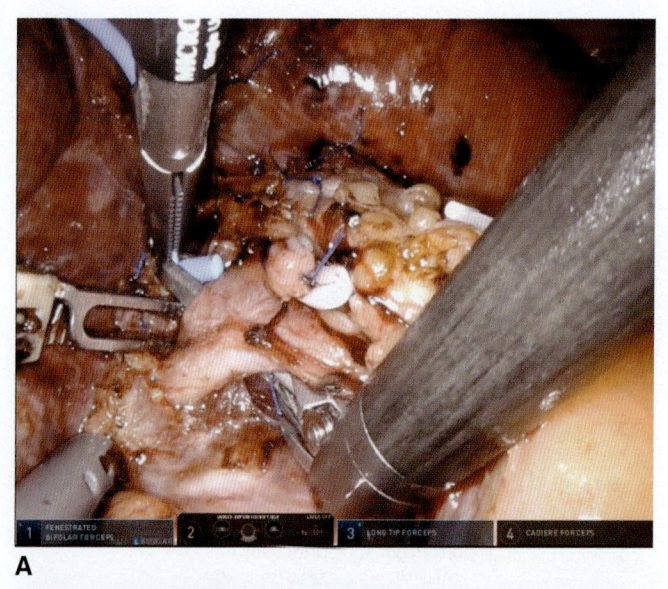

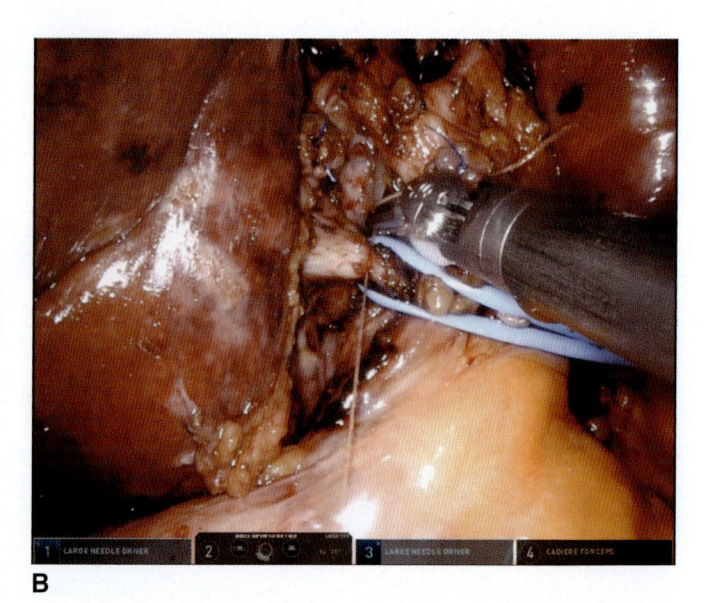

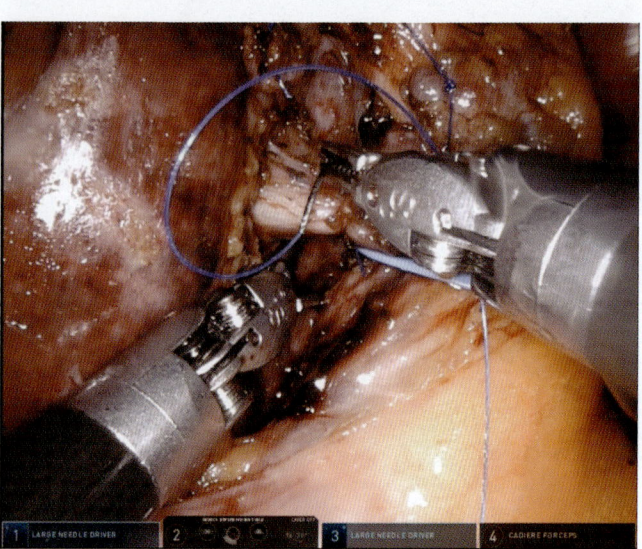

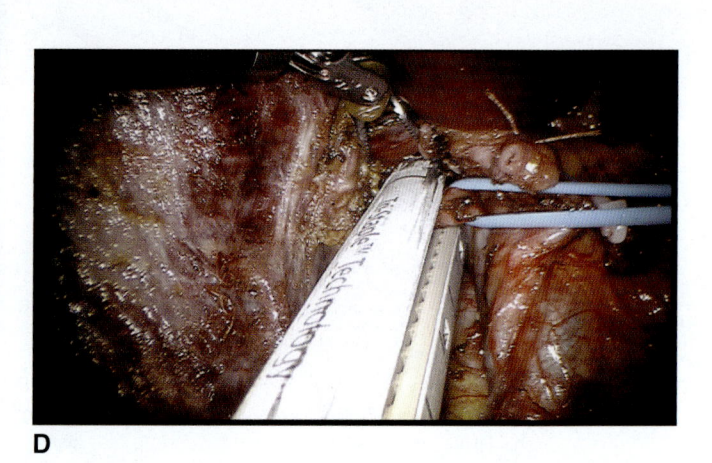

FIGURE 33-15 • Portal vein.

Before proceeding to the right portal vein ligation, a bulldog clamp can be applied to ensure that the line of demarcation obtained correlates with the right hepatic lobe. Portal vein anomalies may result in incomplete or excessive amount of ischemic parenchyma. After having ensured that this is not the case, the right portal vein ligation can take place.

Step 4 average time frame: 20–30 min

> ### 🔎 ANATOMICAL HIGHLIGHTS
> The portal vein anatomical variations can trick even the most experienced surgeon. This situation should be recognized via IOU or preop imaging. A bulldog clamp must be applied on the vein prior to ligation and the demarcation line should be evaluated.

▶ **Video 33-4.** Step 4. Right Portal Vein Ligation

▶ **Video 33-5.** Step 4. Right Portal Vein Stapler

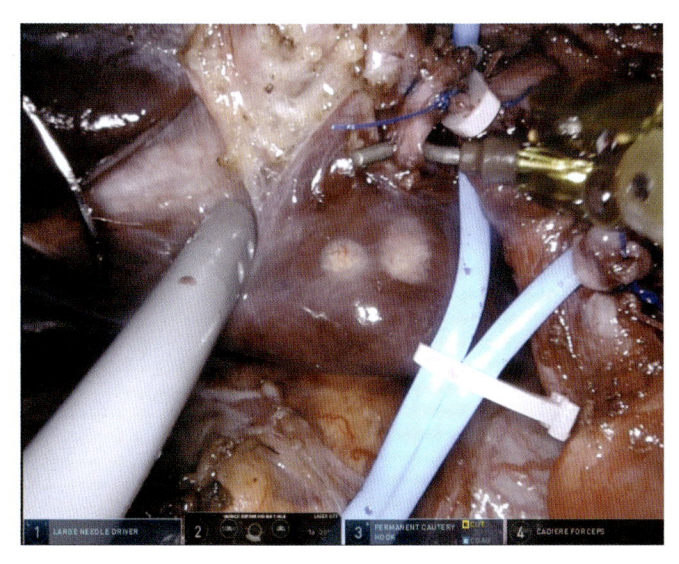

FIGURE 33-16 • Portal vein. Control of small branches for S1.

> **▶▶ TIPS**
>
> The portal vein ligation poses some challenges that are worth explaining. The right portal vein is a short vessel with high flow. Tout-court transfixion can result in significant bleeding through the needle hole. The best way to a safe right portal vein ligation is to start with the application of a simple Vicryl™ or silk 3-0 tie. After the inflow has been interrupted, an additional transfixion stitch can be applied proximally and distally. Only then, can the vein be divided.
>
> Stapling is also a very safe option. When doing so, an adequate length of the vessel should be exposed. Failure to do so may result in tearing of the vein or narrowing of portal vein bifurcation with onset of portal hypertension. An 8-mm vascular stapler with curved tip is a good fit for the space.

Step 5. Right hepatic duct

The right hepatic duct anatomical variations have to be carefully identified; the most clinically significant ones are represented in **Figure 33-17**. (Several other variations can occur, and different classifications are available; for additional information, see suggested readings #20, 21.)

After arterial and portal vein dissection and ligation, the right hepatic duct (**Figures 33-18 A–F**) should be identified. An ICG cholangiogram provides additional help in anatomy identification. The right hepatic duct can be a source of complications (bile leak or strictures of the left duct); therefore, extrahepatic ligation should only be used in cases where (1) no anatomical abnormalities are present and (2) the biliary anatomy is very clear.

In all other cases, especially in the presence of a high bifurcation, the right hepatic duct ligation should be done intracapsularly at the hilar plate during parenchymal transection. Damage to segment 1 drainage ducts should be avoided during this step.

Step 5 average time frame: 15–20 min

▶ Video 33-6. Step 5. Right Hepatic Duct

Step 6. Hepatocaval dissection

The mobilization of the liver is performed at different stages of the operation. A preliminary step consisting in the (at least partial) mobilization of the right triangular and coronary ligaments is carried out, at the beginning of the procedure, to facilitate the assessment of posterior lesions or other anatomically challenging situations (e.g., evaluation of vena cava infiltration of paracaval lesions).

When mobilizing the liver, stable anterior retraction with the R3 over a sponge should be applied to the parenchyma. As the right lobe is retracted upward (anteriorly), hook diathermy is used to dissect the areolar tissue between the liver and the vena cava. Posteriorly, the liver is dissected off the Gerota's fascia. Continuing the dissection superiorly, the adrenal gland and the lateral aspect of the inferior vena cava are encountered. During the dissection, many small tributaries draining directly into the vena are identified. These should be individually ligated with 4-0 or 5-0 braided ties and reinforced with transfixing Prolene™ 4/0 or 5/0 sutures on the cava side. Larger accessory veins draining segments 5, 6, or 7 can be also encountered at times. Is it important to secure these vessels with suture ligation and Hem-o-lok® application (**Figures 33-19 A–F**). After ligation of one or more accessory hepatic veins, there will be an increasing amount of space between the liver parenchyma and the vena cava.

In 70–80% of patients, due to the caudate lobe anatomy that presents a bridge of tissue anterior to the vena cava, it may be difficult to freely open the hepatocaval space. In these circumstances, the caudate lobe and the antecaval tissue can be partially split with an energy-based device. This will provide additional room for maneuvering/retraction/exposure (**Figures 33-20 A–D**).

A complete liver mobilization is achievable in most cases. In ideal circumstances, the entire right lobe of the liver is mobilized and the hepatocaval dissection has been able to free the anterior portion of the vena cava, such that it is possible to create a tunnel between the right and middle hepatic vein anterior to the vena cava. In these instances, it is possible to predispose the classical hanging maneuver (**Figures 33-21 A, B**).

Depending on several factors such as liver size, its relationship to the patient's abdominal conformation, and its

718 The Foundation and Art of Robotic Surgery

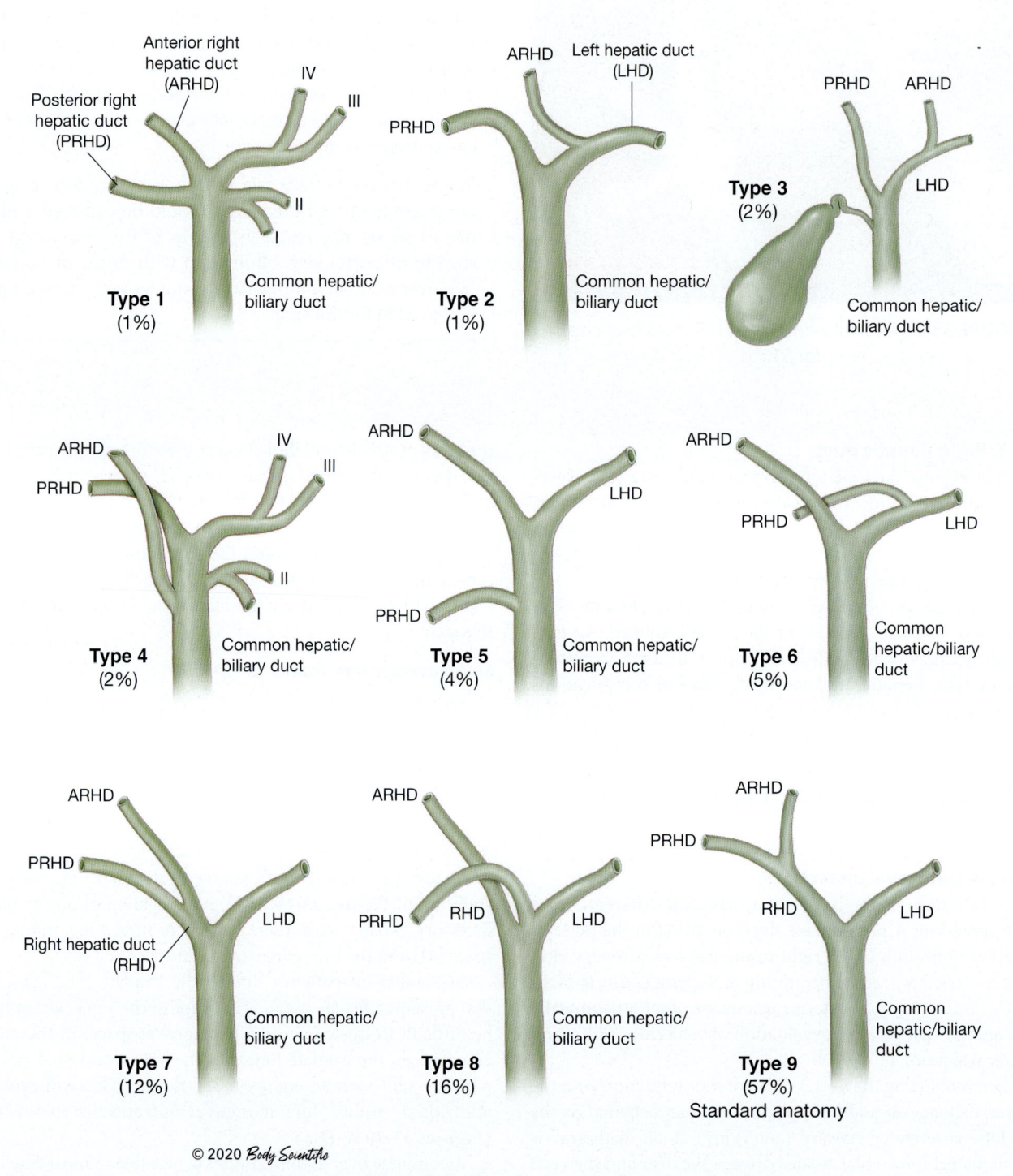

FIGURE 33-17 • Right hepatic duct anatomical variations (**Types 1–9**).

Right Hepatectomy 719

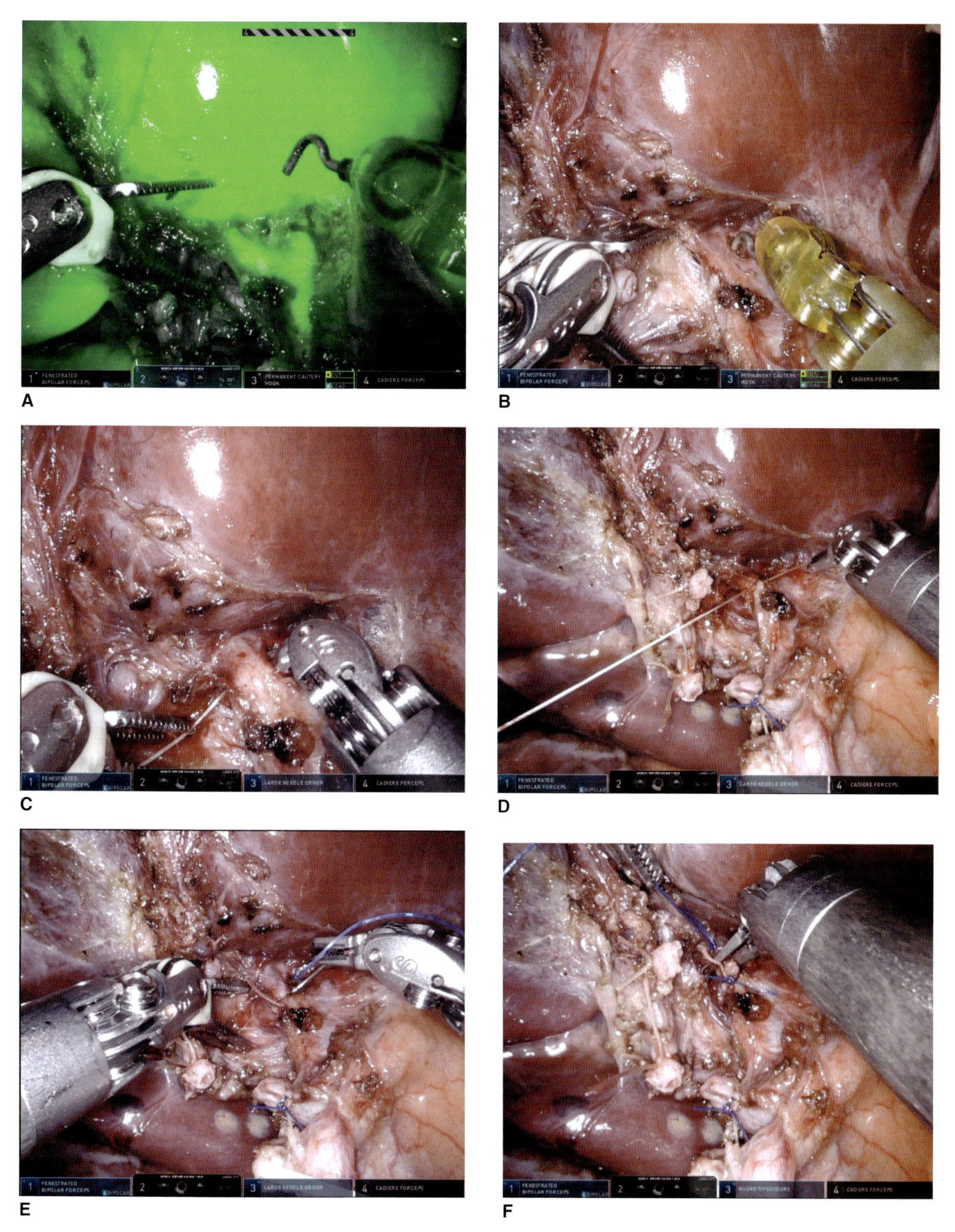

FIGURE 33-18 • Step 5. Right hepatic duct.

720 The Foundation and Art of Robotic Surgery

A

B

C

D

E

F

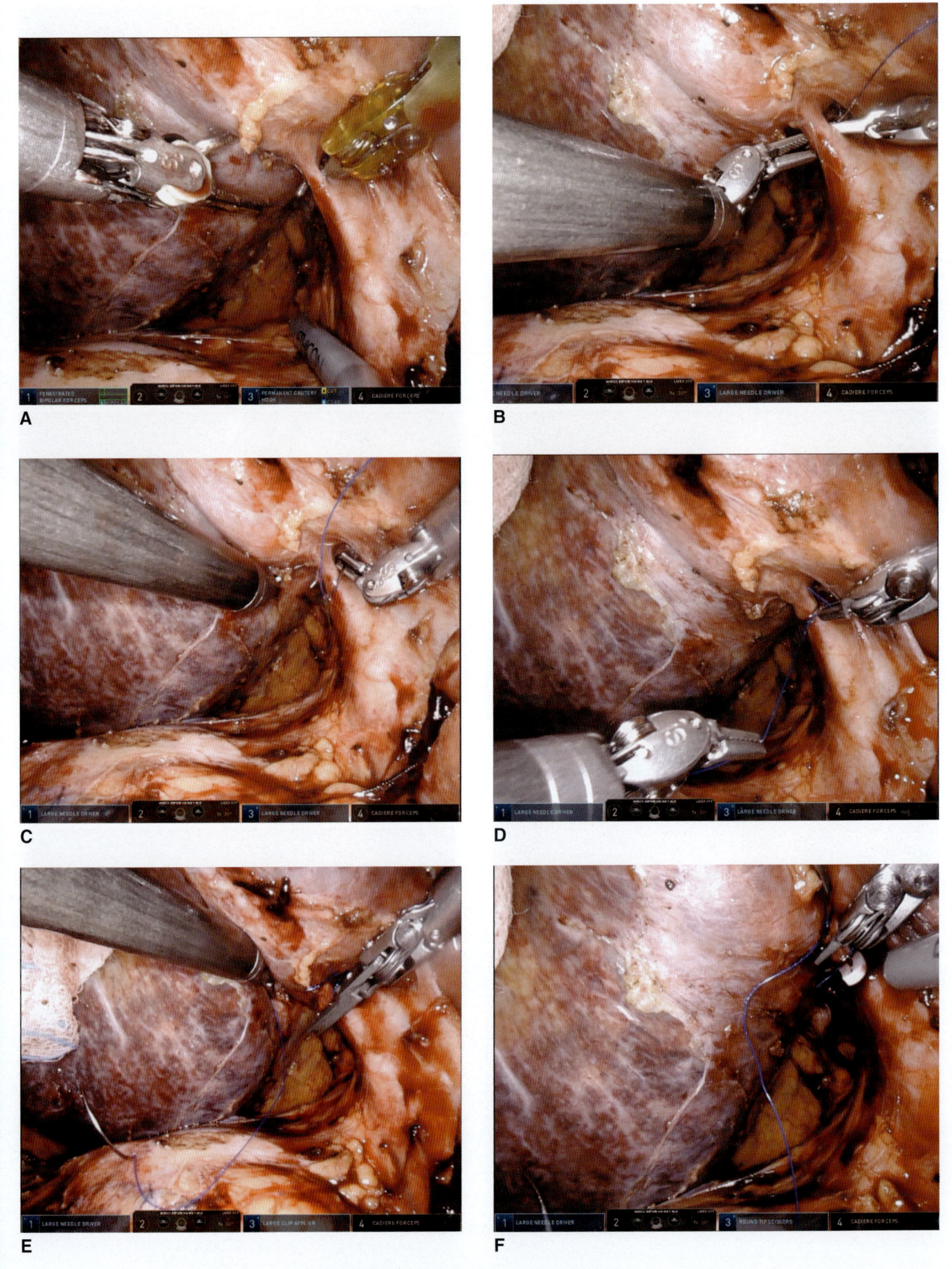

FIGURE 33-19 • Hepatocaval dissection.

Right Hepatectomy

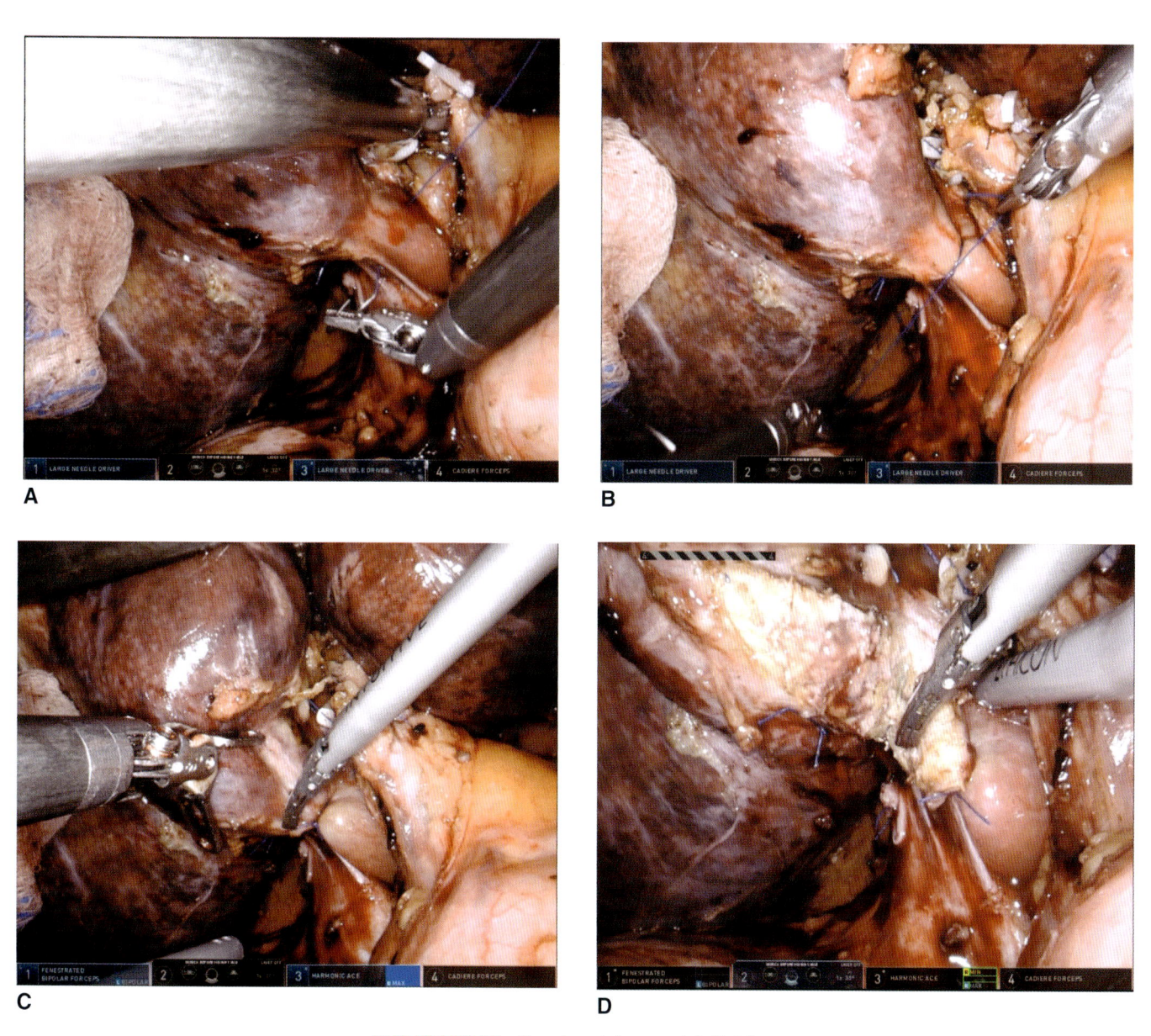

FIGURE 33-20 • Caudate lobe partial division.

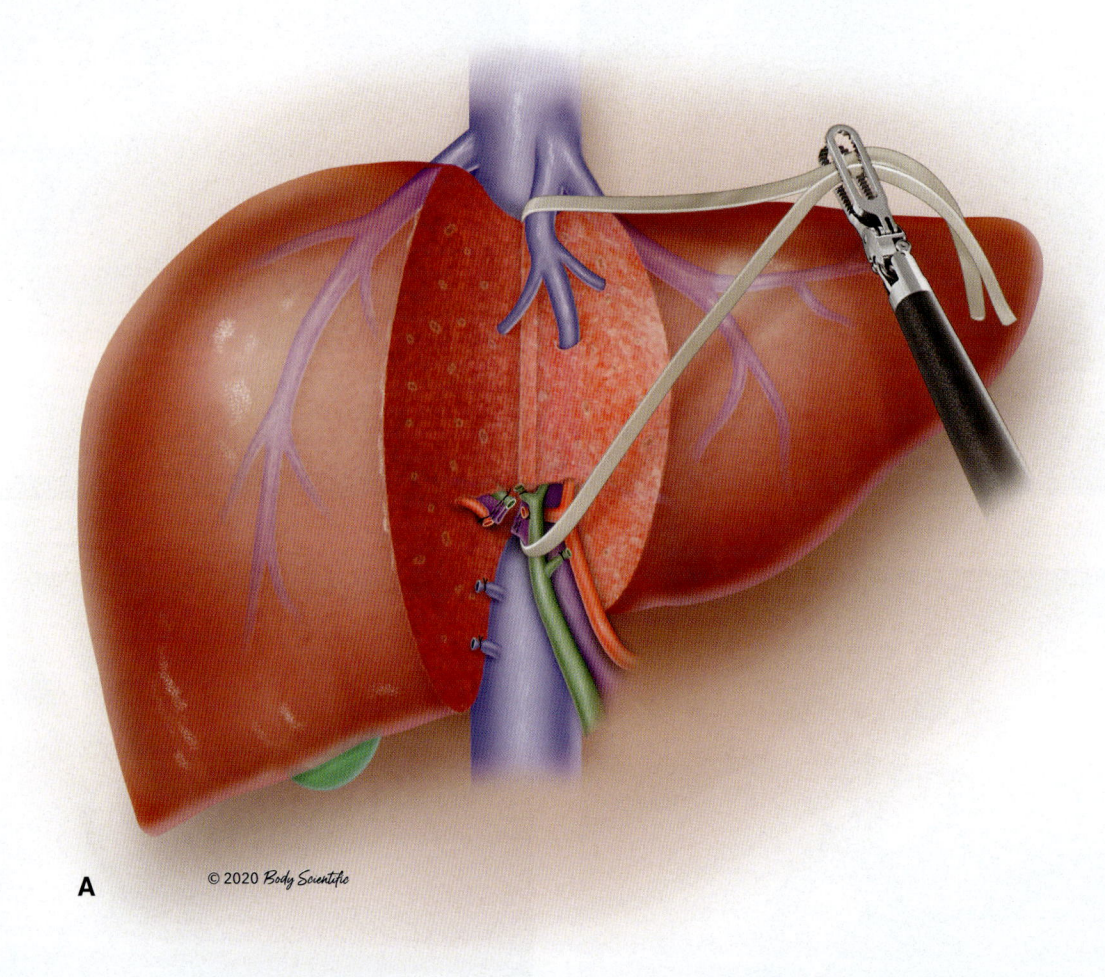

FIGURE 33-21 • Step 6. Hepatocaval dissection: **A.** Hanging maneuver.

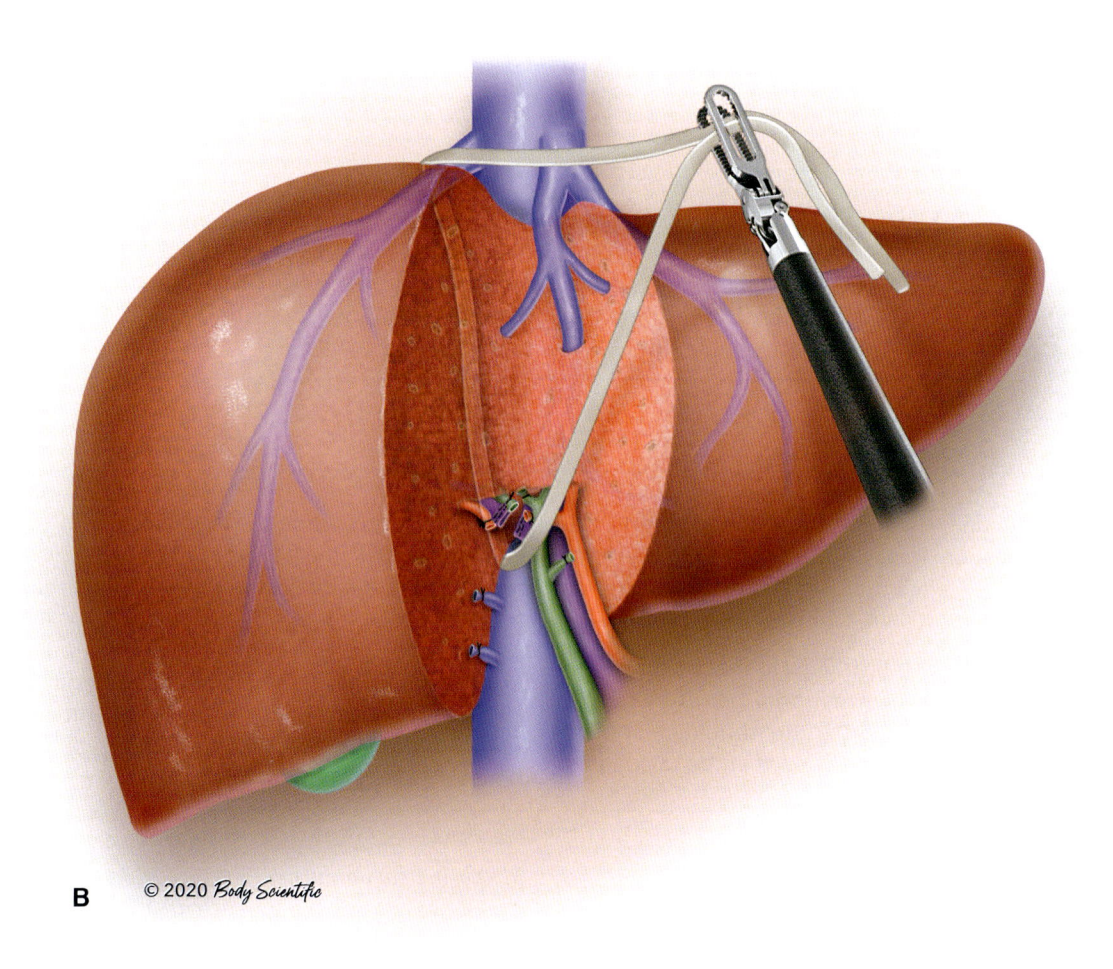

FIGURE 33-21 • (*Continued*) **B.** Modified hanging maneuver.

consistency (steatotic/fibrotic livers are more difficult to retract), this may not be possible. Should the hepatocaval detachment prove too hazardous at the level of its anterior and most cranial portion, the dissection can veer to the right of the vena cava and be continued cranially on this plane (right paracaval plane). At this point, similarly to the classical hanging maneuver, the umbilical tape can be passed in a paracaval fashion to the right of the right hepatic vein and a "modified hanging maneuver" can be achieved.

Although this represents a shortcut to the more traditional hanging maneuver, it is still very useful in helping to guide the parenchymal transection and the final division of the right hepatic vein. At the end of the parenchymal transection, the tape will be lifting the right hepatic vein providing the stapling surgeon an important landmark in the orientation of its course and its relationship with the vena cava (**Figures 33-21 A, B**). By the same principle, the "modified" hanging maneuver will be used to exert "lifting" action during the parenchymal transection (see Step 7) and keep the liver off the vena cava.

Step 6 average time frame: 20–30 min

▶▶ **Video 33-7. Step 6. Hepatocaval Dissection**

> ▶▶ **TIPS**
>
> In order to mobilize the liver, the hook and bipolar instruments can be swapped. Sometimes, the liver dome obstructs the instruments coming from the left side of the patient. The EndoWrist® ability can help overcome this problem to some extent, but in the case of bulky livers, this is not sufficient. In such situations, swapping instruments (placing the hook in R2 and the bipolar in R1) allows better access to the right triangular and coronary ligaments. Needless to say, it is essential to have practiced ambidexterity before doing this.

> ▶▶ **TIPS**
>
> In case short hepatic veins are encountered during the hepatocaval dissection, it may not be possible to perform the standard double ligation due to their short course as they enter the liver parenchyma from the vena cava.
>
> When this is the case, a similar strategy to the one discussed for the control of the segment 1 portal branches can be used. First, a Prolene™ 4-0 or 5-0 suture should be applied on the vena cava side. The vessel can then be divided by cutting it sharply inside the liver capsule. This can be done without ligating the vessel on the liver side. Following portal and arterial inflow control, minimal back-bleeding should occur at this point. This can be controlled with bipolar forceps or a parenchymal stitch. This principle of the "asymmetric cutting technique" is based on the fact that, during the hepatocaval dissection, the central venous pressure (CVP) is kept low. Therefore, the back-bleeding from the specimen side is minimized.

Step 7. Parenchymal transection

Following the inflow control and hepatocaval preparation (that may or may not include full liver mobilization), the parenchymal transection takes place. A surface demarcation of the ischemic area is usually evident, even though at times it might not be so obvious. By this time, full liver mobilization should be completed. If this has not been possible, it is important that at least a "paracaval tunnel" has been created (see Step 6), meaning that no liver parenchyma should be attached to the right side of the vena cava. This *tempo* of the procedure can be subdivided in 2 substeps: an initial "subcortical" parenchyma transection, and a later "core/hepatic vein" step. To safely perform these steps, in-depth knowledge of the anatomy, in particular of the hepatic vein anatomical variations, is essential. (Multiple variations can occur and different classifications are available; for additional information, see suggested readings #22, 23. In **Figure 33-22**, the most relevant ones are presented).

Step 7 average time frame: 40–60 min

a. Subcortical parenchymal transection

The key aspect of the parenchymal transection is to "superficialize" the section line as much as possible. This is called "superficialization technique" (**Figures 33-23 A–F**). This helps identify the intraparenchymal structure and greatly facilitates the management of bleeding if encountered. It is easier to control a bleeding vessel that is well exposed, as opposed to one that bleeds from a deep and not completely visible location. "Superficialization" of the transection line can be achieved with 2 main strategies. One is to apply sequential stay sutures (Prolene™ 2-0) on the free edge of segment 4, while the dissection progresses, making sure that the Glissonian capsule is encompassed. With the R3 grasping the sutures and retracting the liver parenchyma medially, the section line remains well exposed ("superficialized") with the help of the "gravity", since the patient is tilted toward the left. While the parenchyma is divided further, progressive medial traction is applied. Placement of additional stitches along the section line further

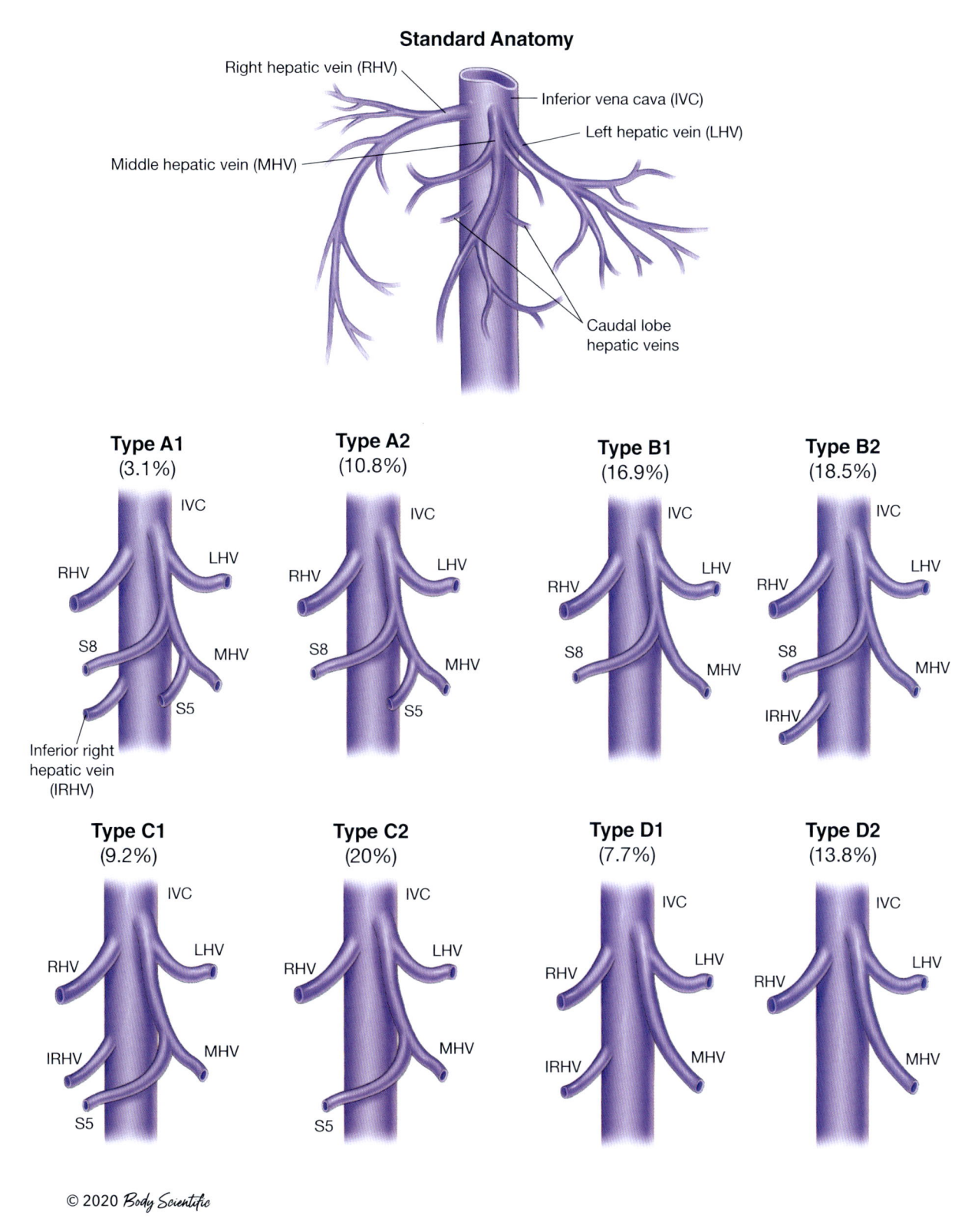

FIGURE 33-22 • Hepatic vein anatomical variations.

Standard Anatomy

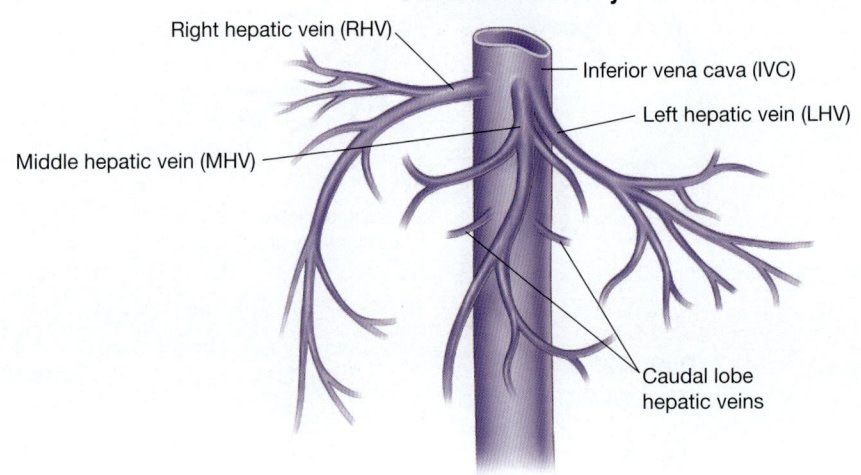

Right hepatic vein (RHV)
Inferior vena cava (IVC)
Left hepatic vein (LHV)
Middle hepatic vein (MHV)
Caudal lobe hepatic veins

Common trunk (61%)
MHV
RHV
LHV
Common trunk between MHV and LHV
IVC

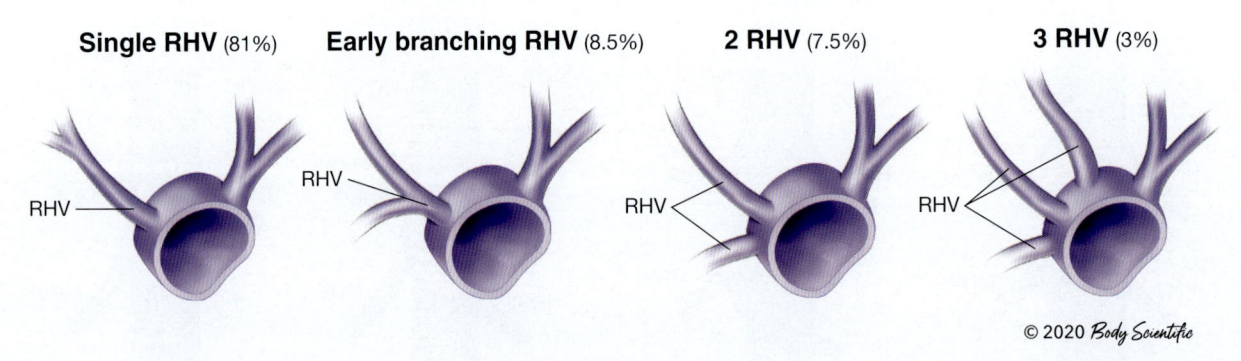

Independent stem (39%)
MHV
RHV
LHV
IVC

Single RHV (81%) — RHV

Early branching RHV (8.5%) — RHV

2 RHV (7.5%) — RHV

3 RHV (3%) — RHV

© 2020 Body Scientific

FIGURE 33-22 • (Continued)

Right Hepatectomy 727

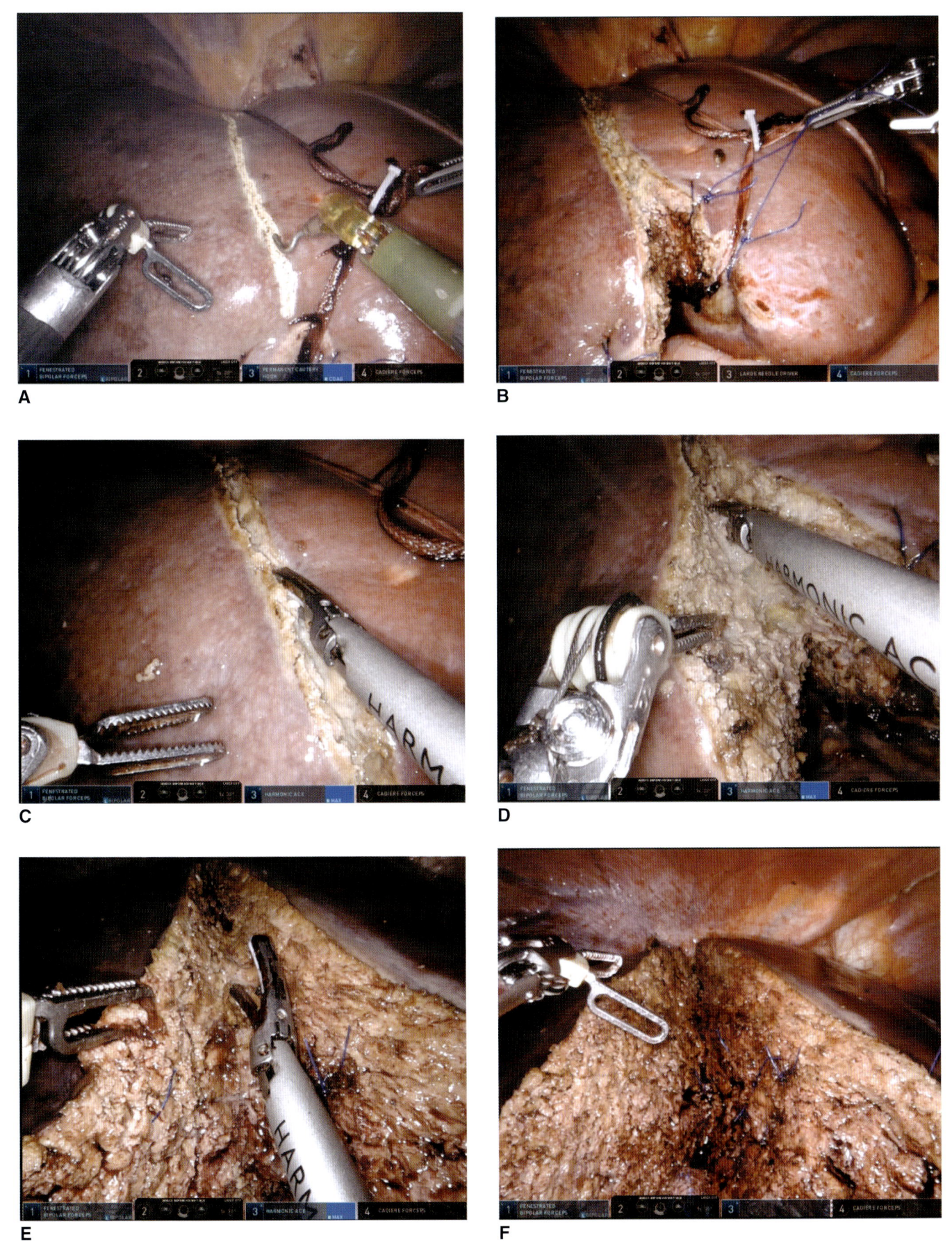

FIGURE 33-23 • **A–F.** Subcortical parenchymal transection.

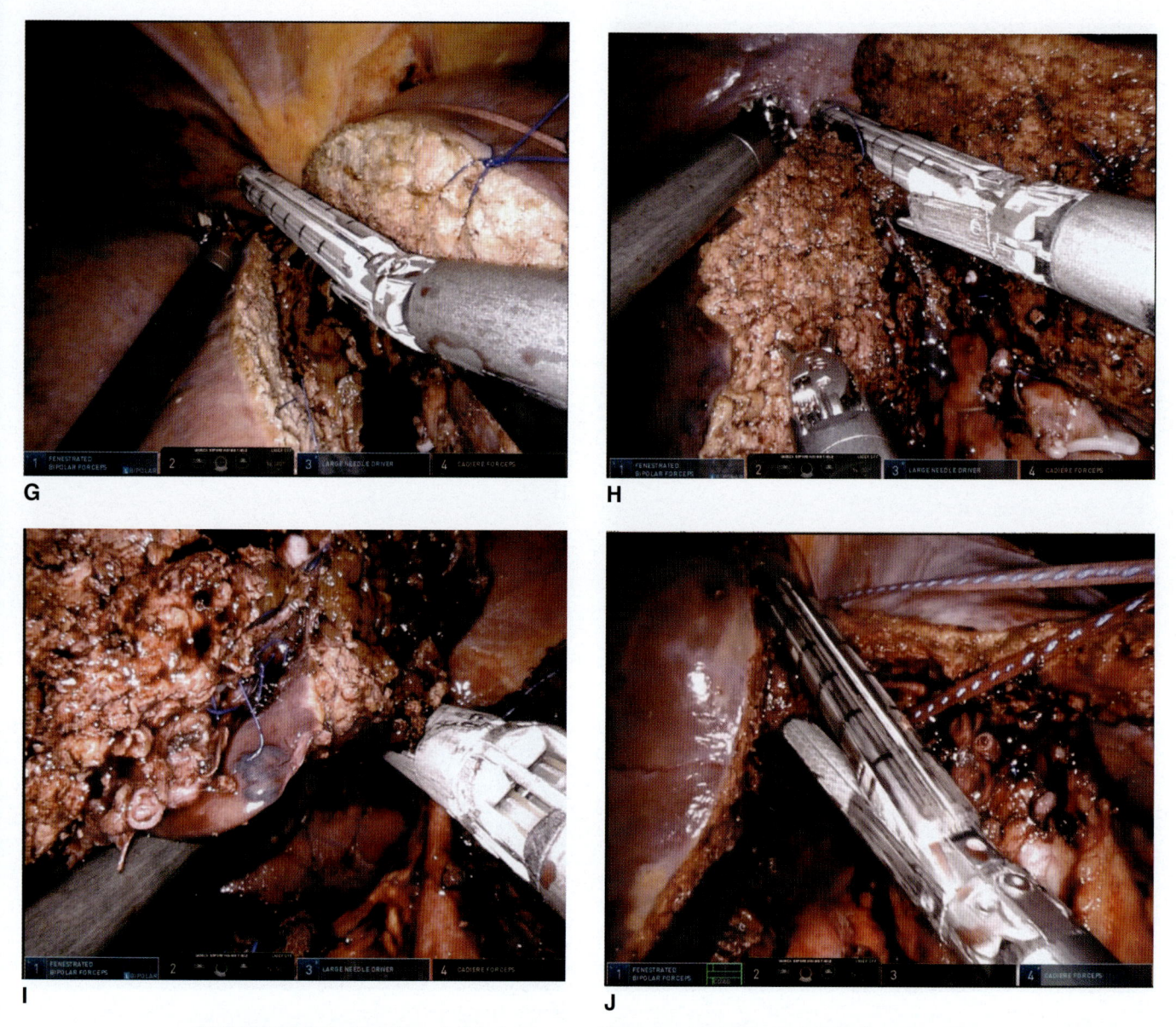

FIGURE 33-23 • *(Continued)* **G-J.** Core parenchymal transection and right hepatic vein.

facilitates the process. The second way to obtain "superficialization" of the section line is provided by the natural gravity effect of the right lobe of the liver, as it falls downward, away, while the dissection progresses.

As far as instrumentation is concerned, Harmonic® shears and bipolar forceps are used. Wise use of the Harmonic® shears with incremental/progressive closure over the parenchyma with low CVP can obtain a rather bloodless transection. If bleeding is encountered, nonabsorbable monofilament sutures can be placed as needed (Prolene™ 3-0 or 4-0 usually with large needles).

b. Core parenchymal transection and right hepatic vein

The transection of the deeper portion of the liver parenchyma (**Figures 33-23 G–J**) can be carried out in the same way as the subcortical step (Harmonic® shears with sequential closure technique). Also, a vascular stapler can be used to complete this part of the procedure in a safe and expedited fashion. When staplers are used, the position of the right, middle hepatic vein as well as the course of the vena cava must be very clear.

The last portion of the "core" part of the parenchymal transection entails the stapling of the right hepatic vein. Care must be taken staying at a safe distance from the middle hepatic vein and vena cava, because improper stapling can easily cause injuries of these large vessels with possible bleeding or CO_2 embolism.

These complications represent a risk, especially if stapling is handled by an inexperienced bedside assistant, and certain principles should be followed in order to avoid them.

A correct application of the stapler depends mainly on two factors:

1. Proper guidance from the console surgeon, who must have a clear mind representation of the main anatomical structures involved, namely the right hepatic and middle hepatic veins, the vena cava, and their relationship with the tumor.

The position of those landmarks has to be clear even in a wet field, which can be the case toward the end of the parenchymal transection.

2. The skills and experience of the bedside surgeon. The introduction of the stapler should happen with gentle but progressive pressure, while making short semirotational movements of the tip of the stapler, to favor the inclusion of the vascular structure in between the jaws to bluntly dissect the liver parenchyma with the tip of the stapler. This "blunt" advancement should continue until the entire width of the vein is encompassed such that no partial stapling can occur with the risk of CO_2 embolization.

At the end of the parenchymal transection, the hemostasis can be checked and additional Prolene™ 3-0 stitches can be applied on bleeding areas. The anesthesia team, at this point, can increase the CVP by resuscitating the patient and performing a Valsalva maneuver. Steps 7 a, b are shown in **Figures 33-23 A–J**.

▶ **Video 33-8.** Step 7. Parenchima Transection with Harmonic Scalpel

▶ **Video 33-9.** Step 7. Parenchima Transection with Stapler

▶▶ **TIPS**

The Harmonic® scalpel has an active vibrating and a "sealing" blade. The effect of this combination is a simultaneous "tissue penetration" followed by hemostatic effect. Such a thin vibrating blade is an ideal tool to be introduced into the liver parenchyma (almost with a "CUSA®-like effect") without causing damages to vascular structures. Once introduced within the tissue, the sealing blade completes the hemostasis and the division of the tissues. When used efficiently, this tool allows fairly bloodless transections. The Harmonic® scalpel should be placed parallel to the dissection line because it does not have EndoWrist® features. To obtain this, an operative 8-mm robotic trocar can be inserted in the assistant 12 mm (telescopic maneuver) and be used for the Harmonic® scalpel. The 12-mm trocar generally has a better alignment with the "Cantlie's line" and therefore is often preferred to the R1 robotic trocar for this part of the procedure. For best hemostatic results, the instrument should meet any vascular structure at a 90° angle and encompass the entire vessel during the application of energy. Incomplete sealing results in bleeding. It is therefore important to have knowledge of the position of the middle hepatic vein and any communicating branches that may be encountered during the parenchymal transection.

The liver microscopic structure also has an effect on the efficacy of the Harmonic® shears. This works rather ineffectively in fibrotic, steatotic, and cirrhotic livers. In normal liver parenchyma, it works at its best when placed on energy setting 5. In other instances, a different energy setting (e.g., level 3 setting) may achieve better coagulation.

One of the known drawbacks of continuous Harmonic® shears usage is overheating of the blades (melting of the plastic coverage of the instrument with loss of sealing efficacy). A few drops of saline irrigation, at regular intervals, prevents this occurrence and extends the instruments life (see Chapter 2, The Basic Principles of Clinical Applications, for additional details). The robotic vessel sealer represents an alternative instrument for the parenchymal transection.

While the Harmonic® shears are more dynamic, the vessel sealer has a more static sealing/cutting type of action. The process of insertion of the instrument inside the parenchyma is, by itself, creating some bleeding (see Chapter 2 for additional details).

One of the open liver surgeon's favorite tools, for the parenchymal transection, is the CUSA®. Unfortunately, there is no robotic adaptation for this instrument that signifies having to delegate the entire step to the assistant surgeon. Furthermore, besides a built-in monopolar cautery within the tip, the CUSA® has no sealing effect, making necessary hand ligation of each and every vessel encountered. Finally, its "cavitation" effect causes a significant "splashing effect" within the field, causing frequent soiling of the camera and need for repeated cleaning. The ideal robotic instrument for the parenchymal transection has yet to be devised, and surgeons have to adapt to the ones available.

> ► ► **TIPS**
>
> The robotic staplers are a valid alternative to the laparoscopic handheld ones. These provide some interesting features, such as an advanced software to give feedback on tissue thickness and also completeness and safety of the stapling. Additionally, they can be operated directly by the primary surgeon without need for delegation of such an important step. The leading surgeon is more able to control details of the action, like precise angle, direction, and length of the stapling. The main disadvantage, however, is that that there is no partially indirect haptic feedback, which is not ideal when navigating the stapler blades within the friable liver core, and even more so, when performing the right hepatic vein division. Another inconvenience of the robotic staplers is that the electronic control of the thickness of the tissue, included in the jaws, usually an advantage, sometimes becomes a disadvantage, not allowing to fire in critical steps. To overcome this situation, multiple clamping/de-clamping and/or changing of the stapler size may be required. If this inconvenience happens in a critical step, with some bleeding, this may increase the difficulty of the vascular control. Another possible disadvantage is the presence of only two lines of stitches, from each side of the staple line.

> ► ► **TIPS**
>
> The Pringle maneuver is not normally required with this technique. In the presence of pneumoperitoneum, low CVP, energy based-devices and proper technique, the Pringle maneuver is not necessary for bleeding control. Nevertheless, it might be wise to predispose a Pringle clamping at the beginning of a surgeon's learning curve.
>
> Good communication with the anesthesia and OR teams by alerting them of the possibility that the robot may need to be undocked to perform urgent maneuvers is key (see Chapter 2, The Basic Principles of Clinical Applications).

> ⚠ **PITFALLS**
>
> During the parenchymal transection, accessory (and sometimes major) hepatic veins may open up. In many instances, the low CVP, and the high intraperitoneal pressure will make the bleeding negligible. However, there is a risk of CO_2 embolization. This event is known to cause hemodynamic instability. Should a major vein open, the first maneuver to do is to close the opening to prevent CO_2 embolization. This can be achieved by compressing the vessel with an instrument or with a sponge. Then, pneumoperitoneum is decreased (but not excessively, because adequate view must be maintained). Lastly, the vessel is closed with a nonabsorbable suture or, if applicable, a Hem-o-lok®. If the patient is hemodynamically unstable, and bleeding control appears difficult, it is advisable to consider an early conversion.

Step 8. Reconstruction of the falciform ligament

The falciform ligament is reconstructed to prevent torsion of the remaining left lobe of the liver toward the right side (**Figures 33-24 A, B**). Such an event can generate an "acute Budd–Chiari-like" syndrome. If the liver left lobe ligaments have not been divided, torsion is less likely. The falciform ligament is reconstructed with interrupted nonabsorbable sutures.

Step 8 average time frame: 5–10 min

Step 9. Specimen extraction

The specimen is placed in an Endobag™ and retrieved through a Pfannenstiel incision. Certain circumstances, such as morbidly obese patients, where this incision may not be practical and carries a risk of wound infection, require a different strategy such as a small midline laparotomy. Additional details on specimen retrieval have been extensively described in Chapter 2, The Basic Principles of Clinical Applications.

Step 9 average time frame: 15–20 min

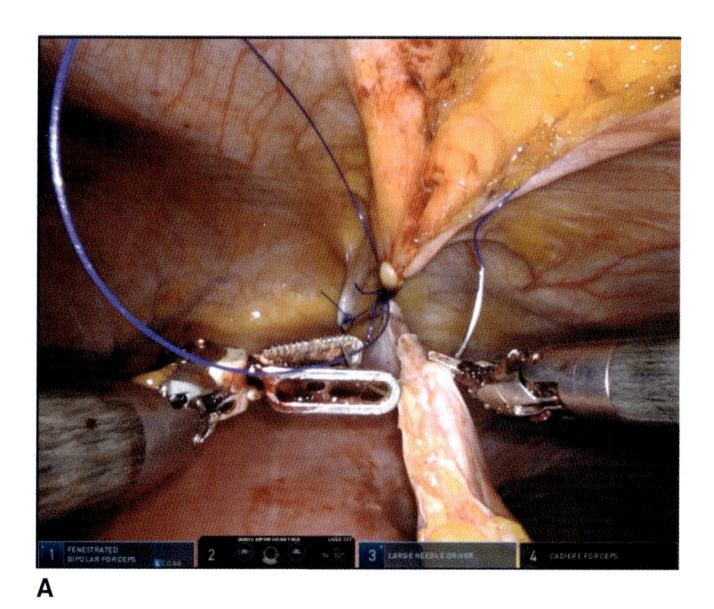

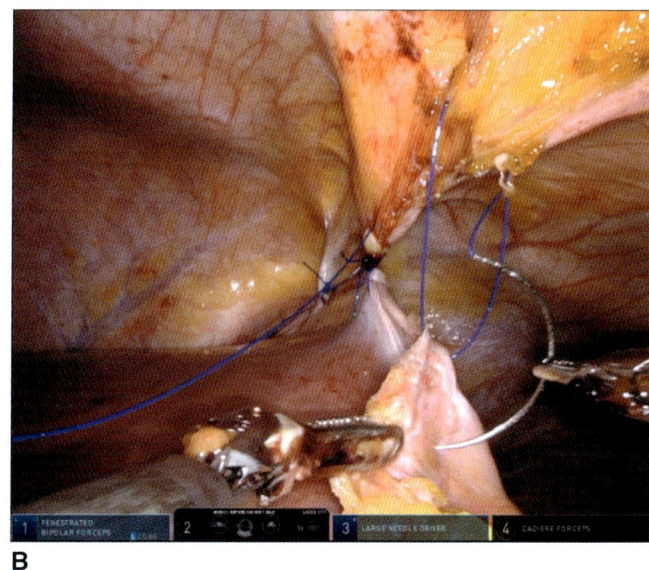

FIGURE 33-24 • Reconstruction of the falciform ligament.

Suggested Readings

1. Fernandes E, Aguiluz G, Bustos R, et al. Chapter 69. Robotic hepatic lobectomies. In: Gharagozloo F, Patel VR, Giulianotti PC, et al., eds. *Robotic Surgery*, 2nd ed. Springer; 2021.
2. Nota CL, Hagendoorn J, Fong Y ASO. Author reflections: the role of robotic surgery in liver resection. *Ann Surg Oncol.* 2019;26(2):591-592. doi: 10.1245/s10434-018-7082-5
3. Guerra F, Di Marino M, Coratti A. Robotic surgery of the liver and biliary tract. *J Laparoendosc Adv Surg Tech A*. 2019;29(2), 141-146. doi: 10.1089/lap.2017.0628
4. Giulianotti PC, Coratti A, Angelini M, et al. Robotics in general surgery: personal experience in a large community hospital. *Arch Surg.* 2003;138(7):777-784. doi: 10.1001/archsurg.138.7.777
5. Giulianotti PC, Coratti A, Sbrana F, et al. Robotic liver surgery: results for 70 resections. *Surgery.* 2011;149(1):29-39. doi: 10.1016/j.surg.2010.04.002
6. Gonzalez-Ciccarelli LF, Quadri P, Daskalaki D, et al. Robotic approach to hepatobiliary surgery. *Chirurg.* 2017;88(Suppl 1): 19-28. doi: 10.1007/s00104-016-0223-0
7. Giulianotti PC, Bianco FM, Daskalaki D, et al. Robotic liver surgery: technical aspects and review of the literature. *Hepatobil Surg Nutrit.* 2016;5(4):311-321. doi: 10.21037/hbsn.2015.10.05
8. Milone L, Daskalaki D, Fernandes E, et al. State of the art in robotic hepatobiliary surgery. *World J Surg.* 2013;37(12): 2747-2755. doi: 10.1007/s00268-013-2276-2
9. Giulianotti PC, Sbrana F, Coratti A, et al. Totally robotic right hepatectomy: surgical technique and outcomes. *Arch Surg.* 2011;146(7):844-850. doi: 10.1001/archsurg.2011.145
10. Giulianotti PC, Sbrana F, Bianco FM, et al. Robot-assisted laparoscopic extended right hepatectomy with biliary reconstruction. *J Laparoendoscop Adv Surg Techniq.* 2010;Part A, 20(2):159-163. doi: 10.1089/lap.2009.0383
11. Mori Y, Nakata K, Aly MYF, et al. Congenital biliary dilatation in the era of laparoscopic surgery, focusing on the high incidence of anatomical variations of the right hepatic artery. *Hepatobil Pancreat Sci.* 2020;27(11):870-876. doi: 10.1002/jhbp.819. Online ahead of print.
12. Giulianotti PC, Mangano A, Bustos RE, et al. Operative technique in robotic pancreaticoduodenectomy (RPD) at University of Illinois at Chicago (UIC): 17 steps standardized technique: lessons learned since the first worldwide RPD performed in the year 2001. *Surg Endosc.* 2018;32(10):4329-4336. doi: 10.1007/s00464-018-6228-7
13. Ho CM, Wakabayashi G, Nitta H, et al Systematic review of robotic liver resection. *Surg Endosc.* 2013;27(3):732-739. doi: 10.1007/s00464-012-2547-2
14. Anwar AS, Srikala J, Papalkar AS, et al. Study of anatomical variations of hepatic vasculature using multidetector computed tomography angiography. *Surg Radiol Anat.* 2020;42(12): 1449-1457. doi: 10.1007/s00276-020-02532-5
15. Yan J, Feng H, Wang H, et al. Hepatic artery classification based on three-dimensional CT. *Br J Surg.* 2020;107(7):906-916. doi: 10.1002/bjs.11458
16. De Blasi V, Makkai-Popa S-T, Arru L, et al. Rare anatomic variation of the hepatic arterial blood supply: case report and literature review. *Surg Radiol Anat.* 2019;41(3):343-345. doi: 10.1007/s00276-018-2163-5
17. Nakamura T, Tanaka K, Kiuki T, et al. Anatomical variations and surgical strategies in right lobe living donor liver transplantation: lessons from 120 cases. *Transplantation.* 2002;73(12):1896-1903 doi: 10.1097/00007890-200206270-00008
18. Cheng YF, Huang TL, Lee TY, et al. Variation of the intrahepatic portal vein; angiographic demonstration and application in living-related hepatic transplantation. *Transplant Proc.* 1996;28:1667-1668.

19. Carneiro C, Brito J, Barreiro C, et al. All about portal vein: a pictorial display to anatomy, variants and physiopathology. *Insights Imaging*. 2019;10(1):38. doi: 10.1186/s13244-019-0716-8
20. Chaib E, Kanas AF, Galvão FHF, et al. Bile duct confluence: anatomic variations and its classification. *Surg Radiol Anat*. 2014;36(2):105-109. doi: 10.1007/s00276-013-1157-6
21. Brunicardi FAD, Billiar TR, Dunn DL, et al. Liver. In: Brunicardi, FC, Andersen DK, Billiar, TR, et al., eds. *Schwartz's Principles of Surgery*, 10th ed. McGraw-Hill Professional Publishing; 2014.
22. Varotti G, Gondolesi G, Goldman J, et al. Anatomic variations in right liver living donors. *Am Coll Surg*. 2004;198(4):577-582. doi: 10.1016/j.jamcollsurg.2003.11.014
23. Fang C-H, You J-H, Lau WY, et al. Anatomical variations of hepatic veins: three-dimensional computed tomography scans of 200 subjects. *World J Surg*. 2012;36(1):120-124. doi: 10.1007/s00268-011-1297-y

"Be less curious about people and more curious about ideas."
—Marie Curie (1867–1934)

Left Hepatectomy

Antonio Cubisino • Carolina Baz • Nicolas Hellmuth Dreifuss • Pier Cristoforo Giulianotti

INTRODUCTION

More than a century after the first open left hepatic lobe resection, Azagra et al. described the first laparoscopic anatomical left lateral segmentectomy. A more favorable anatomy of the left hepatic lobe, with easier access to the main vasculobiliary structures, is the principal factor that facilitated the adoption of minimally invasive approaches for left-sided hepatic resections. Similarly to what was described for the right hepatectomy, the complete inflow control, with the demarcation of the Cantlie's line, allows one to proceed with a clear and anatomical hepatic resection.

PROCEDURES FIRST DESCRIBED BY YEAR

- 1992: First laparoscopic liver resections (segments V and VI)—M. Gagner
- 1994: First laparoscopic left lateral segmentectomy—J.S. Azagra
- 1997: Full laparoscopic hepatic resections (20 cases): First laparoscopic left hepatectomies; frist laparoscopic right hepatectomy—C.G.S. Hüscher
- 2003: First robotic liver resections (segments V–VI and V)—P.C. Giulianotti
- 2006: Full-robotic hepatic resections (31 cases): First robotic left lateral sectionectomies; first robotic left hepatectomy; first robotic right hepatectomies—P.C. Giulianotti

🔍 ANATOMICAL HIGHLIGHTS

Following the Couinaud's classification of the liver anatomy, there are different anatomic left-sided hepatic resections: left lateral sectionectomy (Couinaud's segments 2 and 3), left hemihepatectomy (Couinaud's segments 2, 3, and 4 +/−1), and left hepatic trisectionectomy, which was initially known as "extended left hepatectomy" (Couinaud's segments 2, 3, 4, 5, and 8 +/− 1) (**Figures 34-1 A–C**).

INSTRUMENT REQUIREMENTS

The suggested main robotic instruments/tools can be listed as follows:
- 30°/0° scope
- 2 needle drivers (round tip or macro)
- Cautery hook/monopolar scissors
- Harmonic shears/vessel sealer
- Robotic linear stapler (with different loads)
- Multiple Hem-o-lok™ clips
- Medium–large clip applier
- Bipolar forceps
- Cadière forceps
- Long-tip forceps

The suggested main laparoscopic instruments/tools can be listed as follows:
- Needle drivers
- Scissors
- Graspers
- Endostapler (with different loads)
- Suction-irrigation
- Laparoscopic ultrasound (drop-in probe or laparoscopic handheld)

Supplemental materials:
- Gauzes, sponges
- Penrose drains
- Vessel loops
- Red rubber tube for an eventual internal Pringle maneuver
- Endobag™
- Medium–large clips
- Sutures: Vicryl™ 3-0; Silk 3-0; Prolene™ 2-0, 3-0, 4-0, and 5-0

Photo from George Rinhart, Contributor / Getty Images.
Quote source: ©2022 Marie Curie. Registered Charity, England and Wales.

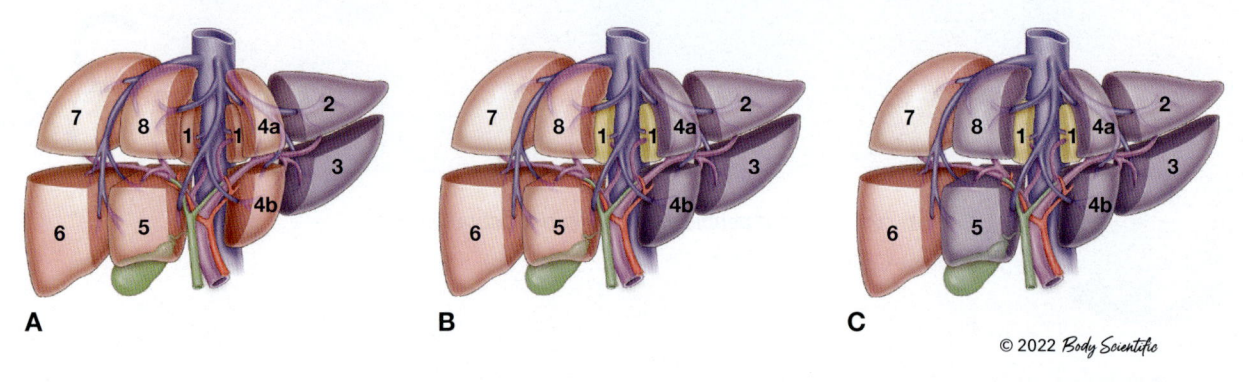

FIGURE 34-1 • Anatomic left-sided hepatic resections. **A.** Left lateral sectionectomy. **B.** Left hemihepatectomy. **C.** Left hepatic trisectionectomy.

A precise preoperative evaluation of the liver anatomy and the tumor relationship with the biliary and vascular structures is essential to optimize the treatment strategy and improve the outcomes. Moreover, an optimal preoperative study is mandatory to assess the risk of postoperative liver failure, especially in case of major liver resections. This risk is related to the volume of the future liver remnant, the quality of the liver parenchyma, and its regenerative capacity. Computed tomography (CT) and magnetic resonance imaging (MRI) are routinely performed preoperatively. Three-dimensional liver reconstructions of CT images can help surgeons in planning with accurate localization of the lesions and the evaluation of possible vascular and biliary anomalies and tumor relationships (**Figure 34-2**).

This chapter will primarily focus on robotic anatomical left hepatectomy with or without caudate lobe resection.

Indications and Relative Contraindications to the Robotic Approach

As for other major procedures, there are no absolute contraindications to left-sided robotic liver resections. There are, however, relative contraindications that may concern the patient's physiological status and their ability to tolerate pneumoperitoneum or characteristics related to the tumor. The latter conditions include bulky lesions with diaphragmatic or major vessels infiltration (inferior vena cava, major hepatic veins, or a segment of the hepatic artery/portal vein, supplying the contralateral lobe, not included in the left-sided resection).

In presence of hepatic lesions with a low risk of vascular invasion and lymph node involvement (e.g., colorectal liver metastasis), a parenchyma-sparing approach that minimizes the sacrifice of functioning liver parenchyma should be the first consideration. However, multiple lesions in difficult locations in the same hepatic lobe may require a formal anatomical resection.

The main indications to perform a standard left hepatectomy are:

- Hepatocellular carcinoma
- Colorectal liver metastases
- Symptomatic hemangioma
- Gigantic symptomatic focal nodular hyperplasia

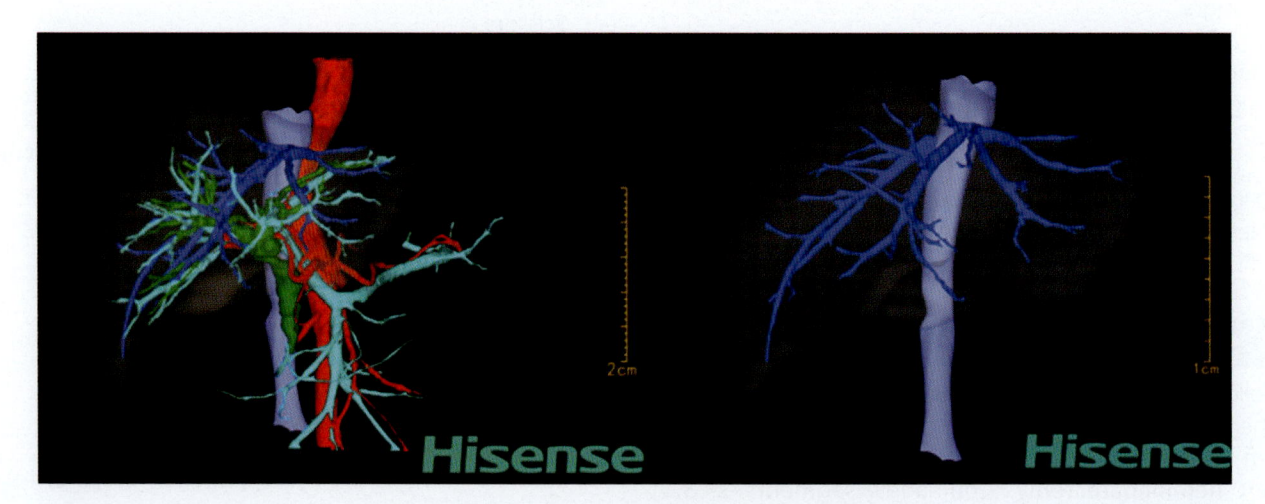

FIGURE 34-2 • Three-dimensional liver reconstruction. The reconstructions were obtained from CAS system (Hisense medical).

- Recurrent, refractory cholangitis associated with intrahepatic lithiasis and chronic abscess
- Giant (>5 cm) symptomatic adenoma
- Peripheral intrahepatic cholangiocarcinoma
- Breast cancer metastases
- Choledochal cyst with dilations/stenosis of intrahepatic ducts, intrahepatic lithiasis, or parenchymal atrophy
- Hepatolithiasis
- Papillary mucinous cystadenoma
- Living donation

EDITORIAL COMMENT

In the presence of potentially resectable cholangiocarcinomas, the surgical procedure is individualized according to the location of the tumor within the biliary tree: intrahepatic, perihilar, or distal.

However, also in case of intrahepatic, centrally located lesions, an extrahepatic bile duct resection with regional lymphadenectomy and Roux-en-Y hepaticojejunostomy reconstruction is required to obtain adequate negative bile duct margins (5 to 10 mm) increasing the possibility of achieving a curative resection.

Patient Positioning, OR Setup, and Port Setting

The patient is placed supine on a beanbag in the French position with arms tucked and parted legs. A 30° reverse Trendelenburg is also given to achieve adequate exposure of the liver (**Figure 34-3**). The assistant surgeon sits between the patient's legs. The OR setup is explained in **Figure 34-4**.

The pneumoperitoneum is induced with the Veress needle at the modified Palmer's point. A diagnostic laparoscopy is usually carried out with a 30° scope through a 5-mm trocar placed in the left upper quadrant. This port is subsequently replaced with an 8-mm robotic trocar. The preliminary diagnostic laparoscopy is performed to rule out any additional incidental findings, unexpected changes in staging, presence of adhesions, or other reasons that may suggest a change in the overall surgical strategy and a more precise tailoring of the port location. Once any contraindications to proceed with the operation have been excluded, the remaining trocars are placed.

A total of 6 ports (four 8-mm robotic, one 10–12 mm, and one 5-mm assistant port) are used during this procedure. The trocar placement line to perform a left-sided hepatic resection is similar to the one described for the right hepatectomy with some specific modifications (see Chapter 33,

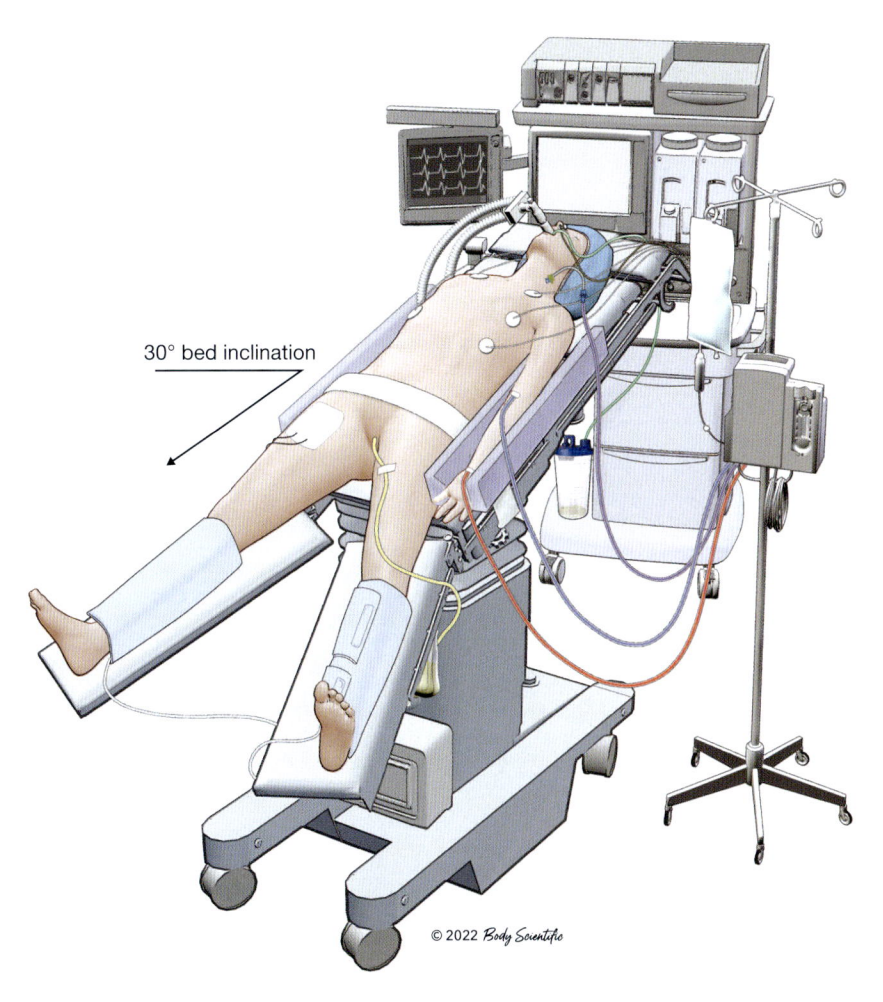

FIGURE 34-3 • Patient positioning.

736 The Foundation and Art of Robotic Surgery

Right Hepatectomy). In this case, the camera can be moved slightly medially keeping the other robotic trocars along a transverse line that usually lies a few centimeters above the transumbilical plane (**Figure 34-5**).

The strategy of trocar placement is of paramount importance for the success of the procedure; however, it may be necessary to adjust the trocar position based on the patient's body habitus (**Figure 34-6**).

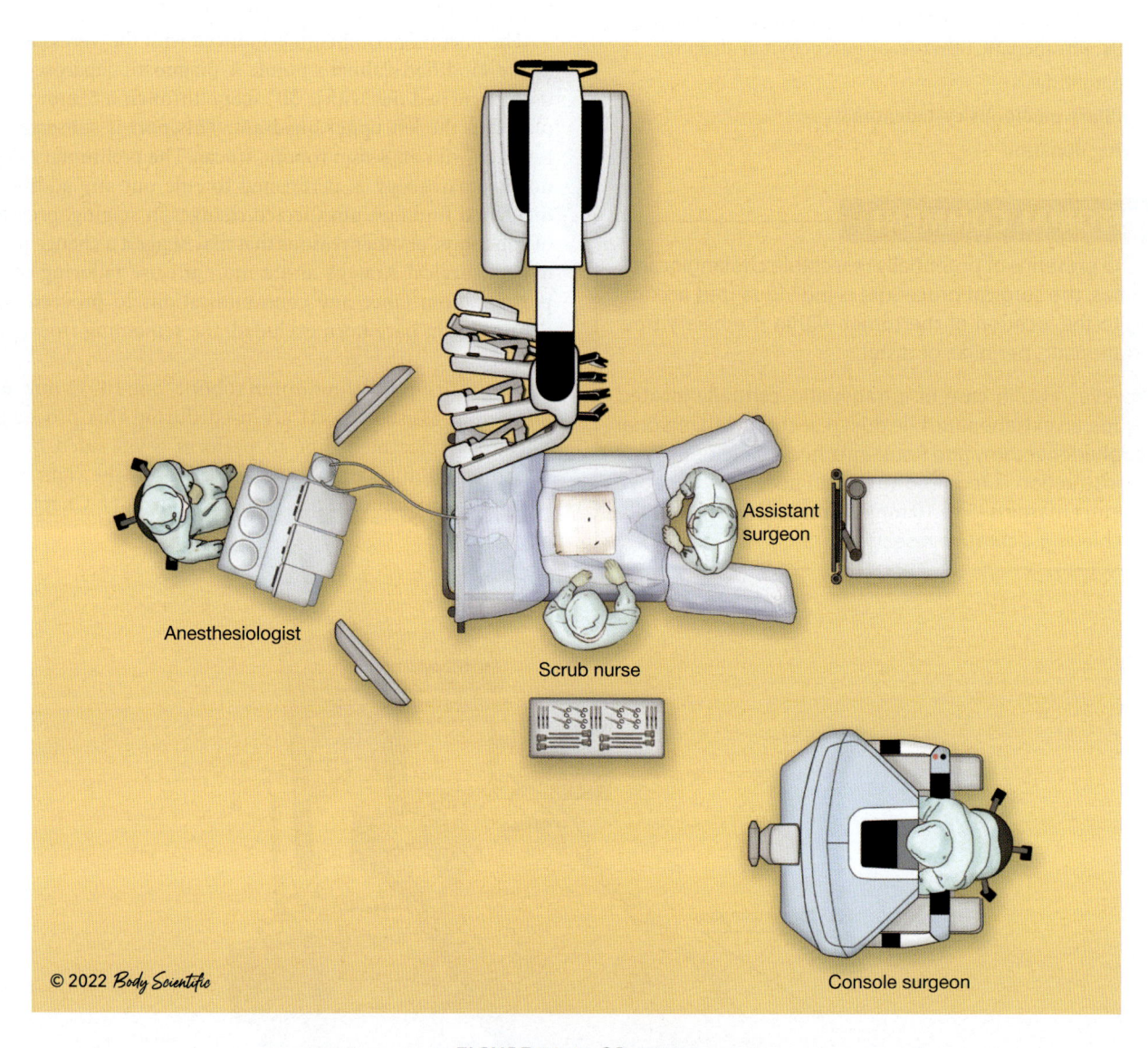

FIGURE 34-4 • OR setup.

FIGURE 34-5 • Port setting normal abdomen.

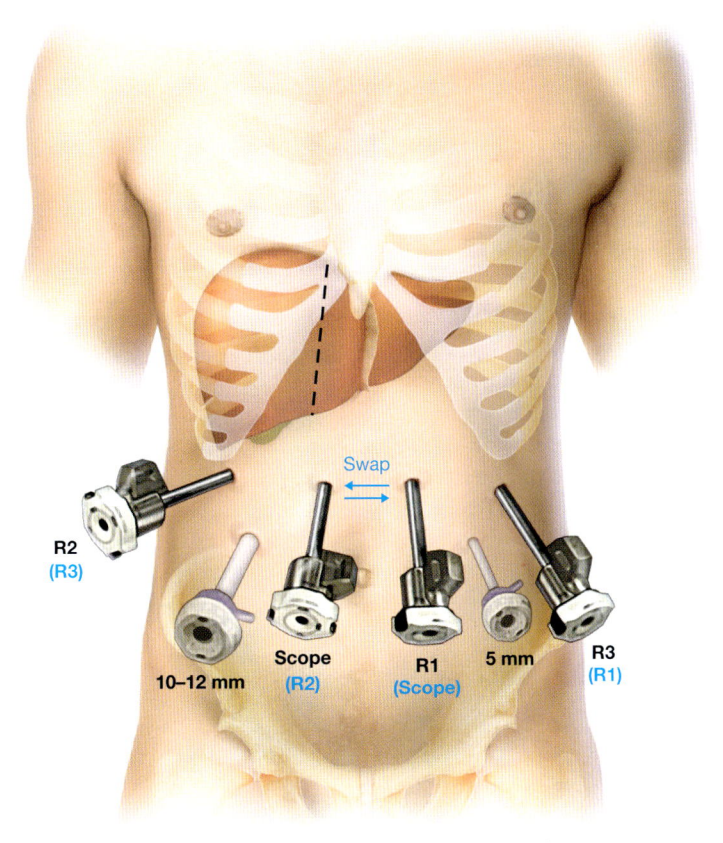

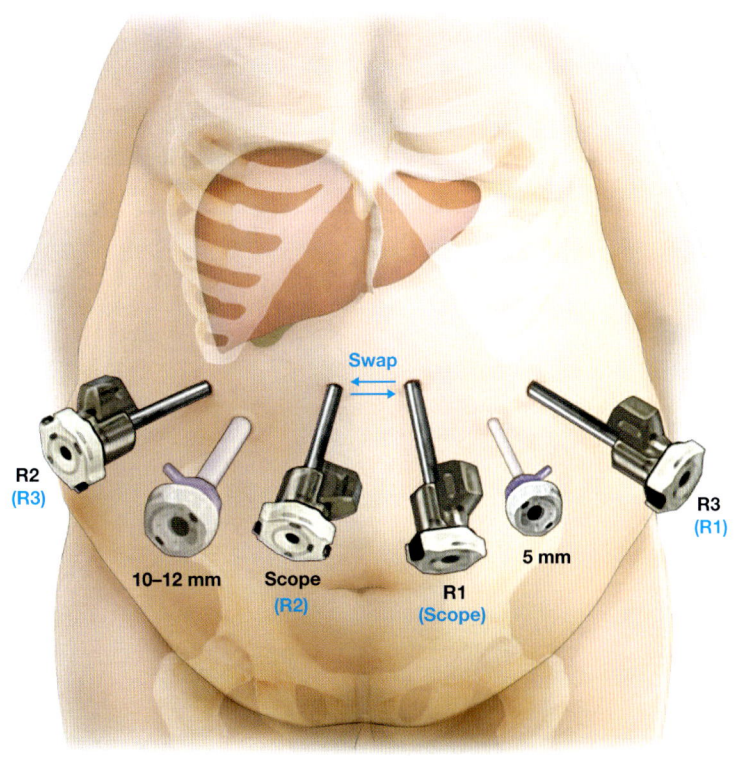

FIGURE 34-6 • Port setting wide abdomen.

Surgical Technique

Step 1. Falciform ligament dissection and mobilization of the left hepatic lobe

Once the preliminary abdominal evaluation has been completed, the falciform ligament is progressively divided by using the monopolar cautery hook. With a smaller and less firmly attached parenchyma to the surrounding structures, the mobilization of the left liver is easier than the one required for the right hepatectomy. This phase of the procedure begins with the division of the left triangular and coronary ligaments to expose the left inferior phrenic vein, the suprahepatic inferior vena cava (IVC), as well as the left and the middle hepatic veins at their confluence with the IVC (**Figures 34-7 A, B**). The mobilization of the left liver is completed by lifting the left hepatic lobe with a grasper in R3 and opening the hepatogastric ligament with the electrocautery hook placed in R1. The division of the lesser omentum is started at the level of the pars flaccida and extended up to the right side of the esophageal hiatus. During the dissection, care should be taken to a possible accessory or replaced left hepatic artery arising from the left gastric artery. In these anatomical settings, the variant vascular structure is carefully prepared and ready to be divided between sutures of Prolene™ 4-0 when the resectability is confirmed.

Step 1 average time frame: 10–15 min

> **EDITORIAL COMMENT**
>
> The falciform ligament should be detached starting from the umbilical ligament without leaving hanging tissue attached to the abdominal wall that may interfere with the scope and obstruct the visualization.

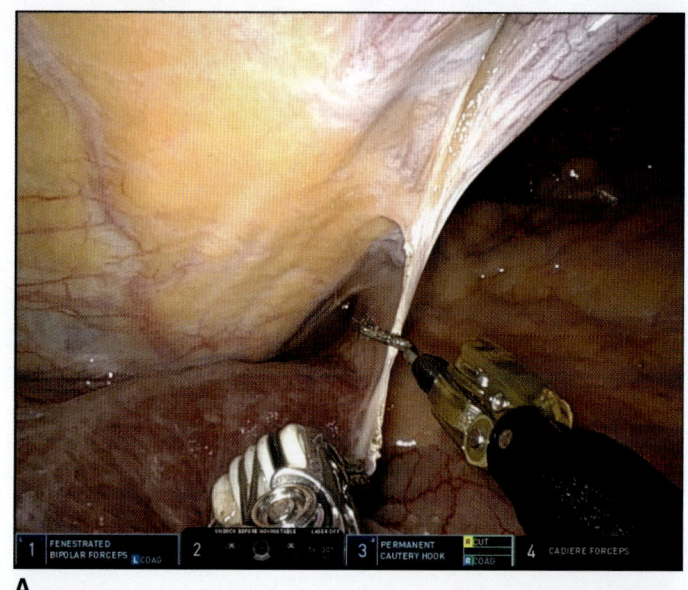

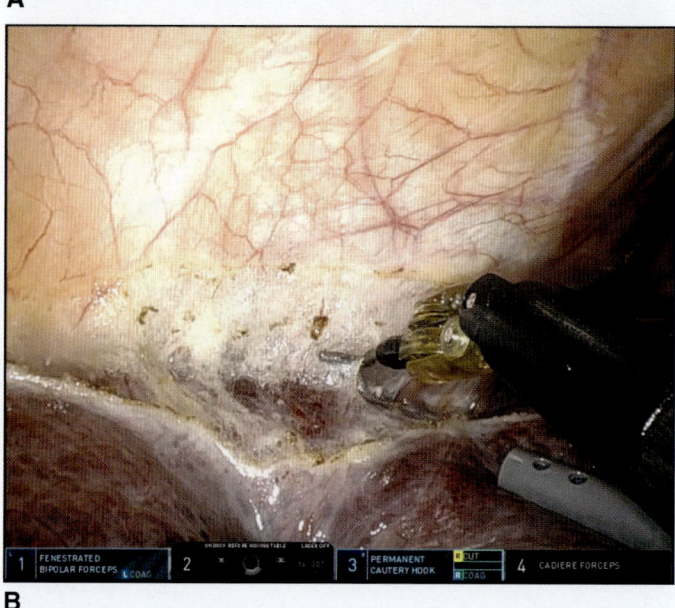

FIGURE 34-7 • **A.** Left triangular ligament dissection. **B.** Left coronary ligament dissection.

Left Hepatectomy

🔍 ANATOMICAL HIGHLIGHTS

Accessory/replaced left hepatic artery (**Figure 34-8**). (For additional information, see suggested readings #8, 9.)

Type 1 (≤ 0.5%)
Right and left hepatic arteries may originate directly from celiac trunk
Proximal bifurcation of common hepatic artery

Type 2 (≤ 1.5%)
Right hepatic artery may cross anterior to common hepatic duct instead of posterior

Type 3 (≤ 2.5%)
Accessory left hepatic artery may originate from right hepatic artery

Type 4 (4.5%)
Gastroduodenal artery
Splenic artery
Replaced common hepatic artery may originate from superior mesenteric artery

Type 5 (7%)
Accessory right hepatic artery may originate from superior mesenteric artery

Type 6 (8%)
Accessory left hepatic artery may originate from left gastric artery

Type 7 (11%)
Replaced right hepatic artery may originate from superior mesenteric artery

Type 8 (10%)
Replaced left hepatic artery may originate from left gastric artery

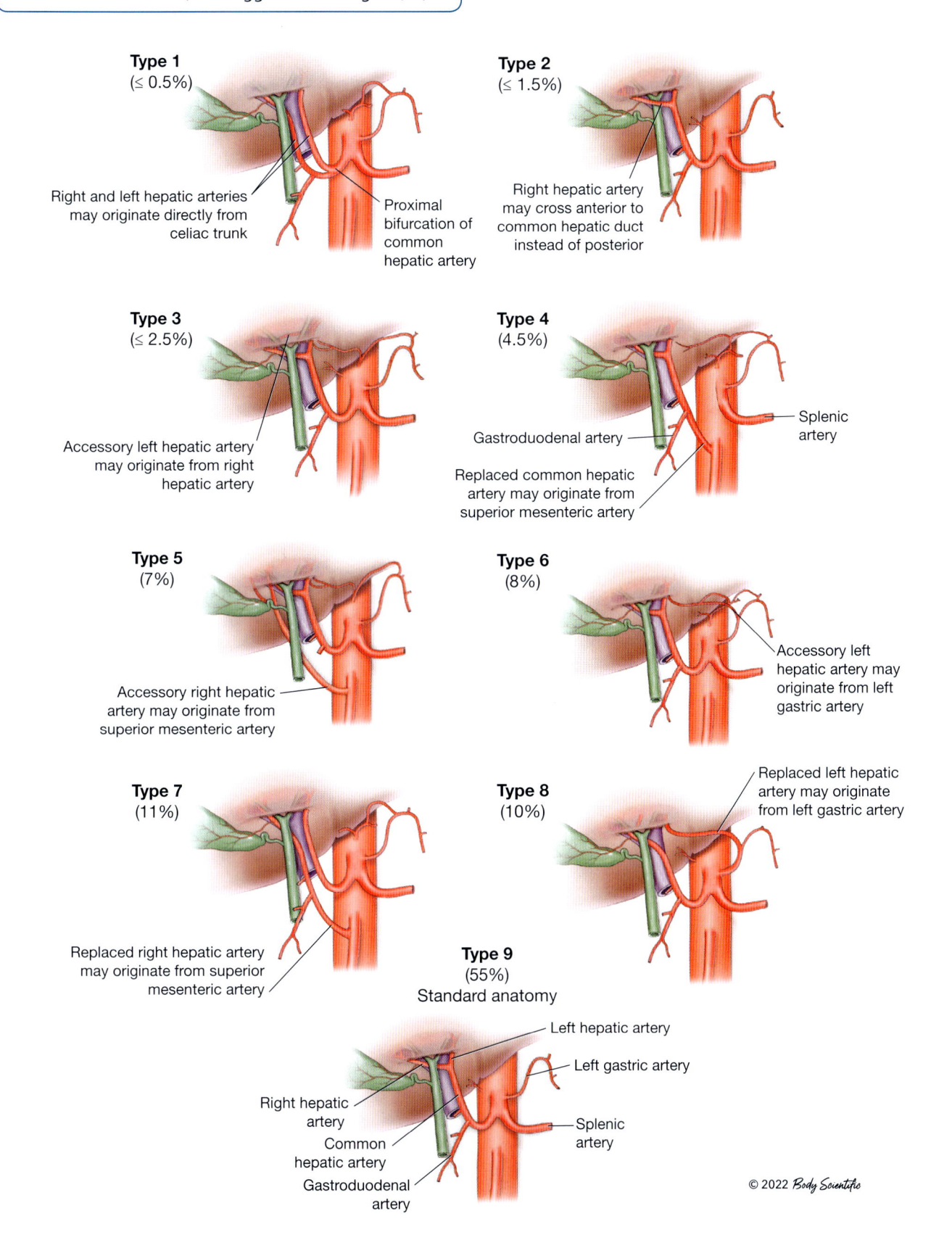

Type 9 (55%)
Standard anatomy
Left hepatic artery
Left gastric artery
Right hepatic artery
Splenic artery
Common hepatic artery
Gastroduodenal artery

© 2022 *Body Scientific*

FIGURE 34-8 • (Type 1-9) Hepatic artery variations.

ANATOMICAL HIGHLIGHTS

The mobilization of the left hepatic lobe is easier than the one required for the contralateral side and can be facilitated by the recognition of two important landmarks: IVC and left inferior phrenic vein.

The left inferior phrenic vein traverses the diaphragm from the left to the right, and it is partially covered by the left triangular and coronary ligaments. This vessel can drain into the IVC below the diaphragm in 37%, the left adrenal vein in 25%, the left renal vein in 15%, the left hepatic vein in 14%, and both the IVC and the left adrenal vein in 9% of the cases (**Figures 34-9 A–E**). (For additional information, see suggested readings #10, 11.)

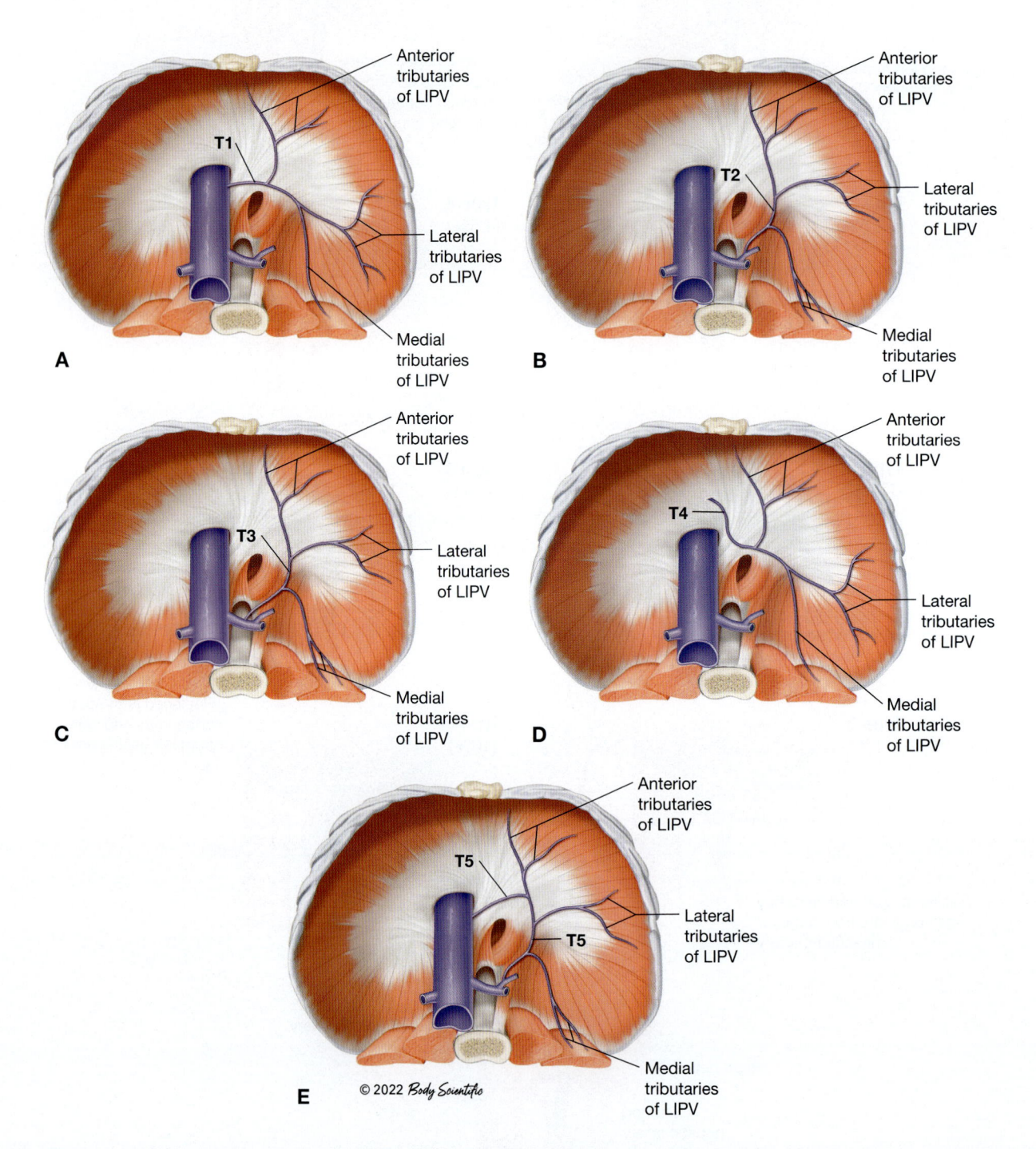

FIGURE 34-9 • Left inferior phrenic vein (LIPV) variations. **A.** T-1 (drainage into infradiaphragmatic IVC). **B.** T-2 (drainage into left adrenal vein). **C.** T-3 (drainage into left renal vein). **D.** T-4 (drainage into left hepatic vein). **E.** T-5 (dual drainage into IVC and left adrenal vein).

Step 2. Intraoperative ultrasonography (IOUS)

The left hepatic lobe mobilization allows for a better access and evaluation of the hepatic parenchyma with an easier positioning of the drop-in or laparoscopic handheld ultrasonographic probe (**Figure 34-10**). The goal of the IOUS study is to confirm the feasibility and adequacy of the planned surgical procedure ruling out possible concomitant lesions and defining the anatomical relationship of the tumor with the main vasculobiliary structures. (For additional information, see Chapter 33, Right Hepatectomy.)

Step 2 average time frame: 3–5 min

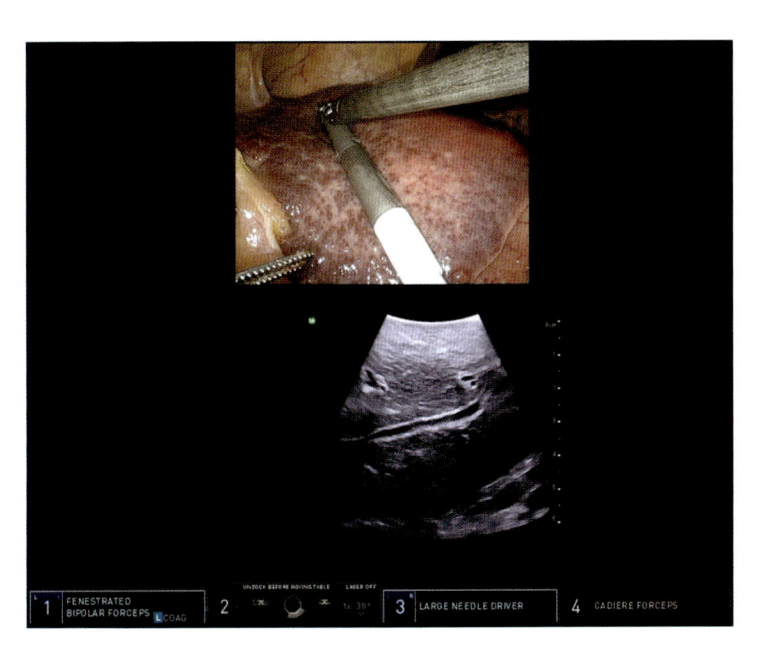

FIGURE 34-10 • IOUS.

Step 3. Cholecystectomy and hilum dissection

A retrograde cholecystectomy is usually performed to lower the hilar plate and achieve a better exposure of the main vasculobiliary structures. The cystic duct is then ligated with Vicryl™ 3-0 ties and divided. The stump of the cystic duct is left long enough to allow a safe injection of radiographic contrast material, if necessary. An intraoperative cholangiography should be carried out any time the biliary anatomy is unclear. With the ProGrasp™ in R3 lifting up the liver (segment 4b), a careful hilar dissection is progressively performed with the monopolar cautery hook in R1 and the bipolar forceps in R2. A preoperative injection of indocyanine green (ICG) may facilitate a preliminary assessment of the hilar anatomy and the identification of anatomical biliary variations. The dissection of the higher portion of the hepatic hilum may allow the exposure of the bile duct bifurcation. To facilitate the vascular anatomy recognition, the lymphatic tissue and lymph nodes encountered during the hilar dissection are gently removed and sent for permanent pathology. The proper hepatic artery and its bifurcation are identified and progressively skeletonized. The right-angle cautery hook allows a precise vascular preparation with a bloodless dissection of the periadventitial plane. In case of malignant lesions requiring a formal lymphadenectomy (e.g., cholangiocarcinoma), the dissection and lymph nodal retrieval are extended at the level of the common hepatic artery in order to obtain the required lymphadenectomy. The exposure of the left portal vein and biliary duct is usually easier than the one required for the right side due to a longer and more horizontal extrahepatic segment.

Step 3 average time frame: 15–20 min

Video 34-1. How to Prepare an Internal Pringle Maneuver

Step 4. Preparation for a possible Pringle maneuver

The complete opening of the gastrohepatic ligament, performed during the first step of the procedure, facilitates the exposure of the hepatoduodenal ligament and the access to the underlying Winslow foramen. The hepatoduodenal ligament is then encircled with an umbilical tape, which is passed through a 5-cm red rubber tube and left in place for a possible internal Pringle maneuver (**Figures 34-11 A, B**). With the left hepatic lobe inflow control (left hepatic artery and left portal vein), a Pringle clamping is not usually required. However, its preparation might be wise at the beginning of a surgeon's learning curve, or in difficult cases.

Step 4 average time frame: 5–10 min

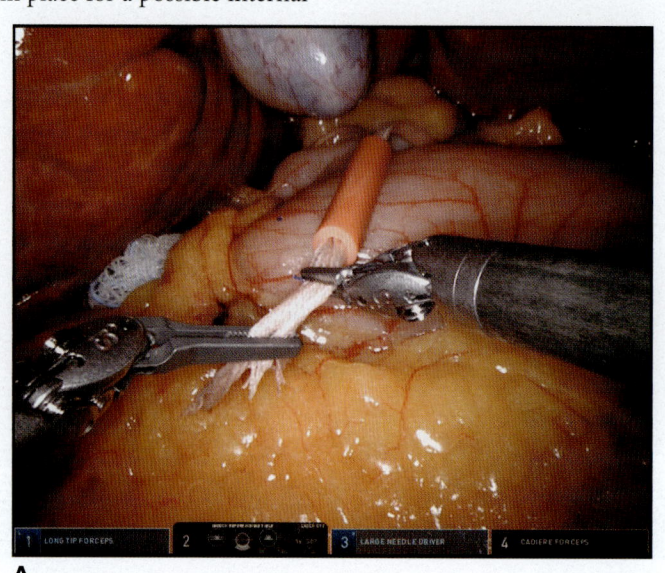

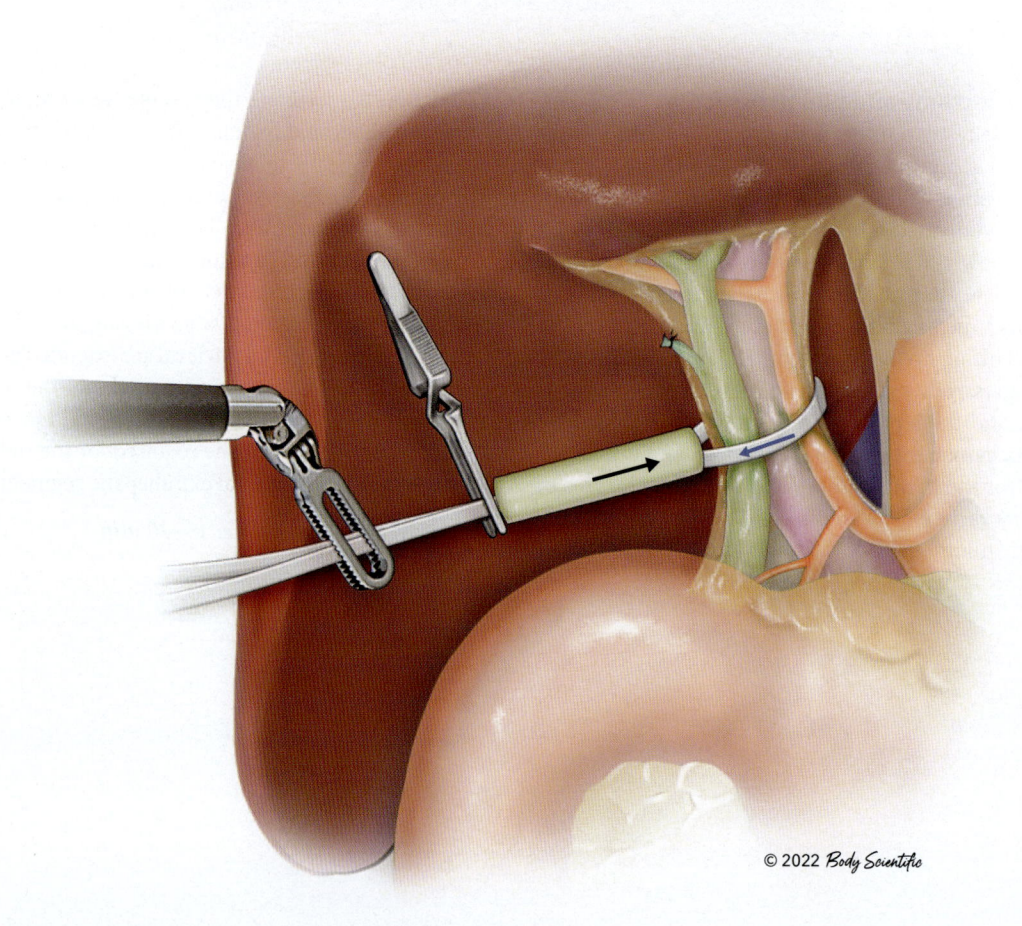

FIGURE 34-11 • **A.** Preparation for a possible Pringle maneuver. **B.** Internal Pringle maneuver.

Left Hepatectomy   743

Step 5. Division of the left hepatic artery

Once isolated, the left hepatic artery is surrounded with a vessel loop to facilitate its atraumatic retraction and further dissection. Before dividing the left hepatic artery, a clamping test is routinely performed with a bulldog clamp to verify the persistence of an intact flow in the right hepatic artery. In case of doubts, a Doppler probing could also be useful (**Figures 34-12 A, B**). Once the arterial anatomy and the presence of a valid inflow in the contralateral right side are assessed, the left hepatic artery is divided with robotic scissors in between Hem-o-lok™ clips or sutures. Also, an 8-mm vascular stapler might be adopted when there is enough space (**Figure 34-13**).

Step 5 average time frame: 5–10 min

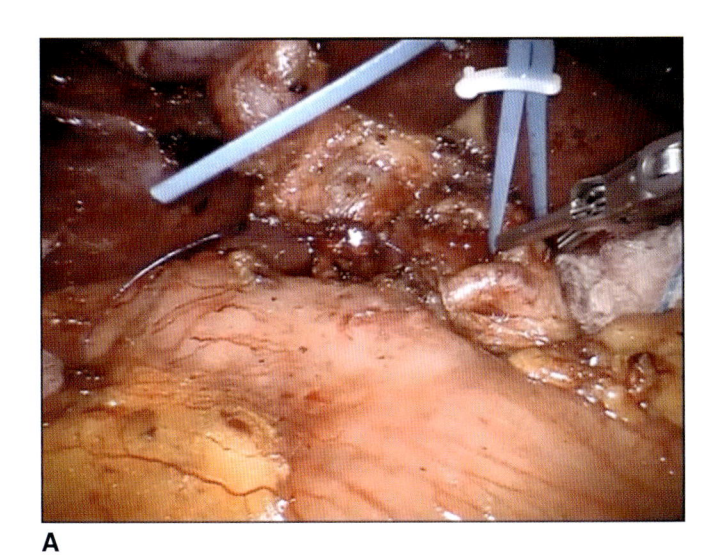

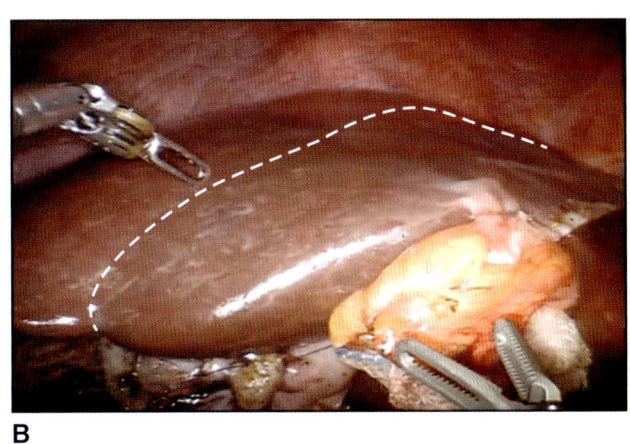

FIGURE 34-12 • **A.** Clamping test of the left hepatic artery. **B.** Initial parenchymal demarcation.

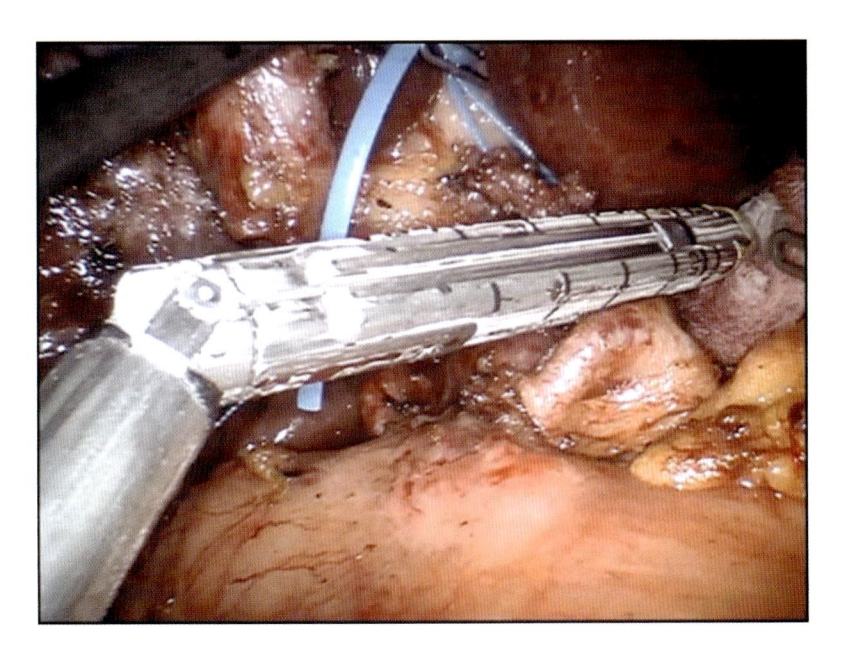

FIGURE 34-13 • Left hepatic artery division.

Step 6. Division of the left portal vein

Once the division of the left hepatic artery is completed, the underlying portal vein and its bifurcation are gently exposed. An adequate preparation of the posteromedial surface of the portal vein may require an extension of the regional lymphadenectomy with the retrieval of station 12p.

While completing the posterior dissection of the left portal vein, extreme care should be taken to avoid any injury to the small portal branches supplying the caudate lobe. These small vessels, interfering with a safe preparation of the portal segment, are individually dissected and divided between Prolene™ 5-0 stitches.

At this point, using a long-tip, atraumatic forceps, it is possible to place a vessel loop around the left portal vein. A clamping test is advisable before proceeding with the transection of the vessel. The color demarcation is usually very clear after this maneuver and confirms the correct inflow evaluation (**Figure 34-14**). As already described for the right hepatectomy, the transection of the portal vein can be made with stapling or using suture-ligation techniques when there is not enough space for the tip of the stapler.

The complete control of the left hepatic lobe inflow produces an evident vascular demarcation along the parenchymal transection plane, which lies along the Cantlie's line.

Step 6 average time frame: 15–25 min

▶▶ **TIPS**

The precise location of the portal vein resection reflects the extension of the planned hepatectomy. A vascular transection close to its bifurcation is necessary when the caudate lobe will be included in the surgical resection. When the segment 1 is spared, and to minimize the risk of vascular/biliary injuries connected with anomalies, the transection of the portal vein is done more distally, before the origin of the glissonian pedicles 3–4 (gate 1–3).

▶▶ **TIPS**

When a proximal and distal control of the small portal vein branches to the caudate lobe is not feasible, only one stitch is placed on the portal vein side allowing a safer vascular transection. The minimal back-bleeding from the parenchyma is easily controlled with bipolar coagulation.

▶▶ **TIPS**

When there is not enough room for the insertion of the stapler, the left portal vein can be divided with a suture-ligation technique. A silk or Vicryl™ 3-0 suture is first tied on the proximal segment of the portal vein to interrupt its flow. After that, it becomes easier to reinforce the proximal stump with Prolene™ 4-0 suturing. The distal segment is controlled with another stitch of Prolene™ 4-0, making sure that there is a safe room for the transection of the vessel with scissors.

Left Hepatectomy 745

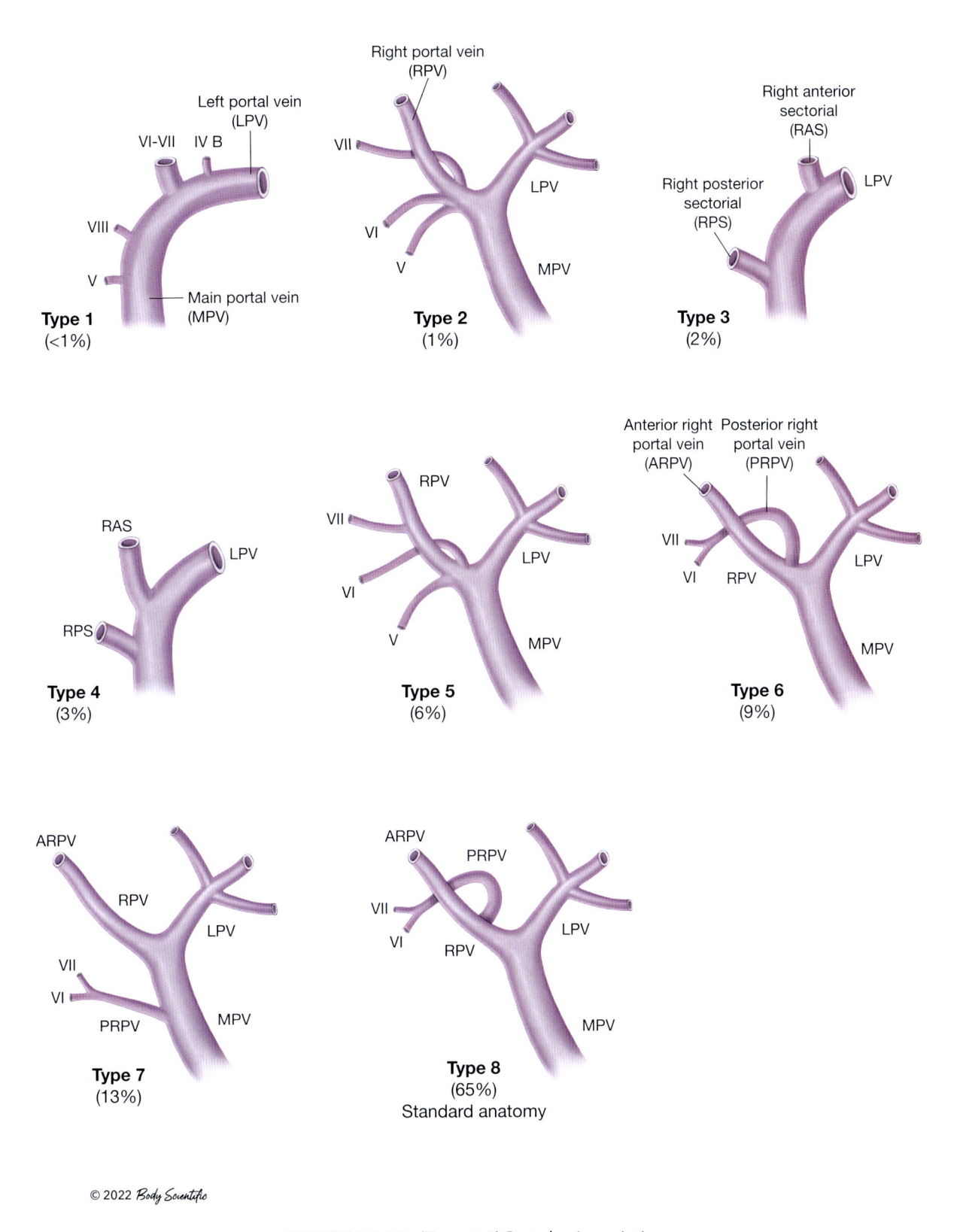

FIGURE 34-14 • (Type 1-8) Portal vein variations.

Step 7. Left hepatic duct transection
Once the normal biliary anatomy is clarified, the left hepatic duct can be controlled and transected completing the hilum dissection. As already described for the portal vein, the level of transection of the bile duct depends on the planned procedure (including or not the caudate lobe). When segment 1 will be preserved, there is no need to divide the bile duct too close to its bifurcation, thus minimizing the risk of postoperative biliary leaks.

The biliary transection is usually performed at the beginning of the liver parenchymal dissection to achieve a clear exposure of the proximal biliary anatomy. Anatomical variations are not infrequently encountered and are described in **Figure 34-15**. (For additional information, see suggested reading #12.)

The proximal stump is sutured-ligated with PDS™ 4-0.

Step 7 average time frame: 15–30 min

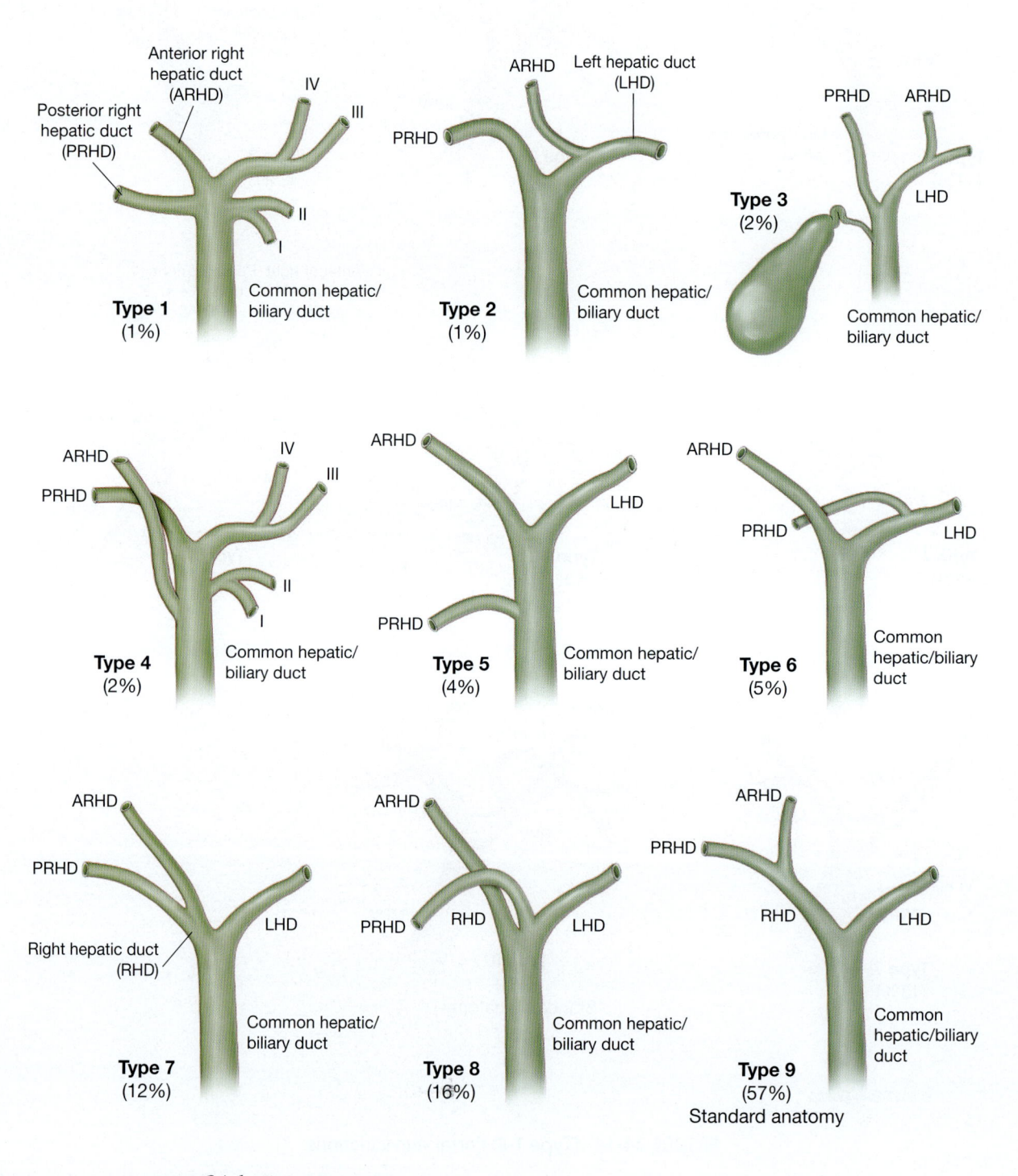

FIGURE 34-15 • **(Type 1-9)** Hepatic duct variations.

Left Hepatectomy 747

> ## 🔍 ANATOMICAL HIGHLIGHTS
>
> **Anatomical Variations of the Right Hepatic Ducts:** it is important to recognize if the right posterior hepatic duct (from segments 6 and 7), or the anterior sectorial bile duct (from segments 5 and 8), empties into the left hepatic duct. A widespread and appropriate knowledge of these anatomical variations is fundamental to avoid major biliary complications. An intraoperative cholangiography may be required to clarify a doubtful anatomy (**Figures 34-16 A–C**). (For additional information, see suggested reading #13.)
>
> **Caudate Lobe Biliary Anatomy:** a careful evaluation of the first segment of the left hepatic duct is also important to avoid major biliary leaks coming from aberrant insertions of sectorial branches emerging from the right caudate lobe segments (**Figure 34-17**). Moreover, some left caudate ducts may drain directly into the left ductal system at various distances from the confluence and, accordingly, also during left hepatectomies without caudate lobe resection, these structures have to be individually controlled with transfixing sutures of Prolene™ 5-0/6-0 to reduce the risk of a postoperative biliary leak (**Figures 34-18 A, B**). (For additional information, see suggested reading #14.)

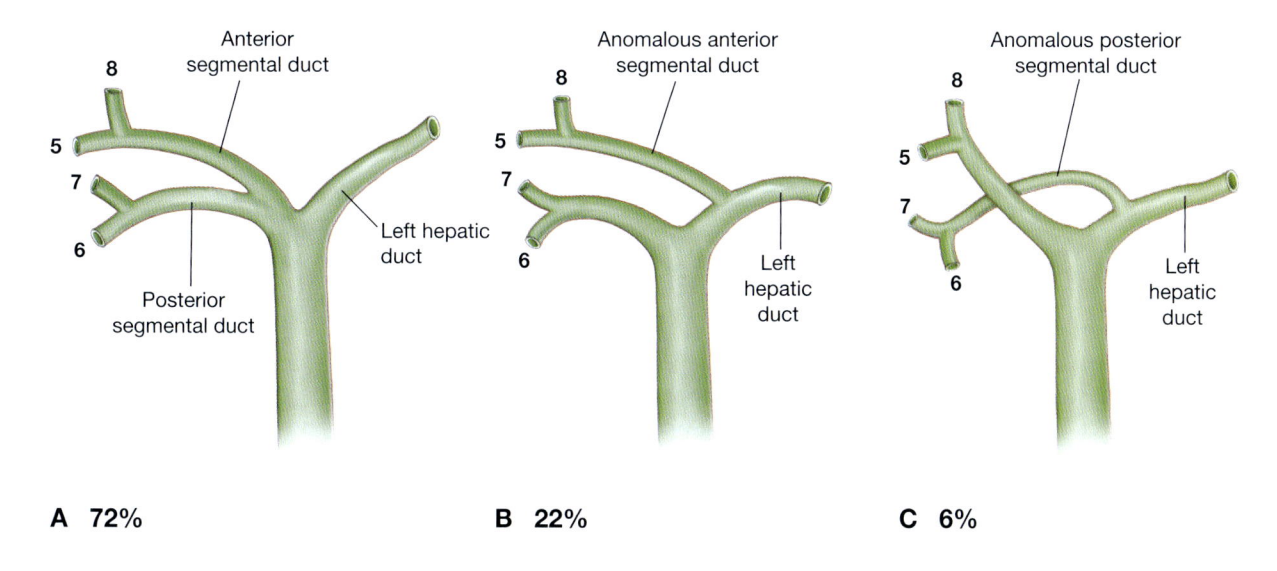

FIGURE 34-16 • Anatomic variations of the right hepatic duct.

748 The Foundation and Art of Robotic Surgery

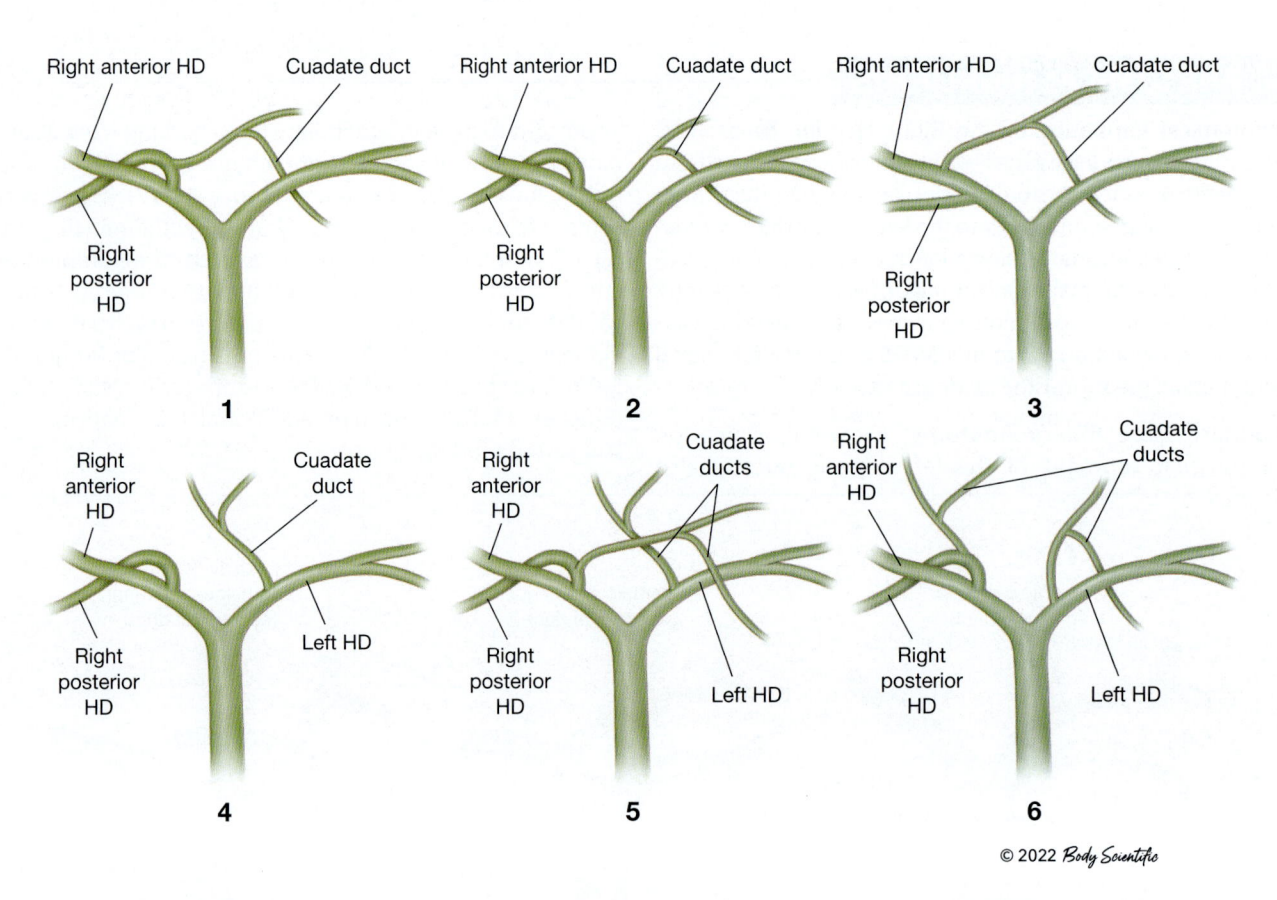

FIGURE 34-17 • **(1-6)** Caudate lobe biliary anatomy. (Type I) left-to-right crossover drainage: (1), (2), and (3) crossover duct is draining into right posterior sectoral duct, right hepatic duct, and right anterior sectoral duct, respectively; (Type II) (4) right-to-left crossover; (Type III) (5) both left-to-right and right-to-left crossovers; (Type IV) (6) no crossover ducts.

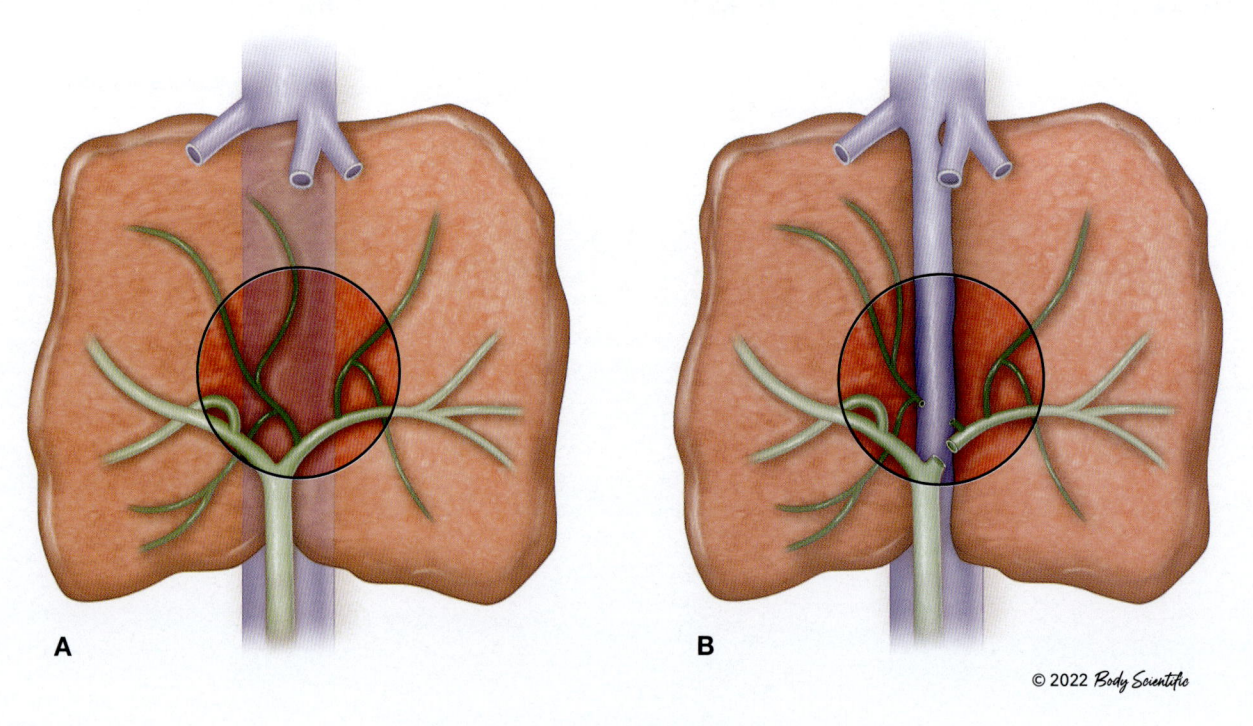

FIGURE 34-18 • Caudate lobe biliary anatomy.

Step 8. Preparation of the left hepatic vein

Once a solid experience in hepatic surgery has been achieved, before starting the parenchymal transection, the left hepatic vein may be prepared extracapsularly. With the grasper in R3 lifting the left hepatic lobe, the *ligamentum venosum* (Arantius' ligament) is localized on the ventral surface of the liver, between the caudate lobe and the main left parenchyma. This structure is the fibrous remnant of the *ductus venosus* of the fetal circulation that is attached to the left branch of the portal vein and connects the umbilical vein to the IVC at the level of the left hepatic vein (**Figure 34-19**). Following this anatomical landmark, along with the complete dissection of the left coronary ligament, the extrahepatic segment of the left hepatic vein is exposed. The thin peritoneal layer covering the left hepatic vein and the suprahepatic IVC is carefully dissected with short and intermittent energy applications of monopolar hook. Once the extrahepatic segment of the left hepatic vein is exposed, before its confluence into the IVC and after clarifying the position of the middle hepatic vein, a vessel loop is placed around this structure. It will help as a landmark for the dissection and will facilitate the final stapling-transection of the vein.

The most relevant anatomical variations involving the hepatic veins are shown in **Figure 34-20**. (For additional information, see suggested reading #15.)

Step 8 average time frame: 5–15 min

> **EDITORIAL COMMENT**
>
> It is useful to remember that, in a considerable number of cases, the left hepatic vein may present a common trunk with the middle hepatic vein. This frequent anatomical setting may increase the risk of vascular injuries that, with an untransected liver parenchyma, are difficult to repair. Moreover, the left hepatic vein may have a very short extrahepatic segment that reduces the possibilities of a safe and complete vascular control. Accordingly, the extracapsular preparation of the left hepatic vein is not routinely performed before the parenchymal transection.

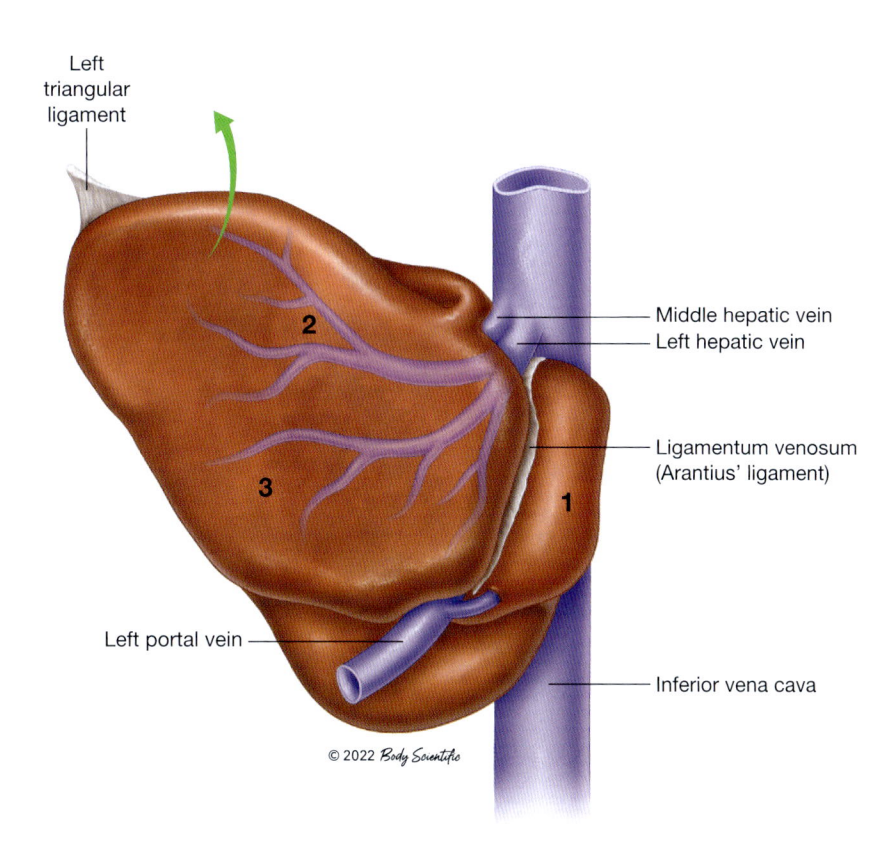

FIGURE 34-19 • *Ligamentum venosum* (Arantius' ligament).

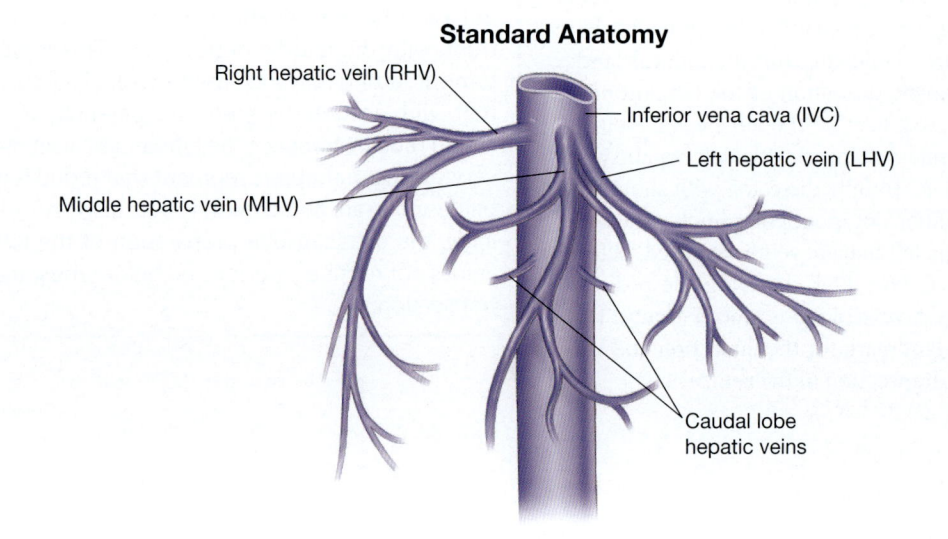

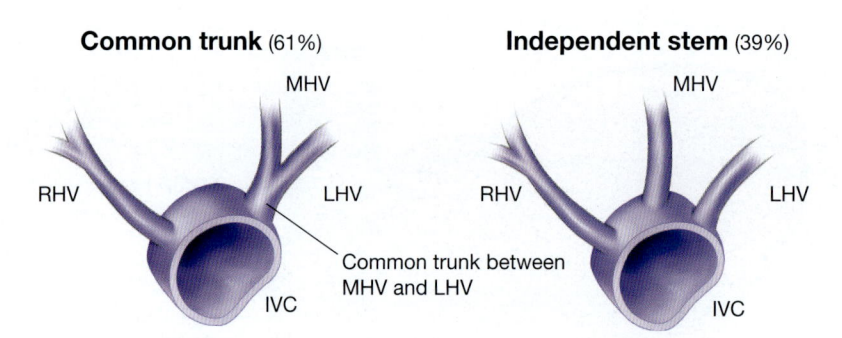

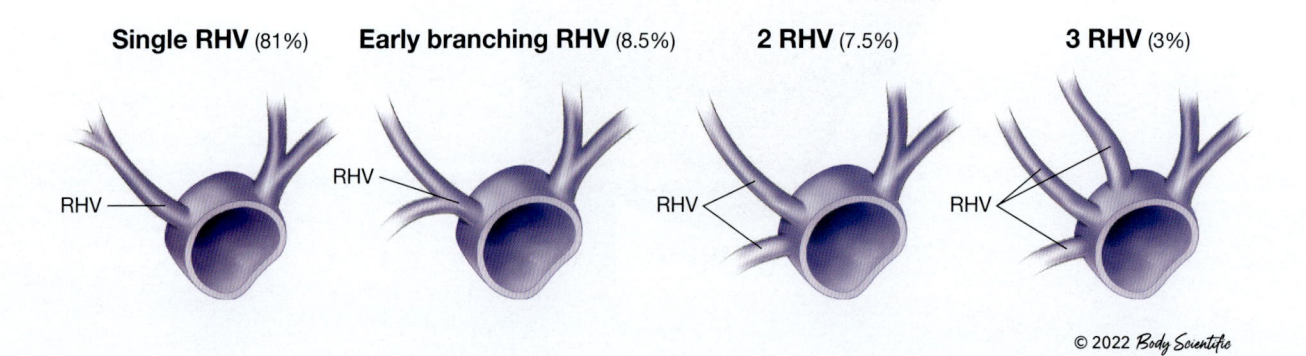

FIGURE 34-20 • Hepatic vein anatomical variations.

▶ **Video 34-2.** Detachment of the Caudate Lobe from the Vena Cava in a Segment 1 Resection

Step 9. Detachment of the caudate lobe from the vena cava

When the planned resection involves the caudate lobe (segment 1) (e.g., perihilar cholangiocarcinoma with involvement of the caudate lobe branches), the division of the left hepatic artery and portal vein is performed at their origin in order to interrupt the blood supply to the caudate lobe. This maneuver should be executed with extreme care, not including the bile duct or the artery supplying the right hemiliver. Moreover, many other short hepatic veins, directly arising from the retrohepatic IVC, are connected to the caudate lobe and should be individually controlled during the left hepatocaval dissection with transfixing sutures of Prolene™ 5-0/6-0 (**Figure 34-21**).

The left lateral approach to the Spiegel's lobe involves a careful dissection of the left IVC ligament. This structure, that on the right side of the IVC is called Makuuchi ligament, encircles and fixes the caudate lobe to the IVC. This fibrovascular structure is preferably ligated with interrupted transfixed stitches of Prolene™ 3-0 and subsequently transected achieving an adequate exposure of the anterior IVC surface and of the short hepatic veins connecting the caudate lobe to the IVC. The caudate lobe dissection is completed, during the final phase of the parenchymal transection, performing the removal of the left side of the caudate lobe.

Step 9 average time frame: 30–40 min

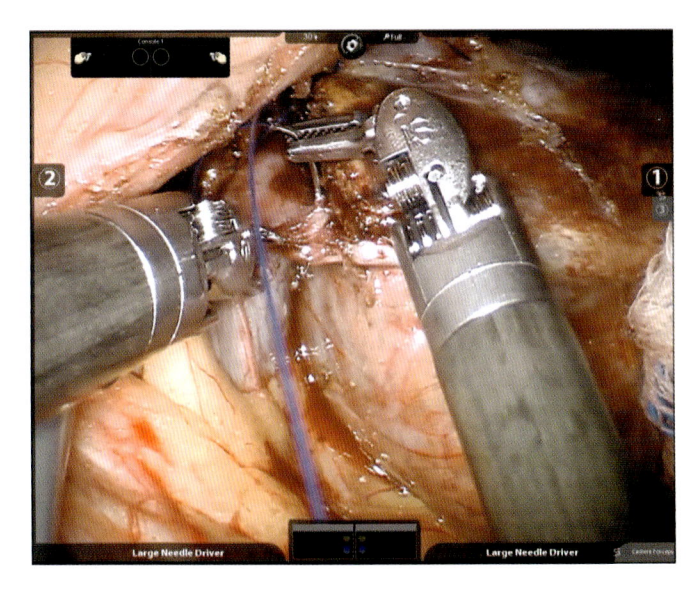

FIGURE 34-21 • Short hepatic vein control.

Step 10. Parenchymal transection

After inflow control, the parenchymal transection margin is marked with the monopolar cautery hook on the liver surface, following the ischemic demarcation line (Cantlie's line) (**Figure 34-22**).

The parenchymal transection begins at the lower margin of the liver and continues with a cephalad direction by following the middle hepatic vein, which represents the main landmark for the left hepatectomy. (The liver parenchymal dissection technique is extensively described in Chapter 33.) The R3 is used to grasp a stay suture of Prolene™ 2-0 that is usually placed on the free edge of segment 4 to maintain an adequate exposure of the parenchymal transection line. As the transection line opens up, additional Prolene™ 2-0 stitches can be applied on the free edge of the left hepatic lobe allowing a better control of the surgical field. The main adopted instruments for this step are the Harmonic shears in R1 and the bipolar forceps in R2. A swap of these instruments may be at some point necessary to maintain the correct alignment of the dissecting tools with the section plane. A Pringle maneuver is not usually performed during a left hepatectomy but may be considered in case of difficult parenchymal transection. The portal and arterial inflow control already achieved in the first steps of the operation reduce the risk of major bleedings during this phase. Minor hemorrhages from the parenchyma or connecting branches of the median hepatic vein can be controlled with bipolar coagulation or selective stitching.

An IOUS is often repeated during the parenchymal transection to evaluate the tumor margins, when necessary, and to localize major tributaries to the middle hepatic vein. These branches encountered during the resection are mainly controlled using interrupted stitches of Prolene™ 3-0/4-0. As described in the previous step, when the caudate lobe has to be included in the resection plan, the parenchymal transection

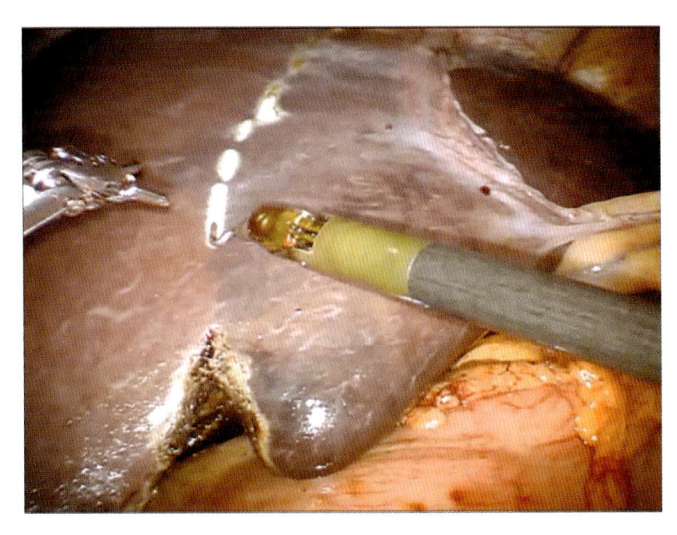

FIGURE 34-22 • Marking the line of perfusion.

runs vertically along the left border of the middle hepatic vein, reaching the anterior surface of the IVC and joining to the hepatocaval dissection previously performed. In case of left hepatectomy without caudate lobe resection, the parenchymal transection is directed vertically and toward the Arantius' ligament, which represents the ventral anatomical landmark of the resection (**Figure 34-23**).

When segments 5 and 8 are included in the resection (left hepatic trisectionectomy), the middle hepatic vein is part of the specimen and the left margin of the right hepatic vein becomes the right limit of the parenchymal transection line.

Step 10 average time frame: 40–120 min

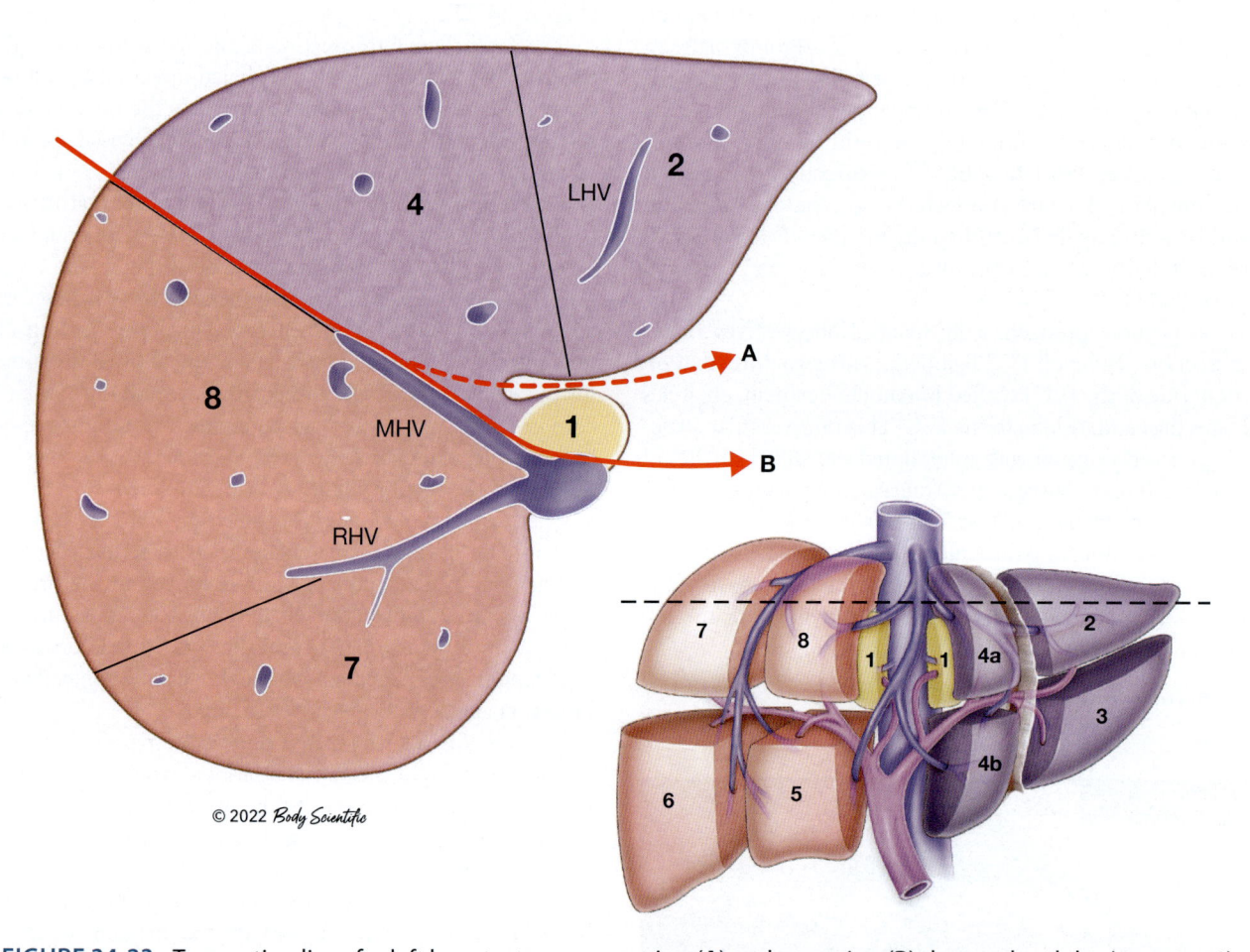

FIGURE 34-23 • Transection lines for left hepatectomy preserving (A) and removing (B) the caudate lobe (segment 1).

Step 11. Stapling of the left hepatic vein

The parenchymal transection proceeds cranially toward the left hepatic vein, which is divided intrahepatically, in an expedited fashion, using a robotic or handheld vascular stapler. The location of the left and middle hepatic veins has been previously verified with the IOUS.

Once the parenchymal transection is completed, meticulous hemostasis and biliostasis are carried out with Prolene™ 3-0 and 4-0 stitches on the remnant transection surface. During the hemostasis verification, the anesthesia team is asked to increase the central venous pressure (CVP), with Valsalva maneuvers, in order to have a reliable assessment of the surgical transection plane.

Step 11 average time frame: 10–15 min

> **EDITORIAL COMMENT**
>
> When the left hepatic vein was prepared extracapsularly, its division is performed by stapling, before starting the parenchymal transection. The advantage of this technique is a decrease in blood loss from the parenchyma.

Step 12. Specimen extraction

At this point, a closed-suction drain is positioned in proximity of the transection margin. The specimen is placed in an Endobag™ and usually retrieved through a Pfannenstiel incision. (Further extraction strategies are described in Chapter 2, The Basic Principles of Clinical Applications.)

Step 12 average time frame: 15–20 min

Suggested Readings

1. Gagner M, Rheault M, Dubuc J. Laparoscopic partial hepatectomy for liver tumor. In: Abstracts of the 1992 Scientific Session of the Society of American Gastrointestinal Surgeons (SAGES). Washington, DC, USA, April 11–12, 1992. *Surg Endosc.* 1992;6:85-110.
2. Azagra JS, Goergen M, Jacobs D. Laparoscopic left lateral segmentectomy (left hepatic lobectomy). *Endosurgery.* 1994;2:7-8.
3. Hüscher CG, Lirici MM, Chiodini S, Recher A. Current position of advanced laparoscopic surgery of the liver. *J R Coll Surg Edinb.* 199;42(4):219-225.
4. Giulianotti PC, Coratti A, Angelini M, et al. Robotics in general surgery: personal experience in a large community hospital. *Arch Surg.* 2003;138(7):777-784. doi: 10.1001/archsurg.138.7.777
5. Giulianotti PC, Coratti A, Bianco F, Sbrana F. Technique de L'Hepatectomie Droite Robottique. *Le Journal de Coelio Chirurgie.* 2006; 59:40-47.
6. Giulianotti PC, Coratti A, Sbrana F, et al. Robotic liver surgery: results for 70 resections. *Surgery.* 2011;149(1):29-39. doi: 10.1016/j.surg.2010.04.002
7. Giulianotti PC, Bianco FM, Daskalaki D, Gonzalez-Ciccarelli LF, Kim J, Benedetti E. Robotic liver surgery: technical aspects and review of the literature. *Hepatobiliary Surg Nutr.* 2016;5(4):311-321. doi: 10.21037/hbsn.2015.10.05
8. Yan J, Feng H, Wang H, et al. Hepatic artery classification based on three-dimensional CT. *Br J Surg.* 2020;107(7):906-916. doi: 10.1002/bjs.11458
9. De Blasi V, Makkai-Popa S-T, Arru L, et al. Rare anatomic variation of the hepatic arterial blood supply: case report and literature review. *Surg Radiol Anat.* 2019;41(3):343-345. doi: 10.1007/s00276-018-2163-5
10. Bonnette P, Hannoun L, Menegaux F, Calmat A, Cabrol C. Anatomic study of the left inferior diaphragmatic vein (vena phrenica inferior sinistra). *Bull Assoc Anat (Nancy).* 1983;67:69-77.
11. Loukas M, Louis RG, Hullett J, et al. An anatomical classification of the variations of the inferior phrenic vein. *Surg Radiol Anat.* 2005;27:566-574. doi: 10.1007/s00276-005-0029-0
12. Chaib E, Kanas AF, Galvão FHF, et al. Bile duct confluence: anatomic variations and its classification. *Surg Radiol Anat.* 2014;36(2):105-109. doi: 10.1007/s00276-013-1157-6
13. Skandalakis JE, Gray SW, Rowe JR. *Anatomical Complications in General Surgery.* New York: McGraw-Hill, 1983.
14. Makki K, Chorasiya V, Srivastava A, Singhal A, Khan AA, Vij V. Analysis of caudate lobe biliary anatomy and its implications in living donor liver transplantation—a single centre prospective study. *Transpl Int.* 2018 May 2. doi: 10.1111/tri.13272
15. Fang C-H, You J-H, Lau WY, et al. Anatomical variations of hepatic veins: three-dimensional computed tomography scans of 200 subjects. *World J Surg.* 2012;36(1):120-124. doi: 10.1007/s00268-011-1297-y

35

"If you find what you are truly passionate about, then finding your career will not be too far away."

—Sir Richard Branson (1950)

Liver Sectionectomies: Left Lateral Sectionectomy

Alberto Mangano • Valentina Valle • Pier Cristoforo Giulianotti

INTRODUCTION

Couinaud classified the liver anatomy into 8 independent functional units (termed segments) rather than detailing the morphological external appearance of the liver. Each segment has its own specific vascular inflow, outflow, and biliary drainage. Other classifications/variations have been published; however, describing those is beyond the scope of this chapter (for more information see suggested readings #1–5).

The anatomical surgical resections are defined by areas (sections) perfused by secondary portal pedicles (see **Figure 35-1**). Based on the size, location, and margins of the lesion that needs to be removed, a sectionectomy could be an alternative to a major resection in order to achieve radical margins and to spare functional liver parenchyma.

INSTRUMENT REQUIREMENTS

The suggested main robotic instruments/tools can be listed as follows:
- 30°/0° scope
- 2 needle drivers (round-tip or macro)
- Cautery hook/monopolar scissors
- Harmonic shears/vessel sealer
- Robotic linear stapler (with different loads)
- Multiple Hem-o-lok™ clips
- Medium/large clip applier
- Bipolar forceps
- Cadière forceps
- Long-tip forceps

The suggested main laparoscopic instruments/tools can be listed as follows:
- Needle drivers

- Scissors
- Graspers
- Endostapler (with different loads)
- Suction-irrigation
- Laparoscopic ultrasound (drop-in probe or laparoscopic handheld)

Supplemental materials:
- Gauzes, sponges
- Penrose drains
- Vessel loops
- Red rubber tube for an internal Pringle maneuver (optional)
- Endobag™
- Medium/large clips
- Sutures: Vicryl™ 3-0; Prolene™ 2-0, 3-0, 4-0, 5-0

Photo from Rob Kim / Stringer.

Quote reproduced with permission from Jachimowicz JM, To C, Agasi S, et al. The gravitational pull of expressing passion: When and how expressing passion elicits status conferral and support from others. Organ Behav Hum Decis Process. 2019;153:41-62.

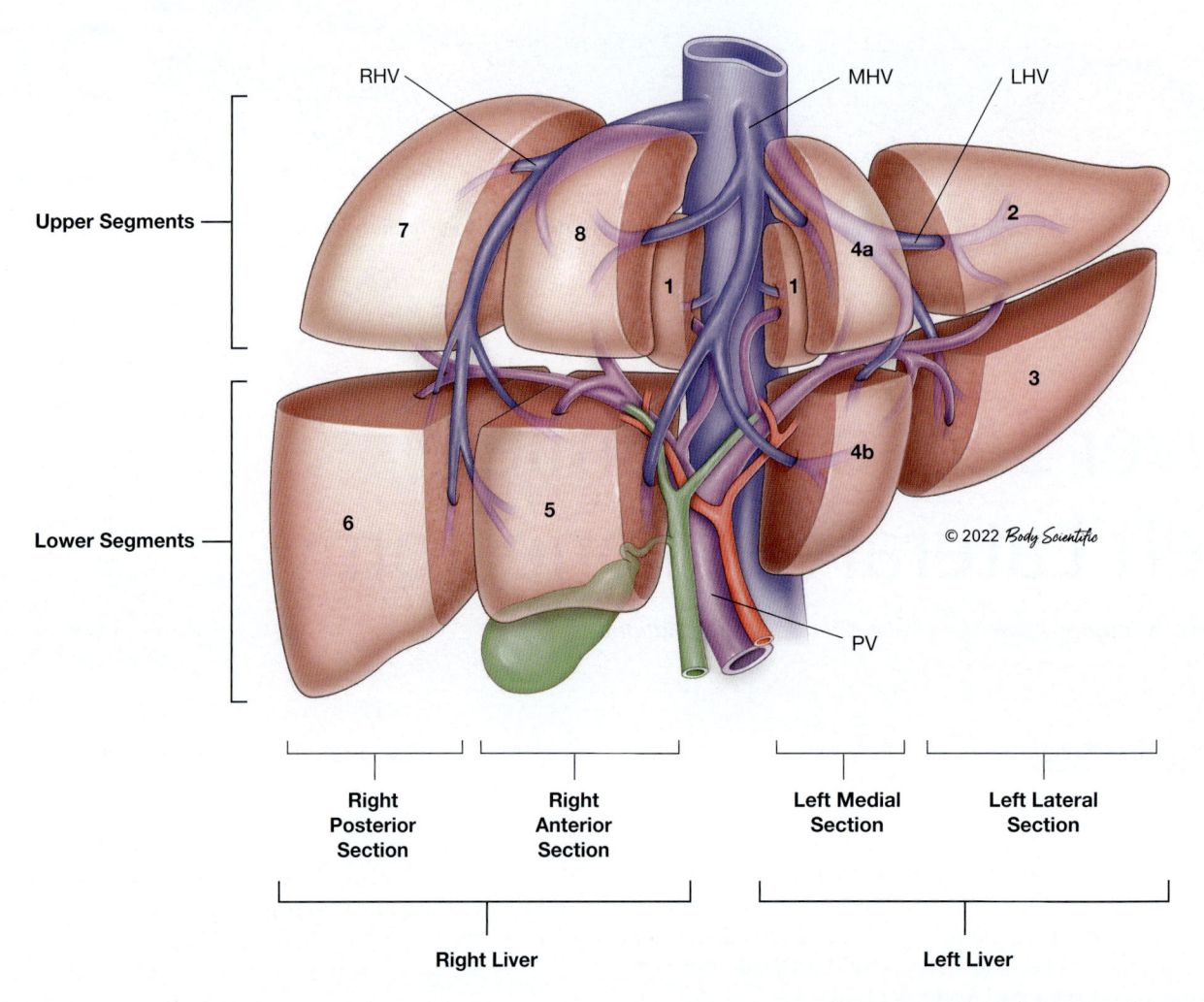

FIGURE 35-1 • Anatomical segments of the liver. The right hepatic vein (RHV) divides the right lobe into anterior and posterior segments. The middle hepatic vein (MHV) divides the liver into right and left lobes (or right and left hemi liver). This plane runs from the inferior vena cava to the gallbladder fossa. The left hepatic vein (LHV) divides the left lobe into a medial and lateral part.

Classification of Sectionectomies

See **Figures 35-2 A–F** for the classification of sectionectomies.

Indications and Relative Contraindications to the Robotic Approach

The main indications can be listed as follows: liver metastasis, hepatocellular carcinoma, and other liver tumors.

Like other surgical procedures, patient selection is of paramount importance. There are currently no absolute contraindications to robotic liver resections; rather, the indications should be based on the surgeon's skills and experience. Particular attention should be paid in assessing risks and benefits of robotic liver sectionectomies in the following circumstances (as already explained in Chapter 33, Right Hepatectomy):

1. Tumor invasion of the major vascular structures. These types of resections are possible, but they require high levels of skills and should be approached only by very experienced surgeons.
2. Bulky lesions that involve the diaphragm, especially in its posterior portion in proximity to the vena cava.
3. Presence of multiple lesions where hybrid techniques of resection are necessary. An open procedure is probably more suitable, in cases where multiple parenchymal sparing resections associated with radiofrequency ablations (RFAs) throughout the liver are required. An exception to these considerations is perhaps represented by large hemangiomas, which feature significant volume reduction after the arterial blood supply is interrupted.
4. Some conditions can also preclude the safety of robotic liver surgery. Patients with cardiorespiratory comorbidities, who are unfit for major surgery, should not be offered a robotic procedure either.

General Concepts about Liver Sectionectomies

1. A preoperative careful evaluation of the patient liver anatomy (portal pedicles and hepatic veins) is necessary: computed tomography (CT) scan, magnetic resonance imaging (MRI), and 3D reconstructions are essential (**Figure 35-3**).
2. Intraoperative ultrasound scanning competence is required (for verification of the vascular anatomy and the definition of margins).
3. Preliminary inflow control is not always required, but it is recommended in difficult sectionectomies. It could be

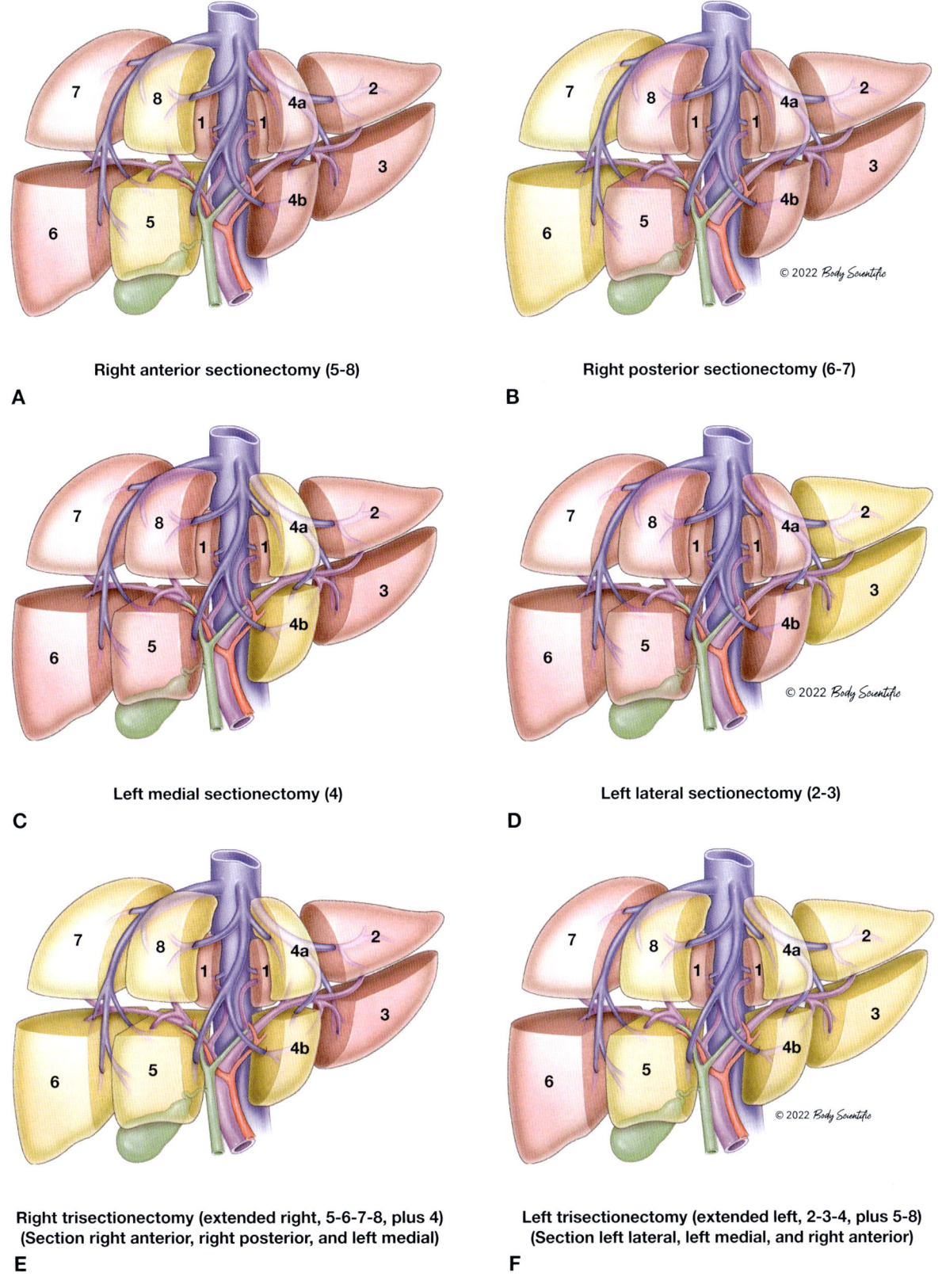

FIGURE 35-2 • **A.** Right anterior sectionectomy (5–8). **B.** Right posterior sectionectomy (6–7). **C.** Left medial sectionectomy (4). **D.** Left lateral sectionectomy (2–3). **E.** Right trisectionectomy (extended right, 5-6-7-8, plus 4) (section right anterior, right posterior, and left medial). **F.** Left trisectionectomy (extended left, 2-3-4, plus 5-8) (section left lateral, left medial, plus right anterior).

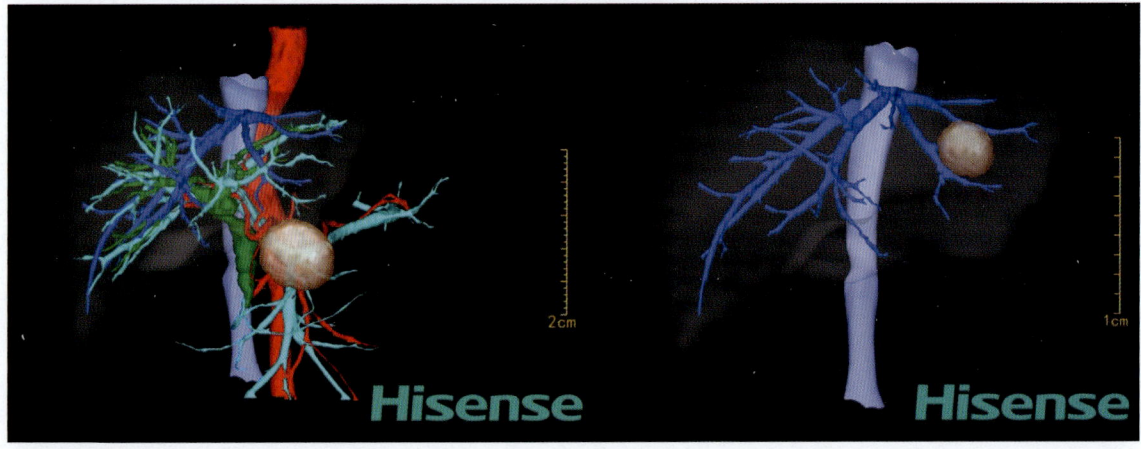

FIGURE 35-3 • CT 3D reconstruction of the anatomy.

selective (Glissonian pedicle clamping and/or division) or general (Pringle maneuver).

4. Extrahepatic outflow preliminary control should be avoided. In some cases, the extracapsular isolation of the hepatic veins could be risky. A low intraoperative central venous pressure (CVP) is essential.
5. Indocyanine green (ICG) fluorescence with selective injection or clamping may help in defining the segments involved (negative or positive images) (**Figures 35-4 A, B**).
6. Some kind of mobilization of the liver (depending on the section involved) is always helpful in obtaining a better retraction/exposure and in favoring the best angle of orientation of the dissecting instruments.
7. The working instrument (Harmonic™, LigaSure™, CUSA®) should be aligned and parallel to the main parenchyma section line. The robotic platform is facilitating the bimanual handling of the instruments, allowing a change in the direction of the tools, and favoring the correct approach to the target line.
8. The subcortical parenchyma of the liver is easily dissected layer by layer (as previously described in Chapter 33, Right Hepatectomy).
9. While dissecting the parenchyma, the intrahepatic vascular anatomy should be anticipated (e.g., connecting hepatic veins, main pedicles, etc.), proceeding with small bites of tissue and being ready to react (suturing/stapling). In this surgery, the future perspectives of the robotic platform with overlapping of preoperative images ("fusion images") on the real-time surgical field is quite interesting because the intraparenchymal approach to the Glissonian pedicles could be facilitated (for more information, see Chapter 6, Implemented Imaging and Artificial intelligence).
10. An effective and dynamic retraction of the segments to be resected is paramount to control the section line (stay sutures, R3, gravity, assistant work).
11. The Glissonian pedicles and the main hepatic veins are better controlled with staplers (laparoscopic or robotic). To be effective, the amount of parenchyma surrounding the pedicles should be minimized.

The description of the details of all types of sectionectomies is beyond the goals of this book. The left lateral sectionectomy will be the focus of this chapter, as it is becoming one of the most commonly performed minimally invasive liver resections and one of the main training models.

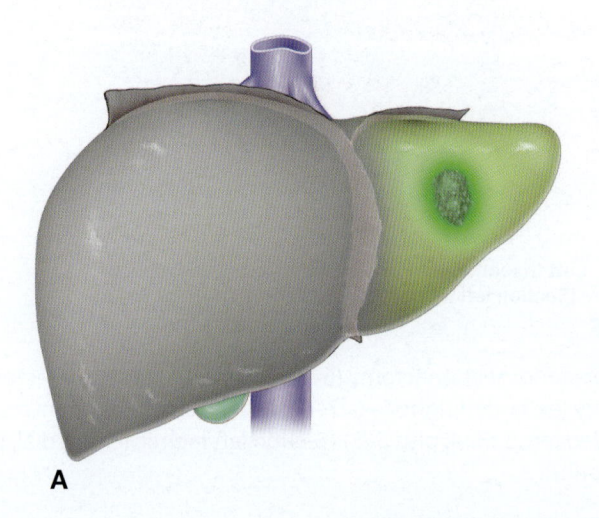

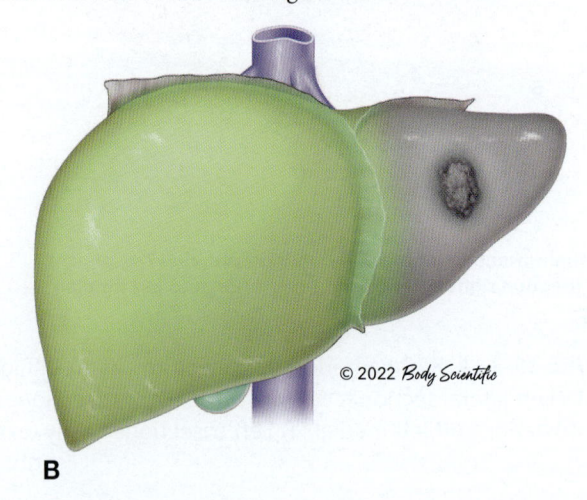

FIGURE 35-4 • Indocyanine green fluorescence.

Left Lateral Sectionectomy

Patient Positioning, OR Setup, and Port Setting

The patient positioning (**Figure 35-5**) and OR setup (**Figure 35-6**) are the same as previously described in Chapter 34, Left Hepatectomy. The port setting (**Figures 35-7 A, B**) is also similar (with some possible minor variations).

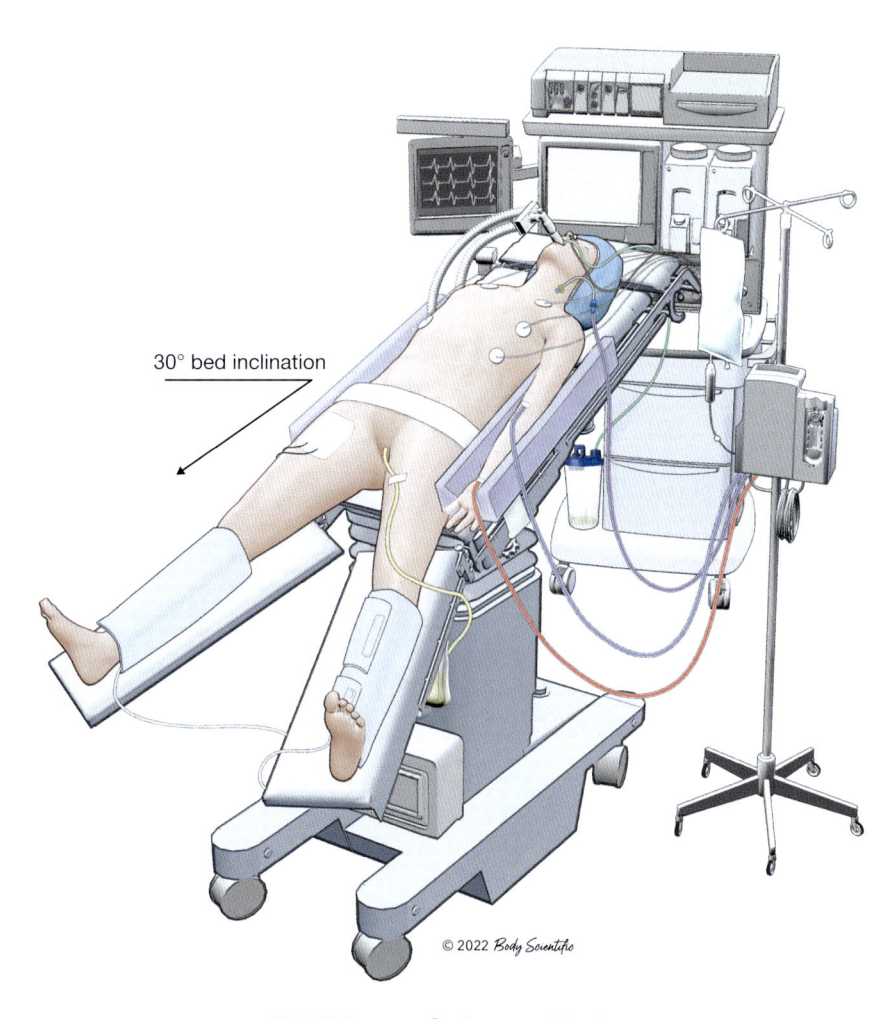

FIGURE 35-5 • Patient positioning.

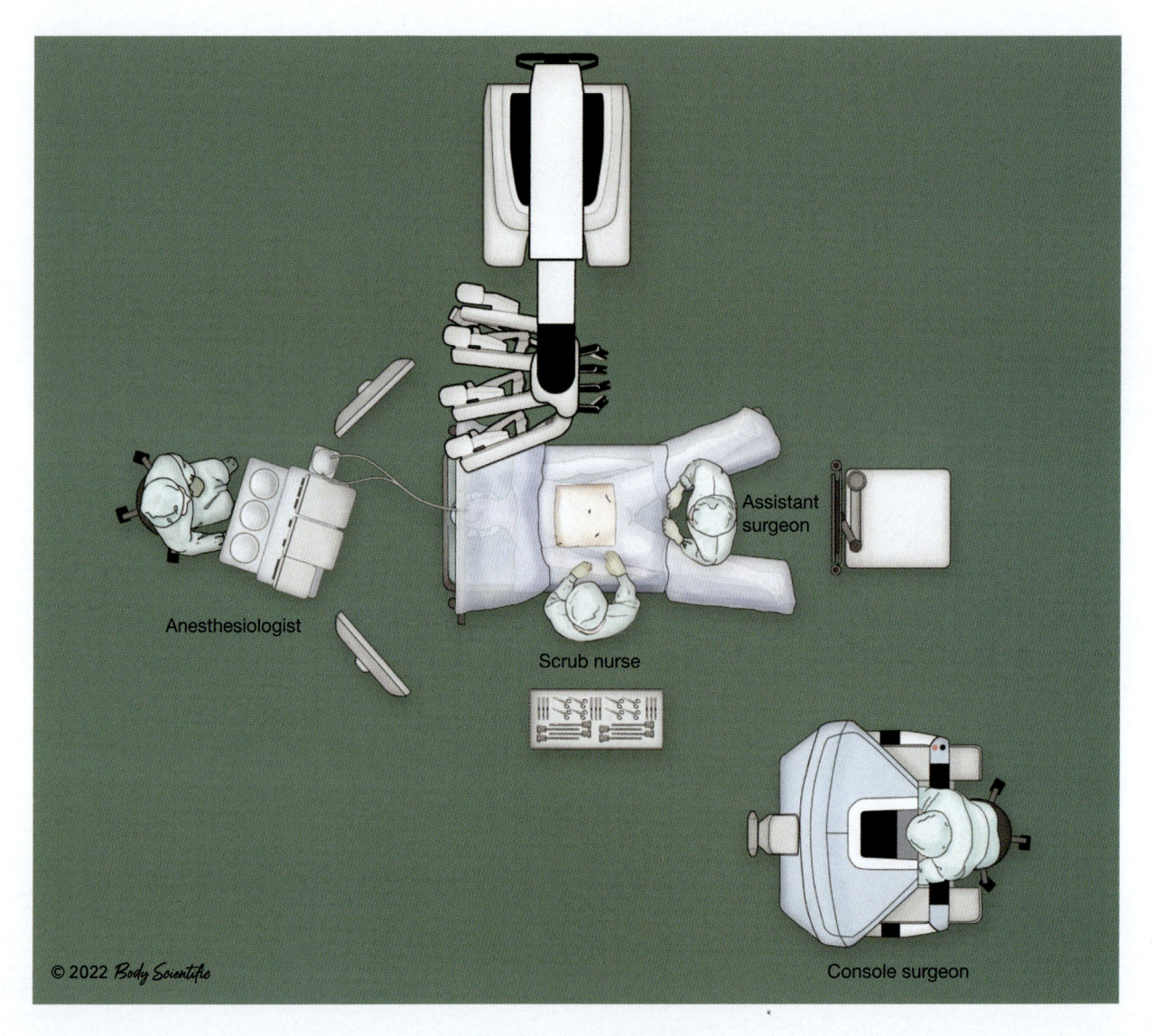

FIGURE 35-6 • OR setup.

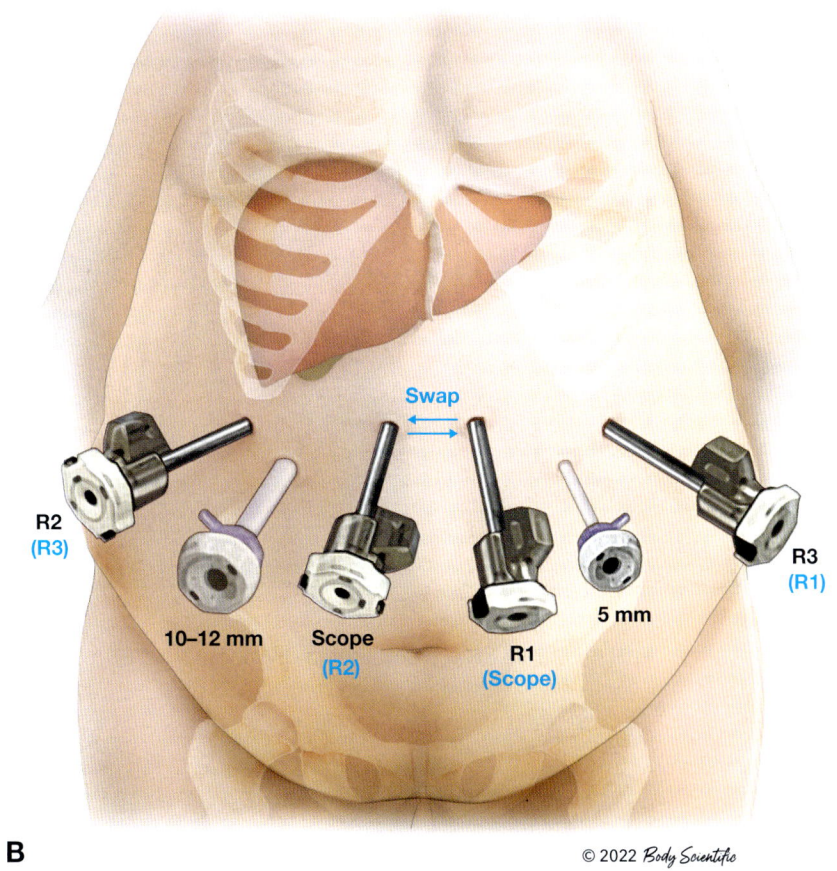

FIGURE 35-7 • Port setting. **A.** Normal abdomen. **B.** Wide abdomen.

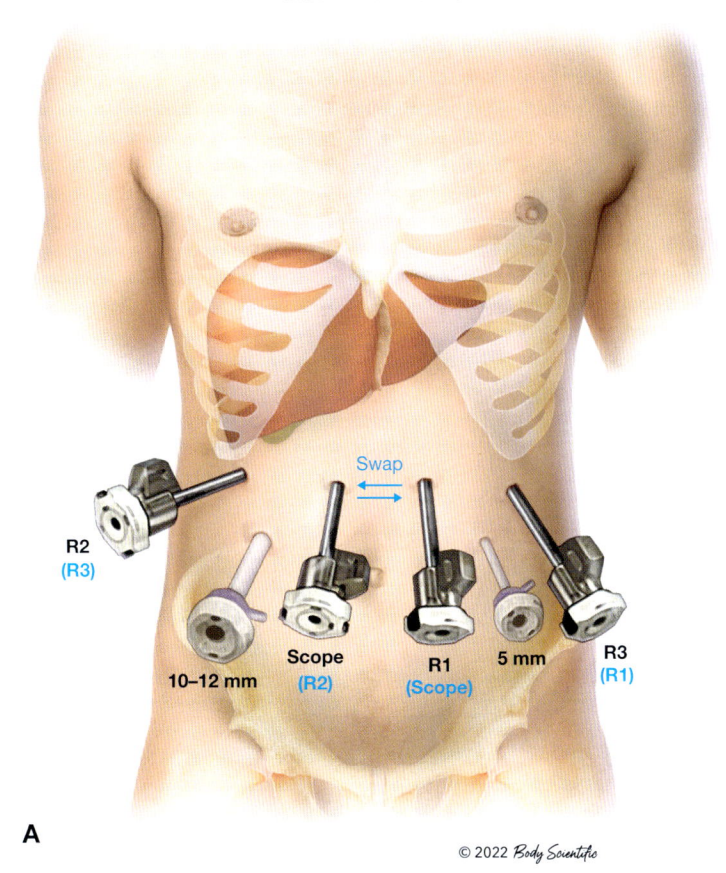

Video 35-1. Left Lateral Sectionectomy – Full Procedure

Left Lateral Sectionectomy Surgical Technique

After the induction of pneumoperitoneum (which is achieved with a Veress needle unless there is a bulky left lobe or other contraindications as already described Chapter 2, The Basic Principles of Clinical Applications), and after the intra-abdominal exploration, the stepwise surgical approach is started.

The main relevant liver anatomy is described in Chapters 33, 34, and 36. Some additional anatomical reminders are provided in **Figure 35-8**.

Step 1. Round and falciform ligaments division

The round and falciform ligaments are taken down to allow a better exploration of the liver (**Figures 35-9 A, B**) and to facilitate the mobilization of the left lateral segments. If there is a small bridge (fibrotic or parenchymal) between segments 3 and 4b, it should be divided.

Step 1 average time frame: 5–10 min

> **▶▶ TIPS**
>
> The round ligament should be entirely divided staying close to the abdominal wall to avoid possible hanging tissue interfering with the visualization (this may be a problem mainly in obese patients who may have a redundant umbilical ligament).

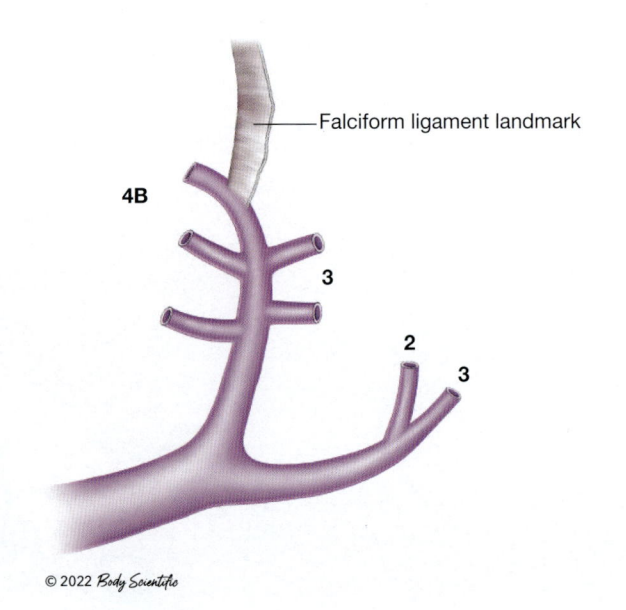

FIGURE 35-8 • Anatomical reminders.

A   B

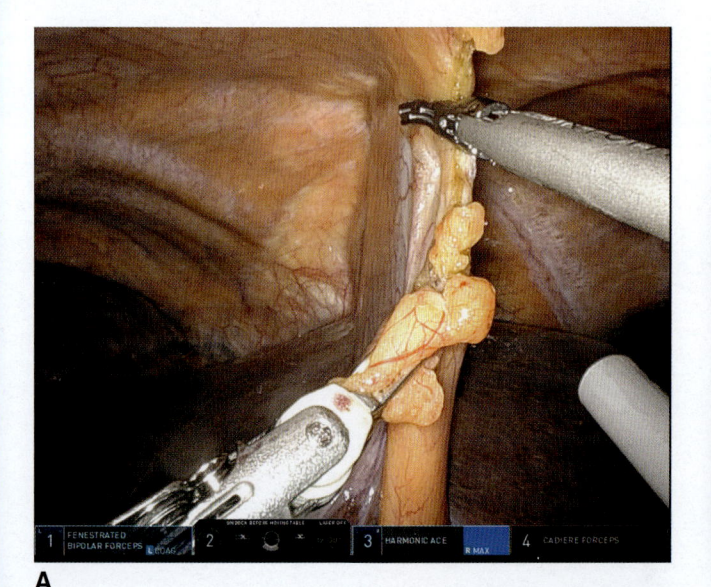

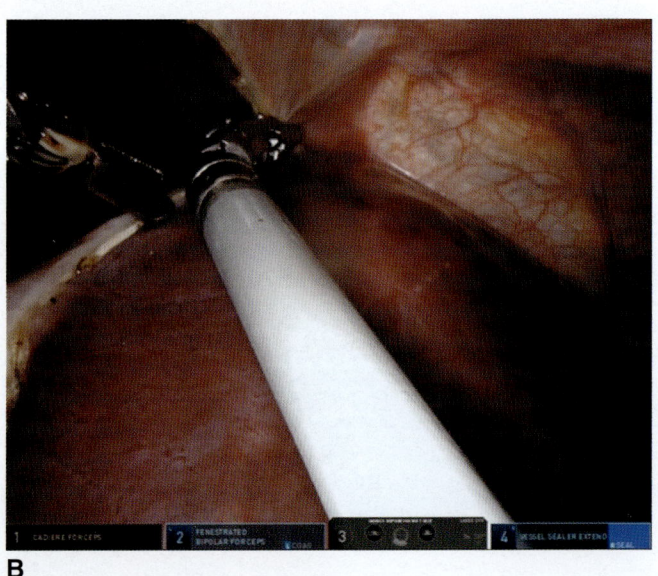

FIGURE 35-9 • Step 1. Ligaments division.

Step 2. Intraoperative ultrasound

The feasibility and the extent of the operation must be evaluated during this step. An adequate surgical plan should be made. In case of malignancy, the peritoneal involvement would have been ruled out during the initial explorative laparoscopy. The intraoperative ultrasound (IOUS) is performed according to the modalities described in Chapter 33 (**Figure 35-10**).

The knowledge of the anatomical relationships of the lesion with the segmental pedicles, the portal vein, the hepatic artery, the hepatic vein, and even the major communicating branches is essential.

Step 2 average time frame: 5–15 min

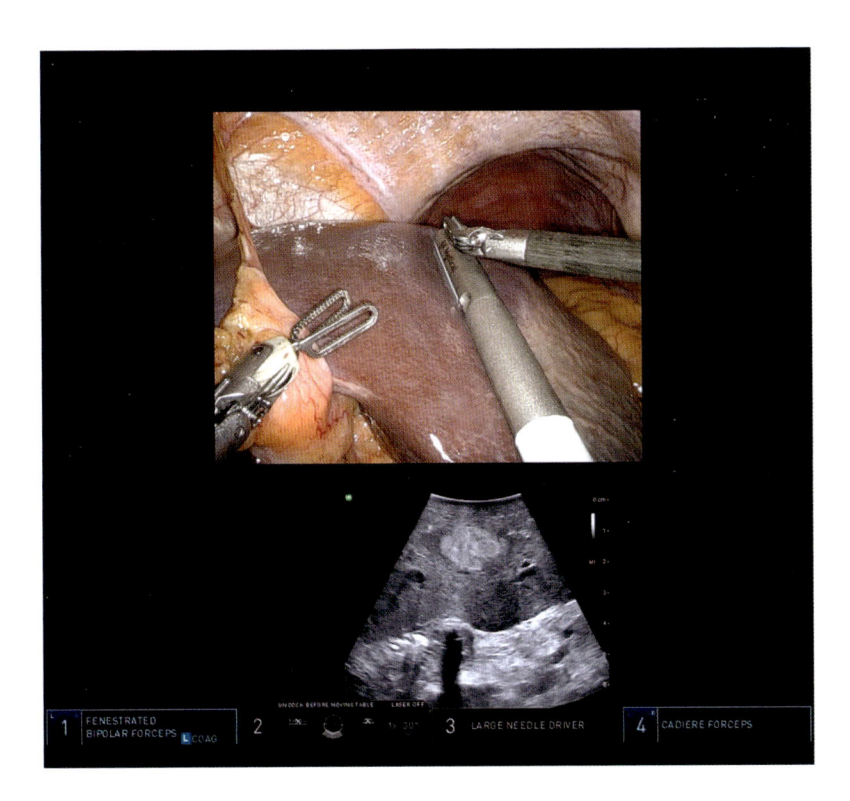

FIGURE 35-10 • Step 2. Intraoperative ultrasound.

> **▶▶ TIPS**
>
> Attention should be paid to the left phrenic vein that is merging into the vena cava. The direction of the phrenic vein is a landmark to be followed to identify the position of the vena cava (see **Figure 35-11**).

> **⚠ PITFALLS**
>
> Lacerations of the splenic capsule can occur while pulling the lateral portion of the triangular ligament. In some patients, the triangular ligament may end up very lateral and close to the spleen and segment 2 of the liver may reach the splenic hilum.

Step 3. Dissection of the triangular ligament and the left side of the coronary ligament

The best instrument to make this dissection (**Figures 35-12 A, B**) is the monopolar hook, with small pick-up of tissue.

Step 3 average time frame: 10–15 min

764 The Foundation and Art of Robotic Surgery

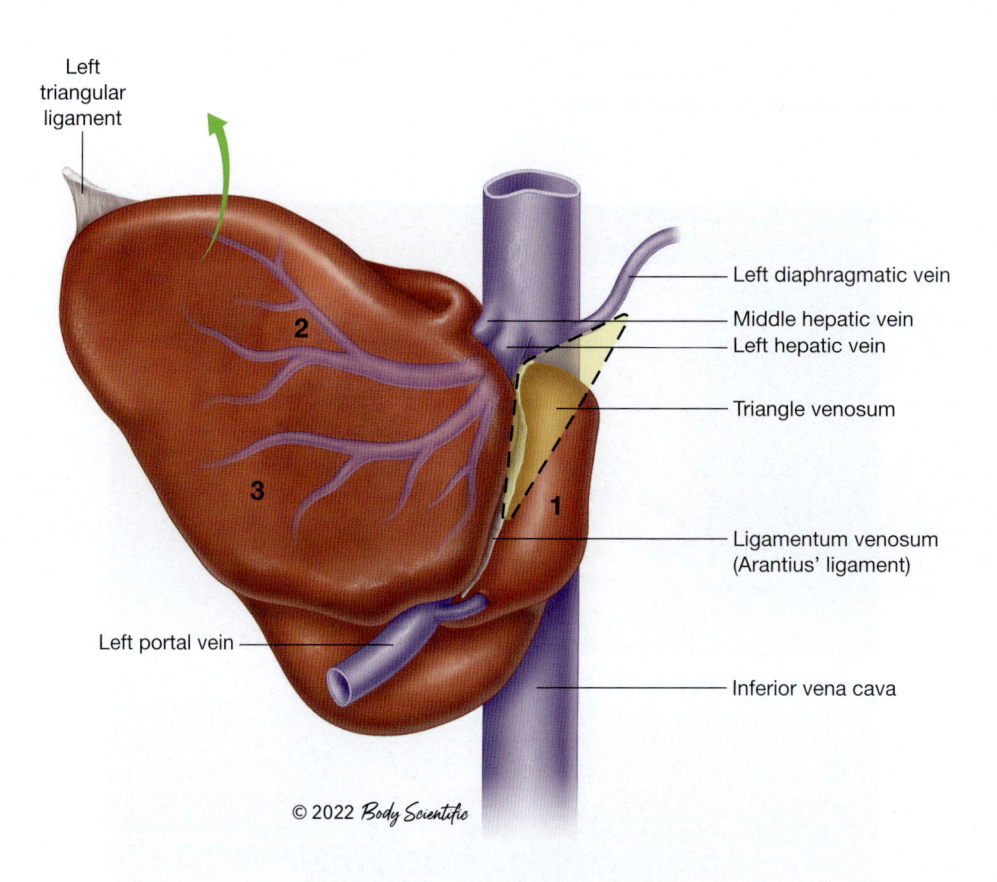

FIGURE 35-11 • Triangle venosum.

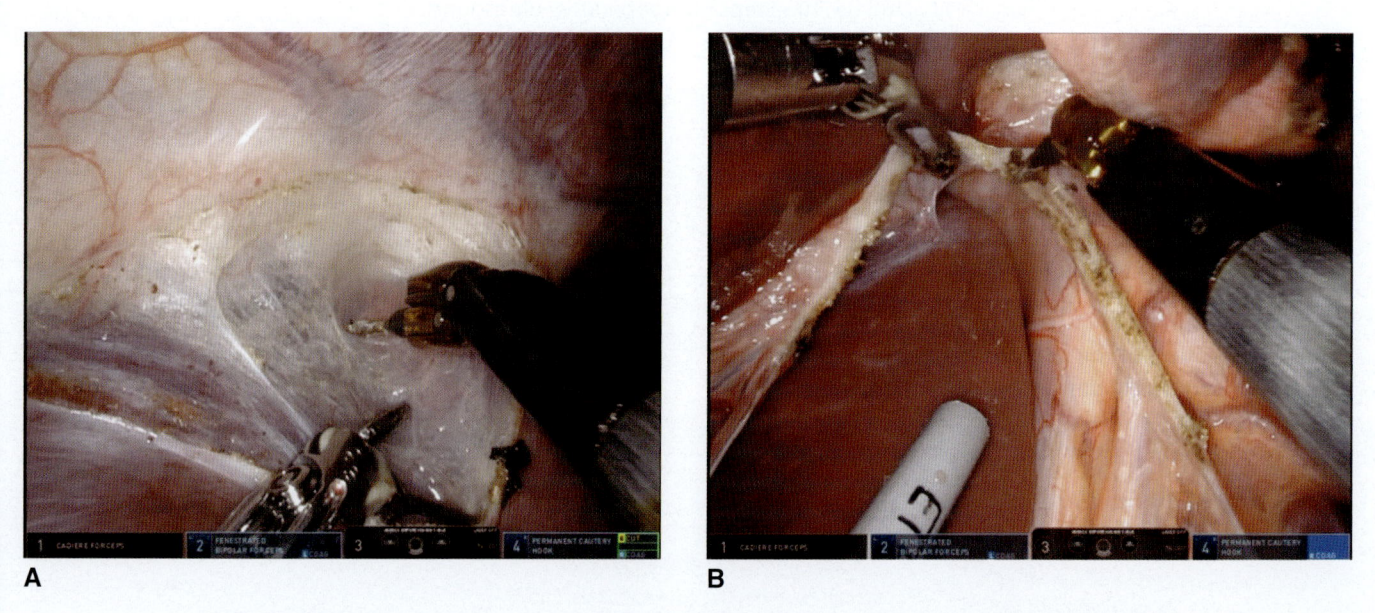

FIGURE 35-12 • Step 3. Dissection of the triangular and left side of the coronary ligaments.

Step 4. Pringle preparation (optional)

If the surgeon is experienced, and the anatomy is favorable, the Pringle maneuver (**Figure 35-13**) is not always necessary for the left lateral sectionectomy. However, at the beginning of the learning curve, or in difficult cases, it could be prudent to prepare for the inflow control.

Step 4 average time frame: 5–15 min

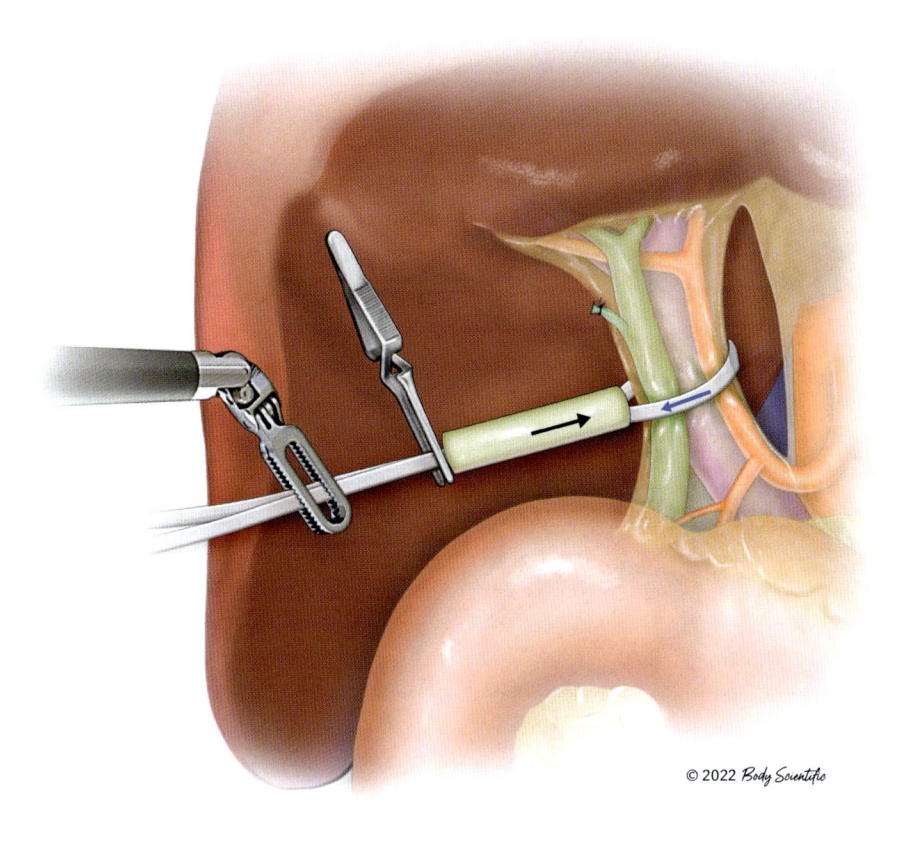

FIGURE 35-13 • Step 4. Internal Pringle maneuver.

Step 5. Dissection of the subcortical parenchyma along a longitudinal line lateral (left side) and parallel to the falciform ligament

The section (**Figure 35-14**) should proceed, following the principles already described and with the following goals:

1. Maintaining adequate oncological margins.
2. Decreasing the amount of tissue around the vascular structures that should be divided with different techniques (staplers, clips, suturing).
3. Minimizing bleeding with anticipation of the anatomy.

The best tool for this dissection is still the Harmonic™ shears, despite the limitations already described (lack of Endowrist).

Step 5 average time frame: 20–40 min

> ▶▶ **TIPS**
>
> The instrument (Harmonic™ shears) should always be kept aligned with the section line, either favoring the alignment, acting on the lateral retraction of the resected segments with the R3, or changing the active port for the instrument.
>
> It is important to learn how to perform a bi-handed work.

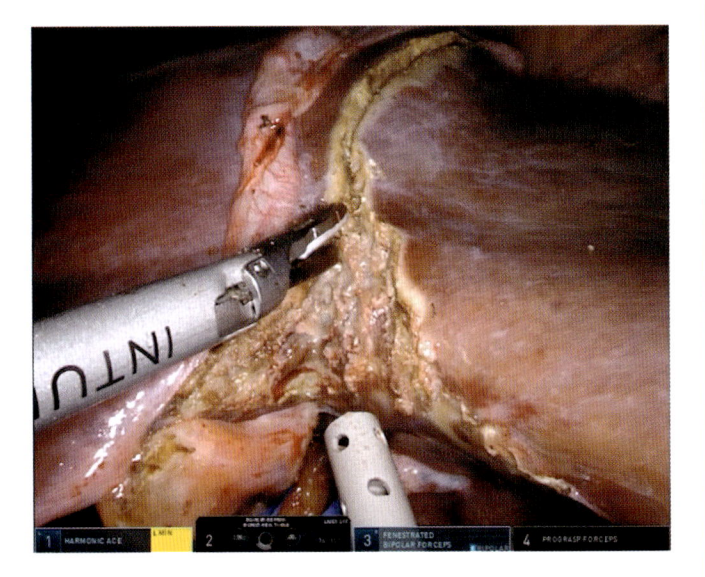

FIGURE 35-14 • Step 5. Dissection of the subcortical parenchyma.

Step 6. Stapling of the portal pedicle (2–3)

Once the thickness of the anterior parenchyma has been decreased enough to get close to the Glissonian pedicle (2–3), a vascular stapler is applied (**Figures 35-15 A, B**). The direction of the stapling should always be from the right toward the left, to avoid the inclusion of inappropriate anatomy.

Step 6 average time frame: 5–10 min

> **ANATOMICAL HIGHLIGHTS**
>
> The left Glissonian pedicle is adjacent to other important structures (e.g., the caudate lobe, the vena cava, the Aranzius ascending portal trunk to segment 4, the main connecting branches draining toward the median hepatic vein) (see **Figure 35-11**).

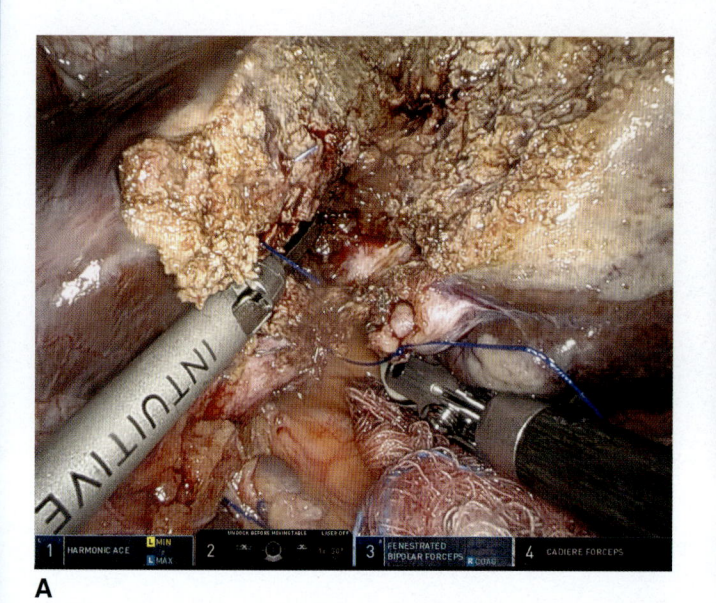

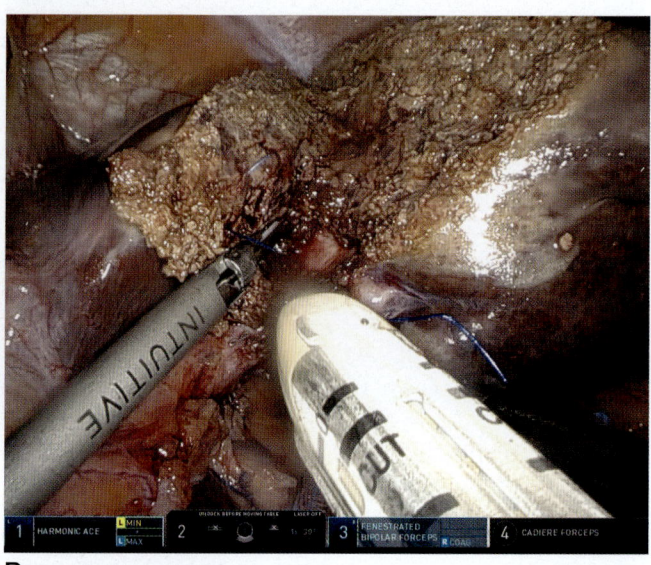

FIGURE 35-15 • Step 6. Stapling of the portal pedicle.

Step 7. Stapling of the left main hepatic vein

Once the Glissonian pedicle is divided, it is easy to retract the lateral segments more toward the left, and to open the angle where the main left hepatic vein is draining into the vena cava. Some parenchymal bridge, before reaching the hepatic vein, can be further divided with the Harmonic™ shears or with a sequence of progressive stapling (**Figure 35-16**).

Step 7 average time frame: 10–15 min

> **ANATOMICAL HIGHLIGHTS**
>
> There are anatomical landmarks guiding toward the base of the left hepatic vein: the confluence of the ligamentum venosum, and the left diaphragmatic vein is pointing exactly at the origin of the left hepatic vein (see **Figure 35-11**).

> **▶▶ TIPS**
>
> As already suggested for the stapling of the left Glissonian pedicle, the direction of the stapler should go away from the vena cava, pointing toward the left side, and using the operative ports located in the right upper quadrant.

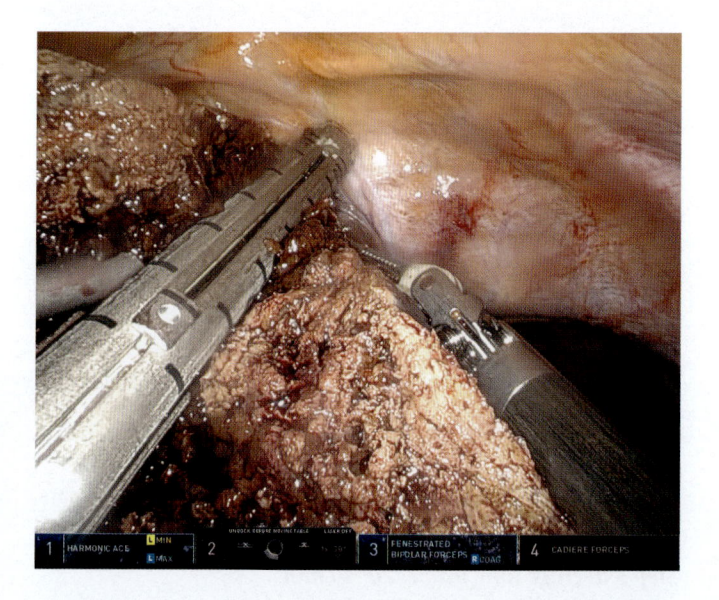

FIGURE 35-16 • Step 7. Stapling of the left main hepatic vein.

Step 8. Hemostasis verification

An accurate intraoperative hemostasis verification is carried out (**Figure 35-17**). This may require restoring a normal CVP and/or Valsalva maneuvers and a decrease of the CO_2 intraperitoneal pressure.

Additional interrupted Prolene™ 3-0 stiches with large needle (SH-MH) may be necessary.

Step 8 average time frame: 5–10 min

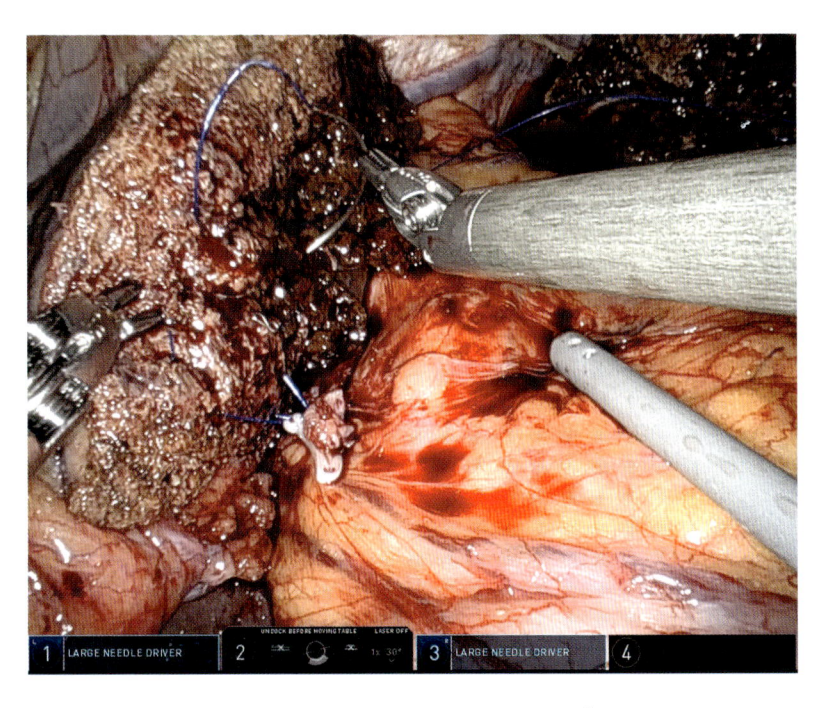

FIGURE 35-17 • Step 8. Hemostasis verification.

Step 9. Specimen extraction

The specimen extraction is carried out in a similar way, as already described in Chapter 34.

Step 9 average time frame: 10–15 min

> **EDITORIAL COMMENT**
>
> The technique that was described in this chapter is the most frequently performed laparoscopically. It is the simplest and the fastest one.
>
> Alternatively, for experienced surgeons, a more detailed and sophisticated technique may be applied involving a selective control of the inflow and outflow. An example of precise devascularization (inflow control) of segment 2 and 3 is shown in **Video 35-2**.

▶ Video 35-2. Left Lateral Sectionectomy – Selective Inflow Control

Suggested Readings

1. Couinaud C. Lobes et segments hepatiques. Note sur l'architectureanatomiques et chirurgicales du foie. *Presse Med.* 1952;62:709-712.
2. Bonnel F, Duparc F. Historical anatomy of hepatic segmentation: about 250 livers corrosions by Rapp (1953) and Couinaud (1953) in the Conservatory of Anatomy in Montpellier. *Surg Radiol Anat.* 2020;42(12):1407-1420. doi: 10.1007/s00276-020-02596-3
3. Couinaud C. The anatomy of the liver. *Ann Ital Chir.* 1992;63(6):693-697.
4. Sibulesky L. Normal liver anatomy. *Clin Liver Dis (Hoboken).* 2013;2(Suppl 1):S1-S3. doi: 10.1002/cld.124
5. Wakabayashi T, Benedetti Cacciaguerra A, et al. Landmarks to identify segmental borders of the liver: a review prepared for PAM-HBP expert consensus meeting 2021. *J Hepatobiliary Pancreat Sci.* 2022;29(1):82-98. doi: 10.1002/jhbp.899
6. Giulianotti PC, Bianco FM, Daskalaki D, Gonzalez-Ciccarelli LF, Kim J, Benedetti E. Robotic liver surgery: technical aspects and review of the literature. *Hepatobiliary Surg Nutr.* 2016;5(4):311-321. doi: 10.21037/hbsn.2015.10.05
7. Mangano A, Valle V, Masrur MA, Bustos RE, Gruessner S, Giulianotti PC. Robotic liver surgery: literature review and future perspectives. *Minerva Surg.* 2021;76(2):105-115. doi: 10.23736/S2724-5691.21.08495-9
8. Mangano A, Valle V, Giulianotti PC. Challenges in robotic liver surgery. In: Horgan S, Fuchs KH (eds) *Innovative Endoscopic and Surgical Technology in the GI Tract.* Springer, Cham; 2021. doi: 10.1007/978-3-030-78217-7_3
9. Gonzalez-Ciccarelli LF, Quadri P, Daskalaki D, Milone L, Gangemi A, Giulianotti PC. Robotic approach to hepatobiliary surgery. *Chirurg.* 2017;88(Suppl 1):19-28. doi: 10.1007/s00104-016-0223-0
10. Giulianotti PC, Coratti A, Angelini M, et al. Robotics in general surgery: personal experience in a large community hospital. *Arch Surg.* 2003;138(7):777-784. doi: 10.1001/archsurg.138.7.777

"There is a particularly striking symmetry between the two livers in segmental disposition and distribution of portal pedicles."

—Claude Couinaud (1922–2008)

Segmental and Atypical Liver Resections

Francesco Guerra • Carolina Baz • Alberto Patriti

INTRODUCTION

Advances in surgical techniques and the availability of growing oncological evidence are progressively reducing the need for major hepatectomies, regardless of tumor location and proximity to important vasculature. In fact, parenchyma-sparing resections (PSRs) are associated with the same oncological outcomes of major hepatectomies for both colorectal liver metastases (CRLMs) and hepatocellular carcinoma (HCC). Moreover, blood loss, operative time, and postoperative outcome measures favor PSRs even in patients with technically challenging tumor locations, where intraoperative ultrasound guidance plays a crucial role.

Especially in case of HCC, the underlying liver function imposes a careful balance between oncological needs and parenchymal preservation. Segment-oriented resections are particularly useful in this setting, as well as for the growing proportion of patients receiving repeated or bilobar resections.

The last decade has seen a dramatic implementation of minimally invasive liver surgery, resulting in excellent outcomes

INSTRUMENT REQUIREMENTS

The suggested main robotic instruments/tools can be listed as follows:
- 30° scope or 0° scope (the latter in few cases when the surgical field is very deep; see Chapter 2, The Basic Principles of Clinical Applications)
- Two needle drivers (round tip or macro)
- Cautery hook/monopolar scissors
- Harmonic shears™/vessel sealer (subcortical layer parenchyma transection)
- Robotic linear staplers (with different loads, for the core parenchymal transection)
- Multiple Hem-o-lok™ clips
- Medium/large clip applier
- Bipolar forceps
- Long-tip forceps
- Maryland bipolar forceps

The suggested main laparoscopic instruments/tools can be listed as follows:
- Needle drivers
- Scissors
- Graspers
- Staplers (with different loads)
- Hemoclips
- Suction-irrigation
- Laparoscopic ultrasound (drop-in probe or handheld laparoscopic)

Supplemental materials:
- Chest tube for the external or red rubber tube for the internal Pringle maneuver
- Gauzes, sponges
- Penrose drains/Jackson Pratt
- Vessel loops
- Endo Bag™
- Medium–large clips
- Sutures: Vicryl® 3-0, Prolene® 2-0/3-0/4-0/5-0

Photo reproduced with permission from Hardy KJ. Liver surgery: the past 2000 years. Aust N Z J Surg. 1990;60(10):811-817.
Quote reproduced with permission from Helling TS, Azoulay D: Historical Foundations of Liver Surgery, 1st ed. Switzerland: Springer Nature; 2020.

in terms of both surgical and oncological results. The need to perform more technically demanding surgeries such as major hepatectomies and/or procedures featuring bilioenteric reconstructions is currently the situation in which the robot may offer technical advantages over conventional laparoscopy. However, as for open and conventional laparoscopic liver surgery, segmentectomies and multiple nonanatomical resections are sometimes more technically demanding than major hepatectomies, owing to the need of intraparenchymal control of blood supply, the careful dissection required to achieve negative margins, and the meticulous identification and repair of intrahepatic bile duct injuries. Currently, conventional laparoscopy as well as robot-assisted laparoscopy are routinely used for segmental liver resection in experienced referral centers.

Indications and Relative Contraindications to the Robotic Approach

As for conventional laparoscopic hepatectomies, there are no absolute contraindications to robotic liver resections (RLR), except for the inability to tolerate pneumoperitoneum for a relatively prolonged time. Similarly, CRLMs and HCC account for the vast majority of indications in most series, although both benign and different malignant conditions are reported quite frequently.

Despite some anecdotal experiences quoting favorable outcomes with RLR, for most patients with large tumors or tumors encroaching on or adjacent to the main portal pedicle or major vasculature such as the inferior vena cava (IVC) or major hepatic veins, an open approach should be preferred. The technical difficulty of the procedure may substantially vary in relation to a number of factors, including the anatomical location of the lesion to be resected and the quality of liver parenchyma (cirrhosis, prior resection, and/or systemic chemotherapy). In the initial phase of the learning curve, limited resections in the so-called "laparoscopic segments" (2–6) of noncirrhotic patients should be considered. These include wedge resection/subsegmentectomy, monosegmentectomy, and left lateral sectionectomy. More complex procedures, such as bi- or trisegmentectomy in the right lobe, or resections in segments 7, 8, and 1 in the cirrhotic patient, are advisable when a specific expertise has been already achieved by the team.

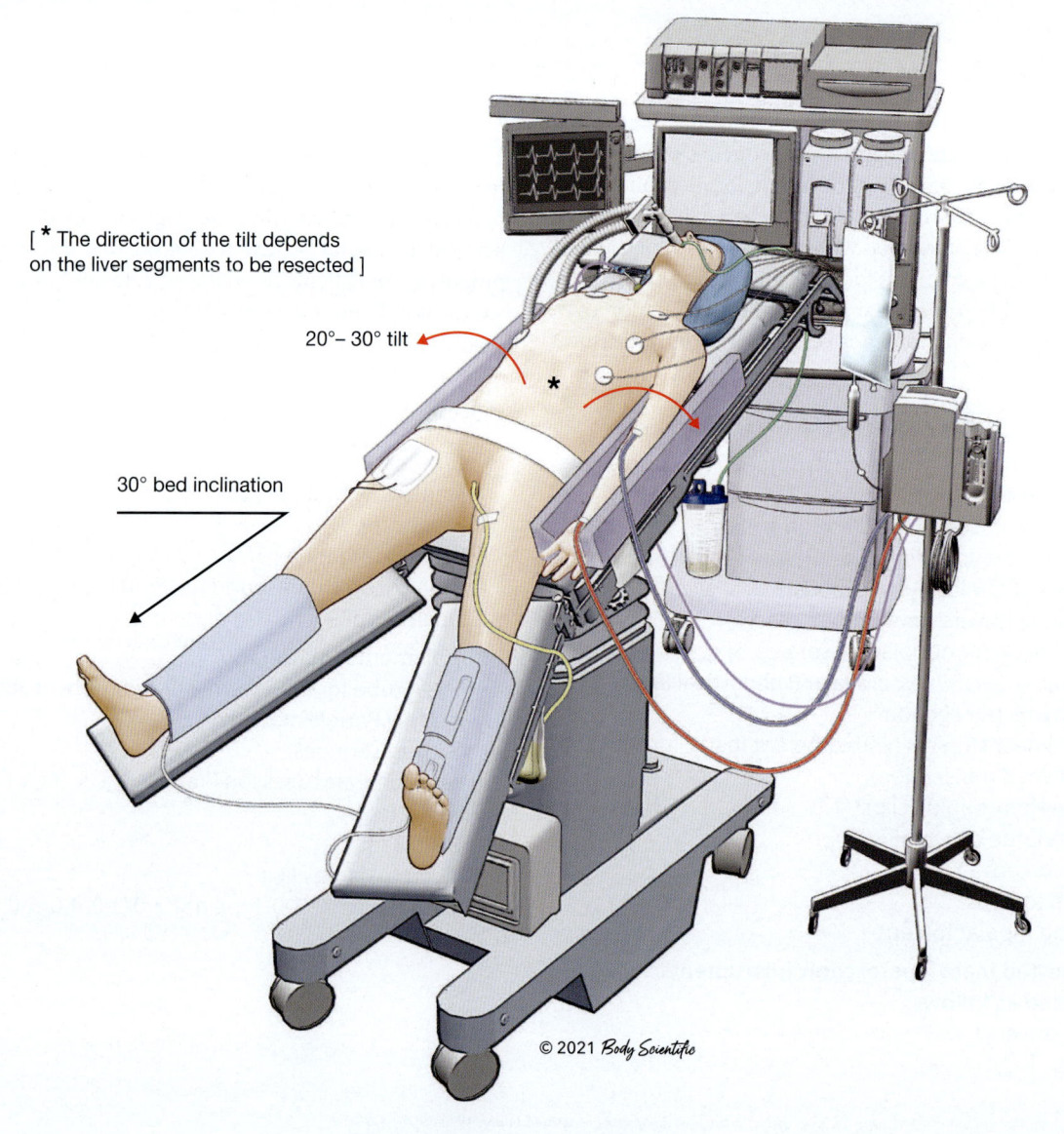

FIGURE 36-1 • Patient positioning.

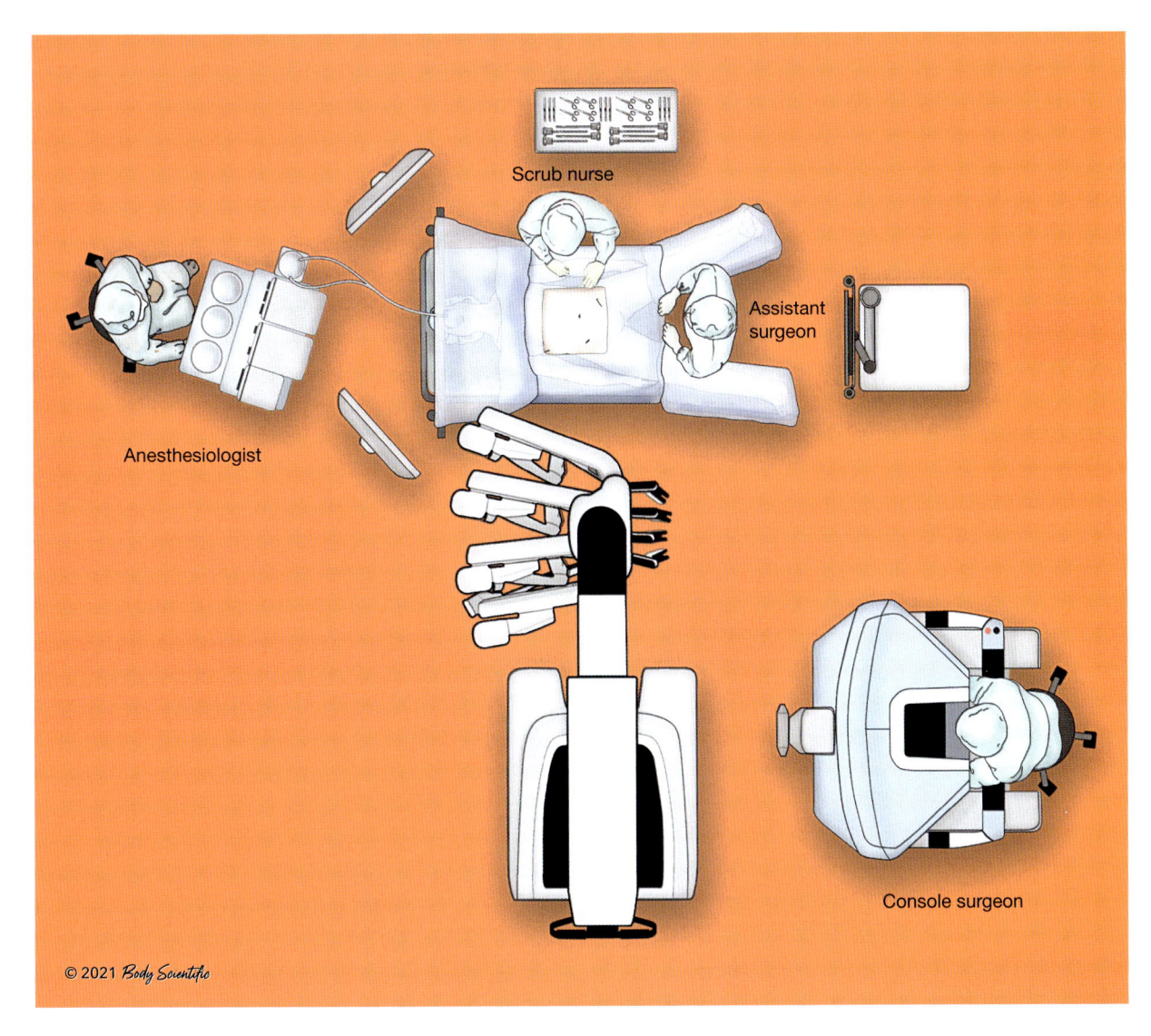

FIGURE 36-2 • OR setup.

Patient Positioning, OR Setup, and Port Setting

Robot docking and patient positioning, as well as the strategy used to dispose surgical accesses, are crucial to ease the approach to the segments to be resected and minimize technical challenges with each phase of the procedure (**Figure 36-1**). The OR setup is described in **Figure 36-2**.

The patient is placed supine, with parted legs. A reversed Trendelenburg, left-side or right-side up position, depending on the lesion location, is given and the robot is preferably docked on the right side of the patient (Xi). The assistant surgeon stands between the patient's legs. Pneumoperitoneum is obtained using the Veress needle in the left hypochondrium. One or 2 assistant ports and 4 standard 8-mm robotic ports are placed. When approaching posterosuperior segments of the right lobe, robotic ports are placed differently, following an oblique line close to the right costal margin and a right-side-up position (15–20°) is given. Occasionally, the right lateral trocar can be inserted with an intercostal, transdiaphragmatic access for tumors located in the hepatic dome and segment 7. In case of resection of anterior segments, robotic ports are positioned transversally, more or less cranially to the transverse umbilical line according to the conformation of the abdomen. The ports line is moved to the left when lesions in segment 2 or 3 are to be approached. The third arm (R3) of the robot is preferably installed on the left side of the patient. Especially when the Harmonic™ scalpel is used for parenchymal transection, an adequate positioning of the ports is of paramount importance due to limited maneuverability of this instrument (**Figures 36-3 A–C**).

772 The Foundation and Art of Robotic Surgery

⚠️ PITFALLS
Suboptimal trocar positioning will significantly hinder the procedure by limiting instrument maneuverability and proper visualization. This is particularly true when approaching the posterosuperior segments. The bedside surgeon must have comfortable access to the surgical field to assist the resection for suctioning, traction, and clip positioning. An incorrectly positioned assistant port may complicate the entire procedure.

EDITORIAL COMMENT
The R3 can be more useful from the left side, also for the left liver resections. It may retract the specimen laterally, keeping open the section line. The right lobe is naturally being laid down by gravity.

▶▶ TIPS
When transdiaphragmatic trocars are placed, ultrasound assessment should be performed to identify respiratory movements of the lower edge of the right lung in order to avoid its injury. Ultrasound exploration can be performed using the laparoscopic probe laid on the right diaphragm or the standard abdominal convex probe. An alternative safe technique is to use an optic trocar for the transdiaphragmatic insertion.

A place for an extracorporeal tourniquet should be identified prior to port placement to avoid collisions with the robotic arms.

Normal abdomen

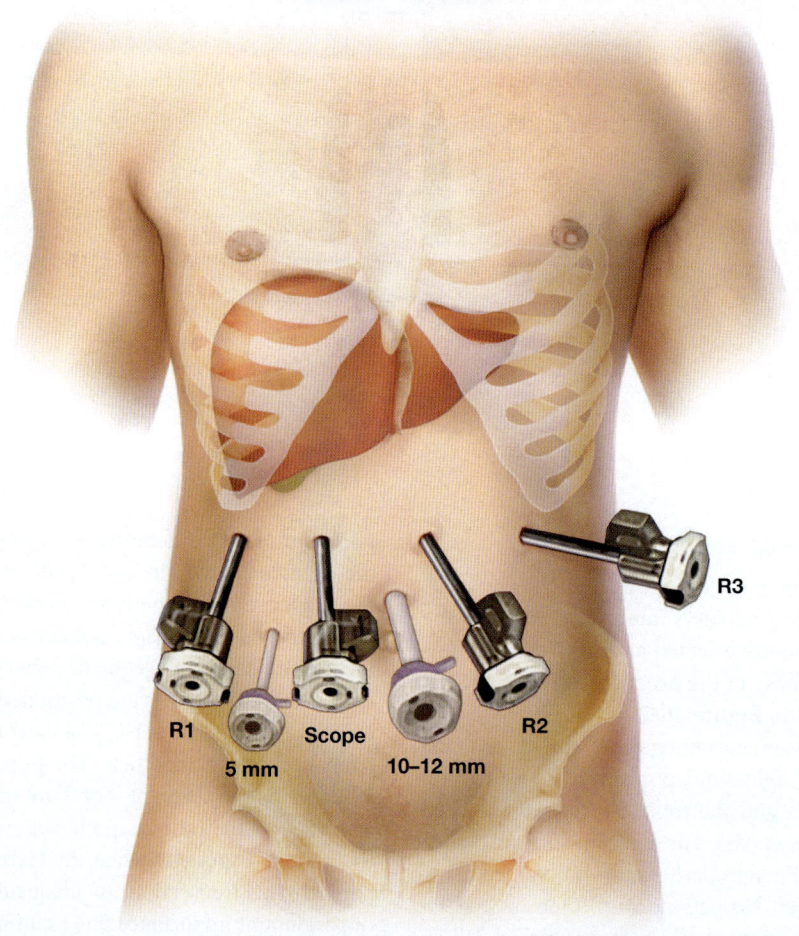

FIGURE 36-3 • Port setting. **A.** Anterior right segments.

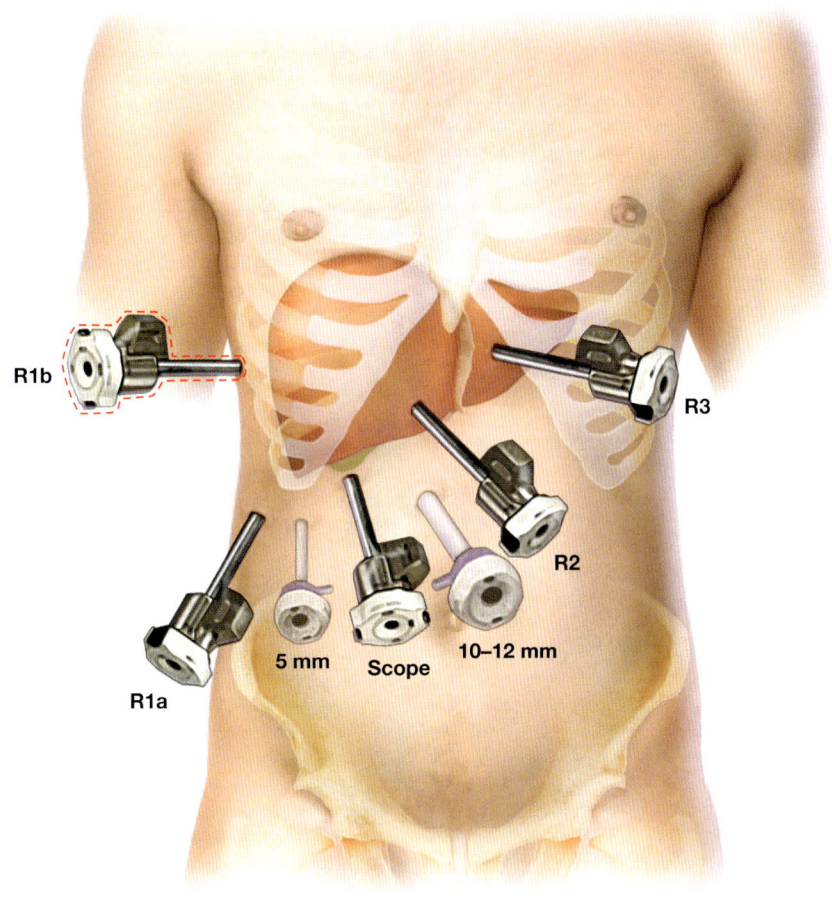

Segmental and Atypical Liver Resections 773

FIGURE 36-3 • (*Continued*) **B.** Posterior right segments.

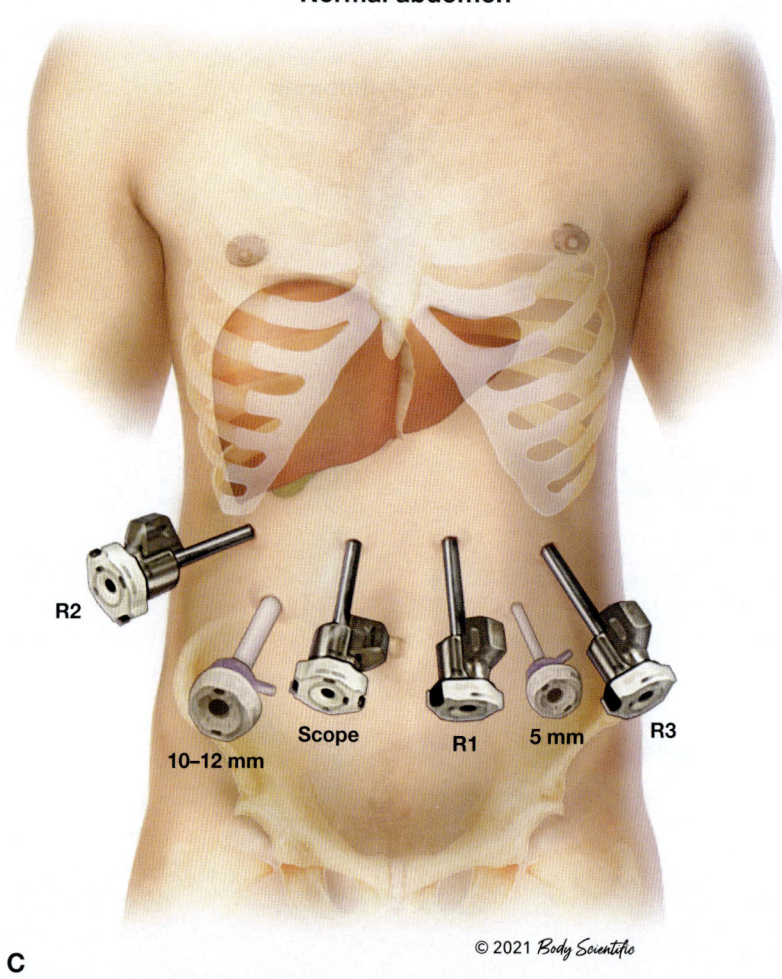

FIGURE 36-3 • (Continued) C. Left segments.

Segmental and Atypical Liver Resections 775

Surgical Technique

Step 1. Abdominal exploration, initial ultrasound assessment

The procedure starts with conventional laparoscopic exploration of the abdominal cavity. The peritoneum, omentum, mesentery, and viscera are inspected for signs of peritoneal disease. Once the presence of contraindication to resectability is ruled out, the robot is brought into the surgical field and the robotic arms are docked. An intraoperative ultrasound (IOUS) inspection of the liver parenchyma follows in order to confirm the preoperative findings and to appropriately define the exact location, size, and specific relationship of the lesion with major biliovascular structures. This phase is performed with conventional laparoscopic probes or with robot-integrated ultrasound systems (drop-in probes). The robotic IOUS probe enters the peritoneal cavity through the standard laparoscopic assistant port and is freely manipulated by the operating surgeon via R1 or R2. Using the da Vinci TilePro™ capability, the operative field and the IOUS video stream are visualized simultaneously (**Figures 36-4** and **36-5 A–I**).

Step 1 average time frame: 15–20 min

> **ANATOMICAL HIGHLIGHTS**
>
> There are 5 main elements to define intrahepatic segmental anatomy:
> - **Direct vascular signs:**
>   1. Hepatic veins
>   2. Portal pedicles
> - **Indirect signs (nearby structures):**
>   3. Vena cava
>   4. Falciform ligament
>   5. Gallbladder

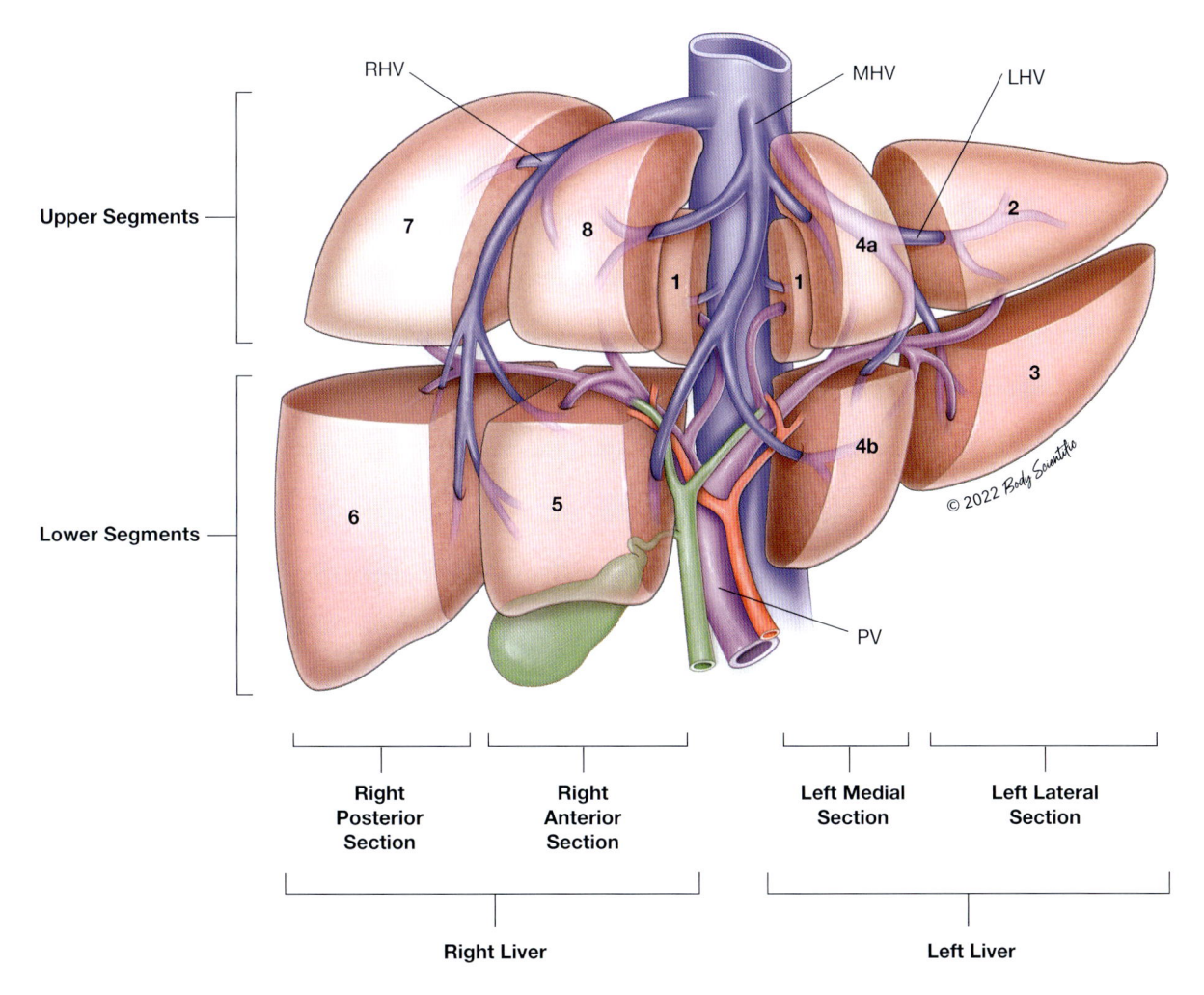

FIGURE 36-4 • Anatomical segments of the liver. Right hepatic vein (RHV): divides the right lobe into anterior and posterior segments. Middle hepatic vein (MHV): divides the liver into right and left lobes (or right and left hemi liver). This plane runs from the IVC to the gallbladder fossa. Left hepatic vein (LHV): divides the left lobe into medial and lateral parts. Portal vein (PV): divides the liver into upper and lower liver segments. There are 8 liver segments (S); S4 is divided into segments 4a and 4b according to Bismuth. S1 (caudate lobe) is located posteriorly and not visible on a frontal view.

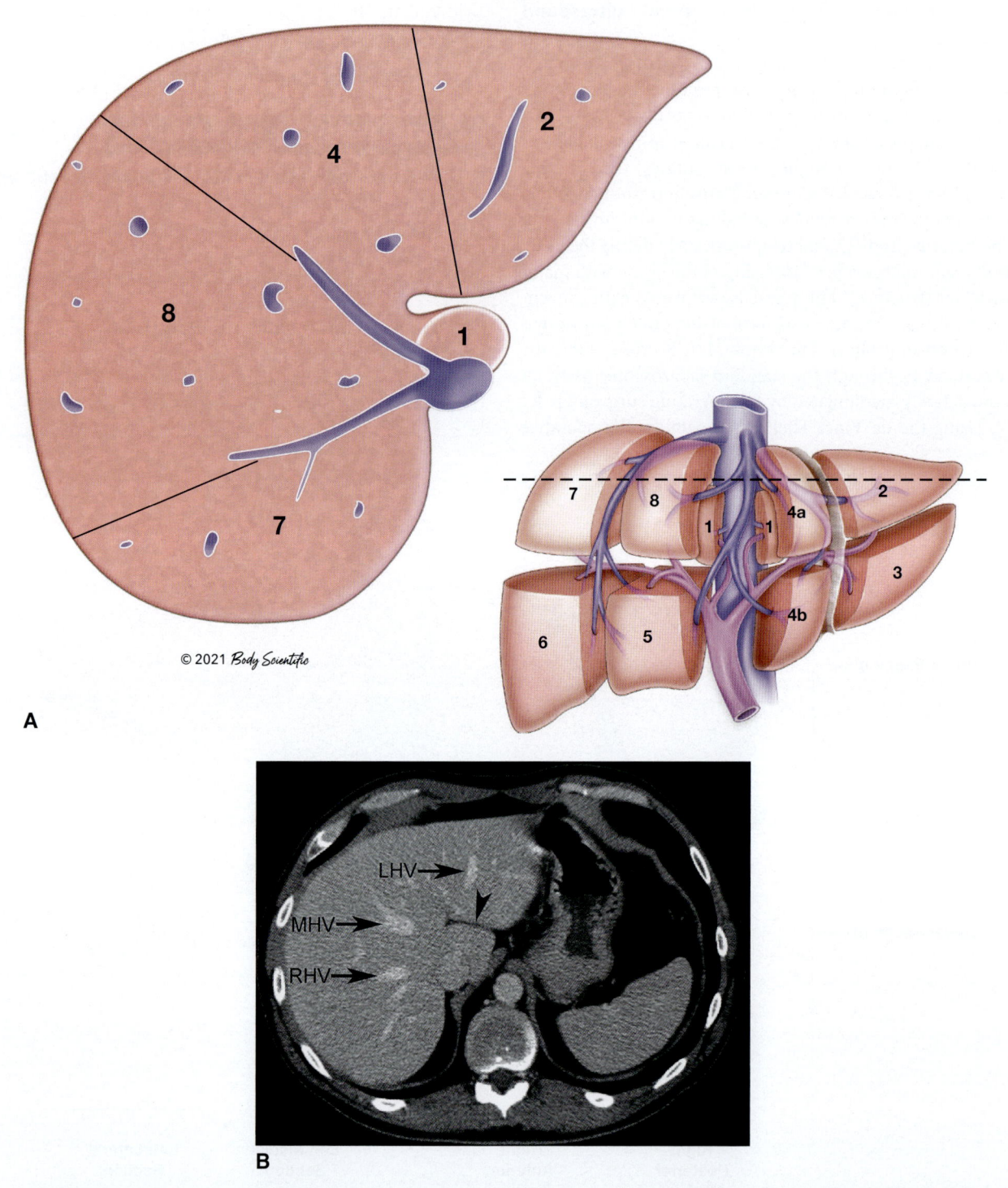

FIGURE 36-5 • Liver segment Illustrations/computed tomography (CT)/magnetic resonance (MR) scan images. **A.** Transverse anatomy: a transverse image through the superior liver segments that are divided by the right hepatic vein (RHV), the middle hepatic vein (MHV), and the falciform ligament. The MHV is dividing the left lobe from the right lobe. To define segment 4a, the vena cava (VC) with the confluence of the RHV should be seen. To define 4b, the portal bifurcation should be seen. The left hepatic vein (LHV) is defining segments 2 and 3. **B.** Cross-sectional imaging anatomy of Couinaud liver segments: hepatic veins depicted on contrast-enhanced axial CT. The fissure for *ligamentum venosum* (arrowhead) demarcates the border of the caudate lobe.

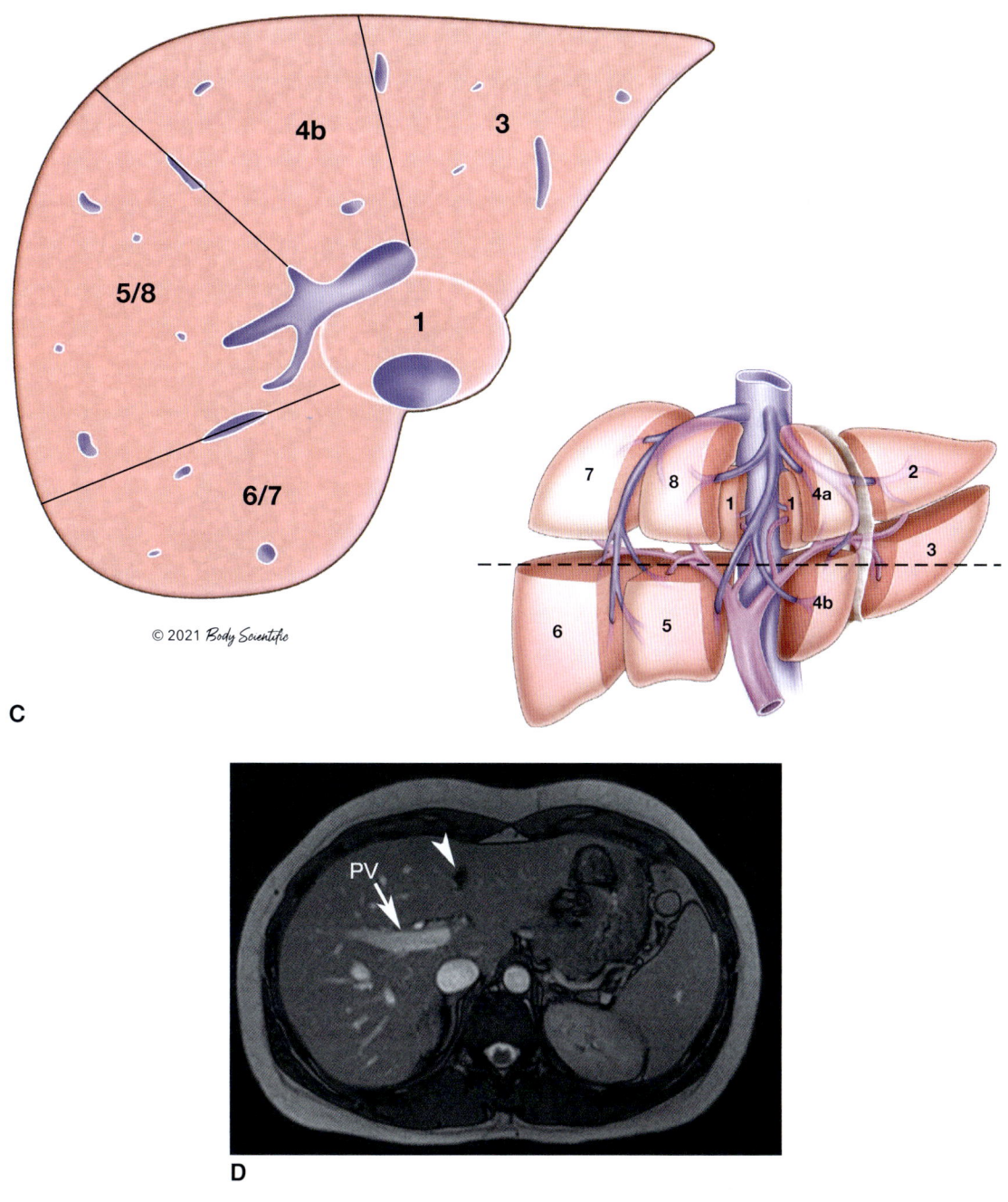

FIGURE 36-5 • (*Continued*) **C.** Level of the right portal vein: the right portal vein separates the right lobe of the liver into the superior segments (7-8) and the inferior segments (5-6). The right portal vein is inferior to the left portal vein. Some segments are better defined by the boundaries of the hepatic veins and others by the portal pedicles. Anterior segments 5-8; posterior segments 6-7. **D.** Noncontrast T2 MR: intrahepatic portal vein imaging scans serve as an anatomic landmark to partition the liver segments craniocaudally. The fissure for *ligamentum teres* (arrowhead) defines the border of the medial and lateral segments of the left hepatic lobe.

778 The Foundation and Art of Robotic Surgery

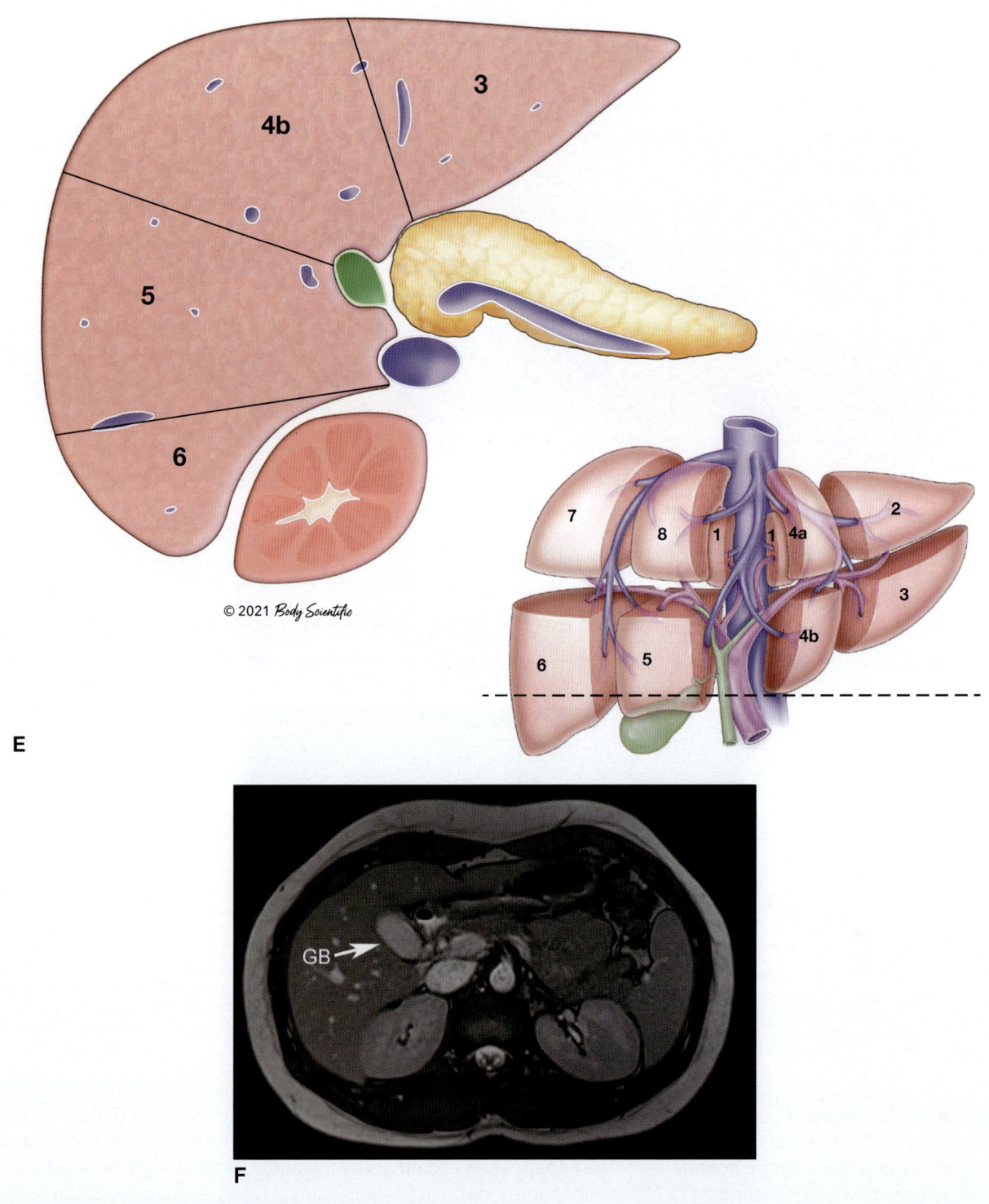

FIGURE 36-5 • (*Continued*) **E.** Below the level of the right portal vein, only the inferior segments can be visualized. **F.** Gallbladder (GB), shown on noncontrast T2 MR imaging scan: serves to delineate the right and left hepatic lobes inferiorly (below intrahepatic portal vein). The GB is a good landmark to differentiate 4b (left) and 5 (right).

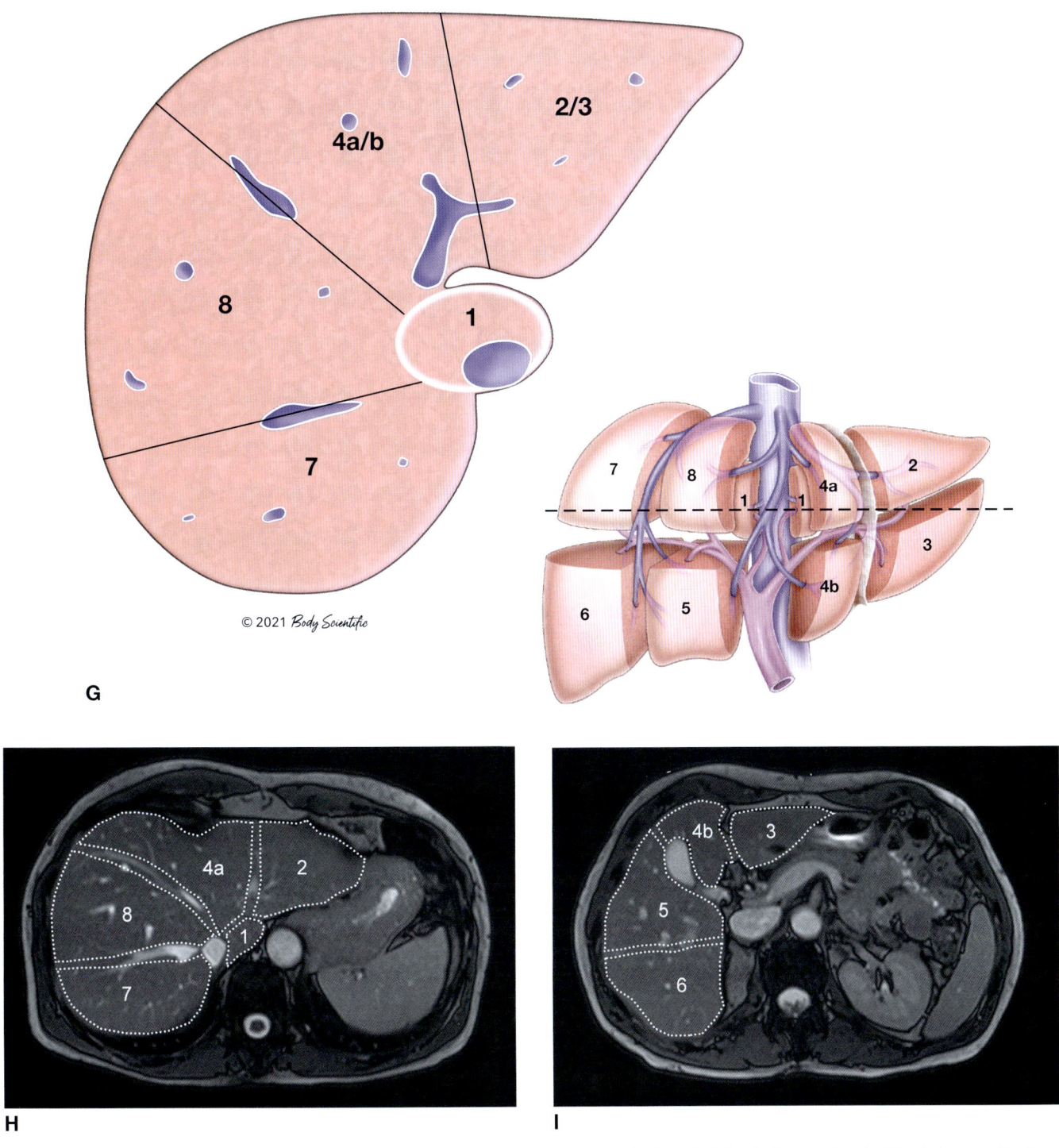

FIGURE 36-5 • (*Continued*) **G.** Transverse anatomy: transverse figure at the level of the left portal vein. The left portal vein divides the left lobe into the superior segments (2-4a) and the inferior segments (3-4b). The left portal vein is higher than the right portal vein. The bifurcation of the left branch of the portal vein is between 4a and 4b. **H.** Noncontrast T2 MR imaging scan: displays Couinaud liver segments. Above the intrahepatic portal vein, these include segments 2, 4a, 8, and 7. **I.** Noncontrast T2 MR imaging scan: displays Couinaud liver segments below the intrahepatic portal vein; these include segments 3, 4b, 5, and 6. The GB defines segments 4b and 5. To differentiate the boundaries between segments 5 and 6, the portal pedicles should be seen. Segment 3 is lateral to the falciform ligament.

Step 2. Preparation for the Pringle Maneuver

In all cases, an extracorporeal tourniquet is used to allow the Pringle maneuver. The lesser sac is accessed by dividing the *pars flaccida* of the lesser omentum. The hepatoduodenal ligament is encircled with an umbilical tape around the Winslow foramen. The tape is then exteriorized from the abdominal cavity through a 20 Ch chest tube in the right upper quadrant (**Figure 36-6**). During the operation, when inflow occlusion is needed, the bedside surgeon performs the intermittent pedicle clamping.

Step 2 average time frame: 10–15 min

> **EDITORIAL COMMENT**
>
> The Pringle maneuver can also be performed endoabdominal with an internal technique, without the need to exteriorize the tourniquet. The advantages are the avoidance of a dedicated incision and the direct control by the console surgeon. The disadvantage is that the maneuver is less strong compared to the external one (**Figures 36-7 A–D**).

> **▶▶ TIPS**
>
> Specific skills in IOUS and minimally invasive IOUS are essential. A complete parenchymal ultrasound assessment is of paramount importance not only to identify biliary and vascular anatomy (and their variations) and their relationship with the lesion(s), but also to guide parenchymal transection and ensure an adequate resection margin.

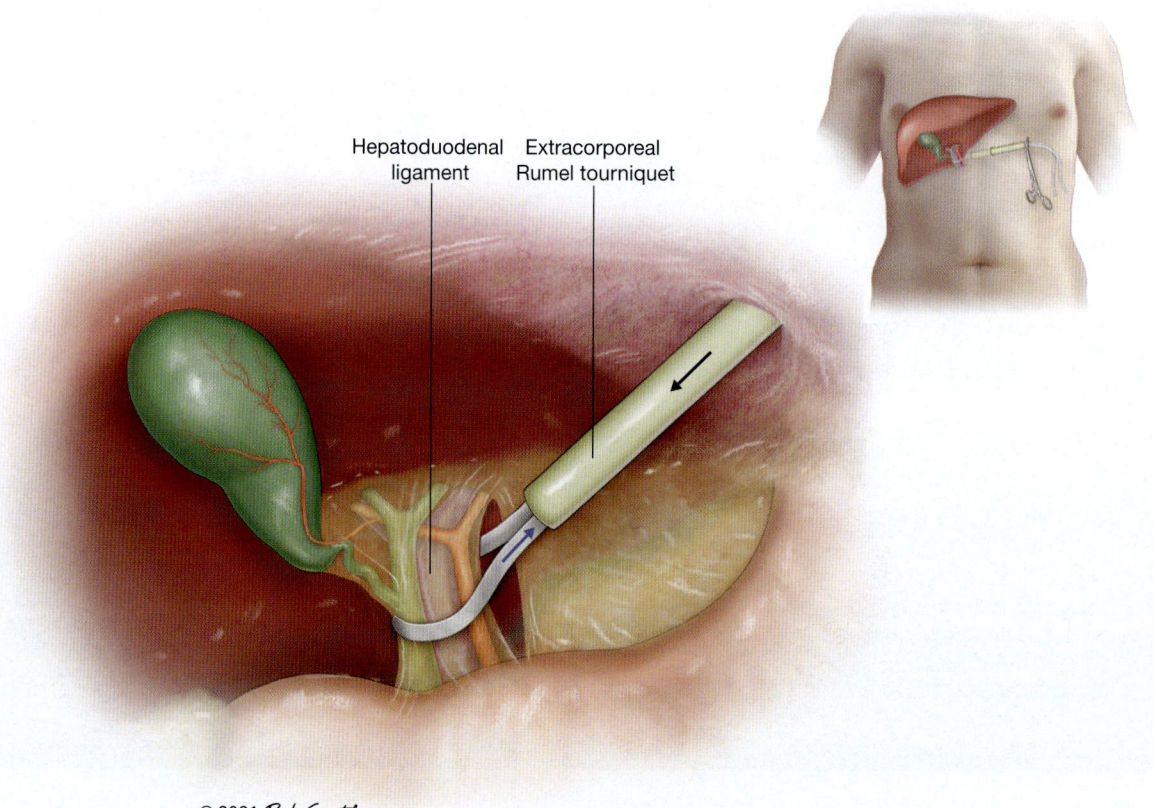

FIGURE 36-6 • External Pringle maneuver.

Segmental and Atypical Liver Resections   781

> ▶▶ **TIPS**
>
> Every step of the procedure and specific anatomy must be clear before surgery. Ultrasound exploration of the liver anatomy should only be a confirmation of what the surgeon learned from preoperative imaging. Careful observation of echogenic characteristics of the lesions is extremely important. Isoechoic liver lesions could be a challenge and cause of conversion to avoid positive margins.

> ⚠ **PITFALLS**
>
> Failure to adequately identify portal pedicles may result in significantly higher blood losses and prolonged time of the Pringle maneuver.

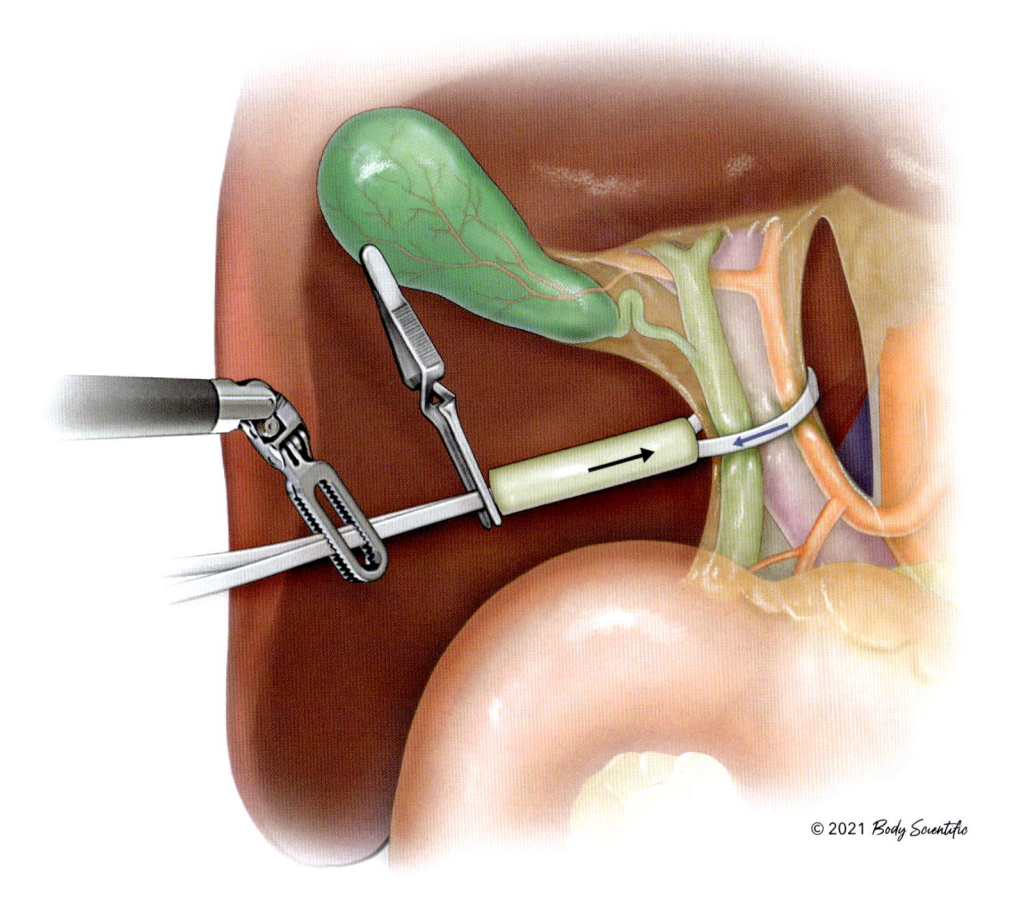

A

FIGURE 36-7 • Internal Pringle maneuver.

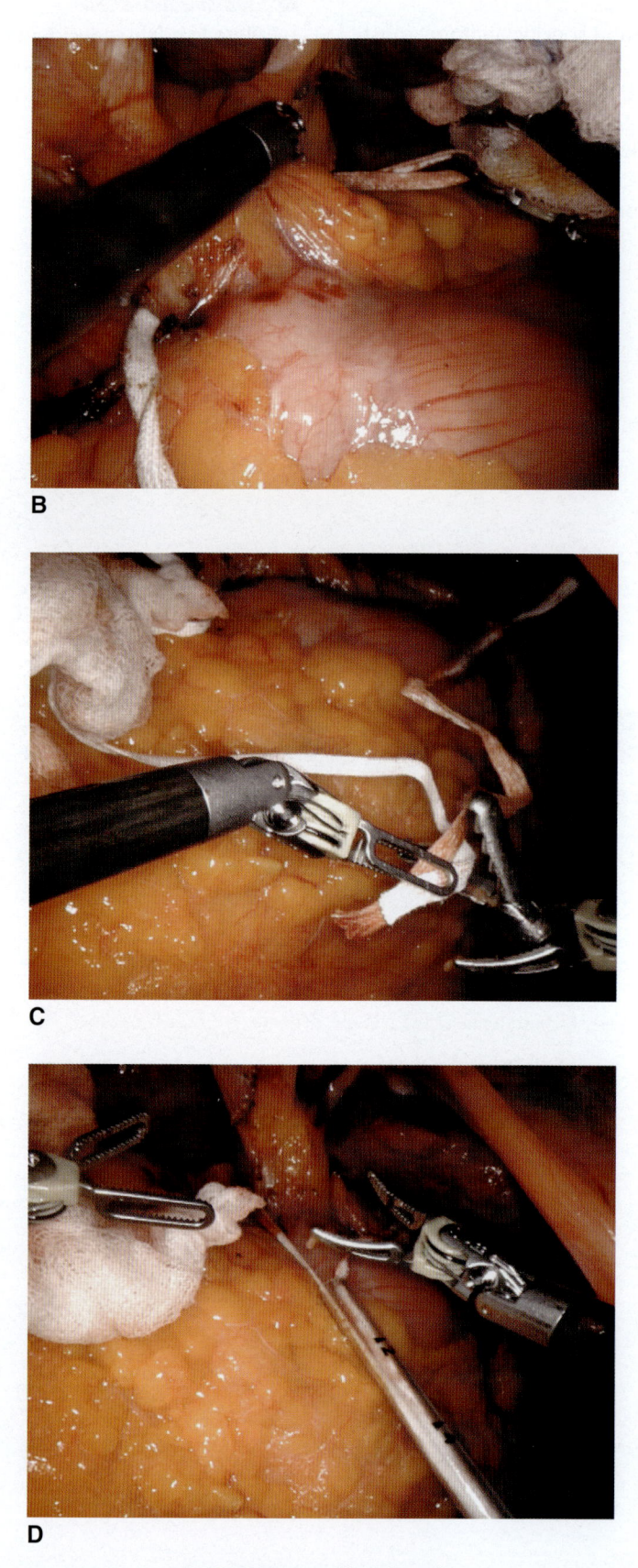

FIGURE 36-7 • *(Continued)*

Step 3. Liver mobilization and segmental demarcation

Depending on the resection to be performed and the conformation of the organ, partial lobar mobilization follows. Usually for right lobe segments, the round and falciform ligament are taken down; also, a partial mobilization of the posterior ligaments, triangular and coronary, may facilitate access to the target segment with a more favorable angle.

▶ **Video 36-1. Step 3. Right Liver Lobe Mobilization**

In case of anatomical, regulated mono- or bisegmentectomies, the relation between the tumor and the portal pedicle is clearly defined with IOUS for precise inflow control. Specific segmental pedicles and the location of the portal scissurae with the hepatic veins are identified. Under IOUS guidance, the Glissonian surface is tattooed with electrocautery to delineate the plane of the intended resection.

▶ **Video 36-2. Step 3. IOUS Guidance**

Sometimes, the projection of the route of major structures (such as the hepatic veins) is also marked to assist with their preservation/isolation. Before initiating the transection, optimal positioning of the instruments and the liver must be achieved. Besides mobilization, retraction and tension are also crucial for further exposure and parenchymal dissection. For resections of anterosuperior segments, including left lateral sectionectomy, stay sutures can be of great help to retract the specimen using the R3 or the assistant grasper (**Figures 36-8 A–C**). A vessel loop held by the R3 arm around the left segments can be of aid to perform a kind of hanging maneuver and facilitate the application of the clamp-crushing technique. In the case of deeply located lesions or when the tumor to be resected is close to major vasculature, the corkscrew technique can be an option.

Step 3 average time frame: 10–45 min

> ⚠ **PITFALLS**
>
> Inadequate mobilization and exposure may create difficulties during parenchymal transection.

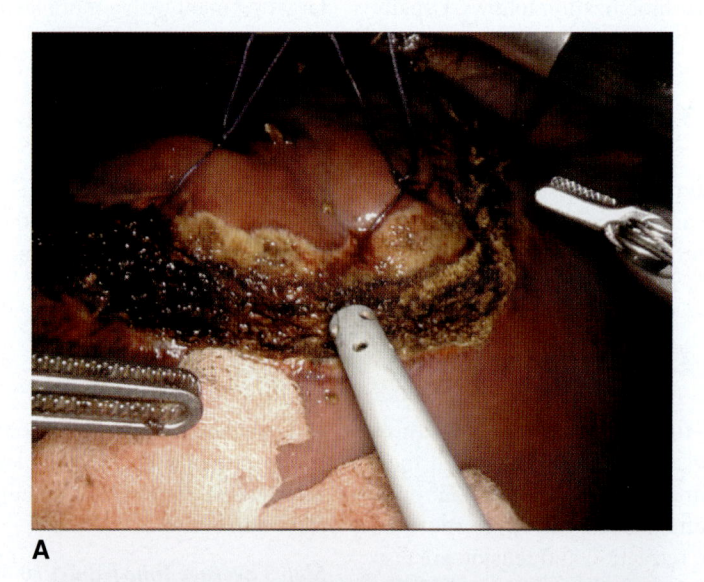

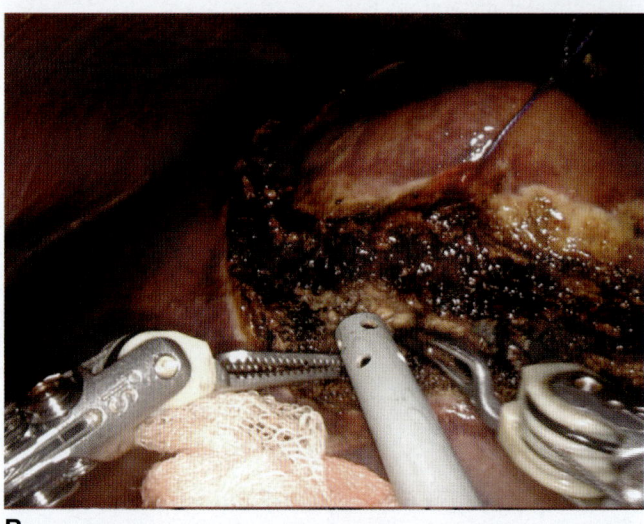

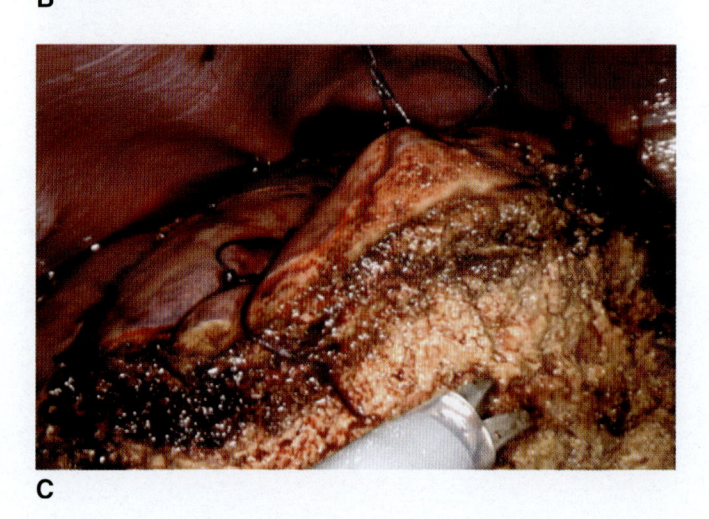

FIGURE 36-8 • Liver stay sutures.

Step 4. Parenchymal transection

Transection starts in a layer-by-layer fashion. Superficial dissection (first 5–10 mm from the Glissonian surface) is usually carried out with monopolar energy. The clamp-crushing technique is then used for deeper parenchymal transection using the Maryland bipolar forceps.

▶ **Video 36-3. Step 4. Parenchymal Transection**

The Maryland bipolar forceps is carried by the arm on the same side of the liver remnant in order to achieve the maximal hemostasis in this side of the resection line; in the other operative arm, monopolar scissors are generally used. Both instruments are set at a high energy level.

The Kelly clamp-crushing technique associated with intermittent Pringle maneuver is still considered the safest and most cost-effective method for parenchymal division in open liver surgery. The main advantages of this technique are the low costs and the ability to fragment the parenchyma preserving the vascular structures that can be ligated and divided or preserved according to the resection plan. This effective technique is not performed laparoscopically on a routine basis due to the lack of dedicated instruments. Robotic surgery has renewed the interest for this approach. Using the EndoWrist® bipolar precise forceps, the parenchyma can be easily fragmented exposing the inner vessels as in open surgery. The bedside surgeon performs the intermittent inflow occlusion, thereby allowing the console surgeon to focus their attention only on the transection line. The EndoWrist® instruments allow the laparoscopic surgeon to perform curved and angled resections in all the liver segments, an ability lost with the rigid laparoscopic tools. Therefore, the robotic clamp-crushing technique allows parenchymal preservation even for deeply located lesions, widening the indications for a minimally invasive approach.

In the case of anatomical resection (segments), liver parenchyma is first dissected toward the specific segmental portal pedicle (or toward the roots of its branches in the case of subsegmentectomies), until its identification and division. The section line follows the boundary of the demarcated region. During this phase, ultrasound is frequently used to check the appropriate line of the parenchymal transection and to verify the tumor margins. Similarly, near-infrared fluorescence (da Vinci Firefly™) with indocyanine green (ICG) dye is used in order to facilitate vascular and biliary identification, even though the background uptake of the colorant has an important masking effect. Hemostasis of small vessels is obtained with bipolar cautery, while biliary ducts and larger vessels are controlled with hemoclips and/or selective monofilament sutures (Prolene® 3-0/4-0).

▶ **Video 36-4. Step 4. Vessel Control with Sutures**

Where needed, major hepatic veins are usually transected with endostaplers. After resection, a final ultrasound inspection is performed to review the residual parenchyma and the specimen to confirm that the excision has been effective. Finally, the transection surface is examined under fluorescent light to detect and manage any evidence of bile leak (water leak test) (**Figures 36-9 A–C**).

When indicated, cholecystectomy is performed in a conventional fashion, usually at the beginning of the parenchymal transection phase.

Step 4 average time frame: in this phase of the procedure, the time frame may significantly vary according to a number of factors. These include the location of the resection to be performed, the width of parenchymal transection, and the quality of liver parenchyma.

▶▶ **TIPS**

Occasionally, temporary outflow control is also achieved to limit blood losses and facilitate parenchymal transection. To do so, depending on the scheduled resection, pertinent hepatic lobes need to be fully mobilized to access the right hepatic vein or the left vein at its confluence with the middle vein or at their common trunk.

▶▶ **TIPS**

A strong Prolene® 2-0 stay suture holding the segment/wedge to be resected may facilitate retraction and exposure of the section line (corkscrew technique). The specimen tends to collapse by gravity, closing the working space.

Once the segmental portal triad is identified, the pedicle is temporarily clamped and divided only after confirming with the ultrasound the normal blood supply distribution in contiguous segments. This process may also be assisted by fluorescence imaging, with extra boluses of intravenous ICG, even though the artifacts of the baseline parenchyma uptake are very disturbing. As transection progresses, IOUS is repeated to assess the relationship with the tumor and major vasculature.

EDITORIAL COMMENT

The transection of the parenchyma can be achieved with other techniques, like the layer-by-layer Harmonic shears transection with open or closed jaws of the instrument, laparoscopic CUSA®, a vessel sealer, and SynchroSeal™. For more details, see Chapter 33, Right Hepatectomy.

Fluorescence water leak test. The surgical field is irrigated with saline. Major bile leaks can be identified, even if the background parenchymal uptake is diffusely fluorescent. The leak is visualized as a stream of color into the transparent saline solution.

Step 5. Specimen extraction
The specimen is placed into a plastic bag and generally extracted enlarging the periumbilical port or via a Pfannenstiel incision for bulky lesions. (See Chapter 2, The Basic Principles of Clinical Applications.) A closed-suction drain is usually positioned adjacent to the resection field.

Step 5 average time frame: 15–20 min

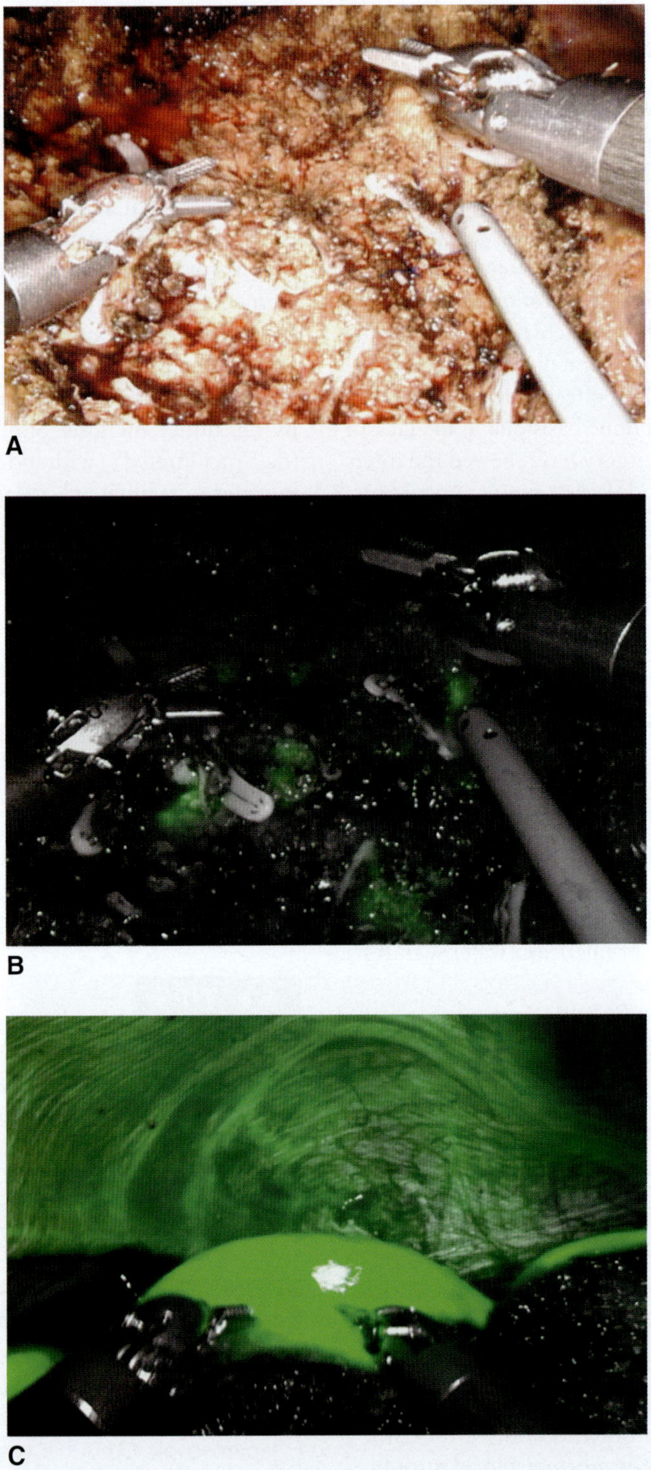

FIGURE 36-9 • Parenchyma transection using ICG. At the end of the procedure, the operative field is viewed under standard and fluorescent light to rule out any evidence of bile leak and to assess the resultant demarcation of parenchymal perfusion after intravenous ICG injection. **A.** Standard light. **B.** Fluorescent light. **C.** Parenchymal perfusion after ICG.

ACKNOWLEDGMENT

The editors thank Dr. Ron Gaba for providing the liver segments CT and MRI scan images and for the descriptions matching each image.

Suggested Readings

1. Billingsley KG, Jarnagin WR, Fong Y, Blumgart LH. Segment-oriented hepatic resection in the management of malignant neoplasms of the liver. *J Am Coll Surg.* 1998;187(5):471-481. doi: 10.1016/s1072-7515(98)00231-2
2. Abu Hilal M, Aldrighetti L, Dagher I, et al. The Southampton Consensus Guidelines for Laparoscopic Liver Surgery: from indication to implementation. *Ann Surg.* 2018;268(1):11-18. doi: 10.1097/SLA.0000000000002524
3. Guerra F, Di Marino M, Coratti A. Robotic surgery of the liver and biliary tract. *J Laparoendosc Adv Surg Tech A.* 2019;29(2):141-146. doi: 10.1089/lap.2017.0628
4. Ishizawa T, Gumbs AA, Kokudo N, Gayet B. Laparoscopic segmentectomy of the liver: from segment I to VIII. *Ann Surg.* 2012;256(6):959-964. doi: 10.1097/SLA.0b013e31825ffed3
5. Giulianotti PC, Bianco FM, Daskalaki D, Gonzalez-Ciccarelli LF, Kim J, Benedetti E. Robotic liver surgery: technical aspects and review of the literature. *Hepatobiliary Surg Nutr.* 2016;5(4):311-321. doi: 10.21037/hbsn.2015.10.05
6. Sucandy I, Gravetz A, Ross S, Rosemurgy A. Technique of robotic left hepatectomy: how we approach it. *J Robot Surg.* 2019;13(2):201-207. doi: 10.1007/s11701-018-0890-6
7. Chiow AK, Lewin J, Manoharan B, Cavallucci D, Bryant R, O'Rourke N. Intercostal and transthoracic trocars enable easier laparoscopic resection of dome liver lesions. *HPB (Oxford).* 2015;17(4):299-303. doi: 10.1111/hpb.12336
8. Guerra F, Amore Bonapasta S, Annecchiarico M, Bongiolatti S, Coratti A. Robot-integrated intraoperative ultrasound: initial experience with hepatic malignancies. *Minim Invasive Ther Allied Techno.* 2015;24(6):345-349. doi: 10.3109/13645706.2015.1022558
9. Torzilli G, Botea F, Donadon M, et al. Criteria for the selective use of contrast-enhanced intra-operative ultrasound during surgery for colorectal liver metastases. *HPB (Oxford).* 2014;16(11):994-1001. doi: 10.1111/hpb.12272
10. Patriti A, Ceccarelli G, Bartoli A, Casciola L. Extracorporeal Pringle maneuver in robot-assisted liver surgery. *Surg Laparosc Endosc Percutan Tech.* 2011;21(5):e242-244. doi: 10.1097/SLE.0b013e31822d7fb4
11. de Santibañes E, Sánchez Clariá R, Palavecino M, Beskow A, Pekolj J. Liver metastasis resection: a simple technique that makes it easier. *J Gastrointest Surg.* 2007;11(9):1183-1187. doi: 10.1007/s11605-007-0227-7
12. Gonzalez-Ciccarelli LF, Quadri P, Daskalaki D, Milone L, Gangemi A, Giulianotti PC. Robotic approach to hepatobiliary surgery. *Chirurg.* 2017;88(Suppl 1):19-28. doi: 10.1007/s00104-016-0223-0
13. Giulianotti PC, Coratti A, Angelini M, et al. Robotics in general surgery: personal experience in a large community hospital. *Arch Surg.* 2003;138(7):777-784. doi: 10.1001/archsurg.138.7.777

SECTION VIII

Biliary Surgery

Chapter 37 • Cholecystectomy 791
Stephan Gruessner • Francesco Bianco • Pier Cristoforo Giulianotti

Chapter 38 • Roux-en-Y Hepaticojejunostomy 809
Eric CH Lai • Chung Ngai Tang

Chapter 39 • Bile Duct Injuries Repair 825
Pier Cristoforo Giulianotti • Antonio Cubisino • Nicolas Hellmuth Dreifuss

Chapter 40 • Management of Intrahepatic Biliary Stones 841
Eric CH Lai • Chung Ngai Tang

Referring to laparoscopic cholecystectomy: "The approach was like magic."
—Erich Mühe (1938–2005)

Cholecystectomy

Stephan Gruessner • Francesco Bianco • Pier Cristoforo Giulianotti

INTRODUCTION

The first open and laparoscopic cholecystectomies were performed in Germany in 1882 by Carl Langebuch, and in 1985 by Erich Mühe, respectively. The first laparoscopic cholecystectomy fell under significant criticism and resistance from the German medical community at the time and only received traction after Philippe Mouret presented his first series starting in 1987. Noting the reduced pain and improved cosmesis of the technique, the idea of a laparoscopic cholecystectomy spread to the United States and was first performed by Barry McKernan and William Saye in June of 1988. On March 3, 1997, Dr. Jacques Himpens performed the world's first robotic cholecystectomy, using an early prototype named the "Mona" (after Leonardo da Vinci's *Mona Lisa*). In contrast to the introduction of laparoscopic surgery, less concern needed to be placed on the feasibility and safety of the approach. However, routine use of the robotic platform for a cholecystectomy was often disregarded due to the associated costs. Recent advances in the technology (e.g., indocyanine green [ICG] fluorescence, single-port access) as well as the development of cost-saving strategies have been increasing the popularity of the robotic technique.

Novices to robotic surgery may find significant benefit in performing them robotically in order to hone their skills. This is also true for the support staff unfamiliar with the robotic platform, because a common surgery can help the team effectively focus on troubleshooting when needed.

Indications and Relative Contraindications to the Robotic Approach

The indications for a robotic cholecystectomy are similar to performing the procedure laparoscopically. The main pathologies include acute or chronic cholecystitis, biliary colic cholelithiasis, biliary dyskinesia (gallbladder ejection fraction less than 35%), acalculous cholecystitis, gallstone pancreatitis, and gallbladder polyps (>1 cm or age >60 years). While basic indications (e.g., biliary colic) can be a great learning opportunity for beginners, the indications can surpass laparoscopy in trained hands. With the improved optics and microsurgical capabilities, the robotic platform can outperform laparoscopy in complex cases, especially ones with dense fibrosis or significant inflammatory changes.

Patient Positioning, OR Setup, and Port Setting

The patient is placed supine and the table is rotated to reverse Trendelenburg and slightly toward the left (**Figure 37-1**).

INSTRUMENT REQUIREMENTS

The suggested main robotic instruments/tools can be listed as follows:
- 30° scope
- Cautery hook/monopolar scissors
- Round-tip scissors
- Medium–large clip applier
- Bipolar forceps
- Cadière forceps

The suggested main laparoscopic instruments/tools can be listed as follows:
- Forceps
- Suction-irrigation device (if needed)
- Needle driver (if needed)

Supplemental materials:
- Endo Bag™
- Hem-o-lok® clips
- Sponges
- Jackson-Pratt (JP) drain (if needed)
- Nylon 2-0
- Vycril or Prolene 4-0 (if needed)

Photo and quote reproduced with permission from Litynski GS. Erich Mühe and the rejection of laparoscopic cholecystectomy (1985): a surgeon ahead of his time. JSLS. 1998;2(4):341-346. Society of Laparoscopic & Robotic Surgeons.

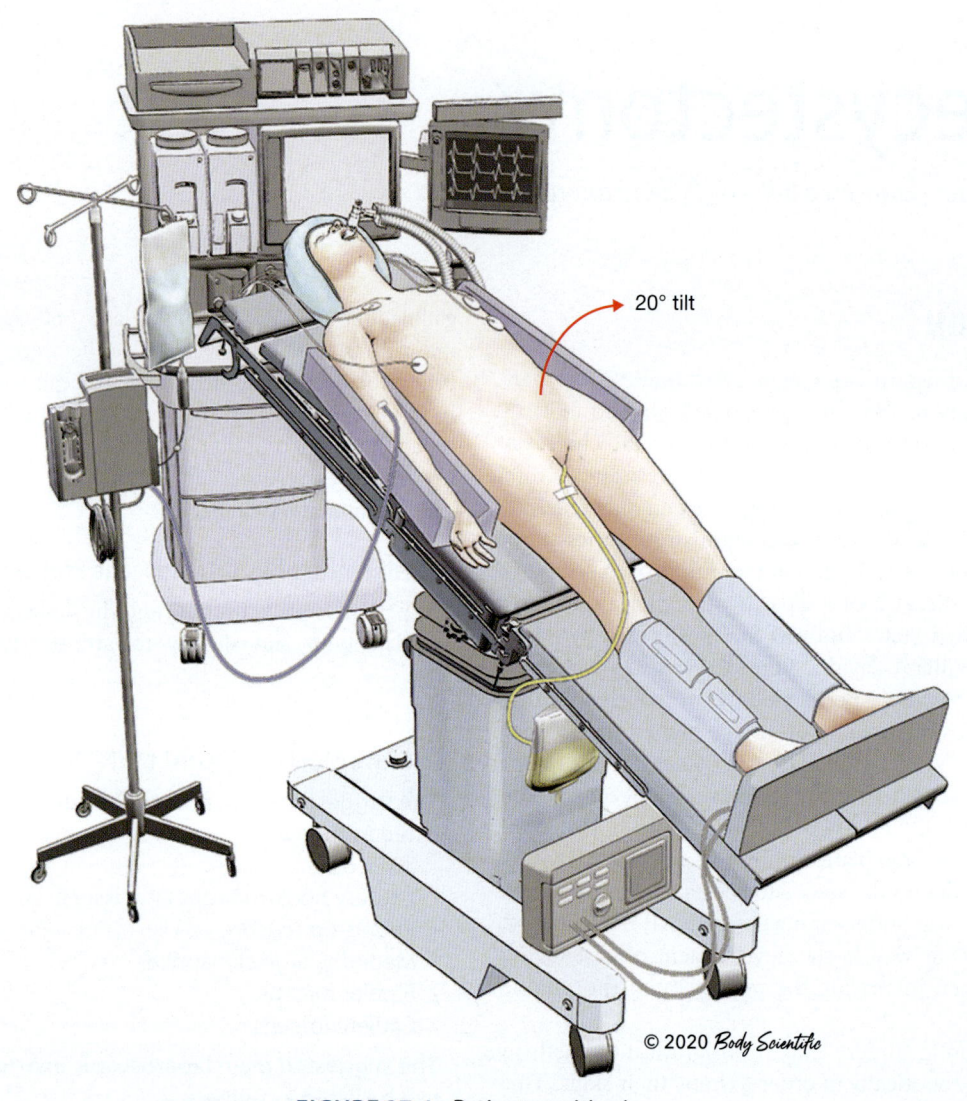

FIGURE 37-1 • Patient positioning.

The patient's arms are tucked to allow better cart maneuverability and access to the patient for the surgical assistant. A footboard should be placed to prevent shifting of the patient during the surgery. Depending on the patient's body habitus, a beanbag may also be used to secure the patient to the table. The positioning should allow intraoperative cholangiogram (IOC) if needed. The assistant surgeon should be standing to the left of the patient with the robotic cart on the right (**Figure 37-2**).

The operation starts with the induction of pneumoperitoneum with the Veress technique at the modified Palmer's point (see Chapter 2, The Basic Principles of Clinical Applications). A 5-mm OptiView™ trocar should be placed in the left upper quadrant, inferior and lateral to the Veress needle. This assessment can be used to rule out possible complications of Veress insertion (such as bleeding or perforation), determine if adhesiolysis is required, and insert the subsequent trocars under direct visualization. When placing the 5-mm port, it is important to keep some distance between the costal margin and the trocar to maintain mobility of the R3 when the trocar is upsized. The 3 subsequent trocars are placed approximately 10 cm apart in a

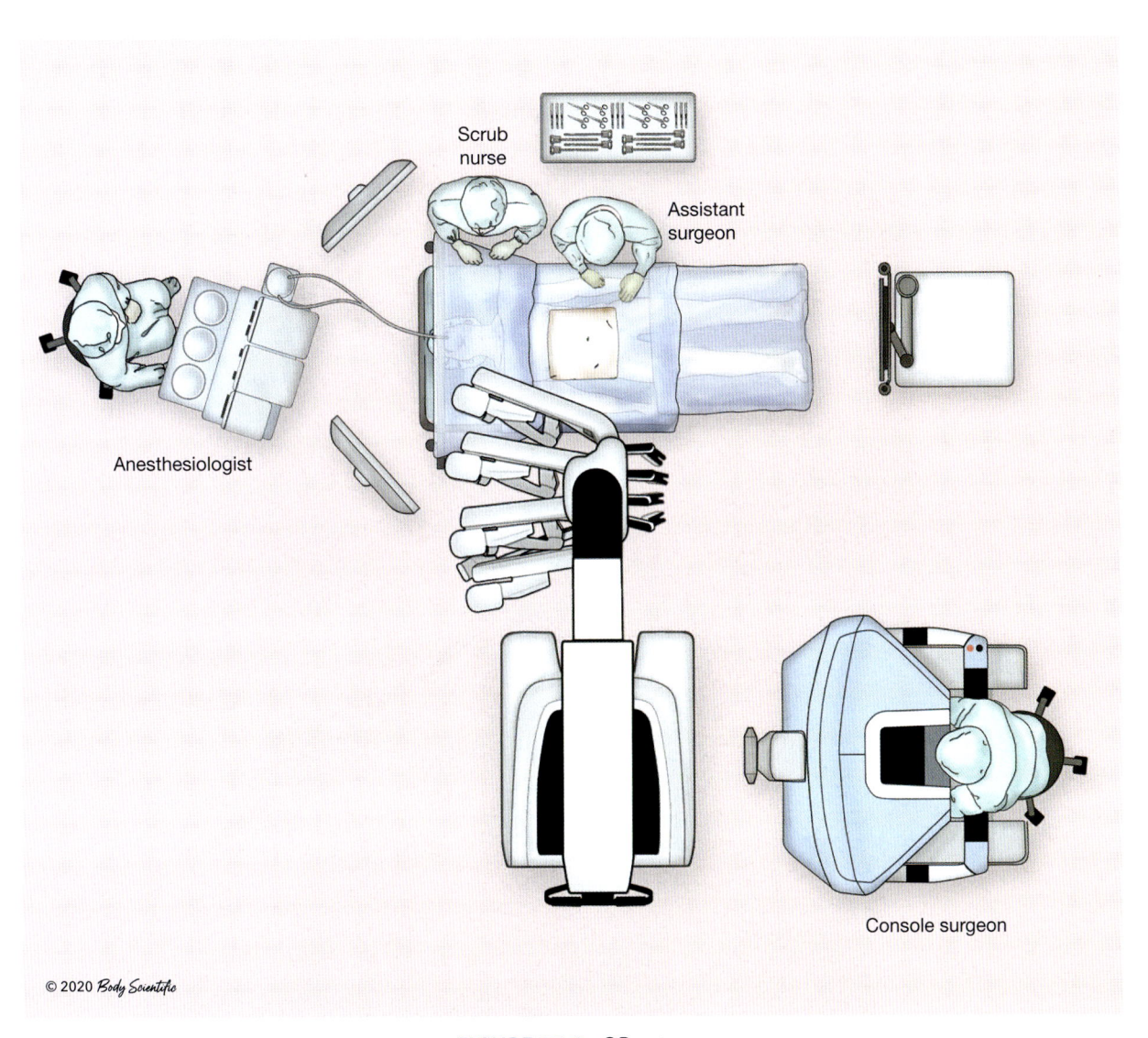

FIGURE 37-2 • OR setup.

straight line along the transverse umbilical line. The port for the scope should be at the intersection of the transverse umbilical line and the right pararectal line. A greater distance between trocars may be needed in high body mass index (BMI) patients. The final port is placed a further 10 cm to the right, forming a straight line with the previous two. When an assistant port is needed, it is optimally placed slightly below the space between the camera and the left working port. A 5-mm assistant trocar is sufficient when only suction is needed, with the 12-mm reserved for complex cases requiring additional retraction, sponge exchange, or stone retrieval. Port setting for normal and wide abdomen is depicted in **Figures 37-3** and **37-4**.

> ▶▶ **TIPS**
>
> In contrast to the laparoscopic approach, where the retraction is achieved from the right side, the R3 is placed in the left upper quadrant. This provides more space for the working ports, thereby lowering the risk of collisions during dissection. The most important action of the R3 is also the upward retraction of the hilar plate underlying the segment 4b. This action is more effectively achieved with the retracting instrument coming from the left side.

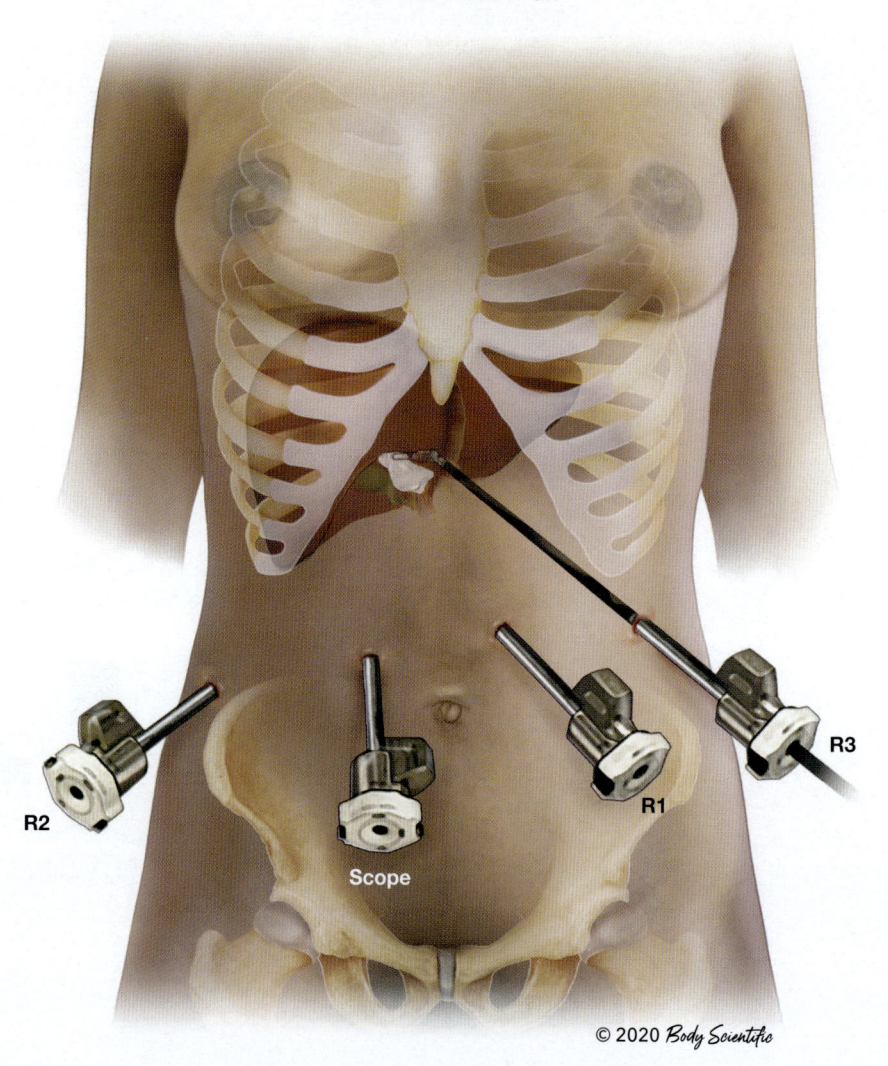

FIGURE 37-3 • Port setting normal abdomen.

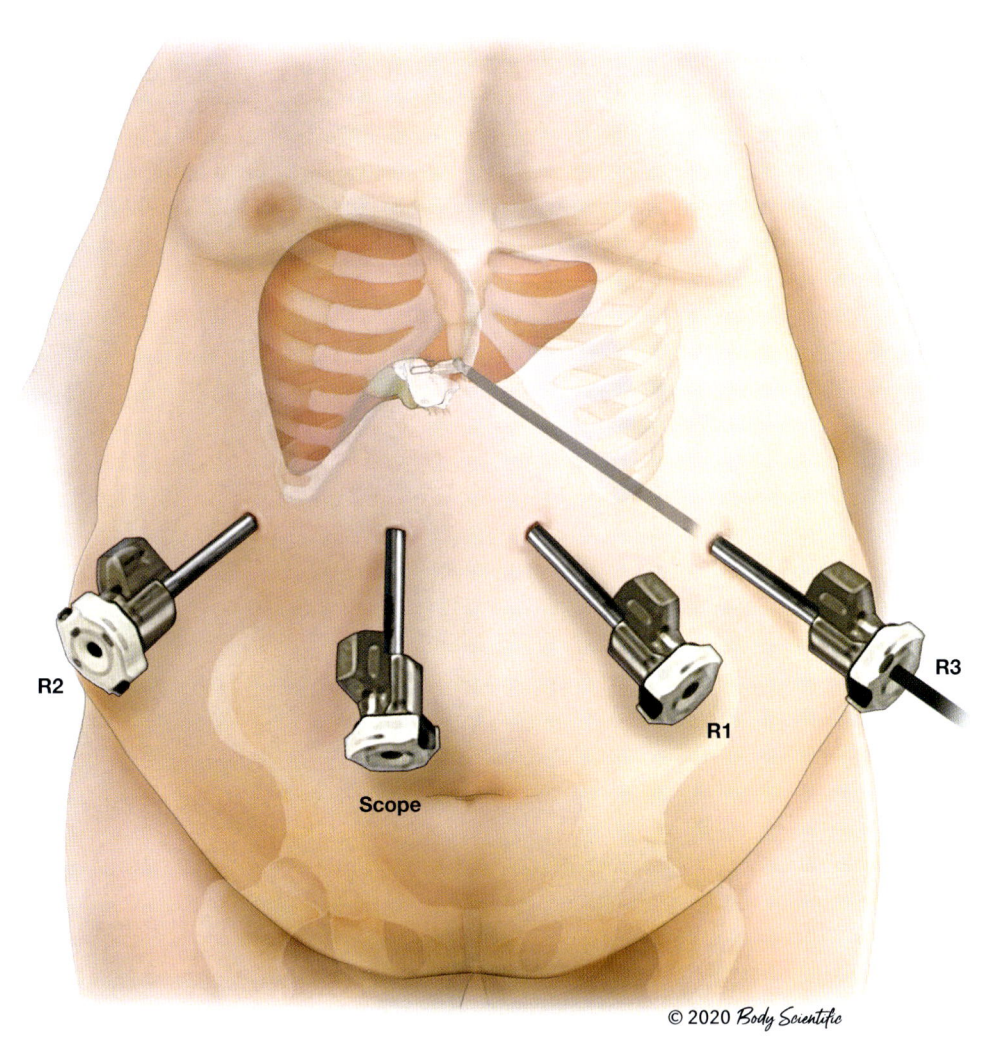

FIGURE 37-4 • Port setting wide abdomen.

Surgical Technique

▶ **Video 37-1. Cholecystectomy – Full Procedure**

Step 1. Exposure of the working area

For optimal exposure of the gallbladder and hilum, the R3 (cushioned by a single RAY-TEC™ gauze) can be advanced from the left to gently retract segment 4b of the liver cranially. If the gallbladder fundus is grasped and retracted cranially as in the laparoscopic approach, the angle between the cystic duct and hepatic duct would be narrowed, increasing the risk of misinterpreting the anatomy.

The primary purpose of retraction is to visualize the major landmarks. Ideally, the gallbladder neck, the cystic artery, the cystic duct, and its confluence with the common bile duct should be recognized. However, patients rarely display the ideal anatomy, and retraction should maximize this exposure without injuring the liver parenchyma (**Figures 37-5 A, B**).

Step 1 average time frame: 2–3 min

> ▶▶ **TIPS**
>
> If the left lobe of the liver is floppy and falling onto the surgical field, the surgeon can orient the R3 at a more horizontal angle, using the shaft of the arm to support the weight of segment 3 while retracting segment 4b with the instrument tip cushioned by a sponge.
>
> When encountering a fatty/bulky round ligament obstructing the view and dissection, the assistant can pass a 2-0 nylon suture with a straight needle through the skin for the surgeon to retrieve and return on the opposite side of the ligament, effectively retracting the round ligament for the duration of the surgery (via suspension effect).

A

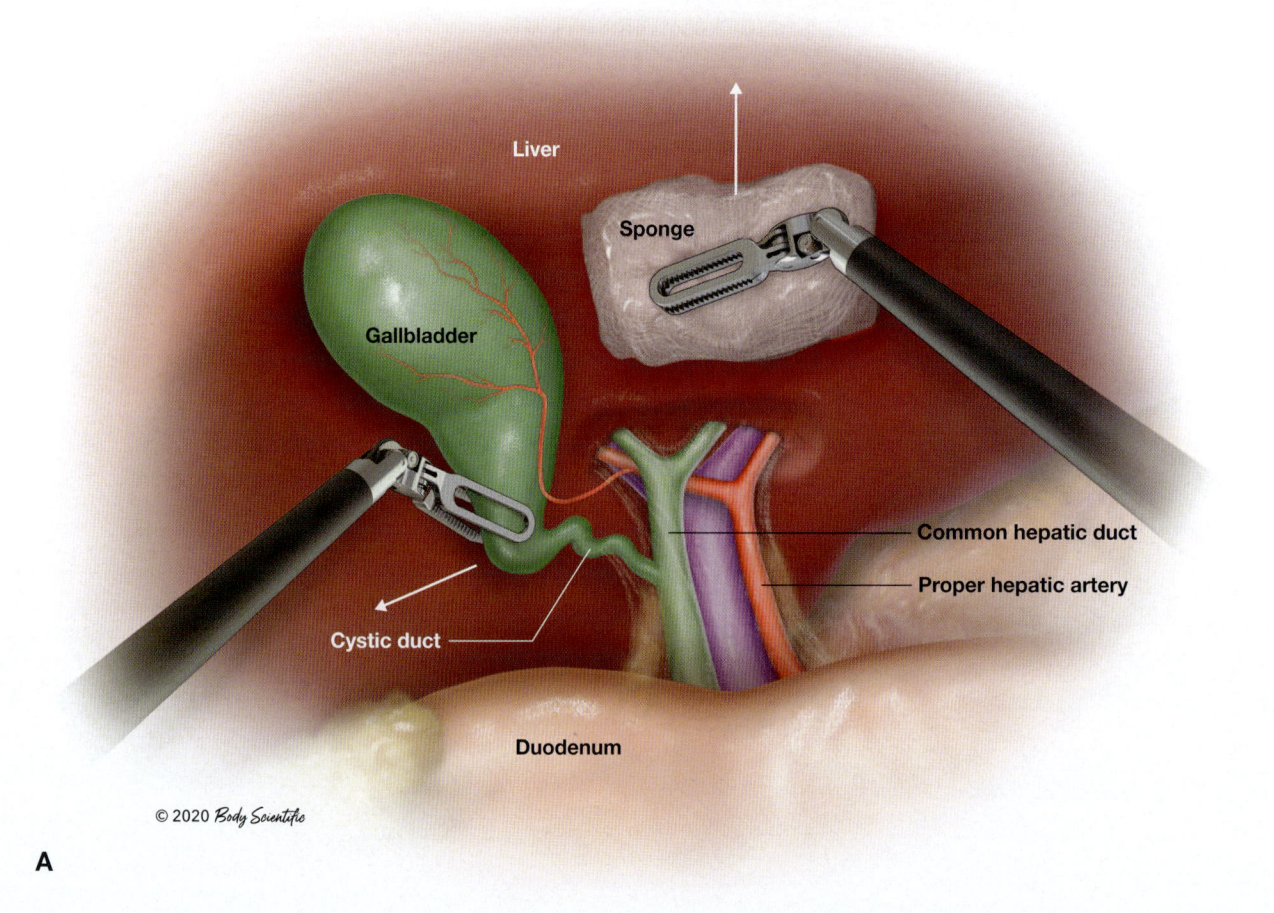

FIGURE 37-5 • A liver hilum exposure.

B

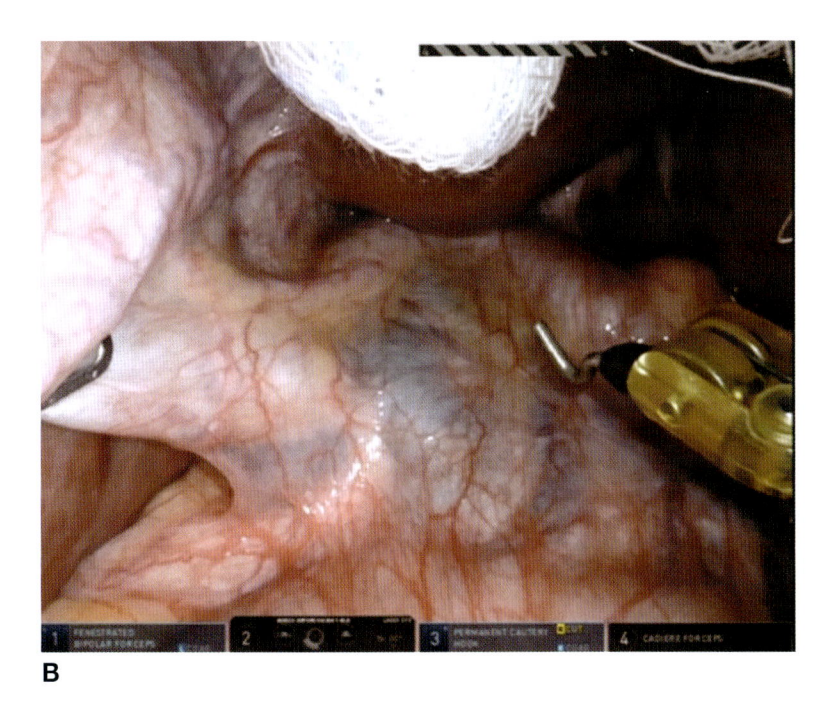

FIGURE 37-5 • (*Continued*)

▶ Video 37-2. Cholecystectomy Exposure

> ⚠ **PITFALLS**
>
> Dissection without clear understanding of the hilar anatomy can be dangerous and a surgeon should recognize the reasons for limited visualization. There are 3 main factors that will limit exposure.
>
> The most common reason is a partial or incomplete mechanical retraction. This can be caused by an inadequate position of the R3, poor countertraction, or overdistension of the gallbladder obstructing visualization. These reasons can be directly influenced by repositioning the R3, maneuvering the angle of R2 traction, or draining the bile from the gallbladder.
>
> The next factor that can limit visualization is from inflammation and fibrosis extending to the hilum. In these cases, slow progression is paramount, but a subtotal cholecystectomy may be considered to prevent biliary injury.
>
> Aberrant anatomy of the liver is the least common reason for inadequate exposure and may require a modification of approach. In cases where the cystic duct has a high insertion with the hepatic duct, an early anterograde dissection of the gallbladder from the liver is advisable. In cases of an intrahepatic gallbladder, hepatic parenchymal transection may be necessary to expose the gallbladder from the surrounding liver.
>
> If exposure of the hilum is difficult, one factor, a combination of factors, or even all these factors may be present. A surgeon should be prudent and try to optimize his approach rather than dissecting blindly. The problem should be approached systematically by reorienting the retraction, modifying the technique, or considering a subtotal cholecystectomy.

Step 2. Retraction of the gallbladder neck

With the gallbladder hilum exposed using the R3, the neck of the gallbladder can be retracted laterally and inferiorly. This maneuver creates tension perpendicular to the cystic duct's confluence with the hepatic duct, thereby widening the angle between the 2 structures.

> ▶▶ **TIPS**
>
> If the gallbladder is distended and difficult to retract, it may be appropriate to decompress it first. The assistant port may be placed for insertion of a suction device. The gallbladder is scored at the level of the fundus, and the suction device is bluntly inserted through the weakened wall to avoid spillage. After decompression, a suture may be placed to limit further bile contents from spilling into the abdomen.

The combination of the retraction of segment 4b and lateral/inferior retraction of the gallbladder neck allows optimal exposure of the triangle of Calot (**Figure 37-6**), which is needed to obtain the critical view of safety. This has 3 key criteria that should be met before dividing structures:

- The triangle of Calot (cystic duct, the common hepatic duct, and the cystic artery) is recognized.
- The lower third of the fibrous ligament connecting the gallbladder and liver (cystic plate) is freed.
- Only 2 structures should be isolated, leaving the hilum toward the gallbladder (cystic duct and artery).

> 🔍 **ANATOMICAL HIGHLIGHTS**
>
> While the modern borders of the triangle of Calot are described as the cystic duct, the common hepatic duct, and the inferior border of the liver, the original borders described in 1891 were the cystic duct, the common hepatic duct, and the cystic artery. As the interpretation of the "inferior border of the liver" can be vague, the original description by Calot will be used.

The expanded microsurgical capabilities and precision of the robotic platform can take this a step further. When possible, the common hepatic and cystic duct bifurcation should be identified. The right hepatic artery runs parallel and posterior to the common hepatic duct, and the branch leading to the cystic artery can be isolated. If the critical view of safety is achieved and these landmark structures are properly identified, the surgeon can confidently proceed with the case.

Step 2 average time frame: 1–10 min (depending on whether decompression of the gallbladder is required)

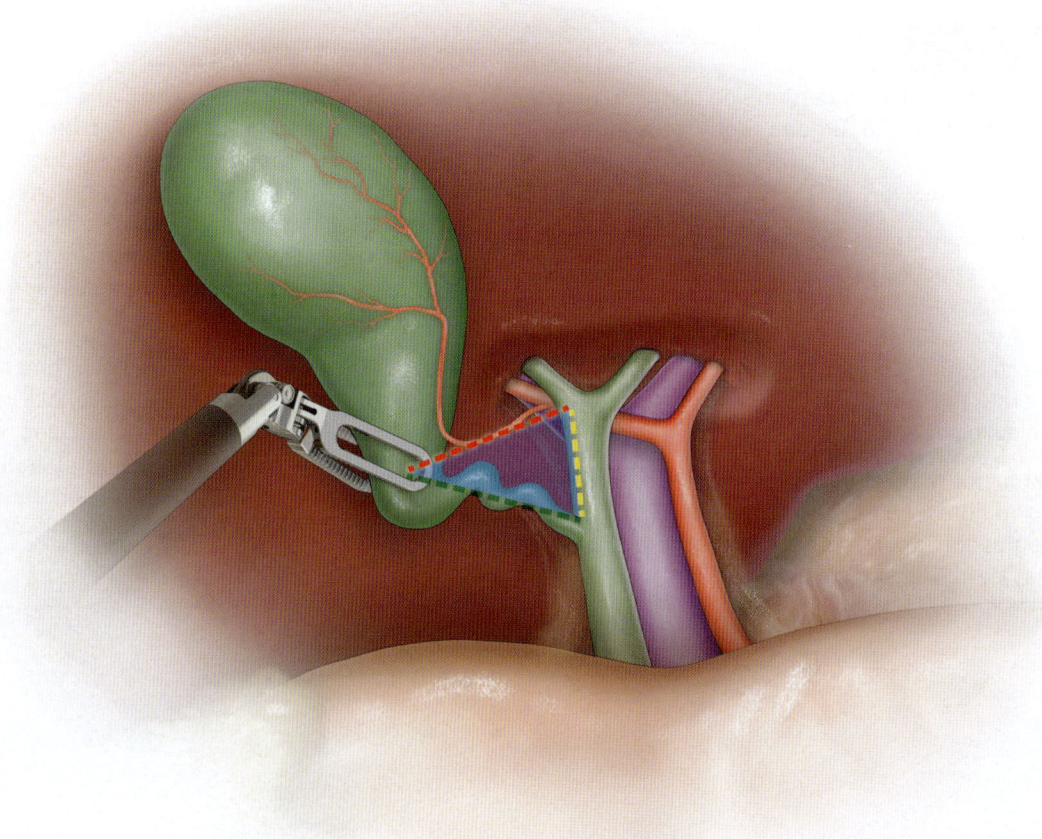

FIGURE 37-6 • Triangle of Calot.

Step 3. Opening the anterior peritoneal layer of the triangle of Calot

With the hilum exposed, the tip of the monopolar hook can be used to lift the anterior peritoneal layer. Brief cautery under traction will open the plane safely and away from critical structures. It is important to begin the dissection laterally and not directly over the hilum. The surgeon should move from known to unknown by following the inferior border of the gallbladder neck and progressing toward the cystic duct. The cystic duct will usually be encountered first; however, the cystic artery is highly variable, and can occasionally be encountered first. In severe and extensive fibrosis/adhesions, the basic landmarks of the colonic flexure and edges of the liver should be visually confirmed. In the hands of an experienced hepatobiliary surgeon, a partial Kocher maneuver may be done to better understand the trajectory of the portal triad.

Step 3 average time frame: 2–3 min

> **ANATOMICAL HIGHLIGHTS**
>
> Normally, there will be a single artery traveling within the triangle of Calot just behind the duct from the right hepatic artery (~70%) (**Figures 37-7 A–F**). (Multiple anatomical variations can occur, and these can be classified in different ways. Here, the most clinically significant are presented. The single artery branches near the neck of the gallbladder for a medial and lateral blood supply. The cystic artery may also arise from a replaced right hepatic artery originating from the superior mesenteric artery (~15%). A second artery may be encountered (~10%) arising from the right hepatic artery separately. The hepatic artery may also originate from a source outside of the triangle of Calot with the gastroduodenal artery as the most common variant (~2%). When the cystic artery seems to be absent from the hilum, there may be an intraparenchymal source supplying the gallbladder through one or more arteries (~2%). While rare, the cystic artery can even originate from the left hepatic artery (<1%). See suggested readings #3, 4.

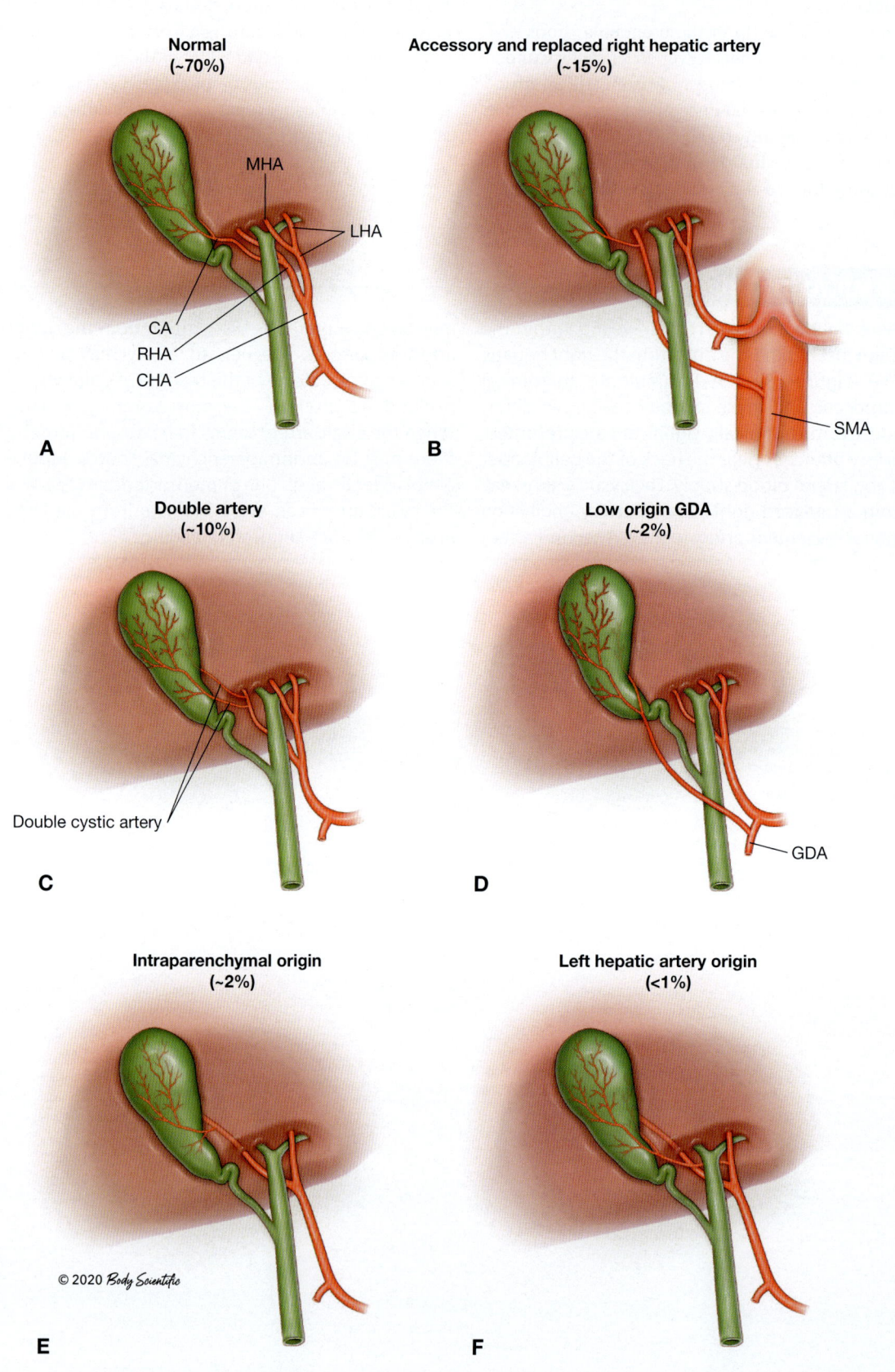

FIGURE 37-7 • Cystic artery anatomy variations. (CA, cystic artery; CHA, common hepatic artery; GDA, gastroduodenal artery; LHA, left hepatic artery; RHA, right hepatic artery; SMA, superior mesenteric artery.)

Step 4. Opening the posterior peritoneal layer of the triangle of Calot

As the anterior cystic plate is cleared, the surgeon can freely retract the neck medially, allowing progressive dissection within tissue planes (**Figures 37-8 A, B**). Through posterior dissection, the surgeon mobilizes the cystic duct and artery from their posterior attachments. It is important to remain close to the gallbladder and not move too deep from the known anatomy to prevent iatrogenic injury of the portal vein, right hepatic artery, right hepatic duct, or common bile duct. If needed, wide detachment of the neck from the liver will provide increased control over the tissue. On some occasions, it may be necessary to move back and forth between the anterior and posterior layers to complete this step.

Step 4 average time frame: 1–3 min

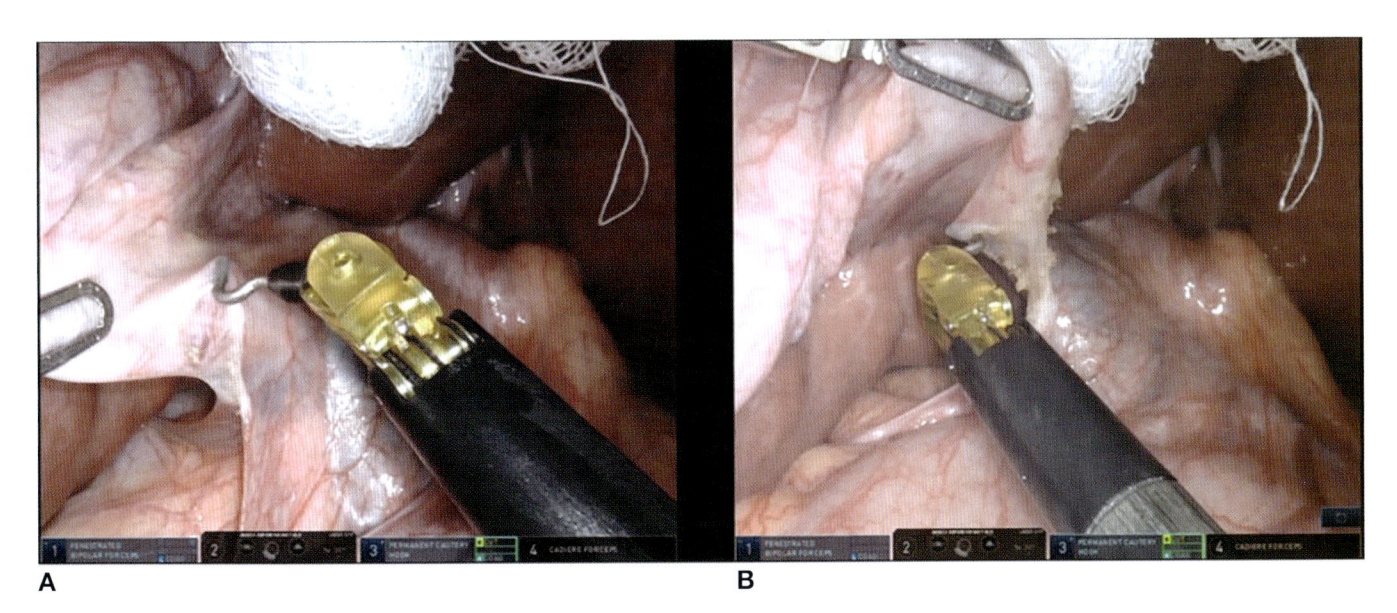

FIGURE 37-8 • Opening the anterior/posterior peritoneal layer.

Video 37-3. Opening the Anterior/Posterior Peritoneal Layer of the Calot Triangle

Step 5. Isolation of the cystic duct

By retracting the neck of the gallbladder, the tension will primarily be transmitted through the cystic duct and aid in identification and dissection. It is essential to fully skeletonize the neck and anterior/posterior connections to the cystic duct when entering the hilum. While aberrant anatomy of the duct is less frequent than that of the artery, anomalies are still common. In the absence of an impacted stone or obstructing mass, ICG can be beneficial in identifying the cystic duct throughout the case. (For more information, see Chapter 7, Fluorescence Imaging: Basics and Clinical Applications.)

ICG should be injected at least half an hour before the surgery. The confluence of the cystic duct and common bile duct is almost always visible, because the fluorescent dye is likely retained behind the cystic duct's Heister valve closest to the common bile duct.

When isolating the cystic duct, the degree of inflammation can vary. The duct can be normal, dilated, or obliterated. In the presence of a dilated duct, there will likely be (or has been) a distal obstruction. The neck should be carefully retracted because stones may be pushed distally when grasping broadly with forceps. Due to the size of the dilated duct, the cystic duct can be confused with the common bile duct (especially in cases with a short cystic duct). If the anatomy is not clear, ICG or even an IOC should be used to identify the key landmarks.

There are cases where the duct has been obliterated due to chronic inflammation, suppurative cholecystitis, hydropic gallbladder, or malignant obstruction. The gallbladder is typically distended in these patients, and early drainage will aid the grasping and retraction of the gallbladder. To safely ligate the duct, the surgeon should dissect the hilum to identify normal tissue with a clear understanding of the anatomy. In some cases, the extent of dissection may need to reach the confluence with the common hepatic duct.

With the enhanced visualization of the robotic camera and the assistance of ICG fluoroscopy, the IOC is rarely used. Historically, IOC was routinely used when there was confusion of the biliary anatomy, doubt of common bile duct stones, or to rule out/document an injury. While the robotic platform can reduce the need for IOC, every surgeon should be able to perform one when needed. This can be achieved by clipping/tying the cystic duct close to the gallbladder and making an anterior incision in the cystic duct. A catheter can then be passed and secured to prevent backflow with a suture or balloon. Once secured, dye can be injected with fluoroscopy active.

🔍 ANATOMICAL HIGHLIGHTS

Anatomic variations of the cystic duct are less pronounced than those of the cystic artery. The insertion of the cystic duct is the most variable (**Figure 37-9**), normally inserting within the middle third of the extrahepatic bile duct (~40.2%). The duct can have a low insertion in the distal third of the common bile duct (~9%) or high insertion in the proximal third (~6.5%). It can rarely join with the right hepatic duct (~0.5%).

The height of the insertion is not the only anomaly to be aware of. The duct can spiral anteriorly or posteriorly toward its insertion in the extrahepatic bile duct (16.1%, 20.2%, respectively). The cystic duct can also run parallel with the common bile duct with a common fibrous sheath (~7.5%). It is extremely rare for a double duct to occur, and when encountered, it should be treated with suspicion until completion of the dissection. (Multiple anatomical variations can occur, and these can be classified in different ways. Here, the most clinically significant are presented. See suggested reading #5.)

Normal anatomy (~40.2%)

Posterior spiral (~20.2%)

Anterior spiral (~16.1%)

Low union with common bile duct (~9%)

Parallel course with fibrous sheath (~7.5%)

High union with common bile duct (~6.5%)

Union with the right hepatic duct (~0.5%)

© 2020 *Body Scientific*

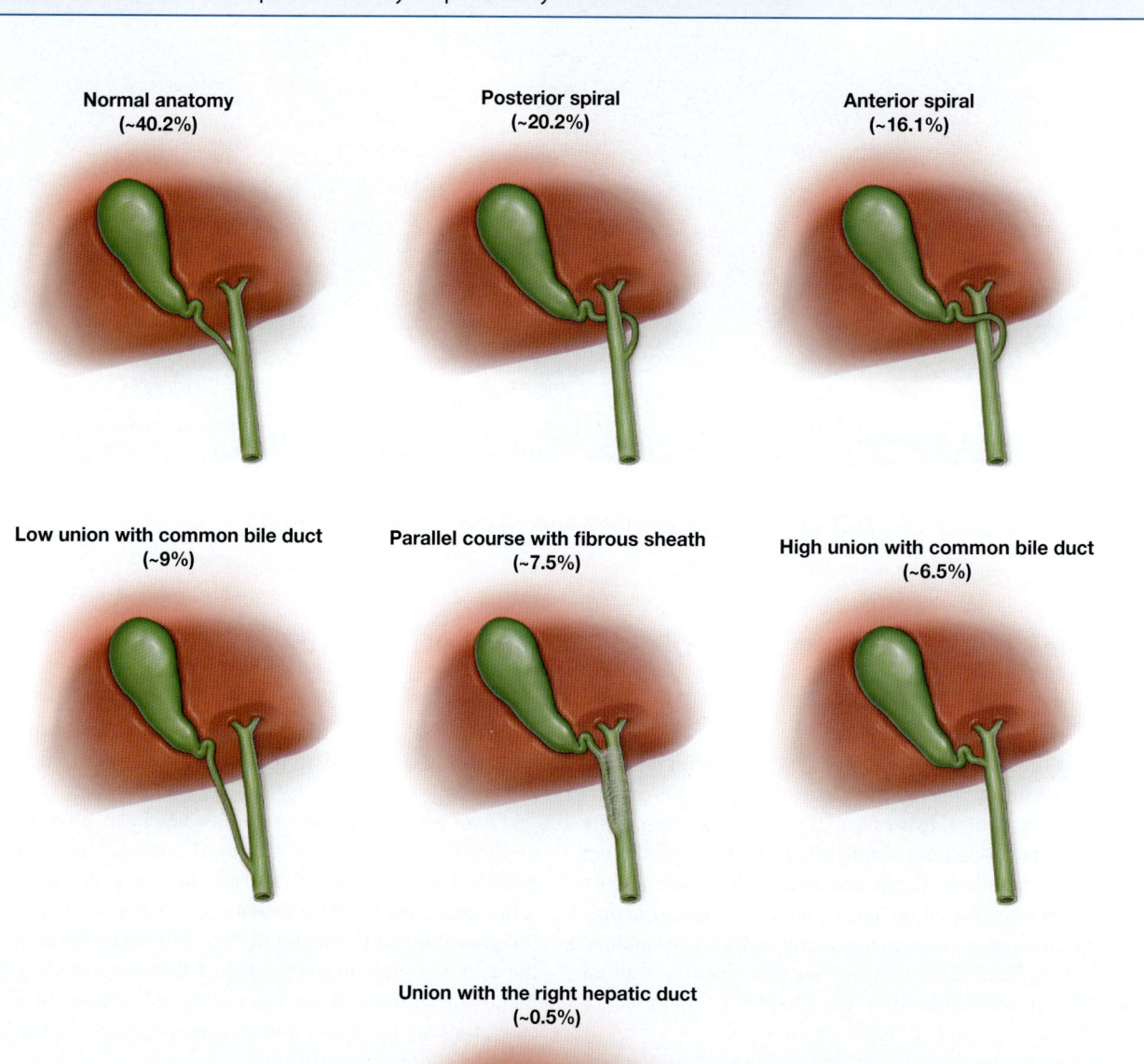

FIGURE 37-9 • Cystic duct anatomy variations.

Video 37-4. Cholecystectomy Difficult IOC

> **▶▶ TIPS**
>
> If the surgeon experiences difficultly entering the cystic duct with the catheter, 2 stay sutures may be placed on both sides of the insertion site to lift and straighten the cystic duct.
>
> When bringing the x-ray toward the table, the robotic cart may not need to be undocked completely. If needed, some robotic instrument and camera may remain in place with the fluoroscopy active.

Even with the enhanced capabilities of the robotic platform, iatrogenic injury to the biliary tree can still occur. There are several ways to categorize the location of biliary trauma; however, the most commonly used is the Strasberg classification, which expanded Bismuth's initial descriptions (**Figure 37-10**). (See suggested reading #9.)

Type A injuries are leaks that occur at the cystic duct or a minor hepatic duct. Type B and C are injuries to an aberrant sectoral duct but are differentiated by leak (Type B) or occlusion (Type C). Type D is a leak from the common hepatic duct, without complete transection or tissue loss. Type E is the incorporation of the Bismuth classification. Types E1 and E2 are differentiated by the level of transection of the common hepatic duct (>2-cm stump vs. <2-cm stump, respectively). E3 is a transection at the confluence of the right and left hepatic ducts, which are in communication. Type E4 is a transection that separates the left and right hepatic ducts. Lastly, Type E5 is a Type C injury with a concomitant hilar injury.

Step 5 average time frame: 5–30 min

> **⚠ PITFALLS**
>
> Excessive use of energy can cause thermal injury to the biliary structures in the hilum. The arteries and veins are relatively better protected from thermal injury than the bile ducts due to the dissipation of heat from the "heat-sink" effect of flowing blood.

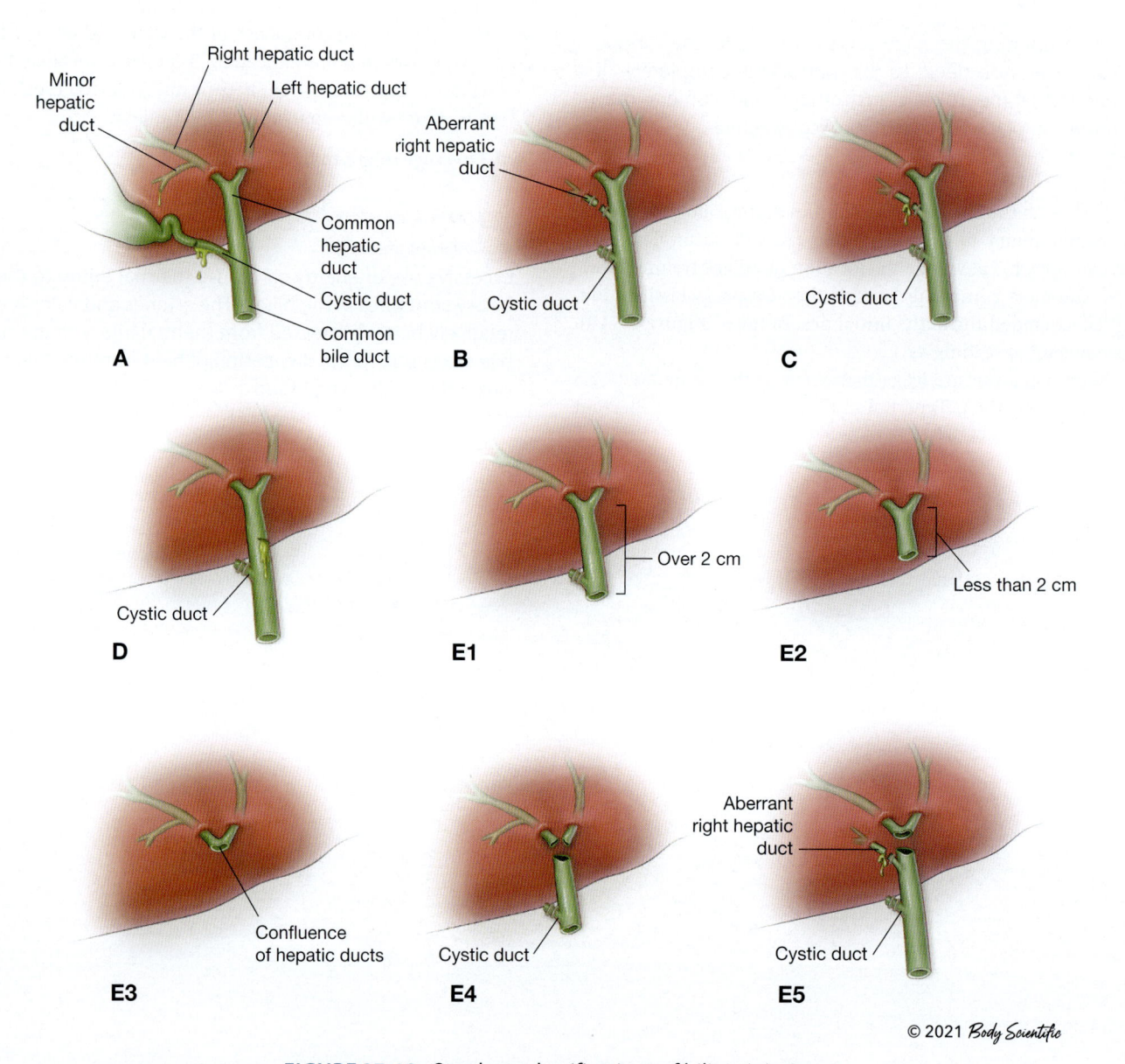

FIGURE 37-10 • Strasberg classifications of biliary injuries.

Step 6. Isolation of the cystic artery

As previously mentioned, it is important to note throughout the hilar dissection that the cystic artery can be highly variable in its origin and path of travel. Obtaining the critical view of safety and assuring that only 2 structures are entering the gallbladder is paramount. If the cystic artery is not adequately isolated, injury to the proper hepatic artery or right hepatic artery may occur. If either of these arteries are ligated, the liver may survive or develop necrosis, but the intrahepatic biliary tree will lose its vascular supply. Consequently, a vanishing biliary tree or intrahepatic strictures resembling sclerosing cholangitis may be seen.

When identification of the artery is difficult, the surgeon should not dissect blindly. By carefully dissecting along the cystic duct, the confluence with the hepatic duct is reached. The common hepatic duct is used as an anterior landmark for the right hepatic artery, and careful dissection within the hilum will lead to the right hepatic artery and subsequently, the branch of the cystic artery. When following the paths of each structure, the surgeon always remains in a safe plane of known tissue and can avoid iatrogenic injury.

Step 6 average time frame: 5–30 min

Step 7. Clipping of the cystic duct

While using the hook, it must be confirmed that the duct is free from all attachments posteriorly and there is ample space to insert a clip (**Figures 37-11 A, B**). If the space created is insufficient, the clip can be easily displaced. The tip should be visible before closing a Hem-o-lok® clip because including unnecessary tissue can reduce the security of the locking mechanism.

One Hem-o-lok® clip is placed on the distal cystic duct and 1 proximally. When placing the distal clip, best practice is to position it close to the confluence with the common hepatic duct when the anatomy is clear. If the surgery is complicated, it may be prudent to leave a longer stump. It is important that cuff of tissue must be present proximal to the distal clip to prevent the clip from dislodging.

When there is concern for stones in the distal cystic duct, the first clip may be placed close to the gallbladder, and the cystic duct can be opened. This maneuver will allow the surgeon to gently milk out any small stones present in the duct.

Step 7 average time frame: 1–3 min

> ▶▶ **TIPS**
>
> The cystic artery may become difficult to isolate when grasping the gallbladder neck due to hilar tissue folding on top of the cystic duct and obstructing the view. The surgeon can release the traction from R2 and attempt a different maneuver. The tip of the forceps can be placed between the liver and gallbladder neck, and the jaws can be opened like a small Weitlaner retractor. By spreading the jaws open, there will be 3 forces in action: lateral retraction of the neck, tension on the cystic duct, and counter-retraction of the hilar tissue. This maneuver can greatly assist the surgeon in opening the triangle of Calot and isolating the cystic artery.

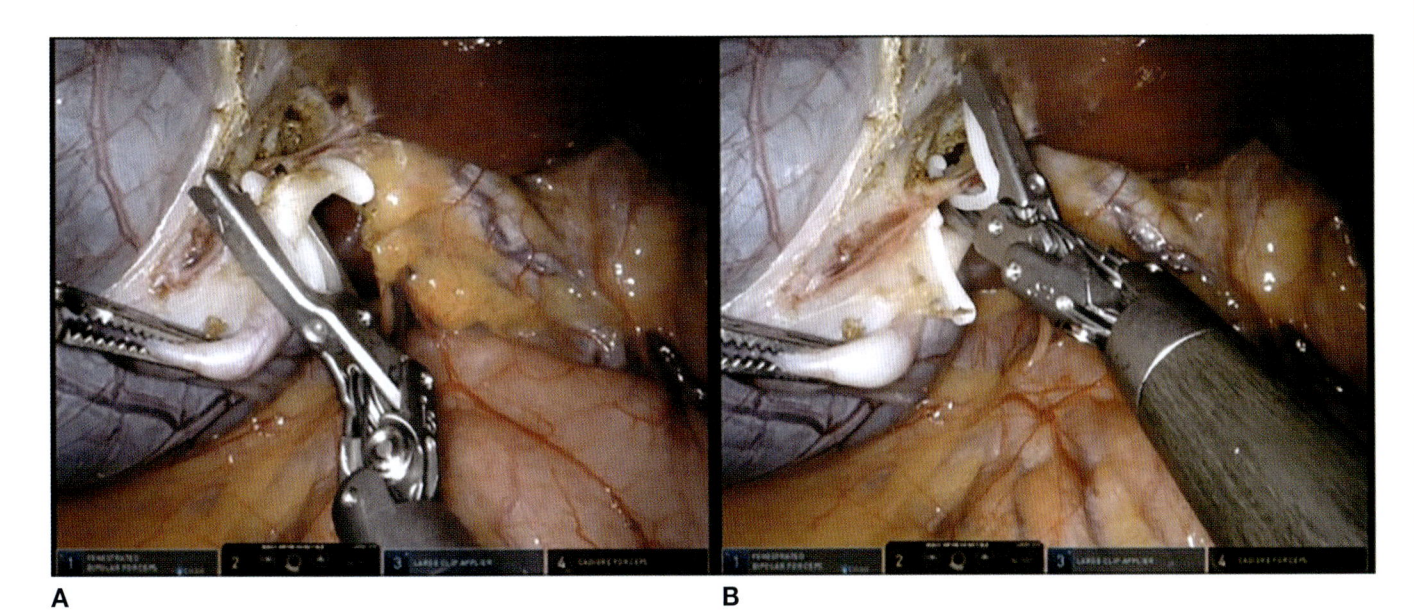

FIGURE 37-11 • Clipping the cystic duct and artery.

Step 8. Clipping the cystic artery

One Hem-o-lok® can be placed distally and proximally on the cystic artery. Metallic clips should be avoided because they have a higher risk of dislodgement.

Step 8 average time frame: 1–3 min

> ⚠️ **PITFALLS**
>
> Sometimes, it may feel safer to place more clips than are necessary. The number of clips used should be limited to 2 for the duct and 2 for the artery. Each time an extra clip is placed, there is a chance that something that does not belong is included.

▶ **Video 37-5. Cholecystectomy Clip and Cut**

Step 9. Division of the cystic duct and artery

Cold scissors are recommended for dividing the cystic duct and cystic artery. The use of monopolar cautery is controversial in transection of the vessels between clips. The cautery can damage the ligation point, destroying the cuff of tissue in front of the clip, and delayed bleeding/bile leak can occur.

Step 9 average time frame: 1–2 min

Step 10. Dissection of the gallbladder from the liver

While maintaining exposure with the R3 retracting segment 4b of the liver, the R2 arm can grasp the neck/fundus of the gallbladder and retract it cranially and laterally. The traction of the R2 arm should shift medially and laterally as dissection progresses to maximize focal tension. It is important not to pull too hard, because the cystic plate can be stronger than the parenchyma of the liver and tearing of the hepatic tissue will lead to bleeding.

The ideal plane of dissection in the cystic plate is the fibroareolar connective tissue layer between the gallbladder wall and liver parenchyma. Maintaining this perfect plane of dissection ("holy plane") allows the best hemostasis and reduces the risk of postoperative hematomas and bilomas.

A physician in training should use this opportunity to master a combination of the "pull" and "push" techniques described in Chapter 2, The Basic Principles of Clinical Applications (**Figure 37-12**). The "pull" technique is best used in situations where there is minimal inflammation of the gallbladder. In these cases, the gallbladder wall is thin, and the connective tissue is more elastic and easier to pull. Alternatively, the "push" technique is best used when there is significant inflammation, because the gallbladder wall is edematous, thickened, and the "holy plane" will not be visible. The line of division will likely be within the gallbladder wall itself (intramural) rather than the "holy plane," because the inflammatory process will make the cystic plate rigid and inelastic while the thickened and edematous wall of the gallbladder will favor the conduction of energy. This intramural technique can be advantageous, because the most external layer of the gallbladder wall provides tissue that can easily conduct monopolar energy for hemostasis and dissection without harming the parenchyma of the liver. This technique should of course be avoided if there is any suspicion of malignancy.

Step 10 average time frame: 5–15 min

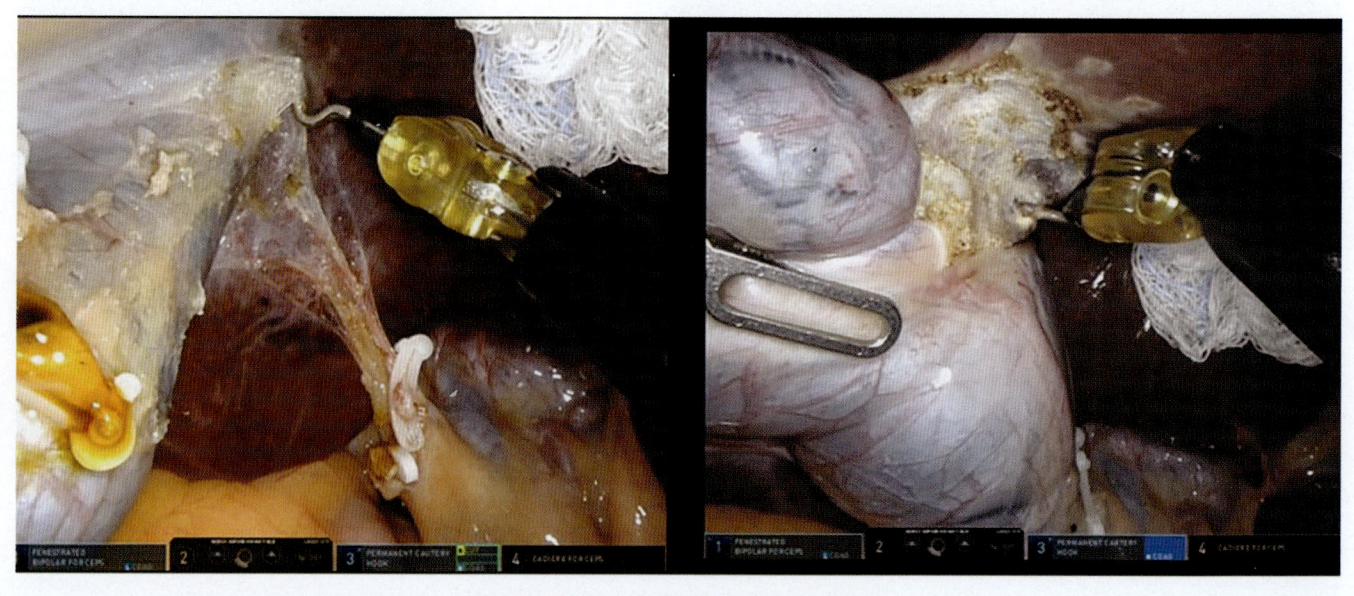

FIGURE 37-12 • Pull and push methods.

▶ **Video 37-6. Dissection of the Gallbladder from the Liver**

Step 11. Specimen retrieval

When the gallbladder has been completely detached from the liver, an accurate review of the hemostasis should be conducted. The supraumbilical port site can be used to retrieve the specimen. If the fascia restricts removal of the Endobag™, the cause of the obstruction should be eliminated. If the obstruction is from impacted stones, ring forceps can be used to crush them within the bag. If the gallbladder is too distended, a suction device to reduce the volume of the bile should be used. Stretching the fascia with a hemostat should be avoided, because enlarging the incision increases the chance of delayed complications like port hernias.

After retrieval of the gallbladder, a final check of the hilum and gallbladder bed is performed ensuring hemostasis is obtained, and that the 2 clips are secure.

Step 11 average time frame: 5–10 min

🔍 ANATOMICAL HIGHLIGHTS

The gallbladder itself can have anatomical variations. It can have a prominent mesentery, which is prone to torsion, and it can be intrahepatic with a small rim of liver parenchyma encapsulating the organ.

The gallbladder can also have ducts of Luschka that communicate with the intrahepatic biliary tree. These can be difficult to identify when dissecting the cystic plate. If ICG was used in the case, the gallbladder bed might be irrigated with saline and active extravasation of ICG will confirm the suspicion. A close inspection of the posterior gallbladder wall may reveal a small hole where the Luschka duct was merging.

▶▶ TIPS

If the gallbladder wall was perforated and stones spill into the peritoneum, these should be retrieved and included in the Endobag™ before extraction.

▶▶ TIPS

The large majority of patients do not need a drain; however, it may be prudent to leave a JP drain for 24–48 hours if the surgery was complex and difficult. The drain can offer the benefit of early recognition of a bile leak that can be managed with an ERCP and stent in the early postoperative period.

▶▶ TIPS

A subtotal cholecystectomy may be necessary in cases where the biliary anatomy is unclear, or if the posterior wall of the gallbladder is necrotic (**Figures 37-13 A–D**). There are variations of the subtotal cholecystectomy that can be done. If the hilar anatomy is distorted and cannot be dissected safely, the gallbladder can be approached at the neck (A). If the tissue is viable, a purse-string suture may be placed to close the gallbladder neck (B). If the posterior wall of the gallbladder is necrotic and bleeds profusely with manipulation, the gallbladder can be drained and only the anterior wall resected. The cystic duct is frequently obliterated in these cases and the lumen can either be closed with a purse-string (C) or left open. If the neck of the gallbladder can be transected, the cystic duct may be closed with sutures (D). It is advised to leave a JP drain for early detection and intervention of a leak with endoscopic retrograde cholangiopancreatography (ERCP) and stenting.

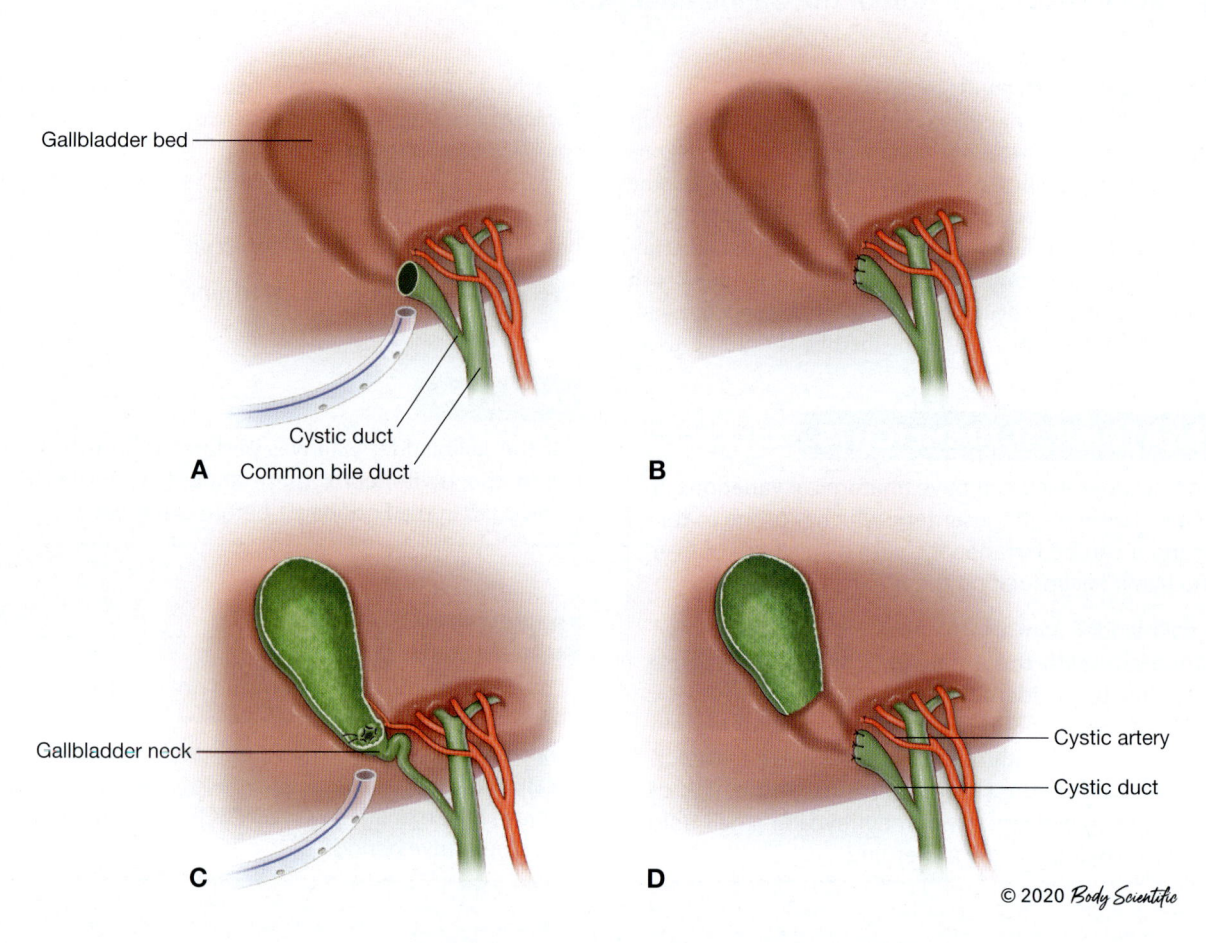

FIGURE 37-13 • Partial cholecystectomy.

Suggested Readings

1. Brunt LM, Deziel DJ, Telem DA, et al. Safe cholecystectomy multi-society practice guideline and state of the art consensus conference on prevention of bile duct injury during cholecystectomy. *Ann Surg.* 2020;272(1):3-23. doi: 10.1097/SLA.0000000000003791
2. Strasberg SM, Brunt LM. Rationale and use of the critical view of safety in laparoscopic cholecystectomy. *J Am Coll Surg.* 2010;211:132-138.
3. Prasoon P, Katada T, Miura K, Hurose Y, Sakata J, Wakai T. Cystic artery variations and associated vascular complications in laparoscopic cholecystectomy. In Qi X, Koroth S, eds., *Digestive System.* IntechOpen: 2018. doi: 10.5772/intechopen.81200
4. Ding YM, Wang B, Wang WX et al. New classification of the anatomic variations of cystic artery during laparoscopic cholecystectomy. *World J Gastroenterol.* 2007;13(42):5629-5634. doi: 10.3748/wjg.v13.i42.5629
5. Sarawagi R, Sundar S, Raghuwanshi S. Anatomical variations of cystic ducts in magnetic resonance cholangiopancreatography and clinical implications. *Radiol Res Pract.* 2016. doi: 10.1155/2016/3021484
6. Daskalaki D, Fernandes E, Wang X, et al. Indocyanine green (ICG) fluorescent cholangiography during robotic cholecystectomy: results of 184 consecutive cases in a single institution. *Surg Innov.* 2014;21(6):615-621. doi: 10.1177/1553350614524839
7. Pesce A, Piccolo G, La Greca G, Puleo S. Utility of fluorescent cholangiography during laparoscopic cholecystectomy: a systematic review. *World J Gastroenterol.* 2015;21(25):7877-7883. doi: 10.3748/wjg.v21.i25.7877
8. Hope WW, Fanelli R, Walsh DS, et al. SAGES clinical spotlight review: intraoperative cholangiography. *Surg Endosc.* 2017;31(5):2007-2016. doi: 10.1007/s00464-016-5320-0
9. Chun K. Recent classifications of the common bile duct injury. *Korean J Hepatobiliary Pancreat Surg.* 2014;18(3):69-72. doi: 10.14701/kjhbps.2014.18.3.69
10. Giulianotti PC, Coratti A, Angelini M, et al. Robotics in general surgery: personal experience in a large community hospital. *Arch Surg.* 2003;138(7):777-784. doi: 10.1001/archsurg.138.7.777

"There is probably no greater surgical tragedy than the production of an extra-hepatic biliary stricture, and there are few surgical procedures quite as gratifying as the successful permanent relief of this condition."

—Kenneth W. Warren (1911–2001)

Roux-en-Y Hepaticojejunostomy

Eric CH Lai • Chung Ngai Tang

Roux-en-Y hepaticojejunostomy (HJ) is the most common surgical reconstruction for a variety of biliary conditions. This procedure has multiple indications, and several technical variations exist depending on the underlying pathology. Historically, Roux-en-Y HJ has been performed through a conventional right subcostal incision. As in other surgical procedures, the minimally invasive approach for HJ offers several advantages. Despite that laparoscopic HJ has been proved safe and feasible, it is a technically challenging operation, and it is not widely adopted by the surgical community. The robotic system has several advantages over conventional laparoscopy, especially in bile duct injury repairs or cholangiocarcinoma resections where precise dissection or more complex reconstructions might be necessary.

Indications and Relative Contraindications to the Robotic Approach

Robot-assisted HJ has several indications such as benign biliary strictures, bile duct injuries, bile duct tumors, choledochal cysts, recurrent cholangitis due to bile duct stones, and palliation of nonresectable periampullary malignancy. There are no absolute contraindications for the robotic approach. The feasibility will largely depend on the surgeon's experience.

Patient Positioning, OR Setup, and Port Setting

The patient is placed supine on a beanbag, with arms tucked and lower limbs parted in the French position, with a 30°

INSTRUMENT REQUIREMENTS

The suggested main robotic instruments/tools can be listed as follows:
- 30° scope
- Needle drivers (round tip or macro)
- Permanent cautery monopolar hook/monopolar curved scissors
- Harmonic shears/vessel sealer
- Bipolar forceps
- Cadière forceps
- Clip applier

The suggested main laparoscopic instruments/tools can be listed as follows:
- Needle drivers
- Scissors
- Graspers
- Suction-irrigation
- Laparoscopic linear staplers (with different loads)
- Laparoscopic ultrasound probe

Supplemental materials:
- Gauzes, sponges
- Sutures: PDS™ 3-0, 4-0, and 5-0
- Hem-o-lok™ clips
- Vessel loops

EDITORIAL COMMENT

With experience, perihepatic adhesions and redo biliary surgery are better managed with the robotic platform than in open surgery. The only adhesions that are difficult to deal with robotically, when massive, are those involving the lower quadrants for the preparation of the jejunal Roux-en-Y loop.

Photo reproduced with permission from Tooouli J. Dr Kenneth W Warren. 1911-2001. HPB (Oxford). 2002;4(3):123-125.

Quote reproduced with permission from Warren KW, McDonald WM: Facts and fiction regarding structures of the extrahepatic bile ducts. Ann Surg. 1964;159(6):996-1010.

reverse Trendelenburg (**Figure 38-1**). The assistant surgeon is sitting between the patient's legs. Six ports (4 robotic and 2 assistant trocars) are used during the procedure. After the creation of the pneumoperitoneum with the Veress technique, a 5-mm trocar is inserted in the left upper, lateral quadrant, and an exploratory laparoscopy is performed with a 30° scope. The four 8-mm robotic cannulas are positioned along a straight line 4–10 cm (depending on the body habitus) above the umbilicus. Additionally, a 12 mm assistant port is placed between the R1 and the scope, and a 5 mm between the scope and the R2. The port placement must be adjusted based on the body habitus of the patient (**Figures 38-2 A, B**). After all the ports are placed, the robotic system is docked into position (**Figure 38-3**).

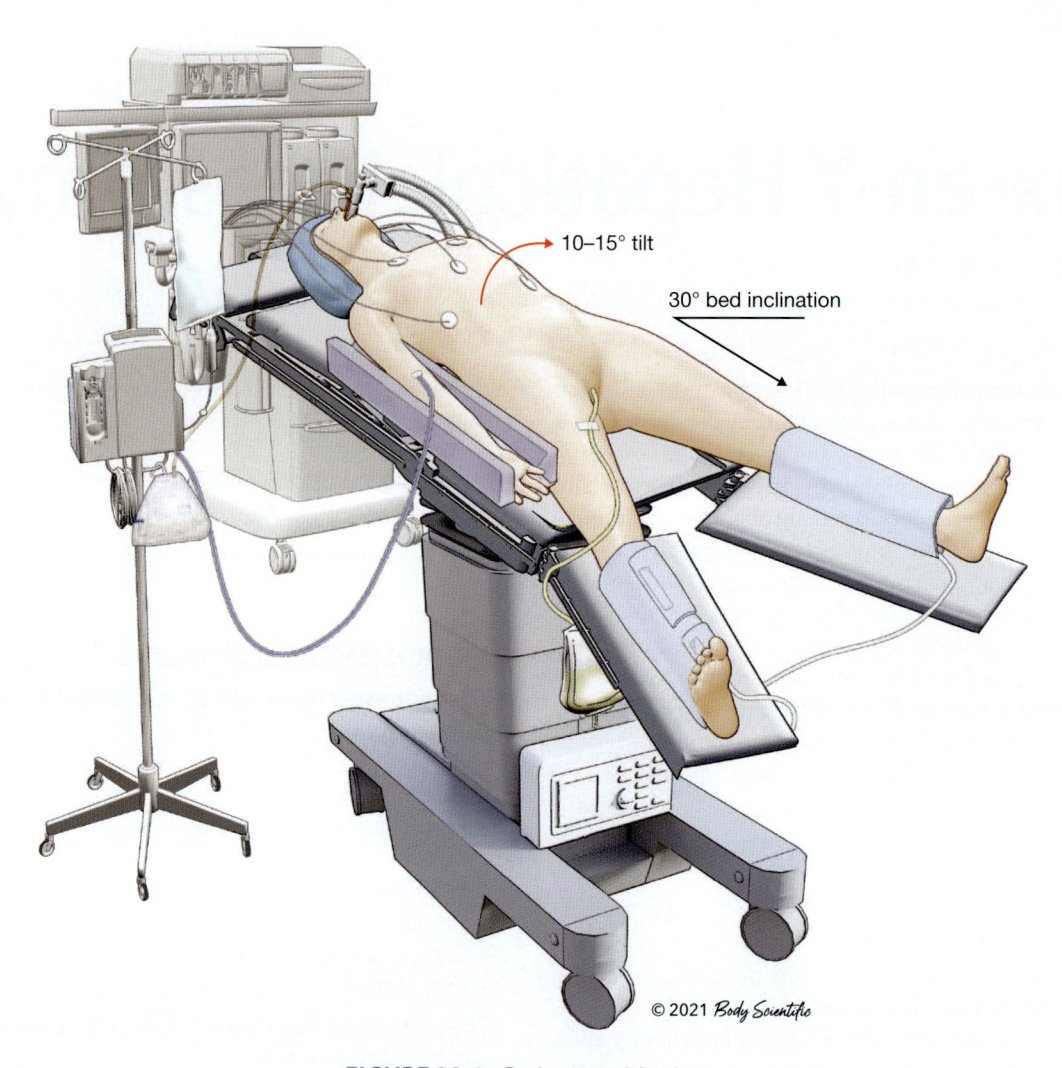

FIGURE 38-1 • Patient positioning.

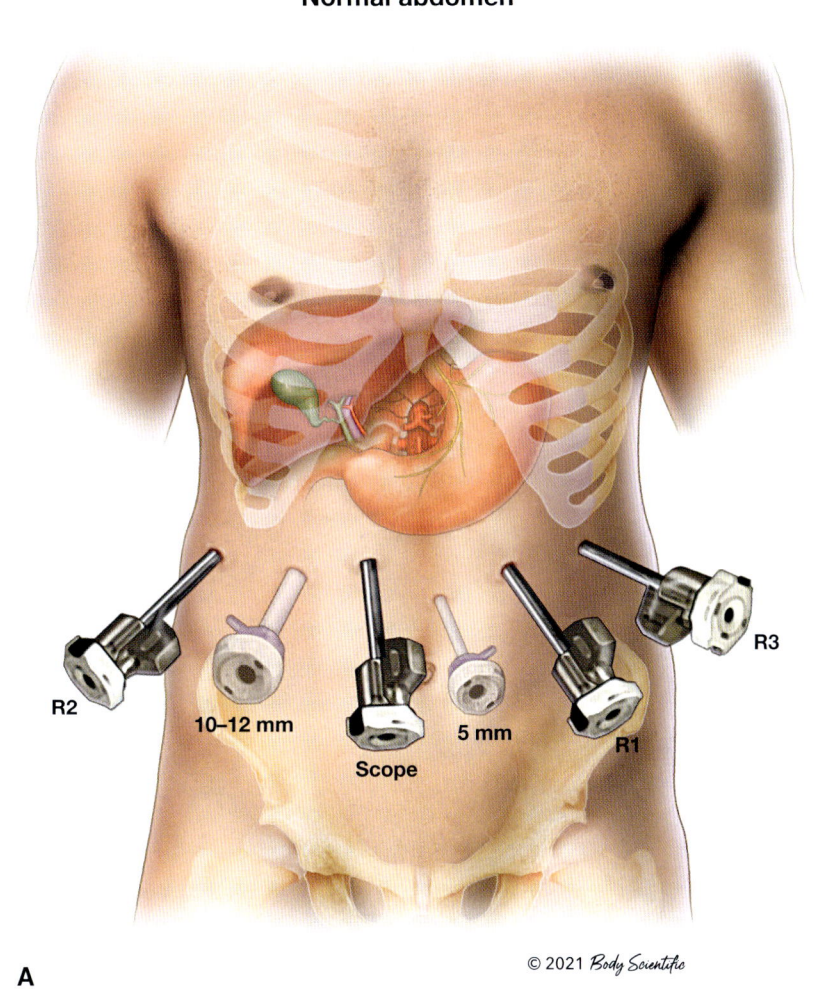

FIGURE 38-2 • **A.** Port setting, normal abdomen.

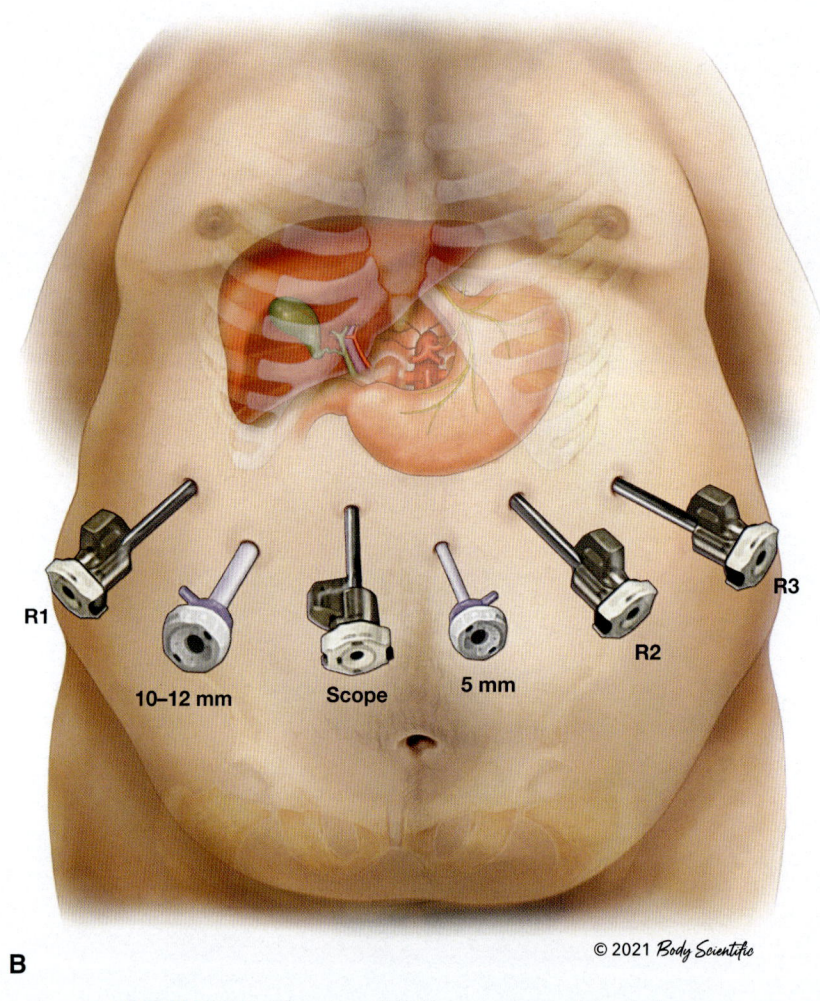

FIGURE 38-2 • (*Continued*) **B.** Port setting, wide abdomen.

Roux-en-Y Hepaticojejunostomy 813

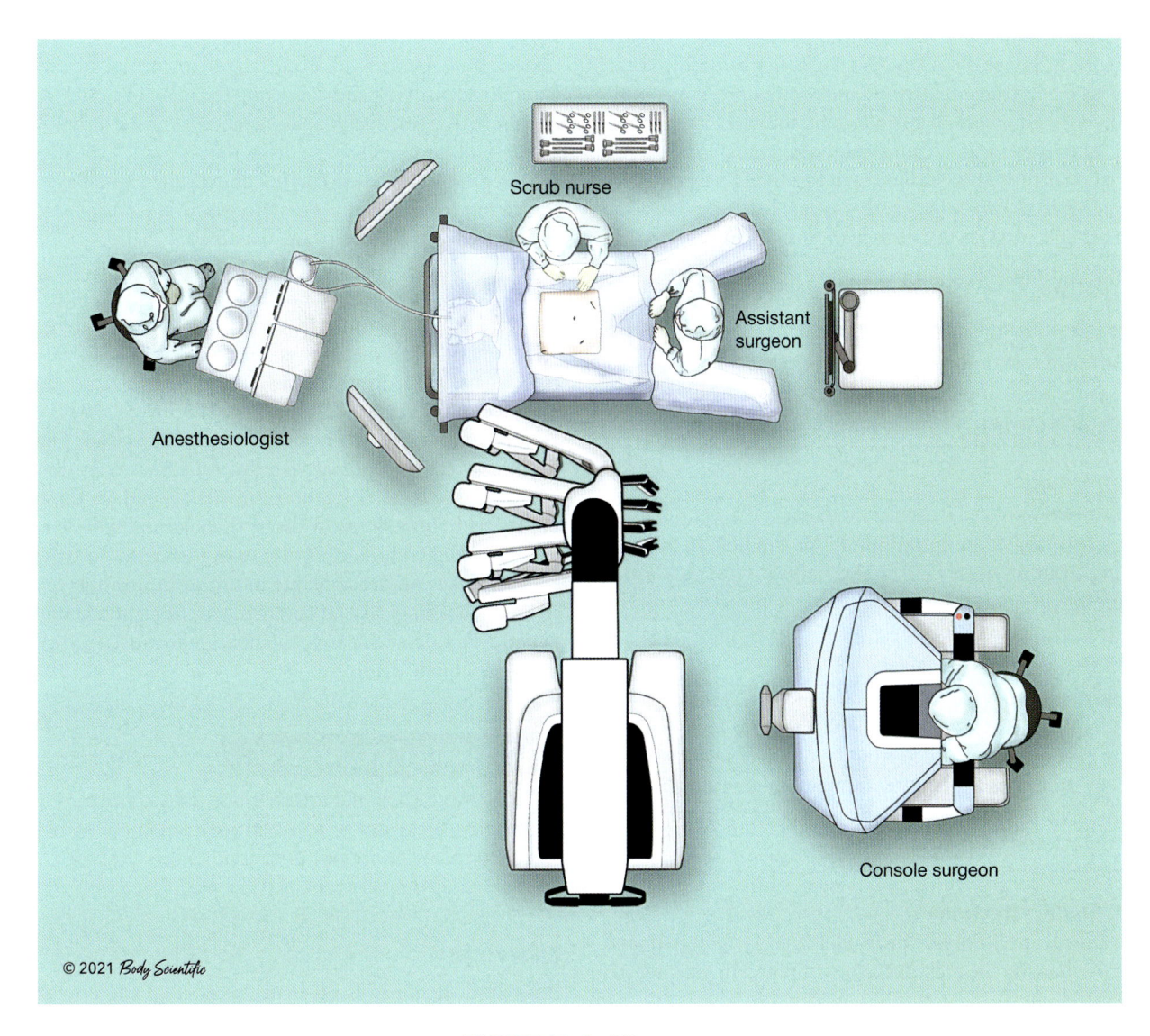

FIGURE 38-3 • OR setup.

Surgical Technique

🎬 **Video 38-1.** Robotic Hepaticojejunostomy (Dr. Tang's Video)

🎬 **Video 38-2.** Robotic Hepaticojejunostomy (Dr. Giulianotti's Video)

Step 1. Exposure of the hepatoduodenal ligament

The first step of the HJ operation is to properly expose the hepatoduodenal ligament and porta hepatis. To do so, segment 4b of the liver is retracted upward with a Cadiére forceps inserted through the R3 port. A sponge is used to protect the liver parenchyma and to increase the instrument grip. Adhesions from previous surgeries involving the stomach, duodenum, and the liver's inferior surface are taken down with a monopolar hook and/or cold scissors. Mobilization of the right colic flexure and a partial Kocher maneuver are performed with electrocautery to gain better exposure and to have better landmarks to approach the liver hilum.

Step 1 average time frame: 15–20 min

> **🔍 ANATOMICAL HIGHLIGHTS**
>
> In **Figure 38-4**, the anatomy of the hepatoduodenal ligament is explained.

> **▶▶ TIPS**
>
> Gauze insertion is recommended. This can help in maintaining a better visual field. It also helps for traction and protection of adjacent organs.

> **EDITORIAL COMMENT**
>
> In redo HJ, massive adhesions encasing the lower face of the liver might be encountered. In such cases, the dissection should be performed from lateral to medial and guided by anatomical landmarks such as the duodenum and the inferior vena cava.

Step 2. Cholecystectomy

If not already performed, the gallbladder is dissected and removed following the technical steps outlined in Chapter 37, Cholecystectomy.

Step 2 average time frame: 10–15 min

> **EDITORIAL COMMENT**
>
> The gallbladder is removed for 3 good reasons:
> 1. To achieve better exposure of the hilum.
> 2. Because the best anastomotic site on the bile duct is above the confluence of the cystic duct.
> 3. Because the defunctionalized gallbladder, if preserved, would increase the risk of recurrent cholecystitis/sludge and stones.

Step 3. Mobilization of the bile duct and identification of the hepatic artery and portal vein

The peritoneal leaf covering the hepatic pedicle is lifted with the grasper and incised with the monopolar hook. The hilum dissection is performed from lateral to medial direction by carefully identifying and dissecting the main bile duct from the hepatic artery (medially) and portal vein (posteriorly). A combination of blunt and sharp dissection is used. The extent and type of dissection depend on the underlying pathology and the indication for the biliary anastomosis. The common bile duct is prepared distally toward the pancreas.

In the case of middle segment stricture, careful dissection is carried out toward the biliary bifurcation, until a normal caliber hepatic duct is identified. Understanding of the extrahepatic biliary anatomy (**Figure 38-5A**), its variations (see Chapter 33, Right Hepatectomy, and Chapter 34, Left Hepatectomy), and its blood supply (**Figure 38-5B**) is of paramount importance to perform a safe dissection. Once the hepatic artery and portal vein are separated from the main bile duct, the level of transection will depend on the type of biliary pathology. In most cases, the jejunum will be anastomosed to the common hepatic duct just distal to its confluence. If this is not feasible due to tumor infiltration or a high stricture, drainage will be obtained via the right hepatic or left hepatic duct. In such cases, the hilar plate must be lowered to secure adequate exposure.

> **EDITORIAL COMMENT**
>
> These more proximal intrahepatic anastomoses require complex techniques, sometimes associated with liver resections. They are not described in this chapter.

Biliary Injury

If a bile duct injury is present, the normal anatomy may be altered and the anatomical elements difficult to recognize. After aspirating serous sanguineous secretions and bile, it is important to identify the main landmark structures. A careful exploration of the bile duct and arterial integrity should be performed to diagnose the bile duct injury type and the presence of an associated vascular injury (which might impact the reconstruction success). To do so, laparoscopic Doppler ultrasound may be helpful to assess the liver blood flow. Moreover, if the biliary anatomy is unclear, an intraoperative cholangiography should be performed. For additional information regarding bile duct injury repairs, see Chapter 39, Bile Duct Injuries Repair.

Malignancy

In case of malignancy, where an associated hepatic resection will be necessary (hilar cholangiocarcinoma), the corresponding artery and portal vein are dissected and addressed as previously described in Chapter 33, Right Hepatectomy, and Chapter 34, Left Hepatectomy. Laparoscopic ultrasound is performed to confirm the location of the lesion, to rule out the presence of other nodules, and to assess the resectability.

Step 3 average time frame: variable depending on the pathology

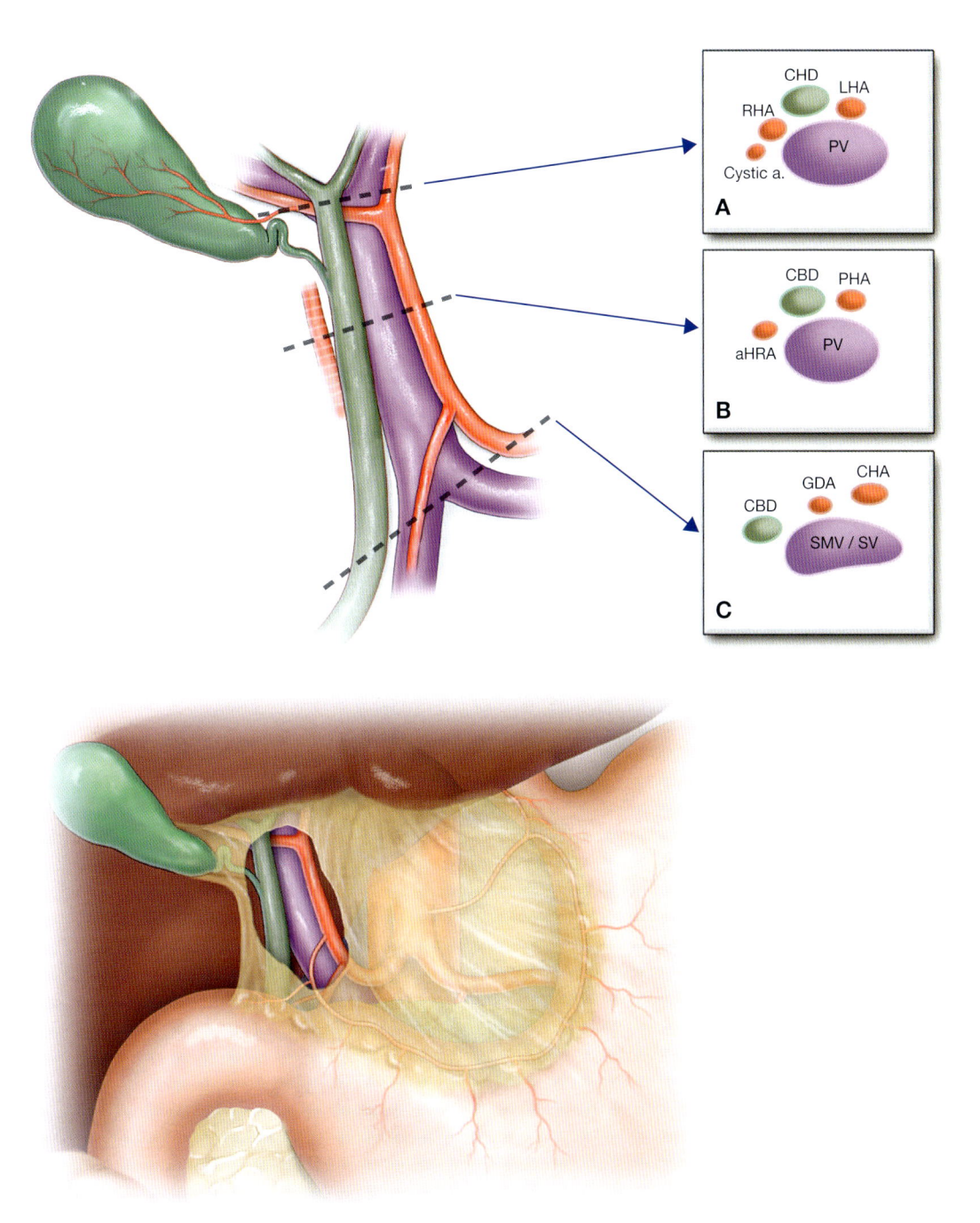

FIGURE 38-4 • Anatomy of the hepatoduodenal ligament.

816 The Foundation and Art of Robotic Surgery

> **ANATOMICAL HIGHLIGHTS**
>
> Extrahepatic bile duct anatomy (**Figure 38-5A**) and blood supply (**Figure 38-5B**).

> ▶▶ **TIPS**
>
> The monopolar hook is the ideal tool for dissection and can also work as a right angle. If severe fibrosis is encountered, cold scissors might also be needed.
>
> Near-infrared indocyanine green (ICG) fluorescence can be used during this step to assess the biliary anatomy. For this purpose, ICG should be injected intravenously 30–45 minutes before the operation (for more details, see Chapter 7, Fluorescence Imaging: Basics and Clinical Applications).
>
> Unfortunately, the background parenchyma uptake of ICG is very disturbing, and if there is a bile leak in the surgical field, it becomes impossible to visualize the biliary tree.

Labels:
- Gallbladder
- Cystic artery
- Cystic duct
- Common bile duct
- Descending part of duodenum
- Hepatopancreatic ampula
- Head of pancreas
- Right and left hepatic ducts
- Common hepatic duct
- Pancreatic duct

© 2021 Body Scientific

A

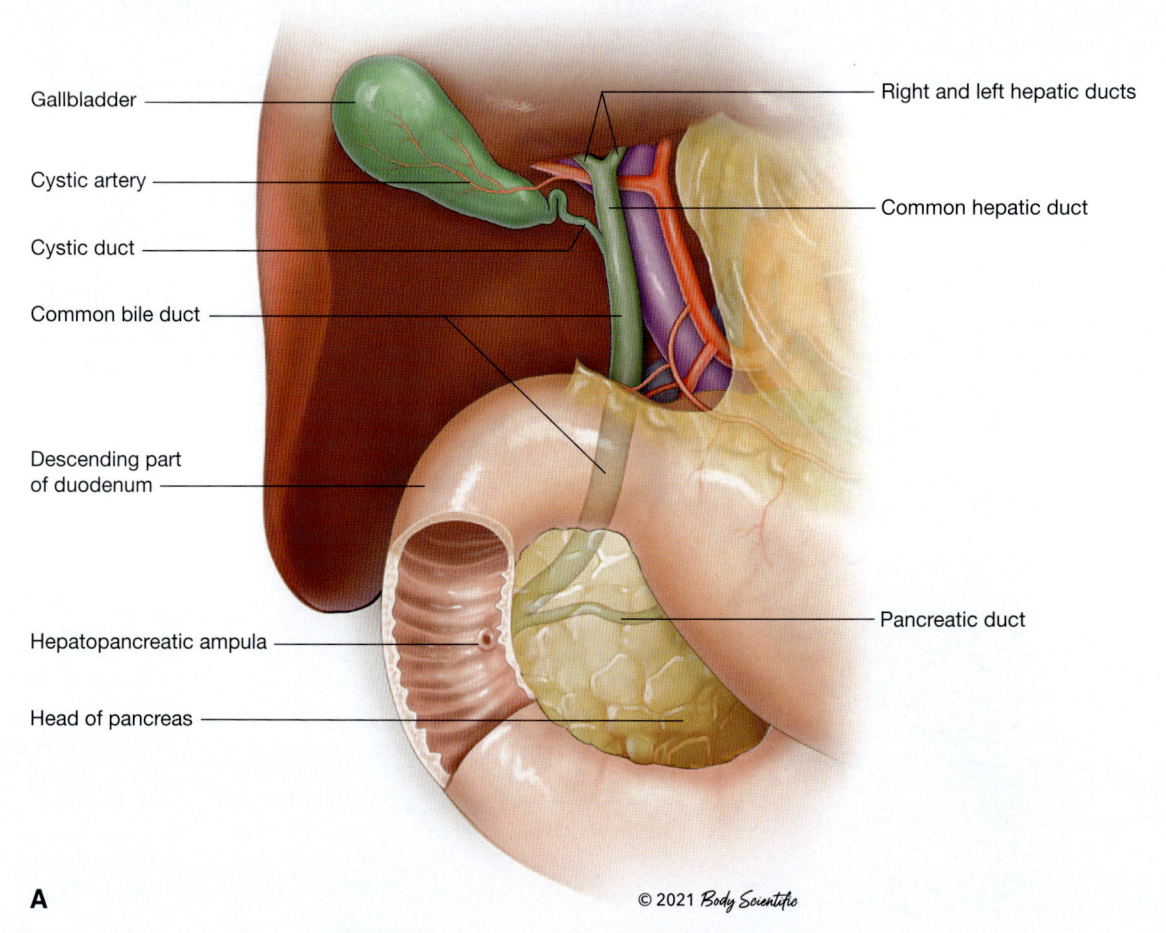

FIGURE 38-5 • **A.** Extrahepatic bile duct anatomy.

> ⚠️ **PITFALLS**
>
> **Thermal injury:** Care must be taken while dissecting the common bile duct with the monopolar hook. Inadvertent injury to the duct or its blood supply due to thermal lateral spread can occur and cause delayed complications.
>
> A lesion of an aberrant accessory right hepatic artery can occur while dissecting the lateral portion of the common bile duct.

B

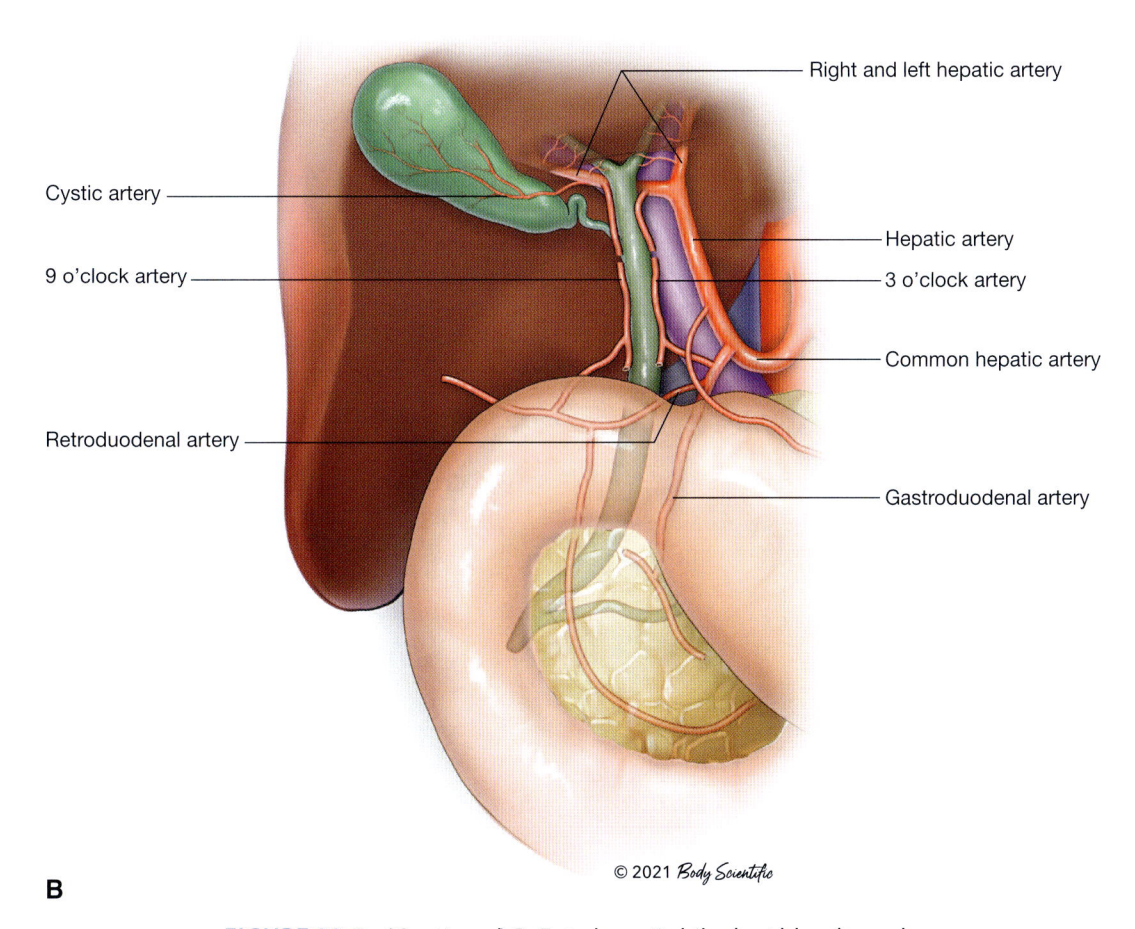

FIGURE 38-5 • (*Continued*) **B.** Extrahepatic bile duct blood supply.

Video 38-3. Bile Duct Dissection-Transection

Step 4. Bile duct transection
The level of bile duct transection will depend on the type/extent of biliary pathology and should be performed on healthy tissue. The most frequent site of transection is located just above the confluence of the cystic duct. The common bile duct (CBD) is divided with cold scissors to reduce the traumatism and to assess the bile duct blood supply (**Figure 38-6**). However, if a very thick CBD is encountered (chronic obstruction, stenting), this can also be divided with the monopolar hook. The anterior wall of the CBD is opened, and afterward, the posterior wall is transected from the inside. If the operation was indicated for recurrent lithiasis, the stones and biliary stent (if present) are retrieved, and the bile duct is flushed with saline. In the case of cholangiocarcinoma, the entire biliary tree should be dissected and reflected cephalad. At first, the CBD is dissected and transected at the superior aspect of the duodenum. A portion of the distal stump is sent for frozen intraoperative pathology analysis to confirm negative margins. The distal stump is then oversewn with PDS™ 3-0. The CBD and the surrounding lymph nodes are, in a cephalad manner, dissected off the portal vein and hepatic arteries up to the hilum. Afterward, the proximal extent of the tumor is evaluated. The hepatic duct(s) are transected and sent for frozen pathology analysis. In rare occasions (middle third cholangiocarcinomas, small type 1 Bismuth-Corlette tumors, or choledochal cysts), bile duct resection and regional lymphadenectomy (if indicated) are sufficient. In most hilar cholangiocarcinomas, an oncological resection will also require a partial hepatectomy with or without caudate lobe excision. At this point, ligation of the appropriate portal and hepatic arterial branch is performed and followed by the hepatic parenchyma transection.

Step 4 average time frame: 10–15 min

> **▶▶ TIPS**
>
> In cases of palliative HJ for advanced malignancy with bulky tumors or the presence of portal hypertension, an anterior bile duct opening and a side-to-side HJ might be performed.

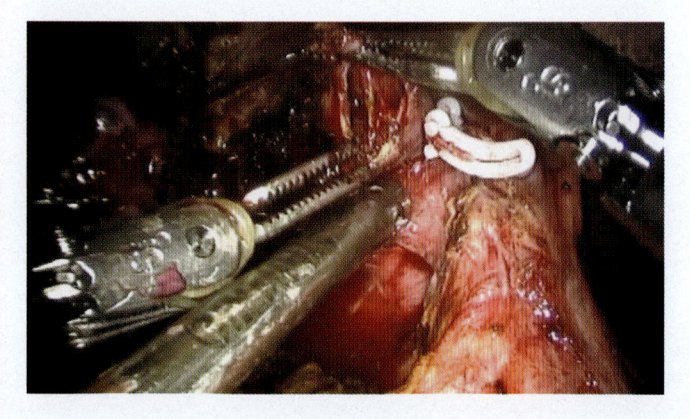

FIGURE 38-6 • Bile duct transection.

> **EDITORIAL COMMENT**
>
> The side-to-side anastomosis should be reserved for exceptional cases where more dissection is risky or impossible. An example is the presence of portal cavernoma of the hepatoduodenal ligament. The side-to-side anastomosis does not work well and the palliation is inferior to the endoscopic or transhepatic one.

> **⚠ PITFALLS**
>
> Excessive dissection of the proximal bile duct stump might create biliary ischemia.

Step 5. Ligament of Treitz identification
Once the bile duct has been transected, the duodenojejunal flexure and ligament of Treitz should be identified. The R3 is used to retract the transverse mesocolon cephalad. The assistant surgeon uses a grasper to retract the small bowel loops and help with exposure. At this point, the ligament of Treitz and inferior mesenteric vein are visualized.

Step 5 average time frame: 5–10 min

Step 6. Creation of the jejunal limb
At this point, the roux limb is created. The second or third jejunal loop is divided with an endostapler at the most suitable level to allow adequate mesenteric mobility to reach the right upper quadrant (**Figures 38-7 A, B**).

Step 6 average time frame: 10–20 min

> **▶▶ TIPS**
>
> ICG fluorescence can be used after the transection to assess perfusion of the small bowel stumps.

Step 7. Assessment of the best pathway for the biliary limb transposition
There are several routes to bring the biliary limb into the right upper quadrant: transmesocolic paraduodenal, transmesocolic anteduodenal, antecolic, and transmesocolic retrogastric (**Figures 38-8 A–D**). The chosen route should ensure a favorable angle to construct a tension-free anastomosis. This decision is based on the surgical indication and the patient's anatomy. In the case of a Whipple procedure, the jejunal limb is brought to the right upper quadrant behind the mesentery root following the native duodenal anatomical course. A similar paraduodenal route can be created using the avascular window between the second portion of the duodenum, the right branch of the middle colic, and the ileocolic vessels. This route will require the mobilization of the right colic flexure (**Figures 38-9 A–C**). In most cases, the paraduodenal pathway is the shortest

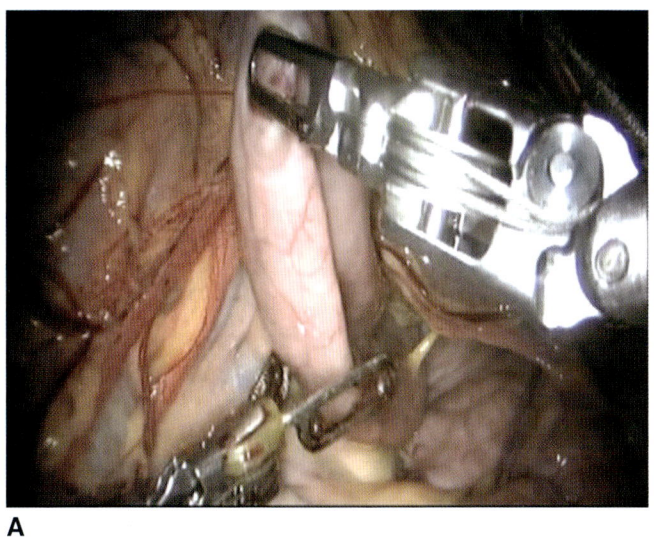

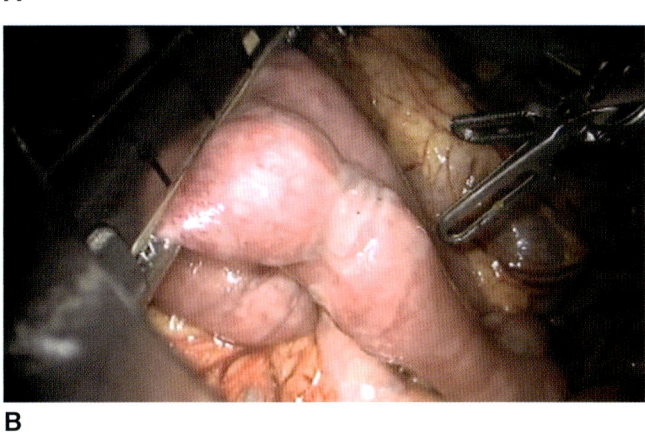

FIGURE 38-7 • Creation of the jejunal limb.

to the right upper quadrant and offers an excellent angle for constructing the HJ.

In the transmesocolic anteduodenal route, the biliary limb is transposed through an avascular window on the right side of the middle colic vessels. The transmesocolic anteduodenal pathway may be useful in cases in which the paraduodenal route is technically challenging due to previous right colonic surgery or adhesions. In the transmesocolic retrogastric route, the jejunal limb is brought to the hepatic hilum through the lesser sac between the pancreas and the stomach passing on the left side of the middle colic vessels. This pathway can be useful in obese patients or in cases where the jejunum needs to be anastomosed with the right intrahepatic ducts (left hepatectomy). Finally, the antecolic route can be useful in advanced malignancy with mesenteric infiltration.

Step 7 average time frame: 15–20 min

> **ANATOMICAL HIGHLIGHTS**
>
> Routes for biliary limb transposition (**Figures 38-8 A–D**).

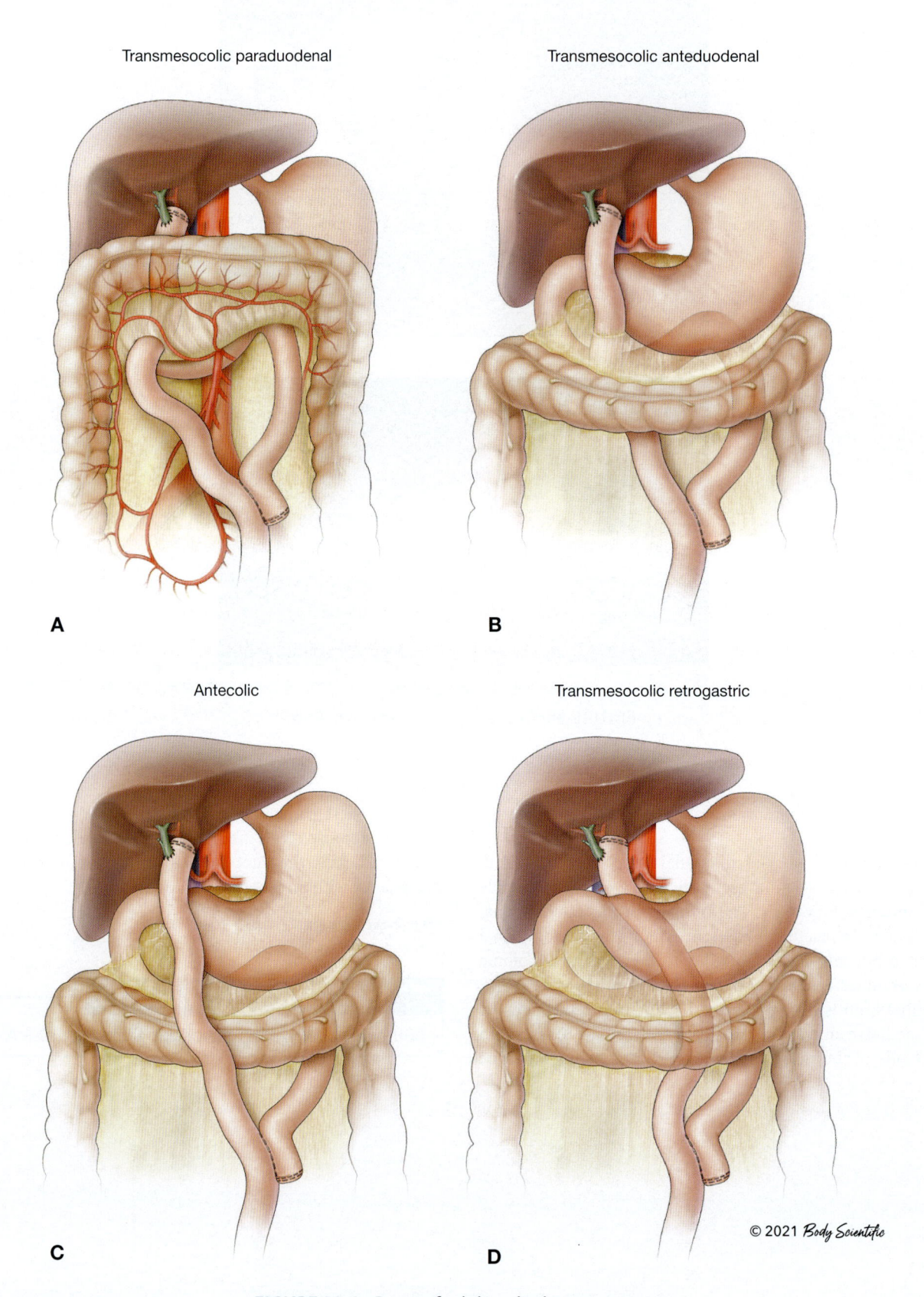

FIGURE 38-8 • Routes for biliary limb transposition.

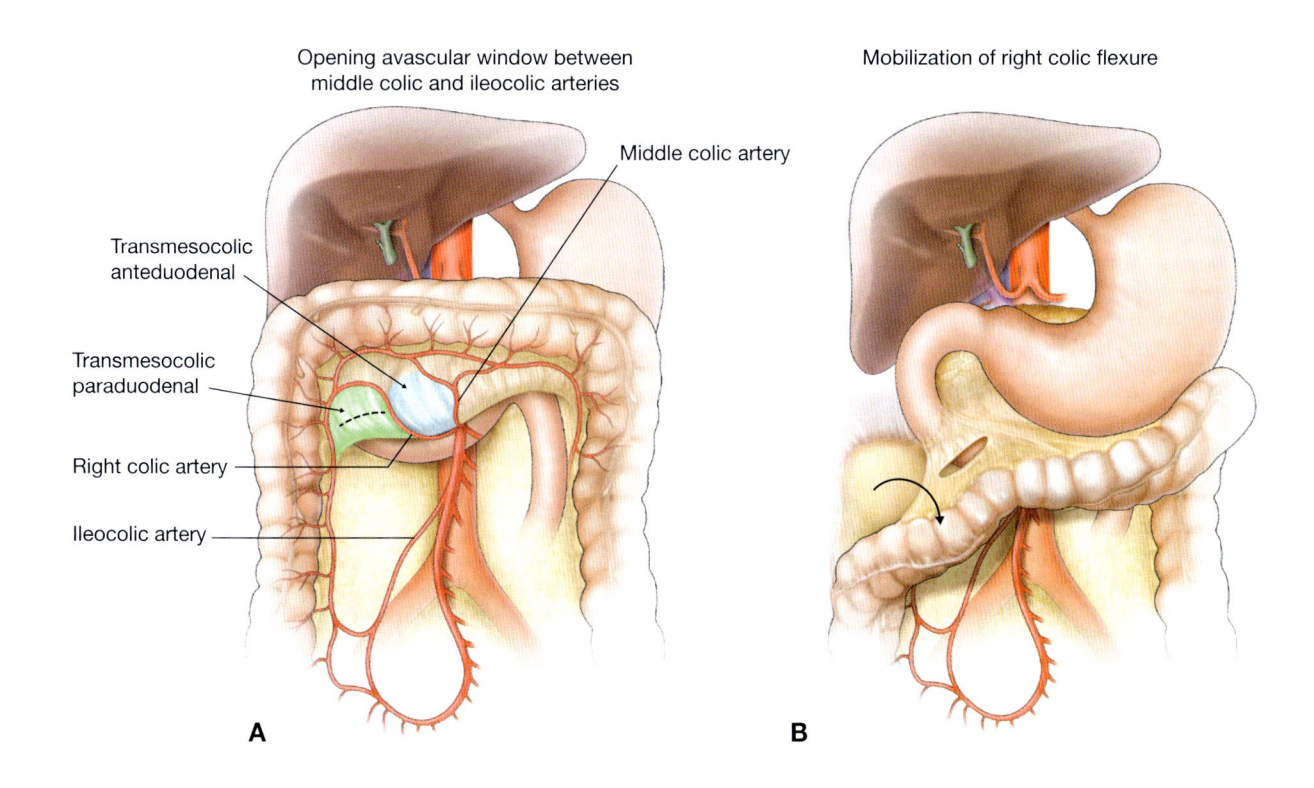

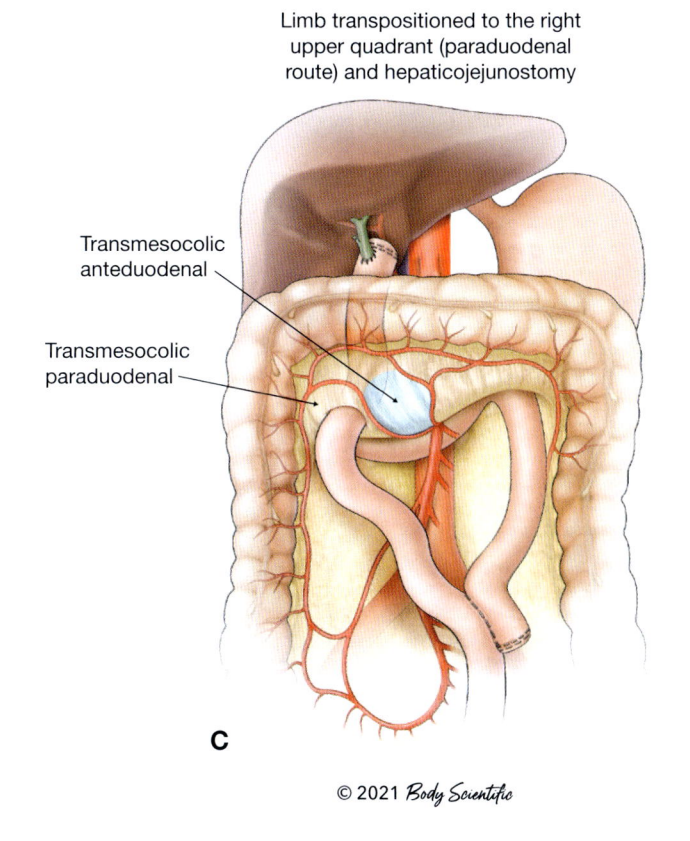

FIGURE 38-9 • Paraduodenal route.

Step 8. Hepaticojejunostomy

▶ **Video 38-4.** Hepaticojejunostomy (Dr. Tang's Video)

▶ **Video 38-5.** Hepaticojejunostomy in Intrahepatic Cholangiocarcinoma (Dr. Giulianotti's Video)

The HJ is usually performed in an end-to-side fashion (**Figures 38-10 A–D**). Depending on the size/thickness of the bile duct, HJ can be of variable complexity. In every case, the anastomosis should be performed using vital and well-vascularized bile duct wall. The enterotomy needs to be created before making the posterior suture line (monopolar hook or Harmonic shears). The posterior anastomotic row (if the surgeon is right-handed) is better started from the 9 o'clock position.

> **EDITORIAL COMMENT**
>
> The 9 o'clock position is preferable for two reasons: (1) in some passages, the suture can be held with the nondominant hand not interfering with the construction of the anastomosis (dominant hand); and (2) when suturing from right to left, there is better visualization of the suture corner because the scope has a more favorable alignment.

The biliary anastomosis is constructed in one layer with interrupted stitches or a running suture depending on the diameter of the bile duct. The preferred technique is to fashion the HJ with a short posterior layer running suture and interrupted stitches for the anterior layer.

Dilated ducts (larger than 1 cm) with thickened walls are usually easier to suture. In these cases, the anastomosis is performed with 2 (posterior and anterior) half running absorbable PDS™ 3-0/5-0 sutures. The HJ for patients with a thin and nondilated bile duct is technically more demanding. The anastomosis should be done with interrupted absorbable 4-0/5-0 PDS™ stitches because they provide less purse-string effect and better patency.

In some circumstances (bile duct injuries with associated arterial injury, hilar cholangiocarcinoma) where the transection of the bile duct is performed at a higher level, the lumen of multiple separate bile ducts may be encountered. In such cases, the walls of adjacent ducts can be sutured together to create a

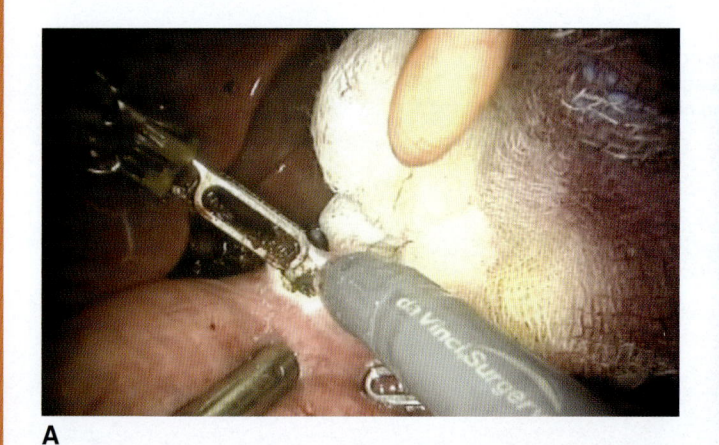

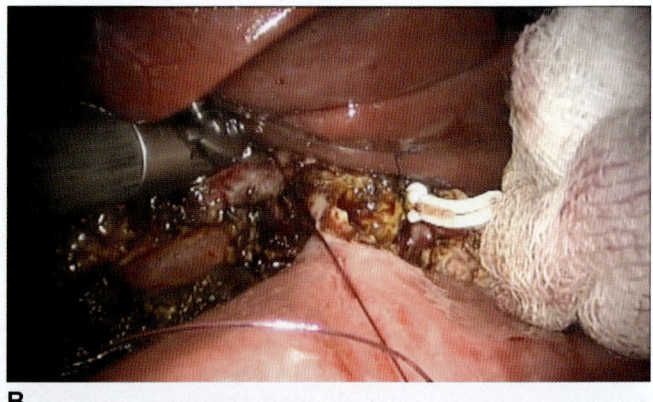

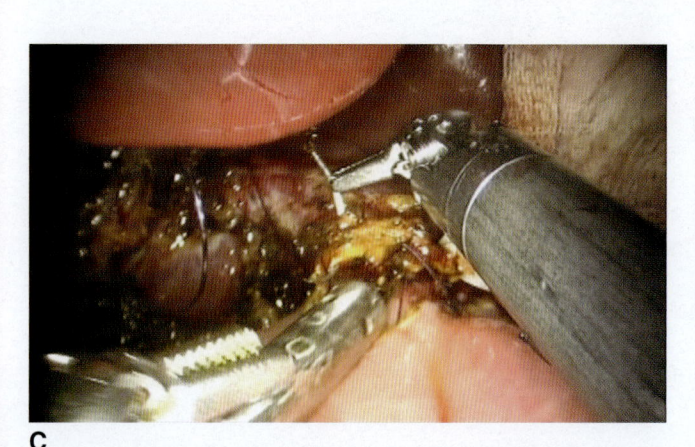

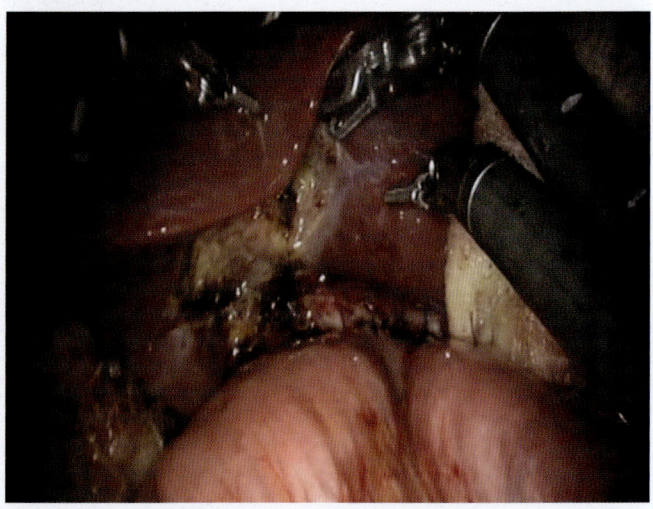

FIGURE 38-10 • Hepaticojejunostomy.

> **EDITORIAL COMMENT**
>
> **SUTURE MATERIALS**
>
> Absorbable monofilament sutures (like PDS™) have the advantage of distributing the tension more homogeneously and of allowing better visual control, because the tension can be released to open the space for difficult passages of the needle.
>
> Barbed sutures, on the other hand, have the advantage of holding the approximation of the anastomotic edges without the help of the assistant or the R3.

single lumen to facilitate the anastomosis construction. Moreover, if the proximal margin is positive (and further resection is not feasible) or the tumor is found to be unresectable after the division of the CBD, a retrograde transhepatic biliary stent could be placed.

Step 8 average time frame: 15–30 min

> **▶▶ TIPS**
>
> During this step, the assistant will use the two assistant ports. Using a grasper, they will help to maintain the jejunal loop in the correct position and to decrease the tension when tying the knots. The other port will be used to pass sutures and needles.
>
> The interrupted stitches of the anterior row are temporarily secured with Hem-o-lok™ clips before tying. After all stitches are placed, they are tied starting from the 3 o'clock position (where the last suture was placed). This allows adequate visualization and approximation of the bile duct and small bowel wall during the last stitches.
>
> Similarly, if a running suture is used on the anterior row, the last passages of the needle are placed without tightening the suture to allow better visualization.

> **⚠ PITFALLS**
>
> Tearing of the bile duct wall while tying the knots. Optimal visual feedback is necessary to adjust the adequate tension of the knots.

Step 9. Jejunojejunostomy

The jejunojejunostomy is constructed 70–80 cm distal to the HJ. After the enterotomies are made in the antimesenteric border, the endostapler is introduced, properly oriented, and fired (**Figure 38-11**). The staple line is checked for hemostasis and the enterotomy site is closed with a PDS™ 3-0 running suture.

Finally, the HJ is covered with a fibrine-based sealant, and a Jackson-Pratt drain is placed next to the biliary anastomosis.

Step 9 average time frame: 15–20 min

> **▶▶ TIPS**
>
> The jejunojejunostomy could be constructed before the HJ, and this sequence is more ergonomic and saves time by avoiding going back and forth in the submesocolic space. However, this requires more experience, because the surgeon must be sure that the loop reaches the hepatic hilum without tension and is well perfused. For less experienced surgeons, it is advisable to do the jejunojejunostomy after the HJ.
>
> Before firing the stapler, the correct orientation and alignment of the small bowel and its mesentery should be checked.

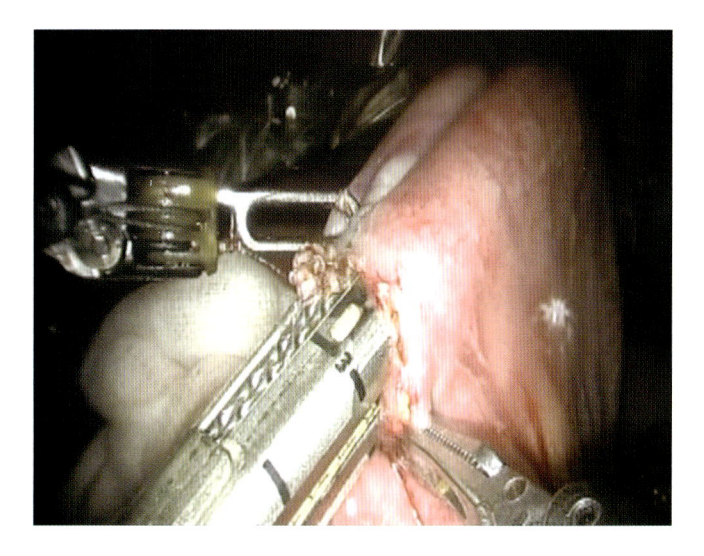

FIGURE 38-11 • Jejunojejunostomy.

Suggested Readings

1. Lai EC, Tang CN. Robot-assisted laparoscopic hepaticojejunostomy for advanced malignant biliary obstruction. *Asian J Surg.* 2015;38:210-213.
2. Lai EC, Tang CN, Yang GP, Li MK. Approach to manage the complications of choledochoduodenostomy: robot-assisted laparoscopic Roux-en-Y hepaticojejunostomy. *Surg Laparosc Endosc Percutan Tech.* 2011;21:e228-31.
3. Chu CC, Lai EC, Chan OC, Chung DT, Tang CN. Robotic left hepatectomy and Roux-en-Y right hepatico-jejunostomy for biliary papillomatosis. *Hong Kong Med J.* 2016;22:78-80.
4. Giulianotti PC, Quadri P, Durgam S, Bianco FM. Reconstruction/repair of iatrogenic biliary injuries: is the robot offering a new option? Short clinical report. *Ann Surg.* 2018;267:e7-e9.
5. Bustos R, Fernandes E, Mangano A, et al. Robotic hepaticojejunostomy: surgical technique and risk factor analysis for anastomotic leak and stenosis. *HPB (Oxford).* 2020;22:1442-1449.
6. Giulianotti PC, Coratti A, Angelini M, et al. Robotics in general surgery: personal experience in a large community hospital. *Arch Surg.* 2003;138(7):777-784. doi: 10.1001/archsurg.138.7.777

"Laparoscopic bile duct injuries have health and litigation consequences beyond what should be expected from a benign condition, and the problem is compounded by the fact that too many of these injuries are managed outside referral centres, with sub-optimal results."

—Henri Bismuth (1934)

Bile Duct Injuries Repair

Pier Cristoforo Giulianotti • Antonio Cubisino • Nicolas Hellmuth Dreifuss

INTRODUCTION

Bile duct injury (BDI) is the most serious complication of open and minimally invasive cholecystectomy. Despite that BDI can occur in multiple operations, it is more frequent after laparoscopic cholecystectomy (LC). BDI's incidence significantly increased when LC was widely adopted by the surgical community. Currently, the estimated incidence of BDI during LC ranges between 0.3% and 0.7% (see suggested reading #7). BDI results in significant morbidity, reduced overall survival, and poor quality of life. Moreover, it is one of the most frequent causes of litigation against surgeons.

Several techniques have been described to enhance the safety of LC and to reduce the risk of iatrogenic BDI. These include the critical view of safety (CVS) method, the infundibular technique, subtotal cholecystectomy, intraoperative cholangiography (IOC), near-infrared fluorescent cholangiography, laparoscopic ultrasound, and judicious conversion to open surgery.

The most common reason for BDI is an incorrect interpretation of the biliary anatomy. Other contributing factors include substantial inflammation, Mirizzi syndrome, anatomical variations, technical pitfalls (imprudent use of clips or electrocautery), and the surgeon's inexperience or overconfidence.

Early recognition of a BDI is of utmost importance. Intraoperative recognition and immediate repair by an experienced surgeon have the highest success rate. If a BDI is recognized intraoperatively but the surgeon is inexperienced, a drain should be placed, and the patient must be immediately transferred to a high-volume hepatobiliary center for repair. This is essential because unsuccessful previous repairs make subsequent attempts more difficult and result in a higher chance of failure. Nevertheless, most BDIs (>70%) are diagnosed postoperatively.

Clinical presentation will vary according to the extent and type of lesion (stricture or leak). Symptoms may initially be subtle, so any deviation of the normal postoperative course should prompt the surgeon to rule out a BDI. In these cases, imaging studies (abdominal ultrasound, computed tomography [CT] scan,

INSTRUMENT REQUIREMENTS

The suggested main robotic instruments/tools can be listed as follows:
- 30° scope
- Needle drivers (round tip or macro/micro)
- Permanent cautery monopolar hook/monopolar curved scissors
- Harmonic shears/vessel sealer
- Bipolar forceps/Maryland forceps
- Cadière forceps
- Clip applier

The suggested main laparoscopic instruments/tools can be listed as follows:
- Needle drivers
- Scissors
- Graspers
- Suction-irrigation
- Laparoscopic linear staplers (with different loads)
- Laparoscopic ultrasound probe

Supplemental materials:
- Gauzes, sponges
- Sutures: PDS™ 3-0, 4-0, 5-0, and 6-0; Prolene™ 4-0 and 5-0
- Hem-o-lok™ clips
- Cholangiogram catheter

Photo reproduced with permission from He VJ. Professor Henri Bismuth: the past, present and future of hepatobiliary surgery. Hepatobiliary Surg Nutr. 2013;2(4):236-238.
Quote reproduced with permission from Bismuth H, Majno PE. Hepatobiliary surgery. J Hepatol. 2000;32(1 Suppl):208-224.

magnetic resonance cholangiopancreatography [MRCP], percutaneous transhepatic cholangiography [PTC], and endoscopic retrograde cholangiopancreatography [ERCP]) are of paramount importance to assess the type and extent of the BDI, presence of bilioenteric continuity, ongoing bile leak, liver atrophy, intra-abdominal collections, and associated complications such as vascular injuries. A multidisciplinary approach with specialized surgeons, endoscopists, and an interventional radiologist is vital for the assessment and management of BDI.

The management of BDI will vary according to the patient's clinical condition and type and extent of injury. Minor bile leaks from the cystic duct or small ducts in the liver bed are usually managed conservatively. ERCP with sphincterotomy, or stenting, reduces the biliary pressure, allowing small fistulas to heal.

If fluid collections/bile peritonitis are detected on imaging studies, percutaneous abscess drainage and percutaneous biliary drainage are required to improve the patient's clinical condition before definitive surgical repair. Surgical repair should be avoided in the presence of uncontrolled infection or sepsis because the bile ducts are friable due to severe local inflammation. Drainage will help to solve the infection and create a well-controlled fistula.

If cholangitis is present, IV antibiotics and biliary drainage are necessary prior to surgical treatment. Patients with long-standing BDI are frequently affected by anemia, coagulation defects, electrolytic disturbances, and malnutrition, all of which should be improved before the definitive repair. Moreover, associated vascular injuries might result in hepatic abscesses or ischemia, requiring preoperative drainage or hepatectomy. Rarely, failure of BDI management might result in chronic liver failure and even the need for liver transplantation.

Several surgical strategies exist for BDI repair. The operative technique will depend on the type and extent of the BDI, the mechanism of injury (thermal vs. cold), and the presence or absence of associated lesions. The most common operations are primary closure with or without T-Tube placement (minor injuries, cold mechanism) and Roux-en-Y hepaticojejunostomy (major injuries). When transection of >50% of the common bile duct (CBD) circumference or strictures are present, bilioenteric anastomosis is the procedure of choice.

Historically, BDI repairs have been performed through conventional open surgery. However, the robotic approach offers an excellent minimally invasive alternative, with a high success rate when performed by experienced surgeons. Fine dissection and microsuturing in the liver hilum are especially useful during this procedure.

In this chapter, the most frequent operative techniques for BDI repair will be detailed.

Indications and Relative Contraindications to the Robotic Approach

BDI repair should always be performed by surgeons with significant experience in both open and minimally invasive hepatobiliary surgery. All BDI could be approached robotically. The feasibility will largely depend on the surgeon's experience. Unless there are specific reasons to postpone the operation (infection or patient condition), the robotic repair should be done as soon as possible. In the past, many open surgeons were deferring the operation with the goal of achieving a larger size of the bile duct to facilitate the anastomosis. The ability of the robot to perform precise microsurgery reconstructions even in presence of very thin ducts has overcome this limitation. The advantage of an early surgery is to reduce the patient disability time and to avoid scar tissue that can complicate the precise recognition of biliary structures and vessels.

Patient Positioning, OR Setup, and Port Setting

The patient is placed supine on a beanbag, with arms tucked and lower limbs parted in the French position, with a 30° reverse Trendelenburg and left-side tilting (**Figure 39-1**).

The assistant surgeon is sitting between the patient's legs. Six ports (4 robotic and 2 assistant trocars) are used during the procedure. After the creation of the pneumoperitoneum with the Veress technique, an exploratory laparoscopy is performed with a 30° scope. The four 8-mm robotic cannulas are positioned along a straight line 4–10 cm (depending on the body habitus) above the umbilicus. The assistant ports are placed on both sides of the scope (**Figures 39-2 A, B**). After all the ports are placed, the robotic system is docked into position (**Figure 39-3**).

Surgical Technique

▶ **Video 39-1.** Bile Duct Injury Repair: Roux-en-Y Hepaticojejunostomy (Case 1)

▶ **Video 39-2.** Bile Duct Injury Repair: Roux-en-Y Hepaticojejunostomy (Case 2)

▶ **Video 39-3.** Bile Duct Injury Repair: Roux-en-Y Hepaticojejunostomy (Case 3)

▶ **Video 39-4.** Kasai Procedure

▶ **Video 39-5.** Delayed Bile Duct Injury Repair

▶ **Video 39-6.** Right Hepatic Duct Injury Repair

▶ **Video 39-7. Bihepaticojejunostomy** (Reproduced with permission from Giulianotti PC, Quadri P, Durgam S, et al. Reconstruction/repair of iatrogenic biliary injuries: is the robot offering a new option? Short clinical report. *Ann Surg.* 2018;267(1):e7-e9.)

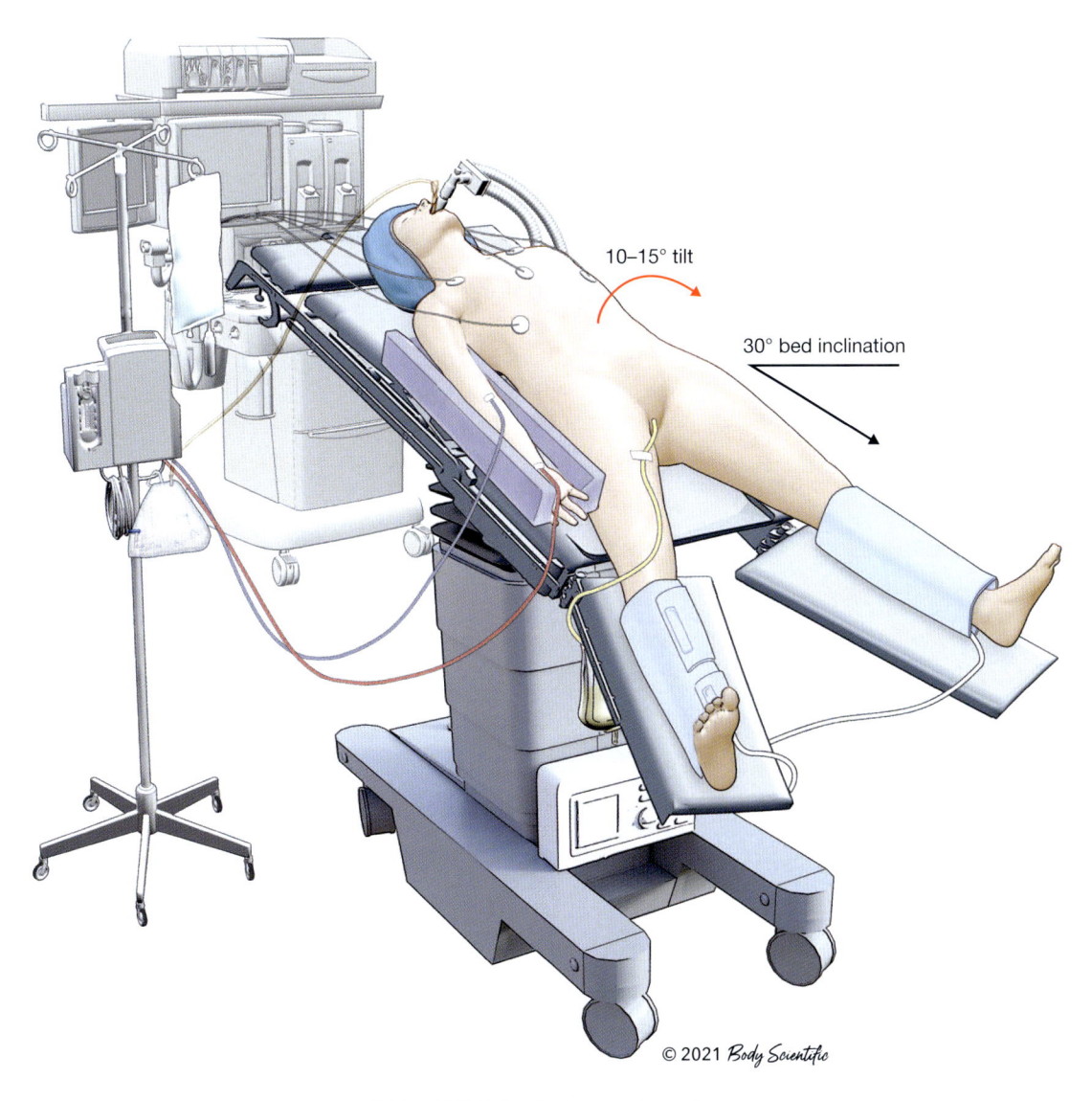

FIGURE 39-1 • Patient positioning.

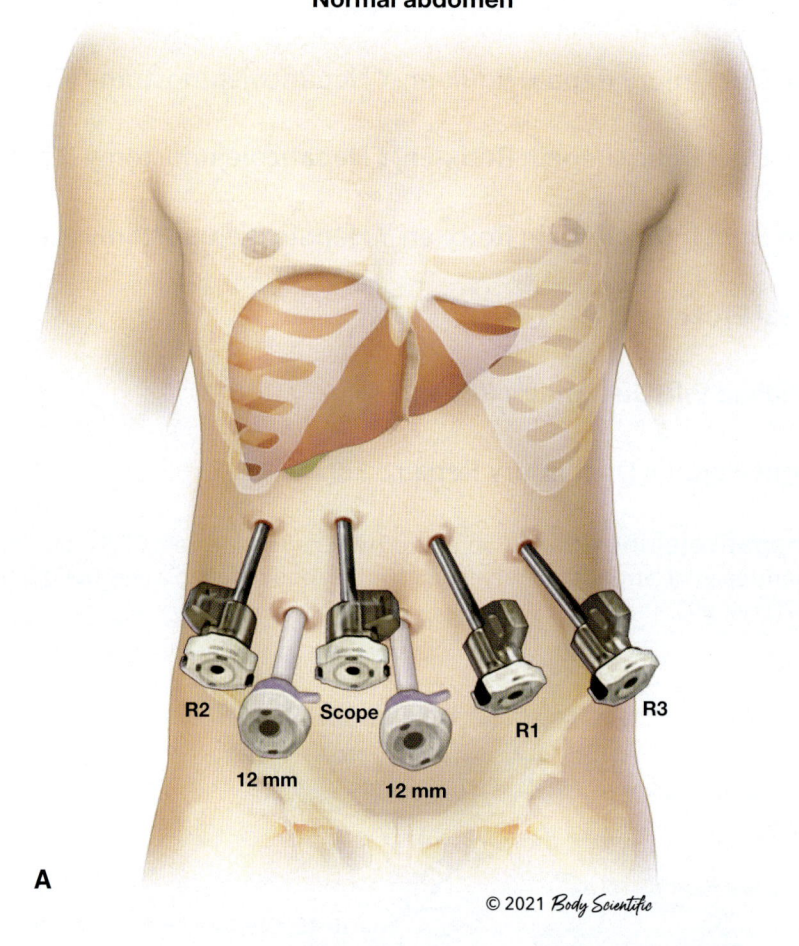

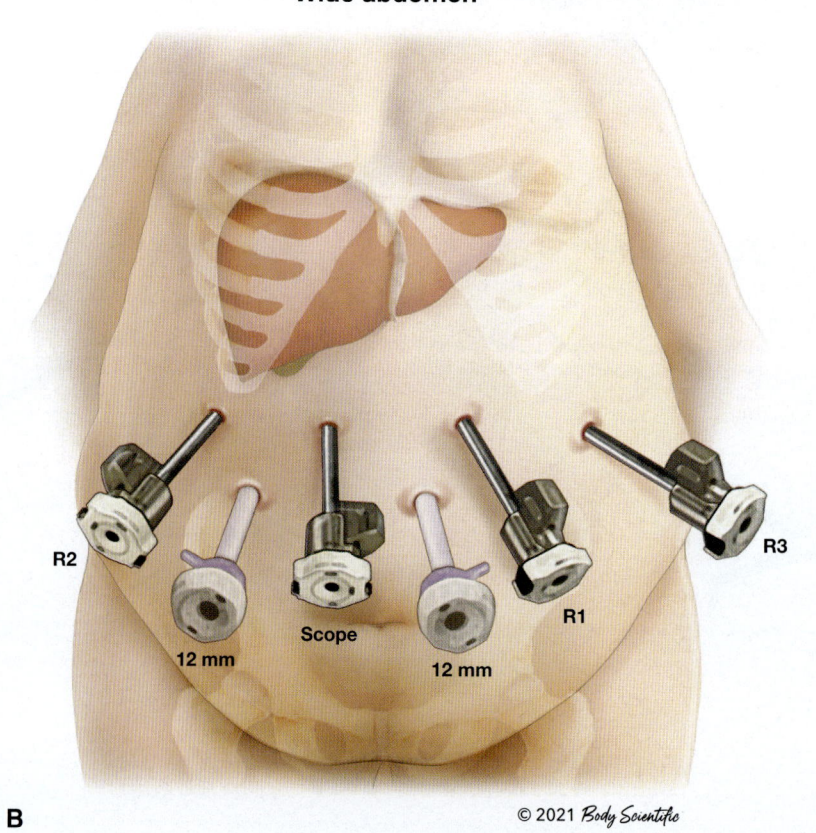

FIGURE 39-2 • Port setting.

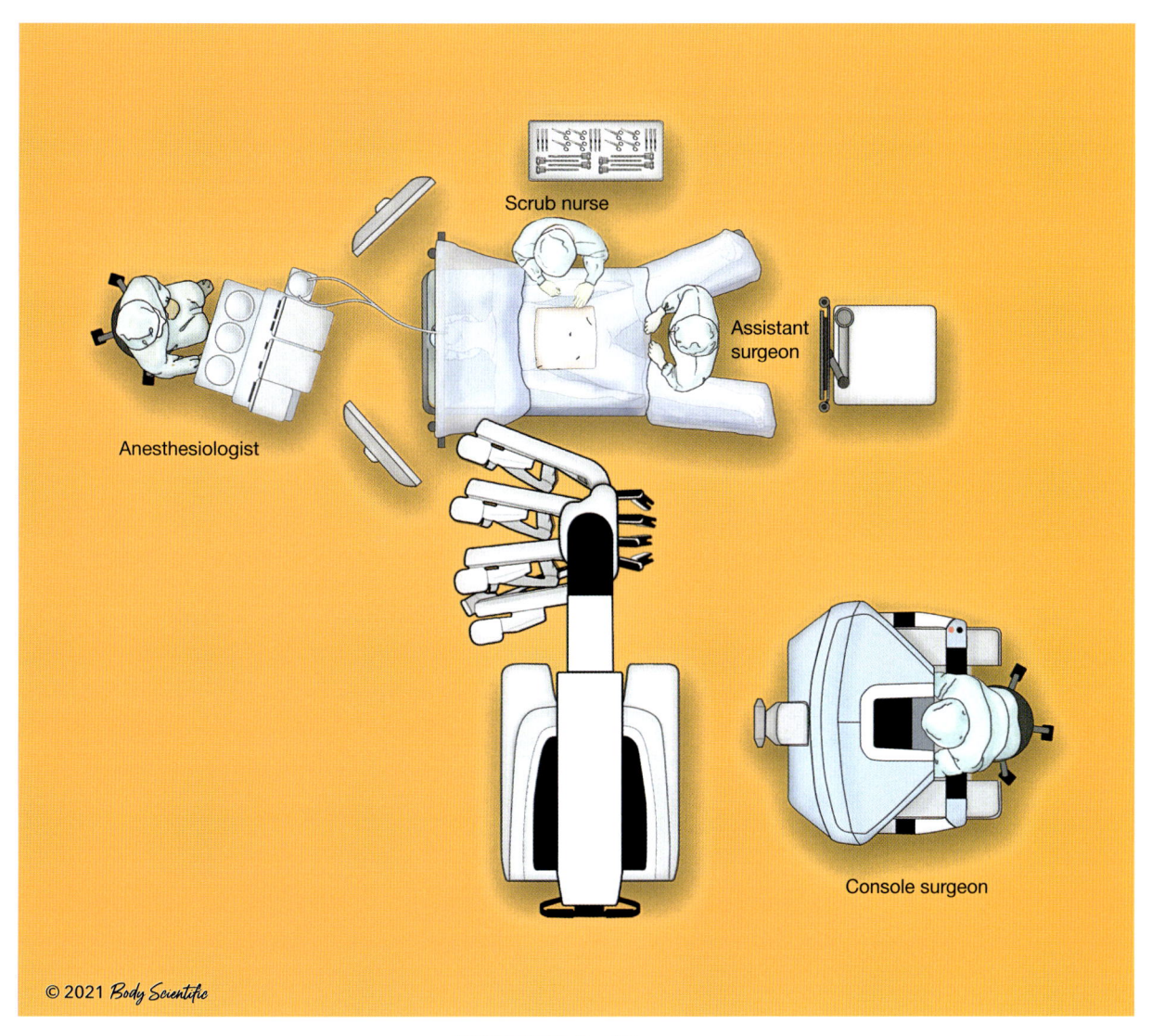

FIGURE 39-3 • OR setup.

Step 1. Exposure of the hilum and anatomical recognition

To expose the hepatoduodenal ligament and porta hepatis, a Cadiére forceps protected with a gauze is inserted through the R3 and used to retract cephalad segment 4b of the liver.

Lysis of adhesions, mainly when they are recent and "fresh", involving the antrum, duodenum, and gallbladder bed, is performed with a combination of blunt dissection and suctioning. Only when there are chronic adhesions is the sharp dissection with the monopolar hook or scissors necessary. The Cadiére forceps and suction-irrigation device are extremely helpful for both blunt dissection and aspiration of serosanguineous fluid and bile during exposure. Also, mobilization of the right colic flexure and a partial Kocher maneuver are sometimes necessary to achieve a better visualization. Before going into the hilum, it is always necessary to get precise landmarks (inferior vena cava, duodenum, Winslow foramen), and the safest way is to proceed from lateral to medial.

After the hepatic hilum is exposed, a meticulous exploration is conducted to achieve a clear understanding of the patient's anatomy, which might be significantly altered and difficult to recognize. Identification of main landmark structures and careful evaluation of the biliary anatomy and the arterial integrity should be performed. In addition, assessment of the surrounding organs to identify associated lesions is warranted.

Step 1 average time frame: 10–20 min

> **🔍 ANATOMICAL HIGHLIGHTS**
> - Anatomy of the hepatoduodenal ligament (**Figure 39-4**).
> - Anatomy of the extrahepatic bile duct (**Figure 39-5**).

> **⚠ PITFALLS**
> Going immediately straight down to the liver hilum without achieving lateral landmarks. It is easy to lose 3-dimensional (3D) perception and, in the attempt to enter into the inflammatory tissue, to injure vascular or biliary structures.

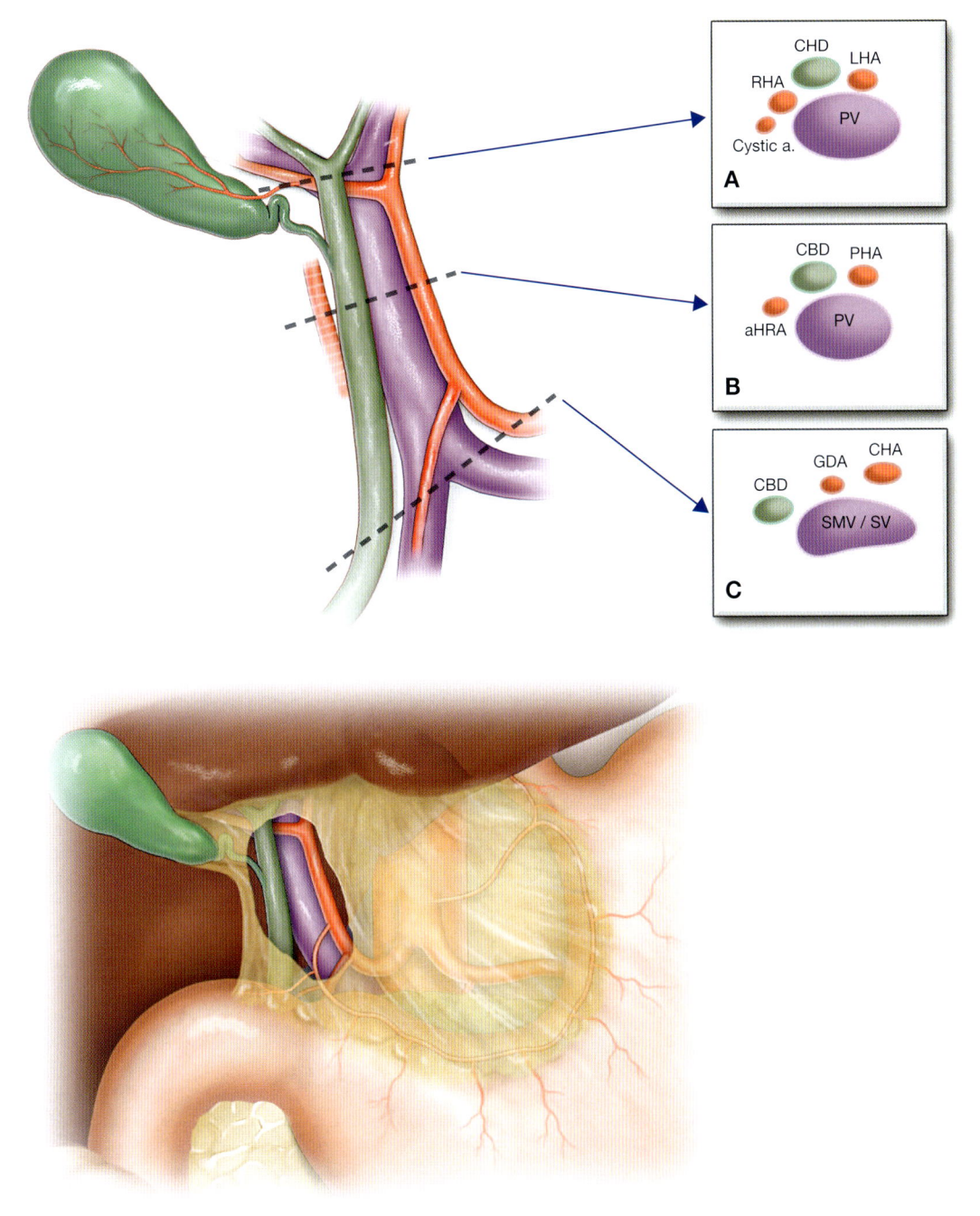

Bile Duct Injuries Repair 831

FIGURE 39-4 • Anatomy of the hepatoduodenal ligament.

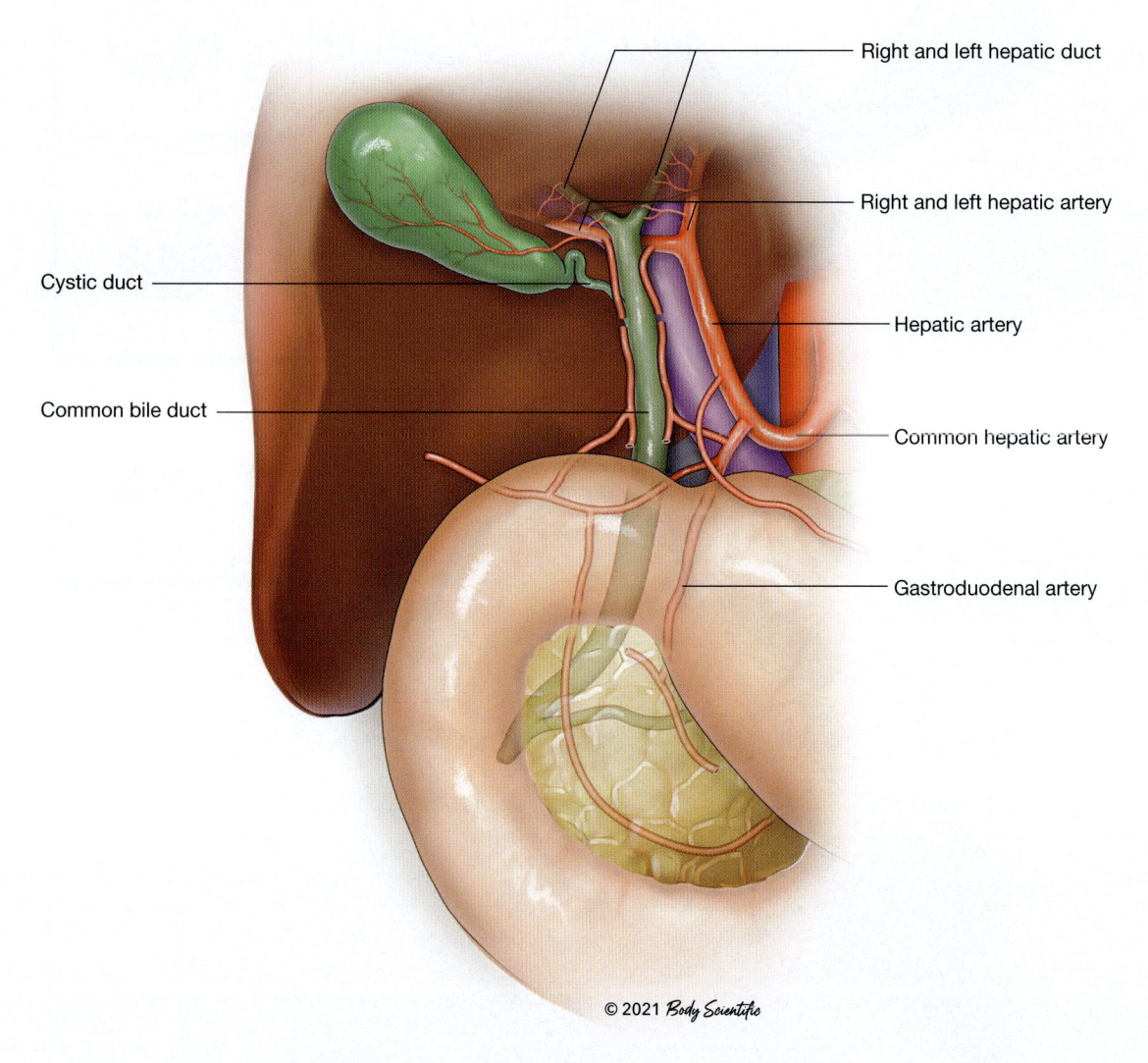

FIGURE 39-5 • Anatomy of the extrahepatic bile duct.

Step 2. Bile duct injury recognition

During this step, near-infrared indocyanine green (ICG) fluorescence might be helpful to recognize the CBD; mainly, in cases without bile leak (strictures, CBD clipping). This could be complemented by traditional cholangiography or laparoscopic ultrasound. Multiple clips from the initial operation might be encountered during the exploration, and careful removal of them may be necessary. Once the CBD has been identified, its integrity should be assessed. The hilum dissection is performed from lateral to medial. Careful identification and dissection of the main bile duct from the hepatic artery and portal vein are performed. Then, the status of the hepatic confluence must be evaluated (**Figures 39-6 A–F**).

Several types of bile duct injuries exist. Partial or total bile duct sections, resection of a bile duct segment, or strictures might be encountered (**Figure 39-7**).

In the classic LC BDI, the CBD is mistaken for the cystic duct, resulting in transection of a variable portion of the CBD. This is frequently associated with a right hepatic artery injury (**Figures 39-8 A, B**).

Once the BDI's type and level have been identified, the blood supply of the bile duct and the integrity of the hepatic artery are evaluated. In some cases the proper hepatic and/or the right hepatic artery has to be prepared on a vessel loop. A laparoscopic Doppler ultrasound may also be helpful to assess the blood flow.

Step 2 average time frame: 20–30 min

> ▶▶ **TIPS**
>
> The 2 most famous classifications of BDI are those proposed by Bismuth and Strasberg. Strasberg's BDI classification combined biliary injuries seen more frequently in the laparoscopic cholecystectomy era (types A–D) with the biliary stricture classification proposed by Bismuth (E1–E5).

> ⚠ **PITFALLS**
>
> Injury of an aberrant accessory right hepatic artery while dissecting the lateral portion of the CBD.

834 The Foundation and Art of Robotic Surgery

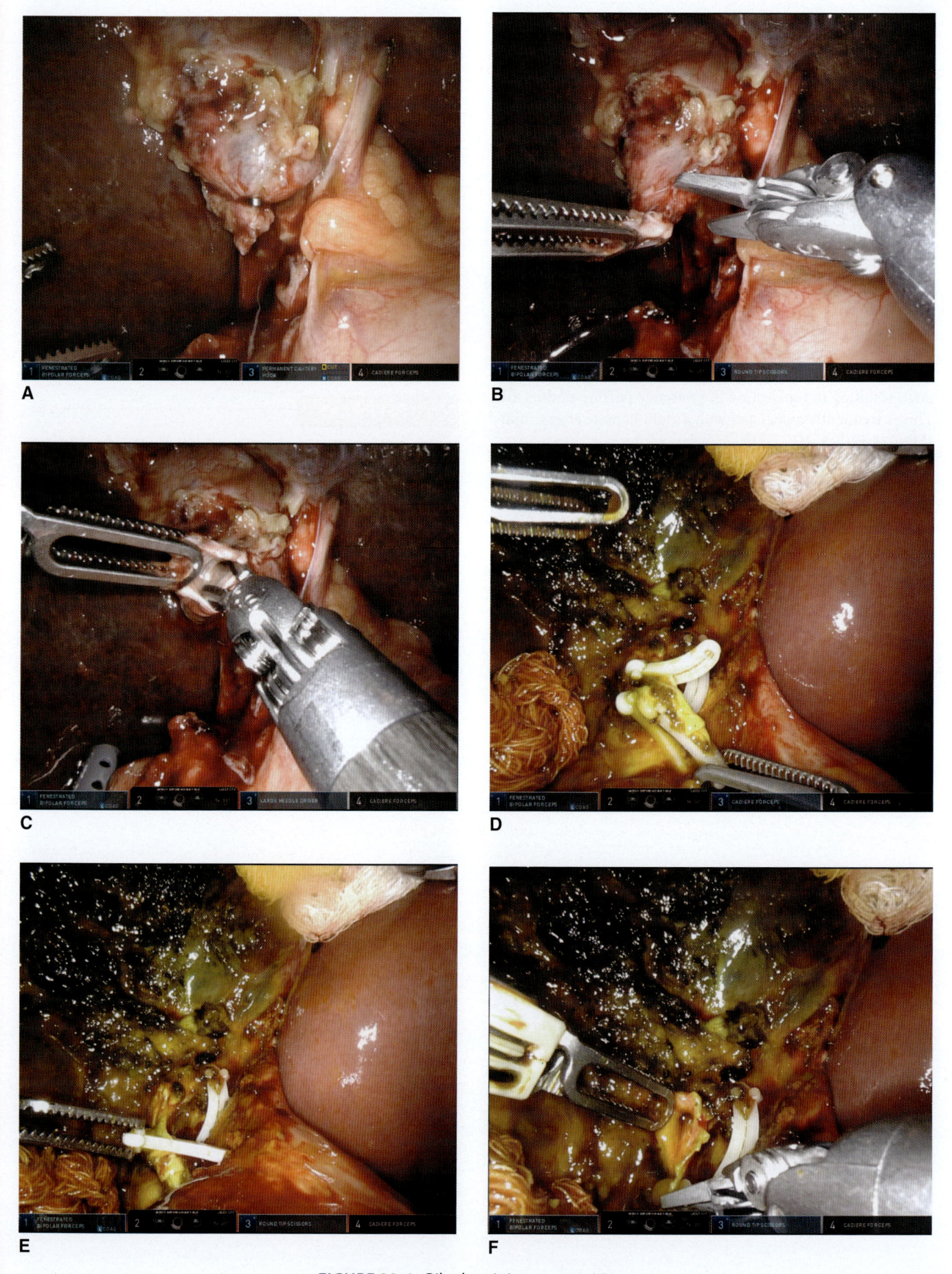

FIGURE 39-6 • Bile duct injury recognition.

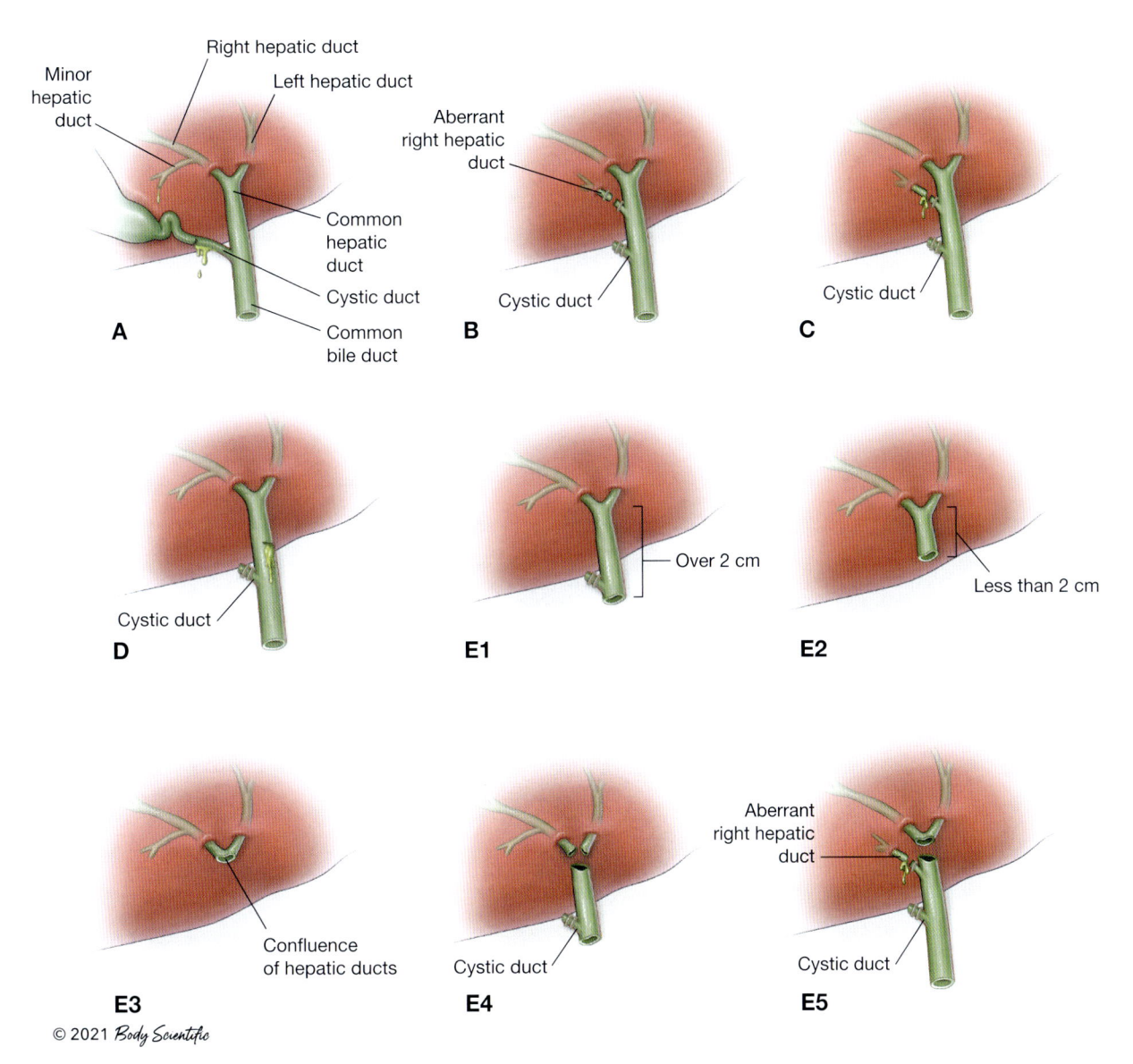

FIGURE 39-7 • Bile duct injury classification.

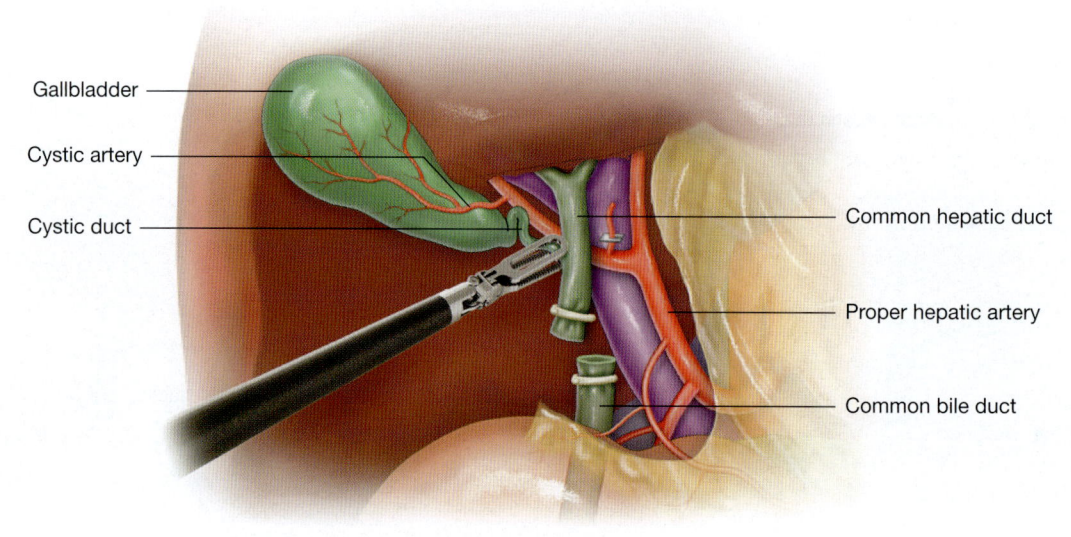

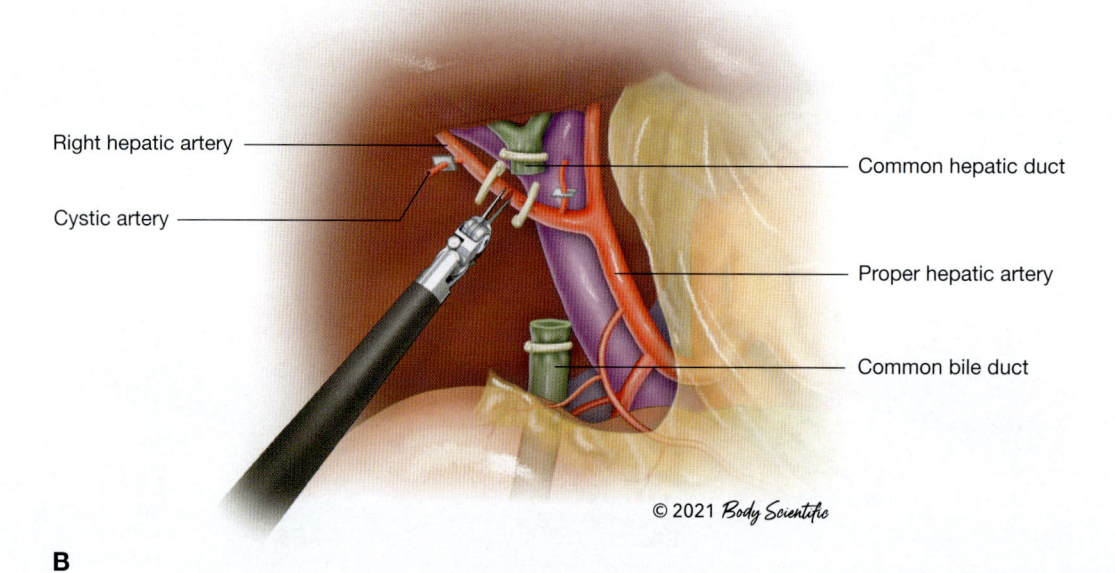

FIGURE 39-8 • Classic LC BDI.

Step 3. BDI repair

Several techniques for BDI repair have been described. However, the most common are primary closure with interrupted stitches and Roux-en-Y hepaticojejunostomy. End-to-end anastomosis after a complete bile duct transection or injuries with loss of a portion of the CBD should be avoided due to the high risk of late stricture formation.

Isolated right posterior hepatic duct injury

Ligation of the right posterior hepatic duct (Strasberg's type B) is difficult to diagnose. Most patients are asymptomatic, and the nondrained liver segments might undergo atrophy. Section without ligation of the right posterior hepatic duct is easily apparent because of the biliary leak. If the lesion is small, primary suture might be attempted. Otherwise, a bilioenteric anastomosis is constructed (**Figure 39-9**).

Minor lateral or anterior CBD injuries

Small lateral or anterior CBD injuries (Strasberg's type D) could be primarily sutured, especially if diagnosed intraoperatively and if the mechanism of injury was not thermal. To do so, interrupted stitches using an absorbable suture (PDS™ 4-0 or 5-0) are placed. In some cases, a T-Tube could be placed to protect the suture and for postoperative biliary access (**Figures 39-10 A, B**).

Major injuries, thermal lesion, biliary resection, and strictures

Most of these BDIs will need to be repaired with a Roux-en-Y hepaticojejunostomy (for more details, see Chapter 38, Roux-en-Y Hepaticojejunostomy). For this purpose, the common hepatic duct or hepatic ducts are dissected to prepare the edges of the proximal stump over healthy and well-perfused tissue. The distal stump is closed with a nonabsorbable suture. In high lesions affecting the confluence, the hilar plate must be dissected to achieve adequate exposure.

Once the bile duct is ready for reconstruction, a Roux-en-Y jejunal loop is prepared. The ligament of Treitz is identified and the mesentery of the second jejunal loop is divided with the vessel sealer. The jejunum is transected with the linear stapler preferably coming from the right-side assistant port. Perfusion of the stumps is checked with ICG fluorescence. A side-to-side jejunojejunostomy is constructed 70–80 cm distal to the future hepaticojejunostomy site. The enterotomy is then closed with a running PDS™ 3-0 suture.

The jejunal loop is then transposed to the right upper quadrant usually through the transmesocolic paraduodenal route. Even though all the possible modalities should be known (see Chapter 38, Roux-en-Y Hepaticojejunostomy) (**Figure 39-11**).

The technique for the hepaticojejunostomy depends on the size, thickness, and quality of the bile duct. In lesions where the transection of the bile duct is performed above the confluence, the medial wall of adjacent ducts can be sutured together to create a single lumen (ductoplasty) that will facilitate the construction of the anastomosis. More frequently, the anastomosis is performed with a short posterior running PDS™ 5-0 suture and anterior interrupted stitches of PDS™ 5-0.

As previously explained in Chapter 38, Roux-en-Y Hepaticojejunostomy, the bilioenteric anastomosis is constructed from the 9 o'clock to 3 o'clock position and the anterior row of interrupted stitches is temporarily secured with Hem-o-lok™ clips before tying. Once all the stitches have been placed, they are tied starting from the 3 o'clock position to facilitate the visualization and approximation of the edges (**Figures 39-12 A–E**).

Finally, fibrin glue is applied to the bilioenteric anastomosis and a Jackson Pratt drain is placed next to the hepaticojejunostomy.

In some cases, a direct mucosa-to-mucosa hepaticojejunostomy is not feasible. This might happen in the case of a very high BDI where thin, fragile, and separated ducts far from each other are encountered. In such circumstances, a jejunal loop might be sutured to the hilar plate surrounding the transected bile ducts (Kasai procedure).

Step 3 average time frame: 30–90 min

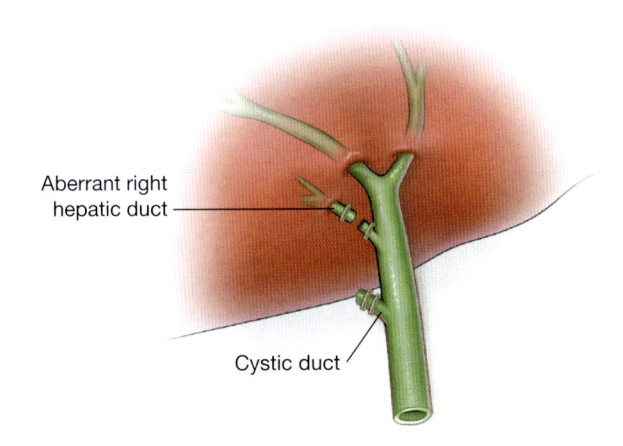

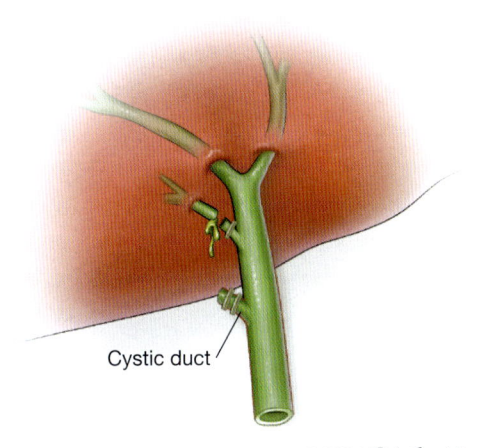

FIGURE 39-9 • Right posterior hepatic duct injury.

838 The Foundation and Art of Robotic Surgery

A   B

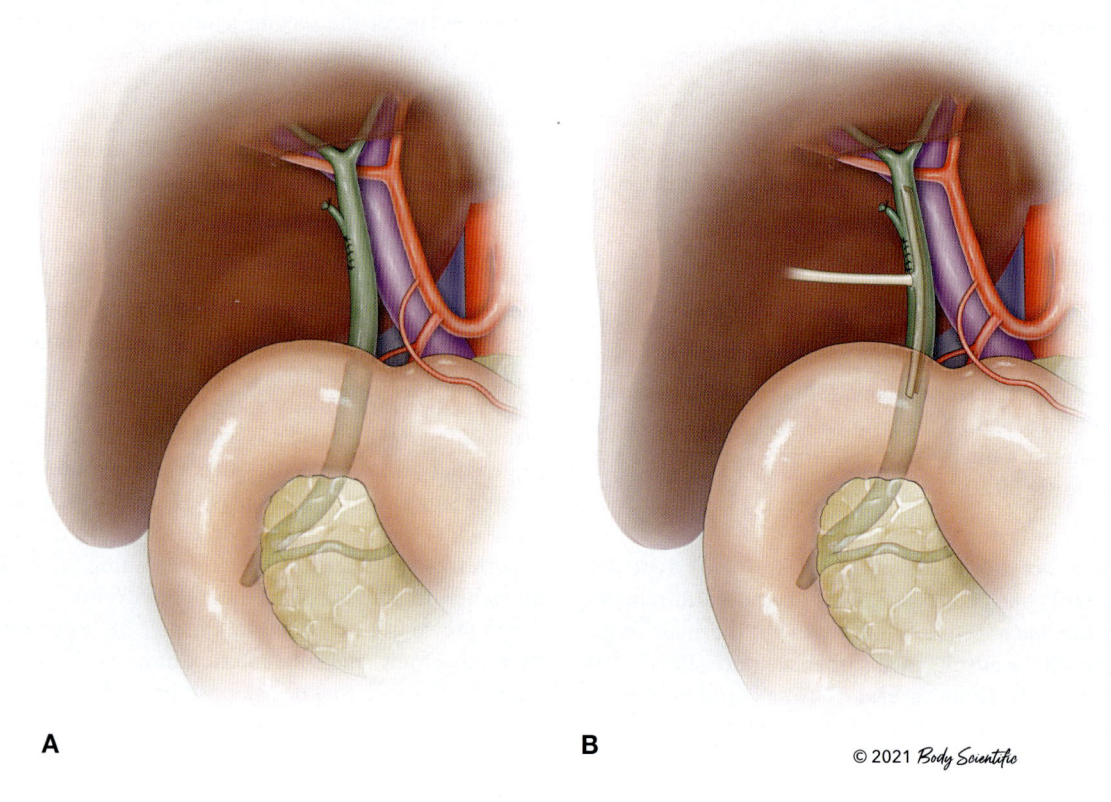

FIGURE 39-10 • Primary repair and T-Tube placement.

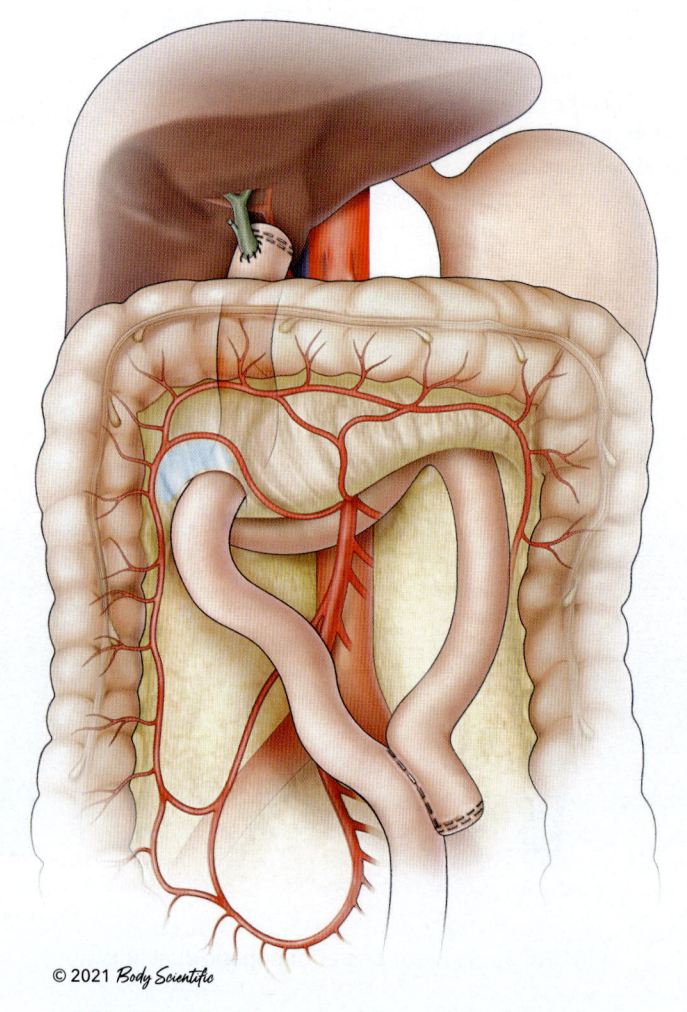

FIGURE 39-11 • Transmesocolic paraduodenal route.

Bile Duct Injuries Repair 839

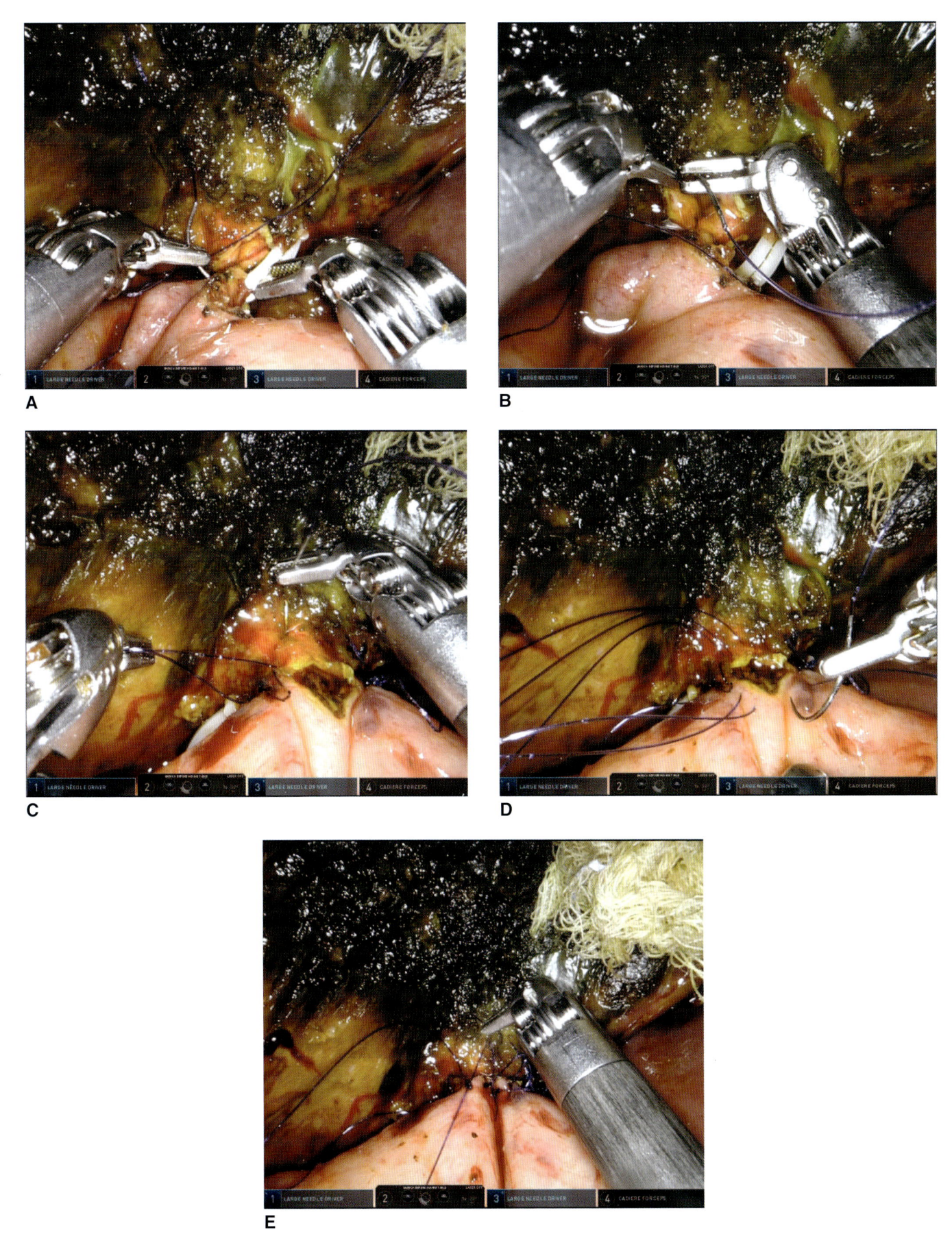

FIGURE 39-12 • Hepaticojejunostomy.

Suggested Readings

1. Bismuth H, Majno PE. Biliary strictures: classification based on the principles of surgical treatment. *World J Surg.* 2001;25(10):1241-1244. doi: 10.1007/s00268-001-0102-8
2. Strasberg SM, Hertl M, Soper NJ. An analysis of the problem of biliary injury during laparoscopic cholecystectomy. *J Am Coll Surg.* 1995;180(1):101-125.
3. Giulianotti PC, Quadri P, Durgam S, Bianco FM. Reconstruction/repair of iatrogenic biliary injuries: is the robot offering a new option? Short clinical report. *Ann Surg.* 2018;267(1):e7-e9. doi: 10.1097/SLA.0000000000002343
4. de'Angelis N, Catena F, Memeo R, et al. 2020 WSES guidelines for the detection and management of bile duct injury during cholecystectomy. *World J Emerg Surg.* 2021;16(1):30. doi: 10.1186/s13017-021-00369-w
5. Strasberg SM, Brunt LM. Rationale and use of the critical view of safety in laparoscopic cholecystectomy. *J Am Coll Surg.* 2010;211(1):132-138. doi: 10.1016/j.jamcollsurg.2010.02.053
6. Giulianotti PC, Coratti A, Angelini M, et al. Robotics in general surgery: personal experience in a large community hospital. *Arch Surg.* 2003;138(7):777-784. doi: 10.1001/archsurg.138.7.777
7. Pesce A, Palmucci S, La Greca G, Puleo S. Iatrogenic bile duct injury: impact and management challenges. *Clin Exp Gastroenterol.* 2019;12:121-128. doi: 10.2147/CEG.S169492

"Few operations give greater satisfaction to patient and to surgeon alike than does a successful operation for gall-stones. And, one may add, few experiences are more distressing than failure of the operation to procure relief."

—Kenelm Hutchinson Digby (1884–1954)

Management of Intrahepatic Biliary Stones

Eric CH Lai • Chung Ngai Tang

INTRODUCTION

Primary hepatolithiasis is formed *de novo* in the intrahepatic ducts (IHDs). This disease is characterized by repeated primary bacterial infection of the biliary system, with subsequent formation of multiple stones and strictures in any portion of the biliary tract. The disease was first described in Hong Kong in 1930 by KH Digby, and it then came to be known as recurrent pyogenic cholangitis (RPC). It is a prevalent disease in Southeast Asia, but rare in Western countries. The definitive management of RPC involves a multidisciplinary approach, aiming to remove all biliary stones, establish adequate drainage to the biliary system, and resect nonfunctioning liver segments that harbor bacteria and serve as foci of infection. Theoretically, partial hepatectomy is the most definitive approach for hepatolithiasis, because it can remove IHD stones and bile duct strictures simultaneously, thus reducing the risk of recurrent stones and the development of cholangiocarcinoma. However, partial hepatectomy in patients with RPC is particularly difficult due to the presence of dense perihepatic inflammatory adhesions from previous infections, multiple previous abdominal operations, and liver abscesses rupturing into the perihepatic space.

The development of minimally invasive surgery over the last three decades has had a great impact on the surgical practice in the world. With the wide application of laparoscopic surgery in biliary diseases, laparoscopic common bile duct (CBD) exploration has been one of the main treatment methods for CBD stones. The technique for stone removal in the CBD can be applied to IHD stones. Laparoscopic liver resection also became possible with the availability of new instruments

INSTRUMENT REQUIREMENTS

The suggested main robotic instruments/tools can be listed as follows:
- 30° scope
- Needle drivers (round tip or macro)
- Permanent cautery monopolar hook/monopolar curved scissors
- Harmonic shears/vessel sealer
- Bipolar forceps
- Cadière forceps
- Clip applier
- Endostapler

The suggested main laparoscopic instruments/tools can be listed as follows:
- Needle drivers
- Scissors
- Graspers
- Suction-irrigation
- Laparoscopic ultrasound probe

Supplemental materials:
- Gauzes, sponges
- Sutures: polydioxanone, V-Lock™, polypropylene 3-0, 4-0, and 5-0
- Hem-o-lok™ clips
- Choledochoscope
- Electrohydraulic lithotripsy (EHL)
- Basket and balloon catheter for biliary stone removal
- Suction catheter with syringe for saline flushing
- T-Tube

Photo source: Courtesy of the Department of Surgery, University of Hong Kong.
Quote reproduced with permission from Digby KH. Observations on the treatment of gallstones. Ann Surg. 1926;83(1):47-54.

that allowed a relatively bloodless liver transection. The potential advantages of the laparoscopic approach are those of minimally invasive surgery, such as early recovery, shorter hospital stay, and better cosmetic outcome. The recently developed robotic platform has gained popularity in hepatobiliary surgery due to its significant advantages over open and conventional laparoscopic techniques. The superior robotic features allow surgeons to perform fine-tissue dissection, precise intracorporeal suturing, and anastomosis. As such, the robotic approach was also applied as one of the options in the management of RPC.

Acute and Elective Management

The basic principle of management of RPC is to control infection during an acute attack of cholangitis and to eradicate all stones, strictures, and destroyed liver segments by elective definitive surgery when the disease is quiescent.

The initial conservative measures for acute cholangitis consist of broad-spectrum antibiotics, intravenous fluids infusion, adequate analgesics, and careful monitoring of abdominal and vital signs. Emergency therapeutic intervention for decompression of the biliary tract, such as endoscopic retrograde cholangiopancreatography (ERCP) or percutaneous transhepatic biliary drainage (PTBD), is necessary for some patients when the acute attack fails to resolve, as evidenced by persistent fever, septicemia, shock, and worsening of peritoneal signs.

The definitive procedure is planned according to the results of all the imaging studies. Preoperative evaluation of the hepatobiliary system includes the use of ultrasonography (US), computed tomography (CT) scan, hepatobiliary iminodiacetic acid (HIDA) scintigraphy, magnetic resonance cholangiopancreatography (MRCP), ERCP, or PTBD. These investigations provide information about the location and extent of stones, biliary strictures, or liver atrophy, which in turn guide the type of operation. Because the disease affects the biliary tract at different sites and with varying degrees of severity, many procedures have been developed to deal with the different circumstances. The choice of surgical procedures includes CBD/common hepatic duct (CHD)/enterobiliary anastomosis exploration with extraction of stones, or partial hepatectomy, with or without bile duct exploration or bilioenteric bypass. In general, RPC can be arbitrarily divided into simple and complicated cases depending on the absence or presence of intrahepatic strictures. For simple cases, cholecystectomy, exploration of the CBD, and choledochoscopy with or without hepaticojejunostomy suffice. For complicated cases, partial hepatectomy, with or without bile duct exploration, or hepaticojejunostomy is needed to circumvent intrahepatic ductal strictures and to eradicate impacted stones.

Indications and Relative Contraindications to the Robotic Approach

Robot-assisted surgery has similar indications as conventional laparoscopic surgery. Contraindications are also similar to those of conventional laparoscopy (e.g., intolerance to pneumoperitoneum, significant intraperitoneal adhesions from multiple prior open abdominal operations, poor visualization, or exposure).

Indications of Bile Duct Exploration

CBD/CHD/enterobiliary anastomosis exploration with extraction of stones is performed for patients with stones filled in the extrahepatic bile duct or proximal bile duct branches.

Indications of Partial Hepatectomy

Indications of partial hepatectomy include biliary stricture, atrophy of the affected liver segments or hemi-liver, presence of a liver abscess, suspected cholangiocarcinoma, and stones filled in peripheral bile duct branches inaccessible from extrahepatic bile duct incision.

Indications of Hepaticojejunostomy

Hepaticojejunostomy is performed in selected patients to eliminate bile stasis and prevent stone recurrence or to tackle strictures in the CHD or CBD. Bile stasis is common when CHD/CBD is dilated (> 2 cm in size).

Patient Positioning, OR Setup, and Port Setting

The patient is placed supine on a beanbag, with arms tucked and lower limbs parted in the French position, with a 30° reverse Trendelenburg (**Figure 40-1**). The assistant surgeon is sitting between the patient's legs. Five to 6 ports (4 robotic trocars and 1/2 assistant ports: 5 mm and 12 mm) are used depending on the procedure. The port settings for a choledochotomy/hepaticojejunostomy and a left hepatectomy/left lateral sectionectomy are presented in **Figures 40-2 A, B**, respectively. The position of the R2 and scope could be exchanged depending on the planned procedure (left hepatectomy or left lateral sectionectomy). The first 8-mm trocar is inserted using open method into the umbilical area, and a pneumoperitoneum is created at 12 mm Hg pressure.

> **EDITORIAL COMMENT**
>
> The Veress technique might be more convenient for the induction of pneumoperitoneum in obese patients or large abdomens where the umbilicus is not a favorable port site in relation to the target.

After all the ports are placed, abdominal exploration and laparoscopic ultrasound assessment are performed. The robotic system is docked into position afterward (**Figure 40-3**).

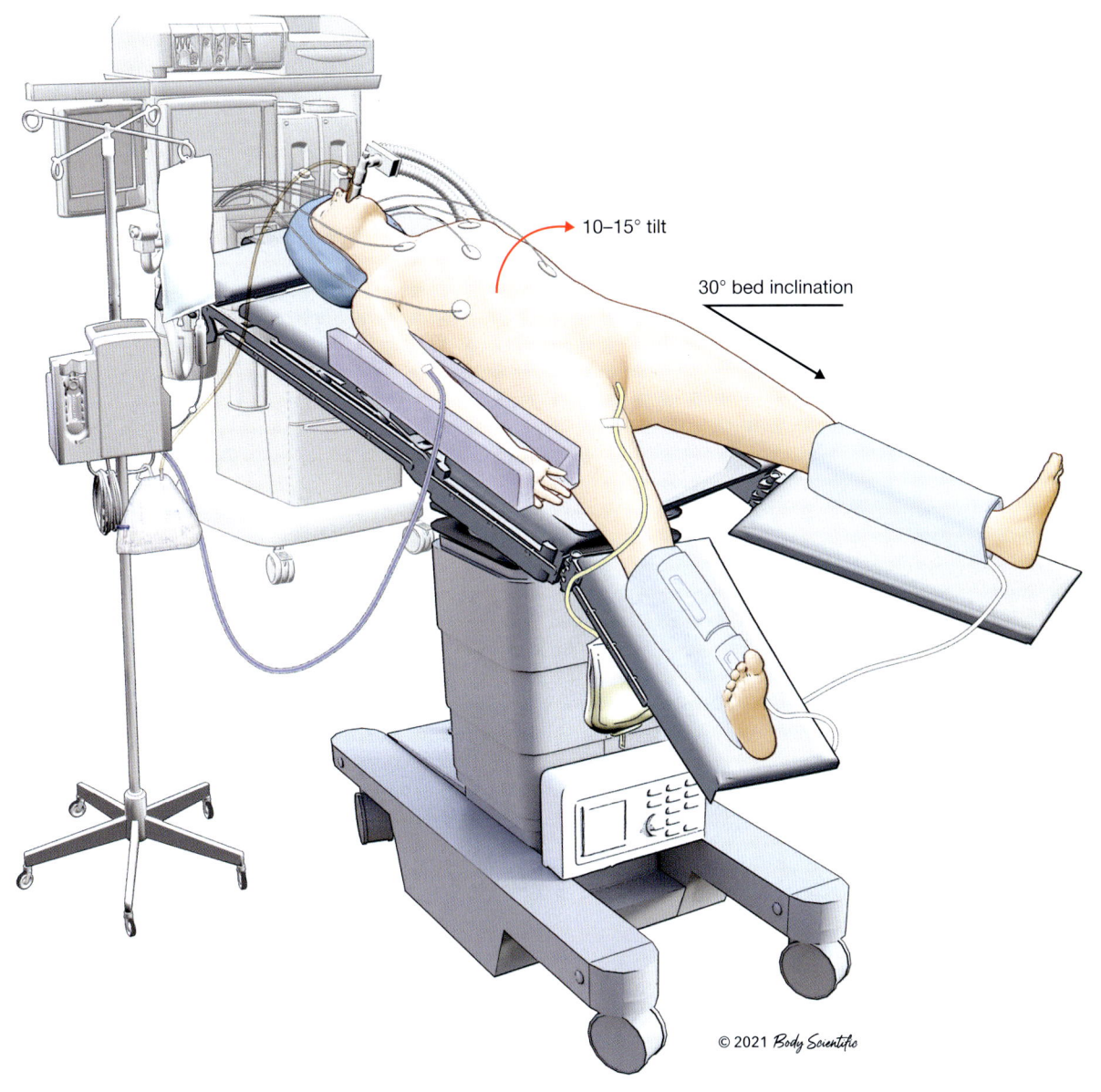

Management of Intrahepatic Biliary Stones 843

FIGURE 40-1 • Patient positioning.

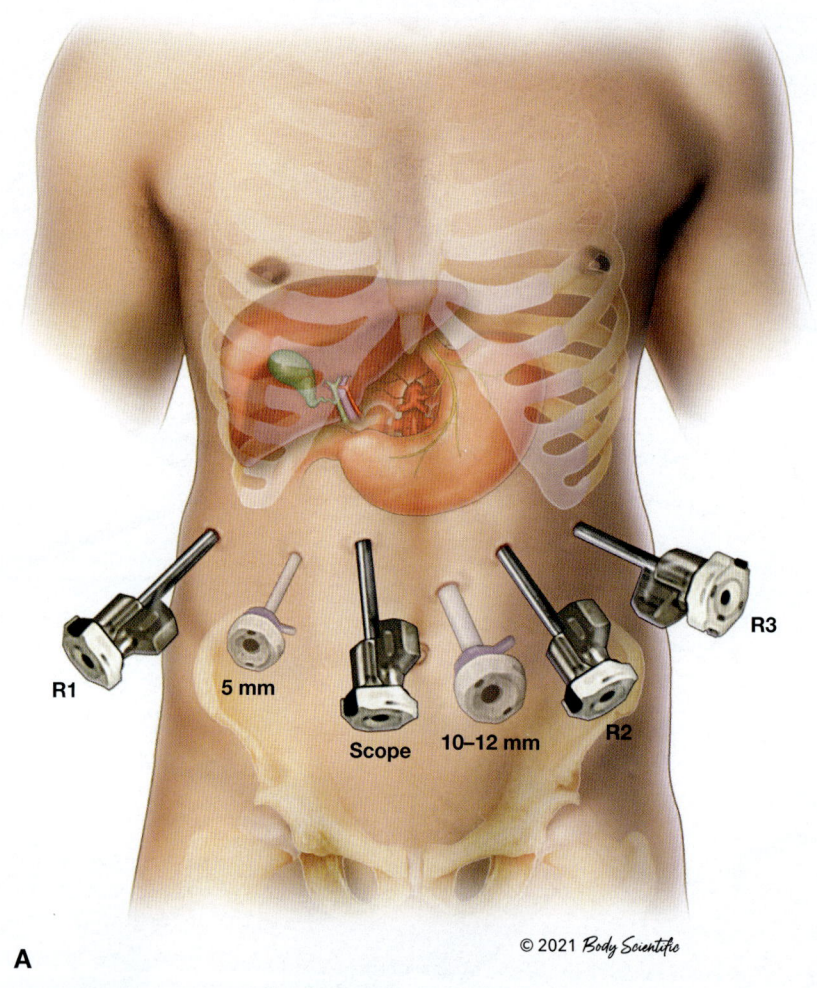

FIGURE 40-2 • **A.** Port setting for choledochotomy/hepaticojejunostomy.

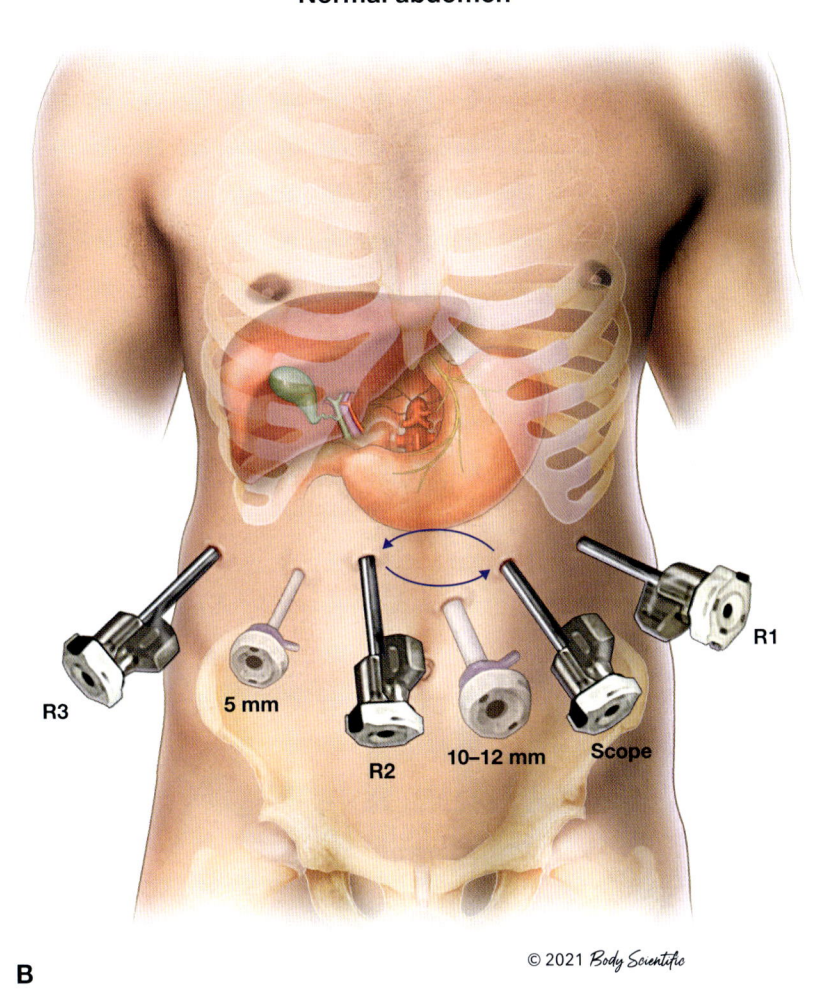

FIGURE 40-2 • (*Continued*) **B.** Port setting for left lateral sectionectomy/left hepatectomy.

846 The Foundation and Art of Robotic Surgery

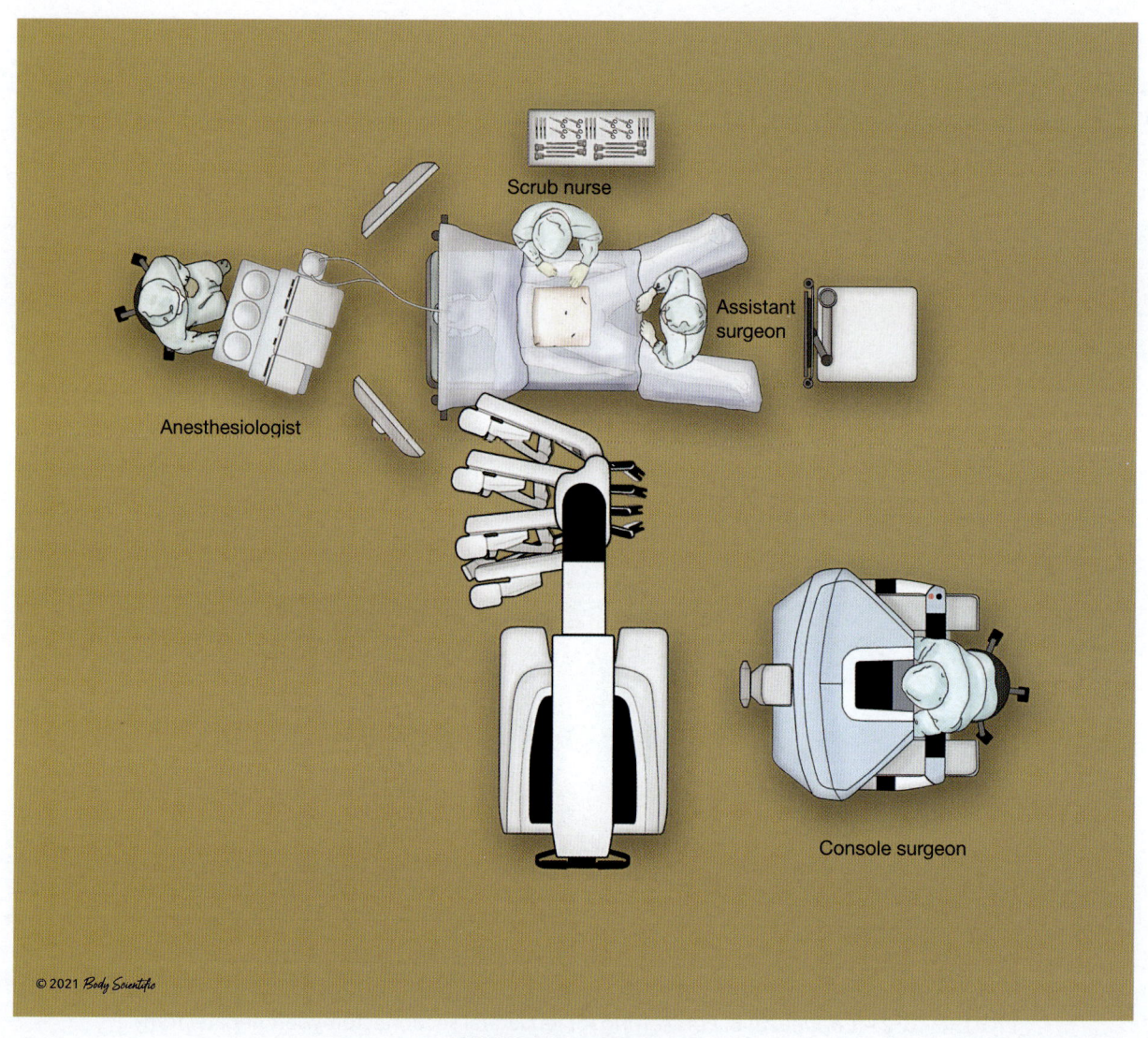

FIGURE 40-3 • OR setup.

Surgical Technique

▶ Video 40-1. Left Hepatectomy and Biliary Duct Exploration

Step 1. Cholecystectomy and cholangiography

To expose the hepatoduodenal ligament and porta hepatis, the liver's segment IVb is retracted upward by a Cadiére forceps inserted through the R3. Afterward, the cholecystectomy is performed using a standardized technique (see Chapter 37, Cholecystectomy). An intraoperative cholangiogram is necessary if preoperative cholangiogram is suboptimal.

Step 1 average time frame: 20–30 min

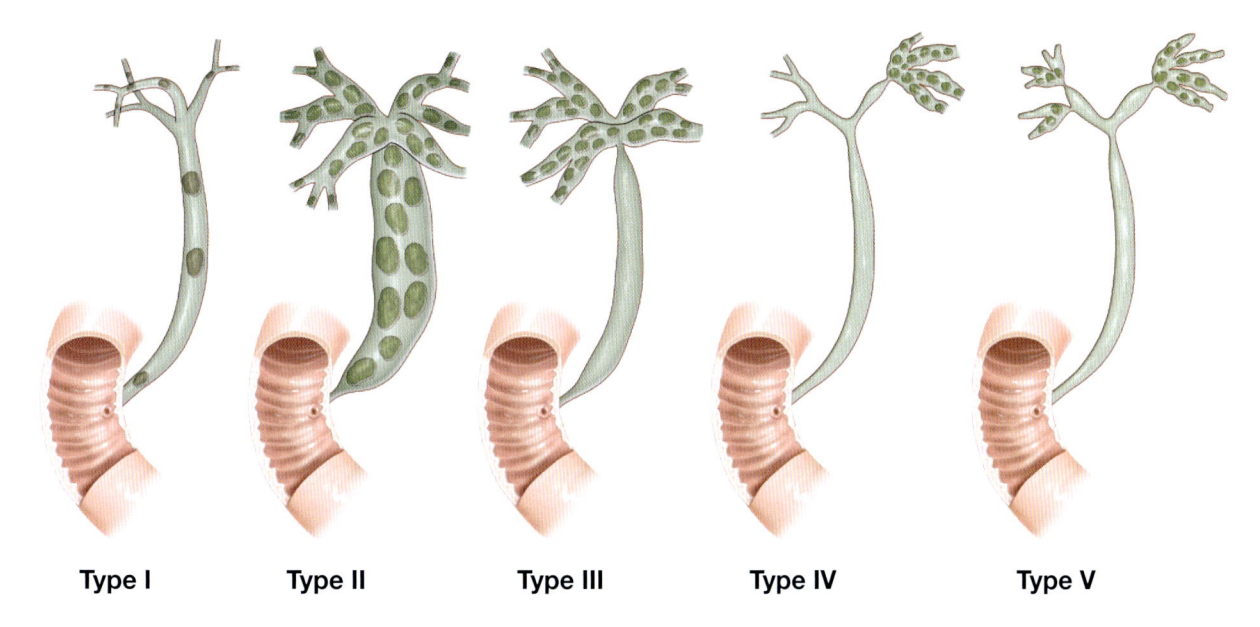

> **🔍 ANATOMICAL HIGHLIGHTS**
>
> Classification of the hepatolithiasis (**Figure 40-4**). See suggested reading #1.
>
> Anatomy of the hepatoduodenal ligament (**Figure 40-5**).

Type I   Type II   Type III   Type IV   Type V

© 2021 Body Scientific

FIGURE 40-4 • Classification of the hepatolithiasis.

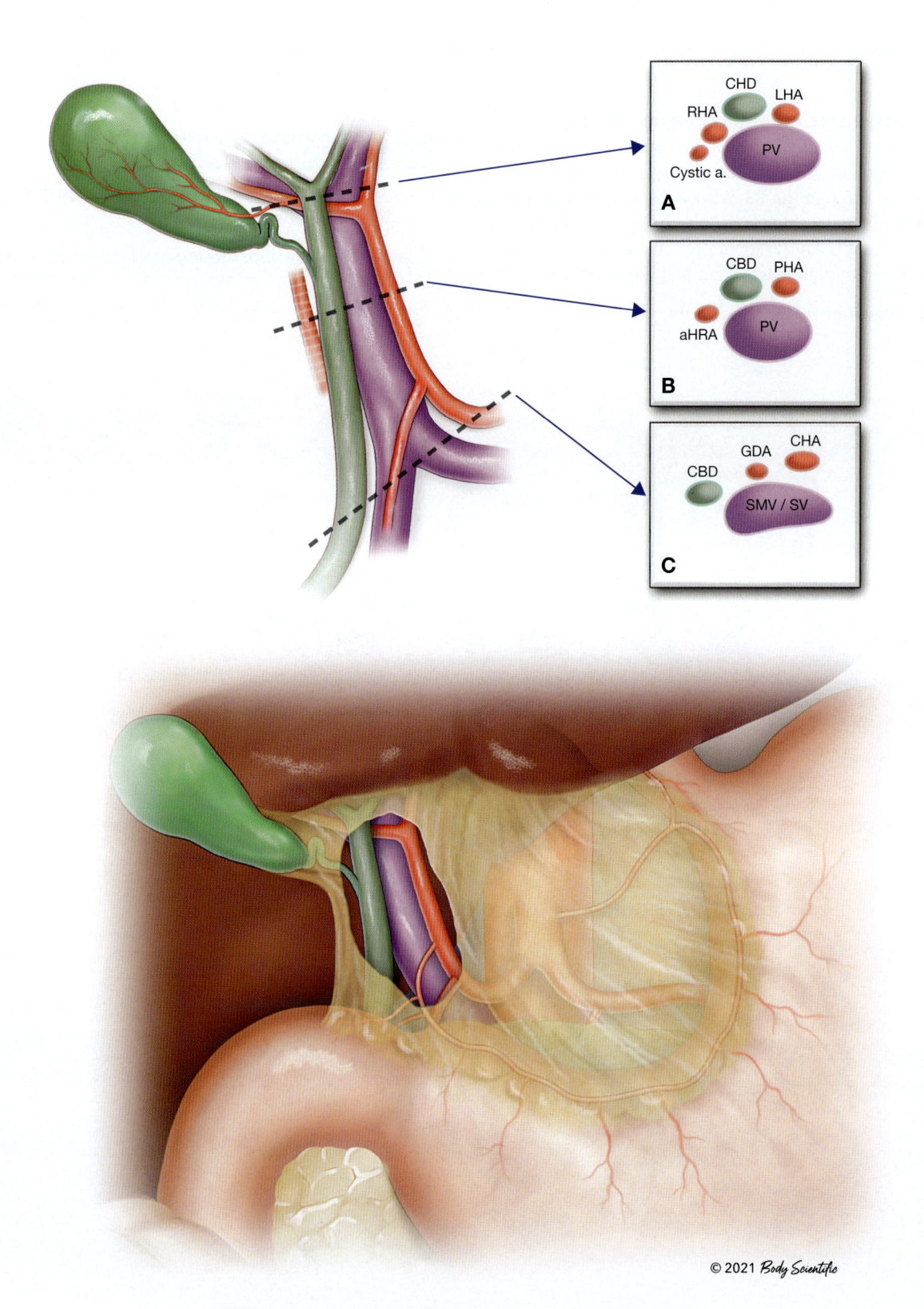

FIGURE 40-5 • Anatomy of the hepatoduodenal ligament.

Step 2. Preparation of the common bile duct and ultrasonograpy

Next, the bile duct is dissected and exposed using the monopolar hook or cold scissors. A partial Kocher maneuver and mobilization of the right colic flexure might be necessary to have better control and exposure of the liver hilum. To confirm the correct structure of the main bile duct (in cases of severe inflammation), a spinal needle might be inserted percutaneously into the CBD for bile aspiration before doing the choledochotomy incision (**Figures 40-6 A, B**). Understanding of the bile duct anatomy and its vascularization is of utmost importance during this procedure (**Figures 40-7 A, B**).

Step 2 average time frame: 15–20 min

> ⚠ **PITFALLS**
>
> Inadvertent CBD injury might happen due to difficult exposure by dense adhesions. This is the result of repeated previous infections, operations, or a pericholedochal venous plexus related to portal vein thrombosis or portal hypertension. On occasion, due to liver atrophy or hypertrophy, the CBD has a different relationship with the hepatic artery and the portal vein.

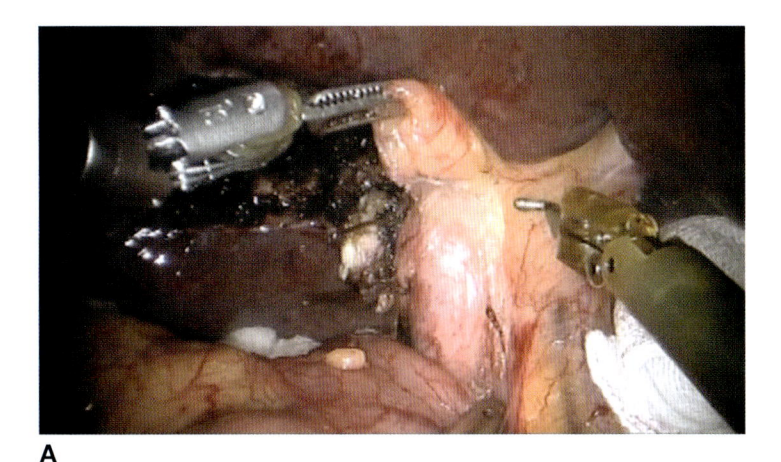

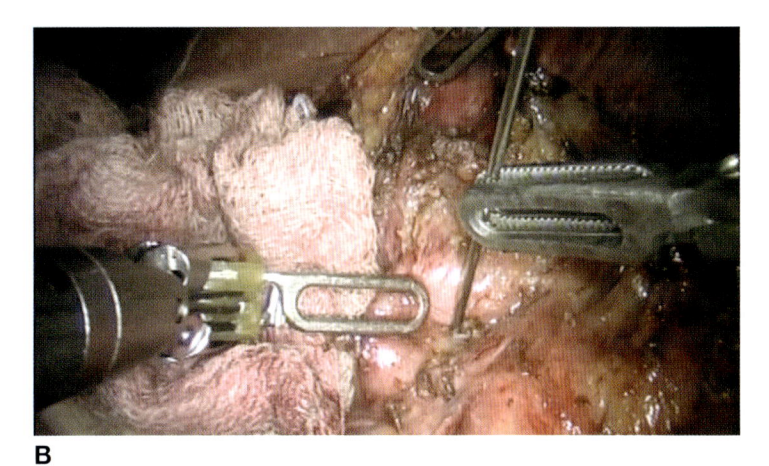

FIGURE 40-6 • Bile duct dissection.

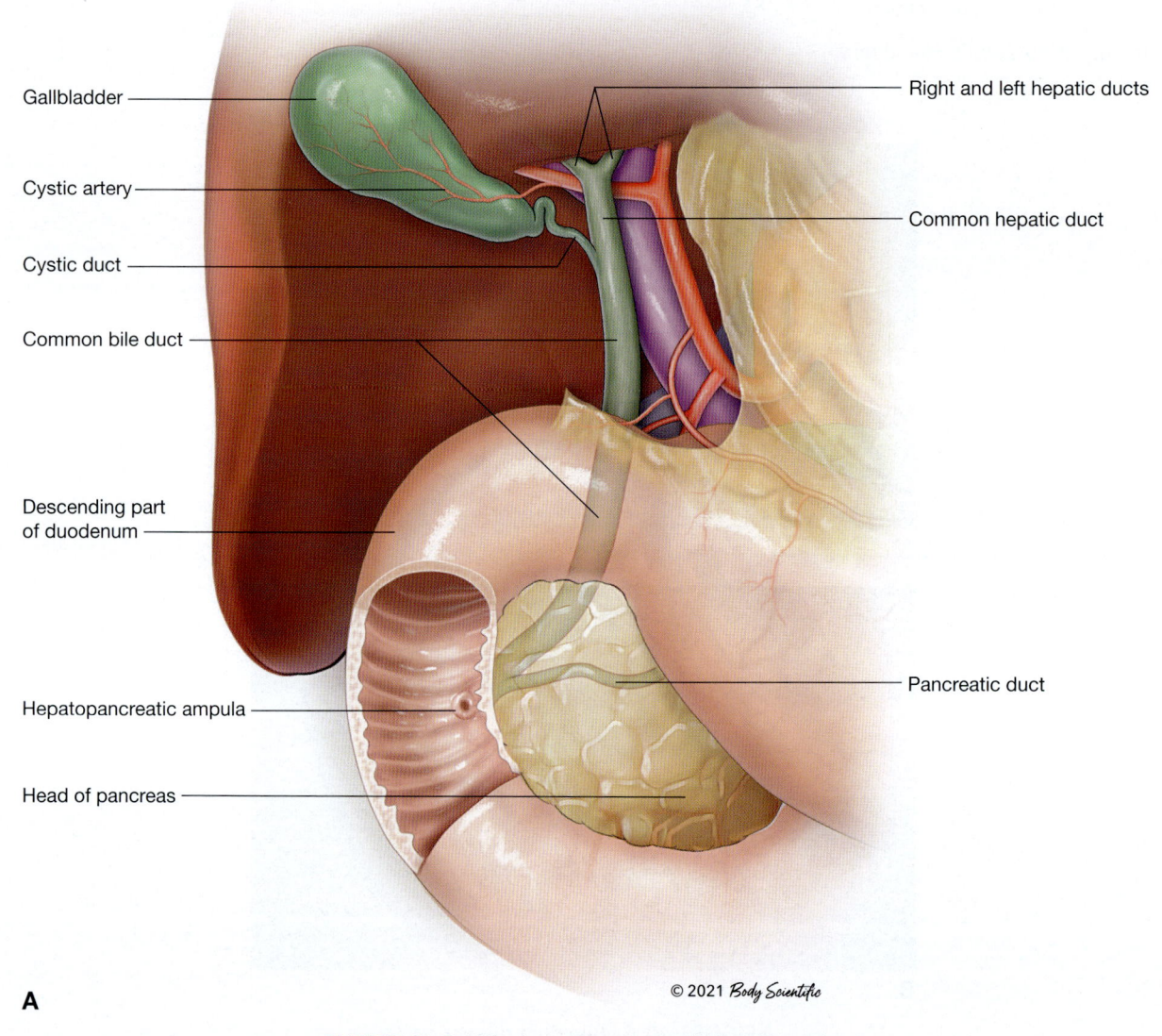

FIGURE 40-7 • Bile duct anatomy and blood supply.

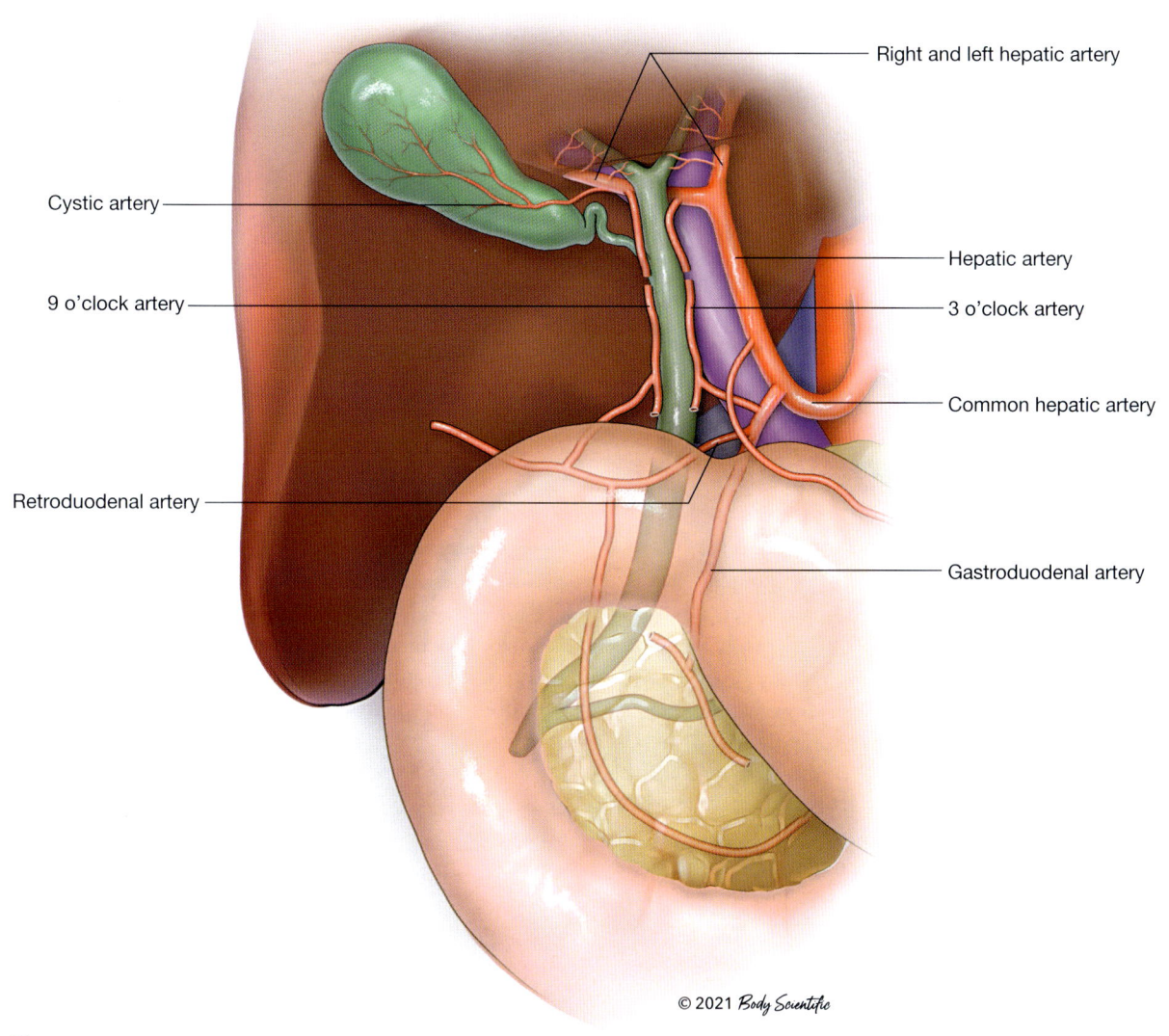

FIGURE 40-7 • (Continued)

Step 3. Choledochotomy

After the CBD is dissected, a 2-cm longitudinal incision is made in the anterior surface just below the cystic duct confluence (**Figure 40-8**). A flexible choledochoscope is then inserted in the CBD through the choledochotomy at a right angle. This could then be maneuvered in the proximal and distal biliary tree. The length and site of the choledochotomy can be modified depending on the stone's size and location. If necessary, the choledochotomy incision can be extended to the CHD.

Step 3 average time frame: 3–5 min

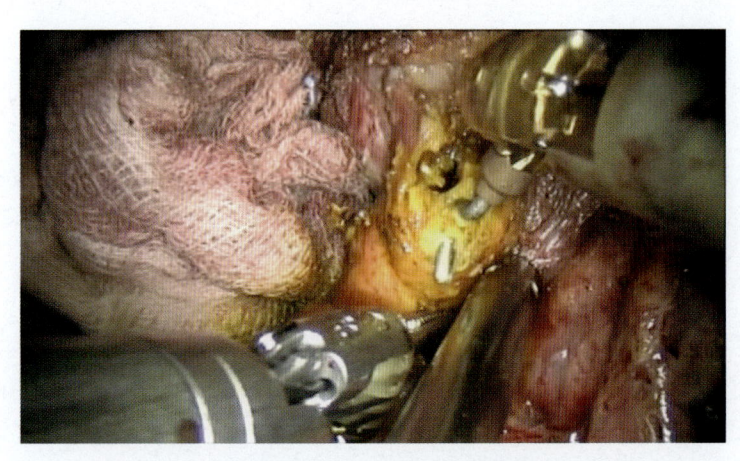

FIGURE 40-8 • Choledochotomy.

▶ Video 40-2. Bile Duct Exploration

Step 4. Choledochoscopy and stone removal

Once the bile duct is opened, stones are removed using the robotic forceps, basket, balloon extraction, or saline flushing under the choledochoscope guidance (**Figures 40-9 A–C**). The choledochoscope should enter the abdomen as close as possible to the entry point in the bile duct to improve the maneuverability of the instrument. In order to apply this principle, a dedicated trocar could be added, or the camera could be swapped to the 10–12 mm assistant port with a trocar in trocar technique and the choledochoscope inserted through the camera port. Electrohydraulic lithotripsy might be used to break large and impacted stones in order to facilitate their removal (**Figures 40-10 A–D**).

Step 4 average time frame: 15–30 min

> ▶▶ **TIPS**
>
> Gauze packing around the subhepatic space for bile soaking is recommended to prevent bile spillage over the peritoneum. A specimen bag is placed over the right subhepatic space for immediate retrieval of stones.

> ⚠ **PITFALLS**
>
> The lithotripter might cause bile duct damage and hemobilia if the tip of the probe is in contact with the bile duct wall.

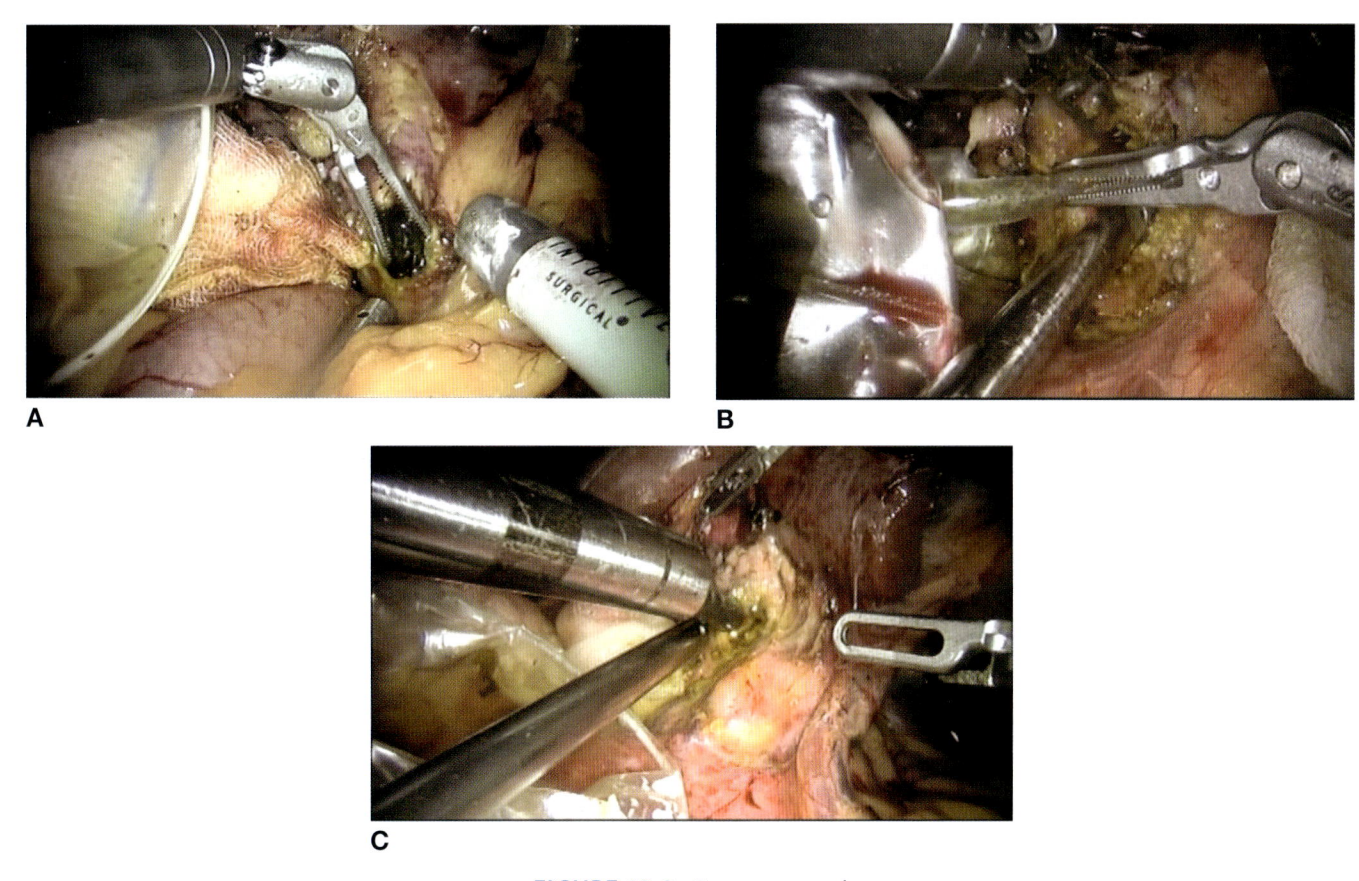

Management of Intrahepatic Biliary Stones **853**

FIGURE 40-9 • Stone removal.

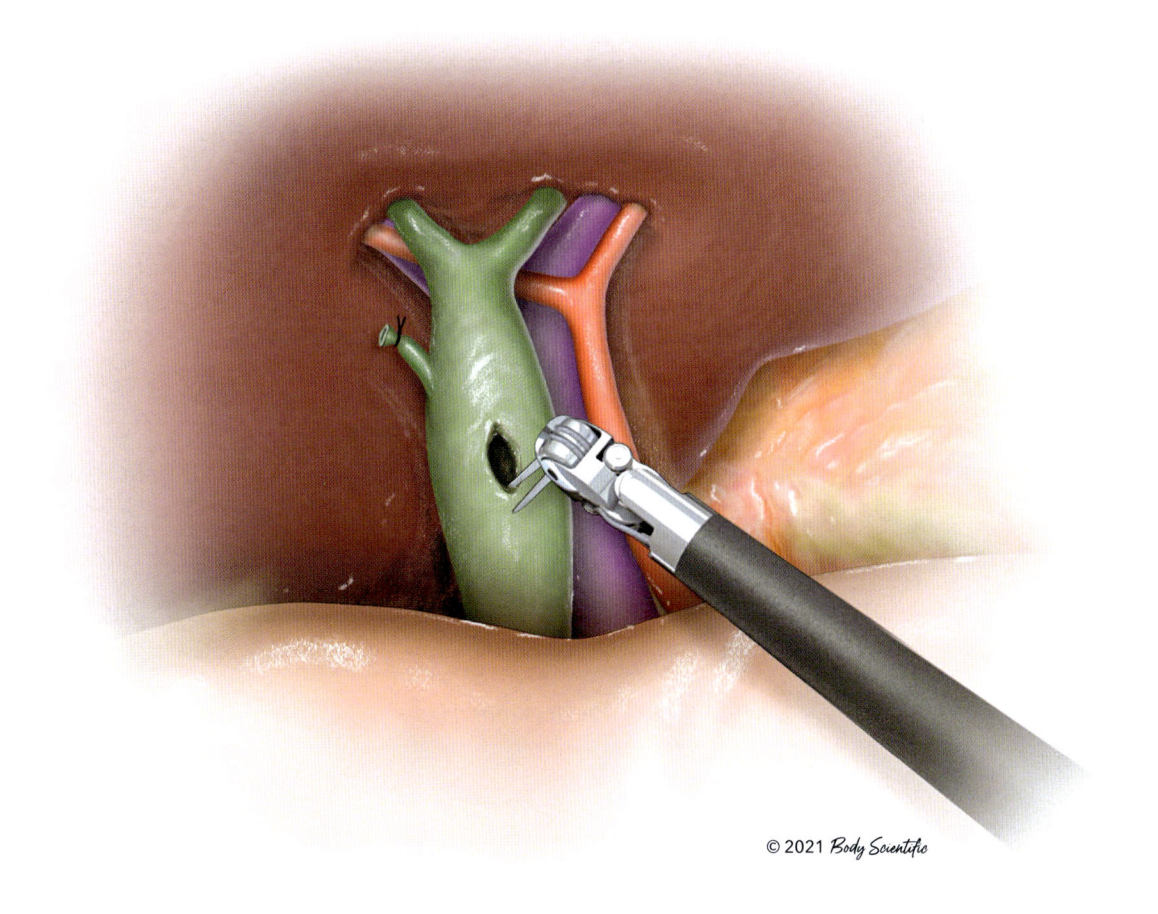

FIGURE 40-10 • Choledochotomy and choledochoscopy.

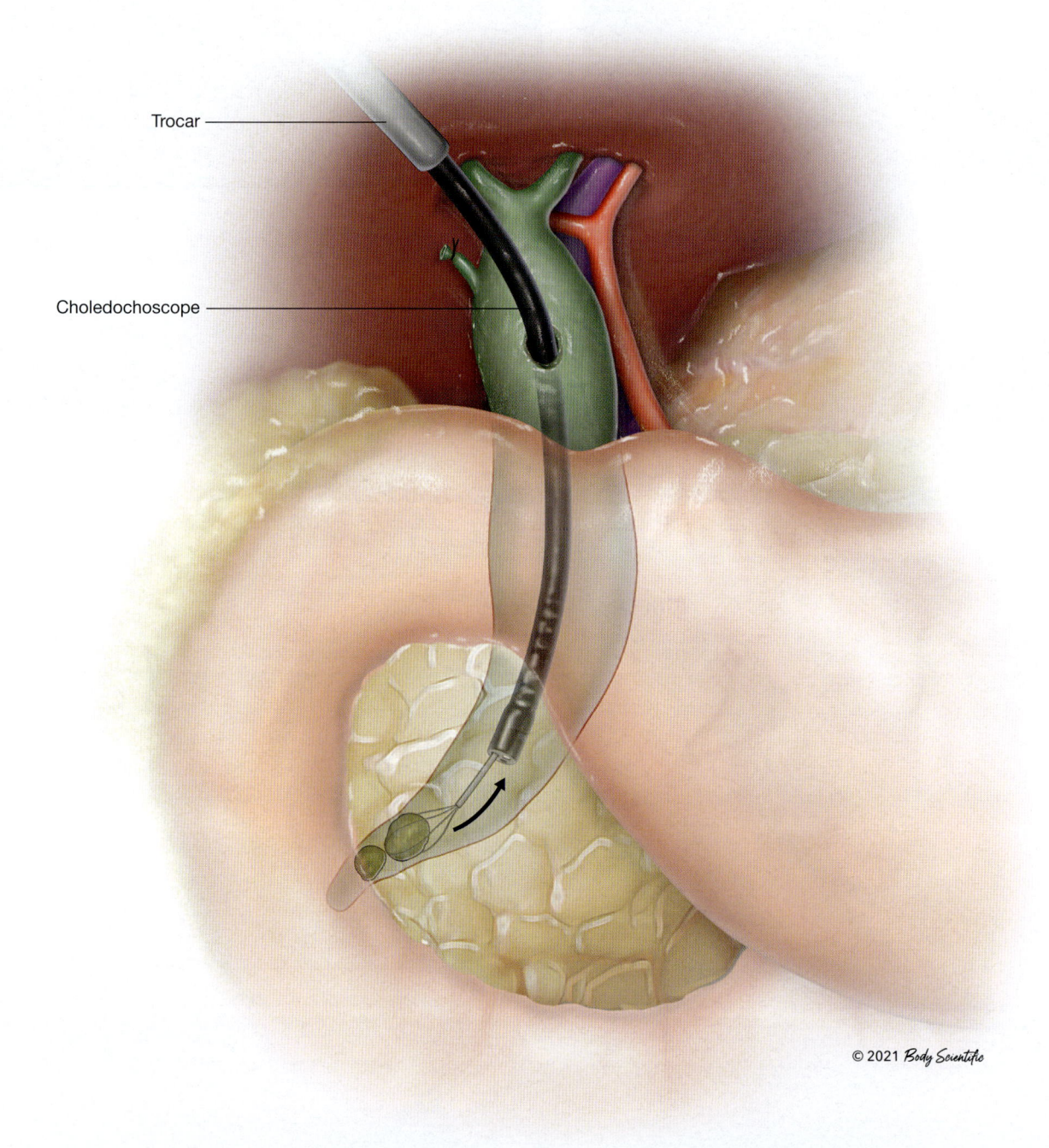

FIGURE 40-10 • *(Continued)*

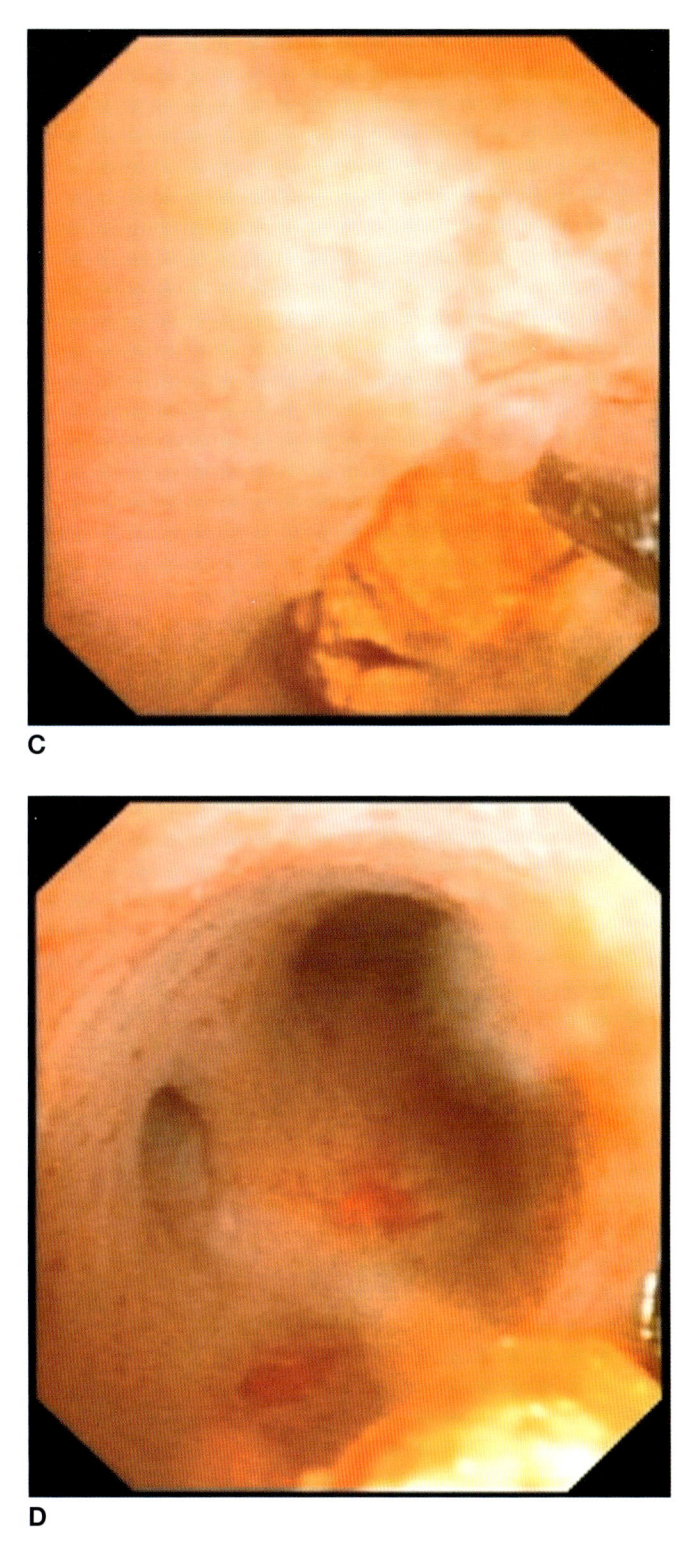

FIGURE 40-10 • (*Continued*)

Step 5. Closure of the choledochotomy

After complete clearance of the extrahepatic duct, the choledochotomy is closed with 3-0 or 4-0 absorbable sutures (**Figures 40-11 A, B**). In selected patients with muddy stones or suspected residual stones, a T-Tube is inserted (**Figure 40-12**). Postoperative cholangiography is performed through the T-Tube about 2–3 weeks after the operation to detect residual stones. If no stones are found, the T-Tube is removed. If residual stones are found on the T-Tube cholangiography, the T-Tube tract is left to mature for 10–12 weeks. Then, a choledochoscopy through the tract is performed for stone extraction.

Step 5 average time frame: 10–15 min

> ⚠ **PITFALLS**
>
> Incorrect placement of the T-Tube (**Figures 40-13 A, B**):
> - Long distal T-Tube limb that extends through the papilla: this could lead to postoperative pancreatitis
> - Long proximal T-Tube limb: this might result in obstruction of one of the hepatic ducts

Robotic Hepatectomy

The left biliary system is more frequently and severely affected by stones than the right biliary system. Left biliary involvement alone is found in 40% of cases of intrahepatic disease, right biliary system involvement alone in 20%, and involvement of both systems in 40%. No satisfactory explanation has been offered for this finding. However, it has been suggested that the left bile duct is more horizontal, and bile in the left duct may not drain as well as bile in the right duct. Therefore, hepatic resection for RPC is usually a left lateral sectionectomy, and sometimes a left hepatectomy when ductal strictures are already near the confluence of the right and left ducts. The technique of partial hepatectomy for RPC is no different from the standardized procedures (see Chapter 34, Left Hepatectomy, and Chapter 35, Liver Sectionectomies) (**Figure 40-14**). Partial hepatectomy for RPC might be technically challenging due to multiple previous operations, repeated infections, perihepatic adhesions, and distorted liver anatomy due to liver hypertrophy and atrophy.

FIGURE 40-11 • Closure of the choledochotomy.

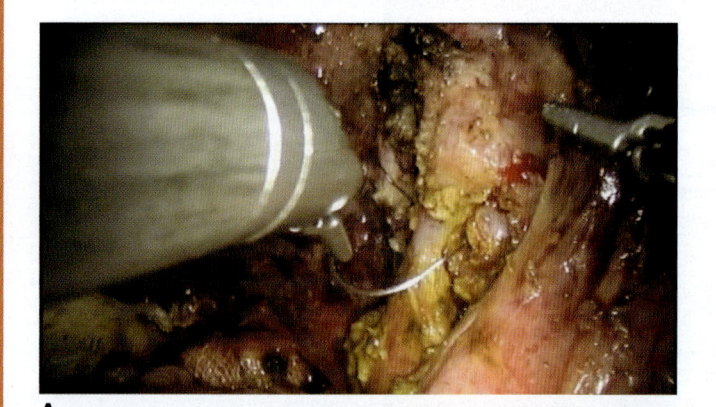

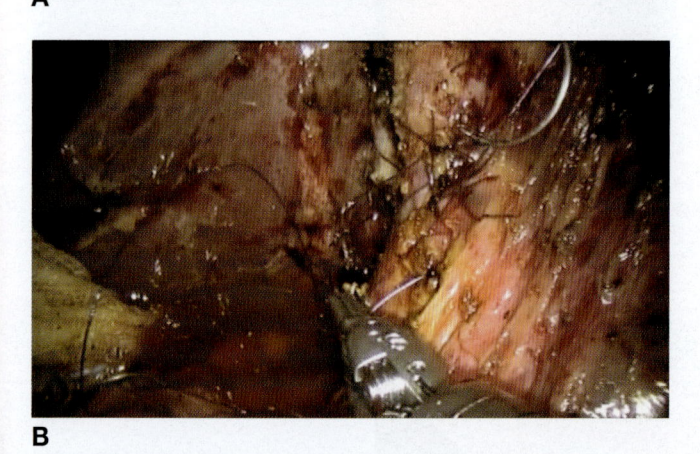

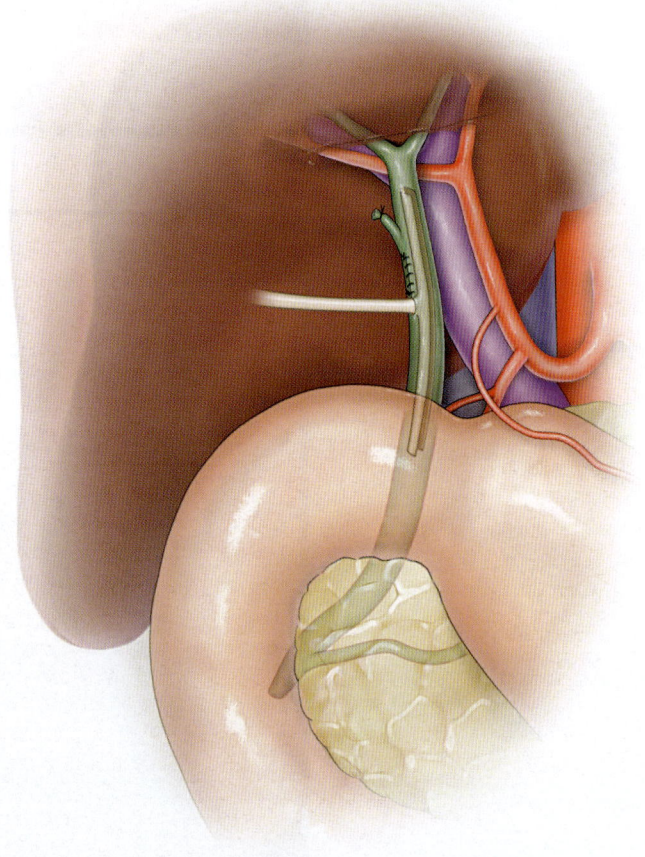

FIGURE 40-12 • T-Tube placement.

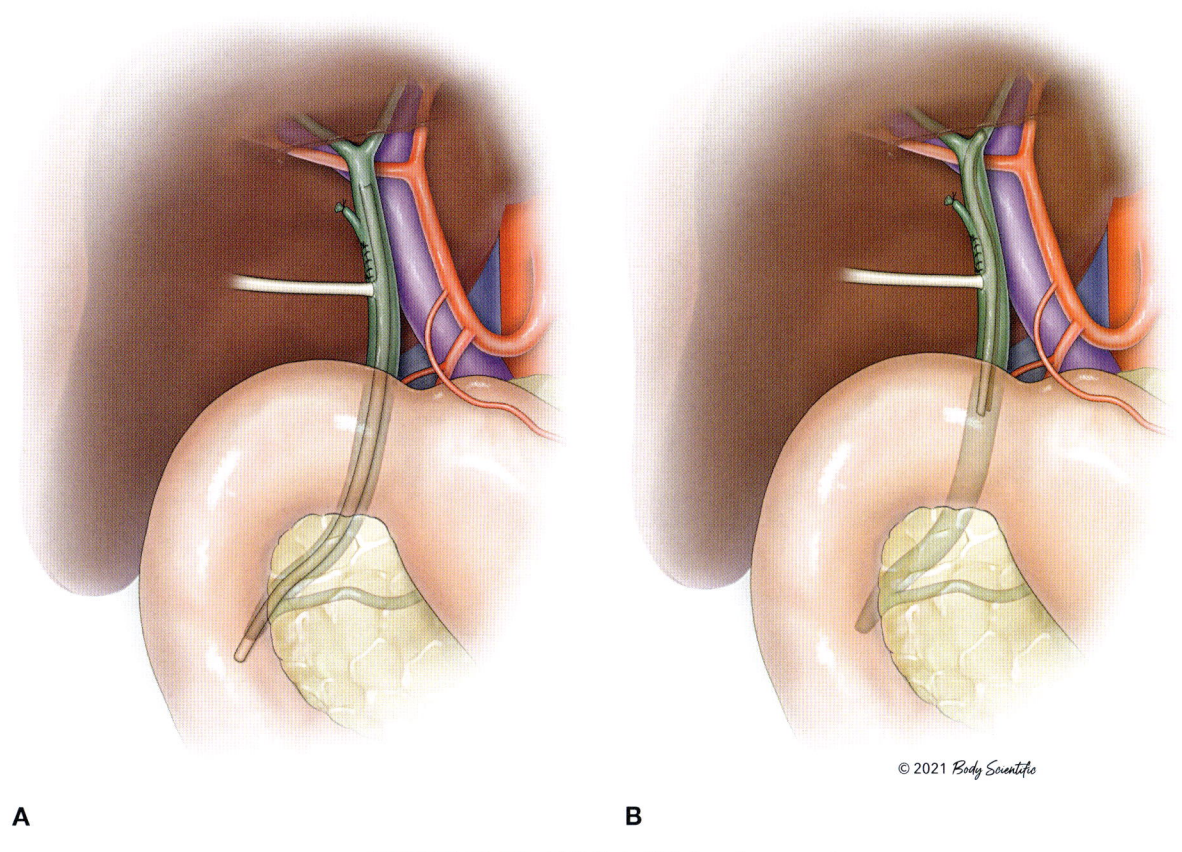

FIGURE 40-13 • Pitfalls in T-Tube placement.

Bile Duct Exploration After Hepatectomy

After the hepatectomy, the choledochoscope can be passed through the main intrahepatic duct over the resection plane to check for any residual stones or strictures (**Figures 40-15 A, B**). The choledochoscope might be inserted through an additional dedicated port or the R2. Biliary stones are removed by robotic forceps, basket, balloon extraction, or saline flushing under choledochoscopic guidance. Large impacted stones are removed after electrohydraulic lithotripsy. After complete clearance of the biliary system, the bile ductal opening of the transection plane is closed with 3-0 absorbable sutures. Perihepatic Jackson-Pratt drains are left close to the resection line.

Hepaticojejunostomy

Hepaticojejunostomy is performed in selected patients to eliminate bile stasis and prevent stone recurrence or to tackle those strictures in the CHD or CBD (see Chapter 38, Roux-en-Y Hepaticojejunostomy). A hepaticojejunostomy is also constructed with the hope of providing adequate passage of newly formed intrahepatic stones. Reoperation for recurrence of stones after hepaticojejunostomy becomes increasingly difficult and risky. Hepaticocutaneous jejunostomy is a possible option for future choledochoscope access. Percutaneous access to the biliary tract may be achieved by flexible choledochoscopy if the Roux-en-Y limb of the hepaticojejunostomy is fixed to the abdominal wall and opened as a stoma. Through the stoma, it is possible to remove recurrent stones and to perform biliary stricture dilatation. The stoma is closed and buried under the skin with radiopaque marking. This will facilitate a new stoma construction (for diagnostic and therapeutic purposes) when recurrence of the disease is suspected (**Figures 40-16 A, B**).

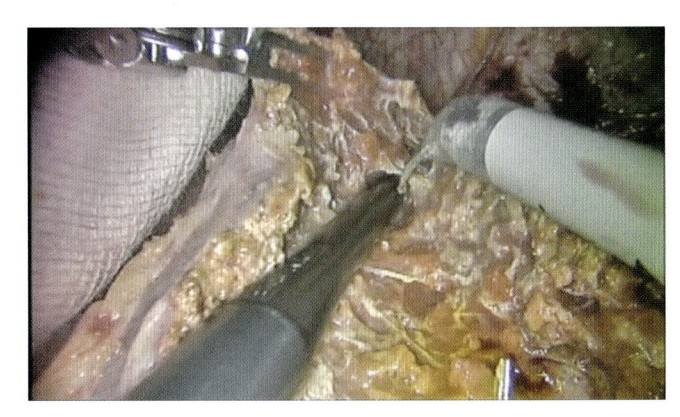

FIGURE 40-14 • Hepatectomy for RPC.

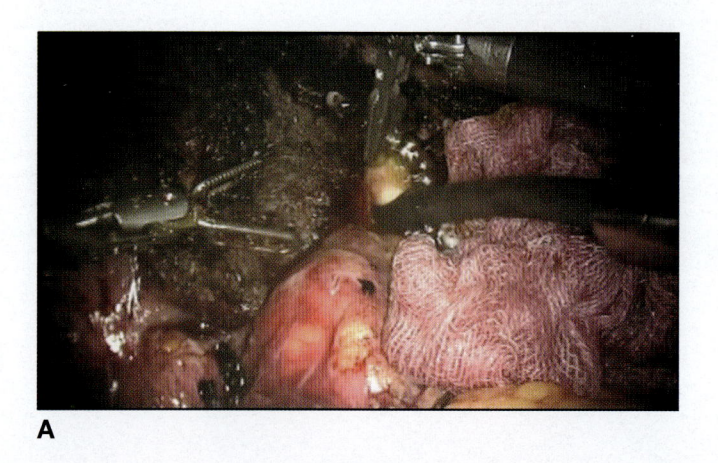

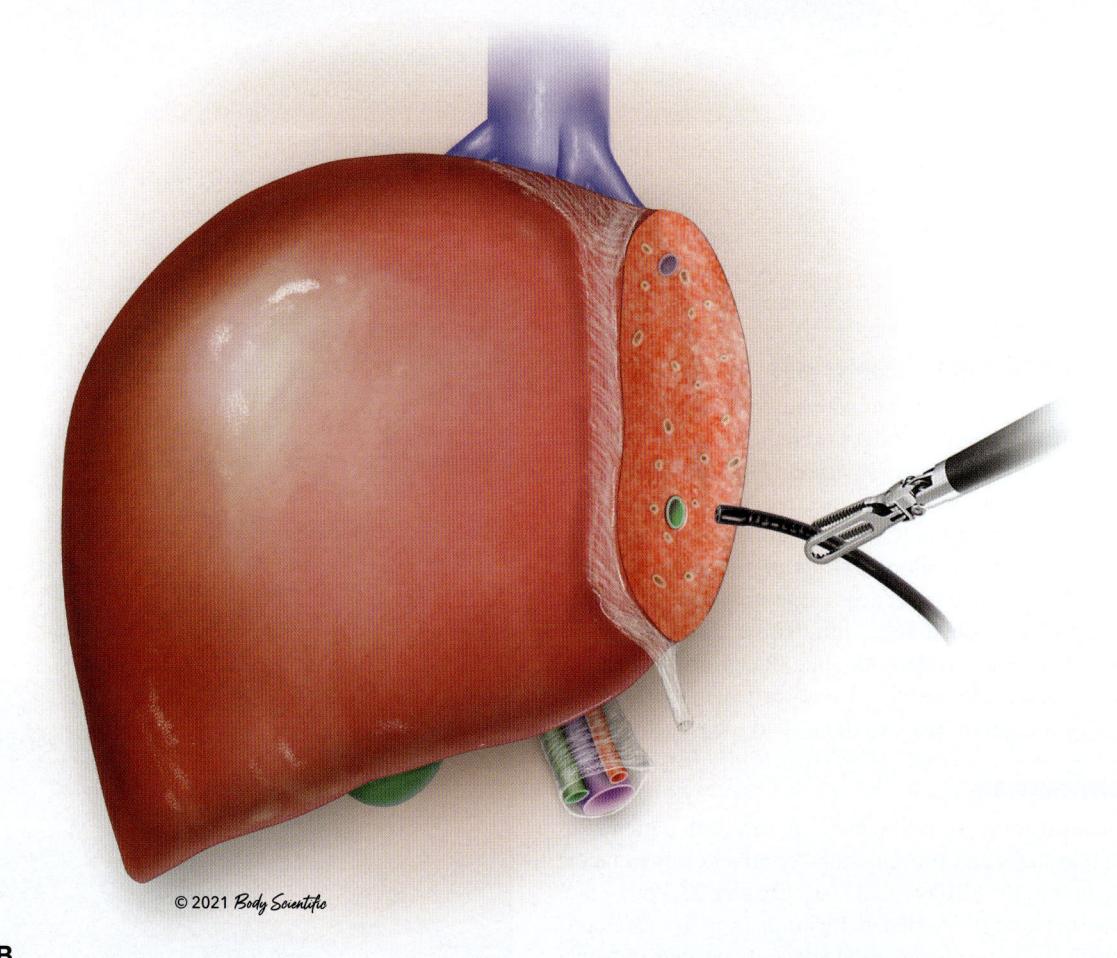

FIGURE 40-15 • Choledochoscopy through the hepatic resection line.

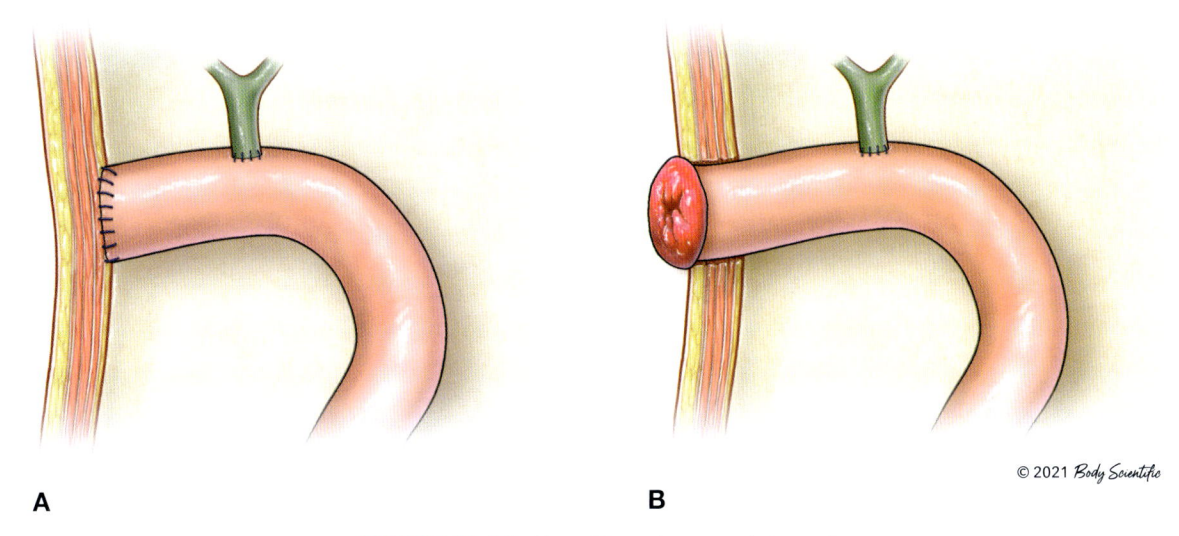

FIGURE 40-16 • Hepaticocutaneous jejunostomy.

Suggested Readings

1. Takada T, Uchida Y, Fukushima Y, et al. Classification and treatment of intrahepatic calcali. *Jap J Gastroenterol Surg.* 1978;11:769-774.
2. Digby KH. Common-duct stones of liver origin. *Br J Surg.* 1930;17:578-591.
3. Cook J, Hou PC, Ho HC, et al. Recurrent pyogenic cholangeitis. *Br J Surg.* 1954;42:188-203.
4. Lau WY, Leow CK. Management of recurrent pyogenic cholangitis. In: Poston GJ, Blumgart LH, eds. *Surgical Management of Hepatobiliary and Pancreatic Disorders.* Martin Dunitz; 2003:237-249.
5. Fan ST, Lai EC, Wong J. Hepatic resection for hepatolithiasis. *Arch Surg.* 1993;128:1070-1074.
6. Fan ST, Mok F, Zheng SS, et al. Appraisal of hepaticocutaneous jejunostomy in the management of hepatolithiasis. *Am J Surg.* 1993;165:332-335.
7. Tang CN, Siu WT, Ha JP, et al. Laparoscopic biliary bypass–a single centre experience. *Hepatogastroenterology.* 2007;54:503-507.
8. Tang CN, Tai CK, Ha JP, et al. Laparoscopy versus open left lateral segmentectomy for recurrent pyogenic cholangitis. *Surg Endosc.* 2005;19:1232-1236.
9. Tang CN, Tai CK, Siu WT, et al. Laparoscopic treatment of recurrent pyogenic cholangitis. *J Hepatobiliary Pancreat Surg.* 2005;12:243-248.
10. Tang CN, Li MK. Hand-assisted laparoscopic segmentectomy in recurrent pyogenic cholangitis. *Surg Endosc.* 2003;17:324-327.
11. Lai EC, Tang CN, Yang GP, et al. Laparoscopic approach of surgical treatment for primary hepatolithiasis: a cohort study. *Am J Surg.* 2010;199:716-721.
12. Lai EC, Tang CN, Yang GP, et al. Approach to manage the complications of choledochoduodenostomy: robot-assisted laparoscopic Roux-en-Y hepaticojejunostomy. *Surg Laparosc Endosc Percutan Tech.* 2011;21:e228-231.
13. Giulianotti PC, Coratti A, Angelini M, et al. Robotics in general surgery: personal experience in a large community hospital. *Arch Surg.* 2003;138(7):777-784. doi: 10.1001/archsurg.138.7.777

SECTION IX

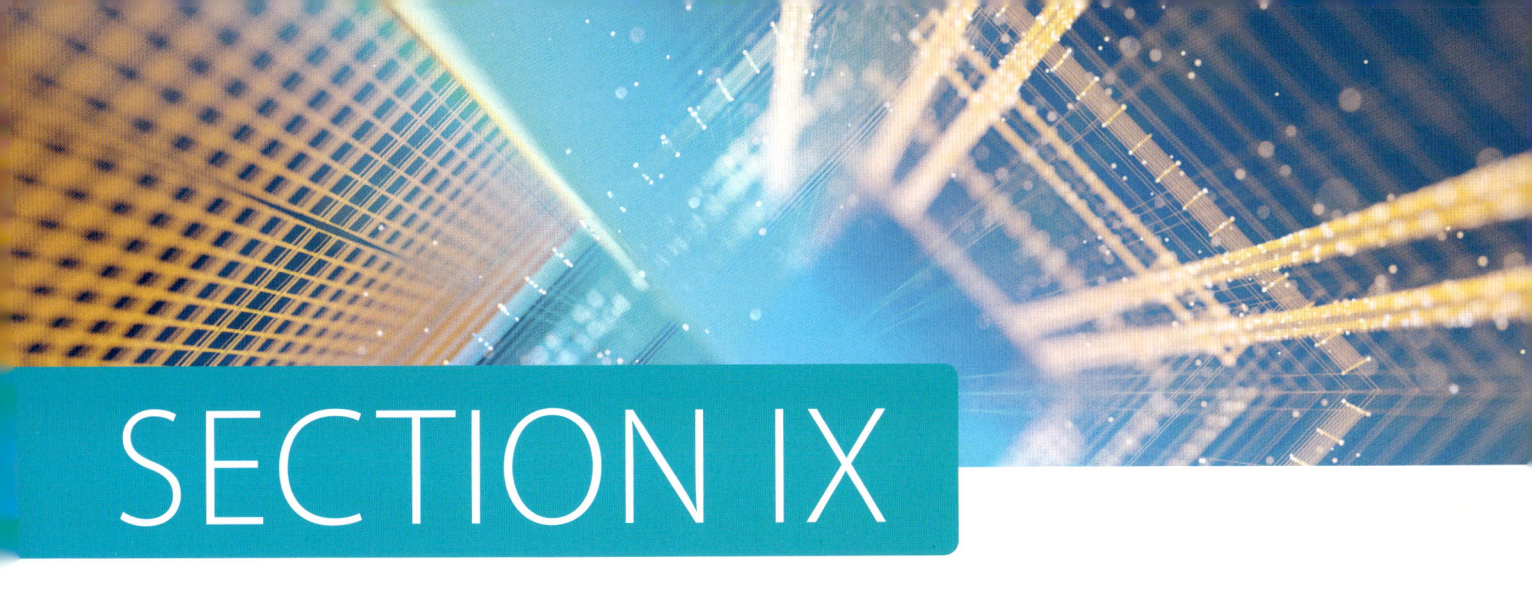

Adrenal Surgery

Chapter 41 • Right Adrenalectomy 863
Francesco Maria Bianco • Yevhen Pavelko • Alberto Mangano • Pier Cristoforo Giulianotti

Chapter 42 • Left Adrenalectomy 879
Francesco Maria Bianco • Yevhen Pavelko • Valentina Valle • Pier Cristoforo Giulianotti

"Regardless of the method, knowledge of anatomy, meticulous hemostasis, and delicate tissue handling are essential in making any form of adrenal surgery successful."

—Michel Gagner (1960)

Right Adrenalectomy

Francesco Maria Bianco • Yevhen Pavelko • Alberto Mangano • Pier Cristoforo Giulianotti

INTRODUCTION

Since the first description of a laparoscopic adrenalectomy by Gagner in 1992, this approach has constantly gained popularity, becoming the gold standard for both benign and selected malignant adrenal lesions. The laparoscopic technique has been shown to be safe and feasible with comparable results to the open approach, also for oncological indications, although controversy persists with regard to adrenal carcinomas.

Multiple studies demonstrate minimal morbidity, shorter hospital stay, excellent cosmesis, and a significantly lower catecholamine surge during pheochromocytoma dissection with a minimally invasive approach. Since the first robotic adrenalectomy performed by Giulianotti in 2000, there has been growing evidence that shows that this approach is safe and effective. The robotic approach presents clear advantages in terms of fine dissection of the vascular structures and when working in a deep narrow space as during adrenalectomies. This allows expansion of the indications for a minimally invasive approach to patients with a higher body mass index (BMI) (>30–35 kg/m^2) or larger tumors or in adrenal-sparing surgery. Different approaches to minimally invasive adrenalectomies have been described: anterior, lateral, and retroperitoneal. In this chapter, the anterior transabdominal approach will be described as the preferred method.

Indications and Relative Contraindications to the Robotic Approach

The indications for the robotic approach are closely related to the surgeon's experience. At the beginning of the learning curve, which is estimated to be around 20 cases, it is important to select smaller nonmalignant lesions. As experience grows for both the surgeon and the surgical team, more complex cases can be performed while maintaining optimal outcomes and cost effectiveness. The robot-assisted approach is appropriate for the treatment of the following benign adrenal masses:

- Aldosteronoma; glucocorticoid, androgen, estrogen-producing adenomas; paragangliomas, and rare lesions such as myelolipomas
- Pheochromocytoma (size of the lesion is based on surgeon's experience)
- Any lesion <4 cm with significant growth (>1 cm) or with hormonal activity
- Any lesion >4 cm

INSTRUMENT REQUIREMENTS

The suggested main robotic instruments/tools can be listed as follows:
- 30° scope
- Cautery hook/monopolar curved scissors
- Bipolar forceps
- Needle driver
- Vessel sealer
- Robotic linear staplers (with different loads)
- Cadiére/ProGrasp
- Round tip scissors
- Medium/large clip applier

The suggested main laparoscopic instruments/tools can be listed as follows:
- Scissors
- Needle driver
- Graspers
- Suction-irrigation

Supplemental materials:
- Sponges
- Clips
- Endo Bags™
- Hem-o-lok® clips
- Sutures: Prolene® 3-0/4-0
- Penrose
- Vessel loops

Photo reproduced with permission from Gagner M, Shikora S. Michel Gagner—Biography. Obes Surg. 2016;26(8):1657-1658.
Quote reproduced with permission from Gagner M, Pomp A, Heniford BT, et al. Laparoscopic adrenalectomy: lessons learned from 100 consecutive procedures. Ann Surg. 1997;226(3):238-246.

Indications regarding malignant tumors and metastases removal are more dependent on the surgeon's experience. Intracapsular primary malignancy, as well as solitary metastases without evidence of local invasion, can be approached robotically. Although there are no strict criteria regarding the size of the lesions, this indication is recommended for an expert high-volume surgeon.

The relative contraindications can be listed as follows:

- Very bulky lesions >12–15 cm
- Extracapsular malignant disease with evidence of minimal invasion to adjacent viscera, lymph nodes, or vascular structures

There are some scenarios that contraindicate the robotic operation:

- Larger infiltrative adrenal tumor
- Mass with local invasion of major vessels and/or nearby organs
- Multiple metastases involving not just the adrenal gland

>> **TIPS**

Pheochromocytomas represent a special challenge. The size and secretory activity of the lesions can increase the complexity of the procedure and require more skills to perform a precise delicate resection.

Patient Positioning, OR Setup, and Port Setting

The patient is positioned supine with both arms tucked as shown in **Figure 41-1A**. The assistant is working from the left side of the patient. The OR setup is explained in **Figure 41-1B**.

Pneumoperitoneum is achieved using a Veress needle placed in the left subcostal space at the modified Palmer's point (see Chapter 2, The Basic Principles of Clinical Applications). After induction of pneumoperitoneum, a 5-mm port is placed with OptiView™ technique in the left upper quadrant. An initial abdominal exploration, using a 5-mm laparoscope, is useful to assess for peritoneal metastases, advanced disease, or other signs of unresectability. This step is also important to assess

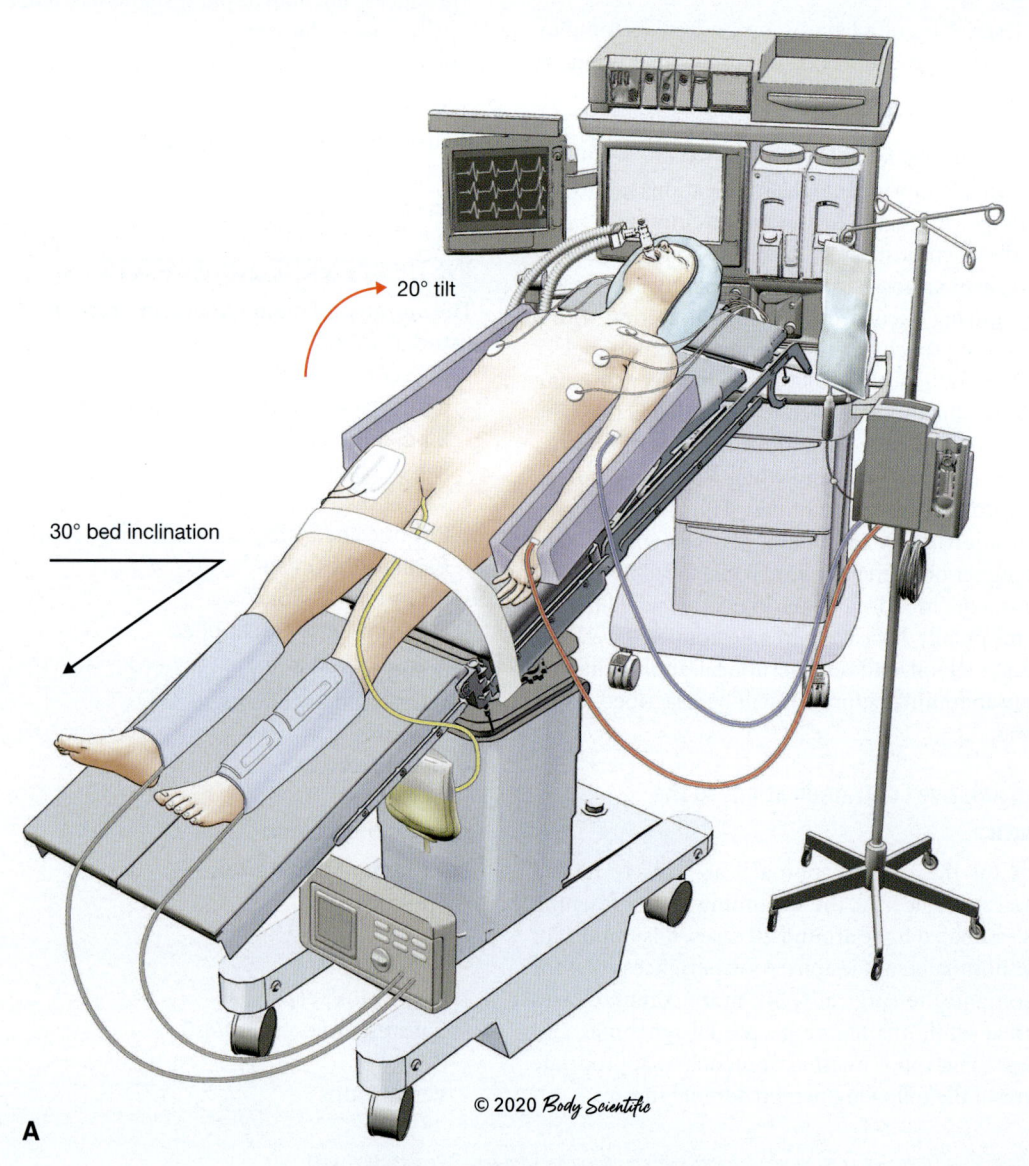

FIGURE 41-1 • A. Patient positioning.

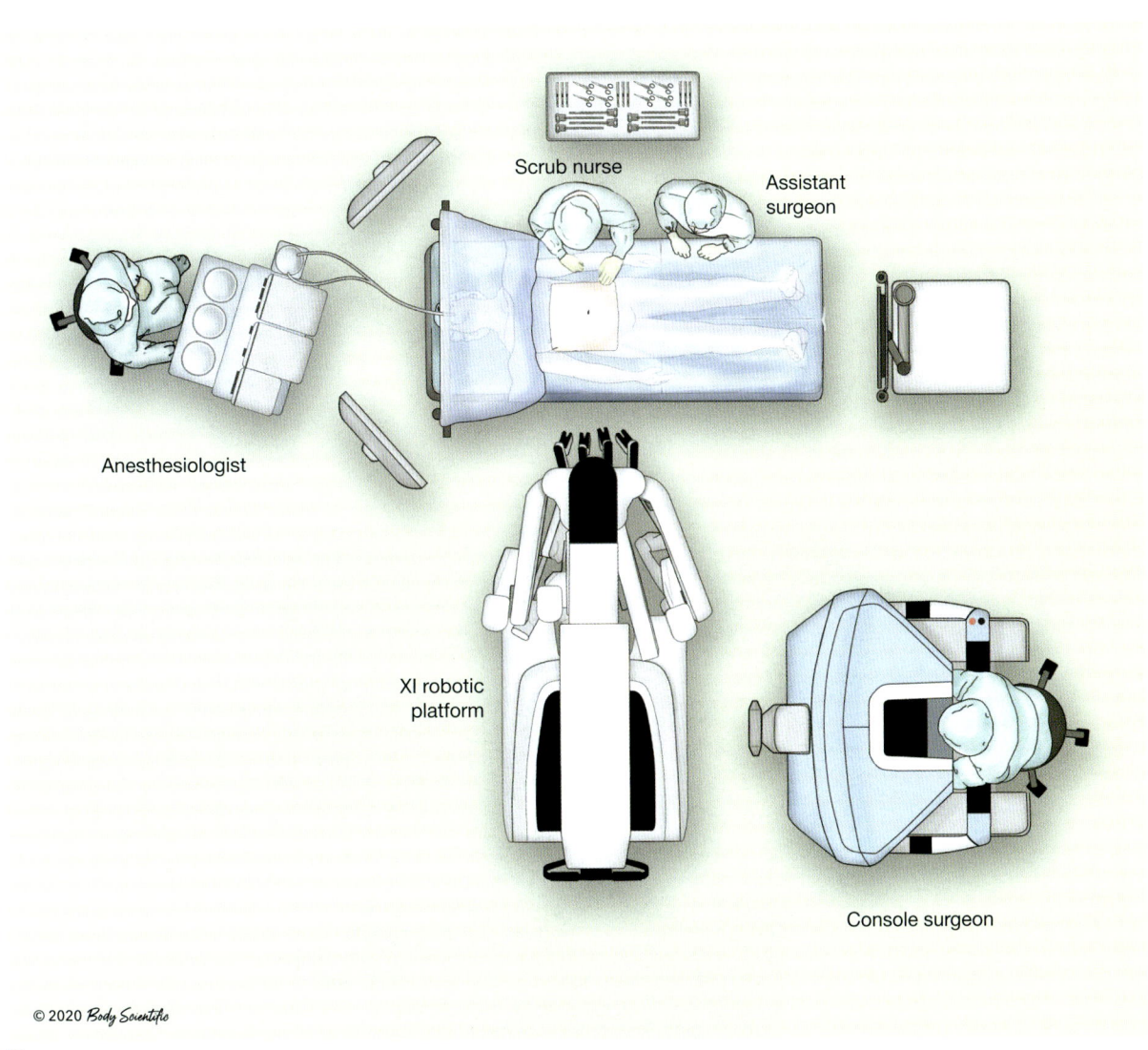

FIGURE 41-1 • *(Continued)* **B.** OR setting.

the anatomy, to address possible peritoneal adhesions, and to understand if the planned technique or the port placement setting needs to be modified. A total of five/six trocars, depending on the complexity of the operation, are inserted under direct visualization, as shown in **Figures 41-2 A, B** for normal and wide abdomen, respectively.

The camera port is placed in the right upper quadrant, along the right pararectal line with an ideal angle of 45° toward the surgical target. Three 8-mm operative ports are located along an oblique line going straight from the upper left to the lower right quadrant. The first 8-mm port is positioned lateral to the camera port on the right side. The second and third working ports are placed in the left upper quadrant. The assistant 12-mm port is introduced at the periumbilical area. The second optional assistant port (5 mm) is positioned slightly lateral and lower to the camera port on the right.

Following the port settings, the bed is placed in reverse Trendelenburg 30° and tilted 20° to the left side. The robotic cart is docked.

> ▶▶ **TIPS**
>
> If adhesions are present at the initial exploration, additional ports may be placed to perform adhesiolysis and clear the working space. (See Chapter 2, The Basic Principles of Clinical Applications, for a comprehensive description of the different operative strategies.)

> ▶▶ **TIPS**
>
> The anterior approach with the patient supine is generally preferred to the one with full lateral decubitus. Although the supine position doesn't allow gravity to retract the colon and requires a more active retraction by the assistant, it has the great advantage to allow better exposure of the retrocaval space between the inferior vena cava (IVC) and the adrenal gland. This space is less accessible with the patient in the lateral position because gravity tends to close it. Opening this space while detaching the gland allows for a safer dissection and better control of the anatomy.

Normal abdomen

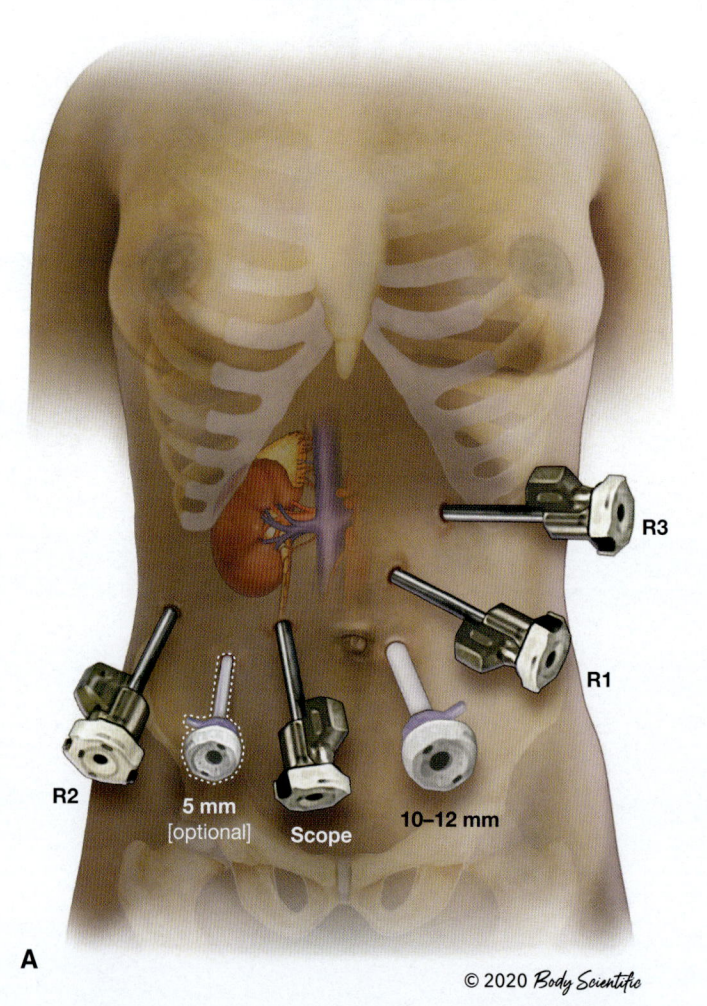

FIGURE 41-2 • **A.** Trocars setting normal abdomen.

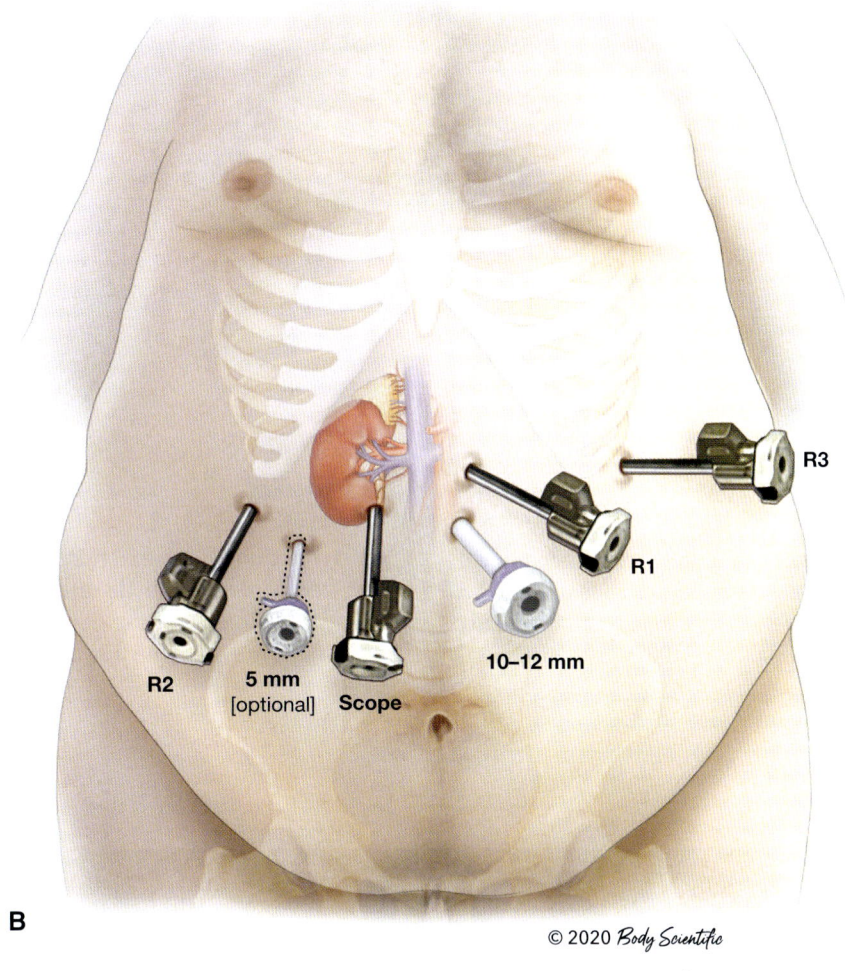

FIGURE 41-2 • *(Continued)* **B.** Trocars setting wide abdomen.

Surgical Technique

▶ **Video 41-1.** Right Adrenalectomy – Full Procedure

▶ **Video 41-2.** Right Adrenalectomy Bulky Lesion

Step 1. Mobilization of the right colonic flexure

The operation starts by retracting the liver cephalad and medially using the third robotic arm (R3). The right colonic flexure is taken down using a combination of monopolar energy and bipolar forceps. The dissection is carried out along the Toldt's fascia, and it is extended inferiorly and laterally to the ascending colon and medially until the second portion of the duodenum is clearly visualized. During this step, the assistant retracts the colon caudally and medially using atraumatic graspers.

Step 1 average time frame: 10–15 min

>> **TIPS**

The liver is retracted using a sponge that is introduced by the assistant at the beginning of the procedure. This is grasped by the R3 in order to apply safe retraction without damaging the hepatic parenchyma. This is particularly helpful in large and soft fatty livers more prone to be injured.

Step 2. Partial Kocher maneuver

The IVC is one of the major anatomical landmarks of the procedure. For this reason, a proper exposure is of critical importance. The second portion of the duodenum can partially cover the IVC or even extend far behind to the right lateral edge. At the very least, a partial Kocher maneuver is necessary in these situations, as shown in **Figure 41-3**.

▶ **Video 41-3.** Step 2. Partial Kocher Maneuver

When the duodenum is in a favorable position, however, the Kocher maneuver might be minimal or rarely avoidable altogether. The monopolar hook or monopolar scissors combined with the bipolar forceps are the main instruments to perform the dissection. The R3 retracts the liver cephalad and medially while the assistant retracts the colon medially. The dissection begins at the duodenum and the head of the pancreas, moving caudally until the right renal vein is identified.

Step 2 average time frame: 5–10 min

>> **TIPS**

When the duodenum extends beyond the IVC, the assistant can facilitate the dissection by gently retracting the second portion of the duodenum medially using an atraumatic grasper with a sponge.

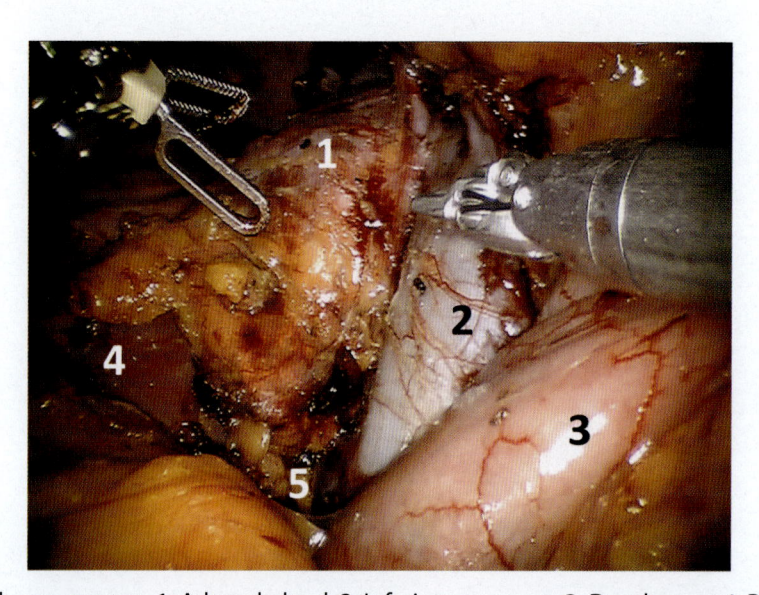

FIGURE 41-3 • Partial Kocher maneuver. 1. Adrenal gland. 2. Inferior vena cava. 3. Duodenum. 4. Right kidney. 5. Renal vein.

Step 3. Mobilization of the liver

The mobilization of the liver is necessary to achieve adequate exposure of the retrohepatic segment of the IVC where the critical anatomy of the adrenal venous drainage is located. The right triangular ligament and the posterior coronary ligament can be partially taken down. The dissection should be extended until an adequate exposure of the IVC is achieved.

Proper mobilization of the liver and visualization of the IVC allow better understanding of the adrenal vein anatomy and recognition of possible anatomical variations.

Step 3 average time frame: 5–10 min

> ▶▶ **TIPS**
>
> Besides providing exposure, a proper mobilization of the liver will reduce the risk of tearing the liver capsule, by pushing and pulling forces on fixed liver parenchyma.
>
> For some large tumors, the mobilization of the liver may be extended all the way up to the diaphragm in order to achieve complete control of the IVC.
>
> The R3 facilitates this step by retracting the right liver. Frequent repositioning of the instrument controlled by the R3 will maintain ideal exposure as the dissection progresses, as shown in **Figures 41-4 A, B**.

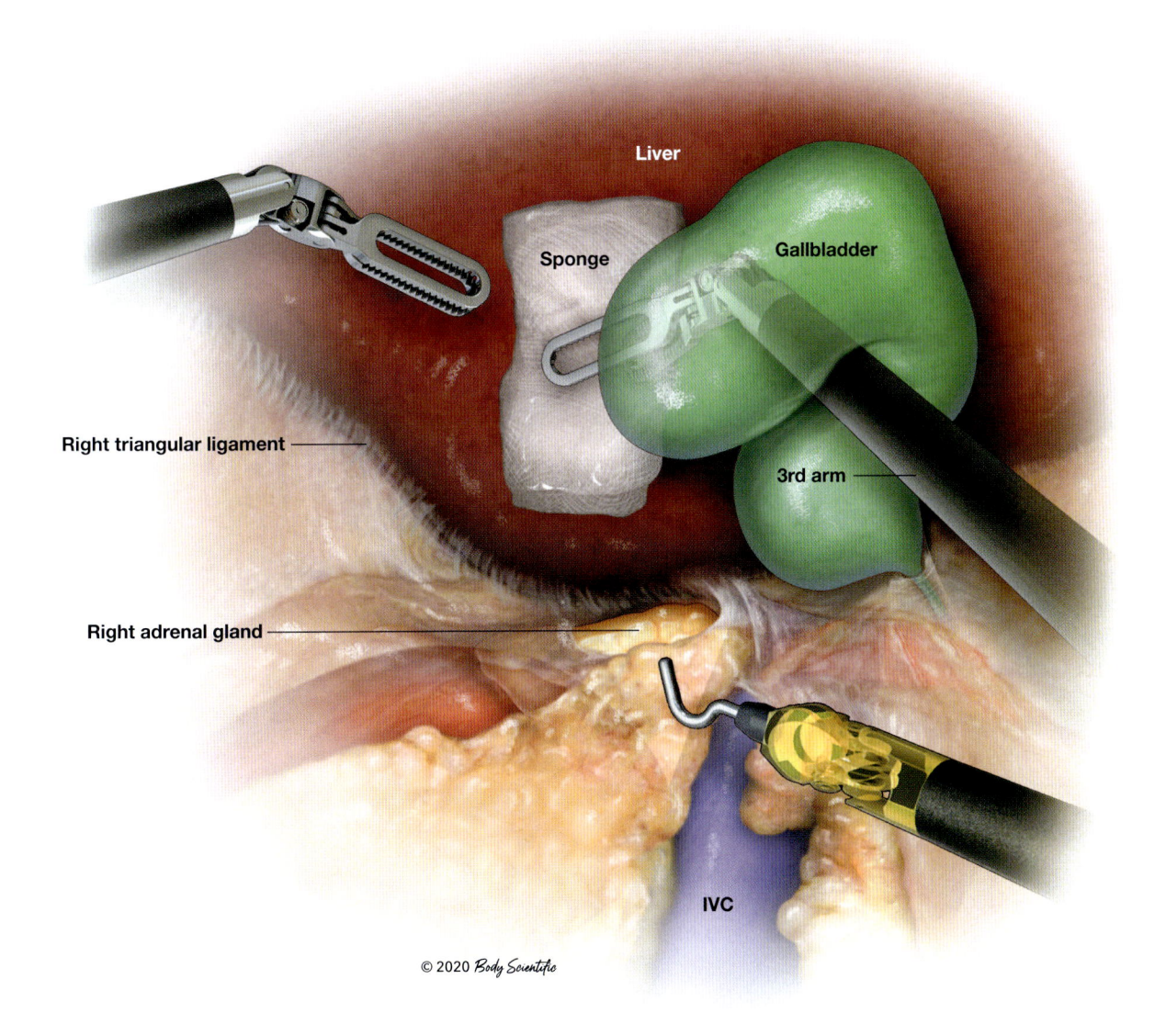

A

FIGURE 41-4 • **A.** Liver retraction.

870 The Foundation and Art of Robotic Surgery

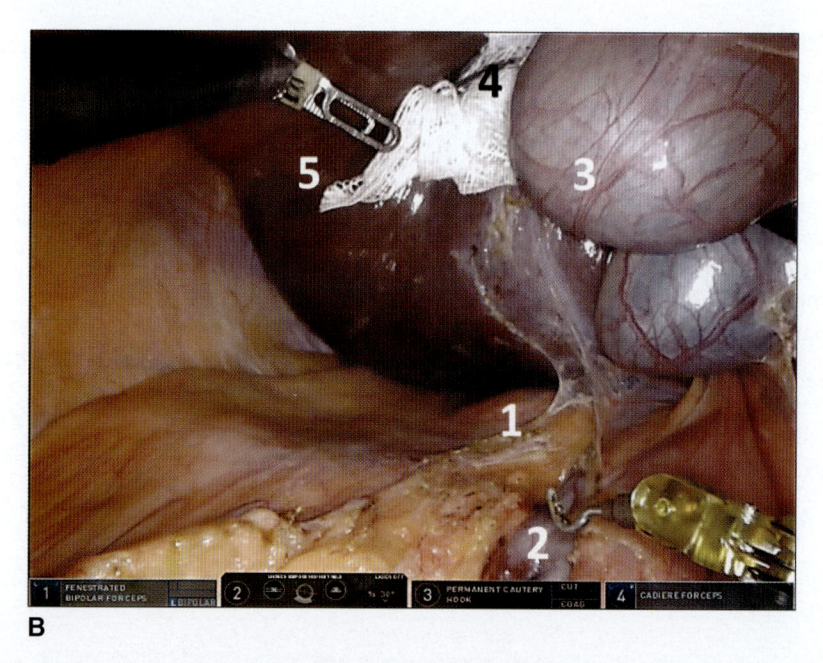

FIGURE 41-4 • (Continued) B. Liver retraction. 1. Adrenal gland. 2. Inferior vena cava. 3. Gallbladder. 4. The area where the R3 is retracting a liver. 5. Liver.

Step 4. Identification of the anatomical landmarks

After completing the mobilization of the liver, it is important to reassess the anatomical landmarks: IVC medially with a good understanding of the retrohepatic space including accessory hepatic veins, the renal vein inferiorly, and the adrenal main vein medial to the adrenal gland, as shown in **Figure 41-5**.

Perirenal adipose tissue between the renal vein and artery can be bluntly separated to better understand the position of the renal artery and the inflow to the gland.

Step 4 average time frame: 5–10 min

▶▶ TIPS

A preliminary evaluation of the anatomy of the kidney and its blood supply should be carefully conducted on the preoperative computed tomography (CT) scan. This allows identification of possible anomalies like multiple renal arteries and veins or an abnormal course.

⚠ PITFALLS

Inadequate exposure of the IVC and/or of the adrenal vein can lead to blind maneuvers during the dissection and control of the vein. This is a dangerous situation that might cause significant bleeding.

The accessory hepatic veins can be close to the adrenal vein. Supernumerary or anomalous adrenal veins can be present as described in **Figure 41-6**. Failure to recognize those structures can be a source of complications.

Right Adrenalectomy 871

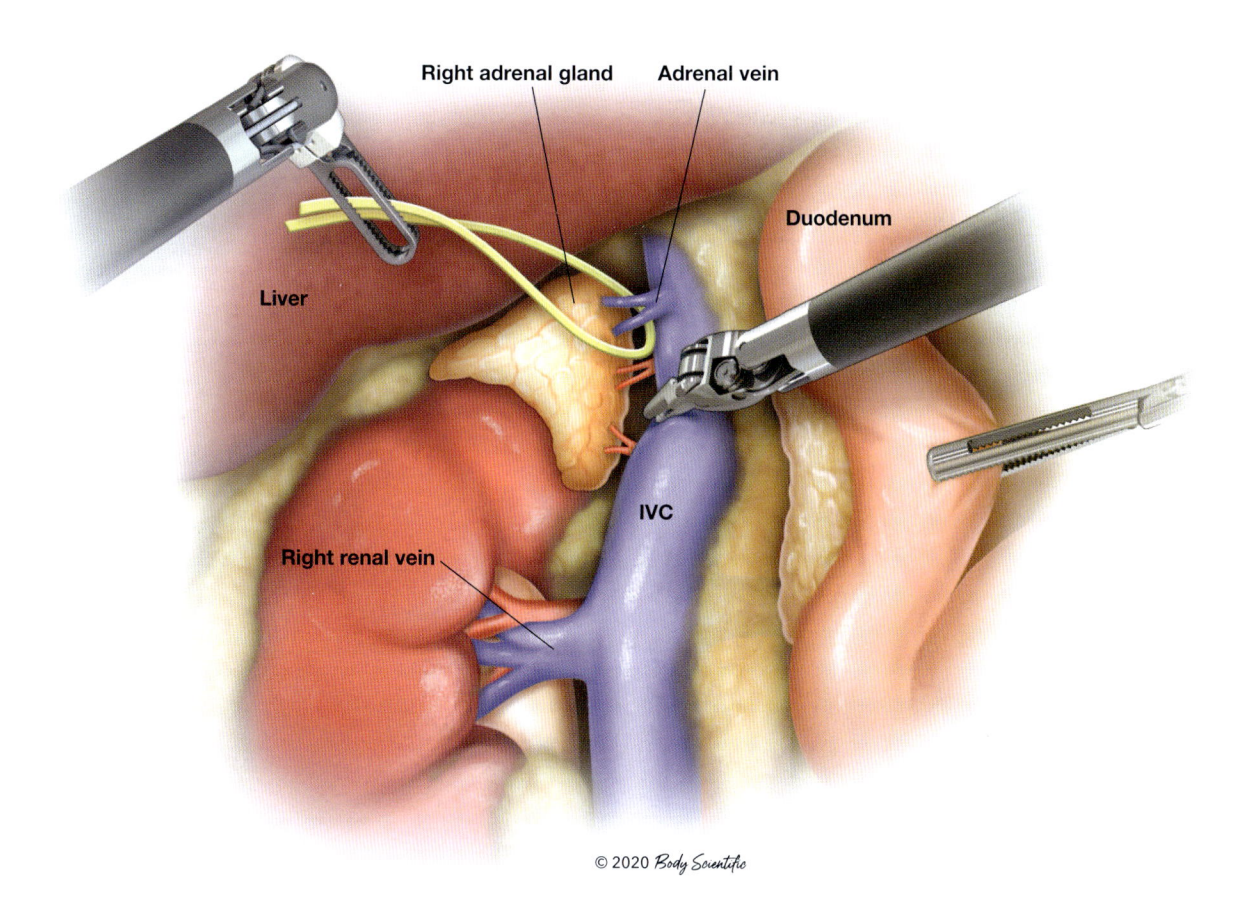

FIGURE 41-5 • Landmark identification.

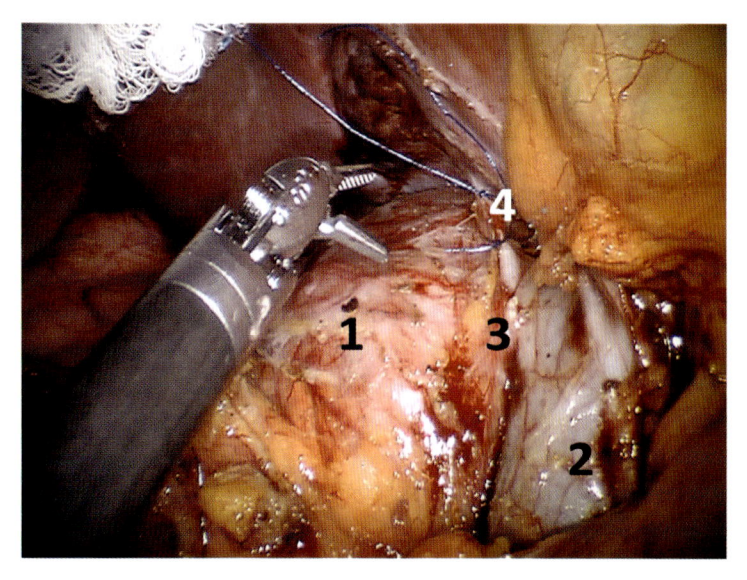

FIGURE 41-6 • Accessory hepatic vein. 1. Adrenal gland. 2. Inferior vena cava. 3. Adrenal vein. 4. Accessory short hepatic vein.

872 The Foundation and Art of Robotic Surgery

> **🔍 ANATOMICAL HIGHLIGHTS**
>
> The right adrenal vein has several potential variations, as described in **Figure 41-7**. Most commonly (80% of cases), it is short and wide and drains directly into the IVC. Other variations include multiple veins with aberrant drainages (2 or 3 veins). In some cases, the adrenal vein can join an accessory hepatic vein and present a common tract going to the IVC. Rarely, the adrenal vein can drain into the right hepatic vein or even the right renal vein. (Multiple anatomical variations can occur, and these can be classified in different ways. Here, the most clinically significant are presented. For more information, see suggested reading #7.)

Type 1 (80%)
- Adrenal vein (AV)
- Inferior vena cava (IVC)
- Right renal vein (RV)
- Right gonadal vein (GV)

Type 2 (9%)
- Right hepatic vein (HV)
- Accessory hepatic vein
- IVC
- AV
- RV

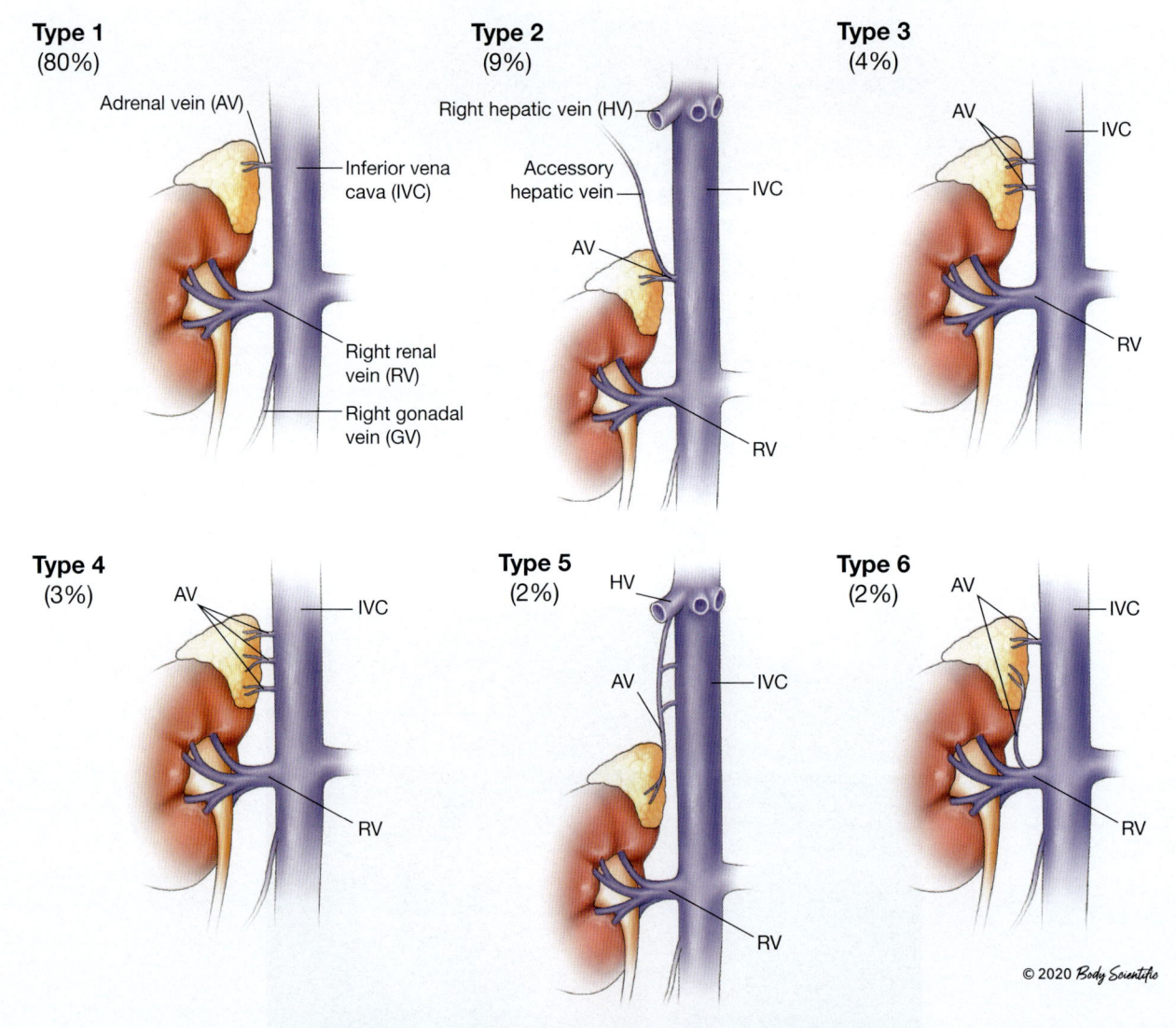

Type 3 (4%)
- AV
- IVC
- RV

Type 4 (3%)
- AV
- IVC
- RV

Type 5 (2%)
- HV
- AV
- IVC
- RV

Type 6 (2%)
- AV
- IVC
- RV

© 2020 Body Scientific

FIGURE 41-7 • Types 1–6. Variations of venous drainage.

Step 5. Exposure of the upper pole of the kidney

The upper pole of the kidney is a safe landmark to start the dissection of the adrenal gland. The attachments between the capsule of the kidney and the adrenal gland are progressively released with a combination of monopolar energy and vessel sealer. The dissection is extended posteriorly underneath the gland, on top of the psoas muscles and laterally, as described in **Figures 41-8 A, B**.

Appropriate exposure of the posterior and lateral planes will facilitate the retraction of the gland during the dissection along the IVC.

Step 5 average time frame: 10–15 min

> ▶▶ **TIPS**
>
> A small amount of adipose tissue can be left attached to the adrenal gland; this tissue can be used for retraction and gentle manipulation. This will also protect the gland better, given the lack of a proper strong capsule.

> ⚠ **PITFALLS**
>
> This step should always follow a clear understanding of the vascular anatomy of the kidney. Some anomalous branches for the upper pole of the kidney could be injured at this point if anatomy is not clear.

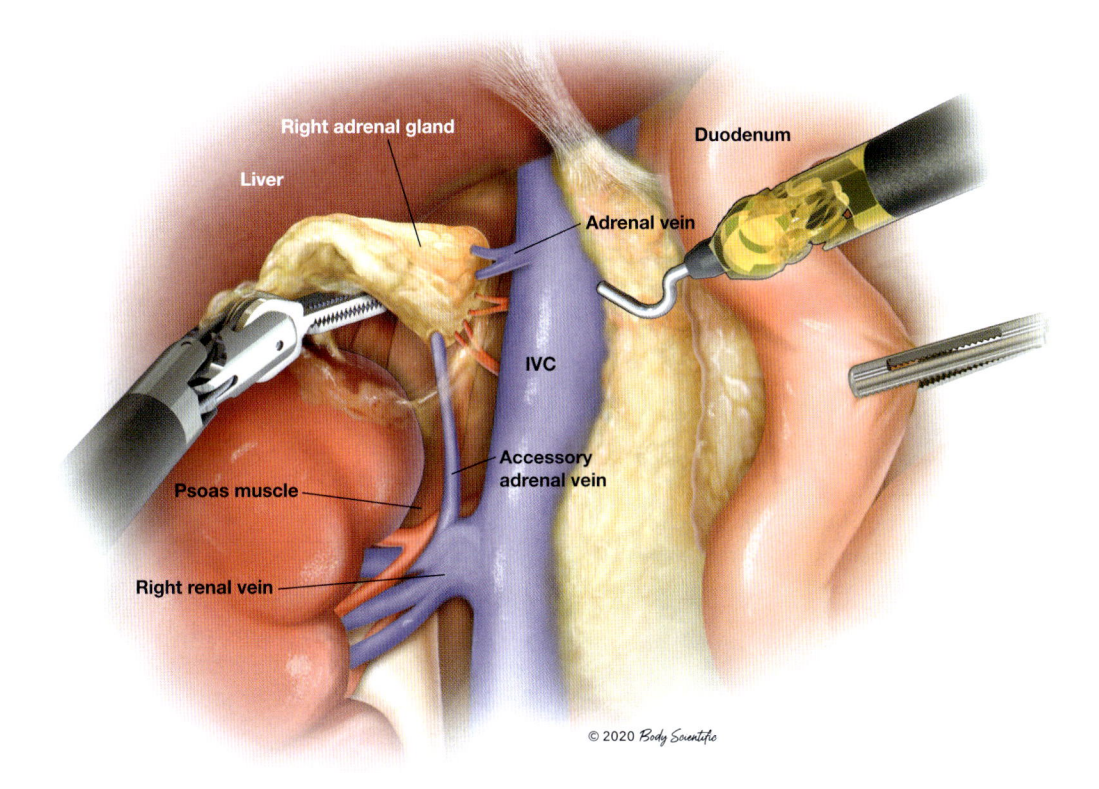

A

FIGURE 41-8 • **A.** Exposure of the upper pole of the kidney.

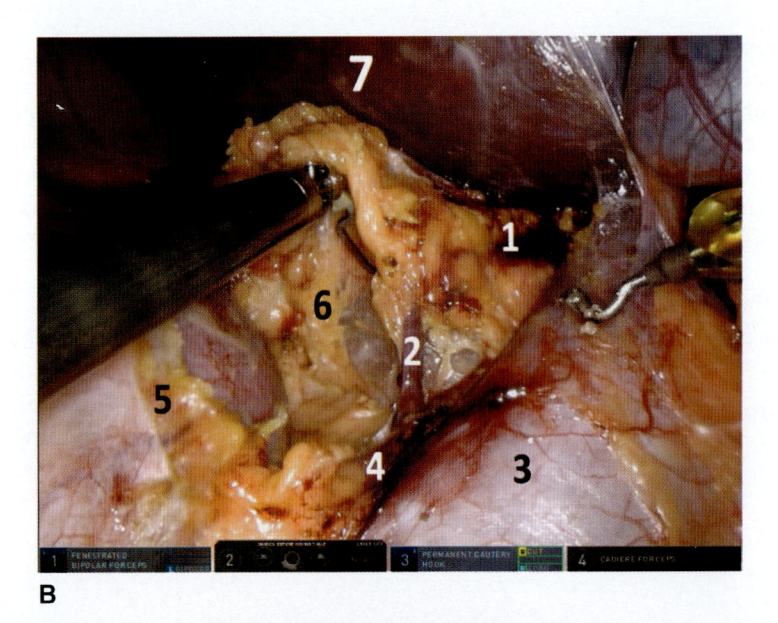

FIGURE 41-8 • (*Continued*) **B.** Exposure of the upper pole of the kidney. 1. Area of the adrenal vein. 2. Accessory adrenal vein merging into the right renal vein. 3. Inferior vena cava. 4. Renal vein. 5. Kidney. 6. Avascular plane on top of the psoas muscle. 7. Liver.

Step 6. Control of inflow

The adrenal gland receives multiple arterial blood vessels originating from the superior suprarenal artery (that comes from the inferior phrenic artery), the middle adrenal artery (from the aorta), and the inferior adrenal arteries (from the renal artery), as described in **Figure 41-9**.

Following the retroperitoneal plane, in front of the psoas muscle, the dissection is extended medially using a vessel sealer that allows good control of the arterial blood supply. The dissection is continued alongside the lateral border of the IVC until the adrenal vein is identified.

Step 6 average time frame: 15–20 min

> ▶▶ **TIPS**
>
> During the dissection along the lateral border of the IVC, an experienced assistant can bluntly retract the vena cava medially, while the console surgeon retracts the adrenal gland laterally holding on to some periadrenal adipose tissue. The careful retraction of the IVC can be performed using a blunt suction device to simultaneously clean the surgical field.

> ▶▶ **TIPS**
>
> During the dissection, some small arterial branches can be accidentally interrupted, causing bleeding. This can be controlled with bipolar coagulation, the vessel sealer, or transfixing sutures.

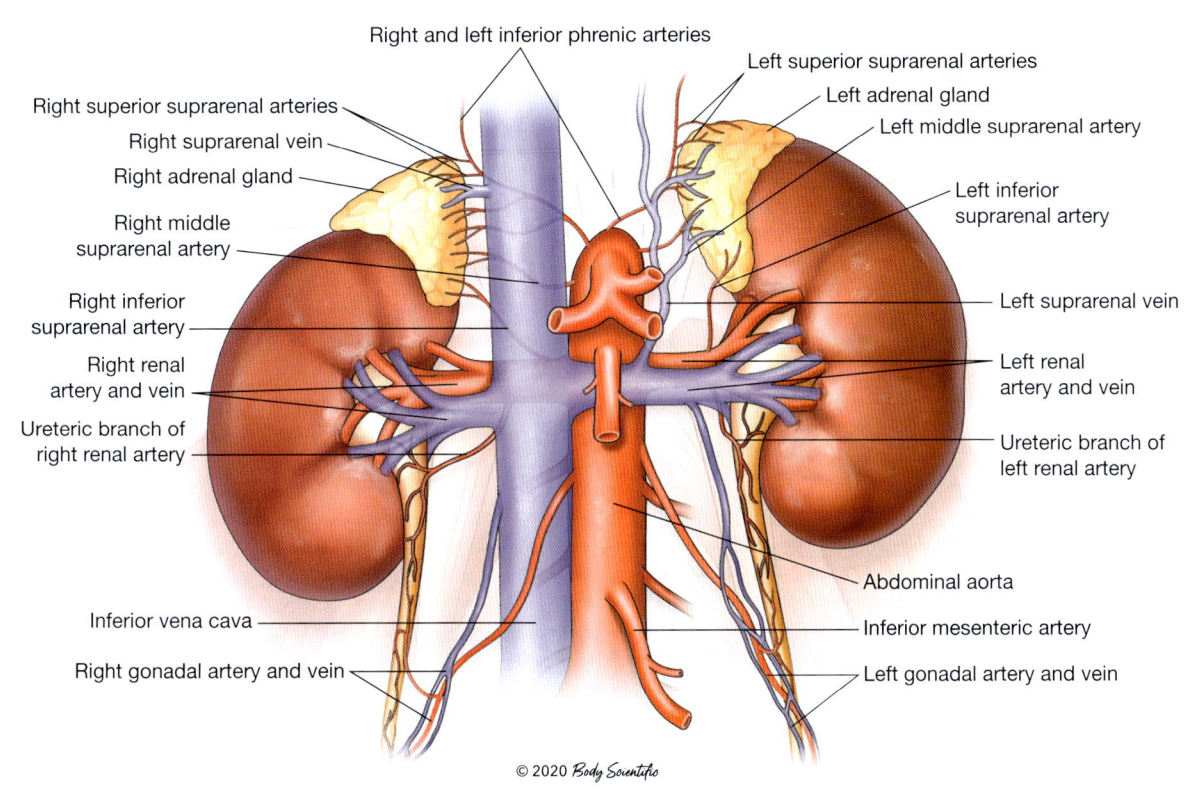

FIGURE 41-9 • Control of inflow.

Step 7. Adrenal vein control

Controlling the adrenal vein prior to gland dissection for pheochromocytomas and hormone-secreting lesions has traditionally been advocated in open surgery where manipulation of the gland cannot be avoided. The robotic technique allows precise and gentle dissection of the gland in a "no touch" fashion. An initial mobilization of the posterior and lateral aspect of the gland facilitates vascular control at the end. A "no touch" dissection can minimize the hormone release in the bloodstream and can delay controlling of the vein until a clear understanding of the anatomy is achieved. Postponing control of the outflow also has the advantage to decrease the congestion of the gland and to reduce backflow bleeding that would reduce visibility. Mastering this technique with easier cases will be fundamental in more challenging situations when dealing with larger or retrocaval lesions.

The dissection of the adrenal vein is meticulously carried out until control of the adrenal vein at the origin of the IVC is achieved.

At this point, the vein is divided between Hem-o-lok® clips or with a stapler, as shown in **Figures 41-10 A, B**, respectively.

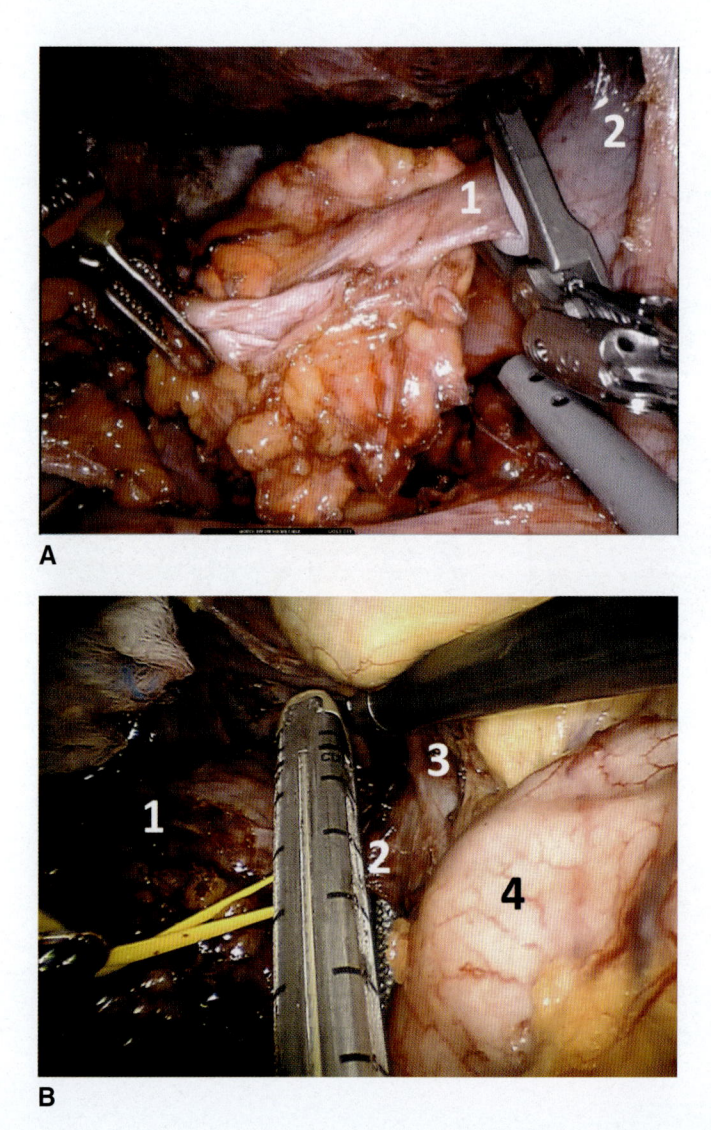

FIGURE 41-10 • **A.** Adrenal vein control with the Hem-o-lok® clip. 1. Adrenal vein. 2. Inferior vena cava. **B.** Adrenal vein control with the stapler. 1. Adrenal gland. 2. Adrenal vein. 3. Inferior vena cava. 4. Duodenum.

▶ **Video 41-4.** Step 7. Adrenal Vein Control with the Hem-o-lok® Clip

▶ **Video 41-5.** Step 7. Adrenal Vein Control with the Stapler

▶ **Video 41-6.** Step 7. Renal Vein Bleeding Control

In some cases, the clip can be reinforced with a suture. The resection of pheochromocytomas or bulky lesions extending into the retrocaval space can be particularly complex because the anatomy is often less clear and achieving adequate retraction can be challenging. In such cases, a "no touch" technique of the posterior and lateral aspect of the gland is the only way to progress with the dissection. This is performed with the vessel sealer while the grasper gently retracts the gland.

Step 7 average time frame: 5–15 min

▶▶ **TIPS**

Bleeding from the IVC during this step can be temporarely controlled by increasing the pressure of CO_2 just enough to overcome the central venous pressure (CVP) and slow down the bleeding (being mindful of the potential small risk of embolism). At this point, a precise suturing with Prolene™ stitches may be necessary. At the end of the procedure, the CO_2 pressure is reduced and the anesthesiologist is making a Valsalva maneuver on the patient in order to increase the CVP and to test the Hemostasis. Hemostasis can be perfected with Prolene™ stitches as shown in **Figure 41-11**.

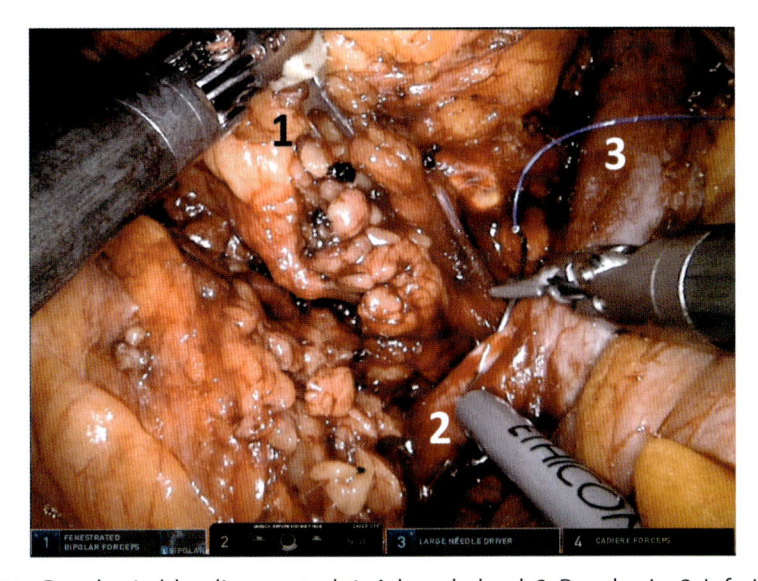

FIGURE 41-11 • Renal vein bleeding control. 1. Adrenal gland. 2. Renal vein. 3. Inferior vena cava.

Step 8. Specimen extraction
After the dissection is completed, the specimen is placed into an Endobag™. The adrenal fossa is irrigated and suctioned for hemostasis verification. The robotic arms are undocked, and the specimen is extracted. For the extraction of a small specimen, it is sufficient to slightly extend the assistant port incision. For larger lesions, the preferred extraction site is a Phannenstiel incision, please refer to the general concepts discussed in Chapter 2, The Basic Principles of Clinical Applications. No drains are usually necessary for this procedure.

Step 8 average time frame: 5–20 min

Suggested Readings

1. Gagner M, Lacroix A, Bolté E. Laparoscopic adrenalectomy in Cushing's syndrome and pheochromocytoma. *N Engl J Med.* 1992;327(14):1033.
2. Brunt LM. Minimal access adrenal surgery. *Surg Endosc.* 2006;20:351-361.
3. Tsuru N, Ushiyama T, Suzuki K. Laparoscopic adrenalectomy for primary and secondary malignant adrenal tumors. *J Endourol.* 2005;19:702-708.
4. Henry JF, Sebag F, Iacobone M, et al. Results of laparoscopic adrenalectomy for large and potentially malignant tumors. *World J Surg.* 2002;26:1043-1047.
5. Stefanidis D, Goldfarb M, Kercher KW, et al. Society of Gastrointestinal and Endoscopic Surgeons. SAGES guidelines for minimally invasive treatment of adrenal pathology. *Surg Endosc.* 2013;27(11):3960-3980. doi: 10.1007/s00464-013-3169-z
6. Lee J, El-Tamer M, Schifftner T, et al. Open and laparoscopic adrenalectomy: analysis of the National Surgical Quality Improvement Program. *J Am Coll Surg.* 2008;206:953-959; discussion 959-961.
7. Scholten A, Cisco RM, Vriens MR, et al. Variant adrenal venous anatomy in 546 laparoscopic adrenalectomies. *JAMA Surg.* 2013;148(4):378-383. doi:10.1001/jamasurg.2013.610
8. Brunaud L, Bresler L, Ayav A, et al. Robotic-assisted adrenalectomy: what advantages compared to lateral transperitoneal laparoscopic adrenalectomy? *Am J Surg.* 2008;195:433-438.
9. Giulianotti PC, Buchs NC, Addeo P, et al. Robot-assisted adrenalectomy: a technical option for the surgeon? *Int J Med Robot.* 2011;7(1):27-32. doi: 10.1002/rcs.364
10. Teo XL, Lim SK. Robotic assisted adrenalectomy: Is it ready for prime time? *Investig Clin Urol.* 2016;57(Suppl 2):S130-S146. doi: 10.4111/icu.2016.57.S2.S130
11. Giulianotti PC, Coratti A, Angelini M, et al. Robotics in general surgery: personal experience in a large community hospital. *Arch Surg.* 2003;138(7):777-784. doi: 10.1001/archsurg.138.7.777. PMID: 12860761.

"We are not making science for science. We are making science for the benefit of humanity."
—Françoise Barré-Sinoussi (1947)

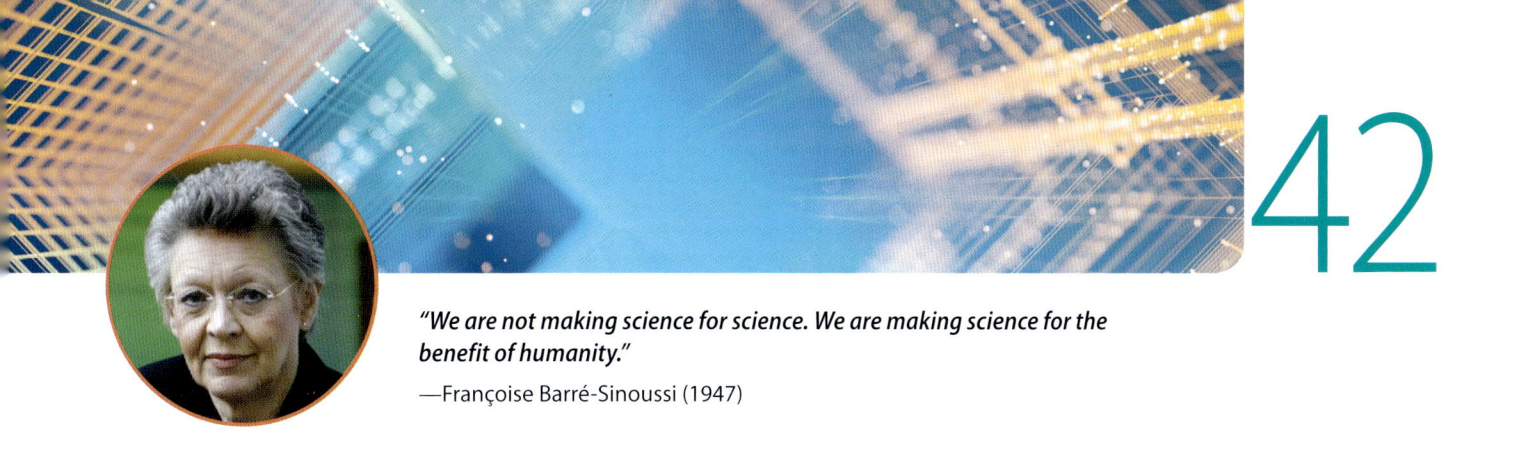

Left Adrenalectomy

Francesco Maria Bianco • Yevhen Pavelko • Valentina Valle • Pier Cristoforo Giulianotti

INTRODUCTION

The adrenal glands are located on both sides of the upper retroperitoneum superior and medially to the kidneys. The left adrenal gland has a semilunar shape with a pyramid conformation and is slightly larger compared to the right adrenal gland. The anatomical relationship of the left gland is also different from the right one. The left adrenal gland is surrounded by the pancreas, aorta, and the left renal vein. Because of this peculiar anatomical position, the technical challenges for left adrenalectomy are different and that is why it is described in a separate chapter from the right adrenalectomy.

Indications and Contraindications to the Robotic Approach

See Chapter 41, Right Adrenalectomy, for a discussion of the indications and contraindications.

INSTRUMENT REQUIREMENTS

The suggested main robotic instruments/tools can be listed as follows:
- 30° scope
- Cautery hook/monopolar curved scissors
- Bipolar forceps
- Needle driver
- Vessel sealer
- Robotic linear staplers (with different loads)
- Cadiére/ProGrasp
- Round tip scissors
- Medium/large clip applier

The suggested main laparoscopic instruments/tools can be listed as follows:
- 5-mm scope
- Scissors
- Needle driver
- Graspers
- Suction-irrigation

Supplemental materials:
- Sponges
- Clips
- Endo Bag™
- Hem-o-lok® clips
- Sutures (Prolene™ 3-0/4-0)
- Penrose
- Vessel loop

Photo reproduced with permission from Institut Pasteur - photo François Gardy.
Quote reproduced with permission from Institut Pasteur.

Surgical Technique

🎥 **Video 42-1.** Left Adrenalectomy – Full Procedure

🎥 **Video 42-2.** Left Adrenalectomy Combined Supra- and Infrapancreatic Approach – Full Procedure

Patient Positioning, OR Setup, and Port Setting

The patient is positioned supine with legs parted and both arms tucked to the side. The stomach is usually decompressed by placing the nasogastric or orogastric tube. A Foley catheter is placed for urinary output control (**Figure 42-1A**).

The assistant sits in between the patient's legs. The OR setup is described in **Figure 42-1B**.

Initial peritoneal access is achieved using the Veress needle technique. The needle is placed in the left subcostal space at the modified Palmer's point (see Chapter 2, The Basic Principles of Clinical Applications). Once the abdomen is insufflated to a pressure of 15 mm Hg, a 5-mm port is placed with the OptiView™ technique in the left upper lateral quadrant where it will be replaced by one of the robotic ports, and an initial abdominal exploration is performed.

A 5-mm 30° laparoscopic scope is inserted, and all 4 abdominal quadrants are assessed for peritoneal metastases, advanced disease, or other signs that might affect the operative plan. The abdominal cavity survey is also important to assess the patient's anatomy and to look for any adhesions prior to the placement

A

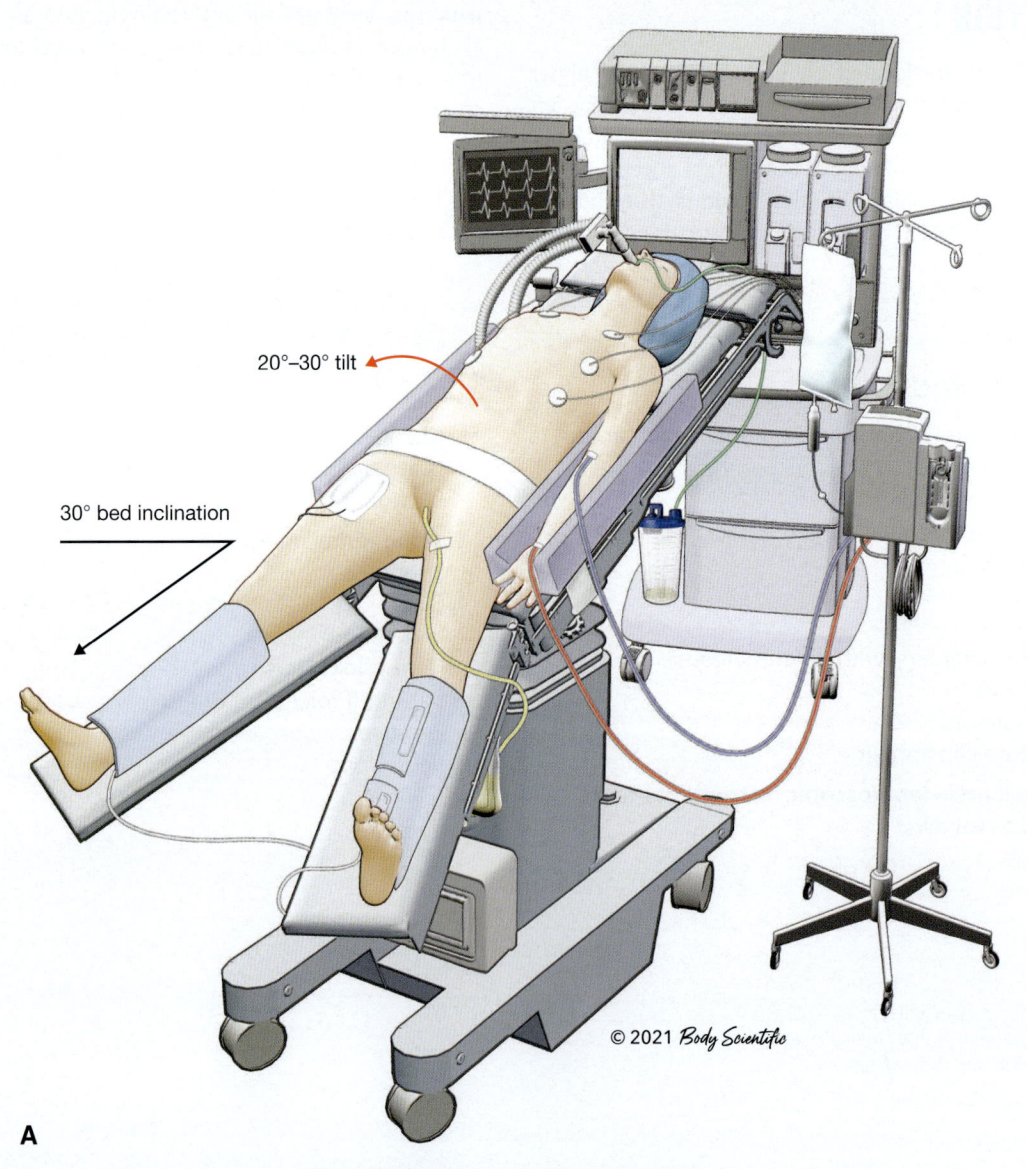

FIGURE 42-1 • **A.** Patient positioning.

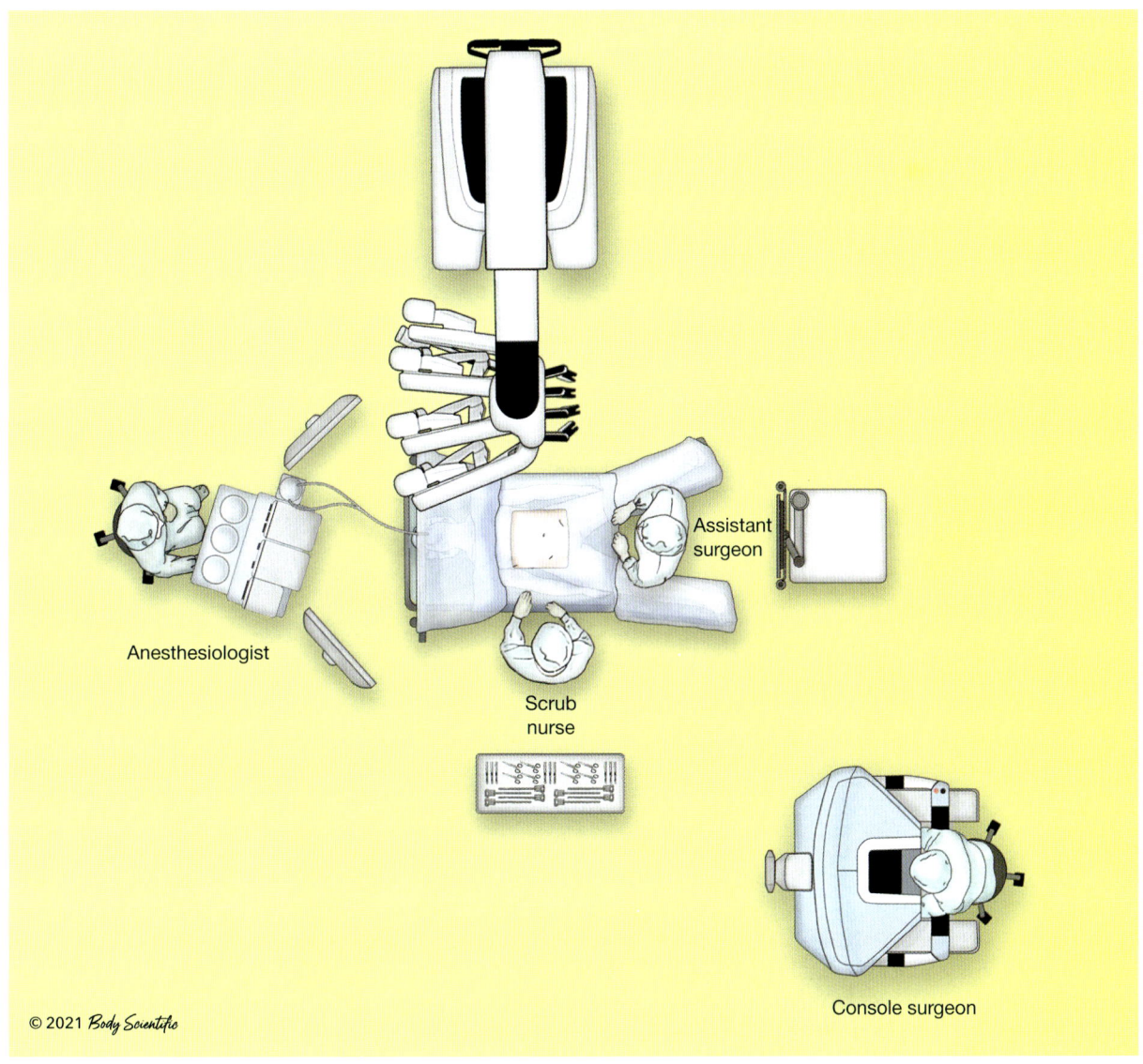

FIGURE 42-1 • (*Continued*) **B.** OR setting.

of the additional ports. For a left adrenalectomy, 4 robotic trocars and 1 to 2 assistant ports are used. **Figures 42-2 A, B** describe the port placement for normal and wide abdomens, respectively.

The camera port is introduced in the left upper quadrant, along the left pararectal line. The height of the camera port position should be optimized so that the scope ideally overlies the target anatomy at an angle of 45°. This can be achieved when placing the port under direct visualization.

Once the anatomy is confirmed, three 8-mm operative ports are placed along a straight line. The 8-mm port for the first robotic arm (R1) is positioned in the left lateral quadrant and slightly cephalad to the camera. The second operative port (R2) is placed on the right side of the camera along the midline, and the port for the third robotic arm (R3) is introduced on the far-right side along the same line. One or 2 assistant ports are placed: 1 in the umbilicus and 1 optional in between the camera and the left operative port a few centimeters lower. The operative table is then moved to the 30° reverse Trendelenburg position and tilted 20–30° to the right side. The robotic cart is docked.

> ▶▶ **TIPS**
>
> If adhesions are present at the initial exploration, additional ports may be placed to perform adhesiolysis and clear the working space. (See Chapter 2, The Basic Principles of Cinical Applications, for a comprehensive description of the different operative strategies.)

> **EDITORIAL COMMENT**
>
> For the robotic procedure, the anterior approach with the patient supine is generally preferred to the lateral approach. The lateral position is favored in laparoscopy because sometimes it is necessary to mobilize the splenopancreatic block. In such a case, gravity facilitates the exposure. The robotic approach allows instead a progressive lifting of the pancreatic body, while opening the retropancreatic avascular plane using the R3 with a grasper holding a sponge. A better exposure of the space between the adrenal gland and aorta is then achieved in the supine position.

Normal abdomen

A

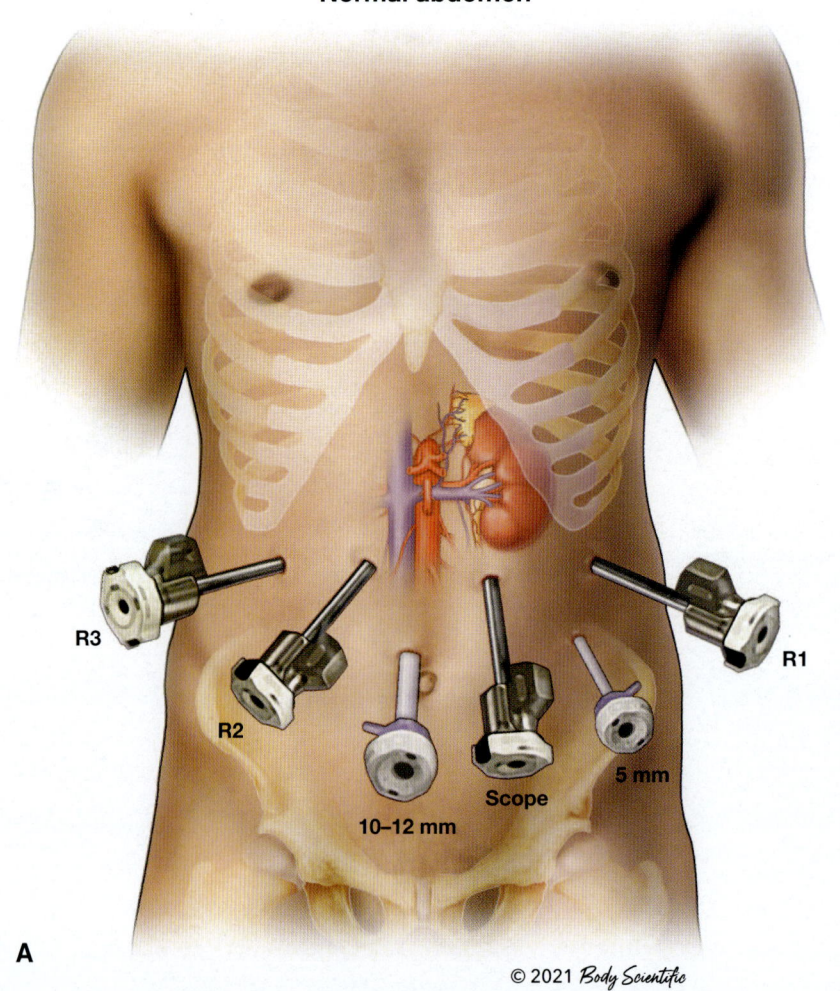

FIGURE 42-2 • **A.** Trocars setting normal abdomen.

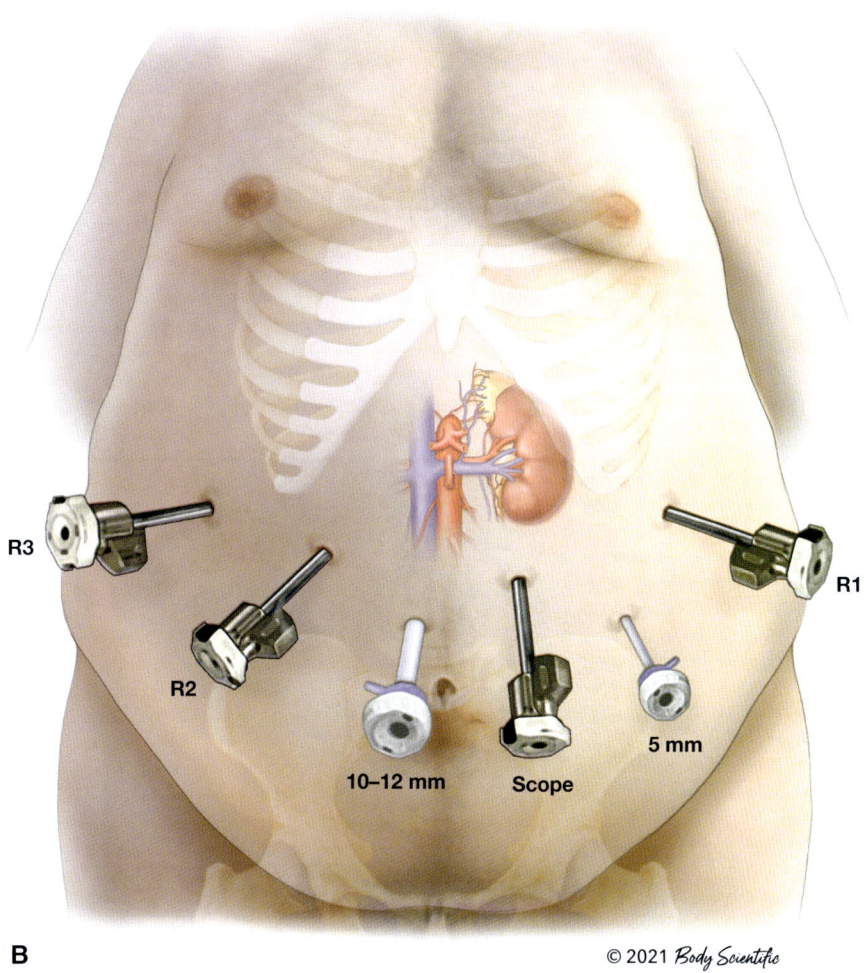

FIGURE 42-2 • (*Continued*) **B.** Trocars setting wide abdomen.

Step 1. Opening of the gastrocolic ligament

The first step is to divide the left portion of the gastrocolic ligament in order to gain access to the lesser sac. The stomach is retracted cephalad and medially using the R3. Proper retraction on the transverse colon inferiorly, putting some tension on the mesentery, allows identification of the Bouchet's zone. The gastrocolic ligament is opened using the cautery hook and the vessel sealer, as described in **Figure 42-3**.

▶ **Video 42-3. Step 1. Opening of the Gastrocolic Ligament**

The dissection is carried out toward the short gastric vessels. The short gastric vessels are generally preserved. A good exposure of the lesser sac facilitates the mobilization of the left colonic flexure and identification of the lower edge of the pancreatic body.

Step 1 average time frame: 5–10 min

> ⚠ **PITFALLS**
>
> When the gastrocolic ligament is adherent to the mesocolon, the vessel sealer tends to fuse the planes, which can lead to a wrong division of vessels going to the transverse colon inside the mesentery.

> ▶▶ **TIPS**
>
> It is advisable to use a monopolar hook for the initial opening of the gastrocolic ligament. This facilitates identification of the anatomical planes. Once the planes are recognized, the vessel sealer can be used to complete the dissection. During this step, the assistant provides countertraction and retracts the colon caudally and medially using atraumatic graspers.

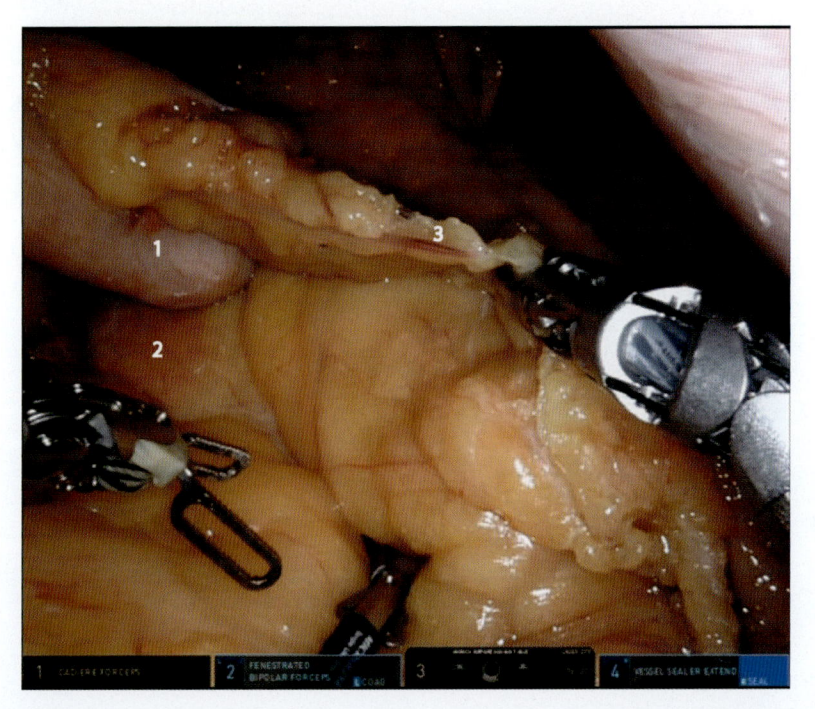

FIGURE 42-3 • Opening of the gastrocolic ligament. 1. Stomach. 2. Pancreas. 3. Gastrocolic ligament.

Step 2. Mobilization of the left colonic flexure

The left colonic flexure and descending colon are mobilized along the Toldt's fascia inferiorly and medially, using the monopolar hook and the bipolar forceps, as shown in **Figures 42-4 A, B**.

▶ **Video 42-4. Step 2. Mobilization of the Left Colonic Flexure**

The splenorenal and splenocolic ligaments are taken down allowing separation of the spleen from the colon. This step is important in order to expose the underlying inferior edge of the pancreas and the left kidney that will lead to identification of the left adrenal gland. The mobilization should be generous and should overcome the renal hilum (see Chapter 24, Left Colectomy).

Step 2 average time frame: 15–20 min

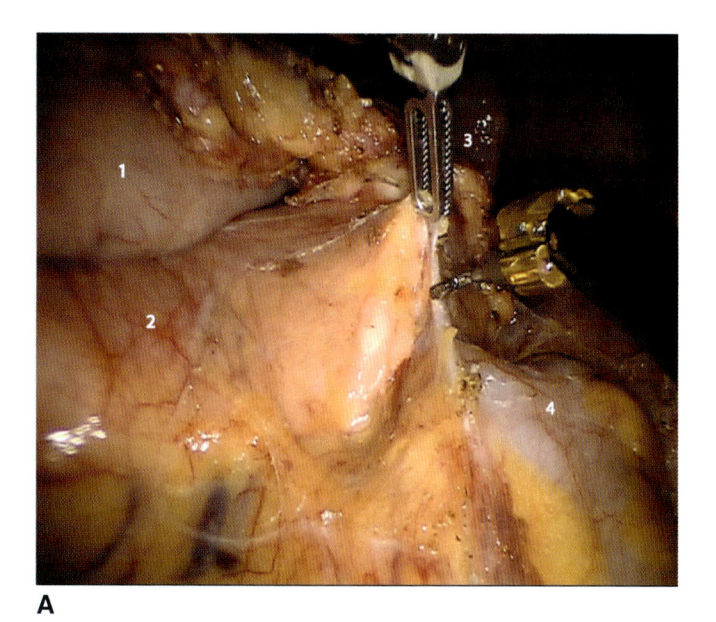

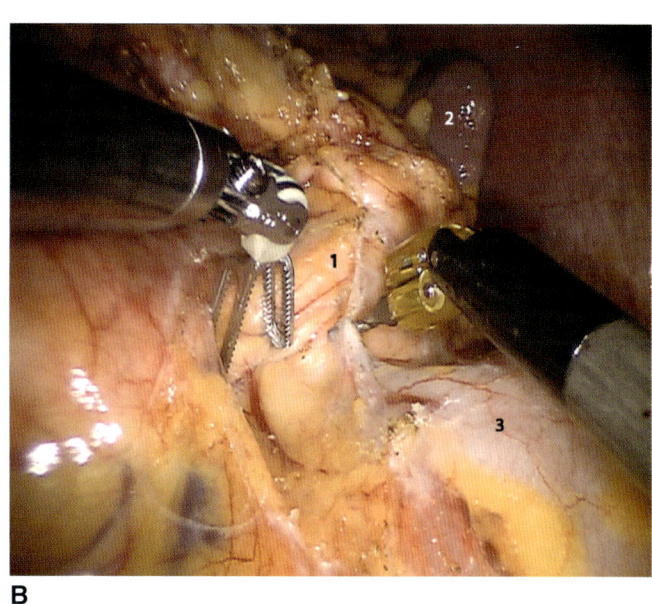

FIGURE 42-4 • **A.** Mobilization of the left colonic flexure. 1. Stomach. 2. Pancreas. 3. Spleen. 4. Left colonic flexure. **B.** Mobilization of the left colonic flexure. 1. Pancreas. 2. Spleen. 3. Left colonic flexure.

886 The Foundation and Art of Robotic Surgery

> ▶▶ **TIPS**
>
> The R3 is very important for retraction of the pancreas when exposing the upper pole of the left adrenal gland. In some cases, redundant or not fully decompressed stomach can cover target anatomy. To facilitate the exposure of the adrenal fossa, the stomach can be temporarily fixed to the anterior abdominal wall with a stitch of Prolene™ 2-0, as described in **Figure 42-5**.

> ⚠ **PITFALLS**
>
> During this step, retraction needs to be made very carefully in order not to pull on some omental adhesions with the spleen that can cause a laceration of the splenic capsule and subsequent bleeding.

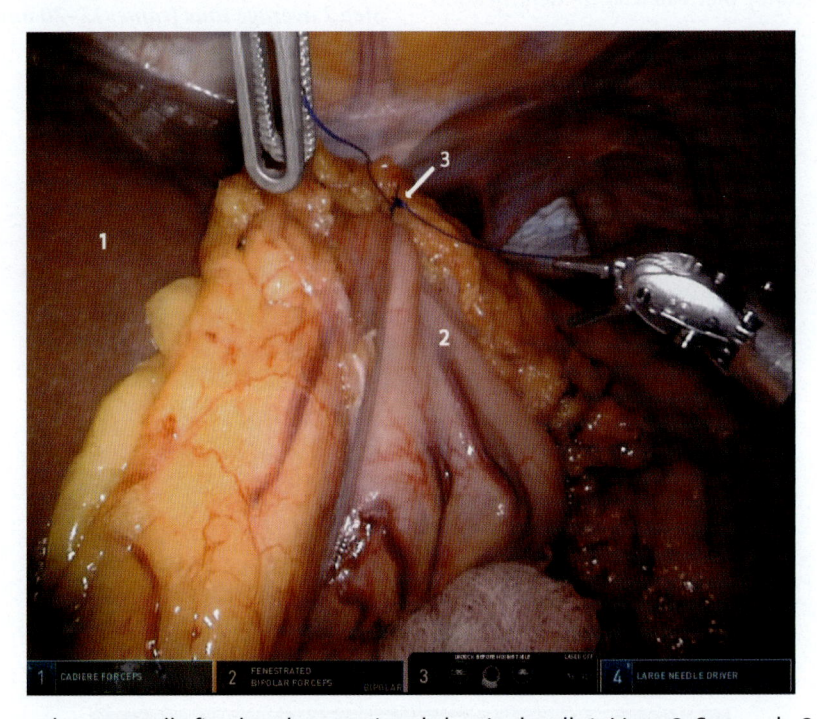

FIGURE 42-5 • Stomach temporally fixed to the anterior abdominal wall. 1. Liver. 2. Stomach. 3. Temporary stitch.

Step 3. Mobilization of the pancreatic body

The partial mobilization of the body and tail of the pancreas is necessary to achieve adequate exposure of the critical anatomy of the adrenal gland. The extent of mobilization also depends on anatomy of the individual and location of the adrenal gland, which can be higher and above the pancreas. In such cases, the body and the tail of the pancreas have to be mobilized completely.

The pancreatic body and tail are progressively dissected with a monopolar hook alternated to bipolar energy. The dissection is extended laterally over the kidney and the adrenal gland on top of the Gerota's fascia. During this step, the pancreas is gently retracted cranially using the R3 with a sponge, as shown in **Figures 42-6 A, B**.

Step 3 average time frame: 20–30 min

Video 42-5. Step 3. Mobilization of the Pancreatic Body

▶▶ **TIPS**

A correct position of the R3 is important in order to avoid collisions and to achieve effective retraction. The R3 port placed too close to the costal margin can make retraction of the pancreas difficult, limiting the vertical range of motion of the instrument. The R3 port placed too low can be cause of collision with the R2.

⚠ **PITFALLS**

Inadequate mobilization and retraction of the pancreatic body and tail may limit the necessary exposure of the underneath anatomy; furthermore, limited mobilization of the pancreas could also increase the risk of injuries of the gland while trying to retract it.

▶▶ **TIPS**

An adequate mobilization of the pancreatic body and tail along the posterior avascular plane is required to expose the Gerota's fascia and the kidney underneath. Sometimes, the dissection should also include the lower splenophrenic ligaments.

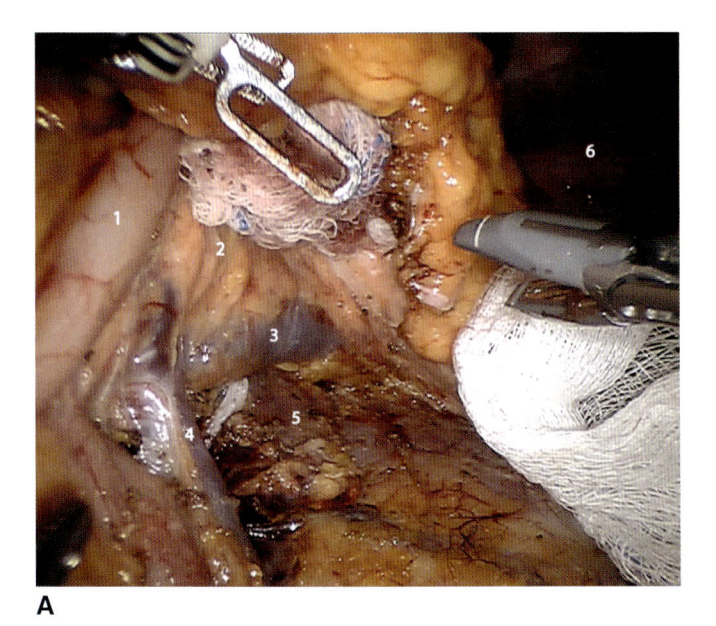

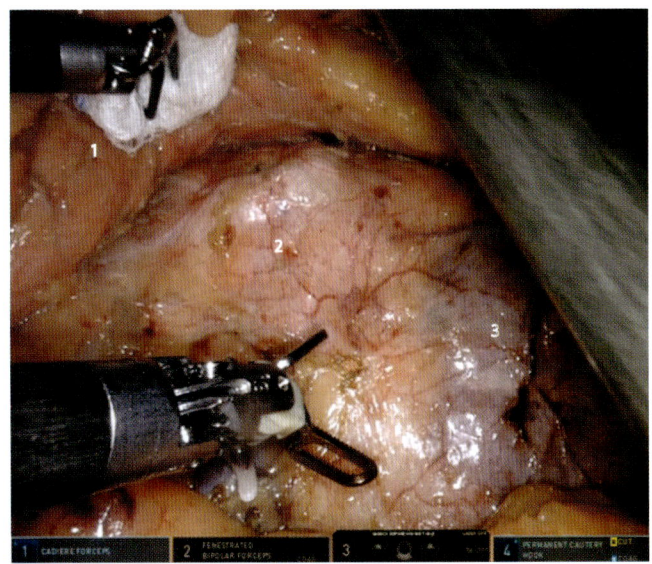

FIGURE 42-6 • **A.** Mobilization of the pancreatic body. 1. Stomach. 2. Pancreas. 3. Splenic vein. 4. Inferior mesenteric vein. 5. Adrenal gland. 6. Spleen. **B.** Mobilization of the pancreatic body. 1. Stomach. 2. Adrenal gland. 3. Left kidney.

Step 4. Identification of the left renal and adrenal vein with exposure of the adrenal gland

The anatomy of the left kidney is identified underneath the Gerota's fascia. The left renal vein is recognized at its intersection with the aorta. Some of the lympho-adipose tissue might cover the vein; this tissue is opened using the monopolar hook and bipolar forceps. The anterior surface of the left renal vein is then partially skeletonized until the insertion of the adrenal vein is detectable, as described in **Figure 42-7**. The recognition of the anatomy of the adrenal vein helps with defining the overall conformation of the adrenal gland.

Step 4 average time frame: 15–20 min

▶ **Video 42-6.** Step 4. Identification of the Left Renal and Adrenal Vein with Exposure of the Adrenal Gland

▶▶ **TIPS**

In case of bleeding, the surgeon must have a precise understanding of the renal vessel anatomy to safely identify and manage the source of the bleeding. Using sutures for hemostasis is usually safer than electrocautery.

⚠ **PITFALLS**

Retraction during this step has to be particularly careful in order to avoid bleeding from the back of the renal vein, which is more dangerous and difficult to control. Optimal access of the adrenal vein should be achieved as soon as possible, mainly in a case of pheochromocytoma.

🔍 **ANATOMICAL HIGHLIGHTS**

There are several potential variations of the left adrenal vein, as described in **Figures 42-8 A–K**. Most commonly, it is a single vein that drains directly into the left renal vein in conjunction with the left inferior phrenic vein. Other variants are duplication of the left adrenal vein, or one adrenal vein and one inferior phrenic vein draining separately into the left renal vein. The least common type is when one adrenal vein drains into the left lumbar vein or in the Azygos system. The retroaortic renal vein itself or in combination with an adrenal gland tumor is a rare anomaly. In such cases, the drainage of the adrenal gland should be evaluated very carefully. There are 2 possible directions of a drainage. One possible drainage is a single long vein that is located more medially and draining directly to the inferior vena cava. The second possible drainage of the gland may be deeper in tissue directly to the retroaortic renal vein.

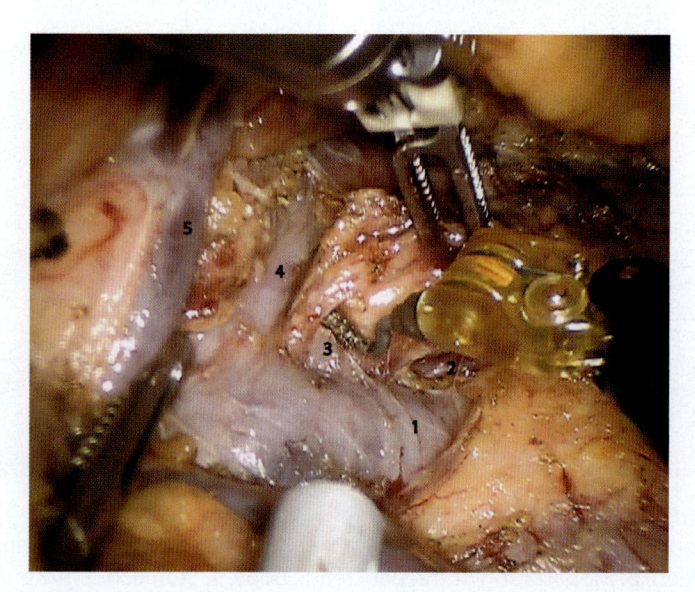

FIGURE 42-7 • Identification of the left renal and adrenal veins with exposure of the adrenal gland. 1. Left renal vein. 2. Left renal artery. 3. Left accessory adrenal vein. 4. Left main adrenal vein. 5. Left phrenic vein.

Left Adrenalectomy 889

> ▶▶ **TIPS**
>
> The main landmark for left adrenalectomy is the left renal vein. Failure to identify the left renal vein should caution a surgeon of possible variation of drainages of the adrenal gland, either to the vena cava or to the retroaortic renal vein. In such an event, a surgeon must proceed very carefully to avoid difficult bleeding.

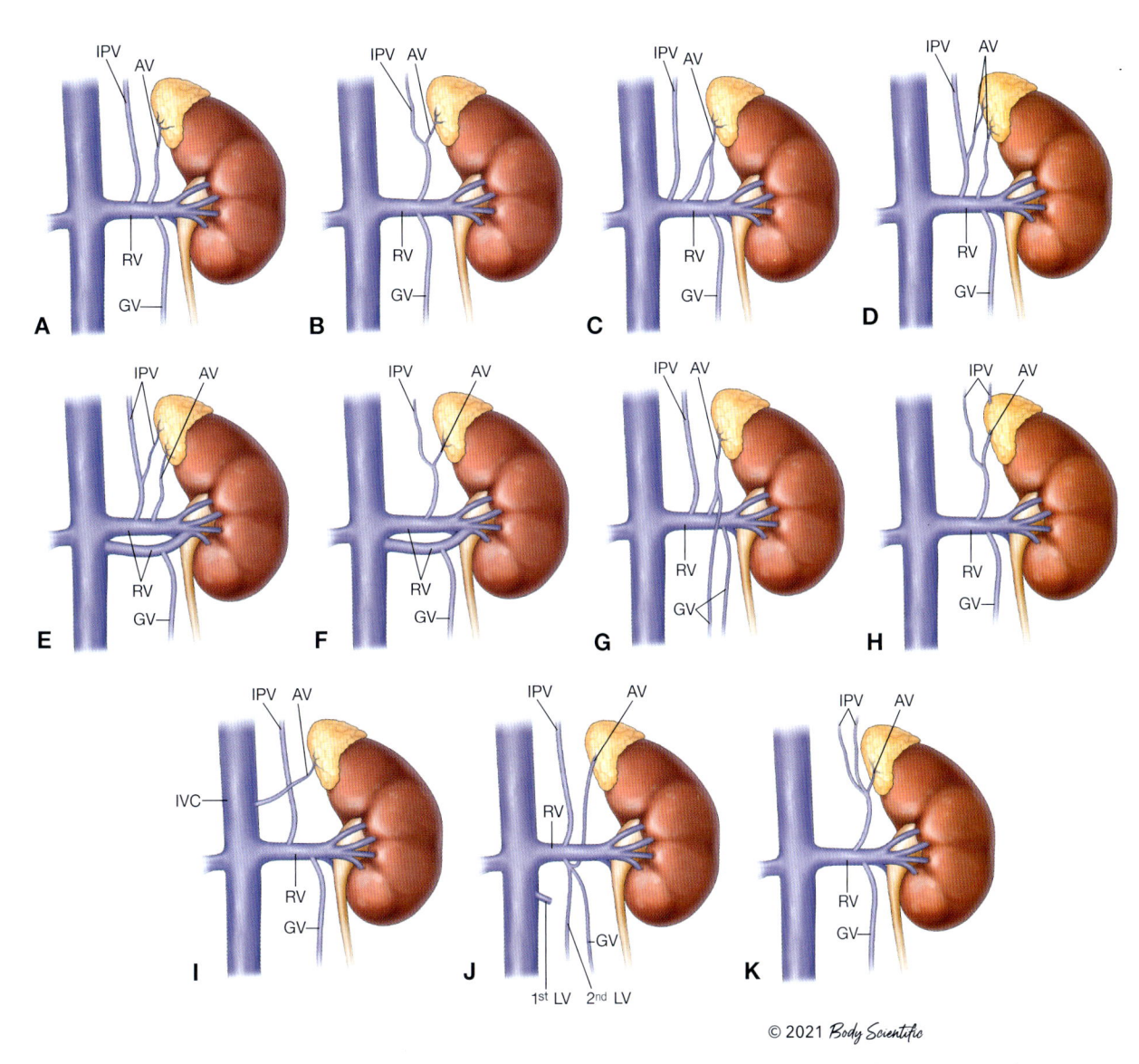

FIGURE 42-8 • Variations of venous drainage. IPV, inferior phrenic vein; AV, adrenal vein; RV, renal vein; GV, gonadal vein; LV, lumbar vein.

Step 5. Left adrenal vein ligation

The left adrenal vein is circumferentially isolated using the monopolar hook and bipolar forceps. The dissection is meticulously carried out until complete control of the vessel is achieved.

A conventional approach, particularly in cases of pheochromocytoma, is that the venous drainage should be ligated prior to the manipulation of the adrenal gland to prevent catecholamine release. The adrenal vein can be divided between suture ligation/Hem-o-lok clips. The "no touch" technique allows a late ligation of the vein, decreasing the backflow bleeding during mobilization (see Chapter 41, Right Adrenalectomy, for a detailed description of the "no touch" technique and different operative strategies) (**Figure 42-9**).

Step 5 average time frame: 10–15 min

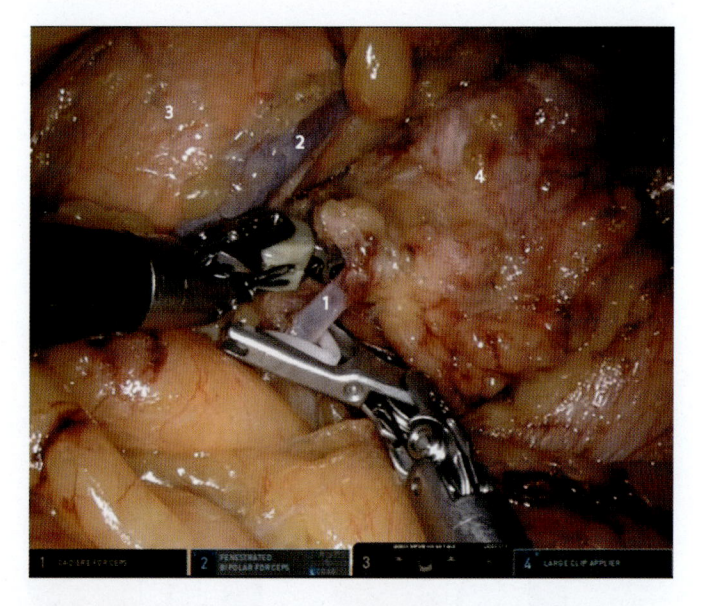

FIGURE 42-9 • Left adrenal vein ligation. 1. Left adrenal vein. 2. Splenic vein. 3. Pancreas. 4. Adrenal gland.

Video 42-7. Step 5. Left Adrenal Vein Ligation

Step 6. Exposure of the upper pole of the kidney with identification of the left renal artery anatomy

Once the venous drainage is controlled, gentle traction on the adrenal gland and countertraction on the kidney by the assistant will help to open the dissection plane. It is of paramount importance to recognize the left renal artery as shown in **Figure 42-10**.

Step 6 average time frame: 10–15 min

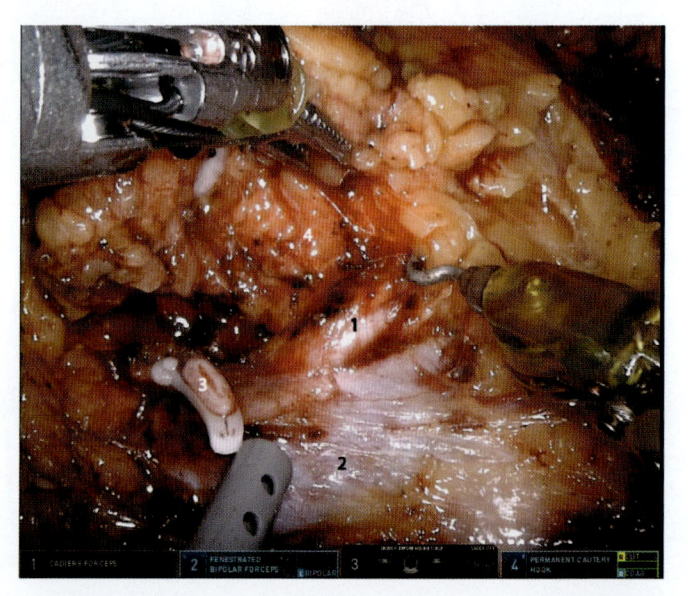

FIGURE 42-10 • Exposure of the upper pole of the kidney with identification of the left renal artery anatomy. 1. Left renal artery. 2. Left renal vein. 3. Left adrenal vein.

Left Adrenalectomy 891

> ▶▶ **TIPS**
> In some cases, upper polar renal arteries may be present. These vessels have to be identified and preserved, as shown in **Figure 42-11**.

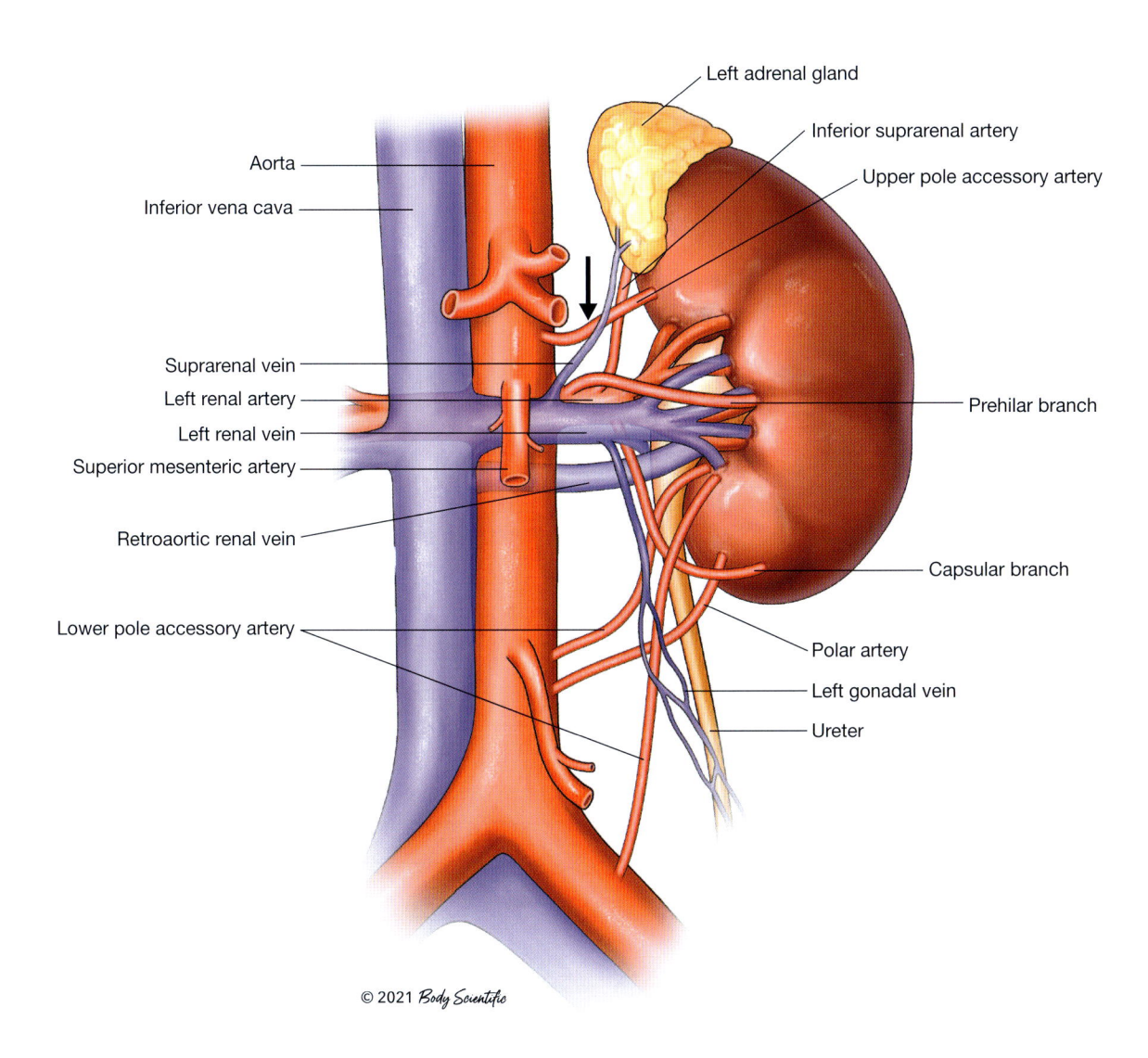

FIGURE 42-11 • Exposure of the upper pole of the kidney with identification of the upper pole accessory left renal artery.

Step 7. Detachment of the adrenal gland from the renal artery and upper pole of the left kidney

The periadrenal tissue is dissected, following the plane along the superior pole of the kidney and the anterior aspect of the psoas muscle. The dissection is extended medially and then progresses in a cranial direction.

The attachments between the renal capsule and the adrenal gland are progressively released with a combination of monopolar energy and the vessel sealer. Some adipose tissue surrounding the adrenal gland is generally left in place in order to be used to move the gland without touching it.

Step 7 average time frame: 15–20 min

> ### ANATOMICAL HIGHLIGHTS
> The left adrenal gland arterial blood supply consists of the superior suprarenal artery taking its origin from the inferior phrenic artery, the middle adrenal artery that originates from the aorta, and the inferior adrenal arteries originating from the renal artery, as described in **Figure 42-12**.

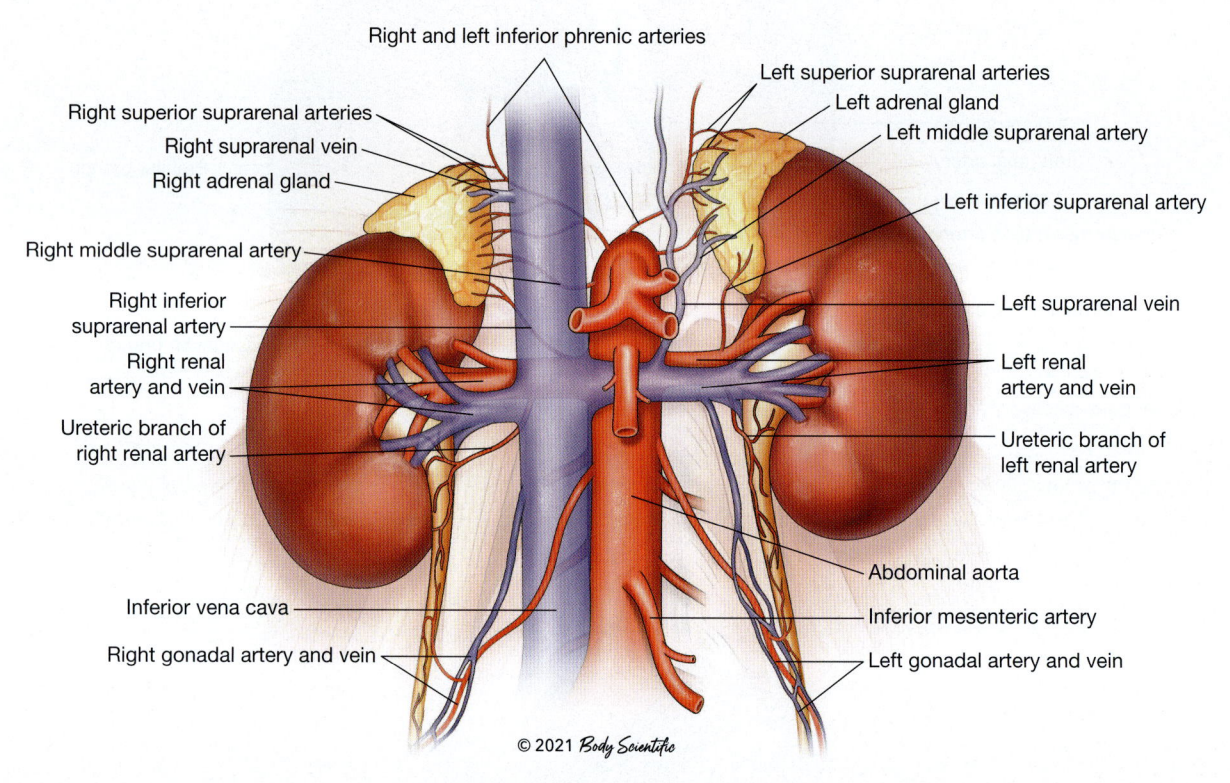

FIGURE 42-12 • Control of inflow.

Step 8. Lifting the adrenal gland and detachment from the aorta and left diaphragmatic pillar

The adrenal gland is elevated anterolaterally, and the posteromedial attachments from the aorta and the left diaphragmatic pillar are taken down, using the vessel sealer as described in **Figures 42-13 A, B**.

> **Video 42-8.** Steps 8–9. Lifting the Adrenal Gland, Detachment from the Aorta and Left Diaphragmatic Pillar, and Completion of the Dissection of the Posterolateral Plane

Care must be taken not to injure the left inferior phrenic vein running caudally along the medial border of the adrenal gland toward the renal vein. The variable arterial supply to the adrenal gland (branches from the inferior phrenic artery and aorta) is controlled using an energy device.

The dissection of the superomedial aspect of the gland over the aortophrenic groove should be cautiously performed. A small superior adrenal artery originating from the inferior phrenic artery can be encountered. This vessel is best controlled with the vessel sealer or clips.

Step 8 average time frame: 15–20 min

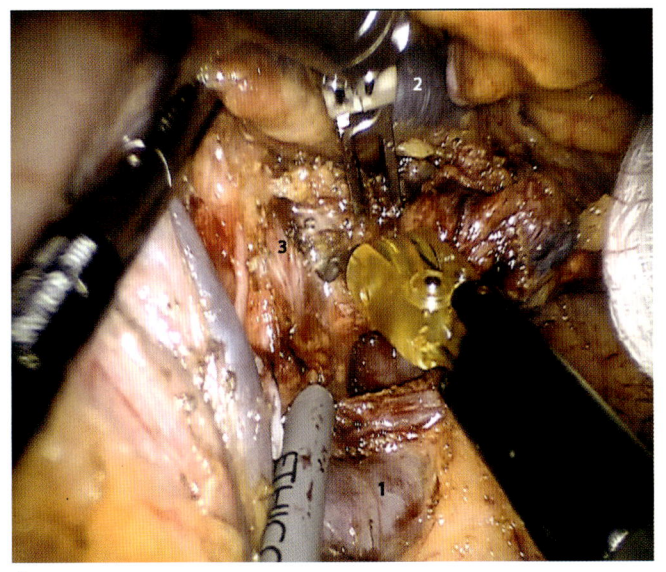

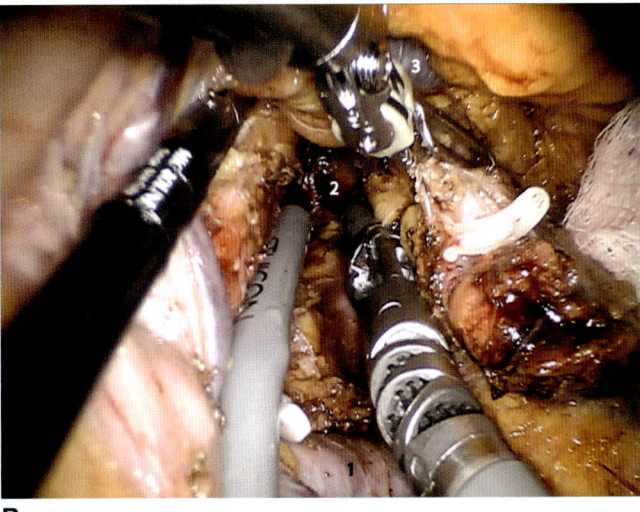

FIGURE 42-13 • **A.** Lifting the adrenal gland and detachment from the aorta and left diaphragmatic pillar. 1. Left renal vein. 2. Splenic vein. 3. Aorta. **B.** Lifting the adrenal gland and detachment from the aorta and left diaphragmatic pillar. 1. Left renal vein. 2. Diaphragm. 3. Splenic vein.

Step 9. Completion of the dissection of the posterolateral plane

The periadrenal fat is fully dissected from the superior pole of the kidney and lateral retroperitoneal tissue using the vessel sealer, as shown in **Figure 42-14**.

Careful dissection of the adrenal gland while avoiding grasping the gland directly can help minimize blood loss.

Step 9 average time frame: 10–15 min

Step 10. Specimen extraction

For the small lesion, an enlargement of one of the port sizes can be sufficient. For a larger mass, a Pfannenstiel incision is preferred. See Chapter 2, The Basic Principles of Clinical Applications, and Chapter 41, Right Adrenalectomy, for a comprehensive description of this step and different operative strategies.

Step 10 average time frame: 5–10 min

> ▶▶ **TIPS**
>
> The resection of bulky lesions can be particularly complex because the anatomy is often less clear and retraction difficult.
>
> In rare cases, when a bulky lesion is in association with the high location of the adrenal gland, the suprapancreatic approach is an alternative to the infrapancreatic one. This approach requires careful mobilization and lowering down of the pancreatic body and upper pole of the spleen. When dissecting the upper edge of the pancreas, care must be taken to avoid injuries of the nearby splenic vessels.

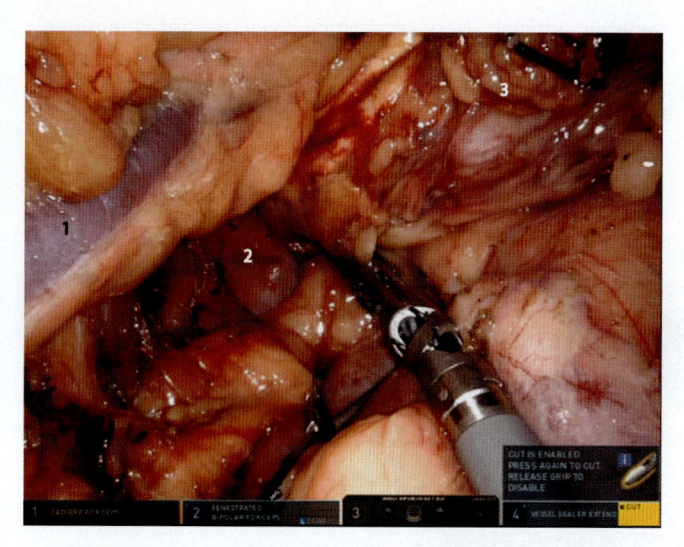

FIGURE 42-14 • Completion of the dissection of the posterolateral plane. 1. Splenic vein. 2. Diaphragm. 3. Adrenal gland.

Suggested Readings

1. Gagner M, Lacroix A, Bolté E. Laparoscopic adrenalectomy in Cushing's syndrome and pheochromocytoma. *N Engl J Med.* 1992; 327(14):1033.
2. Brunt LM. Minimal access adrenal surgery. *Surg Endosc.* 2006;20: 351-361.
3. Tsuru N, Ushiyama T, Suzuki K. Laparoscopic adrenalectomy for primary and secondary malignant adrenal tumors. *J Endourol.* 2005;19:702-708.
4. Henry JF, Sebag F, Iacobone M, et al. Results of laparoscopic adrenalectomy for large and potentially malignant tumors. *World J Surg.* 2002;26:1043-1047.
5. Stefanidis D1, Goldfarb M, Kercher KW, et al. Society of Gastrointestinal and Endoscopic Surgeons. SAGES guidelines for minimally invasive treatment of adrenal pathology. *Surg Endosc.* 2013;27(11):3960-80. doi: 10.1007/s00464-013-3169-z
6. Lee J, El-Tamer M, Schifftner T, et al. Open and laparoscopic adrenalectomy: analysis of the National Surgical Quality Improvement Program. *J Am Coll Surg.* 2008;206:953-959; discussion 959-961.
7. Brunaud L, Bresler L, Ayav A, et al. Robotic-assisted adrenalectomy: what advantages compared to lateral transperitoneal laparoscopic adrenalectomy? *Am J Surg.* 2008;195:433-438.
8. Giulianotti PC, Buchs NC, Addeo P, et al. Robot-assisted adrenalectomy: a technical option for the surgeon? *Int J Med Robot.* 2011;7(1):27-32. doi: 10.1002/rcs.364
9. Teo XL, Lim SK. Robotic assisted adrenalectomy: is it ready for prime time? *Investig Clin Urol.* 2016;57(suppl 2):S130-S146. doi: 10.4111/icu.2016.57.S2.S130
10. Giulianotti PC, Coratti A, Angelini M, et al. Robotics in general surgery: personal experience in a large community hospital. *Arch Surg.* 2003;138(7):777-784. doi: 10.1001/archsurg.138.7.777. PMID: 12860761.

SECTION X

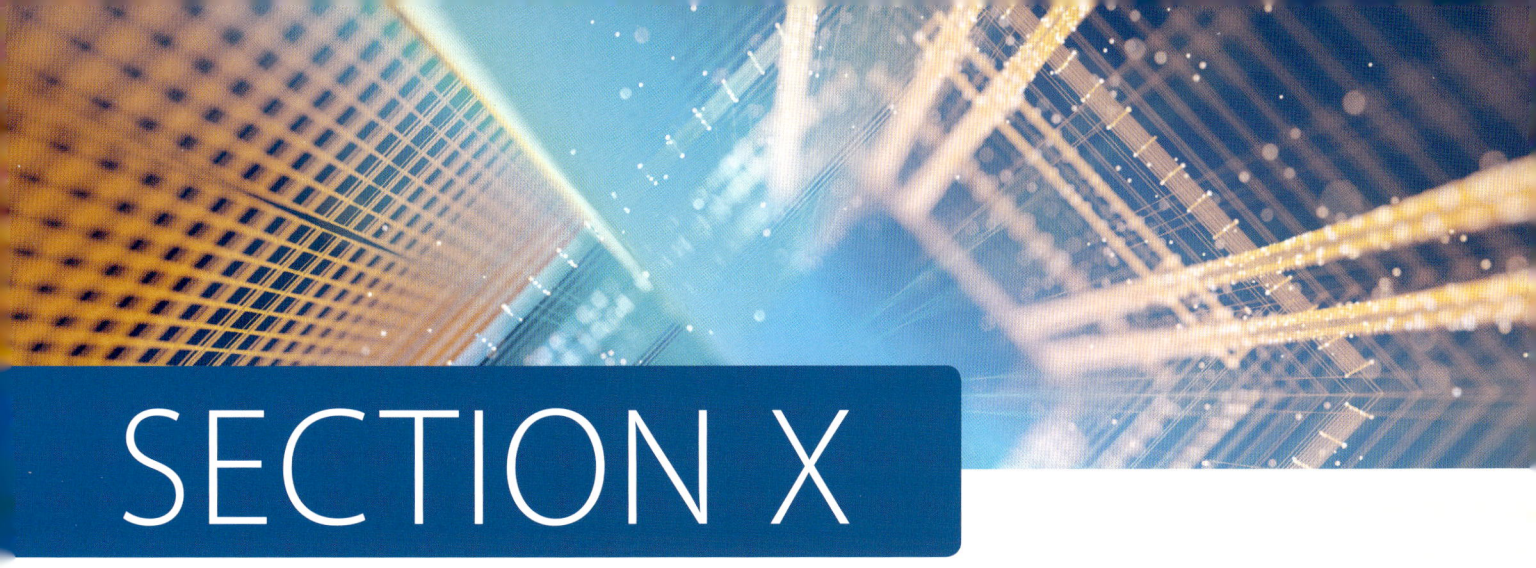

Hernia Surgery

Chapter 43 • Inguinal Hernia Repair 897
Francesco Maria Bianco • Yevhen Pavelko • Pier Cristoforo Giulianotti

Chapter 44 • Ventral Hernia Repair (Intraperitoneal Onlay Mesh with Fascial
 Defect Approximation) 911
Karl LeBlanc • Patrice Frederick • Carolina Baz

Chapter 45 • Robotic Transversus Abdominis Release (roboTAR) 925
Tiffany Nguyen • Ethan Ballecer • Katherine Hoener • Alice Gamble • Conrad Ballecer

"No disease of the human body, belonging to the province of the surgeon, requires in its treatment, a better combination of accurate anatomical knowledge with surgical skills than hernia in all its varieties."

—Sir Astley Paston Cooper (1768–1841)

Inguinal Hernia Repair

Francesco Maria Bianco • Yevhen Pavelko • Pier Cristoforo Giulianotti

Introduction

Minimally invasive techniques have become widely adopted in abdominal wall surgery. The advantages of robotic surgery can be particularly appreciated in this indication where the surgical field is sometimes turned upside down, and in patients with a high body mass index (BMI) or large and/or recurrent hernia defects. Of particular interest is the fact that the system gives the ability for the surgeon to control the camera without relying on assistants and, as a result, to perform a type of solo surgery. When dealing with complex cases, the benefits of robotics can potentially reduce the conversion risk to open surgery. This approach offers additional technical advantages compared to laparoscopy such as the possibility to fix the mesh using hand-sewn sutures as an alternative to tacks. Chronic pain is still a feared complication for hernia repair, with an incidence ranging from 3% to 18%. A precise, dissection may improve long-term outcomes, as approximately 800,000 hernia surgery repairs per year are performed in the United States (see suggested readings #1–3). This number may explain the impact that improved techniques may have on social cost.

With the constant growth of applications in general surgery and the increased need for training, this procedure represents a valid teaching model to develop and retain useful surgical skills. In many institutions, the robotic inguinal hernia repair became part of the curriculum for residents. In this chapter, the standardized technique of robotic transabdominal preperitoneal repair (RTAPP) of inguinal hernias is described.

Indications and Contraindications to the Robotic Approach

The indications are based mostly on the surgeon's experience. The first cases, at the beginning of the learning curve, should consist of smaller defects with pristine anatomy. As the experience grows, more complex cases and recurrent hernias may be considered. The most challenging situations are in patients with a history of previous anterior pelvic surgery (prostatectomy/cystectomy), recurrences, and large chronically incarcerated inguino-scrotal hernias.

Patients with incarcerated hernias without signs of bowel obstruction can also be considered for a robotic repair. Ascites, the presence of a peritoneal dialysis catheter, and extremely large defects are not absolute contraindications, but they require an expert surgeon because of the increased complexity. Strangulated hernias in an emergency setting are still better managed with an open approach.

INSTRUMENT REQUIREMENTS

The suggested main robotic instruments/tools can be listed as follows:
- 30° scope
- ProGrasp™ forceps/bipolar fenestrated grasper
- Monopolar cautery hook/monopolar scissors
- Suture cut needle driver

The suggested main laparoscopic instruments/tools can be listed as follows:
- Needle drivers
- Graspers
- Scissors (optional)
- 5-mm laparoscopic scope (optional)

Supplemental materials:
- Sponges
- Sutures: Prolene™ 2-0/3-0; Vicryl™ 0/3-0
- Mesh (different sizes)

Photo from Mashuk / Getty Images.
Quote reproduced with permission from Coopoer A. The Anatomy and Surgical Treatment of Inguinal and Congenital Hernia. London: Cox; 1804.

> ▶▶ **TIPS**
>
> The ProGrasp™ forceps has higher grasping strength compared to the Cadiére or bipolar forceps, which is why it is effective when more traction is needed on large, thick hernia sacs. However, the bipolar forceps should be preferred for normal cases as a multitask tool. Bipolar coagulation is the safest technique to address minor bleedings in risky zones.

> ▶▶ **TIPS**
>
> The monopolar hook is the preferred instrument for dissection. It can be used for precise energy delivery or blunt dissection. The monopolar scissors are used alternatively, mainly when fibrotic tissue is present, requiring the action of cutting.

Patient Positioning, OR Setup, and Port Setting

The patient is positioned supine with both arms padded and tucked to the side. Shoulders support or an anti-sliding mattress is necessary to prevent shifting when in Trendelenburg position (**Figure 43-1**).

The assistant surgeon is standing at the opposite side of the hernia. The OR setup is shown in **Figure 43-2**.

Pneumoperitoneum is established with the Veress technique (see Chapter 2, The Basic Principles of Clinical Applications) and the first 8 mm port is placed in the left lateral upper quadrant. After insufflation, the 8-mm robotic scope or a laparoscopic camera is used to perform an initial exploration. This step is helpful in evaluating the size of the defect and providing guidance for port placement or ruling out reasons to modify the operative plan. The remaining two 8-mm robotic trocars are inserted under direct visualization along the transverse or oblique umbilical line, in the left and right flanks with a minimum distance from the camera port of approximately 1 fist. The port setup can be different for patients with a short abdomen and for more complex/large hernias. In those cases, the camera port can be placed more cranially in order to achieve a wider view of the surgical field, and the operative ports generally follow the same modification being placed along a transverse line across the camera port. In large hernias, an optional 10–12-mm assistant port may be indicated to enhance the retraction of the sac and can be used to introduce larger meshes and sutures. This port is generally positioned in between the camera and the robotic operative trocar opposite to the hernia side (**Figures 43-3 A–C**). After port placement, the operative table is adjusted to mild Trendelenburg and tilted 20° with the hernia side up. For simple bilateral hernias, the tilt is usually not performed to avoid redocking when approaching the contralateral site.

> ▶▶ **TIPS**
>
> For the ports setting, instead of the transverse line centered on the umbilicus, an oblique one with the operative port ipsilateral to the hernia side, a bit higher, might facilitate the range of motion of the instruments, increasing the distance from the target. Since the anterior superior iliac spine (ASIS) is the landmark for the lateral extent of the peritoneal flap, it is important to have enough space from the ASIS to avoid difficulties during the closure of the peritoneal flap.

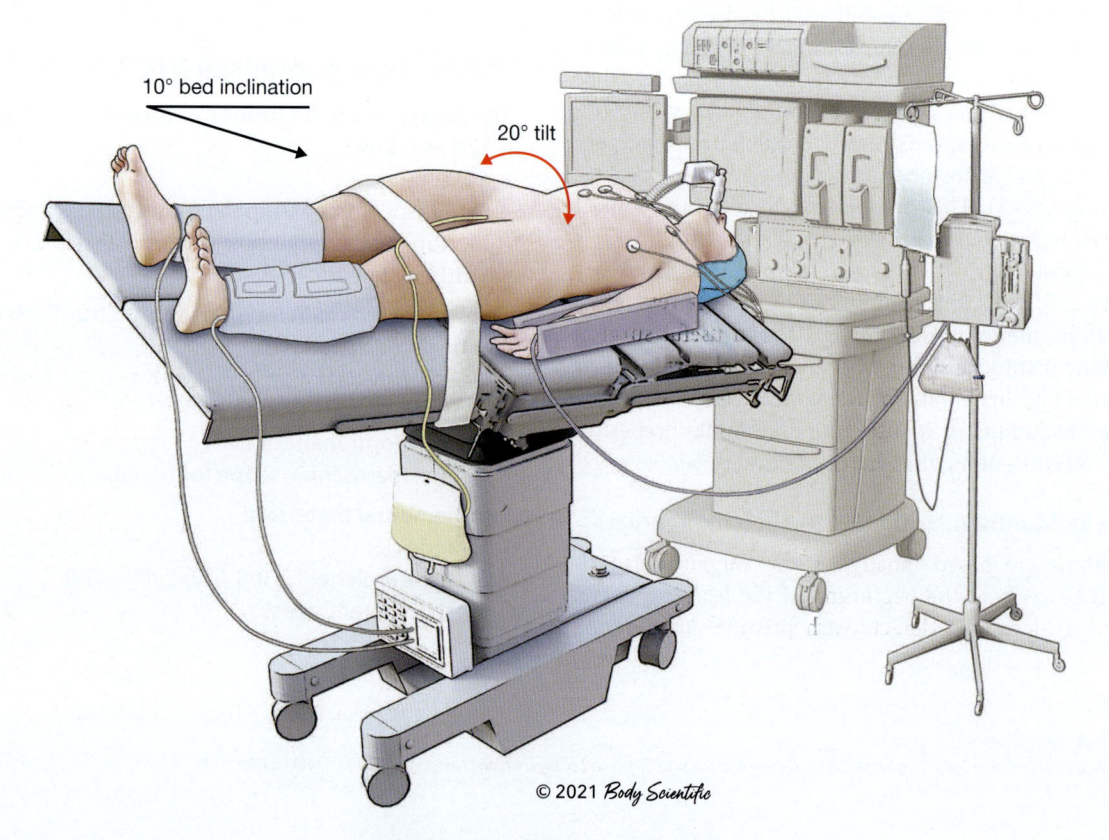

FIGURE 43-1 • Patient positioning.

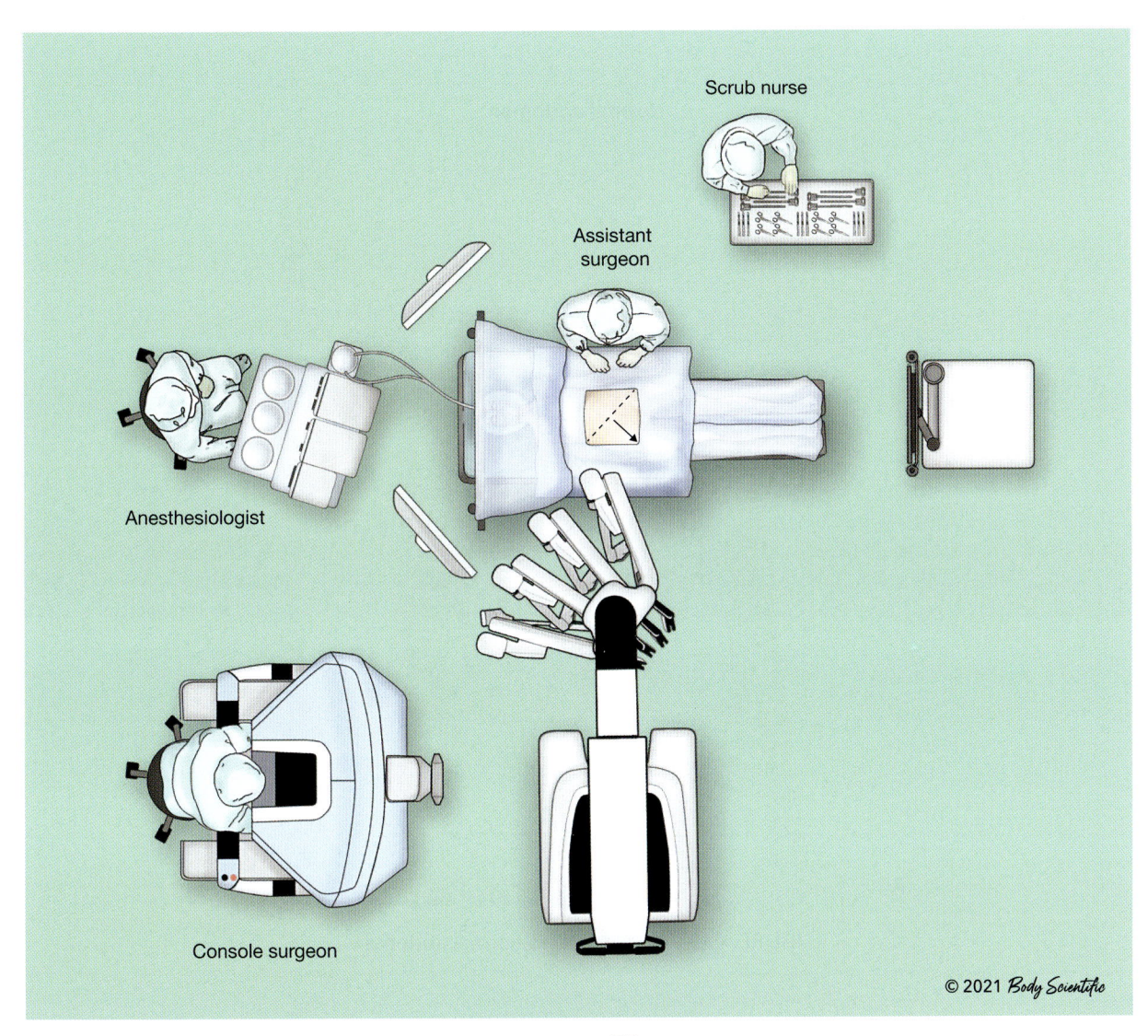

FIGURE 43-2 • OR setup.

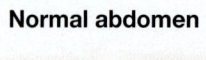

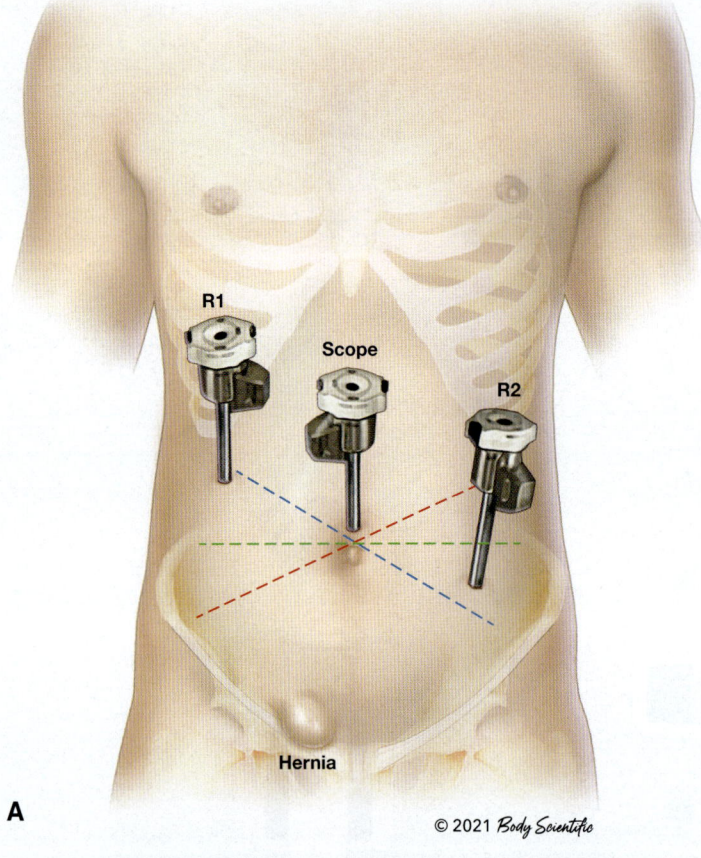

FIGURE 43-3 • **A.** Port setting normal abdomen.

FIGURE 43-3 • (*Continued*) **B.** Port setting complex hernias, early experience. **C.** Port setting obese/short umbilico-pubic distance.

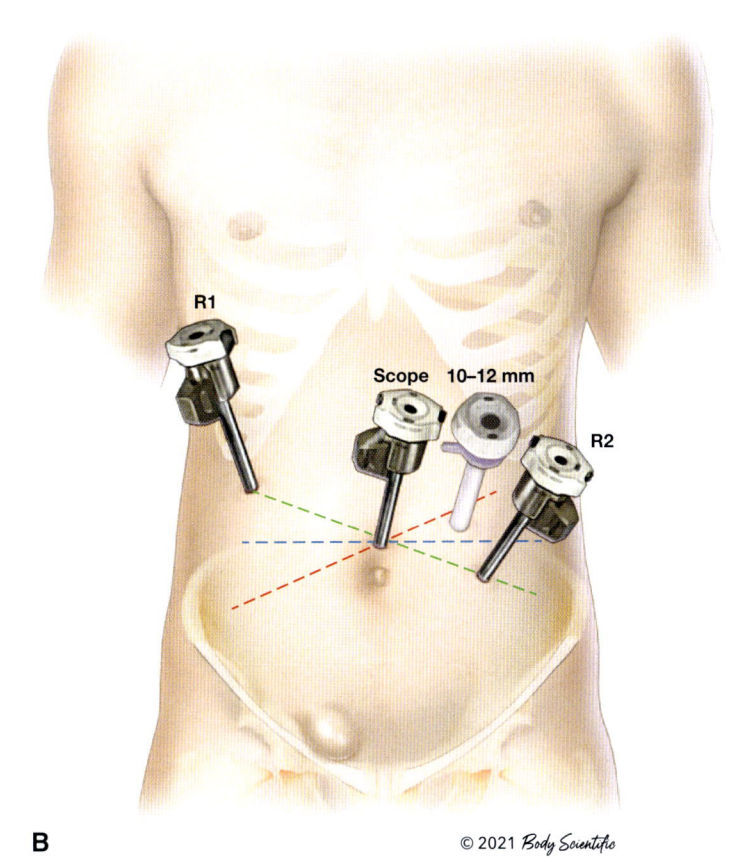

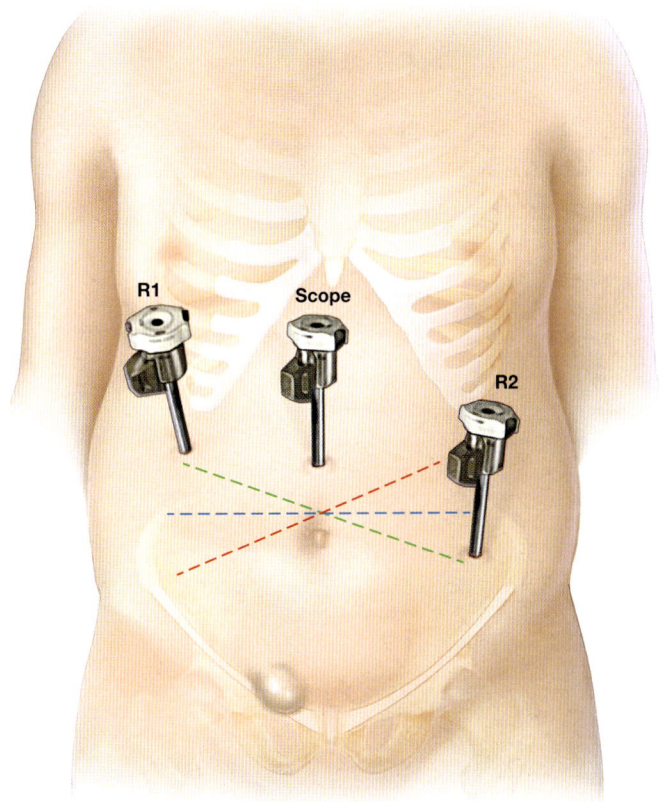

Surgical Technique

Video 43-1. Robotic Inguinal Hernia – Full Procedure

Step 1. Recognition of the anatomical landmarks

Recognition of the predissection anatomical landmarks is an important part of the operation. It is always worthy to spend some time to have a perfect understanding of the anatomy. The ASIS, medial umbilical ligament, inferior epigastric vessels, and deep inguinal ring will give the proper orientation of where to conduct the dissection and the areas to be avoided. A good exploration will also give an idea of the complexity of the dissection, the type of hernia, the size of the defect, the presence of adhesions, anatomical anomalies and variations, and reasons to change the preoperative plan.

Step 1 average time frame: 3–5 min

> **ANATOMICAL HIGHLIGHTS**
>
> Preoperative and intraoperative dissection landmarks: ASIS, medial umbilical ligament, inferior epigastric vessels, iliopubic tract, *vas deferens*, spermatic vessels, deep inguinal ring, Hesselbach's triangle, triangle of doom, triangle of pain, and triangle of femoral hernia (**Figures 43-4** to **43-6**).

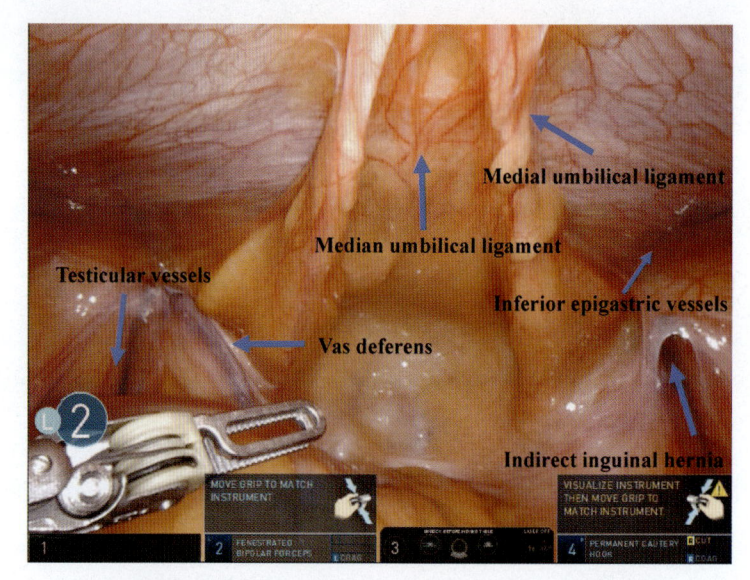

FIGURE 43-4 • Predissection anatomical landmarks.

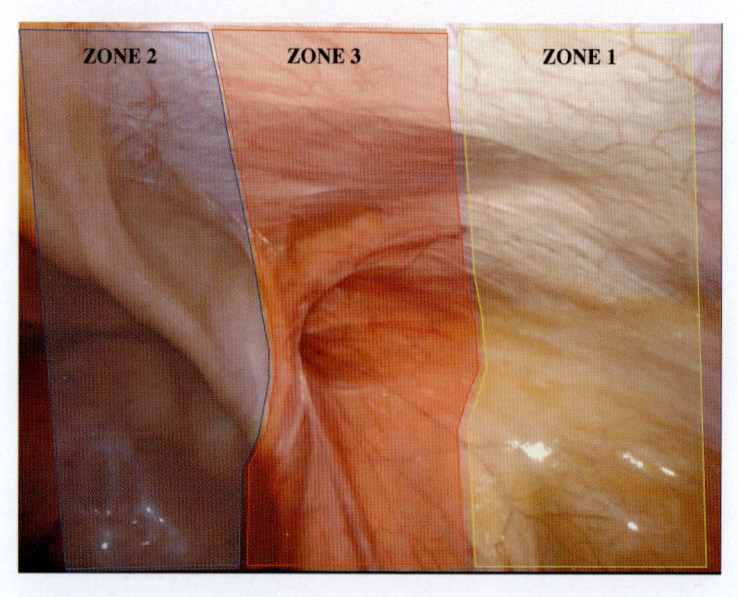

FIGURE 43-5 • Anatomical zones of the inguinal canal region.

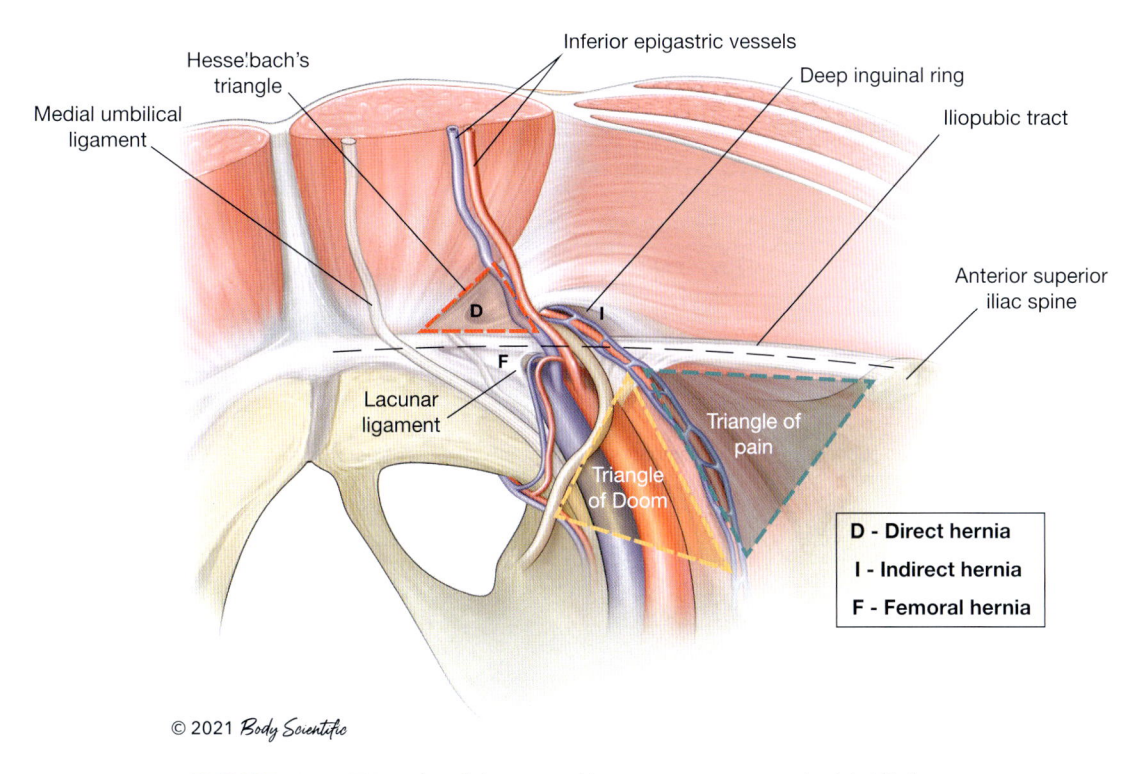

FIGURE 43-6 • Triangle of doom and important topography highlights.

Step 2. Flap dissection

The peritoneum is incised at the level of the internal inguinal ring 3–5 cm above it, with a monopolar hook and a grasper. The grasper is used to hold the flap under tension, while the hook opens the peritoneum along a slightly oblique line toward the medial umbilical ligament, and then downward to the ASIS following the arch of the transverse muscle. The correct plane is created dissecting close to the peritoneum and ensuring that the preperitoneal fat stays attached to the abdominal wall. This will help to avoid entering in a wrong deeper plane. Once the peritoneum is incised, the preparation of the flap is done with blunt gentle diverging actions of the 2 working instruments, favoring spontaneous opening of the space with the CO_2 pressure, until the bottom of the surgical field is reached, on top of the hernia sac. Depending on the structure of the peritoneum, which can be thick and dense or thin and fragile, the preparation of a pure peritoneal flap may be easy, but in other cases, the dissection may include patches of transversalis fascia. If this happens medial to the epigastric vessels, it is less risky than lateral, where a deeper plane may bring directly in contact with muscle and neural fibers of the region. It is important to recognize the presence of the transversalis fascia attached to the flap and reenter in the right plane as soon as possible (**Figure 43-7**).

Step 2 average time frame: 5–10 min

> ▶▶ **TIPS**
>
> The initial opening of the peritoneum starts with measuring a proper distance above the internal inguinal ring. Once incised, the peritoneum is then pulled with the hook, allowing the CO_2 to spread and dissect the preperitoneal space (**Figure 43-8**).
>
> The flap incision is made along a slightly oblique line with the lateral portion being lower than the medial one. This allows an optimal exposure of the surgical field without having the peritoneal flap covering the view. Often, the shaft of the robotic instruments can be used to provide retraction of the flap while simultaneously using the EndoWrist® for fine movements and dissection.

> ⚠ **PITFALLS**
>
> Losing the correct plane is a possible risk when not familiar with the anatomy. When the fibers of the rectus muscle are visible, the plane is too deep. A wrong plane is riskier for neural damage laterally and at the base of the surgical field.

904 The Foundation and Art of Robotic Surgery

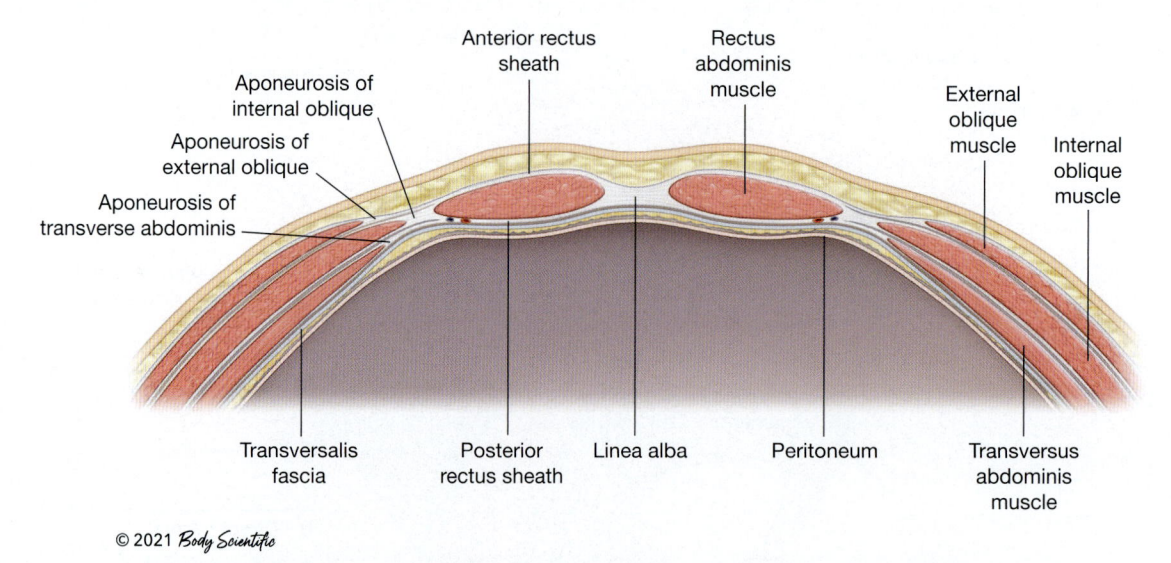

FIGURE 43-7 • Transversalis fascia.

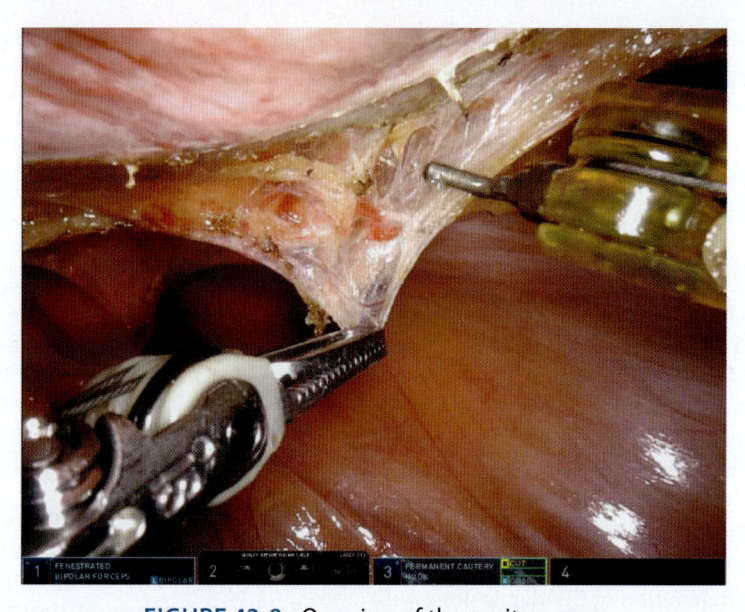

FIGURE 43-8 • Opening of the peritoneum.

▶ **Video 43-2. Medial Dissection**

Step 3. Medial dissection (Zone 2)

Once the upper margin of the preperitoneal flap is opened, the blunt dissection proceeds toward the Cooper's ligament without touching the hernia sac. The peritoneum is dissected medially to and around the medial aspect of the hernia sac. This maneuver allows a better understanding of the anatomy of the preperitoneal space, which will facilitate a safer hernia sac dissection. It is important to follow the correct plane in front of the prevesical fat. When in the proper plane, the dissection is almost bloodless and can be done bluntly with minimal use of energy. The plane is progressively opened until the pubic bone and the Cooper's ligament are identified. Dissection should expose a short segment of the pubic bone to allow a good accommodation of the mesh and to be able to safely apply a fixing stitch (**Figure 43-9**).

A direct hernia defect is located medial to the epigastric vessels and above the pectineal ligament. The direct hernia "pseudo-sac" is characterized by a weakened transversalis fascia and muscles, and its content most frequently consists of preperitoneal fat. This is generally on the way during the medial dissection, and it is easier to dissect medially to it before reducing the hernia. At the end of this step, it is usually possible to recognize the *vas deferens* entering into the inguinal canal in the medial corner of the deep inguinal ring. The Cooper's ligament and the pubis are exposed.

Step 3 average time frame: 5–10 min

Inguinal Hernia Repair   905

> ▶▶ **TIPS**
>
> Frequent lifting of the peritoneal flap and retraction of the hernia sac allows a better recognition of the spermatic vessels and the *vas deferens* underneath. Usually, the spermatic vessels are at the bottom of the hernia sac, and the *vas deferens* is joining the spermatic vessels at the level of the medial corner of the deep inguinal ring.
>
> While dissecting medially to expose the pubic bone, gentle probing of the tissue with a grasper can help identifying this landmark. Although the system has no tactile feedback, it will be easy to notice that the instrument doesn't move when it reaches the bony structure (virtual tactile feedback).

> ⚠ **PITFALLS**
>
> In some cases, a vascular connection between the external iliac vessels or the deep inferior epigastric and the obturator vessels might be present. This anatomical structure was called the *"corona mortis"* by ancient surgeons facing uncontrollable bleeding caused by inadvertent lesion of those vessels. During medial dissection in proximity of the pubic bone, the possibility of this anatomical variant should be kept in mind (**Figure 43-10**).

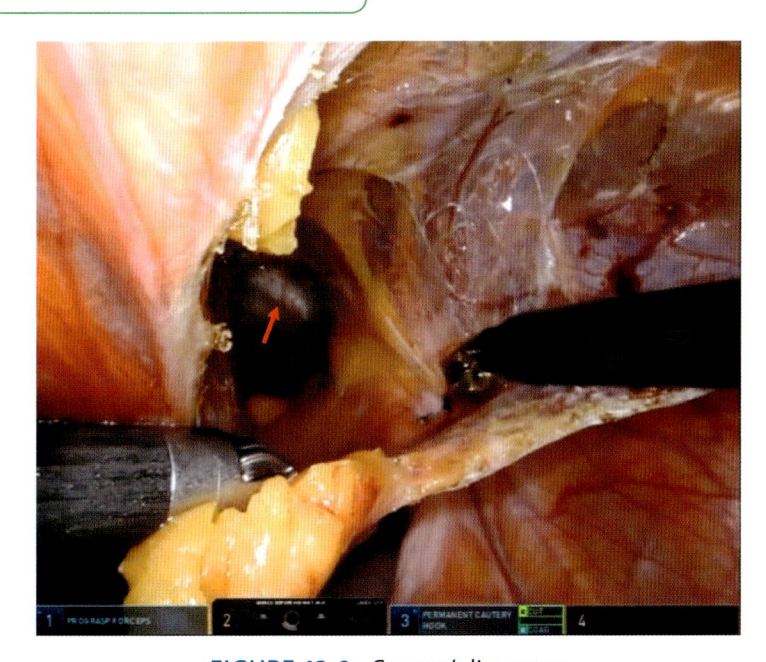

FIGURE 43-9 • Cooper's ligament.

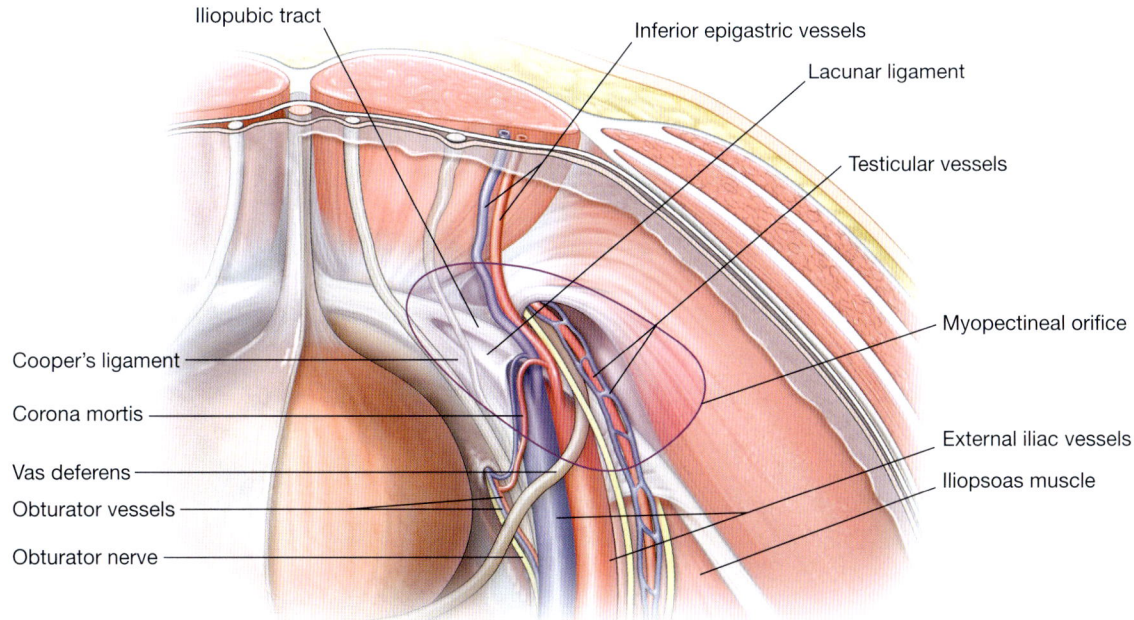

FIGURE 43-10 • *Corona mortis.*

Step 4. Lateral dissection (Zone 1)

The lateral dissection space corresponds to the area located lateral to the inferior epigastric vessels and spermatic cord. Blunt dissection in this area should be performed very carefully because preperitoneal fat covers the lateral cutaneous nerve of the thigh, the femoral nerve, and the branches of the genitofemoral nerve. The monopolar hook or the monopolar scissors combined with the grasper are the main instruments to perform the dissection. The ASIS represents the lateral border of this dissection, and the psoas muscle represents the base. In addition to the psoas muscle, the spermatic vessels should also be identified.

Step 4 average time frame: 3–5 min

> ⚠ **PITFALLS**
> - Risk of damaging the lateral cutaneous nerve of the thigh, the femoral nerve branches, and the genitofemoral nerve.
> - A good understanding of the position of the spermatic vessels should be obtained, at this stage, so that the vessels are not lifted with the sac increasing the risk of their injury.

> ▶▶ **TIPS**
> A thin layer of connective tissue, present in the preperitoneal space, should be kept in contact with the inguinal floor and not with the peritoneum, in order to reduce the risk of nerve damage. Energy levels should be kept low, and blunt dissection should be preferred to monopolar energy in this area. If hemostasis is necessary, bipolar coagulation should be used.

> 🔍 **ANATOMICAL HIGHLIGHTS**
>
> **Nerves in the inguinal region.** The relevant nerves in the inguinal region are the iliohypogastric, the ilioinguinal, the genitofemoral, the lateral femoral cutaneous, and the femoral nerves. These nerves arise from the lumbar plexus, innervate the abdominal musculature, and give sensitive fibers to the skin and the parietal peritoneum. Their entrapment may cause refractory pain (difficult to treat), and their transection results in numbness. These nerves are inconstantly visualized during the laparoscopic procedure. The risk of iatrogenic injury is different in laparoscopy/robotics and open surgery (see **Figures 43-11 A, B**).
>
> These 3 nerves are mainly endangered in laparoscopy:
> 1. Lateral femoral cutaneous nerve
> 2. Genitofemoral nerve
> 3. Anterior branches of the femoral nerve
>
> These 3 nerves are more at risk of injury during open hernia repair:
> 1. Iliohypogastric
> 2. Ilioinguinal
> 3. Genital branches of genitofemoral

Inguinal Hernia Repair 907

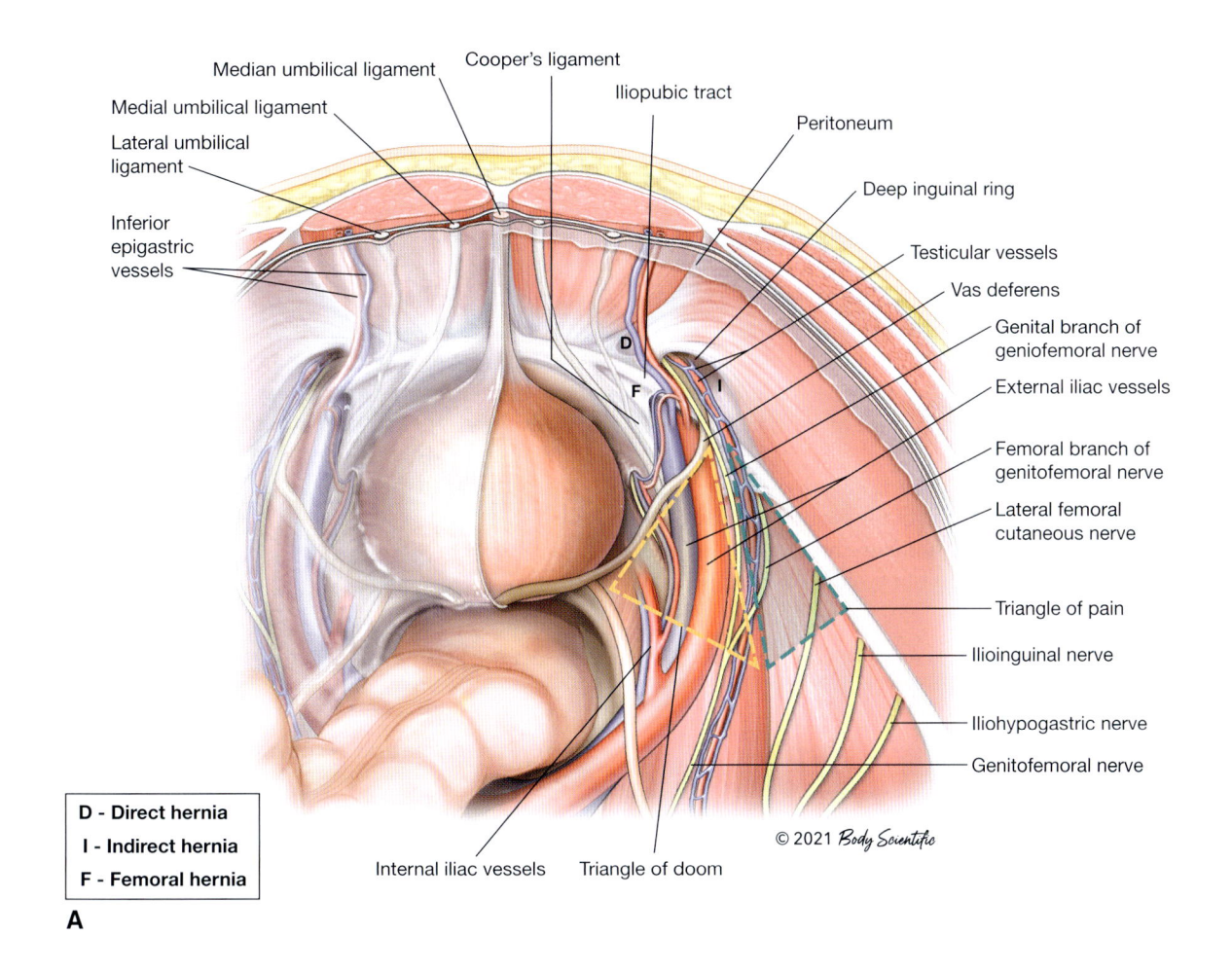

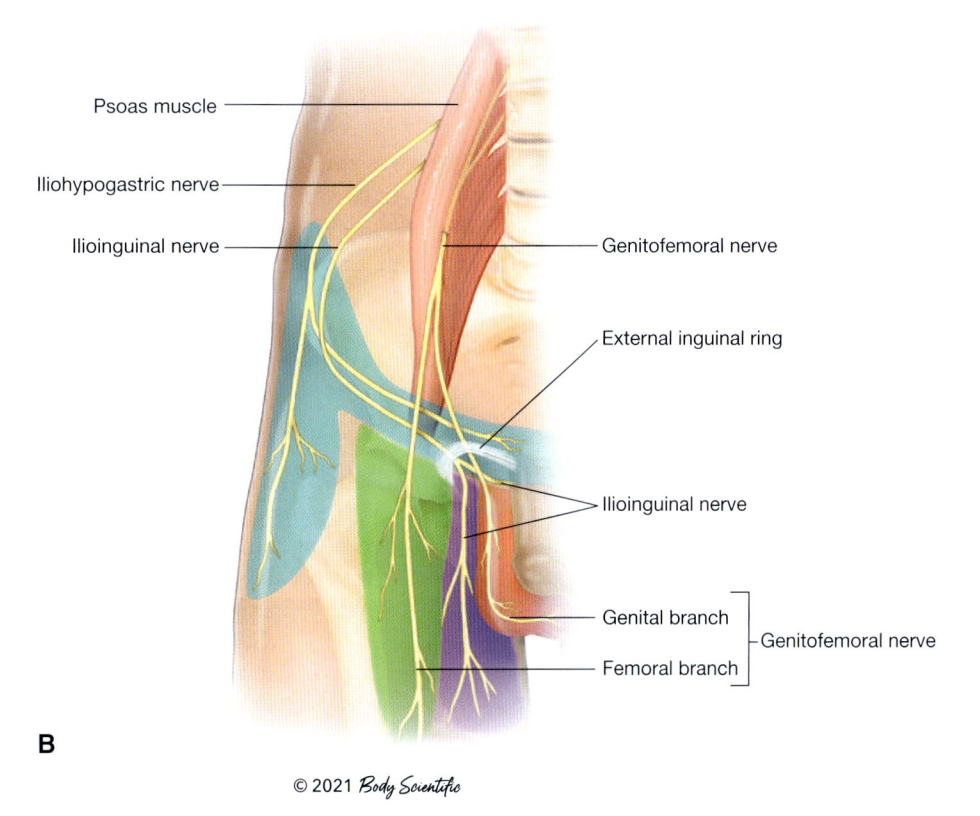

FIGURE 43-11 • Nerves of the inguinal canal.

▶ **Video 43-3. Hernia Sac Dissection**

Step 5. Hernia sac dissection (Zone 3)

The hernia sac is grasped at the superomedial edge. With a combination of blunt traction and monopolar energy, the hernia sac is progressively dissected along its superior border. Holding the superior border of the hernia sac allows to dissect safely, staying away from the cord elements. The dissection is mostly blunt, gently pushing down the spermatic vessels and detaching the hernia sac. Once the tip of the sac is reached, the traction is moved on the tip, and at this point, it is easier to complete the separation of the sac from the spermatic cord.

In rare occasions, when the dissection is particularly difficult and the hernia large, a portion of the sac can be transected and abandoned. In such cases, it is important later on to suture the resulting peritoneal flap defect to avoid a possible internal herniation.

Step 5 average time frame: 10–20 min (or more depending on the anatomy)

> 🔍 **ANATOMICAL HIGHLIGHTS**
>
> The triangle of doom is formed medially by the *vas deferens*, laterally by the spermatic vessels, and inferiorly by the psoas muscle. It is an important region where the external iliac vessels are located.

> ▶▶ **TIPS**
>
> In primary hernias with a smaller hernia sac, a blunt dissection is sufficient in most cases. A suture cut needle driver with stronger grasping action may help in gentle peeling the sac off from the tunica vaginalis and cord structures. However, in large, recurrent, and/or chronically inflamed hernias, the sac can sometimes be thick and fibrotic. In such cases, a combination of sharp and blunt dissection is necessary. The hernia sac inside the inguinal canal may be fused with cremasteric muscle fibers and cremasteric fascia. The separation of the sac may require the division of cremasteric structures. Sharp dissection with the monopolar scissors or the hook is necessary. This dissection is particularly delicate, requires a perfect understanding of the anatomy, and entails the risk of injuring the genital branch of the genitofemoral nerve, the spermatic vessels, and also the testicles. If this dissection becomes too difficult, it is preferable to open the sac, divide it from inside, abandon the distal stump, and reduce the proximal one toward the abdomen.

> ⚠ **PITFALLS**
>
> In female patients, the round ligament of the uterus is an important structure running inside the inguinal canal. Some surgeons advocate its transection to have a better placement of the mesh. In reality, there is no need to divide the ligament if a good preparation of the space is made. There is no proof that by dividing the ligament the hernia recurrence rate will be lower. On the contrary, there is evidence that the division of the ligament, in rare cases, is connected with prolapse of the labium majus and also the uterus.
>
> The possibility of a spermatic cord lipoma should be always taken into account. In many occasions, the hernia defect is quite small, but there can be a significant symptomatic spermatic cord lipoma. Failure to recognize and resect the lipoma can cause persistence of symptoms.

Step 6. Parietalization of spermatic vessels and extension of the horizontal plane

It is essential to extend the dissection to expose the iliopsoas muscle. This maneuver facilitates the creation of a good horizontal space to ensure an adequate positioning of a properly sized mesh. In this process, the spermatic vessels should be progressively detached from the peritoneal flap that, at this point, is containing the hernia sac (parietalization of the spermatic vessels). The separation is performed with a gentle blunt technique, being careful not to damage the veins.

Step 6 average time frame: 3–5 min

> ⚠ **PITFALLS**
>
> **Bleeding from the spermatic veins.** In this case, it is better to avoid coagulation that might entail the risk of obliterating the small spermatic artery. Compression has to be applied first, and it could be enough for minor injuries. If necessary, additional Prolene™ 5-0/6-0 precise stitches can be added.

Step 7. Reinforcement of myopectineal orifice (optional)

This step is controversial and optional. Not all hernia surgeons are in agreement, some claim an increased risk of damaging the nerves. However, the precise closure of the hernia defect may add strength to the reconstruction and decrease the formation of seromas. A clear understanding of the anatomy is paramount. One or 2 interrupted stiches of Prolene™ 2-0 are applied between the ligament and the edge of the defect containing fibers of the internal oblique and the arch of the transvers fascia. When passing the stiches on the ligament, the needle should be seen in transparency during the entire passage, avoiding the risk of going too deep and pinching the nerves or even vessels. Also, the upper passage of the needle on the internal oblique and transverse fibers should be prudent, avoiding including too much tissue and possible neural branches. This step should be avoided if the defect is too large, if it creates too much tension, or if there is a risk of encasing neural branches.

Step 7 average time frame: 3–5 min

Step 8. Mesh placement

The standard mesh used is a 10 × 15-cm polypropylene. This mesh allows for adequate coverage of the hernia site with good overlap in most patients. In rare cases, a larger or smaller mesh may be required, but this occurs in less than 15% of cases. The first step is to roll the mesh on a laparoscopic grasper. Then, the mesh is deployed in the abdominal cavity through one of the robotic ports or the optional 10–12-mm assistant port, if present. The mesh will then be placed to cover the defect.

The stitch is placed at the Cooper's ligament using a 2-0 Prolene™ (**Figure 43-12A**). The needle is first passed through the mesh still suspended, and then to the Cooper's ligament with an unobstructed view and back to the mesh with a U configuration. The shaft of the needle driver, while working, is used to retract the peritoneal flap and to expose the anatomy. A perfect visualization during stitching is important to avoid inadvertent injury of nearby structures created by the needle (*corona mortis*, external iliac vein, retropubic venous plexus). One or 2 stitches at the upper edge of the mesh can be placed on the transversalis fascia to stabilize the mesh and to avoid lateral twisting. In doing that, attention should be paid not to penetrate too deep to avoid including the nerves (**Figure 43-12B**).

Step 8 average time frame: 5–10 min

> ⚠ **PITFALLS**
>
> - There is a risk of the mesh rolling when its edges are not laid completely flat and the peritoneum is pulled up for the final closure.
> - Another potential pitfall is to use a smaller mesh than what is ideal because of lack of adequate dissection. Most patients will need a 10 × 15-cm mesh.

> ▶▶ **TIPS**
>
> The appropriate size of the mesh, and its correct flat positioning, are extremely important to reduce the risk of recurrence. The prosthetic material has to be large enough to cover the most vulnerable recurrence sites (such as the medial aspect over Hesselbach's triangle, the femoral space, the iliac vessels, and the iliopsoas muscle). The final 3D configuration, in a lateral projection, should be L-shaped with equal length of the vertical and horizontal limbs; the vertical being the anterior abdominal wall, and the horizontal being the posterior retroperitoneal muscles. In this configuration, all pressure forces will be distributed on the mesh, keeping it in perfect position against the wall and avoiding recurrences above and below the mesh.
>
> The easiest way to place a mesh is to push the medial end as deep as possible over the pubic symphysis and Cooper's ligament. While keeping the medial end of the mesh in place, the lateral part is placed over the border of the iliopubic tract.
>
> A standard-weight mesh can be challenging for the introduction through the 8-mm port. This maneuver can be facilitated using, for the introduction of the mesh, a smaller diameter instrument, such as a 5-mm laparoscopic needle driver.

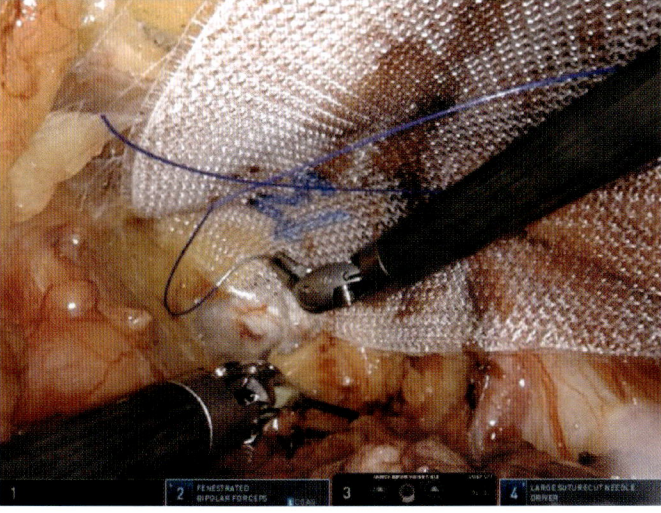

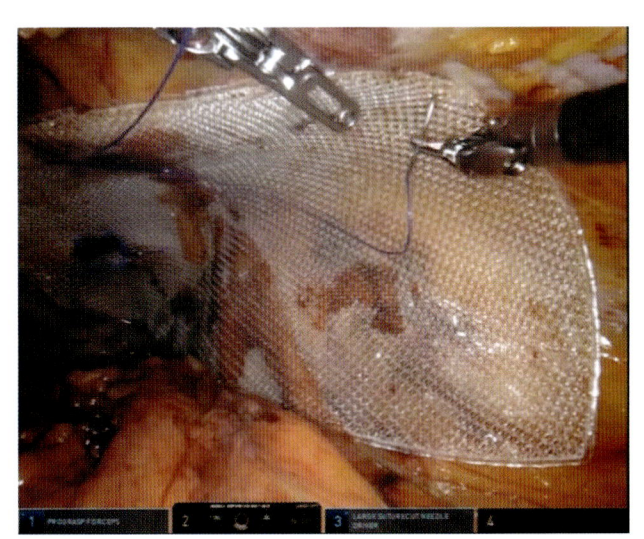

FIGURE 43-12 • **A.** Mesh fixation. **B.** Mesh placement.

Step 9. Flap closure

The last step is the closure of the peritoneal flap. Care must be taken for accurate flap closure to avoid contact between the mesh and the bowel. A Vicryl™ 3-0 suture, 25 cm long, is used in running fashion. The direction of suturing should be lateral to medial for the left side and medial to lateral for the right. In this way, there will be no overlapping in between the function of the 2 hands, the grasper holding the suture, and the needle driver passing the needle (**Figure 43-13**).

Step 9 average time frame: 5–10 min

▶▶ TIPS

- In order to reduce the flap tension, a portion of the umbilical ligament or the hernia sac can be incorporated in the final closure, so that the gaps can be covered without breaking the peritoneum (plasty of the flap).
- The closure doesn't need to be sealed tight. As long as the mesh is not exposed, little imperfections in the flap closure will allow potential drainage of serous fluids in the early postoperative period.

⚠ PITFALLS

The closure of the flap under tension can create an empty space between the flap and the abdominal wall. The flap may break down, creating a risk of postoperative symptomatic small bowel internal herniation. In this situation, it is prudent to consider a plasty of the closure using adjacent tissue (e.g., portion of the hernia sac or median umbilical ligament).

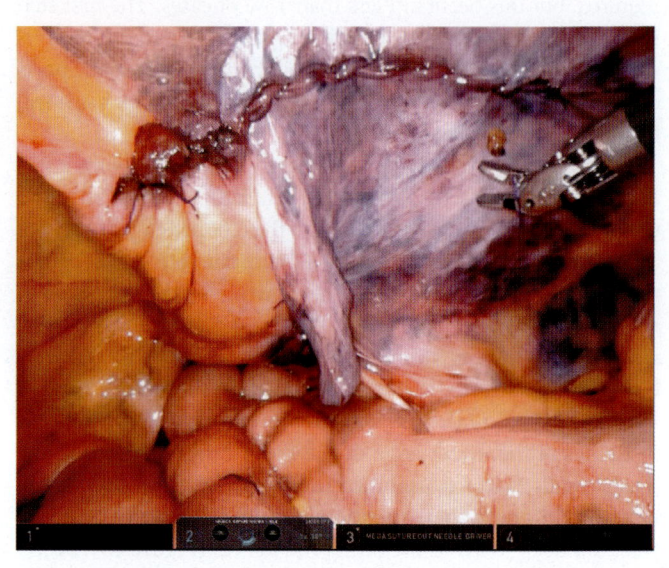

FIGURE 43-13 • Closure of the peritoneal flap.

Suggested Readings

1. Rutkow IM. Demographic and socioeconomic aspects of hernia repair in the United States in 2003. *Surg Clin North Am.* 2003;83(5):1045-1051, v-vi.
2. HerniaSurge. International guidelines for groin hernia management. *Hernia.* 2018;22(1):1-165.
3. Beadles CA, Meagher AD, Charles AG. Trends in emergent hernia repair in the United States. *JAMA Surg.* 2015;150(3):194-200.
4. Ger R. The management of certain abdominal herniae by intra-abdominal closure of the neck of the sac. Preliminary communication. *Ann R Coll Surg Engl.* 1982;64(5):342-344.
5. Arregui ME, Davis CJ, Yucel O, Nagan RF. Laparoscopic mesh repair of inguinal hernia using a preperitoneal approach: a preliminary report. *Surg Laparosc Endosc.* 1992;2(1):53-58.
6. LeBlanc KA. *Evolution of Laparoscopic Ventral Hernia Repair, in Laparoscopic Ventral Hernia Repair.* Springer: 2003:107-114.
7. Simons MP, Aufenacker T, Bay-Nielsen M, et al. European Hernia Society guidelines on the treatment of inguinal hernia in adult patients. *Hernia.* 2009;13(4):343-403.
8. Bittner R, Arregui ME, Bisgaard T, et al. Guidelines for laparoscopic (TAPP) and endoscopic (TEP) treatment of inguinal hernia [International Endohernia Society (IEHS)]. *Surg Endosc.* 2011;25(9):2773-2843.
9. Henriksen NA, Jensen KK, Muysoms F. Robot-assisted abdominal wall surgery: a systematic review of the literature and meta-analysis. *Hernia.* 2019;23(1):17-27.
10. Gamagami R, Dickens E, Gonzalez A, et al. Open versus robotic-assisted transabdominal preperitoneal (R-TAPP) inguinal hernia repair: a multicenter matched analysis of clinical outcomes. *Hernia.* 2018;22(5): 827-836.
11. Muysoms F, Van Cleven S, Kyle-Leinhase I, et al. Robotic-assisted laparoscopic groin hernia repair: observational case-control study on the operative time during the learning curve. *Surg Endosc.* 2018;32(12):4850-4859.
12. Szold A, Bergamaschi R, Broeders I, et al. European Association of Endoscopic Surgeons (EAES) consensus statement on the use of robotics in general surgery. *Surg Endosc.* 2015;29(2):253-288.
13. Ito F, Jarrard D, Gould JC. Transabdominal preperitoneal robotic inguinal hernia repair. *J Laparoendosc Adv Surg Tech A.* 2008;18(3):397-399.
14. Iraniha A, Peloquin J. Long-term quality of life and outcomes following robotic assisted TAPP inguinal hernia repair. *J Robot Surg.* 2018;12(2):261-269.
15. Kolachalam R, Dickens E, D'Amico L, et al. Early outcomes of robotic-assisted inguinal hernia repair in obese patients: a multi-institutional, retrospective study. *Surg Endosc.* 2018;32(1):229-235.
16. Giulianotti PC, Coratti A, Angelini M, et al. Robotics in general surgery: personal experience in a large community hospital. *Arch Surg.* 2003;138(7):777-784. doi: 10.1001/archsurg.138.7.777

"The state of hernial surgery has advanced to the point that one must consider the systematic surgical cure of all diagnosed hernias."

—Rene Stoppa (1921–2006)

Ventral Hernia Repair
(Intraperitoneal Onlay Mesh with Fascial Defect Approximation)

Karl LeBlanc • Patrice Frederick • Carolina Baz

INTRODUCTION

Ventral hernias can be divided into 2 main categories: acquired or congenital. Congenital hernias appear in weak areas of the abdominal wall, whereas acquired hernias protrude through the closure site after a surgical procedure (incisional hernias) or are the consequence of a trauma (posttraumatic hernias).

Among the different types of ventral hernias, the incisional ones represent about 85%. The incidence of these hernias after a midline laparotomy is 2–30%; wound infection may drive the incidence even higher. Umbilical hernias follow in frequency with an estimated incidence of 6–14%, then epigastric hernias (3–5%) and finally spigelian hernias (0.12–2%). See suggested readings #3, 5, 6, 7.

Annually, there are more than 400,000 ventral hernia operations in the United States. The morbidity and the rate of infections connected with the open technique encouraged a progressive adoption of a minimal invasive approach.

Laparoscopic ventral hernia repair was first described by Karl LeBlanc in 1993. This minimally invasive approach became progressively adopted for these kinds of hernias because of its improved outcomes. The application of laparoscopic techniques broadened to include more complex hernias, and eventually, endoscopic and laparoscopic approaches were used for component separation and flap development. As indications for robotic surgery encompassed more procedures, allowing more sophisticated suturing and dissection techniques, those who repaired ventral hernias by laparoscopy became early adopters of the robotic approach. Robotic repair with primary defect closure resulted in improved recovery time and decreased hospital stay in addition of achieving better cosmesis and function. Nowadays, there are innumerable options for robotic repair (**Table 44-1**); however, this chapter will focus on the most frequent, the standard technique of the intraperitoneal onlay mesh (IPOM) plus repair.

Extended totally extraperitoneal (eTEP)—This repair gains access to the abdominal wall with the initial port placement. The plane of dissection is above the posterior rectus sheath. Hernia dissection and repair occur in this space avoiding the mesh placement within the peritoneum.

Transversus abdominis release (TAR)—Also known as the posterior component separation. It is typically reserved for larger defects >10 cm. The procedure begins with accessing the posterior rectus sheath and dissecting it until the neurovascular bundle of the rectus muscle is identified. The transversus abdominis muscle is divided, and the plane between this muscle and the peritoneum is dissected to advance a myofascial

INSTRUMENT REQUIREMENTS

The suggested main robotic instruments/tools can be listed as follows:
- 30° scope
- Fenestrated bipolar forceps
- Cautery hook/monopolar scissors
- Needle holders
- Round-tip scissors (if not using suture cut needle holder)
- Cold scissors (if needed for adhesiolysis)

The suggested main laparoscopic instruments/tools can be listed as follows:
- Needle driver
- Scissors
- Laparoscopic forceps

Supplemental materials:
- Composite mesh
- Sutures: #1 V-Loc™ nonabsorbable, Prolene™ 2-0
- Endo Bag™ (to remove the hernia sac, if excised, or lipomas, if present)

Photo reproduced with permission from Stoppa RE. Wrapping the visceral sac into a bilateral mesh prosthesis in groin hernia repair. Hernia. 2003;7(1):2-12.
Quote reproduced with permission from Arora E, Kukleta J, Ramana B. A detailed history of retromuscular repairs for ventral hernias: a story of surgical innovation. World J Surg. 2022;46(2):409-415.

TABLE 44-1 • Additional Types of Repairs		
Types of Robotic Repairs	**Size of Defect**	**Mesh Placement**
IPOM Plus	<10 cm	Intraperitoneal
eTEP (extended view totally extraperitoneal)	<10 cm	Intraparietal
TAR (transversus abdominis release)	>10 cm	Intraparietal
TAPP (transabdominal preperitoneal)	<10 cm	Intraparietal
Retrorectus Repairs	<10 cm	Intraparietal

ANATOMICAL HIGHLIGHTS

Abdominal wall anatomy

- The abdominal wall is a complex structure involving muscles and aponeurotic fibers intertwined in a matrix of cross-fibers with varying densities. It is conformed by the rectus abdominis, a vertically orientated muscle that originates from the pubic symphysis and inserts into the costal cartilages of the 5th to 7th ribs. Laterally, it is connected with 3 flat muscles, the external oblique, internal oblique, and the transversus abdominis, whose fibers fuse to form the sheath that covers the rectus abdominis, reaching the midline to form the línea alba (**Figure 44-1**).
- The fibers of the external and internal oblique muscles build up the anterior sheath of the rectus, whereas the posterior one is composed by the transversus abdominis and the internal oblique fibers. This conformation of the anterior and posterior sheaths of the rectus abdominis changes once the arcuate line is encountered.
- The arcuate line is located 3–5 cm below the umbilicus. Under this point, the aponeurosis of all the lateral muscles forms the anterior sheath of the rectus abdominis and only the transversalis fascia passes posterior to the muscle.
- The linea semilunaris runs along the lateral edges of the rectus abdominis muscle and extends from the 9th costal cartilage to the pubic tubercle; it is where the lateral abdominal muscles meet the rectus abdominis.
- Hernias are the result of congenital defects, surgical incisions, or trauma (**Figure 44-2**). An understanding of the abdominal wall is paramount to the repair of hernias, especially complex ones that may require component separation. The mesh can be placed in different planes into the abdominal wall according to the type of repair being used (**Figures 44-3 A–D**).

flap to relieve tension and allow fascial reapproximation. The peritoneum serves as a barrier, and the mesh is placed behind the dissected transversus abdominis muscle.

Transabdominal preperitoneal (TAPP)—This repair is performed by dissecting the peritoneum from the abdominal wall; it is an extension of what is routinely done for robotic-assisted inguinal hernia repairs. If an adequate preperitoneal plane can be created around the defect, the mesh is placed above the peritoneum and the peritoneum is closed.

Retrorectus repair—This repair is limited to the retrorectus space. Access to this space can be performed as described via an eTEP or TAPP approach.

EDITORIAL COMMENT

Is not the goal of this chapter to discuss in depth the role of different types of meshes?

Anyway, a commonly used composite mesh in these procedures is one that combines polypropylene with an opposing Sepra® Technology (ST) barrier to minimize adhesions to the bowel. ST combines carboxymethylcellulose and hyaluronic acid and attaches to polypropylene by polyglycolic acid fibers. This hydrogel layer is activated when dipped in saline and expands for adequate barrier protection. It is present for approximately 4 weeks, allowing adequate time for a neoperitoneum to form over the polypropylene portion of the mesh. One of the first meshes used in laparoscopic ventral hernia repair was expanded polytetrafluoroethylene (ePTFE). These flat meshes have both a visceral side and a parietal side and provide a permanent barrier protection. Absorbable meshes, either synthetic or biologic, are not routinely used in the IPOM plus repair because of the risk of hernia recurrence if primary fascial closure fails. These meshes, however, have been described as adjuncts to component separation.

Ventral Hernia Repair 913

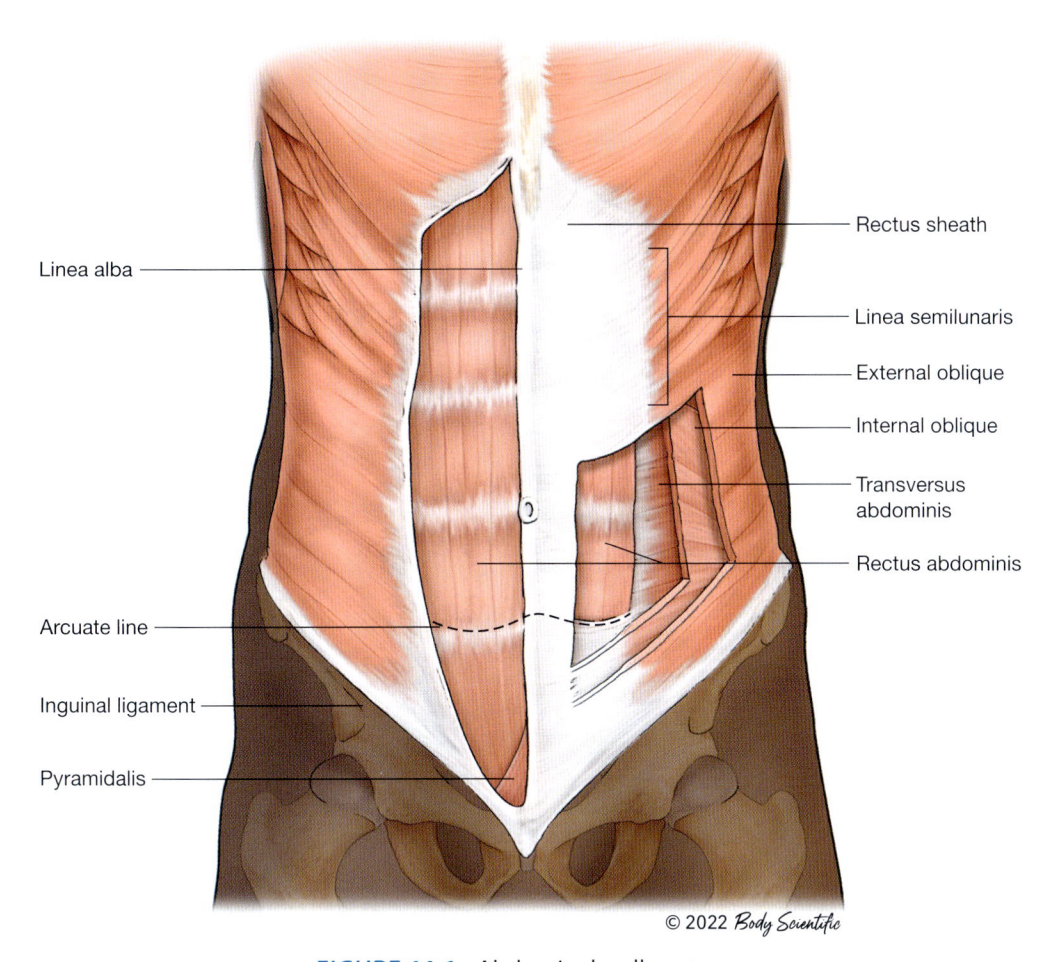

FIGURE 44-1 • Abdominal wall anatomy.

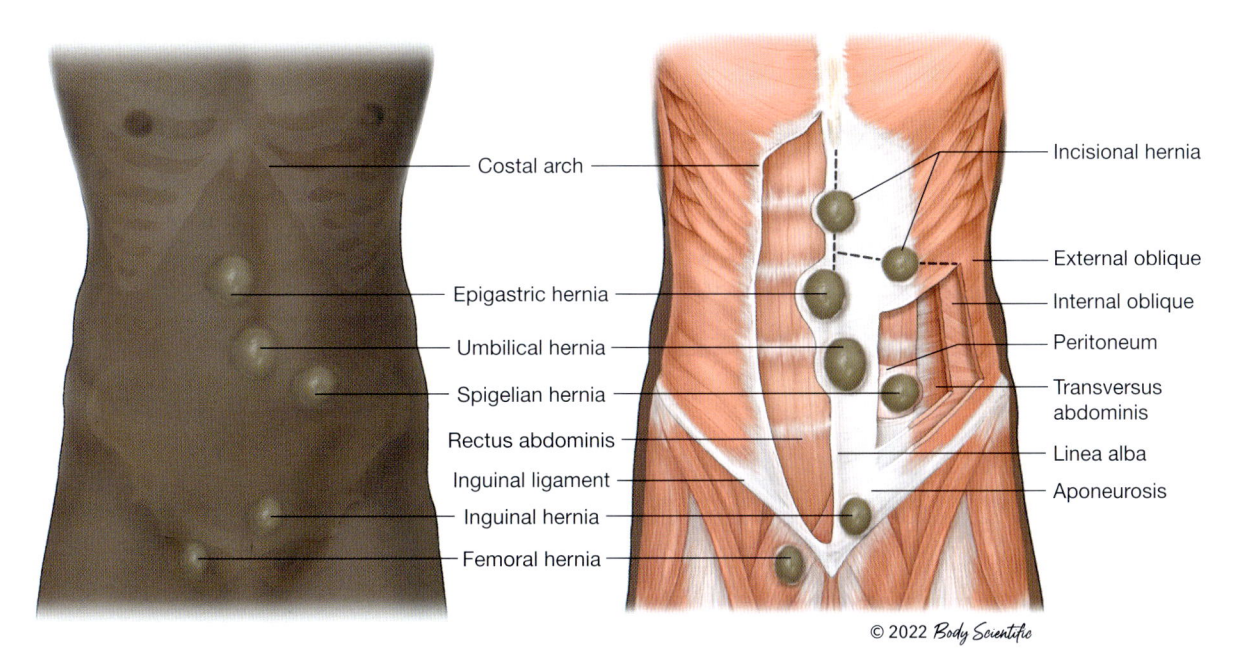

FIGURE 44-2 • Types of ventral hernias.

914 The Foundation and Art of Robotic Surgery

A

B

C

D

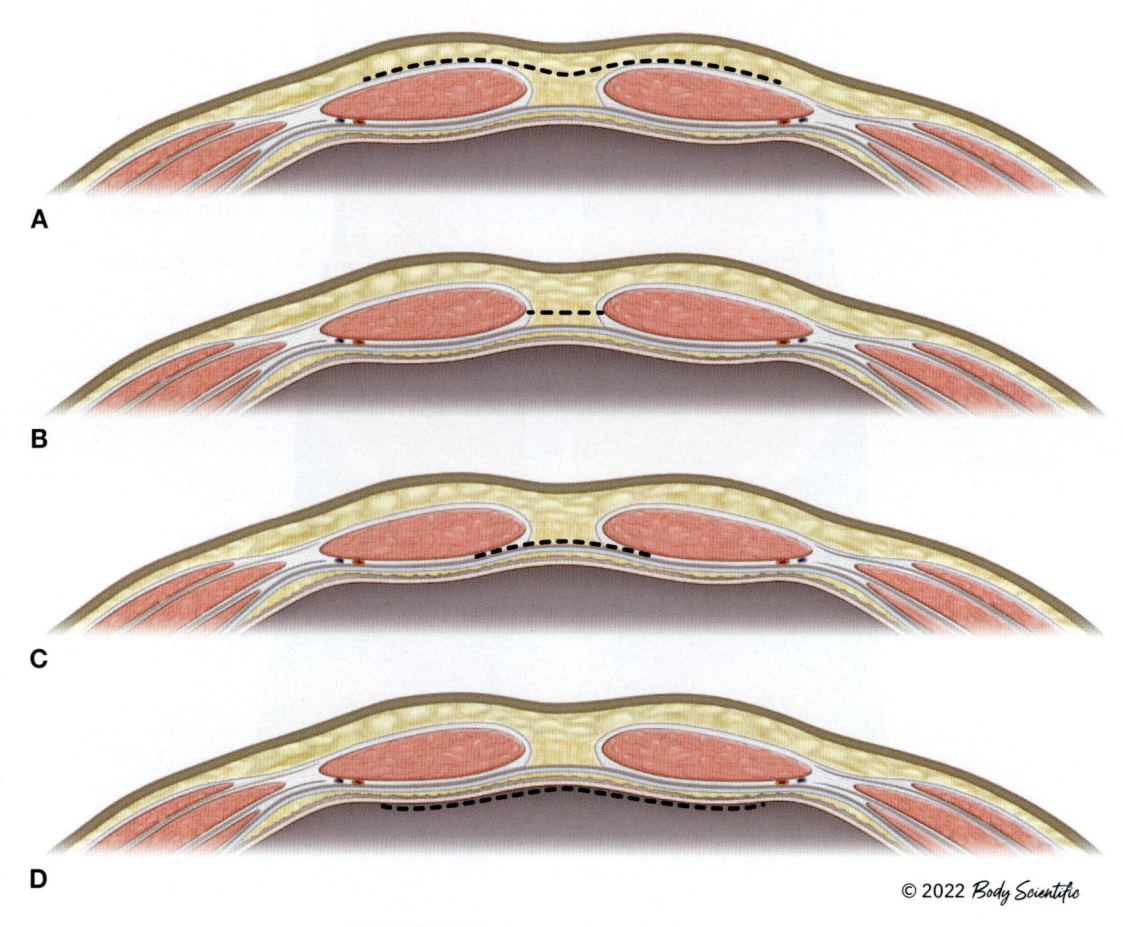

© 2022 Body Scientific

FIGURE 44-3 • Types of mesh placements.

> **EDITORIAL COMMENT**
>
> The mesh can be placed in different planes in the abdominal wall:
>
> A. **Onlay:** on the anterior fascia (premuscular location)
> B. **Inlay:** between the edges of the fascia where the defect is
> C. **Sublay:** in the retrorectus space (posterior to the rectus muscle and anterior to the posterior rectus sheath)
> D. **Intraperitoneal onlay:** over the peritoneum from inside the abdominal cavity

IPOM Plus Robotic Repair

Indications and Relative Contraindications to the IPOM Plus Robotic Approach

Any patient with a ventral defect may be a candidate for robotic repair. Generally, only defects less than 10 cm can be repaired robotically with the IPOM plus technique, because larger defects may require myofascial release to reapproximate. However, the selection should be based also on additional complexities connected with previous abdominal surgery (hostile abdomen), incarceration inside the hernia sac, body mass index (BMI), and multiple associated fascia defects. Additional complexities are not by themselves contraindications, but they can make the procedure more challenging. They are better dealt with once the surgical team has developed a consolidated experience.

General contraindications are the same as per any other laparoscopic procedure. Smoking cessation and weight loss should be encouraged before any elective operation.

> **EDITORIAL COMMENT**
>
> With experience, the improvement of materials (barbed sutures), and tricks such as lowering the intraoperative CO_2 pressure, the indication can sometimes be expanded to include defects >10 cm (**Figures 44-4 A, B**).

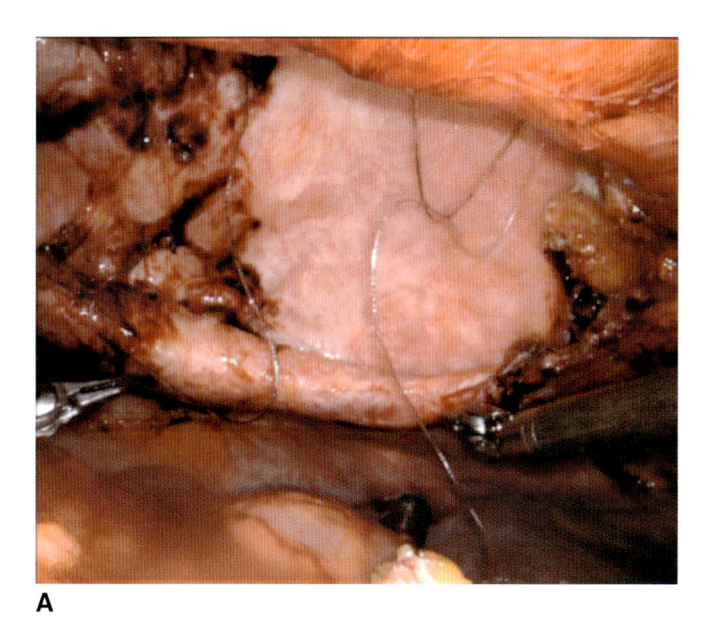

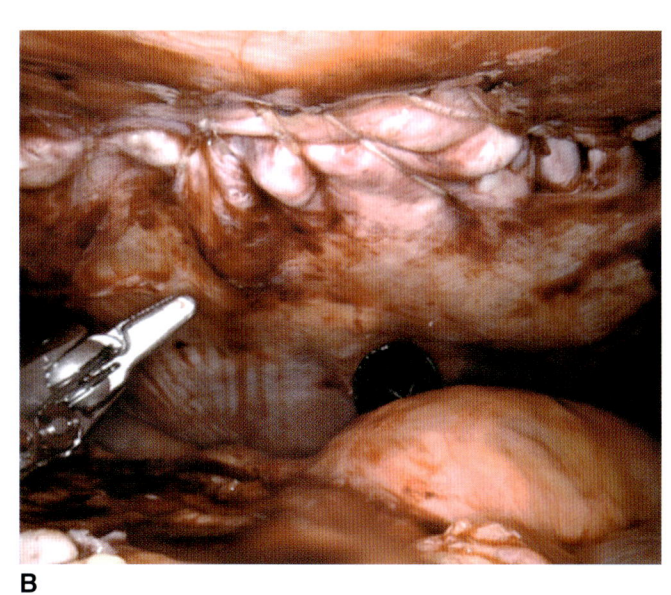

FIGURE 44-4 • Large ventral defect.

Patient Positioning, OR Setup, and Port Setting

The patient is placed in a supine position with both arms tucked to lower the risk of nerve injury. The patient is moved closer to the edge of the surgical bed on the side where the operative trocars will be placed to favor the mechanical movements of the robotic arms going downward to be able to reach up the anterior abdominal wall without restrictions of the instruments (**Figure 44-5**).

The assistant surgeon is standing on the same side of the ports (**Figure 44-6**).

> ▶▶ **TIPS**
>
> Having a full longitudinal relaxation of the rectum muscles is of paramount importance to favor the horizontal approximation when suturing:
> 1. The patient position should favor relaxation (breaking the table may paradoxically increase the tension).
> 2. The anesthesiologist should induce complete pharmacologic muscle release.

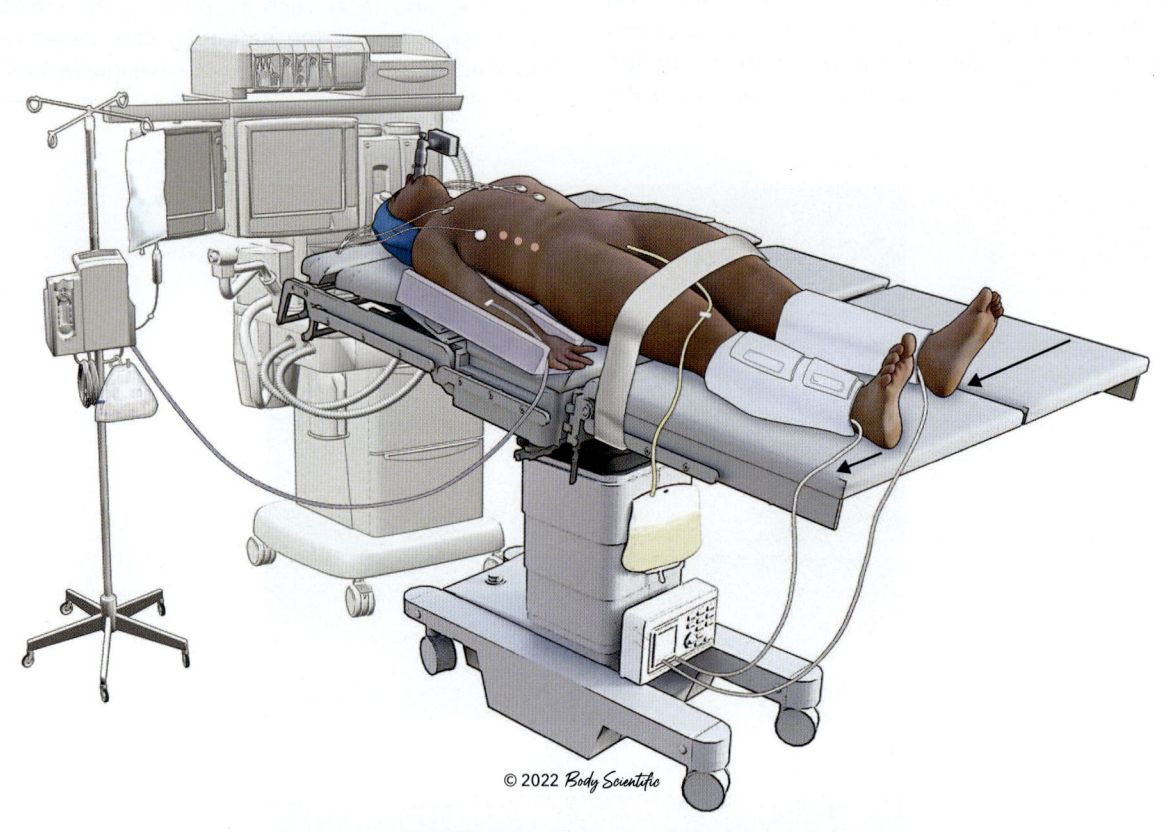

FIGURE 44-5 • Patient positioning.

Ventral Hernia Repair 917

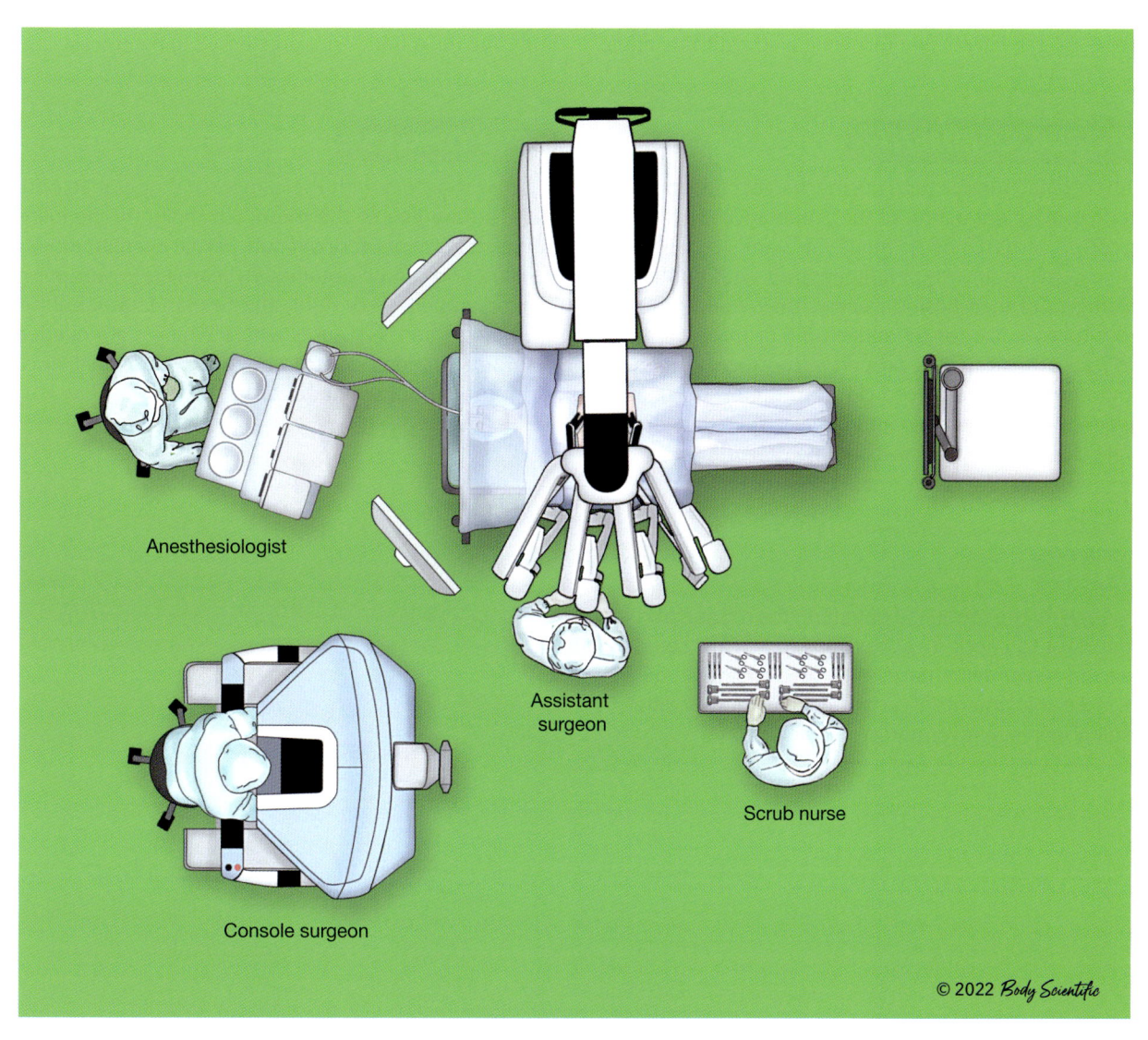

FIGURE 44-6 • OR setup.

Initial access is dependent on previous abdominal surgery and location of the defect. If the defect is centered in the midline, the ports can be positioned on the right or on the left. If defects are not centered, the contralateral side of the abdomen away from the defect may provide the best placement for the ports. Moreover, the bed can be tilted 20–30° lifting the side of the ports. This lateral movement of the surgical bed improves the motion capabilities of the robotic arms and decreases the collision with the surgical bed and the patient body (**Figure 44-7**).

On the right, the initial 5-mm trocar is placed in the middle portion of the lateral side following a straight line along the anterior axillary line and should be at least 8–10 cm away from the defect. Later on, this trocar is replaced with an 8-mm metallic trocar for the scope (**Figure 44-8**). The two 8-mm remaining trocars are placed above and under the first one following the same straight line. Ideally, the ports should be away enough from each other to avoid conflict, and at the same time, it should be kept in mind that the closer the trocars are to the chest or iliac spine, the higher are the chances of instrument collision in some area of the surgical field.

The robot is now placed directly over the midportion of the body and the robotic arms are docked to the trocars.

EDITORIAL COMMENT

It is important to understand the mechanics of the divergent or convergent action of the 2 operative arms and the scope. Learning how to move the 3 arms consensually in a convergent way simultaneously, with frequent adjustments of their position, allows their work even in narrow tunnels like for thyroidectomy or mastectomy. Taking advantage of this property, the trocars for the ventral hernia can be placed closer to the center point between the costal margin and the iliac spine avoiding lateral collision with the chest and the patient's legs.

⚠ PITFALLS

Being too close with the camera and operative ports to the suture line of the mesh can make the handling of the instruments very difficult. Partial overcoming of this restriction can be obtained by learning to suture with 1 hand, either left or right, and to plan strategical points where to tie the sutures where 2 hands are needed. In some situations, a port relocation or a dual docking approach might be required.

▶▶ TIPS

After docking the robot and engaging the robotic ports, is important to check that the robotic arms are able to do all the movements necessary to cover the surgical field. More adjustments of the patient and table position are still possible to favor unrestricted work.

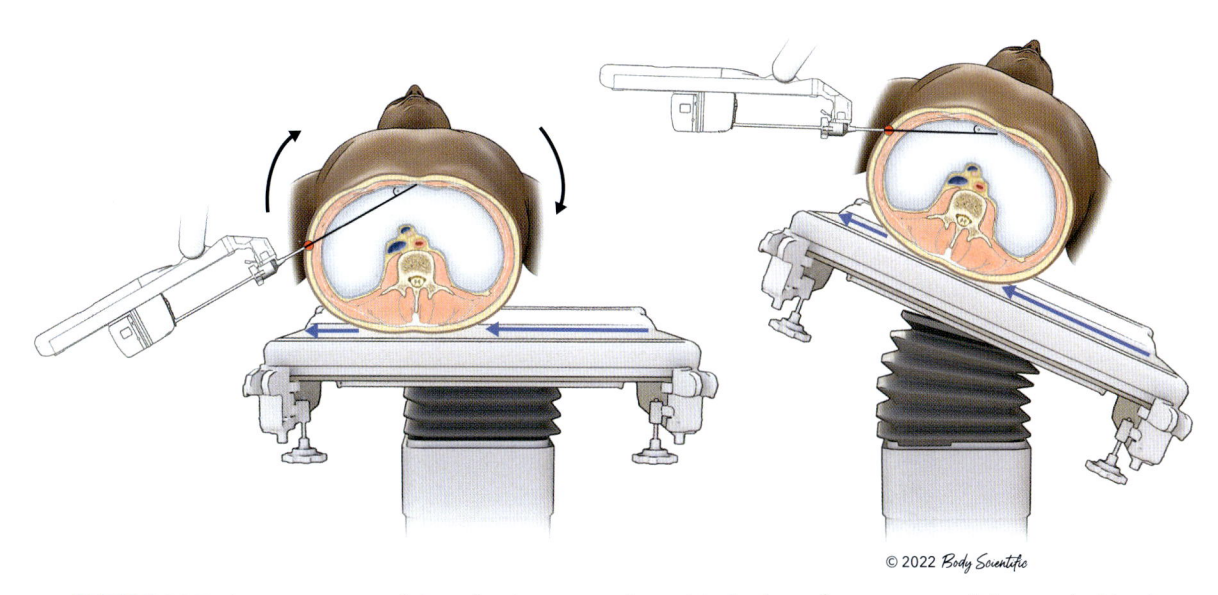

FIGURE 44-7 • Improvement of the robotic arm motion with the lateral movement of the surgical bed.

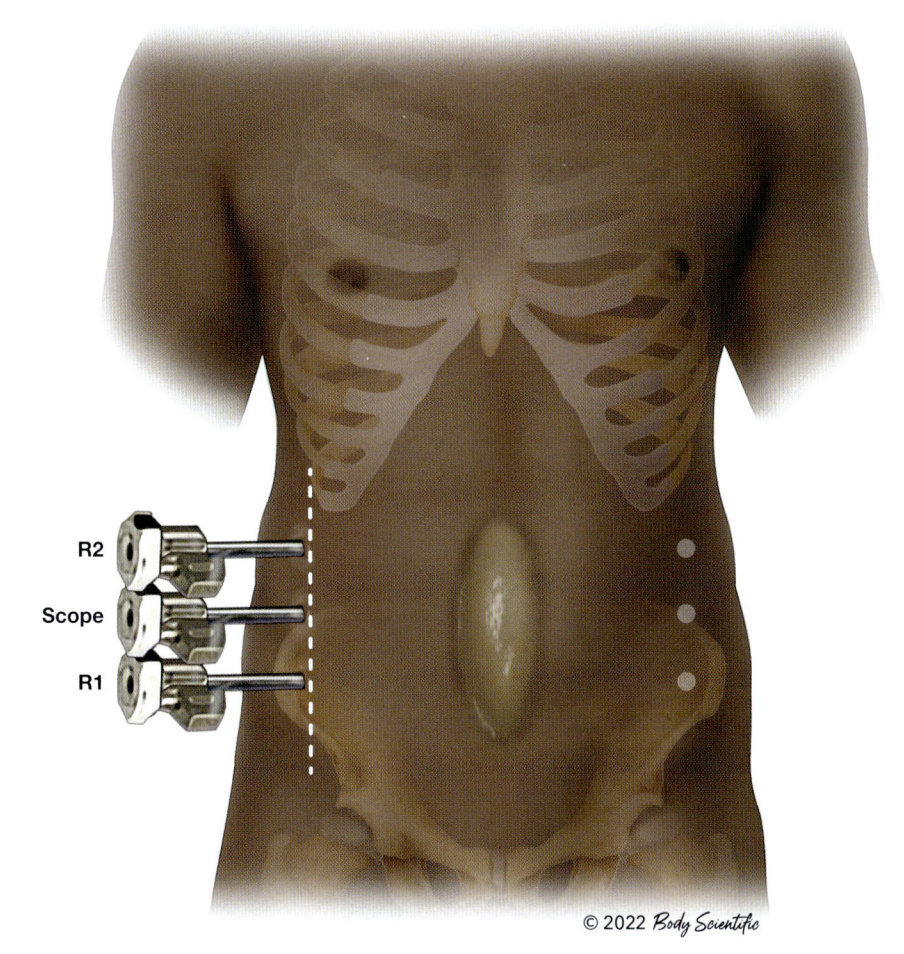

FIGURE 44-8 • Port setting midline hernia.

Surgical Technique

Step 1. Dissection and adhesiolysis

Once inside the abdominal cavity, if adhesions are encountered, adhesiolysis has to be performed. Omental adhesions can be divided with the use of the cautery hook. Adhesions involving the small bowel or colon should be dissected cautiously and ideally with the cold scissors to maintain the correct plane to avoid serosal tears. If deserosalizations happen, it is better to suture them immediately with PDS™ 4-0 because they can be missed if the suture is done later or at the end of the procedure. Minor bleeding from the adhesiolysis is controlled with bipolar coagulation (**Figures 44-9 A, B**). As adhesions are lysed, pneumo-dissection helps to delineate the plane between the portions of adherent bowel and helps to provide a safer bowel dissection with minimal traction.

Step 1 average time frame: 0 min (no adhesions)/60 min (multiple plastered adhesions)

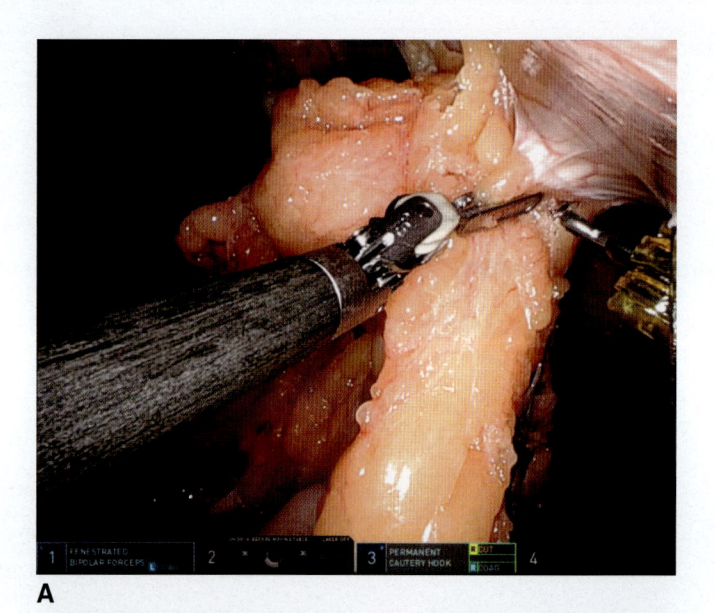

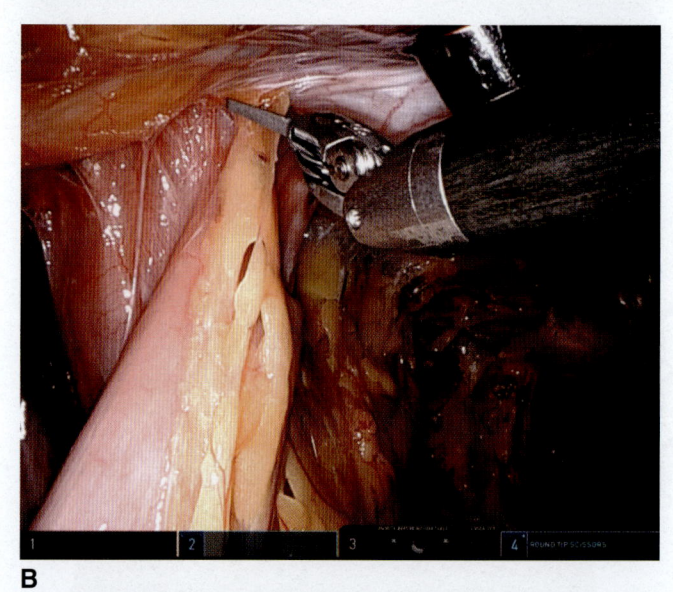

FIGURE 44-9 • Intra-abdominal adhesion resection.

Step 2. Dissection of the abdominal ventral defect

Once adhesions are lysed, hernia contents can be reduced. At times, incarcerated bowel or omentum may require careful dissection for complete reduction. After the reduction of the contents, the hernia sac can be dissected and reduced. The adhesions of the bowel with the hernia sac should be carefully taken down, unless they are extremely difficult, because leaving the sac even though reduced inside the abdominal cavity with the untouched adhesions can be reason of future episodes of bowel obstruction. With traction on the peritoneum, the hernia sac can be dissected from the defect with a peeling technique. A 5-cm fascial clearance around the defect is created for mesh overlap and adequate adherence to the abdominal wall.

Step 2 average time frame: 10–30 min

> **EDITORIAL COMMENT**
>
> The complete removal of the hernia sac can be difficult or contraindicated in some situations such as multiloculation of the sac or close adhesion to the skin with the risk of necrosis or perforation. The only consequence of leaving a portion of the sac is an increased risk of seromas. The majority of postoperative seromas can be managed conservatively.

Step 3. Closure of the fascial defect

Usually, the fascial defect is approximated with a running suture of #1 V-Loc™. The barbed sutures allowed significant progress in the technical ability of closing big gaps under some tension. The suture may start cephalad or from the bottom; it is better to start where the gap is shorter with less tension.

It is advisable to make multiple passages of the needle before adjusting the tension on the suture, pulling each passage loop individually (**Figure 44-10**).

Step 3 average time frame: 5–20 min

▶ **Video 44-1. Closure of the Fascial Defect**

> ▶▶ **TIPS**
>
> Reduction of the pneumo-pressure to 10–12 mm Hg may decrease the tension of the suture and favor the reapproximation of the fascial defect. Also, a complete muscle relaxation induced by the anesthesiologist is necessary.

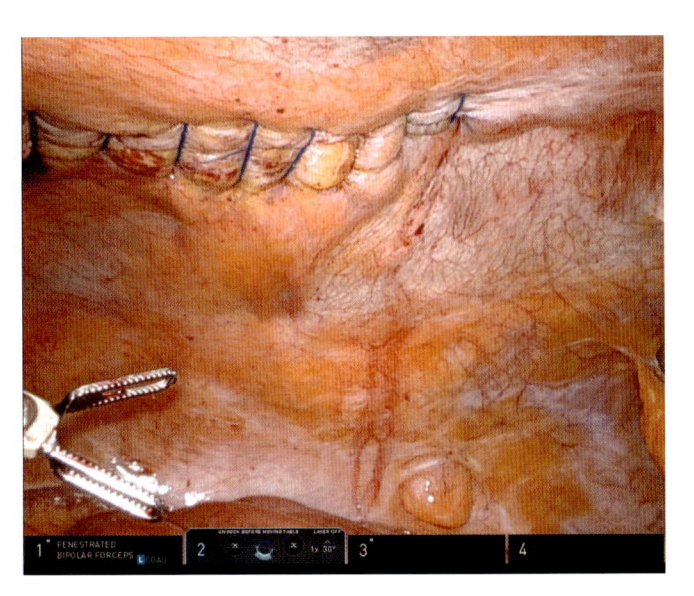

FIGURE 44-10 • Closure of the fascial defect.

Step 4. Mesh placement and fixation

After the defect closure, a composite mesh is routinely used. The mesh is labeled to identify the visceral side and inserted into the abdomen. The size of the mesh is chosen by approximating an overlap of at least 5 cm. Fixation to the abdominal wall is the next step. A straight needle with a 2-0 Prolene™ suture is inserted by the assistant into the abdominal wall at cardinal points. The needle is grabbed by the needle driver of the console surgeon, passed through the mesh, and finally pushed again through the abdominal wall. The assistant now can temporarily tie the suture to the skin anchoring the mesh in a perfect position (**Figures 44-11 A, B**). The console surgeon is suturing the edges of the mesh to the peritoneum and posterior fascia with segments of running sutures of Prolene™ 2-0 (SH). Once the circumferential suturing is complete, the temporary cardinal stiches are removed (**Figure 44-12**).

▶ **Video 44-2. Cardinal Stitches with Straight Needle**

▶▶ TIPS

When making the circumferential fixation of the mesh, it is important to have a strategic plan in mind, knowing where the most difficult segments of the suture are located. It is better to avoid areas of knot tying where 1 of the 2 needle drivers has movement restrictions. The running suture needle can be handled with just 1 hand, left or right, to overcome the difficult segment, but to tie a knot, 2 working hands are necessary.

⚠ PITFALLS

There is a risk of bowel obstruction (internal herniation) if the anchoring running suture has very loose passages allowing the presence of gaps between the anterior abdominal wall and the mesh.

EDITORIAL COMMENT

Mesh Fixation Options

Often, surgeons place "stay" sutures in the mesh prior to its insertion. These sutures are grasped with a transfacial needle, and the mesh is pulled up to the anterior abdominal wall. Additionally, some mesh brands are fitted with a fixation system (**Figure 44-13**).

Another strategy utilizes the V-Loc™ suture that was used for fascial reapproximation. This suture is reversed after the closure of the defect and returned to the center. The suture can then be placed in the center of the mesh, allowing its fixation to the abdominal wall.

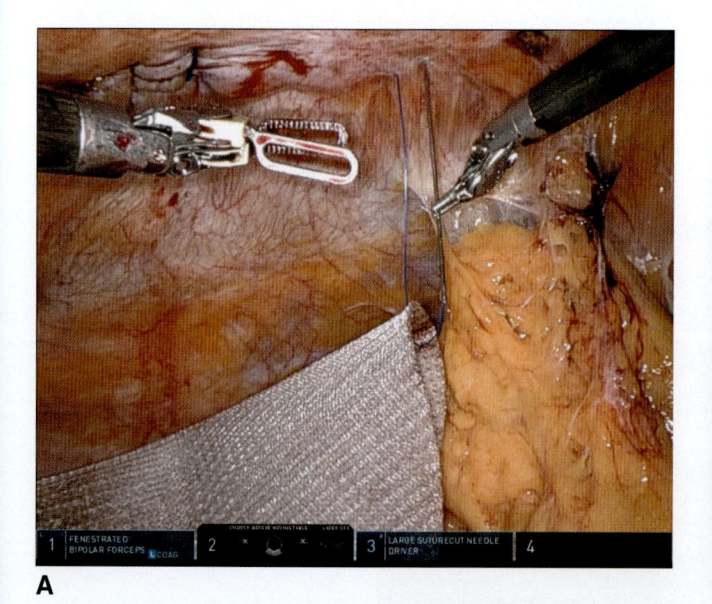

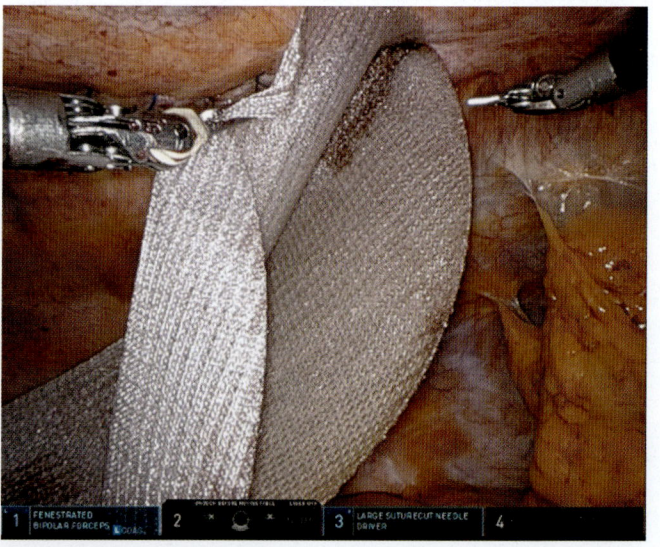

A   B

FIGURE 44-11 • Cardinal stitches with straight needle.

Ventral Hernia Repair 923

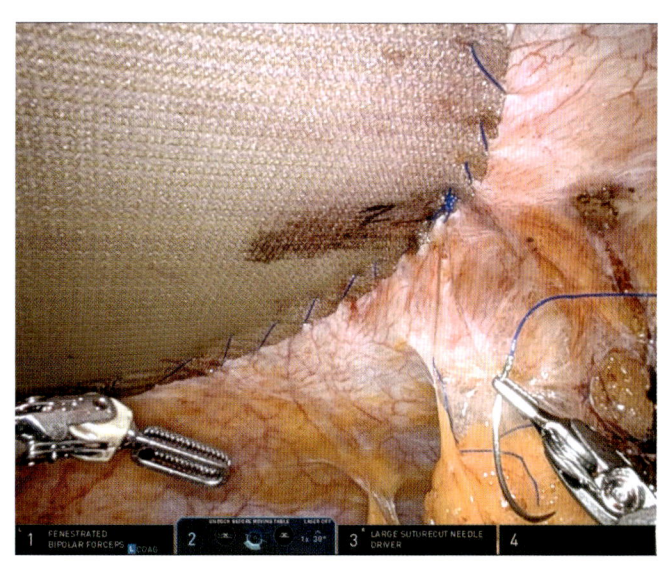

FIGURE 44-12 • Mesh fixation with running sutures.

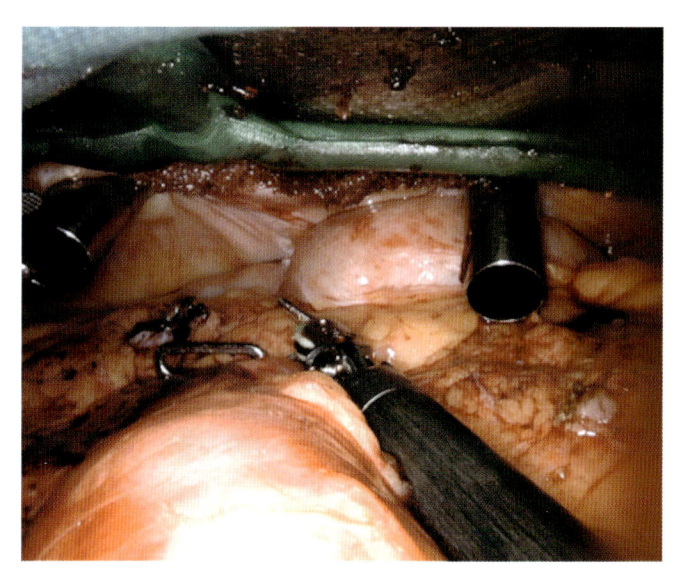

FIGURE 44-13 • Fixation system.

▶ **Video 44-3. Mesh Fixation with Running Sutures**

After the complete mesh fixation, the residual sutures, needles, and hernia sac are removed. The abdomen is inspected and the larger port sites (> 8 mm), if present, are closed with transfascial sutures (suture passer technique).

Step 4 average time frame: 15–30 min

> ▶▶ **TIPS**
>
> For larger mesh placement, consider dual docking. Robotic ports can be placed on both sides of the abdomen to facilitate suturing the mesh to the abdominal wall (**Figures 44-11 A, B**). Once one side of the mesh is secured, the robot is undocked, the boom rotated, and the robot is docked to the contralateral side.

Suggested Readings

1. Muysoms FE, Miserez M, Berrevoet F, et al. Classification of primary and incisional abdominal wall hernias. *Hernia*. 2009;13(4):407-414. doi: 10.1007/s10029-009-0518-x
2. Smith J, Parmely JD. Ventral hernia. *StatPearls*, August 11, 2021. http://www.ncbi.nlm.nih.gov/books/nbk499927
3. Stylianides N, Slade D. Abdominal wall reconstruction. *Br J Hosp Med (Lond)*. 2016;77(3):151-156. doi: 10.12968/hmed.2016.77.3.151
4. Park A, Roth J, Kavic SM. Abdominal wall hernia. *Curr Probl Surg*. 2006;43(5):326-375. doi: 10.1067/j.cpsurg.2006.02.004
5. Huttingear R, Sugumar K, Baltazar-Ford KS. Spigelian hernia. *StatPearls*, June 29, 2021. http://www.ncbi.nlm.nih.gov/books/nbk538290/
6. Huu Nho R, Mege D, Ouaïssi M, Sielezneff I, Sastre B. Incidence and prevention of ventral incisional hernia. *Visc Surg*. 2012;149(5 Suppl):e3-14. doi: 10.1016/j.jviscsurg.2012.05.004
7. Ponten JE, Somers KY, Nienhuijs SW. Pathogenesis of the epigastric hernia. *Hernia*. 2012;16(6):627-633. doi: 10.1007/s10029-012-0964-8
8. Awad ZT, Puri V, LeBlanc K, et al. Mechanisms of ventral hernia recurrence after mesh repair and a new proposed classification. *J Am Coll Surg*. 2005;201(1):132-140. doi: 10.1016/j.jamcollsurg.2005.02.035
9. LeBlanc K. Current considerations in laparoscopic incisional and ventral herniorrhaphy. *JSLS*. 2000;4(2):131-139.
10. Fuenmayor P, Lujan H, Plasencia G, Karmaker A, Mata W, Vecin N. Robotic-assisted ventral and incisional hernia repair with hernia defect closure and intraperitoneal onlay mesh (IPOM) experience. *Robot Surg*. 2020;14(5):695-701. doi: 10.1007/s11701-019-01040-y
11. Gonzalez A, Escobar E, Romero R, et al. Robotic-assisted ventral hernia repair: a multicenter evaluation of clinical outcomes. *Surg Endosc*. 2017;31(3):1342-1349. doi: 10.1007/s00464-016-5118-0
12. Coakley KM, Sims SM, Prasad T, et al. A nationwide evaluation of robotic ventral hernia surgery. *Am J Surg*. 2017;214(6):1158-1163. doi: 10.1016/j.amjsurg.2017.08.022
13. Zahiri H R, Belyansky I, Park A. Abdominal wall hernia. *Curr Probl Surg*. 2018;55(8):286-317. doi: 10.1067/j.cpsurg.2018.08.005
14. Faylona J. Evolution of ventral hernia repair. *Asian J Endosc Surg*. 2017;10(3):252-258. doi: 10.1111/ases.12392
15. Deeken C, Lake S P. Mechanical properties of the abdominal wall and biomaterials utilized for hernia repair. *J Mech Behav Biomed Mater*. 2017;74:411-427. doi: 10.1016/j.jmbbm.2017.05.008
16. Chevrel JP, Rath AM. Classification of incisional hernias of the abdominal wall. *Hernia*. 2000;4:7–11.
17. Muysoms FE, Antoniou SE, Bury K, et al. European Hernia Society guidelines on the closure of abdominal wall incisions. *Hernia*. 2015;19(1):1-24. doi: 10.1007/s10029-014-1342-5
18. Sharbaugh ME, Patel PB, Zaman JA, et al. Robotic ventral hernia repair: a safe and durable approach. *Hernia*. 2021;25(2):305-312. doi: 10.1007/s10029-019-02074-9
19. Kudsi OY, Paluvoi N, Bhurtel P, McCabe Z, El-Jabri R. Robotic repair of ventral hernias: preliminary findings of a case series of 106 consecutive cases. *Am J Robot Surg*. 2015;2(1):22-26. doi: 10.1166/ajrs.2015.1020
20. Giulianotti PC, Coratti A, Angelini M, et al. Robotics in general surgery: personal experience in a large community hospital. *Arch Surg*. 2003;138(7):777-784. doi: 10.1001/archsurg.138.7.777

"The key challenge to this robotic technique is the learning curve…it is crucial that surgeons have a clear understanding and experience performing the open Rives retrorectus repair and TAR before they attempt it robotically."

—Alfredo M. Carbonell (1970)

Robotic Transversus Abdominis Release (roboTAR)

Tiffany Nguyen • Ethan Ballecer • Katherine Hoener • Alice Gamble • Conrad Ballecer

INTRODUCTION

Robotic transversus abdominis release (roboTAR) allows a minimally invasive approach to repairing large, complex ventral hernias, respecting the principles outlined by Rives and Stoppa in establishing a retromuscular preperitoneal approach. Stoppa made minor modifications to Rives's technique of retromuscular mesh placement and, in conjunction with his own technique, authored the concept of the giant prosthetic reinforcement of the visceral sac (GPRVS), which mandates that the mesh should extend well beyond the area of the defect. The advantage of the retromuscular preperitoneal approach is the development of a well-vascularized space for mesh placement that is protected from the visceral space. Although the Rives–Stoppa technique was considered the gold standard for ventral hernia repair, the size of the retromuscular preperitoneal space was limited by the semilunaris, thus making this approach not amenable to repairing large abdominal wall defects.

To overcome this limitation, Novitsky et al. first described the open transversus abdominis release (TAR) as a form of posterior component separation for abdominal wall reconstruction with the avoidance of the neurovascular bundle (NVB) to allow for the reconstruction of the linea alba. This technique does not require the development of large lipocutaneous flaps with a high risk for complications such as skin necrosis and enables the creation of a significantly larger extraperitoneal space accepting a larger mesh. While historically an open approach, recent advances in robotic surgery have made a minimally invasive approach to TAR possible. The enhanced visualization and articulated instruments, lacking in laparoscopy, allow minimally invasive repairs of increasingly complex ventral hernias, thus pushing the boundaries of advanced minimally invasive hernia repair.

Compared to the open approach, roboTAR is associated with a shorter hospital stay, reduced wound morbidity, and decreased postoperative pain, with an expedited return to work and activities of daily living.

INSTRUMENT REQUIREMENTS

The suggested main robotic instruments/tools can be listed as follows:
- 30° scope
- Fenestrated bipolar forceps
- Cautery monopolar hook/monopolar curved scissors
- Needle holders
- Round-tip scissors (if not using suture cut needle holder)
- Round-tip scissors (cold scissors, if needed for adhesiolysis)

The suggested main laparoscopic instruments/tools can be listed as follows:
- Needle driver
- Scissors
- Laparoscopic forceps

Supplemental materials:
- Large-pore polypropylene mesh
- Vicryl™ 0, 2-0, 3-0
- V-Loc™ 1, 2-0, 3-0
- Haemostatic agents: powder or glue
- Jackson-Pratt 19-French drain

Photo reproduced with permission from Dr. Alfredo Carbonell.
Quote reproduced with permission from General Surgery News. Surgeons Abuzz Over New Robotic Hernia Technique. Surgeon Performs Live Robotic TAR to Captive Crowd, July 14, 2015.

The robotic procedure does increase the potential cost for the institution including a prolonged operative time. Despite this, there are many positive advantages already mentioned allowing a positive final balance in favor of robotics. Moreover, even though the learning curve in roboTAR has yet to be determined, a rapidly increasing volume of cases might speed up the surgeon's and team's proficiency. A more efficient operation will translate into faster operative times, adding further value to the technique.

Preoperative Evaluation

As with any surgery, a detailed history and physical exam are essential prior to developing an operative plan. Risk factors for poor wound healing such as uncontrolled diabetes, obesity, smoking, and collagen vascular disease should be carefully evaluated. It is recommended that the patient achieves adequate glucose control (preferably HgbA1C <7), initiates weight loss, and demonstrates smoking cessation at least 4 weeks prior to surgery. In some cases, preoperative weight loss can be difficult. In these patients, a body mass index (BMI) of <40 can be accepted; however, a BMI <35 remains ideal.

Due to the significant reconstruction required for a TAR, all patients need to have preoperative imaging, such as a CT scan, to define the abdominal wall layers and cavity. This workup allows the surgeon to evaluate the defect, identify potentially incarcerated abdominal contents, recognize the placement of a previous mesh in the setting of recurrence, and detect concurrent hernias not detected on the physical exam. (For more information about abdominal wall anatomy, see Chapter 44, Ventral Hernia Repair [Intraperitoneal Onlay Mesh with Fascial Defect Approximation].)

> **ABDOMINAL WALL ANATOMY: TRANSVERSUS ABDOMINIS**
>
> The transversus abdominis muscle (TA) is located on the anterior and lateral sides of the abdominal wall, being the deepest of the 3 anterolateral abdominal wall muscles. Its fibers run horizontally, with a muscular lateral portion, and a medial aponeurotic one. It arises from the lateral third of the inguinal ligament, the anterior two-thirds of the iliac crest, the thoracolumbar fascia, and the lower 6 costal cartilages and their ribs interdigitating with the diaphragm. The TA ends in the linea alba, and inserts into the pubic crest and pectineal line, forming the conjoint tendon with the internal oblique muscle.
>
> Above the arcuate line, the TA is located posterior to the rectus muscles contributing to the posterior rectus sheath. Inferiorly, the aponeurosis contributes only to the anterior rectus sheath.
>
> In the abdominal wall, the NVBs run laterally, within a plane between the internal oblique and the TA muscles, before perforating the posterior rectus sheath (**Figure 45-1**).

> ▶▶ **TIPS**
>
> Accurate knowledge of the abdominal wall anatomy, and comfort with 3-dimensional reconstruction, are of paramount importance for the roboTAR technique.

Indications and Contraindications to the roboTAR

In general, indications for a robotic TAR *versus* open TAR are relatively the same, and they include large ventral hernias with defects greater than 10–12 cm, previous ostomy sites, and lateral wall defects. The Carbonell equation can be used to determine if a patient is an appropriate candidate for the roboTAR; this equation states that if the sum of the widths of the rectus is less than twice the size of the defect, a TAR should be considered. If the sum is greater than twice the size of the defect, a Rives–Stoppa repair is sufficient.

> **EDITORIAL COMMENT**
>
> The width of the defect is not always a reliable measure of indication to perform a component separation. Some patients with smaller defects may have poor abdominal wall compliance, making it difficult to achieve midline fascial reapproximation without it.
>
> Many so-called "frozen abdomens," with plastered adhesions after multiple abdominal surgeries, might still be good candidates for laparoscopic robotic adhesiolysis. With experience, safe access to the abdominal cavity can be obtained, and gradually the anterior adhesiolysis can be completed before addressing the hernia repair. (For more details see Chapter 2, The Basic Principles of Clinical Applications.)

Absolute contraindications to roboTAR are similar to those of laparoscopic surgery. The patient must be able to tolerate pneumoperitoneum, and the abdomen must be safe to enter laparoscopically.

Patients with extensive abdominal surgical history, dense adhesions, or a "frozen" abdomen should not undergo this approach. Similarly to other mesh-based hernia repairs, roboTAR is recommended only in clean cases due to the risk of mesh infection. Relative contraindications to roboTAR include significant loss of domain, defects extending from flank to flank, and poor skin integrity. Patients with open wounds and fistulas should not be offered this approach; oftentimes, the compromised skin receives collateral blood supply from underlying adhesions to the viscera or fat.

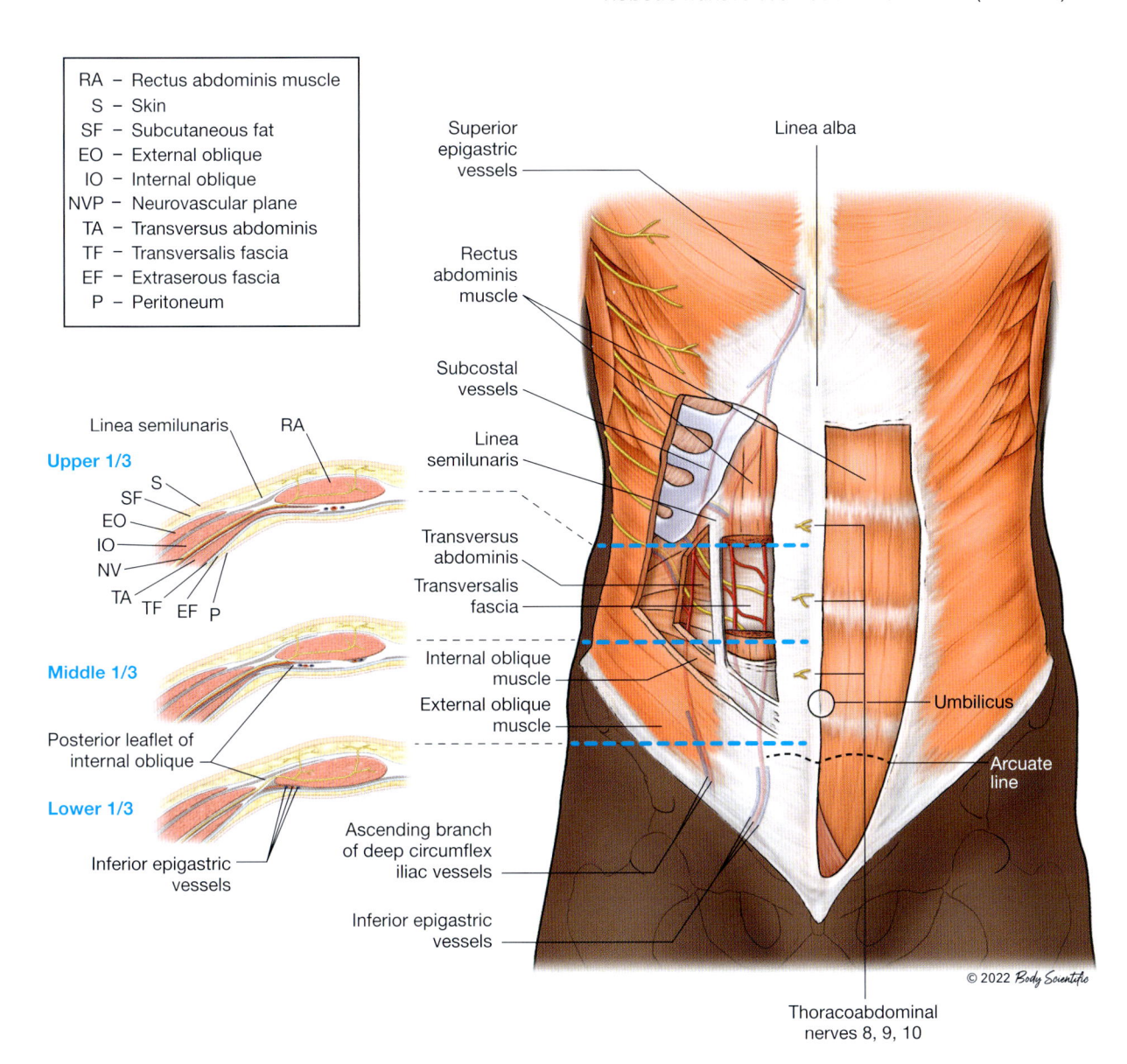

FIGURE 45-1 • Transversus abdominis.

Operative Techniques

There are 3 main techniques to perform a roboTAR: Bottoms-Up, Novitsky, and Top-Down Technique. All 3 techniques can be used interchangeably to initiate the TAR and to proceed with the dissection. All 3 planes will coalesce with the prior Novitsky dissection and can be joined. The critical view of TAR is achieved when the cut edge of the TA is demonstrated on the lateral abdominal wall medial to the preserved NVBs and linea semilunaris, and the other cut edge of the TA is observed on the posterior sheath with no muscular fibers on the posterior elements. The decision to employ either of the 3 techniques to initiate the dissection depends on patient factors. Scarring from prior hernia repair or underlying viscera adhesions will dictate which approach is preferred.

Patient Positioning, OR Setup, and Port Setting

The patient is placed supine on the operating table with the arms tucked, and all pressure points should be adequately padded. The patient should be positioned on the break of the bed, so that measures such as flexing the bed can aid in increasing the distance between the costal margin and the iliac crest to create additional space for trocar placement in the setting of patients with a short torso (**Figure 45-2**). The assistant surgeon stands on the opposite side of the robot (**Figure 45-3**).

Intraabdominal access is achieved under direct laparoscopic visualization in the left upper quadrant lateral to Palmer's point. Then, 8-mm robotic trocars are placed in the left upper quadrant, left lateral mid-abdomen, and left lower quadrant, and the robot is docked over the contralateral abdomen (**Figures 45-4 A, B**).

> **EDITORIAL COMMENT**
>
> Breaking the table may increase the space between the costal margin and the iliac spine. However, it may also increase the longitudinal tension of the rectum muscles, not favoring the horizontal approximation when suturing. A neutral position of the patient on the table seems more favorable.
>
> For dual docking, the patient should be placed in the center of the table.

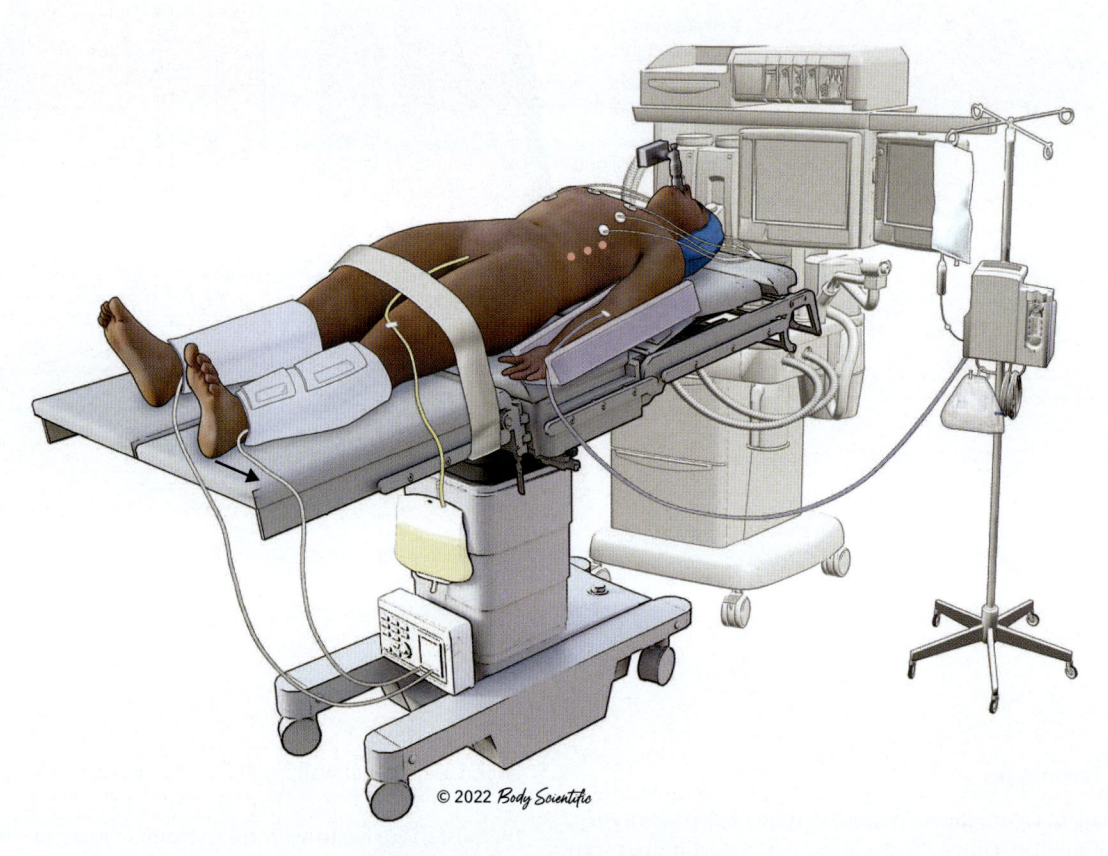

FIGURE 45-2 • Patient positioning.

Robotic Transversus Abdominis Release (roboTAR) 929

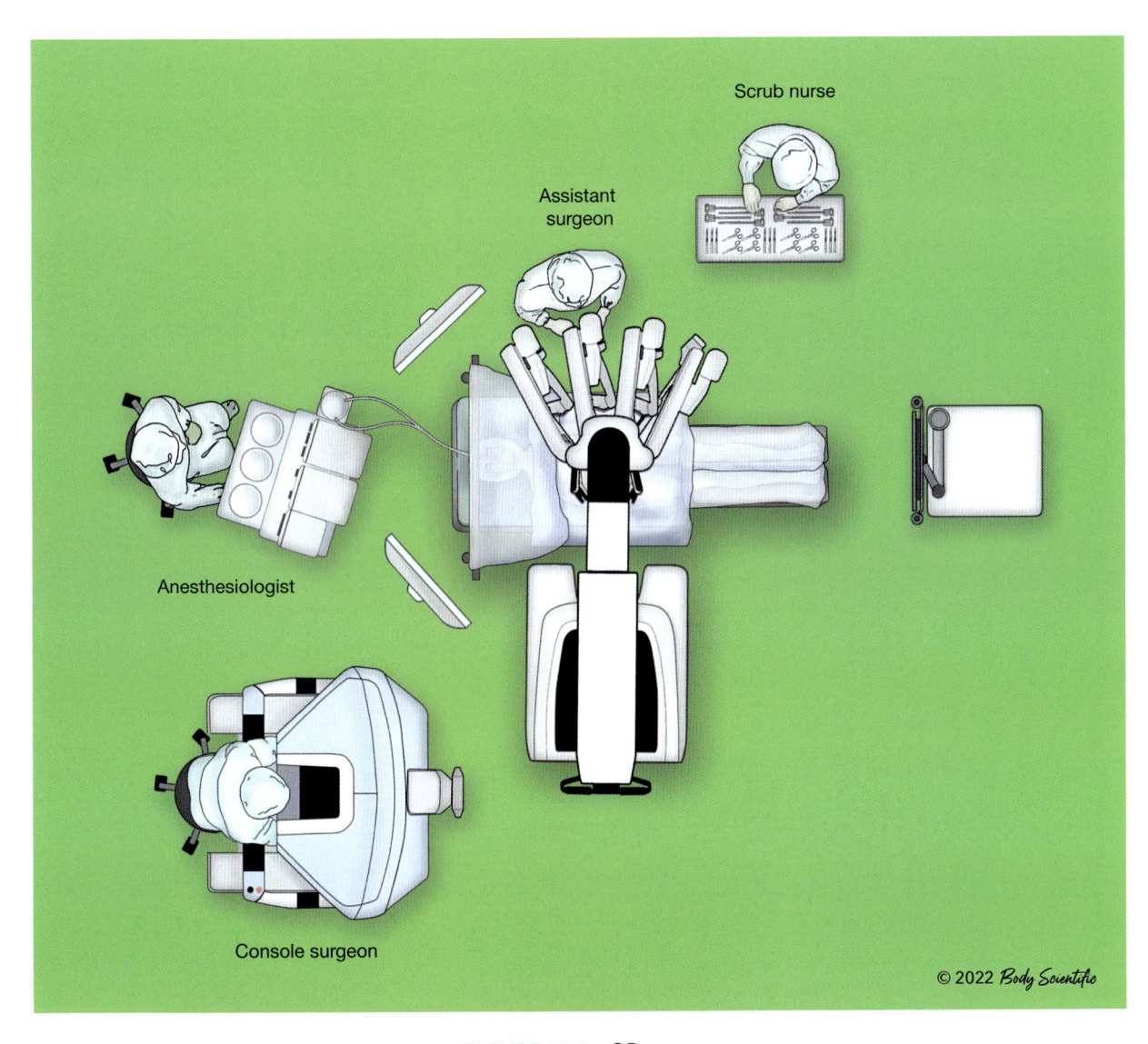

FIGURE 45-3 • OR setup.

A

B

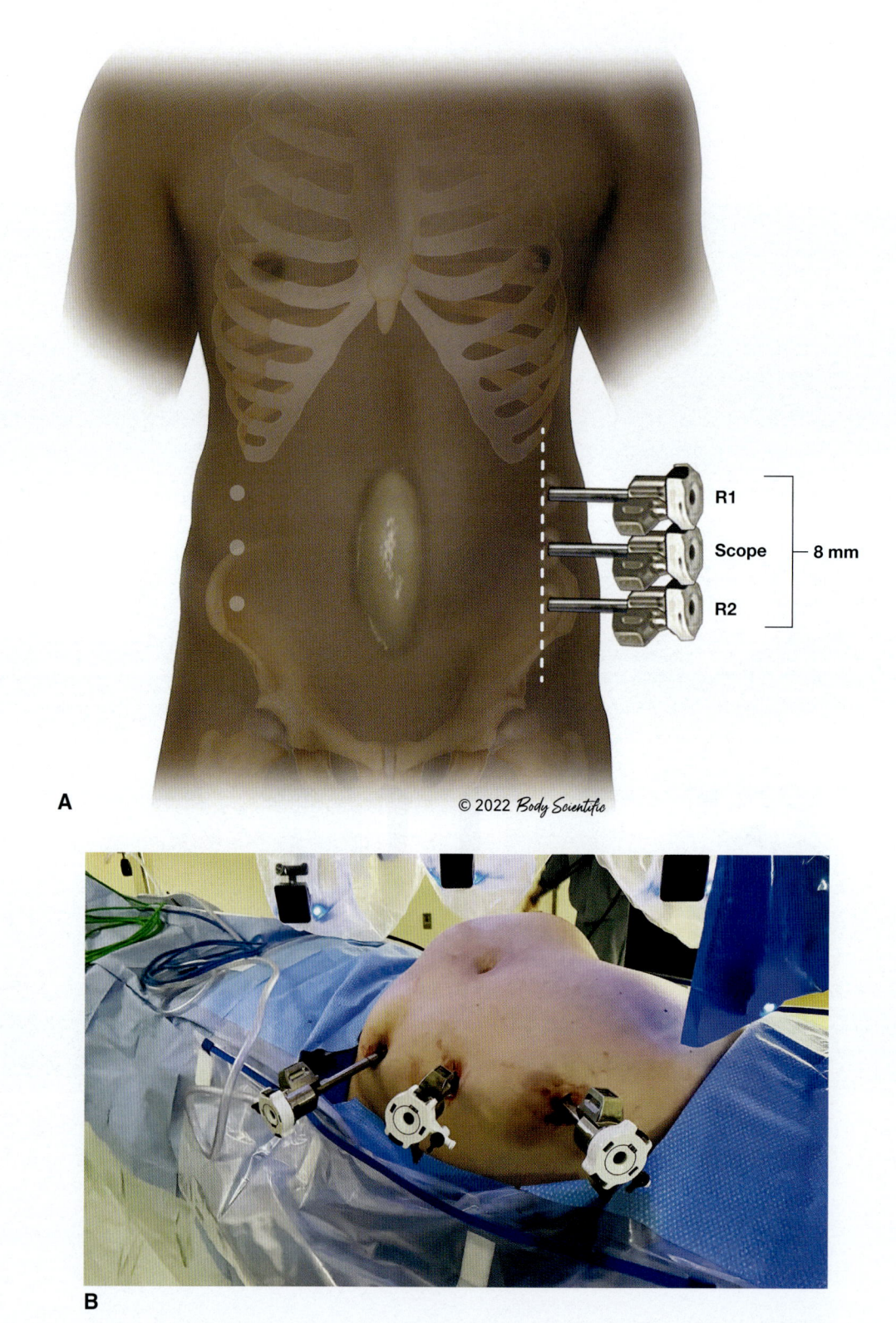

FIGURE 45-4 • Port setting. Initial robotic port setting with the robot docked on the contralateral abdomen.

Surgical Technique

▶ **Video 45-1.** Robotic Transversus Abdominis Release (RoboTAR) – Full Procedure

Step 1. Adhesiolysis and reduction of the hernia

Initially, a laparoscopic exploration of the abdominal cavity is performed. The bowel and underlying viscera are examined to ensure no inadvertent injuries, and the abdominal defects are assessed. Adhesions can be carefully taken down laparoscopically before docking the robotic system or using the robotic approach. In the case of a hostile abdomen, complexity is variable. An incarcerated ventral hernia and complex adhesions inside and outside the hernia sac may be encountered. In this scenario, the robotic technique is recommended since its ability to execute a precise adhesiolysis is superior. This step could be nonexistent if no adhesions are present or extremely time-consuming and complicated. The risk of contamination of the surgical field if an unintended full-thickness bowel tear occurs should always be kept in mind.

Step 1 average time frame: 0 min (no adhesions)–180 min (multiple adhesions)

Step 2. Division of the posterior rectus sheath and subsequent mobilization to the linea semilunaris

The retromuscular space is accessed by incising the posterior sheath approximately 1–2 cm lateral from the linea alba (**Figure 45-5**). This allows for adequate fascial visualization prior to the anterior sheath closure. Muscle fibers

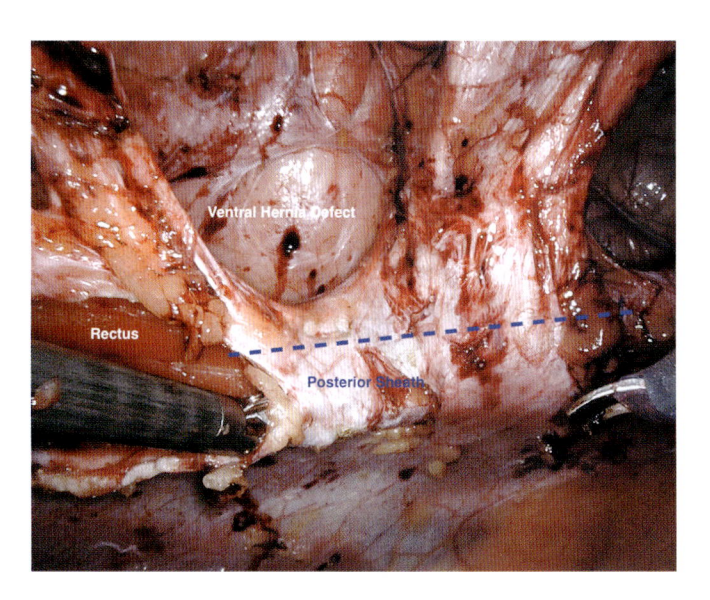

FIGURE 45-5 • Retromuscular space access. The transverse fibers of the rectus abdominis muscle must be recognized, after the incision of the posterior sheath, to ensure that the correct space is entered. The dissection is continued along the dotted line to release the posterior sheath.

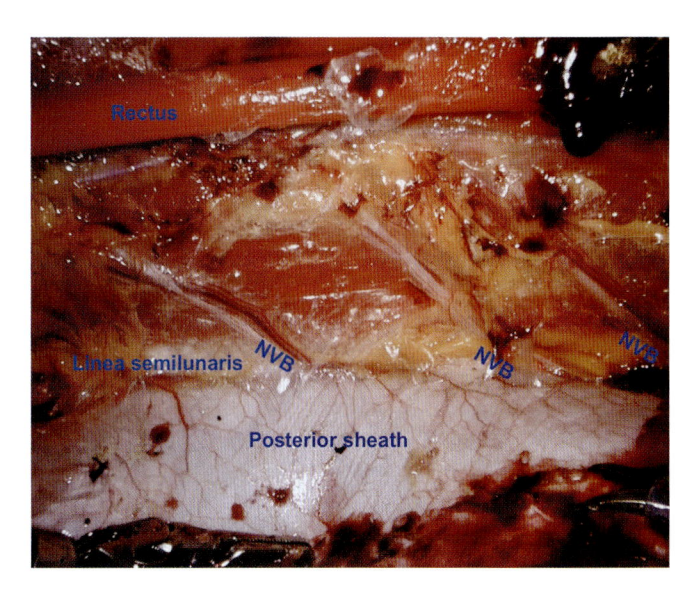

FIGURE 45-6 • Retromuscular dissection to the semilunar line. The semilunar line is reached. The NBVs should be visualized and preserved.

of the rectus must be visualized to verify the correct plane. The rectus abdominis muscle is kept anteriorly up against the abdominal wall, and the posterior elements should be mobilized to the "floor" posteriorly. The dissection is continued laterally until the NVBs are identified and the linea semilunaris has been reached at the lateral border of the rectus (**Figure 45-6**). Care must be taken to preserve the NVBs to avoid devascularization and denervation of the rectus muscle.

> ⚠ **PITFALLS**
>
> Incorrect identification of the linea semilunaris could result in devascularization and denervation of the rectus abdominus muscle.

The epigastric crossover is performed in the preperitoneal plane, typically at the level of the falciform ligament, which is mobilized posteriorly with the flap prepared during the retrorectus dissection (**Figure 45-7**). This flap is the cephalad apex of the visceral sac, which will be subsequently closed during the posterior sheath closure. To ensure that the flap is contiguous with the posterior rectus sheath, the preperitoneal fat should be dissected posteriorly and away from the linea alba. Caudally, the retrorectus dissection is continued below the arcuate line

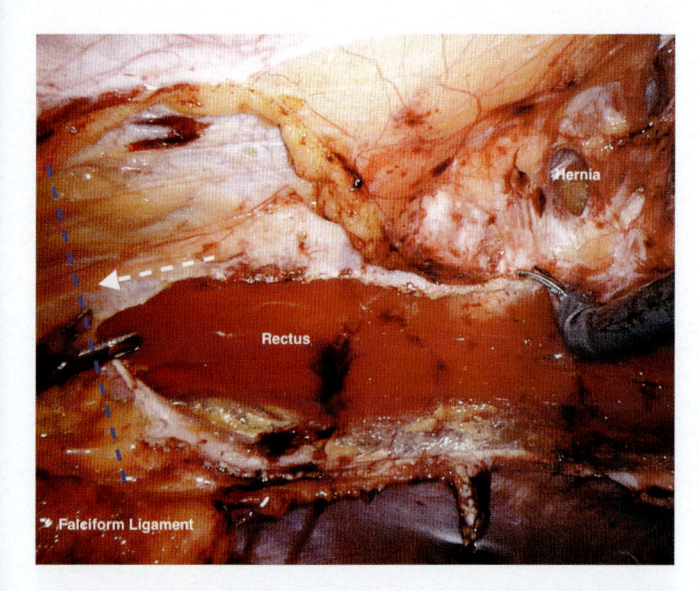

FIGURE 45-7 • Epigastric crossover. The epigastric crossover is performed in the cephalad direction. The blue dotted line denotes the dissection of the epigastric flap needed to reach the preperitoneal space. The falciform ligament is brought down with the flap. The white arrow demonstrates the plane of dissection.

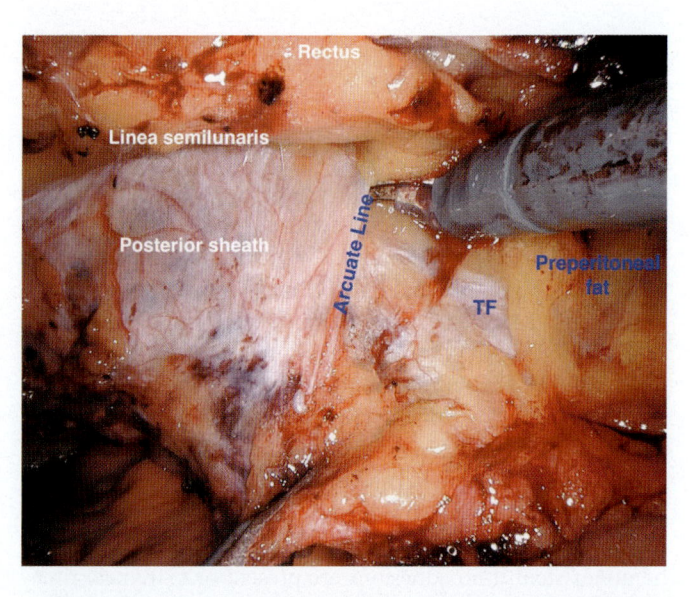

FIGURE 45-9 • Arcuate line. The arcuate line is visualized, at the linea semilunaris, after the lateral dissection. The preperitoneal fat is more prominent in the lower abdomen, which facilitates the mobilization of the posterior elements. To enter the preperitoneal plane, the TF is incised between the arcuate line and the preperitoneal fat.

and the suprapubic crossover is performed (**Figure 45-8**). A preperitoneal flap is created down to the space of Retzius and the dissection is continued laterally until the arcuate line is delineated at the level of the linea semilunaris (**Figure 45-9**). Inferior to the junction between the arcuate line and the linea semilunaris, the transversalis fascia (TF) is incised to enter the preperitoneal plane (**Figure 45-10**).

Once the preperitoneal plane has been entered, the preperitoneal fat is swept downward until the TA is visualized along the lateral abdominal wall and the space of Bogros has been reached. It is bounded anteriorly by the superficial transverse fascia, medially by the inferior epigastric vessels, laterally by the pelvic wall, and posteriorly by the psoas muscle, external iliac vessels, and the femoral nerve. The inferior epigastric vessels and the myopectineal orifice can be used as a key landmark for the suprapubic crossover (**Figure 45-11**). This space is the starting location for the Bottoms-up TAR.

Step 2 average time frame: 10–20 min (posterior sheath release)/60–80 min (TAR)

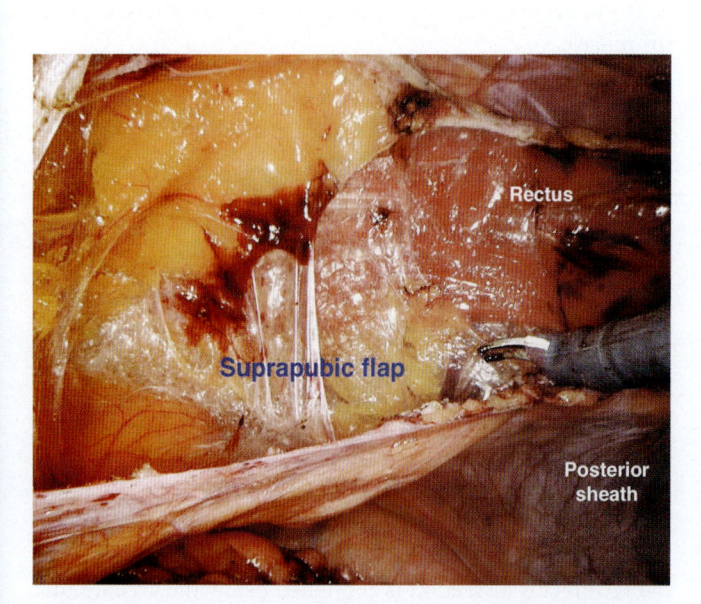

FIGURE 45-8 • Suprapubic crossover. Similarly to the epigastric crossover, the dissection is carried caudally to perform the suprapubic crossover to create a flap in the space of Retzius.

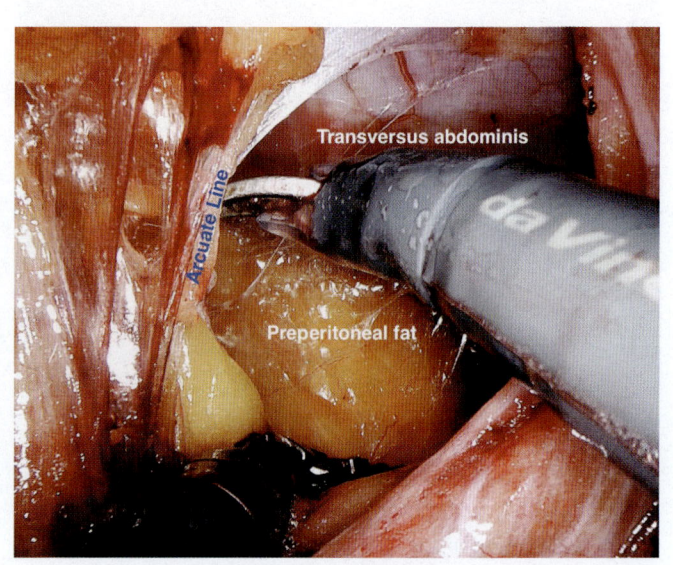

FIGURE 45-10 • Suprapubic preperitoneal dissection. The TA is visualized along the lateral abdominal wall. The preperitoneal fat is swept downward to allow entering into the space of Bogros.

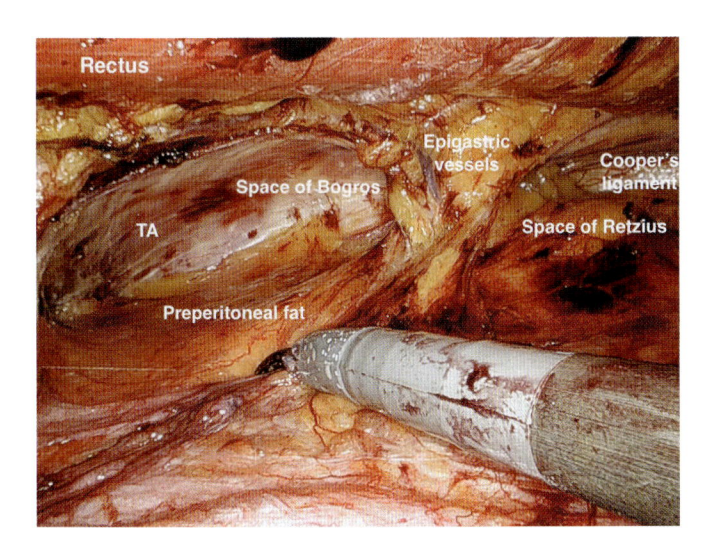

FIGURE 45-11 • Myopectineal orifice. Concurrent inguinal hernias should be repaired at this time.

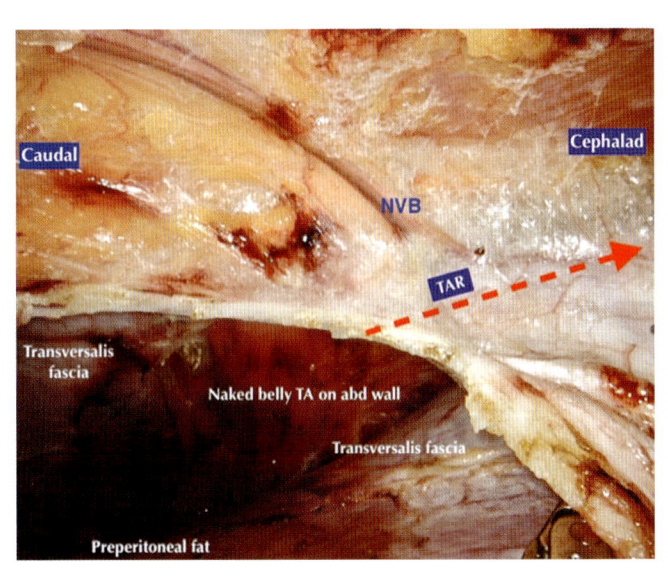

FIGURE 45-13 • Posterior rectus sheath incision. A large preperitoneal cave is created isolating the aponeurotic portion of the TA. The TAR is continued along the dotted line of the TA aponeurosis.

Three Ways to TAR

Bottoms-Up Technique

The Bottoms-up technique begins in the space of Bogros. The posterior elements (i.e., peritoneum, TF, and preperitoneal fat) must be separated from the overlying transverse abdominis (TA) muscle and lateral posterior sheath. This allows for the subsequent division of the aponeurotic TA in the lower abdomen and the muscular TA in the mid to upper abdomen. To aid in orientation, the TA muscle should be visualized on the lateral abdominal wall throughout the Bottoms-up approach. This dissection is executed in a caudal to cephalad direction and a preperitoneal cave is developed (**Figure 45-12**).

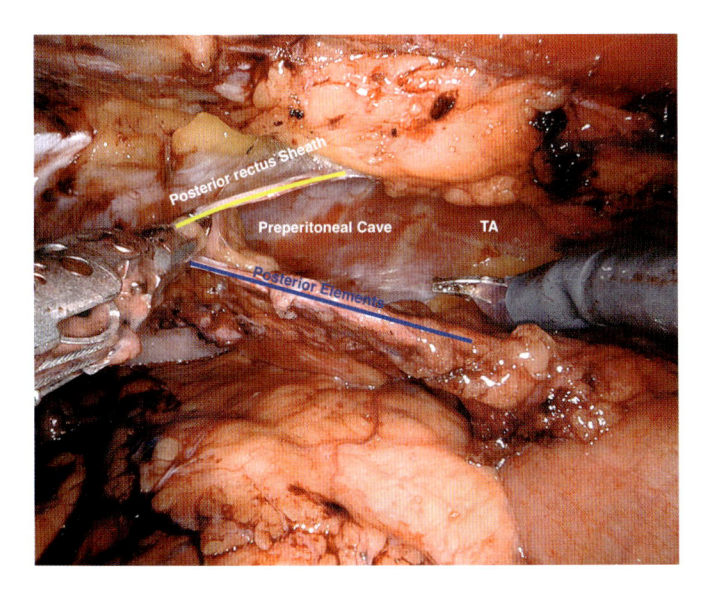

FIGURE 45-12 • Bottoms-up technique. The peritoneum and the preperitoneal fat represent the posterior elements; these structures are separated from the posterior rectus sheath. The TA is on the lateral abdominal wall.

The preperitoneal and retroperitoneal fat is more abundant in the lower and lateral abdomen, allowing for the dissection and preservation of the posterior elements.

Once the lateral extent of the retroperitoneal fat is reached, the dissection is performed in a medial direction along the line of the reflected peritoneum, isolating the aponeurotic portion of the TA. The posterior sheath is retracted in a cephalad and medial direction, creating a "V" shape. The horizon can be changed on the surgeon's console touchpad to allow for better visualization of the preperitoneal cave and its cephalad aspect. By creating the "V," the posterior elements are separated from the aponeurotic portion of the TA as it inserts into the lateral posterior sheath (**Figure 45-13**). This area is now safe to divide medial to the NVBs and semilunar line.

Cephalad to the mid-abdominal region, there is a loss of preperitoneal fat. Care must be taken during the dissection to ensure the integrity of the flap. Here, it is often required to transition between the preperitoneal to the pre-transversalis plane or between the anterior and posterior leaflets of the TF. The aponeurotic portion of the TA also becomes more muscular in this region, and the dissection is more challenging. Once the Bottoms-up technique becomes too difficult, it can be transitioned to either the Novitsky technique or the Top-down approach.

Novitsky Technique

As the dissection turns more cephalad, the muscle belly of the TA inserts more medially on the posterior sheath. The NVBs need to be identified and preserved to avoid denervation of the rectus muscle complex. Medial to the NVBs, the posterior lamella of the internal oblique (PLIO) is incised to expose the

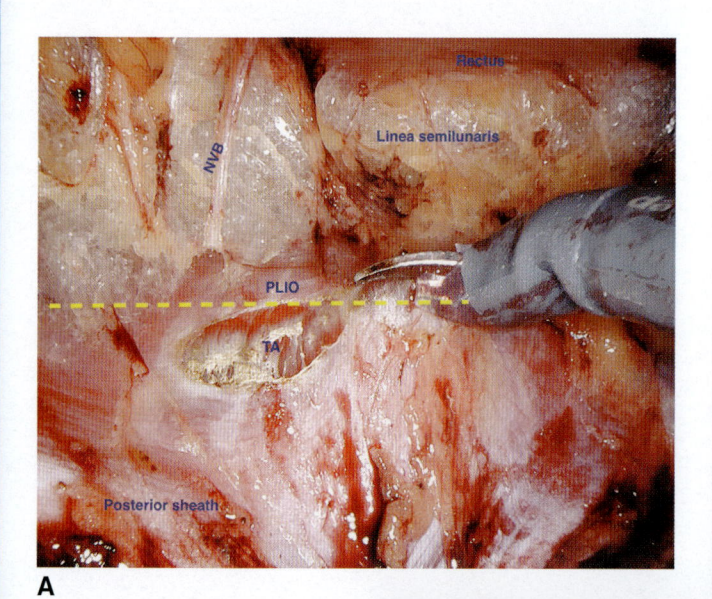

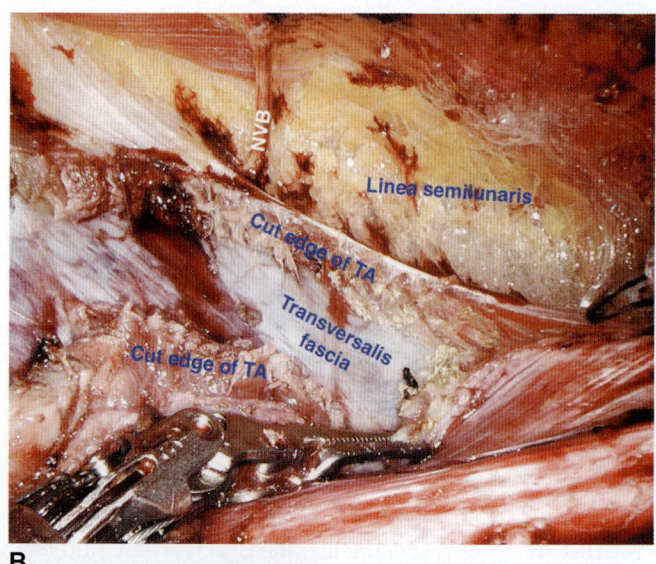

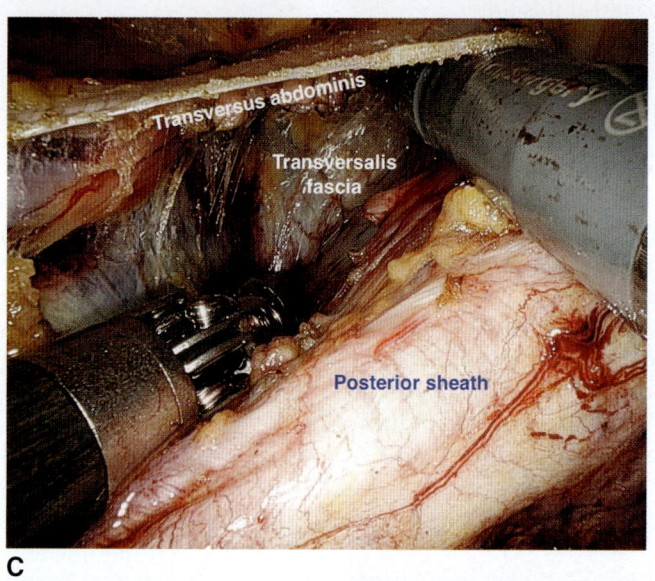

FIGURE 45-14 • A. Novitsky incision. PLIO. The posterior lamella of the internal oblique is incised along the dotted line medial to the NVBs to reveal the underlying muscle fibers of the TA. **B.** Pretransversalis dissection. Monopolar scissors are used to cut the TA muscle to reveal the underlying TF. The cut edge of the TA is up on the abdominal wall and the posterior sheath. The NVBs are carefully preserved. **C.** Transversalis fascia dissection. This dissection extends to the retroperitoneal fat on the lateral abdominal wall. The muscle fibers of the TA should be lifted and the TF brought down with the posterior elements.

TA muscle fibers (**Figure 45-14A**). Next, the TA muscle needs to be carefully divided to reveal the underlying TF (**Figure 45-14B**). The pretransversalis dissection is continued laterally until the retroperitoneal fat pad is identified, similarly to the Bottoms-up approach (**Figure 45-14C**). This technique can be connected with the Bottoms-up and Top-down approaches to complete the TAR dissection.

Top-Down Technique

The dissection begins at the site of the epigastric crossover within the preperitoneal space. Similarly to the lower abdomen, there is a significant amount of preperitoneal fat, which aids in the dissection. The preperitoneal/pretransversalis dissection is carried laterally toward the retroperitoneal fat underneath the diaphragm and the TA on the lateral abdominal wall. Inadvertent dissection into the diaphragm can result in an iatrogenic diaphragmatic hernia and/or entry into the thoracic cavity. The fibers of the diaphragm interdigitate with the fibers of the TA making the dissection difficult; however, there is a sentinel fat pad that can aid in the identification of the position of the overlying diaphragm. The Top-down technique creates a preperitoneal/pretransversalis cave that preserves the posterior elements (peritoneum and TF) while separating them from the overlying TA muscle inserting on the lateral posterior sheath. During this

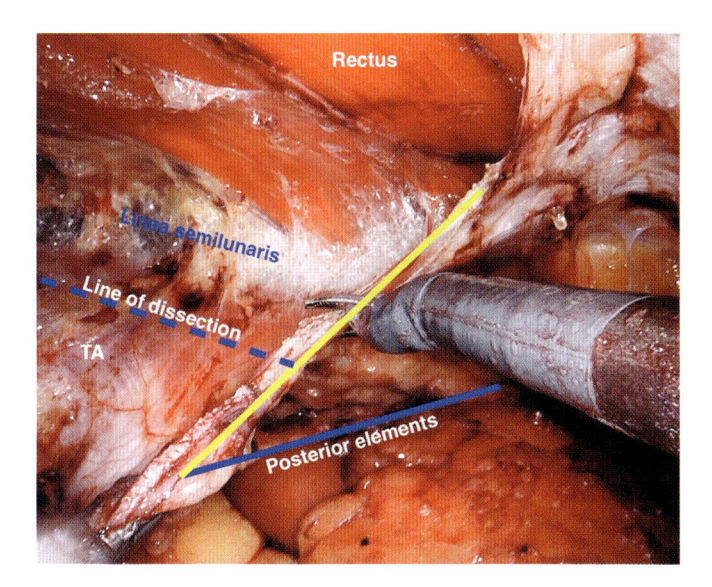

FIGURE 45-15 • Top-down TAR approach. A preperitoneal cave is created. The posterior elements (peritoneum and TF) are separated from the posterior sheath to create a "V." Care is taken to avoid injury at the linea semilunaris and the NVBs. The dotted blue line indicates where the TA is incised.

⚠ PITFALLS

Misidentifying the muscular fibers of the diaphragm can lead to iatrogenic Morgagni hernias and/or entry into the thoracic cavity.

▶▶ TIPS

The 3 techniques (Bottoms-up, Novitsky, and Top down), can be utilized based on the surgeon's comfort and knowledge. Patient factors such as scarring or underlying visceral adhesions may dictate the type of approach used.

dissection, the diaphragm, and TA muscle fibers, should be on the anterolateral abdominal wall, and not on the "floor" of the posterior elements. In parallel to the other approaches, the TA is incised once an adequate preperitoneal cave has been formed (**Figure 45-15**).

All 3 approaches will eventually coalesce with the prior Novitsky dissection (**Figures 45-16 A, B**). As the dissection continues, there will be a single pedicle of TA that can be divided without injuring the posterior elements. This will connect all 3 dissection planes into one. The "floor" now consists of the posterior rectus sheath, TF, and peritoneum, which will provide coverage for the mesh. The critical view, or *sine qua non* of TAR, is achieved when the cut edge of the TA is demonstrated on the lateral abdominal wall medial to the preserved NVBs and linea semilunaris and the other cut edge of TA is observed on the posterior sheath with no muscular layer on

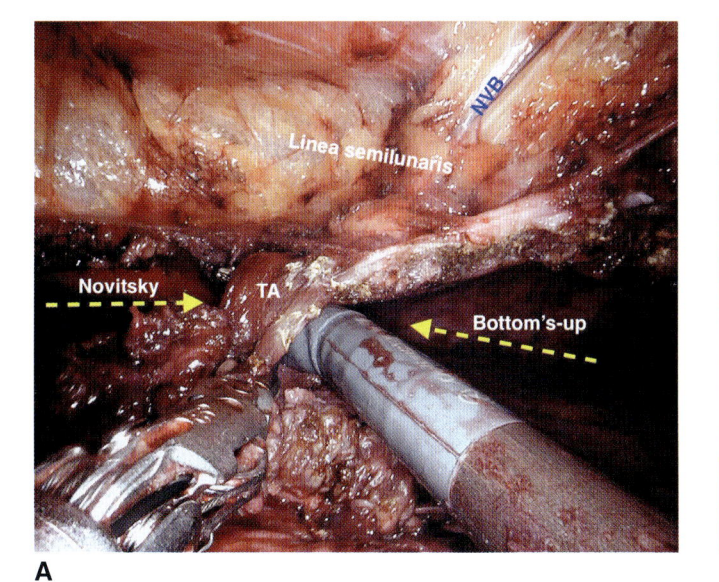

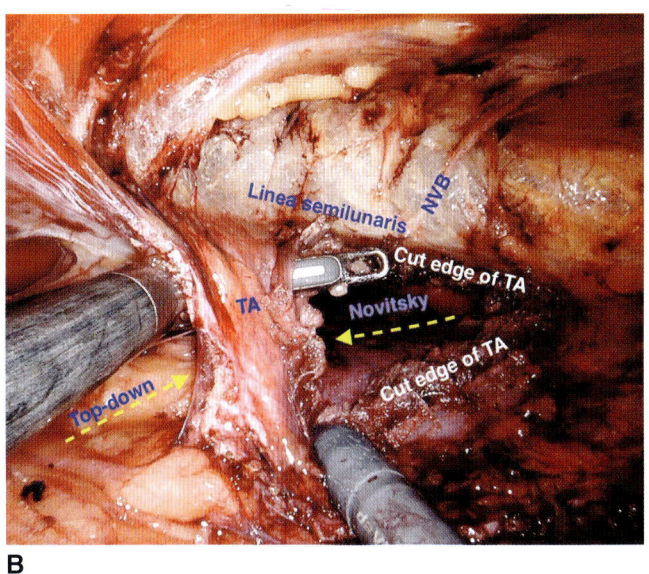

FIGURE 45-16 • **A.** Connection of the Novitsky method and the Bottoms-up. **B.** Connection of the Top-down and the Novitsky method.

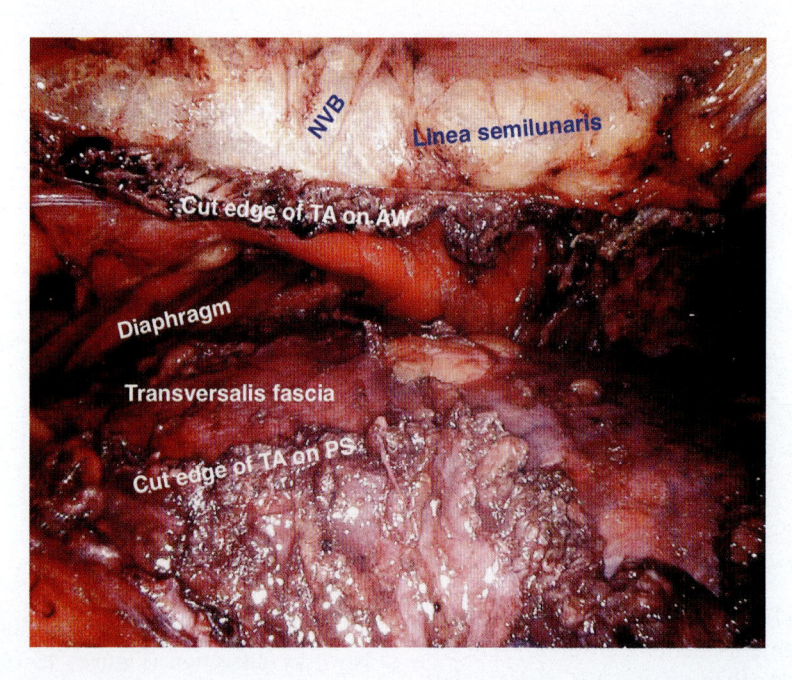

FIGURE 45-17 • *Sine qua non* critical view. Critical view of TAR. In the upper abdomen, there is the cut edge of TA on the abdominal wall, the cut edge of TA on the posterior sheath, and no additional muscle on the posterior elements is seen. The flap should lay nice and flat, on top of the viscera, without any undue tension.

the posterior elements (**Figure 45-17**). To ensure the posterior sheath is closed without tension, the dissection of the posterior layers needs to extend to the retroperitoneal fat or the lateral border of the psoas muscle.

> ▶▶ **TIPS**
>
> The critical view of TAR is obtained when the cut edge of TA is visible on the lateral abdominal wall, and the posterior sheath with no muscular layers present on the posterior sheath elements.

Step 3. Initial deployment and fixation of the mesh
The extent of the cranial-caudal dissection depends upon the longitudinal size of the defect to ensure adequate craniocaudal overlap of the mesh. A minimum of 5 cm of overlap on all sides is recommended, but oftentimes, this overlap is exceeded to ensure a giant prosthetic reinforcement of the entire visceral sac. After the dissection is completed, the abdominal wall is measured to choose an appropriate size for the mesh. To ensure an adequately sized mesh, the dissection sometimes needs to extend inferiorly to the space of Retzius and superiorly to the level of the central tendon of the diaphragm. If there are concomitant groin hernias, these should be reduced and repaired.

The "suture trick" involves the placement of a Vicryl™ 0 suture in the top center of the mesh preserving a long tail that facilitates the unscrolling of the mesh once placed at the top of the posterior sheath. A large-pore polypropylene synthetic mesh is used; it is rolled up and inserted into the abdomen via a preexisting trocar, and it is deployed into the retromuscular and preperitoneal/pretransversalis space (**Figure 45-18**). If a bilateral TAR is performed, contralateral ports are placed above the mesh after its initial deployment on the lateral abdominal wall. The rolled mesh is then fixated with Vicryl™ 2-0 along the posterolateral abdominal wall prior to the contralateral dissection.

Step 3 average time frame: 15–20 min

> **EDITORIAL COMMENT**
>
> **Dual docking method and contralateral dissection.**
> Three 8-mm trocars are placed on the contralateral side of the abdomen, mirroring the initial 3 trocars, and the robot is re-docked. The steps are similar to the ones previously described. Retroxiphoidal or retropubic dissection is performed, as indicated, to achieve sufficient cephalad-caudal overlap of the hernia defect. Completion of an adequate dissection is confirmed when the 2 leaves of the posterior sheath rest flat against the abdominal viscera and can be approximated without undue tension.

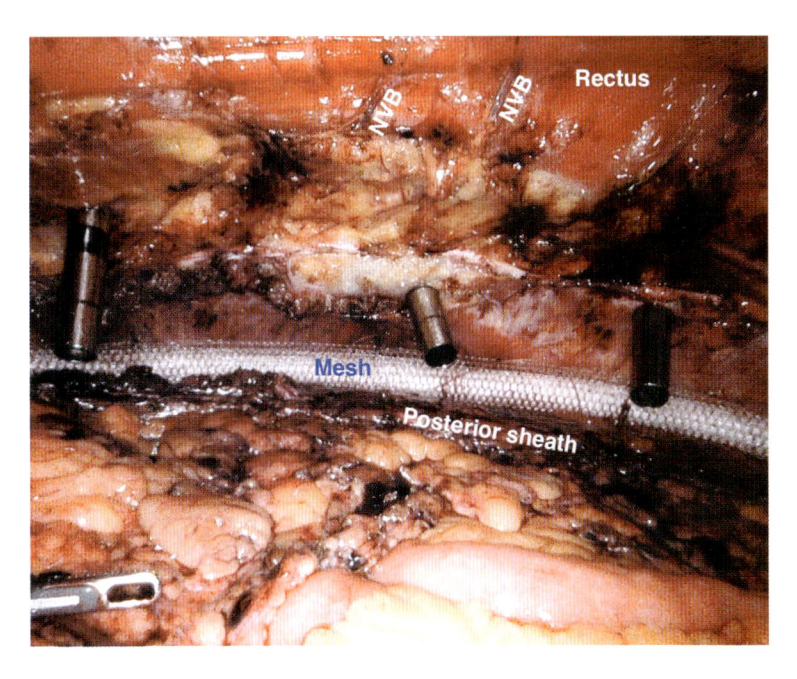

FIGURE 45-18 • Contralateral docking and mesh deployment. The mesh is rolled and inserted into the abdomen. Contralateral trocar placement is seen here for a bilateral TAR.

Step 4. Closure of the posterior and anterior rectus sheath

Peritoneal defects should be closed with absorbable sutures; Vicryl™ 3-0 for small defects (<4 cm) and V-Loc™ 3-0 for large peritoneal defects (>4 cm). Care needs to be taken to avoid injuries to the underlying viscera. The posterior sheath is re-approximated in a running fashion, and the utilization of a V-Loc™ 2-0 suture will facilitate this closure (**Figure 45-19**). A Connell stitch may minimize the contact between the barbed suture and the bowel. The anterior fascia is reapproximated with a barbed suture as well. To aid this process, pneumoperitoneum can be reduced to 6–10 mm Hg to decrease the tension. The dome of the hernia defect is incorporated within the anterior sheath closure to obliterate the dead space. The bilateral rectus muscles are returned to their midline position, and the linea alba is restored via V-Loc™ 1 suture (**Figure 45-20**).

Step 4 average time frame: 30–50 min

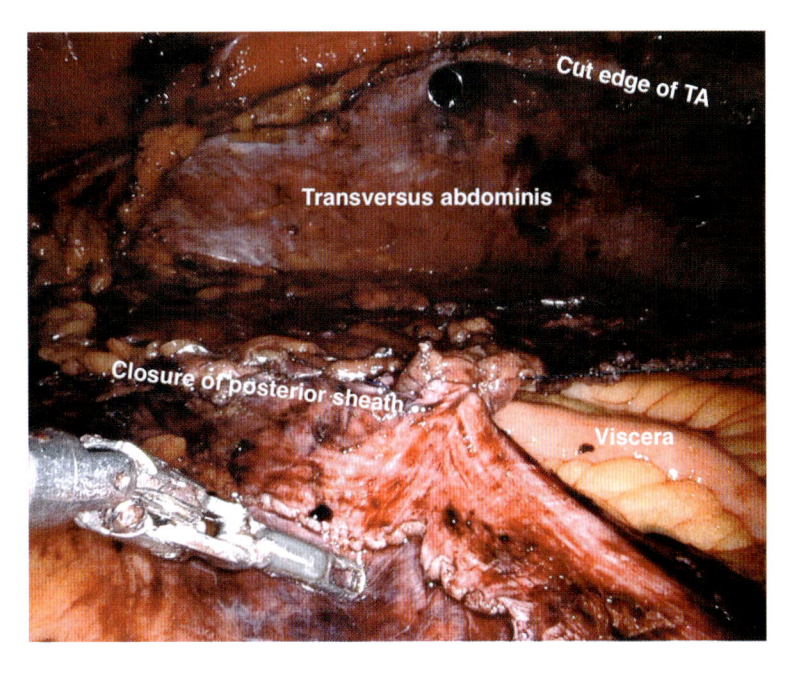

FIGURE 45-19 • Posterior sheath closure.

938 The Foundation and Art of Robotic Surgery

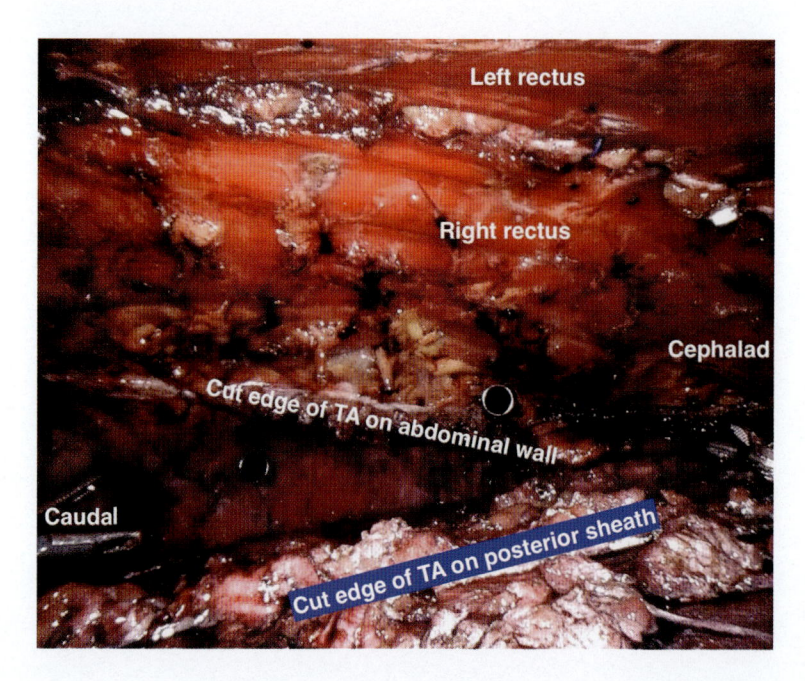

FIGURE 45-20 • Anterior sheath closure. The anterior sheath is closed with an absorbable barbed suture, and the bilateral rectus muscles are returned to their midline position.

Step 5. Final mesh deployment

The mesh is unscrolled by the "suture trick" by pulling on the suture that was placed in the center of the mesh until it lays flat on top of the posterior sheath and the posterior elements (**Figure 45-21**). A single retromuscular Jackson-Pratt 19-French drain is used and is placed using one of the previous port sites. Hemostatic agents such as powder or glue can assist with hemostasis and seroma control.

Step 5 average time frame: 10–15 min

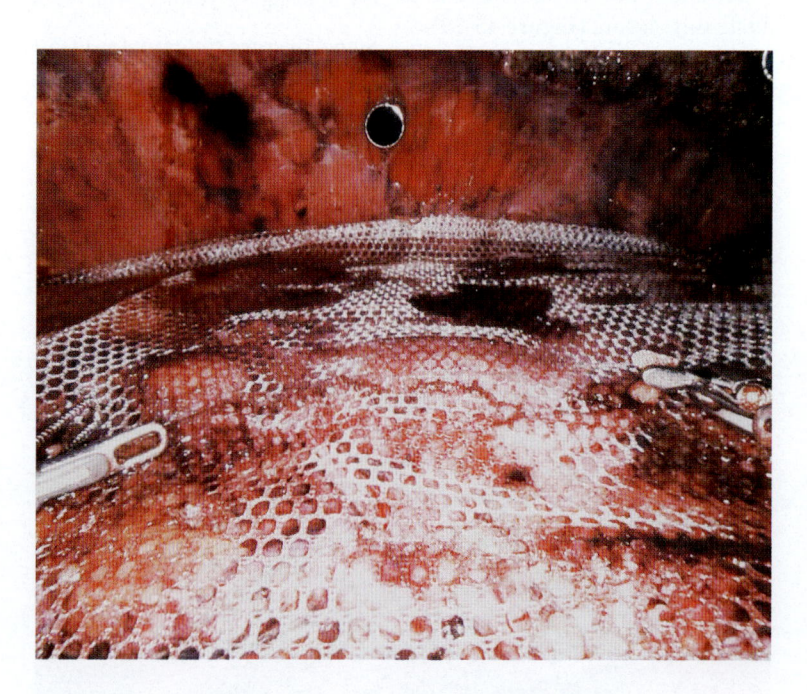

FIGURE 45-21 • Final mesh deployment.

Suggested Readings

1. Carbonell A. Rives-Stoppa retromuscular repair. In: Novitsky Y. *Hernia Surgery: Current Principles*. 1st ed. Springer International Publishing; 2016:107-115.
2. Stoppa RE. The treatment of complicated groin and incisional hernias. *World J Surg*. 1989;13(5):545-554.
3. Novitsky YW, Elliott HL, Orenstein SB, Rosen MJ. Transversus abdominis release: a novel approach to posterior component separation during complex abdominal wall reconstruction. *Am J Surg*. 2012;204(5):709-716.
4. Majumder A, Miller HJ, Del Camo LM, Soltanian H, Novitsky YW. Assessment of myofascial medialization following posterior component separation via transversus abdominis muscle release in a cadaveric model. *Hernia*. 2018;22(4):637-644.
5. Pauli EM, Rosen MJ. Open ventral hernia repair with component separation. *Surg Clin North Am*. 2013;93(5):1111-1133.
6. Carbonell AM, Warren JA, Prabhu AS, et al. Reducing length of stay using a robotic-assisted approach for retromuscular ventral hernia repair: a comparative analysis from the Americas hernia society quality collaborative. *Ann Surg*. 2018;276(2):210-217.
7. Novitsky YW. *Atlas of Robotic General Surgery*. 1st ed. Elsevier Inc; 2022:127-140.
8. Amaral MVFD, Guimarães JR, Volpe P, et al. Robotic transversus abdominis release (TAR): is it possible to offer minimally invasive surgery for abdominal wall complex defects? *Rev Col Bras Cir*. 2017;44(2):216-219.
9. Radu VG, Lica M. The endoscopic retromuscular repair of ventral hernia: the eTEP technique and early results. *Hernia*. 2019;23(5):945-955.
10. Love MW, Warren JA, Davis S, et al. Computed tomography imaging in ventral hernia repair: can we predict the need for myofascial release? *Hernia*. 2021;25(2):471-477.
11. Bracale U, Corcione F, Neola D, et al. Transversus abdominis release (TAR) for ventral hernia repair: open or robotic? Short-term outcomes from a systematic review with met-analysis. *Hernia*. 2021;25(6):1471-1480.
12. Bittner JG, Alrefai S, Vy M, et al. Comparative analysis of open and robotic transversus abdominis release for ventral hernia repair. *Surg Endosc*. 2018;32:727-734.
13. Martin-Del-Campo LA, Weltz AS, Belyansky I, Novitsky YW. Comparative analysis of perioperative outcomes of robotic versus open transversus abdominis release. *Surg Endosc*. 2018;32: 840-845.
14. Giulianotti PC, Coratti A, Angelini M, et al. Robotics in general surgery: personal experience in a large community hospital. *Arch Surg*. 2003;138(7):777-784. doi: 10.1001/archsurg.138.7.777

SECTION XI

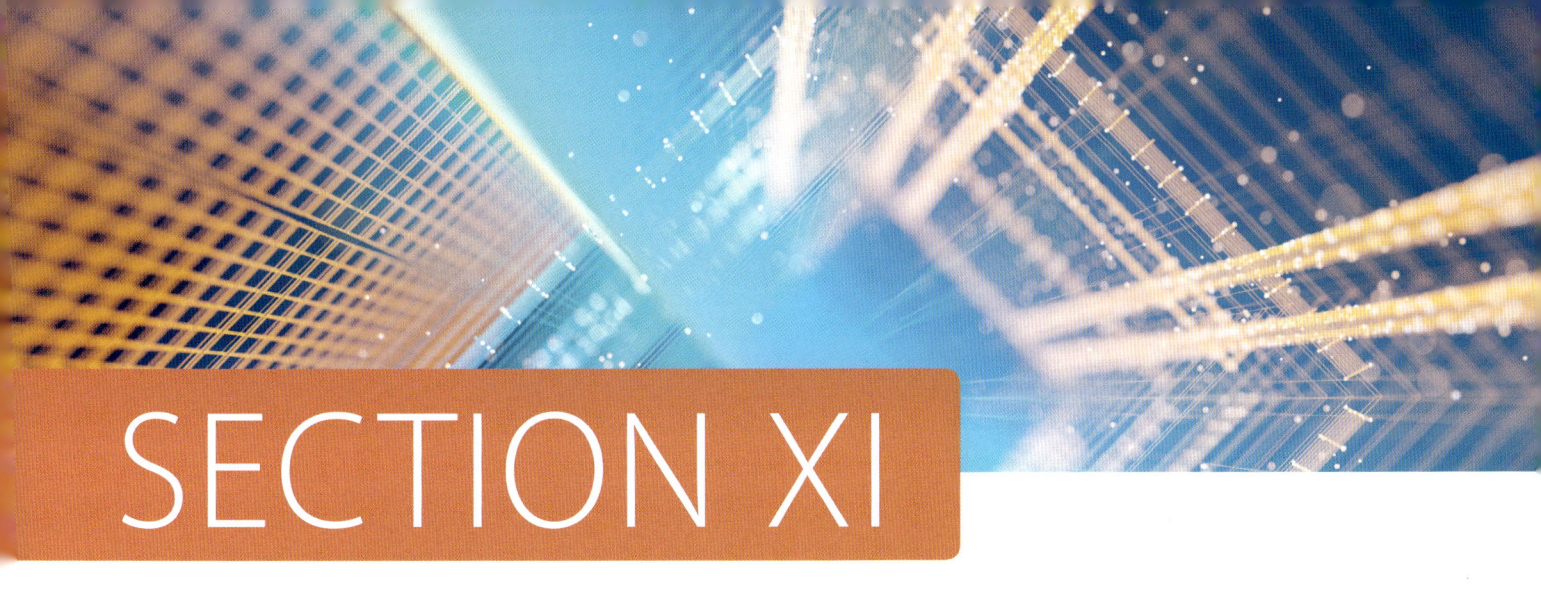

Transplant

Chapter 46 • Donor Nephrectomy 943
Mario Spaggiari • Ivo Georgiev Tzvetanov • Enrico Benedetti

Chapter 47 • Kidney Transplant 963
Pierpaolo Di Cocco • Ivo Georgiev Tzvetanov • Luciano Ambrosini • Enrico Benedetti

Chapter 48 • Pancreas Transplant 983
Pierpaolo Di Cocco • Ivo Georgiev Tzvetanov • Mario Spaggiari • Luciano Ambrosini • Enrico Benedetti

Chapter 49 • Living Donor Hepatectomy 997
Ahmed Zidan • Dieter Broering

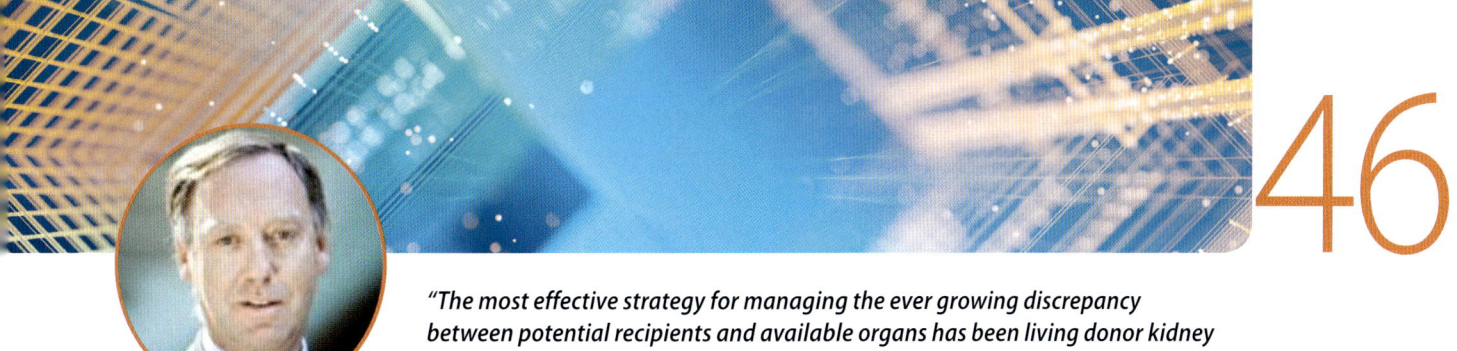

"The most effective strategy for managing the ever growing discrepancy between potential recipients and available organs has been living donor kidney transplantation."
—Santiago Horgan

Donor Nephrectomy

Mario Spaggiari • Ivo Georgiev Tzvetanov • Enrico Benedetti

INTRODUCTION

Living donor nephrectomy represents a unique surgical situation, where an invasive procedure is performed on a healthy individual for the benefit of another human being, rather than a patient accepting surgical risks for their own benefit. Minimizing donor morbidity is of paramount importance because of the altruistic component of live donation and the lack of patient pathology. The surgical technique must be balanced, provide precise and cosmetically appealing results, minimize pain, and ensure optimal functional outcome for the donor without jeopardizing the integrity of the allograft for the recipient. Since the introduction of laparoscopic donor nephrectomy (LDN) by Ratner in 1995, unrelenting efforts have been made in this field and the operative technique is continuously evolving. Long-term studies have confirmed equivalent outcomes compared to open donor nephrectomy (ODN) with all the advantages of laparoscopy, resulting in expansion of the donor pool. These findings have propelled LDN to be the standard of care at most transplant centers. The introduction of laparoscopic techniques has not only facilitated the increase in number of donors, but it has also allowed obese donors to experience recovery comparable to their nonobese counterparts.

Potential advantages of robotic-assisted donor nephrectomy over laparoscopy include safety in complex cases involving vascular anomalies and easier operative management for potential donors with a high body max index (BMI).

In this context, the University of Illinois at Chicago was the first to utilize robotic assistance for LDN in the year 2000 and to adopt this approach as a standard operation.

The described technique is a hand-assisted one. The reasons why it is preferred over a purely minimally invasive technique are as follows:

- Retrieving the kidney graft requires anyway a mini-laparotomy.
- A Pfannenstiel incision performed since the beginning facilitates and speeds up the induction of the pneumoperitoneum and the port placement.

INSTRUMENT REQUIREMENTS

The suggested main robotic instruments/tools can be listed as follows:
- 30° scope
- Two needle drivers
- Cautery hook
- Vessel sealer (optional)
- Scissors
- Multiple Hem-o-lok® clips (medium)
- Clips applier
- Bipolar forceps

The suggested main laparoscopic instruments/tools can be listed as follows:
- Needle drivers
- Grasper
- Suction-irrigation
- Clips and clip applier
- Stapler (Endo GIA/TA™)
- GelPort®, wound protector

Supplemental materials:
- Gauzes, sponges
- Penrose drains
- Vessel loops
- Endo Close™
- Medium/large clips
- Sutures: Prolene™ 4-0

Photo reproduced with permission from Santiago Horgan, MD, FACS.

Quote reproduced with permission from Horgan S, Galvani C, Gorodner MV, et al. Effect of robotic assistance on the "learning curve" for laparoscopic hand-assisted donor nephrectomy. Surg Endosc. 2007;21(9):1512-1517.

944　The Foundation and Art of Robotic Surgery

- Expert hand assistance may decrease the risk of complications and set the threshold for conversion higher. The assistant can temporarily stop a major bleed, and provide exposure and suctioning at the same time while the instruments are exchanged.
- With the growing ratio of obese living donors, purely minimally invasive techniques could become somehow challenging, and hand assistance can facilitate the procedure also under these circumstances.
- The hand retraction is wider and smoother than any other instruments for grasping.

Indications and Relative Contraindications to the Robotic Approach

The selection criteria and evaluation have been previously described (see suggested readings #5, 6). All living donor transplants are approved by a multidisciplinary committee after undergoing a comprehensive medical, psychosocial, and nutritional assessment. A donor advocate assesses all the candidates as part of the preoperative workup to ensure that all ethical standards are upheld. All donors are healthy volunteers without concomitant comorbidities. Imaging evaluation includes computed tomographic (CT) angiogram with three-dimensional reconstruction of the renal vessels and collecting system to evaluate for anomalies (**Figures 46-1 A–C**).

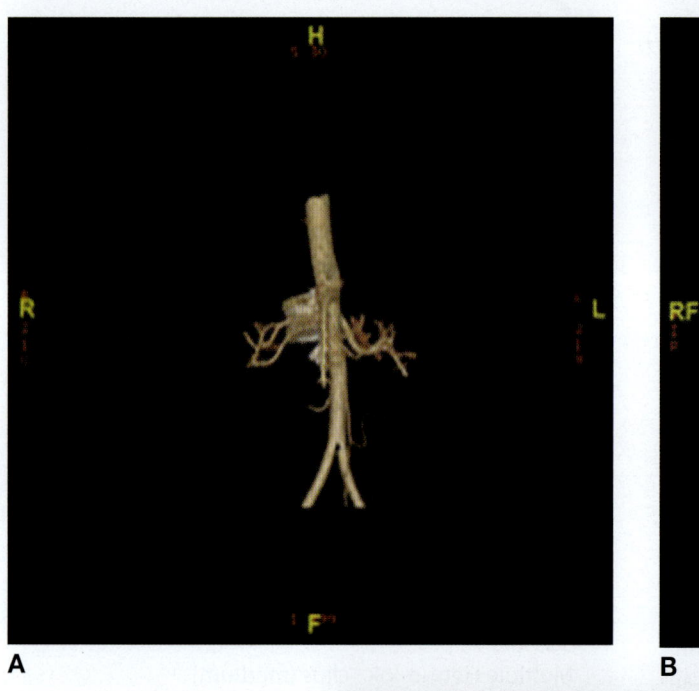

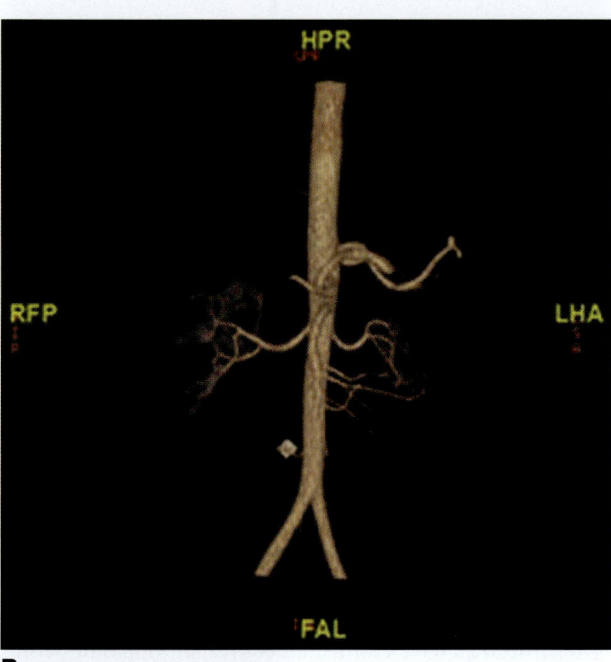

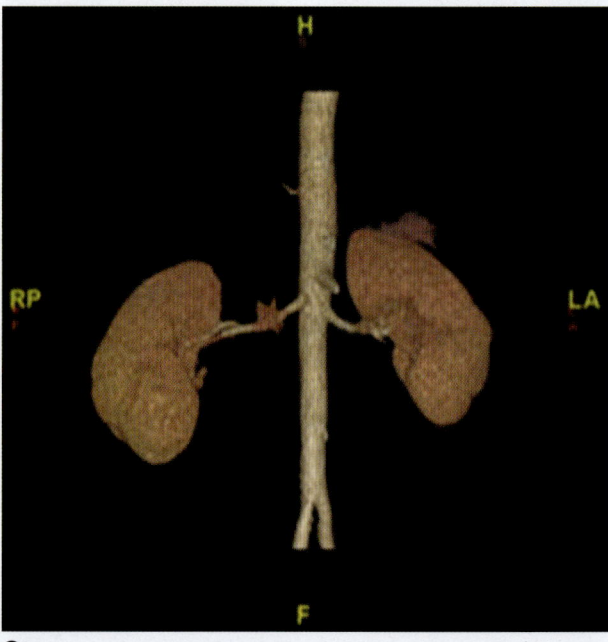

FIGURE 46-1 • CT angiogram with three-dimensional reconstruction.

After review by the multidisciplinary committee, the donors are selected for donor nephrectomy and requested to sign an informed consent for the procedure. The left kidney is routinely preferred for safer donation. However, the right kidney can be chosen in the presence of any anomaly (e.g., vascular variations, benign lesions, worse split function compared to the left kidney, kidney stones), aiming at optimizing donor safety by retaining the "healthiest" kidney for the donor. Once the donor is deemed a suitable candidate from a medical standpoint, a few surgical considerations are yet to be made. In general, there are no absolute surgical contraindications to proceed with the donation; however, the decision to adopt a minimally invasive strategy in the setting of previous abdominal operations, partially calcified vasculature, and multiple arteries or veins should be balanced with the surgeon's expertise.

Patient Positioning, OR Setup, and Port Setting

Left Nephrectomy

The patient is placed in a semilateral position (45–60°): the surgical bed is adjusted (flexed with the left side up) to open the left costophrenic angle (**Figure 46-2**).

A 7-cm Pfannenstiel incision is performed: the linea alba is incised longitudinally, instead of the classical horizontal opening, to allow the extension of the incision proximally and distally, should the kidney graft be particularly bulky and difficult to retrieve.

At this point, with the hand assistance through the Pfannenstiel incision, 4 trocars are placed in the left side of the abdomen.

An 8-mm trocar for a robotic arm is placed close to the left costal margin, at the midclavicular line (R2). The camera trocar (8 mm) is placed about 10 cm lower and more medial than the previous one. Finally, the second robotic arm trocar (R1) (8 mm) is placed about 10 cm lower from the camera port along the midclavicular line. The 12-mm assisting trocar should be placed ideally lower in the left iliac fossa. Using the anterosuperior iliac spine as a landmark, the assistant port site is placed 3–4 cm higher and medially (**Figures 46-3 A, B**).

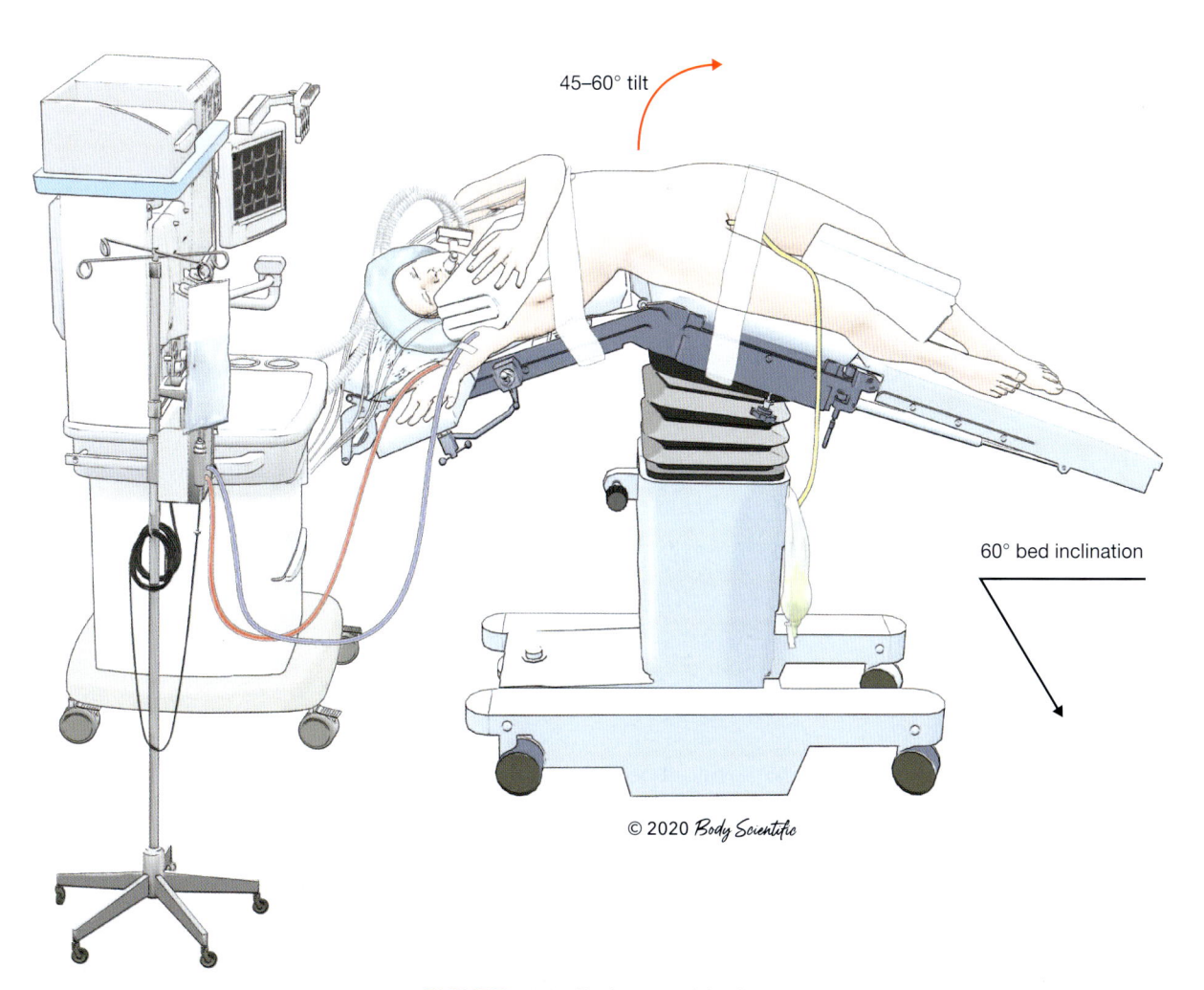

FIGURE 46-2 • Patient positioning.

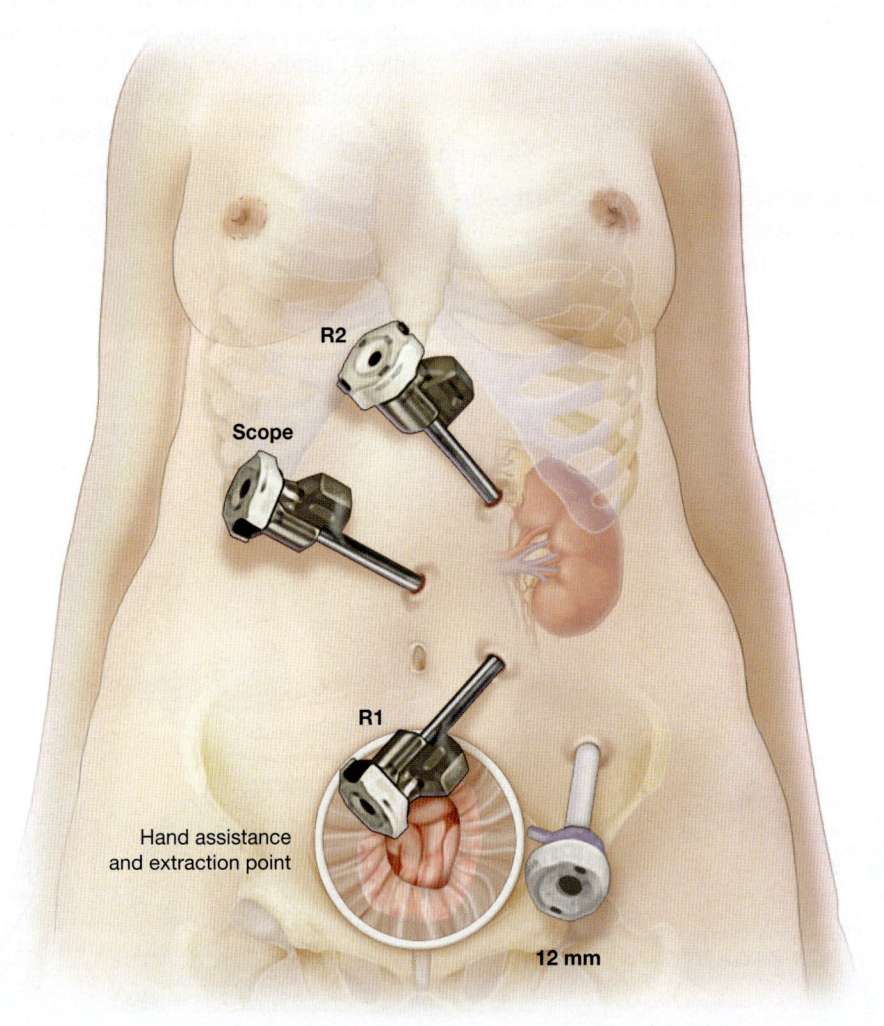

FIGURE 46-3 • A. Left nephrectomy trocar positioning.

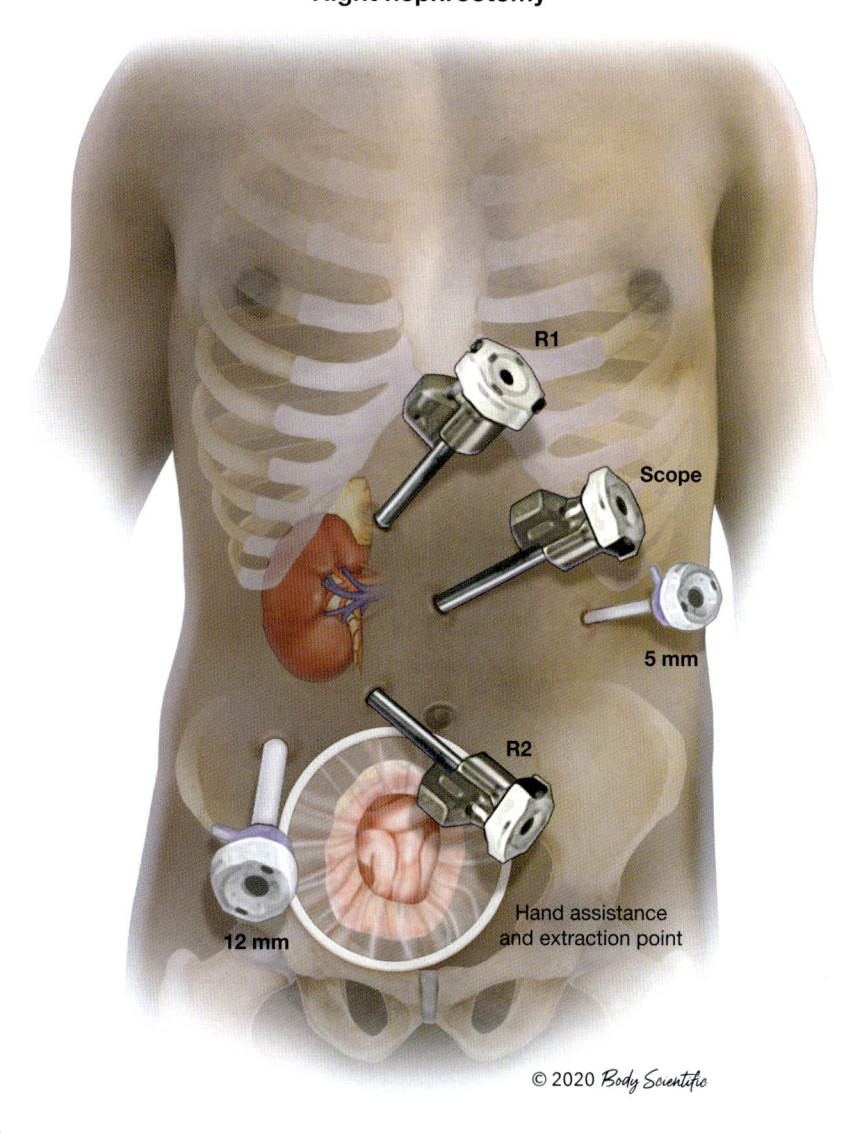

FIGURE 46-3 • (*Continued*) **B.** Right nephrectomy trocar positioning.

948 The Foundation and Art of Robotic Surgery

At this point, the robotic cart is docked to the patient bed, preferably coming from the left side (**Figure 46-4**). The first assistant is sitting on the right side of the surgical bed, and a sterile wrap (Ioban™) is covering the assistant's arm to go through the wound protector via the Pfannenstiel incision. A second assistant will handle the 10–12-mm port (complementary actions/stapling) (**Figure 46-4**).

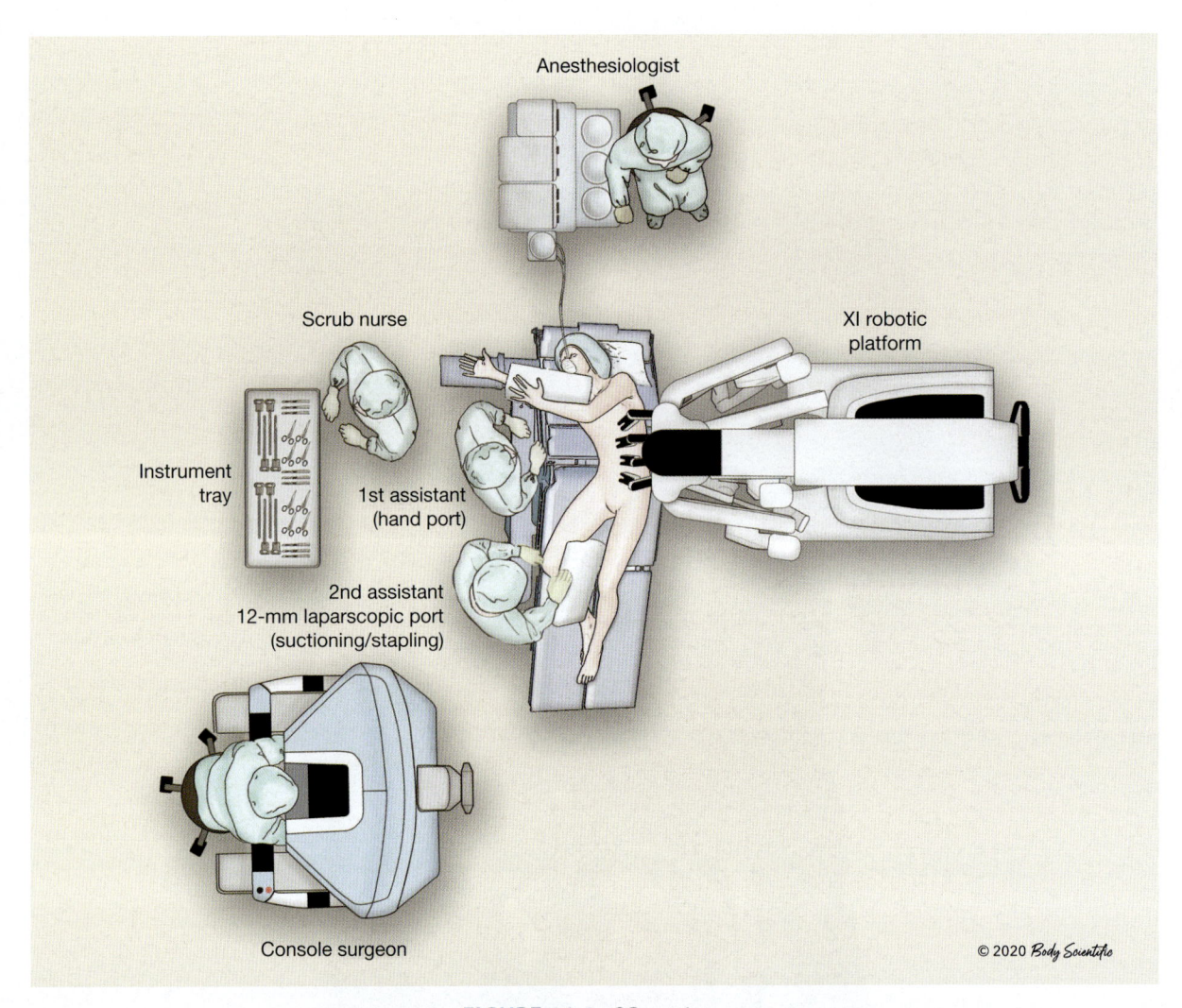

FIGURE 46-4 • OR setting.

Surgical Technique: Left Nephrectomy

▶ Video 46-1. Left Donor Nephrectomy – Full Procedure

Step 1. Mobilization of the descending colon and splenic flexure

The descending colon and splenic flexure are mobilized with a lateral-to-medial approach, keeping the dissection plane in front of the Toldt's fascia. The monopolar hook is the main tool. The splenocolic ligaments are taken down, recognizing the spleen, the lower edge of the pancreatic body, and the pancreatic tail.

Step 1 average time frame: 10–20 min

> ▶▶ **TIPS**
>
> The hand assistance exerts a dynamic retraction on the colon and small bowel loops, optimizing the exposure.
>
> Entering into the Gerota's capsule at an early stage and dissecting from the upper pole of the kidney proceeding with a top-down direction (**Figure 46-5**) decreases the risk of splenic or pancreatic injury.

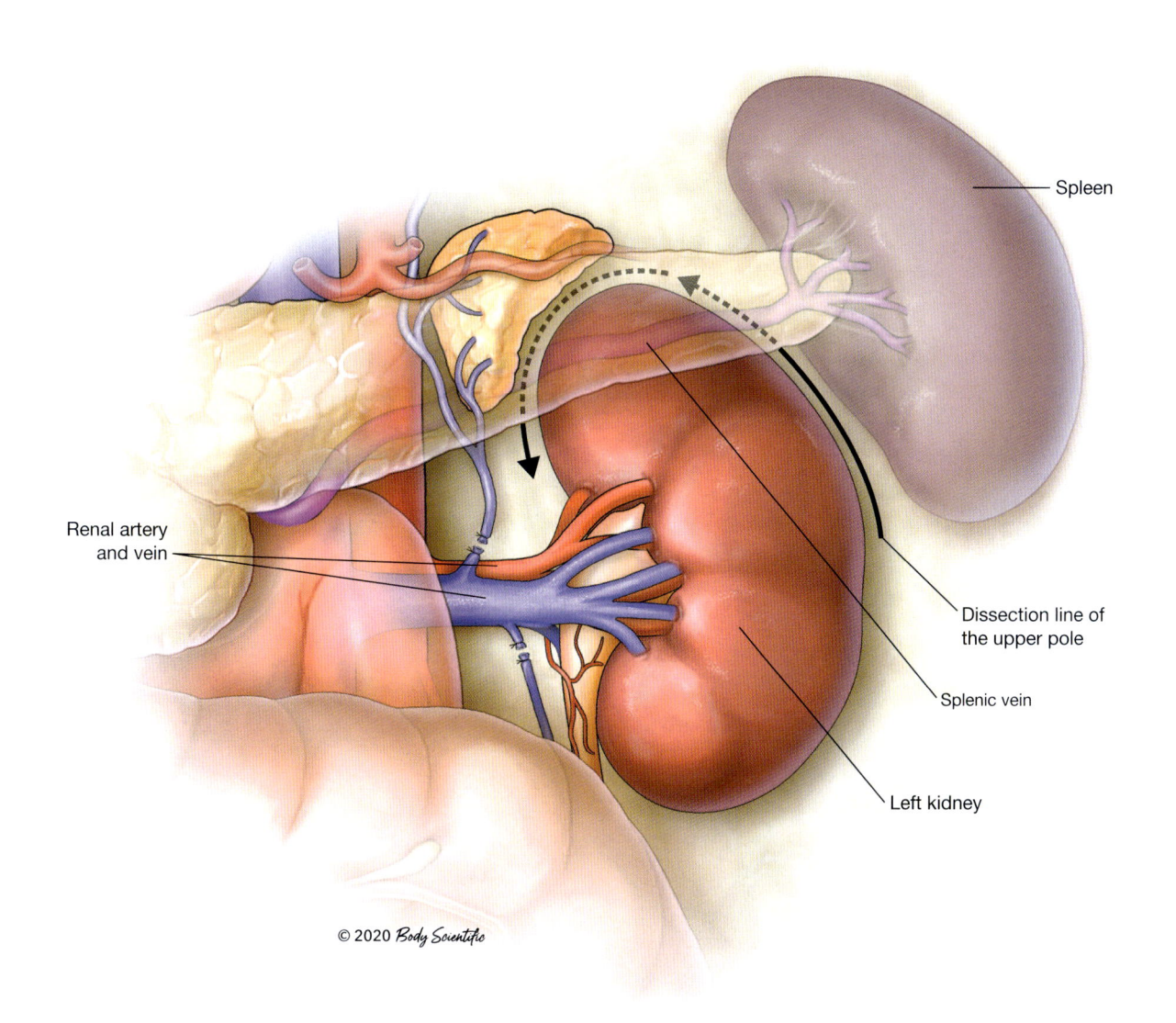

FIGURE 46-5 • Dissection of the kidney upper pole.

Step 2. Preparation of the ureter and the gonadal vein
The left ureter is identified and dissected free at the level of the left iliac vessels (**Figure 46-6**). Care has to be taken to avoid injury of the periureteral vessels. A Penrose drain or a vessel loop is passed around the ureter and used for retraction. The left gonadal vein is exposed (**Figures 46-7 A–C**) where it is still medial to the ureter. The assistant retracts the ureter laterally.

Following and preparing the gonadal vein moving cephalad, the left renal vein is reached and exposed. One or two gonadal arteries are divided on the left side of the aorta using the vessel sealer or in between clips.

Step 2 average time frame: 10–15 min

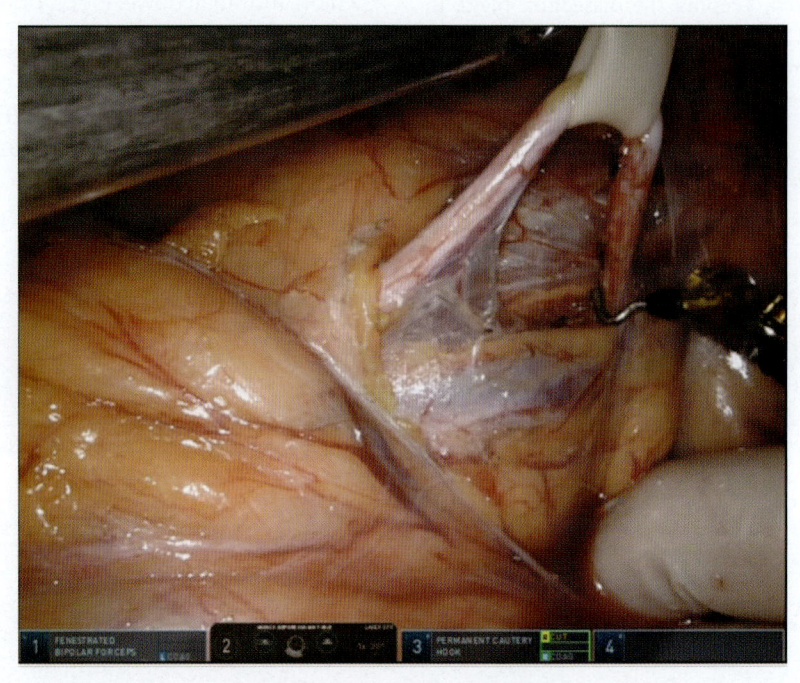

FIGURE 46-6 • Ureter isolation.

Donor Nephrectomy 951

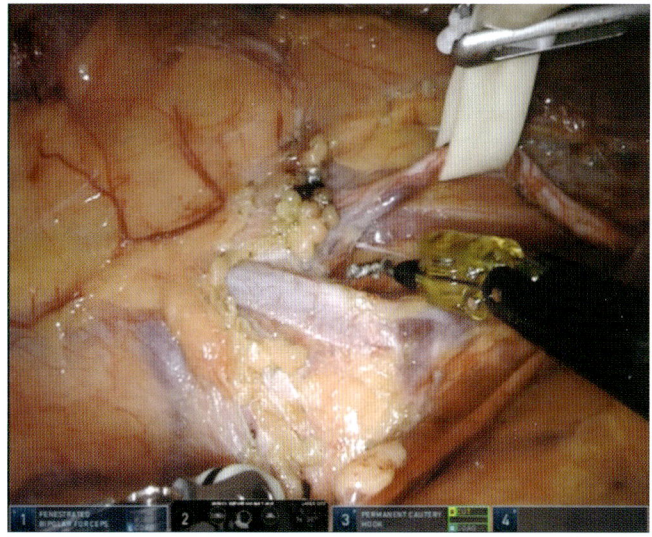

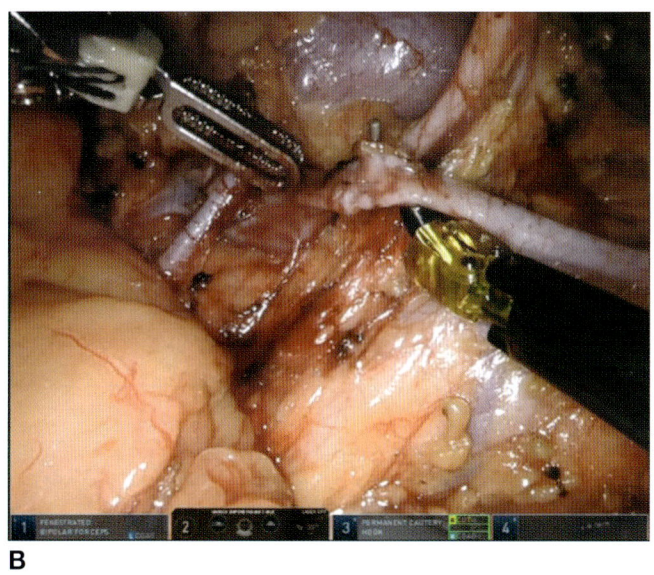

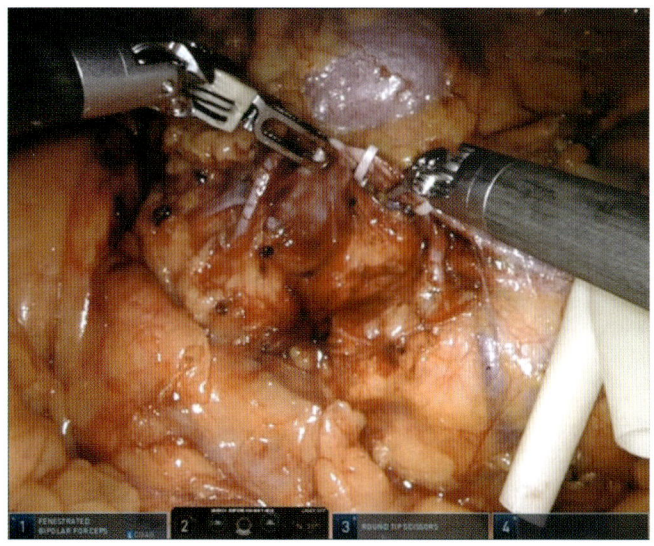

FIGURE 46-7 • Gonadal vein preparation and division.

952 The Foundation and Art of Robotic Surgery

▶ **Video 46-2. Step 2. Preparation of the Ureter and the Gonadal Vein**

> 🔍 **ANATOMICAL HIGHLIGHTS**
>
> The ureter receives its blood supply from multiple arterial branches (aorta, renal artery, iliac). The arterial supply will course longitudinally along the ureter creating a plexus of anastomosing vessels (**Figure 46-8**).

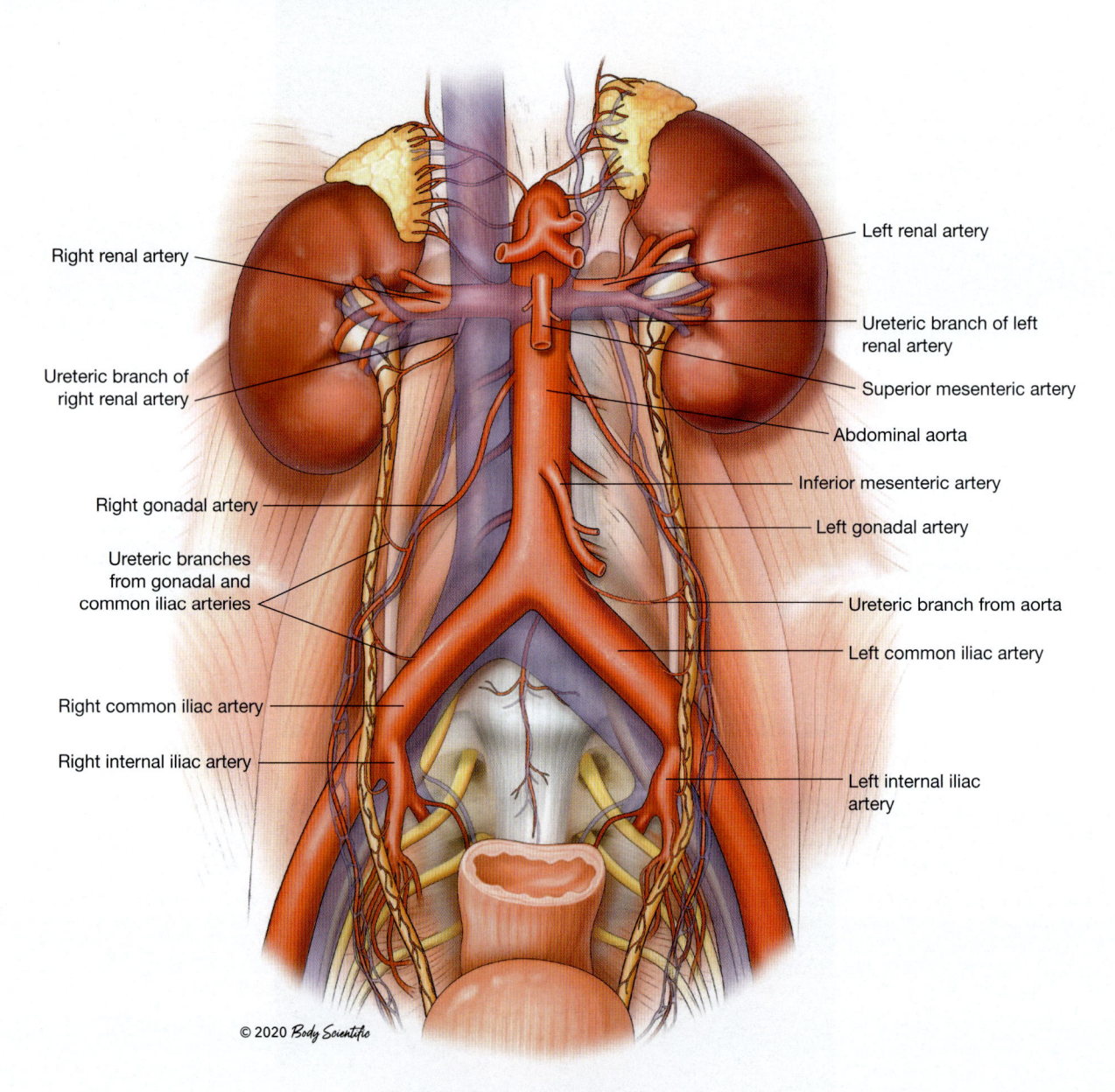

FIGURE 46-8 • Ureter blood supply.

Step 3. Preparation of the left renal vein

At this point, the dissection of the renal vein should be completed (**Figures 46-9 A–G**). The left adrenal vein is identified, and both the adrenal vein and the gonadal vein are divided in between clips or sutures.

The renal vein is prepared. A gentle traction favors the exposure of the posterior aspect of the vein, and it allows the identification of a possible venous reno-hemiazygos lumbar trunk. If present, this trunk should be carefully divided in between clips and/or Prolene™ 4-0 sutures.

Step 3 average time frame: 15–25 min

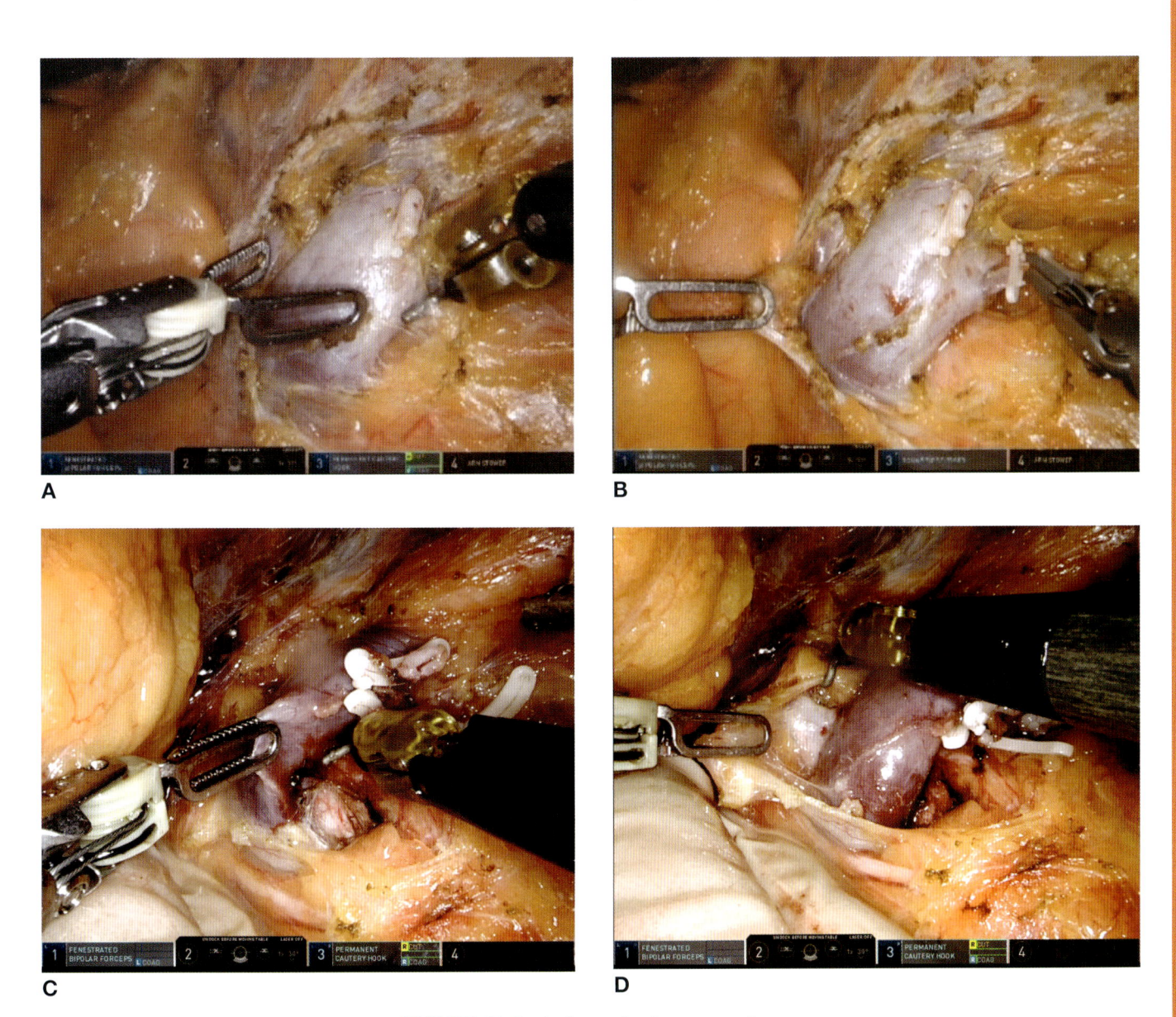

FIGURE 46-9 • Left renal vein preparation.

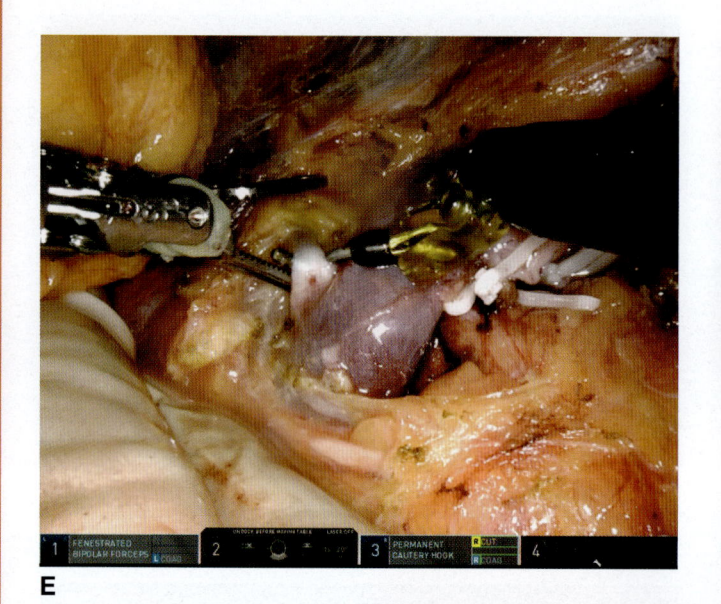

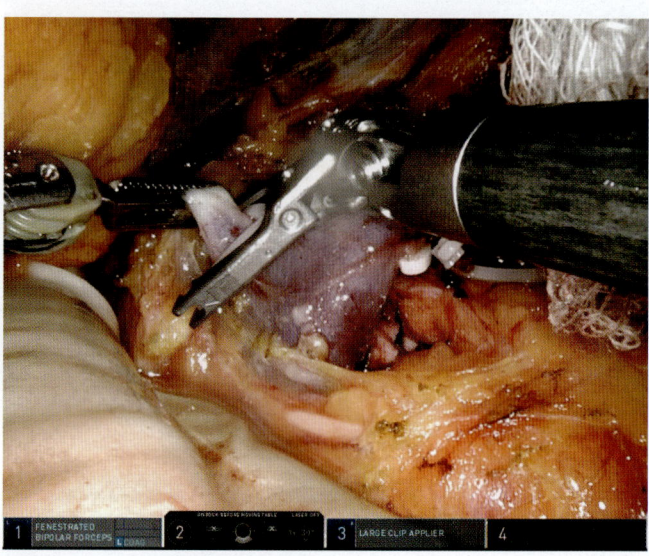

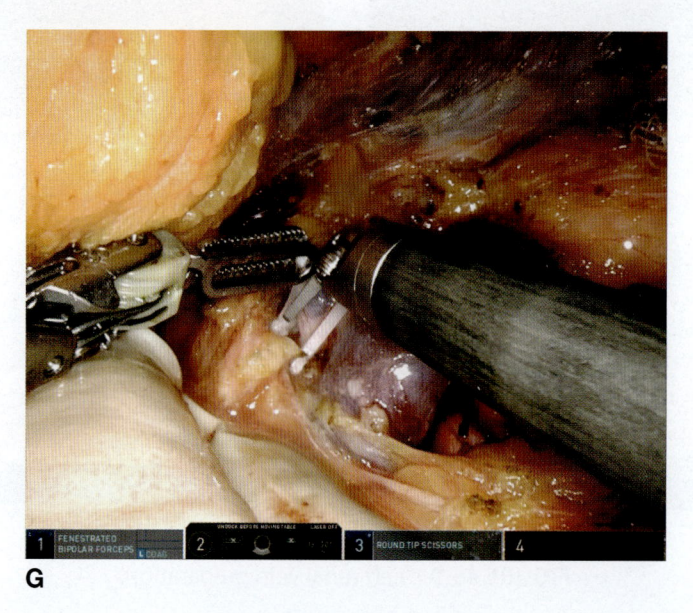

FIGURE 46-9 • (Continued)

▶ **Video 46-3.** Step 3. Preparation of the Left Renal Vein

🔍 **ANATOMICAL HIGHLIGHTS**

The knowledge of the standard anatomy (**Figure 46-10**), and of the multiple anatomical variations that can occur in this region, is paramount.

In **Figures 46-11 A, B**, some relevant anomalies of the renal artery are represented. (Different classifications are described in the literature. For additional information, see suggested readings #7, 8.)

In **Figures 46-12 A–E**, the most significant venous variations are depicted. (For additional information, see suggested reading #9.)

⚠ **PITFALLS**

It is fundamental to avoid injuries of the posterior lumbar tributaries of the left renal vein during the left living donor nephrectomy. The lumbar veins, if injured, might retract into the retroperitoneal fat, with bleeding that is difficult to control. This complication may require transfusions and possible conversions and rarely could cause gas embolism.

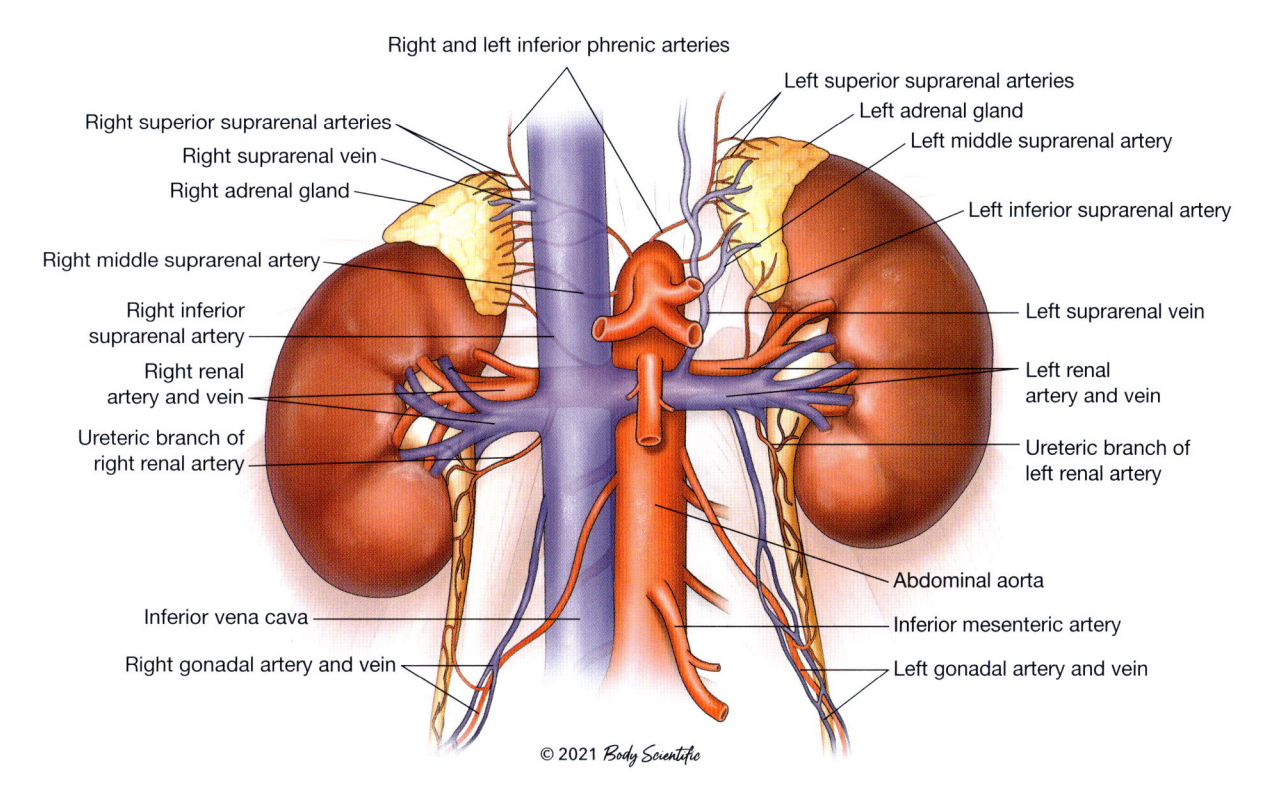

FIGURE 46-10 • Renal vascular standard anatomy.

956   The Foundation and Art of Robotic Surgery

A

- Inferior phrenic artery
- Right renal artery (posterior branch)
- Right renal artery (anterior branch)
- Inferior vena cava
- Accessory right renal artery
- Inferior suprarenal artery
- Right renal artery
- Inferior vena cava

* A caudal accessory right renal artery may course anteriorly (not posteriorly) to the ICV.

** An inferior phrenic artery with superior supra-renal vessels may originate from the renal artery (in the absence of the middle supra-renal artery).

The renal artery can have a proximal subdivision.

B

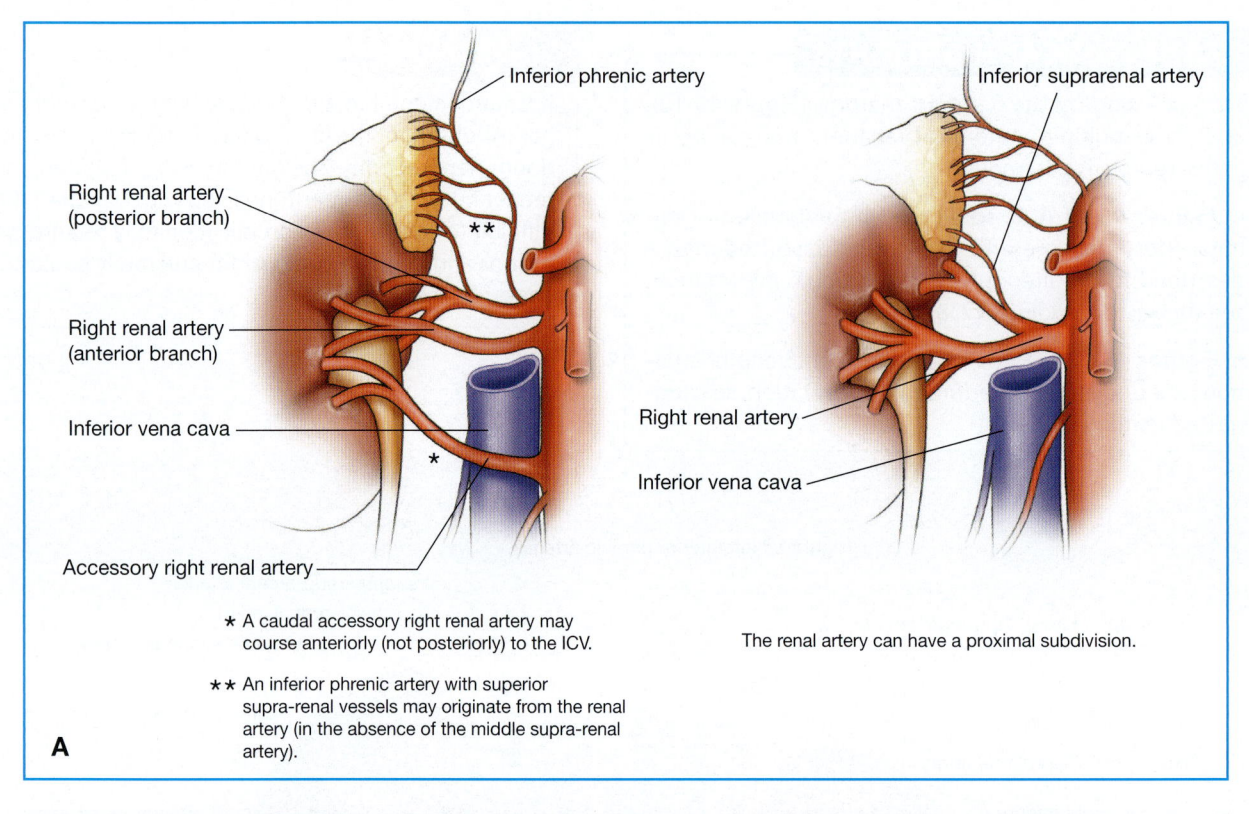

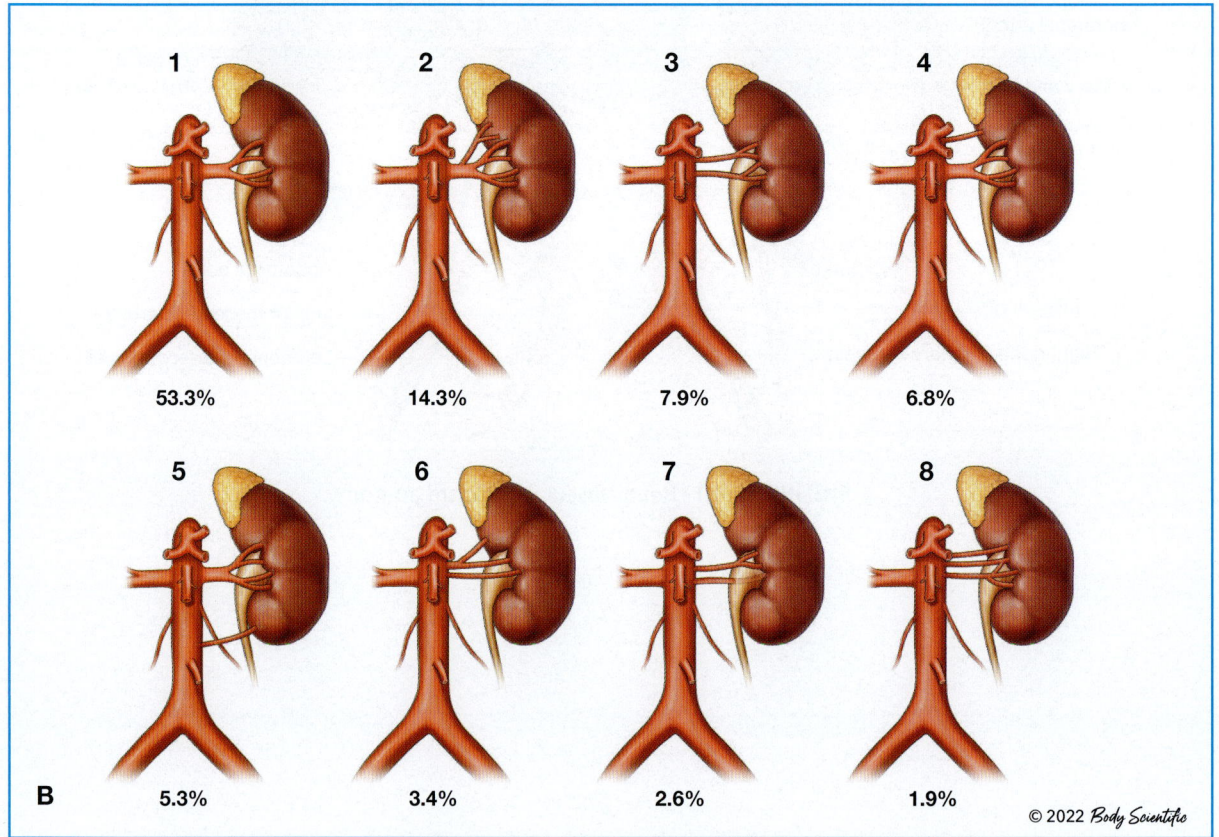

1. 53.3%
2. 14.3%
3. 7.9%
4. 6.8%
5. 5.3%
6. 3.4%
7. 2.6%
8. 1.9%

© 2022 Body Scientific

FIGURE 46-11 • Renal artery variations.

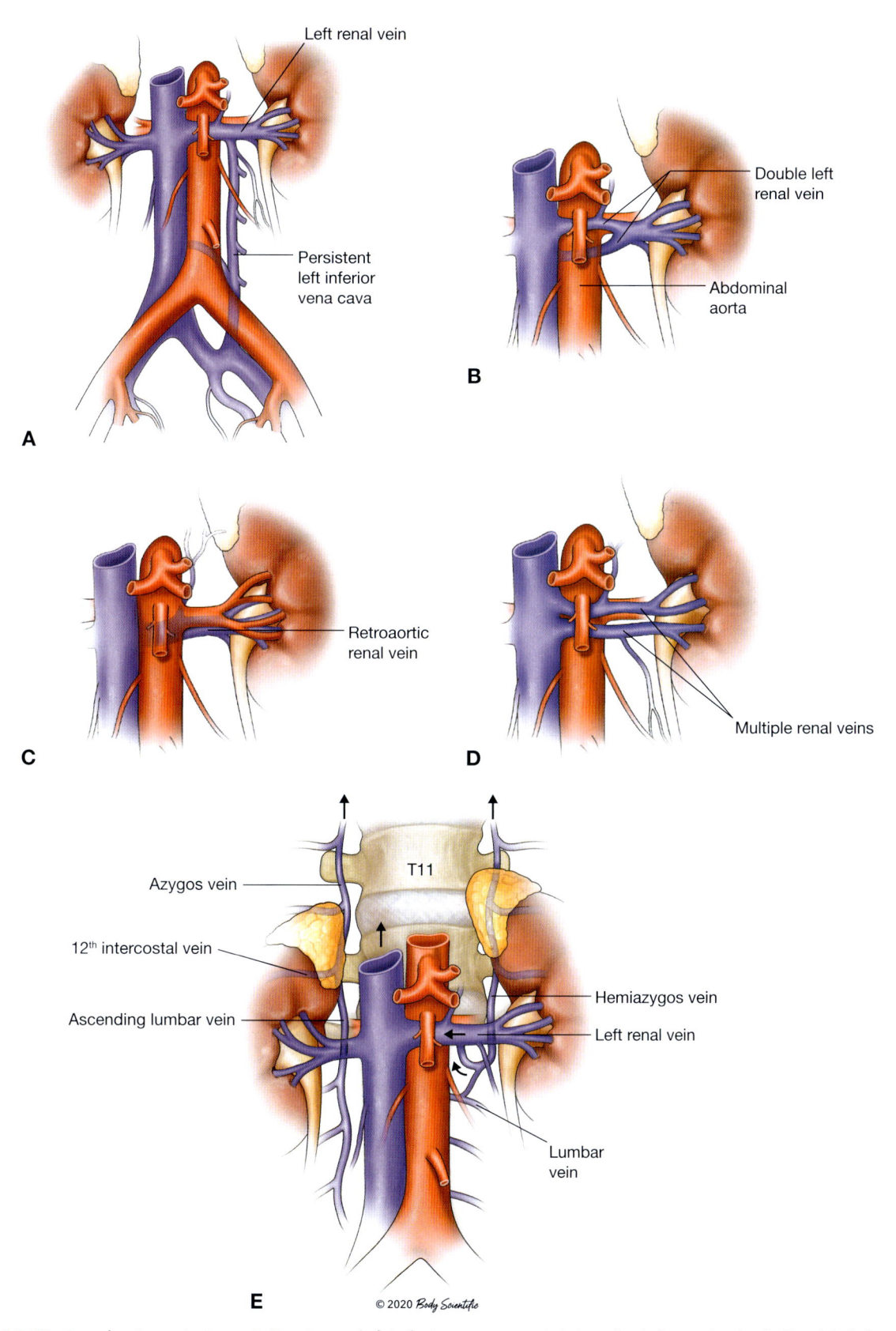

FIGURE 46-12 • Renal vein variations. **A.** Persistent left inferior vena cava joining the left renal vein. **B.** Double left renal vein forming a "ring" around the aorta. **C.** Retroaortic renal vein. **D.** Multiple renal veins. **E.** Renal-azygos-lumbar connection.

Step 4. Identification of the left renal artery

The artery is usually located just behind the renal vein, on the left side of the aorta. Its position may also be higher, or less frequently lower, according to individual variations. Using a gentle dissection with the hook, the anterior part of the artery is exposed, removing some lymphoneural tissue around it.

Step 4 average time frame: 5–10 min

Step 5. Division of the ureter and mobilization of the kidney

Once the anterior portion of the artery is exposed, the left ureter is clipped distally, at the crossing of the iliac vessels, and it is divided with scissors. This maneuver allows a full mobilization of the kidney from the retroperitoneum.

Step 5 average time frame: 5–10 min

Step 6. Preparation of the renal artery

The kidney can be flipped medially by the assistant's hand, and with this exposure, it is easier to complete the preparation of the posterior aspect of the renal artery. The artery is then encircled with a vessel loop.

Step 6 average time frame: 10–15 min

▶ **Video 46-4. Step 6. Preparation of the Renal Artery**

Step 7. Renoadrenal separation

The upper pole of the kidney is completely separated from the adrenal gland. A careful utilization of the vessel sealer is sometimes helpful in controlling tiny arterial branches that may connect the adrenal gland with the renal artery. Starting from the venous stump of the adrenal vein, the lower edge of the gland is followed until reaching the previous dissection of the upper pole of the kidney. At this point, the kidney is completely free from the retroperitoneum.

Step 7 average time frame: 15–20 min

> ▶▶ **TIPS**
>
> The dissection of an accessory artery is usually easier when the kidney is flipped medially. This vessel should be divided first, followed by the main renal artery and vein.

Step 8. Division of the renal artery

Five thousand units of intravenous heparin are administered, and with the kidney medially flipped, the renal artery is stapled by the assistant using an Endo TA™ vascular stapler. The aortic stump is also secured with an additional Hem-o-lok clip®. The distal stump is then transected with scissors.

Step 8 average time frame: 3–5 min

> ▶▶ **TIPS**
>
> In the presence of the retroaortic renal vein, this vessel has a typical caudocranial course. The dissection of the vein should be carefully carried out in a distal to proximal fashion, keeping in mind that the artery may cross the anterior wall of the vein. When this particular anatomical variation occurs, the artery should be divided with the kidney resting in its natural lateral position.

Step 9. Division of the renal vein

With the kidney back in its natural position, the renal vein is divided by the assistant using an Endo GIA™ stapler (**Figures 46-13 A, B**).

Step 9 average time frame: 3–5 min

Step 10. Extraction of the graft

The kidney is then removed through the hand port device. The graft is promptly placed in cold saline, flushed with 250 mL of University of Wisconsin solution through the renal artery, and immediately transplanted into the recipient after a standard back-table preparation. Protamine sulfate may be administered to the donor. The surgical field is carefully inspected to perfect the hemostasis. No drains are left in place. The 12-mm port site is closed with Endo Close™, and the Pfannenstiel incision is sutured layer by layer in the standard way (see Chapter 2, The Basic Principles of Clinical Applications).

Step 10 average time frame: 2–3 min

Patient Positioning, OR Setup, and Port Setting

Right Nephrectomy

The steps described for the left nephrectomy can also be applied, with some minor difference, for the right nephrectomy. The position of the patient mirrors the one previously described for the left nephrectomy (**Figure 46-2**) with the patient tilted 45–60° on the left side. The trocar placement, after Pfannenstiel incision, is described in **Figure 46-3B**.

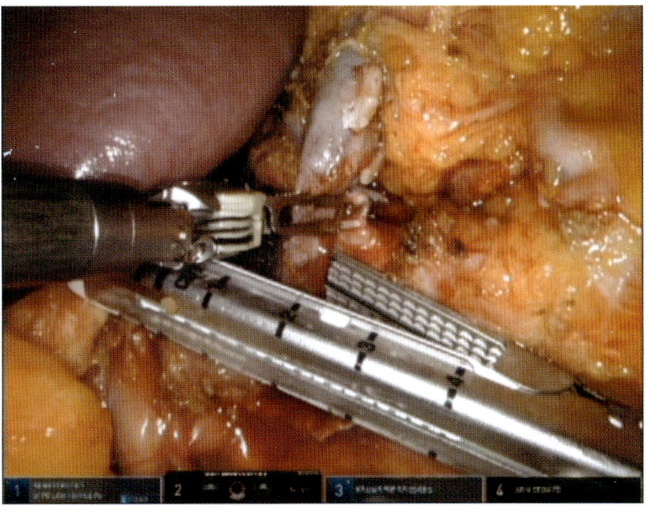

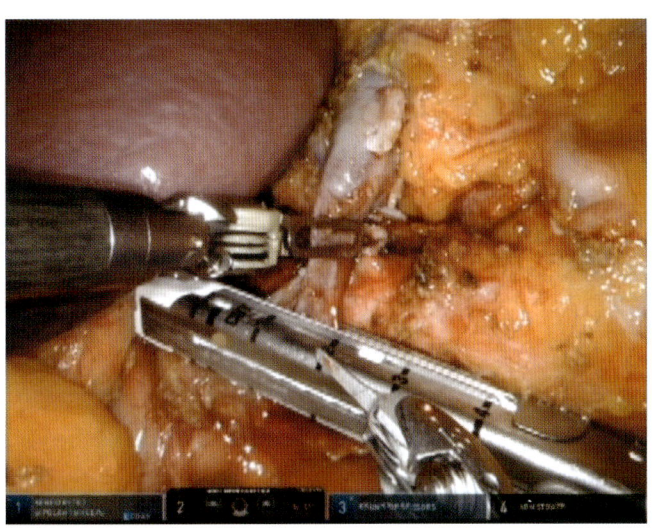

FIGURE 46-13 • Division of the renal vein.

Surgical Technique: Right Nephrectomy

Step 1. Mobilization of ascending colon, hepatic flexure, and duodenum

The ascending colon and the hepatic flexure are mobilized medially, exposing the right kidney and duodenum; the monopolar hook is the main tool needed. The duodenum is then retracted medially to expose the inferior vena cava.

Step 1 average time frame: 15–20 min

> ▶▶ **TIPS**
>
> The assistant's hand will retract the ascending colon and the duodenum dynamically, optimizing the exposure. An additional 5-mm laparoscopic port is placed in the left upper quadrant to facilitate retraction of the liver upward and to clearly expose the upper pole of the right kidney and the right adrenal gland.

Step 2. Preparation of the ureter and anterior exposure of the right renal vein

The right ureter is identified and dissected starting distally and up to the level of right iliac vessels. The dissection must be kept away from the ureter to avoid devascularization. The right gonadal vein is followed up to the entrance into the inferior vena cava. The lateral wall of the inferior vena cava is exposed, and the right renal vein identified. If present, accessory renal veins are recognized and divided between clips. The right adrenal gland is separated by the perirenal tissue.

Step 2 average time frame: 10–15 min

> ▶▶ **TIPS**
>
> It is better not to attempt direct dissection of the right renal vein until the entire dissection, described in Step 2, is completed.

Step 3. Preparation of the right renal vein

The right renal vein is carefully dissected close to its entrance into the inferior vena cava. There are usually no tributaries, but on occasion, small ones must be divided in between sutures (Prolene™ 4-0) to optimize the limited length. Rarely, during this dissection, a precaval lower polar artery coming from the right common iliac artery can be encountered and needs to be dissected free.

Step 3 average time frame: 10–15 min

> ▶▶ **TIPS**
>
> The right renal vein is short and quite delicate; therefore, the dissection must be careful and extremely gentle. The posterolateral wall of the vein may be difficult to dissect; in that case, it is best to complete this step with the kidney retracted medially and the renal artery identified.

Step 4. Division of the ureter and mobilization of the kidney

The ureter is double clipped and divided just passed the junction with the iliac vessels. The right kidney is progressively retracted medially by the hand assistance and completely mobilized laterally and superiorly. The liver is retracted upward by the assistant to facilitate the dissection.

Step 4 average time frame: 10–20 min

> ▶▶ **TIPS**
>
> If there is a large amount of visceral fat surrounding the kidney, it is best to detach it as much as possible at this stage to facilitate extraction. In donors with a high BMI, this maneuver is routinely performed.

> **EDITORIAL COMMENT**
>
> Depending on the anatomy and position of the liver, setting the R3 of the robot with a subcostal-left port may help in improving the exposure of the right kidney in a stable and safe way.

Step 5. Identification of the right renal artery

The renal artery is usually located posteriorly in relation to the right renal vein, and it runs behind the inferior vena cava. This dissection is performed after complete medial mobilization of the kidney. It is important to dissect the lateral wall of the inferior vena cava to facilitate the arterial exposure, as well as the placement of the stapling device later on. If multiple arteries are present, their preparation is completed at this stage.

Step 5 average time frame: 5–10 min

Step 6. Division of the renal artery

Five thousand units of intravenous heparin are given. The kidney is retracted medially exposing the right renal artery which is stapled using a vascular Endo TA™. A robotic clip is applied over the stapler line and the artery is sharply divided with robotic scissors.

Step 6 average time frame: 3–5 min

Step 7. Division of the renal vein

The renal vein is stapled right at the junction with the inferior vena cava with an Endo GIA™ stapler. The kidney is placed in its natural position to facilitate this maneuver.

Step 7 average time frame: 3–5 min

Step 8. Extraction of the graft

The kidney is rapidly removed through the hand port and immediately flushed with 250 mL of University of Wisconsin solution through the renal artery. Protamine sulfate may be administered to the donor (see left nephrectomy). After standard back-bench preparation, the kidney is immediately transplanted.

Step 8 average time frame: 2–3 min

> **ANATOMICAL HIGHLIGHTS**
>
> Common anatomical variations are the presence of accessory arteries (upper, lower pole).
>
> Dissection of an accessory artery is generally easier when the kidney is flipped medially. The accessory artery should be divided first, followed by the main renal artery and vein.

> ▶▶ **TIPS**
>
> A problem, commonly seen in small abdomens, is the collision between the right arm of the robot and the assistant's instruments at the time of the arterial stapling. To avoid this occurrence, the assistant port should be placed as low as possible in the right iliac fossa. However, if that happens, the robotic arm can be disconnected for the time of the stapling and reconnected afterward.
>
> In large abdomens, the Endo TA™ vascular stapler may not reach the target at the time of stapling. The situation may be easily overcome by pushing the assistant trocar all the way inside the abdominal wall. This maneuver may increase by 4–5 cm the reach of the stapler.

Suggested Readings

1. Ratner LE, Ciseck LJ, Moore RG, et al. Laparoscopic live donor nephrectomy. *Transplantation* 1995;60(9):1047-1049.
2. Giessing M. Laparoscopic living-donor nephrectomy. *Nephrol Dialysis Transplant* 2004;19(suppl 4):iv36-40.
3. Eng M. The role of laparoscopic donor nephrectomy in renal transplantation. *Am Surgeon* 2010;76(4):349-353.
4. Leventhal JR, Deeik RK, Joehl RJ, et al. Laparoscopic live donor nephrectomy–is it safe? *Transplantation* 2000;70(4):602-606.
5. Horgan S, Vanuno D, Sileri P, Cicalese L, Benedetti E. Robotic-assisted laparoscopic donor nephrectomy for kidney transplantation. *Transplantation* 2002;73(9):1474-1479.
6. Horgan S, Galvani C, Gorodner MV, et al. Effect of robotic assistance on the "learning curve" for laparoscopic hand-assisted donor nephrectomy. *Surg Endosc.* 2007;21(9):1512-1517.
7. Cases C, García-Zoghby L, Manzorro P, et al. Anatomical variations of the renal arteries: cadaveric and radiologic study, review of the literature, and proposal of a new classification of clinical interest. *Ann Anat.* 2017;211:61-68. doi: 10.1016/j.aanat.2017.01.012
8. Tardo DT, Briggs C, Ahern G, et al. Anatomical variations of the renal arterial vasculature: an Australian perspective *Med Imaging Radiat Oncol.* 2017;61(5):643-649. doi: 10.1111/1754-9485.12618
9. Hostiuc S, Rusu MC, Negoi I, et al. Anatomical variants of renal veins: a meta-analysis of prevalence. *Sci Rep.* 2019;9(1):10802. doi: 10.1038/s41598-019-47280-8
10. Giulianotti PC, Coratti A, Angelini M, et al. Robotics in general surgery: personal experience in a large community hospital. *Arch Surg.* 2003;138(7):777-784. doi: 10.1001/archsurg.138.7.777

"What is to say that patterns of surgical use will be the same 10 years hence?... Will another avalanche of demand, similar to that seen when laparoscopic cholecystectomy became widely available, occur when some new surgical procedure is developed, or will advances in genomics, pharmacology, or other technology replace operations?"

—Olga Jonasson (1934–2006)

Kidney Transplant

Pierpaolo Di Cocco • Ivo Georgiev Tzvetanov • Luciano Ambrosini • Enrico Benedetti

INTRODUCTION

Kidney transplantation provides a clear survival advantage over patients in dialysis with end-stage renal disease; however, this procedure presents several challenges, in some groups of patients, such as the obese.

Access to the external iliac vessels is more difficult in morbidly obese patients; therefore, larger and more extensive incisions are required, increasing the risk of wound infection. Overall, the invasiveness of the procedure may delay early postoperative mobilization and increase the risk of deep vein thrombosis, pulmonary embolism, and respiratory complications.

Surgical innovation has led to the development of minimally invasive approaches in many surgical specialties, which is contributing to improved outcomes. Kidney transplantation, initially not considered feasible with conventional laparoscopic techniques because of its higher complexity and necessary precision, can be performed with robotic technology.

Since the first report by Giulianotti et al. at the University of Illinois Chicago (UIC) in 2009, robot-assisted kidney transplant (RAKT), with its 3-dimensional, higher resolution visual

INSTRUMENT REQUIREMENTS

The suggested main robotic instruments/tools can be listed as follows:
- 30°, 0° scope
- Cadière forceps
- Fenestrated bipolar forceps
- Permanent monopolar cautery hook
- Large clip applier (Hem-o-lok® clips)
- Large needle driver
- Black diamond micro forceps
- Potts scissors
- Round-tip scissors
- Robotic bulldog vascular clamps

The suggested main laparoscopic instruments/tools can be listed as follows:
- Needle drivers
- Scissors
- Graspers
- Large clip applier (Hem-o-lok® clips)
- Suction-irrigation
- GelPort®
- Bulldog clamps

Supplemental materials:
- Gauzes, sponges
- Vessel loops
- Medium-large clips
- Sutures:
  - Prolene™ 3-0, 4-0, 5-0, and 6-0
  - Vicryl™ 3-0, 0
  - Monocryl™ 5-0
- Gore-Tex® 4-0 and 5-0
- PDS™ 3-0, 4-0, 5-0, and 1
- Microvascular clamps (Scanlan® Reliance Bulldog Clamp) (**Figure 47-1**)
- Ureteral stent
- Suture passer

Photo reproduced with permission from Bartholomew A, Ascher N, Starzl T. Tribute: Dr. Olga Jonasson. Born in Peoria, Illinois, August 12, 1934. Died in Chicago, Illinois, August 30, 2006. Am J Transplant. 2007;7(8):1882-1883.

Quote reproduced with permission from Jonasson O. "I prefer old age to the alternative.": Maurice Chevalier, 1962. Ann Surg. 2003;238(2):178-179.

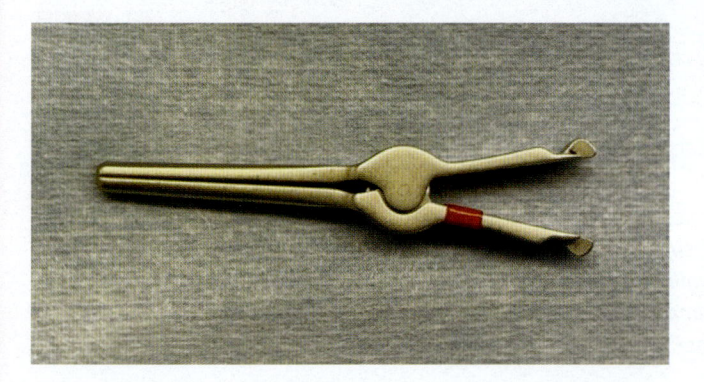

FIGURE 47-1 • Scanlan® Reliance Bulldog Clamp. (Reproduced with permission from Dr. Luciano Ambrosini, author of chapter.)

system and wrist-like, multidimensional instrument motions, became progressively adopted by some institutions.

RAKT in the obese population has been shown to reduce the incidence of surgical complications, offering outcomes comparable to the nonobese counterpart.

Indications and Relative Contraindications to the Robotic Approach

Candidates to RAKT follow the standard guidelines for kidney transplant. Obesity and previous abdominal surgeries are no longer considered contraindications to the robotic approach. Patients with a BMI of 30 kg/m², or above, were once considered not suitable for a kidney transplant. On the contrary, obesity can be regarded as a primary indication for RAKT, because this approach brings lower rates of surgical site infections.

In addition to the classic absolute contraindications of kidney transplantation (see **Table 47-1**), the only exclusion criterion to proceed with the robotic approach is severe atherosclerosis of the recipient iliac vessels. Relative contraindications could be related to previous multiple abdominal/pelvic surgeries (hostile abdomen).

TABLE 47-1 • Absolute Contraindications to Kidney Transplantation
Reversible kidney disease
Severe cirrhosis biopsy proven
Patient noncompliant with medications
Active neoplasm
Severe lung or cardiovascular disease
Active substance abuse or uncontrolled psychiatric disorders
Active infection
Life expectancy less than 1 year

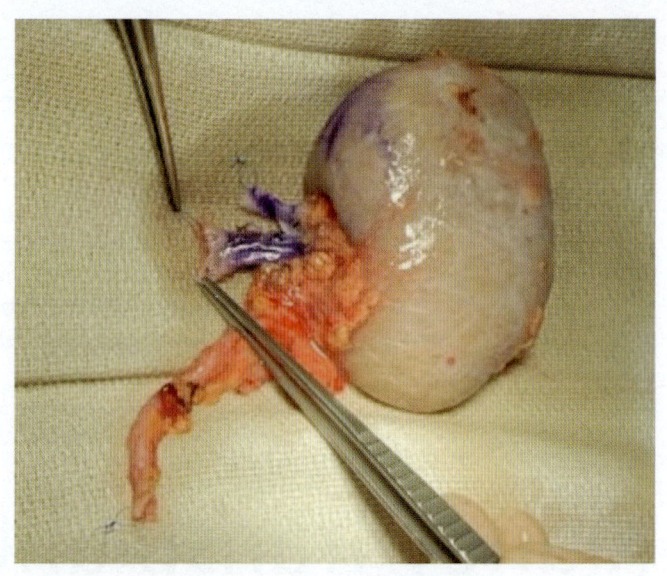

FIGURE 47-2 • Kidney graft.

Backbench Preparation of the Graft

Usually, this part of the procedure is performed by another surgical team, the one that did the living donor nephrectomy. Here, it is worthy to repeat some details, because backbench preparation of the graft for robotic transplantation follows some specific steps that differ from conventional preparation for open surgery. The instruments required are those for standard microsurgical bench surgery. The adipose capsule is dissected, and meticulously ligated with silk or Vicryl® ties during excision, to minimize bleeding from the surface of the kidney after the reperfusion.

Renal vein and artery are dissected toward the hilum and tattooed with a marking pen, depending on the site of implantation, right or left, to facilitate the orientation of the organ before the vascular anastomosis (**Figure 47-2**). The use of a Prolene™ 5-0 stitch placed, as an air knot, on the upper pole of the artery and vein is optional; however, it allows manipulation of the vessels during the anastomosis.

The ureter is appropriately shortened and spatulated. A Prolene™ 5-0 stitch is placed, as an air knot, at the tip of the ureter.

Average time frame: 30–45 min

> ⚠ **PITFALLS**
>
> Extensive dissection of the perihilar fat may potentially cause bleeding, which is difficult to control at reperfusion.
>
> The dissection of the periureteral connective tissue and excessive manipulation of the so-called "golden triangle," must be avoided to minimize the risk of ischemia of the ureter.

Kidney Transplant   965

🔍 ANATOMICAL HIGHLIGHTS

The "golden triangle" is the space between the ureter, the kidney, and the renal artery (**Figure 47-3**).

▶▶ TIPS

Perform meticulous ligation of the adipose capsule, the perihilar vessels, and lymphatics should be performed to minimize bleeding at reperfusion.

Marking the vessels will facilitate their orientation before the vascular anastomosis.

Placing an air knot Prolene™ 5-0 tie at the upper corner of the artery and vein will facilitate the manipulation of the vessels during the anastomosis.

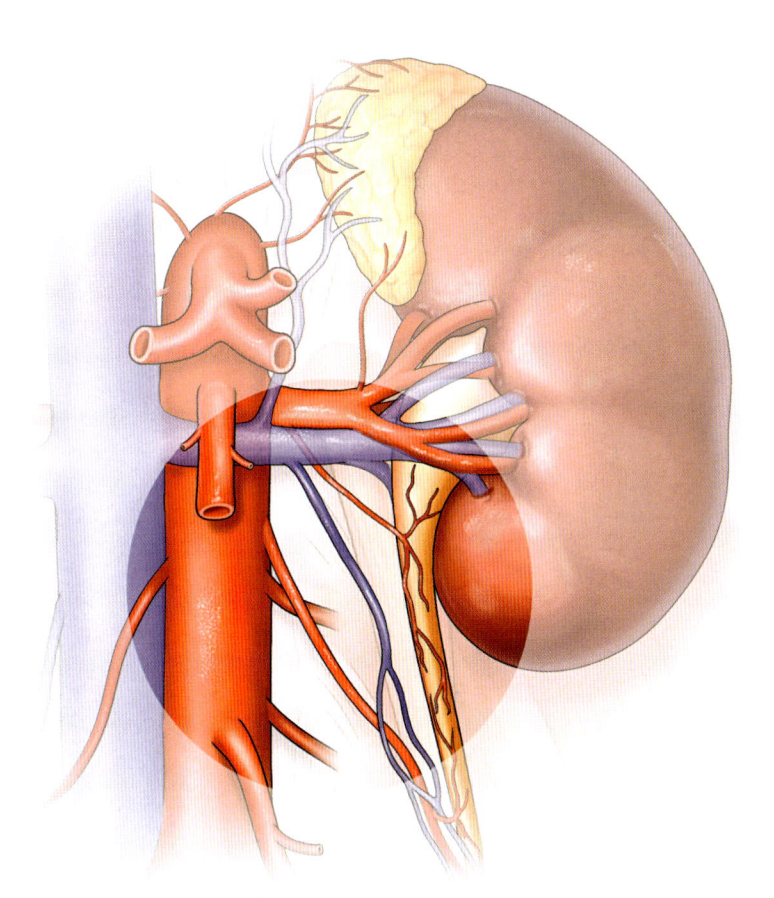

© 2022 Body Scientific

FIGURE 47-3 • General anatomy of the kidney (golden triangle).

Patient Positioning, OR setup, and Port Setting

The patient is positioned supine, with parted and flexed legs. Upper extremities are adducted and tagged to the body. Shoulder block and tape are used to avoid the sliding of the patient during the operation (**Figures 47-4 and 47-5**).

The following description is for kidney transplantation on the right side, which is the most commonly chosen one. However, the technique is symmetrical on the left side, performed in the case of previous transplant on the right side, vascular calcifications, or venous thrombosis on the right iliac vessels.

After induction of general anesthesia, a 3-way Foley catheter is placed and left momentarily on free drainage. This strategy allows filling the bladder later on with 100–150 mL of diluted methylene blue solution after completion of the vascular anastomosis, which facilitates the identification of the bladder. At the beginning of the operation, the empty bladder prevents spatial interference during the vascular dissection and suturing.

After the patient is prepared in the sterile fashion, a 7-cm subxiphoid midline incision approximately 5 cm below the xyphoid process is made and a hand access device is placed (GelPort®). Depending on the body habitus of the recipient, the location of this midline incision could be closer to the umbilicus in order to allow easier access to the surgical field for the bedside hand-assisting surgeon. This evaluation should be done carefully in order to avoid interfering with the robotic arms and cannulas positioned in the lower quadrants.

The induction of pneumoperitoneum (15 mm Hg) is achieved with insufflation through the GelPort®.

The laparoscopic/robotic ports are then inserted under direct laparoscopic visualization. One 8-mm robotic trocar, for the scope, is inserted in the periumbilical region (usually just above the umbilicus), and two 8-mm trocars for the robotic arms are inserted, one in the left iliac fossa and the other more lateral in the right side.

A 12-mm disposable laparoscopic port, for the bedside assistant, is inserted between the umbilicus, and the robotic metallic trocar is placed on the left iliac fossa (**Figure 47-6**).

An 8-mm robotic trocar for the R3 is optional; generally, it is not utilized. If used, it is placed between the 12-mm laparoscopic and the 8-mm robotic port on the left iliac fossa.

> ▶▶ **TIPS**
>
> The R3 (optional) is placed on the left lower lateral position for a more effective retraction of the bladder or the uterus, but it is rarely necessary, and it may create conflicts with the other 2 operative arms.

Once the ports are placed, the patient is positioned in a 30° Trendelenburg, with the right side elevated.

The robotic cart is docked on the right side.

Average time frame: 30–40 min

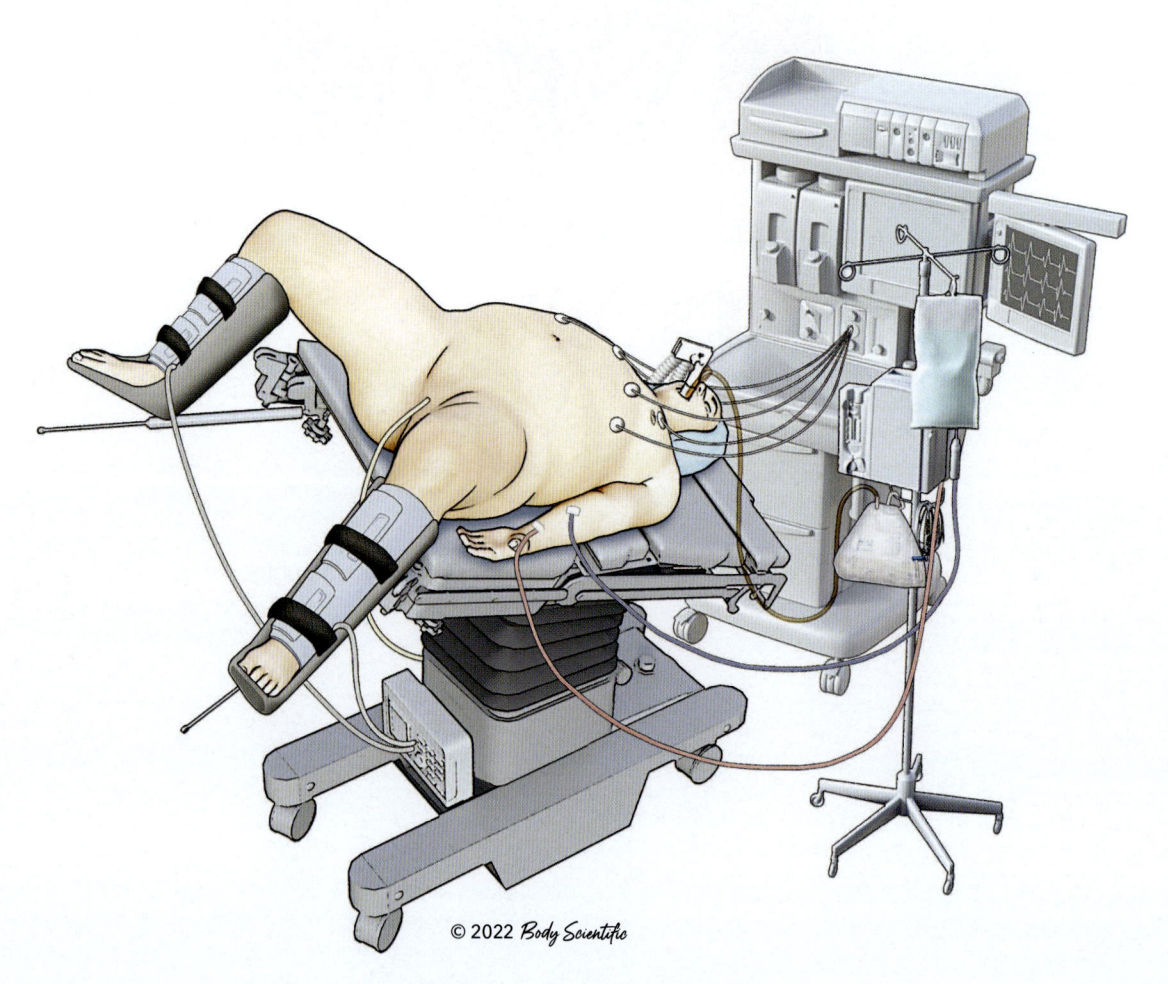

FIGURE 47-4 • Patient positioning.

⚠️ **PITFALLS**

By placing the right flank trocar too low and medial, the instrument will become perpendicular to the vessels making suturing more difficult. On the contrary, if the trocar is too lateral toward the flank, the instrument may collide with the edges of the pelvis, and create problems mainly during the venous anastomosis.

▶▶ **TIPS**

The trocars must be placed under laparoscopic vision in order to avoid accidental injuries of the epigastric vessels or surrounding organs. Also, the direct visualization, during this maneuver, allows a precise identification of the pelvic region; therefore, the placement of the trocars becomes more tailored on the specific anatomy, allowing a better triangulation.

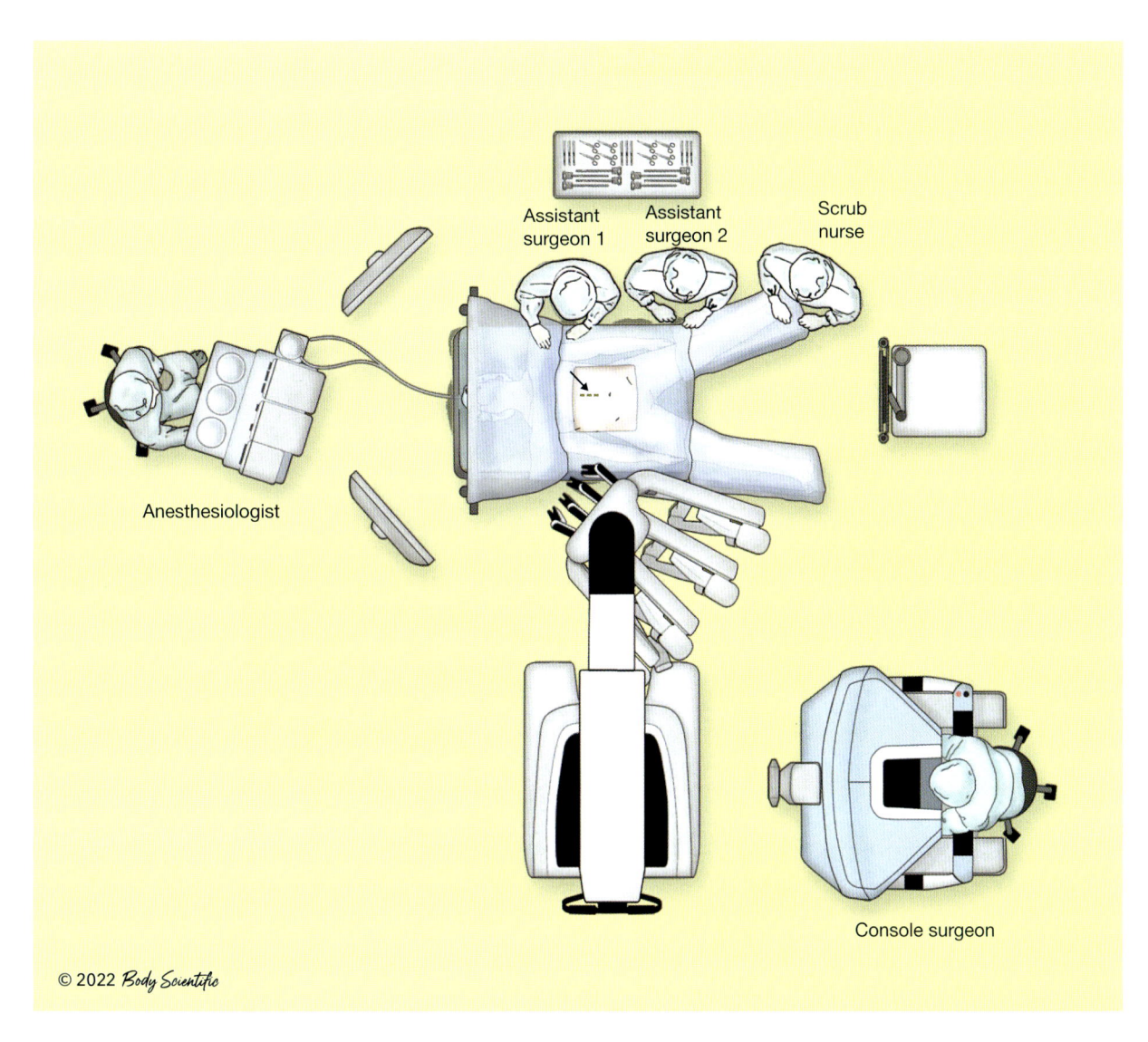

FIGURE 47-5 • OR setup.

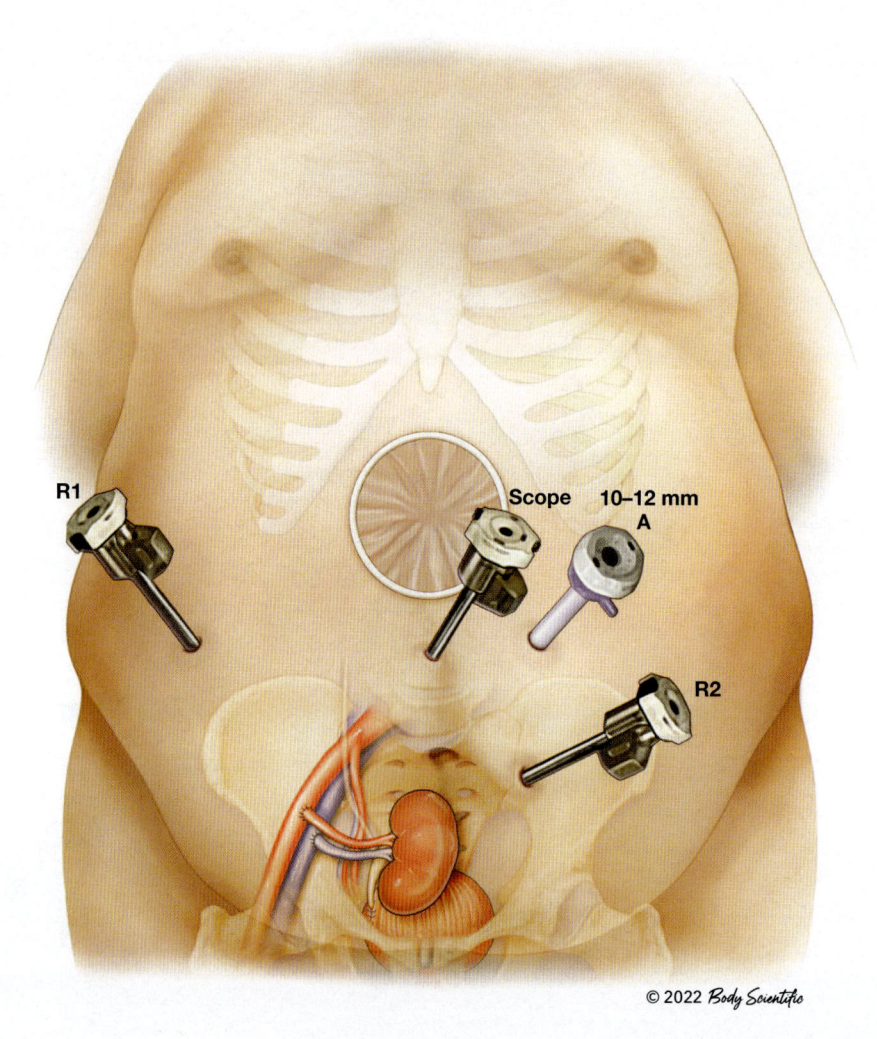

FIGURE 47-6 • Port setting.

▶️ **Video 47-1. Robotic Kidney Transplant – Full Procedure**

Phase A: Vessel Preparation

Step 1. Mobilization of the cecum

The operation starts with the mobilization of the cecum. The amount of the dissection depends on the anatomy and position of the ascending colon.

In the majority of cases, some kind of mobilization of the cecum and the proximal ascending colon may be necessary to have adequate exposure of the iliac region.

The assistant hand will displace the colon medially to maintain tension on the peritoneal reflection, and to allow dissection on an avascular plane. The dissection is conducted using bipolar forceps and hook electrocautery. The native ureter, crossing the common iliac artery in its anatomical location, will be left in place (**Figure 47-7**).

Step 1 average time frame: 5–10 min

> **🔍 ANATOMICAL HIGHLIGHTS**
>
> The retroperitoneum is a virtual space of the abdomen that lies behind the peritoneum.
>
> The structures identified during this phase are the cecum, the appendix, the right gonadal vessels, and the right ureter.

> **▶▶ TIPS**
>
> Asking the assistant to maintain some tension on the mesentery of the colon helps in keeping the avascular dissection plane.

> **⚠ PITFALLS**
>
> Insufficient or incomplete mobilization of the cecum.

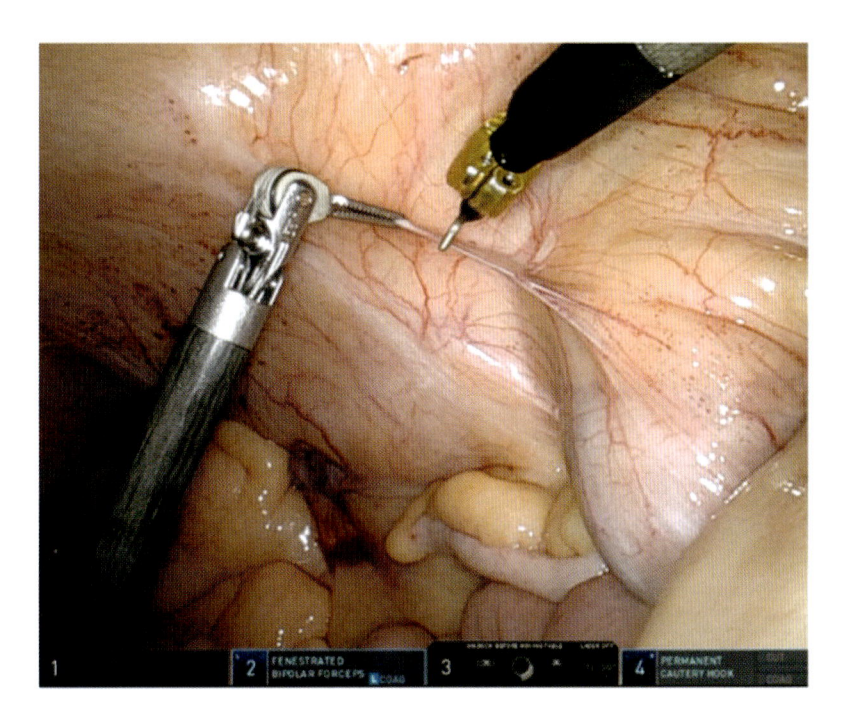

FIGURE 47-7 • Mobilization of the cecum.

970 The Foundation and Art of Robotic Surgery

Step 2. Exposure of the surgical field
During the exposure of the iliac vein and artery, the gonadal vessels are identified (**Figures 47-8 A, B**).

In females, the suspensory ligament of the ovary is incised at the level of the proximal portion of the external iliac artery, and the ovarian vessels are identified and dissected free.

They are mobilized to be able to be retracted medially improving the exposure of the iliac vessels.

In males, the testicular vessels run laterally to the common and external iliac arteries on the body of the psoas major muscle and they usually do not need to be dissected.

Anatomical factors that may limit the exposure of the right iliac axis are a redundant sigmoid colon and/or a bulky uterus. In this situation, the R3 may help in retraction.

Step 2 average time frame: 10–20 min

> ⚠ **PITFALLS**
>
> Insufficient or incomplete exposure of the iliac vessels.

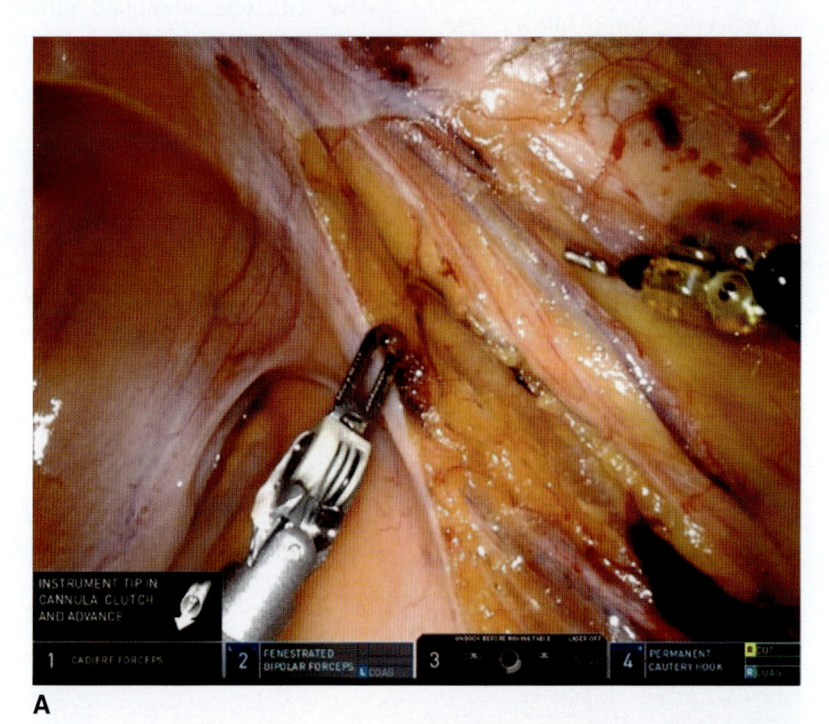

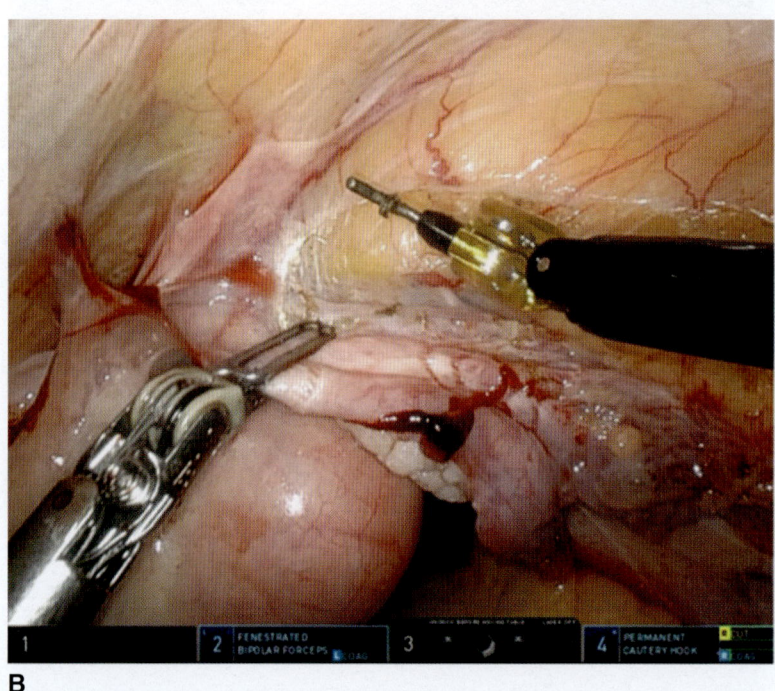

FIGURE 47-8 • Vascular exposure. A. Male. B. Female.

Kidney Transplant 971

> **ANATOMICAL HIGHLIGHTS**
> The suspensory ligament of the ovary is a fold of peritoneum that extends laterally, and cranially, from the ovary to the pelvic wall over the iliac vessels (**Figure 47-9**).

> **▶▶ TIPS**
> A good exposure should include the view of the common and the external iliac vessels until the inguinal ligament.

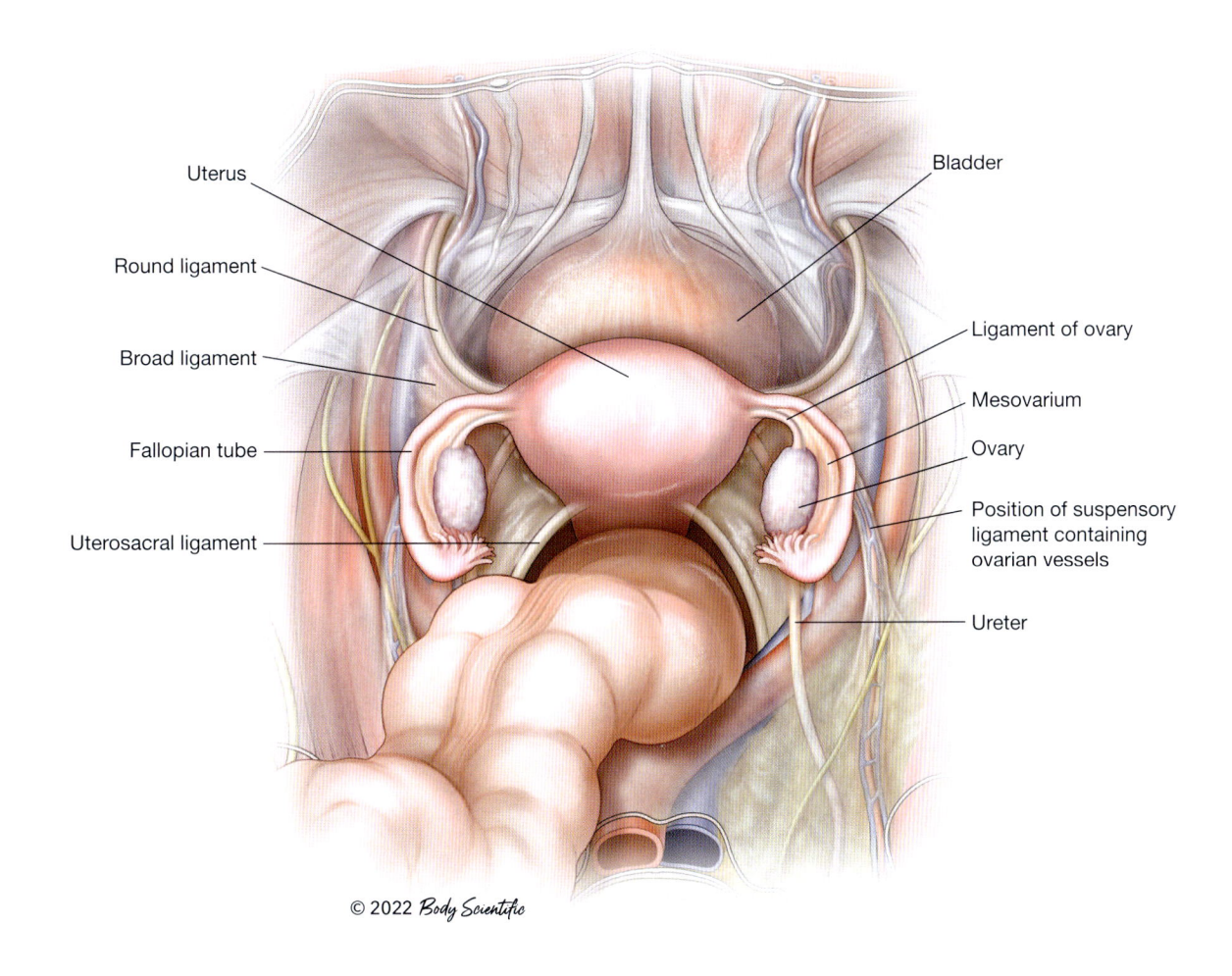

FIGURE 47-9 • Suspensory ligament of the ovary.

Video 47-2. Step 3. Preparation of the External Iliac Artery

Step 3. Preparation of the external iliac artery
The dissection starts proximally from the origin of the external iliac artery up to the level of the inguinal ligament. This maneuver is conducted with the monopolar hook and bipolar forceps, avoiding directly grasping the arterial wall, which could be calcified and fragile. The artery is often surrounded by lymph nodes that could be hyperplastic and enlarged. Sometimes, it is necessary to remove some of these lymph nodes to mobilize the artery.

This artery runs along the medial border of the psoas major muscle and passes beneath the inguinal ligament where it becomes the femoral artery; at the level of the pelvic brim, it gives rise to 2 large branches: the inferior epigastric and the deep circumflex arteries. Those branches are usually very distal and rarely need to be ligated. In order to facilitate the following exposure and dissection around the external iliac vein (Step 4), a vessel loop is used to retract the artery upward.

Step 3 average time frame: 15–20 min

> ⚠ **PITFALLS**
> Insufficient or incomplete mobilization of the external iliac artery.

> 🔍 **ANATOMICAL HIGHLIGHTS**
> The external iliac artery is superior and lateral to the external iliac vein, and it is located along the medial border of the psoas major muscle (**Figure 47-10**).

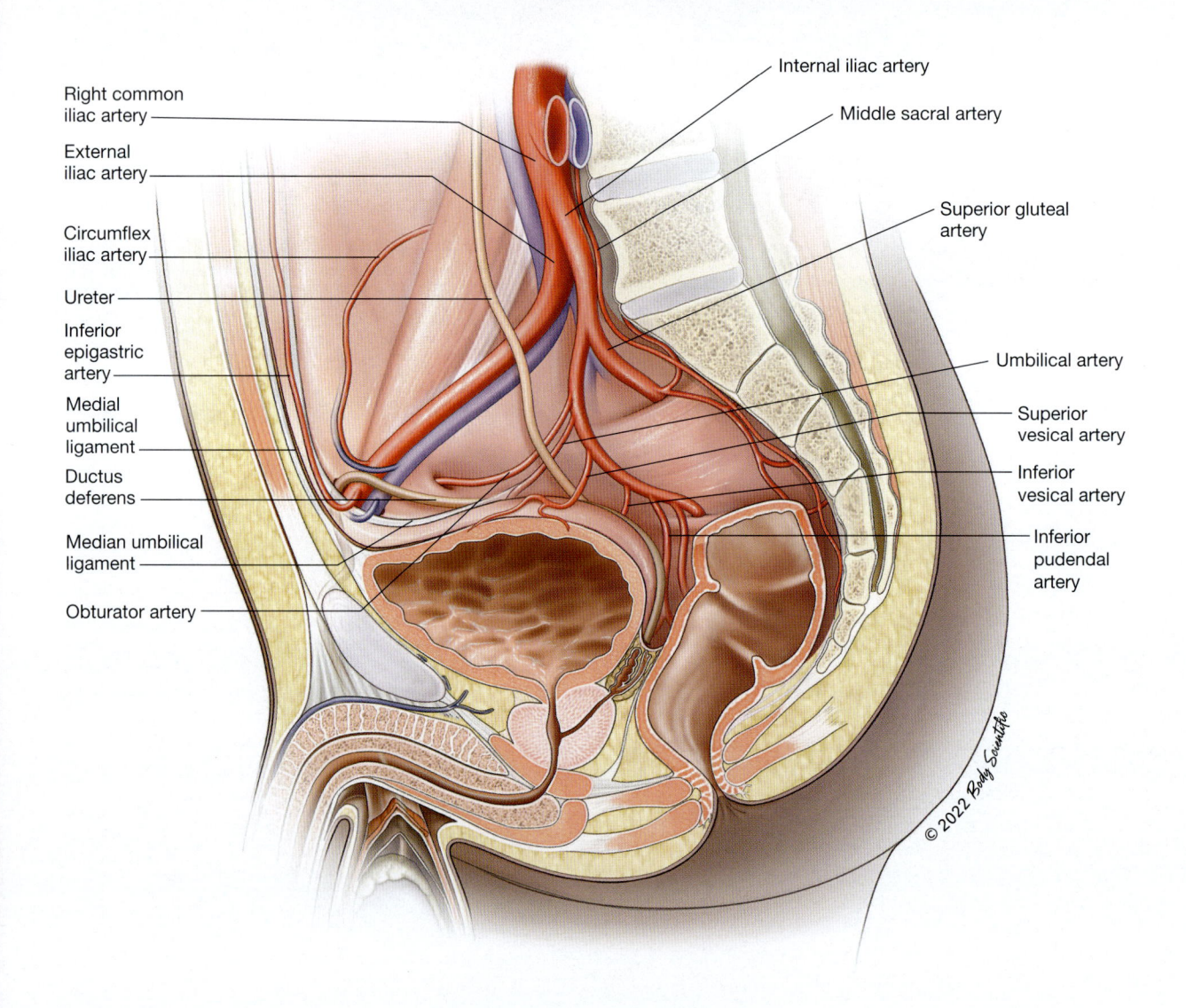

FIGURE 47-10 • External iliac artery.

> > **TIPS**

A vessel loop is placed around the external iliac artery in order to minimize direct manipulation on the vessel itself, and to perform a kind of "hanging maneuver" of the artery (**Figure 47-11**).

This maneuver facilitates the exposure and the dissection of the external iliac vein and, later on, the construction of the venous anastomosis.

In case of possible presence of atherosclerotic plaques, the bedside surgeon may directly palpate the artery through the hand assistant GelPort® to complete the assessment.

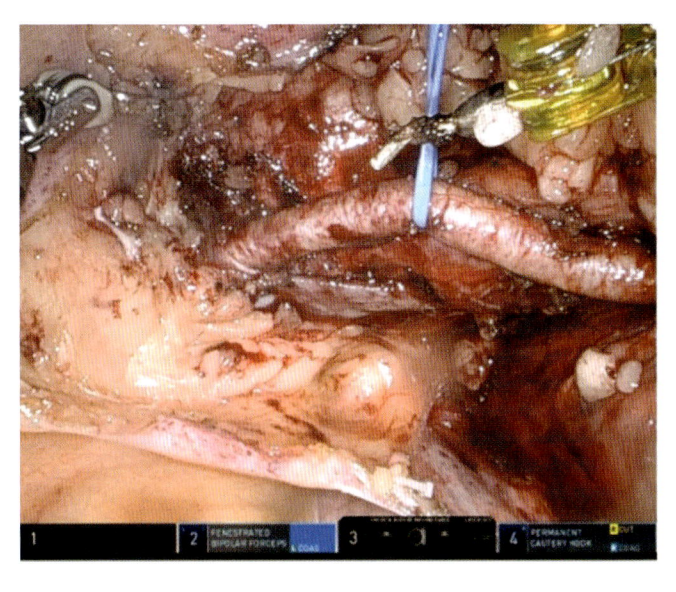

FIGURE 47-11 • Hanging maneuver.

Video 47-3. Step 4. Preparation of the External Iliac Vein

Step 4. Preparation of the external iliac vein

A second vessel loop is placed around the external iliac vein to allow dissection on the posterior aspect of the vein. The dissection is conducted proximally, up to the level of the ureter and the internal iliac artery, and distally up to the inferior margin of the inguinal canal. In males, care must be taken to respect the vas deferens, while in females, the round ligament can be sacrificed. Pubic, inferior epigastric, and deep circumflex iliac veins only occasionally need to be suture ligated and transected (Prolene™ 4-0/5-0).

The length of the external iliac vein is variable: it could be long and easily accessible or short and deep. The vein should be mobilized enough to allow a safe placement of the bulldog clamps and a good segment for the anastomosis. In order to achieve this goal, it is usually necessary to prepare a segment of 6–7 cm.

Step 4 average time frame: 15–25 min

⚠ PITFALLS

Insufficient, incomplete dissection of the external iliac vein.

🔍 ANATOMICAL HIGHLIGHTS

The external iliac vein is medial to the external iliac artery; on the left, it remains medial, but on the right, it runs more posteriorly (**Figure 47-12**).

The external iliac vein is crossed proximally by the ureter and internal iliac artery, and distally by the *vas deferens*, or by the round ligament and ovarian vessels.

▶▶ TIPS

A vessel loop is placed around the vein in order to ease the dissection, minimize the manipulation, and later on, facilitate the application of vascular clamps.

The external iliac vein is usually devoid of collaterals; if these are present, they sometimes need to be divided, and the safest way is to do it in between transfixing sutures (Prolene™ 4-0/5-0).

Dividing the collaterals not only allows a better mobilization of the vein (superficialization), but also avoids backflow of blood during the anastomosis.

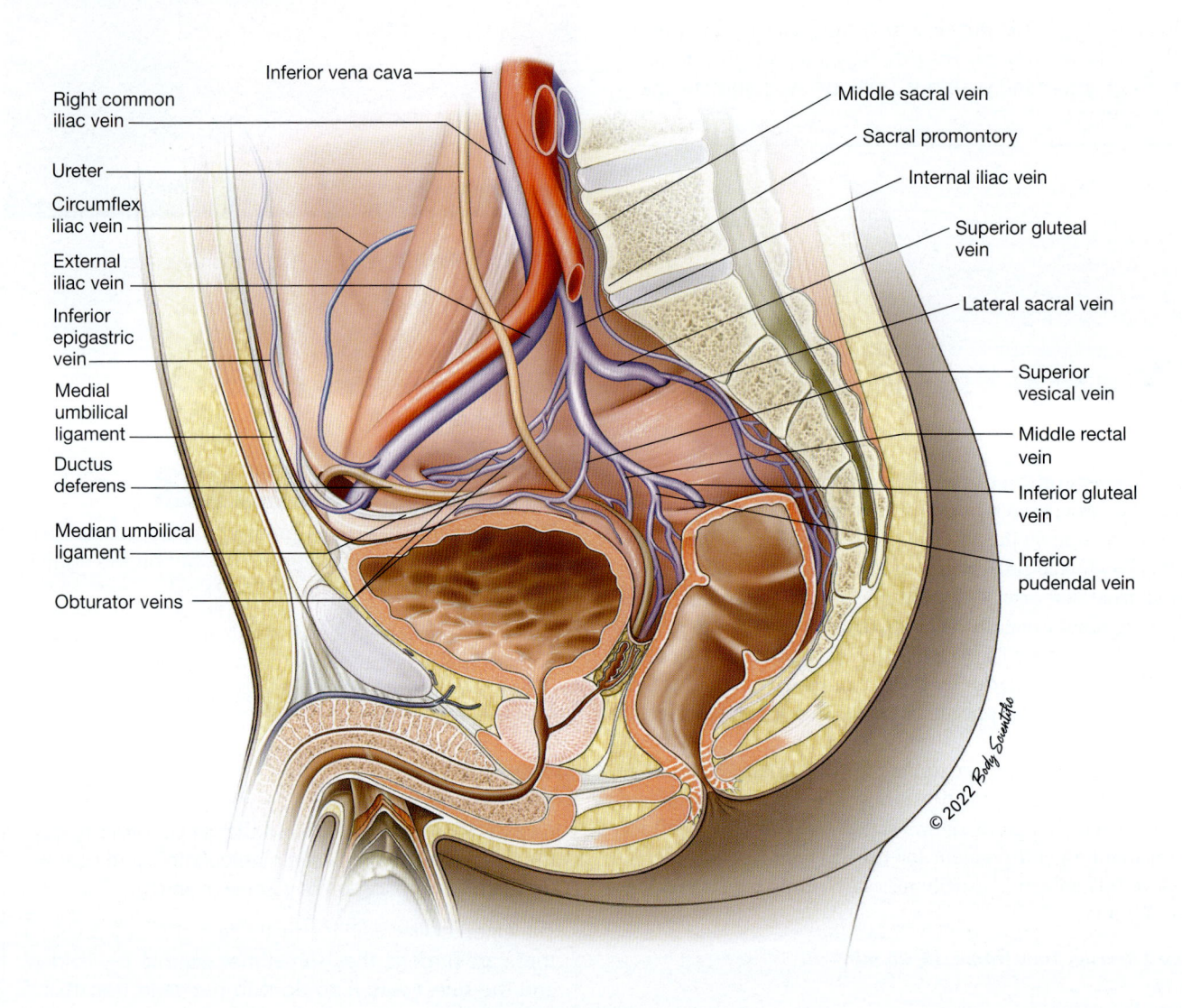

FIGURE 47-12 • External iliac vein.

Kidney Transplant   975

▶ Video 47-4. Step 5. External Iliac Vein Clamping and Venotomy

Phase B: Vascular Anastomosis and Graft Reperfusion

Step 5. External iliac vein clamping

Once the external iliac vessels are completely dissected free, 5 robotic bulldog clamps (**Figure 47-1**) are brought into the field (pelvis) by the assistant. The anesthesiologist is usually injecting heparin IV (2000 IU).

In preparation for the venous anastomosis, the external iliac vein is occluded proximally and distally with 2 robotic bulldog clamps. The remaining bulldog clamps are left aside for the following arterial clamping.

The vessel loop is not removed, but positioned outside the proximal clamp, in order to avoid interference with the anastomosis. The vessel loop is a safety measure in case of sliding of a bulldog clamp during the reconstruction (**Figure 47-13**).

Robotic Potts scissors are used to create a venotomy of about 15 mm, and, if encountered, valve cusps are carefully disrupted.

A 12-cm handmade, double-armed, Gore-Tex® 5-0 suture with a knot in the middle is placed at the corner of the venotomy, ready to start the suture, minimizing the warm ischemia time.

Step 5 average time frame: 3–5 min

> ▶▶ **TIPS**
>
> The 3 bulldog clamps not in use should be hanged to the lateral peritoneum, in a place where they can be easily retrieved, and where they are not interfering with the surgical maneuvers. When the transplanted kidney is brought into the pelvis, finding a missing clamp is an avoidable waste of time.

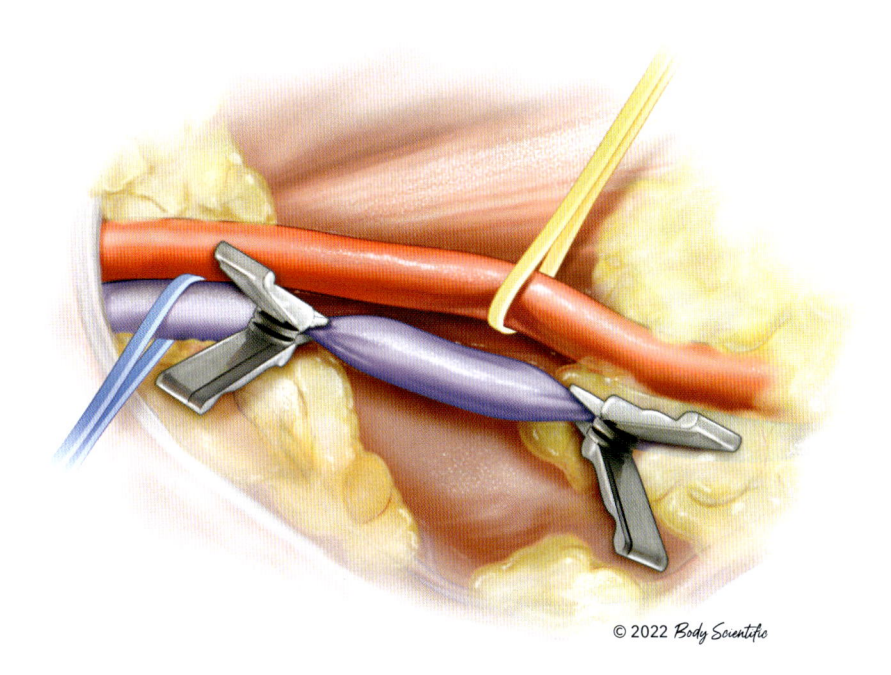

FIGURE 47-13 • Clamping of the external iliac vein.

Video 47-5. Step 6. Venous Anastomosis

Step 6. Insertion of the graft and venous anastomosis

The kidney graft is inserted into the abdominal cavity by the assisting surgeon, and positioned medial and parallel to the dissected iliac vessels. Previous marking tattoos, and a Prolene™ 5-0 stitch placed on the upper edge of the renal vein, facilitate the orientation. At this point, the assistant hand stabilizes the kidney. An end-to-side reno-iliac venous anastomosis is completed with 2 half-running sutures, starting from the posterior wall with a proximal-to-distal direction (**Figures 47-14 A–C**).

The anterior wall is made with the second needle of the same suture following the same direction.

The 2 corners of the anastomosis, where the suture could become loose, are reinforced with 1 interrupted stitch of Prolene™ 5-0 or Gore-Tex® 5-0.

Step 6 average time frame: 15–20 min

>> **TIPS**

The proximal bulldog clamp is positioned first, the vein is lifted with gentle traction on the vessel loop, and the distal bulldog clamp is subsequently placed.

This maneuver allows the correct positioning of the distal bulldog clamp on an empty vein. The vessel loop is then repositioned lateral to the proximal clamp, not interfering with the anastomosis.

After performing the venotomy, a careful check for possible valve cusps has to be done. Usually, the external iliac vein does not have valves, but if they are present, they occasionally need to be disrupted because they can interfere with the anastomosis, and/or the proper outflow from the renal transplant.

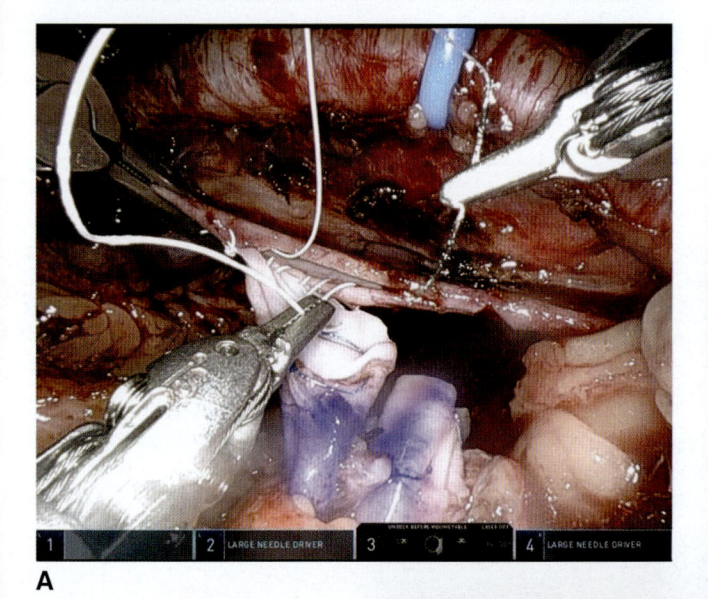

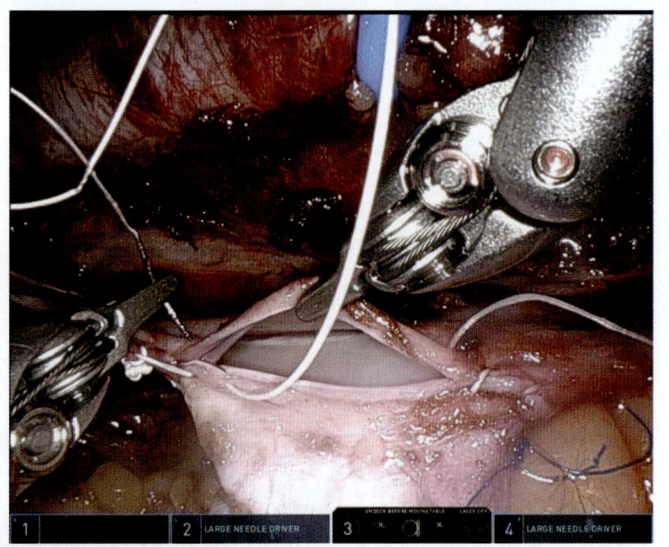

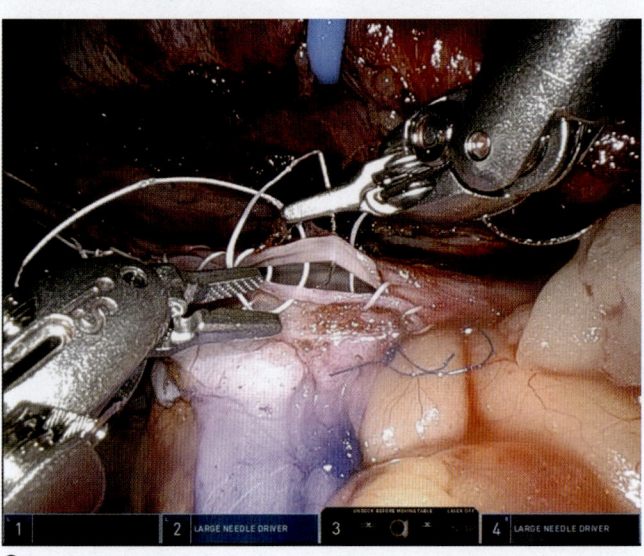

FIGURE 47-14 • Venous anastomosis.

▶ **Video 47-6. Step 7. Arterial Anastomosis**

Step 7. Arterial anastomosis

The external iliac artery, previously lifted with the hanging maneuver, is now freed from the abdominal wall, releasing the clip holding the loop. The artery is then clamped proximally and distally to the flow using the remaining bulldog clamps.

An oval window (proportional to the size of the renal artery of the graft) is made in the anterior-medial wall of the artery with robotic scissors. To facilitate the creation of the arterial opening, a Prolene™ 5-0 stitch is placed exactly where the arterial window will be created. Lifting the suture is easier to create a perfect round opening removing a small patch of the artery.

A 12-cm, handmade, double-armed, Gore-Tex® 6-0 suture, with a knot in the middle, is placed at the corner of the arteriotomy. An end-to-side reno-iliac arterial anastomosis is completed with running suture, starting from the posterior wall (**Figures 47-15 A–C**). The anastomosis can be reinforced with interrupted stitches at the corners, if necessary.

Step 7 average time frame: 15–20 min

> ▶▶ **TIPS**
>
> The proximal bulldog clamp is positioned first, the artery is then lifted with gentle traction on the vessel loop, and the distal bulldog clamp is then placed. If the artery is rigid, a second proximal bulldog clamp may be necessary.
>
> The assistant hand may confirm the absence of pulsations before proceeding to the arteriotomy. Anyway, the arteriotomy has to be started cautiously, understanding immediately if the clamping is incomplete.
>
> The site of the arteriotomy should be carefully selected, keeping in mind the final orientation of the anastomosis. A location too anterior may cause a kinking of the renal artery with decreased flow. An arteriotomy on the anteromedial aspect of the iliac artery usually offers the best angle.

A

B

C

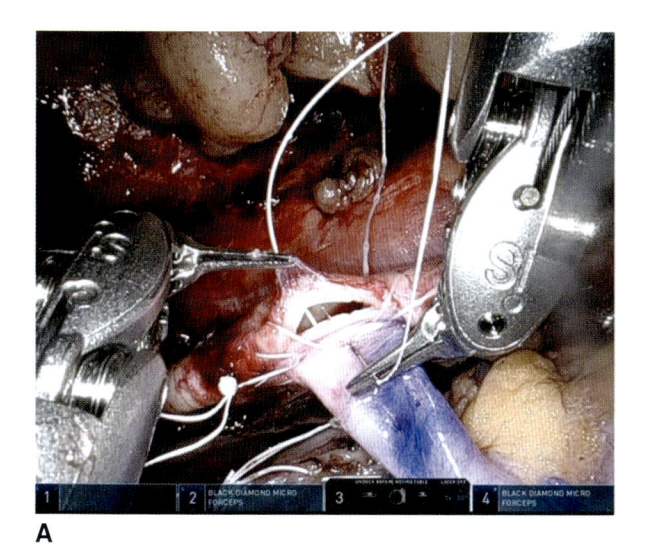

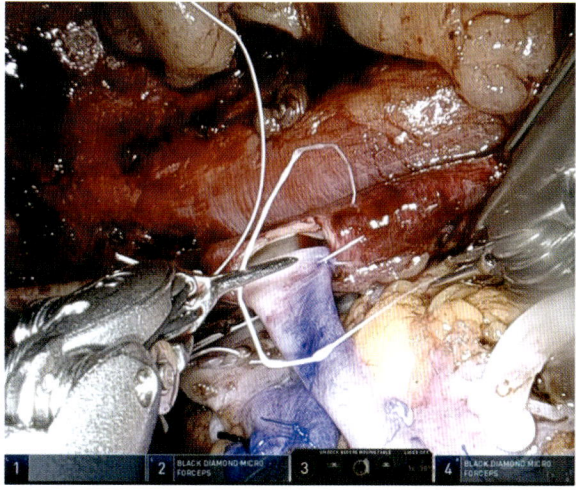

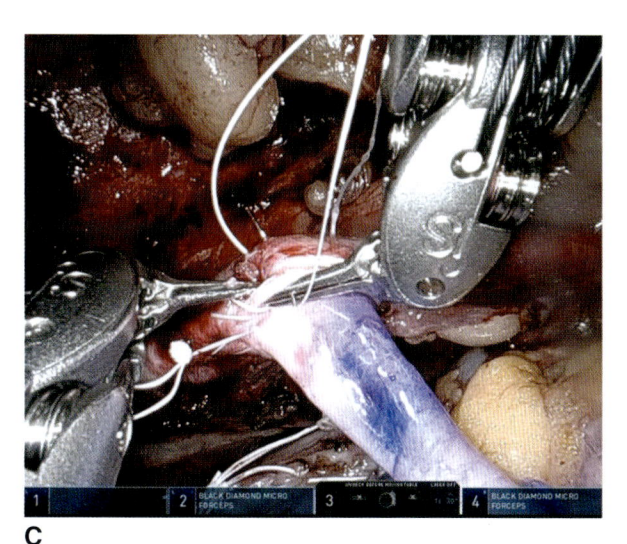

FIGURE 47-15 • Arterial anastomosis.

Step 8. Reperfusion of the graft

Before proceeding to this step, the anesthesiologist injects IV furosemide and mannitol according to the usual transplant protocol. Once the vascular reconstruction is completed, both anastomoses should be tested before reperfusion of the kidney. The venous anastomosis is verified first, putting a small bulldog clamp on the renal vein, and then removing the distal iliac clamp.

If additional stitches are necessary, they are placed without rewarming the graft.

Then, the proximal iliac venous clamp is removed, restoring the iliac venous flow.

The arterial anastomosis is then tested in the same way. When both anastomoses are verified, the 2 small bulldog clamps on the renal vessels are removed, allowing the reperfusion of the organ.

Additional hemostasis may be required on the graft if there are significant bleeding spots.

An intraoperative Doppler with the probe inserted through the assistant port is used to verify the flow. Intraoperative indocyanine green (ICG) (3 mL) is given IV to the patient to confirm the complete and homogeneous reperfusion of the graft (**Figure 47-16**).

The assistant retrieves the bulldog clamps. At this point, the pressure of the pneumoperitoneum is decreased to 10 mm Hg to minimize the possible negative effect of high intraabdominal pressure on the graft microcirculation.

Step 8 average time frame: 10–15 min

>> **TIPS**

For optimal hemostasis, the assistant will gently lift the kidney, after reperfusion, allowing inspection of the posterior wall for eventual bleeding points.

ICG and Doppler will confirm global perfusion and flow, respectively.

EDITORIAL COMMENT

- Intraoperative Doppler provides a direct and real-time quality assessment of the circulation. It allows evaluation of the modality of the flow (systolic, diastolic, speed, and resistance) at the level of the main artery, vein, and parenchyma.
- ICG fluorescence angiography is also an excellent tool for assessment of the renal allograft perfusion (see Chapter 7, Fluorescence Imaging: Basics and Clinical Applications).
- A dose of 0.02 mg ICG per kg of body weight, injected intravenously, is recommended to ensure an optimal visualization (**Figure 47-16**).

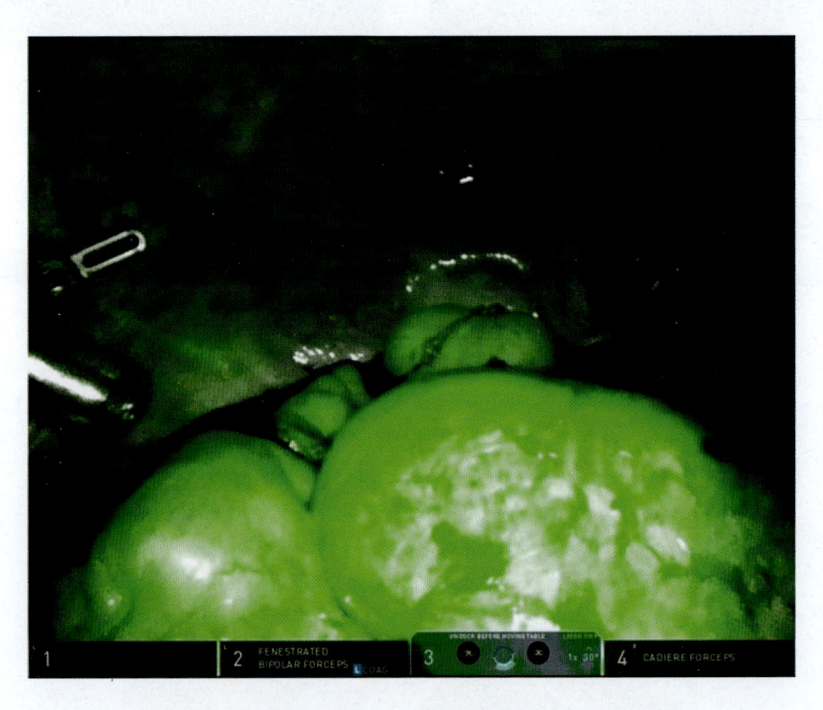

FIGURE 47-16 • Reperfusion of the graft with ICG.

▶ **Video 47-7. Step 9. Ureteroneocystostomy**

Phase C: Urinary Reconstruction

Step 9. Ureteroneocystostomy
The urinary bladder is filled with diluted methylene blue solution in order to facilitate its identification. Once the dome of the bladder is localized, the muscular layers are incised with an inverted "Y" shape with the mucosa opening at the tip of the vertical limb.

One Vicryl® 3-0 stitch is placed at each side of the bladder's muscular layers and fixed at the parietal peritoneum of the anterior abdominal wall to avoid the retraction of the bladder once opened. The bladder mucosa is then incised with robotic scissors (0.5 cm) and the Foley catheter unclamped to empty the bladder. The ureter is then anastomosed, mucosa to mucosa, to the bladder with PDS™ 5-0 or Monocryl® 5-0 running suture.

Using a modified Lich-Gregoir antireflux technique, the reconstruction is completed suturing the bladder muscle layers of oblique limbs of the inverted "Y" (Vicryl® 3-0) on top of the ureter, which is now having an oblique passage through the bladder wall. Utilization of a ureteral stent is optional, and may be required, when the anastomosis is challenging and risky for complications (small size ureter, atrophic bladder) (**Figures 47-17 A–C**).

Step 9 average time frame: 30–40 min

> ⚠ **PITFALLS**
>
> Excessive filling of the bladder may cause its rupture, with infiltration of its layers with methylene blue making the dissection very complex.
>
> In the case of twisting of the ureter with a bad orientation of the anastomosis, before completing the reconstruction, the insertion of an endoluminal stent may clarify the situation, and allow the precise construction of the anastomosis.

> ▶▶ **TIPS**
>
> The mucosa-to-mucosa ureteroneocystostomy should start at the base of the ureter section line, proceeding toward the tip, in order to avoid obstructing the visualization of the anastomotic edges.

> ▶▶ **TIPS**
>
> The assistant will hold the tip of the ureter using the Prolene™ 5-0 stitch previously applied, holding it with a laparoscopic needle driver. This maneuver facilitates the placement of the corner stitch of the ureter.

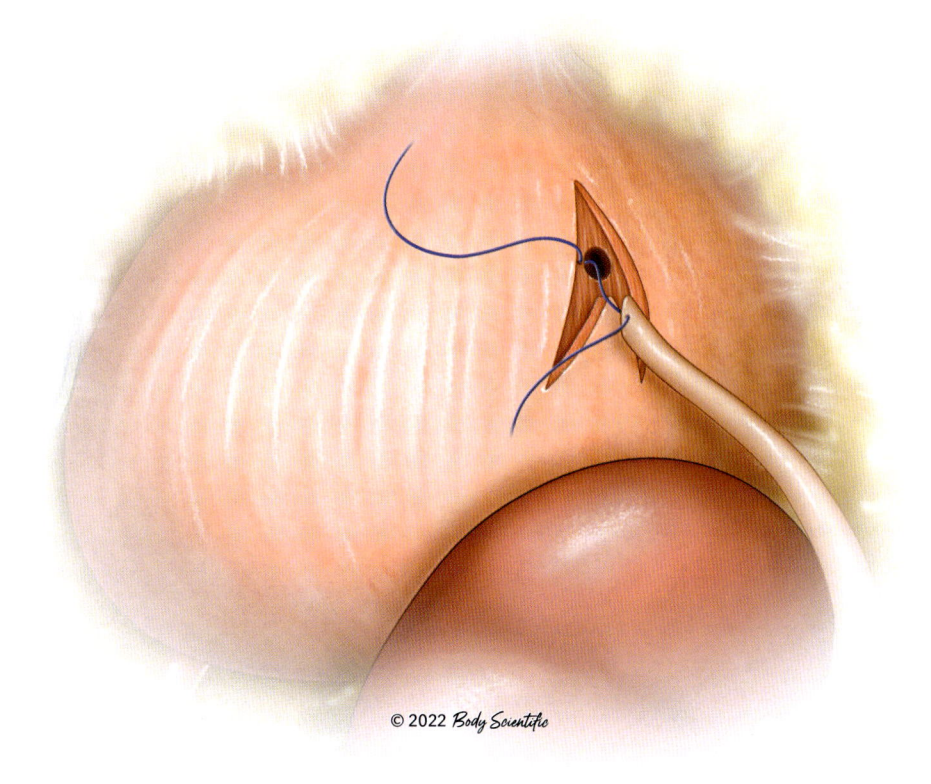

A

FIGURE 47-17 • Ureteroneocystostomy.

980 The Foundation and Art of Robotic Surgery

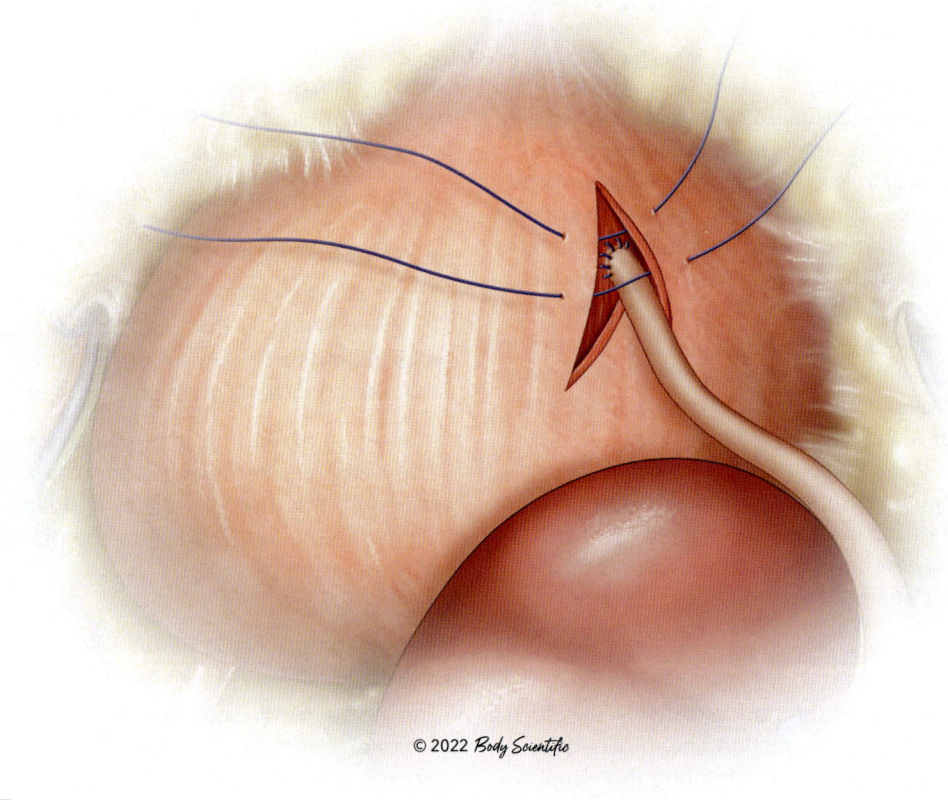

B

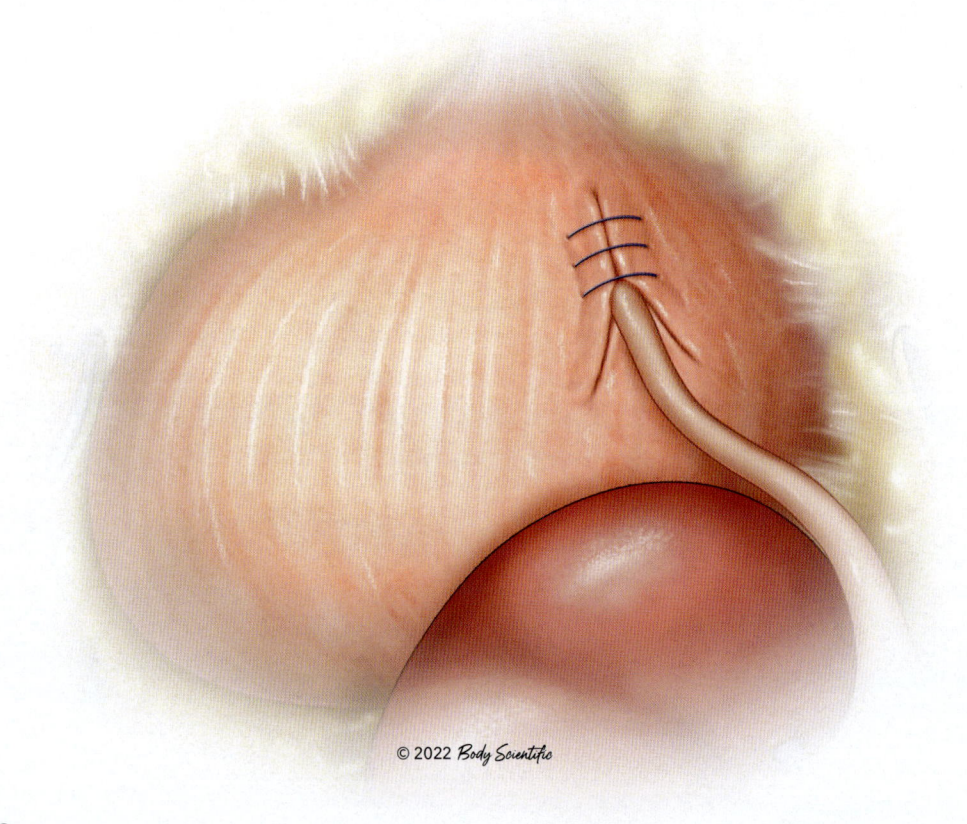

C

FIGURE 41-17 • *(Continued)*

Closure of the minilaparotomy and the port sites

At the end of the procedure, the minilaparotomy is closed with interrupted PDS™ 1, and the 12-mm port site is closed from inside the abdomen with a suture passer needle and Vicryl® 0 suture. Skin incisions are closed cosmetically. Placement of drains is usually not necessary (**Figure 47-18**).

Average time frame: 15–20 min

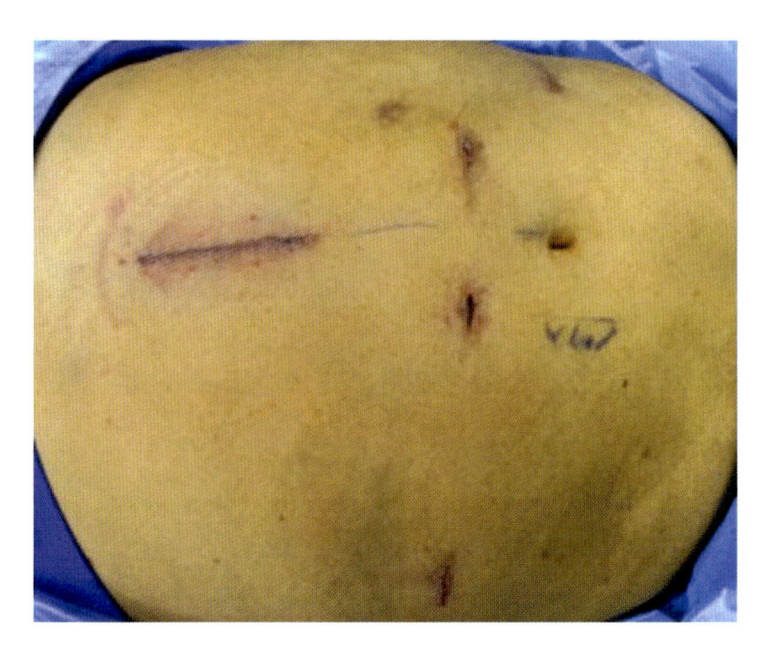

FIGURE 47-18 • Closure.

Suggested Readings

1. Giulianotti P, Gorodner V, Sbrana F, et al. Robotic transabdominal kidney transplantation in a morbid obese patient. *Am J Transplant.* 2010;10(06):1478-1482. doi: 10.1111/j.1600-6143.2010.03116.x
2. Hoznek A, Zaki SK, Samadi DB, et al. Robotic assisted kidney transplantation: an initial experience. *J Urol.* 2002;167(4):1604-1606
3. Gallioli L, Territo A, Boissier R, et al. Learning curve in robot-assisted kidney transplantation: results from the European Robotic Urological Society Working Group. *Eur Urol.* 2020;78(2)239-247. doi: 10.1016/j.eururo.2019.12.008
4. Tzvetanov IG, Spaggiari M, Tulla KA, et al. Robotic kidney transplantation in the obese patient: 10-year experience from a single center. *Am J Transplant.* 2020;20(2):430-440.
5. Segev DL, Simpkins CE, Thompson RE, et al. Obesity impacts access to kidney transplantation. *J Am Soc Nephrol.* 2008;19(2):349-355.
6. Gill JS, Lan J, Dong J, et al. The survival benefit of kidney transplantation in obese patients. *Am J Transplant.* 2013;13(8):2083-2090.
7. Krishnan N, Higgins R, Short A, et al. Kidney transplantation significantly improves patient and graft survival irrespective of BMI: a cohort study. *Am J Transplant.* 2015;15(9):2378-2386
8. Giulianotti PC, Coratti A, Angelini M, et al. Robotics in general surgery: personal experience in a large community hospital. *Arch Surg.* 2003;138(7):777-784. doi: 10.1001/archsurg.138.7.777

"What the field of pancreas transplantation needs is a new wave of creativity."
—David E. R. Sutherland (1940)

Pancreas Transplant

Pierpaolo Di Cocco • Ivo Georgiev Tzvetanov • Mario Spaggiari • Luciano Ambrosini • Enrico Benedetti

INTRODUCTION

Pancreas transplantation is the only treatment for type 1 diabetes that offers insulin independence, and the resulting normoglycemic state confers ultimately superior long-term survival compared to medical treatment.

Pancreatic transplant is most commonly performed in conjunction with renal transplant, in the so-called simultaneous pancreas-kidney (SPK) transplantation, for end-stage renal disease and diabetes.

Pancreas transplant alone (PTA) is done for poorly controlled type 1 diabetes (brittle) with stable renal function.

Only 10% of pancreas transplants are PTA. Its benefits have to be balanced against potential surgical complications. The growing incidence of obesity in potential recipients is responsible for an increased rate of these complications, particularly wound infections. Consequently, obesity is considered a relative contraindication to pancreas transplantation. A minimally invasive surgical approach to transplantation is an alternative to laparotomy and theoretically may lower postoperative morbidity mainly in patients with high body mass index (BMI). Robotic pancreas transplant in these population, performed in selected patients and only in very few centers worldwide, has been shown to be feasible, reducing the incidence of surgical complications and offering outcomes comparable to the nonobese counterpart. The rationale for the robotic pancreas transplantation is related to the reduction of the overall surgical trauma, to decreasing wound complications, and to allowing an earlier recovery.

Indications and Relative Contraindications to the Robotic Approach

Indications include type 1 and selected type 2 diabetes mellitus patients with a BMI of 30 kg/m² or above. PTA is performed for patients with brittle type 1 diabetes with stable renal function (30% of patients receiving a PTA may require a renal transplant in the long-term follow-up).

INSTRUMENT REQUIREMENTS

The suggested main robotic instruments/tools can be listed as follows:
- 30° scope, 0° scope
- Cadière forceps
- Fenestrated bipolar forceps
- Permanent monopolar cautery hook/monopolar scissors
- Large clip applier (Hem-o-lok® clips)
- Large needle driver
- Black diamond micro forceps
- Potts scissors
- Round-tip scissors
- Robotic bulldogs

The suggested main laparoscopic instruments/tools can be listed as follows:
- 30°, 5-mm scope
- Needle holders
- Scissors
- Graspers
- Suction-irrigation device
- Large clip applier (Hem-o-lok® clips)
- Vascular clamps (DeBakey peripheral)

Supplemental materials:
- Sponges
- Vessel loops
- Clips
- Sutures: Prolene™ 4-0, 5-0, and 6-0
- PDS™ 1, 3-0 and 4-0
- GIA™ linear stapler and vascular cartridge
- GelPort®
- Gore-Tex® 5-0 and 6-0
- Vicryl™ 0, 3-0
- Endosuture passer needle
- Closed drain

Photo reproduced with permission from Dr. David Sutherland.

Quote reproduced with permission from Sutherland DE. Extra-renal living donor transplants with special reference to segmental pancreas transplantation. Clin Transplant. 2011;25(1):1-3.

TABLE 48-1 • Absolute Contraindications to Pancreas Transplantation
Active neoplasm
Severe lung or cardiovascular disease
Noncompliance to medications
Active substance abuse or uncontrolled psychiatric disorders
Active infection
Life expectancy of less than 1 year

In addition to the classic absolute contraindications of pancreas transplantation (see **Table 48-1**), the only exclusion criterion to proceed with the robotic approach is severe atherosclerosis of the recipient iliac vessels.

A hostile abdomen with a history of multiple abdominal/pelvic operations may be a relative contraindication and it should be balanced with the experience of the surgical team.

Backbench Preparation of the Graft

The backbench preparation of the pancreas for robotic transplantation has to be done with meticulous attention to details in order to minimize bleeding sources at reperfusion. The splenectomy is performed by ligating the splenic artery and vein at the splenic hilum. The proximal and distal stumps of the duodenum are stapled with a GIA™ linear stapler and the stapler lines are oversewn with a Prolene™ 4-0 running suture. The stapler line on the mesentery of the small bowel is also oversewn with a Prolene™ 5-0 running suture. The following step is the creation of a single arterial inflow using the "Y" graft (donor common, internal and external iliac arteries). The internal iliac artery is anastomosed to the proximal splenic artery stump and the external iliac artery to the superior mesenteric artery with Prolene™ 5-0 sutures. The portal vein is usually extended with a segment of the donor iliac vein, sutured in an end-to-end fashion with a Prolene™ 5-0 running suture. The inflow and outflow vessels are marked with a marking pen, depending on the site of implantation, right or left, to facilitate the orientation of the organ before the vascular anastomosis. The use of a Prolene™ 5-0 stitch placed, as an air knot, on the upper pole of the artery and vein is optional; however, it allows a safer manipulation of the vessels during the orientation of the anastomosis (**Figure 48-1**).

Average time frame: 60–90 min

> ▶▶ **TIPS**
> - Meticulous ligation of all the potential bleeding sources will help to avoid bleeding at reperfusion.
> - Ink marking the vessels will facilitate their orientation before the vascular anastomosis.
> - Placing an air knot Prolene™ 5-0 tie at the upper corner of the artery and vein will facilitate the manipulation of the vessels during the anastomosis.

> ⚠ **PITFALLS**
> Major, diffuse bleeding at reperfusion may be very difficult to control with the robotic approach.

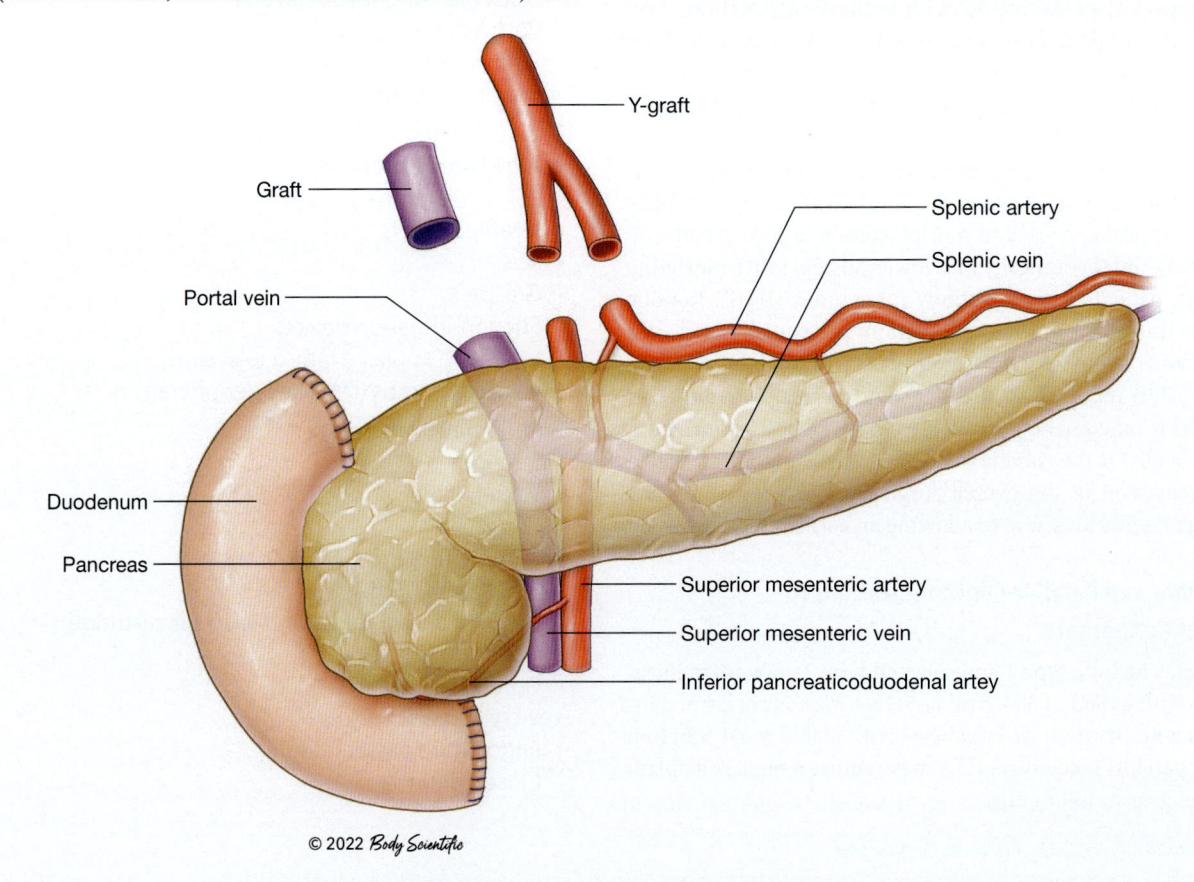

FIGURE 48-1 • Backbench preparation.

Pancreas Transplant

Patient Positioning, OR Setup, and Port Setting

After induction of general anesthesia, a 3-way Foley catheter is placed into the bladder and left on free, gravity drainage. This strategy is applied in case of simultaneous kidney transplant and/or the less frequently performed bladder exocrine drainage of pancreas transplant; it allows filling the bladder with 100–150 mL of diluted methylene blue solution after completion of the vascular anastomosis, which facilitates the identification of the bladder. Also, the drainage of the bladder prevents spatial interference during the vascular suturing, allowing a better exposure.

The patient is positioned supine, with parted and flexed legs on stirrups. Upper extremities are adducted and tagged to the body. Shoulder blocks and tape are used to avoid the risk of the patient sliding during the operation. The following description is for pancreas transplantation on the left iliac side, which is the most commonly performed; however, the technique is symmetrical on the right side, and it is carried out in case of a previous transplant on the left, vascular calcifications, or venous thrombosis on the left iliac vessels (**Figure 48-2**).

After the patient's abdomen is prepared in a sterile fashion, a 7-cm subxiphoid midline incision is made and a GelPort® is placed.

After induction of the pneumoperitoneum (15 mm Hg) through the GelPort®, the laparoscopic/robotic cannulas are inserted under direct vision. One 8-mm robotic trocar, for the 30° robotic scope, is placed in the periumbilical region (usually just above the umbilicus), and two 8-mm trocars for the robotic arms are inserted, one in the right iliac fossa and the other one in the left lateral lower quadrant. Finally, a 12-mm laparoscopic port, for the bedside assistant, is positioned between the umbilicus and the trocar in the right iliac fossa. Once the ports are set, the patient is placed in a 30° Trendelenburg position, with the left side tilted up (20°). The robotic cart is docked into position from the left side (**Figures 48-3** and **48-4**).

Average time frame: 20–30 min

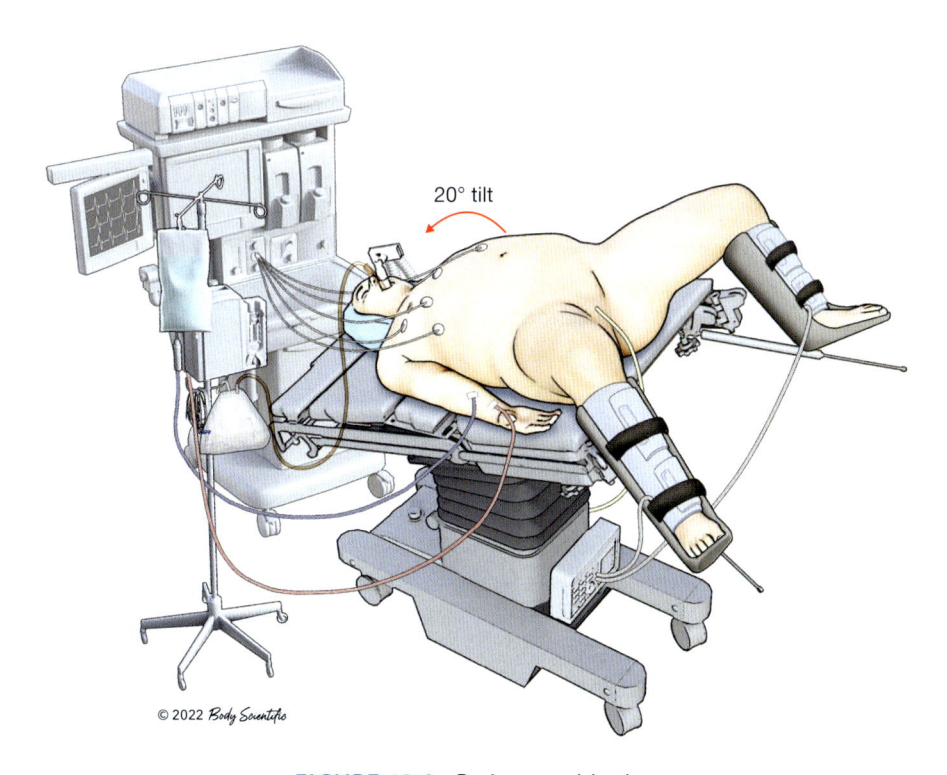

FIGURE 48-2 • Patient positioning.

> ⚠️ **PITFALLS**
>
> If the trocar in the left lower lateral quadrant is placed too low, the cannula will become perpendicular to the vessels, making handling of the instruments more difficult.

> 🔍 **ANATOMICAL HIGHLIGHTS**
>
> Anatomy of the anterior abdominal wall, with the epigastric vessels and pelvic organs.

986 The Foundation and Art of Robotic Surgery

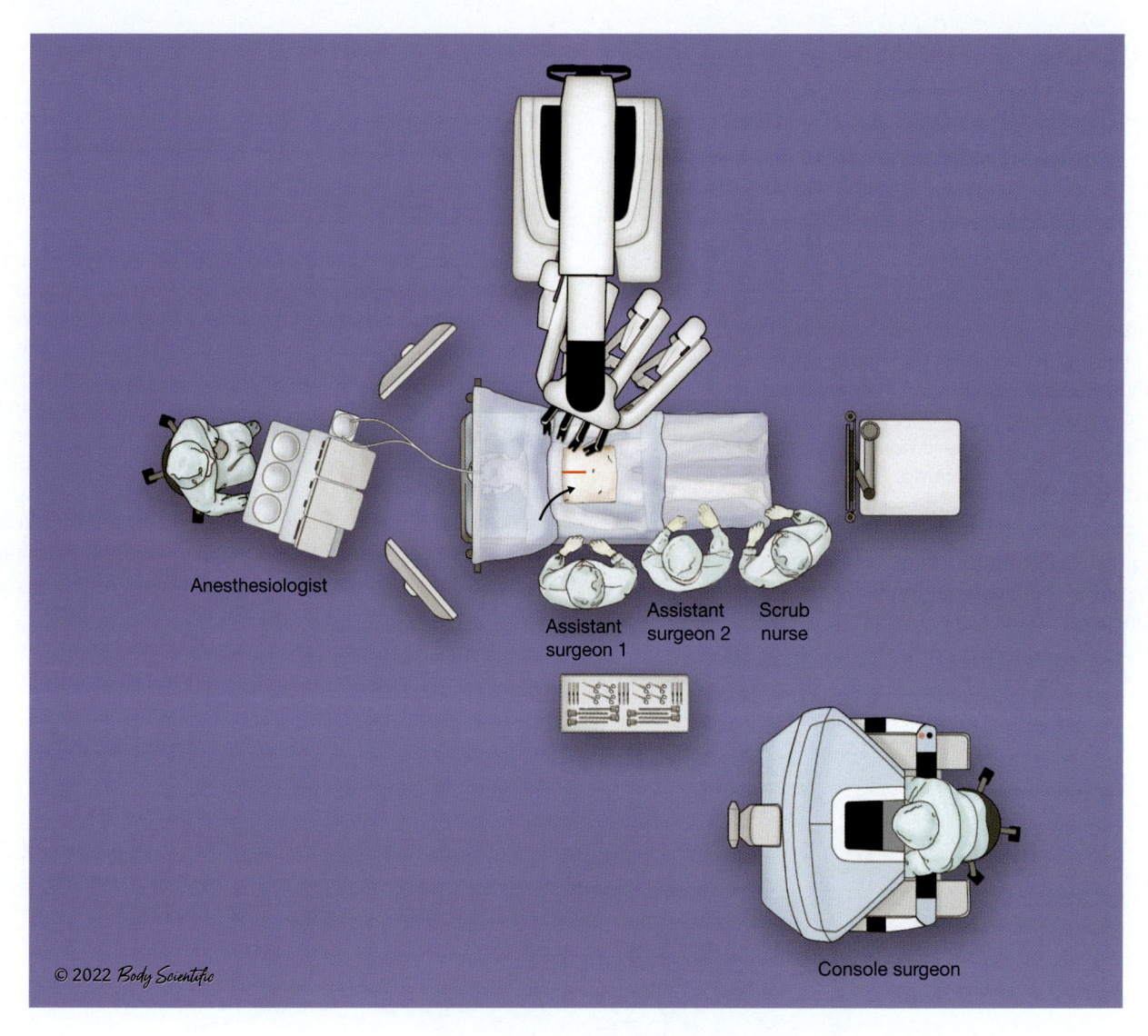

FIGURE 48-3 • OR setup.

▶▶ TIPS

Adapting the trocar positioning under laparoscopic vision allows a precise identification of the pelvic anatomy (width, depth, distance), achieving a better triangulation.

The location of the midline incision (distance from the xyphoid process) depends on the body habitus of the recipient, but is ideally as high as possible, achieving a better spacing for the robotic arms. Also, closer to the xyphoid process, the subcutaneous fat is usually less thick and the risk of infection is lower. Of course, the distance from the iliac area should be carefully evaluated in order to maintain an effective and comfortable interaction with the assistant hand.

EDITORIAL COMMENT

Placing the graft in the left iliac fossa achieves a better orientation of the duodenum for the side-to-side duodenoenterostomy.

Also, there is a more favorable position on the left side for the vascular anastomosis and less risk of kinking.

On the right side, it is sometimes necessary to drain the portal vein into the vena cava and to place the inflow in the common iliac artery.

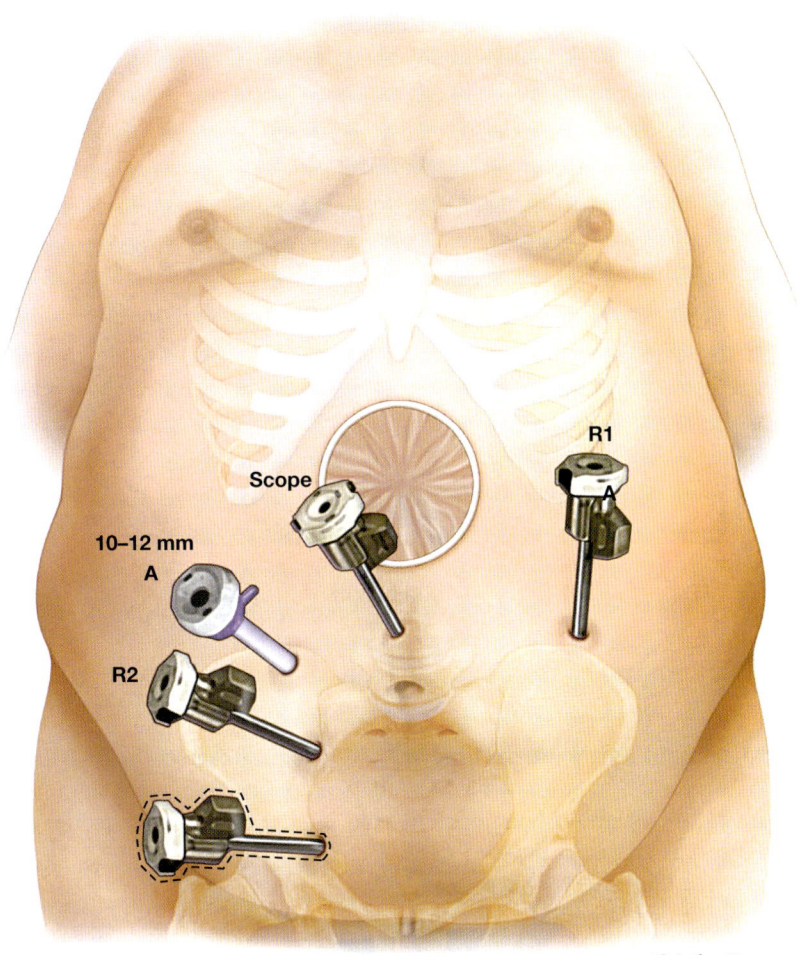

FIGURE 48-4 • Port setting.

▶ Video 48-1. Robotic Pancreas Transplant – Full Procedure

▶ Video 48-2. Step 1. Mobilization of the Colon

Step 1. Mobilization of the colon

The operation starts with the mobilization of the left colon at the junction between the descending and sigmoid colon (**Figure 48-5**). The assistant retracts the colon medially in order to maintain tension on the peritoneal reflection and to allow dissection on an avascular plane. The dissection is conducted with the hook electrocautery and the bipolar forceps. The native ureter, crossing the common iliac artery in its anatomical location, is left in place. It is important to perform a good mobilization of the distal descending and sigmoid colon in order to achieve a good exposure of the left iliac vessels.

Step 1 average time frame: 10–15 min

⚠ PITFALLS

Entering into the colon mesentery, mainly when the sigmoid colon is adherent to the left lateral abdominal wall, as it may happen in patients with diverticular disease.

Insufficient, incomplete mobilization of the left colon.

▶▶ TIPS

Asking the assistant to maintain some tension on the mesentery of the left colon helps in keeping the proper avascular dissection plane.

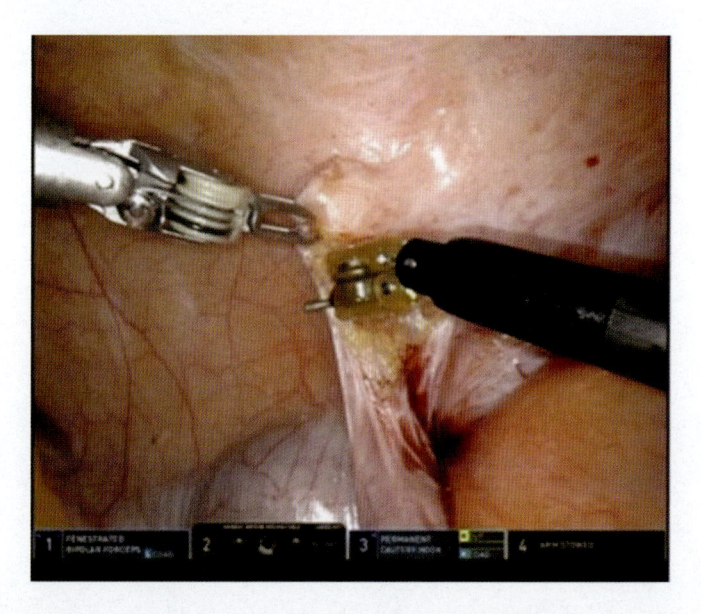

FIGURE 48-5 • Mobilization of the colon.

▶ **Video 48-3. Step 2. Exposure of the Surgical Field**

Step 2. Exposure of the surgical field (left external iliac vessels)

During this step, the gonadal vessels are identified. In females, the suspensory ligament of the ovary is incised at the level of the proximal portion of the external iliac artery. Then, the ovary and the utero-ovarian vessels are mobilized and retracted medially. To achieve a complete exposure of the iliac axis, it may be necessary to dissect the broad ligament of the uterus and divide the left round ligament. These maneuvers allow the medial retraction of the uterus. In males, the testicular vessels run laterally to the common and the external iliac arteries on the body of the psoas major muscle. In the majority of cases, they do not interfere with the preparation of the external iliac artery (**Figure 48-6**).

Anatomical factors that may limit the exposure are a thick mesentery or a redundant sigmoid colon. Also a bulky uterus may interfere with the procedure.

Step 2 average time frame: 10–20 min

> ▶▶ **TIPS**
>
> To facilitate the exposure and retract a bulky uterus, setting the R3 with a grasper may be helpful. The trocar for the R3 is positioned in the right lower quadrant.

> ⚠ **PITFALLS**
>
> Insufficient, incomplete exposure of the left iliac vessels.

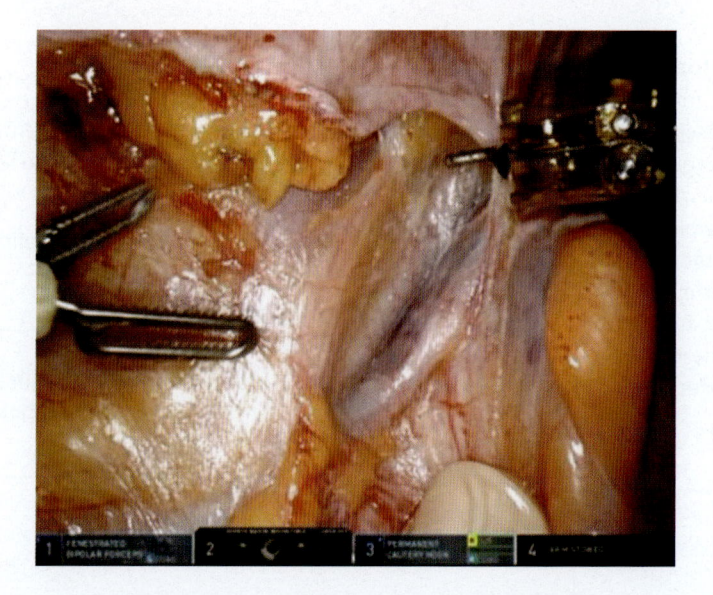

FIGURE 48-6 • Exposure of the surgical field.

Video 48-4. Step 3. Preparation of the Left External Iliac Artery

Step 3. Preparation of the left external iliac artery

The preparation of the external iliac artery on the left side does not differ much from the preparation of the right external iliac artery already described in Chapter 47, Kidney Transplant.

The entire length of the artery should be mobilized from the bifurcation with the common iliac artery to the inguinal canal where the vessel gives origin to collaterals such as the inferior epigastric artery and the deep circumflex. Those branches are usually very distal and rarely need to be ligated and divided. The artery is often affected by plaques and calcifications and should be handled gently and smoothly on the periadventitial layer.

It is sometimes surrounded by enlarged lymph nodes that should be manipulated carefully since they can be source of significant postoperative lymphatic leak.

The mobilization is completed passing a vessel loop around the artery. The loop allows the "hanging maneuver," that is the static, upward lateral retraction of the vessel using a clip anchored to the lateral wall. This maneuver facilitates the exposure of the external iliac vein and, later on, the construction of the venous anastomosis (**Figures 48-7 A, B**).

Step 3 average time frame: 15–20 min

> ⚠ **PITFALLS**
>
> Insufficient, incomplete mobilization of the external iliac artery.

> ▶▶ **TIPS**
>
> The bedside assistant, through the GelPort®, may palpate the artery to confirm the absence or localize the presence of atherosclerotic plaques.

> 🔍 **ANATOMICAL HIGHLIGHTS**
>
> The external iliac artery is superior and lateral to the external iliac vein and is located along the medial border of the psoas major muscle (**Figure 48-8**).
>
> The external iliac artery most commonly gives rise to 2 branches—the inferior epigastric and the deep circumflex arteries—usually at the level of the inguinal ligament.

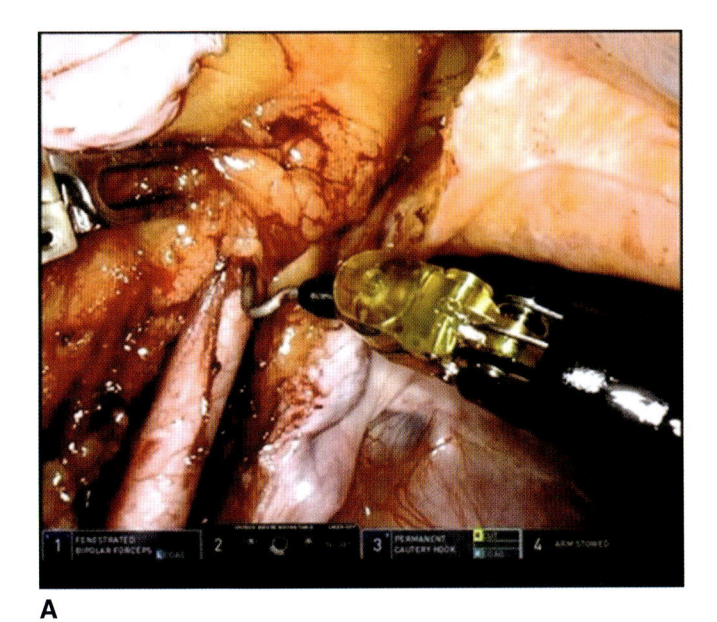

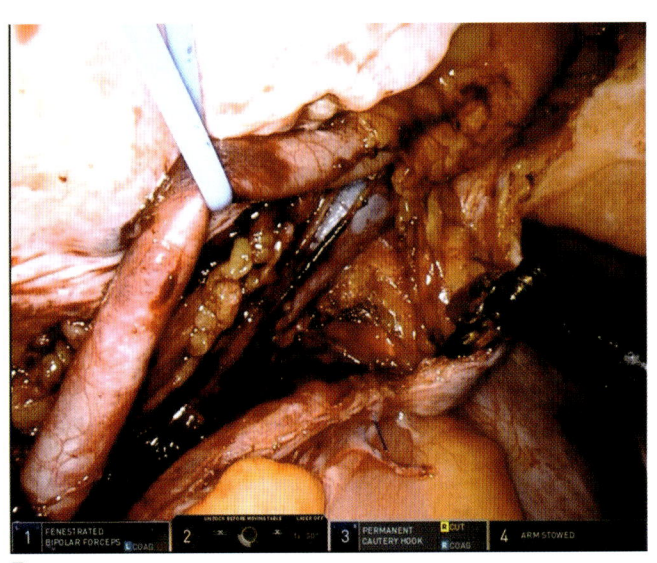

FIGURE 48-7 • Preparation of the left external iliac artery.

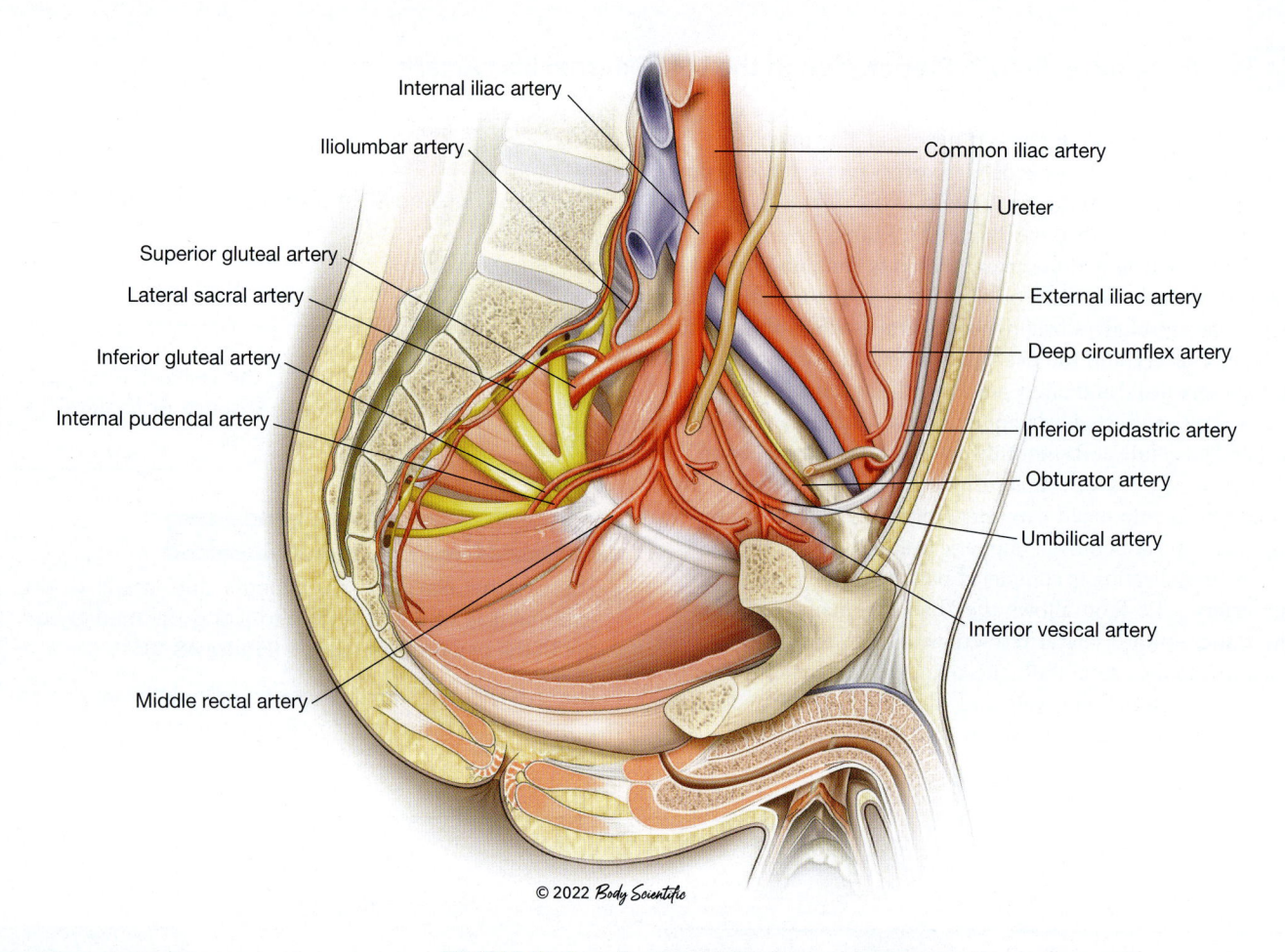

FIGURE 48-8 • Left external iliac artery.

Video 48-5. Step 4. Preparation of the Left External Iliac Vein

Step 4. Preparation of the left external iliac vein

A vessel loop is placed around the external iliac vein to be able to mobilize the posterior, deeper surface of the vessel. The dissection is conducted with the monopolar hook and the bipolar forceps proximally up to the level of the ureter and the internal iliac artery and distally up to the inferior margin of the inguinal canal. In males, care must be taken to respect the *vas deferens*, while in females, the round ligament can be sacrificed. Pubic, inferior epigastric, and deep circumflex iliac veins only occasionally need to be ligated and transected in order to achieve a longer segment of the vein for clamping and anastomosis (**Figure 48-9**).

Step 4 average time frame: 15–25 min

⚠ PITFALLS

Insufficient, incomplete preparation of the external iliac vein. Bleeding from laceration of collateral veins.

🔍 ANATOMICAL HIGHLIGHTS

The left external iliac vein is medial to the external iliac artery and on a deeper plane.

The external iliac vein is crossed proximally by the ureter and internal iliac artery and distally by the *vas deferens* (males) and by the round ligament and utero-ovarian vessels (females) (**Figure 48-10**).

Pancreas Transplant 991

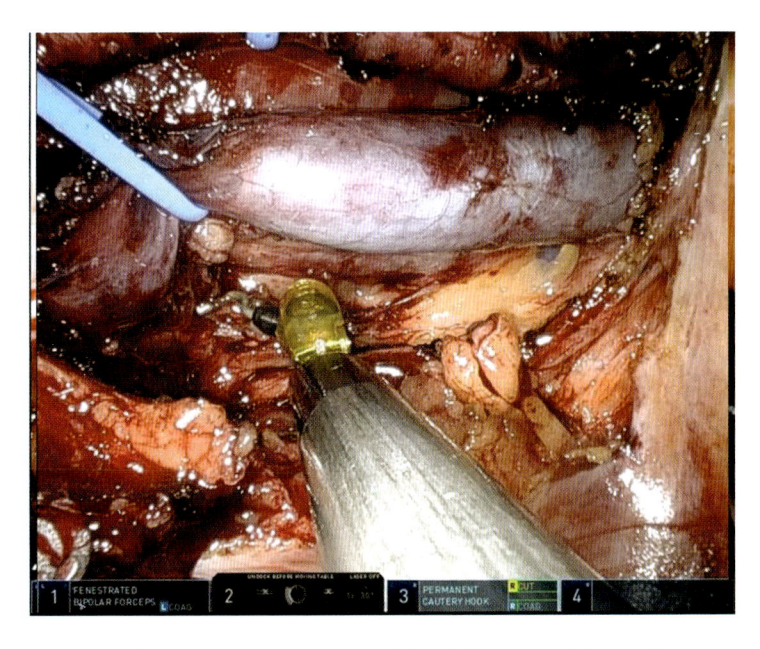

FIGURE 48-9 • Preparation of the left external iliac vein.

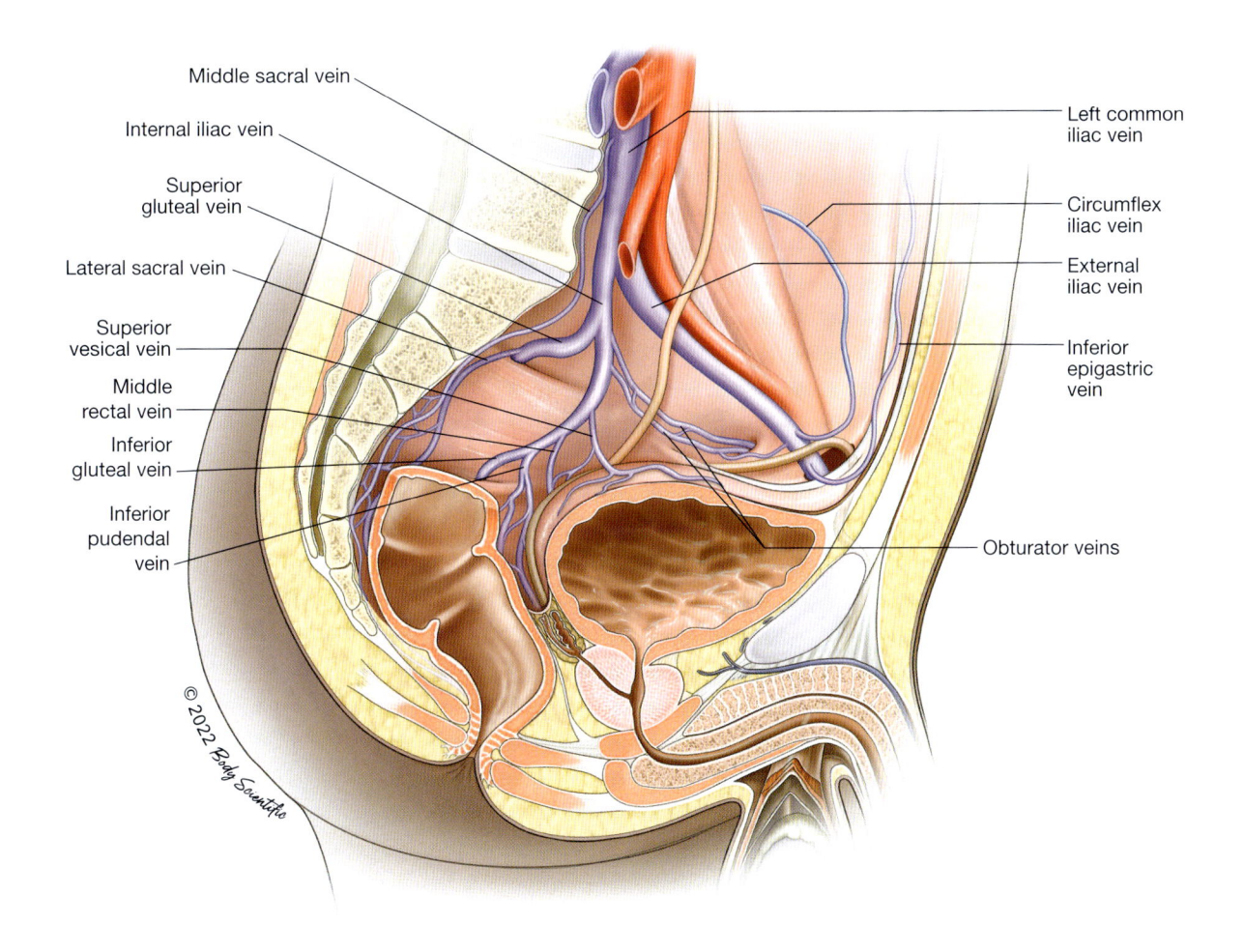

FIGURE 48-10 • Left external iliac vein.

▶ **Video 48-6. Step 5. Venous Clamping and Pelvic Placement of the Graft**

Step 5. Venous clamping and pelvic placement of the graft

Once the external iliac vessels are completely dissected free, 5 robotic bulldog clamps are brought into the field through the GelPort®. Two of them will be used for the venous anastomosis and the 3 remaining ones will be used later on for the arterial reconstruction. The anesthesiologist injects 2000 IU of heparin EV. The external iliac vein is occluded proximally and distally with the robotic bulldog clamps (**Figure 48-11**). The vessel loop is not removed but positioned external to the clamp to avoid interference with the suturing. Robotic Potts scissors are used to create a venotomy of about 15 mm, and eventual valve cusps are carefully disrupted. A 12-cm, handmade, double-armed, Gore-Tex® 5-0 suture with a knot in the middle is placed at the corner of the venotomy. The pancreas graft is inserted in the abdominal cavity by the assisting surgeon and positioned medial and parallel to the dissected iliac vessels with the pancreas head in a deeper pelvic position.

Step 5 average time frame: 15–20 min

▶▶ **TIPS**

The proximal bulldog clamp is positioned first, the vein is then lifted with gentle traction on the vessel loop, and the distal bulldog clamp is subsequently placed. This maneuver allows the correct position of the distal bulldog on an empty vein. The next step is to slightly open the distal bulldog clamp to allow partial refilling of the vein. If the vein becomes partially distended a better orientation of the final distal clamping is achieved. Avoiding distortion of the vessel geometry allows a perfect placement of the venotomy.

The vessel loop on the vein should not be removed, but positioned externally to the proximal bulldog clamp. It is a safety measure in case of accidental sliding of a clamp during the construction of the anastomosis. Just pulling on the loop allows the bleeding to be controlled and the immediate repositioning of the clamp.

🔍 **ANATOMICAL HIGHLIGHTS**

The external iliac vein usually has no valves, but occasionally, they may be present.

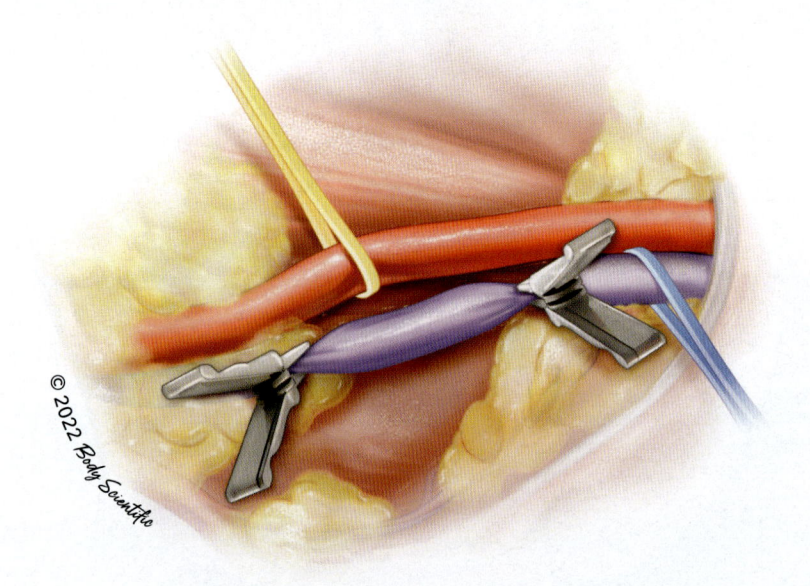

FIGURE 48-11 • Venous clamping.

▶ **Video 48-7.** Step 6. Venous Anastomosis

Step 6. Venous anastomosis

Previous ink marking and a Prolene™ 5-0 stitch placed on the upper pole of the vein facilitate the proper orientation. At this point, the assistant hand stabilizes the pancreas. Also, to avoid twisting of the organ, a grasper inserted from the assisting port is gently placed on top of the head of the pancreas. An end-to-side venous anastomosis (portal vein/iliac vein) is completed with a running suture of Gore-Tex® 5-0, starting from the posterior wall. A second 5-0 Gore-Tex® stitch is then applied at the opposite corner of the venotomy to secure and tighten the anastomosis (**Figure 48-12**).

Step 6 average time frame: 15–20 min

⚠ **PITFALLS**

Breaking the Gore-Tex® 5-0 running suture with the needle driver. The main reason to use the Gore-Tex® is that PTFE is more resistant to instrument manipulation.

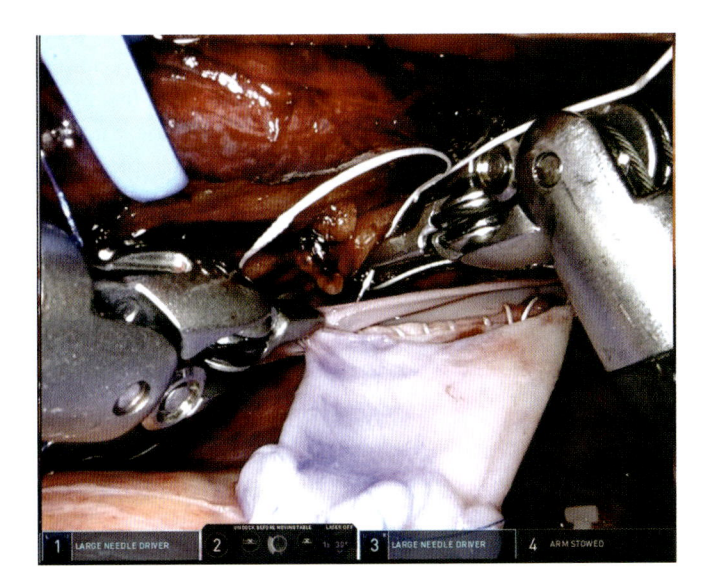

FIGURE 48-12 • Venous anastomosis.

▶ **Video 48-8.** Step 7. Arterial Anastomosis

Step 7. Arterial anastomosis

The external iliac artery, previously lifted and hanged with the vessel loop, is now freed from the abdominal wall and subsequently clamped between robotic bulldog clamps (2 proximal and 1 distal). An oval window (proportional to the size of the graft artery) is made in the anterior-medial wall of the iliac artery with robotic scissors. To facilitate this step, a Prolene™ 5-0 stitch is placed through the anterior wall of the external iliac artery and gentle lifting is applied, removing a small patch of the artery. A 12-cm, double-armed, Gore-Tex® 6-0 suture with a knot in the middle is placed at the corner of the arteriotomy. An end-to-side arterial anastomosis is completed with a running suture, starting from the posterior wall.

A second Gore-Tex® 6-0 stitch is then applied at the opposite corner of the arteriotomy to secure and tighten the anastomosis (**Figure 48-13**).

Step 7 average time frame: 15–20 min

▶▶ **TIPS**

Before doing the complete arteriotomy, it is prudent to verify the effective clamping of the bulldogs. The arterial wall may be rigid and difficult to collapse under the gentle bite of the bulldogs. The assistant may confirm by palpation the absence of pulse. The arteriotomy should, anyway, start with a very small incision and be extended only after confirming the absence of flow.

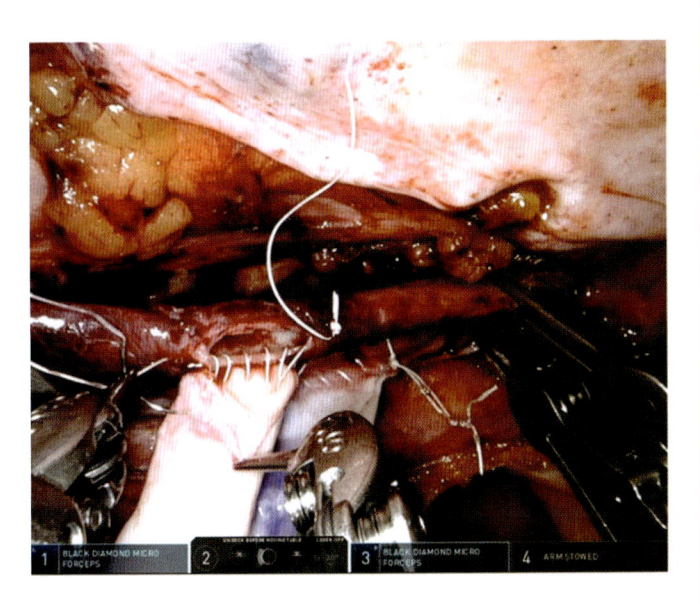

FIGURE 48-13 • Arterial anastomosis.

▶ **Video 48-9. Step 8. Reperfusion**

Step 8. Reperfusion

Once vascular suturing is completed, the anastomosis should be verified before declamping and reperfusing the graft. Anastomotic leaks can be repaired with single stitches with Prolene™ 5-0 without incurring in warm ischemia of the transplant.

In order to do that, a small, soft bulldog clamp is placed on the preanastomotic portal vein and on the proximal arterial inflow conduit. Only after the verification of a good anastomotic construction the clamps are removed and the pancreas is reperfused.

The reperfusion of the organ and the hemostasis are verified and bleeding points controlled with a Prolene™ 6-0 suture. An intraoperative Doppler with the probe inserted through the assistant port verifies the characteristics of the flow. Also, the use of ICG (5 mg) given IV to the patient confirms the complete and homogeneous reperfusion of the graft (see Chapter 7, Fluorescence Imaging: Basics and Clinical Applications).

At this point, the pressure of the pneumoperitoneum is decreased to 10 mm Hg to minimize the possible negative effects of higher intraabdominal pressure on the graft microperfusion (**Figure 48-14**).

Step 8 average time frame: 10–15 min

▶▶ **TIPS**

For optimal hemostasis verification, the assistant gently lifts the pancreas, allowing inspection of the posterior wall for possible bleeding points.

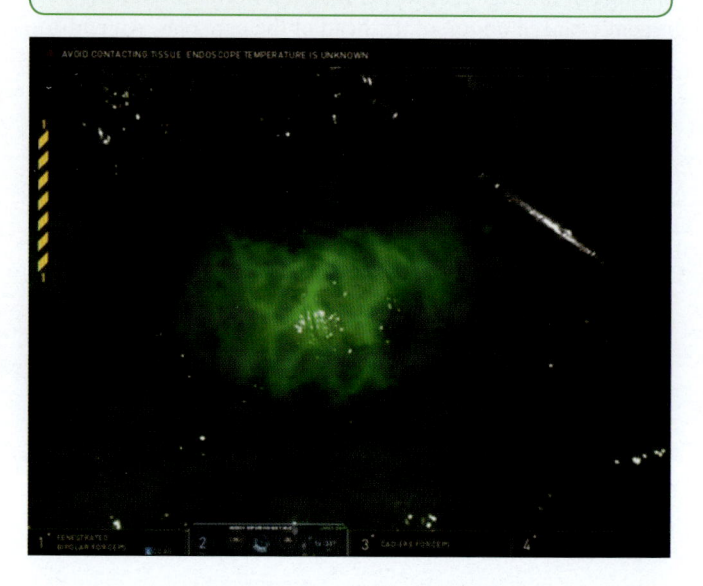

FIGURE 48-14 • Reperfusion.

▶ **Video 48-10. Step 9. Exocrine Drainage (Duodenoenterostomy)**

Step 9. Exocrine drainage (duodenoenterostomy)

The management of the exocrine secretions is now almost exclusively done with an enteric drainage. After the graft is revascularized, a jejunal loop (at least 80 cm from the ileocecal valve) is brought down to the level of the graft duodenum to perform a side-to-side 2-layer duodenoenterostomy (**Figure 48-15**). The outer posterior layer is constructed first with a running Vicryl™ 3-0 suture. The internal layer is done with full-thickness PDS™ 3-0 in a running fashion to achieve thorough hemostasis. The anastomosis is completed with an anterior outer layer with interrupted Vicryl™ 3-0 sutures.

Step 9 average time frame: 30–45 min

⚠ **PITFALLS**

If the duodenoenterostomy is done too close to the ileocecal valve, the chemical effects of the exocrine secretions of the graft may induce a diarrhea difficult to treat.

▶▶ **TIPS**

The small bowel segment selected for the anastomosis should reach the graft duodenum without any tension; a tension-free anastomosis results in a better healing, minimizing the risk of pancreatic leaks.

The papilla of Vater, when observed through the enterotomy, appears as a slight oval elevation of the duodenal mucosa. During the anastomosis, attention must be paid not to include this structure in the suture line.

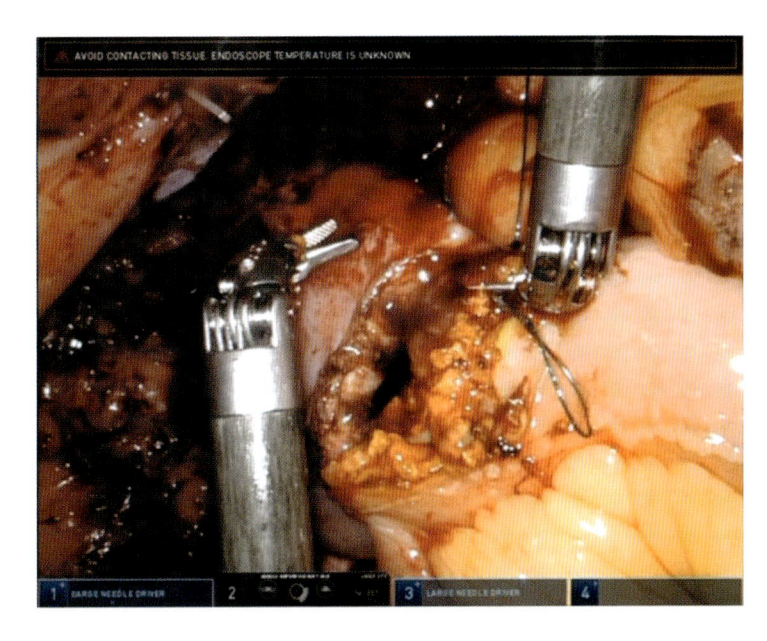

FIGURE 48-15 • Exocrine drainage (duodenoenterostomy).

Step 10. Closure
At the end of the procedure, the minilaparotomy is closed with an interrupted PDS™ 1 and the 12-mm port site is closed with an endosuture passer needle and a Vicryl™ 0 suture. Skin incisions are closed cosmetically. A closed drain is usually left in place.

Step 10 average time frame: 15–20 min

> **EDITORIAL COMMENT**
>
> There are pros and cons in leaving a peritoneal drainage in the surgical field. The most important advantage is that it may allow an early detection of an enteric leak (duodeno-ileal anastomosis). On the other side, an higher risk of infection may be associated with the drain.

Suggested Readings

1. Boggi U, Signori S, Vistoli F, et al. Laparoscopic robot-assisted pancreas transplantation: first world experience. *Transplantation* 2012;93:201-206.
2. Spaggiari M, Tulla KA, Di Bella C, et al. Promising outcomes from 5 robotic pancreas transplants in obese patients. *Transplantation* 2013;96:S1-S155.
3. Chillaron JJ, Benaiges D, Mane L, et al. Obesity and type 1 diabetes mellitus management. *Minerva Endocrinol.* 2015;40:53-60.
4. Bedat B, Niclauss N, Jannot AS, et al. Impact of recipient body mass index on short-term and long-term survival of pancreatic grafts. *Transplantation* 2015;99:94-99.
5. Laurence JM, Marquez MA, Bazerbachi F, et al. Optimizing pancreas transplantation outcomes in obese recipients. *Transplantation* 2015;99:1282-1287.
6. Yeh CC, Spaggiari M, Tzvetanov I, Oberholzer J. Robotic pancreas transplantation in a type 1 diabetic patient with morbid obesity: a case report. *Medicine* 2017;96:e5847.
7. Cantrell LA, Oberholzer J. Robotic pancreas transplantation: the state of the art. *Curr Op Organ Transplant.* 2018;23:423-427.
8. Giulianotti PC, Coratti A, Angelini M, et al. Robotics in general surgery: personal experience in a large community hospital. *Arch Surg.* 2003;138(7):777-784. doi: 10.1001/archsurg.138.7.777

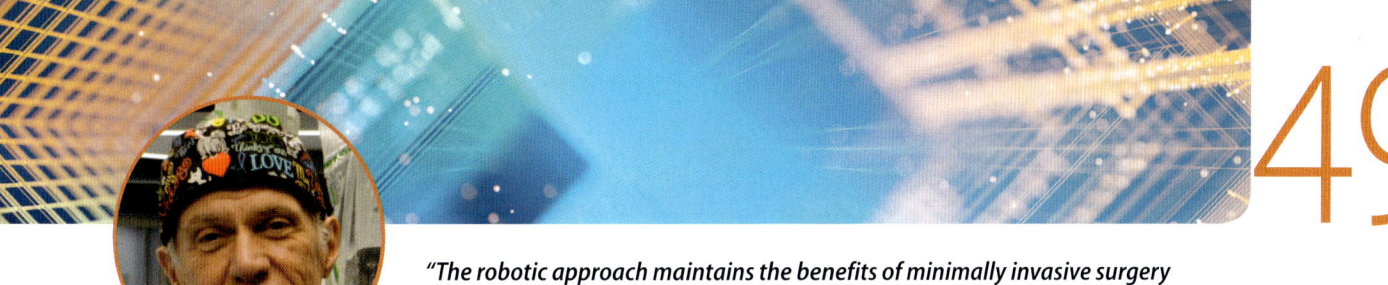

"The robotic approach maintains the benefits of minimally invasive surgery while overcoming the limitations of laparoscopy."

"The advantage of avoiding a painful sub-costal or upper midline incision and the potential for a faster return to normal daily activities for the living donor is significant enough to warrant further evaluation of this innovative strategy."

—Pier Cristoforo Giulianotti (1953)

Living Donor Hepatectomy

Ahmed Zidan • Dieter Broering

INTRODUCTION

Robotic liver surgery evolved after the establishment of laparoscopic techniques, and it is considered to be safe in the hands of experts; however, reports of robotic liver surgery are still limited when compared to their laparoscopic counterparts. With the advancements offered by the robotic platform in a narrow operative field, Giulianotti et al. reported the first-ever robotic live donor right hepatectomy in 2011. Since then, a few countries have successfully incorporated robotic living donor hepatectomy programs (Taiwan, Saudi Arabia, South Korea, and China) with newly established centers in India and the United States. While both left hepatectomies and left lateral segmentectomies have been proven to be feasible for donation, this chapter will primarily focus on living donor right hepatectomies.

Appropriate Donor Selection

It is preferable at the beginning of the learning curve to select donors with standard anatomy (**Figure 49-1**). This will enable the feasibility of the initial experience and result in better outcomes.

Patient Positioning, OR Setup, and Port Setting

The patient is placed supine in the French position with 30–40° reverse Trendelenburg and the right shoulder up slightly (15–20°). The bedside surgeon stands between the patient's legs (**Figure 49-2**).

The OR setup is explained in **Figure 49-3**.

INSTRUMENT REQUIREMENTS

The suggested main robotic instruments/tools can be listed as follows:
- 30°/0° scope
- Needle drivers (large)
- Cautery hook
- Harmonic® shears
- 2 Maryland bipolar dissectors
- Bipolar forceps
- ProGrasp™ forceps
- Round-tip scissors
- Robotic linear staplers (with different loads)
- Multiple Hem-o-lok® clips
- Small/medium/large clip applier

The suggested main laparoscopic instruments/tools can be listed as follows:
- Needle drivers
- Graspers
- Suction-irrigation
- Metal clip applier (optional)
- Laparoscopic staplers

Supplemental materials:
- Gauzes, sponges
- Foley-type catheter
- Endobag™
- Small/medium/large clips
- Titanium metal clips
- Sutures: Prolene™ 2-0, 3-0, 4-0, and 5-0; Vicryl™ 3-0; PDS™ 5-0/6-0
- GelPort® (optional)

Photo reproduced with permission from Dr. Pier Cristoforo Giulianotti.

Quote 1 reproduced with permission from Giulianotti PC, Quadri P, Durgam S, et al. Reconstruction/repair of iatrogenic biliary injuries: is the robot offering a new option? Short clinical report. Ann Surg. 2018;267(1):e7-e9.

Quote 2 reproduced with permission from Giulianotti PC, Tzvetanov I, Jeon H, et al. Robot-assisted right lobe donor hepatectomy. Transpl Int. 2012;25(1):e5-e9.

998   The Foundation and Art of Robotic Surgery

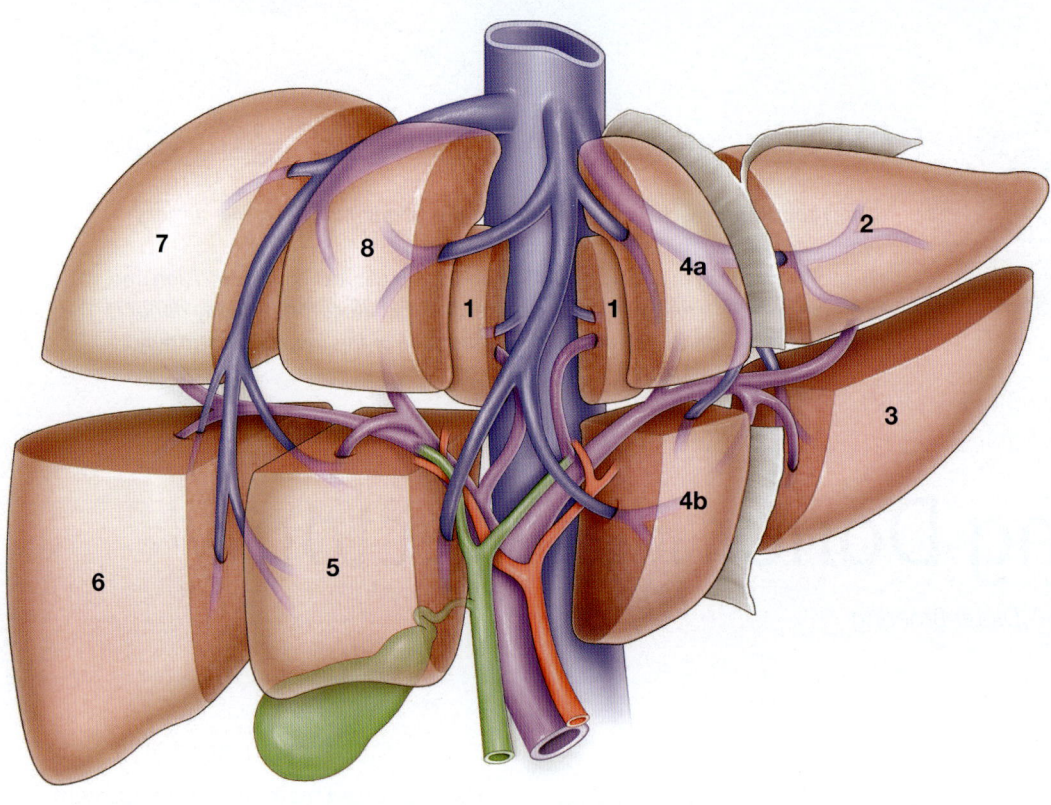

FIGURE 49-1 • Segments of the liver.

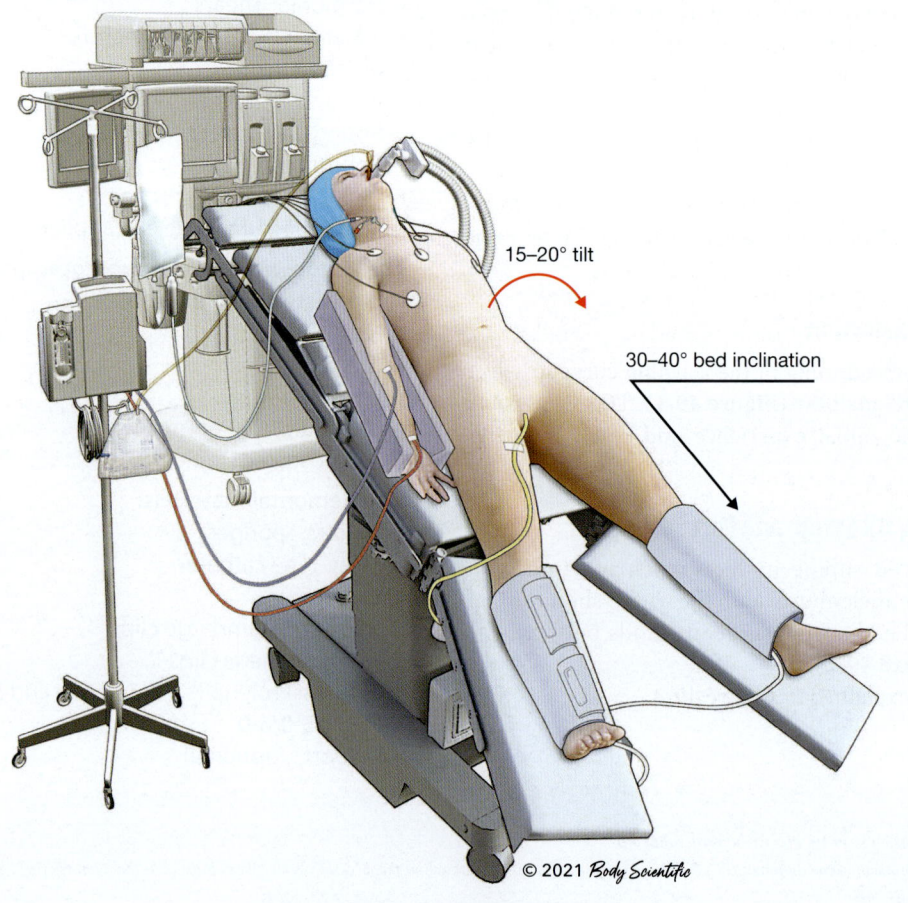

FIGURE 49-2 • Patient positioning.

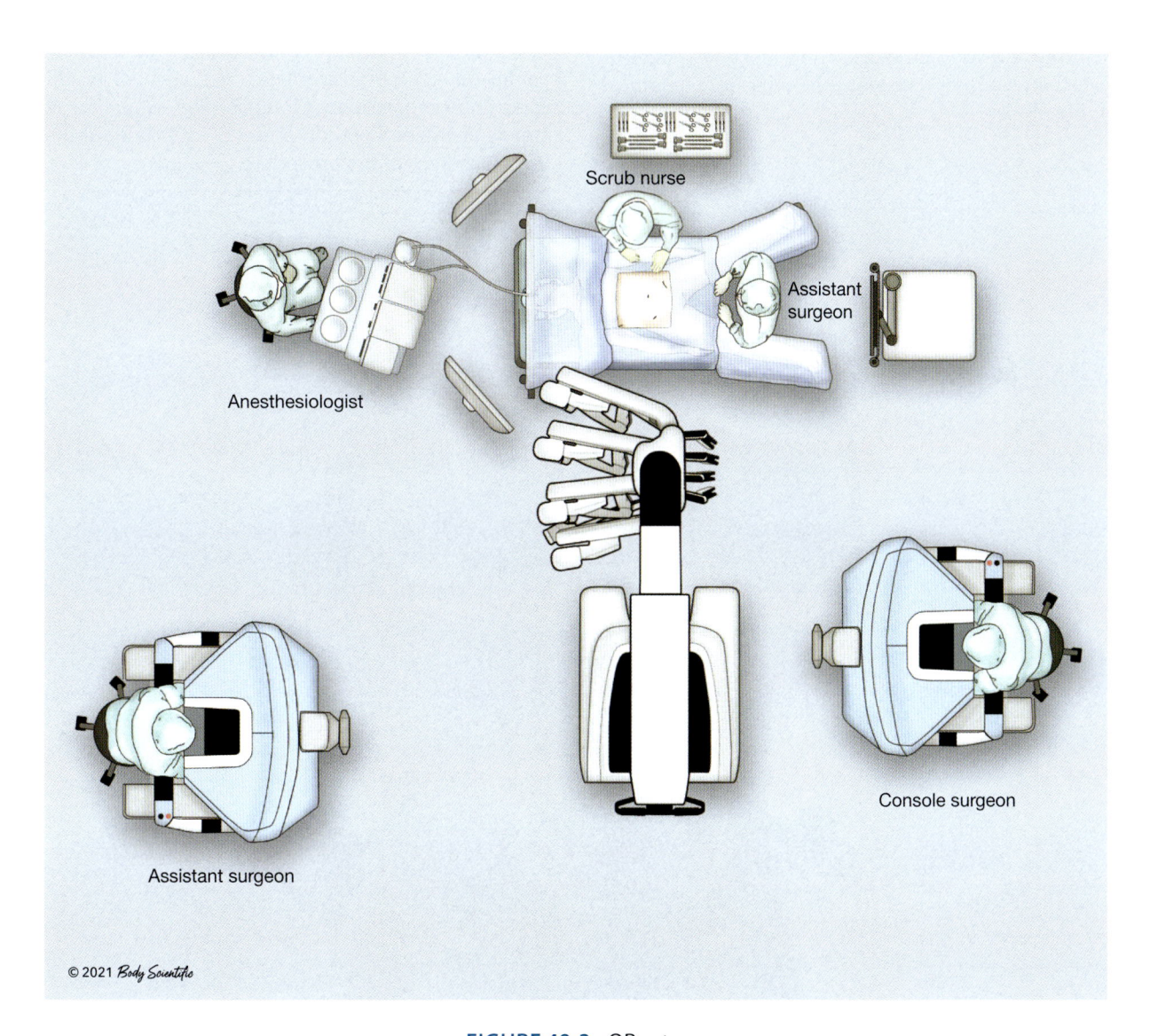

FIGURE 49-3 • OR setup.

> **EDITORIAL COMMENT**
>
> The dual console is not improving the technical performance of the procedure. The best assistant should stay at the patient bedside. The role of the dual console is mainly for teaching and proctoring purposes.

> **EDITORIAL COMMENT**
>
> For major robotic resections, including the living donor hepatectomy, a second assistant port may be helpful, and it doesn't change the minimally invasive nature of the operation. It gives the assistant a full range of surgical capabilities, which is useful in overcoming difficulties and challenges during the operation.
>
> The extraction incision is usually a Pfannenstiel, but in large abdomens, it could be a hypogastric midline. It can be done at the very beginning of the operation. The placement of a GelPort® may facilitate hand assistance or introduction of instruments (e.g., clamps) in difficult steps of the operation. Moreover, the extraction site is ready at the end without need of interrupting the last vascular steps of the procedure.

Pneumoperitoneum with a pressure up to 10–12 mm Hg is established using the open technique through the umbilical assistant port.

Four 8-mm ports are placed, 2 on each side, at the midclavicular line and anterior axillary line, along a straight or slightly curvilinear line 5 cm above the transverse umbilical line (**Figure 49-4**).

FIGURE 49-4 • Port setting normal abdomen.

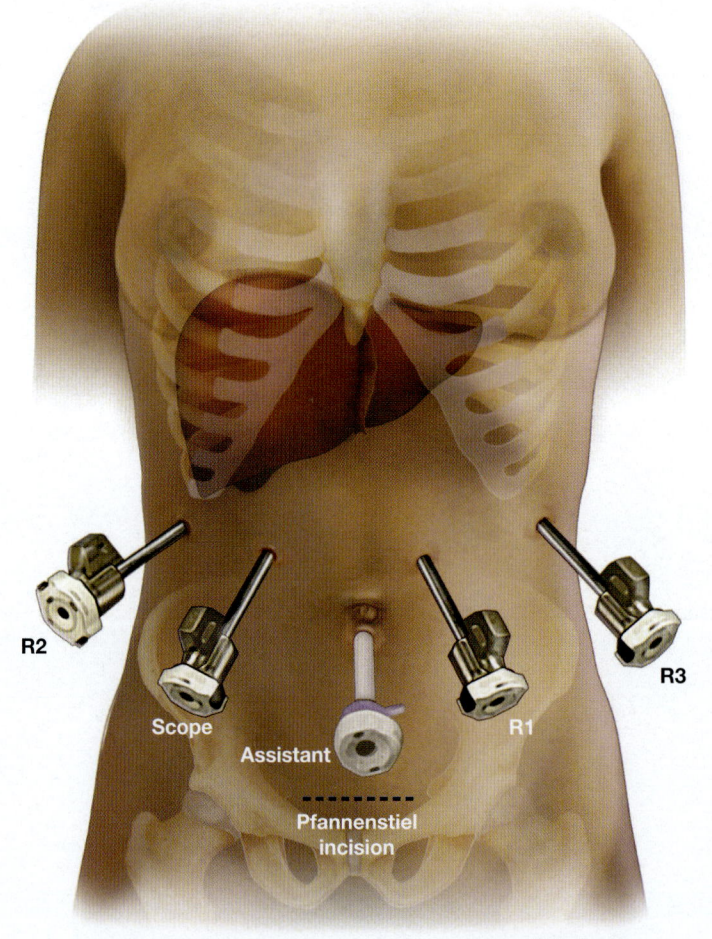

Surgical Technique

▶ **Video 49-1. Living Donor Hepatectomy – Full Procedure**

Liver Mobilization

Step 1. Cutting the falciform and right coronary ligaments

▶ **Video 49-2. Step 1. Cutting the Falciform and Right Coronary Ligaments**

The liver mobilization starts with the transection of the falciform ligament with Harmonic® shears in R1, putting gentle downward pressure and traction with a Maryland in R2. The transection should be completed up to the level of the coronary ligaments. Then, the hepatic veins should be exposed with the robotic hook. Putting a mark with the robotic hook on the left side of the right hepatic vein will help in delineation of the demarcation line later.

The right coronary ligament is exposed by applying traction on the gallbladder from the laparoscopic port toward the left side and downward, and transected either by the monopolar hook in R1 or the bipolar dissector in R2. The right liver lobe is stepwise lifted up by the ProGrasp™ in R3, and the attachments of the right liver toward the diaphragm and the retroperitoneum are cut until the retrohepatic cava is exposed (**Figures 49-5 A–C**). The assistant may help in countertraction by pushing down Gerota's capsule in order to improve the working space of the surgeon.

Step 1 average time frame: 25–30 min

> ▶▶ **TIPS**
>
> - Marking the left side of the right hepatic veins on the liver parenchyma may help in identification of the Cantlie's line later.
> - Using a sponge with the ProGrasp™ in R3 can help to avoid parenchymal injury during traction.
> - Changing the extent and direction of the traction with the ProGrasp™ can help in proper exposure of the right coronary ligament.
> - Gentle and careful dissection between right and middle hepatic veins facilitates tunneling later.

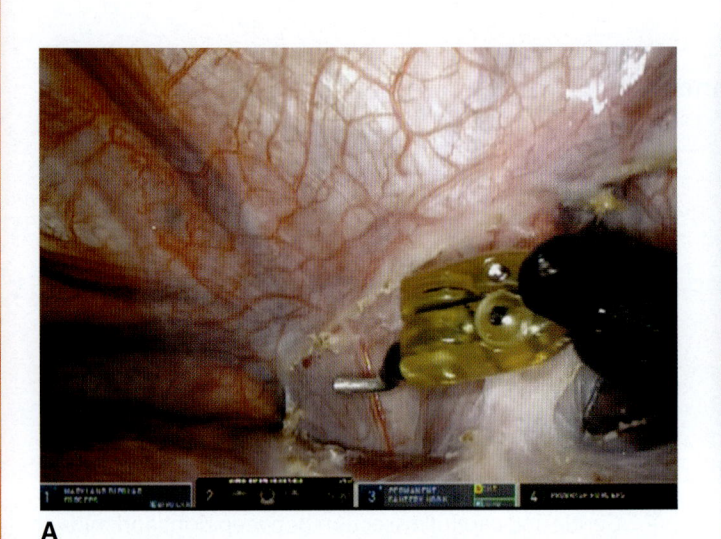

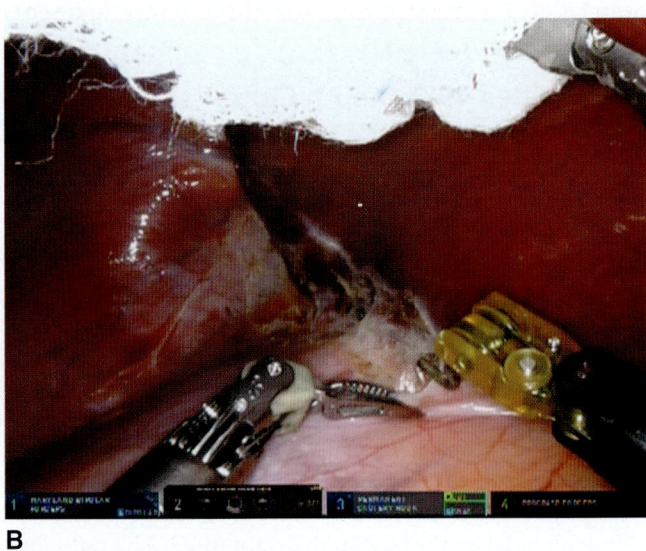

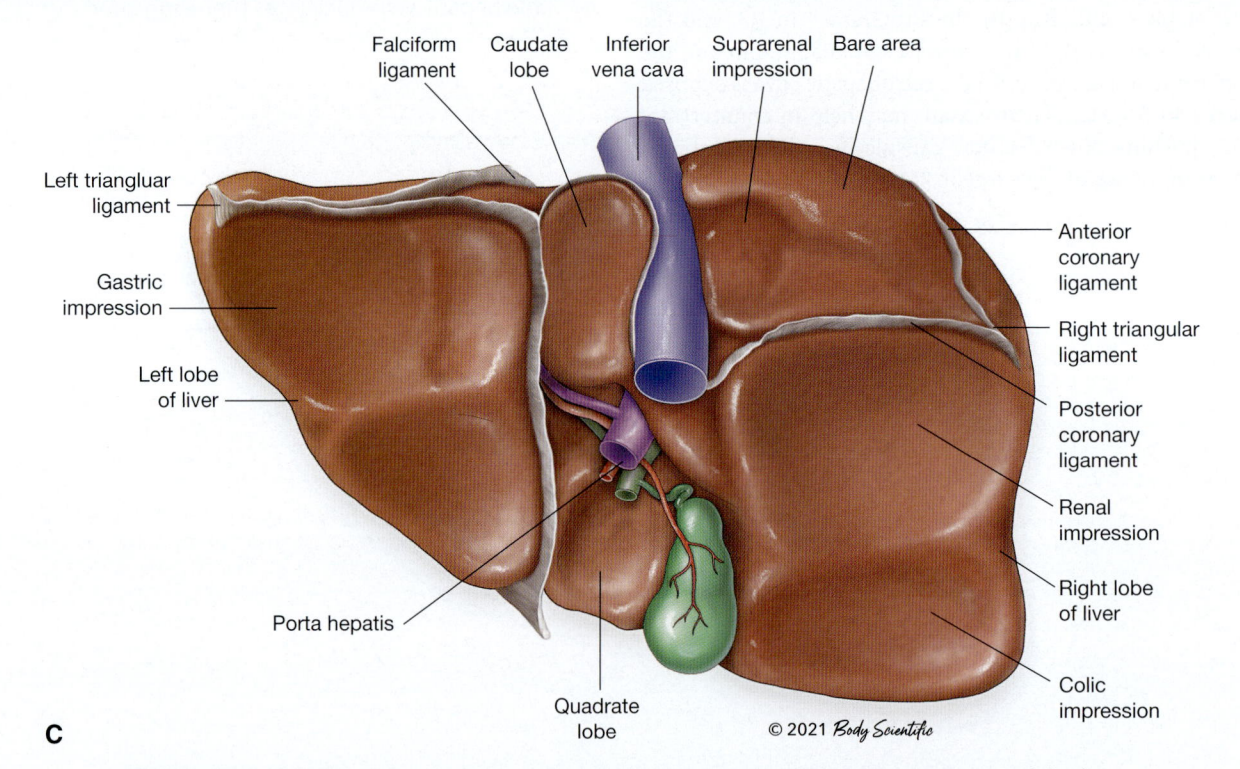

FIGURE 49-5 • **A, B.** Dividing the ligamentous attachments to the liver. **C.** Ligaments of the liver.

Step 2. Cutting short hepatic veins

▶ **Video 49-3.** Step 2. Cutting Short Hepatic Veins

Caudo-cephalad dissection of the short hepatic veins of the inferior vena cava (IVC) is performed using 2 bipolar Maryland forceps in R1 and R2.

Small, short hepatic veins between the IVC and liver are controlled with bipolar coagulation, 5-0 nonabsorbable Prolene™ monofilament sutures, or metallic clips, or coagulated with the robotic Harmonic shears (**Figure 49-6**).

Larger hepatic veins are clipped on the graft side with titanium clips or using a 35-mm articulating vascular stapler.

Dissection is carried up to the right hepatic vein after stepwise takedown of the caval ligament.

Step 2 average time frame: 35–40 min

▶▶ **TIPS**

Hanging a short hepatic vein with a 10-cm 2-0 Vicryl™ suture can help in placing clips or sutures properly.

EDITORIAL COMMENT

Suturing with Prolene™ 4-0/5-0 is always the safest way. There is less risk of sliding, less interference with stapling as with clips, and more secure sealing when compared to bipolar or Harmonic®.

If a large dominant short hepatic vein is present, draining segments 5 and 6, it may require a bench reconstruction once the organ has been perfused with cold solution.

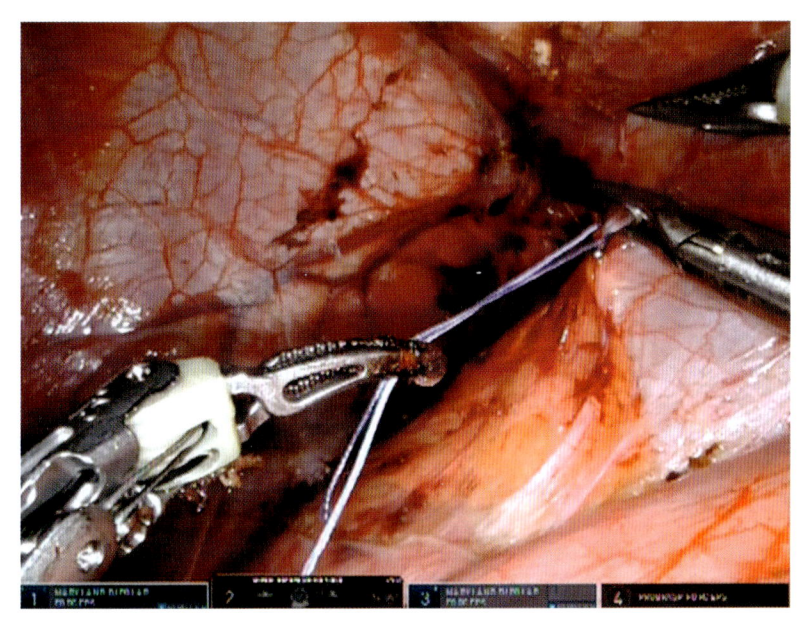

FIGURE 49-6 • Isolating the short hepatic veins.

1004   The Foundation and Art of Robotic Surgery

Step 3. Hanging maneuver

▶ **Video 49-4. Step 3. Hanging Maneuver**

Tunneling is performed between the right and middle hepatic veins with gentle dissection using a Maryland forceps in R2 from below. A 10-Fr silicon Foley catheter is passed through this tunnel to be used later for the hanging maneuver (**Figures 49-7** and **49-8**).

Step 3 average time frame: 10–15 min

> ▶▶ **TIPS**
> After the tip of the Foley is out of the tunnel, putting a Hem-o-lok® clip on the upper end of the Foley catheter will prevent the catheter from slipping downward.

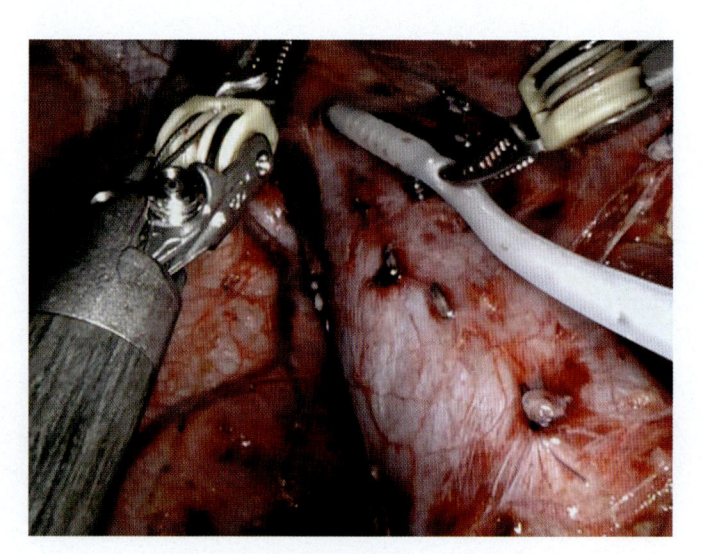

FIGURE 49-7 • Hanging maneuver.

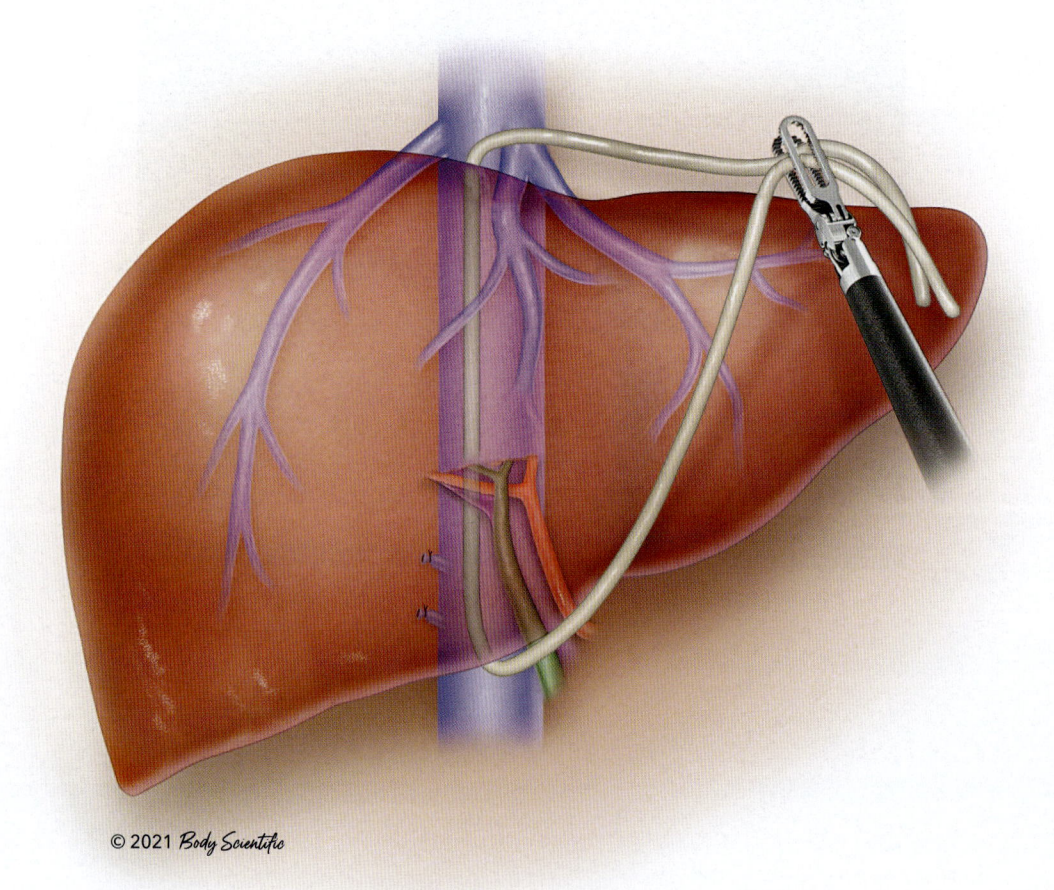

FIGURE 49-8 • Hanging maneuver.

Step 4. Gallbladder dissection

▶ **Video 49-5.** Step 4. Gallbladder Dissection

After the right liver is positioned back in its anatomical position by releasing tension with the ProGrasp™ in R3, the gallbladder is dissected from its fossa in an anterograde fashion with upward pressure from the ProGrasp™ on segment 4 (**Figure 49-9**). The cystic artery and duct are identified, clipped, and cut. The gallbladder is then delivered with an Endobag™ through the umbilical port (or through the GelPort® if present from the beginning).

Step 4 average time frame: 5–10 min

> **EDITORIAL COMMENT**
>
> Leaving a long stump of the cystic duct may allow a better grasping point for retraction. The redundant stump can be resected at the end of the procedure.

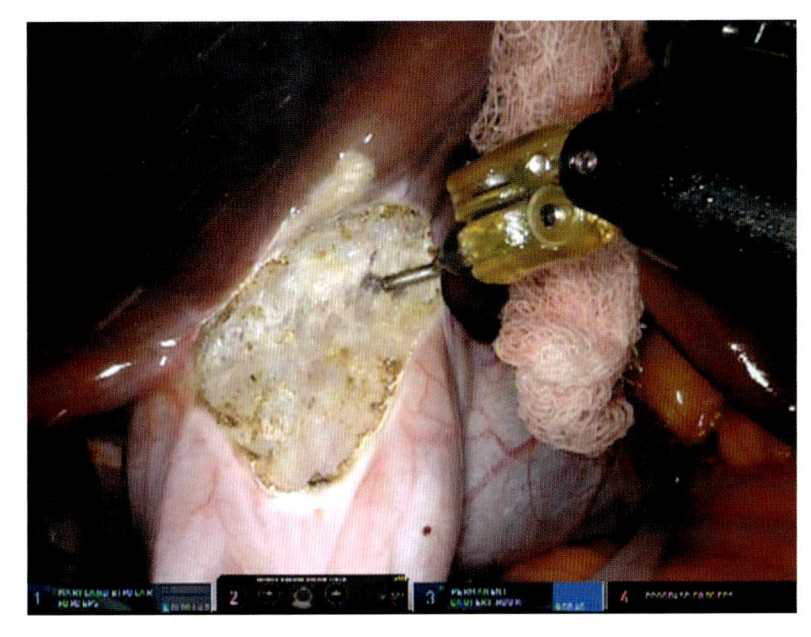

FIGURE 49-9 • Cholecystectomy.

Hilum Dissection

Step 5. Dissection of right hepatic artery and right portal vein

▶ **Video 49-6. Step 5. Dissection of Right Hepatic Artery and Right Portal Vein**

With the cystic duct retracted by the bedside surgeon upward and to the left side, the console surgeon starts to dissect the hilum with Maryland dissectors in R1 and R2 while the Pro-Grasp™ in R3 is supporting segment 4 upward.

The entire hilar dissection stays strictly on the right side of the main bile duct and ends by complete isolation and encircling of both the right hepatic artery and right portal vein with vessel loops.

Meticulous dissection of the right portal vein until identification of the bifurcation is very crucial to avoid encircling the main portal vein (for more details, see Chapter 33, Right Hepatectomy).

Step 5 average time frame: 25–30 min

> ▶▶ **TIPS**
>
> Encircling the right portal vein will help in temporarily applying a bulldog clamp for the demarcation test and later on in applying the stapler to cut the right portal vein.
>
> Gentle handling of the artery is recommended to avoid intimal dissection.

> **EDITORIAL COMMENT**
>
> If bleeding is encountered, having a second assistant port can allow the bedside surgeon to maintain exposure/retraction while simultaneously suctioning.

> 🔍 **ANATOMICAL HIGHLIGHTS**
>
> In some biliary anatomical variation (Types 1, 4 and 5), the right posterior or anterior bile ducts drains into the common bile duct separately and will make the dissection of the portal vein more challenging (**Figure 49-10**). Here, the bedside surgeon can help in improving the exposure by lifting the duct upward with forceps to facilitate dissection and encircling the right portal vein. Early transection of bile ducts is not recommended because indocyanine green (ICG) cannot be used in this situation due to bile leakage out of the biliary system.

Living Donor Hepatectomy 1007

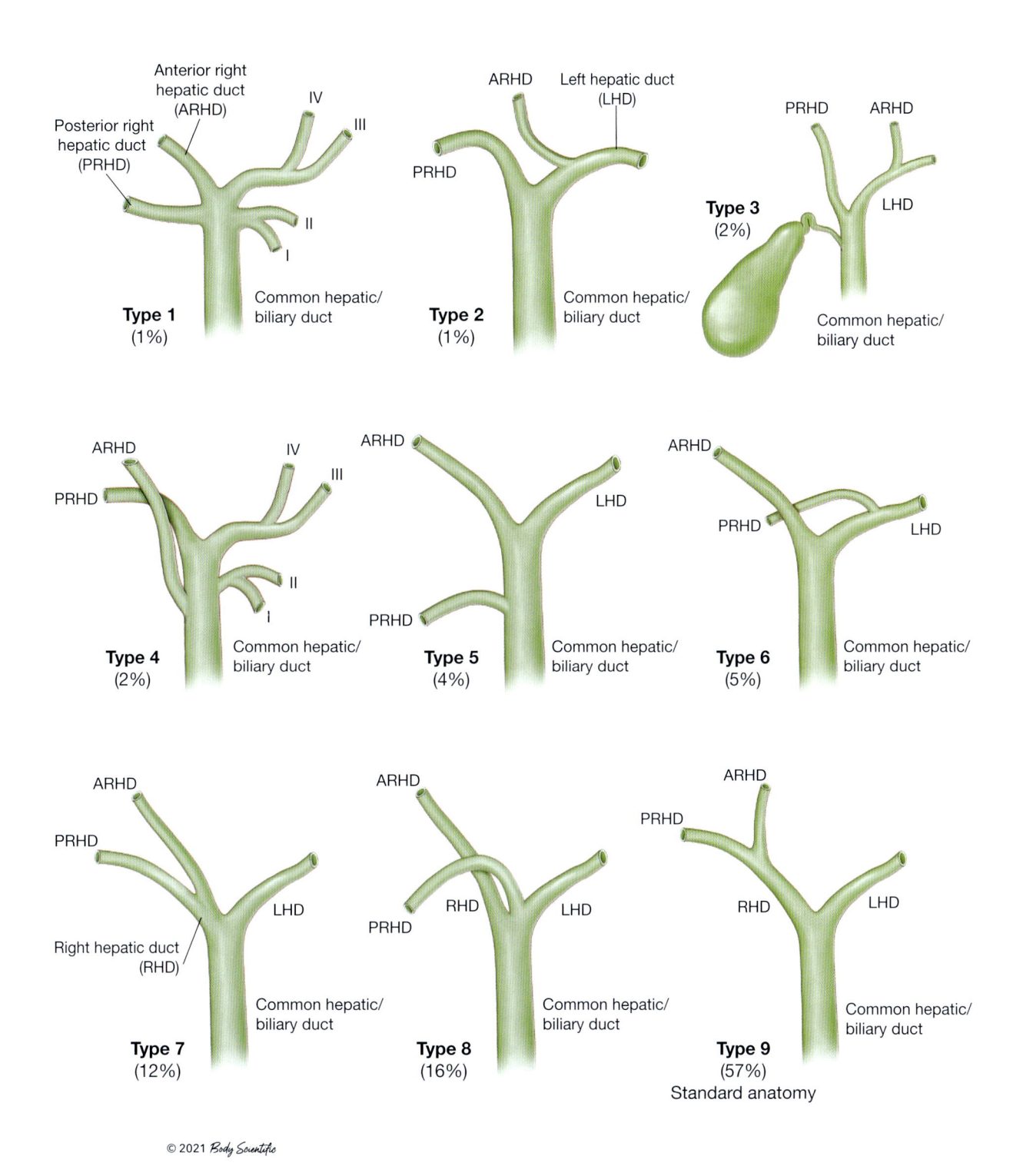

FIGURE 49-10 • Hepatic duct variations.

Step 6. Parenchymal demarcation

▶ **Video 49-7.** Step 6. Parenchymal Demarcation

Both the right hepatic artery and right portal vein are clamped with bulldog clamps introduced via the assistant port, followed by intravenous injection of 2 mg ICG for better identification of the Cantlie's line and for bile duct visualization later (**Figure 49-11**). The liver is positioned back to its anatomical location by releasing tension on the cystic duct and the upward pressure on segment 4. Near-infrared fluorescence view is activated to clarify the demarcation line, which is marked by diathermy from the right hepatic vein to the gallbladder fossa (**Figure 49-12**). Finally, the bulldog clamps are removed, and 2 traction sutures (Prolene™ 2-0) at the edge of the liver on both sides of the demarcation line are used for retraction.

Step 6 average time frame: 10–15 min

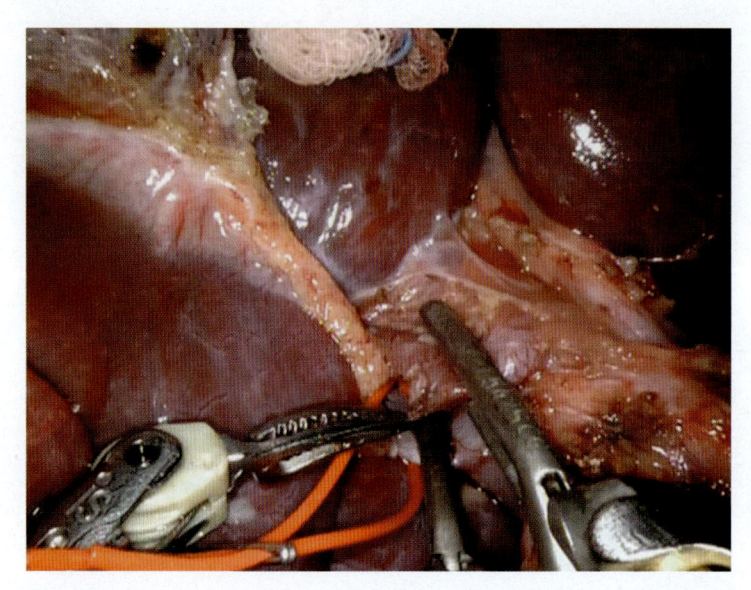

FIGURE 49-11 • Clamping the right hepatic artery and right portal vein.

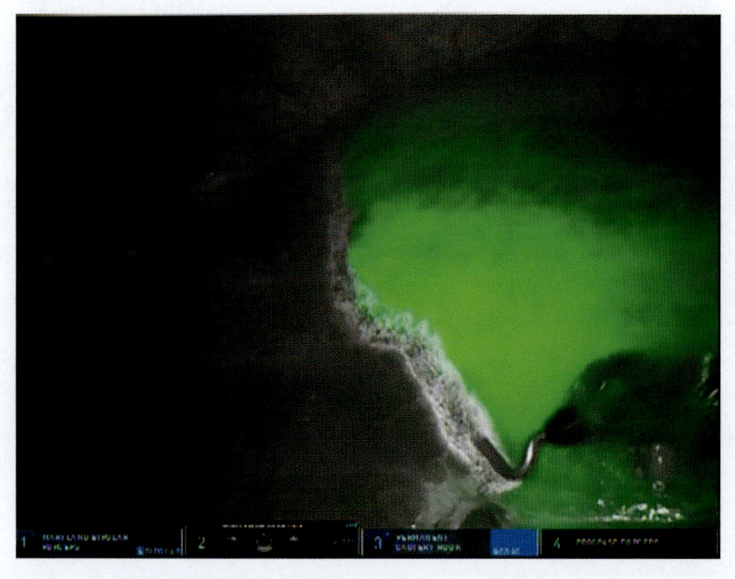

FIGURE 49-12 • Marking the line of perfusion.

Parenchymal Transection

Step 7. Transection of the liver parenchyma

▶ Video 49-8. Step 7. Transection of the Liver Parenchyma

Liver parenchyma transection is performed with Harmonic® shears using open and closed jaw techniques (**Figure 49-13**). Small crossing hepatic veins (<5 mm) are controlled with bipolar coagulation. Large crossing hepatic veins (≥5 mm) are either controlled with sutures (Prolene™ 5-0) or clipped with titanium clips or small vascular staplers.

Step 7 average time frame: 50–60 min

▶▶ **TIPS**

- Adjusting the tension on the traction sutures can help in the exposure of the transection line.
- Hanging large crossing veins with a short segment of Vicryl™ 2-0 suture may help in proper positioning of clips or sutures on both sides.
- Because there is no CUSA™ integrated with the robotic system so far, the bedside surgeon can use suction to clean the field and clear the visualization for the console surgeon.
- The "Open Jaw" technique with the Harmonic® shears is similar to the technique of CUSA™ by only using the active blade to dissect around the vessels and biliary structures in the parenchyma.

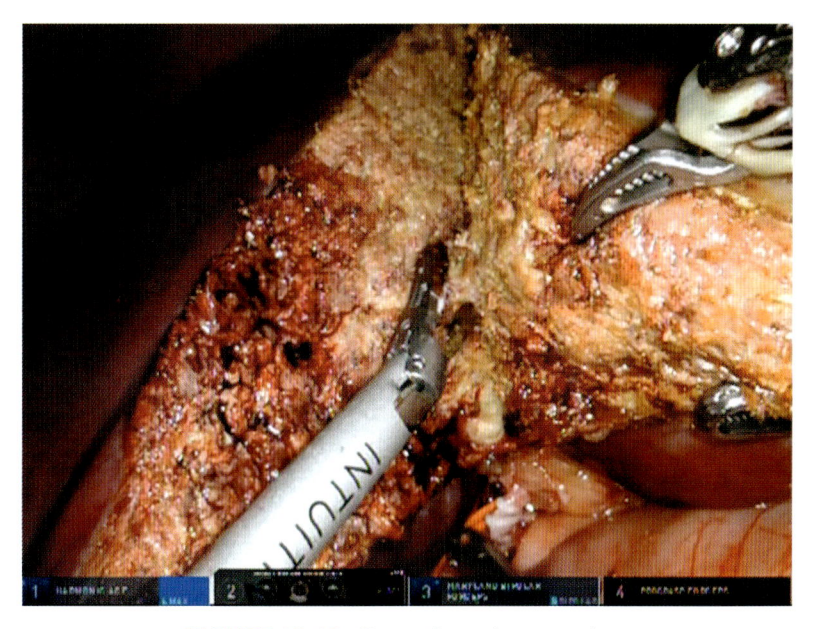

FIGURE 49-13 • Parenchymal transection.

Step 8. Cutting the right hilar plate

▶ **Video 49-9. Step 8. Cutting the Right Hilar Plate**

After completion of 80% of the parenchymal transection, real-time ICG (da Vinci® Firefly™) mode is activated to identify bile duct anatomy, then cutting the right hilar plate including the right bile duct prior to its confluence with the common hepatic duct (**Figure 49-14**). The right bile duct system toward the right lobe should be probed as well as toward the left; the main bile duct should be explored to confirm the biliary anatomy and the presence of a safe passage for further transection of the right hilar plate. Finally, the donor bile duct stump is closed with interrupted monofilament PDS™ 6-0 stitches.

Step 8 average time frame: 25–30 min

▶▶ **TIPS**

The proper position for cutting the right hilar plate is obtained by:
- Lifting segment 4 with the ProGrasp™ in R3.
- Holding the hilar plate with the bipolar Maryland in R2.
- The assistant surgeon should hold the cystic duct in a downward direction to the right.
- Holding the scissors in R1, keeping the right lobe in its anatomical position without tension.

After opening the duct, the biliary system is explored by a lacrimal probe to document integrity of main donor bile duct bifurcation (**Figure 49-15**). Moreover, the probe together with real-time ICG will help in guidance for further cutting of the right hilar plate with right line of transection.

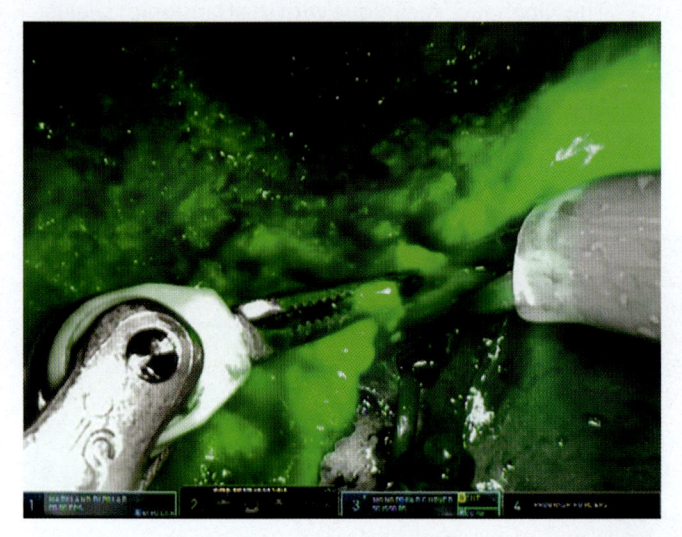

FIGURE 49-14 • Identifying the bile duct anatomy with ICG.

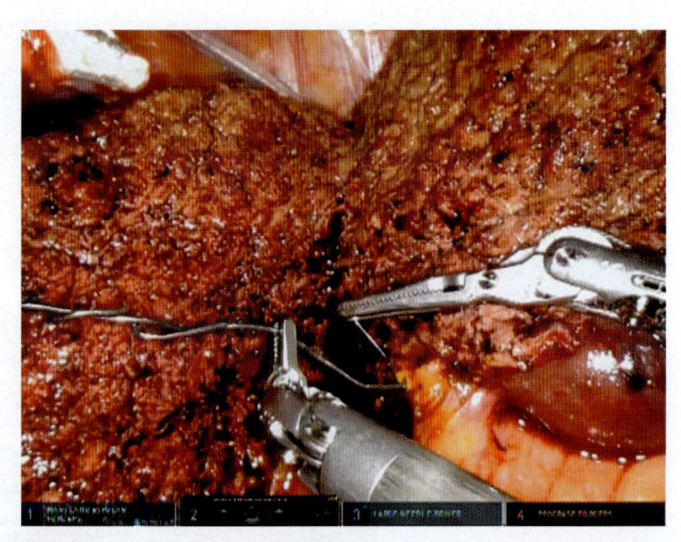

FIGURE 49-15 • Exploring the biliary system with a lacrimal probe.

Step 9. Completion of parenchymal transection

After cutting the hilar plate and closing the bile duct stump on the donor side, completion of the parenchymal transection is achieved by cutting the caudate lobe above the Foley catheter, and then the catheter is placed between the right hilar structure (right hepatic artery and right portal vein) and parenchyma (**Figures 49-16** and **49-17**). Both ends of the catheter are held with a ProGrasp™ in R3, and dissection of the remaining part of liver parenchyma is performed with the bipolar Maryland and Harmonic® shears.

Step 9 average time frame: 30–35 min

> ⚠ **PITFALLS**
>
> Transection of the parenchyma should, at all times, be above or on the right of the Foley catheter to avoid IVC injury.

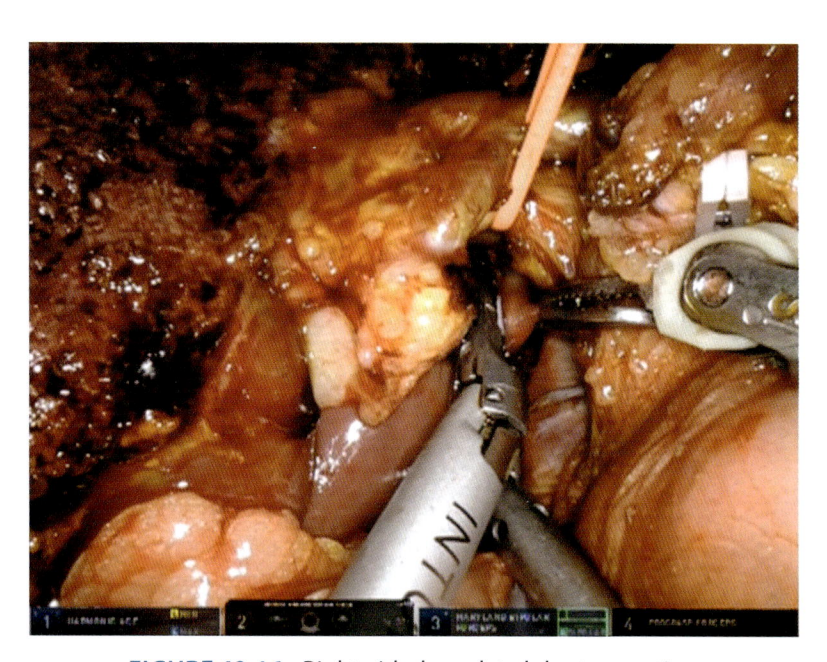

FIGURE 49-16 • Right-sided caudate lobe transection.

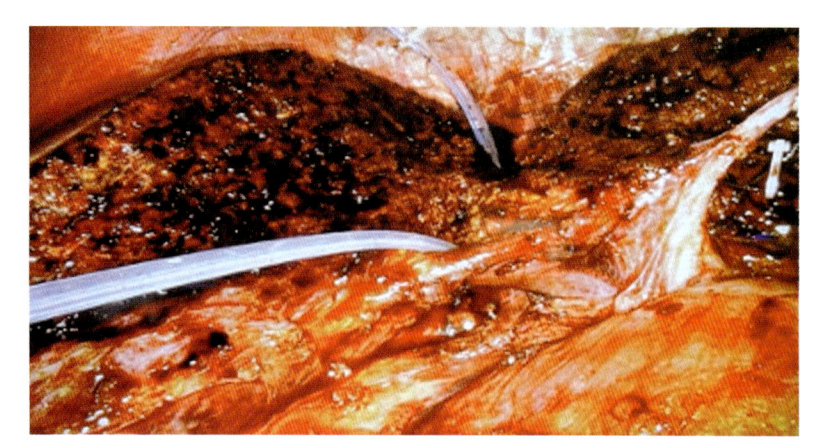

FIGURE 49-17 • Completion of the parenchymal transection with the hanging maneuver.

Step 10. Pfannenstiel incision

Almost 3 cm above the suprapubic bone, a Pfannenstiel incision is performed; the length of the incision is different according to the weight of the liver graft with an average 9–12 cm length. The peritoneum and the posterior rectal fascia are left intact, and a port of 15 mm is inserted into the abdomen. A 15-mm Endo Catch™ retrieval pouch (Medtronic Inc.) is inserted through the cannula. The right lobe, still connected with the inflow and outflow, is partially inserted inside the Endo Catch™ pouch to speed up the final steps.

Step 10 average time frame: 25–30 min

> **EDITORIAL COMMENT**
>
> If a GelPort® is used since the beginning of the operation, the specimen inside the Endo Catch™ pouch is retrieved removing the GelPort® from the wound.

Step 11. Vascular control

▶ Video 49-10. Step 11. Vascular Control

The right hepatic artery is double clipped with Hem-o-lok® clips on the right side of the bile duct; the right portal vein is secured with a 35-mm articulating power vascular stapler (**Figures 49-18 A, B**). The right hepatic vein is controlled with a 60-mm Endo GIA™ curved vascular stapler (**Figure 49-19**).

Step 11 average time frame: 20–25 min

> **▶▶ TIPS**
>
> - Downward traction of the right lobe with R2 should be applied to position the stapler properly.
> - The console surgeon during the stapled division of the main vessels should be ready for additional maneuvers in case of unexpected bleeding or malfunctioning (suturing, clipping).

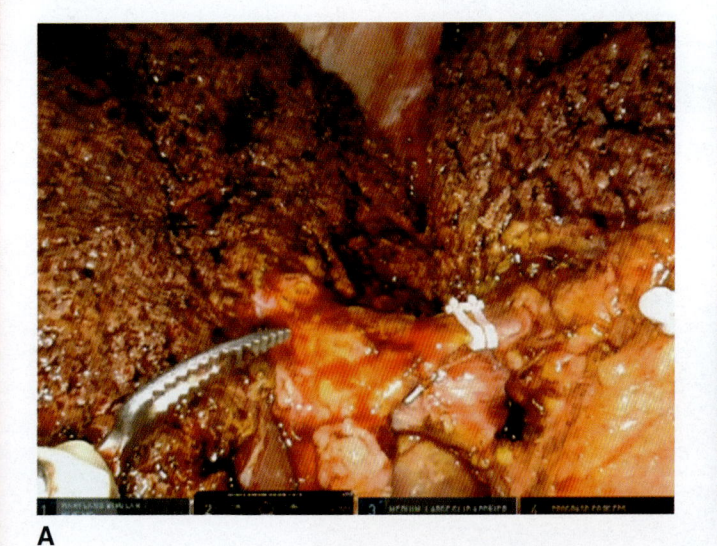

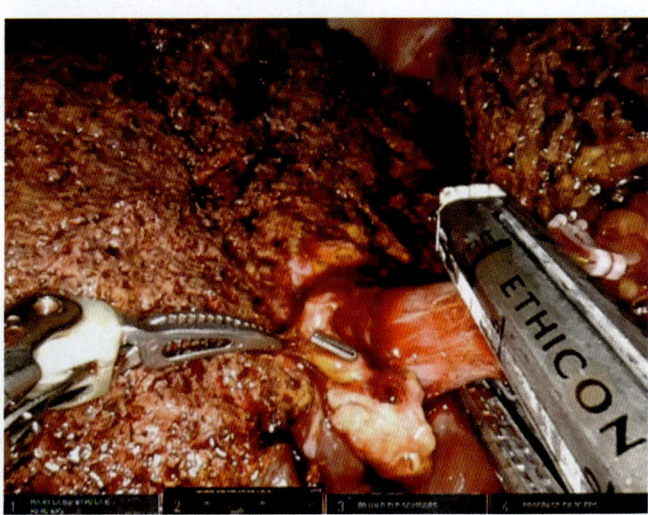

FIGURE 49-18 • **A.** Transecting the hepatic artery. **B.** Transecting the portal vein.

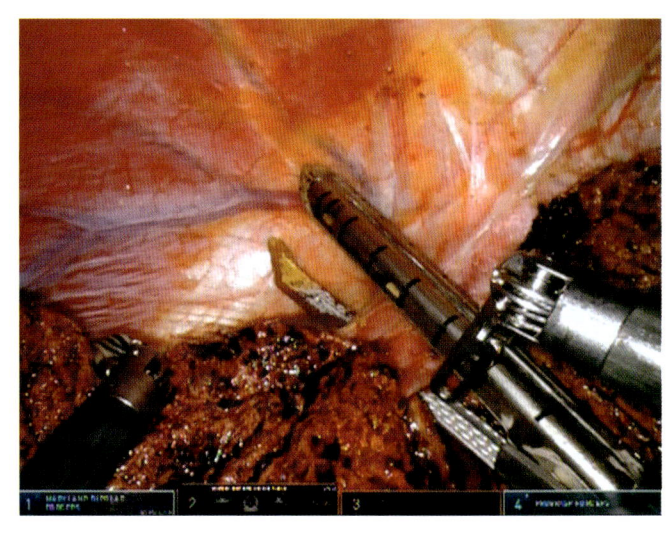

FIGURE 49-19 • Securing the right hepatic vein with a vascular stapler.

Step 12. Retrieval of the right lobe

The Endo Catch™ pouch is closed under vision, and the graft is retrieved enlarging the opening of the fascia and peritoneum at the Pfannenstiel site (**Figure 49-20**). On the back table, the clips and staple line are removed, and perfusion with histidine tryptophan ketoglutarate (HTK) solution (Custodiol®, Franz Köhler Chemie, Germany) is started with a range of 5–8 minutes of warm ischemia time.

Step 12 average time frame: 8–10 min

Step 13. Hemostasis and left lobe fixation

After delivery of the graft and Pfannenstiel incision closure, the cut surface and hilar plate are checked multiple times for hemostasis with any bleeding controlled. All small accessory bile ducts in the hilar plate have to be sutured or clipped as well. Then, the stumps on the right hepatic artery and right portal vein are checked. The falciform ligaments are reconstructed in order to increase the stability of the left hepatic lobe avoiding torsion of the left hepatic vein with possible outflow obstruction (**Figure 49-21**). Finally, a hemostatic agent is placed on the cut surface and a drain placed on the right side.

Step 13 average time frame: 10–15 min

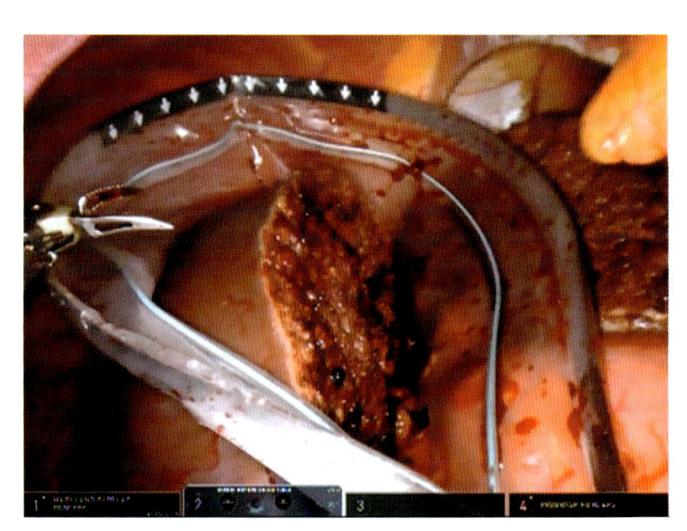

FIGURE 49-20 • Retrieving the right hepatic lobe.

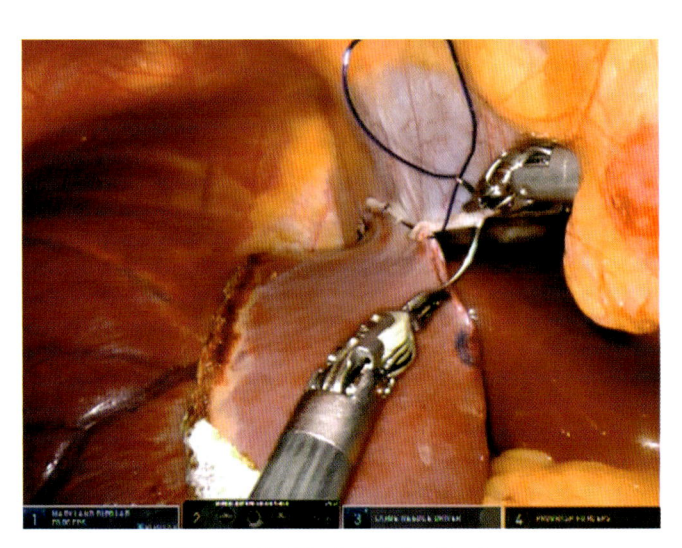

FIGURE 49-21 • Left lobe fixation.

Suggested Readings

1. Broering DC, Elsheikh Y, Alnemary Y, et al. Robotic versus open right lobe donor hepatectomy for adult, living donor liver transplantation: a propensity score-matched analysis. *Liver Transpl.* 2020;26(11):1455-1464.
2. Chen PD, Wu CY, Hu RH, et al. Robotic liver donor right hepatectomy: a pure, minimally invasive approach. *Liver Transpl.* 2016;22(11):1509-1518.
3. Giulianotti PC, Tzvetanov I, Jeon H, et al. Robot-assisted right lobe donor hepatectomy. *Transpl Int.* 2012;25(1):e5-9.
4. Troisi RI, Elsheikh Y, Alnemary Y, et al. Safety and feasibility report of robotic-assisted left lateral sectionectomy for pediatric living donor liver transplantation: a comparative analysis of learning curves and achieved mastery with the laparoscopic approach. *Transplantation.* 2021;105(5):1044-1051.
5. Radtke A, Sotiropoulos GC, Molmenti EP, et al. Transhilar passage in right graft live donor liver transplantation: intrahilar anatomy and its impact on operative strategy. *Am J Transplant.* 2012;12(3):718-727.
6. Giulianotti PC, Coratti A, Angelini M, et al. Robotics in general surgery: personal experience in a large community hospital. *Arch Surg.* 2003;138(7):777-784. doi: 10.1001/archsurg.138.7.777

SECTION XII

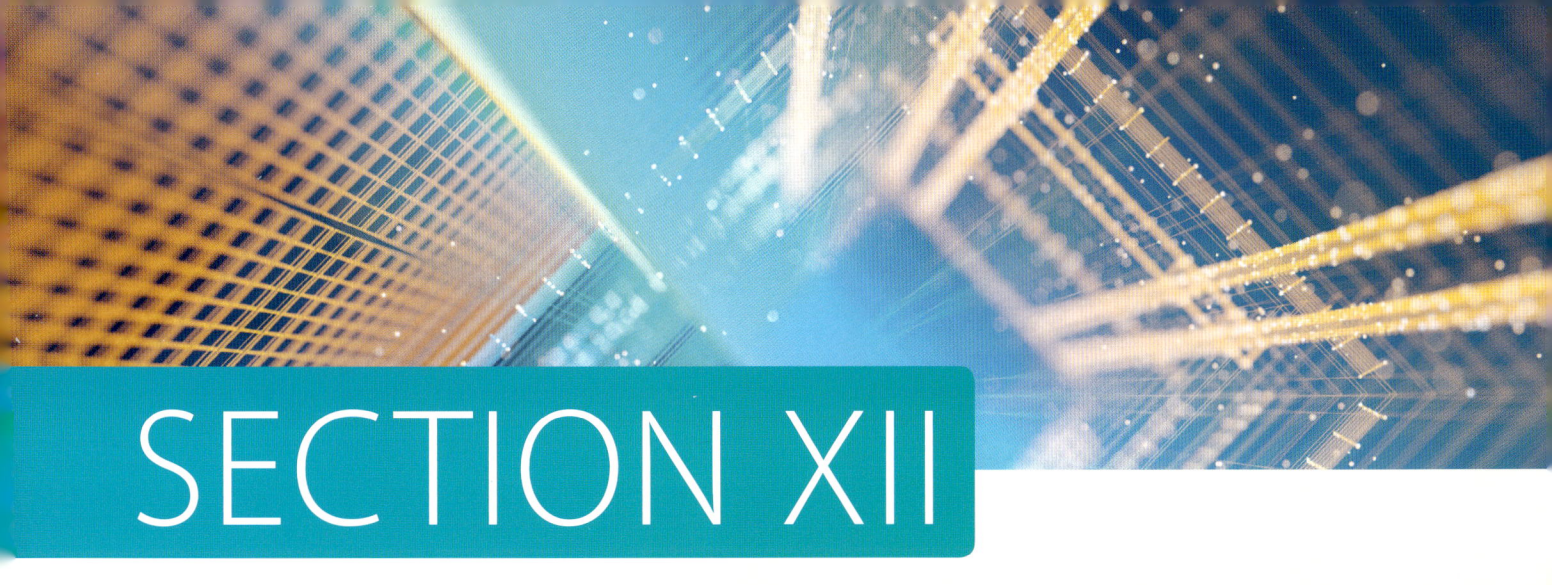

Additional Procedures

Chapter 50 • Renal Aneurysm 1017
Valentina Valle • Stephan Gruessner • Alberto Mangano • Pier Cristoforo Giulianotti

Chapter 51 • Single Port Robotic Surgery: Basic Concepts (Procedures Still
Not FDA Approved/Off-Label Indication) 1037
Nicolas Hellmuth Dreifuss • Antonio Cubisino • Francesco Maria Bianco

"In life, one should never give up, surrender oneself to mediocrity, but rather move out of that 'gray area' where everything is a habit and passive resignation ..."

—Rita Levi Montalcini (1909–2012)

Renal Aneurysm

Valentina Valle • Stephan Gruessner • Alberto Mangano • Pier Cristoforo Giulianotti

INTRODUCTION

Renal artery aneurysms (RAAs) were once considered a rare finding in the general population. However, they have been diagnosed more frequently, in recent years, due to the advancements in imaging technology. In fact, there are interesting contradictory data: the autoptic rates are quite low, in the range of <0.01–0.09%; the computed tomography (CT) rates are about 0.7%; and the arteriogram incidence is even higher, ranging between 0.3% and 2.5% (and up to 9.7% in some reports).

In terms of natural history, studies showed that spontaneous ruptures were not common during a more than 20-year surveillance period. The reported growth ranges between 0.06 and 0.6 mm per year, and the rupture rate is approximately 3–5% (for more information, see suggested reading #1).

RAAs are more frequent in females (up to over 70%), mostly suffering from hypertension, and in the age range 40–60 years old, sometimes in association with fibromuscular dysplasia. In terms of clinical presentation, RAAs are mainly asymptomatic. Symptoms occur in only 4–23% of cases and usually consist of abdominal/flank pain and hematuria; occasionally, a renal bruit can be appreciated at the auscultation. Even though the aneurysms may have different shapes, they are more frequently saccular, and mainly located at the arterial bifurcations, often being multiple, and bilateral in 10–20% of cases. RAAs are often calcified (from 18% to 70%) with a thromboembolism rate ranging from 8% to 11% (for more information, see suggested reading #1).

There has been a significant development in the treatment of RAAs. The guidelines are evolving, and open surgical repair still remains the standard in the majority of institutions, especially with complex RAAs located at a bifurcation and/or involving distal branches. The description of the

INSTRUMENT REQUIREMENTS

The suggested main robotic instruments/tools can be listed as follows:
- 30° scope
- Needle drivers (large or black diamond micro)
- Cautery hook
- Vessel sealer
- Bipolar forceps
- Cadière forceps
- Round-tip scissors
- Robotic linear staplers (with different loads)
- Hem-o-lok® clips
- Medium–large clip applier

The suggested main laparoscopic instruments/tools can be listed as follows:
- Needle driver
- Atraumatic graspers
- Suction-irrigation
- GelPort®, wound protector

Supplemental materials:
- Gauzes, sponges
- Small/medium/large clips
- Robotic bulldog clamps (Scanlan® Reliance Bulldog Clamp)
- Hemostatic agents
- Vessel loops
- Sutures: Prolene™ 4-0, 5-0, and 6-0
- Polytetrafluoroethylene Suture (PTFE-Suture) CV-5/CV-6/CV-7
- Vascular tray (including different clamps for possible hand assistance or conversion)

Photo reproduced with permission from Abbott A. Neuroscience: one hundred years of Rita. Nature. 2009;458(7238):564-567.
Quote reproduced with permission from Melino G, Benedetti B, Bazan N. On Rita Levi-Montalcini. Mol Neurobiol. 2013;47(2):443-445.

open techniques is outside of the scope of this chapter; however, in summary, they can include a wide range of options such as: in situ aneurismectomy and bypass, bench surgery, autotransplant, and nephrectomy, and some of these are very invasive.

Endovascular approaches are growing due to the innovative materials and instrumentations; however, the location of the aneurysm often limits their adoption. Stenting can only be performed when the RAA involves the main renal artery without the side branches. Coil embolization requires a saccular aneurysm with a narrow neck.

The laparoscopic approach has been proposed as a possible option, but it has not gained widespread acceptance, due to its well-known inherent technical limitations. For this reason, only a few laparoscopic cases have been reported.

Since the first robotic RAA repair, which was performed by P.C. Giulianotti in 2002 (and published in 2003), the robotic approach has repeatedly been proven feasible and safe, even for complex repairs. However, to prevent complications and functional damages associated with prolonged warm ischemia, considerable experience and technical proficiency are required.

Indications and Relative Contraindications to the Robotic Approach

The indications of the robotic approach are the same ones valid for the treatment of the aneurysm: aneurysm diameter >2 cm, rapid rate of enlargement, severe hypertension, symptomatic aneurysms (flank/abdominal pain and hematuria), focal renal infarction, and high-risk aneurysms in pregnancy. Obese patients can particularly benefit from the robotic approach. A comprehensive preoperative workup is crucial to establish the most appropriate treatment.

Patient Positioning, OR Setup, and Port Setting

The patient is placed supine on a beanbag, with both arms tucked. When prepping the abdomen, the proximal lower limbs should be included, for femoral access, in case a segment of the greater saphenous vein is needed for grafting (**Figures 50-1 A, B**).

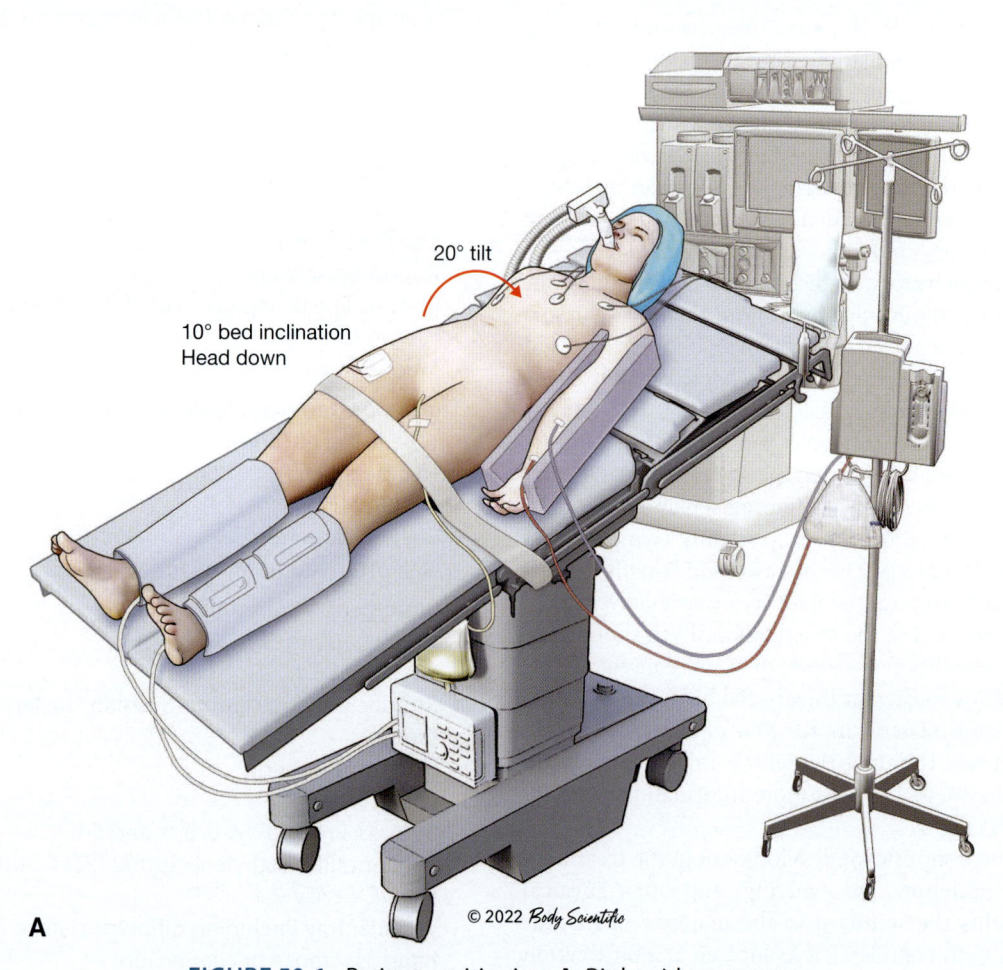

FIGURE 50-1 • Patient positioning. **A.** Right-side aneurysm.

Renal Aneurysm 1019

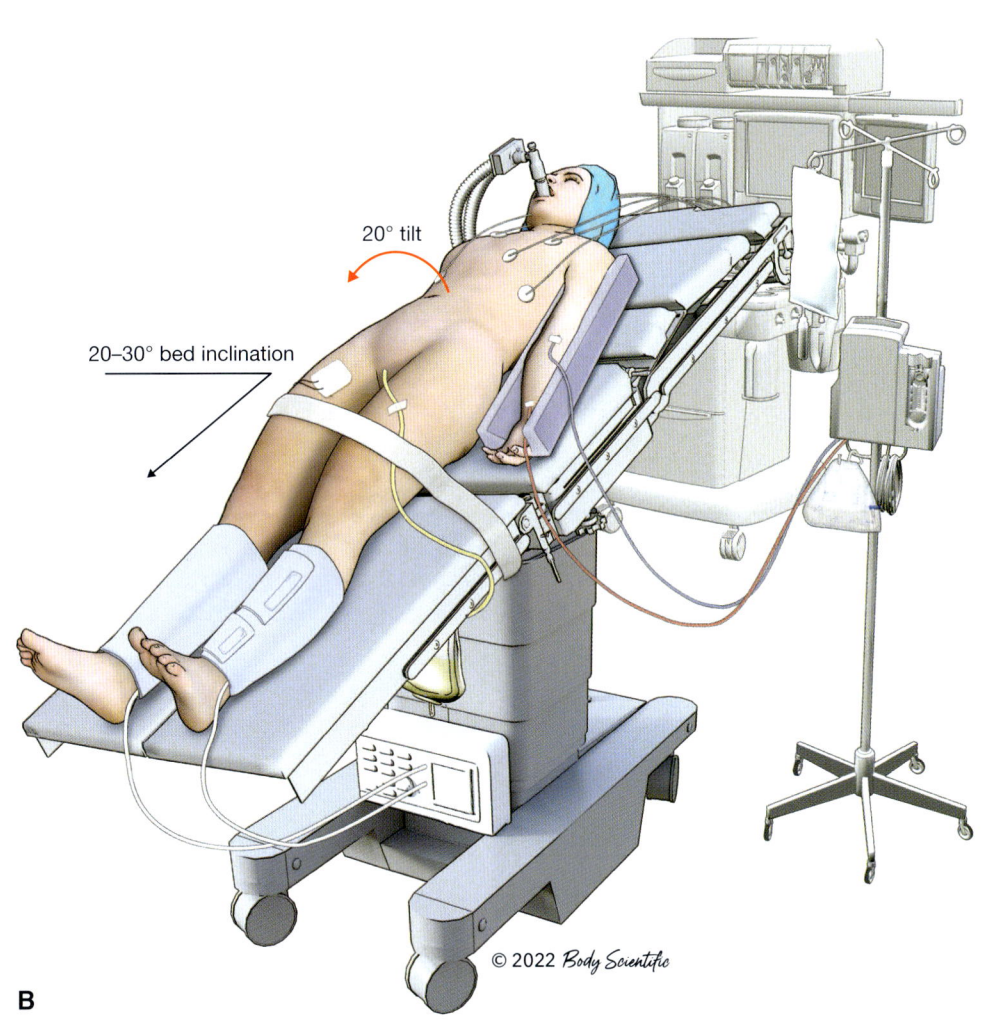

FIGURE 50-1 • (*Continued*) **B.** Left-side aneurysm.

The robotic cart is placed on the same side as the aneurysm. The assistant stays on the opposite side, with a second assistant or a scrub nurse targeting the lesion. The OR setup is depicted in **Figures 50-2 A, B**.

The pneumoperitoneum is achieved by the Veress technique, at the modified Palmer's point.

When the proper pressure is reached, a 5-mm optic trocar is placed in the left or right lateral upper quadrant (opposite to the side of the aneurysm) to access laparoscopically the abdominal space and to allow for the other trocars to be positioned under direct visualization (for more details, see Chapter 2, The Basic Principles of Clinical Applications).

For right RAAs, the trocars are placed along an oblique straight line going from the right lower to the left upper quadrant. For left RAAs, four 8-mm trocars are placed along a similar oblique line from the left lower to the right upper quadrant. Two 10–12-mm assistant ports are required. For right RAAs, one is between the scope and the R1, and the other

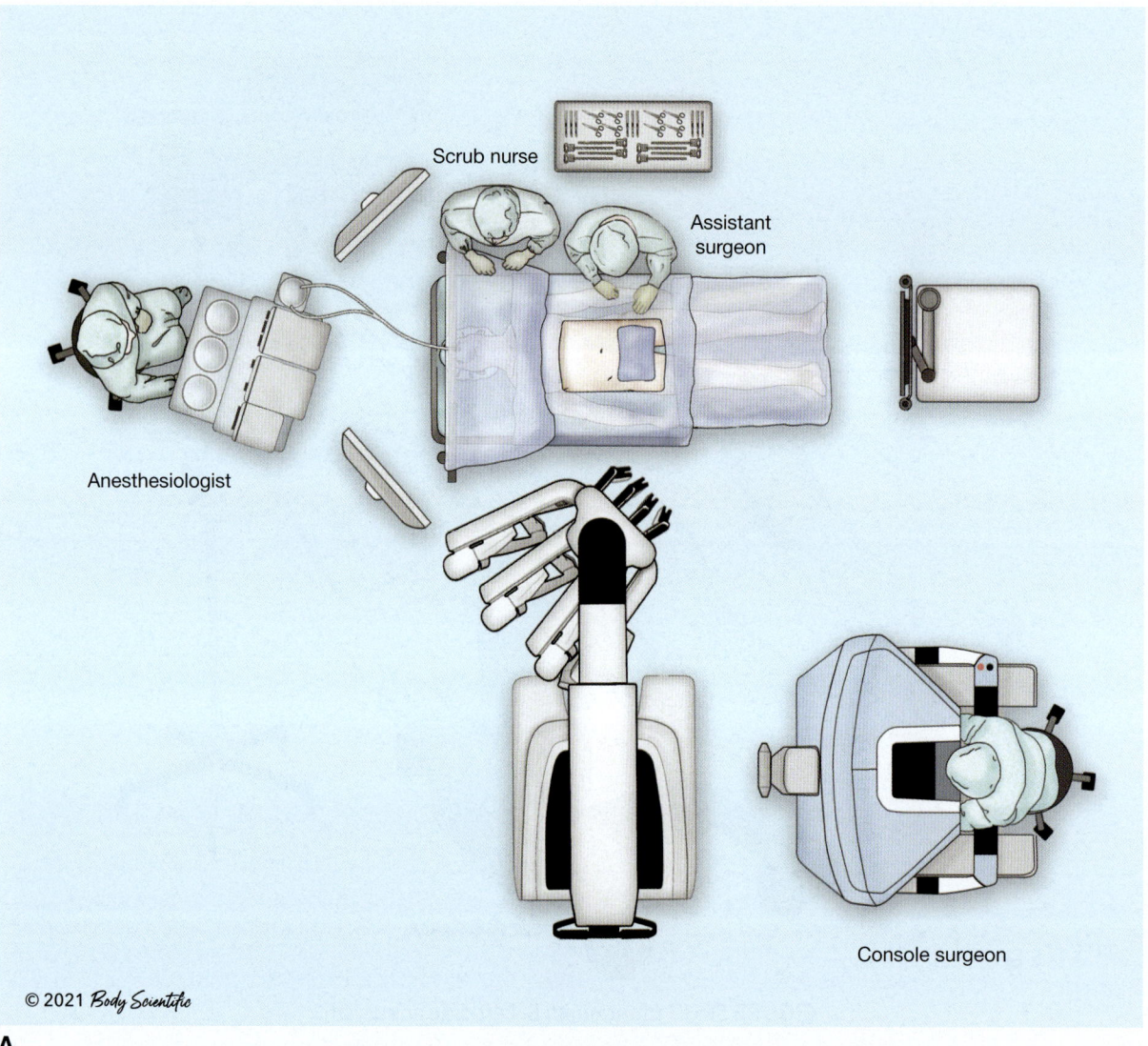

FIGURE 50-2 • OR setup. **A.** Right-side aneurysm.

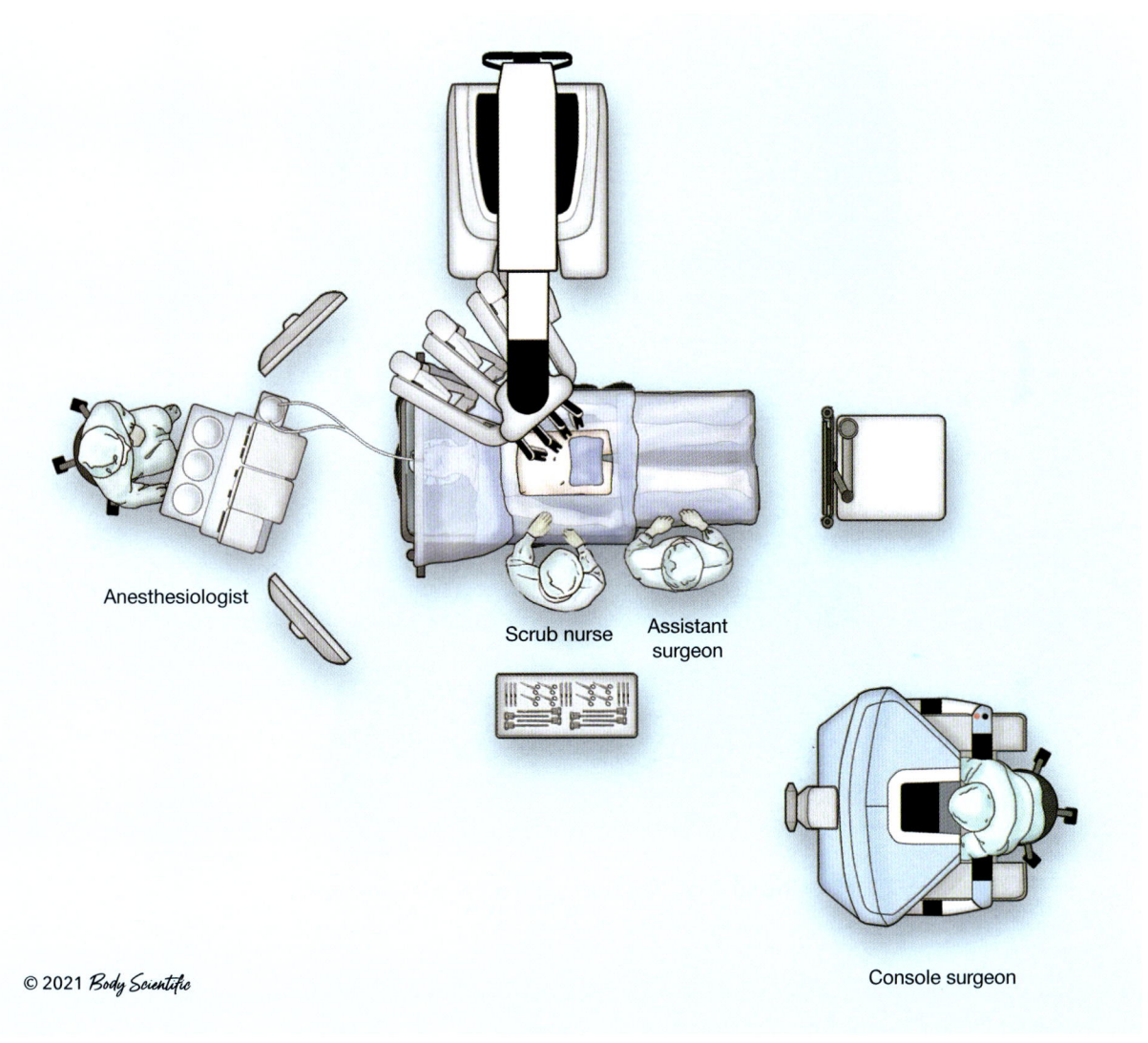

Renal Aneurysm 1021

FIGURE 50-2 • (Continued) B. Left-side aneurysm.

between the R1 and the R3. For left RAAs, one is positioned between the scope and the R2, and the other between the R2 and the R3 (**Figures 50-3 A, B**).

Once all the trocars are in place, the table is laterally tilted, lifting the affected kidney (~20°). For right RAAs, the table is adjusted in slight Trendelenburg (~10°) to aid during the hepatic retraction.

For left RAAs, the table is in reverse Trendelenburg (20–30°) to inferiorly shift the bowel by gravity.

Normal abdomen

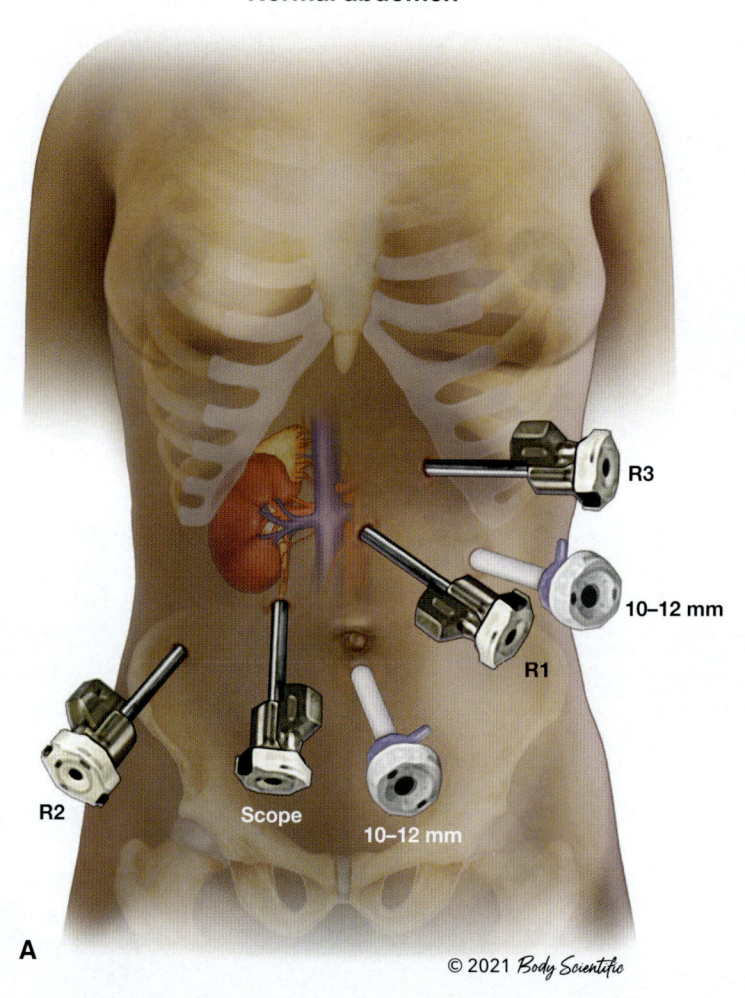

FIGURE 50-3 • **A.** Port setting for right-side aneurysm.

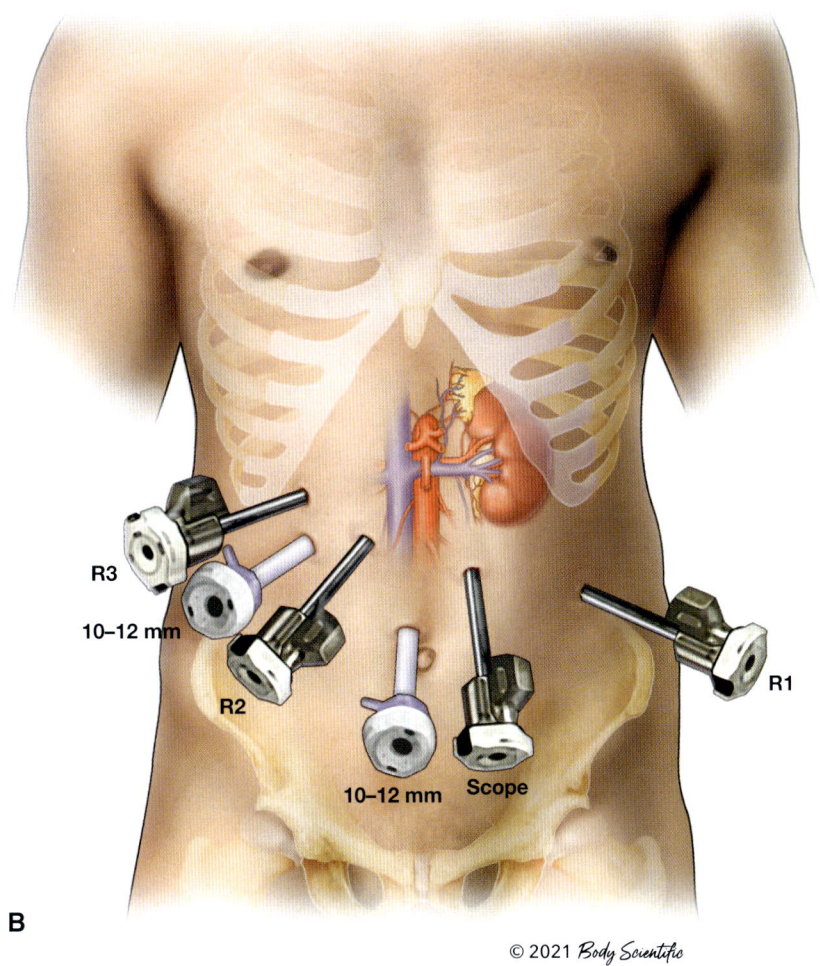

FIGURE 50-3 • (*Continued*) **B.** Port setting for left-side aneurysm.

Surgical Technique

▶ **Video 50-1.** Right Renal Aneurysm – Full Procedure

▶ **Video 50-2.** Left Renal Aneurysm – Full Procedure

Some reminders about the anatomy and the most common locations of RAAs are depicted in **Figures** 50-4 and 50-5, respectively.

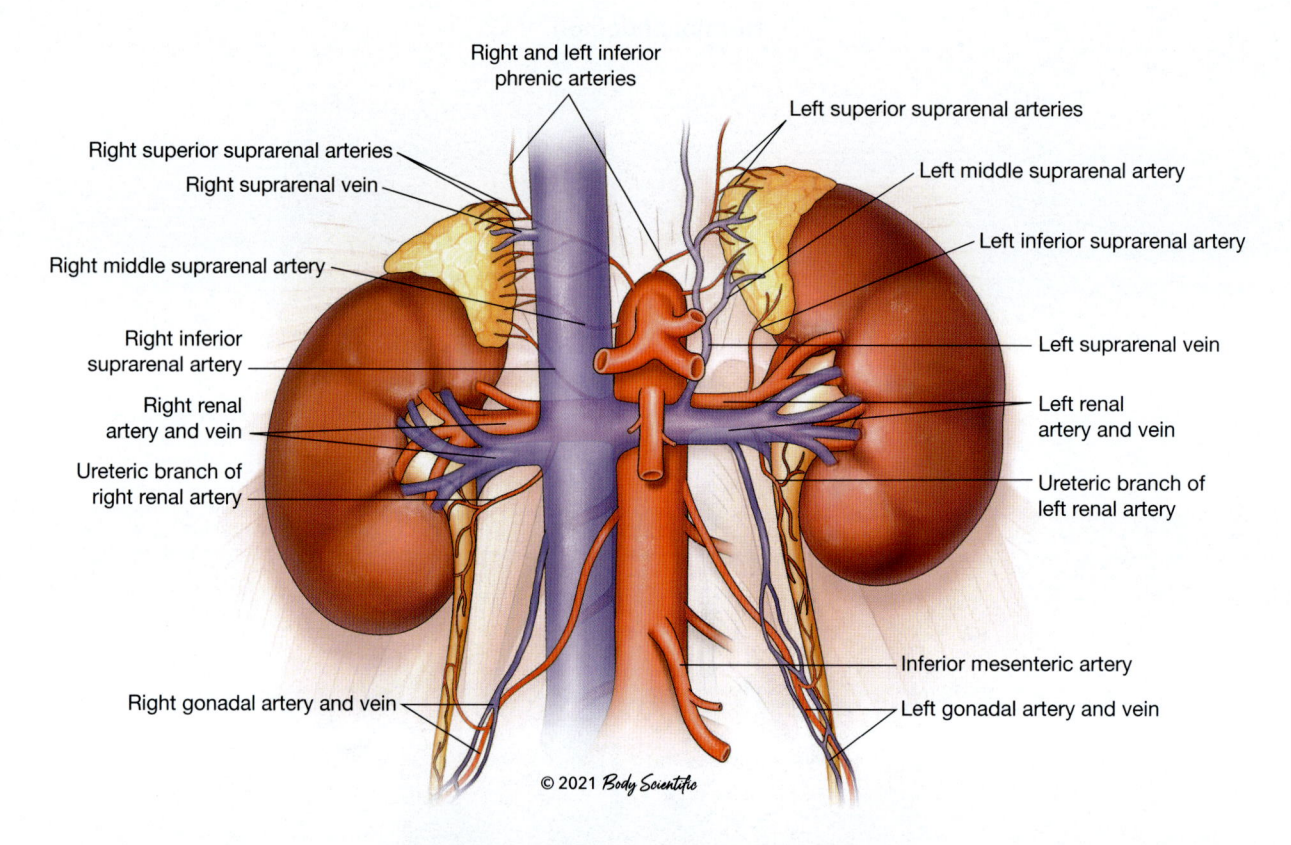

FIGURE 50-4 • Arterial and venous renal anatomy.

Renal Aneurysm 1025

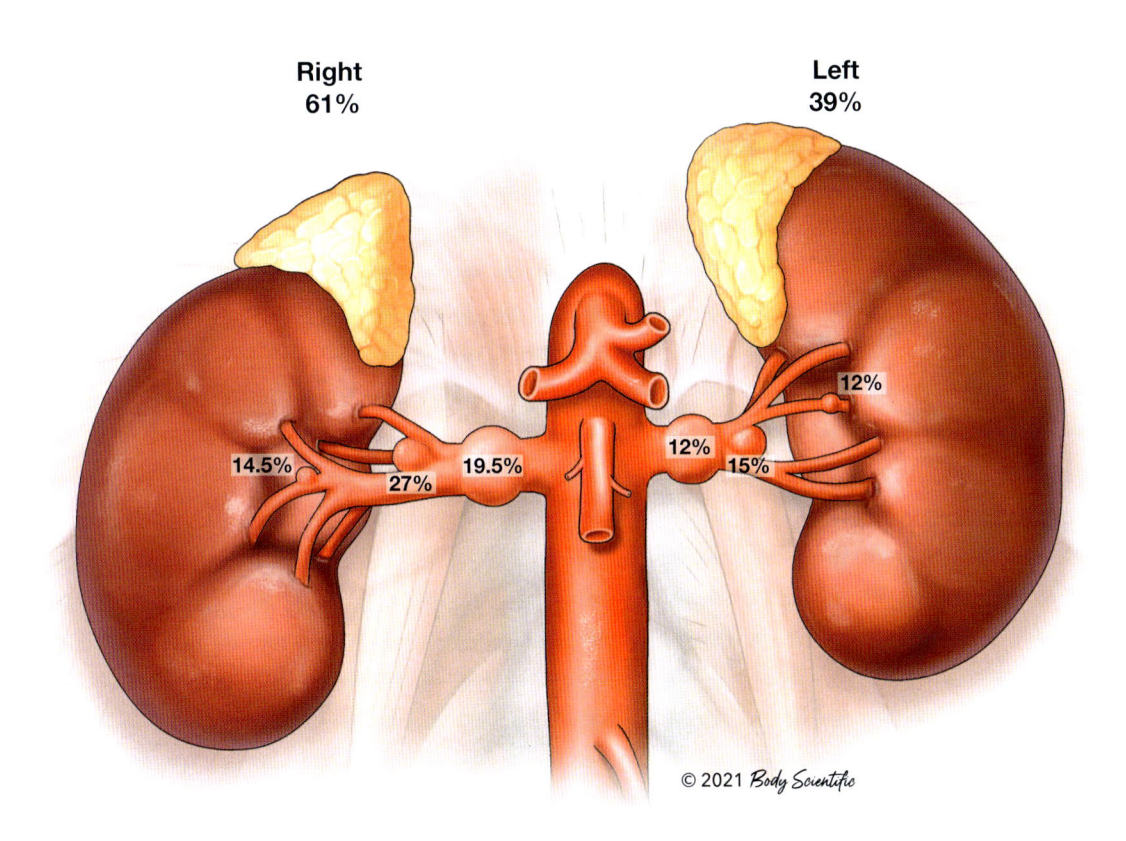

FIGURE 50-5 • Possible locations of RAAs (see suggested reading #2).

▶ Video 50-3. Phase A (Right Side)

PHASE A (EXPOSURE OF THE SURGICAL FIELD)

Right Side

Step 1. Mobilization of the right colon
The dissection is conducted with the monopolar hook in the R1 and the bipolar forceps in the R2. The hepatocolic ligaments are divided. The right colonic flexure is retracted downward, by the assistant, and the Gerota's capsule is exposed. The ascending colon is dissected free, reaching the right iliac vessels, and visualizing the right ureter.

Step 1 average time frame: 20–30 min

Step 2. Mobilization of the liver (right lobe)
The right lobe of the liver is retracted cephalad by a Cadière forceps, positioned in the R3, and holding a gauze to minimize the risk of parenchymal pressure injuries. The right triangular ligament, and the right side of the coronary ligament, are divided to reach the right adrenal gland, which is the upper limit of the surgical field.

Step 2 average time frame: 15–20 min

> ⚠ **PITFALLS**
>
> When retracting the liver with the R3, it is possible to injure the parenchyma or the gallbladder, which is on the way. Usually, injuries depend on poor mobilization of the liver, unfavorable available space below the diaphragm, direction and forces applied to the tip, and the shaft of the retracting instrument.

Step 3. Partial Kocher maneuver and exposure of the right renal vein and vena cava
The second duodenal portion is gently retracted medially and partially mobilized until the vena cava and the right renal vein are adequately exposed. Generally, a complete Kocher maneuver is not necessary, but the relation between the duodenum and the head of the pancreas with the vena cava is quite variable, and this relation may dictate the amount of dissection.

The goal is the wide exposure of the vena cava and of the space between this vessel and the aorta.

After the Kocher maneuver, the medial retraction of the vena cava becomes easier, and can be achieved by the assistant with atraumatic instruments.

Step 3 average time frame: 15–20 min

▶ Video 50-4. Phase A (Left Side)

Left Side

Step 1. Mobilization of the left colonic flexure and descending colon
The dissection is conducted with the monopolar hook in the R1 and the bipolar forceps in the R2.

The omentum is detached from the left side of the transverse colon (alternatively, the left side of the gastrocolic ligament is divided leaving the omentum attached to the colonic flexure) (for more details, see Chapter 24, Left Colectomy). The splenocolic ligaments are divided.

The insertion of the mesocolon, at the lower edge of the pancreatic body, is detached exposing the Gerota's fascia, and the descending colon is fully mobilized reaching the left iliac vessels.

Step 1 average time frame: 20–30 min

Step 2. Mobilization of the body and tail of the pancreas
The pancreatic body and tail are dissected, in the avascular retropancreatic plane, and they are gently lifted, using a grasper in the R3 with gauze support. The left adrenal gland should be fully exposed.

Step 2 average time frame: 10–15 min

Step 3. Exposure of the left renal vein and aorta
The left renal vein is the main landmark of the dissection and must be clearly exposed (**Figure 50-6**).

Sometimes, lymph-adipose tissue has to be removed in order to visualize the left renal vein with its main tributaries (gonadal and adrenal). The vessel sealer is the best tool for this step because it decreases the leak from the divided lymphatic channels.

Step 3 average time frame: 5–10 min

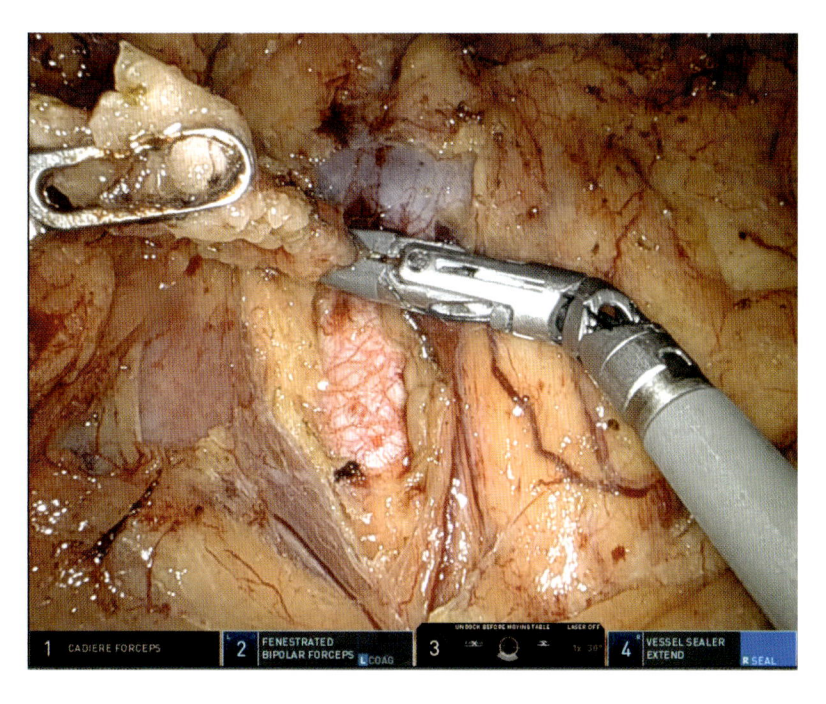

FIGURE 50-6 • Exposure of the left renal vein and aorta.

PHASE B (ANEURYSM CONTROL AND DISSECTION)

Step 4. Intraoperative ultrasonography (IOUS)
At this stage, an IOUS can be very useful. It may confirm the precise position of the aneurysm in relation to the already exposed landmarks. A laparoscopic drop-in probe, which is controlled by the console surgeon, is the best option (**Figure 50-7**).

Step 4 average time frame: 5–10 min

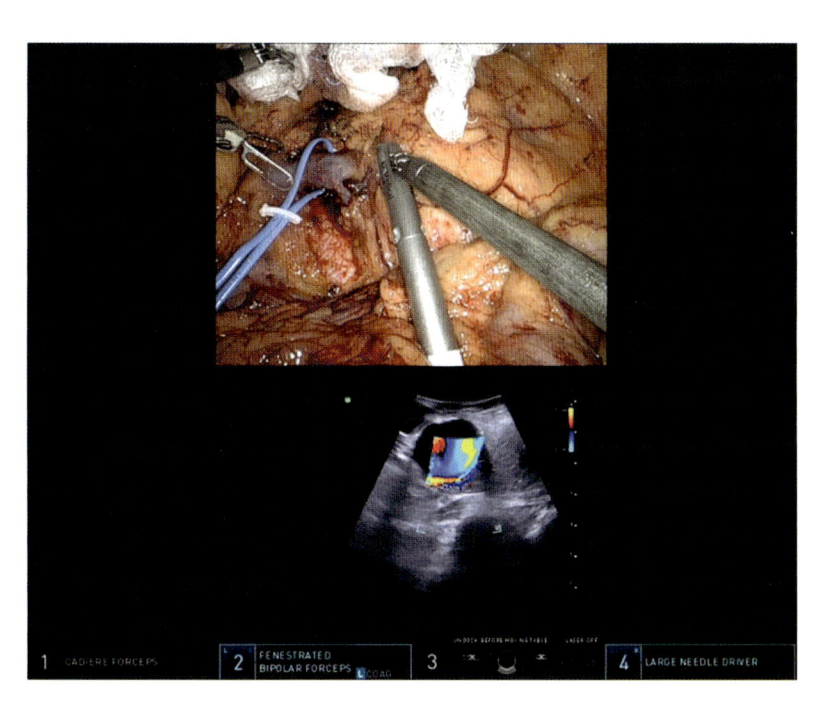

FIGURE 50-7 • Localization of the left renal aneurysm with IOUS.

Step 5. Preparation of the renal vein on a loop

The renal vein can be isolated and encircled with a vessel loop to aid during the retraction.

On the left side, the gonadal vein is merging into the renal vein and must be divided in between sutures of Prolene™ 4-0 or with a stapler (**Figure 50-8**). Attention should be paid to the presence of a posterior lumbar trunk.

On the right side, the gonadal vein is usually merging into the vena cava, and it does not need to be ligated. The use of the vessel loop allows the retraction/manipulation of the vein during the preparation of the artery.

Step 5 average time frame: 10–20 min

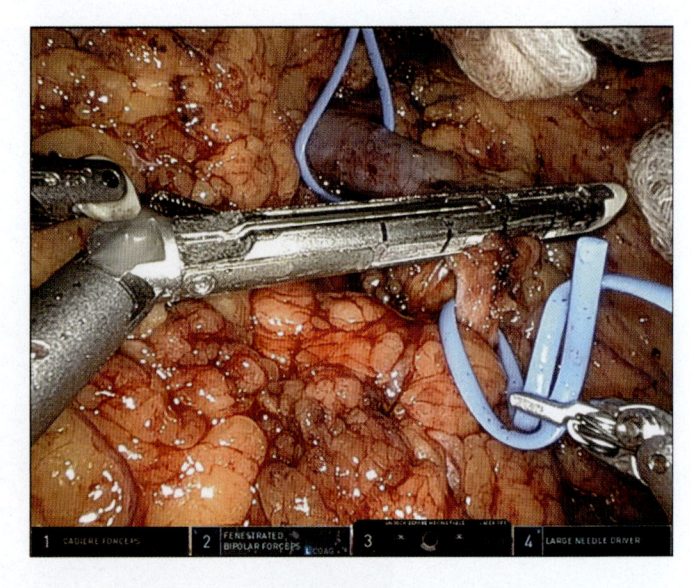

FIGURE 50-8 • Division of the gonadal vein.

▶ Video 50-5. Step 6. Proximal Renal Artery Control (Right Side)

▶ Video 50-6. Step 6. Proximal Renal Artery Control (Left Side)

Step 6. Proximal renal artery control

The proximal control of the renal artery should be addressed before starting the manipulation of the aneurysmatic sac. The dissection and landmarks are different in each side.

On the right side, the proximal segment of the renal artery is behind the vena cava and above the renal vein. Some cooperation, from an experienced assistant, is necessary to improve the retraction of the cava. The proximal artery is controlled with a vessel loop.

On the left side, the proximal segment of the renal artery is located behind (and sometimes above) the renal vein. The assistant may retract the vein while preparing the artery on a vessel loop (**Figures 50-9 A, B**).

Step 6 average time frame: 20–40 min

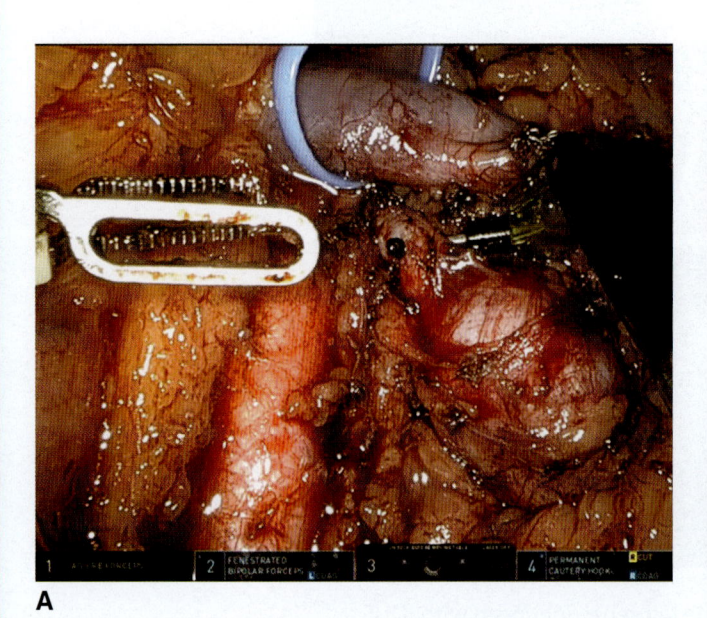

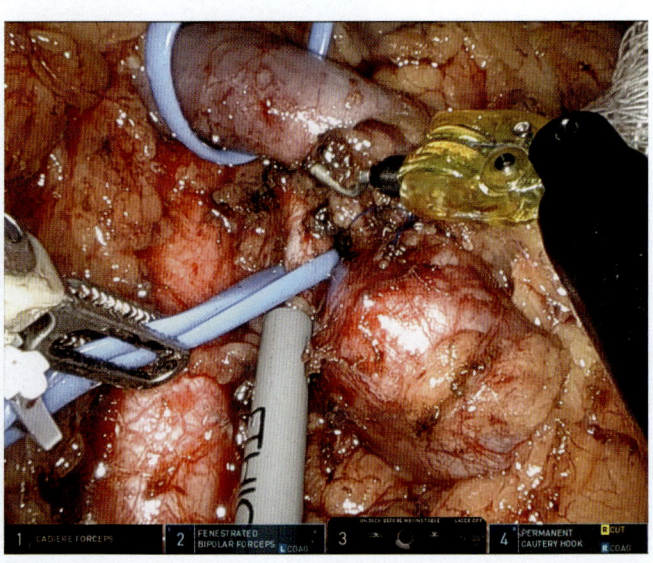

A

B

FIGURE 50-9 • Proximal left renal artery control.

Step 7. Mobilization/isolation of the aneurysmatic sac

A careful dissection of the aneurysmatic sac is usually necessary to localize the efferent artery or the branches that may take origin from the aneurysmatic sac (for more details on types of renal aneurysm, see **Figure 50-10**).

Step 7 average time frame: 15–20 min

> ⚠️ **PITFALLS**
>
> Because the aneurysm wall can be thin and fragile, direct grasping of the aneurysm sac with the robotic forceps increases the risk of rupture. In order to avoid damages, the aneurysm should always be touched indirectly using the side of the instruments.

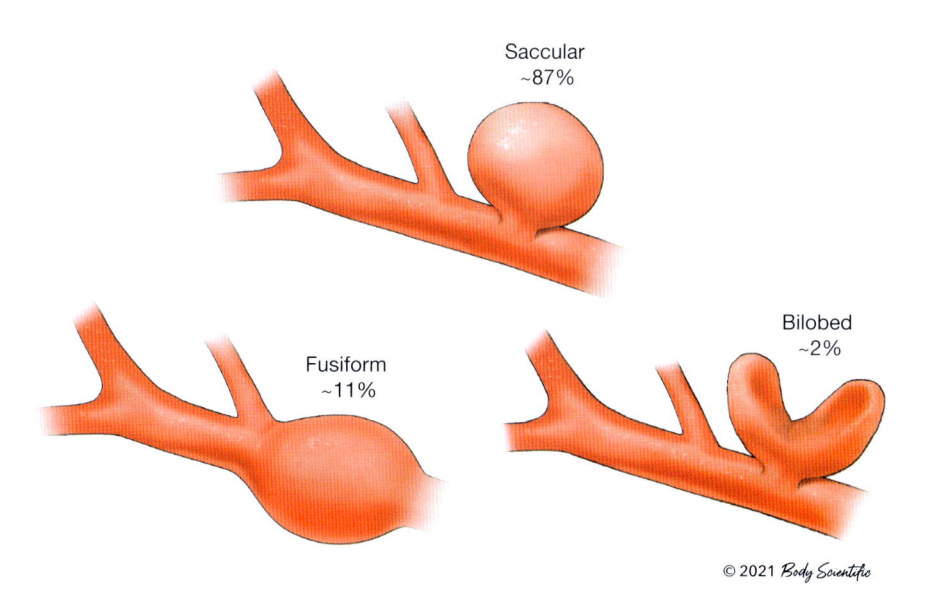

FIGURE 50-10 • Types of renal aneurysms (see suggested reading #2).

▶ **Video 50-7.** Step 8. Preparation of the Distal Branches of the Renal Artery (Right Side)

▶ **Video 50-8.** Step 8. Preparation of the Distal Branches of the Renal Artery (Left Side)

Step 8. Preparation of the distal branches of the renal artery

The complexity of this step depends on the position of the aneurysm and whether there is only an efferent distal segment or multiple branches (**Figures 50-11 A, B**).

The distal segment, or the branches originating from the aneurysm, should be controlled using vessel loops (**Figure 50-12**).

Step 8 average time frame: 20–40 min

> ▶▶ **TIPS**
>
> Gentle and smooth manipulation/lifting of the aneurysmatic sac favors the identification and preparation of the efferent branches.

1030 The Foundation and Art of Robotic Surgery

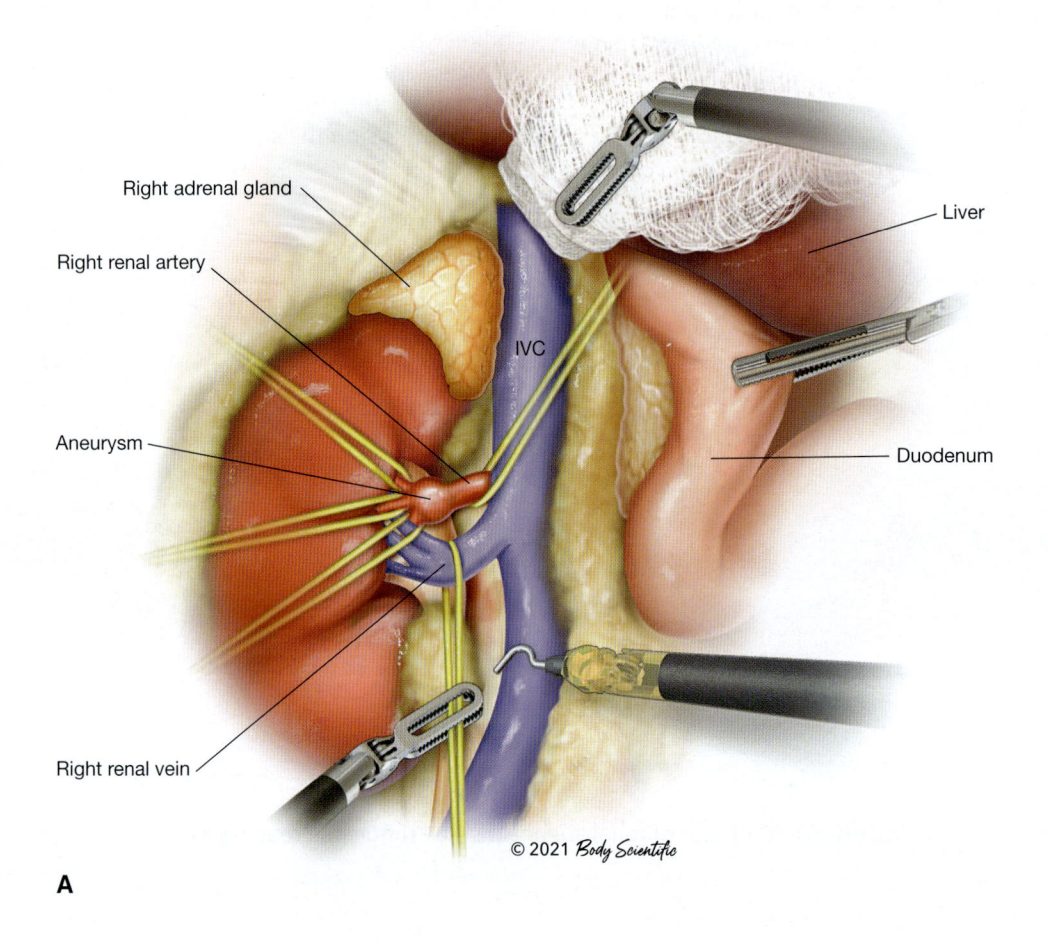

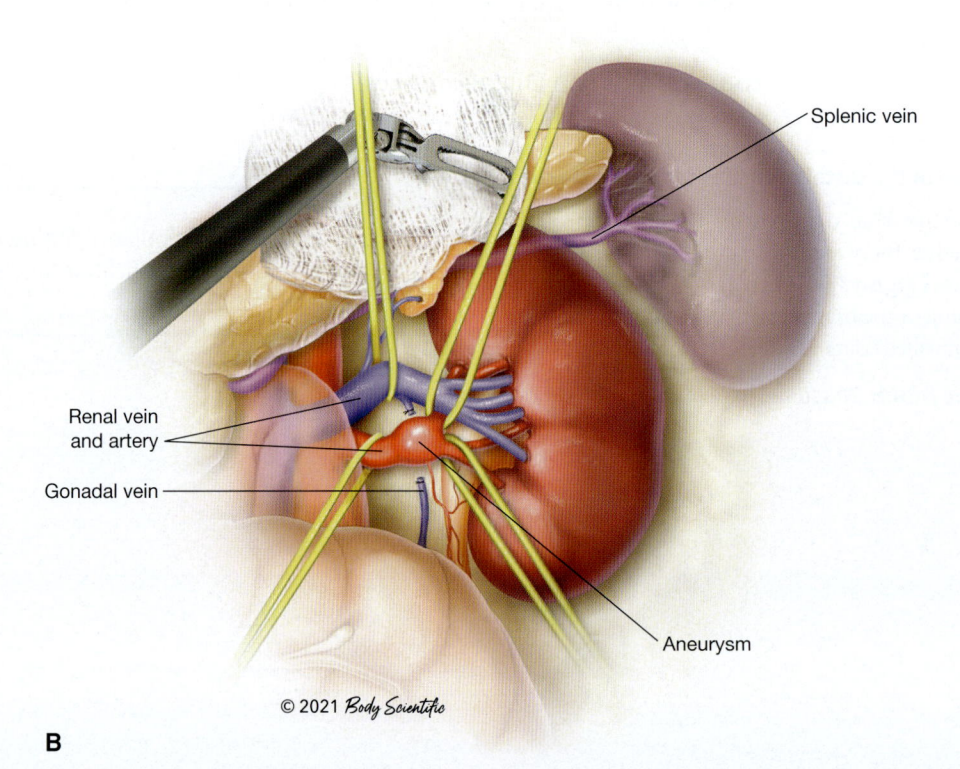

FIGURE 50-11 • **A.** Preparation of the distal branches of the renal artery (right side). **B.** Preparation of the distal branches of the renal artery (left side).

Renal Aneurysm 1031

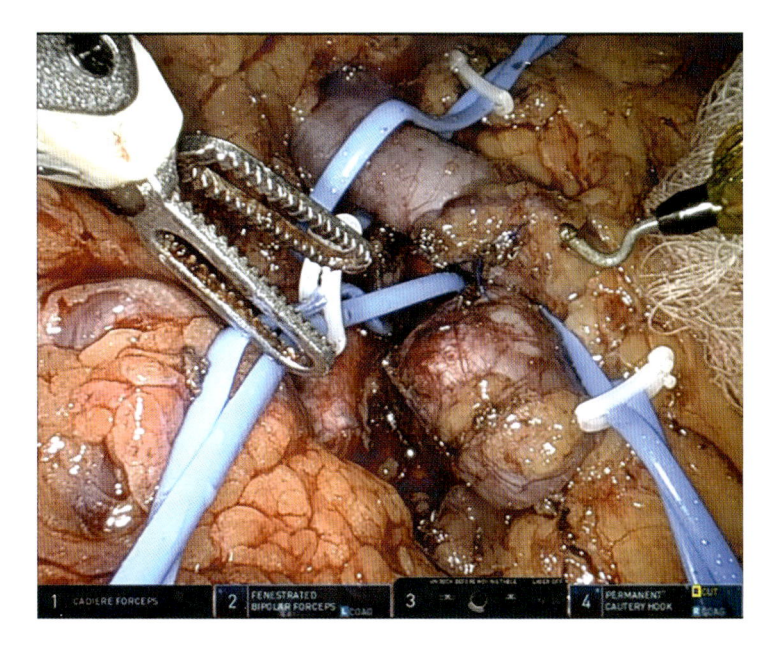

FIGURE 50-12 • Proximal and distal control of the aneurysm (left side).

▶ Video 50-9. Step 9. Clamping and Resecting the Aneurysm

PHASE C (ANEURYSMECTOMY AND RECONSTRUCTION)

Step 9. Clamping of the aneurysm

Prior to clamping, the need for a graft must be assessed. By preparing a graft early, the warm ischemia time of the kidney will be limited. The main reasons for a graft are multiple efferent vessels or if the anastomosis could be under tension. If the aneurysm is saccular and the renal artery redundant, there is a good chance that the stumps distance after the resection will be small, and an end-to-end anastomosis without a graft would be feasible.

After completing the assessment for the reconstruction plan, and before clamping, IV heparin (2000 IU/mg) is administered by the anesthesiologist.

Small bulldogs, controlled by the console surgeon, are applied starting from the proximal artery.

The vessel loops should be maintained external to the clamps, as a safety measure, in case of accidental sliding (**Figure 50-13**).

Step 9 average time frame: 3–5 min

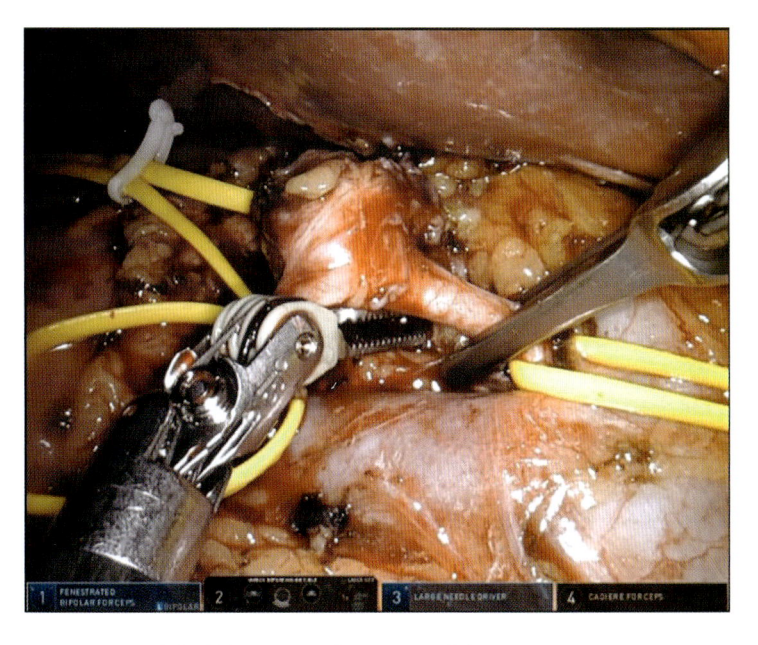

FIGURE 50-13 • Clamping of the aneurysm.

1032 The Foundation and Art of Robotic Surgery

Step 10. Aneurysmatic sac excision
The aneurysmatic sac is completely excised using the robotic scissors. The presence of the sac may, in fact, interfere with the correct approximation of the vascular stumps for the anastomosis (**Figure 50-14**).

Step 10 average time frame: 1–3 min

> ▶▶ **TIPS**
>
> Depending on the quality of the artery, the exposure, and the length of the proximal artery available for clamping, the bulldog may be inadequate or unsafe. In such cases, considering hand assistance with a GelPort® placed on a Pfannenstiel incision could be a wise strategy. Satinsky-like, stronger clamps can be introduced through the GelPort® and applied by hand assistance. This safety assessment should be done before clamping the artery and resecting the aneurysm (**Figure 50-15**).

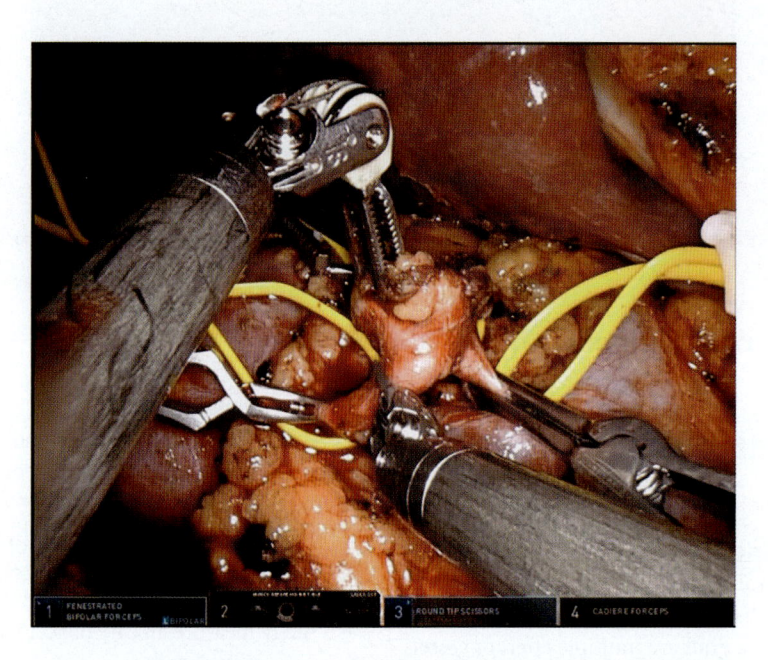

FIGURE 50-14 • Resection of the aneurysm.

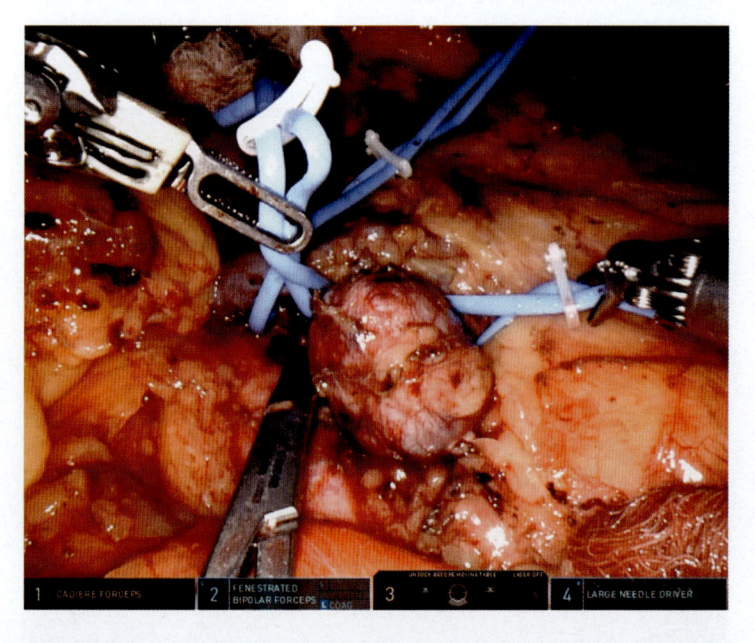

FIGURE 50-15 • Satinsky-like clamp placement (hand assistance).

Video 50-10. Step 11. Anastomosis with a Graft Interposition (Right Side)

Video 50-11. Step 11. Anastomosis Primary Repair (Left Side)

Step 11. Reconstruction

The complexity of this step may be extremely variable, depending on the location of the aneurysm and on the number/position of the efferent branches.

The easiest situation is an end-to-end reconstruction without any graft interposition. The most complex is the use of the saphenous graft previously harvested, from the patient groin, before clamping the renal artery (**Figures 50-16 A–D**).

The saphenous graft can be prepared with microscopic bench surgery techniques and tailored to the patient local anatomy (e.g., Y shape).

A Y reconstruction may allow partial reperfusion of one limb before completing the repair. The proximal anastomosis is done first.

Two vascular needle drivers in the R1 and the R2 are used to make a running suture of double-armed CV-5 PTFE with end-to-end anastomosis (**Figure 50-17**).

The back wall of the anastomosis is carried out first, with the knot outside the lumen of the vessel.

Step 11 average time frame: 20–40 min

> ⚠️ **PITFALLS**
>
> The arterial wall, when manipulating the vessel, should not be grabbed with the needle drivers, because these can easily cause a crushing injury.
>
> The 2 main pitfalls of this anastomosis are the purse string effect (too tight running suture), which can cause stenosis, and the creation of distal dissection/intimal flaps, which may develop thrombosis.

A Main renal artery (primary repair)

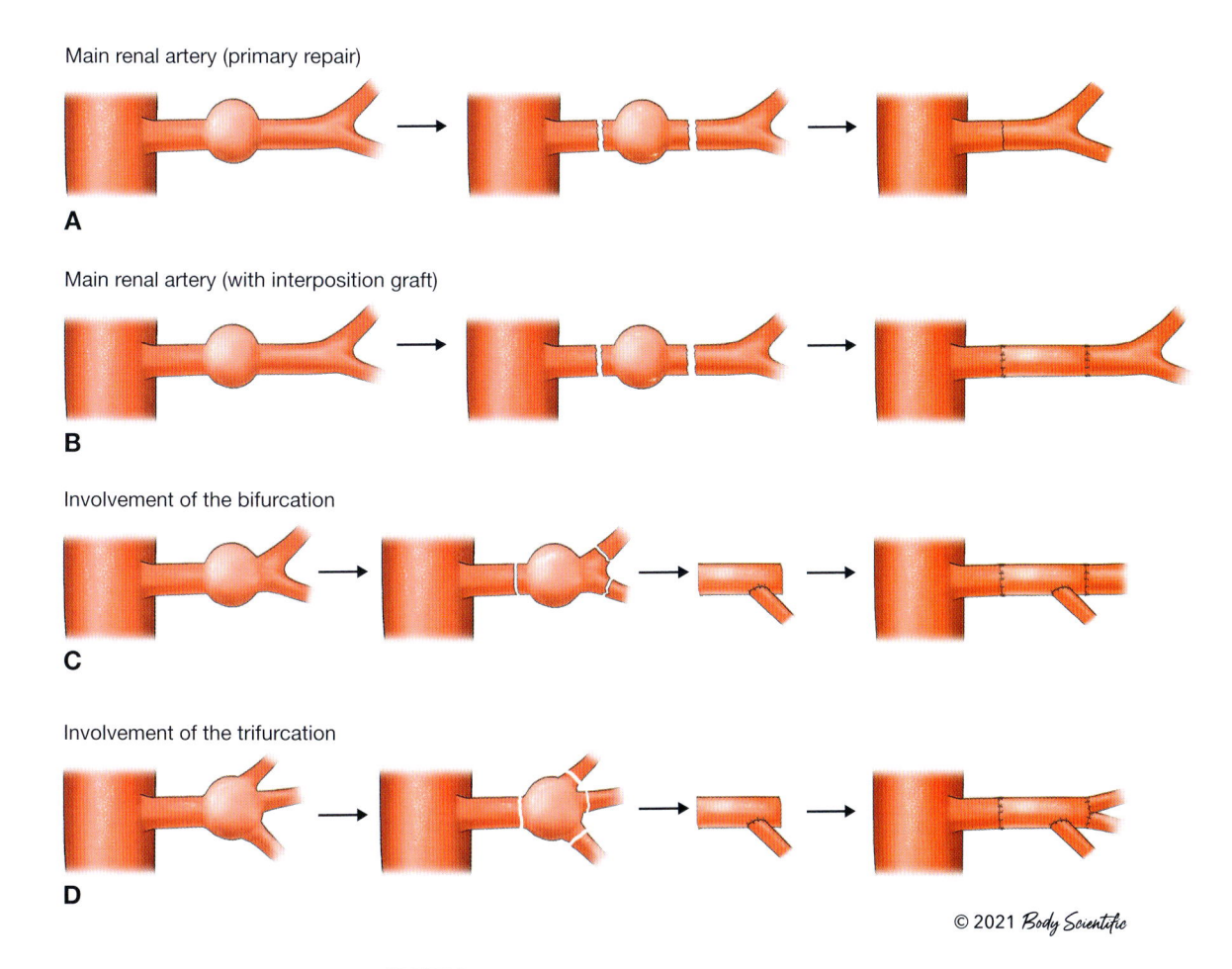

B Main renal artery (with interposition graft)

C Involvement of the bifurcation

D Involvement of the trifurcation

© 2021 *Body Scientific*

FIGURE 50-16 • Common reconstruction types.

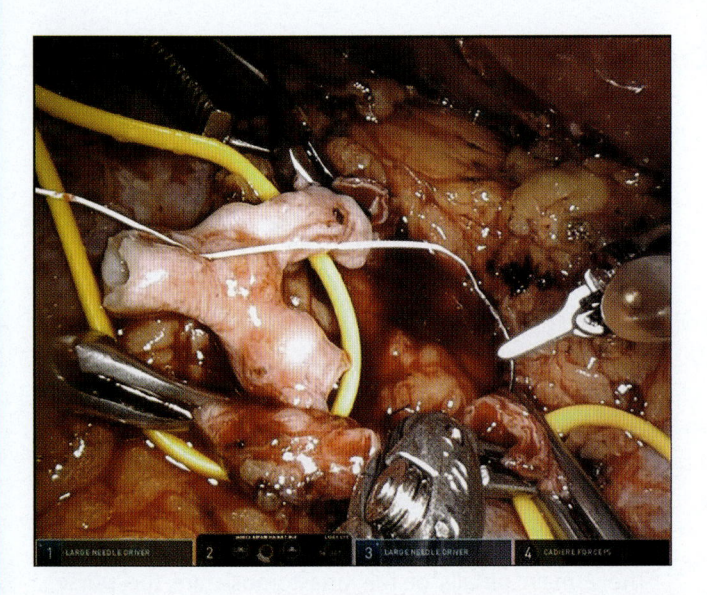

FIGURE 50-17 • Anastomosis with interposition of a graft.

> ▶▶ **TIPS**
>
> When passing the needle for the vascular suture, it is always fundamental to keep in mind the direction of the blood flow. The tip of the needle should puncture the distal arterial wall from inside the lumen going outside. *Vice versa*, when advancing through the artery going toward the lumen, the needle can separate the layers of the wall. Given that the blood flow travels proximal to distal, it has the potential to go between the layers of the arterial wall and dissect them distally (**Figures 50-18 A–D**).

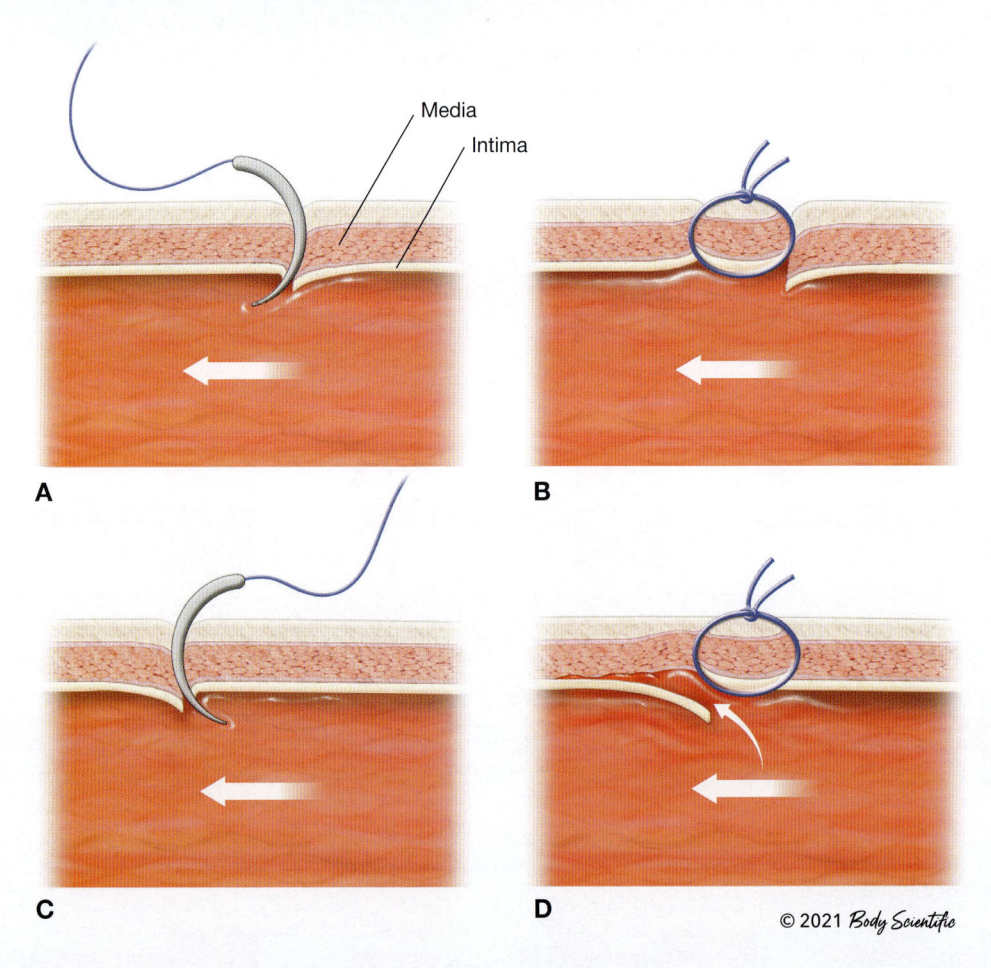

FIGURE 50-18 • Needle-driving technique. **A, B.** Correct technique: inside proximally, outside distally. **C, D.** Flawed technique: inside distally, outside proximally.

▶ **Video 50-12.** Step 12. Reperfusion (ICG) and Hemostasis (Right Side)

▶ **Video 50-13.** Step 12. Reperfusion (ICG) and Hemostasis (Left Side)

Step 12. Reperfusion (ICG/Doppler) and hemostasis

The initial declamping test may require, in case of major bleeding, some additional, interrupted stitches of Prolene™ 5-0/6-0. If the bleeding is minor, a hemostatic agent can be applied to the area of the anastomosis.

Indocyanine green (ICG) and Doppler may finally confirm good renal perfusion (**Figure 50-19**). A final check of the hemostasis is carried out, and the aneurysm sac is retrieved and sent for permanent pathology.

Step 12 average time frame: 5–10 min

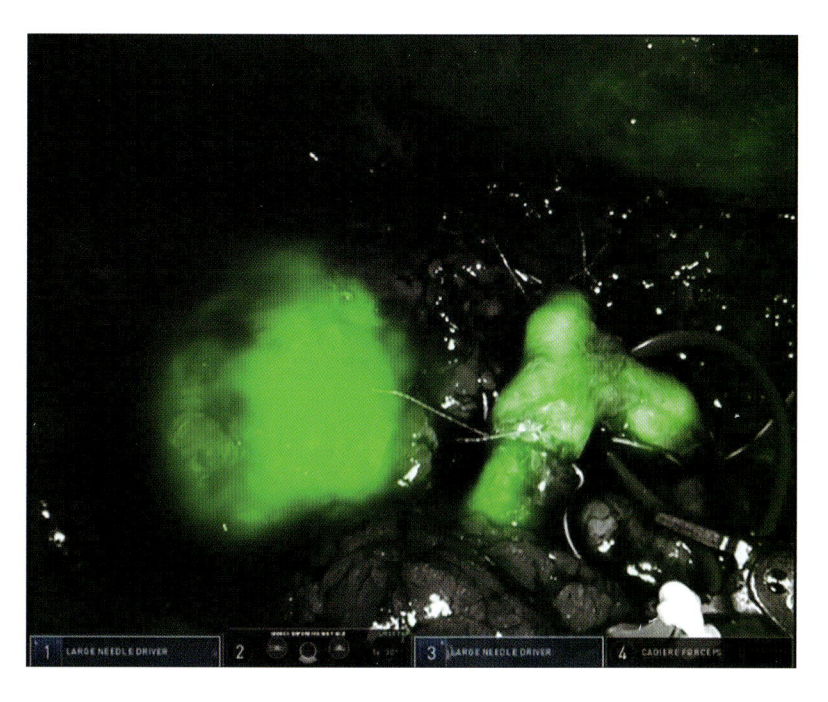

FIGURE 50-19 • Checking the perfusion of the kidney (ICG).

Suggested Readings

1. Coleman DM, Stanley JC. Renal artery aneurysms. *J Vasc Surg.* 2015;62(3):779-785. doi: 10.1016/j.jvs.2015.05.034
2. Klausner JQ, Lawrence PF, Harlander-Locke MP, et al. The contemporary management of renal artery aneurysms. *J Vasc Surg.* 2015;61(4):978-984. doi: 10.1016/j.jvs.2014.10.107
3. Giulianotti PC, Coratti A, Angelini M, et al. Robotics in general surgery: personal experience in a large community hospital. *Arch Surg.* 2003;138(7):777-784. doi: 10.1001/archsurg.138.7.777
4. Le B, Matulewicz RS, Eaton S, Perry K, Nadler RB. Comparative analysis of vascular bulldog clamps used in robot-assisted partial nephrectomy. *J Endourol.* 2013;27(11):1349-1353. doi: 10.1089/end.2013.0367
5. Rod X, Peyronnet B, Seisen T, et al. Impact of ischaemia time on renal function after partial nephrectomy: a systematic review. *BJU Int.* 2016;118:692-705. doi: 10.1111/bju.13580
6. Giulianotti PC, Bianco F, Addeo P, Lombardi A, Coratti A, Sbrana F. Robot-assisted laparoscopic repair of renal artery aneurysms. *J Vasc Surg.* 2010;51(4):842-849. doi: 10.1016/j.jvs.2009.10.104

"There is no doubt that creativity is the most important human resource of all. Without creativity, there would be no progress, and we would be forever repeating the same patterns."
—Edward de Bono (1933–2021)

Single Port Robotic Surgery: Basic Concepts
(Procedures Still Not FDA Approved/Off-Label Indication)

Nicolas Hellmuth Dreifuss • Antonio Cubisino • Francesco Maria Bianco

▶ **Video 51-1.** Da Vinci SP Platform (©Intuitive Surgical Operations, Inc)

DAVINCI SINGLE PORT (SP) BASICS

In 2018, Intuitive released a special platform for single incision surgery, the da Vinci® Single Port (SP). The system features a complete redesign of the surgical platform and the instrument arms architecture. While keeping the same overhead design, the system has a single arm and a drive that hosts 3 robotic multijointed, endowristed instruments and an endoscope that is also, for the first time, multijointed. The significant innovation consists in the fact that the tools are now grouped together to be deployed through a 2.5-cm port or entry guide, as it is generally called (**Figure 51-1**).

The SP operates with the same remote center concept previously described. The arm design allows 360° rotation along the horizontal axis and 120° rotation along the vertical axis, allowing the surgeon to work in every quadrant without the need for redocking. The rotation movements are controlled by the surgeon at the console without the need for a bedside assistant to operate the arm.

The cart has **3 types of clutches**: the **instrument arm clutch** that allows movement of the instrument cluster around the remote center of the cannula, the **port clutch** that allows the care team to move the instrument arm and place it in the desired position to reach the cannula, and the **instrument drive clutch** that allows to advance and retract the instruments and the camera through the port. Each instrument drive also features a dedicated display that shows operational information of the instrument and an emergency instrument disengage button for safety.

The **robotic console and the vision tower** of the SP system appear very similar when compared to the previous robotic platforms. The software is different, and the components are not interchangeable with the previous robotic carts at present time.

The **robotic instruments and the scope** are completely redesigned and are the base of this disruptive technology. Every instrument features a 6-mm shaft, an elbow, a forearm, a wrist, and a tip. The distance from the elbow to the tip is 10 cm and requires the same amount of space beyond the entry guide to deploy (**Figure 51-2**). This special architecture allows creation of the intra-abdominal triangulation of the instruments. Each instrument has 25 lives. The only different one is the clip applier, which has a lifespan of 150 fires. The available instruments for the SP platform can be seen in **Figures 51-3 A, B**.

The **camera** also features a similar multijointed structure. It holds a 3D HD scope with 73° field of view, autofocus, and a dynamic illumination feature that adjusts the light's intensity based on the surgical field conditions. The device allows adjustment of the orientation of the scope, take pictures, and

Photo credit: Roy Zhao.
Quote reproduced with permission from Ahmed ST, Feist GJ. The language of creativity: validating linguistic analysis to assess creative scientists and artists. Front Psychol. 2021;12:724083.

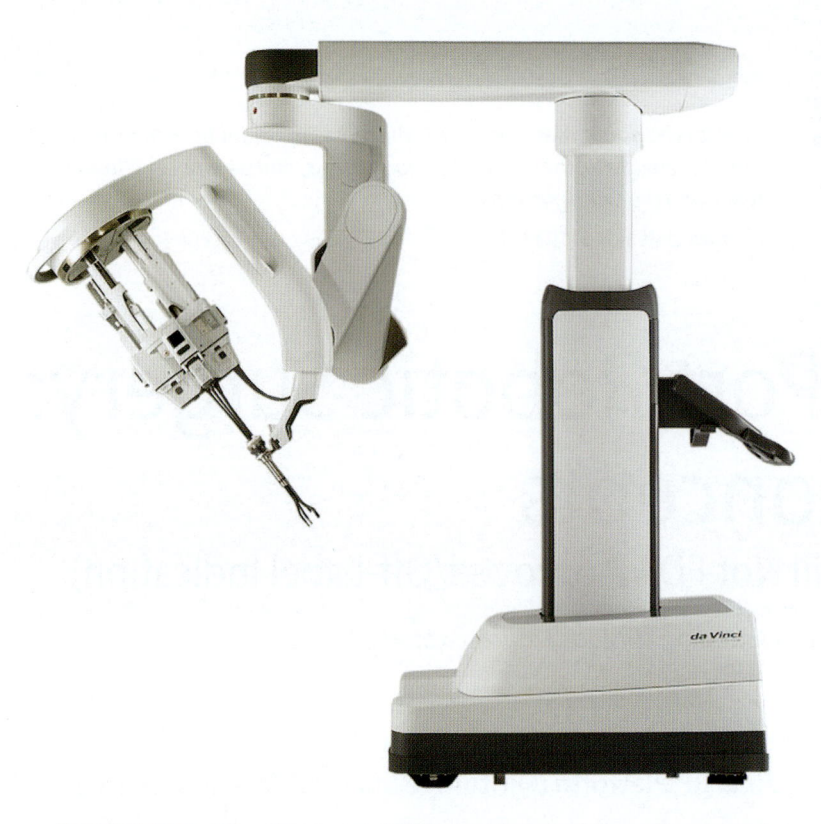

FIGURE 51-1 • SP patient cart. (©Intuitive Surgical Operations, Inc.)

Instrument Housing

Shaft   Tip

Close-up of instrument housing

Release buttons (one on each side)

Close-up of instrument distal end

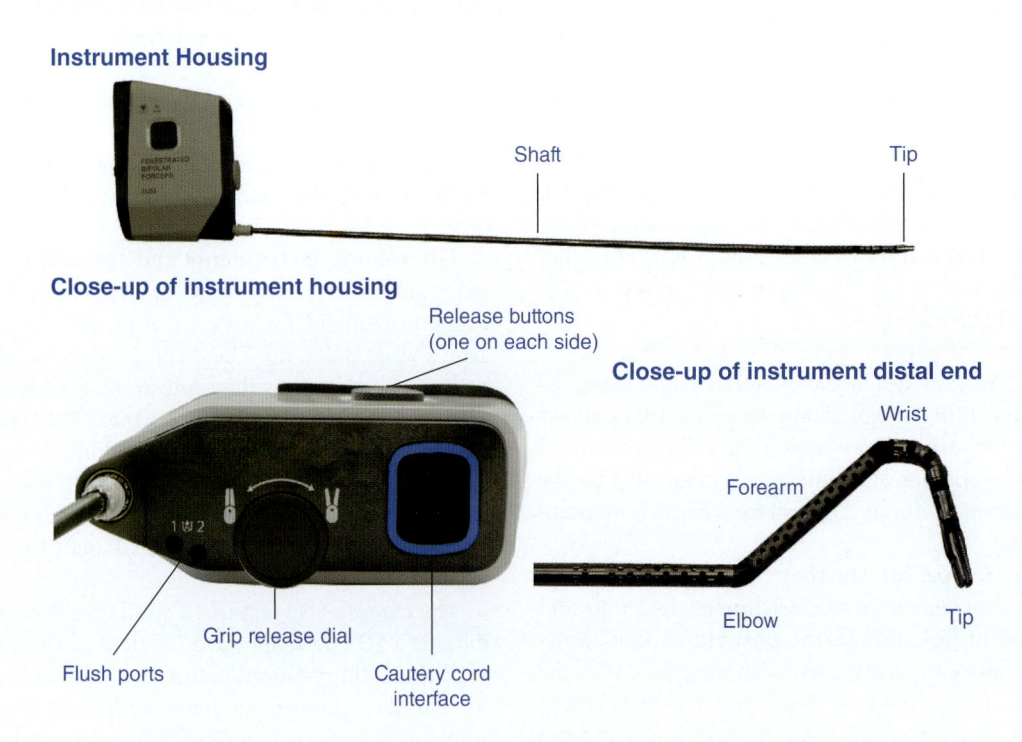

Wrist
Forearm
Elbow   Tip

Grip release dial
Flush ports   Cautery cord interface

FIGURE 51-2 • SP instrument design. (©Intuitive Surgical Operations, Inc.)

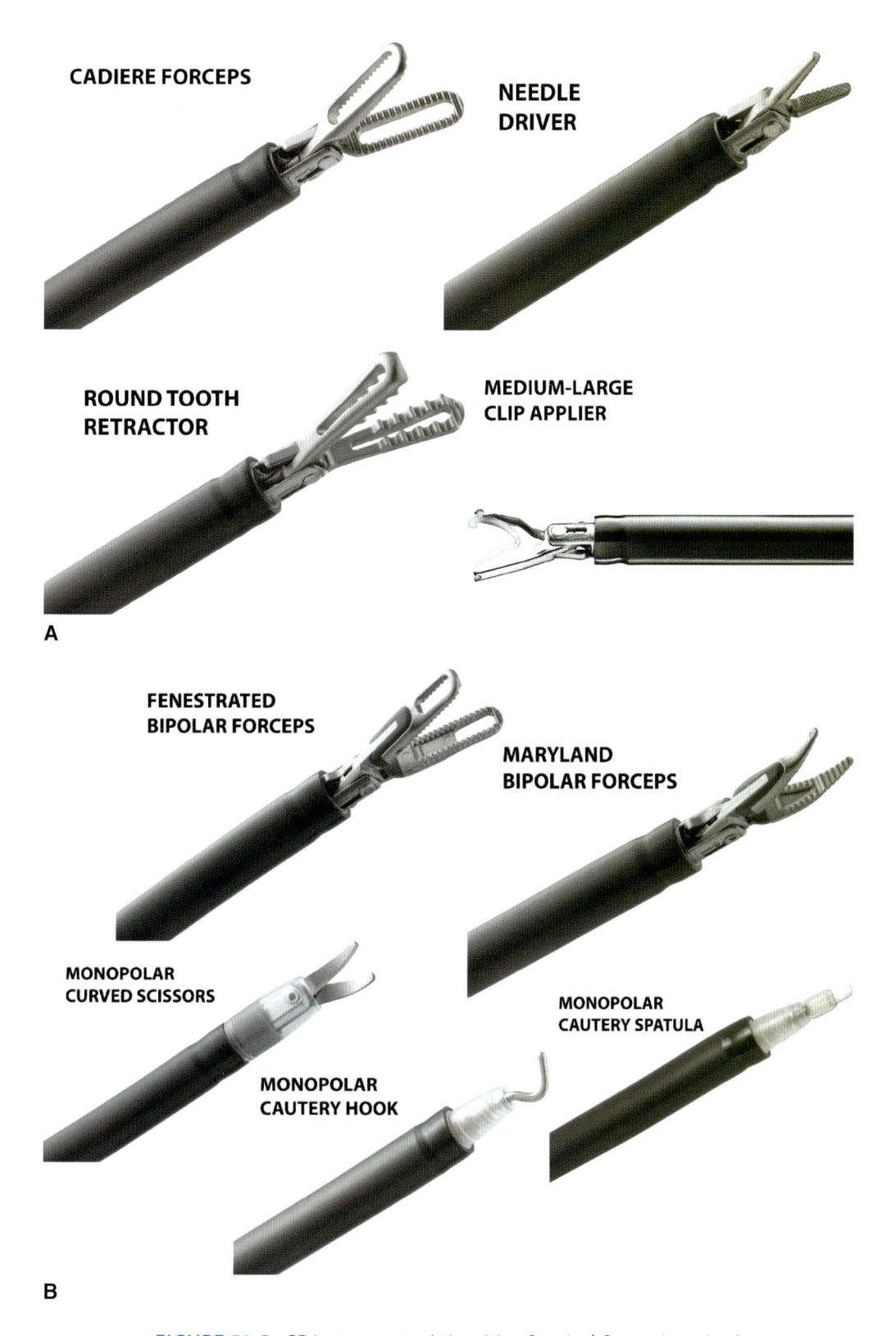

FIGURE 51-3 • SP instruments. (©Intuitive Surgical Operations, Inc.)

1040 The Foundation and Art of Robotic Surgery

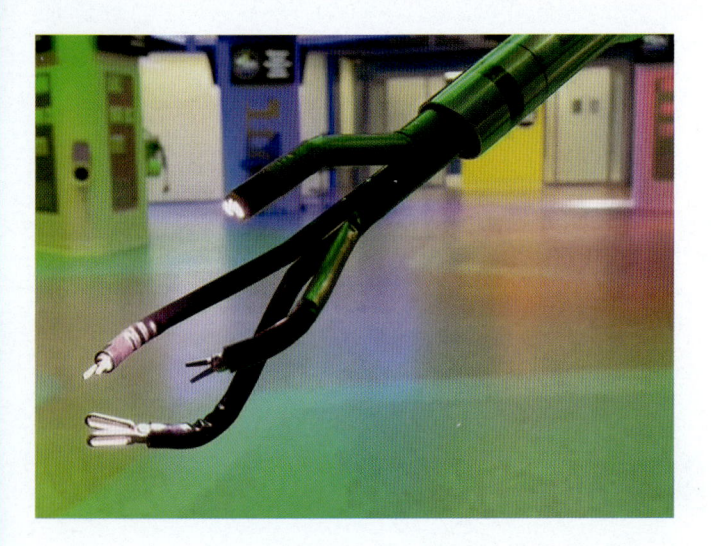

FIGURE 51-4 • SP camera.

turn on and off the light source with dedicated buttons. Each scope can be used 20 times (soon it will be 33) and needs to be reprocessed by the company once all uses have been expended (**Figure 51-4**).

The robotic instruments and endoscope are introduced through either the **access port** or through a **metal cannula**. The access port includes an entry guide and a wound protector, and comes in 2 sizes (small for 2.7–4-cm incisions and large for 2.7–7-cm incisions). The access port enables the robotic instruments to work at the level of the incision by letting them deploy external to the body within a clear plastic chamber (**Figure 51-5**). The chamber maintains insufflation and is also able to store specimens for later retrieval so that the robot can remain docked until the end of the procedure. There are 2 ports to facilitate assistant access and the introduction and removal of equipment: the rotating seal at the top supports equipment 5–12 mm in diameter and rotates to provide the assistant multiple angles of approach to more easily navigate the surgical workspace, and the blue chamber seal on the side accepts equipment 5–10 mm in diameter.

The metal cannula is 25 × 100 mm with an inner entry guide that is placed once the port has been deployed (**Figure 51-6**). Both the access port and metal cannula are used with an entry guide that has 1 oval camera lumen (9 mm) and 3 circular lumens (6 mm) for the instruments. Each seal has a release button that allows evacuation of gas if needed, or to facilitate the extraction of materials such as sutures (**Figure 51-7**).

The **surgical workspace** is the area where the system will need to be able to operate with minimum and maximum reach

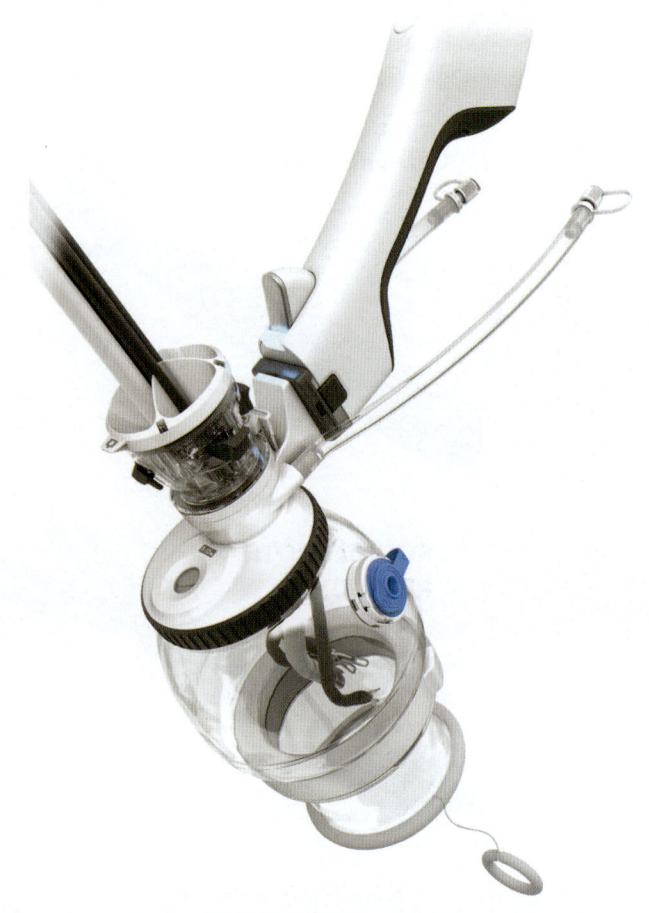

FIGURE 51-5 • Access port. (©Intuitive Surgical Operations, Inc.)

of the instruments. The ideal set up of the port (access port or metal cannula) should be a maximum distance of 25 cm from the furthest edge of the field. Furthermore, the port should have a minimum of 2-cm clearance from any bony prominence and 7 cm from any assistant port. If using the access port, there is no minimum distance from the closest edge of the field as the instruments and camera can deploy outside of the body within the chamber to reach the ideal separation and triangulation to operate (**Figure 51-8A**). If using the metal cannula, a 10-cm distance from the closest edge of the field is needed because the instruments and camera need to be inserted 10 cm into the body before their elbows can clear the tip of the metal cannula (**Figure 51-8B**). The working space is approximately a sphere of 16-cm in diameter, and moving away from this space requires clutching and relocating (**Figure 51-8C**).

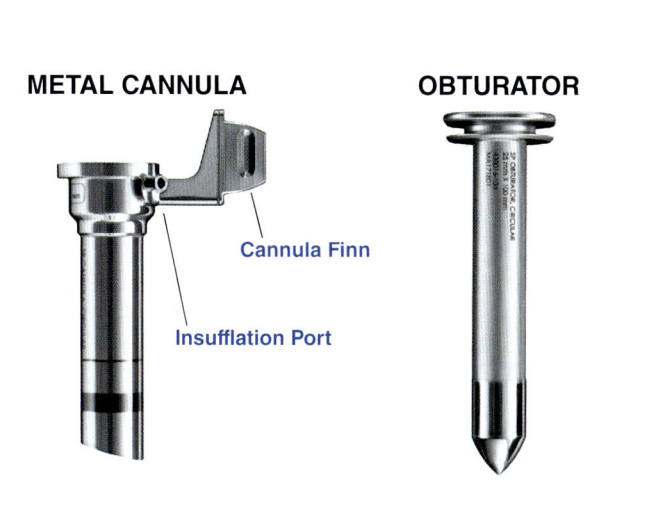

Single Port Robotic Surgery: Basic Concepts   1041

METAL CANNULA
- Cannula Finn
- Insufflation Port

OBTURATOR

FIGURE 51-6 • Metal cannula. (©Intuitive Surgical Operations, Inc.)

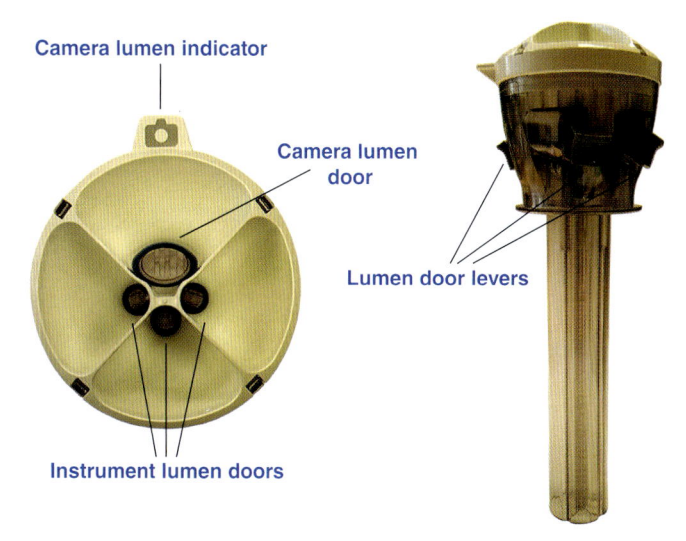

- Camera lumen indicator
- Camera lumen door
- Lumen door levers
- Instrument lumen doors

FIGURE 51-7 • Entry guide. (©Intuitive Surgical Operations, Inc.)

Small access port

6.6 cm
Incision
Internal ring
< 25 cm

Large access port

10 cm
Incision
Internal ring
< 25 cm

© 2022 Body Scientific

A

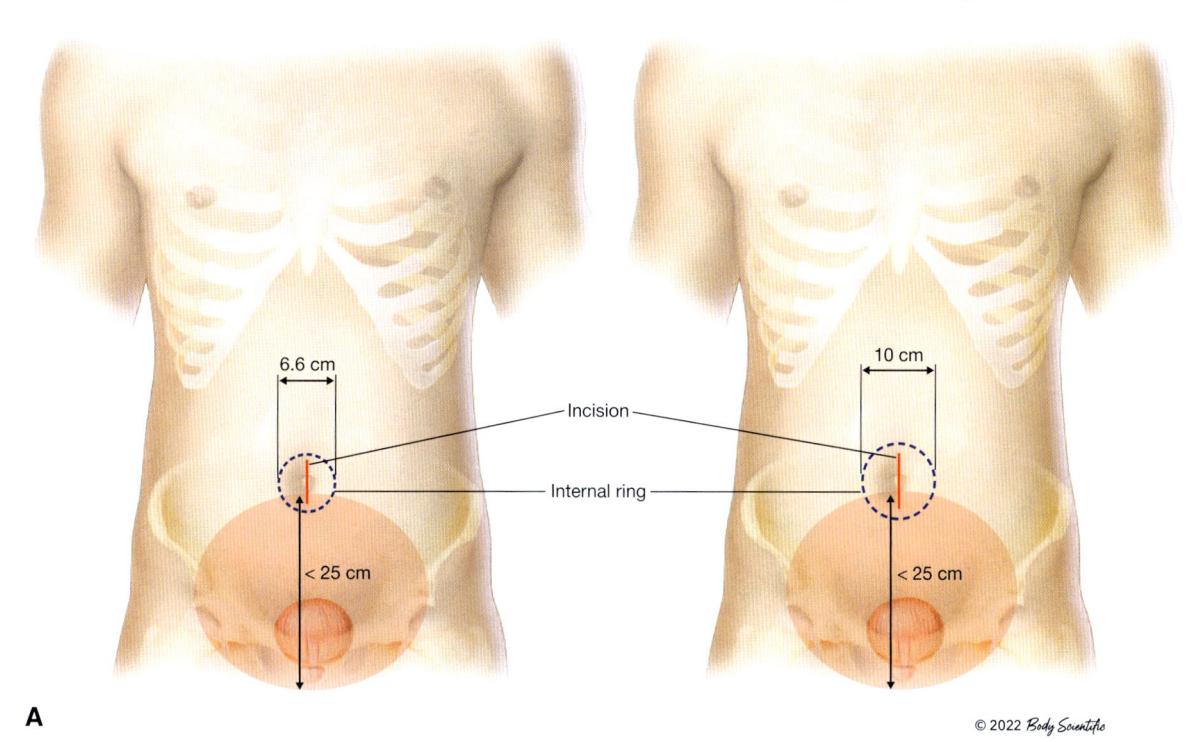

FIGURE 51-8 • **A.** Access port surgical workspace and minimum/maximum distances.

1042 The Foundation and Art of Robotic Surgery

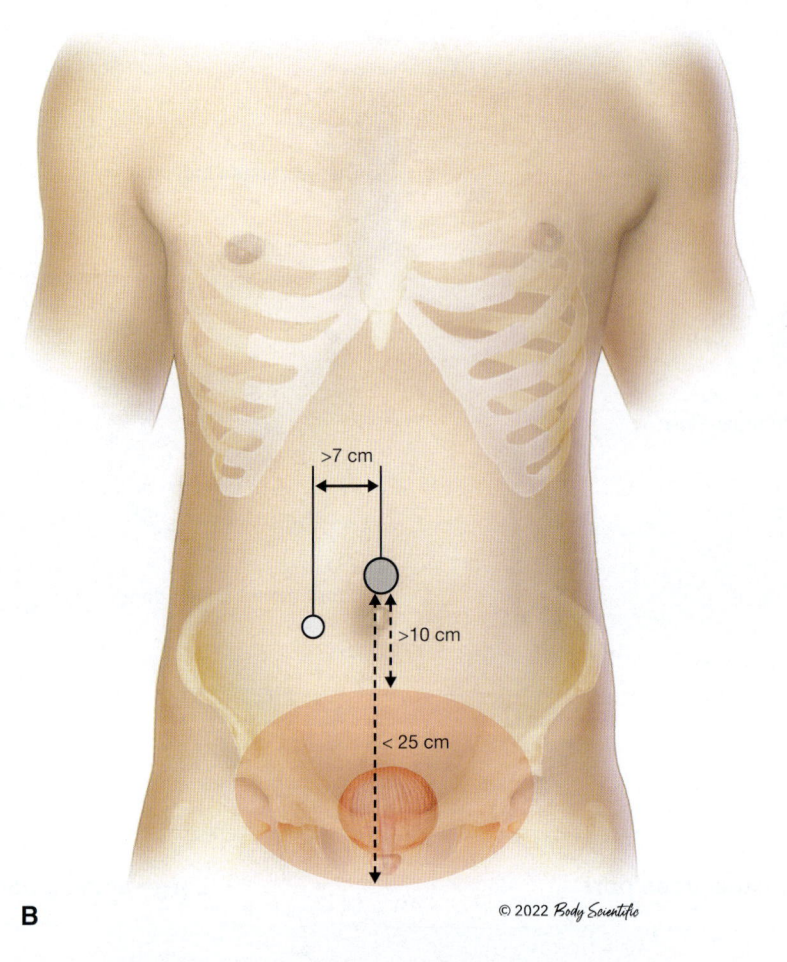

FIGURE 51-8 • (*Continued*) **B.** Metal cannula surgical workspace and minimum/maximum distances.

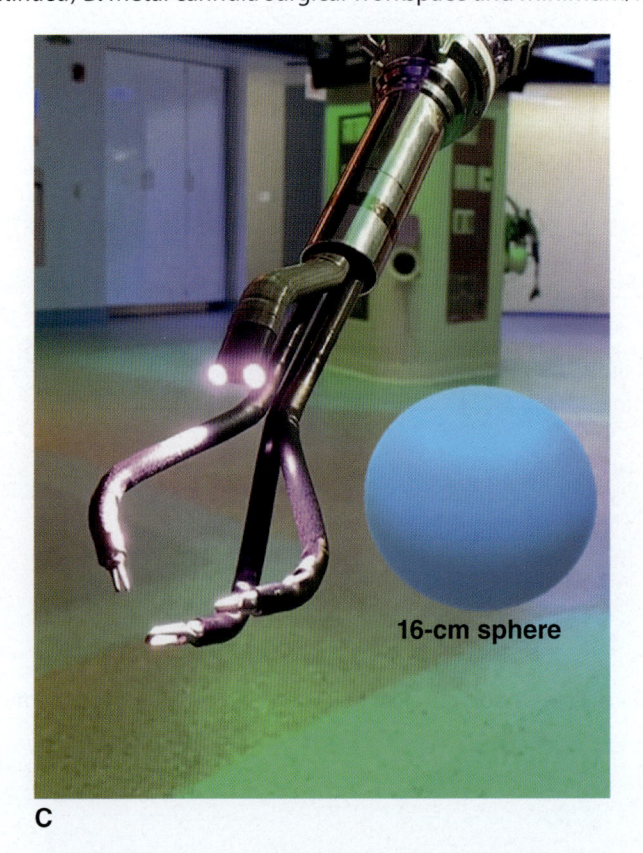

FIGURE 51-8 • (*Continued*) **C.** Surgical workspace.

▶ **Video 51-2. Docking**

Docking: With only 1 instrument arm to be docked, the process is much simpler when compared to the previous platforms. It is important to confirm that the instrument arm and the patient are not located directly under a low hanging ceiling mounted hub to avoid collisions. Once ready, the system is deployed for docking. This will set the boom height, the amount of extension outward from the cart's column, and the instrument arm will move to a vertical position. The cart is positioned by the patient side and the access port or metal cannula is docked to the instrument arm. The last step, after docking is completed, is to set the instrument arm pitch limit. This feature prevents the arm from moving behind a certain vertical angulation to prevent collisions with the patient.

▶ **Video 51-3A. Camera Adjust Mode** (©Intuitive Surgical Operations, Inc)

▶ **Video 51-3B. Camera Control Mode** (©Intuitive Surgical Operations, Inc)

▶ **Video 51-3C. Camera Relocate Mode** (©Intuitive Surgical Operations, Inc)

Camera control modes and relocate mode: While the master clutch operates in a similar way to the previous platforms, the camera clutch activates 3 different modes with different functions. *Adjust mode* allows to move the camera and navigate in the workspace while maintaining the instruments in the same position. This is particularly useful while holding tissue. *Camera control mode* allows to move the camera and the joints without moving the instruments. *Relocate mode* allows to reposition the camera and instruments simultaneously by moving the entire instrument cluster. This last function is useful in multiquadrant procedures to reach different anatomical regions without undocking (**Figure 51-9**).

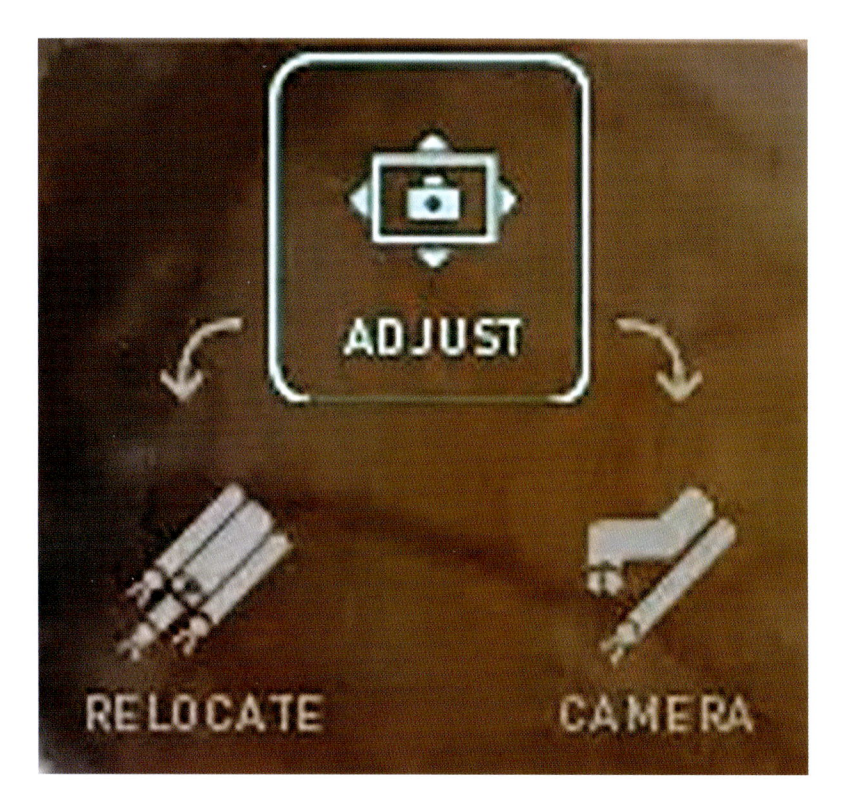

FIGURE 51-9 • Camera modes.

Front view   Top view   Side view

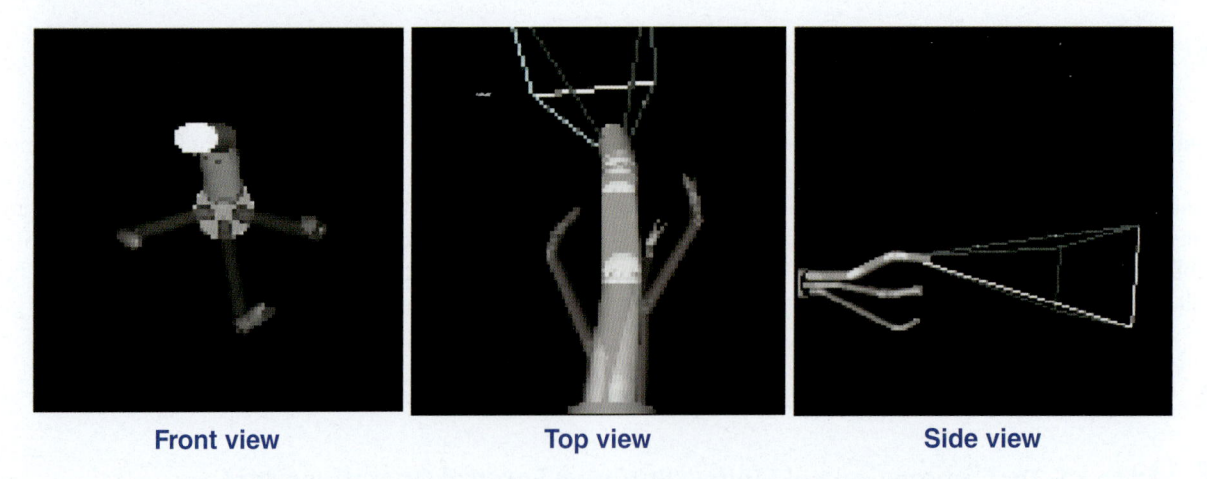

FIGURE 51-10 • Instrument navigator. (©Intuitive Surgical Operations, Inc.)

Instrument navigator: this new feature allows a tridimensional visualization of the instrument's position and the camera. The navigator can provide different angle views including a front, top, and side view. It is useful for general troubleshooting of the instruments and camera. The navigator also allows to set up the camera for the maximum clearance from the instruments and ideal viewing angle. This setup is called the "cobra" pose and it consists in having the camera lifted at a maximum at the elbow with the wrist pointing down. The camera in the navigator turns green to confirm the correct position of the scope. This setup can also be attained with a dedicated button on the touchpad that can toggle in between the "cobra" pose and a totally flat camera setup, which is helpful when retracting the scope (**Figure 51-10**).

Advantages and Limitations of the SP Platform

Performing surgery through a single cannula and with this innovative platform increases the operation's technical complexity. Special training with the SP platform is required before getting privileges for its utilization. This may include simulation and dry lab sessions usually provided by the company, wet lab training, and proctored cases at the beginning of the learning curve. In addition, the OR staff and bedside assistants must also receive adequate SP training.

The SP platform provides some clear **advantages**:

- **Cosmesis and body image:** The 2.5-cm umbilical incision becomes an almost imperceptible scar, which is usually desired. There is a worldwide change in the patient's psychological expectations on the surgical outcomes with a growing emphasis on body image preservation.
- **Opening the way for innovative procedures:** The natural orifices approach to many pathologies and conditions may be reconsidered and relaunched, based on the technical abilities of the endowristed microinstrumentation of the system. Already, transoral and transanal applications have been accomplished, but many other ones will be possible in the future with further development of the platform.
- **Improved postoperative pain control:** Related to the reduced number of ports and incisions with easier release of local anesthesia techniques.
- **Extraction site:** The SP incision is bigger than the regular 8-mm multiport trocar one and it is used to retrieve specimens without the need of creating an additional extraction site.

On the other hand, some **complexities and temporary limitations,** connected to the evolving technology, should be objectively recognized:

- **Limited divergent action of the robotic instruments:** The SP little arms do not allow strong traction and countertraction maneuvers to open up surgical planes (e.g., left colonic mobilization, gastrocolic ligament opening).
- **Small size surgical fields:** The operative field obtained with the SP platform is smaller when compared to the robotic multiport technique. In order to expand the surgical area under control, multiple relocations are usually required.
- **Limitation in the instrument armamentarium:** Currently, advanced energy devices (vessel sealer, harmonic), staplers, and suction-irrigation are not available, which limits the complexity of the procedures that can be performed in a pure SP modality.
- **Role of the assistant:** The work of the bedside assistant is more complicated as they must use a channel that is parallel to the robotic instruments and through the same incision. This geometrical configuration limits the range of movements and actions.
- **Control at the console:** The use of the console and surgical navigation become more sophisticated because they require learning of additional functions and icons.
- **Extra/additional ports:** In some cases, placement of additional assistant ports becomes necessary to perform tasks not easily achieved by the SP instruments only. In such instance, the operation becomes a hybrid SP-multiport, defeating the purpose of the single access surgery and with an increase of costs.
- **Port site incisional hernias:** The increased size of the incision required to introduce the SP may result in higher rates of postoperative incisional hernias.
- **Costs:** The SP instruments are more expensive than the multiport counterparts.

SP General Surgery Applications (Off-Label)

Introduction

Cholecystectomy and inguinal hernia repair are the 2 most frequently performed operations by general surgeons. The minimally invasive approach, for these indications, has become the standard of care due to its known advantages. Multiport laparoscopy and multiport robotic are the validated techniques. Single-incision laparoscopic surgery (SILS) never achieved great popularity in the surgical community due to the reduced ability to triangulate, internal and external clashing, and ergonomic discomfort. Almost a decade ago, specialized instruments for the da Vinci® surgical system (da Vinci® Single-Site: "Vespa") were developed to perform single-incision procedures with robotic assistance and overcome some of the known limitations. However, the increased flexibility, lack of endowrist, and limited strength of the instruments prevented a widespread adoption. The new da Vinci® SP platform has been specifically designed for single-incision surgery and reignited the interest in this approach. The technology is at an early stage and there is not yet an FDA approval for this application.

In this section, the technical aspects of the robotic SP cholecystectomy and transabdominal preperitoneal (TAPP) inguinal hernia repair will be described. For a more detailed description of the specific techniques, please refer to Chapter 37, Cholecystectomy, and Chapter 43, Inguinal Hernia Repair.

SP Cholecystectomy (Off-Label)

Indications and Relative Contraindications to the SP Robotic Approach

The SP cholecystectomy is mainly indicated for symptomatic gallstones in patients who desire an improved cosmetic outcome. Due to intrinsic limitations of the platform and lack of instrumentation (advance energy devices and suction-irrigation), complex cases should be avoided. Patients with super obesity, multiple previous operations, or acute cholecystitis are relative contraindications.

INSTRUMENT REQUIREMENTS

The suggested main robotic instruments/tools can be listed as follows:
- Scope
- Cautery hook/monopolar scissors
- Bipolar forceps
- Cadière forceps
- Clip applier

The suggested main laparoscopic instruments/tools can be listed as follows:
- Grasper
- Needle driver
- Suction device (optional)

Supplemental materials:
- Argyle tracheal canula (used as suction device, optional)
- Hem-o-lok™ clips
- Endobag™ (used in selected cases)
- Army Navy retractor
- PDS™ 1, 3-0
- Vicryl™ 3-0
- Access port (optional)

▶ **Video 51-4. Port Placement**

Patient Positioning, OR Setup, and Port Setting

After the endotracheal intubation, the patient is positioned supine with both arms tucked to the sides. The operation starts by creating a single access in the periumbilical area through a vertical 2.5-cm skin incision. The subcutaneous space is dissected along the umbilical stalk, and the fascia is identified and lifted with Kocher clamps. The fascial plane is well exposed to simplify the closure at the end. The fascia and the peritoneum are opened with a combination of blunt dissection and monopolar energy. The wound is lifted with an Army Navy retractor and the SP device is introduced, advancing it tangentially to the abdominal wall. The abdomen is insufflated, and an exploratory laparoscopy is performed with the manually handled SP scope (**Figures 51-11 A, B**). At this point, the patient

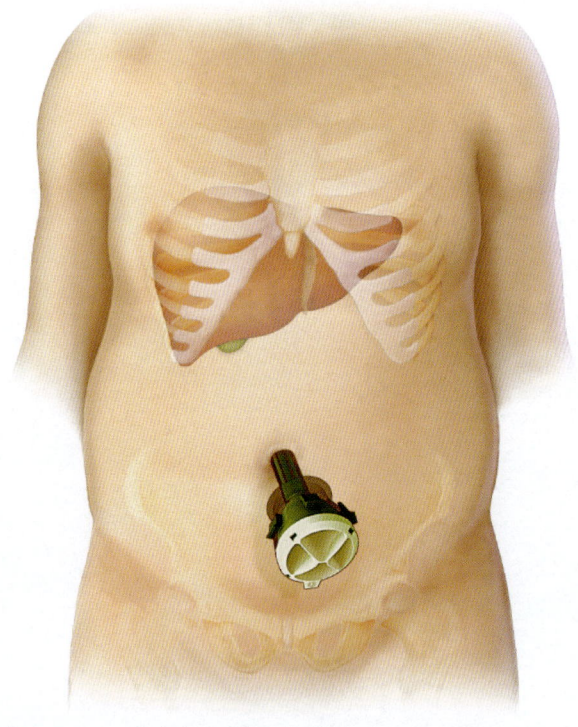

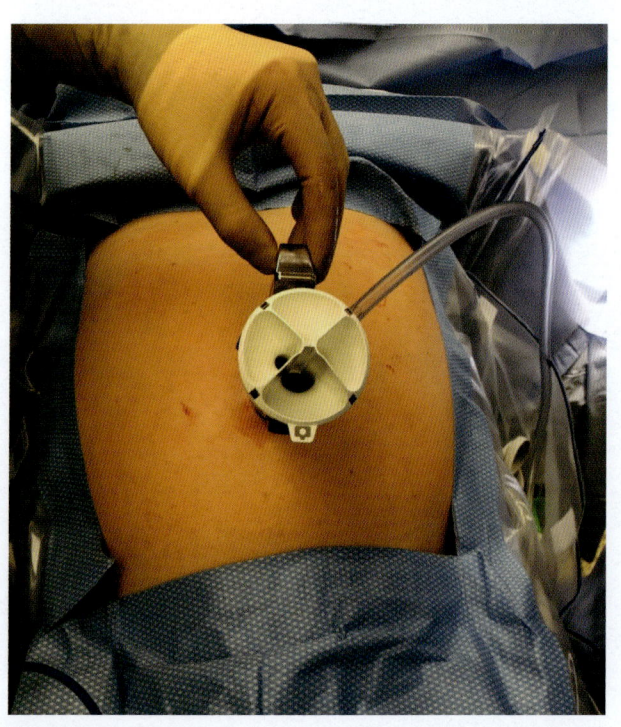

FIGURE 51-11 • Port setting.

Single Port Robotic Surgery: Basic Concepts   1047

is positioned in 30° reverse Trendelenburg with a 20° tilt to the patient's left side (**Figure 51-12**). The robotic cart is docked over the patient's right flank and the assistant surgeon is placed on the patient's left side. The OR setup is described in **Figure 51-13**. The robotic arm is connected to the access port or metal cannula, and the instruments and camera are inserted in the entry guide. The 3D articulating scope is introduced through the inferior oval cannula lumen. The monopolar hook (R1) and the Cadière forceps (R2) are introduced through the right and left circular cannula lumens, respectively. Finally, another Cadière forceps (assisting grasper, R3) is inserted through the upper cannula lumen.

▶▶ **TIPS**

The lower camera configuration will allow a proper retraction of the gallbladder using a Cadière forceps through the upper SP lumen. This will allow to recreate a setup similar to conventional laparoscopy with an adequate vision.

In order to reduce the tangential vision, the port can be pulled up so that the abdominal wall is lifted.

Whenever suction is needed, an Argyle tracheal cannula can be introduced through one of the access port seals or, when using the metal port, before the port placement. In this way, the cannula sits in between the skin and the port, and it is ready to be used by the operating surgeon.

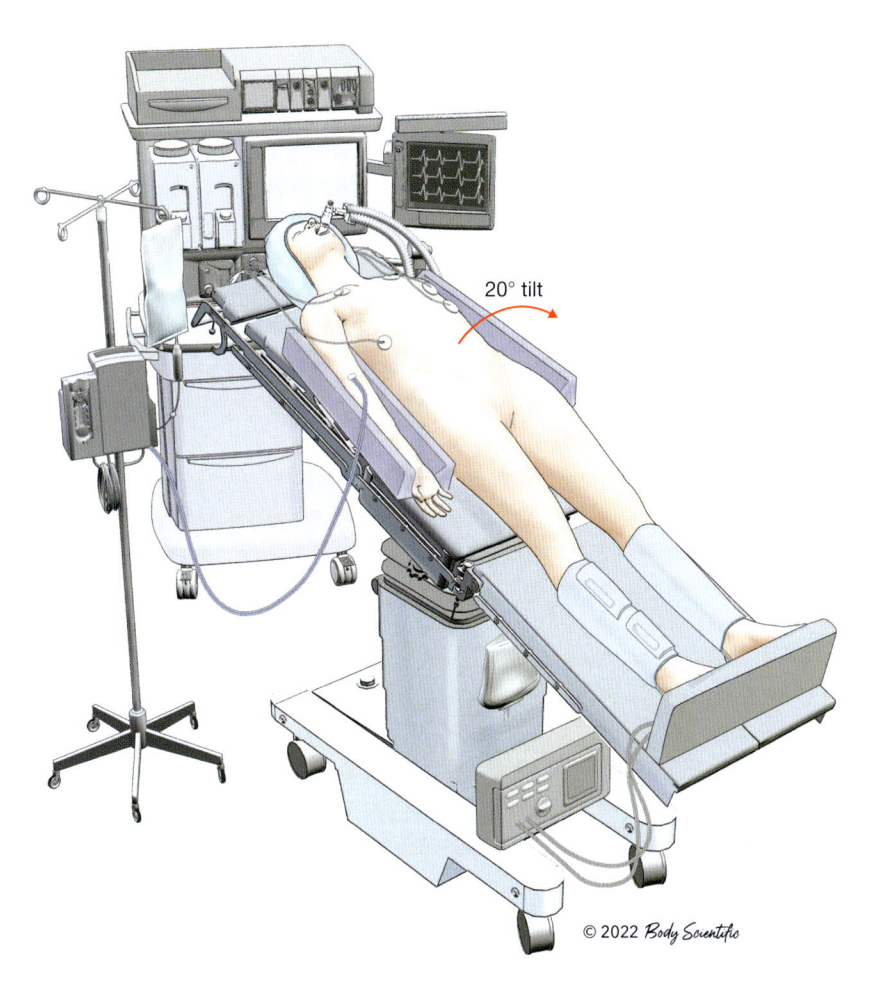

FIGURE 51-12 • Patient positioning.

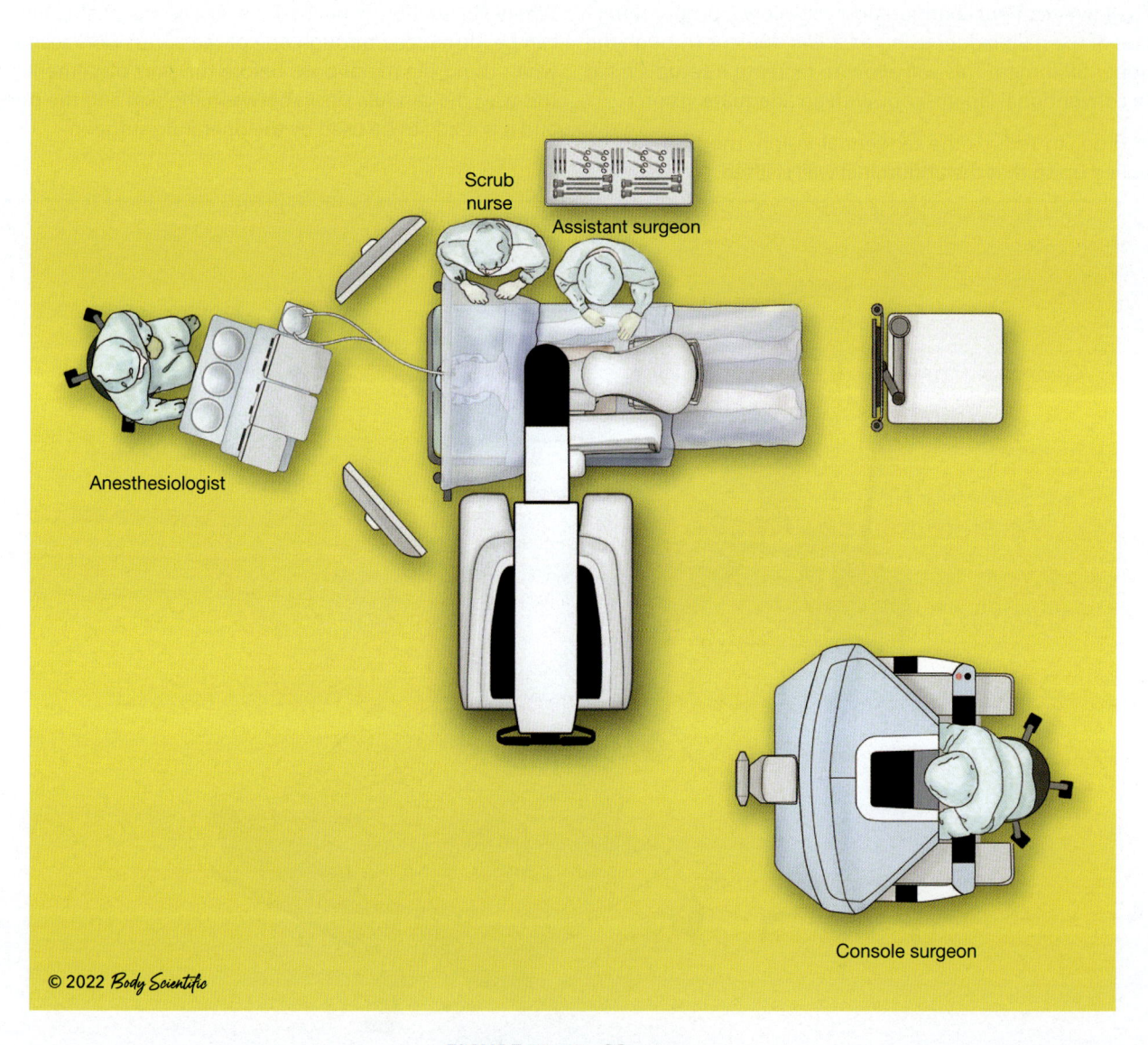

FIGURE 51-13 • OR setup.

Surgical Technique

▶ **Video 51-5.** SP Cholecystectomy

Step 1. Exposure of the working area

After the instruments are introduced and deployed in the abdominal cavity, lysis of omental adhesions (if present) is performed using the monopolar hook or scissors. The first step of the procedure is to expose the gallbladder neck and liver hilum. Using a Cadière forceps (R3) through the upper entry guide lumen, the gallbladder is grasped and retracted cranially. This maneuver will also raise the liver edge and facilitate the exposure of the liver's hilum even though the space between the cystic duct and the common hepatic duct can become narrower. This has to be kept in mind while interpreting the anatomy (**Figures 51-14 A, B**).

Step 1 average time frame: 1–2 min

> ▶▶ **TIPS**
>
> In some cases, retraction of the gallbladder from the middle body, instead of the fundus, is necessary to achieve proper exposure. The ideal working space of the SP platform is more limited (approximately the size of a baseball). Sometimes, to keep all the instruments in the working space, the gallbladder needs to be retracted close to the infundibulum.

> ⚠ **PITFALLS**
>
> **Inadequate exposure:** The exposure achieved with the SP platform is, in some way, similar to the laparoscopic technique. In contrast to the divergent segment IVb retraction achieved with the multiport technique, the gallbladder is retracted cranially in the laparoscopic/SP technique. This might close the angle between the cystic and hepatic duct, increasing the risk of anatomy misinterpretation.

A

B

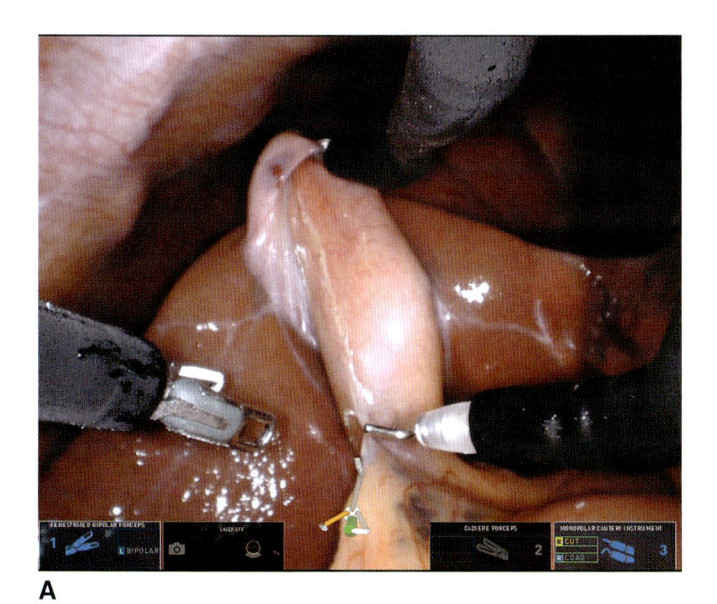

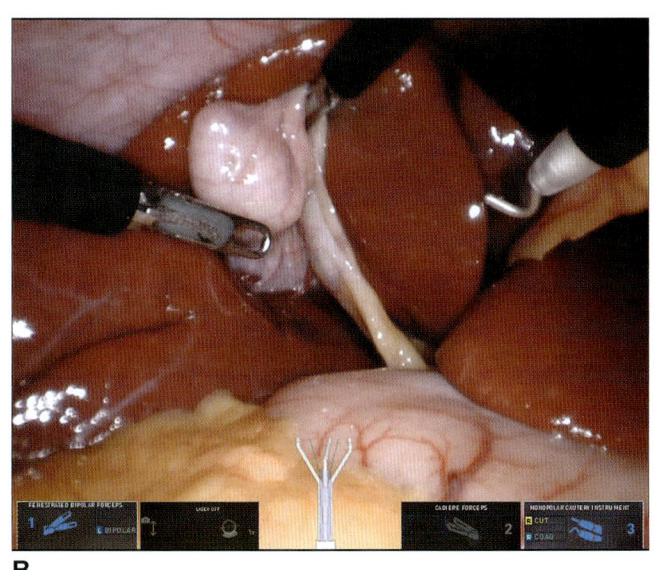

FIGURE 51-14 • Liver hilum exposure.

1050　The Foundation and Art of Robotic Surgery

Step 2. Retraction of the gallbladder neck

Afterward, the gallbladder neck is retracted laterally and inferiorly with a Cadière forceps (R2) (**Figure 51-15**). This maneuver will open the angle between the cystic and the hepatic duct. Moreover, it will allow the exposure of the triangle of Calot and the recognition of the landmark structures (gallbladder neck, cystic artery, cystic duct, and its confluence with the common bile duct [CBD]).

Step 2 average time frame: 2–3 min

> 🔍 **ANATOMICAL HIGHLIGHTS**
> Triangle of Calot (**Figure 51-16**).

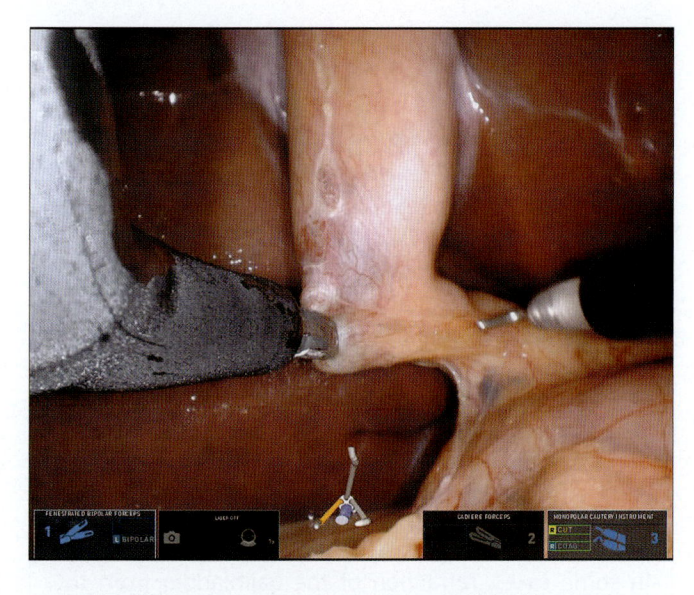

FIGURE 51-15 • Retraction of the gallbladder neck.

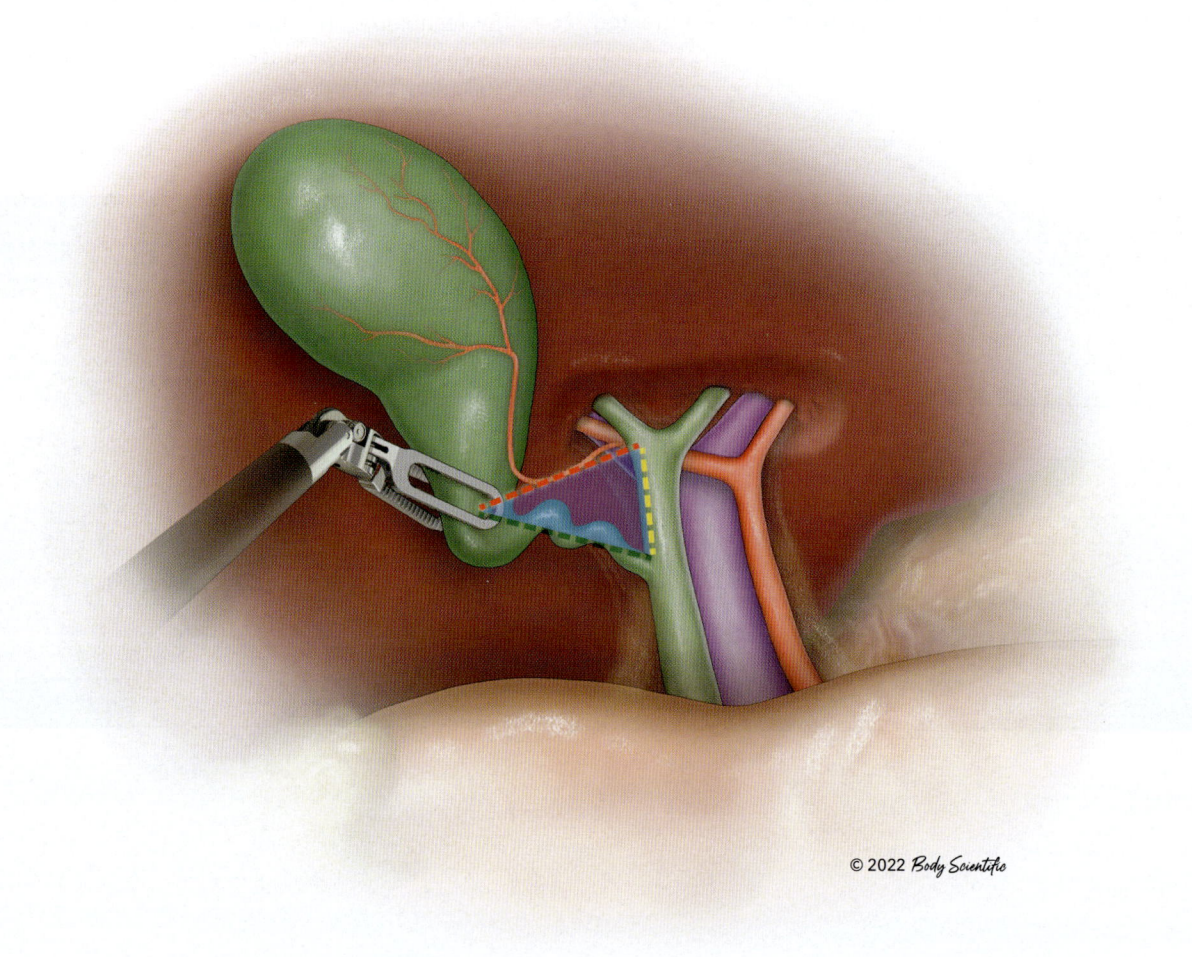

FIGURE 51-16 • Triangle of Calot.

▶▶ TIPS

In cases of unexpected gallbladder distention, when drainage is needed, an Argyle cannula may be inserted through one of the access port seals or one of the operative lumens (after the gallbladder's wall has been partially scored). The cannula is then advanced to perforate and to drain the gallbladder. After the drainage is completed, a stitch is placed to minimize the contamination of the field and spillage of stones (**Figures 51-17 A, B**).

⚠ PITFALLS

Insufficient exposure and poor understanding of the anatomy could lead to bile duct/vascular injury. Limited exposure might be caused by a difficult gallbladder retraction, inadequate positioning of the R3, and inflammation/fibrosis around the hilum. In some cases of unclear anatomy or severe inflammation, conversion to a robotic multiport/laparoscopic/open approach or a subtotal cholecystectomy may be necessary (see Chapter 37, Cholecystectomy). Patient safety is always the number one priority. Structures should never be divided without a clear understanding of the anatomy.

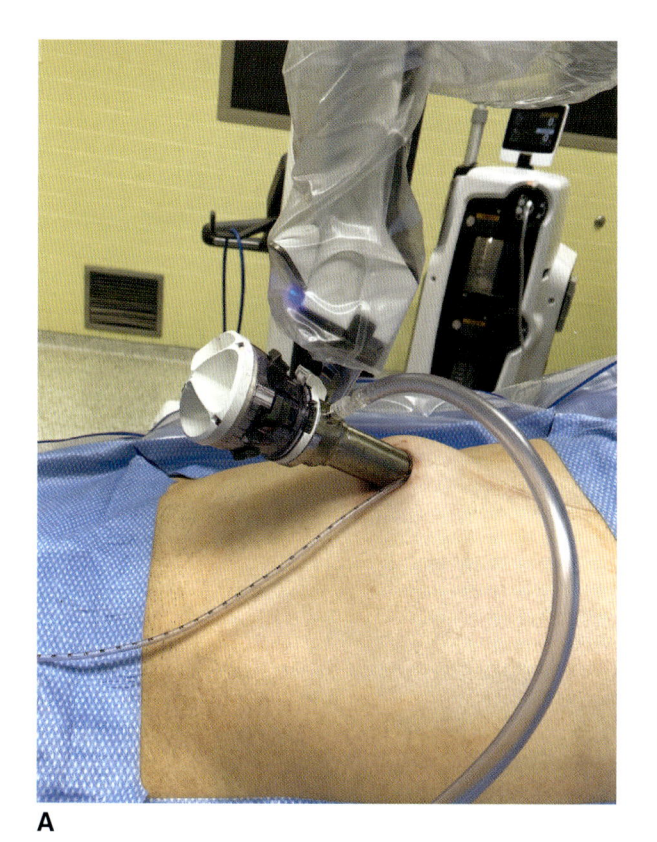

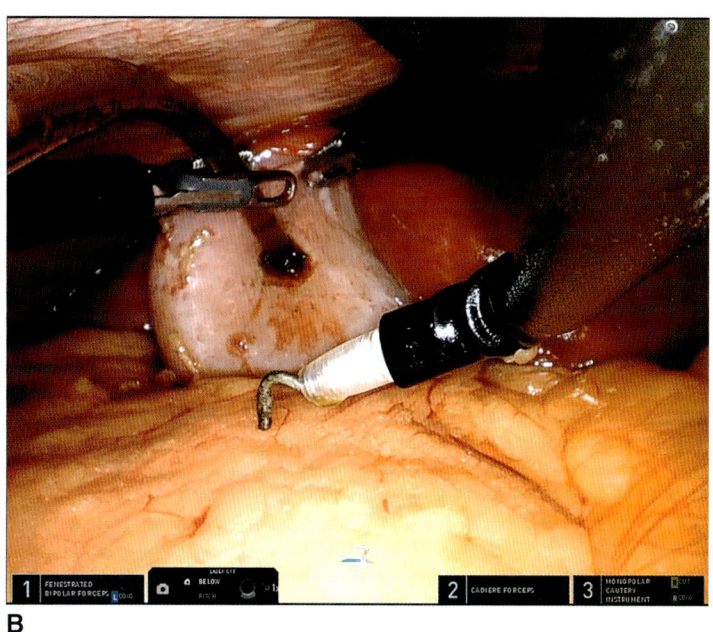

FIGURE 51-17 • Gallbladder drainage.

Step 3. Opening of the anterior peritoneal layer of the triangle of Calot

The anterior peritoneal layer of the triangle of Calot is lifted and incised with the tip of the monopolar hook. The dissection should start after having a preliminary understanding of the location of the cystic duct and artery. The direction of the dissection should proceed either medial-to-lateral or lateral-to-medial depending on the specific anatomy privileging the safest dissection. The goal of this step is to facilitate the following preparation of the cystic duct and artery allowing the creation of more space and completing the anatomical understanding. Short and low-energy cautery bursts (2–3 seconds), under proper gallbladder's neck retraction, will help to open the peritoneal layer and to avoid thermal injury of the cystic duct or artery (**Figure 51-18**).

Step 3 average time frame: 3–5 min

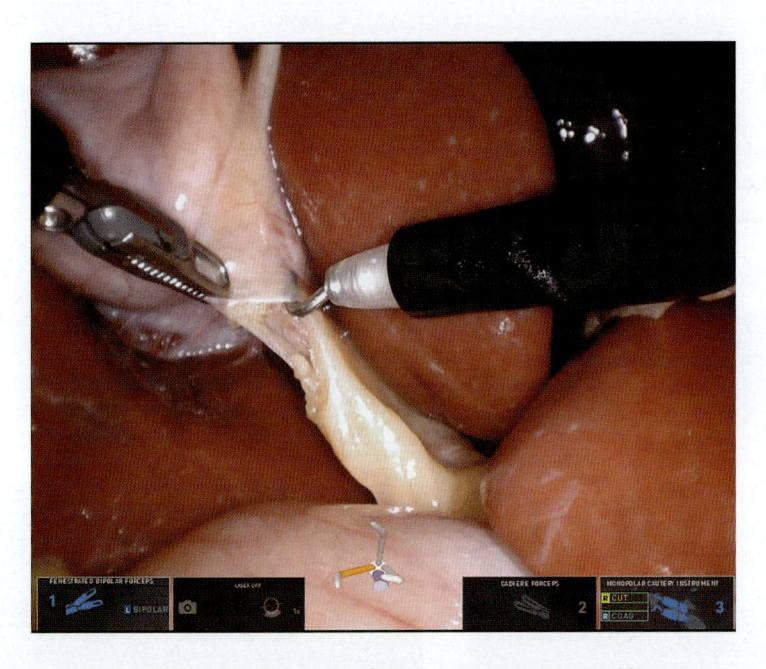

FIGURE 51-18 • Opening of the anterior peritoneal layer.

Step 4. Opening of the posterior peritoneal layer of the triangle of Calot

Once the anterior side of the triangle of Calot is cleared, the gallbladder neck is medially retracted, and attention is focused on the posterior surface. The dissection is performed in a similar fashion and close to the gallbladder wall to release the posterior attachments of the cystic duct and artery (**Figure 51-19**).

Step 4 average time frame: 3–5 min

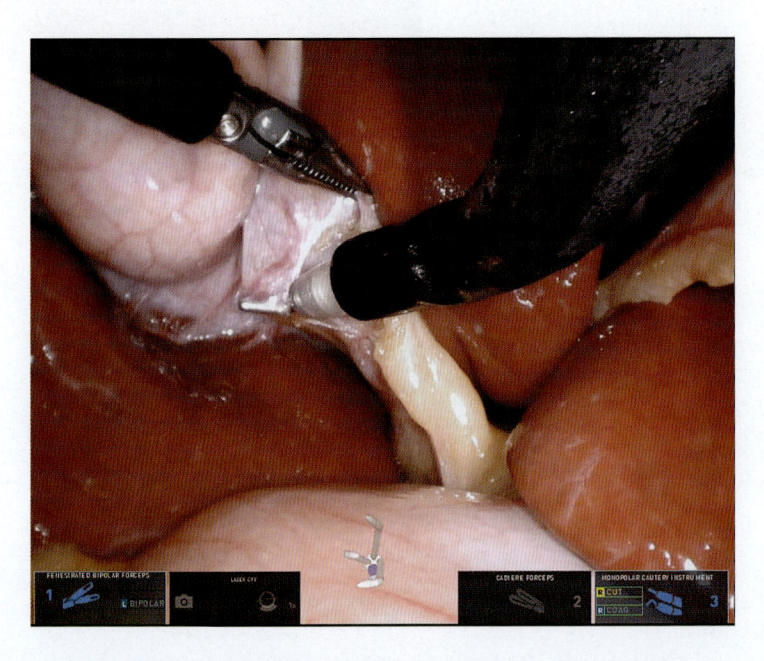

FIGURE 51-19 • Opening of the posterior peritoneal layer.

Step 5. Isolation of the cystic duct

Once the peritoneum is opened on both sides of the triangle of Calot, a window of dissection is developed to achieve the "critical view of safety." Using a combination of blunt and cautery sharp dissection, the attachments surrounding the neck of the gallbladder are addressed until the cystic duct is isolated. Appropriate gallbladder neck retraction is particularly important during this step because this transmits tension to the cystic duct making the dissection easier. Knowledge of the cystic duct normal anatomy and its variants is critical for a safe cholecystectomy (for more details, see Chapter 37, Cholecystectomy).

Step 5 average time frame: 5–8 min

Step 6. Isolation of the cystic artery

In most cases, the cystic artery will be encountered posteriorly and medially to the cystic duct. Once identified, the cystic artery is dissected from its anterior and posterior attachments. Afterward, the gallbladder wall is dissected from the cystic plate. Once all the fat and fibrous tissue are cleared from the triangle of Calot, the surgeon should be able to see only 2 structures entering the gallbladder, and behind these, the cystic plate on the liver. At this point, the critical view is achieved, and it is safe to divide the cystic artery and duct.

Step 6 average time frame: 5–8 min

> **ANATOMICAL HIGHLIGHTS**
>
> Critical view of safety (**Figure 51-20**).

> **▶▶ TIPS**
>
> The making of 2 windows (clearing a small area of the triangle of Calot between the cystic duct and artery, and around the artery) does not necessarily achieve the critical view of safety. In some cases where the gallbladder neck is attached to the liver plate, it has to be partially detached to achieve a complete critical view of safety.

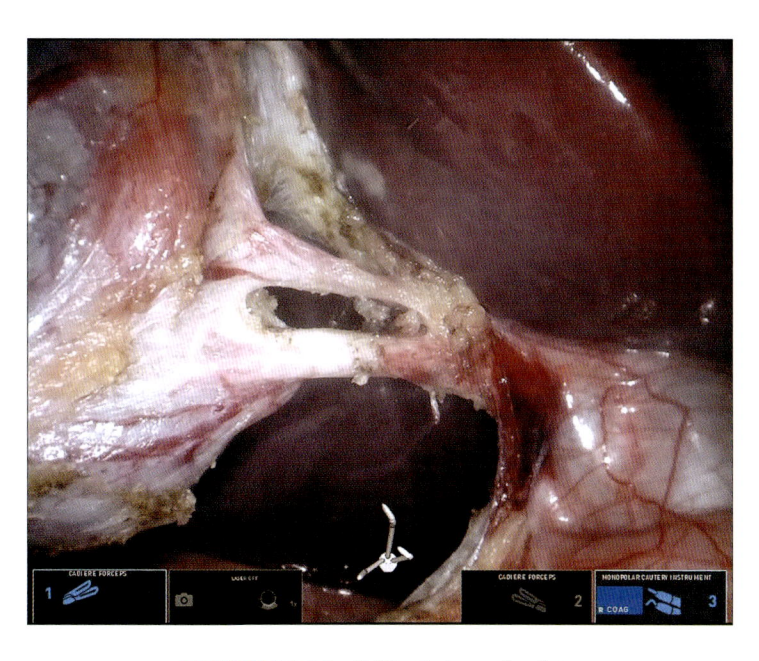

FIGURE 51-20 • Critical view of safety.

> **⚠ PITFALLS**
>
> **Bleeding:** Blind application of clips, sutures, or electrocautery to control bleeding in the triangle of Calot should be avoided because this is the recipe for bile duct and vascular injuries.
>
> **Bile duct injury:** Misidentifying the CBD as the cystic duct is responsible for most of the bile duct injuries during cholecystectomies. Certain situations such as aberrant biliary anatomy, severe inflammation, inexperience, overconfidence, and an inadequate surgical technique are also contributing factors.
>
> Upward retraction of the gallbladder neck results in parallel alignment of the cystic duct and CBD. This facilitates the misidentification of the CBD as the cystic duct and results in dissection and clipping of the CBD. This situation might be associated with a right hepatic artery injury, which is mistaken for the cystic artery.

Step 7. Clipping of the cystic duct

Once the cystic duct is circumferentially dissected and the critical view of safety is achieved, the cystic duct is clipped. It is important to check that enough space is available to place the clips. One or 2 Hem-o-lok™ clips are placed on the distal cystic duct and 1 clip is placed on the proximal side (**Figure 51-21**). Care must be taken to avoid clipping too close to the junction because it can compromise the lumen of a nondilated CBD.

Step 7 average time frame: 2–3 min

> ⚠ **PITFALLS**
>
> **Loose clips:** Clips must be properly applied so they do not come off. When placing a Hem-o-lok™ clip, be sure that the tips of the clip are visible before closing the clip and avoid including tissue in the locking mechanism.

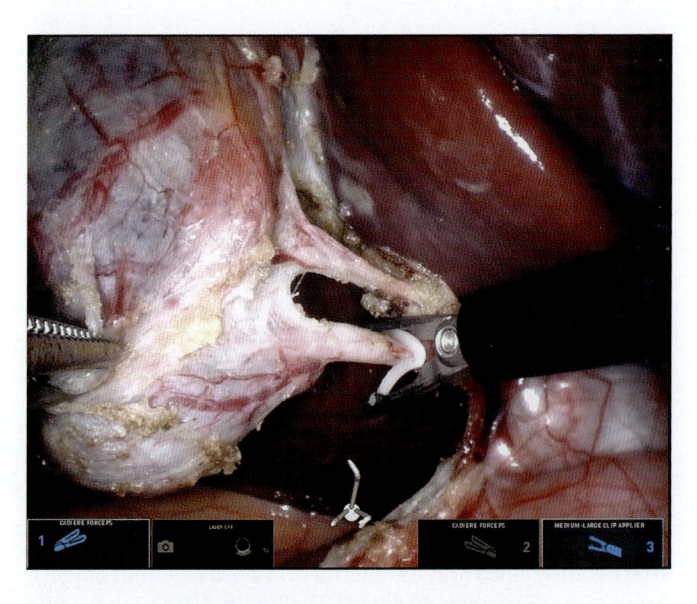

FIGURE 51-21 • Cystic duct clipping.

Step 8. Clipping of the cystic artery

Two Hem-o-lok™ clips, 1 proximal and 1 distal, are placed in the cystic artery in a similar fashion. On some occasions, a very short cystic artery might be encountered, and care must be taken to avoid damage to the right hepatic artery (**Figure 51-22**).

Step 8 average time frame: 1–2 min

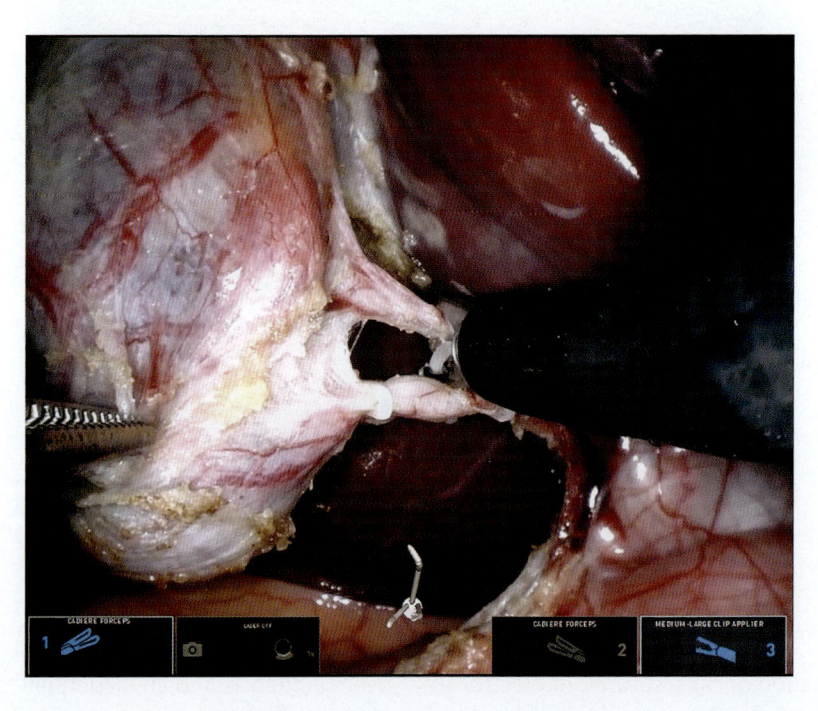

FIGURE 51-22 • Cystic artery clipping.

Step 9. Division of the cystic duct and artery

The cystic duct and artery are preferably divided with cold scissors. It is recommended to leave a bigger cuff of tissue attached to the distal clip to prevent accidental dislodgement. Division with cautery should be avoided mainly if the space between the 2 clips does not allow the transection without burning or compromising the stability of the stump.

Step 9 average time frame: 1–2 min

Video 51-6. Top-Down Dissection

Step 10. Dissection of the gallbladder from the liver

Following the division of the cystic duct and artery, retrograde dissection of the gallbladder from the liver bed is performed. The best tool to perform the gallbladder dissection is the monopolar hook using the "pull" and "push" technique described in Chapter 37, Cholecystectomy. The dissection should be carried out following the plane of areolar connective tissue between the gallbladder's wall and the liver's parenchyma. Appropriate retraction by pulling the gallbladder medially and laterally will facilitate the visualization and maintain tension on the dissection line. If this "holy plane" is not respected, gallbladder perforation with bile/stone spillage or entry into the liver bed with bleeding/bile leak may occur.

In some cases, it might be necessary to perform a top-down dissection after the elements of the hilum have been divided (antegrade dissection). In this case, the peritoneal reflection between the gallbladder fundus and the capsule of the liver is retracted cephalad with the R3, and the gallbladder is dissected down using the 2 operative arms (R1 and R2). The grasper applies uniform tension while the hook dissects the "holy plane." This setup allows completion of the dissection with minimal adjustments of the camera or the instruments (**Figures 51-23 A–C**).

Step 10 average time frame: 20–30 min

> ⚠ **PITFALLS**
>
> **Gallbladder perforation:** Special attention should be paid to avoid perforating the gallbladder during the dissection. Picking up and collecting the stones spilled in the abdominal cavity is harder than with the multiport approach.

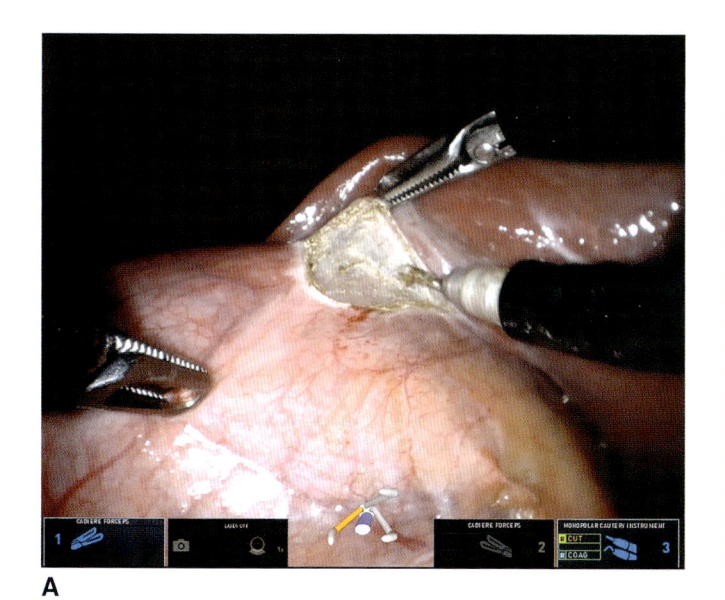

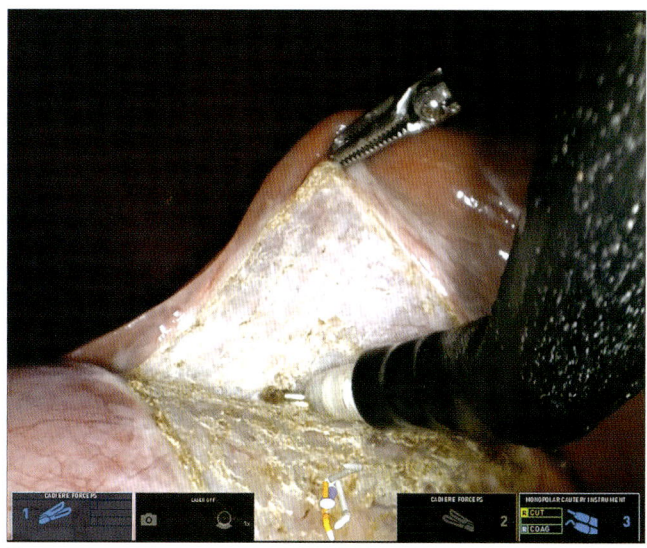

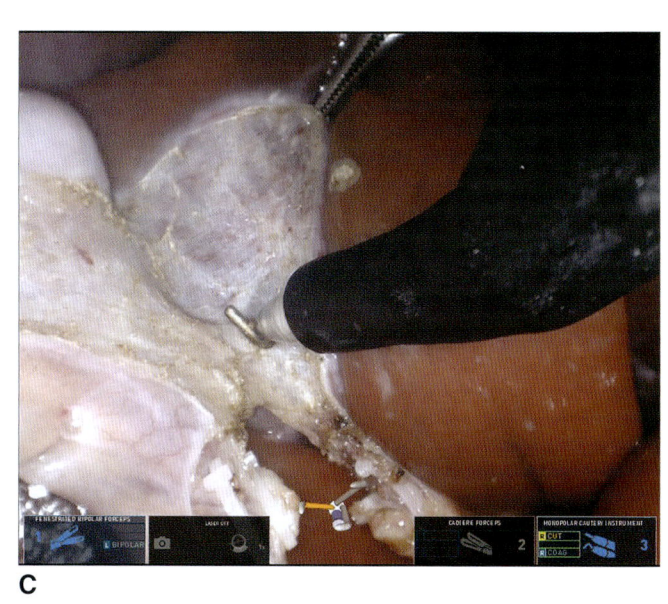

FIGURE 51-23 • Gallbladder bed dissection.

Video 51-7. Gallbladder Extraction

Step 11. Hemostasis review and specimen retrieval

Before completely detaching the gallbladder from the liver's bed, a final inspection for hemostasis is performed using the gallbladder for retraction to expose the dissected area. After the cholecystectomy is completed, a laparoscopic locking grasper is introduced to hold the gallbladder. At this point, the robotic instruments are removed and the cart is undocked. The grasper is gently pulled out until resistance is encountered (this is the sign that the gallbladder is close to the cannula). After that, the gallbladder and the metal cannula are retrieved together.

If the gallbladder was opened during the procedure, a 5-mm Endobag™ is inserted through the access port rotating seal (or R2 port if using the metal cannula) and then retrieved using the same method described above. In some cases, the incision will not be large enough to easily retrieve the gallbladder. In those cases, the same tips used in Chapter 37, Cholecystectomy, will be applied. Abdominal drains are not routinely placed in this operation.

Right exposure of the fascia is the key for an appropriate closure. The 2 fascial edges are lifted up with Kocher clamps, and 3 or 4 figure-8 PDS™ 1 stitches are placed. The subcutaneous plane is closed with Vicryl™ 3-0 sutures to orient the wound. Finally, the skin is closed with subcuticular interrupted stitches (**Figure 51-24**).

Step 11 average time frame: 3–5 min

> ▶▶ **TIPS**
>
> The gallbladder extraction is easier than with the multiport technique due to the bigger umbilical incision used to introduce the SP cannula.

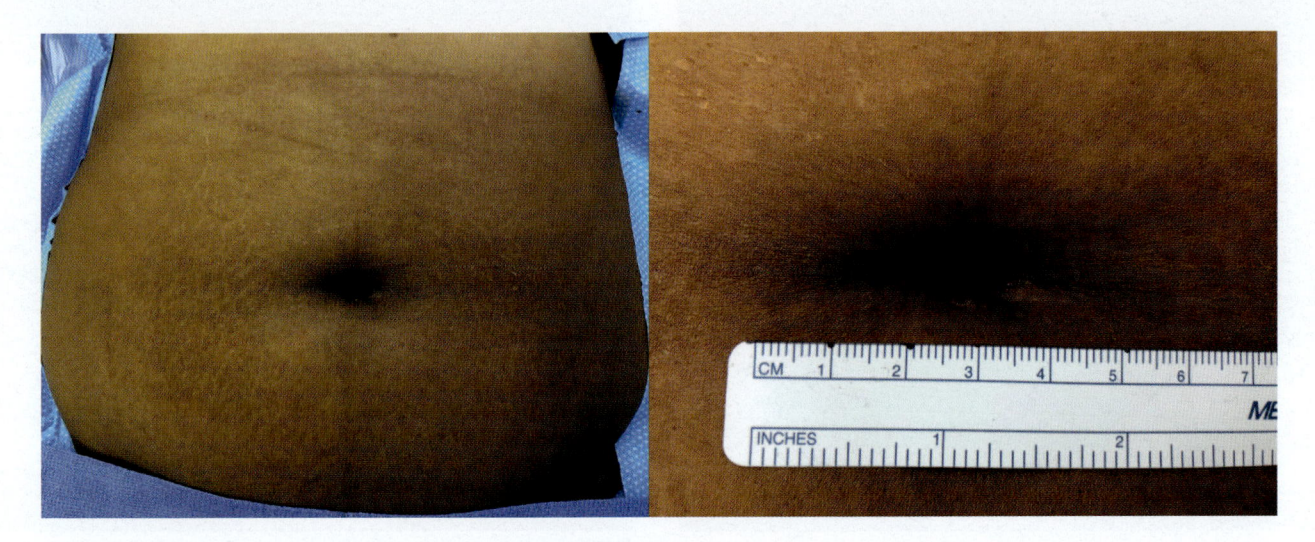

FIGURE 51-24 • Skin closure.

SP Transabdominal Preperitoneal (TAPP) Inguinal Hernia Repair (Off-Label)

Indications and Relative Contraindications to the SP Robotic Approach

SP TAPP inguinal hernia repair has the same indications as the laparoscopic technique. However, large inguinoscrotal, recurrent hernias, patients with previous pelvic surgery, and super obesity are relative contraindications.

INSTRUMENT REQUIREMENTS

The suggested main robotic instruments/tools can be listed as follows:
- Scope
- Cautery hook/monopolar scissors
- Bipolar forceps
- Cadière forceps
- Needle driver

The suggested main laparoscopic instruments/tools can be listed as follows:
- Grasper
- Needle driver

Supplemental materials:
- Mesh
- Sutures: Prolene™ 3-0/4-0, Vicryl™ 3-0
- Access port (optional)

Patient Positioning, OR Setup, and Port Setting

After the endotracheal intubation, the patient is positioned supine with arms tucked. The operation starts by creating a single access in the periumbilical area through a vertical 2.5-cm skin incision as previously described. A dedicated SP device is introduced, the abdomen insufflated, and an exploratory laparoscopy is performed (**Figures 51-25 A, B**). At this point, the patient is positioned in 30° Trendelenburg and tilted down 20° to the contralateral side of the hernia (**Figure 51-26**). The robotic cart is docked over the patient's flank with no preferred side since the system allows for 360° rotation around the abdominal wall access. The OR setup is explained in **Figure 51-27**. The robotic instrument arm is connected to the access port or metal cannula and the instruments and camera are inserted in the entry guide. The 3D articulating scope is introduced through the inferior oval cannula lumen. The monopolar hook (R1) and the Cadière forceps (R2) are introduced through the right and left cannula lumen, respectively. If using the metal cannula, the remaining upper lumen will be used by the assistant to introduce sutures.

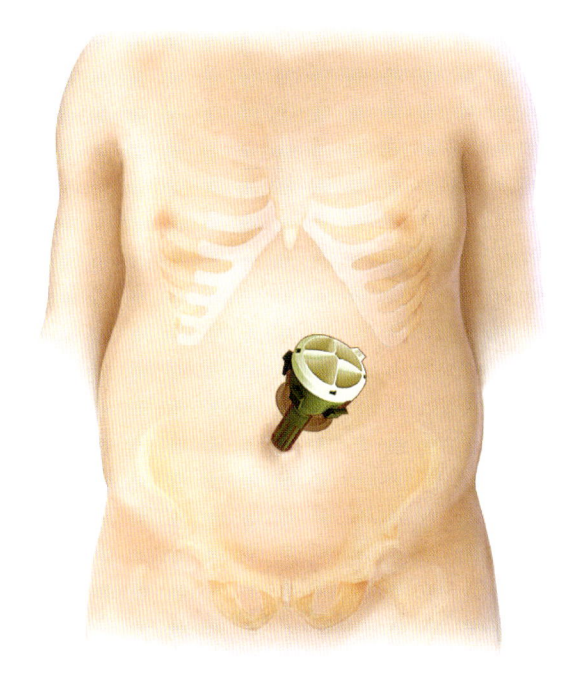

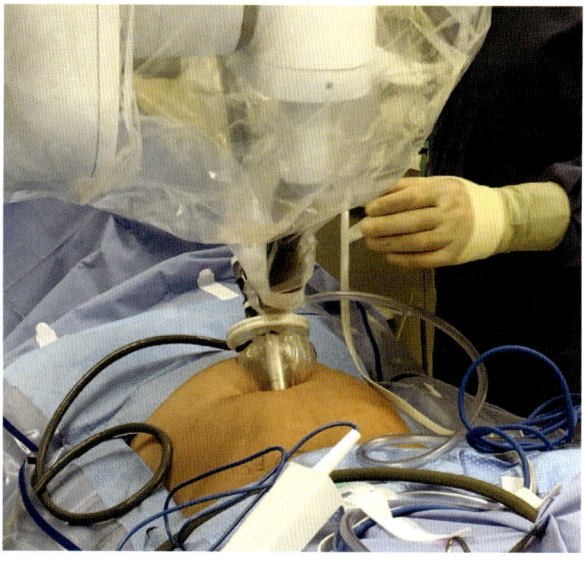

FIGURE 51-25 • Single port placement.

1058   The Foundation and Art of Robotic Surgery

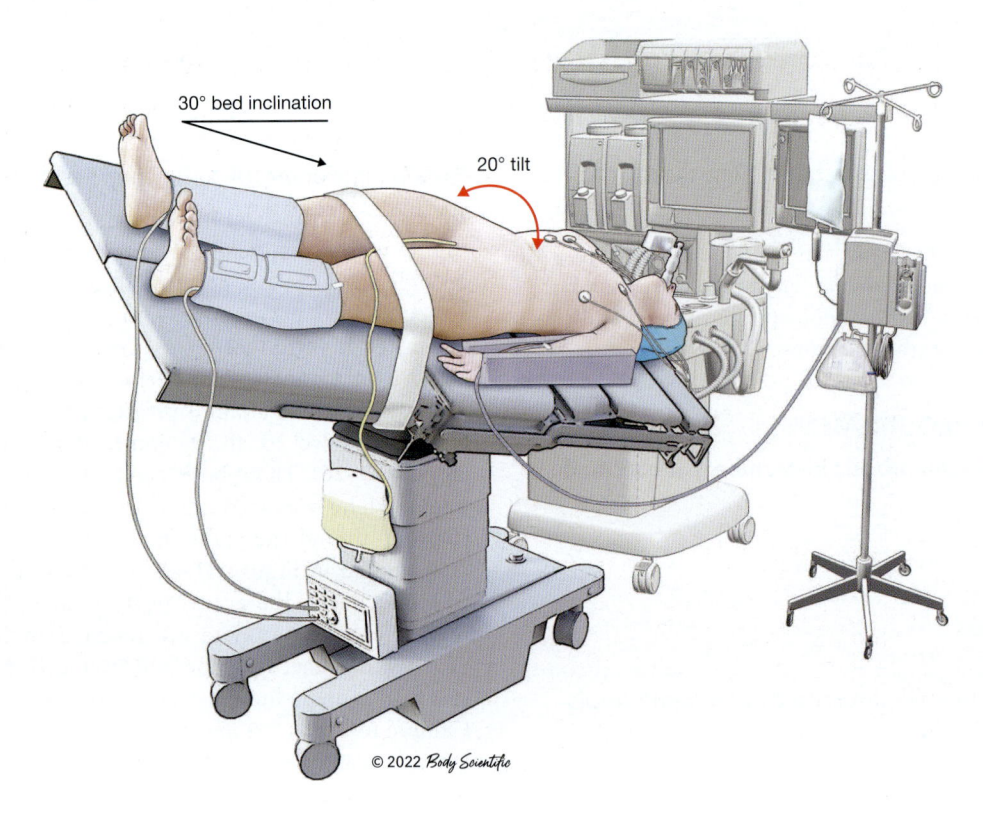

FIGURE 51-26 • Patient positioning for right-sided hernia.

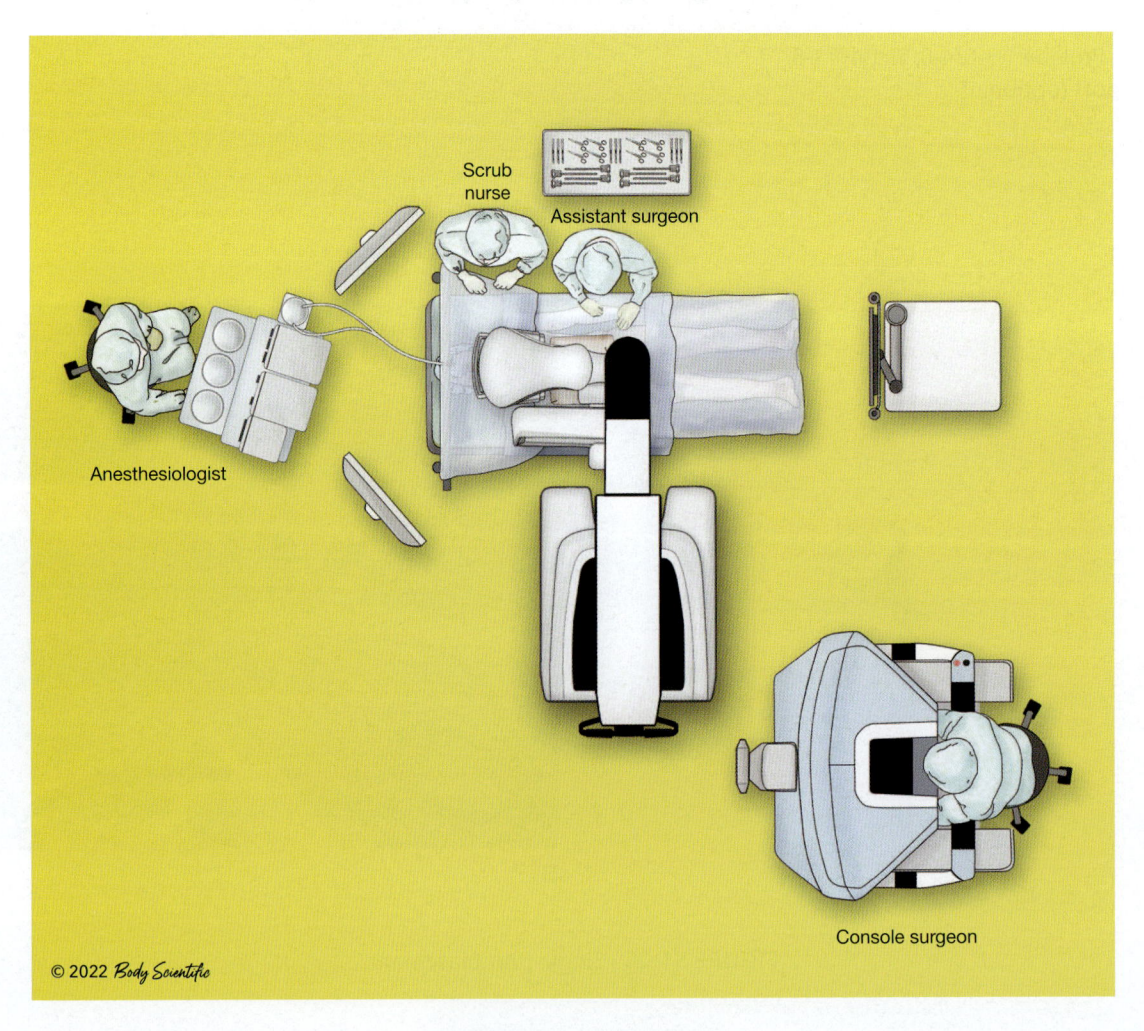

FIGURE 51-27 • OR setup.

Single Port Robotic Surgery: Basic Concepts

> ▶▶ **TIPS**
>
> **Floating Port Technique:** In patients with a short abdomen, a floating dock is used to facilitate the flap closure, because a minimum distance of 10 cm from the target anatomy is required to fully deploy the instruments. This may be also achieved by using the access port by port clutching the instrument arm away from the body until there is sufficient room to deploy the instruments to their desired location.
>
> If using the SP metal cannula (instead of the access port), a plastic wound retractor is placed before inserting the cannula. The metal cannula is then introduced through the wound retractor and secured with a large silk suture tied to maintain the pneumoperitoneum. With this setup, the SP cannula can be pulled out of the abdominal cavity and "float" within the wound retractor. This increases the distance from the target anatomy and allows the instruments' deployment (**Figure 51-28**).
>
> Emptying the urinary bladder might improve exposure and reduce the risk of injury. If a long or complex procedure is expected, a Foley catheter should be placed.

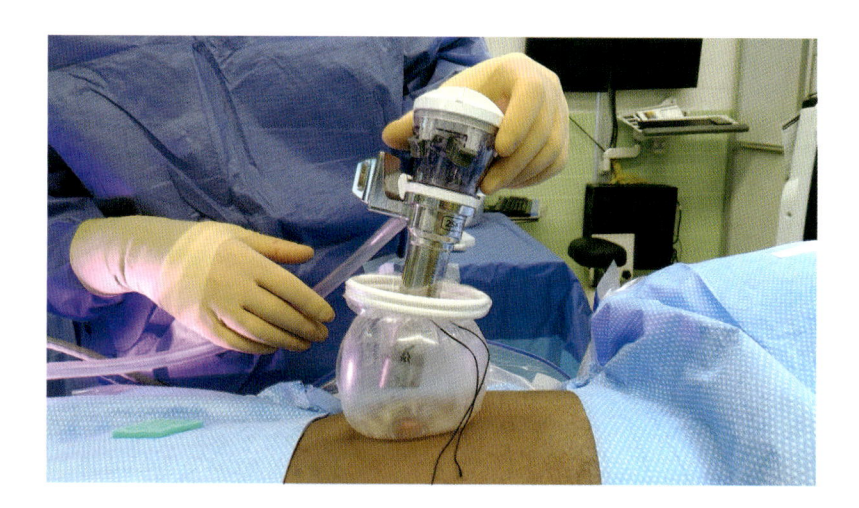

FIGURE 51-28 • Floating port.

Surgical Technique

▶ **Video 51-8.** SP Inguinal Hernia Repair

Step 1. Recognition of the anatomical landmarks
After the instruments are introduced and deployed in the abdominal cavity, lysis of adhesions is performed (when needed) using the monopolar hook or cold scissors. Exploration of both inguinal regions is then carried out to detect potential contralateral defects and to recognize the patient's anatomy.

Afterward, careful identification of the groin anatomical landmarks is performed. The anterior superior iliac spine, medial umbilical ligament, deep/internal inguinal ring, inferior epigastric vessels, *vas deferens*, and spermatic vessels should be recognized.

Step 1 average time frame: 1–5 min

> 🔍 **ANATOMICAL HIGHLIGHTS**
> - Zones of the inguinal region (see Chapter 43, Inguinal Hernia Repair).
> - Inguinal region topography highlights (**Figure 51-29**).

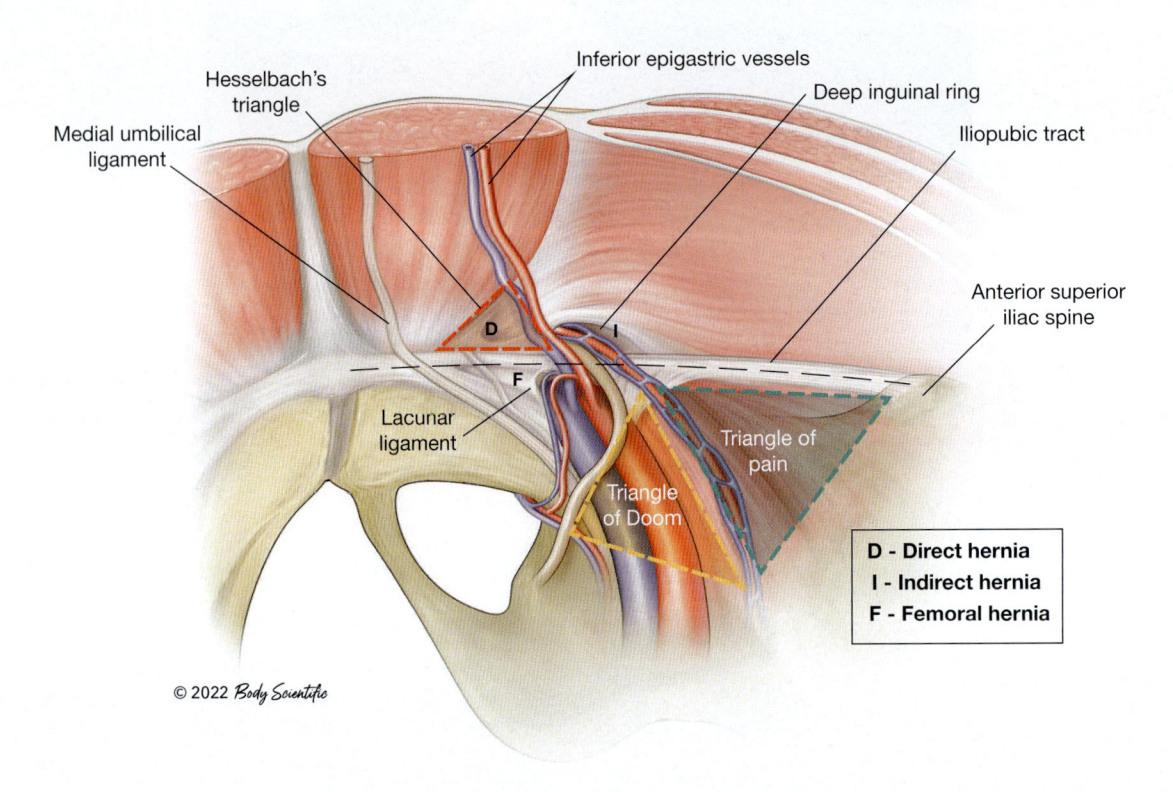

FIGURE 51-29 • Inguinal region topography highlights.

Video 51-9. Flap Dissection

Step 2. Flap dissection

The peritoneum incision is performed following a slightly oblique line (arch of the transverse muscle) from the medial umbilical ligament to the anterior superior iliac spine. This line should be at least 2–4 cm above the deep inguinal ring to allow a proper mesh overlap. The peritoneal opening can be performed either from lateral-to-medial or medial-to-lateral direction, after the preliminary identification of the inferior epigastric vessels that should not be injured while opening the flap. The peritoneum is gently grasped with the Cadière forceps and retracted downward. This maneuver separates the peritoneum from the transversalis fascia. Sometimes, the peritoneum is very thin, and this separation becomes impossible without tearing it. In this situation, it is convenient to leave a patch of transversalis fascia attached to the peritoneum, reentering in the proper plane once the critical area is overcome. The inferior edge of the peritoneal flap is grasped and pulled upward while making counterpressure on the preperitoneal tissue progressively opening the space. The CO_2 is spreading into the preperitoneal space, further facilitating the dissection. The peritoneal incision is then extended to the above-mentioned landmarks (**Figures 51-30 A, B**).

Step 2 average time frame: 2–5 min

> ▶▶ **TIPS**
>
> In contrast to the totally extraperitoneal (TEP) technique, the TAPP approach allows identification of occult contralateral defects or concomitant intraperitoneal pathologies.
>
> It is advisable to obtain consent before surgery for possible bilateral repair in case a contralateral hernia is identified during this step.

A   B

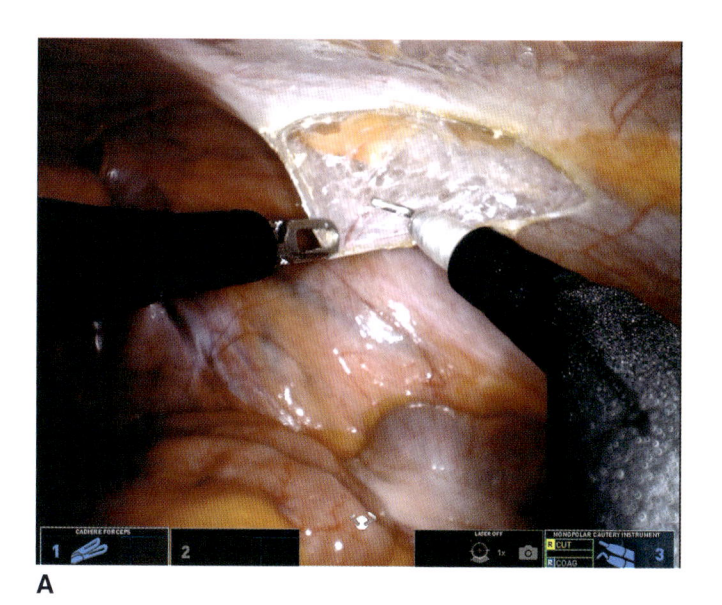

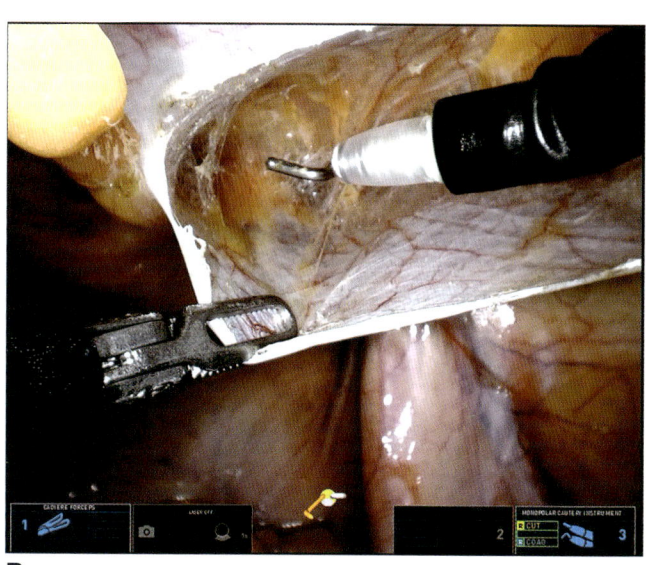

FIGURE 51-30 • Flap dissection.

▶ **Video 51-10. Medial Dissection**

Step 3. Medial dissection (zone 2)
The next step is to perform a wide dissection of the preperitoneal space that will allow the placement of a prothesis that covers all the potential hernia defects with an adequate mesh overlap and posterior coverage. The preperitoneal space dissection starts medially to the epigastric vessels. The areolar tissue in this area is easily dissected with blunt maneuvers. The prevesical space is exposed until the Cooper's ligament and pubic symphysis are identified (**Figure 51-31**). At this point, a direct hernia could be encountered above the pectineal ligament. In that case, if the direct hernia is small, it can be separated from the transversalis fascia and completely reduced. If the direct hernia is bigger, it is advisable to complete the dissection after the lateral aspect of the peritoneal flap has been completed. This will provide more space for traction of the peritoneum during the hernia sac dissection.

Step 3 average time frame: 2–5 min

> ⚠ **PITFALLS**
>
> - *Corona mortis* injury during medial dissection close to the pubic bone.
> - If during the dissection excessive bleeding is encountered, it means that there is a wrong surgical plane.

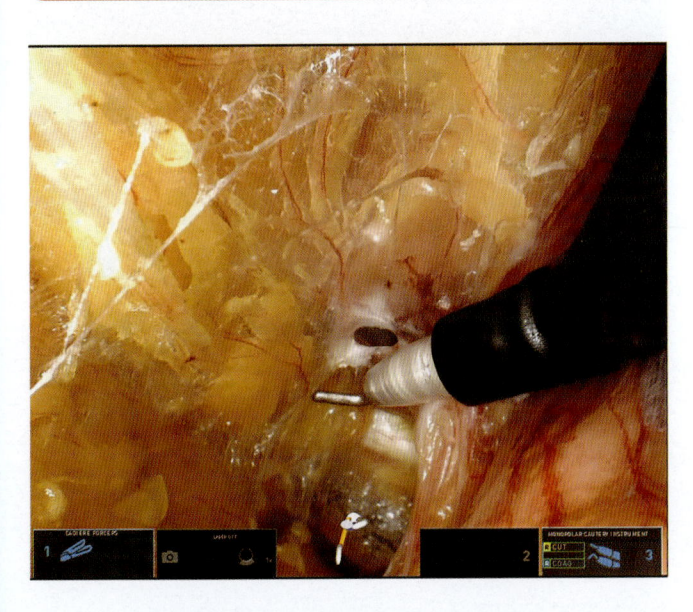

FIGURE 51-31 • Medial zone dissection.

Step 4. Lateral dissection (zone 1)
Dissection continues in the area lateral to the spermatic and inferior epigastric vessels. Lateral dissection is performed using horizontal retraction of the peritoneum and countertraction on the preperitoneal fat. The fatty tissue should be dissected off the peritoneum and kept attached to the abdominal wall. This is the key to avoid damage to the nerves present in this zone. The lateral dissection should be extended as much as possible on the medial side to see the spermatic vessels, posterior to the internal ring (**Figure 51-32**).

Step 4 average time frame: 2–10 min

> 🔍 **ANATOMICAL HIGHLIGHTS**
>
> Nerves of the inguinal region (**Figure 51-33**).

> ▶▶ **TIPS**
>
> During this part of the dissection, the electrocautery should be used cautiously. Blunt tissue separation and selective use of bipolar coagulation are advisable to minimize the risk of nerve damage.

> ⚠ **PITFALLS**
>
> Damage to the lateral cutaneous nerve of the tight, femoral nerve, or femoral branch of the genitofemoral nerve due to excessive dissection or injudicious electrocautery use.
>
> Peritoneal tears due to excessive traction or misidentification of the correct dissection plane.

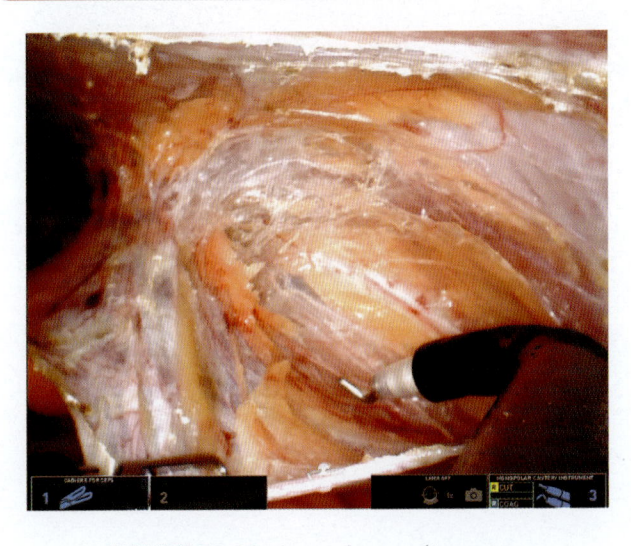

FIGURE 51-32 • Lateral zone dissection.

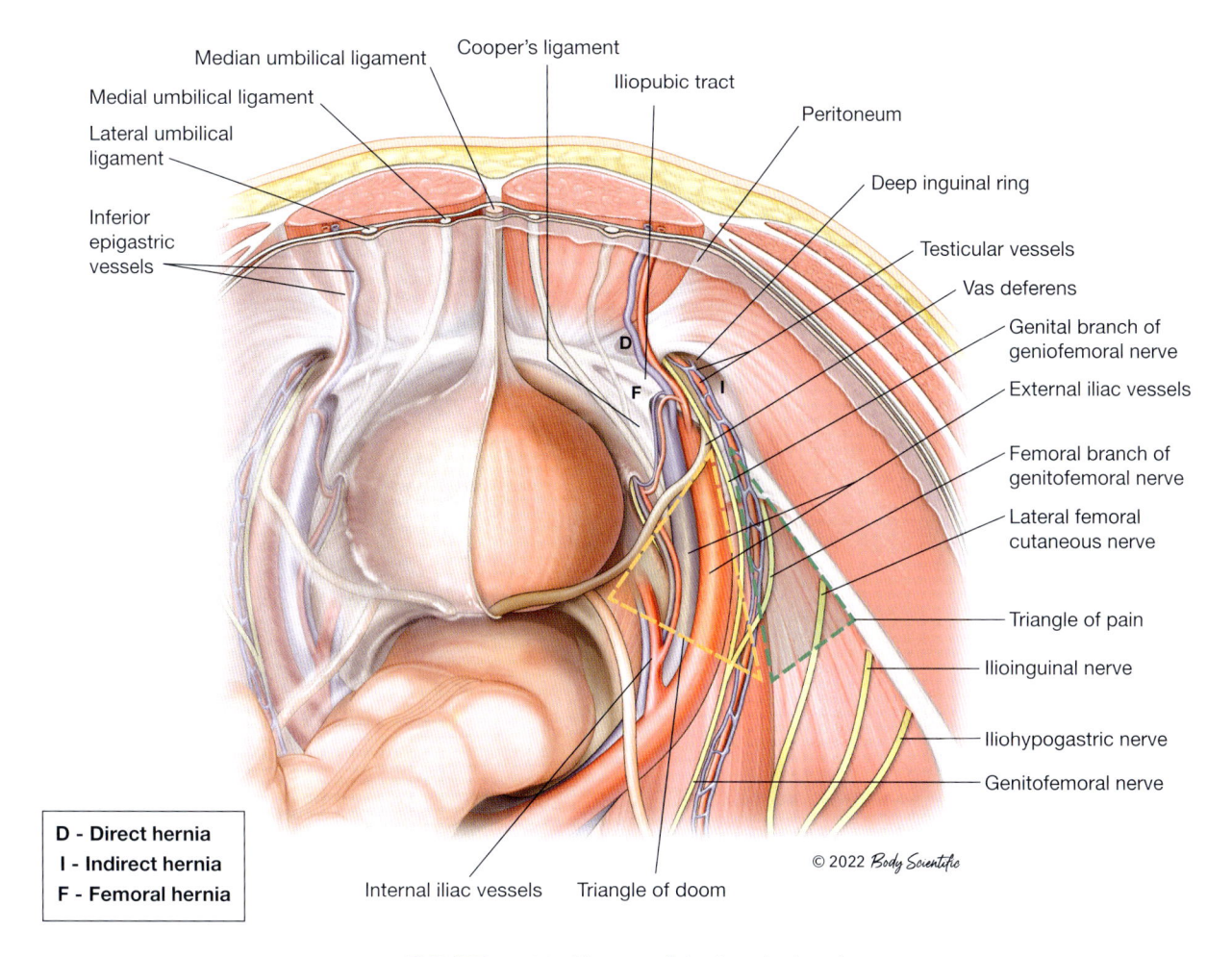

FIGURE 51-33 • Nerves of the inguinal region.

Step 5. Central (zone 3) and indirect hernia sac dissection

In this step, the peritoneum over the spermatic cord and *vas deferens* is mobilized and the sac of an indirect hernia is dissected. The spermatic vessels and *vas deferens* delineate the "triangle of doom" where the external iliac vessels will be found. Deep dissection between these elements and the peritoneum must be done very carefully to avoid major complications. The peritoneal flap and the indirect hernia sac are retracted and dissected away from the elements of the spermatic cord. The hernia sac is grasped at the superomedial edge and dissected along its superior border. A combination of blunt and sharp dissection with the electrocautery is used for this purpose. At last, the spermatic cord is inspected looking for possible lipomas that should be completely reduced to avoid persistence of the symptoms (**Figures 51-34 A, B**). When the surgeon can identify the hernia defect, Cooper's ligament, pubic symphysis, inferior epigastric vessels, spermatic cord, *vas deferens*, and psoas muscle, the dissection is completed.

Large direct hernias are approached as well during this phase after the dissection of the lateral and central zone.

Step 5 average time frame: 5–30 min

> ▶▶ **TIPS**
>
> Central dissection (zone 3) should be carefully performed, usually after the other zones have been completely dissected. This is the most delicate part of the operation, where the elements of the inguinal cord, *vas deferens*, and an indirect sac are dissected. Preparing the other zones allows identification of all landmarks before starting the central zone dissection.
>
> A combination of sharp and blunt maneuvers are used to dissect the hernia sac. In some cases, a needle driver may be used to peel the sac off the *tunica vaginalis* and cord elements.

> ⚠ **PITFALLS**
>
> Damage to the *vas deferens* or vascular elements of the spermatic cord.

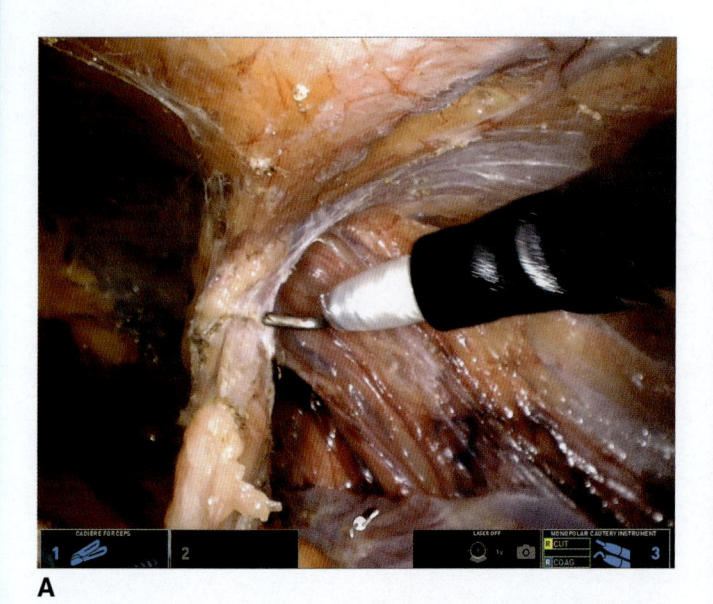

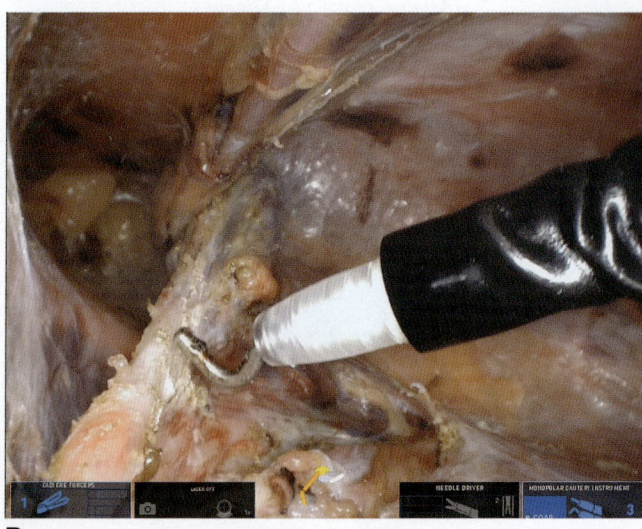

FIGURE 51-34 • Central zone dissection.

▶ Video 51-11. Mesh Placement

Step 6. Parietalization of the spermatic vessels and extension of the horizontal plane

To create a horizontal space to properly place the mesh, the dissection plane is extended until the psoas muscle is exposed. To do so, the spermatic vessels must be carefully separated from the peritoneal flap and the hernia sac with blunt dissection.

Step 6 average time frame: 3–5 min

Step 7. Mesh placement

Once the preperitoneal dissection is completed, a polypropylene mesh of at least 10 × 15 cm is placed to cover all potential hernia sites (direct, indirect, and femoral) with at least 3–4 cm of overlap. The mesh is rolled on a laparoscopic grasper and it is inserted through the rotating seal at the top of the access port (which is the largest seal) or through the camera lumen. Once deployed in the abdominal cavity, the medial end of the mesh is placed over the pubic symphysis and Cooper's ligament. While keeping the medial end of the mesh in place, the lateral part is adapted to the abdominal wall (**Figure 51-35**). The mesh is fixed in place using a nonabsorbable suture to the Cooper's ligament and 1 or 2 stitches to the transversalis fascia. The suture can be easily introduced through the third operative lumen on the top part of the port.

Step 7 average time frame: 2–10 min

> ⚠ **PITFALLS**
> - Inguinal hernia recurrence due to a small, incorrectly placed, or dislodged mesh. This is usually related to an incomplete preperitoneal dissection mostly in the medial and posterior aspect.
> - Injury to vascular structures during mesh fixation.

> ▶▶ **TIPS**
> If using the metal cannula instead of the access port, laparoscopic instruments produce a gas leak when entering the robotic port because of a 1-mm difference in size. A wet sponge wrapped around the shaft of the laparoscopic instrument can significantly reduce this leak.

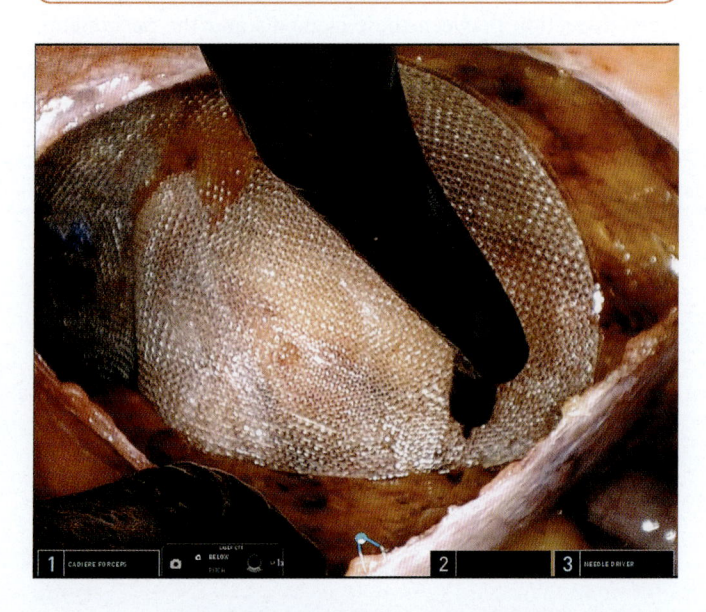

FIGURE 51-35 • Mesh placement.

▶ Video 51-12. Closure of the Peritoneum Flap

Step 8. Closure of the peritoneum flap
This step is the most difficult when using the SP platform. This is mainly due to the limited distance between the target and the instruments, which restrict the movements. Using the access port or a floating dock can overcome these difficulties.

The peritoneum flap is closed with a running PDS™ or Vicryl™ 3-0 absorbable suture. In order to avoid conflicting actions between the 2 operative arms (forceps and needle driver), the direction of suturing for "right-handed surgeons" should be lateral-to-medial for left groin hernias and medial-to-lateral for the right side. A complete peritoneum closure is the key to avoid contact between the synthetic mesh and the small bowel. To avoid tension during the flap closure, the hernia sac or a portion of the umbilical ligament could be included (**Figures 51-36 A, B**).

Step 8 average time frame: 2–10 min

> ⚠ **PITFALLS**
>
> A peritoneal flap closed under tension, mainly when there is partial resection of the peritoneal sac, might create a real empty space in front of the peritoneum closure. The suture may breakdown and this can favor the herniation of small bowel loops in the preperitoneal space with possible obstruction.

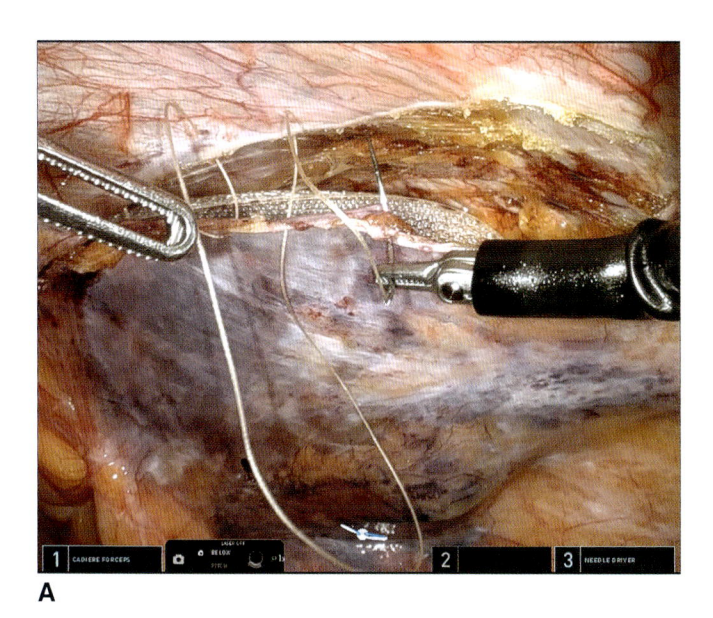

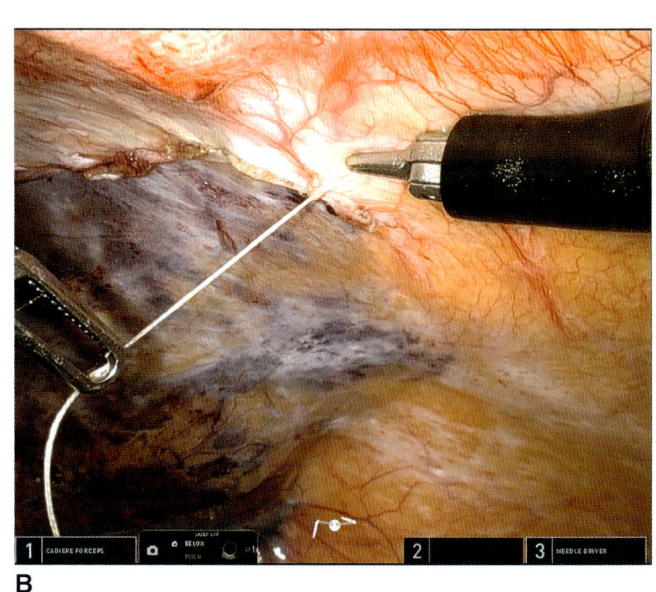

FIGURE 51-36 • Closure of the peritoneal flap.

Suggested Readings

1. Navarra G, Pozza E, Occhionorelli S, Carcoforo P, Donini I. One-wound laparoscopic cholecystectomy. *Br J Surg.* 1997;84(5):695.
2. Sajid MS, Khawaja AH, Sayegh M, Baig MK. A systematic review comparing single-incision versus multi-incision laparoscopic surgery for inguinal hernia repair with mesh. *Int J Surg.* 2016;29:25-35. doi: 10.1016/j.ijsu.2016.02.088
3. Lurje G, Raptis DA, Steinemann DC, et al. Cosmesis and body image in patients undergoing single-port versus conventional laparoscopic cholecystectomy: a multicenter double-blinded randomized controlled trial (SPOCC-trial). *Ann Surg.* 2015;262(5):728-735. doi: 10.1097/SLA.0000000000001474
4. Pietrabissa A, Sbrana F, Morelli L, et al. Overcoming the challenges of single-incision cholecystectomy with robotic single-site technology. *Arch Surg.* 2012;147(8):709-714. doi: 10.1001/archsurg.2012.508
5. Perivoliotis K, Tzovaras G, Sarakatsianou C, Baloyiannis I. Current status of single-port versus multi-port approach in laparoscopic inguinal hernia mesh repair: an up-to-date systematic review and meta-analysis. *Hernia.* 2019;23(2):217-233. doi: 10.1007/s10029-018-01876-7
6. Cruz CJ, Huynh F, Kang I, Lee WJ, Kang CM. Initial experiences of robotic SP cholecystectomy: a comparative analysis with robotic Si single-site cholecystectomy. *Ann Surg Treat Res.* 2021;100(1):1-7. doi: 10.4174/astr.2021.100.1.1
7. Kim D, Lee CS. Single-port robotic totally extraperitoneal (TEP) inguinal hernia repair using the da Vinci SP platform: a video vignette. *Asian J Surg.* 2022;45(10):2062-2063. doi: 10.1016/j.asjsur.2022.04.101
8. Bianco FM, Dreifuss NH, Chang B, et al. Robotic single-port surgery: preliminary experience in general surgery. *Int J Med Robot.* 2022;18(6):e2453. doi: 10.1002/rcs.2453
9. Dreifuss NH, Chang B, Schlottmann F, et al. Robotic inguinal hernia repair: is the new Da Vinci single port platform providing any benefit? *Surg Endosc.* 2023;37(3):2003-2013. doi: 10.1007/s00464-022-09737-2
10. Giulianotti PC, Coratti A, Angelini M, et al. Robotics in general surgery: personal experience in a large community hospital. *Arch Surg.* 2003;138(7):777-784. doi: 10.1001/archsurg.138.7.777

Index

Note: Page numbers followed by *f* and *t* refer to the page location of figures and tables respectively.

A

Abdominal insufflation, 46, 47*f*
Abdominal lymph nodes
   dissection of, 256
   list of, 243*t*
Abdominal wall
   anatomy of, 912, 913*f*, 926
   stomach fixation to, in left adrenalectomy, 886*f*
   transversus abdominis muscle, 926, 927*f*
Absorbable monofilament sutures, 823
Academics, 63
Achalasia, 299
ACS. *See* American College of Surgeons
Acute cholecystitis, biliary leaks in, 97*f*
Adhesiolysis
   for adhesions, 29–31, 830, 866
   in robotic transversus abdominis release, 931
   in small bowel, 444
Adhesions
   adhesiolysis for, 29–31, 830, 866
   intra-abdominal, 920*f*
Adrenal glands
   anatomy of, 879
   arterial supply to, 874
   left, 879
   right, 879
Adrenal surgery, 118, 118*f*
Adrenal veins
   anatomical variations of, 888, 889*f*
   in left adrenalectomy, 888, 888*f*, 890, 890*f*
   in right adrenalectomy, 872, 872*f*, 876–877
Adrenalectomy
   laparoscopic, 863
   left. *See* Left adrenalectomy, robotic
   right. *See* Right adrenalectomy, robotic
AI. *See* Artificial intelligence
ALA. *See* 5-Aminolevulinic acid
Albumin, indocyanine green binding to, 91, 92*f*
American College of Surgeons, 33
American Statistical Association, 86
5-Aminolevulinic acid, 93
Anaglyph glasses, 9
Anastomosis
   bilio-digestive, 631
   cervical, 257
   end-to-end, 227
   end-to-side, 257
   enterobiliary, 842
   esophagogastric, 227, 230*f*–231*f*
   gastrojejunal, in Roux-en-Y gastric bypass, 430, 430*f*
   ileocolic isoperistaltic, 477
   leakage of, during gastric surgery, 108
Anesthesiologist, 27
Aneurysmectomy, 1031, 1031*f*
Angle of His, 425, 425*f*
Animal models, for robotic training, 50–51
Annotation, 83–84
Anterior phrenoesophageal membrane, 305, 306*f*
Anterior pleural reflection at hilum, 336, 336*f*
Anterior superior iliac spine, 898, 906
Anterolateral parenchymal bridge, 340, 340*f*
Aortic lymph nodes, 322*f*
Aortocaval groove, 207, 207*f*
Aortopulmonary window, 198, 201, 204, 204*f*
APMs. *See* Automated performance metrics
Arantius' ligament, 749, 749*f*
Arc of Riolan, 503*f*, 505*f*
Arcuate line, 912, 931, 932*f*
Arterial anastomosis
   in kidney transplant, 977, 977*f*
   in pancreas transplant, 993, 993*f*
Artificial intelligence
   barriers to adoption of, 82–86
   benefits of, 73
   definition of, 12
   explainable, 84–86, 85*f*
   fluorescence imaging applications of, 121
   indocyanine green perfusion analysis, 73
   intraoperative applications of, 12–13, 78–82
   limitations of, 13
   reproducibility of, 86
   robotic training uses of, 52
   scientific articles regarding, 12*f*
   segmentation, 68*f*
   software, 52
   surgery workflow analysis uses of, 78, 80
   surgical applications of, 12, 78–82
   surgical data acquisition, 83
   surgical education applications of, 82
   surgical skills application of, 80–82
   3D measurements and, 80*f*
   trustworthy, 84, 86
Ascending colon mobilization, in right colectomy with complete mesocolic excision, 461–462
ASIS. *See* Anterior superior iliac spine
Assistant
   active, 43
   bedside, 62
   docking by, 40–41, 41*f*
   ergonomic positioning of, 38*f*
   exposure by, 27
   instrumentation review by, 37, 39*f*
   laparoscopic assisting by, 43–44
   operating room preparation by, 33–36, 34*f*–35*f*
   passive, 43
   prepping of patient by, 36–37
   targeting by, 40
   training of, 44
   troubleshooting by, 39–40
Augmented reality
   description of, 9–10, 10*f*, 73–74
   liver surgery application of, 78*f*
   surgical, 74
   workflow, 74–75
Automated performance metrics, 52
Automation bias, 82, 86
Azygos vein
   anatomy of, 241*f*
   division of, in Ivor-Lewis esophagectomy, 225

B

Barety's lodge lymph node dissection, 357*f*
Bariatric surgery
   Roux-en-Y gastric bypass. *See* Roux-en-Y gastric bypass
   sleeve gastrectomy. *See* Sleeve gastrectomy
Bedside assistant, 62
Berry ligament, 152
Bias, automation, 82, 86
Bihepaticojejunostomy, 827
Bile duct. *See also* Common bile duct
   anatomy of, 816*f*, 850*f*, 1010*f*
   blood supply to, 833, 850*f*–851*f*
   mobilization of, in Roux-en-Y hepaticojejunostomy, 814, 817*f*
   transection of, 818, 818*f*

1067

Bile duct injuries
  in cholecystectomy, 1053
  classification of, 835f
  laparoscopic cholecystectomy for, 836f
  recognition of, 833, 834f
  repair of
    bihepaticojejunostomy for, 827
    contraindications for, 826
    delayed, 827
    end-to-end anastomosis in, 837
    extrahepatic hepatic duct, 832f
    hepatoduodenal ligament, 831f
    hilum exposure in, 830
    incidence of, 825
    indications for, 826
    instruments for, 825
    Kasai procedure for, 827
    near-infrared indocyanine green fluorescence imaging in, 833
    operating room setup for, 826, 829f
    overview of, 825
    patient positioning for, 826, 827f
    port setting for, 826, 828f
    Roux-en-Y hepaticojejunostomy for, 827, 839f
    techniques, 837, 837f–839f
    transmesocolic paraduodenal route, 838f
Biliary anastomosis, 822
Biliary leaks, in acute cholecystitis, 97f
Biliary limb transposition, in Roux-en-Y hepaticojejunostomy, 818–819, 820f
Biliary structures, in cholecystectomy, 95f, 96–97
Bilio-digestive anastomosis, 631
Bilioenteric anastomosis, 837
Biofluorescence, 27
Bipolar cautery instruments, 25f
Bipolar coagulation, 337
Bleeding
  anticipation of, 29
  control of, 29
  prevention of, 28–29
  repair of, 29
Body image scale, 179
Bottoms-Up technique, for robotic transversus abdominis release, 927, 933, 933f
Bowel surgery
  fluorescence imaging uses for, 102–107, 103f–107f
  perfusion assessment, 102, 103f
Breast
  anatomy of, 178f, 190f–192f
  lymphatic drainage of, 184f
  vascularization of, 193f–194f
Breast surgery, robotic
  indications for, 179
  nipple-sparing mastectomy. See Nipple-sparing mastectomy
BREAST-Q, 179

Bronchial arteries, 246f
Bronchial tree, 319f
Bronchoscopy, robotic, 330f
Bronchus, left upper, 362, 363f
Bulldog clamp, 964f, 976, 992
"Burping," 41

C
Cadaver models, for robotic training, 51–52
Cadière forceps, 24, 25f, 213, 391, 393, 425, 523
Camera port adjustment, 41f
Carbon dioxide insufflation, for robotic-assisted thymectomy, 200–201
Carotid sheath, 149, 149f
Case volume, 55
Caudate lobe
  biliary anatomy of, 747, 748f
  detachment of, from vena cava, 751
  partial division of, in right hepatectomy, 721f
Cavitron Ultrasonic Surgical Aspirator, 27, 729
CCND. See Central compartment node dissection
Cecum mobilization
  in kidney transplant, 969, 969f
  in right colectomy with complete mesocolic excision, 461–462
Celiac lymphadenectomy, 218
Celiac trunk, 647f
Central compartment node dissection
  in gasless transaxillary robotic thyroidectomy, 149, 149f–150f
  in transoral thyroidectomy, 173–174
Central pancreatectomy
  contraindications for, 674
  distal pancreatic transection, 686
  distal pancreaticojejunostomy in, 687
  gastrocolic ligament in, 678
  history of, 673
  indications for, 674
  instruments for, 673
  intraoperative ultrasonography in, 678, 679f
  operating room setup for, 675, 676f
  pancreatic neck preparation in, 680, 680f
  patient positioning for, 675, 675f
  peripancreatic arteries in, 681
  port setting for, 675, 677, 677f
  proximal pancreatic body mobilization in, 684
  proximal pancreatic transection in, 683, 683f
  reconstruction, 687
  retropancreatic neck dissection in, 680, 680f
  retropancreatic tunnel completion in, 682
  Roux-en-Y jejunal loop, 687, 687f
  sample lymphadenectomy in, 681
  small bowel viability during, 103f
  specimen extraction in, 688

splenic artery dissection in, 681f
surgical technique for, 678–688
Cernea classification, of external branch of superior laryngeal nerve, 144f, 172f
Certified registered nurse anesthetist, 27
Certified surgical assistants, 33
Certified surgical first assistants
  description of, 33
  laparoscopic assisting by, 43
Cervical anastomosis, in radical esophagectomy with extended mediastinal lymphadenectomy, 257
Cervical lymph nodes, 242t
Chemical pyloroplasty, 222
Cholangiography, for intrahepatic biliary stones, 847
Cholangitis, 826
Cholecystectomy, laparoscopic, 791, 794, 825, 836f
Cholecystectomy, robotic
  anomalies during, 96f
  biliary injuries in, 804f
  biliary structures in, 95f, 96–97
  contraindications for, 791, 1046
  cystic artery in, 799, 800f, 805–806, 1053–1054
  cystic duct
    clipping of, 805, 805f, 1054, 1054f
    complications involving, 95
    division of, 1054
    isolation of, 801, 802f, 1053
  da Vinci SP system for, 1045–1056, 1046f–1056f
  difficult IOC, 803
  fluorescence imaging uses in, 95f–98f, 95–98
  gallbladder in
    dissection of, from liver, 806, 1055, 1055f
    drainage, 1051f
    perforation of, 1055
  gallbladder neck retraction, 798, 798f, 1050, 1050f
  hemostasis review in, 1056
  hepatic artery in, 799
  hilum exposure in, 796, 796f–797f, 1049, 1049f
  history of, 791
  iatrogenic injury after, 97f
  indications for, 791, 1046
  indocyanine green fluorescence imaging in, 95, 801
  instruments for, 791, 1046
  for intrahepatic biliary stones, 847
  in left hepatectomy, 741
  in living donor hepatectomy, 1005f
  operating room setup for, 791, 793, 793f, 1046–1047, 1048f
  in pancreaticoduodenectomy, 616, 616f
  partial, 807f

patient positioning for, 791–793, 792f, 1046, 1047f
pneumoperitoneum in, 793
port setting for, 79f–795f, 791, 793–794, 1046f, 1046–1047
pull and push methods in, 806, 806f
retraction for, 21
retraction in, 796–797
in Roux-en-Y hepaticojejunostomy, 814
simulation of, 46, 49–50, 50f
skin closure in, 1056f
specimen retrieval in, 808, 1056
subtotal, 807, 1051
surgical technique for, 796–808
top-down dissection, 1055
triangle of Calot in, 798f, 798–799, 801, 1050f, 1052
in Whipple procedure, 616
working area for, 796, 796f–797f, 1049
Choledochoscope, 857
Choledochoscopy, 852, 853f–855f
Choledochotomy, 844f, 852, 852f–856f, 856
Clinical Robotic Surgery Association, 52
CME. See Complete mesocolic excision
CNNs. See Convolutional neural networks
Code blue algorithm, 31f
Code training, 60, 60f
Colonic arteries, 470f–471f
Colonic mesentery, 987
Colorectal liver metastases, 769
Colorectal surgery
iatrogenic nerve injuries during, 107
nerve imaging during, 107, 107f
Common bile duct. See also Bile duct
anatomy of, 850f
anterior, injuries to, 837
blood supply to, 850f–851f
cystic duct versus, 833
dissection of, 849f
exploration of, 841–842, 852
imaging of, 97f
injuries to, 837, 838f, 849, 1053
laparoscopic exploration of, 841
preparation of, 849, 849f–850f
thermal injury during dissection of, 817
transection of
in pancreaticoduodenectomy, 617, 617f
in Roux-en-Y hepaticojejunostomy, 818
Communication, in robotic surgery, 44
Complete mesocolic excision, right colectomy with
anatomy of, 473f
ascending colon mobilization in, 461–462
cecum mobilization in, 461–462
contraindications for, 456
ileocolic isoperistaltic anastomosis in, 477
ileocolic vessel division, 468
illustration of, 460f
indications for, 456
instruments for, 455
lymph node anatomy in, 475f
medial-to-lateral dissection, 468

mesentery of terminal ileum, division of, 474
omental division, 460, 460f
operating room setup for, 456, 459f
overview of, 455
patient positioning for, 456, 456f
pneumoperitoneum in, 456
port setting for, 456, 457f–458f
reconstruction after, 477, 477f
right colonic flexure mobilization, 464, 465f–467f
specimen extraction in, 477
surgical technique for, 460f–477f, 460–478
terminal ileum division, 474
transverse colon division, 474, 475f
transverse colon mesentery division, 476
trocar placement in, 457f–458f
venous anatomy in, 467f, 469f
Computer
as interface, 6
computer-aided imaging analysis, 121
computer-enhanced system, 6, 7f
CONDOR. See Connected Optimized Network and Data in Operating Rooms
Cone visualization, 77
Connected Optimized Network and Data in Operating Rooms, 83
Continued surgical education, robotic simulators for, 49–50
Convolutional neural networks, 73, 78, 82
Cooper's ligament, 904, 905f, 909
Core parenchymal transection, 728f, 728–729
Corona mortis, 905, 905f, 909
Coronary ligament
in left lateral sectionectomy, 763, 764f
right, in living donor hepatectomy, 1001, 1002f
Cost tracking, 57t, 57–58
Couinaud liver segments, 779f
Credentialing, 53
Crests of Duret, 189, 193f
Cricothyroid muscle, 148
Critical View of Safety, 82, 1053f
CRLM. See Colorectal liver metastases
Crowdsourcing, 82
CRSA. See Clinical Robotic Surgery Association
Cruroplasty
in Nissen fundoplication, 293, 293f
in paraesophageal hernia repair, 270, 271f
CSAs. See Certified surgical assistants
CSFAs. See Certified surgical first assistants
Curricula, 52
CUSA. See Cavitron Ultrasonic Surgical Aspirator
CVS. See Critical View of Safety
Cy5 fluorophore, 93
Cyanine dyes
aggregation of, 90, 91f
indocyanine. See Indocyanine green

Cystic artery, 799, 800f, 805–806, 1053–1054
Cystic duct
anatomical variations of, 802, 802f
clipping of, 805, 805f, 1054, 1054f
common bile duct versus, 833
division of, 806, 1054
isolation of, in cholecystectomy, 801, 802f
retraction of, in right hepatectomy, 709, 711f

D

D2 total gastrectomy, robotic
contraindications for, 387, 388t
dissection of distal portion of splenic artery, 401
distal esophagus transection, 402
duodenal transection, 400
gastrosplenic ligament division with short gastric vessels division, 395, 398f
indications for, 387, 388t
instruments for, 387, 391f
intracorporeal Roux-en-Y esophagojejunostomy for, 403, 403f–404f
left paracardial lymph node retrieval, 395
liver retraction in, 392, 392f
omentectomy in, 393, 393f–394f
operating room setup for, 387, 389f, 389–390
patient positioning for, 387, 388f, 389–390
port setting for, 387, 389–390, 390f–391f
right gastric artery ligation, 400
right gastroepiploic vessels, infrapyloric dissection and ligation of, 399
specimen extraction in, 405
splenic hilum dissection, 399
suprapancreatic dissection, 400
suprapyloric dissection, 400
surgical technique for, 392f–404f, 392–405
da Vinci S system, for total mesorectal excision for rectal cancer, 518, 519f
da Vinci Si system
gasless transaxillary robotic thyroidectomy, 135
nipple-sparing mastectomy, 180, 187f
operating room setup for, 389
for total mesorectal excision for rectal cancer, 518, 519f
transoral robotic thyroidectomy, 168f, 168–169, 170t
da Vinci Skills Simulator, 46, 48f
da Vinci SP system
access ports, 1040, 1040f, 1041f
advantages of, 1044
camera, 1037, 1040, 1040f
camera control modes, 1043, 1043f
cholecystectomy, 1045–1056, 1046f–1056f
cholecystectomy using, 1045–1056, 1046f–1056f
disadvantages of, 1044
docking of, 1043

1070 Index

da Vinci SP system (Cont.):
   entry guide in, 1040, 1041f
   gasless transaxillary robotic
      thyroidectomy, 137, 153
   general surgery applications of, 1045
   history of, 1037
   instrument arm clutch, 1037
   instrument drive clutch, 1037
   instrument navigator feature of, 1044, 1044f
   instruments, 1037, 1038f–1039f
   metal cannula used in, 1040, 1041f–1042f, 1064
   patient cart, 1037, 1038f
   port clutch, 1037
   relocate mode in, 1043, 1043f
   robotic console of, 1037
   surgical workspace in, 1040, 1041f–1042f
   total mesorectal excision for rectal cancer, 545f–548f, 545–547
   transabdominal preperitoneal repair using, 1057f–1065f, 1057–1065
   vision tower of, 1037
da Vinci system
   Firefly, 71
   Food and Drug Administration approval of, 6
   illustration of, 4f–5f
da Vinci Xi system
   gasless transaxillary robotic thyroidectomy, 136
   nipple-sparing mastectomy, 180, 187f
   pancreatic tumor enucleation, 691
   total mesorectal excision for rectal cancer, 520, 521f–522f
   transoral robotic thyroidectomy, 169f, 170, 170t
Data
   annotated, 84
   kinematic, 81
   labeled, 84
   quality of, 83–84
   surgical, 83
Data collection, 83
Data labeling, 83–84
Deep learning, 78, 82
Delphi process, 60
Denonvilliers' fascia, 540, 540f
Descending colon, mesentery of, 507, 507f
DICOM standard, 83
Differential privacy, 83
Digital interaction, 6–8
Direct volume rendering, 67
Discharge, remote monitoring for complications after, 60
Disposable instruments, 57–58
Distal pancreatectomy
   spleen-preserving
      contraindications for, 654
      description of, 116, 116f
      gastrocolic ligament division in, 659, 659f

"hanging" maneuver in, 665, 665f
      history of, 654
      indications for, 654
      indocyanine green fluorescence splenic inflow and outflow check in, 671
      instruments for, 653
      intraoperative ultrasonography in, 663
      Kimura technique for, 653
      lateral-to-medial dissection in, 669, 669f
      left colonic flexure mobilization in, 662, 662f
      medial-to-lateral dissection in, 668f
      operating room setup for, 654, 656f, 657
      pancreatic body mobilization in, 667, 667f–668f, 670f
      pancreatic division in, 666, 666f
      pancreatic neck preparation in, 665, 665f
      pancreatic tail mobilization in, 667, 667f–670f
      patient positioning for, 654, 655f
      pneumoperitoneum for, 654
      port setting for, 654, 657, 657f–658f
      retropancreatic tunnel creation in, 665, 665f
      short gastric vessels in, 663
      specimen extraction in, 671
      splenic artery in, 664f
      splenic artery preparation in, 661, 661f
      splenic vein in, 664f
      surgical technique for, 659f–670f, 659–671
      Warshaw technique for, 653
   with splenectomy, 635
Distal pancreaticojejunostomy, 687
Docking
   assistant's role in, 40–41, 41f
   for modified radical neck dissection, 158
   in nipple-sparing mastectomy, 187, 187f–188f
   robotic arms, 40–41, 41f
   training of, 51
   in transoral robotic thyroidectomy, 167–170
DOME, 45, 46f
Donor nephrectomy, laparoscopic, 943
Donor nephrectomy, open, 943
Donor nephrectomy, robotic
   computed tomographic angiogram in, 944, 944f
   contraindications for, 944–945
   donor selection in, 945
   indications for, 944–945
   instruments for, 943
   left
      descending colon mobilization, 949
      gonadal vein in, 950, 951f
      graft extraction in, 958
      left renal artery in, 958
      left renal vein in, 953, 953f–954f

      operating room setup for, 945, 948f
      patient positioning for, 945, 945f
      port setting for, 945, 946f
      renal artery preparation in, 958, 959f
      renoadrenal separation in, 958
      splenic flexure mobilization, 949
      surgical technique for, 949f–959f, 949–959
      ureter preparation, 950, 950f, 952f, 958
   operating room setup for, 945, 948f
   overview of, 943–944
   patient positioning for, 945, 945f
   port setting for, 945, 946f–947f
   right
      operating room setup for, 945, 948f, 958
      patient positioning for, 945, 945f, 958
      port setting for, 945, 947f, 958
      renal artery, 960
      surgical technique for, 960–961
      ureter preparation in, 960
Dor fundoplication. See Modified Dor fundoplication, Heller myotomy with
Dorsal pancreatic artery, 471f
Ducts of Luschka, 808
Duodenoenterostomy, in pancreas transplant, 994, 995f
Duodenojejunal flexure, 623
Duodenum, 616, 616f
DVR. See Direct volume rendering

E
EBSLN. See External branch of superior laryngeal nerve
Echo-endoscopy, 690
Emergencies, preparation for, 60
Emergency codes, 31
En bloc mesoesophagus, 225
Endo Catch™ pouch, 1013
Endobag, 22, 878
Endoscopic cameras, white-light imaging used by, 89
Endoscopic retrograde cholangiopancreatography, 842
Endostapler, 354
EndoWrist
   description of, 10, 11f, 600, 785
   instruments, 25f
   unrestricted working arms for, 19
End-to-end anastomosis, 227
End-to-side anastomosis, 257
End-to-side pancreaticojejunostomy, 628, 628f
Enos single access surgery system, 55, 57f
Enterobiliary anastomosis, 842
Epigastric crossover, 931, 932f
ERCP. See Endoscopic retrograde cholangiopancreatography
Error, 82

Esophageal cancer
　Japanese classification of, 244f
　lymph nodal stations for, 218f
　radical esophagectomy in. See Radical esophagectomy with extended mediastinal lymphadenectomy
Esophageal surgery, 109f–110f, 109–111
Esophagectomy, robotic-assisted
　Ivor-Lewis. See Ivor-Lewis esophagectomy, robotic
　radical esophagectomy with extended mediastinal lymphadenectomy. See Radical esophagectomy with extended mediastinal lymphadenectomy
　stomach blood supply visualization in, 110f
　thoracic duct injury caused by, 111
Esophagogastric anastomosis, 227, 230f–231f
Esophagogastric junction, 213
Esophagojejunostomy, Roux-en-Y, 403, 403f–404f
Esophagus
　anatomy of, 284f
　distal, transection of, 402
　perforation of, 314
　wall of, 314f
Expanded polytetrafluoroethylene, 912
Expert panels, 53
Explainable artificial intelligence, 84–86, 85f
Exposure, retraction levels for, 21–22
Extended thymectomy (robotic), for myasthenia gravis and thymoma
　carbon dioxide insufflation for, 200–201
　instruments for, 197
　operating room setup for, 198f, 198–199
　overview of, 197
　patient positioning for, 198, 199f
　port setting for, 198–199
　surgical technique for, 200f–207f, 200–208
　trocar placement for, 199f
Extended totally extraperitoneal repair, 911
External branch of superior laryngeal nerve, 138, 144f, 172, 172f
External iliac artery
　in kidney transplant, 972, 972f
　left, in pancreas transplant, 989, 989f–991f
External iliac vein, in kidney transplant, 973, 974f–975f, 975
Extrahepatic hepatic duct, 746f, 832f

F
Face validity, 46
Falciform ligament
　dissection of
　　in left hepatectomy, 738, 738f
　　in living donor hepatectomy, 1001, 1002f
　　in right hepatectomy, 707, 708f
　division of, in left lateral sectionectomy, 762, 762f
　in left hepatectomy, 738, 738f
　in right hepatectomy
　　dissection of, 707, 708f
　　reconstruction of, 730, 731f
Feedback
　haptic, 6, 22, 24, 24f
　virtual tactile, 22, 24
　visual, 24
Feeding jejunostomy, 222
Femoral artery cannulation, 51f
Femoral vein cannulation, 51f
^{18}F-fluorodeoxyglucose, 690
FIGS. See Fluorescence image-guided surgery
Financials, of robotic program, 55–58, 57t
FIRST. See Fundamental Inanimate Robotic Skills Tasks
First assistants
　description of, 33
　laparoscopic assisting by, 43
　robotic training for, 44
Flex Robotic System, 55, 57f
Floating port technique, 1059, 1059f
Fluorescence
　definition of, 89–90
　dye molecules, 90
　excitation light versus, 90
　nerve imaging using, 93
　target tissue properties, 92
Fluorescence enhancement, 9
Fluorescence image-guided surgery
　benefits of, 72
　description of, 70–73
　fluorophores, 70
　indocyanine green, 70
　3D VR/AR models with, 73
Fluorescence imaging
　adrenal surgery uses of, 118, 118f
　apparatus for, 93–94
　artificial intelligence in, 121
　basics of, 89–93
　blood perfusion assessments, 102, 103f
　bowel surgery applications of, 102–107, 103f–107f
　cholecystectomy uses of, 95f–98f, 95–98
　esophageal surgery uses of, 109f–110f, 109–111
　gastric surgery uses of, 108f–109f, 108–109
　indocyanine green. See Indocyanine green fluorescence imaging
　kidney surgery uses of, 112, 112f–113f
　liver surgery applications of, 98f–101f, 98–101
　lymph node mapping uses of, 105, 106f
　pancreatic surgery uses of, 114–117
　parathyroid surgery uses of, 118
　perspective on, 121
　robotic surgery applications of, 94–120
　sentinel lymph node identification using, 105, 106f
　short-wave infrared, 121
　spleen vessel imaging uses of, 116, 116f–117f
　strategies for, 92–93
　thoracic surgery uses of, 119–120, 120f
　thoracic tumor uses of, 119–120
　white-light imaging and, 121
Fluorescence inducer, 93
Fluorescence probes
　development of, 121
　monitoring of, 92–93
Fluorescence tracer, 92
Fluorescence water leak test, 785
Fluorophores, 70, 92–93
Force feedback, 22, 24f
Frenulum labii inferioris, 164
"Frozen abdomen," 926
FRS. See Fundamentals of Robotic Surgery
Fulcrum effect, 3, 4f
Fundamental Inanimate Robotic Skills Tasks, 45–46
Fundamentals of Robotic Surgery curricula, 52
Fundoplication
　modified Dor. See Heller myotomy, with modified Dor fundoplication
　Nissen. See Nissen fundoplication, selective
　in paraesophageal hernia repair, 274, 275f
　Toupet, 275f

G
Gallbladder
　anatomical variations of, 808
　anatomy of, 778f
　dissection of
　　from liver, 806, 1055, 1055f
　　in living donor hepatectomy, 1005, 1005f
　distension of, 1051
　ducts of Luschka, 808
　perforation of, 1055
Gallbladder neck retraction, in cholecystectomy, 798, 798f, 1050, 1050f
Gallbladder surgery, precision multimodal, 71f
Gasless transaxillary robotic thyroidectomy
　anatomy involved in, 138, 139f–147f
　central compartment node dissection, 149, 149f–150f
　contraindications for, 127–129
　contralateral lobectomy, 152, 152f
　da Vinci S, Si system, 135
　da Vinci SP system, 137, 153
　da Vinci Xi system, 136
　incision lines, 130, 131
　indications for, 127–129
　instruments for, 127, 128f
　ipsilateral lobectomy, 151, 151f
　operating room setup, 129
　patient positioning, 129

Gasless transaxillary robotic thyroidectomy (*Cont.*):
  port setting, 129
  upper pole dissection, 148
  working space for, 130*f*–134*f*, 130–134
Gastrectomy, robotic
  D2 total. *See* D2 total gastrectomy, robotic
  sleeve. *See* Sleeve gastrectomy
Gastric artery
  posterior, 592*f*
  right
    division of, 614, 614*f*
    ligation of, 400
Gastric bands, 407
Gastric conduit
  in Ivor-Lewis esophagectomy, 219, 220*f*–221*f*
  in radical esophagectomy with extended mediastinal lymphadenectomy, 257
Gastric fundus, posterior
  anatomy of, 416, 418*f*
  dissection of, in Nissen fundoplication, 291, 291*f*
  mobilization of, in sleeve gastrectomy, 416, 416*f*–418*f*
Gastric pouch, in Roux-en-Y gastric bypass, 425, 425*f*–426*f*, 431*f*
Gastric pull-up, 228*f*
Gastric surgery
  anastomotic leakage during, 108
  D2 total gastrectomy. *See* D2 total gastrectomy
  fluorescence imaging uses for, 108*f*–109*f*, 108–109
  near-infrared fluorescence imaging for, 401, 401*f*
Gastric vein, left, 684, 685*f*
Gastrocolic ligament
  dissection of, 527*f*
  division of
    in pancreaticoduodenectomy, 604, 604*f*
    in radical anterograde modular pancreatosplenectomy, 641, 641*f*
    in spleen-preserving distal pancreatectomy, 659, 659*f*
    in splenectomy, 581, 581*f*
  in Ivor-Lewis esophagectomy, 214, 216
  opening of
    in central pancreatectomy, 678
    in left adrenalectomy, 884, 884*f*
    in pancreatic tumor enucleation, 694
  in sleeve gastrectomy, 414, 414*f*
Gastroduodenal artery
  anatomical variations of, 619, 621*f*
  anatomy of, 619, 620*f*
  transection of, in pancreaticoduodenectomy, 618, 619*f*, 622*f*
Gastroepiploic arcade, 214, 215*f*, 615
Gastroepiploic artery, left
  anatomy of, 216, 217*f*
  division of
    in radical anterograde modular pancreatosplenectomy, 645
    in spleen-preserving distal pancreatectomy, 659
Gastroesophageal junction, 282, 304, 312
Gastroesophageal reflux disease, 277
Gastrohepatic ligament, 213, 283, 286*f*, 305*f*, 425
Gastrojejunal anastomosis, in Roux-en-Y gastric bypass, 430, 430*f*
Gastrojejunostomy, 631
Gastropancreatic fold, 256
Gastrophrenic ligament, 427
Gastrosplenic ligament division
  with short gastric vessels division, 395
  in sleeve gastrectomy, 415
GERD. *See* Gastroesophageal reflux disease
Gerota's capsule, 490, 949, 1001
Gerota's fascia, 888
Giant prosthetic reinforcement of the visceral sac, 925
Glissonian pedicle, 766
Global Operative Assessment of Laparoscopic Skills rating system, 82
GOALS rating system. *See* Global Operative Assessment of Laparoscopic Skills rating system
"Golden triangle," 964–965, 965*f*
Gonadal vein, 889*f*, 950, 951*f*, 1028
Grasper, needle driver versus, 39
Gravity, rectal dissection use of, 21
Greater omentum, 393

H
Hanging maneuver
  in kidney transplant, 973, 973*f*
  in living donor hepatectomy, 1004, 1004*f*, 1011*f*
  in pancreas transplant, 989
  in right hepatectomy, 722*f*–723*f*
  in spleen-preserving distal pancreatectomy, 665, 665*f*
Haptic feedback, 6, 22, 24, 24*f*
Haptics-assisted procedure-specific learning, 50*f*
Harmonic curved shears, 135, 728, 1009
Harmonic scalpel, 729
Hasson technique, 17–18, 410
Head-mounted displays, optical see-through, 37, 38*f*
Heller myotomy
  with modified Dor fundoplication
    anterior partial fundoplication, 315, 315*f*
    anterior phrenoesophageal membrane division, 305, 306*f*
    contraindications for, 299
    gastrohepatic ligament division in, 305*f*
    hiatus in
      anatomy of, 307*f*
      exposure of, 304, 304*f*
    indications for, 299
    instruments for, 299
    intraoperative endoscopy in, 315
    left vagal trunk identification in, 309, 309*f*–310*f*
    mediastinal dissection in, 308
    myotomy, 312, 312*f*–313*f*
    operating room setup for, 299–300, 301*f*
    overview of, 299
    patient positioning for, 299–300, 300*f*
    pneumoperitoneum for, 299–300
    port settings for, 299–300, 302*f*–303*f*
    surgical technique for, 304*f*–315*f*, 304–315
    vagal trunk in, 309, 309*f*–310*f*
  port placement for, 20*f*
Hemihepatectomy, left, 734*f*
Hem-o-lok clip, 876
Hemostasis verification
  in left lateral sectionectomy, 767, 767*f*
  in pancreatic tumor enucleation, 696
Henle's trunk, 474, 476*f*
Hepatectomy, 770
  bile duct exploration after, 857
  left. *See* Left hepatectomy
  living donor. *See* Living donor hepatectomy
  for recurrent pyogenic cholangitis, 856, 857*f*
  right. *See* Right hepatectomy
Hepatic artery
  anatomical variations of, 618, 618*f*, 713*f*, 739*f*
  in cholecystectomy, 799
  left, 743, 743*f*
  right
    anatomy of, 618*f*
    clipping of, 1012
    dissection of, in living donor hepatectomy, 1006
    in right hepatectomy, 712, 713*f*–714*f*
    in Roux-en-Y hepaticojejunostomy, 814
    transection of, 1012*f*
Hepatic duct
  anatomical variations of, 1007*f*
  extrahepatic, 746*f*, 832*f*
  left, 97*f*, 746, 746*f*
  right. *See* Right hepatic duct
Hepatic flexure mobilization, 605, 605*f*
Hepatic segments, 98–99
Hepatic vein
  accessory, 870, 871*f*
  in left hepatectomy, 750*f*, 752
  in right hepatectomy, 725*f*–726*f*
Hepaticocutaneous jejunostomy, 857, 859*f*
Hepaticojejunostomy, 631, 631*f*, 842, 857, 859*f*
Hepaticojejunostomy, Roux-en-Y
  bile duct injuries repair, 827, 839*f*
  bile duct mobilization, 814, 817*f*
  bile duct transection in, 818
  biliary injury, 814

biliary limb transposition in, 818–819, 820f
bilioenteric anastomosis, 837
cholecystectomy in, 814
contraindications for, 809
hepatic artery in, 814
hepatoduodenal ligament exposure in, 814, 815f
indications for, 809
instruments for, 809
in intrahepatic cholangiocarcinoma, 822–823
jejunal limb creation in, 818, 819f
jejunal loop, 837
jejunojejunostomy in, 823, 823f
ligament of Treitz in, 818
malignancy, 815
operating room setup for, 809–810, 813f
paraduodenal route in, 821f
patient positioning for, 809–810, 810f
port setting for, 809–810, 811f–812f, 844f
portal vein in, 814
surgical technique for, 814–823
Hepatocarcinoma, 769
fluorescence imaging of, 100f
organic anion transporters in, 101
Hepatocaval dissection, 717, 720f–722f
Hepatoduodenal ligament
anatomy of, 831f, 848f
exposure of, in Roux-en-Y hepaticojejunostomy, 814, 815f
Hepatolithiasis, 847f
Hepato-pancreatic-biliary surgery, 701
Hepatosplenomegaly, 17
Hernia repair
inguinal. See Inguinal hernia repair, robotic
ventral. See Ventral hernia repair
Hesselbach's triangle, 902, 903f, 909
Hiatal hernia
classification of, 259, 260f
postoperative, 213
type I, 259, 260f
type II, 259, 260f
type III, 259, 260f
type IV, 259, 260f
High-resolution manometry, 299
Hilar lymph nodes, 346, 354
Hilar lymphadenectomy, splenic, 399
Hilum
biliary structures in, thermal injury to, 803
dissection of, 99, 741
exposure of, in bile duct injuries repair, 830
fluorescence imaging of, 98–99
Hominis, 55, 57f
Horizontal mattress, 47f
HSA. See Human serum albumin
Hugo Robotic-assisted surgery, 8, 8f
Human error, 82

Human serum albumin, indocyanine green binding to, 91, 92f
Hybrid operations, 57

I
Iatrogenic injuries, patient positioning to prevent, 36
Ileocecal region, 463f
Ileocolic isoperistaltic anastomosis, 477
Ileocolonic anastomosis, during left colectomy, 103f
Image-based registration, 76, 77f
Imaging
fluorescence. See Fluorescence imaging
3D reconstruction, 67–69, 68f–69f
Implemented imaging, 66–67
Incision
Pfannenstiel. See Pfannenstiel incision
planning of, 22
Incisional hernias, 911
Incisura angularis, 219
Indexity, 84, 85f
Indocyanine green
aggregation of, 90, 91f
description of, 70, 90
fluorescence quantum yield of, 90
H-aggregates of, 90, 91f
human serum albumin binding of, 91, 92f
intraoperative tissue classification, 73
J-aggregates of, 91, 91f
liver retention of, 98
peritumoral injection of, 401
preparation of, 94
reconstitution of, 94
Indocyanine green angiography, 72
Indocyanine green fluorescence imaging
advantages of, 105
in cholecystectomy, 95, 801
liver segments, 758, 758f
liver tumors, 99, 101f–102f
lymph node mapping uses of, 105, 106f
in pancreatic tumor enucleation, 694, 695f
pancreatic tumor imaging and margining uses of, 114
parathyroid glands, 119f
partial nephrectomy uses of, 112
perfusion assessment, 109
sentinel lymph node identification, 105
thoracic duct identification, 111f
Inferior mediastinal lymph nodes, 322f
Inferior mesenteric artery
anatomical variations of, 504f
anatomy of, 499f–501f
control and division of, 502, 502f
laparoscopic ligation of, 520
ligation of, 523f–524f, 546f
superior hypogastric plexus around, 107
Inferior mesenteric vein
anatomical variations of, 649f
description of, 492

division of, in radical anterograde modular pancreatosplenectomy, 649, 649f
exposure of, 645
laparoscopic ligation of, 520
ligation of, 525f
Inferior thyroid artery, recurrent laryngeal nerve and, 138, 143f
Inferior vena cava, bleeding from, 877
Inguinal canal
anatomy of, 902f
nerves of, 906, 907f
Inguinal hernia repair, robotic
advantages of, 897
anatomical landmarks in, 902, 902f–903f
contraindications for, 897
description of, 897
flap closure in, 910, 910f
hernia sac dissection in, 908
indications for, 897
instruments for, 897
lateral dissection in, 906, 907f
medial dissection in, 904, 905f
mesh placement in, 909, 909f
myopectineal orifice, 908
operating room setup for, 898, 899f
patient positioning for, 898, 898f
pneumoperitoneum for, 898
port setting for, 898, 900f–901f
spermatic vessels, 908
Inguinal region, 1060f
Innominate vein, 204f
Instrument(s). See also Laparoscopic instruments; Robotic instruments; specific instrument
assistant's role with, 37, 39f
disposable, 57–58
optimization of, 57
standby, 37
Instrument arm clutch, 1037
Instrument drive clutch, 1037
Instrument navigator, 1044, 1044f
Internal jugular vein, 132, 132f
Intersegmental plane, 120
Intraductal papillary mucinous neoplasms
central pancreatectomy for, 674
enucleation of, 689–696
spleen-preserving distal pancreatectomy for, 654
Intrahepatic biliary stones
cholecystectomy for, 847
choledochoscopy for, 852, 853f–855f
choledochotomy for, 844, 852, 852f–855f, 856, 856f
common bile duct preparation, 849, 849f–850f
description of, 841–842
hepatectomy for, 856, 857f
hepaticojejunostomy for, 842, 844, 857, 859f
instruments for, 841
operating room setup for, 842, 846f
partial hepatectomy for, 842

Intrahepatic biliary stones (*Cont.*):
  patient positioning for, 842, 843*f*
  port setting for, 842, 844*f*–845*f*
  removal of, 852, 853*f*
  surgical procedures for, 841
  surgical technique for, 847*f*–859*f*, 847–859
  T-Tubes for, 856, 856*f*–857*f*
Intrahepatic cholangiocarcinoma, Roux-en-Y hepaticojejunostomy in, 822–823
Intraoperative period, artificial intelligence applications in, 12–13
Intraoperative ultrasound
  in central pancreatectomy, 678, 679*f*
  in left lateral sectionectomy, 763, 763*f*
  in liver resections, 775, 783
  in pancreatic tumor enucleation, 694, 696
  in radical anterograde modular pancreatosplenectomy, 643
  in renal artery aneurysm repair, 1027, 1027*f*
  in right hepatectomy, 707, 708*f*
  in spleen-preserving distal pancreatectomy, 663
Intrapericardial pneumonectomies, 346
Intraperitoneal onlay mesh and ventral hernia repair
  abdominal ventral defect dissection, 921
  adhesiolysis, 920, 920*f*
  cardinal stitches with straight needle, 922, 922*f*
  contraindications for, 915
  fascial defect closure, 921, 921*f*
  indications for, 915
  mesh placement and fixation, 922, 923*f*
  operating room setup for, 916, 917*f*, 918
  patient positioning for, 916, 916*f*
  port setting for, 919*f*
  surgical technique for, 920*f*–923*f*, 920–923
Intuitive Firefly camera, 94
Intuitive Surgical, 3, 6
Ion platform, 55, 56*f*
IPMN. *See* Intraductal papillary mucinous neoplasms
IRCAD, 72
Isthmus division, in transoral robotic thyroidectomy, 171, 171*f*
Ivor-Lewis esophagectomy, robotic
  abdominal phase of
    celiac lymphadenectomy, 218
    esophageal hiatus dissection, 213
    feeding jejunostomy, 222
    gastric conduit creation, 219, 220*f*–221*f*
    gastrocolic ligament, 214
    Kocher maneuver, 214, 216
    lesser curvature division, 219
    operating room setup for, 210, 212*f*
    patient positioning for, 210, 210*f*
    port setting for, 210–211, 211*f*
    pyloric release, 222
    right colonic flexure mobilization in, 214, 216
    short gastric vessel dissection, 216
    surgical technique for, 213–222
    transhiatal mediastinum dissection, 219
  indications for, 209
  instruments for, 209
  pneumoperitoneum for, 210
  thoracic phase of
    azygos vein division, 225
    en bloc mesoesophagus removal, 225
    esophageal dissection, 225, 226*f*
    esophageal transection, 227, 229*f*
    esophagogastric anastomosis, 227, 230*f*–231*f*
    inferior pulmonary ligament mobilization, 225
    mediastinal pleura, 225
    omental patch, 231*f*
    operating room setup for, 223, 224*f*
    patient positioning for, 223
    port setting for, 223, 223*f*
    specimen extraction, 232
    subcarinal mediastinal lymphadenectomy, 225
    supracarinal lymphadenectomy, 227
    thoracic duct ligation, 226

J

Jackson-Pratt drain, in transoral thyroidectomy, 174
Jejunal loop, Roux-en-Y, 687, 687*f*
Jejunojejunostomy
  in Roux-en-Y gastric bypass, 429, 429*f*
  in Roux-en-Y hepaticojejunostomy, 823, 823*f*
JIGSAWS. *See* John Hopkins University and Intuitive Surgical Inc. Gesture and Skill Assessment Working Set
John Hopkins University and Intuitive Surgical Inc. Gesture and Skill Assessment Working Set, 82

K

Kasai procedure, 827
Kelly clamp-crushing technique, 785
Ki-67 index, 690
Kidney
  anatomy of, 955, 955*f*, 965*f*, 1024*f*
  perfusion of, 1035*f*
  upper pole of
    in left adrenalectomy, 890, 890*f*–891*f*, 892
    in right adrenalectomy, 873, 873*f*–874*f*
  vascular anatomy of, 955, 955*f*
Kidney surgery
  fluorescence imaging uses in, 112, 112*f*–113*f*
  renal artery identification in, 112, 112*f*–113*f*
  selective arterial clamping in, 112*f*

Kidney transplant, robot-assisted
  arterial anastomosis in, 977, 977*f*
  cecum mobilization in, 969, 969*f*
  contraindications for, 964, 964*t*
  external iliac artery preparation, 972, 972*f*
  external iliac vein in
    clamping of, 975, 975*f*
    preparation of, 973, 974*f*
  "golden triangle," 964–965, 965*f*
  graft in
    backbench preparation of, 964, 964*f*
    insertion of, 976
    reperfusion of, 978, 978*f*
  hanging maneuver in, 973, 973*f*
  history of, 963–964
  indications for, 964
  indocyanine green fluorescence imaging in, 978
  instruments for, 963, 964*f*
  minilaparotomy closure in, 981, 981*f*
  operating room setup for, 966, 967*f*
  patient positioning for, 966, 966*f*
  pneumoperitoneum for, 966
  port setting for, 966, 968*f*
  port site closure, 981
  surgical field in, 970, 970*f*
  suspensory ligament of the ovary, 971, 971*f*
  testicular vessels, 970
  ureteroneocystostomy in, 979, 979*f*–980*f*
  urinary reconstruction in, 979, 979*f*–980*f*
  venous anastomosis in, 976, 976*f*
Kimura technique, 653
KindHearth™, 51
Kinematic data, 81
Kocher maneuver
  description of, 695, 849
  in Ivor-Lewis esophagectomy, 214, 216
  in pancreaticoduodenectomy, 607, 608*f*–609*f*
  partial, 868, 868*f*, 1026

L

Lack of tremor, 10
Lacrimal probe, 1010*f*
Laimer-Bertelli membrane, 213
Laparoscopic cholecystectomy
  outcomes of, 3
  safety alerts, 82
Laparoscopic instruments
  disadvantages of, 3
  robotic instruments versus, 11*f*
Laparoscopic splenectomy, 575
Laparoscopic stapler, 27
Laparoscopic stapling
  description of, 43
  sleeve gastrectomy, 419, 419*f*
Laparoscopic surgery
  adrenalectomy, 863
  assisting in, 43–44
  cholecystectomy, 791, 825, 836*f*
  common bile duct exploration, 841
  disadvantages of, 3

donor nephrectomy, 943
fluorescent markers in, 76
history of, 3
incorporating knowledge of, 15
open surgery conversion, 30f, 30–31
pancreaticoduodenectomy, 599
robotic surgery versus, 59
sewing in, 58
single-incision, 1045
spleen-preserving distal pancreatectomy, 653–654
surgeon injuries during, 59
ventral hernia repair, 911
Laparoscopy
  diagnostic, in small bowel resection, 442
  image segmentation uses of, 79f
  small bowel evaluation, 442, 444
  total mesorectal excision, 517
  value of, to patients, 59
LARs. *See* Low anterior resections
Left adrenalectomy, robotic
  adrenal gland in
    detachment of, 892–893, 893f
    exposure of, 888
    lifting of, 893, 893f
  adrenal veins in, 888, 888f, 890
  contraindications for, 879
  gastrocolic ligament in, 884, 884f
  indications for, 879
  inflow control in, 892f
  instruments for, 879
  landmarks for, 889
  left adrenal vein in, 890, 890f
  left colonic flexure mobilization in, 885, 885f
  left diaphragmatic pillar in, 893, 893f
  left renal artery in, 890, 890f–891f
  left renal vein in, 888, 888f
  operating room setup for, 880, 881f
  pancreatic body mobilization in, 887
  patient positioning for, 880, 880f
  port setting for, 880, 882, 882f–883f
  posterolateral plane dissection in, 894, 894f
  retroperitoneum dissection with, in radical anterograde modular pancreatosplenectomy, 651, 651f
  specimen extraction in, 894
  splenocolic ligament in, 885
  splenorenal ligament in, 885
  stomach fixation to anterior abdominal wall in, 886f
  surgical technique for, 880f–893f, 880–894
  upper pole of kidney in, 890, 890f–891f, 892
Left colectomy
  contraindications for, 480
  ileocolonic anastomosis during, 103f
  indications for, 480
  instruments for, 479
  mesenteric lymphography during, 106f, 107
  operating room setup for, 480, 481f, 494, 495f, 511, 513
  overview of, 479–480
  patient positioning for, 480, 482f, 494, 496f, 511f, 513f
  phase A
    lateral-to-medial dissection, 484, 485f, 490
    left omentum-colic detachment in, 489
    medial-to-lateral dissection, 484, 486f, 492, 493f, 494
    operating room setup for, 481f
    patient positioning for, 482f
    port setting for, 483f
    splenic flexure mobilization in, 484, 492
    splenocolic ligament dissection, 489, 489f
    top-down approach with gastrocolic ligament opening, 484, 488f
    top-down dissection with omental-colonic detachment, 484, 487f
    transverse colon mesenteric root detachment from pancreatic body, 491
    venous anatomy in, 493f
  phase B
    colonic division in, 511
    descending colon mesentery, 507, 507f
    indocyanine green perfusion check in, 511
    inferior mesenteric artery control and division, 502, 502f
    left ureter identification, 498
    lymph nodes in, 507, 509f–510f
    operating room setup for, 494, 495f
    overview of, 494
    patient positioning for, 494, 496f
    port setting for, 494, 497f
    promontory in, 498
    retrograde preaortic dissection, 498
    sigmoid colon mesentery, 498
    sigmoid colon mobilization, 502
    sigmoidal-rectal transection, 506, 506f
  phase C
    operating room setup for, 495f, 511
    patient positioning for, 511f
    port setting for, 511, 512f
    specimen extraction in, 513
  phase D
    end-to-end transanal stapled anastomosis, 515
    operating room setup for, 495f, 513
    patient positioning for, 513f
    port setting for, 513, 514f
  port setting for, 480, 483f, 494, 497f, 511, 512f, 513, 514f
  surgical technique for, 481f–514f, 481–515
Left colon resection, 34f
Left colonic flexure mobilization
  in left adrenalectomy, 885, 885f
  in radical anterograde modular pancreatosplenectomy, 642, 642f
  in spleen-preserving distal pancreatectomy, 662, 662f
  in splenectomy, 582
Left crus dissection
  in Nissen fundoplication, 288, 288f
  in paraesophageal hernia repair, 264, 264f–265f
Left donor nephrectomy, robotic
  descending colon mobilization, 949
  gonadal vein in, 950, 951f
  graft extraction in, 958
  left renal artery in, 958
  left renal vein in, 953, 953f–954f
  operating room setup for, 945, 948f
  patient positioning for, 945, 945f
  port setting for, 945, 946f
  renal artery preparation in, 958, 959f
  renoadrenal separation in, 958
  splenic flexure mobilization, 949
  surgical technique for, 949f–959f, 949–959
  ureter preparation, 950, 950f, 952f, 958
Left gastric vein, 684, 685f
Left gastroepiploic artery
  anatomy of, 216, 217f
  division of
    in radical anterograde modular pancreatosplenectomy, 645
    in spleen-preserving distal pancreatectomy, 659
Left hemihepatectomy, 734f
Left hepatectomy
  caudate lobe detachment from vena cava, 751
  cholecystectomy in, 741
  falciform ligament dissection in, 738, 738f
  hepatic vein in, 750f
  hilum dissection in, 741
  history of, 733
  indications for, 734–735
  instruments for, 733
  intraoperative ultrasonography in, 741, 741f
  left hepatic artery, 743, 743f
  left hepatic duct transection in, 746, 746f
  left hepatic lobe mobilization, 738, 740
  left hepatic vein in
    preparation of, 749
    stapling of, 752
  left inferior phrenic vein in, 740, 740f
  left portal vein, 744, 745f
  operating room setup for, 735, 736f
  parenchymal transection, 751f–752f, 751–752
  patient positioning for, 735f, 735–736
  port setting for, 735–736, 737f, 845f
  preoperative evaluation for, 734
  Pringle maneuver, 742, 742f
  specimen extraction in, 752
Left hepatic duct transection, in left hepatectomy, 746, 746f

1076 Index

Left hepatic lobe mobilization, in left hepatectomy, 738, 740
Left hepatic vein
  in left hepatectomy
    preparation of, 749
    stapling of, 752
  in liver resections, 775f
Left inferior phrenic vein, in left hepatectomy, 740, 740f
Left lateral sectionectomy
  anatomy of, 734f, 757f
  contraindications for, 756
  coronary ligament in, 763, 764f
  falciform ligament division in, 762, 762f
  hemostasis verification in, 767, 767f
  indications for, 756
  instruments for, 755
  intraoperative ultrasound in, 763, 763f
  left main hepatic vein stapling in, 766
  left phrenic nerve in, 763, 764f
  operating room setup for, 759, 760f
  patient positioning for, 759, 759f
  pneumoperitoneum in, 762
  port setting for, 759, 761f, 845f
  portal pedicle stapling in, 766
  Pringle maneuver in, 765, 765f
  round ligament division in, 762, 762f
  specimen extraction in, 767
  subcortical parenchyma dissection in, 765, 765f
  surgical technique for, 762f–767f, 762–767
  triangular ligament dissection, 763, 764f
Left lower lobectomy, robotic
  bronchus isolation and section, 382, 382f
  fissure division, 382, 382f
  left inferior pulmonary artery isolation, 382, 382f
  left inferior pulmonary vein, isolation and section of, 380, 380f–381f
  lymph nodal dissection, 383, 383f
  mediastinal lymph nodes dissection, 383
  operating room setup for, 378, 378f
  patient positioning for, 378
  port setting for, 378, 379f
  pulmonary ligament dissection, 380
  surgical technique for, 380f–383f, 380–383
Left main hepatic vein stapling, 766
Left medial sectionectomy, 757f
Left phrenic nerve, 201, 889f
Left portal vein, 744, 745f, 779f
Left renal artery
  in left adrenalectomy, 890, 890f–891f
  in left donor nephrectomy, 958
Left renal vein
  in left adrenalectomy, 888, 888f
  in left donor nephrectomy, 953, 953f–954f
Left trisectionectomy, 734f, 757f
Left upper lobectomy, robotic
  anterior pleural reflection at hilum, opening of, 336, 336f
  anterolateral parenchymal bridge transection, 340
  apical pulmonary artery branches, 342, 342f
  bronchus, 342, 343f, 362, 363f
  contraindications for, 332, 345–346
  fissure dissection, 338, 338f, 365, 365f
  indications for, 332, 345–346
  inferior pulmonary ligament dissection with station 8–9 lymphadenectomy, 335
  instruments for, 345
  lymph node dissection in, 327f, 360, 365–366, 366f
  lymphadenectomy, 335, 344
  operating room setup for, 332, 333f, 358f, 358–359
  patient positioning for, 332, 332f, 358–359
  port setting for, 324f, 332, 334f, 358–359, 359f
  posterior pleural reflection at hilum, opening of, 337, 337f
  posterolateral parenchymal bridge transection, 340, 340f, 343f
  pulmonary artery branches, 338, 339f, 361, 361f–362f, 364, 364f
  pulmonary vein preparation and division, 341, 341f, 360, 360f
  specimen extraction in, 344, 344f, 365–366, 366f
  surgical technique for, 335–344, 360f–366f, 360–366
Lesser curvature, 219
Ligament of Berry, 172
Ligament of Treitz
  identification of, 818
  transection of, 623, 623f
Ligamentum venosum, 749, 749f, 776f
LIME. *See* Local Interpretable Model-Agnostic Explanations
Linea alba, 912, 913f
Linea semilunaris, 912, 932f, 935f
Linitis plastica, 108
Liver
  anatomy of, 702f–703f, 734, 756f, 775f, 998f
  exposure of, Nissen fundoplication, 282, 282f
  indocyanine green fluorescence, 98, 758f
  ligaments of, 1002f
  pars condensa of, 392
  pars flaccida of, 392
  retraction of
    in D2 total gastrectomy, 392, 392f
    in right adrenalectomy, 868, 869f–870f
  segmental anatomy of, 702f, 776f–779f, 998f
  three-dimensional reconstruction of, 734f
  transection line of, 703f
  vasculature of, 74f
Liver metastases
  fluorescence imaging of, 100f
  rectal carcinoma as cause of, 100f
Liver resections, robotic
  abdominal exploration in, 775
  as outpatient surgery, 60
  atypical, 769–786
  contraindications for, 770
  fluorescence water leak test in, 785
  indications for, 770
  intraoperative ultrasound in, 775, 783
  liver mobilization in, 783
  operating room setup for, 771, 771f
  parenchymal transection in, 785, 786f
  patient positioning for, 770f, 771
  pneumoperitoneum in, 771
  port setting for, 771, 772f–774f
  Pringle maneuver in, 780, 780f–782f
  segmental, 769–786
  segmental demarcation in, 783
  specimen extraction in, 786
  stay sutures in, 783, 784f, 785
  surgical technique in, 775–786
  vessel control with sutures in, 785
Liver retractor, in sleeve gastrectomy, 413, 413f
Liver sectionectomies
  classification of, 757f
  contraindications for, 756
  description of, 755
  indications for, 756
  instruments for, 755
  left medial sectionectomy, 757f
  left trisectionectomy, 757f
  right anterior sectionectomy, 757f
  right posterior sectionectomy, 757f
  right trisectionectomy, 757f
Liver surgery, 98f–101f, 98–101
Liver tumors
  fluorescence imaging of, 99, 100f
  indocyanine green fluorescence imaging of, 99, 101f–102f
Living donor hepatectomy
  anatomy of, 998f
  cholecystectomy in, 1005f
  donor selection for, 997
  falciform ligament in, 1001, 1002f
  gallbladder dissection in, 1005, 1005f
  hanging maneuver in, 1004, 1004f, 1011f
  hemostasis in, 1013
  left lobe fixation in, 1013, 1013f
  operating room setup for, 997, 999f
  parenchymal demarcation in, 1008, 1008f
  parenchymal transection in, 1009, 1009f, 1011, 1011f
  patient positioning for, 997, 998f
  Pfannenstiel incision in, 1012
  pneumoperitoneum in, 1000
  port setting for, 997, 1000f
  right coronary ligament in, 1001, 1002f
  right hepatic artery dissection, 1006
  right hilar plate in, 1010
  right lobe retrieval, 1013, 1013f
  right portal vein dissection, 1006
  short hepatic veins in, 1003, 1003f

surgical technique for, 1001–1013, 1002f–1012f
vascular control in, 1012, 1012f–1013f
Lobectomies, robotic lung. *See* Lung lobectomies, robotic
Local Interpretable Model-Agnostic Explanations, 86
Low anterior resections, 479, 520
Lower esophageal lesions, 213
Lower quadrant abdominal surgery, patient positioning for, 16f
Lumbar vein, 889f
Lung(s)
  anatomy of, 318f–319f
  bronchial tree of, 319f
  left, 318f, 321f
  lobes of, 318f
  lymph node distribution, 322, 322f
  pleural adhesions, 325, 325f
  pulmonary vasculature, 320f
  right, 318f
  segments of, 319f
Lung cancer, 317
Lung lobectomies, robotic
  anterior approach, 327
  approaches for, 326–327
  instruments for, 317
  left lower
    bronchus isolation and section, 382, 382f
    fissure division, 382, 382f
    left inferior pulmonary artery isolation, 382, 382f
    left inferior pulmonary vein, isolation and section of, 380, 380f–381f
    lymph nodal dissection, 383, 383f
    mediastinal lymph nodes dissection, 383
    operating room setup for, 378, 378f
    patient positioning for, 378
    port setting for, 378, 379f
    pulmonary ligament dissection, 380
    surgical technique for, 380f–383f, 380–383
  left upper
    anterior pleural reflection at hilum, opening of, 336, 336f
    anterolateral parenchymal bridge transection, 340
    apical pulmonary artery branches, 342, 342f
    bronchus, 342, 343f, 362, 363f
    contraindications for, 332, 345–346
    fissure dissection, 338, 338f, 365, 365f
    indications for, 332, 345–346
    inferior pulmonary ligament dissection with station 8–9 lymphadenectomy, 335
    instruments for, 345
    lymph node dissection in, 327f, 360, 365–366, 366f
    lymphadenectomy, 335, 344

operating room setup for, 332, 333f, 358f, 358–359
    patient positioning for, 332, 332f, 358–359
    port setting for, 324f, 332, 334f, 358–359, 359f
    posterior pleural reflection at hilum, opening of, 337, 337f
    posterolateral parenchymal bridge transection, 340, 340f, 343f
    pulmonary artery branches, 338, 339f, 361, 361f–362f, 364, 364f
    pulmonary vein preparation and division, 341, 341f, 360, 360f
    specimen extraction in, 344, 344f, 365–366, 366f
    surgical technique for, 335–344, 360f–366f, 360–366
  right lower
    instruments for, 367
    lymph node excision in, 323f
    mediastinal lymphadenectomy in, 373
    operating room setup for, 367, 368f
    patient positioning for, 367
    port setting for, 367, 368f
    pulmonary artery isolation and section, 370, 370f–372f
    pulmonary bronchus isolation and section, 372, 372f
    pulmonary ligament preparation, 369
    pulmonary vein isolation, 369, 369f
    surgical technique, 369f–373f, 369–373
  right middle
    arterial branches, isolation and division of, 376, 377f
    arterial vascularization, 376
    bronchus isolation and division, 376, 376f
    fissure division, 377, 377f
    instruments for, 367
    middle lobe artery, 374f
    middle lobe pulmonary vein, 374, 374f–375f
    operating room setup for, 367, 368f
    patient positioning for, 367
    port setting for, 367, 368f
  right upper
    arterial anatomy of, 353f
    bronchus isolation and division, 354, 355f–356f
    contraindications for, 345–346
    fissure division, 356, 356f
    indications for, 345–346
    instruments for, 345
    mediastinal lymph nodes dissection, 357
    operating room setup for, 347, 347f
    patient positioning for, 347, 348f
    peribronchial lymph node dissection, 354, 355f
    pleural cavity isolation in, 350
    port setting for, 347–349, 349f

pulmonary artery branches, isolation and division of, 352, 352f–353f
    right upper pulmonary vein division, 350, 350f–351f
    specimen extraction, 356, 356f
    surgical technique for, 350f–357f, 350–357
  robotic, 326, 326f
  stapling vessel technique in, 328, 328f
  transfissure approach, 327
Lung nodules, 120f
Lung surgery, 318–331
Lymph node(s)
  abdominal, 243t
  cervical, 242t
  hilar, 346, 354
  inflamed, 323
  in left colectomy, 507, 509f–510f
  lung distribution of, 322, 323f
  mediastinal distribution of, 322, 323f
  pancreatic, 646f
  paraesophageal, 245
  peribronchial, 354, 355f, 362
  rectum, 539f
  in right colectomy with complete mesocolic excision, 475f
  supradiaphragmatic, 245
  thoracic, 242t
Lymph node mapping
  in esophageal surgery, 111
  fluorescence imaging for, 105, 106f, 108
  in gastric surgery, 108
Lymphadenectomy
  anatomical landmarks for, 502
  celiac, 218
  incomplete, 651
  paratracheal, 373f
  in small bowel resection, 444
  splenic hilar, 399
  station 8–9, 335
  station 12, in pancreaticoduodenectomy, 610, 613f
  technique for, 323, 323f
Lymphatic drainage
  of breast, 184f
  of small bowel, 448f

M
Machine learning algorithms, 52
Machine-learning-based tumor margining, 121
Mako SmartRobotics, 55, 56f
Mammary gland. *See also* Breast
  anatomy of, 190f–191f
  vascularization of, 193f–194f
Marginal arcade, 507
Marginal artery, 471f
Marker-based registration, 76
Maryland forceps, 24, 167, 323, 785
Mastectomy, nipple-sparing
  anatomy involved in, 178f
  bilateral, 180, 181f–182f
  contraindications for, 179–180

Mastectomy, nipple-sparing (Cont.):
  da Vinci Si system for, 180, 187f
  da Vinci Xi system for, 180, 187f
  docking in, 187, 187f–188f
  indications for, 179–180
  instruments for, 177, 179
  international studies on, 178–179
  local recurrence risks, 177
  monoport placement in, 186, 186f
  nipple-areola complex in, 177, 178f
  open approach versus, 177, 179
  open axillary access for, 183, 184f
  operating room setup for, 180, 181f–182f
  overview of, 177–179
  patient positioning for, 180, 180f
  patient satisfaction with, 179
  port placement in, 186, 186f
  postoperative outcome evaluation, 195, 195f
  retropectoral reconstruction after, 195, 195f
  robotic dissection in, 189, 189f–194f
  robotic reconstruction after, 195, 195f
  subcutaneous flap dissection in, 183, 184f
  subcutaneous tunnels in, 185, 185f
  surgical technique for, 183f–195f, 183–195
  trocar placement in, 186
  tumescent injection in, 185, 185f
  tunneling technique in, 185, 185f
MAUDE database, 53
Mayo stand, 39
Mediastinal dissection, in Heller myotomy with modified Dor fundoplication, 308
Mediastinal lymph nodes dissection
  in left lower lobectomy, 383
  in right upper lobectomy, 357
Mediastinal lymphadenectomy
  in right lower lobectomy, 373, 373f
  subcarinal, 225, 373f
Medical Image Computing and Computer-Assisted Intervention, 86
Medtronic EleVision IR Platform
Mental nerve, in transoral thyroidectomy, 165, 166f
Mesenteric dissection, in small bowel resection, 444, 449f
Mesenteric gap closure
  in Roux-en-Y gastric bypass, 434, 434f
  in small bowel resection, 454, 454f
Mesenteric lymphography, 106f, 107
Mesentery
  anatomy of, 450f, 461f, 491f
  descending colon, 507, 507f
  detachment of, 461
  hematoma of, 454
  mobilization of, in right colectomy with complete mesocolic excision, 463
  sigmoid colon, 498
  of terminal ileum, division of, 474
  transverse colon, division of, 476

Mesoesophagus
  definition of, 245
  en bloc, 225
  mobilization of, 238f–245f, 238–245
Mesorectum, 535f
Metal cannula, in da Vinci SP system, 1040, 1041f–1042f, 1064
MIC-CAI. See Medical Image Computing and Computer-Assisted Intervention
Midclavicular point, 17
Middle adrenal artery, 874
Middle colic artery, 470f–472f, 505f
Middle hepatic vein, 775f–776f
Middle mediastinal lymph node dissection, 245f, 245–246
Mimic dV-Trainer, 48f
Mimic X-experience, 50f
Minimally invasive surgery
  description of, 66–67
  intraoperative guidance during, 73
  intraoperative ultrasound in, 707, 708f
  liver, 701
  robotic surgery as, 60
  splenectomy, 575
MLAs. See Machine learning algorithms
Modified Dor fundoplication, Heller myotomy with
  anterior partial fundoplication, 315, 315f
  anterior phrenoesophageal membrane division, 305, 306f
  contraindications for, 299
  gastrohepatic ligament division in, 305f
  hiatus in
    anatomy of, 307f
    exposure of, 304, 304f
  indications for, 299
  instruments for, 299
  intraoperative endoscopy in, 315
  left vagal trunk identification in, 309, 309f–310f
  mediastinal dissection in, 308
  myotomy, 312, 312f–313f
  operating room setup for, 299–300, 301f
  overview of, 299
  patient positioning for, 299–300, 300f
  pneumoperitoneum for, 299–300
  port settings for, 299–300, 302f–303f
  surgical technique for, 304f–315f, 304–315
  vagal trunk in, 309, 309f–310f
Modified Palmer's point, 17, 17f
Modified radical neck dissection
  anatomy involved in, 153, 154f
  contraindications for, 153
  indications for, 153
  level II dissection, 161, 161f
  level III dissection, 159, 160f
  level IV dissection, 159, 160f
  level Vb dissection, 159, 161f
  operating room setup for, 155
  patient positioning for, 155, 155f
  port setting for, 155

robot positioning and docking for, 158
  specimen extraction, 161
  working space for, 155–161, 157f
  wound closure, 161
Molecular imaging, 121
MONARCH, 120
Monarch platform, 55, 56f
Monopolar cautery instruments, 25f
Monopolar curved scissors, for nipple-sparing mastectomy, 179
Monopolar hook, 24, 27, 313, 816, 898
MRND. See Modified radical neck dissection
Mucinous cystadenomas, 674
Myasthenia gravis, extended thymectomy for
  carbon dioxide insufflation for, 200–201
  instruments for, 197
  operating room setup for, 198f, 198–199
  overview of, 197
  patient positioning for, 198, 199f
  port setting for, 198–199
  surgical technique for, 200f–207f, 200–208
  trocar placement for, 199f
Myopectineal orifice, 908, 933f
Myotomy. See Heller myotomy, with modified Dor fundoplication

N
Nano surgery, 12
Nathanson retractor, 413, 422
Near-infrared fluorescence imaging
  biliary anatomy assessments using, 816
  description of, 71f
  for gastric cancer surgery, 401, 401f
Near-infrared indocyanine green fluorescence
  bile duct injuries recognition using, 833, 834f
  description of, 9, 9f
  small bowel assessment, 452f
Near-infrared spectrum, 70
Neck zones, 154f
Needle driver, 39, 1033
Nephrectomy. See Donor nephrectomy
Nerve imaging
  during colorectal surgery, 107, 107f
  fluorescence for, 93
Nipple, 190f–191f
Nipple-areola complex, 177, 178f
Nipple-sparing mastectomy, robotic
  anatomy involved in, 178f
  bilateral, 180, 181f–182f
  contraindications for, 179–180
  da Vinci Si system for, 180, 187f
  da Vinci Xi system for, 180, 187f
  docking in, 187, 187f–188f
  indications for, 179–180
  instruments for, 177, 179
  international studies on, 178–179
  local recurrence risks, 177
  monoport placement in, 186, 186f

Index **1079**

nipple-areola complex in, 177, 178*f*
open approach versus, 177, 179
open axillary access for, 183, 184*f*
operating room setup for, 180, 181*f*–182*f*
overview of, 177–179
patient positioning for, 180, 180*f*
patient satisfaction with, 179
port placement in, 186, 186*f*
postoperative outcome evaluation, 195, 195*f*
retropectoral reconstruction after, 195, 195*f*
robotic dissection in, 189, 189*f*–194*f*
robotic reconstruction after, 195, 195*f*
subcutaneous flap dissection in, 183, 184*f*
subcutaneous tunnels in, 185, 185*f*
surgical technique for, 183*f*–195*f*, 183–195
trocar placement in, 186
tumescent injection in, 185, 185*f*
tunneling technique in, 185, 185*f*
NIS. *See* Near-infrared spectrum
Nissen fundoplication, selective
anatomy involved in, 284*f*–285*f*
construction of, 293–296
contraindications for, 278
cruroplasty in, 293, 293*f*
dissection, 282*f*–291*f*, 282–291
failures of, 296*f*
fundoplication in, 294, 294*f*–295*f*
gastrohepatic ligament opening, 283, 286*f*
hiatus exposure in, 282, 282*f*
indications for, 278
instruments for, 277
left crus dissection in, 288, 288*f*
liver exposure in, 282, 282*f*
operating room setup for, 278, 279*f*
overview of, 277
in paraesophageal hernia repair, 274, 275*f*
patient positioning for, 278, 278*f*
Penrose drain for, 289, 290*f*
pneumoperitoneum in, 280
port setting for, 278, 280*f*–281*f*
posterior gastric fundus dissection in, 291, 291*f*
retroesophageal window, 289, 289*f*
right crus dissection in, 283, 286*f*
slipped, 296*f*
wrap
failures involving, 296*f*
testing of, 292, 292*f*
Nonrecurrent laryngeal nerve, 138, 142*f*, 252*f*
Novitsky technique, for robotic transversus abdominis release, 927, 933–934, 934*f*–935*f*
NRLN. *See* Nonrecurrent laryngeal nerve

O
OATPs. *See* Organic anion transporting polypeptides
OATs. *See* Organic anion transporters
Omental bursa, 256

Omentectomy
in D2 total gastrectomy, 393, 393*f*–394*f*
left side, 393
Omohyoid muscle, 132, 132*f*
Open surgery
haptic feedback in, 22, 24, 24*f*
laparoscopic surgery conversion to, 30*f*, 30–31
Operating room
hourly cost of, 58
layout of, 33, 34*f*
preparation of, by assistant, 33–36, 34*f*–35*f*
Operating room coordinator, 61–62, 63*t*
Operating room tables
integrated, 17, 36, 66
lowering of, 36–37
Optical see-through head-mounted displays, 37, 38*f*
OR 4.0, 83
ORB-SLAM, 76
Organic anion transporters, 101
Organic anion transporting polypeptides, 101

P
PA. *See* Physician assistants
Pancreas
distal, transection of, 686
division of, in spleen-preserving distal pancreatectomy, 666, 666*f*
lymph node mapping of, 646*f*
transection of
in central pancreatectomy, 683, 683*f*
in radical anterograde modular pancreatosplenectomy, 648, 648*f*
Pancreas transplant, robotic
arterial anastomosis in, 993, 993*f*
closure of, 995
colon mobilization in, 987, 988*f*
contraindications for, 983–984, 984*t*
duodenoenterostomy in, 994, 995*f*
graft in
backbench preparation of, 984, 984*f*
pelvic placement of, 992
hanging maneuver in, 989
indications for, 983–984
instruments for, 983
left external iliac artery preparation in, 989, 989*f*–991*f*
operating room setup for, 985, 986*f*
patient positioning for, 985, 985*f*
port setting for, 985, 987*f*
reperfusion in, 994, 994*f*
surgical field exposure, 988, 988*f*
trocar positioning in, 985–986, 987*f*
venous anastomosis in, 993, 993*f*
venous clamping in, 992, 992*f*
Pancreas transplant alone, 983
Pancreatectomy
central. *See* Central pancreatectomy
distal. *See* Distal pancreatectomy
small bowel viability during, 103*f*

Pancreatic body
anatomical variations of, 594*f*, 670*f*
anatomy of, 660*f*
arterial supply of, 643*f*
mobilization of
in left adrenalectomy, 887
in renal artery aneurysm repair, 1026
in spleen-preserving distal pancreatectomy, 667, 667*f*–668*f*, 670*f*
venous supply of, 644*f*
Pancreatic cystic neoplasms, 689–690
Pancreatic neck
antegrade dissection of, 682
preparation of
in central pancreatectomy, 680, 680*f*
in radical anterograde modular pancreatosplenectomy, 643, 643*f*
in spleen-preserving distal pancreatectomy, 665, 665*f*
transection of, 624, 624*f*
Pancreatic neuroendocrine tumors
central pancreatectomy for, 674
enucleation of, 689–696
functional, 690–691
imaging and margining of, 115*f*
nonfunctional, 690
spleen-preserving distal pancreatectomy for, 654
Pancreatic nodules, 690*f*, 691
Pancreatic parenchyma
anatomy of, 666
lesions of, 491
Pancreatic surgery, 114–117
Pancreatic tail
anatomical variations of, 594*f*, 670*f*
arterial supply of, 643*f*, 660*f*
mobilization of
in renal artery aneurysm repair, 1026
in spleen-preserving distal pancreatectomy, 667, 667*f*–670*f*
retraction of, 592, 592*f*–593*f*
venous supply of, 644*f*, 660*f*
Pancreatic tumor enucleation
contraindications for, 690–691
da Vinci Xi system for, 691
drain in, 696
enucleation, 696
gastrocolic ligament opening in, 694
hemostasis verification in, 696
indications for, 690–691
indocyanine green fluorescence imaging in, 694, 695*f*
instruments for, 689
intraoperative ultrasound in, 694, 696
operating room setup for, 691, 693*f*
overview of, 689
pancreatic gland exposure in, 694
patient positioning for, 691, 692*f*
pneumoperitoneum in, 691
port setting for, 691, 693*f*
retropancreatic tunnel in, 695
specimen extraction in, 696

Pancreatic tumor enucleation (Cont.):
  surgical technique for, 694–696
  uncinate process in, 695
Pancreatic tumor imaging and margining, 114, 115f
Pancreaticoduodenectomy, laparoscopic, 599
Pancreaticoduodenectomy, robotic
  anatomy of, 612f
  cholecystectomy, 616, 616f
  common bile duct transection, 617, 617f
  contraindications for, 599
  duodenal derotation, 623
  duodenum transection, 616, 616f
  gastrocolic ligament division in, 604, 604f
  gastroduodenal artery transection, 618, 619f, 622f
  hepatic flexure mobilization, 605, 605f
  hepatic hilum in, 610, 610f–611f
  history of, 599
  indications for, 599
  instruments for, 599
  Kocher maneuver in, 607, 608f–609f
  ligament of Treitz transection, 623, 623f
  operating room setup for, 600, 601f
  pancreatic neck transection, 624, 624f
  patient positioning for, 600, 600f
  pneumoperitoneum in, 600
  port setting for, 600–601, 602f–603f
  pylorus-preserving, 604
  reconstruction after
    bilio-digestive anastomosis, 631
    description of, 627
    end-to-side pancreaticojejunostomy, 628, 628f
    gastrojejunostomy, 631
    hepaticojejunostomy, 631, 631f
    pancreaticogastrostomy, 629, 630f
    pylorojejunostomy, 632f–633f
  right colonic vein, 606f
  right gastric artery division, 614, 614f
  right gastroepiploic artery division, 615, 615f
  right hepatic artery, 618f
  specimen extraction, 634
  station 12 lymphadenectomy in, 610, 613f
  surgical technique for, 604f–633f, 604–634
  uncinate process dissection, 625, 626f–627f
  visual feedback in, 24
Pancreaticogastrostomy, transgastric, 629, 630f
Pancreaticojejunostomy
  distal, in central pancreatectomy, 687
  end-to-side, 628, 628f
Pancreatosplenectomy, robotic radical anterograde modular
  contraindications for, 635–636
  da Vinci Si system, 638f, 639
  da Vinci Xi system, 638f, 639
  gastrocolic ligament division in, 641, 641f
  history of, 635

indications for, 635–636
inferior mesenteric vein division, 649, 649f
instruments for, 635–636
intraoperative ultrasound in, 643
left colonic flexure mobilization in, 642, 642f
left gastroepiploic artery division, 645
operating room setup for, 636, 637f
pancreas transection in, 648, 648f
pancreatic neck preparation in, 643, 643f
patient positioning for, 636, 636f
pneumoperitoneum for, 636
port setting for, 636, 638f–640f
resectability assessments, 643, 645
retroperitoneum dissection with left adrenalectomy in, 651, 651f
short gastric vessels, 645, 645f
specimen extraction, 651
splenic artery control and division in, 646, 647f
splenic vein division, 650, 650f
surgical technique for, 641–652
Paracardial lymph nodes, 213
Paracolic gutter, 462, 524, 526f
Paraesophageal hernia repair
  contraindications for, 259
  cruroplasty in, 270, 271f
  dissection in, 264f–270f, 264–270
    left crus, 264, 264f–265f
    mediastinal, 266f–269f, 266–269
    right crus, 270
  esophagogastric mobilization, 270
  fundoplication in, 274, 275f
  indications for, 259
  instruments for, 259
  mesh reinforcement in, 272, 272f–273f
  operating room setup for, 260, 261f
  overview of, 259
  patient positioning for, 260, 261f
  pneumoperitoneum in, 260
  port setting for, 260, 262f–263f
  reconstruction after, 270–275, 271f–273f
Paraesophageal lymph nodes
  cervical, dissection of, 250, 250f, 253, 253f–254f
  description of, 245
Parallax, 78
Parathyroid glands
  anatomy of, 138, 145f–147f
  autofluorescence of, 92, 118, 119f
  identification of, 118
  inferior, 150f, 152
  superior, 172, 173f
  variants of, 146f–147f
Parathyroid surgery, 118
Parenchymal demarcation, in living donor hepatectomy, 1008, 1008f
Parenchymal tissue, 27
Parenchymal transection
  core, 728f, 728–729
  hepatic veins in, 730

intraoperative ultrasonography during, 751
  in left hepatectomy, 751f–752f, 751–752
  in liver resections, 785, 786f
  in living donor hepatectomy, 1009, 1009f, 1011, 1011f
  in right hepatectomy, 724–729, 727f–728f
  subcortical, 724, 727f, 728
Parenchyma-sparing resections, 769
Parietal pleura, 270
Partial cholecystectomy, 807f
Patient positioning. See also specific procedure, patient positioning for
  description of, 15–17
  supine, 36f
Patient prepping, 36–37
Patient-surgeon interface, 6, 7f
PCNs. See Pancreatic cystic neoplasms
Pelvic cavity, 534f
Pelvic floor muscles, 541f
Pelvic plexus, in total mesorectal excision, 107, 107f
Pelvic surgery, 36
Pelvis
  anatomy of, 529f
  autonomic nerves of, 528, 530f
  fasciae of, 530f
  neural anatomy of, 530f
Penrose drain, in Nissen fundoplication, 289, 290f
Percutaneous transhepatic biliary drainage, 842
Perfusion assessment
  in bowel surgery, 102, 103f
  in esophageal surgery, 109
  in gastric surgery, 108
Peribronchial lymph node dissection, 354, 355f, 362
Perihilar fat, 964
Peripancreatic arteries, in central pancreatectomy, 681
Peritoneal flap, 910, 910f, 1065, 1065f
Per-oral endoscopic myotomy, 299
Petersen space, 434
Pfannenstiel incision, 405, 454, 634, 943, 948, 1000
  description of, 22
  illustration of, 23f
  in living donor hepatectomy, 1012
Phase recognition, 80
Pheochromocytoma
  fluorescence imaging identification of, 118, 118f
  right adrenalectomy for, 863–864
Phrenic nerve
  left, 201, 889f
  right, 207
Phrenogastric ligament, 589, 591f
Phrenosplenic ligament, 589, 591f
Physician assistants, 33
Pleural adhesions, 325, 325f
PNETs. See Pancreatic neuroendocrine tumors

Index 1081

Pneumoperitoneum
    in cholecystectomy, 793
    establishing of, 17f–18f, 17–18
    in Heller myotomy with modified Dor fundoplication, 299–300
    in Ivor-Lewis esophagectomy, 210
    in kidney transplant, 966
    in left lateral sectionectomy, 762
    in liver resections, 771
    in living donor hepatectomy, 1000
    in pancreatic tumor enucleation, 691
    in pancreaticoduodenectomy, 600
    in paraesophageal hernia repair, 260
    pressure of, 21
    in radical anterograde modular pancreatosplenectomy, 636
    in right adrenalectomy, 864
    in right colectomy with complete mesocolic excision, 456
    in right hepatectomy, 704
    in robotic transabdominal preperitoneal repair, 898
    in Roux-en-Y gastric bypass, 422
    in selective Nissen fundoplication, 280
    in sleeve gastrectomy, 409–410
    in small bowel resection, 438
    in spleen-preserving distal pancreatectomy, 654
    in splenectomy, 578
    Veress technique for, 842
Pneumothorax, 308
POEM. See Per-oral endoscopic myotomy
Polarized glasses, 9
POPF. See Postoperative pancreatic fistula
Port clutch, 1037
Port placement
    for D2 total gastrectomy, 389–390, 390f–391f
    for Heller myotomy, 20f
    for Ivor-Lewis esophagectomy, 210–211, 211f
    in obese patients, 20
    for right upper lobectomy, 349
    targeting, 40
    triangulation principle for, 18–20, 19f
Portal pedicle stapling, in left lateral sectionectomy, 766
Portal vein
    anatomical variations of, 715f, 745f
    left, 744, 745f, 779f
    ligation of, 714–716, 715f–716f
    resection of, 744
    right
        anatomy of, 777f
        dissection of, in living donor hepatectomy, 1006
        in right hepatectomy, 714–716, 715f–716f
        in Roux-en-Y hepaticojejunostomy, 814
Posterior axillary line, 237
Posterior gastric fundus
    anatomy of, 416, 418f
    dissection of, in Nissen fundoplication, 291, 291f
    mobilization of, in sleeve gastrectomy, 416, 416f–418f
Posterior lamella of the internal oblique, 933, 934f
Posterior mediastinal lymph nodes, 255f, 255–256
Posterior pleura, 380
Posterior pleural reflection at hilum, opening of, 337, 337f
Posterior rectus sheath incision, in robotic transversus abdominis release, 933f
Posterolateral parenchymal bridge, 340, 340f, 343f
Postoperative pancreatic fistula, 689
Postoperative period, artificial intelligence applications in, 13
Potts scissors, 975
Prehabilitation, monitored, 61f
Prepping of patient, 36–37
Primary hepatolithiasis, 841
Pringle maneuver, 730
    in left hepatectomy, 742, 742f
    in left lateral sectionectomy, 765, 765f
    in liver resections, 780, 780f–782f
Privileging, 53
Proctors, 81
ProGrasp™ forceps, 24, 151, 898
Promontory, 498
Prostatectomy, 60
Protoporphyrin IX, 93
Proximal bulldog clamp, 976, 992
Proximal pancreatic duct, 683f
Proximal pancreatic transection, in central pancreatectomy, 683, 683f
Pseudo-omega technique, 432, 432f–433f
PTA. See Pancreas transplant alone
PTBD. See Percutaneous transhepatic biliary drainage
Pull and push technique, 27
Pulmonary artery
    apical, 342, 342f
    branches of, 338, 339f, 352, 352f–353f, 361, 361f–362f, 364, 364f
    description of, 321
    dissection along, 321f
    left inferior, 382, 382f
    right lower, isolation and section of, 370, 370f–372f
Pulmonary vasculature, 320f
Pulmonary veins
    anatomical variants of, 350, 351f
    left inferior, isolation and section of, 380, 380f–381f
    left upper, 360, 360f
    middle lobe, 374, 374f–375f
    right lower, 369, 369f, 371f
    right upper, 350, 350f–351f
Pylorojejunostomy, 632f–633f
Pylorus-preserving pancreaticoduodenectomy, 604

Q
Quantitative fluorescence imaging, 72

R
Radical anterograde modular pancreatosplenectomy, robotic
    contraindications for, 635–636
    da Vinci Si system, 638f, 639
    da Vinci Xi system, 638f, 639
    gastrocolic ligament division in, 641, 641f
    history of, 635
    indications for, 635–636
    inferior mesenteric vein division, 649, 649f
    instruments for, 635–636
    intraoperative ultrasound in, 643
    left colonic flexure mobilization in, 642, 642f
    left gastroepiploic artery division, 645
    operating room setup for, 636, 637f
    pancreas transection in, 648, 648f
    pancreatic neck preparation in, 643, 643f
    patient positioning for, 636, 636f
    pneumoperitoneum for, 636
    port setting for, 636, 638f–640f
    resectability assessments, 643, 645
    retroperitoneum dissection with left adrenalectomy in, 651, 651f
    short gastric vessels, 645, 645f
    specimen extraction, 651
    splenic artery control and division in, 646, 647f
    splenic vein division, 650, 650f
    surgical technique for, 641–652
Radical esophagectomy with extended mediastinal lymphadenectomy
    abdominal lymph node dissection, 256
    bronchial arteries, 246f
    cervical anastomosis in, 257
    cervical dissection, 234–235
    cervical paraesophageal lymph node dissection, 250, 250f, 253, 253f–254f
    contraindications for, 234
    "double bipolar" method, 238
    extracorporeal gastric conduit creation, 257
    indications for, 234
    instruments for, 233
    mesoesophagus mobilization, 238f–245f, 238–245
    middle mediastinal lymph node dissection, 245f, 245–246
    nerve monitoring, 234–235
    operating room setup for, 235, 235f
    overview of, 233
    patient positioning for, 235, 237, 237f
    port setting for, 235
    posterior mediastinal lymph node dissection, 255f, 255–256
    recurrent laryngeal nerve dissection in
        left, 253, 253f
        right, 250, 250f

Radical esophagectomy with extended
    mediastinal lymphadenectomy
    (*Cont.*):
  specimen extraction in, 257
  stomach mobilization in, 256
  thoracic phase of, 235–237
  three dissectable layers, 247*f*, 247–248
  tracheobronchial lymph node dissection,
    255*f*, 255–256
  upper esophagus mobilization, 248*f*–249*f*,
    248–249
RAMPS. *See* Radical anterograde modular
    pancreatosplenectomy
RAT. *See* Robotic-assisted thymectomy
RATS. *See* Robotic-assisted thoracoscopic
    surgery
Rectal artery, 506, 506*f*
Rectal cancer, total mesorectal excision for
  anatomy, 528, 528*f*–530*f*
  anterior dissection, 540
  anterolateral dissection, 540
  autonomic nerves, 528
  circular concentric dissection of distal
    mesorectum, 541, 541*f*
  colorectal/coloanal anastomosis,
    544
  contraindications for, 517
  da Vinci S system docking, 518, 519*f*
  da Vinci Si system docking, 518, 519*f*
  da Vinci SP system, 545*f*–548*f*,
    545–547
  da Vinci Xi system docking, 520,
    521*f*–522*f*
  deep posterior dissection in, 542, 542*f*
  Denonvilliers' fascia, 540, 540*f*
  distal rectum division, 543
  endoscopic ultrasound in, 518
  fasciae, 528, 530*f*
  fascial adhesions, 528
  full robotic approach, 523–525
  hybrid laparoscopic-robotic approach,
    523
  indications for, 517
  instruments for, 517
  operating room setup for, 520, 522*f*
  orogastric tube in, 518
  overview of, 517
  patient positioning for, 518, 518*f*
  pelvic dissection, 534, 534*f*, 547*f*
  port setting for, 518, 519*f*, 521*f*
  posterior dissection, 534, 534*f*–535*f*
  postero-bilateral dissection, 535–536,
    536*f*
  proximal colon preparation, 544
  retraction levels, 528, 531, 531*f*–533*f*
  specimen extraction in, 544
  splenocolic ligament dissection in, 525,
    527*f*
  surgical techniques, 523–527
Rectal carcinoma
  liver metastases from, 100*f*
  rectum resection for, rectosigmoid
    anastomosis after, 104*f*

Rectal dissection, gravity in, 21
Rectosigmoid anastomosis, after rectum
    resection for rectal carcinoma,
    104*f*
Rectum
  anatomy of, 528*f*
  anterior side dissection of, 541*f*
  arterial anatomy of, 537*f*
  cancer of. *See* Rectal cancer
  dissection of, 534, 534*f*–536*f*
  lymph nodes of, 539*f*
  resection of, for rectal carcinoma,
    104*f*
  venous anatomy of, 538*f*
  washing of, 543*f*
Recurrent laryngeal nerve
  anatomy of, 138, 141*f*, 150*f*, 251*f*
  counterlateral, 153
  course of, 141*f*
  damage to, 173
  inferior thyroid artery and, 138, 143*f*
  left
    damage to, 383
    dissection of, 253, 253*f*
    preservation of, 172–173, 173*f*
  right
    anatomy of, 251*f*
    dissection of, 250, 250*f*
  in transoral robotic thyroidectomy, 173,
    173*f*
Recurrent neural networks, 82
Recurrent pyogenic cholangitis
  description of, 841–842
  hepatectomy for, 856, 857*f*
  partial hepatectomy for, 856
Registered nurse first assistants, 33
Registration
  algorithms for, 76
  challenges for, 77–78
  image-based, 76, 77*f*
  marker-based methods, 76
  rigid, 77–78
Relative value units, 58
Remote monitoring, 60
Renal artery
  anatomical variations of, 955, 957*f*
  anomalies of, 955, 956*f*
  distal branches, 1030*f*
  identification of, in kidney surgery, 112,
    112*f*–113*f*
  left
    in left adrenalectomy, 890, 890*f*–891*f*
    in left donor nephrectomy, 958
  right, aneurysm repair of, 113, 113*f*
Renal artery aneurysms
  clamping of, 1031, 1031*f*
  distal control of, 1031*f*
  endovascular approaches, 1018
  gender and, 1017
  instruments for, 1017
  location of, 1025*f*
  overview of, 1017–1018
  proximal control of, 1031*f*

  robotic repair of
    anastomosis with, 1034*f*
    aneurysmatic sac, 1029, 1032, 1032*f*
    aneurysmectomy, 1031, 1031*f*
    aorta exposure in, 1026
    contraindications for, 1018
    descending colon mobilization in, 1026
    hemostasis, 1035
    history of, 1018
    indications for, 1018
    intraoperative ultrasonography in,
      1027, 1027*f*
    left colonic flexure mobilization in,
      1026
    left renal vein exposure, 1026
    left-side aneurysm, 1018, 1020, 1021*f*
    liver mobilization in, 1026
    needle-driving technique, 1034*f*
    operating room setup for, 1018, 1020,
      1020*f*–1021*f*
    overview of, 1017–1018
    pancreatic body and tail mobilization,
      1026
    partial Kocher maneuver in, 1026
    patient positioning for, 1018,
      1018*f*–1019*f*
    pneumoperitoneum in, 1020
    port setting for, 1018, 1022,
      1022*f*–1023*f*
    proximal renal artery control, 1028,
      1028*f*
    reconstruction, 1033, 1033*f*–1034*f*
    renal artery preparation, 1030*f*
    renal vein preparation, 1028
    reperfusion, 1035
    right colon mobilization in, 1026
    right-side aneurysm, 1018, 1020, 1020*f*
    saphenous graft after, 1033
    surgical field, 1026
    surgical technique, 1024–1035
  types of, 1029*f*
Renal transplantation
  illustration of, 114*f*
  perfusion confirmation in, 113
  vascular flow in, 114*f*
Renal vein
  left. *See* Left renal vein
  middle, 957*f*
  retroaortic, 889, 957*f*, 958
Renal-azygos-lumbar connection, 957*f*
Renoadrenal separation, 958
Reproducibility, 86
Retraction
  levels of, for exposure, 21–22
  liver
    in D2 total gastrectomy, 392, 392*f*
    in right adrenalectomy, 868, 869*f*–870*f*
Retroaortic renal vein, 889, 957*f*, 958
Retroesophageal window, in Nissen
    fundoplication, 289, 289*f*
Retrograde cholecystectomy, 709
Retromuscular space, in robotic transversus
    abdominis release, 931, 931*f*

Retropancreatic neck dissection, in central pancreatectomy, 680, 680f
Retropancreatic tunnel
    in central pancreatectomy, 682
    in pancreatic tumor enucleation, 695
    in spleen-preserving distal pancreatectomy, 665, 665f
Retroperitoneum
    definition of, 969
    dissection of, with left adrenalectomy in radical anterograde modular pancreatosplenectomy, 651, 651f
Retrorectus ventral hernia repair, 912, 912t
Return on investment, 28
Reverse Trendelenburg position, 37f
Right adrenalectomy, robotic
    adrenal vein in, 872, 872f, 876–877
    anatomical landmarks in, 870, 871f
    contraindications for, 863–864
    indications for, 863–864
    inflow control in, 874, 875f
    instruments for, 863
    liver mobilization in, 869
    liver retraction in, 868, 869f–870f
    operating room setup for, 864, 865f, 866f
    partial Kocher maneuver in, 868, 868f
    patient positioning for, 864, 864f
    pneumoperitoneum for, 864
    port setting for, 866, 866f–867f
    right colonic flexure mobilization, 868, 868f
    specimen extraction in, 878
    trocar placement for, 866f–867f
    upper pole of kidney in, 873, 873f–874f
Right anterior sectionectomy, 757f
Right colectomy
    with complete mesocolic excision
        anatomy of, 473f
        ascending colon mobilization in, 461–462
        cecum mobilization in, 461–462
        contraindications for, 456
        ileocolic isoperistaltic anastomosis in, 477
        ileocolic vessel division, 468
        illustration of, 460f
        indications for, 456
        instruments for, 455
        lymph node anatomy in, 475f
        medial-to-lateral dissection, 468
        mesentery of terminal ileum, division of, 474
        omental division, 460, 460f
        operating room setup for, 456, 459f
        overview of, 455
        patient positioning for, 456, 456f
        pneumoperitoneum in, 456
        port setting for, 456, 457f–458f
        reconstruction after, 477, 477f
        right colonic flexure mobilization, 464, 465f–467f
        surgical technique for, 460f–477f, 460–478
        terminal ileum division, 474
        transverse colon division, 474, 475f
        transverse colon mesentery division, 476
        trocar placement in, 457f–458f
        venous anatomy in, 467f, 469f
        right colon stump during, 103f
Right colic artery, 470f
Right colonic flexure mobilization
    in right adrenalectomy, 868, 868f
    in right colectomy with complete mesocolic excision, 464, 465f–467f
    in right hepatectomy, 711
Right colonic vein, 606f
Right crus dissection
    in Nissen fundoplication, 283, 286f
    in paraesophageal hernia repair, 270
Right donor nephrectomy, robotic
    operating room setup for, 945, 948f, 958
    patient positioning for, 945, 945f, 958
    port setting for, 945, 947f, 958
    renal artery, 960
    surgical technique for, 960–961
    ureter preparation in, 960
Right gastric artery
    division of, 614, 614f
    ligation of, 400
Right gastroepiploic artery, 214, 615, 615f
Right hepatectomy, robotic
    anatomy of, 702f–703f
    caudate lobe partial division in, 721f
    contraindications for, 702
    cystic duct retraction in, 709, 711f
    falciform ligament in
        dissection of, 707, 708f
        reconstruction of, 730, 731f
    "hanging" maneuver, 722f–723f
    hepatic artery, 712, 713f–714f
    hepatic hilum exposure/evaluation in, 709, 709f–710f
    hepatic vein in, 725f–726f
    hepatocaval dissection, 717, 720f–722f
    indications for, 702
    instruments for, 701
    intraoperative ultrasound in, 707, 708f
    operating room setup for, 704, 706f
    parenchymal transection, 724–729, 727f–728f
    patient positioning for, 704, 705f
    pneumoperitoneum in, 704
    port setting for, 704, 707f–708f
    portal vein in, 714–716, 715f–716f
    retrograde cholecystectomy in, 709
    right colonic flexure mobilization in, 711
    right hepatic duct in, 717
    specimen extraction in, 730
    surgical technique for, 704–731
Right hepatic artery
    anatomy of, 618f
    clipping of, 1012
    dissection of, in living donor hepatectomy, 1006
Right hepatic duct, 97f
    anatomical variations of, 718f, 747, 747f
    anatomy of, 719f
    posterior, 837f
    in right hepatectomy, 717
Right hepatic vein, 728, 775f–776f
Right lower lobectomy, robotic
    instruments for, 367
    lymph node excision in, 323f
    mediastinal lymphadenectomy in, 373
    operating room setup for, 367, 368f
    patient positioning for, 367
    port setting for, 367, 368f
    pulmonary artery isolation and section, 370, 370f–372f
    pulmonary bronchus isolation and section, 372, 372f
    pulmonary ligament preparation, 369
    pulmonary vein isolation, 369, 369f
    surgical technique, 369f–373f, 369–373
Right middle lobectomy, robotic
    arterial branches, isolation and division of, 376, 377f
    arterial vascularization, 376
    bronchus isolation and division, 376, 376f
    fissure division, 377, 377f
    instruments for, 367
    middle lobe artery, 374f
    middle lobe pulmonary vein, 374, 374f–375f
    operating room setup for, 367, 368f
    patient positioning for, 367
    port setting for, 367, 368f
Right portal vein
    anatomy of, 777f
    dissection of, in living donor hepatectomy, 1006
Right posterior sectionectomy, 757f
Right trisectionectomy, 757f
Right upper lobectomy, robotic
    arterial anatomy of, 353f
    bronchus isolation and division, 354, 355f–356f
    contraindications for, 345–346
    fissure division, 356, 356f
    indications for, 345–346
    instruments for, 345
    mediastinal lymph nodes dissection, 357
    operating room setup for, 347, 347f
    patient positioning for, 347, 348f
    peribronchial lymph node dissection, 354, 355f
    pleural cavity isolation in, 350
    port setting for, 347–349, 349f
    pulmonary artery branches, isolation and division of, 352, 352f–353f
    right upper pulmonary vein division, 350, 350f–351f
    specimen extraction, 356, 356f
    surgical technique for, 350f–357f, 350–357
Rigid registration, 77–78
Rives-Stoppa technique, 925
RLN. *See* Recurrent laryngeal nerve

1084 Index

RNFAs. See Registered nurse first assistants
RNNs. See Recurrent neural networks
Robot(s), 53, 54f
Robotic arms
  collisions involving, 40
  docking of, 40–41, 41f
  repositioning of, 40
Robotic cannulas
  placement of, 42, 42f
  remote center placement of, 42, 42f
Robotic certification, 49–50
Robotic instruments
  damaging of, 41
  illustration of, 25f–26f
  laparoscopic instruments versus, 11f
  Mayo stand for, 39
  types of, 25f–26f
  understanding of, 24–27, 25f–26f
Robotic platforms
  description of, 27, 67
  design of, 36
  overview of, 65–66
Robotic program
  academic contributions of, 63
  case volume of, 55
  cost tracking of, 57t, 57–58
  financials of, 55–58, 57t
  keys for success, 55–63, 57t
  profitability of, 58
  reimbursement of, 58
  utilization of, 55
  value of, 58–59
Robotic simulators
  for cholecystectomy, 46, 49–50, 50f
  continued surgical education uses of, 49–50
  description of, 46, 48f
  proficiency of, 49
  Simbionix RobotiX Mentor, 46f, 48f, 50f
  team training, 46
Robotic staplers
  description of, 27
  features of, 730
  sleeve gastrectomy, 419f, 420
Robotic surgeons
  credentialing of, 63
  proctoring of, 63
  training of, 60–61, 63
Robotic surgery
  bleeding control during, 29
  case volume for, 55
  code training in, 60, 60f
  communication during, 44
  credentialing in, 53
  diverging models of, 27
  evolution in, 67
  exposure in, 21–22
  fluorescence imaging applications in, 94–120
  history of, 3–13, 55
  instruments for. See Robotic instruments
  intraoperative guidance during, 73
  laparoscopic surgery versus, 59

  outcomes of, 60
  privileging in, 53
  safety of, 60
  scientific articles regarding, 6, 6f
  staff members involved in, 27
  team members in. See Robotic team
Robotic systems
  advancements in, 60–61
  lack of tremor with, 10
  mechanical enhancements of, 10–12, 11f
  new types of, 60–61
  return on investment, 28
  stability of, 10–12
  troubleshooting of, 39–40
  vision enhancements of, 8–10
Robotic team
  bedside assistant, 62
  communication among, 62–63
  nursing/technician team, 62
  operating room coordinator, 61–62, 63t
Robotic training
  animal models for, 50–51
  artificial intelligence in, 52
  for assistants, 44
  cadaver models for, 51–52
  curricula for, 52
  inanimate models for, 45–46, 46f
  role of, 28
  simulators for. See Robotic simulators
  virtual reality models for, 45–46, 48f
Robotic transabdominal preperitoneal repair
  anatomical landmarks in, 902, 902f–903f
  central zone dissection, 1063, 1064f
  contraindications for, 897, 1057
  description of, 897
  flap closure in, 910, 910f, 1065, 1065f
  flap dissection in, 1061
  floating port technique, 1059, 1059f
  hernia sac dissection in, 908, 1063
  indications for, 897, 1057
  instruments for, 897, 1057
  lateral dissection in, 906, 907f
  medial dissection in, 904, 905f
  mesh placement in, 909, 909f, 1064, 1064f
  myopectineal orifice, 908
  operating room setup for, 898, 899f, 1057, 1058f
  patient positioning for, 898, 898f, 1057, 1058f
  peritoneal flap closure in, 910, 910f, 1065, 1065f
  pneumoperitoneum for, 898
  port setting for, 898, 900f–901f, 1057, 1057f
  spermatic vessels, 908, 1064
Robotic transversus abdominis release
  abdominal wall in, 926
  adhesiolysis in, 931
  advantages of, 925
  anterior rectus sheath closure, 937, 938f
  arcuate line in, 931, 932f
  Bottoms-Up technique, 927, 933, 933f

  contraindications for, 926
  description of, 925
  disadvantages of, 926
  dual docking method in, 936
  epigastric crossover in, 931, 932f
  hernia reduction in, 931
  indications for, 926
  instruments for, 925
  intraabdominal access in, 928
  mesh deployment and fixation, 936, 937f–938f, 938
  myopectineal orifice in, 933f
  Novitsky technique, 927, 933–934, 934f–935f
  operating room setup for, 928, 929f
  operative techniques for, 927, 931–938, 933f–935f
  patient positioning for, 928, 928f
  port setting for, 928, 930f
  posterior rectus sheath closure, 937, 937f
  posterior rectus sheath incision in, 933f
  preoperative evaluation, 926
  retromuscular space access in, 931, 931f
  Rives-Stoppa technique, 925
  suprapubic crossover in, 931, 932f
  Top-Down technique, 927, 934–936, 935f
Robotic-assisted thoracoscopic surgery, 318
Robotic-assisted thymectomy
  carbon dioxide insufflation for, 200–201
  instruments for, 197
  operating room setup for, 198f, 198–199
  overview of, 197
  patient positioning for, 198, 199f
  port setting for, 198–199
  surgical technique for, 200f–207f, 200–208
  trocar placement for, 199f
ROI. See Return on investment
RoSS II, 48f
Round ligament division, in left lateral sectionectomy, 762, 762f
Roux-en-Y esophagojejunostomy, in D2 total gastrectomy, 403, 403f–404f
Roux-en-Y gastric bypass, robotic
  advantages of, 421
  alimentary limb of, 431f
  anatomy of, 431f
  angle of His dissection in, 425, 425f
  biliopancreatic limb of, 431f
  contraindications for, 421–422
  endoscopic evaluation in, 434
  gastric pouch in, 425, 425f–426f, 431f
  gastrojejunal anastomosis in, 430, 430f
  indications for, 421–422
  instruments for, 421–422
  jejunojejunostomy in, 429, 429f
  mesenteric gap closure, 434, 434f
  operating room setup for, 422, 423f
  patient positioning for, 422, 422f
  Petersen space closure, 434
  pneumoperitoneum for, 422
  port setting for, 422, 424f

pseudo-omega technique in, 432, 432f–433f
Roux-en-Y limb, 428, 428f
surgical technique for, 425f–434f, 425–434
Roux-en-Y hepaticojejunostomy
bile duct injuries repair, 827, 839f
bile duct mobilization, 814, 817f
bile duct transection in, 818
biliary injury, 814
biliary limb transposition in, 818–819, 820f
bilioenteric anastomosis, 837
cholecystectomy in, 814
contraindications for, 809
hepatic artery in, 814
hepatoduodenal ligament exposure in, 814, 815f
indications for, 809
instruments for, 809
in intrahepatic cholangiocarcinoma, 822–823
jejunal limb creation in, 818, 819f
jejunal loop, 837
jejunojejunostomy in, 823, 823f
ligament of Treitz in, 818
malignancy, 815
operating room setup for, 809–810, 813f
paraduodenal route in, 821f
patient positioning for, 809–810, 810f
port setting for, 809–810, 811f–812f
portal vein in, 814
surgical technique for, 814–823
Roux-en-Y jejunal loop, 687, 687f
RPC. See Recurrent pyogenic cholangitis
RTAPP. See Robotic transabdominal preperitoneal repair
RVUs. See Relative value units

S
SA-Cs. See Surgical assistant certified
Safety alerts, 82
SAGES. See Society of American Gastrointestinal and Endoscopic Surgeons
Saline drop test, 18, 18f
Satinsky-like clamp, 1032f
Scanlan Reliance Bulldog Clamp, 964f
SCDs. See Sequential compression devices
Scissors, EndoWristed, 26f
ScopEYE, 39f
Sectionectomy, left lateral
anatomy of, 734f, 757f
contraindications for, 756
coronary ligament in, 763, 764f
falciform ligament division in, 762, 762f
hemostasis verification in, 767, 767f
indications for, 756
instruments for, 755
intraoperative ultrasound, 763, 763f
left main hepatic vein stapling in, 766
left phrenic nerve in, 763, 764f
operating room setup for, 759, 760f
patient positioning for, 759, 759f
pneumoperitoneum in, 762
port setting for, 759, 761f, 845f
portal pedicle stapling in, 766
Pringle maneuver in, 765, 765f
round ligament division in, 762, 762f
specimen extraction in, 767
subcortical parenchyma dissection in, 765, 765f
surgical technique for, 762f–767f, 762–767
triangular ligament dissection, 763, 764f
Selective Nissen fundoplication
anatomy involved in, 284f–285f
construction of, 293–296
contraindications for, 278
cruroplasty in, 293, 293f
dissection, 282f–291f, 282–291
failures of, 296f
fundoplication in, 294, 294f–295f
gastrohepatic ligament opening, 283, 286f
hiatus exposure in, 282, 282f
indications for, 278
instruments for, 277
left crus dissection in, 288, 288f
liver exposure in, 282, 282f
operating room setup for, 278, 279f
overview of, 277
in paraesophageal hernia repair, 274, 275f
patient positioning for, 278, 278f
Penrose drain for, 289, 290f
pneumoperitoneum in, 280
port setting for, 278, 280f–281f
posterior gastric fundus dissection in, 291, 291f
retroesophageal window, 289, 289f
right crus dissection in, 283, 286f
slipped, 296f
wrap
failures involving, 296f
testing of, 292, 292f
Semilunar line, 931
Senhance, 55, 57f
Sentinel lymph node identification
in esophageal surgery, 111
fluorescence imaging for, 105, 106f, 108
in gastric surgery, 108
Sentinel node biopsy, 183, 184f
Sepra, 912
Sequential compression devices
in sleeve gastrectomy, 408
in total mesorectal excision for rectal cancer, 518
SHAP. See Shapely Additive Explanations
Shapely Additive Explanations, 86
Short gastric vessels
division of
gastrosplenic ligament division with, in D2 total gastrectomy, 395, 398f
in radical anterograde modular pancreatosplenectomy, 645, 645f
in sleeve gastrectomy, 415, 415f
in spleen-preserving distal pancreatectomy, 663
Short hepatic veins, in living donor hepatectomy, 1003, 1003f
Short-wave infrared, 121
Short-wavelength infrared band, 90
Shutter 3D glasses, 9
Side-to-side esophagogastric anastomosis, 227, 230f
Side-to-side small bowel anastomosis, 453, 453f
Sigmoid colon
mesentery of, 498
mobilization of, 502
Sigmoidal-rectal transection, in left colectomy, 506, 506f
SILS. See Single-incision laparoscopic surgery
Simbionix RobotiX Mentor, 46f, 48f, 50f
SimNow™ simulator, 49
Simple adhesiolysis, 29–30
Simulators
applications of, 80
robotic training uses of. See Robotic simulators
Simultaneous localization and mapping, 76
Single-incision laparoscopic surgery, 1045
SLAM. See Simultaneous localization and mapping
Sleeve gastrectomy
bariatric table extenders used in, 408
contraindications for, 407
gastrocolic ligament division in, 414, 414f
gastrosplenic ligament division in, 415
indications for, 407
instruments for, 407
laparoscopic, 407
laparoscopic stapling technique for, 419, 419f
liver retractor placement in, 413, 413f
operating room setup for, 408–409, 410f
patient positioning for, 408f–409f, 408–409
pneumoperitoneum in, 409–410
port setting for, 410–411, 412f
posterior gastric fundus mobilization in, 416, 416f–418f
robotic stapling technique for, 419f, 420
sequential compression device indications in, 408
short gastric vessels division, 415, 415f
specimen extraction in, 420
stapling of, 419, 419f
surgical technique for, 413f–419f, 413–420
Sliding hernia, 293
Small bowel
arterial anatomy of, 445f–446f
lymphatic drainage of, 448f
near-infrared indocyanine green fluorescence perfusion assessment of, 452f

1086 Index

Small bowel (*Cont.*):
  robotic resection
    anatomy of, 445*f*–448*f*
    contraindications for, 437
    diagnostic laparoscopy in, 442
    distal small bowel segments, 440*f*–441*f*
    docking time in, 444
    indications for, 437
    instruments for, 437
    laparoscopic evaluation of, 442, 444
    lymphadenectomy in, 444
    mesenteric dissection in, 444, 449*f*
    mesenteric gap closure, 454, 454*f*
    mesentery, 450*f*
    operating room setup for, 438, 439*f*, 441*f*
    overview of, 437
    patient positioning for, 438, 438*f*, 440*f*, 444
    perfusion assessment and transection, 451, 451*f*–452*f*
    pneumoperitoneum in, 438
    port setting for, 438, 442*f*–443*f*
    proximal small bowel segments, 438*f*
    reconstruction, 453
    side-to-side small bowel anastomosis in, 453, 453*f*
    specimen extraction in, 454
    surgical technique for, 442*f*–454*f*, 442–454
    trocar positioning in, 442, 442*f*–443*f*
  side-to-side anastomosis of, 453, 453*f*
  transection of, 451, 451*f*
  venous anatomy of, 447*f*
Small bowel stump, 104*f*
SMV. *See* Superior mesenteric vein
Society of American Gastrointestinal and Endoscopic Surgeons, 52
Software, artificial intelligence, 52
Spermatic cord lipoma, 908
Spermatic veins, 908
Spiegel's lobe, 751
Spinal accessory nerve, 157
Spleen
  accessory, 598*f*
  anatomy of, 582*f*–584*f*
  ligaments of, 589*f*–590*f*
  mobilization of, 589, 591*f*, 597, 597*f*
  venous anatomy of, 595*f*–596*f*
Spleen-preserving distal pancreatectomy, laparoscopic, 653–654
Spleen-preserving distal pancreatectomy, robotic
  contraindications for, 654
  description of, 116, 116*f*
  gastrocolic ligament division in, 659, 659*f*
  "hanging" maneuver in, 665, 665*f*
  history of, 654
  indications for, 654
  indocyanine green fluorescence splenic inflow and outflow check in, 671
  instruments for, 653
  intraoperative ultrasonography in, 663

  Kimura technique for, 653
  lateral-to-medial dissection in, 669, 669*f*
  left colonic flexure mobilization in, 662, 662*f*
  medial-to-lateral dissection in, 668*f*
  operating room setup for, 654, 656*f*, 657
  pancreatic body mobilization in, 667, 667*f*–668*f*, 670*f*
  pancreatic division in, 666, 666*f*
  pancreatic neck preparation in, 665, 665*f*
  pancreatic tail mobilization in, 667, 667*f*–670*f*
  patient positioning for, 654, 655*f*
  pneumoperitoneum for, 654
  port setting for, 654, 657, 657*f*–658*f*
  retropancreatic tunnel creation in, 665, 665*f*
  short gastric vessels in, 663
  specimen extraction in, 671
  splenic artery in, 664*f*
  splenic artery preparation in, 661, 661*f*
  splenic vein in, 664*f*
  surgical technique for, 659*f*–670*f*, 659–671
  Warshaw technique for, 653
Splenectomy, robotic
  anatomy of, 582*f*–584*f*
  contraindications for, 576
  diagnostic uses of, 576*t*
  gastrocolic ligament division in, 581, 581*f*
  history of, 575
  indications for, 576
  instruments for, 575
  left colonic flexure mobilization, 582
  operating room setup for, 576, 578, 578*f*
  pancreatic tail, 592, 592*f*–593*f*
  patient positioning for, 576, 577*f*
  phrenogastric and phrenosplenic ligament take-down with splenic mobilization, 589, 591*f*
  pneumoperitoneum in, 578
  port setting for, 576, 579, 579*f*–580*f*
  short gastric vessels in, 588, 588*f*
  specimen extraction in, 597
  splenic anatomy, 582*f*
  splenic artery control in, 585, 585*f*
  splenic hilum exploration, 592
  splenic mobilization, 589, 591*f*, 597, 597*f*
  splenic vessels, transection of, 595, 595*f*–596*f*
  surgical technique for, 581*f*–598*f*, 581–597
  therapeutic uses of, 576*t*
Splenic artery
  anatomy of, 664*f*
  aneurysm repair of, 117, 117*f*
  control of
    in radical anterograde modular pancreatosplenectomy, 646
    in splenectomy, 585, 585*f*
  dissection of
    in central pancreatectomy, 681*f*
    in D2 total gastrectomy, 401

    distal portion, dissection of, 401
  division of
    description of, 645–646
    in radical anterograde modular pancreatosplenectomy, 646, 647*f*
  preparation of, in spleen-preserving distal pancreatectomy, 661, 661*f*
  variations of, 586*f*–587*f*
Splenic flexure
  mobilization of, 480, 546*f*
  takedown of, 525, 527*f*
Splenic hilar lymphadenectomy, 399
Splenic vein, 585
  anatomy of, 664*f*
  division of, in radical anterograde modular pancreatosplenectomy, 650, 650*f*
Splenocolic ligament
  dissection
    in left colectomy, 489, 489*f*
    in total mesorectal excision for rectal cancer, 525, 527*f*
    in left adrenalectomy, 885
Splenogastric ligament, 416, 417*f*
Splenopancreatic ligament, 416, 417*f*
Splenorenal ligament, 885
Sponges, for bleeding control, 29
SR. *See* Surface rendering
Standard of care, 65
Stapling
  automated, 65
  laparoscopic, 43
  sleeve gastrectomy, 419, 419*f*
Stay sutures, 783, 784*f*, 785
Stomach
  anatomy of, 284*f*
  arterial supply of, 214*f*, 284*f*, 395*f*, 427*f*
  blood supply of, in robotic-assisted esophagectomy, 110*f*
  lesser curvature of, 219
  lymph node stations, 395, 397*f*
  mobilization of, 256
  venous drainage of, 395, 396*f*
Strap muscles, 132, 132*f*
Strasberg classification, of biliary injuries, 803, 804*f*, 833
Subcarinal mediastinal lymphadenectomy, 225
Subcortical parenchymal transection
  in left lateral sectionectomy, 765, 765*f*
  in right hepatectomy, 724, 727*f*, 728
Subcutaneous emphysema, 42
Subcutaneous flap dissection, in nipple-sparing mastectomy, 183, 184*f*
Subplatysmal skin flap, 131, 131*f*, 157
Subtotal cholecystectomy, 807, 1051
Suction irrigator, 26*f*
Suctioning, of surgical field, 43
Superior hypogastric plexus, around inferior mesenteric artery, 107
Superior laryngeal nerve, external branch of, 138, 144*f*, 172, 172*f*
Superior mediastinal lymph nodes, 322*f*

Superior mesenteric artery
  lesion of, 651
  in pancreaticoduodenectomy, 625
  in right colectomy with complete mesocolic excision, 472f
Superior mesenteric vein
  lesion of, 651
  in right colectomy with complete mesocolic excision, 464, 468, 474
Superior parathyroid gland, 172, 173f
Superior pole dissection, in transoral robotic thyroidectomy, 172
Superior thyroid artery, 148, 148f
Superior thyroid vein, 148, 148f
Supracarinal lymphadenectomy, 227
Suprapubic crossover, 931, 932f
Surface rendering, 67
Surgery workflow analysis, artificial intelligence for, 78, 80
Surgical artificial intelligence, 12, 78–87
Surgical assistant
  definition of, 33
  exposure by, 27
Surgical assistant certified, 33
Surgical augmented reality
  components of, 75f
  definition of, 74
  liver surgery application of, 78f
  registration, 76–78
Surgical competence
  credentialing–privileging in, 53
  procedure-specific, 53
Surgical data acquisition, 83
Surgical decision-making, 86
Surgical field, suctioning of, 43
Surgical monitors, 37
Surgical planning
  description of, 9
  virtual reality models for, 69, 70f
Surgical procedures, competence in, 53
Surgical robots, 53, 54f
Surgical skills
  artificial intelligence applications, 80–82
  automatic assessment of, 82
Surgical step recognition, 80, 81f
Surgical technician, 27
Suspensory ligament of the ovary, 971, 971f
SutureCut™ needle drivers, 24
SWIR band. See Short-wavelength infrared band

T
Tactile feedback, 22, 24f
Target tissue, 92
Targeting, 40
Telemanipulation, 6–8
Telemedicine, 60
Tenting maneuver, 41
Terminal ileum tumors, 451
Thoracic duct
  anatomy of, 240f–241f
  in esophageal surgery, 111

  esophagectomy-related injury of, 111
  variants of, 241f
Thoracic duct ligation, 226
Thoracic lymph nodes, 242t
Thoracic surgery, 119–120, 120f
Thoracic tumor, 119–120
Thoracoscopy
  history of, 317
  robotic-assisted, 318
  value of, to patients, 59
3D image reconstruction, 67–69, 68f–69f
Thymectomy
  extended. See Extended thymectomy
  transsternal, 197
Thymic veins, 207
Thymoma, extended thymectomy for
  carbon dioxide insufflation for, 200–201
  instruments for, 197
  operating room setup for, 198f, 198–199
  overview of, 197
  patient positioning for, 198, 199f
  port setting for, 198–199
  surgical technique for, 200f–207f, 200–208
  trocar placement for, 199f
Thymus
  anterior, 200f–201f
  cervical, 206
  ectopic, 204, 205f
  right, 203f
Thymus surgery
  nerve imaging in, 119
  vasculature in, 119
Thyroid gland
  anatomy of, 140f
  cricothyroid muscle, 148
  exposure of, 132, 132f
  landmarks of, 134
  left lobectomy of, 174
  lobectomy of, 174
  upper pole of, 148, 148f
Thyroidectomy
  gasless transaxillary robotic
    anatomy involved in, 138, 139f–147f
    central compartment node dissection, 149, 149f–150f
    contraindications for, 127–129
    contralateral lobectomy, 152, 152f
    da Vinci S, Si system, 135
    da Vinci SP system, 137, 153
    da Vinci Xi system, 136
    incision lines, 130, 131
    indications for, 127–129
    instruments for, 127, 128f
    ipsilateral lobectomy, 151, 151f
    operating room setup, 129
    patient positioning, 129
    port setting, 129
    upper pole dissection, 148
    working space for, 130f–134f, 130–134
  parathyroid glands in, 118
  transoral robotic
    advantages of, 163

    axillary arm for, 167
    central neck dissection in, 173–174
    contraindications for, 163–164
    da Vinci Si docking in, 168f, 168–169
    da Vinci Xi docking in, 167, 169f, 170, 170t
    docking stage in, 167–170
    flap creation in, 164, 165f–166f
    incisions in, 164, 165f–166f
    indications for, 163–164
    instruments for, 163, 170
    isthmus division in, 171, 171f
    mental nerve in, 165, 166f
    midline incision in, 171, 171f
    operating room setup for, 164
    patient positioning for, 164, 164f
    port setting for, 164
    recurrent laryngeal nerve in, 173, 173f
    right lobectomy in, 173–174
    specimen removal, 173–174
    superior pole dissection, 172
    surgical technique in, 171–174
    trocar insertion in, 165, 165f–166f
    working space for, 165, 165f–166f
Thyrothymic ligament, 206f–207f
Toldt's fascia, 490f, 491, 498, 524, 582, 642, 949
Top-Down technique, for robotic transversus abdominis release, 927, 934–936, 935f
TORT. See Transoral robotic thyroidectomy
Total mesorectal excision
  pelvic plexus identification in, 107, 107f
  for rectal cancer. See Total mesorectal excision for rectal cancer
Total mesorectal excision for rectal cancer
  anatomy, 528, 528f–530f
  anterior dissection, 540
  anterolateral dissection, 540
  autonomic nerves, 528
  circular concentric dissection of distal mesorectum, 541, 541f
  colorectal/coloanal anastomosis, 544
  contraindications for, 517
  da Vinci S system docking, 518, 519f
  da Vinci Si system docking, 518, 519f
  da Vinci SP system, 545f–548f, 545–547
  da Vinci Xi system docking, 520, 521f–522f
  deep posterior dissection in, 542, 542f
  Denonvilliers' fascia, 540, 540f
  distal rectum division, 543
  endoscopic ultrasound in, 518
  fasciae, 528, 530f
  fascial adhesions, 528
  full robotic approach, 523–525
  hybrid laparoscopic-robotic approach, 523
  indications for, 517
  instruments for, 517
  operating room setup for, 520, 522f
  orogastric tube in, 518
  overview of, 517

Total mesorectal excision for rectal cancer (*Cont.*):
   patient positioning for, 518, 518*f*
   pelvic dissection, 534, 534*f*, 547*f*
   port setting for, 518, 519*f*, 521*f*
   posterior dissection, 534, 534*f*–535*f*
   postero-bilateral dissection, 535–536, 536*f*
   proximal colon preparation, 544
   retraction levels, 528, 531, 531*f*–533*f*
   specimen extraction in, 544
   splenocolic ligament dissection in, 525, 527*f*
   surgical techniques, 523–527
Toupet fundoplication, 275*f*
Tracheobronchial lymph node dissection, 255*f*, 255–256
Trainees, robotic surgery value for, 59
Transabdominal preperitoneal repair, robotic
   anatomical landmarks in, 902, 902*f*–903*f*, 1060, 1060*f*
   central zone dissection, 1063, 1064*f*
   contraindications for, 897, 1057
   da Vinci SP system for, 1057*f*–1065*f*, 1057–1065
   description of, 897
   flap closure in, 910, 910*f*, 1065, 1065*f*
   flap dissection in, 1061
   floating port technique in, 1059, 1059*f*
   hernia sac dissection in, 908, 1063
   indications for, 897, 1057
   instruments for, 897, 1057
   lateral dissection in, 906, 907*f*, 1062, 1062*f*
   medial dissection in, 904, 905*f*, 1062, 1062*f*
   mesh placement in, 909, 909*f*, 1064, 1064*f*
   myopectineal orifice, 908
   operating room setup for, 898, 899*f*, 1057, 1058*f*
   patient positioning for, 898, 898*f*, 1057, 1058*f*
   peritoneal flap closure, 910, 910*f*, 1065, 1065*f*
   pneumoperitoneum for, 898
   port setting for, 898, 900*f*–901*f*, 1057, 1057*f*
   spermatic vessels, 908, 1064
Transabdominal preperitoneal repair, robotic floating port technique, 1059, 1059*f*
Transabdominal preperitoneal ventral hernia repair, 912, 912*t*
Transaxillary robotic thyroidectomy, gasless
   anatomy involved in, 138, 139*f*–147*f*
   central compartment node dissection, 149, 149*f*–150*f*
   contraindications for, 127–129
   contralateral lobectomy, 152, 152*f*
   da Vinci S, Si system, 135
   da Vinci SP system, 137, 153
   da Vinci Xi system, 136
   incision lines, 130, 131
   indications for, 127–129
   instruments for, 127, 128*f*
   ipsilateral lobectomy, 151, 151*f*
   operating room setup, 129
   patient positioning, 129
   port setting, 129
   upper pole dissection, 148
   working space for, 130*f*–134*f*, 130–134
Transfer learning, 84
Transgastric pancreaticogastrostomy, 629, 630*f*
Transmesocolic anteduodenal route, 819
Transmesocolic paraduodenal route, 838*f*
Transoral robotic thyroidectomy
   advantages of, 163
   axillary arm for, 167
   central neck dissection in, 173–174
   contraindications for, 163–164
   da Vinci Si docking in, 168*f*, 168–169
   da Vinci Xi docking in, 167, 169*f*, 170, 170*t*
   docking stage in, 167–170
   flap creation in, 164, 165*f*–166*f*
   incisions in, 164, 165*f*–166*f*
   indications for, 163–164
   instruments for, 163, 170
   isthmus division in, 171, 171*f*
   mental nerve in, 165, 166*f*
   midline incision in, 171, 171*f*
   operating room setup for, 164
   patient positioning for, 164, 164*f*
   port setting for, 164
   recurrent laryngeal nerve in, 173, 173*f*
   right lobectomy in, 173–174
   specimen removal, 173–174
   superior pole dissection, 172
   surgical technique in, 171–174
   trocar insertion in, 165, 165*f*–166*f*
   working space for, 165, 165*f*–166*f*
Transplants
   donor nephrectomy. *See* Donor nephrectomy
   kidney. *See* Kidney transplant
   pancreas. *See* Pancreas transplant
Transversalis fascia, 904*f*
Transverse cervical artery, 159, 160*f*
Transverse colon
   division of, in right colectomy with complete mesocolic excision, 474, 475*f*
   mesenteric root detachment from pancreatic body, 491
Transversus abdominis, 926, 927*f*
Transversus abdominis release
   open, 925–926
   robotic. *See* Robotic transversus abdominis release
   in ventral hernia repair, 911–912
Trastuzumab, 93
Treitz ligament, 428
Tremor, lack of, 10
Triangle of Calot, 22*f*, 71, 798*f*, 798–799, 801, 1050, 1052
Triangle of doom, 902, 903*f*, 907*f*, 908, 1063
Triangle venosum, 764*f*
Triangular ligament dissection, 763, 764*f*
Triangulation, 18–20, 19*f*
Tridimensional vision, 8–9
"Triple two" procedure, 480
Trisectionectomy, left, 734*f*
Trocar placement
   animal models for training in, 51
   in nipple-sparing robotic mastectomy, 186
   in pancreas transplant, 985–986, 987*f*
   in right adrenalectomy, 866*f*–867*f*
   in right colectomy with complete mesocolic excision, 457*f*–458*f*
   in small bowel resection, 442, 442*f*–443*f*
   transdiaphragmatic, 772
   in transoral thyroidectomy, 165, 165*f*–166*f*
Troubleshooting, 28, 39–40, 43
T-Tubes, 856, 856*f*–857*f*
Tumescent injection, in nipple-sparing mastectomy, 185, 185*f*
Tunneling technique, in nipple-sparing mastectomy, 185, 185*f*

U

Ultrasound, intraoperative
   in central pancreatectomy, 678, 679*f*
   in left lateral sectionectomy, 763, 763*f*
   in liver resections, 775, 783
   in pancreatic tumor enucleation, 694, 696
   in radical anterograde modular pancreatosplenectomy, 643
   in renal artery aneurysm repair, 1027, 1027*f*
   in right hepatectomy, 707, 708*f*
   in spleen-preserving distal pancreatectomy, 663
Umbilical hernias, 911
Uncinate process
   dissection of, 625, 626*f*–627*f*
   in pancreatic tumor enucleation, 695
Universal standard of care, 65
Upper esophagus mobilization, 248*f*–249*f*, 248–249
Upper quadrant abdominal surgery, patient positioning for, 16*f*
Ureter
   blood supply to, 952, 952*f*
   preparation of, in left donor nephrectomy, 950, 950*f*, 952*f*
Ureteroneocystostomy, 979, 979*f*–980*f*

V

Vagal trunk
   anatomy of, 285*f*, 310*f*
   left, in Heller myotomy with modified Dor fundoplication, 309, 309*f*–310*f*
Vagus nerve, 287*f*, 311*f*
VATS. *See* Video-assisted thoracoscopic surgery

Venous anastomosis
 in kidney transplant, 976, 976f
 in pancreas transplant, 993, 993f
Ventral hernia repair
 extended totally extraperitoneal repair, 911
 incisional hernias, 911
 instruments for, 911
 intraperitoneal onlay mesh and
  abdominal ventral defect dissection, 921
  adhesiolysis, 920, 920f
  cardinal stitches with straight needle, 922, 922f
  contraindications for, 915
  fascial defect closure, 921, 921f
  indications for, 915
  mesh placement and fixation, 922, 923f
  operating room setup for, 916, 917f, 918
  patient positioning for, 916, 916f
  port setting for, 919f
  surgical technique for, 920f–923f, 920–923
 mesh placements in, 914f
 retrorectus, 912, 912t
 transabdominal preperitoneal, 912, 912t
 transversus abdominis release, 911–912
 types of, 912t, 913f, 915f
 umbilical hernias, 911
Ventral hernia repair, laparoscopic, 911
Veress needles, extra-long, 412
Veress technique
 description of, 17–18
 modified Palmer's point for, 17, 17f
 for pneumoperitoneum, 842
Vicarious Surgical System, 55, 57f
Video-assisted thoracoscopic surgery
 description of, 317–318
 robotic, 326, 326f
Virtual fixtures enhancement, 13
Virtual reality
 description of, 9–10, 67
 robotic training models, 45–46
Virtual reality models, 69, 70f
Virtual reality simulators
 animal models versus, 50
 robotic training uses of, 45–46, 48f
Virtual tactile feedback, 22, 24
Visible Patient, 67
Vision enhancements
 augmented reality, 9–10
 fluorescence, 9, 9f
 tridimensional vision, 8–9
 virtual reality, 9–10
VisiPort, 578
Visual feedback, 24

W

Warshaw technique, 653
Whipple procedure, 616
White-light imaging, 89, 121

Z

Zuckerkandl tubercle, 148